NEONATAL MEDICINE

NEONATAL
MEDICINE

Edited by

Leo STERN, M. D.

Professor and Chairman of Pediatrics
Brown University
Providence, RI (USA)

Paul VERT, M. D.

Professeur de Pédiatrie
Université de Nancy I
Nancy (France)

Distributed by
YEAR BOOK MEDICAL PUBLISHERS • INC.
35 EAST WACKER DRIVE, CHICAGO

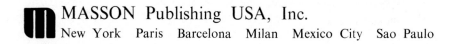 MASSON Publishing USA, Inc.
New York   Paris   Barcelona   Milan   Mexico City   Sao Paulo

ISBN: 0-89352-229-5

Library of Congress Catalog Card Number 86-33290

Printed in France

Contributors

Claudine AMIEL-TISON, M.D.
Maître de Recherche
INSERM Unité 162
Maternité Baudelocque
Hôpital Port-Royal
Paris (France)

Monique ANDRÉ, M.D.
Médecin des Hôpitaux
Service de Médecine Néonatale
Maternité Régionale Universitaire
Nancy (France)

Cynthia T. BARRETT, M.D.
Associate Professor of Pediatrics
University of California
School of Medicine
Los Angeles, CA (USA)

Geneviève BARRIER, M.D.
Professeur d'Anesthésiologie
Hôpital des Enfants-Malades
Paris (France)

Arié L. BENSOUSSAN, M.D.
Professeur agrégé de clinique en chirurgie
Université de Montréal
Hôpital Sainte-Justine
Montréal, Québec (Canada)

Élisabeth BENZ-LEMOINE, M.D.
Praticien Hospitalier
Service d'Hématologie
Université de Poitiers
Poitiers (France)

Jean-Claude BERLINGUET, M.D.
Chirurgien
Centre Hospitalier Lanaudière
Joliette, Québec (Canada)

Hervé BLANCHARD, M.D.
Professeur Titulaire de Chirurgie
Université de Montréal
Hôpital Sainte-Justine
Montréal, Québec (Canada)

Pierre BORDIGONI, M.D.
Médecin des Hôpitaux
Université de Nancy I
Hôpital d'Enfants
Nancy (France)

Pierre BOUDROS GHOSN, M.D.
Chirurgien
Hôpital Saint-Luc
Montréal, Québec (Canada)

André BOUE, M.D.
Professeur de Biologie
Université de Paris-Ouest
Groupe de Recherche de Biologie Prénatale
INSERM Unité 73
Château de Longchamp
Paris (France)

Gérard BRÉART, M.D.
Maître de Recherche
Groupe de Recherches Épidémiologiques sur
    la Mère et l'Enfant
Unité INSERM 149
Hôpital de Port-Royal
Paris (France)

André CALAME, M.D.
Professeur de Pédiatrie
Médecin-Chef du Service de Néonatologie
Centre Hospitalier Universitaire Vaudois
Lausanne (Switzerland)

William J. CASHORE, M.D.
Associate Professor of Pediatrics
Brown University
Rhode Island Hospital
Providence, RI (USA)

Pierre-Paul COLLIN, M.D.
Professeur Titulaire de Chirurgie
Université de Montréal
Hôpital Sainte-Justine
Montréal, Québec (Canada)

Jacques COUVREUR, M.D.
Laboratoire de Sérologie Néonatale
et de Recherche sur la Toxoplasmose
Institut de Puériculture
Paris (France)

Richard M. COWETT, M.D.
Associate Professor of Pediatrics
Brown University
Rhode Island Hospital
Providence, RI (USA)

Maria DELIVORIA-PAPADOPOULOS, M.D.
Professor of Pediatrics and Physiology
University of Pennsylvania
Hospital of the University of Pennsylvania
Philadelphia, PA (USA)

Jean G. DESJARDINS, M.D.
Professeur Titulaire de Chirurgie
Université de Montréal
Hôpital Sainte-Justine
Montréal, Québec (Canada)

Georges DESMONTS
Laboratoire de Sérologie Néonatale
et de Recherche sur la Toxoplasmose
Institut de Puériculture
Paris (France)

Victor DUBOWITZ, M.D., Ph.D., F.R.C.P.
Professor of Pediatrics
University of London
Department of Pediatrics and Neonatal Medicine
Hammersmith Hospital
London (UK)

Gabriel DUC, M.D.
Professor of Neonatology
Universitätsspital
Zurich (Switzerland)

Jacques-Charles DUCHARME, M.D.
Professeur Titulaire de Chirurgie
Université de Montréal
Hôpital Sainte-Justine
Montréal, Québec (Canada)

Claude DUPUIS, M.D.
Professeur de Pédiatrie
Université de Lille II
Chef du Service de Cardiologie Infantile
Hôpital Cardiologique
Lille (France)

Pierre FENDER, M.D.
Médecin Épidémiologiste
Groupe de Recherches Épidémiologiques sur
  la Mère et l'Enfant
INSERM Unité 149
Hôpital de Port-Royal
Paris (France)

Maguelone G. FOREST, M.D.
Maître de Recherche
Unité de Recherches Endocriniennes et Métaboliques
  chez l'Enfant
INSERM Unité 34
Hôpital Debrousse
Lyon (France)

Fernand GEUBELLE, M.D.
Professeur de Pédiatrie
Université de Liège
Hôpital de Bavière
Liège (Belgium)

Hélène GRANDJEAN, M.D.
Chargé de Recherche
Groupe de Recherche en Physiologie Obstétricale
  et Pharmacologie Périnatale
INSERM Unité 168
Hôpital La Grave
Toulouse (France)

Jean-Pierre GUIGNARD, M.D.
Professeur Associé
Médecin-Adjoint de Néphrologie Pédiatrique
Centre Hospitalier Universitaire Vaudois
Lausanne (Switzerland)

Frank M. GUTTMAN, M.D.
Professor of Surgery
McGill University
Montreal Children's Hospital
Montréal, Québec (Canada)

Vincent C. HARRISON, M.D.
Associate Professor
Department of Pediatrics and Child Health
University of Cape Town
Mowbray Maternity Hospital
Cape Town (South Africa)

Jean KACHANER, M.D.
Professeur de Pédiatrie
Université de Paris V
Service de Cardiologie Infantile
Hôpital des Enfants-Malades
Paris (France)

Rutger LAGERCRANTZ, M.D.
Professor of Pediatrics
Karolinska Institute
Stockholm (Sweden)

Luc LARGET-PIET, M.D.
Professeur de Pédiatrie
Centre Hospitalier Universitaire
Angers (France)

Annick LARGET-PIET, M.D.
Centre Hospitalier Universitaire
Angers (France)

Jeanne-Claudie LARROCHE, M.D.
Maître de Recherche au CNRS
Unité INSERM 29
Hôpital de Port-Royal
Paris (France)

Malcom I. LEVENE, M.B., M.R.C.P.
Senior Lecturer
Department of Child Health
University of Leicester
School of Medicine
Leicester (UK)

† John LIND, M.D.
Professor Emeritus of Pediatrics
Karolinska Institute
Stockholm (Sweden)

Lewis P. LIPSITT, M.D.
Professor of Psychology
Director, Child Study Center
Brown University
Providence, RI (USA)

Atties F. MALAN, M.D.
Associate Professor and Head of Newborn Services
Department of Pediatrics and Child Health
University of Cape Town
Cape Town (South Africa)

Claire MALBRUNOT
Assistante de Microbiologie
Hôpital Ambroise-Paré
Boulogne-Billancourt (France)

François MARCHAL
Assistant de Physiologie
Université de Nancy I
Laboratoire d'Exploration Fonctionnelle
Hôpital d'Enfants et Maternité Régionale
Nancy (France)

Michel MANCIAUX, M.D.
Professeur d'Épidémiologie, Économie
de la Santé et Prévention
Département de Santé Publique
Université de Nancy I
Faculté de Médecine
Nancy (France)

Pierre MONIN, M.D.
Professeur de Pédiatrie
Université de Nancy I
Service de Médecine Néonatale
Maternité Régionale Universitaire
Nancy (France)

Alain MORALI, M.D.
Médecin des Hôpitaux
Université de Nancy I
Hôpital d'Enfants
Nancy (France)

Paolo L. MORSELLI, M.D.
Directeur de la Recherche Clinique
LERS Synthélabo
Paris (France)

Christian MOSSAY, M.D.
Résident Spécialiste
Université de Liège
Hôpital de Bavière
Liège (Belgique)

André J. MOULAERT, M.D.
Consultant in Pediatric Cardiology
Wilhelmina Kinderziekenhuis
Utrecht (Nederland)

William OH, M.D.
Professor of Pediatrics and Obstetrics
Brown University
Rhode Island Hospital
Providence, RI (USA)

Danièle OLIVE, M.D.
Professeur de Pédiatrie
Université de Nancy I
Hôpital d'Enfants
Nancy (France)

Alain OUIMET, M.D.
Professeur Adjoint de clinique en chirurgie
Université de Montréal
Hôpital Sainte-Justine
Montréal, Québec (Canada)

Émile PAPIERNIK, M.D.
Professeur de Gynécologie-Obstétrique
Université de Paris-Sud
Hôpital Antoine-Béclère
INSERM Unité 187
Clamart (France)

Claude PERNOT, M.D.
Professeur de Cardiologie
Université de Nancy I
Hôpital de Brabois
Nancy (France)

François PLENAT, M.D.
Anatomo-Pathologiste
Maître de Conférence Universitaire
Université de Nancy I
Faculté de Médecine
Nancy (France)

Georges PONTONNIER, M.D.
Professeur de Clinique Gynécologique et Obstétricale
INSERM Unité 168
Hôpital de la Grave
Toulouse (France)

Jean PRÉVOT, M.D.
Professeur de Chirurgie Infantile
Université de Nancy I
Hôpital d'Enfants
Nancy (France)

Jean-Pierre RELIER, M.D.
Professeur de Pédiatrie
Service de Médecine Néonatale
Hôpital de Port-Royal
Paris (France)

Jack S. REMINGTON, M.D.
Chairman
Department of Immunology and Infectious Diseases
Palo Alto Medical Foundation
Research Institute
Palo Alto, CA (USA)

J. Stephen ROBINSON, M.D.
Division of Neonatology
University of California
School of Medicine
Los Angeles, CA (USA)

Claude C. ROY, M.D.
Professeur de Pédiatrie
Université de Montréal
Hôpital Sainte-Justine
Montréal, Québec (Canada)

Claude RUMEAU-ROUQUETTE, M.D.
Directeur du Groupe de Recherches Épidémiologiques
  sur la Mère et l'Enfant
Unité INSERM 149
Hôpital de Port-Royal
Paris (France)

Bernard SALLE, M.D.
Professeur de Néonatologie
Université Claude-Bernard
Hôpital Édouard-Herriot
Lyon (France)

Michel SCHMITT, M.D.
Professeur de Chirurgie Infantile
Université de Nancy I
Hôpital d'Enfants
Nancy (France)

Robert SCHWARTZ, M.D.
Professor of Pediatrics
Director, Division of Pediatric Metabolism and
  Nutrition
Brown University
Rhode Island Hospital
Providence, RI (USA)

Jacques SENTERRE, M.D.
Professeur Associé de Pédiatrie
Centre de Néonatologie
Hôpital de la Citadelle
Liège (Belgium)

Mervin SILVERBERG, M.D.
Professor of Pediatrics
Cornell University
Chairman Department of Pediatrics
North Shore University Hospital
Manhasset, NY (USA)

Mildred T. STAHLMAN, M.D.
Professor of Pediatrics and Pathology
Director, Division of Neonatology
Vanderbilt University
School of Medicine
Nashville, TE (USA)

Leo STERN, M.D.
Professor and Chairman of Pediatrics
Brown University
Pediatrician in Chief
Rhode Island Hospital
Providence, RI (USA)

Paul R. SWYER, M.D.
Professor of Pediatrics
University of Toronto
Director, Department of Neonatology
The Hospital for Sick Children
Toronto, Ontario (Canada)

Michel C. SZALAY, M.D.
Department of Pediatrics and Child Health
University of Cape Town
Mowbray Maternity Hospital
Cape Town (South Africa)

Jean-François THIERCELIN, P.D.
LERS Synthélabo
Paris (France)

Antonio TORRADO, M. D.
Professeur de Pédiatrie
Hospital Pediatrico
CHC-CELAS
Coimbra (Portugal)

Bernard VAUDAUX, M.D.
Chef de Clinique
Centre Hospitalier Universitaire Vaudois
Lausanne (Switzerland)

Paul VERT, M.D.
Professeur de Pédiatrie
Université de Nancy I
Chef du Service de Médecine et Réanimation Néona-
  tales
Maternité Régionale Universitaire
Unité INSERM 272
Nancy (France)

Michel VIDAILHET, M.D.
Professeur de Pédiatrie
Université de Nancy I
Hôpital d'Enfants
Nancy (France)

C. Göran WALGREN, M.D.
Professor of Pediatric Cardiology
Karolinska Institute, St Goran's Hospital
Stockholm (Sweden)

Marietta XANTHOU
Associate Professor of Pediatrics
Athens University
Director, Neonatal Intensive Care Unit
« Aghia Sophia » Children's Hospital
Athens (Greece)

Salam YAZBECK, M.D.
Professeur Adjoint de Clinique en Chirurgie
Université de Montréal
Hôpital Sainte-Justine
Montréal, Québec (Canada)

Sami YOUSSEF, M.D.
Professeur Adjoint de Clinique en Chirurgie
Université de Montréal
Hôpital Sainte-Justine
Montréal, Québec (Canada)

Alvin ZIPURSKY, M.D.
Professor of Pediatrics
University of Toronto
Director, Division of Haematology/Oncology
Department of Pediatrics
The Hospital for Sick Children
Toronto, Ontario (Canada)

Introduction

In this, the english language counterpart of Médecine Néonatale, *we signal the completion of the original undertaking of a group of international colleagues in the preparation of a work in two languages that deals in a physiological and developmental manner with the neonatal patient and his or her surroundings.*

It should be stressed once again that this english edition is not simply a translation from the french version whose earlier appearance is the result only of a sequential advantage in the publishing process. All of the contributions were originally submitted by the authors in both languages, to accomplish this goal. In addition to several chapter differences, there has also been an upgrading of additional new information for example, a section on AIDS in the chapter on Viruses Diseases and mention of some of the newer CNS radiographic imaging techniques in the chapter on Central Nervous System Pathology.

It has been the intent of the authors to present an approach based on an understanding of the basic physiologic and biochemical foundations of neonatal medicine. Thus a subject is less often considered as "what to do" but hopefully more often "why it may be so". We would prefer to leave the implementation of the presented concepts to both the enterprise and imagination of those who will explore and adapt them to the individuality of the care and management of the newborn.

We are grateful to our publishers for their unfailing help and collaboration as well as to a number of agencies in France whose fiscal assistance has permitted the appearance of the work in both editions. These include:

Ministère de la Culture, Direction du Livre; Ministère de l'Éducation Nationale, Direction des Bibliothèques, des Musées et de l'Information Scientifique et Technique; Ministère des Relations Extérieures; Institut National de la Santé et de la Recherche Médicale; Association des Amis des Universités de Lorraine; Association Obstétrico-Pédiatrique de Médecine Périnatale, Fondation pour la Recherche Médicale, Comité Lorraine.

We can only hope that the reader will find in these chapters the knowledge and information necessary and helpful for an approach to the care and management of the patients and their families.

Leo STERN, Providence, Rhode Island USA
Paul VERT, Nancy France
September 26, 1986

Contents

Introduction (64); The neonatal nervous system and the effects of experience (65); Sensation and perception in the newborn (66); Learning processes of the newborn (68); Neonatal habituation (70); The significance of early human cognition (71); Approach-avoidance, and the hedonic basis of behavior development (72); Critical conditions of infancy: a psychological perspective and an example (73).

The pregnancy, a period of change and strain (78); Preparation for birth and parenthood (79); Education for tomorrow's youth (79); Courses for parents during pregnancy (80); The expectant father's participation in labor, delivery and care of the newborn (80); The birth of the family (81); The climate of hospital care and co-operation (81); The needs of the sick newborn (82); An example of psychological problems in the neonatal period (82); The parents and premature baby (83); The deformed child and its parents (84); Brothers and sisters at home (85); Caring for parents of infants who die (85); The importance of continuity in medical care (86); The work of the psychologist on the maternity ward and the neonatal ward (86); two examples of the significance of psychosocial factors in pregnancy, childbirth and early parenthood (87).

History (88); Definition (89); Necessity of prevention (89); Epidemiology of premature birth (90); From epidemiology to prevention (90); Analysis by cause of preterm birth (96); Organization of a preventive program (97); Results of prevention (98); Quality control (100); Conclusion (101).

PART TWO

NEONATAL NEUROLOGY

PART THREE

CARDIOCIRCULATORY AND RESPIRATORY DISEASES

PART FOUR

NEONATAL INFECTIONS

PART FIVE

HEMATOLOGY. ONCOLOGY

PART SIX

METABOLISM AND ENDOCRINOLOGY

PART NINE

HEREDITARY AND CONGENITAL DISORDERS

1

The normal newborn and perinatal risk factors

1

The normal newborn and perinatal risk factors

Perinatal morbidity and mortality
An epidemiologic approach

M. MANCIAUX, C. RUMEAU-ROUQUETTE, P. FENDER and G. BREART

Introduction

Since the end of World War II, perinatal morbidity and mortality have been considerably reduced in most of the industrialized countries. According to WHO [76], the rate of late fetal deaths declined by two-thirds between 1940 and 1970, and that of early neonatal deaths by one-half.

This improvement is clearly encouraging, but we are far from having resolved all the problems. For example, our understanding of perinatal morbidity is still inadequate, as is our knowledge of its relationship to mortality. A number of questions confront us: Have the mortality rates in certain countries attained an irreducible minimum? Does such a minimum exist? If so, at what rate should it be fixed? Have all mothers, and all children, benefited equally from this remarkable progress? On a worldwide basis, certainly not. Where do we stand in our own countries? And, above all, what must be done to continue, to amplify, to generalize this progress? How should we pursue the decline in rates? This appears to be all the more important since perinatal mortality—even though considerably reduced—remains significant and the number

of permanently handicapped greater than in any other period of man's existence. At the end of the 1960s, it was estimated that as many human beings in Great Britain died during the 15 weeks of the average perinatal period as among those between the ages of zero and 35 years. Even though these numbers have since declined considerably, the perinatal period remains one of high risk, indeed.

Also, the media and the public in general are ever more demanding in terms of the quality of services and a successful outcome of pregnancy. Pressure groups, for example, have been created in the United Kingdom challenging and criticizing the government and the National Health Service because the reduction in perinatal mortality has been less striking than in other countries of equivalent socioeconomic level. The question is all the more important because zero population growth makes every new life more precious.

In the developed countries, the objective is thus evident: to ensure that the newborns live, without sequelae, whatever their initial pathological problems. As WHO [76] has observed: "Mere survival does not suffice—if the reduction in perinatal mortality were to be accompanied by an increase in the number of survivors condemned to short and miserable lives, its advantages would be illusory".

The situation in the developing countries is less clear. Perinatal mortality may seem relatively minor in the overall context of infant and child mortality. The special problems posed by this period of life may seem to lack priority importance. But when the risks associated with inadequate birthweight are considered, the situation is in fact worrisome. Each year, 22 millions out of the world's 125 millions newborns come into the world underweight [78]: these 22 millions are almost exclusively children born in the developing countries. This low birthweight, which generally reflects malnutrition of the fetus during pregnancy, is a source of increased

mortality and is at the origin of many handicaps among the survivors—on the world scale, it is a true catastrophe. It is definitely linked to maternal malnutrition, insufficient spacing of births, and to a whole complex of factors which medical action alone will not be able to resolve in the predictable future. This problem merits the attention of public health planners, as well as of those responsible for social development, in the developing countries.

Thus, from every point of view, perinatal morbidity and mortality are problems of great significance, and of capital importance, for individuals, families, and all countries. In the following pages, we will review successively perinatal morbidity and mortality, the complex factors that link them, and the measures susceptible of helping to improve—in various contexts—a situation that remains disturbing in most countries of the world.

Perinatal morbidity

DEFINITIONS
AND SOURCES OF INFORMATION

Definition problems. — The notion of morbidity is difficult to explain: the pathological condition is defined socially and is characterized as a divergence from a norm. The concept of disease is evolutive, dependent upon the degree of medical knowledge; the structure of morbidity changes with time [10, 73, 94].

Furthermore, it is necessary to distinguish perinatal morbidity (that is, morbidity manifested during the perinatal period) and morbidity resulting from perinatal causes, but discovered later, though having its origins in the period.

With a view to unifying disease concepts that vary by country, and over a period of time, WHO periodically organizes international conferences to establish an "International Classification of Diseases" (ICD) [74]. The ICD presently in use is the 9th revision. A special list concerns perinatal questions. But varying national usages cause the same condition to be classified under different categories of the ICD. Although some pathological situations are clearly circumscribed—e. g., feto-maternal incompatibility—others are not: for example, feto-maternal infection, acute fetal distress,

or neonatal asphyxia. These imprecisions greatly complicate the study of morbidity and its evolution in time and space. They account for approaches based on therapeutics (including preventive ones) peculiar to this age group, on weight criteria (birthweight), on chronological factors (gestational age), on biological parameters (acidosis, hypoglycemia, etc.), more than on well-defined clinical patterns. Such procedures, though eminently pragmatic, mix indicators and risk factors, symptoms and syndromes—unification often appears problematic.

In addition to the diversity of terminology and classification, there are differences in methods of reporting and registration. Sometimes tied to medico-social circumstances, but above all to the rapid growth of knowledge in this ever-developing area, these variations singularly complicate the task of establishing a reliable body of statistics.

In this chapter, we have chosen to make frequent reference to a multicountry study by WHO [1] in 1973, because it succeeded in achieving the greatest possible uniformity [76]. It proposed

---

[1] Eight countries participated in the study: England and Wales, Austria, Cuba, Hungary, Japan, New Zealand, Sweden, and the United States (six states: Hawaii, Oklahoma, Rhode Island, Utah, Vermont, and Washington).

a classification by four principal causes of morbidity and mortality: maternal causes (P_{1-20}), obstetrical causes ($P_{21-43,45,47-49}$), fetal causes (P_{53-100}, with the exception of feto-maternal causes), feto-maternal causes ($P_{44,46,50,52,57-60,61,63,67,68,94}$) (List **P** of the ICD, eighth revision).

This method of approaching the problem, however, has its limits, It rests on an arbitrary choice of the causes and groupings. It fails to include certain risk factors linked to the condition of the newborn that nonetheless have a strong correlation with perinatal morbidity and mortality; for example, birthweight and length of gestation, which will be discussed in detail below (See "Abnormalities in duration of Pregnancy and in Birth-Weight").

Sources of information. — The industrialized countries have recently established a system of registration that may be classified under four groups:

— The establishment of *health certificates* for all newborns was made mandatory in France in 1970 [62], and a similar practice exists in several European countries. These certificates span the whole range of perinatal pathology, but remain limited to a few basic elements (birthweight, gestational age, neonatal distress, congenital malformations). The routine use of the certificates sometimes has a negative effect on the quality of the information.

— *Registration of congenital malformations* has become widespread since 1963; the aim is to monitor the frequency of these abnormalities in order to reveal eventual changes in rates and discover their causes. Coordination of these registrations has been undertaken in the framework of the European Economic Community: the EUROCAT system (European Registration of Congenital Abnormalities and Twins) consists of 16 centers in 10 countries where the same study methods are applied. WHO, the Council of Europe, and private organizations such as the "International Clearinghouse for Birth Defects Monitoring System" have also contributed to the standardization of registrations and dissemination of the results.

— A number of *surveys* of representative birth samples on a country level have been conducted: the American "Collaborative Perinatal Study" [99], the "British Perinatal Survey" [13], and, in France, the nationwide studies conducted in 1972, 1976, and 1981 under the auspices of INSERM (*Institut national de la Santé et de la Recherche médicale* [89]). The British studies also included follow-up of the children. Such surveys make it possible to obtain more detailed information than that offered by registrations concerning overall births and serve as a useful supplement to the latter.

— *Registrations* using identical formats have been employed in *maternity clinics* in certain parts of the United States and Europe. Although the samples are not rigorously representative on a national level, they nonetheless constitute an important tool for information and evaluation.

It must not be forgotten, however, that all these systems are dependent not only on the quality of the registrations, but also on the state of knowledge at the time the data are collected. Comparisons between countries and between periods are thus hazardous. They must also take into consideration sociocultural changes and demographic crosscurrents that account for a number of the differences observed.

These reservations explain why we will limit our approach here to the main perinatal problems: abnormalities in the length of gestation and in weight constitute the two most frequent causes of perinatal pathology. Next come congenital malformations, which are increasingly important because of the stability of their incidence, while other pathologies regress. Fetal distress, the result of hypoxia in the course of pregnancy and/or during delivery, can constitute a complication in other causes of morbidity or can occur accidentally in a perfectly normal fetus. Finally, infection represents a frequent cause of morbidity and of mortality during the neonatal period. For each of these major problems, we will note the risk factors so far identified and the problems of epidemiological methodology that they raise—without exploring the pathological details, which will be the subject of a number of the following chapters.

ABNORMALITIES IN DURATION OF PREGNANCY AND IN BIRTH-WEIGHT

Definitions. — According to internationally recognized norms, a premature infant is one born less than 37 full weeks (259 days) after the first day of the last menstruation. Imprecision in the determination of the beginning date of the last menstrual period means that the *gestational age* often remains uncertain, or must sometimes be corrected by taking into account the morphologic and neurologic condition of the infant. Such criteria are difficult to use in international surveys and the determination of the gestational age often lacks precision.

Birthweight is more accurately measured and more often available; thus, the 2,500-gram limit continues to be very much used, even though the group of infants weighing less than 2,500 g includes both premature infants and those born after a normal length of gestation but having experienced a delay in intrauterine growth—and sometimes a combination of these two conditions.

The study of birthweight in relation to gestational age enables us to investigate hypotrophy (or "small-for-date" babies): one establishes for infants born in the same gestational week the distribution of birthweight and calculates the indices that characterize this distribution (the average and the mean deviation if the Laplace-Gauss law is followed; the median and percentiles, if not).

These data are generally shown separately for girls and boys: Table I and Figures I-1a and I-1b are illustrative. They represent the results of a survey conducted in France on a representative sampling of 11,200 births chosen at random in public and private maternity centers— the centers also being chosen at random among all the childbirth centers [89].

To designate "small-for-date" babies, one generally isolates those whose weight is under the 10th or the 5th percentile; this is an arbitrary limit that can vary from one study to another.

Birthweight remains the leading indicator used in international comparisons. However, it is interpreted differently according to country. In the developing countries, more than two-thirds of the infants with low birthweight are "small-for-date"; in the developed countries, the majority of the newborns with low weight are true premature babies. Moreover, as Rooth [85] remarks, average birthweight and the distribution of birthweight must be differently interpreted according to the countries concerned: the 1,501- to 2,000-gram group does not have the same significance in India as in the United States. That further complicates inter-country comparisons; but, despite these reservations, birthweight remains by far the best indicator of health or sickness at birth—easier to measure than size, more reliable than gestational age, and more often documented than those two parameters. "WHO efforts to have weight adopted as the general criterion must therefore be energetically supported" [42].

International comparisons. — The international study organized under the auspices of WHO

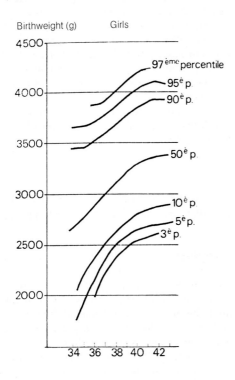

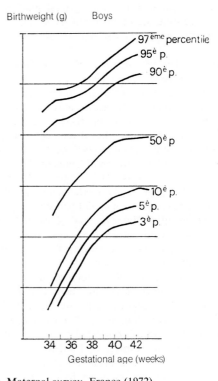

Gestational age (weeks)

Fig. I-1. — *Birthweight by gestational age.* Maternal survey, France (1972), smoothed curves after exclusion of stillbirths, twins, malformed infants (Source: [89]).

TABLE I. — Birthweight (percentiles and means) by gestational age. Nationwide study, France, 1972 (Data smoothed after exclusion of stillborns, twins, infants with malformations or of uncertain gestational age) (Source: Rumeau-Rouquette [89]).

a) *Girls.*

| Gestational age (weeks) | Number | Percentiles | | | | | | | Mean |
		03	05	10	50	90	95	97	
34	48			2,056	2,697	3,447			2,722
35	84		1,995	2,226	2,786	3,452	3,649		2,802
36	125	2,031	2,156	2,357	2,888	3,498	3,701	3,853	2,903
37	219	2 205	2,318	2,475	2,982	3,549	3,754	3,890	2,997
38	495	2,341	2,448	2,584	3,077	3,635	3,823	3,951	3,092
39	978	2,455	2,551	2,687	3,182	3,730	3,904	4,034	3,195
40	1,214	2,534	2,633	2,775	3,277	3,830	4,012	4,131	3,288
41	870	2,579	2,678	2,825	3,327	3,910	4,092	4,206	3,349
42	329	2,621	2,698	2,850	3,357	3,938	4,123	4,218	3,381
43	104			2,868	3,372	3,928			3,392

b) *Boys.*

| Gestational age (weeks) | Number | Percentiles | | | | | | | Mean |
		03	05	10	50	90	95	97	
34	39			2,021	2,706	3,533			2,759
35	87		2,043	2,228	2,861	3,642	3,855		2,913
36	131	2,091	2,233	2,406	2,979	3,689	3,890	3,975	3,023
37	271	2,280	2,399	2,564	3,102	3,748	3,916	4,004	3,126
38	541	2,413	2,525	2,694	3,212	3,808	3,961	4,066	3,227
39	1,074	2,538	2,647	2,812	3,325	3,888	4,049	4,160	3,334
40	1,258	2,618	2,748	2,907	3,414	3,989	4,162	4,273	3,423
41	894	2,648	2,801	2,956	3,452	4,060	4,243	4,364	3,482
42	384	2,662	2,811	2,973	3,465	4,104	4,295	4,459	3,511
43	145			2,970	3,476	4,124			3,527

TABLE II. — Rates of prematurity, birthweight < 2,500 g, and perinatal mortality in 7 countries in 1973 (Source: WHO [76]).

Country	Gestational age <37 weeks %	Weight <2,500 g %	Perinatal mortality °/oo
Hungary . . .	19.8	10.8	29.1
Cuba	11.2 *	10.8	26.9
Austria . . .	10.8 **	5.7	21.4
U. S. A. (in part).	7.3	6.0	14.9
Sweden . . .	5.0	3.9	12.6
New Zealand. .	4.5	5.2	17.3
Japan	2.6 **	5.3	17.0

* Calculated on births with duration of gestation stated.

** Before 10th lunar month.

in 1973 carried data on gestational age and birthweight [76]. The prematurity rates varied significantly (Table II). Hungary, Cuba and Austria had rates above 10 %. These three countries also had the highest rates (above 20 °/oo) of perinatal mortality. Furthermore, Hungary and Cuba had a high percentage of infants with a birthweight below 2,500 grams; the Austrian percentage, on the contrary, was close to that of the countries having an average or low rate of prematurity.

In France, prematurity rates were measured during the same period in a national survey covering a representative sampling of births [89]. In 1972, the prematurity rate was 8.2 %, thus higher than the rate obtained in Great Britain (5.3 % in 1970) or in the United States (7.2 % in 1973). Infants born with a weight equal to, or below, 2,500 grams constituted 7 % of the sample in 1972, halfway between the American rate (7.5 %) and the English rate (6.5 %).

TABLE III. — Percentage of infants in different countries weighing less than 2,500 g at birth
(Source: Boldman [7]).

Country	Population	1950-1959	1960-1969	1970-1976
Africa				
Ethiopia	Total		16.5	8.8-16.5
Rhodesia	Total	16.6	11.0	—
Sudan	Total	—	17.3	—
Zaire	Total	—	10.0-24.4	—
Asia				
China	Total	11.3	—	—
India	New Delhi	29.0	40.0	—
	Agra	—	26.0	—
	Kanpur	—	45.0	—
Japan	Total	8.0	11.3	5.3
America				
Canada	Total	—	—	6.3
U. S. A.	All	—	7.8	7.5
	Whites	6.9	7.0	6.4
	Non-Whites	11.6	12.5	12.5
	Indians	—	6.0	—
Mexico	Mexico City	11.0	—	—
Europe				
Austria	Total	—	6.0	—
Denmark	Total	4.6	5.6	—
Finland	Total	—	4.7	—
Greece	Total	—	9.5	—
Hungary	Total	—	10.2	—
Italy	Total	17.0	5.1	—
No. Ireland	Total	—	5.9	—
Norway	Total	—	5.2	4.9
Poland	Total	6.7	5.8	—
United Kingdom	England and Wales	—	7.5	—
	Great Britain	6.7	6.2-7.4	6.5
Sweden	Total	4.8	4.9	4.1
Czechoslovakia	Total	6.7	6.0	
Middle East				
Iran	Total	—	14.2	—
Israel	Total	—	5.5	—
Syria	Total	—	19.9	—
Oceania				
Australia	Queensland	—	6.4	—

The percentage of infants weighing less than 2,500 grams at birth is often very high in the developing countries. In 1977, Boldman and Reed published a bibliographic survey [7] from which Table III has been extracted. The highest rates were observed in Asia; they were over 40 % in some parts of India, but much lower in Japan (11.3 % for the same period, 1960-1969). Africa and the countries of the Middle East had rates varying between 10 % and 20 %; European rates fluctuated between 5 % and 10 %. It is in this range that the Canadian rates and those of the white population in the United States were situated.

Recently, an attempt was made to assess on a worldwide basis the number of infants with low birthweight [51]. The authors made a series of estimates based on the countries where the frequency was known, taking into account the distribution of social classes. They arrived at the following results for 1975:

Africa	:	2.8 millions
North America	:	0.4 million
South America	:	1.5 million
Asia	:	16.5 millions
Europe	:	0.5 million
Oceania	:	0.1 million
USSR	:	0.2 million

More recent figures, collected by WHO [78], are, respectively:

Africa	:	3.2 millions (15 % of births)
North America	:	0.3 million (7 % of births)
Latin America	:	1.4 million (11 % of births)
Asia	:	14.8 millions (20 % of births)
Europe	:	0.5 million (8 % of births)
Oceania	:	0.06 million (12 % of births)
USSR	:	0.4 million (8 % of births)

Even if the total number of low-weight newborns is underestimated, these results nevertheless give an idea of the magnitude of the problem.

Regional differences. — Regional differences are found to be relatively important in very large countries like the United States, even if only the white population is studied (Fig. I-2) [82]. But differences exist even in middle-size countries like France, where there also exists a certain similarity between the distribution of perinatal mortality and prematurity [89].

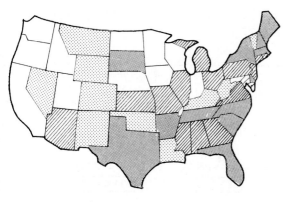

% of L.B.W.

☐ 4,7 à 5,9 (13 states)

▨ 6 à 6,3 (15 ")

▨ 6,4 à 6,6 (12 ")

▨ 6,7 à 8,8 (11 ")

Fig. I-2.

Chronological differences. — Information concerning changes in prematurity rates is scanty and sometimes difficult to interpret, due to the confusion that has for a long time prevailed between prematurity and hypotrophy. A clear-cut decline in rates is evident in France: 8.2 % in 1972 v. 6.3 % in 1981 [1]; the same is true for the United States, at least for the white population: 6.7 % in 1950; 5.9 % in 1967. On the other hand, the rates are stable and high among black Americans (10.4 % and 11 %), stable and low in England (5.2 % in 1958; 5.3 % in 1970) [13, 21, 89].

Concerning low birthweight, information is more plentiful, although for Table III we have only a limited body of older statistics (1950-1959) and recent data (1970-1976). The percentage of infants born alive and weighing under 2,500 grams declines clearly in Rhodesia (now Zimbabwe), Japan, and Italy. It varies little in the United States, Denmark, France, Norway, Great Britain, and Sweden. An increase is noted in India between 1950-1959 and 1960-1969 [7].

Risk factors. — In the industrialized countries, a relatively minor portion of prematurity cases have a precise origin (cervical incompetence, multiple pregnancies, placenta praevia, etc.); in the other cases, one can only detect risk factors that, while failing to explain the origin of the prematurity, do permit its anticipation and prevention. A number of studies have made it possible to describe them.

One observes, first, that premature births have a tendency to recur in the same women: a premature antecedent doubles the probability of having another premature child. Moreover, premature deliveries are more frequent among those under 20 years of age and over 35; this frequency increases with parity.

Economic and cultural factors such as the level of education, profession of the father, family income, play an important role in the causes of prematurity. In some countries, particularly in France, professional women are less likely to have a premature child; in general, they are younger, better educated and better informed than others. However, strenuous working conditions influence the duration of the gestation: the rate of prematurity increases with the number of hours worked per week and with the fatigue index (Fig. I-3) [33].

Taking these factors into account, the population of pregnant women was divided into subgroups having different *prematurity risks*. Figure I-4

---

[1] From C. Rumeau-Rouquette et al.: Naître en France : 10 ans d'évolution 1972-1981. Paris, Doin et INSERM, 1984.

illustrates a segmentation analysis performed on a representative sample of 11,200 births in France [89]. Risk coefficients can also be calculated by using statistical or empirical methods, for example, the "Coefficient of Risk of Premature Delivery" (Papiernik [79]).

Such an approach also makes it possible to study the factors of risk of small-for-date babies. Maternal antecedents have primary importance here: hypotrophy tends to repeat itself; but is decreases with parity (unlike prematurity). It is linked to smoking and, possibly, to the consumption of alcohol.

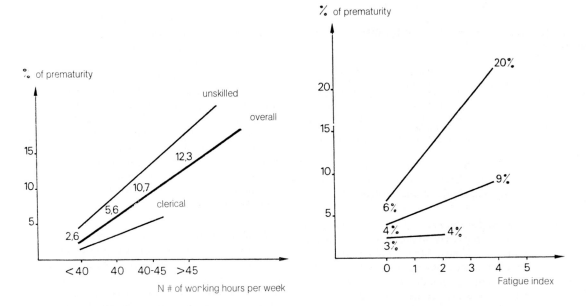

FIG. I-3. — *Prematurity rate by employment in 1972* (Source: Ministère du Travail [33]).

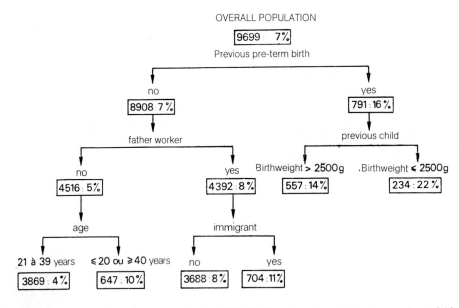

FIG. I-4. — *Prematurity: results of segmentation in 1972* (Each rectangle contains the number of births and the prematurity rate in the sub-group concerned, after exclusion of twins, stillborn, and infants with malformations.) (Source : Rumeau-Rouquette [75]).

The role of social factors varies considerably from one country to another; that of maternal malnutrition is paramount in the developing countries.

The concept of risk has been widely used by the medical profession and even by government authorities [80]. But it has become evident that the concept has had little influence on the public [89].

The difficulties encountered in trying to determine gestational age are such that the indicator most widely used on an international level for studying risk factors remains *birthweight under 2,500 grams*. Its link to maternal antecedents, to family situation, and to socioeconomic characteristics, as well as to the weight and height of the parents, is evident. Surveys conducted in the United States show, for example, that the percentage of infants weighing 2,500 grams or less is only half as great among white children (6.1 %) as among the others (12.1 %) (Fig. I-5) [103]. The percentage diminishes as the duration of education increases, whatever the ethnic origins of the parents might be (Table IV). Finally, closely spaced pregnancies contribute to low birthweight, which is also linked to the age of the mother (Fig. I-5).

Nutrition plays an important role. The effects of the famine in the Netherlands during World War II demonstrated this convincingly. Conditions just as dramatic are still frequent in the Third World [50]. The example of the Sahel drought (1972-1976) remains vivid in our minds: Average birthweight declined, and perinatal and infant mortality increased, in the areas affected. In reviewing a whole series of studies of the effects on fetal growth of changes in the supply of protein and calories during pregnancy, Rush concludes that nutritional supplementation does not always have the desired effect: supplements high in protein content are constantly associated with a decline in birthweight; those with low protein content

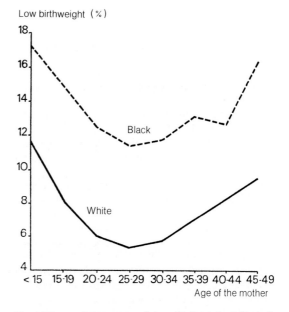

FIG. I-5. — *Percentage of low birthweight infants by maternal age and race of the infant, U. S. A., 1976* (Source: NCHS [84]).

usually bring about an increase in birthweight—but a very moderate one (an average of 50 g), and always less significant than hoped for. These effects vary little in terms of the conditions under which the experiments are conducted [115].

Future research must concentrate on subgroups of women among whom a positive result is most likely to be observed (for example, among heavy smokers). It must also specify whether the minimal gains in birthweight attained are accompanied by a significant reduction in perinatal morbidity and mortality, and by an improvement in the growth and development of the infant.

TABLE IV. — Percent of infants of low birth wright (≤ 2,500 g) by marital status and educational attainment of mother and race of child (U. S. A., 1976) (Source: NCHS [103]).

Years of education completed by mother	Married women			Unmarried women		
	All races	White	Black	All races	White	Black
Total	6.4	5.8	11.1	12.7	9.8	14.8
0-8 years	8.7	8.2	13.0	13.6	10.8	16.4
9-11 years	8.6	7.9	12.7	13.2	10.3	15.4
12 years.	6.1	5.5	10.7	11.7	9.0	13.6
13-15 years.	5.4	5.0	10.0	11.7	9.2	13.3
16 years or more.	4.8	4.4	9.0	9.9	7.5	12.0

CONGENITAL MALFORMATIONS

These include malformations of genetic origin induced before birth, as well as chromosomal abnormalities, and malformations that occur during the first three months of pregnancy. Their frequency is approximately 2 % at birth, but only one-half of them are diagnosed during the early neonatal period.

A number of sources clearly indicate important differences in the frequency and, most of all, in the distribution of congenital malformations from one country to another. This is shown in Table V, taken from a WHO survey conducted from 1961 to 1964 in 16 countries [96]. For all malformations, frequency varied from 1.02 per 100 births (the Japanese rate [71]) to 12.33 % in Australia. Malformations of the central nervous system had a particularly high frequency in Ireland and in the United Kingdom, with a notable predominance of anencephaly: 4.6 $^o/_{oo}$ of births in Ireland at the end of the 1950s [95], and of *spina bifida*: 4.1 $^o/_{oo}$ of births in Wales [49]. Very high rates were obtained in Egypt [52]. The frequency of malformations of muscle and of bone structure was found to be two to three times higher in South Africa, Brazil, and Colombia, than in other countries. The highest

frequency of harelip appeared among Asian populations: in Japan and Malaysian [52].

The evolution of malformations in time and space has been widely studied since 1963, for the most part in regional centers linked through international systems: "European Registration of Congenital Abnormalities and Twins" (EUROCAT) and "The International Clearinghouse for Birth Defects and Monitoring System." The latest report of the International Clearinghouse notes a particularly sharp diminution of anencephaly in England and Northern Ireland; it is presently recognized that this could be due to prenatal diagnosis, but could also represent a diminution of prevalence, independent of prenatal diagnosis. The frequency of *spina bifida* has also diminished, but to a lesser extent. For Down's syndrome, the same source indicates an increase in frequency among young women and a decline among those over 35. The latter phenomenon might be attributable to the steadily expanding practice of prenatal diagnosis for women above 35. The increased frequency of the syndrome among young women has yet to be explained.

These geographic and age differences in congenital malformations have given rise to numerous hypotheses, specifically implicating ethnic origins and *living conditions*, especially eating habits. On this subject, Wynn [112] reminds us that, on the basis of a historical study in Europe, "epidemics" of malformations often follow famine periods and epide-

TABLE V. — FREQUENCY OF MALFORMATIONS BASED ON A WHO STUDY OF MATERNITY CENTERS IN 16 COUNTRIES (Rates per 10,000 live births) (Source: STEVENSON [96])

Country	Number of births	Overall frequency		Central nervous system	Cardiovascular system	Harelip and cleft palate	Digestive system	Genitourinary system	Muscles, bone structure	Various
		Number	Rate							
South Africa	24,242	407	168	25	13	10	7	5	42	11
Australia	11,765	216	180	36	15	11	13	5	25	18
Brazil	14,421	231	160	29	6	13	10	7	48	6
Chile	23,720	224	94	13	1	14	3	3	19	3
Colombia	39,271	544	138	10	7	14	2	2	46	9
Egypt	9,598	111	116	79	1	9	4	0	7	5
Spain	19,714	264	134	18	33	10	5	4	15	6
Hong Kong	9,872	114	113	22	9	16	5	2	24	15
India	58,689	399	68	26	2	11	4	2	9	4
No. Ireland	28,091	544	194	104	11	13	6	2	19	6
Malaysia	55,620	510	92	15	0.07	17	4	5	15	4
Mexico	38,783	519	134	21	10	7	6	3	20	12
Panama	15,852	329	208	24	1	7	1	1	41	8
Philippines	29,669	252	85	10	7	15	3	2	16	10
Czechoslovakia	20,074	348	173	25	17	11	11	5	27	15
Yugoslavia	17,304	278	161	18	9	8	6	4	36	10

mics of infectious diseases associated with them. After the thalidomide drama, it was proved experimentally that vitamin deficiencies significantly increased the toxicity of that product, and the same was also demonstrated for other toxic substances —for certain xenobiotics in particular. Among humans, vitamin supplementation initiated before conception may reduce the risk of malformations of the neural tube [93]. The differences in the incidence of congenital malformations varying by country and socioeconomic class can thus be linked to nutritional deficiencies—to which pregnant women are, we know, particularly vulnerable. Assuming increasing degrees of maternal malnutrition, the following sequence is plausible: fetal hypotrophy, congenital malformations, miscarriage, sterility. Nevertheless, exogenous risk factors are still rather poorly understood.

Drugs, however, have been intensively studied following the discovery of the teratogenic role of thalidomide. For certain products, the teratogenic effect is very probable, even certain; the group includes, in addition to thalidomide, hormones whose androgenic effect produces the masculinization of female fetuses (here, it is a question not only of testerone, but also of certain synthetic progestins [53, 109]); diethylstilbesterol has been identified since 1971 with the development of vaginal cancer among females exposed to it *in utero* (*in* [88], p. 104); aminopterin causes severe craniofacial malformations (anencephaly, hydrocephalus, cleft palate) [53]; other antitumor drugs have also been incriminated, busulfan and chlorambucil among others.

Concerning other drugs, there exists a significant increase in the frequency of congenital malformations, but their causal relationship has not been fully demonstrated. Drugs used for the central nervous system have often been incriminated in etiologic studies during the last 15 years. The most persuasive results concern antiepileptic drugs—and, above all, the hydantoins—though their role has not been entirely separated from that of the epilepsy itself [34]. Tranquilizers, both carbamates and benzodiazepines, have also been implicated, but the results have been inconsistent from one survey to another [68]. Some phenothiazines are also suspect, following a French study revealing an excessive frequency of malformations in a group of infants exposed to them *in utero* [87].

Sex hormones, and more especially the estroprogestins contained in some pregnancy tests, are associated with an increase in the frequency of malformations and have been proscribed [36]. Diethylstilbesterol, used in pregnancies for therapeutic purposes, is identified with an excessive frequency of genital abnormalities in men and women exposed to it *in utero*. Isolated results have led to the suspicion that oral contraceptives have a teratogenic effect, but this is far from proven [9]. In fact, the great diversity of products used, doses given, and of the conditions of use makes such an evaluation extremely difficult.

Chemicals that constitute a part of the pregnant woman's environment have been studied to a considerably lesser degree: anesthetics, hexachlorophine, vinyl chloride, certain organic solvents, and pesticides are thought to have a teratogenic role, although this has not been fully demonstrated [12]. The mutagenic, teratogenic, and cancerous effects of X rays and radioactive substances have long been known, but the impact of small doses hat not been clearly assessed.

Some *viral infections* have a teratogenic effect: all have been suspected, but special mention must be made of cytomegalovirus and, above all, German measles (Rubella) [11].

In sum, it is the total environment in which we live that can—through the mother—have harmful effects on the products of conception. Theoretical studies, surveys [88], experimental models, experimentation on animals, in vitro studies are the subject of much research all over the world. A recent general review by H. Kalter and J. Warkany sums up the present state of knowledge in this area. The authors emphasize that the etiology of this pathology—presently responsible for 21 % of infant mortality in the United States—remains unknown in most cases, and resists preventative efforts and treatment attempts [114]. "Echotoxicology" applied to the pregnant woman and to the fetus [81] will undoubtedly clarify many points still obscure concerning the etiology of malformations which remain a major cause of perinatal morbidity and mortality.

ACUTE FETAL DISTRESS

For a long time, fetal hypoxia was detected by clinical examination done at delivery and during the neonatal period. The electronic recording of fetal heartbeat, the study of the blood pH of the fetus, have made possible great progress in the diagnosis of distress at the end of pregnancy and during delivery. However, this kind of examination is far from being the norm, even in industrialized countries (electronic monitoring of fetal heartbeat accompanied only 6.4 % of deliveries in France in 1972, 31 % in 1976, and 68 % in 1981 [89]). These factors explain why the diagnostic criteria of fetal distress are very different from one country to another, with results that are difficult to compare. It can be estimated *grosso modo* that 5 to 7 % of infants born in Western countries show signs of fetal distress of varying importance during delivery. However, available information is insufficient to enable us to establish as international distribution of this cause of morbidity.

While some perinatal distress is directly traceable to obstetrical trauma, most of it is linked to risk factors, some of which have been known for a long time: toxemia of pregnancy, severe disease of the mother, twin pregnancies, premature delivery, non-occiput presentations, placental abnormalities, tight coiling of the umbilical cord, etc. More recently, epidemiologic studies have made it possible to determine the role of sociocultural characteristics. Thus, we know that in France fetal distress is more frequent when the mother is an immigrant, or a native of one of the overseas administrative departments or territories, or when her socioeconomic level is low [89].

PERINATAL INFECTION

Perinatal infection is a well-known cause of mortality and morbidity in the developing countries. The cooperative study of the Pan American Health Organization has shown that deaths due to this cause were as frequent in Argentina, Bolivia, and Colombia as those due to congenital malformations; the facts are very different in Canada and in the United States [83]. Perinatal infections are, however, far from negligible in the industrialized countries. Contamination of the fetus by toxoplasmosis can occur at any time during the pregnancy. If no antibiotics are administered, the infant will be born with congenital toxoplasmosis which can result in severe neurological abnormalities [29]. Cytomegalic inclusion disease is of growing importance among severe fetal illness [8]. Congenital Rubella, also, constitutes a grave risk in the second part of pregnancy [11].

Other maternal infections—specific ones like listeriosis, or others caused by unidentified organisms (frequently the case in urinary infections associated with pregnancy)—trigger severe perinatal infections. Recent French studies have shown that serious infections (meningitis, enterocolitis, septicemia)

affected approximately 5 % of the infants transferred from maternity units to neonatal centers [35], and that the rate of neonatal infections, for all births in a high-risk maternity center, remained stable, at about 1 % [5]. Recent epidemics of necrotizing enterocolitis in highly specialized maternity centers have drawn attention to this problem. These epidemics most frequently affect premature infants, or those who have suffered from fetal distress [63]. They generally do not affect breast-fed newborns, although we are unable to determine the role played by this form of feeding, which is obviously less frequent when the infants are transferred to a neonatal center because of prematurity or fetal distress.

OTHER CAUSES OF MORBIDITY

In the industrialized countries, the frequency of *feto-maternal blood incompatibility* has become minor. As a result of systematic typing and the use of anti-D gamma globulin after an incompatible pregnancy—whether it terminates in childbirth or abortion—prophylaxis should completely eliminate incompatibility in the Rhesus system, at least in its most severe form. Incompatibilities in the ABO system, and the other hyperbilirubinemias of the neonatal period, are less amenable to prevention: but their treatment follows rules by now well established.

Chronic fetal distress, whose diagnosis has been facilitated by technical progress, is a syndrome having multiple causes, by no means all of which have been identified. It presents difficult problems of decision making concerning the action that must be taken [101] and the entire obstetric-pediatric team must participate in such decisions.

The other causes of morbidity are rarer: they are examined in the various chapters of this book. They are often associated with maternal pathology —which complicates their prevention—and are often linked to each other, a factor that complicates accurate reporting. It would be desirable, in order to have surveys viable from the epidemiological viewpoint, to record morbidity in the same way as perinatal deaths (see the model certificate recommended by WHO: Figure I-6), clearly showing the maternal pathology, the pathology of the fetus or of the infant and, perhaps, other relevant factors, while differentiating—in the first two groupings— the main disease and, as the case might be, the other diseases or difficulties present.

CERTIFICATE OF CAUSE OF PERINATAL DEATH

To be completed for stillbirths and live born infants dying within 168 hours (1 week) from birth

(Identifying Particulars)

☐ This child was live born on   at   hours
       and died on   at   hours

☐ This child was stillborn on   at   hours
and died Before labour ☐ During labour ☐ Not known ☐

Mother

Date of birth ☐☐☐☐
or, if unknown, age (years) ☐☐

Number of previous pregnancies:
Live births ☐☐
Stillbirths ☐☐
Abortions ☐☐

Outcome of last previous pregnancy:
Live birth ☐
Stillbirth ☐
Abortion ☐
Date ☐☐☐☐☐

1st day of last menstrual period ☐☐☐☐☐☐
or, if unknown, estimated duration of pregnancy (completed weeks) ☐☐

Antenatal care, two or more visits
Yes ☐
No ☐
Not known ☐

Delivery:
Normal spontaneous vertex ☐
Other (specify) ....

Child

Birthweight: ...... grammes
Sex:
Boy ☐ Girl ☐ Indeterminate ☐
Single birth ☐ First twin ☐
Second twin ☐ Other multiple ☐

Attendant at birth

Physician ☐ Trained midwife ☐
Other trained person (specify) ....
Other (specify) ....

CAUSES OF DEATH

a. Main disease or condition in fetus or infant

b. Other diseases or conditions in fetus or infant

c. Main maternal disease or condition affecting fetus or infant

d. Other maternal diseases or conditions affecting fetus or infant

e. Other relevant circumstances

The certified cause of death has been confirmed by autopsy ☐

Autopsy information may be available later ☐

Autopsy not being held ☐

I certify ....
....
....
Signature and qualification

FIG. I-6.

Perinatal mortality

GENERAL

Perinatal mortality is defined as the sum of the deaths occurring during the late fetal period and the early neonatal period (the first 7 days of life).

But differences in definitions and in the calculation of rates, the varying methods used in national registration systems, and the absence of data for many countries, complicate the study of the overall rate of perinatal mortality and its components, as well as comparisons in time (for the same country or the same region) or in space (comparisons within or between countries). These problems will be examined, to the extent possible, in the context of the World Health Organization's recommendations.

Definitions and recommendations. —
The 9th revision of WHO's International Classification of Diseases (ICD) cites the definitions of live birth and fetal death [74]:

1. **Live birth.** — Live birth is the complete expulsion or extraction from its mother of a product of conception, irrespective of the duration of the pregnancy, which, after such separation, breathes or shows any other evidence of life, such as beating of the heart, pulsation of the umbilical cord, or definite movement of voluntary muscles, whether or not the umbilical cord has been cut or the placenta is attached; each product of such a birth is considered live born.

2. **Fetal death.** — Fetal death is death prior to the complete expulsion or extraction from its mother of a product of conception, irrespective of the duration of pregnancy; the death is indicated by the fact that after such separation the fetus does not breathe or show any other evidence of life, such as beating of the heart, pulsation of the umbilical cord, or definite movement of voluntary muscles.

In its recommendations, WHO sets out certain data for the establishment of perinatal mortality statistics:

It is recommended that *national* perinatal statistics should include all fetuses and infants delivered weighing at least 500 g (or, when birthweight is unavailable, the corresponding gestational age (22 weeks) or body length (25 cm crown-heel))...
... it is recommended that countries should present, solely for *international* comparisons, "standard perinatal statistics" in which both the numerator and denominator of all rates are restricted to fetuses and infants weighing 1,000 g or more (or, where birthweight is unavailable, the corresponding gestational age (28 weeks) or body length (35 cm crown-heel)).

Unfortunately, these recommendations have not been adopted in most countries. In a recent study, Höhn has stressed the disparity of criteria used in collecting and processing statistical data in 8 European countries (West Germany, Austria, France, Great Britain, Luxembourg, Netherlands, Sweden and Switzerland) [42]. This situation makes inter-country comparisons very difficult.

A better-coordinated approach would make it possible to avoid significant distortions. Two studies have illustrated the importance of uniform definitions for international comparisons. The first, conducted in Sweden, concerns the differences in the

concept of life and death at birth. The second is a Dutch study comparing the mortality rates of live newborns when those born before 28 weeks of gestation were included in the calculation, and when they were excluded. In 1956, in Sweden, it was customary to report the non-viable products of delivery as stillborn whether they showed signs of life or not; the study, designed to measure the impact of application of WHO's definitions on rates, dealt with approximately 100,000 births. Results for perinatal mortality did not change overall, but the rates of stillbirths and of early neonatal mortality were affected (Table VI) [20]. The Dutch study proved that breaking down the statistics by births occurring during the early fetal period (before 28 weeks of gestation) and by those occurring during the later fetal period, also affected rates. Stillborn rates remained unchanged, but the overall perinatal mortality rate increased by almost 2 $^o/_{oo}$ when live births among infants with a gestational age under 28 weeks were taken into account (Table VII) [70].

TABLE VI. — Effect of the definition of live births on the components of feto-infantile mortality, Sweden, 1956 (Source: Chase [20]).

	Swedish definition		WHO definition	
	Number	Rate	Number	Rate
Live births . . .	107,960	...	108,081	...
Perinatal deaths [1] . .	3,106	28.3	3,106	28.3
Stillbirths [1] . . .	1,836	16.7	1,715	15.6
Deaths under 1 week [2].	1,270	11.8	1,391	12.9
Deaths under 28 days [2].	1,427	13.2	1,548	14.3
Deaths under 1 year [2].	1,871	17.3	1,992	18.4

[1] Rate per 1,000 total births (live births and stillbirths).
[2] Rate per 1,000 live births.

More recently, Höhn determined that the perinatal mortality rate in West Germany for 1976, which was 17.1 $^o/_{oo}$ according to the criteria used in that country, would change to 16.7 $^o/_{oo}$ if the WHO definition for national statistics were used, and to 14.4 $^o/_{oo}$ if WHO recommendations for international comparisons were followed (infants weighing under 1,000 g excluded from the numerator and from the denominator) [42].

Application of the definitions and recommendations proposed by the 9th revision of the ICD

TABLE VII. — EFFECT OF THE INCLUSION OF INFANTS BORN ALIVE, BUT HAVING A GESTATIONAL AGE OF LESS THAN 28 WEEKS (GA < 28 w), ON THE COMPONENTS OF PERINATAL MORTALITY (Source: WHO [74]).

	GA < 28 w excluded		GA < 28 w included	
	Number	Rate	Number	Rate
Live births	245,739	...	246,150	...
Perinatal mortality [1]. .	6,004	24.1	6,415	25.7
Stillbirths [1]	3,645	14.6	3,645	14.6
Early neonatal mortality [2]	2,359	9.6	2,770	11.3

[1] Rate per 1,000 total births (stillbirths and live births).
[2] Rate per 1,000 live births.

should reduce these disparities among national statistics. But for such application to be useful, it would have to be accompanied by a uniformity of definitions. We are far from that goal. A Council of Europe study [24], involving 14 European countries, has shown that the difficulties are of two kinds:

1. In Belgium and France, an infant who has died by the time the birth is registered (during the three days following the birth) is generally considered to be stillborn. It is nonetheless possible to correct these rates by taking into account the information contained in the death certificate, but this information is lacking in 5 to 10 % of the cases.

2. The definition of viability represents, as we have seen above, a more serious problem. Thus, in Sweden, a stillborn infant is a product of conception having a gestational age of 28 weeks or more, or measuring 35 centimeters or more; in Belgium, France and Italy, viability begins at 180 days; in Denmark, it begins at 28 weeks, with 1,000 g as the equivalent.

In the study mentioned above, Höhn summed up in the form of tables, for the 8 countries surveyed, the legal definitions of live newborns and stillbirths, as well as the criteria used in the registration of births and deaths [42]. The differences are significant and comparisons require delicate corrections and adjustments.

Registration of deaths. — *Registration methods* are often unsatisfactory—and not only in the developing countries. A recent study [27], focused

on three states in the United States, stresses the inadequacies of the perinatal mortality registration (especially for the underprivileged population groups) and notes the errors and imprecisions in the reporting of data, the lack of consistency and liaison between birth and death statistics, etc. Further, improvements in reporting, particularly concerning stillbirths, can temporarily mask a decline in mortality rates. Despite the different methods used in assembling data in the developed countries—especially concerning the prescribed time for registering births and deaths (which vary greatly from one country to another)—the registrations are well complied with and quantifiable; the effects of these differences are virtually negligible as far as births are concerned, but are more serious in the measurement of stillbirth rates and, therefore, of perinatal mortality [42]. It is thus useful to link the data from birth and death registrations. This practice, which is already routine in certain states of the United States—and which is soon to be so in England and Wales [30]— also permits mortality comparisons in terms of the length of gestation, birthweight, age of the mother, parity, and pathologies observed both in the mother and in the child.

Calculation and interpretation of rates.
— The method of calculating rates has altered over the years and the study of change at national levels requires adjustments. Depending on the period and the country, the denominator used in the calculation of perinatal mortality rates has been either the total number of live births, or the sum of live births and stillbirths. In both cases, the rates are generally expressed by the thousand. Until 1980, world statistical annuals published rates calculated using, as the denominator, exclusively live births—these same rates being established on the basis of information furnished by national statistical offices which used their own definitions for the elaboration of the data. For the future, the 9th revision has recommended that the denominator be the sum of live births and stillbirths.

The interpretation of rates sometimes differs. Many authors consider neonatal mortality as an excellent health indicator. It represents a defined event having a minimal risk of under registration which is not the case for stillbirths. As a matter of fact, it is advisable to give particular attention to the changes in the different components of perinatal and infant mortality. Shifting phenomena have become significant, due to improvements in obstetrical techniques and neonatal intensive care. They modify to some extent the classic profiles of mortality.

The shift may affect only the distribution of the deaths between the two components of perinatal mortality without changing the overall figures: stillbirths becoming early neonatal deaths. But it can also include prolonged neonatal survivals, with death beyond the 8th day: perinatal mortality appearing decreased at the expense of later mortality rates.

Many arguments have emerged in support of this hypothesis. In a recent study concerning the European Economic Community (EEC), it was shown that, while perinatal mortality continues to decline, late neonatal mortality (7 to 27 days) and post-neonatal mortality (27 to 365 days) have been stable for several years in most of the EEC countries, and have diminished only in Italy or Greece, where they were particularly high. Moreover, the proportion of perinatal deaths occurring after 27 days increased between 1970 and 1978 in France, Italy, West Germany, and Great Britain [1]. In a study of post-neonatal mortality in the state of New York during the period 1968-1979 (120,000 births per year, on the average), Zdeb [113] found that it had increased among infants weighing under 1,500 g, and diminished among those weighing over 2,000 g, with fluctuations among the infants weighing between 1,501 g and 2,000 g. But in view of the significant proportion of mortality among infants of very low weight, post-neonatal mortality increased for the group as a whole.

Opinions differ about the reality of this phenomenon and, above all, about its magnitude. But the studies lead us to think that perinatal mortality should no longer be examined without simultaneously considering late neonatal and post-neonatal mortality rates [61].

It would also be necessary to take birthweight into account in the presentation of results. To that effect, WHO has long recommended the use of subgroups of 500 g each, beginning with 501 to 1,000 g, 1,001 to 1,500 g, etc. [72]. This method has been used more and more widely.

Finally, in *the interpretation of international comparisons*, it is necessary to take into account the sources of available information. We have most often turned to statistics established by WHO, even though they cover only those countries with which agreements have been made, because many countries lack a valid body of vital statistics. Accord-

ing to Vallin [104], only 29 % of the world's population are fully "covered" by birth certificates and records of deaths occurring during the first year of life: there is almost total coverage in the European countries, Canada, the United States, the USSR, Australia, Japan and New Zealand; 11 % of Latin America; 2.7 % of South Asia; 0.3 % of Africa. Even in countries where the tradition of keeping statistics is well established, data are often published with considerable delay. Finally, not all available data are sent to WHO, and some countries do not always publish them.

If these circumstances make the validity of conclusions more relative, they nevertheless do not make the conduct of scientific studies impossible, as long as the components of feto-infantile mortality are understood in the light of the concepts that have so far governed practice.

In order to better understand perinatal mortality, we will first analyze the levels and the changes in rates while underscoring national and regional disparities; then, we will consider the immediate causes and related conditions; finally, we will specify their ties to certain demographic and socio-economic factors. This analysis of perinatal mortality will use data published by WHO (in its World Health Statistics Annual) and certain national statistics. The international survey conducted by WHO in 1973 will be a frequent reference [76].

THE SITUATION IN 1979-1980

Table VIII indicates the distribution of a number of industrialized countries in terms of different components of fœtal and infant mortality: late fetal mortality, early neonatal mortality and mortality occurring between 7 and 365 days after birth [77].

1) Scandinavia, Switzerland and the Netherlands have the lowest infant mortality in the world (< 10 °/$_{oo}$); the same is true for perinatal mortality (10 to 15 °/$_{oo}$). Canada is in the same group, but its infant mortality is 10.9 °/$_{oo}$.

2) There follow the majority of European Countries, Australia and New Zealand with rates of infant mortality below 15 °/$_{oo}$, and rates of perinatal mortality varying between 12 and 15 °/$_{oo}$.

3) Greece, Hungary, Poland and Portugal, have the highest rates among the countries considered here. In the absence of overall statistics—there are available, in fact, only some hospital studies—the experience of those who practice in the Third

[1] These data are extracted from an unpublished report at the EEC Statistical Office: « La mortalité des jeunes de 0 à 24 ans dans les pays de la communauté européenne », by M. Kaminski, B. Blondel, M. H. Bouvier-Colle, P. Darchy, M. Maujol.

TABLE VIII. — RATES OF STILLBIRTHS, AND PERINATAL, INFANT MORTALITY IN SEVERAL COUNTRIES, 1979-1980
(Rates for 1,000 live births) (Source: WHO [77])

Country	Mortality				
	fetal $^o/_{oo}$	infant $^o/_{oo}$	neonatal $^o/_{oo}$	post-neonatal $^o/_{oo}$	perinatal $^o/_{oo}$
Sweden (1980)	4.5	6.9	4.9	2.0	8.7
Denmark (1980)	4.4	8.4	5.6	2.9	9.0
Finland (1979)	4.2	7.7	5.9	1.7	9.4
Switzerland (1979)	5.7	8.5	5.9	2.6	10.8
Norway (1979)	7.4	8.8	5.4	3.4	11.9
Netherland (1979)	7.1	8.7	5.9	2.8	12.0
Canada (1979)	5.7	10.9	7.2	3.7	11.9
West Germany (1980)	5.3	12.6	7.8	4.8	11.6
New Zealand (1979)	6.7	12.8	6.9	5.9	12.1
East Germany (1980)	6.7	12.1	8.6	3.4	13.6
France (1980)	8.7	10.0	5.6	4.3	13.6
Belgium (1979)	7.9	12.3	8.3	4.0	14.7
United Kingdom, England and Wales (1979)	8.0	12.8	8.2	4.9	14.8
Scotland (1979)	6.9	12.8	8.7	4.2	14.2
Northern Irland (1978)	9.3	15.9	10.5	5.4	18.3
Austria (1980)	12.1	14.3	9.3	5.1	14.2
Australia (1979)	7.9	11.4	7.6	3.8	14.3
Greece (1979)	9.8	18.7	14.5	4.3	21.2
Poland (1979)	6.7	21.2	13.8	7.3	17.2
Hungary (1980)	7.8	23.2	17.8	5.3	23.1
Portugal (1979)	13.4	26.0	15.7	10.3	25.9

World indicates that perinatal and maternal mortality are very high, especially in rural areas, because of the lack of appropriate care when there are complications during delivery, and, also, sometimes, because of harmful practices during the neonatal period; the determining factor seems, however, to be the high rates of newborns with low birthweight (Fig. I-7).

TRENDS

Evolution since 1953 in four countries (England and Wales, Denmark, the United States, France). — The *World Health Statistics Annual* began to carry perinatal mortality rates only in 1967. Thus, national annuals must be used to trace the evolution of rates over a long period. We have chosen four countries because they have published statistics over an extended span of time [25, 26, 38, 102]. Numerous conclusions can be drawn from an examination of these data:

— Improvement is general. If the 1953 perinatal mortality rate is chosen as a base of 100, the rates

thus calculated become, for 1976: 36 for Denmark, 51 for the United States, 47 for England and Wales, 47 for France. The Danish rates prove, moreover, that the lowest limits have not been reached by the other countries (Fig. I-8).

— The components of perinatal mortality do not always develop in a parallel fashion: perinatal mortality has diminished in France because early neonatal mortality declined while the rate of stillbirths remained stable; the decrease in English rates has been primarily due to a decline in late fetal mortality (Fig. I-9 and I-10).

— The diminution of rates has not been uniform over the years and in different countries: compared to other countries, the situation has improved less rapidly in the United States; the early neonatal mortality rate curve in France begins to drop from 1968 onward.

— With the exception of Denmark, the difference between the extremes is less marked.

Evolution since 1967. — Among the EEC countries and Sweden (Fig. I-11), one notes that the groups cited earlier have differed for a number of years. The countries with low perinatal mortality

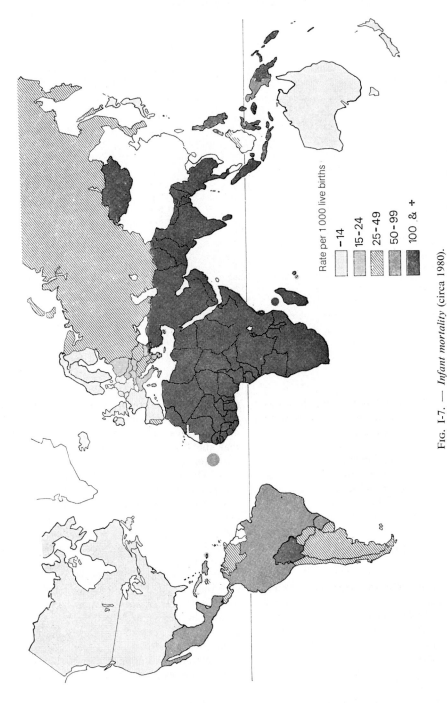

FIG. I-7. — *Infant mortality* (circa 1980).

Source: Population Division, Department of International Economic and Social Affairs, United Nations, New York.

Note: For China, the infant mortality rate is 12 ‰ in urban area and 15-30 ‰ in rural area. According to national authorities the estimated rate is 34,7 ‰ in Vietnam.

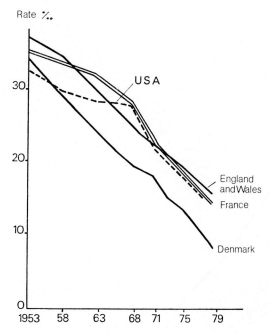

FIG. I-8. — *Perinatal mortality rates in 4 countries 1953-1979 (per 1,000 livebirths)* (Source: WHO [77]).

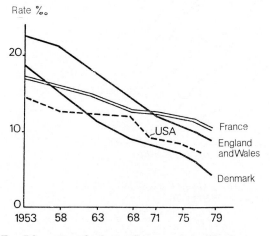

FIG. I-9. — *Late fetal mortality rates (or stillbirth rates) in four countries 1953-1979 (per 1,000 livebirths)* (Source: WHO [77]).

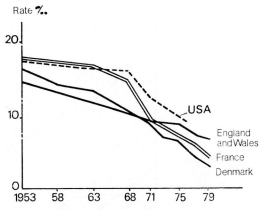

FIG. I-10. — *Eearly neonatal mortality rates in four countries 1953-1979 (per 1,000 livebirths)* (Source: WHO [77]).

their relative positions have changed. Italy continues to have high rates, though the gap has been considerably reduced.

In Eastern Europ (Fig. I-12), the rank order of the countries has remained practically unchanged since 1967. Overall and continuous improvement of the rate is not an invariable process: from 1967 to 1976, perinatal mortality has changed little in Bulgaria and Czechoslovakia, and the decline has been irregular in Hungary and Yugoslavia.

In non-European countries (Fig. I-13), while Japan has shown constant progress, some rates have been stationary, with, even, temporary ups and downs: the Australian rate, after peaking in 1972 and 1973, resumed the same level in 1975 as that of 1971. As for Mexico, its very irregular progress may be due to variations in the system of registering deaths.

The United States. Overall, in the United States, neonatal mortality decreased from 20 $^o/_{oo}$ in 1950 to 11.6 $^o/_{oo}$ in 1975, despite minimal changes in birthweight distribution. The advances achieved—of which 75 % occurred during the final decade of the 25-year period—are attributable to an improvement in one or several birthweight groups [54]. In this regard, California is a good example. There, perinatal mortality—particularly its neonatal component—declined considerably during the 1970's. The diminution in the rates of specific mortality by birthweight categories alone represented 81 % of the total decrease; only 19 % of the decline was due to an improvement in the distribution of birthweight. But there was little progress overall, and no change in birthweights, among the black population.

(Denmark, the Netherlands, Sweden) have had the lowest rates since 1967. But we saw, in Figure 9, that this was not always the case—in Denmark, the rate began to drop sharply in 1960 compared to countries with average rates. The latter have remained grouped very close together since 1967, as, indeed, have France and Great Britain since 1963, though

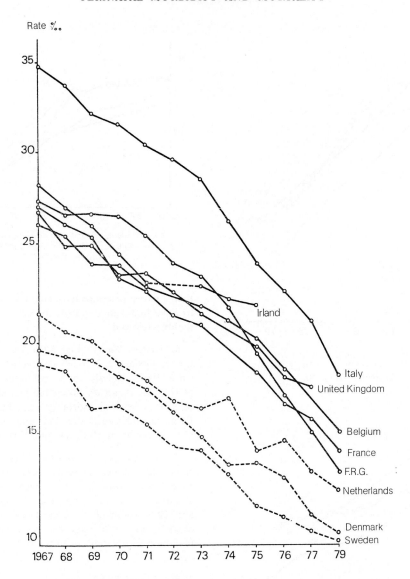

Fig. I-11. — *Evolution of perinatal mortality rates in countries of the EEC and in Sweden 1967-1979* (Rate per 1,000 live births) (Source: WHO [77]).

Mortality dropped more rapidly among the infants born by Caesarean section: it is now at the same level as for infants born by vaginal delivery [110].

REGIONAL DIFFERENCES

Figure I-14 illustrates strong regional disparities among the EEC countries in perinatal mortality [15].

The high rates for southern Italy, with its rural character and low economic level, are evident. But the rates are also high in the heavily industrialized zones of northern Italy, in the north and east of France, as well as in Scotland. In 1973, the extremes ranged from 17.7 $°/_{oo}$ to 23.8 $°/_{oo}$ in England and Wales, from 17.6 $°/_{oo}$ to 24.5 $°/_{oo}$ in France; from 13.3 $°/_{oo}$ to 19.5 $°/_{oo}$ in the Netherlands. The uniformly low levels obtained in Denmark show that it is not impossible to reduce these inequalities.

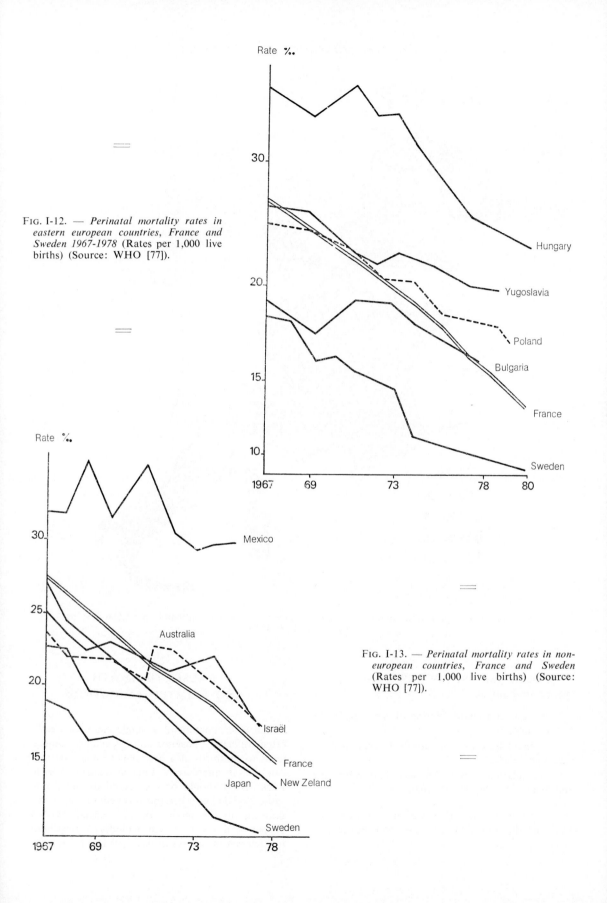

Rate ‰.

30

20

15

10

1967 69 73 78 80

Hungary

Yugoslavia

Poland

Bulgaria

France

Sweden

FIG. I-12. — *Perinatal mortality rates in eastern european countries, France and Sweden 1967-1978* (Rates per 1,000 live births) (Source: WHO [77]).

Rate ‰.

30

25

20

15

Mexico

Australia

Israël

France

Japan   New Zeland

Sweden

1967 69 73 78

FIG. I-13. — *Perinatal mortality rates in non-european countries, France and Sweden* (Rates per 1,000 live births) (Source: WHO [77]).

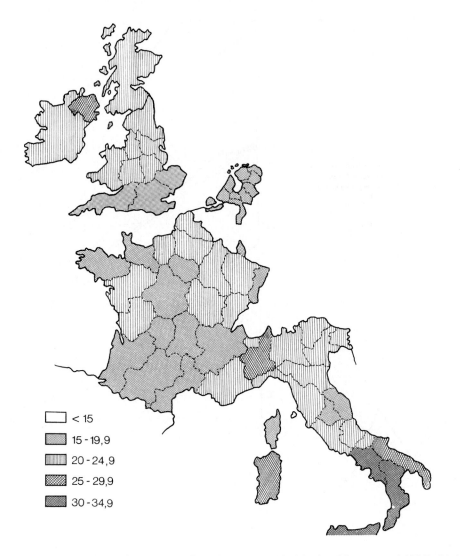

FIG. I-14. — *Perinatal mortality rates in 5 E. E. C. countries, 1974* (regional figures per 1,000 livebirths)
(Source: E. E. C. [15]).

During the years 1973, 1974, 1975, three types of change were noted:

— a slow, continuous closing of the gaps in the Netherlands;
— conversely, an accentuation of regional differences in France;
— irregular changes in Denmark, and in England and Wales [25, 26, 38, 73, 102].

This confirms that no situation is stable once and for all, and that progress can be jeopardized.

CAUSES OF DEATH AND RELATED CONDITIONS

The determination of a single cause of death is often difficult. Toxemia of pregnancy generally leads to the birth of a low-weight baby; the infant can die of intercurrent infection during the first week. What should be considered as the primary cause? WHO has taken this problem into account in drawing up the model for the special certificate of perinatal death, which includes 5 possibilities for defining the causes of death. WHO recommends that this certificate be used for the establishment of national perinatal mortality statistics (Fig. 1-6). In fact, few countries have followed this recommendation, perinatal deaths being declared, registered, collected and categorized by cause, using criteria often different from one country to another. The methods of registration and collection are linked to local conditions and to the level of development of statistical services: ordinary or special death certificates, collection effected by different agents and ministries; moreover, the declarations are not always filled out by doctors [86]. Even when this is the case, the determination of the cause of death depends upon the training, the experience, and the habits of the doctor.

In the WHO certificates of perinatal death, the causes are listed under 5 categories: *a*. Main disease or condition in the fetus or infant; *b*. Other diseases or conditions in the fetus or infant; *c*. Main maternal disease or condition affecting fetus or infant; *d*. Other maternal diseases or conditions affecting fetus or infant; *e*. Other relevant circumstances.

Main causes. — In the WHO study mentioned earlier [76] and based on the classification used therein, the following distribution of causes appears.

Maternal causes are minor, ranging from 7 % in the United States to 19 % in New Zealand. The responsability of *obstetrical causes* varies from 23 % in the United States to 34 % in Japan. Separate mention must be made of Hungary, where deaths due to obstetrical causes are particularly numerous: three times as great, for example, as in the United States. The portion of deaths due to *strictly fetal causes* varies little from one country to another: from 22 % in the United States to 28 % in England and Wales. Finally, as the rate of perinatal mortality increases, the role of *feto-maternal causes also increases* (Fig. I-15).

Discrepancies between some countries are probably linked to the reservations mentioned above: 0.8 % of perinatal deaths in Austria are due to toxemia of pregnancy, while this cause is responsible for 10.8 % of deaths in New Zealand.

It is necessary to break down *specific causes* in order to understand some of the health policies practiced in certain countries and to perceive the risk concepts. Hemolytic diseases of the newborn account for a minor portion of perinatal mortality (Table IX). Infections are still responsible for a great deal of morbidity in the developed countries, and for many deaths in the developing countries: Cuba has the highest proportion among the 8 countries included in the study. In Mexico, 27 % of

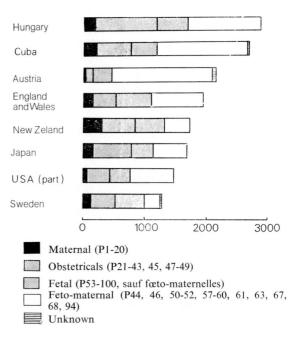

Maternal (P1-20)

Obstetricals (P21-43, 45, 47-49)

Fetal (P53-100, sauf fœto-maternelles)

Feto-maternal (P44, 46, 50-52, 57-60, 61, 63, 67, 68, 94)

Unknown

FIG. I-15. — *Perinatal mortality rates by four principal causes. Rates per 100,000 total births* (Source: WHO [76]).

early neonatal deaths are due to infectious diseases. Maternal-fetal infection remains a worrisome cause of perinatal morbidity and mortality in the industrialized countries. Congenital malformations are responsible for from 5.4 to 20.2 % of deaths, depending on the country.

As promising as it is, this classification is not universally applied. Many authors prefer simpler and more easily usable groupings. Thus, at Hammersmith Hospital in London, Wigglesworth has developed a classification consisting of 5 pathologic groups, to which most perinatal deaths can be tentatively attributed, even in the absence of an autopsy:

— normally formed macerated stillbirth;
— congenital malformations;
— conditions associated with immaturity;
— asphyxial conditions developing in labor;
— specific conditions other than the above.

By matching these diagnoses with birthweight groups, one obtains information immediately usable in concerted, efficient action at the hospital and regional levels [108]. The 5 groups used by Hein et al. [41] in their inter-hospital study in Iowa (U. S. A.) are almost the same, and include 90 % of neonatal deaths.

TABLE IX. — RELATIVE FREQUENCY OF CERTAIN PERINATAL MORTALITY CAUSES IN 8 COUNTRIES IN 1973
(per 100 deaths) (Source: WHO [76])

Causes of death	Country							
	Hungary	Cuba	Austria	England and Wales	New Zealand	Japan	U. S. A. (partial)	Sweden
P12-17 Toxemia	5.8	6.1	0.8	5.3	10.8	9.1	2.3	9.1
P27-29 Difficult labour, with malposition.	8.1	1.5	0.5	1.8	3.6	5.2	1.2	2.0
P42-43 Placenta previa and placental separation	9.6	1.6	1.5	6.4	7.5	6.4	8.5	9.3
P47-49 Umbilical cord conditions .	6.6	8.3	1.7	5.6	6.1	9.8	8.6	4.7
P53-56 Haemolytic disease of the newborn.	2.6	1.9	1.0	2.3	2.4	0.4	1.3	1.0
P69-80 Congenital anomalies. .	11.7	5.4	8.7	20.2	18.0	10.5	14.1	16.9
P58-60 Anoxia and hypoxia. . .	15.0	30.8	10.5	10.6	6.1	5.5	9.9	6.5
P61 Immaturity unqualified. . .	3.0	6.0	24.1	7.5	2.1	6.0	9.5	5.3
P67 Maceration	2.3	1.7	10.3	2.7	1.4	0.9	0.4	11.8
P18-20, 81-88 Maternal infection and infection of the fetus and of the newborn	0.6	3.0	—	0.4	2.2	0.8	2.3	1.0

Related conditions: birthweight and gestational age. — The factor most clearly tied to infant mortality is birthweight. In Sweden, the mortality rate of infants under 1,000 g was still, in 1979, 220 times higher than that of newborns weighing 2,500 g or more (Table X) [86]. On the world level, the phenomenon is of particular concern since it is probably at the origin of millions of deaths annually, with underweight deaths 20 times more numerous in the developing countries than in the industrialized nations [78].

TABLE X. — PERINATAL MORTALITY RATES BY BIRTH-WEIGHT, SWEDEN, 1978 (Rate per 1,000 births) (Source: ROOTH [85]).

Birthweight (g)	Perinatal mortality rate °/oo
—999	750.0
1,000-1,499	405.0
1,500-1,999	171.0
2,000-2,499	52.0
2,500+	3.4

As McFarlane notes, there is a strong correlation between the frequency of low birthweight and unfavorable socioeconomic factors, and the frequency is little influenced by the quality of medical care [56]. Nevertheless, it is through progress in this area, more than through improved distribution of birthweight or through socioeconomic changes—always slow to develop—that perinatal mortality is apt to decline rapidly [47, 54, 100, 110].

The importance of birthweight has led to the establishment of international comparisons by standardizing the results of this variable. In the WHO study, the calculation of standardized rates—taking the New Zealand population as the reference group—notably improves the position of Hungary and reduces the rate spread (Table XI) [76]. In the same study, the calculation of the standardized rate by *length of gestation* significantly modifies the Swedish and Hungarian rates.

It is in fact recognized that, for a given weight, life expectancy varies according to the length of gestation at birth: for infants from 501 to 1,500 g, the survival rate—according to Ritchie [84] in Belfast—increases from 0 (for a gestational age of under 26 weeks) to 50 % (for a gestational age of between 26 and 28 weeks), to 71 % (for a gestational age of between 29 and 31 weeks) and to 96.4 % (for a gestational age of over 32 weeks).

This brief summary of the birthweight/gestational age relationship with mortality rates illustrates the importance of preventive policies whose objectives are the diminution of the number of premature and low-weight newborns, as well as the improvement in their care at all stages, beginning with primary health care [78].

TABLE XI. — PERINATAL MORTALITY RATES: CRUDE AND STANDARDIZED RATES BY BIRTHWEIGHT (B. W.) AND GESTATIONAL AGE (G. A.) IN 7 COUNTRIES IN 1973 (Rates per 1,000 total births) (Source: WHO [76]).

Country	Crude rates $^o/_{oo}$	Standardized rates by B. W. $^o/_{oo}$	by G. A. $^o/_{oo}$
Austria. . . .	21	18	—
Cuba	27	20	24
Hungary . .	29	17	14
Japan	17	19	—
New Zealand . .	17	17	17
Sweden. . . .	13	14	12
U. S. A. (in part).	15	12	9

INFLUENCE OF DEMOGRAPHIC AND SOCIOECONOMIC FACTORS

The rate of perinatal mortality is a good indicator of disparities, revealing, as it does, geographic and socioeconomic inequalities, which are subject to erratic changes over the years and in different places. This property leads us to search for correlations between perinatal mortality and demographic, medical, and socioeconomic factors involved in macro-sociologic analysis [76].

Demographic factors. — Correlations have been calculated on the basis of a limited sample of countries: practically all of them are in the Western industrialized world, or among the Socialist regimes. We have here used the coefficient of rank correlation [91], to permit minimizing annual variations. Table XII shows that there is no significant corre-

TABLE XII. — RELATIONSHIP BETWEEN THE PERINATAL MORTALITY RATE, POPULATION DENSITY AND TOTAL POPULATION IN A NUMBER OF COUNTRIES

Country	Perinatal mortality (1975) Rate %	Rank	Sum of fertility rates Value	Rank	Density of population (1975) Inh./ km²	Rank	Population in millions (1975)
Sweden	11.3	1	1.87	3	18	5	8.3
Denmark	13.4	2	1.91	6	118	14	5.1
Finland	13.9	3	1.49	1	14	4	4.8
Netherlands.	14.0	4	1.89	4	341	22	14.0
Japan	16.0	5	2.13	10	311	20	115.9
Canada	16.5	6	1.92	7	2	2	23.7
New Zealand	16.5	7	2.76	15	12	3	3.2
U. S. A.	16.9	8	1.89	5	23	6	20.3
Bulgaria.	17.6	9			80	9	8.9
France	18.3	10	2.29	12	98	11	53.4
Australia.	19.2	11	2.49	14	2	1	14.3
West Germany. . . .	19.4	12	1.54	2	245	19	61.2
Czechoslovakia. . . .	19.6	13			118	15	15.2
Poland	19.6	14			113	12	35.4
Belgium	19.7	15	1.97	8	316	21	9.8
United Kingdom. . . .	20.2	16	2.03	9	229	18	55.8
Israel.	20.9	17			181	16	3.8
Ireland	21.8	18	3.79	16	47	8	3.3
Yugoslavia	21.9	19	2.34	13	87	10	22.2
Italy	24.1	20	2.27	11	189	17	56.9
Mexico	29.5	21			34	7	67.7
Hungary.	31.6	22			115	13	10.7
Coefficient of rank correlation.			+0.57		+0.20		+0.21

lation between perinatal mortality and *population density* ($r = 0.20$), or the number of inhabitants ($r = 0.21$). Without intimating a direct causal link, the positive relationship existing between fertility rates and the rate of perinatal mortality ($r = +0.57$, significant at 5 %) must be stressed. But this relationship can be indirect and derive from the association of low fertility, majority of births between 20 and 30 years, low parity, planning of births, socio-cultural factors, etc. [76].

The distribution of births in relationship to the *age of the mother* was studied in the countries listed in Table XII. There were few differences among the EEC countries, Japan, and the other industrialized countries, except for Ireland (older mothers). In Hungary and Cuba, there were many births among young women: 22.1 % of mothers in Cuba and 16.5 % in Hungary were under 20 years of age. For most countries, the distribution mode is in the 25-29 age-group, with a concentration around this mode, except for Cuba, Hungary and Ireland [76].

The mortality rates by maternal age are shown in Table XIII; they are usually higher under the age of 20, over 30, and, most pronouncedly, over the age of 35; the widest variations were in Japan, and the narrowest in Sweden. The calculation of the standardized rate shows that the structure of those populations by maternal age has only a minor influence on their perinatal mortality rates, except in Japan, where the low rate partly stems from a particularly favorable age structure. This rate was calculated by applying the national perinatal mortality rates to the New Zealand population, divided according to the age of the mother at the time of birth.

The 1973 WHO study [76] shows a classic U-curve, in relating perinatal mortality to the mother's

parity (Table XIV). Mortality was rather high among women who had no previous pregnancy; it is minimal in those who have had 1 pregnancy and rose thereafter. The English studies seem to show that these differences tend to decline with time [17].

As is shown by the comparison between the rates standardized on the referenced Swedish population and the crude rates of the different countries, parity differences do not explain the differences in perinatal mortality rates between countries, except for Cuba and the United States (Table XV). The fact that the sample of countries is so small calls for prudence, however, in interpreting the results.

In longitudinal studies limited to comparisons over a period of time for a single country, some authors have imputed to these factors a responsibility ranging from 25 to 50 % in the diminution of perinatal and infant mortality. On the other hand, Meirik attributes to them only a limited role (1.4 %) in the 16 % decline occurring in Sweden between 1953-1955 and 1973-1975 [65]. That nonetheless represents 9 % of the overall gain, age modifications accounting for 8 %, and those of parity accounting for 4 %. The combined influence of the two factors is less than the sum of the partial improvements: it is generally equal to this sum, minus approximately 50 % of the weakest factor. For the period 1968-1977, in England and Wales, 17 % of the decline in stillbirth rates is thus attributable to a more favorable distribution of ages and parities, the respective improvements being 13.1 % for parity, and 7.2 % for age [30]. However, these gains are not uniform. In the English study, Edouard et al. estimated them to be over 23 % for mortality linked to anoxia, to hemolytic diseases of the newborn, and to maternal pathology; less than 10 % for multiple pregnancies, obstetrical trauma and feto-

TABLE XIII. — PERINATAL MORTALITY RATES BY AGE OF THE MOTHER AT BIRTH IN 9 COUNTRIES IN 1973
(Rates per 1,000 total births) (Source: from [70, 76])

Country	Maternal age						All ages
	<20	20-24	25-29	30-34	35-39	40+	
England and Wales. . .	23.9	17.9	17.0	20.7	28.1	43.8	18.9
Austria	25.9	17.9	19.5	21.7	31.8	34.2	21.4
Cuba.	27.3	23.1	25.6	29.7	37.3	41.3	26.9
Hungary.	28.1	23.4	30.3	39.6	52.3	55.4	29.1
Japan	36.7	17.5	14.4	18.0	29.3	75.5	17.0
New Zealand	20.1	16.6	14.7	18.0	23.2	43.1	17.3
Netherlands (1975). . .	8.6	6.9	7.0	8.3	12.0	26.1	17.6
Sweden	14.8	11.7	11.8	12.6	19.2	33.2	12.6
U. S. A.	16.9	13.3	13.5	16.1	22.1	36.4	14.9

TABLE XIV. — Rates of perinatal mortality by parity in 9 countries in 1973
(Rates per 1,000 total births) (Source: from [70, 76])

Country	Parity					Total
	0	1	2	3	4+	
England and Wales [1]	20.1	15.3	19.0	24.6	32.3	18.9
Austria	22.0	17.8	19.9	21.2	30.6	21.4
Cuba	24.5	21.7	24.4	28.0	39.5	26.9
Hungary	25.8	27.2	40.2	44.3	47.5	29.1
Japan	17.9	14.1	16.6	32.6	62.5	17.0
New Zealand [1]	18.9	11.8	15.1	16.7	25.1	17.3
Netherlands [2]	8.9	5.3	7.7	11.4	16.2	7.6
Sweden	13.2	10.8	13.1	20.1	21.3	12.6
U. S. A. (in part)	12.6	11.1	12.6	14.4	20.0	14.9

[1] Legitimate births.
[2] Stillbirths only.

TABLE XV. — Perinatal mortality rates: crude and standardized rates by parity in 8 countries in 1973 (Rates per 1,000 total births) (Source: WHO [76]).

Country	Perinatal mortality rates	
	Crude $^o/_{oo}$	Standardized $^o/_{oo}$ [1]
England and Wales	18.9	18.7
Austria	21.4	20.4
Cuba	26.9	23.9
Hungary	29.1	29.3
Japan	17.0	17.7
New Zealand	17.3	16.0
Sweden	12.6	12.6
U. S. A. (some states)	14.9	12.3

[1] Rates obtained by direct standardization, using Sweden's distribution as reference.

maternal infection; and intermediary percentages for the other causes of death.

Legitimacy, immigration, ethnic origin, sex of the child.

— Many studies have stressed the importance of these variables as risk factors. *Illegitimacy* was responsible for an excess of mortality in all countries taking part in the WHO study, but its impact depends upon the social context peculiar to each country: in Hungary, where 6 % of births were illegitimate, the excess of perinatal mortality in the group was 49 %, while in Cuba, where 36 % of births were illegitimate, the excess was only 12 %.

The *foreign origin of mothers* in countries of high immigration has a significant statistical relationship to excess mortality: 18.4 $^o/_{oo}$ among the immigrants in France in 1972, against 8.6 $^o/_{oo}$ among mothers native to the country [44, 89].

The *ethnic factor* has been principally studied in the United States. It is an important risk factor, since a study of American perinatal mortality for the years 1955-1966 showed rates of 34 $^o/_{oo}$ among whites, 51 $^o/_{oo}$ among blacks, 41 $^o/_{oo}$ among Puerto Ricans, and 23 $^o/_{oo}$ among Asians [67]. Despite recent progress, the gap between whites and blacks persists [110].

Sex: males have a higher death risk than female newborns. In all 8 countries included in the WHO study, there was excess masculine mortality. But it is not of the same relative importance in each country. The ratio varied from 113/100 in England and Wales, to 129/100 in Hungary (100 = female perinatal mortality) [76].

Socioeconomic and cultural environment.

— The more underprivileged the *socioprofessional category*, the higher the perinatal mortality rate. All the studies on industrialized countries highlight this relationship. In the United Kingdom, for example, the gradient in 1970 went from a rate of 7.1 $^o/_{oo}$ for social class I, to 27.6 $^o/_{oo}$ for class V [17-105]. The underprivileged population groups (ethnic minorities, immigrants, members of the "Fourth World"), who are also the most fertile, contribute heavily to obstetrical pathology, and to perinatal morbidity and mortality [22, 23, 44, 60, 89, 110]. However, the socioeconomic differences between countries do not by themselves explain the perinatal mortality differences, because, at any given socioeconomic level, significant differences exist (Table XVI).

TABLE XVI. — RATES OF PERINATAL MORTALITY BY OCCUPATION OF FATHER IN 4 COUNTRIES IN 1973 (Rate per 1,000 total births) (Source: WHO [76]).

Occupation of father	England and Wales	Aus- tria	Hun- gary	New Zea- land
Professionals and up- per-level manage- ment	14.7	17.2	25.4	13.6
Civil service . . .	15.3	18.4	17.4	12.1
Clerical	18.5	17.9	30.6	15.5
Trade	17.1	18.0	31.2	13.8
Service	18.6	18.9	29.8	17.3
Farmers	18.7	20.4	31.7	15.8
Industrial workers. .	20.8	20.5	29.2	18.0
Unknown	17.2	32.4	20.5	25.9
Total . . .	18.9	21.4	29.1	17.3

The *level of education* has the same impact: the rate of perinatal mortality declines as the mother's level of education increases. For example, in France, in 1972, the stillbirth rate declined from 13.1 $\%_{oo}$ for mothers who had no education, or only primary school education, to 2.7 $\%_{oo}$ for those with university-level education [89]. At the same level of education, national differences persist (Table XVII) [76, 89]. This criterion is often more discriminatory than profession.

In capitalist countries, the negative rank correlation between the *GNP (Gross National Product) per capita* and the perinatal mortality rate is statistically significant [18]. It continues when one studies countries with very different systems and economic levels (developed capitalist countries, developing countries, socialist countries) with a significant correlation coefficient of − 0.67 ($p < 0.01$) (Table XVIII). High GNP *growth levels* have also been linked to the rapid improvement in perinatal mortality rates in some countries (France, Finland, Japan, West Germany) [3]. National wealth partly determines the level of perinatal mortality.

TABLE XVII. — RATES OF PERINATAL MORTALITY IN HUNGARY AND THE UNITED STATES BY EDUCATION OF THE PARENTS, IN 1973 (Rates per 1,000 total births) (Source: WHO [76]).

	Mother		Father	
	Hun- gary	U.S.A. (in part)	Hun- gary	U.S.A. (in part)
Primary education in- complete	40.6	20.7	39.9	21.9
Primary education com- pleted	31.5	20.6	32.4	14.3
Secondary education incomplete . . .	26.7	16.0	26.3	15.6
Secondary education completed	25.8	13.5	25.9	13.0
Higher education . .	22.0	12.0	23.8	11.3
Unknown	—	17.1	52.2	18.2
Total . . .	29.1	14.9	29.1	14.9

In the developing countries, maternal malnutrition—particularly during periods of food shortages—often constitutes an important risk factor, because of the consequent reduction in birthweight [78]. According to Winick [111], the fetal hypotrophy observed in such cases combines reduction of weight and size with a parallel reduction of various organs, including the brain: thus the risk, in case of survival, of cerebral sequelae with manifestations of retardation.

Socioeconomic level influences the outcome of pregnancy directly and through such factors as maternal age, marital status, and parity: there are twice as many cases of low birthweight in underprivileged groups, and prematurity in such groups is more frequent [22, 23, 76]. However, as indicated earlier, social changes do not alone explain the rapid decline in perinatal mortality experienced in many countries during the last 10 or 20 years [54, 100, 107, 110], although some studies do not specify possible changes in social stratification [30, 97]. In support of this assertion, Mednick et al. recount that 2 university hospitals—one, American; the other, Danish—were able to achieve among pregnant adolescents a perinatal mortality rate lower than at any other age [64]. Such pregnancies generally occur among adolescents from underprivileged socioeconomic groups, and the risk is rather more social than medical [28]. The excellent results obtained in these 2 hospitals were not due to the absence or to the reduction of the unfavorable

TABLE XVIII. — RELATIONSHIP BETWEEN RATES OF PERINATAL MORTALITY, AND THE GROSS NATIONAL PRODUCT (GNP) PER CAPITA AND NUMBER OF DOCTORS, MIDWIVES AND NURSES, IN A NUMBER OF COUNTRIES IN 1975 (Source: WHO [77])

Country	Perinatal mortality Rate °/oo	Rank	GNP per capita $ U.S.	Rank	Doctors per 10,000 inhabitants No.	Rank	Midwives+nurses per 10,000 inhabitants No.	Rank
Sweden	11.3	1	8,439	22	17.1	9	76.5	2
Denmark	13.4	2	6,937	20	19.5 [1]	6	60.5 [1]	5
Finland. . . .	13.9	3	5,508	13	14.2	14	84.2	1
Netherlands . . .	14.0	4	5,890	14	16.0	12	32.9	13
Japan	16.0	5	4,357	12	11.7	18	35.7	12
Canada.	16.5	6	6,664	18	17.1	8		
New Zealand . . .	16.5	7	4,044	10	13.3	15	60.8	4
United States . . .	16.9	8	7,098	21	16.5	11		
Bulgaria.	17.6	9	1,930	3	21.5	2	47.9	9
France	18.3	10	6,418	16	14.7	13	51.9	7
Australia	19.2	11	6,142	15			37.0	11
West Germany. . .	19.4	12	6,831	19	19.9	5		
Czechoslovakia. . .	19.6	13	3,400	8	23.9	1	64.1	3
Poland	19.6	14	2,620	6	17.1	10	42.3	10
Belgium.	19.7	15	6,516	17	18.9	7		
United Kingdom . . .	20.2	16	4,110	11				
Israel	20.9	17	3,570	9				
Ireland	21.8	18	2,520	5	12.1	17	59.8	6
Yugoslavia	21.9	19	1,480	2	12.4	16	28.8 [1]	14
Italy.	24.1	20	3,069	7	20.6 [2]	3		
Mexico	29.5	21	1,190	1	5.4 [2]	19	7.2 [2]	15
Hungary	31.6	22	2,440	4	20.0	4	49.5	8
Coefficient of rank correlation.			−0.67		−0.46		+0.47	

[1] 1976.
[2] 1974.

social factors, but rather to a uniformly high level of prenatal and perinatal care.

It is important to consider other factors—psychosocial and cultural in nature—less easily quantifiable: attitudes toward pregnancy and the infant, toward preventive care, etc. [2]. Thus, not every study should be limited to privileging economic factors among determinants. For example, in Nigeria, in 1977, rapid inflation, drought, and the rapid decline of food consumption had unfavorable effects on perinatal mortality. But in this country, the sociological weight of the environment also plays a role: the populations studied were rural and nomadic, with the women living in semi-isolation. Traditions and customs of early marriage and child-bearing play a role in the health of both mothers and infants [39]. Repeated pregnancies at brief intervals

are a factor in excess perinatal mortality. The WHO study [76] sets the optimal interval between 18 months and 3 years; the risk of perinatal death is 3.5 times higher for infants born within 12 months of a previous pregnancy than for those born during the optimal interval.

Health systems and prenatal care. — In the industrialized countries, the structures of *health systems* do not appear to have an important influence on perinatal mortality rates: the rates do not differ according to health systems, as Table XVIII illustrates. Juxtaposed in that table are the socialized medical systems of Eastern Europe and the United Kingdom; private medical care, free of charge, in West Germany, Denmark, and the Netherlands; the French and Belgian private medical systems, with costs partly covered; and the private medical system of the United States.

The rank correlation between *public health expenditures per capita* and the rates of perinatal mortality is statistically significant ($r = -0.92$, $p < 0.01$) (Table XIX). But the magnitude of these expenditures is directly related to GNP (the coefficient of rank correlation for the 9 countries of the table $= +0.95$). The relative portion of wealth that these countries contribute to health budgets varies little (4.4 to 6.7 %). The policy differences among the countries have not eliminated the negative ratio between GNP per capita and the rate of perinatal mortality [16, 75].

TABLE XIX. — RELATIONSHIP BETWEEN PERINATAL MORTALITY RATES AND PUBLIC HEALTH EXPENDITURES IN 9 EUROPEAN COUNTRIES IN 1975 (Source: CEE [15]).

Country	Perinatal mortality Rate °/₀₀	Perinatal mortality Rank	Public health expenditures per capita (in $ U. S.) Amount	Public health expenditures per capita (in $ U. S.) Rank
Belgium. . . .	19.7	6	198	4
Denmark . . .	13.4	2	345	8
France	18.3	4	254	6
West Germany. .	19.4	5	269	7
Ireland	21.8	8	101	1
Italy.	24.2	9	121	2
Netherlands . .	14.0	3	228	5
United Kingdom .	20.2	7	141	3
Sweden. . . .	11.3	1	420	9
Coefficient of rank correlation . .				−0.92

The coefficient of rank correlation for 19 countries between the *number of doctors* per 10,000 inhabitants and perinatal mortality is significant to a minor degree ($p = 0.05$). There is no significant correlation between perinatal mortality and the density of *paramedical personnel* (Table XVIII).

Along with Butler [13], a number of authors have emphasized, in different countries, the correlation between the *number of prenatal examinations* and the rates of perinatal mortality and prematurity [80]. A more recent study (conducted in Belgium, Denmark, France, the Netherlands, and Sweden) correlates the average number of prenatal visits and the rate of perinatal mortality—the relationship is almost linear [15]. In a population

homogeneous in socioeconomic and racial terms, Ryan et al. have compared two groups of women carefully matched: the first, with an average of 1.43 prenatal examinations, had a significantly higher rate of mortality than the second, whose average number of visits was 12.8: the rates were, respectively, 47.4 °/₀₀ and 13.2 °/₀₀ [90]. It is, however, necessary to note that this ratio is difficult to interpret, because the number of prenatal visits is determined by the duration of the pregnancy (shorter, when there is premature delivery), by the possible existence of gravidic pathology (in this case, more frequent checkups, but higher risks of perinatal mortality)—and not merely by observation of the regulations. Moreover, this purely quantitative parameter does not enable one to judge the content and quality of prenatal supervision.

As early as the end of the 1960's, the existence of a strong link between perinatal mortality and the size of the *maternity services* was made evident. Thus it was that in Quebec—for the year 1970, and for newborns with a weight above 1,000 g—perinatal mortality was 16.9 °/₀₀ for 14,700 births occurring in maternity centers having over 2,000 births per year, but 21 °/₀₀ for 14,400 births in institutions where births averaged only between 251 and 500 [6]. This finding, since confirmed by other studies [1], led a number of countries to close, by administrative action, those maternity centers where the number of deliveries (less than 250 per year) did not justify facilities and personnel compatible with an adequate level of perinatal care.

Some authors are of the opinion that it is essential for obstetrical and pediatric facilities to be located together [98]. Others are less categoric, stressing primarily the possibility of rapid transfer, at all times, between centers offering different levels of care [41, 106]. In fact, what should be studied in detail are the *overall structures of perinatal care* of a country, or, still better, a region.

Improved organization of services, better circulation of information among the different units, and good obstetrical-pediatric coordination make their effects felt rapidly in terms of reduced perinatal morbidity and mortality: the experience of Stormi et al., in Trieste, is a good example of this truth [98].

Regionalization of services makes it possible to better plan and orient improvements at the different levels. Based on the calculation of an optimal

[1] It is to be noted, however, that in France, in 1975, the coefficient of rank correlation calculated by region did not reveal a statistically significant relationship between the maternity centers with fewer than 15 beds and the perinatal mortality rate ($r = 0.18$ for 22 regions [39]).

rate of neonatal mortality—and therefore of an estimate of deaths potentially avoidable at each level—Hein et al. were thus able to show that, in the state of Iowa, small rural maternity centers, with a mere 6.6 $\%_{oo}$ rate of perinatal mortality, were nonetheless the ones where 55 % of the theoretical gain could be achieved; while the university intensive care center, despite a rate of 17.8 $\%_{oo}$, was not far from its optimal level of operation. The authors deduced from this that educational efforts are probably more important than regulations [40, 41] and must concentrate first of all on the peripheral units, services, or centers.

It is just as essential to perfect *a service of rapid transfer* and superior technical quality for high-risk pregnant women, and for newborns requiring special care [35]. Vogt et al. studied the impact of such a regional transfer service: the improvement in the neonatal mortality rate was, between 1975 and 1977, 6 times greater—for the different categories of birthweight—for the hospitals served by the rapid transfer program than for the others [106].

In the continuing evaluation of progress, regional perinatal study committees [61] and the perinatal audit committees [4] play a capital role.

From these several elements of reflection, it is evident that technical progress in obstetrical and neonatal care has been important in the reduction of perinatal mortality during the last 15 or 20 years in the industrialized countries [54, 100]. Persisting differences in the levels of perinatal mortality are to a large degree attributable to the institution of preventive care for pregnant women and newborns [42] and to the use that is made of such services, which is largely influenced by socioeconomic factors. But, according to Kleinman et al. [47], technical progress has proved most important for low-weight newborns; it has been a less evident, and probably less important, element in the reduction of mortality among the newborns of 2,500 g or over, which rather appears to be the continuation of a secular trend. All of which proves, once again, the importance of the "birthweight" indicator in the entire area of perinatal study.

Relationships between perinatal morbidity and mortality

The relationships between perinatal morbidity and mortality are extremely important, but also complex, because, if it is difficult enough to study morbidity and mortality separately during the perinatal period, it is still more difficult to relate them to each other; to determine their mutual evolution over the years; and to compare this evolution country-by-country. These analyses are nevertheless necessary in order to measure progress and to prepare a "de-escalation strategy". There are two essential difficulties, one linked to the methodological problems of evaluation of long-term morbidity, and the other, to the relationships between mortality and morbidity.

METHODOLOGICAL PROBLEMS

The heart of the matter probably lies in the long-term effects of perinatal morbidity and in the apprai-

sal of handicaps left by pathological states during this period. Many surveys have attempted to provide the elements of an answer. Unfortunately, they have often been weakened by methodological shortcomings that render their results questionable —sometimes, even, empty of significance—despite the investment of time and money they require. The principal flaws concern:

— an inadequate initial sample that, given inevitable erosion, further diminishes over the years and becomes "slanted" and too limited to permit evaluation;

— the fact that they are often hospital based studies, conducted in transfer centers, that do not constitute an approach to the phenomenon in the overall population;

— the frequent absence of control groups;

— a lack of initial precision about the pathological problems affecting the subjects studied (their nature, duration, links, etc.);

— lack of precision in the evaluation criteria, especially in the neuropsychiatric field;

— inadequacy of lapsed time, which prevents taking into account late-appearing handicaps: for example, motor disorders, or difficulties encountered when the subjects first go to school;

— interactions, difficult to separate, between the consequences of neonatal distress and the positive, or negative, influences of the milieu or milieus in which the infant lives.

If certain handicaps seem to be significantly associated with a specific perinatal pathological state (or to a circumstance): indirect hyperbilirubinemia and choreoathetosis, hyperoxygenation and blindness due to retrolental fibroplasia, asphyxia, and cerebral palsy—others are more difficult to associate with disorders occurring in this period In order to better target the changing relationships between morbidity and mortality, it is therefore essential that a valid methodology be used: it is indeed because of methodology employed that prospective studies such as the American "Collaborative Perinatal study" [99] and the "British Perinatal Mortality Survey" [13] have provided results of the highest interest.

According to Thompson and Reynolds [100], new studies are needed in order to appraise the long-term development of low-weight newborns, using valid control groups, separating the groups by weight and gestational age, and evaluating the effects of prenatal, perinatal, and postnatal events on all aspects of the child's later development. The list of elements to take into consideration is impressive: no fewer than 24 parameters, certain of which are difficult to evaluate. Such long-term studies can thus only be based on multivariate analysis. The authors insist, moreover, on the need to standardize the criteria for physical and neurological examinations in order to better assess possible handicaps among low birthweight infants. They also stress the usefulness of planning longitudinal studies of sufficient duration to detect minor disabilities that may later develop in hearing, language, behavior, and education—this being the only way to determine possible minor brain damage which becomes only tardily manifest. The divergence of opinions concerning the syndrome of minimal brain damage (MBD) is well known. It is clear that studies very carefully planned and conducted are indispensable to a better understanding of this ambiguous concept. They require impeccable epidemiologic methodology, refined examination techniques, and very sophisticated statistical analyses.

At the community level, there must also be taken into consideration changes in social status, demographic trends, the increase in legal abortions, better education of mothers, economic progress, improvement in prenatal care and nutrition [48], or, on the contrary, the deterioration of socioeconomic conditions. In an area of study with so many aspects, the number of parameters to consider is necessarily high.

Such studies are becoming more and more difficult as, in the industrialized countries, the decline in births, and the improvement of prenatal care and obstetrical and neonatal techniques, diminish the number of infants and newborns shownning pathological incidents of sufficient severity during the perinatal period. In these countries, one is ever more often reduced to studying problems of average or minor importance, whose evolution is very closely related to sociocultural levels and medicosocial measures. Added to that are the difficulties inherent in all longitudinal studies. Moreover, the lack of precision in the pathologies, and the very probable weakness of certain associations, raise questions about the cost-effectiveness of studies of this kind. It makes good sense, therefore, to question the practical lessons that can be learned from them. In this sense, Chalmers [37] notes that the recommendations of the first English perinatal study (in 1946) have lost nothing of their relevance, but that, unfortunately, a number of them have not even begun to be applied. In the face of such a situation, some go so far as to doubt the very utility of expensive and rigorous longitudinal surveys.

If studies of this nature do remain necessary, they should be few in number and limited to groups of infants posing special problems (very early premature babies, for example), paired with carefully defined control groups. On the other hand, it seems to us unreasonable to have these studies deal with large populations. For the latter, methods of surveillance should be available that do not involve a longitudinal study, but, rather, the cross-references of existent records. It would thus be possible to link the registrations of pregnancies existing in many maternity centers with registers of handicapped, or malformed, or even cancerous infants, etc. In the same way, certain transverse studies effected on a group of infants could be enriched by observations registered in the maternity centers. These techniques imply at once good quality registration and the use of methods permitting due respect for medical confidentiality and for the confidentiality of data.

LONG-TERM RELATIONSHIPS
BETWEEN MORBIDITY AND MORTALITY

Is it exact, as is sometimes claimed, that the reduction of perinatal mortality can be accompanied by an increase—at least temporarily—in morbidity and related handicaps? The experience of specialists in neonatal care, as well as a number of studies recently reviewed by Thompson [100], seem to argue against these assertions. After an initial phase of variable duration, but generally short, when the diminution of mortality is accompanied by a stagnation of morbidity, mastery of techniques, and better awareness of the need for, and the limits of, neonatal intensive care, also improve all the parameters: immediate and delayed mortality, morbidity (frequency and length), handicaps (in particular, cerebral palsy, mental disorders, convulsions) [14]. Thompson's conclusions merit detailed enumeration:

— With the establishment and operation of intensive care units, marked improvement in newborn survival rates is noted. This is chiefly due to the increase in survival rates of children of low birthweight and/or insufficient gestational age. This rapid progress cannot be explained by changes in the other parameters—socioeconomic conditions, educational level, prematurity rate, etc.

— Simultaneously, an improvement in long-term evolution is observable, especially for newborns of low birthweight. The growth and development of these infant is, on the whole, satisfactory. There is a clear-cut decline, among the survivors, of such handicaps as mild or severe mental deficiency, cerebral palsy, epilepsy, deafness, blindness. This is explained by the fact that the measures that bring about the avoidance of death also result in the prevention of cerebral damage.

— Obstetricians and perinatal specialists have made considerable progress in understanding and correcting perinatal factors that contribute to the morbidity and mortality of the fetus and of the newborn. They have raised their standards of surveillance and care and understand better how to prevent, or quickly—and very efficiently—correct most of these harmful factors, thus increasing the survival chances of newborns who are thereafter normal in their physical and mental development.

If these remarks conform, on the whole, to the evolution observed in most of the industrialized countries over the last 15 years, and emphasize the remarkable progress achieved in the struggle against perinatal mortality and morbidity, they must be somewhat tempered as far as the prognosis for newborns of very low weight is concerned. In New York, Zdeb found, in a group of 158 infants weighing from 751 to 1,500 g at birth, and reexamined after a year, a 23 % incidence of major abnormalities and a 16 % incidence of minor neuropsychiatric abnormalities, mostly among those weighing 1,000 g or less at birth [113]. Kitchen et al. [46], in Melbourne, between 1966 and 1978, studied 3 groups of newborns weighing 1,500 g and less, 90 % of whom were examined again after a period of from 2 to 8 years. If the improvement in the survival rates is encouraging (they increased from 37.1 % in 1966 to 68.3 % in 1978); if the decline in sensory handicaps is clear-cut; and if the average quotient of mental development at 2 years of age advanced from 75.4 for the second group to 91 for the third—the prevalence of cerebral motor disability appears to have increased by 2.6 % for the 1966 group, by 4.5 % for that of 1973, and by 11.9 % for that of 1978. These differences are not significant for groups numerically small (from 72 to 169 subjects) and are thus difficult to interpret, but they nonetheless show that the increase in the rate of survival is not always accompanied by an overall reduction in handicaps.

The excellent general review of Stewart et al. [97], in examining the worldwide literature on the subject, analyzed 22 studies selected on the basis of the following criteria: precise data on the population of reference, follow up for at least 12 months; indication of the percentage of the sample lost track of; specification of the percentage and nature of observed handicaps. In spite of diversity in the selection, the results were coherent: in the industrialized world, the survival chances of infants of very low weight (1,500 g and less) has tripled since 1960, and the rate of residual handicaps has remained stable, and relatively low: from 6 to 8 %. This evolution, very clear for the group between 1,001-1,500 g, is reproduced, if with some slippage, for those weighing 1,000 g and less. The possible conclusions, in terms of action, are easy to deduce [92].

In fact, this crucially important problem remains unresolved. Recent epidemiologic analyses show divergent tendencies among Western countries [45]: while the prevalence of motor disabilities of cerebral origin (cerebral palsy) has diminished in certain countries (e. g., England and Denmark) in recent decades, it has increased in others (Ireland and, more recently, Australia). Elsewhere, the trend, though downward, is not significant. Many of these variations are due to the lack of uniform criteria for the diagnosis, selection, and follow-up of cases, and any conclusions would be premature. It is possible that the diminution of morbidity and handicaps is less rapid than that of mortality, especially for very low-weight infants. Thus, "although more healthy survivors will result from

newborn intensive care, a modest increase in the prevalence of handicaps may also ensue". Analyzing data from California, Budetti (in a personal communication) notes that, between 1960 and 1976, the mortality rate for newborns of 1,500 g and less diminished by 60 %, while the percentage of healthy survivors multiplied 6 or 7 times; minor handicaps declined by 20 %, while severe residual handicaps increased by 9 %.

From fact-finding to action: some strategies

Epidemiology is obviously not an end in itself: it must be used as a cornerstone of public health programs; it must create impetus for their activities; it must evaluate the results. In perinatal matters, it must encourage strategies that, whatever the starting point may be, have as their purpose the diminution of morbidity and mortality, the reduction of handicaps to a minimum, the attenuation of the socioeconomic cost of this pathology, even if significant investments are necessary in the prenatal and perinatal periods [4, 61]. This is now taking place in many industrialized countries.

DEVELOPED COUNTRIES
WITH LOW BIRTH RATES

In 1971, WHO [72], and, in 1976, the Council of Europe [24], proposed measures whose application would, without any doubt, diminish the incidence of perinatal pathology. The measures concerned conception (genetic counselling, spacing of pregnancies), surveillance of pregnancies for the purpose of detecting those that are high-risk in nature, delivery procedure, examination of the newborn and care of high-risk newborns, health education of the public, training of health care personnel, and research.

It is interesting to recall that as early as 1946, following the first British perinatal study, a series of very concrete recommendations had been elaborated: not all were put into practice. Probably, awareness of the importance of the problem on the part of the public, the authorities, the medical profession, health and social welfare personnel was not yet sufficiently developed to gain acceptance

—not merely for the financial investments, but, most of all, for the distribution of tasks and the changes in practices that these recommendations implied.

The context has changed. Research progress has made possible better surveillance of pregnancy and delivery, as well as more efficient control of reproduction. At the same time, the industrialized countries entered a period marked by a decline in births, and by zero population growth. They realized the heavy socioeconomic costs of the handicaps resulting from perinatal pathology, and the importance of "survival, free of handicaps" as the best indicator of progress in the area. The general public has properly become more demanding, as a result of its becoming better informed.

Strategies of de-escalation have therefore become technically possible and politically desired. Thus, in France, in 1971, a program was established to improve a situation recognized as unsatisfactory. The results have been positive and it is perhaps useful to briefly review this program, often cited abroad as an example [80].

The french perinatal program. — A program of concerted action was instituted with, as its objective, a reduction in the number of perinatal deaths and in the incidence of handicaps. Perinatal mortality was then 26 °/$_{oo}$. Each year, 22,000 infants died during the 15-week perinatal period, and it was estimated that another 40,000 suffered from handicaps acquired or manifested during this period; among these, 25,000 had mental deficiencies.

Based on the results of a study of the "*rationalisation des choix budgétaires*" (RCB), analogous to the Planning, Programming, Budgeting System (PPBS) in the United States, the financial cost of perinatal

TABLE XX. — Estimate of cost-effectiveness of the French perinatal program's health measures (1970)
(Source: *Périnatalité* [80])

Health measures	Cost envisioned over 15 years (in francs)	Number of deaths avoided over 15 years	Number of handicaps avoided over 15 years	Cost of a life without handicaps (in francs)
Training	12,100,000			
Information, studies, research.	28,200,000			
Rubella immunization . . .	48,000,000	2,100	1,000	15,500
Prenatal supervision. . . .	582,000,000	32,000	60,000	6,300
Improved conditions of delivery.	29,000,000	3,700	4,000	3 800
Intensive care of new-borns in delivery room	10,600,000	25,500	25,500	200
Intensive-care centers for new-borns	173,000,000	37,500	5,100	5,600
Total	882,900,000	100,800	95,600	

handicaps was evaluated in 1969 at 15 billion francs per year, or 2.5 % of the Domestic Gross Product. Then, taking into account the technical possibilities, a list of measures designed to improve the situation was drawn up, with the objective of reducing the rate of perinatal mortality to 18 $^{o}/_{oo}$ by 1980 and of reducing the rate of handicaps comparably. It was then possible to calculate the necessary investments and, taking into consideration the foreseeable financial benefit, to establish a cost-effectiveness ratio: the unit of cost used was the "price of death avoided, free of handicaps". The options finally adopted, with their cost-effectiveness ratio, are shown in Table XX; this index is expressed by the ratio:

cost of action undertaken over a 15-year period
_____
number of lives saved, free of handicaps,
during 15 years

If all the subprograms have not been completely realized, the activities as a whole have had a considerable impact on the specialized milieus and have sensitized public opinion to the causes of perinatal mortality and to the means for reducing it.

The effects of the program are being evaluated, especially in the framework of national studies cited earlier [19, 89]. But it is already possible to assert that, for mortality, the objective set for 1980 was attained as early as 1975, permitting France to catch up with, then surpass, some neighboring countries—such as England—initially in a better situation. The revised objective for 1980 was set at 14 $^{o}/_{oo}$: it was attained in 1979. By the same token, the prematurity rate declined from 8.2 % in 1972 to 6.3 % in 1981, while birthweight remained stable between 1972 and 1976, and increased between 1976 and 1981.

At the same time, surveillance of pregnancies and deliveries has improved: the percentage of women having more than four prenatal visits increased from 49 % in 1972, to 80 % in 1981—with checkups more frequently performed by specialists. The closing of a large number of small maternity centers permitted the centralization of deliveries in institutions better equipped in personnel and materials. These improvements have not been achieved without setbacks, due to a sometimes excessive "medicalization" of pregnancies, to insufficient consideration of the sociocultural risk, and to an increase in social inequalities between the well-to-do classes (large consumers of medical care, though they are low risks) and the underprivileged classes who are ignorant of, or cannot always benefit from, the possibilities of preventive care.

These results are obviously encouraging, but it is difficult to claim that there is a cause-effect relationship between specific preventive measures (even when they are a part of an overall program) and progress recorded in the field of mortality, morbidity, and prematurity. The general evolution of attitudes toward reproduction certainly has an important influence in this area: the planning of births, their occurrence at more favorable age periods, the disappearance of multiple pregnancies, the desire to give birth to a normal infant—all are important factors in the progress achieved.

Future challenges. — The challenges we still face are no less significant than those of the last decade. Two observations are called for:

First, the mechanism of and the primary preventive measures against certain perinatal pathologies are still poorly understood. It is too often necessary to be satisfied with a secondary or even tertiary form of preventive care. Thus it is that, because of our inability to better ascertain the cause of congenital malformations, frequently the only available way to prevent them is to interrupt the pregnancy. Similarly, a delivery provoked prematurely is a means of preventing handicaps stemming from hypotrophy. Therefore, research is called for —biological, clinical, epidemiological—in order to understand the causes and development of diseases and determine the means of prevention.

Second, when preventive means exist, they are very unequally applied among the population. Inequality in the use of benefits and services and the inadequacy of social measures—especially for women from underprivileged socioeconomic groups —are at least partially responsible for the inequality of children in the face of death and disease [105]. That is a sociological problem that goes far beyond studies concerned with the perinatal period: the most vulnerable are—in general—those who least frequently seek out the services placed at their disposal. Certain women—adolescents [28, 64], single women, women from underprivileged socioeconomic groups [22, 23], wives of immigrant workers [45, 89], women from ethnic minorities [67, 110]—have a reproductive life which begins early; they also have repeated pregnancies, which are poorly supervised if at all; and they are not fully covered socially (home assistance, prenatal allowances) or medically, despite frequent pregnancy pathologies. The rates of prematurity, fetal and infant mortality, hospital transfers, are singularly high in this population, in comparison with national averages [35, 60, 89, 111]. Here, too, research is needed in order to better determine the reasons for this lag, and to better understand the mechanism of penetration of medical and social improvements in the population. It is equally necessary to seek out the reasons behind resistance and to study the psychological reactions of women and couples.

Such research should be at the origin of new activities designed to improve preventive care through specific programs focused on certain pathologies, risk factors, social groups [58]. These programs should be based, first of all, on a better statistical knowledge of the situation and of the risk factors, and on a vigorous search for the most effective methods of preventive care. They must be based on very careful planning, including: the definition of quantifiable objectives, estimates of the

measures necessary and their costs, and a determination of evaluation methods. Evaluation must be continuous in nature, in order to facilitate, when necessary, the modification of certain aspects of the program. The planning must be effected at all echelons. While the choice of strategies belongs at the national level, it is, on the other hand, desirable that a number of plans be decentralized at the regional level [55, 61, 106] in order to respond to local problems and to permit a more effective participation of the various teams involved. In this regard, the English model, with its several levels of planning and appraisal, might be considered.

DEVELOPING COUNTRIES
WITH HIGH BIRTH RATES

Although data are inadequate, it is certain that perinatal pathology in the developing countries is very significant, and is a source of many deaths and handicaps imposing heavy burdens on individuals, families and communities [1, 69].

Many developing countries are establishing neonatal centers consisting of a few dozen beds in hospitals located in their capitals and other large cities. But this is only one part of the solution—neither the most important part, nor, probably, the most urgent. Perinatal morbidity and mortality will be meaningfully reduced, on national levels, only through very decentralized organization, starting with primary health services oriented to the detection of high-risk pregnant women with a view to transferring them to properly equipped regional centers. Uncomplicated pregnancies and deliveries can be handled locally where modest resources do not rule out a satisfactory quality of technical competence. It would seem that the strategy most likely to improve the situation rapidly is to integrate maternal and child care in primary health-care centers. Cooperation between health services personnel trained in modern methods and those with local status using customary practices—traditional midwives adequately recycled and supervised, for example—should make it possible to proceed more rapidly toward making access to care available to all.

There exists, however, another problem, that of uncontrolled fertility—close, in certain countries, to "natural" fertility. A diminution of parity, a better spacing of births, a later beginning and an earlier end of the reproductive period, are thus indispensable if it is hoped to reduce perinatal pathology and its consequences: all of that falls within the domain of family planning. But many studies [31] have proven that family planning programs are acceptable only to the extent that the survival chances of infants already born are satisfactory. What is more, an interval of 20 to 25 years is necessary for a significant decline in infant mortality to lead, in turn, to a diminution of the birthrate —it is as if the collective mentality needed a generation in order to digest the fact that a new situation has been created, and to adapt its reproductive behavior to it. However, this time gap can be considerably reduced if, along with progress in health care—and especially with improvement in the survival chances of newborns—economic and social development occurs, bringing about an improvement in living conditions. Just as in industrialized countries, though for different reasons and by different mechanisms, it is through socioeconomic development, better nutrition, and, most of all, through generalized access to education, that decisive progress can be realized in reducing perinatal mortality and morbidity. In evaluating this progress, the percentage of newborns of insufficient weight (and the mortality rate due to this factor) is certainly the most relevant indicator, and its evolution should be followed with attention: for the surest way to improve the present situation lies in the prevention of such births.

CONCLUSION

Stewart et al. [97], analyzing the evolution of perinatal situations in the industrialized countries since the end of World War II, identify four successive periods:

— during the first, in the 1940s and 1950s, premature, fragile, small-for-date newborns aroused only slight interest, and most died quickly;

— the second period coincided with the beginning of the 1960s. A better knowledge of fetal physiology and physiopathology made it possible to deal more effectively with a number of problems, but still in a very groping way. Iatrogenic pathology is important: retrolental fibroplasia is one of its unfortunate examples;

— a little later, increased knowledge, growing sophistication of obstetrical techniques and neonatal intensive care, as well as a better organization of perinatal care, led to decisive progress, beginning in a few very specialized centers, but spreading gradually to other centers and other levels;

— during the fourth period, it is recognized that

the causes of mortality and of handicaps are identical (ventricular hemorrhages, cerebral necrosis, etc.). New technologies (scanners, ultrasonic exploration) make it possible to detect these causal factors and to better understand how the brain functions. Operational prognosis becomes possible, permitting—with due attention to the ethical dimensions of the problem —a distinction between cases where the struggle to preserve life is justifiable, and where ceasing intensive care efforts appears more reasonable: therapy thus has an ever more solid foundation.

In this rapidly-changing context, epidemiology is fundamental for three reasons. It permits the determination of the frequency of perinatal pathologies, and the evaluation of the sociocultural environment and of available resources and technology. It is thus possible to trace the evolution of these indicators, showing that countries—or regions within a given country—are in different stages of the process described by Stewart et al.

Epidemiology also contributes to etiologic research, whether it be a matter of determining causes (teratogenic factors, for example), or risk factors and favorable circumstances.

Finally, epidemiology constitutes a methodology of primary importance to the evaluation of new technologies, so numerous in this area, and to that of policies and systems of care. Moreover, it contributes to the study of the spread of these practices in the different social strata, together with sociology, psychology, and health economics.

REFERENCES

[1] L'accouchement prématuré en Afrique. (Série d'articles). *Afr. méd.*, *19*, 307-364, 1980.
[2] ADELSTEIN (A. M.), MACDONALD DAVIES (I. M.), WEATHERALL (J. A. C.). — Perinatal and infant mortality: social and biological factors 1975-1977. Her Majesty's Stationery Office, London, 1980.
[3] ALBERMAN (E.). — Facts and figures. *Clin. Develop. Med.*, *64*, 1-17, 1977.
[4] ALEXANDER (D.). — Progress in perinatal medicine. In: *Perinatal medicine today*. B. K. YOUNG (ed.). Alan R. Liss, New York, 205-223, 1980.
[5] AMIEL-TISON (C.) et coll. — Mortalité et morbidité à la période néonatale. Les objectifs actuels de la prévention. *Arch. Fr. Pédiat.*, *37*, 87-92, 1980.
[6] BERNARD (J. M.). — Analyse de la mortalité infantile et périnatale au Québec, 1965-1974. Ministère des Affaires sociales, Québec, 1979.
[7] BOLDMAN (R.), REED (D. M.). — Worldwide variations in low birth weight. In: *The epidemiology of prematurity*. D. M. REED and F. J. STANLEY (eds.). Urban and Schwarzenberg, Baltimore, 39-52, 1977.
[8] BOUÉ (A.), CABAU (N.). — Épidémiologie des infections par le cytomégalovirus. *Nouv. Presse Méd.*, *7*, 3135-3139, 1978.

[9] BRAKEN (M. B.) et coll. — Role of oral contraception in congenital malformations of offspring. *Int. J. Epidem.*, 7, 309-317, 1978.

[10] BREART (G.), FENDER (P.). — Mortalité et morbidité dans l'enfance. *Cah. Méd.*, 5, 1815-1821, 1980.

[11] BRICOUT (F.). — La rubéole. In : *Médecine périnatale, 7es Journées nationales, Aix-les-Bains, 1977.* Arnette, Paris, 117-124, 1977.

[12] BUFFLER (P. A.). — Some problems involved in recognizing teratogens used in industry. *Contr. Epidem. Biostatist.*, 1, 118-137, 1979.

[13] BUTLER (N. R.), ALBERMAN (E. D.). — Perinatal problems. The 2nd report of the 1958 British périnatal mortality survey. E. and S. Livingstone, Edinburgh, 1969.

[14] CALAME (A.), PROD'HOM (L. S.), VAN MELLE (G.). — Outcome of infants of very low birthweight treated in neonatal intensive care unit. *Rev. Épidém. Santé Publ.*, 25, 21-32, 1977.

[15] CEE. — La santé publique et les premières années de la vie. 2e séminaire européen sur les politiques de santé, Ispra, 1979 (non publié).

[16] CERC. — Le coût de l'hospitalisation, comparaisons internationales. Documents du Centre d'Étude des Revenus et des Coûts, Paris, no 48, 1979.

[17] CHAMBERLAIN (R.) et coll. — British births 1970. A survey under the joint auspices of the National Birthday Trust Fund and the Royal College of Obstetricians and Gynaecologists. Vol. 1: *The first week of life.* W. Heinemann Medical Books, London, 1978.

[18] CHAMBERLAIN (G.). — Background to perinatal health. *Lancet*, 2, 1061-1063, 1979.

[19] CHAPALAIN (M. T.). — Perinatality: French cost-benefit studies and decisions on handicap and prevention. In: *Major mental handicap, methods and costs of prevention.* Elsevier-Excerpta Medica-North Holland, Amsterdam, 193-206, 1978.

[20] CHASE (H. C.). — International comparison of perinatal and infant mortality: The United States and six west European countries. *Vital and Hlth. Statist.* (US Government Printing Office, Washington, DC), Ser. 3, no 6, 1-97, 1967.

[21] CHASE (H. C.). — Time trends in low birth weight in the United States, 1950-1974. In: *The epidemiology of prematurity.* D. M. REED and F. J. STANLEY (eds.). Urban and Schwarzenberg, Baltimore, 17-37, 1977.

[22] COLIN (C.). — Maternité et extrême pauvreté. Étude sur les conditions de la grossesse et de la naissance en Quart Monde dans une ville de l'Est de la France. *Thèse Méd.* Nancy, Faculté A et B, 1980.

[23] COLIN (C.). — La maternité en milieu québecois francophone très défavorisé. *Mémoire en Santé communautaire*, Montréal, 1982.

[24] COUNCIL OF EUROPE. — European Commettee of Public Health. Perinatal morbidity and mortality in Council of Europe Member States and Finland. Report presented by M. MANCIAUX. Council of Europe (Strasbourg), 1977.

[25] CROZE (M.). — Tableaux démographiques et sociaux. INSEE-INED, Paris, 1976.

[26] DANMARKS STATISTIKS. — *Statistik Arbog*, vol. 82, 1978.

[27] DAVID (R. J.). — The quality and completness of birthweight and gestational age data in compu-terized birth files. *Amer. J. Publ. Hlth.*, 70, 964-973, 1980.

[28] DESCHAMPS (J. P.). — *Grossesse et maternité chez l'adolescente.* Le Centurion, Paris, 1976.

[29] DESMONTS (G.). — La toxoplasmose de la femme enceinte. In: *Mises à jour en gynécologie et obstétrique. 3es Journées nationales, Collège national des Gynécologues et Obstétriciens français.* Vigot, Paris, 1979.

[30] EDOUARD (L.), ALBERMAN (E.). — Changing maternal age, parity and causes of fetal wastage. *Rev. Épidém. Santé Publ.*, 30, 355-362, 1982.

[31] Family formation patterns and health. An international collaborative study in India, Iran, Lebanon, Philippines and Turkey. A. R. OMRAN and C. C. STANDLEY (eds.). WHO, Geneva, 1976.

[32] FARRER (J. F.), MACKIE (I. J.). — Survey of possible causes of congenital malformations. *Med. J. Australia*, 2, 702, 1964.

[33] FRANCE-MINISTÈRE DU TRAVAIL. — Groupe de travail du Conseil Supérieur de la Prévention des Risques professionnels. Activité professionnelle de la femme enceinte et issue de la grossesse. Ministère du Travail, Paris, 1980.

[34] GOUJARD (J.), HUEL (C.), RUMEAU-ROUQUETTE (C.). — Antiépileptiques et malformations congénitales. *J. Gynécol. Obstét. Biol. Reprod.*, 3, 831-842, 1974.

[35] GOUJARD (J.) et coll. — Les transferts dans la période néonatale. *Arch. Fr. Pédiat.*, 36, 827-835, 1979.

[36] GOUJARD (J.), RUMEAU-ROUQUETTE (C.), SAUREL-CUBIZOLLES (M. J.). — Tests hormonaux de grossese et malformations congénitales. *J. Gynécol. Obstét. Biol. Reprod.*, 8, 489-496, 1979.

[37] GREAT BRITAIN. — National Perinatal Epidemiology Unit. *Annual report for 1979.* Churchill Hospital-Research Institute, Oxford, 1979.

[38] GREAT BRITAIN, OFFICE OF POPULATION CENSUSES AND SURVEYS. — Mortality statistics, 1977. Her Majesty's Stationery Office (Series DH1, no 5), London, 1979.

[39] HARRISON (K. A.). — Better perinatal health, Nigeria. *Lancet*, 2, 1229-1232, 1979.

[40] HEIN (H. A.). — Evaluation of a rural perinatal care system. *Pediatrics*, 66, 540-546, 1980.

[41] HEIN (H. A.), BROWN (C. J.). — Neonatal mortality review: A basis for improving care. *Pediatrics*, 68, 504-509, 1981.

[42] HOHN (C.). — Les différences internationales de mortalité infantile : illusion ou réalité? *Population*, 36, 791-816, 1981.

[43] INSERM. — Statistiques des causes médicales de décès, 1973, 1974, 1975. Tome II : *Résultats par région.* Éditions INSERM, Paris, 1977, 1978, 1979.

[44] KAMINSKI (M.) et coll. — Issue de la grossesse et surveillance prénatale chez les femmes migrantes. Enquête sur un échantillon représentatif des naissances en France en 1972. *Rev. Épidém. Santé Publ.*, 26, 29-46, 1978.

[45] KIELY (J. L.), PANETH (N.), STEIN (Z.), SUSSER (M.). — Cerebral palsy and newborn care. I. Secular trends it cerebral palsy, 533-538. II. Mortality and neurological impairment in low birthweight infants, 650-659. III. Estimated prevalence rates of cerebral palsy under differing rates of mortality and impairment of low birthweight infants, 801-807. *Develop. Med. Child Neurol.*, 23, 1981.

[46] KITCHEN (W. H.), RYAN (M. M.), RICKARDS (A.), ASTBURY (J.), FORD (G.), LISSENDEN (J. V.), KEITH (C. G.), KEIR (E. H.). — Changing outcome over 13 years of very low birth weight infants. *Sem. Perinatol.*, 6, 373-389, 1982.

[47] KLEINMAN (J. G.), KOVAR (M. G.), FELDMAN (J. J.), YOUNG (C. A.). — A comparison of 1960 and 1973-1974 early neonatal mortality in selected states. *Amer. J. Epidemiol.*, 108, 454-469, 1978.

[48] KNOBLOCH (H.), MALONE (A.), ELLISON (P.), STEVENS (F.), ZDEB (M. S.). — Outcome for infants weighing less than 1,501 g. *Pediatrics*, 69, 285-295, 1982.

[49] LAURENCE (K. M.), CARTER (C. O.), DAVID (P. A.). — Major central nervous system malformations in South Wales. 1. Incidence, local variations and geographical factors. *Brit. J. Prev. Soc. Med.*, 22, 146-160, 1968.

[50] LECHTIG (A.) et coll. — Influence of maternal nutrition on birth weight. *Amer. J. Clin. Nutr.*, 11, 1223-1233, 1975.

[51] LECHTIG (A.) et coll. — Low birth weight babies: worldwide incidence, economic cost and program needs. In: *Perinatal care in developing countries.* Based on a workshop held at Gimo, 1976, jointly sponsored by the WHO and the 5th European Congress of Perinatal Medicine. G. ROOTH and L. ENGSTRÖM (eds.). Perinatal Research Laboratory Univ. of Uppsala, Uppsala, 17-29, 1977.

[52] LECK (I.). — Descriptive epidemiology of common malformations (excluding central nervous system defects). *Brit. Med. Bull.*, 32, 54-52, 1976.

[53] LECK (I). — Teratogenic risks of disease and therapy. *Contr. Epidem. Biostatist.*, 1, 23-43, 1979 (Karger, Basel).

[54] LEE (K. S.), PANETH (N.), GARTNER (L. M.), PEARLMAN (M. A.), GRUSS (L.). — Neonatal mortality: An analysis of the recent improvement in the US. *Amer. J. Publ. Hlth.*, 70, 15-21, 1980.

[55] MCCORMICK (M. C.). — The regionalization of perinatal care. *Amer. J. Publ. Hlth.*, 71, 571-572, 1981.

[56] MCFARLANE (A.). — The derivation and uses of perinatal and neonatal mortality rates. *J. Pediatrics*, 98, 61-62, 1981.

[57] MAC VICAR (J.), KERR (M. M.). — Better perinatal health, maternal disease, infection, trauma, Rhesus iso-immunisation. *Lancet*, 2, 1284-1286, 1979.

[58] MANCIAUX (M.). — Organisation of perinatal care in Europe. Methodology of evaluation. In: *Perinatal medicine, 3rd European congress, Lausanne, April. 1972.* H. BASSART et al. (eds.). Hans Huber Publ., Bern, 13-28, 1973.

[59] MANCIAUX (M.). — Perinatal morbidity and mortality in Council of Europe members States and Finland. In: *Perinatal medicine, 5th European congress, Uppsala, June, 1976.* G. ROOTH and L. E. BRATTEBY (eds.). Almquist and Wiksell, Stockholm, 18-25, 1976.

[60] MANCIAUX (M.). — Children of disadvantaged families: Contemporary studies in Western Europe. *UNESCO.* Reports/Studies, ChR18, 1981.

[61] MANCIAUX (M.). — Périnatologie et pédiatrie sociale. *Arch. Fr. Pédiatr.* 40, 443-448, 1983.

[62] MANCIAUX (M.), DESCHAMPS (J. P.). — *Santé de la mère et de l'enfant : de la PMI à la santé de la famille.* Flammarion Médecine-Sciences, Paris, 1978.

[63] MARIA (B.) et coll. — Étude des facteurs de risque pré- et per-nataux de l'entérocolite ulcéro-nécrosante du nouveau-né. *Méd. et Hyg. (Genève)*, 38, 1712-1714, 1980.

[64] MEDNICK (B. R.), BAKER (R. L.), SUTTON-SMITH (B.). — Teenage pregnancy and perinatal mortality. *J. Youth Adol.*, 8, 343-351, 1979.

[65] MEIRIK (O.), SMEDBY (B.), ERICSON (A.). — Impact of changing age and parity distributions of mothers on perinatal mortality in Sweden 1953-1975. *Int. J. Epidem.*, 8, 361-364, 1979.

[66] MEYER (M. B.). — Effects of maternal smoking and altitude on birth weight and gestation. In: *The epidemiology of prematurity.* D. M. REED and F. J. STANLEY (eds.). Urban and Schwarzenberg, Baltimore, 81-104, 1977.

[67] NAEYE (R.). — Causes of fetal and neonatal mortality by race in a selected US population. *Amer. J. Public Hlth.*, 69, 857-861, 1979.

[68] NAHAS (G.), GOUJARD (J.). — Phenothiazines, benzodiazepines and the fœtus. *Rev. Perinat. Med.*, 3, 243-280, Raven Press, New York, 1979.

[69] NASAH (B. T.), DROUIN (P.). — La surveillance prénatale, postnatale et l'accouchement. *Enf. Mil. trop.*, 105, 3-42, 1976.

[70] NEDERLAND. — Centraal Bureau voor de Statistick. Jaaroverzicht bevolking en volksgezondheid 1977. *Maandstatistick van bevolging en volksgezondheid*, vol. 26, supplement, Staatsuitgeverij, 'gravenhage, 1979.

[71] NEEL (J. V.). — A study of major congenital defects in Japanese infants. *Amer. J. Hum. Genet.*, 10, 338-445, 1958.

[72] OMS. — La prévention de la morbidité et de la mortalité périnatales. Rapport sur un séminaire, Tours, 22-26 avril 1969. *OMS Cah. Santé Publ.*, 42, 1-102, 1971.

[73] OMS. — Aspects sanitaires des tendances et perspectives démographiques. *Rapp. Statist. Sanit. Mond.*, 27, 200-229, 1974.

[74] OMS. — *Manuel de la classification statistique internationale des maladies, traumatismes et causes de décès.* 9e rév. OMS, Genève, 2 vol., 1977.

[75] OMS. — Personnels de santé et établissements hospitaliers. In: *Annuaire de statistiques sanitaires mondiales.* OMS, Genève, vol. 3, 1978.

[76] OMS. — Principaux résultats de l'étude comparative des effets des facteurs sociaux et biologiques sur la mortalité périnatale. *Rapp. Trim. Statist. Sanit. Mond.*, 31, 74-83, 1978.

[77] OMS. — Mouvement de la population et causes de décès. In : *Annuaire de statistiques sanitaires mondiales.* OMS, Genève, vol. 1, 1978, 1979, 1980, 1981, 1982.

[78] OMS. — Division de la Santé de la Famille. Fréquence de l'insuffisance pondérale à la naissance : étude critique des données. *Rapp. Trim. Statist. Sanit. Mond.*, 33, 197-224, 1980.

[79] PAPIERNIK-BERKHAUER (E.). — Coefficient de risque d'accouchement prématuré (CRAP). *Presse Méd.*, 77, 793-794, 1969.

[80] *Périnatalité*, par un groupe de spécialistes obstétriciens et pédiatres. Masson édit., Paris, 1972.

[81] Pharmacologie anté- et post-natale. Table ronde sous la dir. de P. Royer. In: *25e congrès Ass. Pédiat. Langue franç.*, Tunis, 29-31 mai 1978. Expansion scientifique française, Paris, vol. 2, 5-84, 1978.

[82] PRATT (M. W.), JANUS (Z. L.), SAYAL (M. C.).
— National variations in prematurity (1973
and 1974). In: *The epidemiology of prematurity.*
D. M. REED and F. J. STANLEY (eds.). Urban and
Schwarzenberg, Baltimore, 53-80, 1977.

[83] PUFFER (R. R.), SERRANO (C. V.). — Patterns
of mortality in childhood. Report of the Inter-
American investigation of mortality in childhood.
PAHO, Washington, Scientific publ. n° 262, 1973.

[84] RITCHIE (K.), McCLURE (G.). — Prematurity.
Lancet, 2, 1227-1229, 1979.

[85] ROOTH (G.). — Better perinatal health, Sweden.
Lancet, 2, 1170-1172, 1979.

[86] RUMEAU-ROUQUETTE (C.), BREART (G.), PADIEU (R.).
Méthodes en épidémiologie. Flammarion, Paris,
1981.

[87] RUMEAU-ROUQUETTE (C.), GOUJARD (J.), HUEL (G.).
— Possible teratogenic effect of phenothiazines
in human beings. *Teratology, 15,* 57-64, 1977.

[88] RUMEAU-ROUQUETTE (C.) et coll. — *Malformations
congénitales. Risques périnatals. Enquête prospective.* Éditions INSERM, Paris, 1978.

[89] RUMEAU-ROUQUETTE (C.) et coll. — *Naître en
France.* Enquêtes nationales sur la grossesse et
l'accouchement (1972-1976). Éditions INSERM,
Paris, 1979.

[90] RYAN (G. M.), SWEENEY (P. J.), SOLOLA (A. S.).
— Prenatal care and pregnancy outcome. *Amer.
J. Obstet. Gynecol., 737,* 876-881, 1980.

[91] SCHWARTZ (D.). — *Méthodes statistiques à l'usage
des médecins et des biologistes.* Flammarion,
Paris, 1963.

[92] SHAPIRO (S.). — New reductions in infant mortality:
The challenge of low birth weight. *Amer. J. Publ.
Hlth., 71,* 365-366, 1981.

[93] SMITHELLS (R. W.) et coll. — Possible prevention
of neural-tube defects by periconceptional vitamin
supplementation. *Lancet, 1,* 339-340, 1980.

[94] STEUDLER (F.). — *Sociologie médicale.* A. Colin,
Paris, 1972.

[95] STEVENSON (A. C.), WARNOCK (H. A.). — Observations on the results of pregnancies in women
resident in Belfast. 1. Data relating to all pregnancies ending in 1957. *Ann. Hum. Genet., 23,* 382-391,
1959.

[96] STEVENSON (A. C.) et coll. — Congenital malformations: a report of a study of series of consecutive births in 24 centres. *Bull. Wld. Hlth. Org.,
34,* 9-127, 1966.

[97] STEWART (A. L.), REYNOLDS (E. D. R.), LIPS-
COMB (A. P.). — Outcome for infants of very
low birth weight: Survey of world literature.
Lancet, 8228, 1038-1040, 1981.

[98] STORMI (M.), DE VONDERWEID (U.), FERTZ (C.),
GARDINI (A.), LEVI (N.), DI GIACOMO (B.), NOR-
DIO (S.). — L'organizzazione dei servizi di assis-
tenza al neonato. L'esperienza nella provincia
di Trieste. *Riv. Ital. Ped., 5,* 823-840, 1979.

[99] *The Collaborative Perinatal Study of the National
Institute of Neurological Diseases and Stroke.*

Johns Hopkins University Press, Baltimore, 1979.

[100] THOMPSON (T.), REYNOLDS (J.). — The results
of intensive care therapy for neonates. 1. Overall
neonatal mortality rates. 2. Neonatal mortality
rates and long term prognosis for low birth weight
neonates. *J. Perinat. Med., 5,* 39-75, 1977.

[101] TREISSER (A.), SUREAU (C.). — Moyens actuels
de surveillance du fœtus. Le concept de souffrance
fœtale chronique. *Rev. Prat. (Paris), 31,* 329-341,
1981.

[102] US DEPARTMENT OF HEALTH, EDUCATION, AND
WELFARE. *Health, United States, 1978. US DHEW,*
Hyattsville, Md (Publ. n° (PHS) 78-1232), 1978.

[103] UNITED STATES. — National Center for Health
Statistics. Factors associated with low birth weight,
United States, 1976. *Vital and Hlth. Statist.* Ser. 21,
n° 37 (US Department of Health, Education,
and Welfare, Hyattsville, Md), 1979.

[104] VALLIN (J.). — La mortalité infantile dans le
monde. Évolution depuis 1950. *Population, 31,*
801-837, 1976.

[105] VALLIN (J.). — *L'inégalité des enfants devant la
mort.* Communication presented at the Meeting
of the Perinatal and Infant Mortality sub-com-
mittee of the European Collaborative Committee
for Child health, Paris, 20 février 1980.

[106] VOGT (J. F.), CHAN (L. S.), WU (P. Y. K.),
HAWES (W. E.). — Impact of regional dispatch
center on neonatal mortality. *Amer. J. Publ.
Hlth., 71,* 577-582, 1981.

[107] WALLACE (H. M.). — Selected aspects of perinatal
casualties. *Clin. Pediatr., 18,* 213-223, 1979.

[108] WIGGLESWORTH (J. S.). — Monitoring perinatal
mortality: A pathophysiological approach. *Lancet,
196,* 684-686, 1980.

[109] WILKINS (L.). — Masculinization of female fetus
due to use of orally given progestins. *J. Amer.
Med. Ass., 172,* 1028-1032, 1960.

[110] WILLIAMS (R. L.), CHEN (P. M.). — Identifying
the sources of the recent decline in perinatal
mortality rates in California. *New Engl. J. Med.,
306,* 207-214, 1982.

[111] WINICK (M.). — *Malnutrition and brain development.* Oxford Univ. Press, New York, 1976.

[112] WYNN (M.), WYNN (A.). — Historical associations
of congenital malformations. *Intern. J. Environ.
Stud., 17,* 7-12, 1981.

[113] ZDEB (M. S.). — Differences in trends of post-
neonatal mortality by birth weight in Upstate
New York 1968-1979. *Amer. J. Publ. Hlth., 72,*
734-736, 1982.

[114] KALTER (H.), WARKANY (J.). — Congenital malformations: etiologic factors and their role in
prevention. *New Engl. J. Med., 308,* 424-431,
1983.

[115] RUSH (D.). — Effects of changes in protein and
calorie intake during pregnancy on the growth
of the human fetus. In *Effectiveness and satisfaction
in antenatal care.* M. ENKIN and I. CHALMERS
(eds.). London, Philadelphia, 1982.

2

The normal newborn

V. C. HARRISON

CARE AT BIRTH

Onset of breathing. — A full-term baby who is born per vaginum often grimaces as his face is delivered. Small amounts of fluid may ooze from the nostrils and mouth and crying commences as soon as the chest has been extruded. The initial breaths are vigorous and are characterised by deep inspiratory and expiratory movements. Transpulmonary pressures up to −70 cm water may be generated at this stage. Within a minute of birth the blue mucous membranes become pink in colour and crying is followed by a more regular and shallow pattern of breathing. A baby can normally clear fluid from his upper airways by crying and swallowing. The nose and pharynx need not be suctioned for this can result in damage to the mucous membranes. Suctioning is only indicated in abnormal circumstances such as meconium staining and birth asphyxia.

Cessation of the fetal circulation. — An infant's blood volume after birth is related to the time of cord clamping [1]. The umbilical arteries constrict immediately after birth whereas the vein remains patent. This enables fetal blood from the placenta to enter the baby after delivery. This transfusion is dependent on gravity and can increase the infant's blood volume by fifteen percent within 60 seconds

of birth. A further increase in volume caused by "milking" the cord would be considered unphysiological and can result in polycythaemia.

The cord is clamped a minute after birth. Two Spencer Wells forceps are applied 5 and 6 cm from the umbilicus and the cord is divided between them. At a later stage a sterile disposable plastic clamp is applied about 1 cm above the umbilicus and closed by pressure with the fingers. The excess cord is cut about 1 cm beyond the clamp and is discarded.

The establishment of a neonatal circulation depends on the cessation of umbilical cord blood flow and on normal spontaneous breathing.

Prevention of hypothermia. — A newly born infant can lose heat rapidly particularly through evaporation.

The delivery suite should be maintained at a temperature of 24-25° C and be free from drafts. The infant is delivered into a sterile towel and dried. The towel is discarded and another is wrapped around the baby to cover the head as well as the body.

Bonding. — The bond of affection between and mother and her baby commences during pregnancy. It can be enhanced by encouraging the mother to share in the delivery of her infant. Once the head and shoulders have been delivered she can be supported in the sitting position by her husband. She grasps

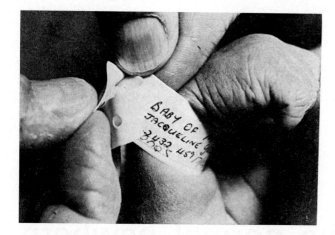

FIG. I-16. — *An identification band
is placed round the wrist immediately after birth.*

her infant under his arms and assists in the delivery of the trunk and legs. She receives her dry and warmly wrapped infant to be fondled and suckled.

This early bond has a number of physiological advantages. It enables the baby to establish a pattern of sucking and also promotes the flow of colostrum. The infant's sterile gut and skin can be colonized by the mother's organisms and the risk of post-partum haemorrhage is reduced as oxytocin is released from the pituitary during sucking to contract the uterus.

Identification. — The infant's name and sex are printed on two cards which are inserted into transparent plastic bracelets. This information is checked by the mother and one bracelet is clipped round the infant's wrist (Fig. I-16) and the other round an ankle. The mother signs the record form indicating that she has identified her infant and has witnessed the procedure. Other methods of identification include finger and foot printing.

Gonococcal ophthalmia prophylaxis. — Eye care is recommended in regions where antenatal attention has been inadequate. It is preferably avoided in areas where good antenatal care exists.

In certain countries the law prescribes that the eyes be treated with a 1 % silver nitrate solution. This is instilled shortly after birth and provides effective prophylaxis. It has the disadvantage of causing chemical conjunctivitis which can lead to superimposed bacterial infection.

One drop of 1 % silver nitrate is instilled into the inner margin of the lower eyelid while the eyelids are held open with the thumb and forefinger of the opposite hand. The eyes become puffy and reddened after this procedure but usually clear within a few days.

Physical examination. — The parent's first question, "Is our baby normal?" needs to be answered before the baby leaves the delivery suite. It is placed on a resuscitation table which is kept warm by infra-red heating and briefly examined in the presence of the parents. Care is taken to exclude congenital abnormalities, respiratory distress, anaemia and birth trauma.

Caesarean section. — When the umbilical cord has been clamped and cut, the infant is carried in a sterile towel to a resuscitation table. This is warmed by an overhead heater. If the baby is vigorous and breathes normally, it is dried, then wrapped in a warm towel and transferred to the nursery. Identification particulars are checked by two staff members who witness and record the attachment of the bracelets. The identified infant is shown to the father.

A normal baby occasionally requires resuscitation particularly if general anaesthesia has been used.

Transfer to the nursery. — The baby is placed in a crib and covered with warm blankets. It is accompanied by a member of the nursing staff who is also responsible for delivering the record chart. This contains details of the mode of delivery, condition of the infant at birth, identification data, drugs given to the mother, her blood group and WR, and a brief summary of pregnancy and labour.

Cord blood. — Samples of cord blood are required for blood grouping and Coomb's test. These are recommended in all deliveries and are essential when the mother's blood group is rhesus negative or unknown.

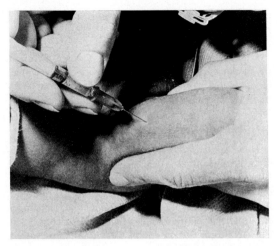

FIG. I-17. — *Vitamin K_1 is injected into the anterior thigh muscles, never into the buttock.*

CARE IN THE NURSERY

The period of separation from a mother should be as short as possible.

An injection of Vitamin K_1, 1 mg is given into the anterior thigh muscle to prevent haemorrhagic disease (Fig. I-17).

MEASUREMENTS

The baby is weighed and length is measured.

Length: crown-heel length is determined by placing the baby in a special measuring crib. He lies on his back with the head touching the upper board and in line with the trunk and limbs. The legs are fully extended and the lower movable board is brought up to the feet which are at right angles to the surface.

Bathing. — Vernix, clotted blood and meconium need to be removed after birth. A bland liquid soap is poured onto sterile cotton swabs and the material is washed off by bathing the baby in water at 39° C. The plastic crib can be used as a bath. The infant is dried and axillary temperature is checked. Hexachlorophene soap is not used as the antiseptic can be absorbed into the circulation and is neurotoxic.

Cord. — The efficiency of the cord clamp is checked and the cord is swabbed with 95 % alcohol. It is left exposed to promote drying.

Dress. — The infant is clothed in a cotton vest and a short gown which ties at the back. A disposable diaper is fitted and the baby is placed in a crib and wrapped in two woollen blankets. These should be arranged so as not to impede movement.

Temperature. — The environmental temperature in the nursery is maintained at 22°-23° C. The infant's axillary temperature is recorded on a low reading mercury thermometer and should be in the range of 36.5°-37° C. A cold infant will need to be warmed. A plastic coated metal cradle is placed over the clothed baby in the cot. It is covered with a heating pad and blankets (Fig. I-18). Care is taken to use a pad which heats to a fixed temperature only. This must not exceed 40° C and the temperature inside the cradle should be approximately 32° C. The device can be removed when the axillary temperature has returned to normal.

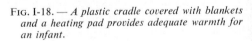

FIG. I-18. — *A plastic cradle covered with blankets and a heating pad provides adequate warmth for an infant.*

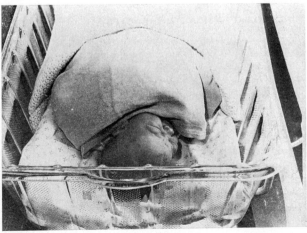

Crib. — A transparent plastic bassinet is suitable. It can be designed to serve as a cot and as a bath. Its metal frame is supported on castors and contains cupboard space for toilet requirements. These include clean clothing, diapers, linen, towels, cotton swabs, soap, a jar of sterile petroleum jelly and a mercury thermometer.

A label is attached to the crib detailing the name, weight, sex and date of birth of the infant.

The baby is taken to his mother's bedside in a crib once it has been bathed and has a stable temperature.

PHYSICAL EXAMINATION

The initial full examination is conducted by a doctor in the presence of the mother so that she can be made aware of various normal characteristics. She also has the opportunity to express any fears or doubts about features which she considers to be abnormal.

The doctor studies the record chart details and washes his hands before touching the infant. The examination is conducted in a good light on a flat surface. A plastic sheet may be placed at the end of the mother's bed and covered by a clean towel for this purpose.

Certain features are best assessed before the baby is disturbed and starts to cry. These include observations on the sleep pattern, response to auditory stimuli, examination of the eyes, auscultation of the heart, observation of respiration and palpation of the abdomen and femoral pulses.

Gestational age can be assessed by means of the Dubowitz or equivalent scoring system.

NORMAL PHYSICAL CHARACTERISTICS

Weight. — Most babies have a weight in the range of 2,700 to 4,000 g. A suitable percentile chart for weight is useful so that the mother can be shown that her baby is of normal size.

Normal variation of weight. — Male babies tend to weigh more than females. Those born at sea level tend to be heavier than those born at high altitudes. First-born babies are often heavier than subsequent ones. Large gains in weight during pregnancy are associated with heavier babies.

Large parents tend to produce large babies. Various ethnic groups show differences in intra-uterine growth which may be related to socioeconomic factors.

Length. — Most normal babies range from 48 to 55 cm in length. Males tend to be longer than females and those born at sea level may be taller than their counterparts born at high altitudes.

Head.

Head circumference. — This important measurement is an indirect reflection of the size of the brain. It is best estimated on the second or third day once swelling and scalp œdema have subsided. A tape measure is placed around the maximum circumference in the occipito-frontal plane (Fig. I-19). This averages 35 cm in the full-term baby with a range of 33 to 37 cm.

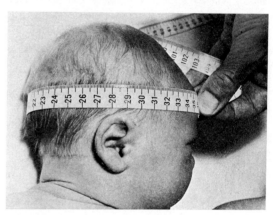

FIG. I-19. — *A tape measure is placed round the most prominent points on the occipital and frontal bones.*

Males tend to have larger heads than females and those born at sea level may have bigger heads than those born at high altitudes.

Moulding. — The shape of the skull depends on the mode of delivery and the degree of head flexion during labour. The head is lengthened in the mento-vertical axis in a vertex presentation, and in the fronto-occipital axis in a breech delivery (Fig. I-20). It is often rounded in the infant who is born electively by caesarean section.

Fontanelles. — These membranous openings are found at the junction of two or more sutures.

The anterior and posterior fontanelles lie at either end of the sagittal suture. The anterior fontanelle is normally concave and varies in size. This diamond shaped opening may admit the tip

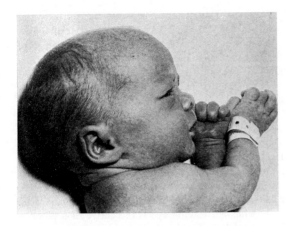

FIG. I-20. — *The typical head of a breech baby.*

of a forefinger or it may be broad enough to admit three finger-tips.

Sutures. — Individual bones are separated from each other by membranous openings. After birth the sutures may be impalpable due to overriding of bones, or they may be separated by 0.5 cm or more. A persistent metopic suture is commonly felt as a depression running forward from the anterior fontanelle.

Hair. — The full-term infant usually has a good growth of scalp hair. Individual strands do not adhere together as in the pre-term infant. In lighter skinned babies the colour of the hair is no guide to its future shade.

Craniotabes. — Areas of skull often indent on palpation. These parchment-like regions are usually situated in the parietal and temporal bones adjacent to the sutures, but can occur anywhere on the cranium. The phenomenon occurs in 10 to 35 % of full-term babies and is probably related to delayed ossification. It corrects itself within weeks or months.

Caput succedaneum. — The presenting area of scalp is often bruised and oedematous. This subsides within days after birth.

Cephalhaematoma. — Blood may accumulate between a cranial bone and its overlying periosteum. Bleeding occurs slowly from damaged capillaries so that a swelling is not obvious at birth.

The injury is likely to occur in primiparous vertex deliveries and there is a higher incidence in forceps or vacuum births. The underlying bone may have a linear fracture. The fluctuant swelling commonly occurs over one or both parietal bones.

It never crosses a suture line as the periosteum is adherent to the edge of the bone. An occipital cephalhaematoma has to be distinguished from other midline swellings in that region. Healing occurs rapidly and the outer edge may calcify to form a firm rim. No treatment is needed and the swelling disappears within 4 to 8 weeks.

Scalp abrasions. — These lesions are frequently seen due to techniques which are used to monitor the fetus and to rupture membranes during labour. Multiple blisters or abrasions can result from a vacuum cup. If the skin has been broken, the surrounding hair ought to be shaved off and a 1 % aqueous mercurochrome solution is painted on the lesion to prevent infection.

Subaponeurotic bleeding. — Extensive bleeding can occur beneath the epicranial aponeurosis as a result of a traumatic delivery. The head is swollen and oedematous and may be increased in size. On the second or third day, blue discolouration may be noted over the upper eyelids and over the skin behind the ears. The swelling subsides without therapy. Severe bleeding can cause anaemia and jaundice.

Face. — Features vary in the different races and it is advisable to know the facial characteristics of the parents before considering a baby's face to be abnormal.

Fetal posture may produce asymmetry of the face particularly when the jaw has been compressed against a shoulder. The lips are asymmetrical and the mandible appears to be angulated. This subsides with growth.

Common facial blemishes include:

(*a*) Milia: these raised white popules are seen on the nose, cheeks and chin (Fig. I-21). They are retention cysts of the sebaceous glands and disappear within a few weeks.

(*b*) Stork bite naevi: capillary haemangiomata are often seen on the upper eyelids, in the midline of the forehead, and at the nape of the neck. These purple naevi fade within several months.

Bruising and purpura. — Traumatic bruising commonly occurs over the mouth and nose in a facial presentation. It can be distinguished from cyanosis by the fact that the lips and tongue are pink. Traumatic petechiae may be seen on the forehead and face especially when there has been difficulty in delivering the shoulders. The lesions rarely extend below the level of the shoulders unlike purpura due to other causes.

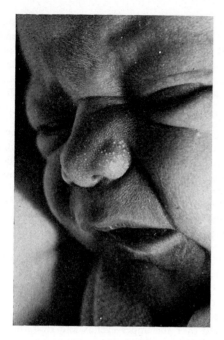

FIG. I-21. — *Milia commonly occur on the nose.*

Ears. — The helix meets the cranium above a horizontal line through the corner of the orbit. It may be incompletely folded. Pre-auricular skin tags may be seen anterior to the ear (Fig. I-22). Those with a narrow pedicle can be tied off.

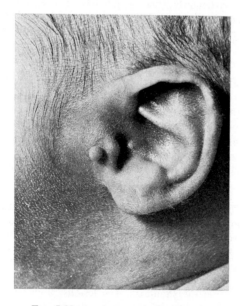

FIG. I-22. — *A pre-auricular skin tag with a thick pedicle.*

Eyes. — The distance between the inner canthi ranges from 1.5 to 2.5 cm in the full-term baby.

Epicanthic folds or slanting of the palpebral fissure can occur as a variation of normal, particularly if present in other members of the family.

The eyes are best examined when the baby is awake and supported in a sitting position. Subconjunctival haemorrhages are seen as red streaks on the eyeball. They disappear within a few weeks. When the retina is examined through an ophthalmoscope small flame shaped haemorrhages may be seen. They resorb without therapy. It is important to assess eyeball size in order to exclude glaucoma, and to visualize the cornea to exclude cataracts.

A persistent tearing eye is indicative of a blocked lachrymal duct. This is relatively common and usually resolves itself within weeks to months. The duct does not require probing in most cases and care must be taken to treat episodes of conjunctivitis.

Nose. — The nose is somewhat saddle shaped at birth. Patency can be determined by listening over each nostril with a stethoscope. The newborn is an obligate nose breather and air is heard to rush out during expiration. Sneezing is common after birth and does not necessarily signify infection.

Mouth. — "Sucking" callouses are often seen on the lips at birth. These patches of thickened epithelium are continually replaced by new ones for several weeks.

Natal teeth are uncommon. They are usually lower incisors which are poorly formed and loose, and can fall out. Small cysts may be seen on the gums. They resolve spontaneously.

Tongue. — This muscle is pink and mobile and tends to stick to the palate if the jaw is forced open. In so-called "tongue-tie" the frenulum from the floor of the mouth is inserted into the anterior portion of the tongue (Fig. I-23). A dimple may be

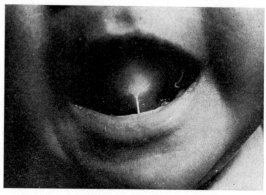

FIG. I-23. — *Mild tongue-tie.*

seen above the point of insertion. Sucking is rarely impaired and there is usually no interference with speech later in life. The anterior position of the tongue tends to grow forwards and the frenulum recesses.

Palate. — Small grey white papules are often seen in the midline of the hard palate. They are termed "epithelial pearls". The posterior pharynx is difficult to visualise even with the aid of tongue depressor. It is best observed during a spell of crying. The soft palate effectively closes off the nasopharynx and the uvula is intact.

Neck. — The short neck of a newborn baby is inspected by extending or rotating the head.

A sternomastoid "tumour" may be seen in the muscle. This firm painless swelling is not obvious at birth and only appears after several weeks. Aetiology is obscure, but may be related to pressure and to bleeding particularly in a breech delivery. Physiotherapy is needed to keep the muscle stretched in order to prevent torticollis in later life.

The clavicles are palpated for crepitus or tenderness which may result from a fracture of that bone.

Chest. — The nipples are situated in the midaxillary line. Their areolae are well developed and breast nodules are palpable.

One or both breast may enlarge and fill with milky secretions. These swellings can occur in male and female babies and may be uni- or bilateral. They persist for weeks to months and must not be squeezed as this can lead to infection.

Accessory nipples may be seen along the nipple line.

Respiration. — Breathing is observed while the baby is quiet. The abdomen rises in inspiration and there is very little movement of the chest cage. The rate averages 30 to 40 breaths per minute. Air entry should be heard equally on both sides of the chest.

Cardiovascular system.

Heart. — The apex beat is difficult to palpate, but may be localised in the 3rd or 4th left intercostal space in the nipple line.

Heart sounds are of equal intensity and a systolic murmur may be audible for the first few days of life. This is often heard as an ejection murmur over the pulmonary area and along the left sternal border. In some cases it is localised to the pulmonary area. It may be caused by the increased flow of blood across the pulmonary valve or in some cases by a patent ductus arteriosus.

Pulses. — The radial artery is easy to locate. The femoral is palpable with the hip abducted. It is felt about a fingerbreadth medial to the anterior superior iliac spine.

Pulse rate ranges from 70 to 180 beats per minute in the first few days of life, with an average of 130.

Blood pressure. — This is best determined by the Doppler ultrasound technique. A 5 cm cuff is suitable for the newborn. The inflatable bag must extend round the full circumference of the upper arm. The systolic blood pressure is approximately 60-65 mm Hg for the first two days of life.

Abdomen. — The abdomen is moderately protuberant. The liver can be palpated in the epigastrium and its edge extends about 2 cm below the costal margin. The kidneys and spleen tip can be felt in thin infants. The bladder is an abdominal organ and when full is felt as a globular mass above the pelvis. It should not be palpable after micturition.

Umbilicus. — The cord normally contains two arteries and one vein. In 0.2 to 1.0 % of births a single artery may be present. This can occur as a variation of normal but should alert one to the possibility of other congenital abnormalities.

Genitalia.

Male. — The scrotum is well developed and covered with transverse skin folds. Testes should be palpable in the sac. They may be retractible in which case they can be brought down without difficulty into the scrotum.

(*a*) Hydrocoele. — The processus vaginalis may persist after birth so that fluid can track from the peritoneal cavity into the tunica vaginalis around the testis. This occurs more frequently on the right side, but can be bilateral. The hydrocoele usually subsides within days or weeks.

(*b*) Penis. — The size varies considerably. The foreskin is adherent to the glans and cannot be retracted (Fig. I-24). The urinary stream is strong and there should be no ballooning of the prepuce.

Female. — The labia minora and clitoris are prominent. A hymenal skin tag may protrude from the vagina. It regresses after a few weeks. A white vaginal discharge may be present. This normally persists for several days and actual bleeding may occur as a result of endometrial shedding.

Anus. — The anus must be inspected to determine patency. This can be done by retracting

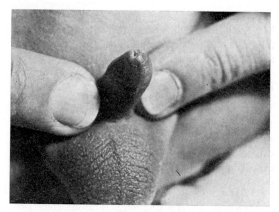

FIG. I-24. — *The foreskin is often tight and cannot be retracted to expose the glans.*

the buttocks. The passage of meconium usually occurs within 24 hours of birth. Anal skin tags are occasionally seen and they resolve within a few weeks. Hemorhoids can occur in breech delivery as a result of pressure. They subside without therapy.

Limbs. — Fingers and toes are counted and inspected for webbing or syndactyly. Minor defects include syndactyly of the 2nd and 3rd toes and poly-dactyly of the fingers. The extra digits are usually attached to the little fingers by narrow pedicles which can be tied off.

Palms. — A single palmar crease is seen in about 4 % of normal babies.

Legs. — Asymmetrical skin creases of the thigh occur in about 5 % of normal babies.

Hips. — The baby is laid on his back with hips flexed to 90° and knees fully bent. The length of the thighs can be determined by noting the position

of the knees, they should be of equal height. There should be no resistance to full abduction of the hips.

Barlow test: the femur and pelvis on one side are steadied between the examiner's thumb and fore-finger while the opposite leg is moved into mid-abduction. It is flexed as described and gripped between the middle finger on the outer side of the thigh and the thumb on the inner side (Fig. I-25). The tips of these fingers rest opposite the greater and lesser trochanters. The middle finger exerts forward pressure behind the greater trochanter. There should be no movement of the femoral head during this procedure. If it is felt to slip forward into the acetabulum the hip has been dislocated. This may be accompanied by a "clunk" like sound.

The thumb applies backward pressure on the inner side of the thigh. If the femoral head slips over the posterior lip of the acetabulum and springs back when pressure has been released, the hip is said to be unstable. It is dislocatable, but not dislocated. The opposite hip is examined in a similar manner.

An audible click is often heard during these manipulations. It is considered to be normal if the hip is stable and the click sound usually disappears within days or weeks. Unstable or dislocated hips ought to be assessed by an orthopaedic surgeon.

Back. — A sacro-coccygeal dimple may be noted at the base of the spine (Fig. I-26). An underlying sinus can be excluded by retracting the skin margins and inspecting the base through an auroscope.

Skin. — Vernix caseosa covers the skin at birth. This greyish-white substance acts as a lubricant during delivery and contains epithelial cells and sebaceous secretions. Fine hair, lanugo, may be seen over the back, especially on dark skinned babies.

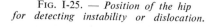

FIG. I-25. — *Position of the hip for detecting instability or dislocation.*

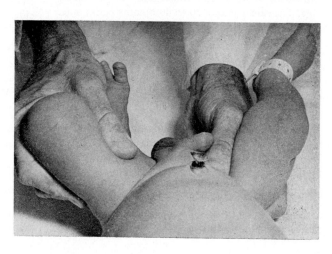

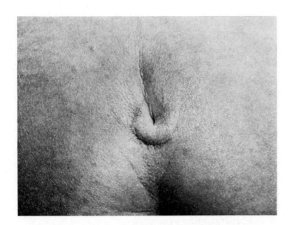

Fig. I-26. — *A deep pilonidal dimple.*

Erythema toxicum. — This papular rash appears on the trunk or face within hours to days after birth. A base of red skin surrounds a central yellowish papule. Lesions fade rapidly and may reappear at other sites.

Harlequin colour change. — This characteristically occurs in a pre-term baby, but is occasionally observed in a full-term infant. One side of the body turns red and a distinct demarcation of skin colour is noted along the midline. This flushing phenomenon has no serious significance.

Mongolian spots. — Blue grey patches of pigment may be seen over the buttocks, thighs or back of dark skinned babies.

Heat rash. — Fine red papules may occur over the chest and neck as a result of overheating. They are probably caused by dilated sweat glands.

Jaundice. — Yellow staining of the skin is commonly seen after the third day of life.

Peeling. — Exfoliation of the skin may occur after a few days. This is commonly seen in post-mature babies and is likely to involve the hands and feet.

Peripheral cyanosis. — The hands and feet of a newborn baby may remain blue for one or two days after birth. This is unrelated to hypothermia and is probably due to a sluggish peripheral circulation.

Subcutaneous fat necrosis. — Indurated areas may be felt under skin which has been traumatized These nodules are not commonly seen until the end of the first week. They are painless and do not fluctuate. The overlying skin is often red and cannot be lifted up between the finger tips. Common areas

include the cheek where forceps have been applied, the scalp, behind the ears, the back and the thighs. The swellings subside within a few weeks time and do not require treatment.

NEUROLOGICAL FUNCTIONS

Movements. — When a baby is awake and on his back the limbs show alternating flexion and extension in reciprocal fashion on both sides. When lying on his abdomen he is able to rotate the head from side to side and may briefly lift it off the surface.

Posture. — In the supine position the arms and legs are semiflexed and the head turns to one side. On occasions the limbs extend on the side to which the face is turned while those on the other side flex. This is the so-called "fencer's" position caused by the asymmetrical tonic neck reflex. In the prone position flexion becomes more marked. The hips are tucked under the abdomen, the arms are flexed and the head is turned to one side.

Muscle tone. — Tone is assessed by extending the elbows and the knees. When the arms are extended and suddenly released they return to their flexed position. Similar flexion is noted in the legs when the knees and hips are extended and then released.

In ventral suspension the spine and limbs flex and the neck may momentarily extend. When the infant is brought to a sitting position the heads tends to lag. It can actively be brought forward in the upright position so that the chin comes to rest on the chest.

Reflexes. — A number of primitive reflexes are present at birth. Several such as the glabellar tap and the pupil reflex have been used as guides to gestational age while others such as the Moro indicate the over-all neurological status.

Grasp reflex: this is elicited by placing a finger against the palm or sole. A traction response can be elicited by bringing the infant to a sitting position while supporting his wrists. The elbows flex and there is an attempt by the baby to hold the head in line with the trunk.

Moro reflex: this can be elicited by a sudden movement such as gently extending the arms then releasing them, or allowing the head to fall back unsupported for a short distance. The hands fly open, arms fling out and legs extend. This is followed by a slow return to the flexed position. The response is symmetrical and disappears between 3 and 4 months of age.

Rooting reflex: when the cheek is touched the infant's head turns towards the side of the stimulus in the hope of finding a nipple.

Stepping reflex: when a baby is held in the standing position and angled forwards with the feet on the ground, the legs make stepping movements as in walking.

Deep tendon reflexes can be elicited, but have limited value unless abnormal reactions are consistently obtained.

Behavioural functions.

SLEEPING AND WAKING. — A newborn infant sleeps for most of the day but requirements vary from baby to baby. Deep sleep is characterised by a state in which the eyes remain closed, breathing is regular and reflex responses to external stimuli are partially suppressed. Light sleep is associated with rapid eye movements which can be observed under the closed lids. Breathing is irregular and sucking and facial movements such as smiling may be noted. This pattern occurs every 45 to 50 minutes and occupies fifty percent of total sleeping time.

Waking is characterised by a state of drowsiness in which the infant may open and shut the eyes and can respond to sensory detail. When fully awake the eyes remain open, the face appears alert and the infant will focus on attractive stimuli. Motor activity increases and crying may occur.

A baby may wake of necessity when the diaper is soiled. He will go off to sleep as soon as the unpleasant stimulus has been removed. He may also wake out of choice and wish to be stimulated. This stage is not frequently observed in noisy bright nurseries, but is more likely seen in a quiet room at the mother's bedside. In this state the baby lies in the crib looking around and can be roused by the appropriate stimuli.

MOTOR BEHAVIOUR. — A full-term baby has the capacity to perform complex motor feats. In the face of hunger or cold he will attempt to calm himself by bringing his hands to his mouth and vigorously sucking his fingers. Defensive action can also be demonstrated. If a cloth is placed over the face, he will attempt to remove it by twisting the head from side to side and finally will bring up his arms to push it away.

SENSORY BEHAVIOUR.

Sight response. — A baby is capable of shutting out noxious stimuli and responding to pleasant stimuli. When a bright light is shone into the eyes, a blink is elicited, the pupils constrict and a startle reflex may be initiated. If this is done repeatedly, the response will diminish and cease. The infant habituates and shuts out the unpleasant stimulus.

An appealing stimulus evokes a different response. When a bright red ball is brought into the line of vision the infant will stare intently at it and then start to track it if it is moved from side to side [2]. Eye movements become smooth and the head turns to follow the object to the side. Other body movements and reflexes are suppressed during this phase of concentration.

Auditory response. — A pleasant auditory stimulus such as the mother's voice is associated with an attempt of the infant to turn his head towards the source of sound. Noises such as a rattle may evoke facial movements or a startle reflex. If an unpleasant sound is repeated the infant will habituate and show no response.

Taste and tactile responses. — Taste is well developed at birth and the baby can distinguish sweetness from sourness. A sweet taste elicits vigorous sucking. Tactile stimuli such as gentle patting, holding the hand or stroking the face can soothe an upset baby.

WARD CARE

Rooming-in. — Ideally the mother and baby are kept together in a single room. Larger wards can also be utilised to accommodate four to eight mothers with their babies. A minimum space of 7.5 sq metres is required for each pair. Rooming-in has distinct advantages. The baby is cared for by the mother and consequently the risk of cross infection is limited. Breast feeding on demand is more readily initiated and nursing staff are available to instruct mothers in the care of their babies.

Equipment. — Each room should be supplied with elbow-controlled wash basins, paper towelling, soap and plastic lined bins which are foot controlled.

Visitors. — Many maternity institutions have unrestricted visiting. The other children in a family are allowed to visit their mother and new sibling. This makes the acceptance of a new baby more easy and does not appear to increase the chances of cross infection. Persons with colds or other infectious diseases must be barred from visiting or touching the newborn baby.

Daily observations.

Cord: the umbilicus is swabbed three times a day with 95 % alcohol. This keeps it dry and free from infection. The clamp is removed after 24 hours (Fig. I-27) and the cord usually separates between the sixth and tenth day.

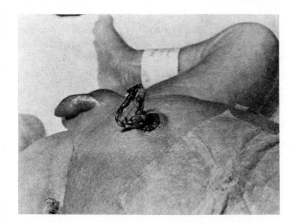

FIG. I-27. — *Appearance of the umbilical cord after the plastic clamp has been removed.*

Buttocks: soiled diapers are discarded as soon as possible. The buttocks are cleaned with soap and water and a small amount of petroleum jelly is applied to the anal region.

Temperature: axillary temperature is checked and recorded twice a day.

Weight: daily weighing gives a good guide to normal growth. A baby loses 3 to 5 % of birth-weight over the first three days. This is thought to be due to a small fluid intake, the loss of meconium and lung fluid and the utilisation of glycogen stores. Birthweight is regained within six to eight days after birth.

Stools: the bowel may contain up to 200 g of meconium at birth. The first stools are usually passed within 24 hours and by the second or third day this sticky black material is replaced by greenish brown changing stools. Normal milk stools are established by the fourth to fifth day or age.
Breast milk stools are bright yellow in colour and of watery consistency. At times they may be frothy and green. They contain very little solid matter and are passed five to eight times a day. The frequency varies greatly and a baby may have ten or more stools a day whereas another normal one may have one stool every few weeks. These patterns can be considered normal provided the infant is gaining adequate weight. Cow's milk stools are of firmer consistency and light yellow in colour. Four or five stools may be passed each day and they tend to be malodorous. The bottle fed infant can become constipated.

Urine: the bladder contains about 50 ml urine at birth. This may be passed at the time of delivery or within the next 24 hours. Occasionally the delay may extend to 48 hours. The frequency and quantity of urine passed each day varies with age. By the end of the first week, wet diapers need to be changed ten or more times a day. A pink or brick red stain may be noted on the diaper. This is caused by urates and is considered to be normal. It should not be confused with haematuria.

Record chart. — Each infant is provided with a chart in which written records are accurately and promptly completed. Hospital forms differ but all should have prominent headings for the baby's name, sex, hospital number and ward. Details of maternal health, antenatal events, labour, birth and placenta are completed in the delivery suite.
Information concerning the physical and neurological examinations, measurements, blood group and gestational age is entered in the chart. Daily notes are made on axillary temperature, pulse rate and weight and these can be displayed on a graph. Details are kept on the nature, frequency and duration of feeds, and on the output of stools and urine.

Minor problems.

Vomiting. — An infant may vomit after the first few feeds as a result of having swallowed blood, pus or meconium at birth. The vomitus contains mucus and the swallowed material. If it persists for more than two feeds then it is advisable to wash out the stomach with 2 % sodium bicarbonate. Ten millilitres of this solution are injected into the stomach through a nasogastric tube. This amount is with-drawn and the injection is repeated until the return is clean. A total of 100 ml is usually sufficient to remove the irritating material.
Excessive air may be swallowed as a result of a blocked nose, extreme hunger or an inadequate teat hole in the case of the bottle fed infant. Regurgitation of milk and air occurs after one or more feeds. The condition is not progressive and does not usually occur after each feed. Care must be paid to eliminating the cause. The mother is also instructed to "wind" her baby during and after each feed. She

holds him upright against her chest with the head resting on her left shoulder. The palm of her right hand rubs his back with a rotary motion until the air in the stomach has been expelled.

Unusual causes of vomiting in the normal baby include chalasia and hiatus hernia.

Jaundice. — Many healthy babies develop a degree of jaundice on the third or fourth day of life. This is probably due to a temporary functional immaturity in the liver conjugation mechanism and can be aggravated by drugs such as oxytocin which are used to induce labour. The total serum bilirubin seldom exceeds 200 µmol/l and usually subsides by the fifth day. Prolonged jaundice may be associated with breast feeding. It is likely that some substance in the milk interferes with the conjugation of bilirubin, but its nature remains uncertain. At one stage it was thought to be 3α 20β pregnanediol. Bilirubin levels should not reach a dangerous level and usually average about 150 µmol/l. It is not necessary to discontinue breast feeding and the jaundice subsides after several weeks.

Crying. — The only eagerly awaited cry is undoubtedly that which initiates lung expansion at birth.

Hunger: no healthy baby will keep quiet for long when hungry. Crying may consist of a few sobs or may be loud and persistent, and associated with vigorous sucking of the fingers or hand.

Loneliness: infants who are kept in nurseries may cry without specific reason for up to two of the 24 hours [3]. This problem is considered to be due to loneliness and can be avoided by having the baby with its mother.

Dissatisfaction: infants complain vocally if they are uncomfortably hot or cold, too tightly wrapped up, or lying in damp or soiled diapers. They also resent sudden bright light, being undressed and being placed in a bath of water.

Pain: high pitched screaming is indicative of pain. This can be caused by a pin, colic or a fractured bone.

Colic: the infant who is likely to develop colic can usually be detected in the first week. He settles with difficulty after feeds, often wakes up after short periods of sleep and is easily roused. By the end of the second week the full-blown picture of colic is established. Feeding is interrupted by bouts of high pitched crying during which the legs are drawn up and the back is arched. This may continue from one feed through to the next so that mother and child

get very little rest. In mild cases the pattern commonly occurs in the evenings only, usually between 6 and 10 p. m.

Factors which cause colic are unknown. Recent evidence points to a possible milk protein allergy [4]. Cow's milk consumed by a mother can be traced into her own breast milk and back into the infant. The elimination of cow's milk from the mother's diet has been associated with marked improvement in many cases.

If this treatment is not possible or effective then an antispasmodic, dicyclomine hydrochloride, may be used for each feed. A dose of 10 mg may be given and is usually sufficient to produce relief. The condition usually subsides after three months of age.

Perianal soreness. — Many babies, especially if bottle fed, develop redness of the skin in the perianal region. This is aggravated if the skin is in contact with stools and actual excoriation can occur. Soiled diapers should be changed as soon as possible, the region is washed with soap and water and petroleum jelly is smeared around the anus. In severe cases it is advisable to expose the buttocks to the air with the baby in the prone position.

Breast feeding.

Antenatal preparation. — Breast feeding is best promoted before the birth of a baby. The pregnant mother is instructed in the practice of feeding and in the care of her breasts. The normal nipple should protrude when the areolar region is gently squeezed between a thumb and forefinger. A nipple which retracts will be unsuitable for breast feeding. This difficulty can be overcome in most cases by a series of simple exercises which are conducted in the last few months of pregnancy [5]. The woman places her thumbs on either side of the base of the nipple and moves them towards the areolar margin to firmly stretch the skin. This manoeuvre is repeated in both the horizontal and vertical planes and gradually breaks down adhesions which anchor the nipple to the underlying tissue. The flow of milk after birth can be enhanced by emptying the breasts during the last few weeks of pregnancy. A breast is gently compressed between two hands which are then moved towards the alveolar region. This pressure impels milky secretions from the small ducts into the larger ducts and sinuses. This is repeated about ten times. The areola is then held between the thumb and forefinger and pressure is exerted backwards towards the centre of the breast. This squeezes secretion out of the milk sinuses.

Lactation. — Milk production is inhibited during pregnancy when the levels of progesterone and estrogen are high. After birth these hormones decrease and prolactin from the anterior pituitary stimulates the alveolar cells of the breast to manufacture milk. The initial secretions of colostrum are thick and yellow and contain about 8 % protein. Daily production amounts to approximately 50 ml. This gradually increases during the transition to mature milk in the first week.

Milk drainage is dependent on the action of oxytocin from the posterior pituitary. This hormone is released during sucking to constrict myoepithelial fibres around the alveola. This results in a forceful ejection of milk down the ducts to empty the breasts. Milk which is secreted before the "let down" reflex is known as foremilk and it contains little fat or protein and has a bluish tinge. That which is released by oxytocin is termed hindmilk and is rich in fat with a creamy appearance. These variations probably satisfy an infant's thirst and hunger. They may play a role in the control of appetite and thus prevent obesity.

Properties of breast milk. — Human milk contains numerous factors which inhibit infection. Immunoglobulin: IgG, IgM and IgA antibodies are found in relatively high concentrations, particularly in colostrum. Secretory IgA has a specific action in the gut against various pathogenic bacteria and viruses. Cells: macrophages comprise 90 % of the leucocyte content of milk and can phagocytose bacteria. Lymphocytes are believed to synthetize IgA. Enzymes: lysozyme occurs in a high concentration. It is stable in an acid environment and can cleave the peptidoglycans of bacterial cell walls. Other protective factors include the C3 and C4 fractions of complement, lactoferrin which inhibits the growth of staphylococci and *E. coli*, Lactoperoxidase and bowel flora regulants. Protection from allergy is thought to reside in the IgA immunoglobulin. This is believed to react with various food allergens in the intestine and to prevent their absorption through the relatively porous gut wall. A low phosphate load prevents hypocalcaemic tetany while a low sodium content protects against hypernatraemia. The small quantity of iron is efficiently absorbed and utilized to prevent iron deficiency and the Vitamin D protects against rickets.

Maintenance of lactation. — The delicate balance between secretion and milk drainage must be maintained to ensure successful breast feeding [6]. Two factors are of prime importance, an adequate suck reflex of the infant, and effective emptying of the breasts.

(*a*) Sucking: an infant should be able to suck the nipple well back into his mouth so that his lips come to lie at the level of the areolar margin. He is unable to grasp a nipple which is engorged or retracted. In such cases the nipple lies at the front of the mouth and bears the brunt of sucking. This can lead to redness, pain and excoriation of the skin. Sucking difficulties may also arise if the infant has a nasal obstruction or if he is excessively lethargic due to oversedation. Inadequate sucking results in incomplete emptying of the breasts.

(*b*) Emptying of the breasts. — A "let down" reflex usually occurs after two or three minutes of sucking. This may happen sooner as a result of emotional stimuli such as crying, but it is wise to allow the infant to suck at the breast until an adequate ejection of milk has occurred. A poor "let down" will result in engorgement. The breast and nipple become œdematous and thus unsuitable for adequate sucking. Eventually the alveolar cells may cease to produce milk due to back pressure.

Milk production is influenced by other factors. It can be reduced by contraceptive tablets which contain œstrogen and progesterone and also by fatigue caused by lack of sleep. The smooth operation of the "let down" reflex is favoured by a tranquil mind. It can be hindered by the tensions and fears which so commonly occur in a new mother during the early post-partum period. Such anxiety can often be dispelled by adopting a sympathetic attitude, and by giving her an adequate explanation for her particular problem.

Sleep is essential for success and provision must be made for the mother who is having to demand feed three hourly. She requires undisturbed rest between feeds and to this purpose may require a single room, restricted visiting, alteration of ward routine such as cleaning and the provision of meals at suitable times.

Techniques of feeding. — Breast feeding commences immediately after delivery. This provides an early stimulus for milk secretion and drainage. Sucking is again encouraged after the period of attention and bathing in the nursery. This does not usually exceed three hours from the time of birth, but it may have to be extended after Caesarean deliveries depending on the condition of the mother and infant.

Demand feeding: a baby is put to the breast when he appears to be hungry. In the first few days he may cry to be fed three hourly or more frequently. The mother must be reassured that the frequency will diminish and care must be taken to determine whether the infant is really hungry or is crying for some other reason. By the third or fourth day a more convenient routine ought to have been established. Some babies, particularly bigger ones, may continue to demand their feeds at three hour intervals.

A mother feeds her baby in the position which she finds most comfortable. She may wish to feed while lying or sitting in bed, or she may prefer to sit in a chair. Care is taken to keep the baby warm during feeds.

The nipples may be washed with soap and water once a day and with water only before feeding. They are wiped dry after the feed and can be kept soft by massaging in a small quantity of lanolin. The breasts are supported in a well-fitting bra which does not compress the nipples.

When putting the baby to the breast use is made of the rooting reflex. The nipple is readily grasped if lightly touching the corner of the mouth. The breast is prevented from covering the infant's nostrils by supporting the areolar base between the second and third fingers.

Optimum drainage of milk is achieved by using both breasts at each feed. The infant initially suckles the breast from which he was taken off at the previous feed. This ensures that at least one side is completely emptied at each nursing session. The infant can be switched from one breast to the other when the initial vigorous sucking and swallowing becomes weaker and less frequent. He may remain on the alternative side until he uses the nipple as a pacifier only.

The duration of feeding varies and can range from about five minutes sucking at each breast on the first day to approximately fifteen minutes by the third or fourth day. The longer interval is to be favoured if the breasts show signs of engorgement. At the end of a feed the mother inserts an index finger into the mouth alongside the nipple to release the suction. In most cases the maximum volume of milk is taken within the first four to five minutes of sucking [7].

The intake of colostrum often does not exceed 50 ml in the first two days. By the end of the first week the volume has increased to provide an infant with approximately 150 ml/kg/day and an energy intake of 420 kJ a day.

Minor problems:

(*a*) Sore nipples. — Mothers often experience a tingling sensation in the nipples when a baby starts sucking. This is normal. A truly sore nipple is reddened and can become cracked. This problem is more likely to occur in fair-skinned women. Soreness in most cases can be prevented by adequate attention to the nipples between feeds and by the correct "fixing" of an infant on the breast. Suction on the nipple should always be released at the end of the feed.

Healing can be encouraged by keeping the nipple dry and by massaging it with lanolin. Short exposures to sunlight or ultra-violet light will also assist in the healing process. A cracked nipple should be rested for 24 hours. Milk can be manually expressed and given to the infant by cup and spoon or in a bottle.

Red inflamed nipples can be the result of a monilial infection. The fungus is usually present in the infant's mouth. Nystatin ointment is applied to the nipples after each feed and nystatin drops are used to treat the mouth infection.

(*b*) Breast engorgement. — Engorgement may occur on the third or fourth day especially in a primip. Portions of the breast become tense and tender and the overlying skin may be œdematous. In a mild case the mother is advised to take a hot shower before putting the infant to the breast. In a more severe case, sucking may not be possible owing the swelling of the nipple and breast. Portions of the breast are red and œdematous. Warm compresses are placed on the affected areas. The breasts are then manually expressed to relieve tension. Once flow has been established the infant may assist by sucking.

Severe engorgement presents with grossly œdematous and painful breasts. The nipples are buried in swollen tissue which renders sucking impossible.

A rapidly acting diuretic may relieve tension and sublingual oxytocin can initiate a flow of milk. Breasts are emptied by means of a mechanical pump as they may be too tender to manipulate by hand.

(*c*) Overfeeding. — Most breast-fed babies can regulate their requirements accurately and it is doubtful whether this entity exists. A rapid flow of milk may certainly occur at the beginning of a feed to cause coughing or vomiting. Milk flow can be controlled by compressing the areola between the second and third finger.

(*d*) Underfeeding. — A poor gain in weight is the most accurate indication of underfeeding, in fact it may be the only sign as the infant may appear content after feeds. Other features include excessive crying, persistent sucking of the fingers, a reduced output of stools and urine or vomiting due to swallowing of air.

Factors which lead to underfeeding include engorgement of breasts, inadequate milk production particularly in the first few days after birth and poor sucking due to oversedation. The amount of milk taken by the baby is best estimated by means of test-weighing. The fully clothed infant is weighed before and after a feed. Care is taken not to change soiled or wet diapers between the weighing. The procedure is repeated after each feed for a day in order to get an accurate estimate of the total milk intake.

The underfed infant will require extra feeds. If the problem is related to engorgement of breasts, it is given milk which has been expressed from the mother. If milk production is inadequate then pooled breast milk can be used until lactation has improved.

Complementary bottle feeds of cow's milk are preferably avoided, but occasionally may have to be used when breast milk is unavailable.

Bottle feeding. — Modified cow's milk is an acceptable substitute for human milk and bottle feeding is relatively simple and safe in privileged communities. It remains a hazardous procedure amongst those of low socio-economic status.

Raw cow's milk is unsuitable for the newborn baby because of its bacterial contamination, casein load, low lactose content, excessive solutes and small quantity of fluoride, iron and vitamins.

A variety of suitable milk products are commercially available. These include evaporated milk, powdered full-cream milk and modified milk. Babies will thrive on most varieties, but the modified group is preferable, although it is the most expensive. Cow's milk is separated into its main components which are then altered and reconstituted to resemble breast milk. No degrees of modification can reproduce the unique nutritional and immunological properties of human milk. The correct casein-lactalbumin ratio is obtained by mixing whey with skimmed milk. Excessive minerals are removed by dialysis and the carbohydrate content is increased by adding a sugar. Fat droplets are decreased in size by homogenisation and the ratio of saturated to unsaturated fatty acids is adjusted by means of vegetable fats. Vitamins are added to most, and iron to some products.

Preparation of feeds. — In many hospitals the feeds are available as a sterile liquid which is pre-packed in bottles ready to use. The milk is stored on a shelf in the nursery and bottles and teats are discarded after use. Facilities are required for the preparation of sterile feeds if such milks are unavailable.

Milk kitchen. — A milk kitchen consists of one section for cleaning and another for the preparation, sterilization and refrigeration of feeds. These areas are separated by a full length wall or partition and communicate only by means of a two-way autoclave oven. Bottles and teats are thoroughly washed before use and then autoclaved for 10 minutes. They are transferred through to the clean side to cool and then filled with prepared milk. Each bottle is fitted with a teat and capped down to the neck with a paper bag held in place by an elastic band. The bottles are placed in racks and re-autoclaved for five minutes at a pressure of 0.7 kg/cm^2 and a temperature of 100° C. They are immediately transferred to a large refrigerator to be rapidly cooled and they remain here until required in the nurseries.

Each bottle must be identified with the baby's name and number and a feed list is kept in both the milk kitchen and the nursery. Personnel employed in the milk kitchen should be free from infection and must be familiar with aseptic procedures.

Feeding recommendations. — An infant can be fed on demand and usually establishes a four-hourly pattern by the third or fourth day. Fluid requirements are variable and range from about 60 ml/kg/day in the first few days to 150 ml/kg/day by the end of the first week.

Technique: the warmly wrapped baby is placed on his mother's lap and held close to the body. Feeds are given at body temperature and can be warmed in an electric bottle warmer or in a sterile metal container of warm water. The temperature of the milk is tested by allowing a few drops of milk to fall on the back of the mother's hand. The hole in the teat should be large enough to allow the milk to drop out steadily when the bottle is inverted. It should not flow out as a stream.

Discharge instruction. — A mother should be familiar with the preparation of feeds. She receives written instructions concerning the nature and amount of ingredients. This includes volume of milk powder in measures or teaspoonfuls, water in millilitres, the quantity of milk per feed and the number of feeds in 24 hours.

A scoop is usually provided with each tin of milk. This is specific for the particular product and cannot be used to measure the volume of other milk products. It is filled by heaping the powder and levelling it with the edge of a knife to the rim. No effort must be made to pack the powder by patting it down, or packing the scoop against the side of the tin as this can result in an overconcentrated feed.

Supplementary iron and vitamins. — Iron is not recommended for the first month or two of life. If not added in the milk it can be prescribed from two months of age as a liquid solution. Most milks contain added vitamins. If not, these should be added

Discharge examination. — A second full examination is conducted towards the end of the first week at the time of discharge. At this stage the baby should be feeding well and gaining weight.

Metabolic screening tests. — Blood is taken by a heel prick and collected onto absorbent paper for specific metabolic tests. The most widely recommended tests screen for hypothyroidism and phenylketonuria. The labelled paper strips are posted to a central laboratory for examination. Radioimmunoassay is used to detect the level of T4 which should be above 6 μg/dl in the euthyroid infant. The Guthrie or equivalent test may be used to estimate the level of phenylalanine which is normally less than 2 mg/dl at this age.

The normal pre-term baby

Fetal maturation is related to gestational age rather than to body size and most infants have been prepared for extrauterine life by 38 weeks of gestation. A baby of less than 37 completed weeks (259 days) is considered to be pre-term. Sixty percent of these weigh 2,000 g or more and many are on the borderline of maturity. Those over 1,500 g without respiratory distress, recurrent apnoea or intraventricular haemorrhage are usually normal and do not necessarily require special care facilities.

CLINICAL FEATURES

The following characteristics may be observed in normal pre-term babies who weigh more than 1,500 g (Fig. I-28).

Head. — The size appears to be disproportionately large in relation to the body, but head circumference is within the normal range for gestation. The skull bones are soft and mobile and fontanelles are relatively small. The hair is silky and its individual strands tend to adhere to one another. The ears are soft, pliable and easily folded. They do not recoil as rapidly as those of a full-term infant.

Skin. — Vernix caseosa may be sparse and lanugo is plentiful, especially over the back. The thin skin is pink and smooth and underlying vessels are visible. Subcutaneous fat is absent or scanty and bony structures can be clearly seen. Oedema may be present over the lower legs. Transverse skin creases on the soles of the feet are poorly developed. Breast nodules are small or absent before 36 weeks of gestation.

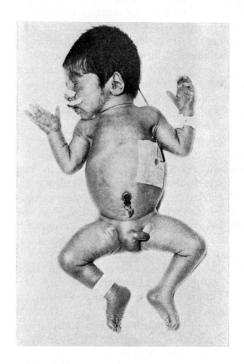

FIG. I-28. — *Characteristic appearance of a pre-term infant of 1,800 g weight.*

Respiratory system. — The chest cage is relatively small and the ribs are prominent. Breathing is diaphragmatic in type and may be irregular or periodic at times. Overdistension of the stomach with milk may hinder movement of the diaphragm and impair respiratory function. Birth asphyxia is more likely to occur than in the full-term infant.

The nostrils are small and can easily be blocked. A cough reflex is absent or poorly developed. The cry may be weak.

Gastrointestinal system. — Sucking is present, but may be inadequate for breast or bottle feeding before 36 weeks of gestation. The gastro-oesophageal junction may be lax and result in regurgitation of milk into the pharynx. The abdomen is relatively large and the underlying muscles are thin. Gut lipase is deficient and fat absorption may be diminished resulting in poor weight gain and excessive amounts of fat in the stools.

Liver. — Glycogen stores are inadequate prior to 36 weeks gestation and the pre-term baby can develop hypoglycaemia after birth especially if starved.

Glucuronyl transferase activity may be inadequate and jaundice is likely to occur.

Haematological system. — Physiological anaemia tends to be more severe than in the full-term infant and can be exaggerated by a deficiency of folic acid and Vitamin E.

Immunological system. — Humoral and cellular immunity is not fully established. Levels of maternal IgG immunoglobulin are reduced and there is a decreased production of IgG, IgM and IgA antibody. These factors render the pre-term infant susceptible to infection.

Genitalia. — The testes may be felt in the inguinal canal by 32 weeks of gestation and in the scrotum by 36 weeks. In females the labia minora are more prominent than the labia majora and the clitoris is well developed.

Neurological function.

Tone: muscle tone is poorly developed before 32 weeks of gestation and at this stage the infant often lies with arms and legs extended. Thereafter the legs become flexed and by 34 weeks the arms and legs are flexed. Neck control is poorly developed.

Primitive reflexes such as the Moro, grasp and placing are well established after 34 weeks of gestation.

Behaviour: the pre-term infant sleeps for the major part of the day and has a well established pattern of rapid eye movement (REM) sleep after 34 weeks. Yawning and stretching are observed at this stage.

ASSESSMENT OF GESTATIONAL AGE

Characteristic physical and neurological signs can be scored to evaluate the gestational age [8]. In order to ensure accuracy, the same person should examine each baby within five days of birth. The unclothed infant must be kept warm and should not be crying as this would alter the colour of the skin.

Eleven physical features are assessed (Table I) and each is assigned a score ranging from 0 to 4. Low scores imply immature features.

Ten neurological signs are scored (Fig. I-29) and the combined score is read off a graph (Fig. I-30).

NEUROLOGICAL FEATURES
(Fig. I-29)

Methods of assessment.

Posture: an infant maintains his limbs in characteristic positions while quiet or asleep on his back. The postures of the arms and legs are noted.

Square window: the infant's hand is gently flexed as far as possible on the forearm by the examiner's forefinger. The angle formed between the hypothenar eminence and the ventral aspect of the forearm is determined.

Ankle dorsiflexion: the foot is gently dorsiflexed as far as possible onto the leg with the examiner's thumb on the sole and other fingers behind the leg (Fig. I-31). The angle between the dorsum of the foot and the anterior surface of the leg is measured.

Arm recoil: the forearms are flexed for 5 seconds, fully extended by pulling on the hands and then released. If they return to full flexion a score of 2 is given. A sluggish or incomplete response is graded as 1 and persistent extension or random movements would score 0.

Leg recoil: the hips and knees are fully flexed for 5 seconds then extended by traction on the feet and released. A return to full flexion scores 2, partial flexion scores 1 and minimal or no movement is given 0.

Popliteal angle: the infant lies on his back with the pelvis flat. A hip is fully flexed and the knee is gently extended as far as possible while the thigh is kept in the knee-chest position by the examiner's forefinger and thumb. The popliteal angle is measured.

Heel to ear manoeuvre: the infant lies on his back and a foot is gently brought up as close as possible to the head. The degree of knee extension is measured.

TABLE I. — PHYSICAL CRITERIA.

External sign	0	1	2	3	4	Method of assessment
Oedema	Hands and feet show obvious oedema. Pitting over tibia.	No obvious oedema of hands and feet. Pitting over tibia.	No oedema.			Skin over lower tibia is depressed by a finger for a few seconds.
Skin texture	Very thin, gelatinous.	Thin and smooth.	Smooth. Medium thickness. Superficial peeling or rash.	Slight thickening, superficial cracking and peeling esp. of hands and feet.	Thick and parchment like. Superficial or deep cracking.	Inspection and palpation.
Skin colour	Dark red.	Uniformly pink.	Pale pink, varies over body.	Pale. Pink over ears, lips, palms or soles only.		Observed while baby is quiet or sleeping. Crying alters the colour.
Skin opacity	Numerous veins and venules clearly seen esp. over abdomen.	Veins and tributaries seen.	A few large vessels clearly seen over abdomen.	A few large vessels indistinctly seen over abdomen.	No blood vessels visible.	Veins over abdomen are inspected in a good light.
Lanugo	Nil present.	Abundant, long and thick over whole back.	Hair thinning esp. over lower back.	Small amount of lanugo. Bald patches.	At least half of back devoid of hair.	Infant is held up to a good light and hair on back is inspected.
Plantar creases	No skin creases present.	Faint red transverse marks over anterior half of sole.	Definite red marks over more than anterior half. Indentations over less than anterior third.	Indentations over more than anterior third.	Deep indentations over more than anterior third.	Toes are extended and transverse marks or creases are inspected.
Nipple formation	Nipple barely visible. No areola.	Nipple well defined. Areola smooth and flat. Diam. < 0.75 cm.	Areola stippled. Edge not raised. Diam. < 0.75 cm.	Areola stippled. Edge raised. Diam. > 0.75 cm.		Nipple and areola inspected.
Breast size	No breast tissue palpable.	Breast tissue on one or both sides. Diam. < 0.5 cm.	Breast tissue both sides. Diam. 0.5-1.0 cm.	Breast tissue both sides. Diam. > 1.0 cm.		Breast tissue palpated between forefinger and thumb.
Ear form	Pinna flat and shapeless, little or no incurving of edge.	Incurving of part of edge of pinna.	Partial incurving of whole of upper pinna.	Well defined incurving of whole of upper pinna.		Inspection of upper portion of ear above external meatus.
Ear firmness	Pinna soft. Easily folded. No recoil.	Pinna soft. Easily folded. Slow recoil.	Cartilage to edge of pinna but soft in places, ready recoil.	Pinna firm. Cartilage to edge. Instant recoil.		Edge of pinna is rolled between finger and thumb to feel cartilage.
Genitalia Male	Testes not in scrotum.	At least one testis high in scrotum.	At least one testis right down.			Testes are palpated with a finger starting at inguinal canal and working towards scrotum to detect a retractile testis.
Female	Labia majora widely separated. Labia minora protruding.	Labia majora almost cover labia minora.	Labia majora completely cover labia minora.			Legs are abducted to inspect labia.

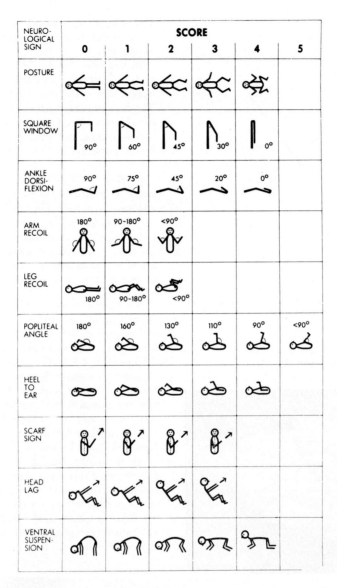

NEURO-LOGICAL SIGN	SCORE					
	0	1	2	3	4	5
POSTURE						
SQUARE WINDOW	90°	60°	45°	30°	0°	
ANKLE DORSI-FLEXION	90°	75°	45°	20°	0°	
ARM RECOIL	180°	90-180°	<90°			
LEG RECOIL	180°	90-180°	<90°			
POPLITEAL ANGLE	180°	160°	130°	110°	90°	<90°
HEEL TO EAR						
SCARF SIGN						
HEAD LAG						
VENTRAL SUSPEN-SION						

Fig. I-29. — *Neurological score for gestational age.*

Scarf sign: a hand is brought across the body as far as possible towards the opposite shoulder. The elbow is supported in this manœuvre and its position is graded in relation to the midline.

Head lag: the infant is slowly pulled by the arms from supine to sitting. The position of the neck in relation to the trunk is noted.

Ventral suspension: the infant is supported under the chest and held prone. The degree of limb, back and neck flexion is noted.

MANAGEMENT

Birth. — Provision must be made for the immediate resuscitation, oxygenation and temperature regulation of a pre-term baby.

Nursing care. — The normal infant over 2,200 g in weight can usually be nursed in a crib at the mother's bedside providing there is no difficulty

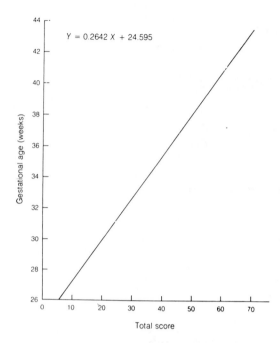

$Y = 0.2642 X + 24.595$

FIG. I-30. — *Gestational age can be determined from the total score.*

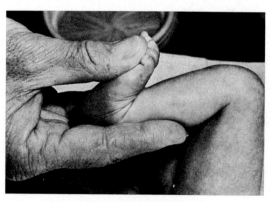

FIG. I-31. — *Position of the foot for determining the degree of ankle dorsiflexion.*

with feeding. A room temperature of 22-24° C is usually adequate to maintain warmth if the infant is clothed in a vest, gown and diaper and wrapped in two woollen blankets. The head can be covered with a bonnet.

Temperature readings are taken in the axilla (normal range 36.5-37° C) using a low reading mercury thermometer or on the skin of the abdomen (normal range 36.2-36.8° C) by means of a thermistor probe. Recordings are made at three hour intervals for the first 24 hours and six hourly thereafter.

The risk of hypothermia is ever present and likely to occur during bathing, weighing or transportation of the infant.

Babies who are unable to maintain a normal body temperature and those of less than 2,000 g weight are preferably kept warm in incubators. The conventional single-walled models are suitable for this purpose. Parents are encouraged to assist in the nursing and feeding of their immature baby in the nursery.

Feeding. — Early feeding is recommended in order to prevent hypoglycaemia and to reduce the chance of hyperbilirubinaemia. Infants on the borderline of maturity can usually cope with breast or bottle feeding whereas many of those below 36 weeks gestation will require nasogastric gavage. Feeds are commenced within 3 hours of birth and consist of breast milk or a modified cow's milk formula.

Nasogastric feeds. — The length of feeding tube to be passed into the stomach can be calculated by measuring the distance from the suprasternal notch to the xiphisternum, doubling this and adding 2.5 cm (Fig. I-32). The infant's head is supported in order to slightly flex the neck and the required length of catheter is gently passed through a nostril into the stomach. No attempt is made to force the tube down and it is changed to the other nostril if the passage is difficult. The catheter is fixed to the nose and cheek by means of strapping. When 2 ml of air is rapidly injected into the tube a loud noise can be heard through a stethoscope placed over the stomach. This confirms the position of the catheter tip. A sample of gastric fluid can be obtained for pH which is usually acidic within six hours of birth. The catheter is replaced every third day by one passed through the opposite nostril.

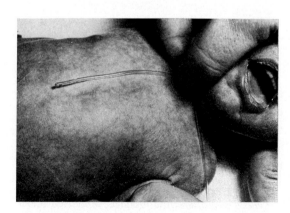

FIG. I-32. — *Method for measuring the length of a naso-gastric tube (see text).*

Amount. — During the first week of life 60-100 ml/kg/day would suffice most normal pre-term babies. Overfeeding must be avoided at this stage as it can cause abdominal distension, impairment of respiration, vomiting and aspiration. Feeds may be given as a continuous drip through an infusion pump if there is excessive abdominal distension or vomiting.

Over the next few weeks the volume is increased to 180-200 ml/kg/day. Feeds are initially given at three hour intervals and by the time the infant has reached 2,000-2,300 g in weight a four hour schedule may be tried. At this stage most babies can suck adequate amounts of milk from the breast or bottle.

Transition from tube to breast or bottle: a baby can usually be weaned from tube feeds after 36 weeks gestation or once the weight has reached 2,000-2,300 g. At this stage the breast or bottle is offered and the required amount of milk should be taken within 20-25 minutes sucking time. If this is not the case then tube feeding is preferably continued for several days before another attempt is made at sucking. The technique used to breast- or bottle-feed a pre-term baby is similar to that used for the full-term infant.

Supplements.

Iron. — Physiological anaemia cannot be prevented by iron therapy and the early introduction of this supplement may enhance the chances of bacterial infection. Daily requirements (1.5 to 2.0 mg/kg) of elemental iron may be given from a month of age as ferrous gluconate drops. Medication is continued until the infant has been established on a mixed diet.

Vitamins. — The pre-term infant has a shortfall of vitamins particularly Vitamin D. Daily requirements of Vitamin A 1,500 IU, C 50 mg and D 800 IU can be given from birth as a water soluble multi-vitamin preparation.

Other requirements include folic acid 50 μg and alpha tocopherol 10 IU per day.

OUTCOME

The overall prognosis for normal pre-term babies has improved dramatically in recent years. Early complications such as birth asphyxia, hypoglycaemia, hypothermia, hyperbilirubinaemia and infections can be prevented or effectively treated. Late complications, such as iron deficiency anaemia and rickets are also preventable.

A mother must be able to handle her infant with confidence before discharge. She should be competent in bathing and in feeding her baby and must be given written instructions regarding iron and vitamin supplements. Most infants will be ready for discharge at 2,300-2,500 g weight.

REFERENCES

[1] USHER (R.), SHEPARD (M.), LIND (J.). — The blood volume of the newborn infant and placental transfusion. *Acta Paediat. Scand.*, *52*, 497-512, 1963.
[2] BRAZELTON (T.), SCHOLL (M.), ROBEY (J.). — Visual responses in the newborn. *Pediatrics*, *37*, 284-290, 1966.
[3] ILLINGWORTH (R.). — *The normal child*, 7th ed., Churchill Livingstone, London, 1979.
[4] JAKOBSSON (I.), LINDBERG (T.). — Cow's milk as a cause of infantile colic in breast-fed infants. *Lancet*, *2*, 437-439, 1978.
[5] HOFFMAN (J.). — A suggested treatment for inverted nipples. *Am. J. Obstet. Gynecol.*, *66*, 346-348, 1953.
[6] APPLEBAUM (R.). — The modern management of successful breast feeding. *Paediat. Clin. N. Amer.*, *17*, 203-225, 1970.
[7] LUCAS (A.), LUCAS (P.), BAUM (J.). — Pattern of milk flow in breast-fed infants. *Lancet*, *2*, 57-58, 1979.
[8] DUBOWITZ (L.), DUBOWITZ (V.). — *Gestational age of the newborn*. Addison-Wesley Publishing Co., Mass., 1977.

3

Cognition and behavior
of the newborn

Lewis P. LIPSITT

INTRODUCTION

Recent research advances in the field of infant behavior and development have resulted in some new understandings of (1) the sensory and learning capabilities of the very young infant, (2) the role of stress or perinatal risk factors in compromising the cognitive capacities of newborns and other infants, and (3) the possibility that experiential and environmental manipulations may have important consequences for the psychological development of the baby, deleterious in some instances and salubrious in others.

This chapter reviews some of the salient findings recently obtained pertaining to each of these considerations. It is not intended to present here an exhaustive survey of the empirical literature on each of these matters, or to provide a complete review of conclusions or theoretical inferences from

Preparation of this chapter was begun while the author was a Fellow at the Center for Advanced Study in the Behavioral Sciences at Stanford, California, where he was supported in part by funds from the Spencer Foundation. The author is indebted as well to the March of Dimes Birth Defects Foundation and the Harris Foundation for support of his research and writing on perinatal medicine during the preparation of this chapter.

the available data. Rather, the purpose is to present a sufficiently detailed overview of the research area of neonatal cognition and behavioral development as to enable the reader to have a reasonable conception of the character of the research now carried out in this relatively new field, and facilitate access to further information on any of these topics in other major contemporary references.

Until quite recently, the psychophysiological and behavioral characteristics, and the learning potential, of young infants had not been extensively explored, nor well utilized for diagnostic and intervention purposes. There were perhaps three or four major works until two decades ago on the behavioral development of infants, and these generally covered the entire age range of infancy. One of these was the classic volume of the German pediatrician Albrecht Peiper (1963), still used as an historic compendium of valuable information, summarizing virtually all of the world's literature on benavioral and neurological development available to that time. Perhaps the major review and critical synthesis of research relating to the sensory and behavioral functioning of newborns was K. C. Pratt's chapter, "The neonate", published in Murchison's (1933) second edition of *A handbook of child psychology* (no chapter on the neonate and infancy appeared in the first, 1931, edition), which was then carried forward and revised for Carmichael's first edition of the *Manual of Child Psychology* (1946). None of these works used the word "cognition" in their descriptions of the capacities, traits, or behavioral outputs of the infant. Cognitive psychology is a relatively recent specialty field, involving the study of information processing strategies and of memorial processes.

The term "cognition" relates to the act, capacity, faculty, or process of knowing. Somewhat loosely, cognition refers to "mental processes" or operations by which organisms become aware of objects of thought or perception. That the term is even used today in a text such as the present one implies acknowledgement that even the newborn has a mind. That assumption has not been long in vogue. Of course, the assertion that the newborn is capable of mental operations ideally requires considerable clarification and qualification. Suffice it to say here that with the recent advent of a wealth of information indicating that at birth all sensory systems are functioning with a modicum of maturity, and with our new understanding that experiential inputs can produce perseverative or lasting changes in the behavior of the baby, it is reasonable to speak of the neonate as a cognitive being.

Because much of our information about the baby's cognitive capacities is derived from the documentation of behavioral changes in the presence of diverse sensory inputs, the examination of cognition inevitably entails study of behavioral development. By the same token, much of the behavior observed in infants is mediated by psychobiological responses of the baby to the pleasures and annoyances of various sensory experiences. Thus our review here will necessitate discussion of hedonic aspects of infantile reactivity as well.

THE NEONATAL NERVOUS SYSTEM AND THE EFFECTS OF EXPERIENCE

All behavioral processes of humans are mediated by the nervous system, and the nervous system is a changing entity with maturation. A very pronounced brain growth spurt occurs just prior to term birth and shortly afterwards (Dobbing, 1975), and within two months or so brain cell division, or formation of new cells, diminishes and probably ceases by about two years of age (Winick and Rosso, 1975). Brain growth continues after such cell division ceases, however, due to cellular growth, the branching of dendrites, and the proliferation of dendritic spines (Pribram, 1971; Purpura, 1975). The typical child developmentalist of the early

20th century believed that the relationship between maturation and environment was a one-way street, with all experiential effects waiting upon maturational changes which would permit the experience to have an effect, or the behavior to occur. It is now well accepted on the basis of early-experience studies, some of which have shown profound neural tissue changes as a function of early experience, that the maturation-environment relationship is a two-way street (Jacobson, 1978; Jeffrey, 1980). Environmental enrichment, or the imposition of special experiences, can alter maturation rates in certain spheres, such as visual cortex development, which in turn can alter the readiness of the organism to appreciate or assimilate further stimulation in that sphere. Visual deficits of children, due to early strabismus and the consequent amblyopia usually accompanying this, apparently can never be properly compensated, regardless of anatomical correction.

Concerning the growth of dendrites and their spines up to the age of two years, there is considerable evidence in the recent literature to support the proposition that experience itself increases dendritic proliferation. In a study, for example, involving restriction of rabbits' vision, Globus and Scheibel (1967) showed that the apical dendritic spines became deformed. By the same token, Schapiro and Vukovich (1970) enhanced the formation of cortical spines and neurons by administering newborn rats about 30 minutes of handling, noise, and visual stimuli for eight days. Now-classic experiments by Hubel and Wiesel (e. g., 1970) showed that a visual deprivation experience in cats, imposed by suturing one eyelid, would, especially if carried on between the fourth and eighth week "critical period", diminish the number of visual cortical neurons that would react to stimulation later in the previously occluded eye.

While it is not a foregone conclusion that impairment effects imposed by experiential constraints will be matched eventually by similarly convincing data showing brain growth enhancement effects from experiential enrichment procedures, it is an exciting prospect that such effects are possible. As suggested by Wittrock (1980), the bold implication that experience can contribute through neural growth to increased ability to learn and remember is worth testing, because an "... increase in brain size and weight, the increased density of arborization of dendritic spines, the profusion of intercellular connections, and changes in neurotransmitters might indicate a greater store of information in the brain, an increased ability to learn, or an increase in the neural substrates of the ability to learn and to remember" (p. 378).

Some degree of confidence can already be placed in this eventuality, through the work of Rosenzweig and his colleagues (see, for example, Rosenzweig and Bennett, 1976). Comparing

— (1) rats reared in groups of three for 25 to 105 days under standard laboratory conditions with

— (2) comparable animals raised singly in a relatively isolated, impoverished condition, and with

— (3) rats raised in groups of 12 in an "enriched" environment involving a cage with a complicated variety of changing apparatus, with which to play and run, they found, upon sacrifice and autopsy of the animals under blindassessment conditions, that the enrichment group exceeded the others in brain size, thickness of the cortex, concentrations of acetylcholine, and number of glial cells.

The chemical events taking place in brain cells, and the manner in which memories are stored in the brain, are exceedingly complex. These topics and their behavioral and developmental implications are reviewed in McGuinness and Pribram (1980) and Thompson, Berger and Berry (1980). Our major concern here is with the sensory capacities of infants, and the permissions and constraints that these capacities confer on the neonate. What can the newborn hear, smell and see, and how does information processing proceed in the normal neonate as opposed to the infant born under varying conditions of risk?

SENSATION AND PERCEPTION IN THE NEWBORN

It is now well accepted that the newborn comes into the world with all sensory channels functioning to an extent determined by both genetic and congenital factors. Determination of just what the newborn senses has been one of the principal challenges of the field of neonatal psychophysiology and psychophysics (Kessen, Haith and Salapatek, 1970). Whereas adults can articulate to an investigator when they see a stimulus or find one visual stimulus brighter or redder or more horizontal than another (as in an optometric examination), other indicator responses must be devised for the study of infants. The challenge has been met, in part, by utilizing such indicator responses as respiratory changes, heart rate accelerations and decelerations, bodily movements recorded on a stabilimeter, sucking behaviors, and the like. The multi-channel polygraph has been exceptionally valuable in this work, as this provides a permanent recording for the assessment of interobserver reliability and for fine-grain

analysis of responses whose features are very frequently quite subtle. The multichannel polygraph has the same advantages over simple observation of a behavior pattern, or naked counts of sucking responses, as the electrocardiogram has over the stethoscope.

Some illustrative procedures and findings follow (Lipsitt, 1979). A typical polygraph record obtained from a normal two-day-old newborn is presented as Figure I-33, in which is shown, among other things, the change that takes place in an infant's sucking behavior and heart rate when the incentive is shifted from a less sweet fluid to a sweeter fluid. It may be seen that the sucking rate slows down within bursts, but that the heart rate nonetheless soars to a higher rate within bursts, even controlling for the differential number of sucks within the burst. In fact, one of the consequences of increased sucrose concentration, even though in this instance the amount of fluid delivered by pump into the infant's mouth is only .02 ml per criterion suck, is extension of the length of the sucking burst, both in temporal terms and in terms of the number of sucks emitted. The normal newborn thus takes fewer and shorter rest periods (interburst intervals) per minute and so manages to engage in more responses, even though sucking more slowly when sucking, thereby demonstrating through several parameters or indices that the sweeter fluid is the more savory substance (Lipsitt, Reilly, Butcher and Greenwood, 1976). The quickening of the heart rate further substantiates the hedonic substrate of this differential responding in the presence of discriminatively different fluids (Lipsitt, 1976).

Figure I-34 shows an infant in the testing situation described, from which it is possible to obtain data from newborns in the presence of stimulation through any of the sensory modalities. Infants have been observed, and their behavior quantified, in response to olfactory, tactile, auditory, and visual stimulation, in addition to gustatory stimulation as in the example (Rovee-Collier and Lipsitt, 1982). Moreover, it has been demonstrated that the discriminability and differential response to fluids differing in sweetness is compromised in infants who are premature, and further compromised in infants whose medical course during the neonatal period has been severe (Cowett et al., 1978).

Behavioral investigation of the newborn is a relatively young enterprise. Until very recently, with the upsurge of interest in the premature and other high-risk infants, and the advent of technological refinements making it increasingly possible for the seriously ill or injured newborn to survive, behavioral studies of the infant with a background

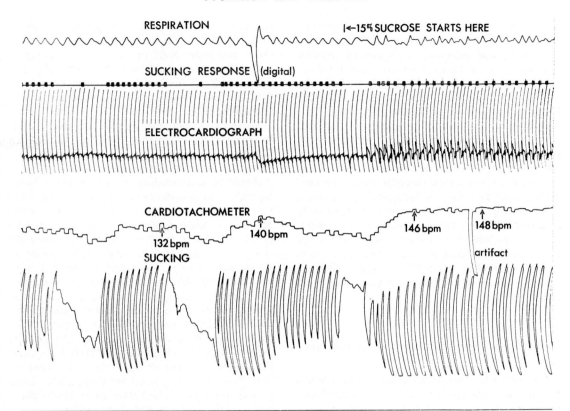

FIG. I-33. — *Polygraphic recording of 2-day-old infant's respiration, heart rate and sucking.* The baby is switched from no-fluid sucking to 15 % (0.02 ml drops) sucrose at the arrow. Record shown is of about 1 min duration, with polygraph running at 5 mm/sec. Electrocardiogram is transformed by cardiotachometer into a beat-by-beat readout ranging from 80 to 180 bpm. The second pen from top gives a digital recording of the criterion sucks shown on the lowest channel.

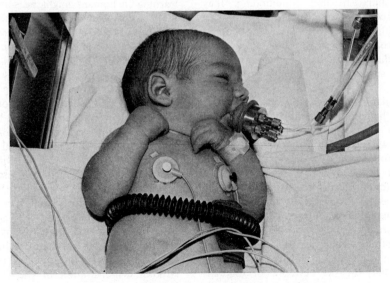

FIG. I-34. — *Infant two days of age, in stabilimeter,*
prepared for recording of heart rate, respiration, and sucking behavior.

of physical jeopardy and intensive care have been virtually non-existent. Thus our knowledge about the sensory and behavioral correlates of physical risk factors in the perinatal period is still minimal, although enormous inroads have been made in the past ten years (see, for example, Field et al., 1979; Friedman and Sigman, 1980; Smeriglio, 1981).

Because of the dearth of comparative behavioral data on the normal and high-risk newborn until very recently, rather little is known also about the relevant brain-behavior relationships that clearly underlie the psychological sequellae during the neonatal period and the developmental dysfunctions that frequently manifest themselves later, apparently as a result of the adverse perinatal circumstances. More will be said later, however, about some of the most promising psychobiological findings which seem to separate the high-risk babies from the essentially normal, and about the predictive validity of these measures.

LEARNING PROCESSES OF THE NEWBORN

Not long ago it was thought that cortical innervation was developed to such an insignificant extent that no learning or memorial process could possibly exist. As reported by Lipsitt (1963), Soviet investigators who tended to be the most sophisticated behavioral researchers with infants made this conclusion or drew this inference quite early in their attempts to demonstrate conditioning in the newborn child. Failing to find conditioning, they reasoned that the brain was not sufficiently mature to permit it. With advances in knowledge about conditioning processes *per se*, however, it can now be concluded that neonates are in fact responsive to stimulation suggestive that memory traces are present.

The pediatrician-psychologist Papousek was one of the first, at the Institute for the Care of Mother and Child in Czechoslovakia, to demonstrate learning in newborns using a modified classical conditioning procedure (Papousek, 1967). His several studies included the finding that older infants require fewer trials to reach a preset learning criterion, but learning nonetheless takes place in the infant under 30 days of age. Using his conditioned headturning response, with milk "rewards" used as the reinforcer, Papousek was able to adapt the conditioning technique for purposes of assessing the discriminability by the newborn of different tones. Obviously, the procedure has valuable implications for demonstrating that a given newborn

can hear and that discriminative ability (within the range of tones used) is possible. The technique is quite elaborate and time-consuming, however, and will be superceded ultimately by evoked potential procedures which can now yield satisfactory data in one session (Schulman-Galambos and Galambos, 1979).

While it is not the purpose of this chapter to provide an exhaustive survey of all infancy literature that capitalizes upon conditioning techniques for assessing sensory capacities of newborns, it should be acknowledged in passing that pediatric ingenuity was in evidence very early after the discovery of conditioning techniques for the possible detection of auditory deficits in newborns. Aldrich (1928) sounded a small bell while stimulating the sole of the infant with a pin-prick. Following 12 to 15 such pairings, the sound of the bell alone was found by Aldrich to be effective in eliciting the response. Although the use of aversive conditioning techniques like these has not been popular among child psychologists, in part because a relatively intense unconditioned prior stimulus must be used in order to effect the conditioned response, the apparent success of this little study suggested that classically conditioned behavior could indeed provide important information as to the auditory acuity of the newborn, and about deafness.

The aforementioned Papousek techniques for establishing conditioned responses in the newborn were important for a number of reasons, not the least of which was the empirical demonstration that the most effective techniques for obtaining learning in humans might be some elaboration of the classical Pavlovian techniques (Rovee-Collier and Lipsitt, 1982). Papousek introduced the technique of "guidance" on trials when the unconditioned (or usually effective congenital response) did not occur to the tactile stimulus at the corner of the infant's mouth. Following the guidance of response in the ipsilateral direction, the reinforcer, involving delivery of milk from a bottle, was given. Thus the infant received the conditioning stimulus, the unconditioned stimulus, and the reward on every trial.

Siqueland and Lipsitt (1966) used a similar procedure but with a dextrose solution as the reinforcer and as many as thirty trials per day, and found that infants as young as 48 to 96 hours of age could reach a substantial conditioning criterion in a training session of less than one hour. Of the three studies they carried out, the third provided the most striking demonstration of the conditionability of normal newborns, in that they were able to show, in the same subjects at the same time, enhanced

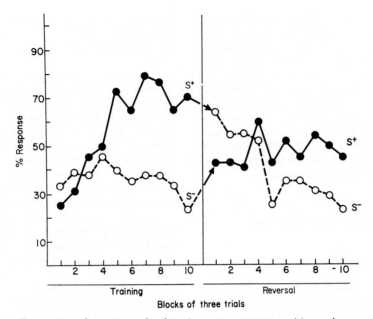

FIG. I-35. — *Comparison of percentage head-turning responses to a positive and a negative stimulus during 60 trials of training and 60 trials of reversal* (SIQUELAND and LIPSITT, 1966).

interest and response to one set of stimuli and disinterest or diminished response to another. Sixteen newborn infants were presented with pairings of either a buzzer or a tone, along with a tactile stimulus delivered to the right cheek. One of the auditory stimuli was paired with dextrose (this stimulus constellation being called S+), which was delivered from a bottle immediately following an "appropriate" right head-turn. It may be seen in Figure I-35 that responding to S+ increased while that to S− (representing the other auditory stimulus paired with the same type of touch to the cheek) remain the same. After thirty minutes of such training, in which there occurred a reliable difference between S+ and S− responding, the stimulus compounds were reversed, such that the previous S+ constellation now became S− and *vice versa*, and the infant's response patterns accordingly shifted. Thus both basic conditioning and reversal learning were demonstrated in newborns within an hour-long training and reversal-training session.

Cross-species validation of this sort of learning, which involves elements of classical Pavlovian and operant (Skinnerian) procedures, is found in work with newborn rat pups carried out by Johanson and Hall (1979). Newborn rat pups were placed in a styrofoam cup with a terry-cloth lever which, if pushed upward, caused 3-4 ml of milk to be infused into the pup's mouth through a cannula which was implanted 30 minutes earlier. Prior to testing, the

pups had been allowed 6-8 hours of post-natal sucking. Compared with litter mate controls of two types, one which received the lever experience and reinforcement non-contingently and the other being a deprivation group which received the lever experience but no reinforcement, the experimental newborns pushed the lever significantly more often during the acquisition phase, and continued responding significantly longer when no further reward was available.

In another study, the same researchers introduced two levers into the container and saturated terry-cloths beneath each with different odors (S+, S−). Six of the eight newborn rats in the experimental group acquired the discrimination within twelve hours. The yoked controls did not acquire this discrimination and, in addition, responded less than the experimental subjects. As in Siqueland and Lipsitt (1966), S+ and S− were then reversed for some animals, and their behavior changed accordingly. This study, and those of Siqueland and Lipsitt, suggest that if the environmental arrangements are so structured as to capitalize upon congenital response repertoires and naturalistic contingencies, learning tends to be more effective in the sense that it occurs sooner and faster. This is as Nobel Laureate Tinbergen suggested when he cautioned that we ought to "approach learning phenomena from a more naturalistic standpoint than is usually done and to ask, not what can an animal learn, but what does it actually learn under natural conditions?" (Tinbergen, 1951, p. 142). Most of the major successes using conditioning techniques with infants have resulted from using experimental paradigms which approximate the conditions of stimulation which have been experienced by the species for many generations, even eons. This may be one reason that the claims of the proponents of naturalistic perinatal conditions (for example, Klaus and Kennell, 1976), seem to be at once both plausible and difficult to confirm under well-controlled experimental constraints.

NEONATAL HABITUATION

Habituation is a stimulus-response phenomenon well known to even the casual observer of every day behavior, in humans and other organisms. Defined as a "stimulus specific response decrement resulting from repeated or constant exposures to the response eliciting stimulus" (Wyers, Peeke and Herz, 1973, p. 12), the definition excludes those response waning processes which result from maturation, sensory adaptation, illness or aging, drugs, or diurnal changes. Habituation is the means through which organisms eliminate superfluous or redundant responses to stimuli which are biologically irrelevant, thus permitting the organism to conserve energy and maintain alertness to pleasant and annoying stimulation, i. e., those aspects of the environment which are to be approached for sustenance or avoided to assure safety.

If habituation is not a primitive type of learning process, it is at least a mechanism whereby information storage is relevant and at least short-term memory is operative. Recent discussions of human infant habituation are contained in the works of Clifton and Nelson (1976), Jeffrey and Cohen (1971), and Tighe and Leaton (1976). In habituation, early presentations of a stimulus evoke greater response than subsequent presentations, suggesting that the organism retains an internal representation of the stimulus event, and responses to subsequent presentations are in inverse relationship to the goodness-of-match between the stored representation and the subsequent stimulus. Thus the procedure which produces habituation to a constant stimulus is one which may be appropriated for the discovery of an organism's capacity for discriminating between stimulus episodes. For example, Stimulus A may be administered ten times in succession, with the effect that over trials response strength will diminish appreciably. Following these ten presentations,

an eleventh trial may be administered, this time of Stimulus B. If response recovery occurs, this signifies discriminability of the two stimuli by the respondent, whereas no change in response signifies lack of discriminability of the two stimuli. The process of habituation thus takes its place, along with classical and operant conditioning, as one which can inform the neonatal investigator about the extent to which cortical functioning is present. To the extent that the infant is deficient in habituation, and may thus be the victim, either temporary or permanent, of cortical dysfunction, this test of central nervous system deficit may enable a more definitive diagnosis and/or ameliorative interventions.

A pioneer in the study of visual interest and visual discrimination processes of newborns, Robert Fantz (1961, 1964) showed that the newborn infant's gaze duration can be observed objectively and repetitively over a series of trials to document the waning of interest in specific visual stimuli. One of Fantz's earliest studies indicated that the habituation process, and thus visual discrimination, becomes more acute over the first ten weeks of life. Subsequent studies, such as that by Friedman, Nagy and Carpenter (1970) showed that even newborns demonstrate a response decrement over trials.

To the extent that habituation is associated with memory function mediated by the brain, the habituation process should be subject to compromise in infants with clear central nervous system impairment. In fact, Brackbill (1971) and Wolff (1969) have shown that neither hydrocephalic nor anencephalic infants habituate, and Lewis (1967) showed that impaired habituation is found in infants with low Apgar scores and other indices of perinatal stress and consequent brain dysfunction. For these reasons, Brazelton (1973) has included habituation measures in his Neonatal Behavioral Assessment Scale which was designed to document the behavioral maturity and well-being of newborns following varying degrees of perinatal distress.

Soviet investigators as early as 1958 used a habituation technique in association with sucking behavior to demonstrate that babies born under conditions of excessive cranial pressure or with the cord around the neck show habituation deficiencies (Bronshtein, Antonova, Kamenetskaya, Luppova and Sytova, 1958). Their infants were presented with an exteroceptive stimulus such as a sound while sucking. Normal, full-term infants would interrupt their sucking upon such stimulus presentations, but then show a waning of such interruptions, or habituation, on subsequent and repetitive presentations of the same stimulus. Infants born at risk, however, required many more stimulus presentations to habituate the response of sucking-suppression.

Among the promising techniques for recording sensory responsivity, stimulus discrimination, and habituation processes is the averaged evoked response technique, which has been refined greatly in the past ten years (Schulman-Galambos and Galambos, 1979). In a study of auditory evoked responses in Down syndrome infants who were compared with normal infants, matched in age from 8 days to 13 months, the Down syndrome babies showed no reliable response decrement over habituation trials (Barnet, Olrich and Shanks, 1974). In the same study it was shown that no babies, normal or not, showed evoked response habituation within the first month of life. As in other studies, the capacity for habituation increased reliably over the first weeks of life.

Cognitive or memorial capacities, signifying information storage and processing capabilities, are affected by obstetrical anesthesia. Using habituation techniques, Bowes, Brackbill, Conway and Steinschneider (1970) studied infants at 2 and 5 days of age. Infants whose mothers had received high dosages of anesthesia during childbirth took as many as four times more trials to habituate than mothers who received little or no medication. Most interestingly, this differentiation between the two groups persisted at least until the infants were one month of age. More systematic studies are required to link perinatal contingencies to such behavioral processes as habituation, to assure that the anesthesia has compromised the infant's response rather than some obstetrical condition or fetal distress dictating the increased dosage of anesthesia, simultaneously diminishing response habituation to environmental stimulation.

THE SIGNIFICANCE OF EARLY HUMAN COGNITION

Much early human behavior is endogenously generated. However, some aspects of behavioral functioning are caused and altered by stimulation provided for the infant by the environment. Although we tend to regard the infant as an independent organism in a world of experiential forces that impinge upon him or her in well-organized regimens of stimulation. The baby's caretakers are actually very much in the picture as providers of that stimulation. The baby and its caretakers form "dyads", which is to say that the caretaker and child systematically reciprocate one another's behaviors,

so that each is simultaneously a stimulant for and a responder to the other. While it is a biological truism that the baby is the more dependent of the two members of such dyads, the image of the infant as simply a passive recipient of environmental inputs must now be regarded as quite inappropriate (Thoman, 1979). Individual differences abound in infants with respect to their physiognomic characteristics, their psychophysiological tempos, and their behavioral propensities, and these all help to determine the reactions of other people to them. The reciprocating transactions which engage the infant from the earliest moments after birth form the context within which the infant will proceed to acquire coping maneuvers and skills, social gestures, and environmental manipulations designed to enable the baby to satisfy needs as these occur. It might be said that the early weeks and months of life are a kind of proving ground for the adequacy of the infant's inherited and congenital response repertoire the embellishment of which will be the by-product of early practice. Learning disabilities and other developmental problems have their earliest origins, in this view, in the interplay between the constitutional "givens" (that is, the behaviors with which the infant comes equipped at birth as a gift of the species and of the fetal environment) and the environmental inputs accorded to or imposed upon the baby from the earliest moments of life (Lipsitt and Werner, 1981).

A great deal of new data from the field of pediatric psychology or behavioral pediatrics indicates that some cognitive deficiencies, representing early signs of developmental disability, are already apparent in the first few days of life. Hazardous events surrounding birth, such as oxygen deficiency, hyperbilirubinemia, or maternal anemia can in some instances have lasting influences upon the infant enduring these stresses (Field, 1979). From actuarial and clinical studies (Drillien, 1964; Sameroff and Chandler, 1975), it is apparent that infants born prematurely, who are small and require oxygen at birth, or who are either hypertonic or hypotonic, do less well during the first year of life and in later years, behaviorally as well as physically. Some perinatal risk factors produce their greatest debilitating effects upon the sensory systems and on central nervous system functioning, with the consequence that behavioral insufficiencies in general, and learning disorders particularly, are not uncommon in high-risk infants.

Summarizing extensive data on the relationship between early behavioral characteristics of the infant and later competencies, Appleton, Clifton, and Goldberg (1975) concluded explicitly that early manifestations of sensory and behavioral incompetence do cause later sensory motor and intellectual deficiencies: "... the competence of the older child in manipulating and comprehending the environment is probably based on interactions with the environment which are dependent upon processing sensory information. Through development of perceptual and sensory motor abilities the infant can learn about his or her surroundings and can develop a practical understanding of reality. Early learning of skills and expectations appears to contribute to further learning and development" (p. 104). For example, poor habituation during the neonatal period is suggestive of later developmental lag, and absence of habituation is now seen as a concomitant of cognitive deficiencies (Lewis, Goldberg and Campbell, 1969).

APPROACH-AVOIDANCE, AND THE HEDONIC BASIS OF BEHAVIOR DEVELOPMENT

It will be apparent to any sophisticated observer of the psychobiological character of infancy that much of early behavior is based upon positive and negative reactions *(taxes)* to stimuli of different types and of varying degrees of attractiveness and repellency. These initial approach and avoidant responses, congenitally given behavioral patterns, are the stuff of which the acquisition of positive and negative cathexes are made. It is through simple association of a neutral stimulus with a strong positive or negative reaction that learned behavior arises. The smell, for example, accompanying the coveted feeding opportunity in the presence of hunger will soon become cathected for itself by the infant. By the same token (but on the other side of the coin), a strong but essentially neutral stimulus, such as a red light, will produce an eye blink if it is paired sufficiently often and judiciously with an air puff to the eyelid, which causes lid closure in even very immature babies. It works for both classical and operant learning, and it has become apparent in recent times that most naturalistic learning situations probably involve both kinds of process.

There does not seem to be any question that the hedonic features of stimulating conditions are rather like stimulus imperatives in these situations. The more pleasurable the feeding situation, the greater will be the effect of contextual cues. The greater the emotional aversion involved in any negatively tainted experience, the more likely will the surrounding stimulation take on aversive pro-

perties. The infant is "prewired", as it were, to respond with approach and avoidance responses to promote survival (for example, to gain sustenance in the presence of hunger, or to flee in the presence of tissue damage), but these basic neurologically mediated adaptive behaviors are primed and embellished by hedonic overtones. It is of no mere passing interest that the hedonic backdrops for these response processes are the rudiments, in humans, of aesthetics, of narcissistic investments, and of the "social graces".

Aversive or avoidance behavior can be noted, then, in the first few days of life. Observers are generally more fascinated, of course, with the positive hedonic patterns of behavior than with the negative or "angry" responses of the baby, as in crying. Crying and other "mad" behaviors are nonetheless very compelling, often including emission of a very noxious auditory stimulus reaching the intensity of 100 decibels. Such behavior has been known to drive parents, for want of a better expression, "to distraction", which means that it elicits a very unfavorable, usually angry, and often retributively hurtful behavior in exchange. Regardless, adults who find themselves in the presence of intensively negative hedonic responses of the infant are urged thereby to turn the behavior off, i. e., supply the appropriate contingencies that will suppress, diminish, or obliterate the objectionable behavior. The successfully appropriated response on the part of the infant's caretaker will become reinforced. Diminution of the infant's behavior will reinforce the parent, who will be more likely to utilize this tactic in the future when the same conditions present themselves again. Thus the parent or other caretaking person presents the infant with some satisfying state of affairs which is effective in altering the behavior, and the altered behavior serves as a rewarding event for the successful caretaker. This is reciprocating interaction at its best, following all of the sound principles of conditioning in naturalistic situations.

The "angry" responses of babies have considerable adaptive significance, and are probably effective on frequent occasions in removing potentially life-threatening stimulation. The English pediatrician, Mavis Gunther, suggested two decades ago, before such interpretations were at all popular (Gunther, 1961) that the "feeding couple" (as she called the mother-neonate pair) can affect one another in subtle ways that have to be clearly understood in order to help both overcome the tensions of their earliest minutes and weeks together. She said that it is quite natural for the newborn to become, at least for brief moments, smothered during the course of feeding. Of course, she was not talking about a lethal condition of hypoxia, or even sustained respiratory occlusion. She was referring to an essentially behavioral interaction between the mother and infant. In newborns, the nostrils come very close to the mother's breast, and breathing is sometimes compromised appreciably while the infant has a tight latch on the nipple. This causes brief difficulty in breathing which the infant, in turn, will resist. The normal newborn turns his head to and fro and pulls back from the nipple, when this circumstance arises. As in a fixed action pattern, the arms will next flail, the face will then redden, and the arms will come to the mouth and nose as if to fight the offending object away. As a last resort if the blockage continues, there will occur a burst of crying, which throws the nipple from the baby's mouth abruptly. Mothers are often offended by this eventuality, becoming quite exasperated after a few occasions, and will report that they consider themselves failures in coping with their newborn's needs and frustrations (Gunther, 1961; Newton, 1955). From extensive observations of newborns with their mothers, Gunther provides a few simple suggestions to mothers to help them adjust themselves posturally or to insert the nipple in a more felicitous manner, in order to prevent occlusion from occurring.

It should be noted that actual respiratory occlusion is not essential for the response pattern just described to occur. The infant's facial network, particularly the neuromusculature in the perioral area, seems particularly sensitized even to the *threat* of respiratory occlusion, and thus the awkward and angry resistance which normal newborns manifest to stimulation approximating occlusion can be effective in generating the aversive behavior described. Many casual observers of newborns, as well as those with theoretical investments in noting that acceptant behaviors often look like avoidant responses (e. g., Spitz and Wolf, 1946) have been aware that often when infants are rooting (that is, moving their mouths quickly in the direction of a tactile stimulus near the mouth), first to one side, then the other, they frequently look as if they are engaging in negatively hedonic behavior. Their side to side head waving looks very much like a "no-no" response, until they center on, strike at, and latch upon the nipple; it is easy to suppose that the simultaneous elicitation of the approach and avoidance components of this maneuver constitute the rudiments of ambivalent behavior (Lipsitt, 1976). In fact, even a bottle-fed newborn sometimes manifests the behavior described, for it is not unusual for the nipple shield to come against the baby's

nostrils while feeding, especially when the commercial nipple is short and stubby. In addition, the neonate's lips are fatty, and the nostrils close to the upper lip. This tends to assure some respiratory blockage during feeding. When actual respiratory occlusion occurs, or when there is the threat, of it, newborns will often execute the described pattern of behavior, ending in a release from the nipple, taking in oxygen, and thereby regaining physical and behavioral stability. This is what psychologists call a high-incentive, or reinforcing, consequence of behavior. Uncoupling from the breast is thereby rewarded, and thus the next time the infant is put to the breast this position will be found by the baby to be less desirable than previously. That is the way learning goes. The negative consequences of contact with the breast override the initially positive features.

As Gunther (1961) has indicated, simple instructions to the mother, by special caretaking personnel concerned with the necessity of helping the infant cope in the first few days of life, can frequently effect rapid changes in the mother's behavior in relation to her infant. This information comes from clinical observation rather than systematic research. There have been, in fact, too few studies providing information about the critical transactional moments between mother and infant in the first few days of life, and about the possibly enduring effects of these early critical experiences. Currently available information does suggest that mother and infant are powerfully important to one another in conditioning subsequent interactions (Korner, 1974).

CRITICAL CONDITIONS OF INFANCY: A PSYCHOLOGICAL PERSPECTIVE AND AN EXAMPLE

The sudden infant death syndrome (SIDS) is responsible for about 8,000 deaths of babies in America each year in the first year of life, excluding the especially hazardous first few days of life. While there is some variation from one country to another, depending in part upon the adequacy of prenatal and early developmental care, on socio-economic circumstances, and on methods of reporting causes of death, there is reason to believe that the real incidence of "death without apparent cause" following expert autopsy is approximately two per 1,000 births. Grief and despair in the thousands of close survivors compound the tragedy of crib death immeasurably. Crib death is especially difficult for parents to accept, because of the absence of definitive answers regarding the basic mechanisms in the final pathway to death. Until recent times, in which confusions about the causes of deaths in infants have abounded, "uncaused" or inexplicable deaths in babies were quite normative. With the gradual diminution of death by obscure diseases, however, the spotlight has been directed, rather by exclusion, to the residual deaths "from no known cause". The historical neglect of research attention to this type of infant death, and the very frequent confusion of SIDS with child abuse, have only recently abated. The fact is that we need to know much more about the precursors of crib death, actuarially, epidemiologically, and in terms of the pathways or processes leading to the demise of such infants.

Two decades ago, there was no thought at all about the behavioral and psychophysiological implications of the crib death syndrome. One of the major tasks of modern behavioral pediatrics is to understand better the psychobiological features of infantile dysfunctions which may play critical roles in the eventual destinies of these infants, perhaps even to the point of disposing the infant to lethal conditions of jeopardy.

Psychophysiological factors might well be involved in the final pathway to the condition that ultimately causes certain infants to succumb between the ages of two and four months. The possibility must be considered that experience, and the subsequent effects that prior experience may have on the infant, are factors in creating the ultimate condition of jeopardy which results in the SIDS baby's demise. A study by Lipsitt, Sturner and Burke (1979) examined the perinatal and pediatric records of 15 crib death cases, all of those which occurred in the context of the National Collaborative Perinatal Project as carried out at Brown University in Providence, Rhode Island. Two control groups were composed, one of these consisting of the next birth into that study of the same sex, and the second control group consisting of the next birth into that study of the same sex and race. It was found that the deceased group of 15 SIDS cases varied from the two control groups in a number of ways, all in a direction suggesting the occurrence of greater perinatal distress and psychobiological hazard in the deceased infants. Reliable differences occurred in Apgar scores, for example, in the first few minutes of life. When it is appreciated that these Apgar scores were registered by specially trained personnel in the delivery room before the life-outcomes of these infants could possibly be predicted, it is remarkable that there should have occurred large differences between the target SIDS infants, on the one hand, and the two control groups on the other. The data indicate clearly that there

was a real difference in vital signs between the to-be-SIDS infants and the infants who were not to become eventual victims of this mysterious syndrome. Diminished Apgar scores in the deceased group indicate that these infants had inadequacies of respiration and heart rate, poor pallor and muscle tone, and were regarded by delivery-room personnel as "in trouble". As it turned out, many other signs pointed toward developmental risks of various sorts. Infants in the deceased group significantly more often were identified as having respiratory abnormalities during the neonatal period. More of the deceased group had mothers with anemia, and required intensive care than the controls. Infants who eventually succumbed to SIDS had been hospitalized longer as newborns, and required more resuscitative measures. We need to know about the fragility of these infants who subsequently succumbed, and about the developmental processes that apparently transform seemingly minor deficits into morbid crises just a few weeks later.

A suggestion worth pursuing is that a basic learning disability is implicated in crib death (Lipsitt, 1976, 1979). This has been based upon the observation that crib deaths have a peak period of occurrence in the range between 2 and 4 months of age, a critical time during development when many basic reflexes are in transition. These responses, like the grasp reflex of the newborn, are strong at birth, begin to weaken soon thereafter, and are often gone by five months of age. Turning the head to a touch near the mouth, grasping at a tactile stimulus in the palm of the hand, and swimming movements when placed in water go through easily observable and fairly quantifiable changes over time. Response progressions in all of these modalities indicate that the behaviors are quite obligatory at the outset and gradually become more deliberative, more "voluntary", as time and experience progress (McGraw, 1943). In McGraw's careful observations of the ontogeny of several reflexes during the first two years of life, she was able to show that the transitional period between reflexive and voluntary phases of these responses usually takes place around the ages of 100 to 150 days, just the age period when infants are most at risk for crib death. McGraw went so far as to call the transitional phase, between the reflexive, obligatory stage and the eventual voluntary and well-controlled stage, the period of "disorganized behavior" or "struggling activity".

It is within the realm of possibility that if the infant's transition does not go smoothly from the condition of basic, congenital, reflexive responding to the more intentional and reflective mode of responding, a condition of jeopardy might arise in

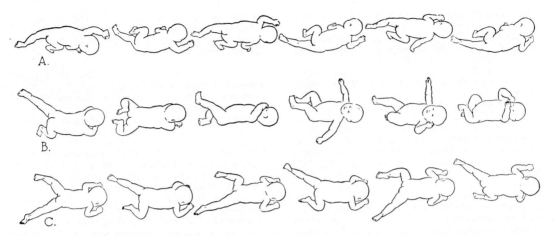

FIG. I-36. — *Typology of aquatic behaviors as identified by* McGraw (1943).

Type A: behavior is reflexive swimming. Type B: is disorganized and ineffective behavior. Type C: behavior is manifest, type B behavior, the so-called disorganized, "confused" behavior replaces the earlier reflexive ("A") behaviors and could place the infant in jeopardy until such time as the learned behaviors are in place.

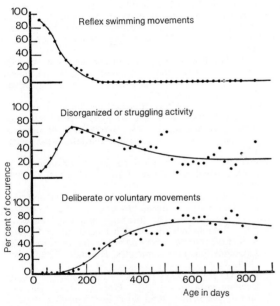

FIG. I-37. — *The incidence of three phases in the aquatic behavior of infants.*

over the first two months or so of life. As can be seen in Figures I-36 and I-37, with respect to aquatic behavior as documented by McGraw (1943), the topology of behavior changes considerably within the first few months of life, and the infant must evolve a mode of response in the second phase (three or four months of age) whereby a deliberative, voluntary, learned, cortically mediated behavior comes to supplant the initially effective sub-cortically mediated behavior characteristic of the newborn.

One concludes on the note, then, that cognition is exceedingly important for the development of normal, thoughtful behavior, and that cognitive and learning processes may in fact be critical for human survival. It may at first seem strange to suppose that a newborn's thought processes may have something to do with whether he or she survives the first year of life. However, when one considers, that most deaths in childhood and adolescence are attributable to experiential circumstances, e. g., non-caring accidents, suicide, and homicide, it is not so wild a dream to suppose that psychobiological factors are important to the survival of newborns and older children (Richmond, 1979).

which the infant will not be able to adequately defend against threats to respiration. There are numerous naturalistic circumstances in which such threats arise, and adults are well-prepared, through throat-clearing mechanisms, coughing, head-turning, and so on, to unocclude the respiratory passages when blocked. Neonates seem relatively well equipped at birth to deal with respiratory threats, with responses well-designed to facilitate survival

REFERENCES

ALDRICH (C. A.). — A new test for hearing in the newborn: The conditioned reflex. *Amer. J. Dis. Child.*, 35, 36-37, 1928.
APPLETON (T.), CLIFTON (R. K.), GOLDBERG (S.). — The development of behavioral competence in infancy. In F. D. HOROWITZ (Ed.), *Review of child development*

research (Vol. 4). University of Chicago Press, Chicago, 1975.

BRACKBILL (Y.). — The role of the cortex in orienting: Orienting reflex in an enencephalic human infant. *Develop. Psychol.*, *5*, 195-201, 1971.

BRAZELTON (T. B.). — *Neonatal behavioral assessment scale*. William Heinemann Medical Books, Philadelphia, 1973.

BRONSHTEIN (A. T.), ANTONOVA (T. G.), KAMENET-SKAYA (N. H.), LUPPOVA (V. A.), SYTOVA (V. A.). — On the development of the functions of analyzers in infants and some animals at the early stage of ontogenesis. In *Problems of evolution of physiological functions*. USSR, Academy of Science, 1958. US Department of HEW, Translation Service, 1960.

CARMICHAEL (L.). — *Manual of child psychology*. Wiley, New York, 1946.

CLIFTON (R. K.), NELSON (M. N.). — Developmental study of habituation in infants: The importance of paradigm, response system, and state. In T. J. TIGHE and R. N. LEATON (Eds.), *Habituation*. Lawrence Erlbaum Associates, Hillsdale, N. J., 1976.

COWETT (R. M.), LIPSITT (L. P.), VOHR (B.), OH (W.). — Aberrations of sucking behavior in low-birth-weight infants. *Develop. Med. Child Neurol.*, *20*, 701-709, 1978.

DOBBING (J.). — Human brain development and its vulnerability. *Mead Johnson symposium on perinatal and developmental medicine: Biological and clinical aspects of brain development*, No. 6, 1974.

DRILLIEN (C. M.). — *The growth and development of the prematurely born infant*. Williams and Wilkins, Baltimore, 1964.

ENGEN (T.), LIPSITT (L. P.). — Decrement and recovery of response to olfactory stimuli in the human neonate. *J. Comparat. Physiol. Psychol.*, *59*, 312-316, 1965.

ENGEN (T.), LIPSITT (L. P.), KAYE (H.). — Olfactory responses and adaptation in the human neonate. *J. Comparat. Physiol. Psychol.*, *56*, 73-77, 1963.

FANTZ (R.). — The origin of form perception. *Scient. Amer.*, *204*, 66-72, 1961.

FANTZ (R.). — Visual experiences in infants: Decreased attention to familiar patterns relative to novel ones. *Science*, *146*, 668-670, 1964.

FIELD (T. M.), GOLDBERG (S.), STERN (D.), SOS-TEK (A. M.). — *High-risk infants and children: Adult and peer interactions*. Academic Press, New York, 1980.

FIELD (T. M.), SOSTEK (A. M.), GOLDBERG (S.), SHU-MAN (H. H.). — *Infants born at risk: Behavior and development*. Spectrum, New York, 1979.

FRIEDMAN (S. L.), SIGMAN (M.). — *Preterm births and psychological development*. Academic Press, New York, 1980.

FRIEDMAN (S.), NAGY (A. N.), CARPENTER (G. C.). — Newborn attention: differential response decrement to visual stimuli. *J. Experim. Child Psychol.*, *10*, 44-51, 1970.

GLOBUS (A.), SCHEIBEL (A. B.). — The effect of visual deprivation cortical neurons: A Golgi study. *Experiment. Neurol.*, *19*, 331-345, 1967.

GUNTHER (M.). — Infant behaviour at the breast. In B. Foss (Ed.), *Determinants of infant behavior*. Methuen, London, 1961.

HUBEL (D. H.), WIESEL (T. N.). — The period of susceptibility to the physiological effects of unilateral eye closure in kittens. *J. Physiol.*, *206*, 419-436, 1970.

JEFFREY (W. E.). — *The developing brain and child development*. In M. C. WITTROCK (Ed.), The brain and psychology. Academic Press, New York, 1980.

JEFFREY (W. E.), COHEN (L. B.). — Habituation in the human infant. In H. W. REESE (Ed.), *Advances in child development and behavior* (Vol. 6). Academic Press, New York, 1971.

JOHANSON (I. B.), HALL (W. G.). — Appetitive learning in 1-day old rat pups. *Science*, *205*, 419-421, 1979.

KAGAN (J.), KEARSLEY (R. B.), ZELAZO (P. R.). — *Infancy: Its place in human development*. Harvard University Press, Cambridge, Mass., 1978.

KEARSLEY (R. B.), SIGEL (I. E.). — *Infants at risk: Assessment of cognitive functioning*. Lawrence Erlbaum Associates Hillsdale, New Jersey, 1979.

KESSEN (W.), HAITH (M. M.), SALAPATEK (P. H.). — *Human infancy: A bibliography and guide*. In P. H. MUSSEN (Ed.), Carmichael's Manual of Child Psychology. Vol. 1, Wiley, New York, 1970.

KLAUS (M. H.), KENNELL (J. H.). — *Maternal-infant bonding*. Mosby, St. Louis, 1976.

KORNER (A.). — The effect of the infant's state, level of arousal, sex, and ontogenic stage on the caregiver. In M. Lewis and L. ROSENBLUM (Eds.), *The effect of the infant on its caregiver*. Wiley, New York, 1974.

LEWIS (M.), GOLDBERG (S.), CAMPBELL (H.). — A developmental study of information processing within the first three years of life: Response decrement to a redundant signal. *Monogr. Soc. Res. Child Develop.*, *34* (Whole No. 133), 1969.

LEWIS (M.). — The meaning of a response, or why researchers in infant behavior should be oriental metaphysicians. *Merrill-Palmer Quarterly*, *13*, 7-18, 1967.

LIPSITT (L. P.). — Learning in the first year of life. In L. P. LIPSITT and C. C. SPIKER (Eds.), *Advances in child development and behavior*, Vol. 1. Academic Press, New York, 1963.

LIPSITT (L. P.). — Developmental psychobiology comes of age: A discussion. In L. P. LIPSITT (Ed.), *Developmental psychobiology: The significance of infancy*. Lawrence Erlbaum Associates, Hillsdale, New Jersey, 1976.

LIPSITT (L. P.). — Critical conditions of infancy: A psychological perspective. *Amer. Psychol.*, *34*, 973-980, 1979.

LIPSITT (L. P.). — Infants at risk: perinatal and risk factors. *Intern. J. Behav. Develop.*, *2*, 23-42, 1979 a.

LIPSITT (L. P.). — The pleasures and annoyances of infants: Approach and avoidance behavior. In E. THO-MAN (Ed.), *Origins of the infant's social responsiveness* Lawrence Erlbaum Associates, Hillsdale, New Jersey 1979.

LIPSITT (L. P.), WERNER (J. S.). — The infancy of human learning processes. In E. GOLLIN (Ed.), *Developmental plasticity: Behavioral and biological aspects of variations in development*. Academic Press, New York 1981.

LIPSITT (L. P.), REILLY (B. M.), BUTCHER (M. J.), GREEN-WOOD (M. M.). — The stability and interrelationships of newborn sucking and heart rate. *Develop. Psychobiol.*, *9*, 305-310, 1976.

McGRAW (M. B.). — *The neuromuscular maturation of the human infant*. Columbia University Press, New York, 1943.

McGUINESS (D.), PRIBRAM (K.). — The neuropsychology of attention: Emotional and motivational controls. In M. C. WITTROCK (Ed.), *The brain and psychology*. Academic Press, New York, 1980.

MURCHISON (C.). — *A handbook of child psychology* (2nd edition, revised), Clark University Press, Worcester, Mass., 1933.

NEWTON (N.). — *Maternal emotions.* Part B. Hoeber, New York, 1955.

OSOFSKY (J.). — *Handbook of infant development.* Wiley, New York, 1979.

PAPOUSEK (H.). — Conditioning during early postnatal development. In Y. BRACKBILL and G. G. THOMPSON (Eds.), *Behavior in infancy and early childhood.* Free Press, New York, 1967.

PEIPER (A.). — *Cerebral function in infancy and childhood* (first edition, in German, 1949), Consultants Bureau, New York, 1963.

PRATT (K. C.). — The neonate. In L. CARMICHAEL (Ed.), *Manual of Child Psychology,* 1954.

PRIBRAM (K. H.). — *Languages of the brain.* Prentice-Hall, Englewood Cliffs, New Jersey, 1971.

PURPURA (D. P.). — Neuronal migration and dendritic differentiation: Normal and aberrant development of human cerebral cortex. In *Mead Johnson Symposium on Perinatal and Developmental Medicine,* No. 6, December 8-11, 1974.

RICHMOND (J. B.). — *Healthy people: The Surgeon General's Report on health promotion and disease prevention.* U. S. Dept. of HEW, DHWE (PHS) Publication No. 79-55071, Washington, D. C., 1979.

ROSENZWEIG (M. R.), BENNETT (E. L.). — *Neural mechanisms of learning and memory.* MIT Press, Cambridge, Mass., 1976.

ROVEE-COLLIER (C. K.), LIPSITT (L. P.). — Learning, adaptation, and memory in the newborn. In P. STRATTON (Ed.), *Psychobiology of the human newborn,* Wiley, New York, 1982.

SAMEROFF (A. J.), CHANDLER (M. J.). — Reproductive risk and the continuum of caretaking casualty. In F. D. HOROWITZ (Ed.), *Review of child development research,* Vol. 4. University of Chicago Press, 1975.

SCHAPIRO (S.), VUKOVICH (K. R.). — Early experience effects upon cortical dendrites; A proposal model for development. *Science, 167,* 292-294, 1970.

SCHULMAN-GALAMBOS (C.), GALAMBOS (R.). — Assessment of hearing. In T. M. FIELD, A. M. SOSTEK, S. GOLDBERG, H. H. SCHUMAN (Eds.), *Infants born at risk: Behavior and development.* Spectrum Publications, New York, 1979.

SCHAFFER (D.), DUNN (J.). — *The first year of life: Psychological and medical implications of early experience.* Wiley, New York, 1979.

SIQUELAND (E. R.), LIPSITT (L. P.). — Conditioned head-turning in human newborns. *J. Experim. Child Psychol., 3,* 356-376, 1966.

SMERIGLIO (V.). — *Newborns and parents: Parent-infant contact and newborn sensory stimulation.* Lawrence Erlbaum Associates, Hillsdale, New Jersey, 1981.

THOMAN (E.). — *Origins of the infant's social responsiveness.* Hillsdale, Erlbaum, New Jersey, 1979.

THOMPSON (R. F.), BERGER (T. W.), BERRY (S. D.). — An introduction to the anatomy, physiology, and chemistry of the brain. In M. C. WITTROCK (Ed.), *The brain and psychology.* Academic Press, New York, 1980.

TIGHE (R. J.), LEATON (R. N.) (Eds.). — *Habituation.* Lawrence Erlbaum Associates, Hillsdale, New Jersey, 1976.

TINBERGEN (N.). — *The study of instinct.* Oxford University Press, Oxford, 1951.

WERNER (J. S.), LIPSITT (L. P.). — The infancy of sensory processes. In E. GOLLIN (Ed.), *Developmental plasticity: Behavioral and biological aspects of variations in development.* Academic Press, New York, 1981.

WINICK (M.), ROSSO (P.). — Malnutrition and central nervous system development. In J. W. PRESCOTT, M. S. READ, D. B. COURSIN (Eds.), *Brain function and malnutrition.* Wiley, New York, 1975.

WITTROCK (M. C.). — Learning and the brain. In M. C. WITTROCK (Ed.), *The brain and psychology.* Academic Press, New York, 1980.

WOLFF (P. H.). — What we must and must not teach our young children from what we know about early cognitive development. In *Planning for better learning.* Spastics International Medical Publications, William Heinemann Medical Books, London, 1969.

WYERS (E. J.), PEEKE (H. V. S.), HERZ (M. J.). — Behavioral habituation in invertebrates. In H. V. S. PEEKE and M. J. HERZ (Eds.), *Habituation.* Academic Press, New York, 1973.

4

The parents
of sick newborn infants

R. LAGERCRANTZ and J. LIND †

The pregnancy,
a period of change and strain

The circumstances regarding pregnancy and early parenthood have changed in many respects during the last half-century. Most parents today have their children during the years in which they are completing their education or beginning their first jobs. The double work that this implies, especially for the woman, can be a difficult burden to bear and a hindrance to the establishment of a good parent-child relationship.

In today's time of recession there are many young parents who are unemployed, and they must also deal with the problems which that entails.

Many young parents have just recently moved away from their home environs and have become isolated in impersonal suburbs. They therefore lack support and stimulation from their relatives and friends who have children.

In many industrialized countries, a woman today has only one or two children. Both hers and the father's experience with pregnancy, childbirth, and parenthood is therefore limited, while at the same time it becomes increasingly important that the newborn child be nice and healthy.

In spite of contraception and free-abortion laws in many countries, there are still children born who are undesired or unaccepted. The ambivalence and guilt feelings which are the lot of many parents increase if the child is sick or deformed.

Under these circumstances, pregnancy, childbirth, and early parenthood imply a big adjustment in the life of the woman and the man. Many experience this period in life as a time of great happiness. They are able to muster up the energy and strength necessary for solving any problems and conflicts that may arise. They can acquire mental strength from each other and from their environment. They invest feelings and thoughts in the coming baby, prepare themselves for the birth and for parenthood, and are ready to satisfy the needs of the child.

Other parents are reticent about their feelings and experiences. They seem to experience the pregnancy, birth, and early parenthood less intensively, and their physical and mental balance is disturbed only very slightly. Some conceal the problems and conflicts which arise when the baby is born.

For a third group of parents even the "standard" crisis becomes traumatic. The changes in their physical, emotional, and social circumstances evoke an anguish to which they don't always manage to adapt. These men and women often have poor

† Professor John Lind died in Stockholm on January 7, 1983. This chapter which he co-authored represents his last published work in a career which spanned such studies as those of his classic ones on the perinatal circulation. His work is one of the foundations of modern neonatal medicine. His interests were multiple and varied and included cardio-pulmonary physiology neonatal adaptation, crying behaviour and neonatal responses to music. His interest in psycho-social adaptation and neonatal behaviour is reflected in this chapter. Above all he was an individual of goodwill, wisdom and charity.

R. L.

relationships with their own parents (especially the mother). Their psychosomatic health both before and after the pregnancy has often been unsatisfactory, with long periods of sick leave in the picture. Their relationship with each other has often been poor and deteriorates during the pregnancy, not uncommonly resulting in separation. They cannot manage to prepare themselves for the childbirth, which contributes to the fact that it is marked not only by pain but by apprehension and anxiety as well.

They find it difficult to draw the attention of doctors and midwives to their needs for help. This is due to the fact that they have difficulty in expressing their thoughts and feelings. They often use imprecise or incorrect words. The background of these women is characterized by one or, most often, several of the following negative conditions:

(1) Unsatisfactory circumstances during childhood, especially in regard to the relationship to one's mother [13].

(2) Age < 18 and > 38 years.

(3) Disharmonious relationship to the child's father or a single parent.

(4) Unplanned *and* undesired pregnancy, often with the experience of shock upon being informed of her pregnancy.

(5) Poor mental health with anxiety, obsessions, abnormal fatigue, and other psychosomatic symptoms during pregnancy, as well as insufficient preparation for childbirth and motherhood [10].

(6) Previous child that was sick, deformed, or had died.

(7) Fertility problem: prolonged unintentional childlessness.

(8) Somatic complication, e. g. Rh-immunization, diabetes, etc.

The handicaps which have been described in points 1-8 exist in all social classes. If in addition the woman has social problems (is single, has a low-paying occupation, inadequate housing conditions, etc.) the risk for a troubled motherchild relationship is increased [10, 13]. This series of reasons often produces a painful and shocking, agonizing childbirth experience. Such a delivery serves to further aggravate the woman's adjustment to the child, as well as her ability to care for, comfort, and stimulate it.

These parents—in need of psychosocial help (we prefer to use this term rather than "psychosocial risk families") often have premature, deformed, or sick children. It is easier for the neonatologist to help them if he is familiar with their background and psychosocial situation. Many doctors (and nurses) hesitate to touch upon these subjects, as

they are afraid of arousing tears and lamentation. Nevertheless, grief, guilt feelings, ambivalence, and anger ought to be expressed. If the personnel can deal with these emotions tactfully, the parents can find solace. In this way they are thus able to achieve a more realistic confrontation with their problems.

Preparation for birth and parenthood

Psychologists as well as psychiatrists are now convinced that the foundations for the individual's confidence—or lack of confidence, as the case may be—are laid during the very first years of life, the years which most children spend in their homes. If the parents are incapable of taking proper care of their children during these years, then no measures taken by society at a later time can be of significant help. It becomes somewhat like mixing in the yeast when the bread is already baked. It is particularly the changes within western society, quite contrary to what one might believe, that have, in certain respects, impaired the possibilities of the infant to have its needs met with proper care.

Education for tomorrow's youth

As early as during the compulsory school years, children, who are the parents of tomorrow, need instruction that will give them a basic knowledge of the family and of children.

They must be taught and have the opportunity to discuss and to think through what it means to live in a family, what babies really are, how they develop, what they require, and what it means to have children.

In all industrialized countries today, schooling for young people is being lengthened, good foundations are being laid for career education and general knowledge within certain sectors is increasing rapidly.

But professional life is, of course, only one component of our existence. Most people find a partner with whom to live together, and most want to have and do have children. Nevertheless, most young people complete the compulsory school years without having received any instruction to speak of concerning that large part of life that is lived within the family.

It is said that one learns not for school but for life, and that is of course correct, that is how it should be. The life that school has taught for up until now is to a large extent the life of education, the life of career.

Now it is time to also educate for the family life. Teaching must be improved in regards to, among other things, explaining how one *avoids* building a family before one wants to do so.

Many pregnancies are unexpected and unwelcome. According to a Swedish investigation only 50 % of those questioned had planned their children, and six months after the child's birth roughly 20 % still considered parenthood as a more or less serious handicap. Substantially improved sexual education and more effective advice about contraception could probably prevent a great many of the undesired pregnancies.

Courses for parents during pregnancy

During pregnancy all parents-to-be need help and support in several areas. "Parent", here, is intended to mean fathers as well.

Once and for all we must get away from the point of view that it is the woman who gives the man a child, and that it is she who continues to be the one who automatically takes care of the child, while he, more or less, stands alongside and watches. All concerned lose out on this point of view. The woman alone takes on all work and responsibility for the child, the man becomes excluded from all dealings with the child, and the child develops an insufficient contact with the father—something which has been shown to be potentially ill-fated, especially when this concerns boys.

Instead, we ought to strive to establish as early as possible a feeling of shared responsibility and participation in all that concerns the expected baby.

When a woman becomes pregnant she generally goes alone to the doctor and, later, to check-ups with the doctor or midwife. The expectant father ought to be present at such visits. He, too, needs to hear the instructions which the mother gets, and the progression of the pregnancy concerns, of course, him to a great extent.

All expectant parents ought to attend courses during the pregnancy in order to increase their knowledge about the development of the unborn child the course of events in the actual pregnancy and birth, and elementary child care. In this way, the various stages of pregnancy become less mysterious. The delivery becomes not a frightening prospect of the future, but one is instead able to

look forward to the birth of the baby whose development one has followed, and the foundations are laid for at least some theoretical knowledge in child care.

Childbirth must not be looked upon as something that the woman is going to eventually undergo, but rather as work that must be carried out and for which one can prepare oneself, both man and woman. Pre-natal exercises, relaxation training, and above all the more fundamental preparation which psycho-prophylaxis offers, have been shown to be an effective help towards the work which the birth process represents. Both partners ought to have the opportunity to visit the maternity ward during the pregnancy so that one knows where one will be headed when the important day arrives, and so that one doesn't feel at the time as though one were on a visit in some foreign country.

The expectant father's participation in labor, delivery, and care of the newborn

We know less about how the father experiences pregnancy, childbirth, and early parenthood. For him, too, this can be a time marked by worry, anxiety, and uncertainty. In a close investigation of 64 men who were expecting their first child, it was found that pregnancy and early parenthood were often problematic for them as well [11].

Sixty-five per cent had symptoms during the pregnancy which were similar to the woman's pregnancy difficulties: fatigue, nausea, headache, vomiting, and back pains. Many worked overtime, ate and drank more and had more accidents than usual. The man's ability to support and help the mother is related to his constitution, the circumstances of his own childhood and youth, his mental, physical, and social health, and his attitude towards the mother and to the pregnancy. He can feel excluded from the biological symbiosis between mother and baby.

He can find it difficult to feel warmth towards the newborn and may react by escape to his work, urgent demands for sexuality, or infidelity. The father-child relationship is improved if the father and mother together prepare for birth and parenthood in a course during the pregnancy, if the father is present at the birth and participates from the very beginning in the care of the baby.

A properly prepared and instructed father who is well-guided can contribute on the maternity ward by

— making the delivery calmer by being with the

mother and helping her to avoid any feelings of panic,

— sharing the experience of the birth with her, and by seeing what she undergoes, better understand her sensitivity and need for help later on,

— talking over the birth experience with her afterwards and by generally acting as her conversational partner in discussions of all that happens to her and the baby on the maternity ward,

— giving her a sense, even in the most primary stages, that they will both make decisions about the child and will share the responsibility,

— having this experience and in this way feeling an increased significance in his own role.

In other words: a more reasonable and just division of roles, and a more reasonable and just meaning for these roles for both of the new parents.

The birth of the family

It is the custom in many countries to announce the birth of a baby in the newspapers. A son has been born, one reads, or a daughter. On the other, one never sees a notice announcing that *a family has been born*. And yet it is actually just that which happens when a couple has their first child [9].

On the maternity ward, too, interest is centered around the birth of the *child*. It doesn't come as naturally to think about the *newborn family* as being just as delicate, and with just the same need for care and concern in order to be able to begin functioning. Nevertheless we believe that it is of the very greatest significance for all of the individual members of the family to be able to begin to live as a family from the very outset, and that the interaction begins as smoothly as possible.

The climate of hospital care and co-operation

The atmosphere on the ward ought to be democratic and kindly optimistic but not overly-brisk. The parents should be encouraged to take initiative, to question and—as much as possible—to take part in caring for the newborn. Passivity and babying must be prevented. The neonatologist is warned against being authoritarian or brusque. He should inform the parents in several interviews, and not be afraid of silent pauses (He often thinks that he speaks less than he does). Leading questions should be omitted. If personal questions are brought up he should be ready to give support and explanations. *It is desirable that the neonatologist should be guided by an experienced psychologist or psychiatrist.*

Parents should also have another contact in the ward, preferably the child's nurse—experienced in life and in her profession. It is very important that these persons can give continuous support, help, and information.

In order to promote this atmosphere and improve the mental hygiene of the personnel, to help and to support them in conflict situations, group discussions should be held regularly (see below).

Electronic supervision and medical monitoring of childbirth frightens many women. Some will deliver in their own home. Most neonatologists are opposed to this.

They feel that one must have the resources of the hospital in order to deal with any unexpected complications. They want to stand up to the criticism of technology in hospital care with better information and by attempting to activate the parents. Some important measures to improve the psychological climate are:

(1) If the mother is capable and so desires, she should have the baby close immediately following the birth. The baby should be naked but careful measures should be taken so that it doesn't become chilled for any length of time. The child often sucks hard at the nipple. Occasionally it has its eyes open and can look into the eyes of the parents, something which they experience with great joy. It is appropriate that the new family be alone for a while—it can be an important part in the intensive experience of this period. If the mother is exhausted or in shock after the delivery, she must have the chance to recover before she can manage to see the baby.

(2) The Credé prophylaxis should be postponed an hour or so, accordingly.

(3) The father, who has helped the mother during the delivery, should also have the chance to hold the baby in his arms, as well as to bathe it and care for the umbilical cord, if he so desires.

(4) On the wards there should be rooming-in, if possible (with single and possibly double rooms) even at night. The parents should be encouraged to attend to the baby as much as they feel capable. They should, at the same time, have access to the help of the nurses on the ward. Breastfeeding should take place in accordance with the needs of the baby, which can mean every hour or every other hour. It is important that the baby gets a proper grip around the areola, otherwise small cracks can easily appear. Supplements of breast milk or substitutes for mother's milk should only be given on the strictest indications as these can jeopardize the breastfeeding. Test weighing should not be recommended.

(5) Mothers ought to remain on the ward for rest and instruction for 5-6 days as a rule. Those women for whom it is not the first birth, who have sufficient help at home, and who would like to go home earlier should of course be permitted to do so. Nevertheless it ought to be pointed out to them that fatigue, as on those "blue days", is common. In a broad Swedish investigation approximately 20 % of women who had recently given birth were troubled by several and often severe psychic symptoms such as anxiety, insomnia, nightmares, and psychosomatic pain. One must not neglect to point out to the father how common these symptoms are, and how they can be alleviated if the mother gets help, support, and understanding. If the father can help in this way then his own jealousy can also be counteracted. Jealousy is often more or less manifest in the older brothers and sisters and can be dealt with by giving them the opportunity to talk about it and to participate as much as possible in the formation of the new family.

(6) The neonatologist ought to be readily available to parents and personnel. He should be on the ward during a large part of the day and have fixed telephone and visiting hours. Unnecessary waiting arouses irritation and anger in all concerned. It is also desirable that the neonatologist speaks with both parents at the same time so as to prevent misunderstanding and to increase the possibilities that they will support one another. The parents' anxiety and fatigue decreases their ability to understand the information that the doctor provides (example: a 32-year old woman who had given birth for the first time cried over her three-day old, slightly icteric baby and lamented: ordinary I'm a competent bureau secretary in the housing administration. Now I'm just washed out). One should therefore repeat the information about the baby several times and by means of counter-questions check and see that the parents have understood correctly. The parents often get upset over even unimportant changes in the baby's condition and over such trivialities as a blood test. In other words, there is a discrepancy between changes in the baby's condition or treatment and the anxiety of the parents. Often there exist good grounds for trying to prevent the parents from paying too much attention to the laboratory results, the significance of which they are not able to evaluate.

The needs of the sick newborn

"The mother's inner reality becomes the child's outer", a wise child psychologist (Anna Freud) has said. Everything that can be done so that the parents will feel well and less worried will be to the benefit of the child both now and in the future.

New investigations have shown that newborn babies react to speech, music, caresses, and other sensory impressions. They need to be tended with closeness and tenderness. The time immediately following the birth is important for the foundation of the mother-child (as well as father-child) relationship (bonding). The premature or sick newborn often misses out on the initial close contact with the mother. The disadvantages with this can, most likely, be completely or partially compensated for later, as the human being has a great ability to adapt. Nevertheless, one ought to try to also satisfy the sick infant's need for contact, fondling, and other sensory impressions. The parents and personnel should touch and fondle the baby in the incubator, and should talk with it when it is awake and responsive. Washings should be done slowly and with gentle movements. As soon as the child can suck it should be given the chance to do so, taken up into the mother's arms and breastfed. Tranquil music and singing seem to have a pleasing effect.

On some wards the newborn is given more food than its appetite demands. The motive here may be that one wants to convince oneself that the infant really can eat, or that one wants to prevent symptoms of illness, such as icterus. This leads to immediate risks for vomiting and other gastrointestinal symptoms and, later, for appetite disorders (anorexia or obesity). There ought therefore to exist only strict indications for giving more calories than the infant's appetite demands.

Examples of psychological problems in the neonatal period

A 21-year old woman becomes unplannedly pregnant and breaks her relationship with the father of the child. Delivery is in the 33rd week of pregnancy. The infant contracts IRDS, is treated with CPAP and a respirator, improves relatively quickly, is vital and lively throughout this time.

The mother comes to the ward on the third day. The personnel attempt to give their support and consolation. The mother tells later about how she had been offended by a doctor who was brusque. It is difficult for her to see the baby at first and she will not touch him. Later, she comes every day and gradually begins to want to touch her son. She develops good contact with a baby nurse and another mother who also has a premature baby on the ward. When her milk begins to flow the mother pumps her breasts and comes with her milk to the ward every day. She thinks that it feels right and important.

After the baby is discharged from the hospital the mother is still uneasy but can enjoy the baby. The nurse from the child health center makes several visits, praises the mother and arranges for her to get in touch with other mothers with children of the same age. When the boy is one year old he is lively and happy. The mother feels quite well, plans for a profession.

Commentary. — In this case there are many factors which could have unfavorably influenced mother and child and their relationship. Some of these could be counteracted during the caretaking process: support and help from personnel and mothers in the same situation. The future will tell whether this family can continue to develop well to avoid, among other things, overprotection, and to compensate for social and intellectual disadvantages.

A 25-year old doctor gives birth to her first child two weeks ahead of the expected time. The boy is fine and healthy up until the fourth day of life when pathologic icterus is detected—due most likely to ABO—immunization. The boy is transferred to the infant ward for light-treatment. The mother cries but is told by a doctor that, "it's a good thing we have a children's ward". The mother is very upset, almost inconsolable—no matter how her husband and the personnel try. The mother speaks of the path between the puerperal ward and the children's ward as a "path to Golgotha". The infant is treated for three days on the children's ward. The mother cannot be persuaded to touch him. She nurses but with severe pains and stops breast-feeding quite soon after. When the child comes back to the mother they need a great deal of help and support from the personnel. Despite this the mother is very upset, has attacks of crying and is not capable of tending to the baby without help. For the next half a year the mother is often tired, unhappy and upset.

Commentary. — Somatically a "banal" case history of illness marked by the mother's distress, anxiety and helplessness. The personnel did not realize how great her need for help actually was. She was in need of psychological support or psychotherapy. Brusque retorts should have been avoided and the woman's anxiety recognized. She would have benefitted from contact, help, and support from motherly women in the same situation as herself.

The parents and the premature baby

Periodically, all parents are more or less ambivalent and burdened with guilt feelings toward their children. Especially in crisis situations they need the chance to talk about their feelings and to find out that they are common and normal. This applies especially to parents of premature children. They often have inaccurate and superstitious notions about the cause of the prematurity. The neonatologist

and other personnel can comfort them by listening, informing, and elucidating. Many parents probably need more help than they are presently receiving —this is best provided by the psychologist or social worker.

The separation from the newborn is often prolonged which can be difficult for the parents. This can be compensated for by (1) having the newborn, even if it has been put in an incubator, if possible with the parents until it is transferred to the premature ward. The parents ought to, in any case, be permitted to see the baby before it is taken from them. Furthermore, the parents should be allowed to come to the ward every day and, as soon as possible, get the chance to fondle the baby and take part in caring for it. There are no epidemiological arguments against this; (2) The mother ought to be encouraged to pump out her breast milk and freeze it. Once defrosted it can be given without pasteurization to the baby. This strengthens the bond between mother and child and increases the motivation to breastfeed.

The parents often find help and pleasure in having the opportunity to speak with others in the same situation. This can be done individually or in groups, preferably led by a psychologist or social worker.

Premature children are over-represented in much of the material on child abuse and negligence. The reason is probably the psycho-social strain under which many of the parents of premature children live. These people have more difficulties than other parents in accepting and enjoying their baby. They often feel strong ambivalence and oscillate between irritation and overprotection. If the infant becomes sick and cries inconsolably, maltreatment can be incited. These families need a great deal of psychosocial support and help.

The risk for overprotection of the child should be discussed early. This can be a consequence of the ambivalence and guilt feelings mentioned above. It can decrease if the parents get the chance to discuss their feelings. They gain knowledge from some of the many popular science books on the subject but they need to be able to discuss their contents with experts.

In the intensive care of premature infants it is a matter of combinding a highly technically developed treatment of these babies with direct human forms of interaction between personnel and parents. The baby should have a name from the very beginning and the parents should be helped in every way to see their baby as a little person with sight and all its senses developed, and who therefore reacts positively to the presence of the parents and to stimulation. The parents must be helped to break away from the role of helpless, outside observers and to be actively included by the members of the treatment team. One must nevertheless be aware of the fact that they have special difficulties in identifying the baby as their own and that this first occurs often after the child has been brought home. The long-range effect of the hospital care depends upon the accuracy of the diagnostic data and the therapy which that data suggest, but also to a large extent upon the ability of the personnel to imagine themselves in the parents' complex of problems, as well as the possibilities for individualizing the guidance of the parents. The parents of the smallest premature infants are a vulnerable clientele. It is often very young people who are in question here, with alcohol and narcotic problems not uncommon. Access to psychological or psychiatric consultation is necessary.

The frequency of child abuse has been shown to be disproportionately high in families where the child has been born prematurely and in need of care at a children's hospital [12].

An example of some of the problems in families with premature babies is given below:

A 19-year old primipara delivered a girl, weighing 1,200 g in the 31st gestational week. The child needed resuscitation and was referred to the neonatal ward. She was treated with CPAP and later received phototherapy. She made an uneventful recovery and left the ward after six weeks. She was checked in the outpatient department and the well-baby clinic.

During the first weeks the mother complained that she could not realize that she had gotten a baby. She was very tense and had difficulty to sleep and eat. She visited the girl after two days but hesitated to touch her.

The mother had several supporting talks with the psychologist who tried to strengthen her self-esteem and reduce her guilt feelings. The neonatalogist stressed all positive signs and gave a favorable long-term prognosis. The mother also was supported and taught by a motherly nurse, who had two children of her own.

Gradually the mother became more optimistic and self-confident. During the child's first year of life the mother was often anxious and tended to overprotect, especially when the child had upper respiratory tract infections. She appreciated joining a parent group in the well-baby clinic to discuss mutual problems. She also received more help from the girl's father, who had been passive.

Comments. — Parents of prematures often have difficulties to realize that they have had a baby. They hesitate to visit, touch, and care. They need much help, praise and stimulation to come, to participate, to give the child a name, etc. They need to discuss their anxiety, guilt feelings, and fears. Neonatologist, psychologist, and nurse must collaborate and give continuous support. The parents also benefit from group discussions with other parents of newborns.

The deformed child and its parents

Most of the ideas presented here can also be applied to parents of children with congenital handicaps. In these situations pediatricians—on maternity wards and at child health centers—have a great responsibility that is not always accepted, especially in those cases where it is a matter of helping the parents to decide how the child should be cared for in the future.

The parents ought to be given information about the baby's handicap starting early during the maternity ward stay so that there is time for at least three or four conversations before mother and child leave the hospital. We believe that it is important to have the child present at the first discussion, with both the mother and the father. There are so many drawbacks, so much deprecation in people's view of different handicaps, that it may be necessary for the doctor to merely hold the baby in his arms and show, personally, clearly, that he accepts this baby just like other babies.

It is important that the doctor endeavor to speak a simple language that is easily understood, free of diagnostic and other technical terms. He or she must, in addition, set aside ample time and give the parents the opportunity to ask questions. Time after time one should emphasize the positive, healthy, and vital qualities of the child.

In most cases, it is often not only the fact that the child has a deformity which so distresses the parents, but rather it is also the consideration of what others will think which is frightening. For the parents themselves it can probably seem conceivable to accept the child's deformity and be just as fond of him or her—but what will other people think? It is then that one must remember that the reactions of those around you depend to a large degree upon how you yourself behave. The more relaxed one is oneself, the less embarrassed others feel. This applies in other situations where we confront people with something to which they are not accustomed. The more one explains oneself, the less there is for others to wonder about.

There is no model, after which a conversation of this kind can be conducted. Every discussion must be adapted to those individuals one is speaking with, and one must "feel out" the situation. We wish to take up several points here which we think ought to be included in the conversation in one way or another. It is necessary to later repeat these things in following discussions, as much of what is said at first is not fully comprehended until somewhat later.

It is not uncommon that newborns with handicaps are moved from the maternity ward to children's hospitals without strict indications. This ought to be avoided.

It is very common that it may take several days for the mother to reach the point where she sees her baby as her own. It is therefore devastating if the baby is separated from the mother in order to be put in a children's hospital. If the newborn absolutely must be moved to a children's hospital, then the mother should, if possible, be provided with an opportunity to visit the baby even during her time on the maternity ward, and the importance of regular visits after she has come home from the hospital ought to be emphasized. On the ward where the baby is being cared for, the personnel should be instructed to allow the mother to help to attend to the baby during her visits to the utmost possible extent. There must be sleeping accommodations for those mothers who live a distance from the hospital or, preferably, possibilities for the mother to live at the hospital.

It is, in other words, extremely important that the contact between parents and child not be broken during this first, delicate time, unless pressing medical reasons exist. The reactions of sorrow which can quite likely not be avoided in situations such as these follow a smoother course if the parents receive opportunities to give vent to them in a natural way, during several days' time and in co-operation with medical personnel.

Brothers and sisters at home

If the newborn baby has deformities then the other children at home should be told. Otherwise they create their own, frightening interpretation of what has happened. If necessary, the parents can receive help in presenting the information in such a way that it is suitable for the child's developmental level.

The situation is the same if the baby is born prematurely or sick and needs to be cared for at a children's hospital. The child or children at home are affected by the increased absence of the parents, by their distress, and anxiety. They are consequently in need of explanations which the parents, however, are often afraid of giving. They can be afraid of starting to cry, which they believe can have a strongly disquieting effect. It is, however, important that they show their feelings openly and speak with the children at home. Children have a great ability to cope with reactions of sorrow.

Caring for parents of infants who die

If the child dies, one should act upon the assumption that the parents should see the dead infant even if it is deformed. Nothing can be worse than dread-filled fantasies. To see the dead child can ease the strain of sorrow.

Immediately following the death of the infant, that member of the personnel who has been closest to the family should stay with them for a while and try to express their sympathy. The parent's tears and lamentation are important components of their mourning. Should they restrain themselves in stiff despair, it can often mean a more prolonged and more complicated sorrow.

Those parents who have religious ties should meet with a clergyman. Even those who are not actively religious may be able to find solace in a clergyman and in the symbols of funeral and burial.

The neonatologist ought to meet with both the parents together several times. The first time, the parents' consciousness is dominated by deep sorrow and it is difficult for them to take in information about the cause of death, etc. It is thus advisable to wait with such things and express only sympathy immediately after the death. Later, when the results of the autopsy are ready, the parents should be informed in clear and simple terms. Due to the parents' discomposure and fatigue, the information needs to be repeated several times. The doctor must be prepared to encounter superstitious notions, irrational guilt feelings, and even aggression towards personnel, including the doctor himself. The situation demands a factual and kind explanation, without any display of contempt, irritation, or anger. Justified complaints about the hospital care should be admitted and apologized for.

The risk for illness in later children-to-come should be discussed and genetic counseling arranged, if necessary. The parents ought to have worked through their sorrow thoroughly before having a new baby.

Attention must be directed towards the brothers and sisters of the dead infant. The doctor or psychologist should volunteer to speak with them as well. The parents should be informed that children often need to "work through" their sorrow in funeral and death games.

Restriction should be practiced in prescribing sedatives and tranquilizers. It must be explained to the parents that they will eventually want to be able to remember this time clearly and distinctly, and that the pain and sorrow can be surmounted most quickly if encountered with full consciousness.

Large amounts of psychopharmacologic drugs involve a risk for suicide.

The neonatologist and other personnel who encounter death among their patients have a need for support and solace in group discussion (see below). This is a prerequisite if they are going to be able to manage their often difficult work and maintain the ability to feel sympathy.

A five-day old boy suddenly died from a complicated cardiac lesion. The parents saw the dead boy. They sat mostly silent with a nurse. The father wept but the mother was stiff and silent. The neonatologist tried to contact her. Two days later he met the parents again and tried to give them information about the disease and cause of death. The mother was still silent and controlled. A week later the parents were told the results of the post mortem. The father seemed to understand and he put some questions about symptoms and therapy. Alone with the neonatologist he spoke about his concern about his wife's state. It was arranged that the mother should see a psychiatrist experienced in the field. During several one-hour long sessions the mother learned to speak of her sorrow and to weep. The parents were also helped to accept that their 5-year old girl played with her doll in digging a grave and speaking about heaven and angels.

The importance of continuity in medical care

In the often dramatic and rapidly changing course of illness, it is often desirable that the same doctor be responsible for the treatment and for contact with the parents. If the doctor must entrust a colleague with responsibility then he ought to inform the parents of this and confer with the doctor taking charge, preferably with the parents present. The doctor should preferably take on the responsibility for the check-ups after the baby has left the hospital as well. His familiarity with the course of the illness and with the parents' situation and manner of reacting makes it easier for him to help them with psycho-social problems as well, possibly referring them to experts within this field. Changing doctors increases the risks for misunderstanding and weakened confidence.

(The neonatologist ought to be responsible for the health care and treatment of the patient during the first years of life. In this way he acquires direct knowledge of the significance of different symptoms and examination results for the long-range prognosis.)

The work of the psychologist on the maternity ward and the neonatal ward

Background. — In modern health care and medical treatment, the patients, relatives, and personnel are encouraged to be open, take initiative, and express constructive criticism. More now than previously, attention is being paid to feelings of distress, sorrow, and anger which should be expressed and met with understanding. Personnel who have been educated in a previously more authoritarian system can, in this more open atmosphere, become uneasy and aggressive towards each other and towards the parents. They need instruction and support in their partially changing role. The many seriously ill or dying children and their parents provoke sorrow and anger among the personnel. These feelings can be suppressed, which usually implies that one is unable to become sympathetically involved and becomes instead tired and irritable. To counteract this, the personnel must have the opportunity to speak about their feelings with experts.

Competence. — The psychologist (social worker) should preferably be trained in therapy and have special knowledge and experience in neonatology with regard to the psychology of parents and personnel. They should have preferably been taught by an experienced psychologist or neonatologist and they should have access to qualified supervision.

The psychologist's (social worker) work should be drawn up in co-operation with the personnel. Below follow several suggestions for work assignments.

(1) The reactions and needs of the parents and personnel faced with the prospect of, e. g., a death, a deformed or seriously sick infant should be discussed at personnel conferences once a week (more often when necessary). The discussion should be carefully structured, everyone should be encouraged to express their opinion. Feelings of anger, guilt, and sorrow should be able to be expressed if the group feels "secure" in and of itself.

(2) Participate in the planning and initial help for parents in need of psycho-social support. There ought to be a prepared organization with possible referral to other helpful authorities (psychiatrists, family counselling bureaus, organizations for mentally handicapped children and youth, etc.).

(3) Information and support for the parents when the efforts of the neonatologist and other personnel does not suffice.

(4) Research and developmental work: the psycho-social problems in the care of newborns must become the object for more research, method development, and evaluation.

Examples
of the significance of psycho-social factors
in pregnancy, childbirth,
and early parenthood

Following are two examples of how different pregnancy, childbirth, and early parenthood can be, and how they are connected with the background, health, and social situation of the parents. The role of health care personnel is discussed in brief.

(1) A 22-year old woman who has undergone two pregnancies visits a maternity clinic in her 10th week. She feels quite well and is taking a course with her husband in psycho-prophylaxis. The delivery is painful but she co-operates well and takes the infant into her arms immediately after the birth. On its third day of life the infant develops hyperbilirubinemia, probably in conjunction with ABO-immunization. It is transferred to the neonatology ward, along with the parents. They are worried but are able to comprehend the information and calming advice. The mother continues to breastfeed. She describes the year immediately after the baby's birth as one of the happiest in her life. The whole family feels, for the most part, very well. The baby develops well and steadily.

Comments. — This family's background was advantageous to parenthood: the mother had a good relationship with her own mother. She had a good profession, with which she was happy. She had many friends. She had a good relationship with the husband, who supported her and participated in the care of the child. This family needed relatively little help from society.

(2) Another woman of the same age visits the maternity clinic in her sixth month of pregnancy. She has had troublesome menstrual periods and difficult psychic symptoms (insomnia, fear, anxiety and psycho-somatic difficulties). She cannot manage to prepare herself for the birth, which becomes traumatic with severe anxiety. The mother does not want to hold the baby. The baby develops difficulty in breathing and must be transferred to the neonatology ward. The mother becomes very upset and has a difficult time understanding and accepting information and reassuring reports. The child has an adaptation syndrome and improves quickly, and can return to the maternity ward two days later. The mother experiences many difficulties in caring for him on the maternity ward, breastfeeding is painful. The infant cries a great deal and the personnel must help the mother to comfort him. After discharge from the hospital the mother continues to have a difficult time despite help from the child-health center and social worker. The child has many respiratory infections and psycho-somatic difficulties such as colic and constipation.

Comments. — This woman had a completely different and less advantageous background to her pregnancy and parenthood. She had a poor relationship with her own mother, with whom she quarreled often. She had had lingering psycho-somatic problems (constipation, colic, stomach pains, etc.).

She had been educated as a baby nurse but was often unhappy at her various places of work. She had a conflict-filled reaction to the child's father and had considered having an abortion. Their relationship did not improve during the pregnancy or the first year after the baby's birth. The nurse at the child-care center and a social worker tried to help the mother, and a psychiatrist prescribed psycho-pharmacologic drugs. Nevertheless the help was not sufficient and it was difficult for the mother to co-operate. When the child was one-year old he was enrolled in a day-care center which was a great relief for the mother. Every time the boy had a respiratory infection, which happened often, the mother became very upset and sought medical help. She told the doctors that, as a newborn the boy "nearly died of breathing difficulties".

The prognosis for the child's and the family's development is dubious.

Readers interested in further reading on the subject are referred to the following list of references.

REFERENCES

[1] BENEDEK (I.). — *Motherhood and Nurturing. Parenthood. Its Psychology and Psychopathology.* Little Brown and Co., Boston, 1970.

[2] BIBLING (G.). — A study of the psychological process in pregnancy of the earliest mother-child relationship. *Psychoanal. Stud. Child.,* 16, 1961.

[3] CAPLAN (G.). — *Concepts of mental health and consultation, their application in public health social work.* Dept. of Health, Education and Welfare, Washington, 1959.

[4] ERIKSEN (E. H.). — *Identity and the Life Cycle.* Int. Nat. Press, New York, 1959.

[5] GRIMM (E.), GRUENBERG (E.), ILLSLEY (R.) et al. — *Child Bearing, its Social and Psychological Aspects.* William and Wilkins, New York, 1967.

[6] KAPLAN (D. N.), MASON (E. A.). — Maternal reactions to premature birth viewed as an acute emotional disorder. *Am. J. Orthopsych.,* 30, 539, 1960.

[7] KLAUS (M.), KENNELL (J.). — *Maternal-infant Bonding.* C. V. Mosby, St. Louis, 1976.

[8] LAGERCRANTZ (E.). — *The Mother and her First Born.* Acad. Diss. in Swedish with an English summary. Wahlström and Widstrand, Stockholm, 1979 (To be published in English).

[9] LIND (J.). — Die Geburt der Familie in der Frauenklinik. *Med. Klin.,* 68, 1597, 1973.

[10] NILSSON (Å.). — Paranatal emotional adjustement. A prospective investigation of 165 women. *Acta Psych. Scand. Suppl.,* 220, 1970.

[11] SHERESHEFSKY (P.), JARROW (L.). — *Psychological Aspects of a First Pregnancy and Early Postnatal Adaptation.* Raven Press Publ., New York, 1973.

[12] KLEIN (M.), STERN (L.). — Low birth weight and the battered child syndrome. *Amer. J. Dis. Child.,* 122, 15, 1971.

[13] UDDENBERG (N.). — Reproductive adaptation in mother and daughter. *Acta Psych. Scand., Suppl. 254,* 1974.

5

Prevention of preterm birth

Analysis of the problem. Preventive methods. Results

Emile PAPIERNIK

In this book on neo-natal medicine, the editors have asked an obstetrician to discuss prematurity. This is not to envisage the problems of the prematurely-born infant, those will be dealt with in several later chapters. The aim of this chapter is to show that very early delivery can be less frequently observed: preventative measures exist to avert pre-term births.

It is necessary for the pediatricians responsible for infants born prematurely to acquaint themselves with the principle causes that result in premature childbirth. This information can also be useful in the initial care of the newborn. Problems presented in previous pregnancies must be elucidated with the parents, followed by open discussion of the risks involved and precautionary measures available to prevent pre-term deliveries in future pregnancies.

A preventive blueprint is not easily put into effect: it is not a recipe. The difficulty arises from the necessity to develop a coherent and well-coordinated program. This can be approached in three main stages. First, the population at risk must be defined and identified by means of epidemiological studies. Second, a preventative policy can be proposed based upon an analysis of the principle causes of premature births and those preventative techniques

available (*i. e.*, information, rest, betamimetic drugs and progesterone). This type of program requires a particular organization of special services: prenatal care and counselling; prenatal hospital beds, and eventually local facilities for the care of high risk patients. Third, the results obtained must be evaluated. The preventative measures must be reviewed and the interventions analyzed in terms of their benefits afforded or not. On the basis of this information, subsequent programs can be designed to minimize the limitations revealed and to maximize the advantages obtained.

HISTORY

The idea of preventing premature childbirth is not new. Folk medicine has for a long time advised pregnant women against travelling or lifting heavy laundry and hanging it out to dry on the line with their arms raised.

During the late 1800's, Adolphe Pinard [105], a Parisian obstetrician, showed that workers in the Vaugirard laundry factories often delivered prematurely, but that they could indeed sustain full-term pregnancies if they could avail themselves of sufficient rest during the final weeks of pregnancy. With this study, he was able to show the social nature of the "problem", and by demonstrating its link with physical exertion, also able to suggest a possible effective means of its prevention.

A multicentric European study was undertaken by the Society of Nations [25] and Debré et al., 1933, to determine the medical and social causes of perinatal mortality, among these being premature birth. This study demonstrated that preterm delivery was a disease of profound social origin and character, affecting mostly the poor, the working class, and young and multiparous women. Physical over-exertion was held to be the primary cause of preterm labor, with economic factors themselves providing only a secondary explanation. Death during the first week of life, following premature birth, existed at a much lower incidence in those European communities having good prenatal care systems, as in Oxfordshire, U. K., even when the socio-economic situation was not more favorable.

These important findings figured highly in the development of generalized guidelines for the protection of pregnant women and children. Prior to World War II, they provided the basis for the policies proposed in Scandinavia and Holland, and were later used in the formation of similar programs in England, France, and eastern Europe. These systems allowed for a complete work leave, of varied duration, as determined by the parent nation; in France at the end of the 34th week, and after 28 weeks in the United Kingdom and northern Europe. Prenatal care clinics were also established, the use of which was further encouraged by monetary inducements or gifts for the child [111].

DEFINITION

It is necessary to carefully define the terminology involved when comparing the rates of prematurity, the rates of perinatal mortality and the role played by preterm birth in the latter, since the definition may vary with each study.

Premature birth is defined as occurring before 37 weeks after the start of the last normal menstrual period, e. g. 36 weeks and 6 days or 259 days. Unfortunately, definition by the length of gestation is not perfect, since it can only be correctly determined if the date of the last menstrual cycle is accurately known. Defining prematurity by birth weight under 2,500 g leads to confusion in the various reasons for a lower birth weight, such as,

prematurity or retarded fœtal growth. Definition of prematurity by weight has surely obscured, for a long time, the clear and necessary distinction between these two mechanisms resulting in low birth weight. It is therefore essential to completely separate shortened gestation and restricted fœtal growth.

One can further reduce the imperfections inherent in this definition by improving our knowledge concerning the true beginning of pregnancy and by prenatal examinations. The actual fœtal age can be determined by charting a temperature curve, prior to impregnation, since the day of ovulation is denoted by a low point followed by a rise in the basal body temperature; or by calculations based on an echogram performed before the 20th week in cases where the date of the last menstrual cycle is unknown or in cases of irregular or long cycles. Finally, the examination of the newborn can be used to obtain a better knowledge of the length of pregnancy. Physical and neurological examination may permit the correction of gross errors in the determination of gestational time should they persist until birth.

Some definitions, such as those of Fedrick [34] or Johnston [57], combine several variables, for example, less than 37 weeks and less than 2,500 g. Unfortunately, this serves only to combine the disadvantages of the two individual definitions and compounds that with an asymmetrical bias.

The lower limit of the definition of premature birth is not usually specified and this presents a problem in distinguishing between miscarriage and birth; this baseline varies with each country, being defined as 20 weeks for some, 24 weeks for others and even 28 weeks elsewhere.

The International Federation of Obstetricians and Gynecologists has proposed a minimal birth weight of 1,000 g as the lower limit in defining very early deliveries and this, hopefully, will enable the statistical comparison of accumulated data. However, it becomes necessary as well to have a 500-1,000 g class for those countries recording these pregnancies as births or even 400 g for Australia, which has chosen this as the lowest acceptable weight in the definition of birth.

NECESSITY OF PREVENTION

The progress made in recent years has reduced the seriousness of premature deliveries by improvements in neo-natal care, by better techniques of fœtal monitoring, and by an increase in the number of caesarian-section births performed [57]. New medications have brought renewed hope, as well as unquestionable advancement in the treatment of prematurity. Corticosteroids have reduced both the frequency and gravity of hyaline membrane disease, and betamimetic drugs have prevented premature labor for several hours, days or sometimes even longer [13, 39, 75, 76, 92, 119, 133]. This progress has opened new risks for the mother [67], related to the use of these drugs. Prostaglandin synthetase inhibitors may induce risks to the fœtus [68, 121].

Unfortunately, the advances have not resulted in the disappearance of premature birth. On the contrary, specialists in neonatal medicine who find themselves responsible for infants more and more immature and weighing less and less at birth, stress that indeed these problems have not been resolved. In addition, the sharp increase in hospital costs is a further limiting factor [106]. In spite of the brilliant successes achieved, this development can go no further.

At present, most of the medications are used too late to truly be preventative. Without wanting to diminish the accomplishments to date, we do not think they have reached their true goal which is to decrease the rate of desease and sequalæ related to premature delivery [12, 14, 31, 61, 99, 110, 113, 124-125].

EPIDEMIOLOGY OF PREMATURE BIRTH

Epidemiologic knowledge of premature births is already well-documented. Donnely [26] submitted a good analysis and publications [55] are quite similar, but report a small amount of progress made against preterm deliveries.

It is an unfortunate fact that earlier epidemiological studies are difficult to interpret since they often define a premature baby as having a birth weight of less than 2,500 g. The majority of these studies present their results according to the principle risk factors exhibited by the mother and they are then correlated with an analysis of the previous medical history [1, 2, 4, 7, 10-11, 16, 17, 19, 28, 31, 37, 38, 41, 43, 44, 52, 58, 60].

These studies end with a list of factors that increase the risk of premature birth, but fail to offer any insight as to possible preventative measures.

The principle factors contributing to an increased risk of premature birth are as follows:

(*a*) Medical history:

— premature birth,
— stillbirth.

(*b*) Characteristics of the women:

— low socio-economic level,
— young (less than 18 years),
— older (more than 35 years),
— multipara (4 or more children),
— unmarried,
— smoker.

(*c*) Variables arising during pregnancy:

— uterine bleeding,
— multiple pregnancy,
— placenta praevia,
— toxemia,
— urinary infection,
— vaginal infection.

The weight afforded each factor can be varied to reflect the population concerned. Whereas a previous preterm delivery doubles the risk for successive pregnancies according to many publications, Keirse [63] found a recurrence rate of 40 % in Oxford. In our population at Clamart, the rate of repeated premature births is only 14 %.

A prior history of a stillbirth or of a neo-natal death increases the risk of preterm birth for pregnancies to follow. A precedence of perinatal death (155 cases) was associated with a preterm birth rate of 14.6 %, as opposed to 5.6 % for the rest of the population. Far more, 42.6 % of the cases, of perinatal deaths are related to previous histories of premature delivery or perinatal death.

The lack of agreement among different studies persists and may be attributable to different approaches, as in prospective compared to retrospective studies. However, it seems that certain inconsistencies depend upon local conditions, such as the predictive value of a previous abortion which has greater significance in a population where the frequency of abortion is much higher [90, 91].

FROM EPIDEMIOLOGY TO PREVENTION

The previous epidemiological studies quoted appear to be incomplete; however, it seems that some improvements have indeed been made. First is the elucidation of those daily events that result in the triggering of uterine contractions. Secondly, a system for the measurements of the risk of preterm delivery based on a variety of clinical observations has been defined. The observations can provide a basis for calculating a score of probable risk of preterm labor. The third advance was the application of a policy of preventive action to a segment of the French population within a defined geographical area and with readily accessible hospital services. The results of these improvements have been measured.

Physical exertion and preterm birth

The relationship between the circumstances of daily life and preterm birth is described below.

Physical exertion can trigger uterine contractions and therefore initiate preterm labor. This fact was known to Pinard [105], in the guise of work-associated activity and clearly demonstrated by Debré [25], in the form of physical over-exertion as a result of either salaried or domestic work and also cited by Mayer [80] and Stewart [123]. Raiha [107] proposed rest and restricted physical activity as a basic method for the prevention of preterm delivery. Papiernik [100] again found that certain physical activities, such as those associated with a change of residence or overly demanding physical efforts required at work were more prevalent among those women who delivered preterm. The analysis was carried even further and demonstrated that certain work-related activities, especially the lifting of heavy objects, or working with machines that vibrate, augment the risk of preterm delivery [98].

A survey was carried out on a working class population in the town of Haguenau. Of the 1,193 working women followed, 210 lifted heavy objects and 31 (14.8 %) gave birth before the 37th week of pregnancy as opposed to 68 (6.9 %) out of the remaining 983 who did not do heavy lifting as part of their work ($p < 0.01$) (Table I). Within this sample same, 73 women worked with vibrating machines (mainly in textiles) and 14 delivered prematurely, that is 19 % compared with 7.5 % who did not work with these machines ($p < 0.01$) (Table II).

TABLE I. — PERINATAL STUDY OF HAGUENAU (PAPIERNIK, 1973)

	Work without heavy lifting	Work with heavy lifting	Total
N	983	210	1,193
Full-term delivery .	915	179	1,094
Preterm delivery . .	68	31	99
% preterm delivery .	6.9 %	14.8 %	8.3 %
			$p < 0.01$

TABLE II. — PERINATAL STUDY OF HAGUENAU (PAPIERNIK, 1973)

	Work without vibrating machinery	Work with vibrating machinery	Total
N	1,120	73	1,193
Full-term delivery.	1,035	59	1,095
Preterm delivery .	85	14	99
	7.5 %	19 %	8.3 %
			$p < 0.01$

The risk linked to physical activity compounds that attributed to prior gynecological and obstetrical problems.

There is a cumulative effect associated with the lifting of heavy objects and previous premature births. For those women who had already sustained full-term pregnancies, work requiring heavy lifting increased the rate of preterm deliveries from 5 % (without) to 12.4 % (with) ($p < 0.01$). When a previous premature birth was recorded, the preterm birth rate presented by heavy lifting jumped from 19 % (without) to 50 % (with) ($p < 0.01$) (Table III).

TABLE III. — PERINATAL STUDY OF HAGUENAU (PAPIERNIK, 1973)

	Work without heavy lifting	Work with heavy lifting	
Previous history of full-term delivery.	5.1 %	12.4 %	$p < 0.01$
Previous history of premature delivery . . .	19.2 %	50.0 %	$p < 0.01$

The relationship between arduous work and preterm delivery has been demonstrated in a survey of the nursing staff at Saint-Antoine Hospital in Paris (Estryn, 1978). Of the 204 women included in this study, 13 % delivered prematurely, while the rate for the overall Parisian population was 8 %. In 22 % of the cases, the women were hospitalized due to threatened preterm birth as compared with 12 % of the control population. The frequency of painful uterine contractions, of uterine bleeding during pregnancy, and of preterm births were studied with regard to working conditions and life style. Birth prior to the 37th week of gestation was significantly correlated with the work load, as measured by the number of patients for which the nurse was directly responsible, and the rate of preterm deliveries was 22 % when this number was elevated ($p < 0.05$).

The incidence of uterine bleeding was increased when the nurses used public transportation. The abnormal sensation of painful uterine contractions was further increased when the women worked standing up continuously ($p < 0.01$), when standing without freedom of mobility ($p < 0.01$) and when they used public transportation ($p < 0.01$) and had a daily commuting time of more than 90 minutes ($p < 0.01$).

This information regarding the harmful effect of hard work on preterm births was expanded and completed by Mamelle [79] in a prospective study of 3,000 pregnancies; who studied the "hardness" of work by precisely describing the movements entailed. Thus, was proposed an index of the "hardness of work" established by the addition of gestures and tiring positions. Preterm births are precisely correlated with the level of heavy labor demanded by the woman's work. This analysis also showed that work-associated fatigue, coupled with a past history of maternity problems, multiplied the risk of a preterm delivery. In the sample population of pregnant women studied, in a large city (Lyon, pop. 1,000,000) and in a small city (Haguenau, pop. 25,000), an increase in the number of preterm deliveries was not associated with the use of public transportation nor with a lengthy commutation time. This is contrary to the observations of Papiernik [100] and Estryn [33], however, their survey populations were located in Paris, a major metropolitan center (pop. 10,000,000).

Mamelle discovered a correlation between preterm births and the number of work-hours per week; finding the rates clearly elevated for more than 40 hours per week and even more markedly so, for more than 45 hours per week.

It must also be mentioned that women not working outside the home also present elevated rates of preterm deliveries, but the mechanism for this risk increase has never been really studied. However, Papiernik [100] has noted the significance of certain indicators of continuous physical fatigue, such as having 3 children at home; 3 or more flights of stairs without an elevator; or the role played by occasional fatigue resulting, for example, from a change of residence. These factors are often noted in the clinical history during pregnancy of those women who later deliver preterm babies.

This information only serves to confirm the long-standing observations which led to the policy of maternity leave for working women. As previously mentioned, in France, this prenatal leave begins only at the 34th week of gestation, whereas in northern Europe, particularly England, Sweden and Holland, it starts with the 28th week. It seems to us that the extremely small rate of preterm births in northern Europe may be related to the longer duration of their prenatal leave.

Clinical manifestations as predictors

Clinical manifestations during pregnancy provide another avenue of approach for predicting the possibility of an early delivery. The observations of Wood [142] have enabled us to recognize the importance of two principle variables: one being the length of the cervix, the other, the presence of uterine contractions. The latter is a well-known threat to preterm labor. It seems important to elucidate the predictive value of both shortening and dilatation of the cervix. Anderson and Turnbull [3] have brought forth arguments with a study of preterm cervical dilatation in 77 nullipara in which they demonstrate that those who delivered prematurely also displayed preterm cervical dilatation at 32 weeks.

Papiernik [93] proposed the measurement of cervical shortening and dilatation as one of the essential factors to be considered in predicting the risk of preterm delivery. This value was used in the prospective study by Papiernik and Kaminski [97]. The prevalence of preterm labor associated with these early cervical changes is known to be greater. However, a large scale study was indispensible in establishing the true value of this precocious clinical manifestation as a valid indicator of the risk of preterm delivery. Tables IV and V present the results observed in the Perinatal Study of Haguenau on 2,874 women. The observation of a shortened cervix is associated with a higher rate of preterm birth from 25 weeks to 36 weeks ($p < 0.001$) (Table IV). The rates of preterm birth were higher when an opening of the cervical inner os has been observed ($p < 0.001$) (Table V).

The thinning of the lower segment of the uterus and the descent of the head of the foetus were also recognized as strong indications of risk of preterm birth (Papiernik [93, 100]). This was verified by Weekes and Flynn [138]. Butler and Bonham [11] have noted the high incidence of uterine bleeding during the pregnancies of those women who had

TABLE IV. — RATES OF PREMATURE DELIVERY ASSOCIATED WITH A SHORTENED CERVIX. Study of 2,874 women examined prior to the 37th week of pregnancy. Study of the rates of premature births associated with a shortened cervix. Measurements were made at 6 different times during gestation (Perinatal study of Haguenau, PAPIERNIK, 1979).

Time of examination (weeks)		18	19 24	25 28	29 31	32 34	35 36
Shortened cervix	No . .	7.0	7.4	7.0	9.0	6.1	3.3
	Yes . .	15.0	13.3	18.4	21.4	18.6	11.6
Significance		N. S.	N. S.	xxx	xxx	xxx	xxx

xxx $p < 0.001$.

TABLE V. — STUDY OF 2,874 WOMEN EXAMINED PRIOR TO THE 37TH WEEK OF GESTATION. Study of the rates of premature delivery associated with early cervical dilation, as measured at 6 different times during pregnancy (Perinatal study of Haguenau, PAPIERNIK, 1979).

Time of examination (weeks)		<18	19 24	25 28	29 31	32 34	35 36
Cervical dilation	No . . .	7.0	7.5	7.3	8.6	5.3	2.9
	Yes . . .		18.5	22.2	37.1	28.8	15.1
Significance.				x	xxx	xxx	xxx

x $p < 0.05$.
xxx $p < 0.001$.

TABLE VI. — STUDY OF 2,874 PREGNANT WOMEN EXAMINED PRIOR TO THE 37TH WEEK OF GESTATION. Study of the rates of preterm deliveries associated with episodes of uterine bleeding as determined at 6 different times during pregnancy (Perinatal study of Haguenau, PAPIERNIK, 1979).

Time of examination (weeks)	Less than 18	19/24	25/28	29/31	32/34	35/36
Uterine bleeding						
No	6.7	7.5	7.2	10	7.4	5.4
Yes	14.8	12.9	25.0	33.3	27.4	12.5

delivered preterm babies. The significant value of these developments in predicting preterm deliveries has been confirmed by our own prospective study (Table VI).

Other omens of preterm birth are difficult to classify objectively, such as refusal on the part of the woman to accept her pregnancy. Wenner and Young [139] found that the risk was increased in those cases where the women were unable to recall the date of their last menstrual cycle. Papiernik and Schneider [98] showed that those women who sought medical attention later in their pregnancies, and who then refused medical recommendations for rest or medications, were often among those women who delivered preterm infants. Maternal attitudes to pregnancy has a tremendous influence on outcome [70]. Finally, Weidinger and Wiest [140] demonstrated that a relationship exists between uncontrollable vomiting and preterm labor.

Thus, there exist well-documented clinical signs present during pregnancy that warm of the possibility of a preterm delivery. The difficulty is to make the transition from these generalized, large-scale, epidemiological tendencies to the individual, and

TABLE VII. — Preterm birth risk score (Papiernik, 1969)

Pts				
1	— 2 or more children without household help. — Low socio-economic level.	— 1 curetage. — Short interval between previous pregnancies (1 yr between del + 2 nd preg.).	— Work outside the home.	— Unusual fatigue.
2	— Not married. For unwed mothers: — less than 20 years, — more than 40 years.	— 2 curetages.	— More than 3 flights of stairs without elevator. — More than 10 cigarettes/day.	— Less than 5 kg (11 lbs) weight gain. — Albuminuria. — Hypertension: > 140 mm Hg S, > 90 mm Hg D.
3	— Very low socio-economic level poverty. — Less than 1.50 cm (5'2"). — Less than 45 kg (99 lbs).	— 3 or more curetages. — Cylindrical uterus.	— Long daily commutation. — Unusual exertions. — Tiring work. — Extensive travel.	— Bleeding during 1st trimester. — Thinned lower segment of uterus. — Breech presentation at 7 months.
4	— Less than 18 years.	— Pyelonephritis.		— Bleeding during 2nd trimester. — Shortered cervix. — Cervical dilation. — Uterine contractions.
5		— Uterine malformation. — 1 late-term abortion. — 1 premature delivery.		— Multiple pregnancy. — Placenta praevia. — Hydramnios.

apply the data to the forecast of her own possible risk of preterm delivery.

The calculation of risk

Rantakallio [108] and Butler [10, 11] have shown the value of using a score, developed by means of a rigorous technique of statistical analysis, to calculate the probable risk of premature birth [1]. Both methods were based upon retrospective studies. Nesbitt [88] also proposed using a semi-quantitative scoring system to calculate, during the pregnancy, the risk of perinatal mortality. Papiernik [93] suggested a scoring "formula", specifically designed to predict premature births, which was based upon the evidence already available in the literature (Table VII). Saling [116] was able to distinguish between the risk of early delivery and that of retarded fetal growth due to the fact that only some, but not all "predicting" factors are shared by these 2 conditions. Thalhammer [13] proposed an equally well balanced type of scoring system.

The principle advantage of a scoring system is that it makes it possible to correlate and thereby simplify all the varied information which presents at prenatal examinations. The Papiernik scoring system is simple. It is based upon 35 factors, which, when they exist, are assigned a value of 1-5 points. Hence, one can weigh the level of influence exerted by each factor by viewing it in terms of various givens, such as: previous medical history, mother's build, uterine anomalies, smoking habits, as well as life style and clinical manifestations arising during the course of the pregnancy. The score calculated in this manner is called the "preterm birth risk score".

A prospective inquiry demonstrated its usefulness as a tool for predicting premature births. This method for predicting problem pregnancies was compared with a computer analysis of probable risk based upon statistical calculations. The comparison revealed only a slightly better "success" rate on the part of the computer. Thus, this quick, handy score card method of determining the risk of premature birth presented by each pregnancy has proven itself to be a valuable and reliable tool for the obstetrician in his daily practice (Kaminski and Papiernik [59]).

The use of this scoring method is widespread

[1] Defined as less than 2,500 g.

in France, and its predicative value has been demonstrated in other hospitals as well as on various segments of the population (Melchior [85]). Lambotte [69] has suggested a change in the point system, assigning 10 rather than 5 points to the most threatening variables, and this modified system is in use in Belgium. Creasy [22] has again demonstrated the value of this method of calculating the risk of preterm delivery based upon a population in northern California.

Since its publication, this system has been improved upon in an attempt to better analyse the possible risks existing at different stages during gestation. It was clearly demonstrated by the perinatal study of all recorded births in the Alsatian town of Haguenau, from 1971 that this scoring method is readily adaptable to the particular characteristics presented by a local population [29].

Using a computer, an overall risk coefficient was calculated based upon the 14 most predictive variables on a randomly chosen sample, equal to 75 % of the total population. The resultant probability score was then applied to the remaining 25 % of the population and its predictive value measured by the correlation between the calculated score and the actual number of preterm births (Table VIII).

The criticism by Anderson [2] of the validity of scoring systems for nullipara is based on her experience with retrospective data, including only sparse information gained during pregnancy, such as bleeding, but nothing else.

In the study at Haguenau, the correlation of the risk coefficient for nulliparous women shows that the ability to foresee preterm births exists and increases as the pregnancy advances (Table IX).

The correlations determined for parous women indicate that their previous medical history is important at the onset of pregnancy, but that the ability to perceive the risk of preterm labor is clearly augmented when one considers the clinical manifestations arising during gestation (Table X).

The analysis of the predicative value of the 14 best variables was made in a step by step regression analysis conducted for each of the 6 examination periods during gestation. The table gives the average values and the classification of the best variables for predicting preterm delivery, and also shows the extreme importance of those abnormal clinical signs arising during pregnancy. These manifestations are given a greater significance than the prior obstetrical history (Table XI).

A danger exists in transferring a group probable tendency and assigning it to an individual. That is to say, a woman thought to present a high risk of preterm delivery, may be exposed to a course of treatment which in itself threatens the woman whose individual case has been misinterpreted. In our daily obstetrical practice, we do not use this scoring system any more. The entire staff is acquainted with the "score card", and employs it under the appropriate circumstances, but it is not a formalized procedure.

During the perinatal study of Haguenau, a controlled inquiry was made to monitor the change in medical decisions as a result of having calculated the coefficient of risk. A prospective score was determined for only half of the women, who were chosen at random. The differences in the medical decisions taken for the two groups became non-

TABLE VIII. — RELATIONSHIP BETWEEN CALCULATED RISK SCORE AND PRETERM DELIVERIES. CORRELATION COEFFICIENT AT 6 DIFFERENT EXAMINATIONS DURING PREGNANCY: The score calculation being based upon the other 75 %. Test group was 25 % of the population.

Time of examination (weeks)	<18	19/24	25/28	29/31	32/24	35/36
N	176	138	179	96	241	141
Correlation	0.17	0.12	0.22	0.41	0.34	0.30

TABLE IX. — CORRELATION COEFFICIENT BETWEEN CALCULATED RISK AND PRETERM DELIVERY AMOUNG NULLIPAROUS WOMEN (Perinatal study of Haguenau, PAPIERNIK, 1979)

Time of examination (weeks)	<18	19 24	25 28	29 31	32 34	35 36
Clinical manifestations during pregnancy.	0.04	0.03	0.23	0.16	0.21	0.30

TABLE X. — CORRELATION COEFFICIENTS BETWEEN CALCULATED RISK. THE SCORE AND ACTUAL NUMBER OF PRETERM BIRTHS BY PAROUS WOMEN MEASURE BASED UPON THE TEST SAMPLE (25 % OF THE POPULATION). The score was calculated based upon 75 % randomly selected population and applied to the remaining 25 % (Perinatal study of Haguenau, PAPIERNIK, 1979).

Time of examinations (weeks)	< 18	19 24	25 28	29 31	32 34	35 36
Previous history only	0.17	0.16	0.22	0.14	0.09	0.09
Clinical manifestations during pregnancy	0.05	0.11	0.15	0.20	0.32	0.11
Previous history+clinical manifestations	0.17	0.19	0.25	0.24	0.33	0.15

TABLE XI. — RANKING OF VARIABLES USED IN PREDICTING PRETERM BIRTHS. Average rank obtained in the step by step regression analysis made for the 6 examination periods (Perinatal study of Haguenau).

	Average rank
Shortened cervix	3.6
Dilated cervix	3.9
Menorrhagia (uterine bleeding). . .	5.7
Cervical incompetence.	5.8
Previous premature birth	6.0
Fetal descent	7.6
Age: less than 19; more than 35. . .	8.1
Worker or farmer	8.6
High blood pressure.	9.2
Previous stillborn	9.2
Pyelonephritis	9.8

measurable within 3 weeks. This gave a yardstick for the time required for the medical staff to assimilate and act upon the data that comprised the score. The score remains, however, a useful educational tool for the less experienced members of the medical team, as well as for the pregnant woman, allowing her a self-appraisal of the possible risk of an early delivery [51].

ANALYSIS BY CAUSE OF PRETERM BIRTH

Even though we do not yet know the physiological mechanisms triggering labor, it is necessary to go beyond the descriptive epidemiological data, and appraise several mechanisms of preterm birth against which preventive action is possible, such as cervical incompetence, infection, uterine distention, and placenta praevia. The importance of progesterone in inhibiting contractions is not well understood [21, 23, 53].

It is known that cervical incompetence is present in many preterm deliveries [127], but it is difficult to determine its exact role. One of the difficulties being that this condition can only be diagnosed when the woman is not pregnant, but the majority of decisions must be made while she is expectant. The notion of probable incompetence has been proposed [64, 73, 103, 135, 141]. Several methods have been suggested to resolve this difficulty; for example, calibration of the cervix at the beginning of pregnancy [35] or the demonstration of an abnormal internal opening of the cervix as revealed by echography [74, 117]. Pregnancy after a cone biopsy of the cervix may be shortened [54].

Concerning cervical competence, certain epidemiological conclusions can be regrouped within the framework of this mechanism: previous preterm birth, a miscarriage, an abortion late in pregnancy, uterine bleeding not related to a low-lying placenta and cervical irregularities. Furthermore, we have shown that women exhibiting a history of probable cervical incompetence do indeed deliver preterm when they have physically demanding careers [97]. This is another example that helps to further understand the relationship between arduous work and preterm deliveries.

The current hypothesis is that the physical efforts stimulate uterine contractions. The contractions are unimportant in the normal woman, but threaten the woman with cervical incompetence. In this latter case, the self-perpetuating phenomenon of labor is set into motion.

Cervical and vaginal infections have more recently

been recognized as possible factors resulting in preterm births. Hawkinson and Schulman [46] have suggested that they may, with or without concomitant foetal infection, cause preterm rupture of the chorio-amniotic membranes. Amnionitis can also develop while the membranes are still intact and it is possible that foetal infection triggers preterm labor by adrenal stimulation [86]. Bacteria can be a local source of phospholipase in chorionic membranes [6] leading to the synthesis of prostaglandins by the placental membranes.

For women from the lower socio-economic classes, this manifestation of cervical infection appears to be the most often used explanation for perinatal deaths subsequent to premature birth [86]. Most probably, a relationship exists between a cervical abnormality and the predilection for cervicovaginal infections. In the case of cervical incompetence, the endocervical mucus is incapable of fulfilling its antibacterial role due to the immunoglobulin A secreted by the internal mucosa of the cervix [109].

It is known that the frequency of bacterial colonization of the cervical mucosa and vagina is augmented during gestation [5]. In addition, streptococcal B infections are present in 14.8 % of the patients during the second trimester and in 25.4 % of them during the final trimester of pregnancy.

The role of these endocervical infections seems important in the etiology of serious preterm deliveries, but they have continuously been poorly investigated and misinterpreted by epidemiological studies. It is interesting to note that in a retrospective study of the 749 mothers of infants admitted to a neonatal care unit, copious leucorrhagia was observed in 48 % of those women delivering prematurely as compared with 17 % of the full-term babies mothers [20]. This clinical manifestation is not sufficiently monitored. Examinations of the cervix using a speculum must be performed as well as bacteriological studies which are usually omitted because of practical difficulties such as more pressing demands imposed upon bacteriology laboratories [36, 83, 87].

Preterm labor triggered by an infection could be the result of a blood-stream transmitted microbial contamination of the foetus such as a listeria infection. In this instance, the responsible microbe is found in blood cultures and not in vaginal smears. Fever can initiate preterm labor without directly affecting the foetus, and acute cholecystitis without bacteremia can be the sole stimulus inducing preterm labor. Maternal pyelonephritis can stimulate preterm labor via a direct bacterial dissemination or by an indirect effect of fever.

There exist other mechanisms causing preterm deliveries, such as uterine distention which is generally put forth as an explanation for prematurity in the case of twins and hydramnios. Here again, uterine distention alone is not sufficient to explain preterm labor, since it is well-known that adequate prenatal rest can often prevent preterm birth in the case of twins [8]. What is truly dangerous is the very real risk associated with uterine distention and physical exertion [53, 137, 144].

One should not forget placenta praevia, which is the oldest-known cause of preterm delivery. Finally, we wish to mention the maternal cardiac volume [62, 107] which seems to have no influence on the duration of the pregnancy, but which offers an interesting measurement for interpreting the risk of retarded foetal growth [29]. Teenage pregnancy has a specific risk of preterm labor [18, 50, 144].

ORGANISATION
OF A PREVENTIVE PROGRAM

Prevention of preterm births can only be realised by a well-organised medical and social program. The first attempt by Kauppinen [62], based upon the suggestions of Raiha [107], clearly showed the requisite involvement of the entire population of pregnant women.

The important points are:

— education of physicians and associated medical personnel,
— education of the public, both men and women,
— organisation of prenatal clinics,
— availability of prenatal hospital facilities.

Education is the essential ingredient. Doctors, as well as the public, must learn that the majority of preterm deliveries are not inevitable, and that in many cases, the risk can be predicted and avoided.

Education of the medical community is the first goal to achieve. In France, we have succeeded in disseminating this information by campaigns in professional journals and later by a series of conferences. All doctors must be given the opportunity to comprehend the risk involved in preterm deliveries and to respond by using techniques to measure this risk and to initiate elementary preventive procedures. A great deal of energy has also been directed towards informing the public, via the press and the television, precisely describing those circumstances triggering premature labor, such as excessive physical exertions, changes of residence or prolonged automobile trips.

The showing of educational films to pregnant women when they come for their prenatal care visits has produced great interest. The practice in France of the Lamaze method of preparation for natural childbirth has further allowed for the diffusion of educational films on the risks of premature delivery and possible methods of prevention.

At the level of prenatal visits, an initial improvement would be to change the current structure and to augment the number of prenatal examinations. Our experience and that of many others in northern Europe, has shown that the ideal number of prenatal visits is at least 10. However, the number is not the crucial issue. Concerning prenatal examinations 3 major points are important:

First: A concerted effort must be made to identify, during the first trimester of pregnancy, those women with cervical incompetence. This is one reason why it is important for pregnant women to consult well-trained obstetrical teams from the beginning of their gestations. It is necessary to analyse the previous medical history, to determine the length of the cervix, to look for exocervicitis, an enlarged isthmus, a cervical scar bearing witness to an hidden tear. But the treatment is not clear. We have demonstrated with a randomized trial that more cerclage does not help reduce the rates of preterm deliveries [71]. This goes against previous proposals [77].

Second: During the course of prenatal care, regular examinations should uncover those signs strongly indicative of risk of preterm labor. It is this method as well, that stresses the appearance of painful uterine contractions; uterine bleeding, even minor spotting; or a shortening of the cervix or an open cervix. This approach must also attempt to search for those circumstances of daily life that trigger preterm labor, such as long daily commuting, physically demanding work, travels or changes of residence. We find at least one of these elements in 29 % of the women undergoing prenatal care in our hospital.

Third: Preventive action is as much social as medical; the primary therapeutic recommendation, therefore, is that of reduced physical exertion and of rest. The possibility of prescribing a leave from work is an effective tool for the population in France where 79 % of the women work outside the home. This work leave allows the interruption of daily commuting to and from the place of work and other directly associated activities. It is more difficult to offer true rest to those mothers with large families at home. In this instance, the preventative measure depends upon the possibility of obtaining household help. Such a social service

system does exist in France, but it lacks sufficient personnel. The husband and/or other members of the family must assume some of the responsibilities for household tasks. We have often succeeded in obtaining sufficient rest for the pregnant woman by arranging for the assistance of a grandmother or a sister.

Medical therapies provide only a second line of defense, with the use of progesterone [56], and rarely, betamimetic drugs, and also by the discovery and treatment of cervico-vaginal infections.

The most serious cases of threatened preterm deliveries must be hospitalized. Hospitalization assures complete bed rest and allows intravenous and subsequent intramuscular treatment with betamimetic drugs. It also provides an educational experience, as the woman understands very rapidly the true threat posed by preterm birth and sees for herself the benefits gained by rest. It is impossible, for reasons of cost, or the availibility of local hospital facilities, as well as for the family life style, to recommend a prolonged hospital stay.

Since 1974, we have used a system of follow-up care at home which involved 9 % of our maternity patients in 1978. The woman returns home and each week a midwife attached to the obstetrical service visits her at home to check up on the situation as far as rest and medications are concerned. She particularly monitors that the return to daily activity is free of physical exertion. This protocol seems to be well accepted by the patients as well as being effective when measured by a controlled therapeutic trial of the number of premature births in women from the lowest socio-economic strata [122].

There are however, threats to preterm delivery which indeed require hospitalization for longer periods, such as the discovery of a placenta praevia. When the placenta is marginal, simple rest or short-term hospitalization followed by rest is sufficient. The same is true in the case of twins [47].

This action at the service level must be associated with a centralization of prenatal care, with the responsibility for the threatened premature birth taken over by those facilities and teams best equipped to handle the crisis presented by preterm delivery of tiny infants.

RESULTS OF PREVENTION

The effectiveness of the prevention has been demonstrated in France. The entire country was reached by the modified aims and technics of prenatal care. The prevention of preterm births was one of the several programs included in the National Perinatal Program implemented by the French Health Authority [15], following our propositions [93]. The national program was evaluated and three successive national representative samples were studied to answer the questions about the diffusion of a modified type of care and about the results [115]. This study shows that prenatal care has been dramaticaly changed in France over the observed 10 years. Women did come early in the first trimester, for the first visit, their mean number of prenatal visits rose from 3 to 7. The main provider of prenatal care, the general practionner at the beginning 1972, did not play major role in 1981, the women coming early and often to a specialized type of care provided by obstetricians themselves in private settings, by teams of midwives under obstetrical control in the public hospitals dealing with half the pregnancies. A major differences is observed with work leave. Work leave given to all pregnant women six weeks before expected date of delivery was not completely used in 1972, only five weeks at the mean. This was extended by prescriptions of workleave for women at risk for preterm delivery, and the mean for all working women became ten weeks.

Preterm deliveries were reduced by one third when all live births are considered of less than 37 weeks, and by one half when livebirths of less than 34 weeks are considered (Table XII). The rates of preterm births were 8.2 % in 1972, 6.8 % in 1976 and 5.6 % in 1981 when all births are considered. After exclusion of stillbirths, twins, major malformations, and exclusion of those births with a birth weight discrepancy with gestational age the rates became 6.3 % in 1972, 5.4 % in 1976 and 4.2 % in 1981, all significantly different. When

births weights are considered as a control for gestational age, the French representative studies demonstrate a decrease in low births weight (less than 2,500 g) related to preterm babies and not to term babies, with rates of 6.2 % in 1972, 6.5 % in 1976 and 5.2 % in 1981, when all births are considered, when stillbirths, twins and malformed were excluded, the rates are 5.5 % in 1972, 4.8 % in 1976 and 3.7 % in 1981. Here also the major improvement was in the very low births weights more than in the global group of low birth weights, with rates of VLBW (less than 1,500 g) of 0.8 % in 1972, 0.7 % in 1976 and 0.4 in 1981.

Perinatal mortality was reduced in both components, but more for neonatal deaths than for stillbirths. The stillbirth rate was 10 °/oo in 1972, 11 in 1976 and 5 in 1981. Babies were transferred more often to neonatal intensive care units, but the rate of hyaline membrane disease was significantly reduced from 4 °/oo in 1972 to 2 °/oo births in 1981.

The Haguenau survey was an added way of evaluation of the effects of care on the observed results. This specific study was designed in 1970 to measure the effects of a national policy on a local district hospital and on the information and behavior of the pregnant women of this population. The same basic observations were made. The women did modify the way they were seeking prenatal care. They came earlier and more often to a specialized care provider, they accepted to reduce their physical activity, their hard jobs during the pregnancy when a risk factor was present. This study allowed us to have a better understanding of the way a new technic is accepted by the population and how pregnant women seek it. Obviously, social class and years of schooling describe groups with different behaviors. The more educated group (13 or more years of schooling) did accept the new care and followed the proposed prescriptions in less than two years. The middle class group (10-12 years) took four years to reach the same behaviour, and the lower class level women (up to 9 years of school) took eight years to reach the level reached by the first at the beginning of the intervention. The results in less preterms is very similar to that for total France [102] with a reduction by 1/3 for all preterm births, a reduction by 1/2 of all livebirths before 34 weeks and a reduction of 2/3 for livebirths before 31 weeks. Fewer babies were transferred to a neonatal intensive care unit. The neonatal mortality is described in Table XIII, the observed rates were 8.5°/oo livebirths in the 1971-1974 period, 6.3 °/oo in the 1975-1978 period and 2.7 °/oo in the 1979-1982 period. We proposed to separate in that improvement the part played

TABLE XII. — FRENCH REPRESENTATIVE STUDIES (Rumeau-Rouquette and coll., 1984)

	Gestational age distribution %		
G. A. (wks)	1972	1976	1981
34	2.4	1.7	1.2
34-36	5.8	5.1	4.4
37-39	37.0	34.9	37.9
40-42	50.8	54.0	53.1
43 +	4.0	4.3	3.4
p. value		0.01	0.01

by better care (the trend observed in all countries and related to technical improvements in obstetric and pediatric care) or by better babies (a better distribution of gestational ages and birth weights when fewer preterm births are observed. Table XIII describes the statistical way to analyse this question. This was done by putting the neonatal risks for death observed in each of the periods 1975-1978 and 1979-1982, but with a non modified distribution of gestational ages, similar to that observed in the first period 1971-1974.

TABLE XIII. — NEONATAL MORTALITY $°/_{oo}$ LIVEBIRTHS BY TIME PERIOD

Period	1971-1974	1975-1978	1979-1982
Neonatal deaths $°/_{oo}$ live births	8.5 47/5,548	6.3 30/4,787	2.7 16/5,808
Standardized rates for gestational age distribution in period 1971-1974 and confidence level	8.5	7.2 4.8-9.6	5.3 3-7.6

This means that in 1979-1982, if the distribution of gestation durations would not have changed, the neonatal mortality rate would have been of 5.3 $°/_{oo}$ (confidence level 3 to 7.6): also that half the improvement in neonatal mortality from 8.5 to 2.7 $°/_{oo}$ is related to better care (from 8.5 to 5.3) but the second half is related to better babies and less preterms (from 5.3 to 2.7 $°/_{oo}$). We have found in this population that many less days were needed in neonatal intensive care units per 1,000 births (from 425 days per 1,000 births in 1971-1974 to 182 days per 1,000 births in 1979-1982). This was not due to a different policy of transfers, as less days were needed in the local pediatric ward as well (from 437 days per 1,000 births in 1971-1974 to 223 days per 1,000 births in 1979-1982). We have not been able to measure the long term effects of this policy on numbers and rates of handicaps in the population, even if this is included in our program in the Haguenau population, as well as in the national data. But nevertheless, it is obvious that less babies are exposed to the most dangerous circumstances. If only gestation age or bith weight are considered with the measured risks for handicaps related to very low birth weight or to very short gestation births, can expect a major reduction in handicapping conditions for the neonates and the children.

QUALITY CONTROL

The establishment of a preventive program is difficult. It requires the active participation of all those involved. For doctors and midwives who are responsible for prenatal examinations, we have organised a system of "retro-control" or internal audit. Such a practice enables a critical analysis of all the cases of premature birth by presenting the evidence of those warning signs neglected or of available information neither pursued nor used.

We wanted to use the pregnant women's participation and therefore, a good proportion of our educational efforts are centered upon those circumstances triggering uterine contractions. It is very probable that both of these approaches have been effective but, needless to say, the effect was not immediate. Taking into account the education of both the medical personnel and the patients, we had to wait for nearly 4 years after the beginning of such a program to achieve those results predicted and anticipated from the onset (Table XIV).

From our study conducted on the entire population of the city of Haguenau, we were able to discern the greatest stumbling block to the establishment of such a program; that being the patients low level of education. However, the rate of preterm deliveries was lowered even under those circumstances, and even more that with better educated women. It is the number of school years which is used to define groups. The rate of prematurity in the more favored group is the same as that observed at Clamart for a better educated population. The investigation showed that for the underprivileged, the rate of preterm delivery could be reduced when clinical manifestations were present or when an ominous medical history existed. But it could only be slightly lowered when the sole indicators of risk were social, such as tiring work or simply being a member of a lower socio-economic class.

Thus, the most significant obstacle in establishing an effective program of prevention is the inadequacy of the education of the population, compounded by the inadequacy of dissemination of pertinent information. The only temporary but efficient protocol elucidated was the attempted therapeutic trial supervised by midwives and conducted at home. For those women with a high risk of preterm delivery, the weekly home visit by a midwife did not alter the rate of prematurity when medically defined risks existed. On the other

TABLE XIV. — EVOLUTION OF PERINATAL MORTALITY, OBSTETRICAL SERVICE, PAPIERNIK, 1981
(Hôpital Antoine-Béclère, Clamart, France)

Year	Number of births	Number of deaths	Perinatal mortality (°/oo)	Perinatal mortality infants ≥ 1,000 g (°/oo)
1974	2,004	33	16.70	16
1975	2,200	29	13.20	11
1976	2,352	32	13.60	10.60
1977	2,428	42	17.30	15.70
1978	2,546	34	13.35	11
1979	2,489	25	10.04	8.40
1980	2,428	22	9.06	8.26

hand, the presence this frequently of a midwife, clearly succeeded in reducing the rate of premature births in those cases where the primary component of the risk was social.

Based on the findings elaborated above, we have attempted to establish a preventative program against preterm delivery on a nationwide basis. Education was one of the principle themes in the health policy proposed to the French government in 1970, following a realistic study of budgetary choices [136]. The idea was to inform both the women and the physicians of those factors presenting a risk of preterm labor. The financial justification was relatively simple, as the cost of this program was extremely small [15], consisting mainly of the dissemination of information.

The nationwide results, based on two representative surveys, have been positive, with a decrease in preterm deliveries from 8.2 % in 1972, to 6.8 % in 1976 and 5.2 % in 1981. Some part of this improvement may be related to a modification in the reproductive habits especially the number of births to multiparous women (3 or more children at home) which have been reduced from 14.9 % to 9.9 %. But at the same time, some important changes have occurred in the prenatal follow-up. The number of prenatal visits which was as low as 3 has been improved to a of 6 per pregnancy. The frequency of early prenatal leave from work has risen. A reduction of working hours has been offered to 11 % of the employed pregnant women.

We have no way to determine which proposed specific action was followed by a calculable effect, however, France is one of the few countries to have enacted this type of policy recently and to have observed a result in preterm births in such a short period of time.

CONCLUSION

We would like the pediatricians to be convinced of the importance of their role in the possible prevention of preterm delivery and not only in the domain of the newborn child. They can be active in the diffusion of information to the mothers of preterm infants and to the team of obstetricians and midwives with whom they work. The pediatrician must warn the mothers that preterm births are occurences that are repetative and that a strict program of prevention must be established. To others, they must stress the exactness of systems for the prevention of preterm birth. Obstetrical teams must be convinced to better analyse the previous medical history and life style of each patient, and especially, to take the time necessary to teach the women those preventative measures available; a role that may be delegated either to the midwives or to specially-trained nurses. They must further be convinced that prevention of preterm birth is part of the critical evaluation performed by the obstetrician. Lastly, pediatricians must act in conjunction with the civil authorities and help to convince them that a program of prevention of preterm births is possible and attainable.

REFERENCES

[1] ALBERMAN (E.), ELLIOT (M.), CREASY (M.), DHADIAL (R.). — Previous reproductive history in mothers presenting with spontaneous abortion. Brit. J. Obstet. Gynaec., 82, 366-373, 1975.
[2] ANDERSON (A. B. M.). — Individual prevention of preterm labor. Perin. Med. Sixth Europ. Congress, Vienne, 1978. Thieme P., Stuttgart, 1979.

[3] ANDERSON (A. B. M.), TURNBULL (A. C.). — Relationship between length of gestation and cervical dilatation. Uterine contractility and other factors during pregnancy. *Am. J. Obstet. Gynecol.*, *105*, 1207-1214, 1969.

[4] BAIRD D. — Environmental and obstetrical factors in prematurity: with special reference to experience in Aberdeen. *Bull. Wld. Hlth. Org.*, *26*, 291, 1962.

[5] BAKER (C. J.), BARRETT (F. F.) YOW (M. D.). — The influence of advancing gestation on group B streptococcal colonisation in pregnant women. *Am. J. Obstet. Gynecol.*, *122*, 820-823, 1975.

[6] BEJAR (R.), CURBELO (V.), DAVIS (C.), GLUCK (L.). — Premature labor. II. Bacterial sources of phospholipase. *Obstet. Gynecol.*, *57*, 479, 1981.

[7] BOLDMAN (R.), REED (D. M.). — *Worldwide variations in low birth weight. Epidemiology of prematurity.* URBAN and SCHWARZENBERG. Baltimore, Munich, 39-50, 1977.

[8] BROWN (E. J.), DIXON (H. G.). — Twin pregnancy. *J. Obstet. Gynecol.*, 251-252, 1963.

[9] BUTLER (N. R.). — Perinatal mortality survey. *Brit. Med. J.*, *2*, 1463-1465, 1962.

[10] BUTLER (N. R.) , ALBERMAN (E. D.). — In: *Perinatal problems* (1 vol.). Livingstone, Edinburgh and London, 1969.

[11] BUTLER (R. R.), BONHAM (D. G.). — In: *Perinatal mortality* (1 vol.). Livingstone, Edinburgh and London, 1963.

[12] CALAME (A.), REYMOND GONI (E.), MAHERZI (M.), ROULET (J.), MARCHAND (C.), PROD'HOM (L. S.). — Psychological and neurodevelopmental outcome of high risk newborn infants. *Helv. Paediat. Acta*, *31*, 287-297, 1976.

[13] CARITIS (S. N.), EDELSTONE (D. I.), MUELLER HEUBACH (E.). — Pharmacologic inhibition of preterm labor. *Am. J. Obstet. Gynecol.*, *133*, 557-578, 1979.

[14] CARLSSON (J.), SBENNINGSEN (N. W.). — Respiratory insufficiency syndrome (RIS) in preterm infants with gestational age of 32 weeks and less. *Acta Paediat. Scand.*, *64*, 813-821, 1975.

[15] CHAPALLAIN (M. T.). — Perinatality: French cost-benefit studies and decisions on handicap and prevention. In: *Ciba Foundation Symposium 59* (new series). Elsevier, Excerpta Medica, North Holland, Amsterdam, Oxford, New York, 193-206, 1978.

[16] CHASE (H. C.). — Time trends in low birth weight in the United States 1950-1974. *Epidemiology of Prematurity.* URBAN and SCHWARZENBERG, Baltimore, Munich, 17-37, 1977.

[17] CLEWELL (W. H.). — Prematurity. *J. Reprod. Medicine*, *23*, 237-244, 1979.

[18] COATES (J. B.). — Obstetrics in the very young adolescent. *Am. J. Obstet. Gynecol.*, *108*, 68-72, 1970.

[19] CORADELLO (H.), POLLAK (A.), SCHEIBENREITER (S.), THALHAMMER (O.). — Verhütung von Frühgeburtlichekeit und pränatalar Dystrophie II : Vor läufige Ergebnisse mit einem einfachen System zur Vorausberechnüng des Frühgeberurysrisikos. *Zeitschrift für geburtsch. Perinat.*, *178*, 19-22, 1974.

[20] COUCHARD (M.), LEFEBVRE (C.), SPIRA (N.), JAEGER (J.), PAPIERNIK (E.), MINKOWSKI (A.). — Difficultés périnatales particulières aux femmes immigrantes à partir des caractéristiques des mères de nouveau-nés au centre de soins intensifs Florence Geller. *Ann. Péd.*, *25*, 521-528, 1971.

[21] COUSIN (L. M.), HOBEL (C. J.), CHANG (R. J.), OKADA (D. M.), MARSCHALL (J. R.). — Serum progesterone and estradiol 17 β levels in premature and term labor. *Am. J. Obstet. Gynecol.*, *127*, 612-615, 1977.

[22] CREASY (R. K.). — System for predicting spontaneous preterm birth. *Obstet. Gynecol.*, *55*, 695-696, 1980.

[23] CSAPO. — The "seesaw" theory of the regulatorymechanism of pregnancy. *Am. J. Obstet.*, *121*, 578-581, 1975.

[24] CURRIE (B. W.). — Physiology of uterine activity. *Clinical Obstet. Gynecol.*, *23*, 32-33, 1980.

[25] DEBRÉ (R.), JOUANNON (P.), CREMIEU-ALAN (M. T.). — In: *La mortalité infantile et la mortinatalité.* Résultats de l'enquête poursuivie en France et dans cinq pays d'Europe sous les auspices du Comité d'Hygiène de la Société des Nations. Masson et Cie, Éditeurs, Paris, 1933.

[26] DONNELLY (J. F.), FLOWERS (C. E.), CREADICK (R. N.), WELLS (H. B.), GREENBERG (B. G.), SURLES (K. B.). — Maternal, fœtal and environmental factors in prematurity. *Am. J. Obstet. Gynecol.*, *88*, 918-931, 1964.

[27] DOTT (A. B.), FORT (A. T.). — Medical and social factors affecting early teenage pregnancy: a literature review and summary of the findings of the Louisiana Infant Mortality Study. *Am. J. Obstet. Gynecol.*, *125*, 532-536, 1976.

[28] DOUGLAS (J. W. B.). — Some factors associated with prematurity; the results of a national survey. *J. Obstet. Gynecol. Brit. Emp.*, *57*, 143, 1950.

[29] DREYFUS (J.), LAZAR (P.), PAPIERNIK (E.), GUEGUEN (S.). — Facteurs communs et différentiels de prévision de la prématurité, de la postmaturité, de l'hypotrophie du nouveau-né. *4th Europ. Congress of perinatal medicine*, Prague, 28-31 août 1974 (in abstracts).

[30] DREYFUS (J.), LAZAR (P.), PAPIERNIK (E.), GUEGUEN (S.). — Individual prediction of premature delivery and insufficiency of new-born weight. *4th Congress of European Society of Perinatal Medicine*, Vol. 1, Stuttgart, 447, 1975.

[31] DUNN (P. M.). — Premature delivery and the preterm infant. *J. Irish Med. Assoc.*, *69*, 246-254, 1976.

[32] EMIG (O. R.), NAPIER (J. V.), BRAZIE (J. V.). — Inflammation of the placenta: correlation with prematurity and perinatal death. *Obstet. Gynecol.*, *17*, 743-750, 1961.

[33] ESTRYN (M.), KAMINSKI (M.), FRANC (M.), FERMAND (S.), GERSTLE (F.). — Grossesse et conditions de travail en milieu hospitalier. *Rev. Franç. Gynécol.*, *73*, 625-631, 1978.

[34] FEDRICK (J.), ANDERSON (A. B. M.). — Factors associated with spontaneous preterm birth. *Brit. J. Obstet. Gynecol.*, *83*, 342-350, 1976.

[35] FOURNIL (C.) HIDDEN (J.), LAJOUX (P.). — Évaluation du calibre de l'isthme utérin en début de grossesse. *La nouvelle presse médicale*, *6*, 523-533, 1977.

[36] GAMSU (H.). — *Intrauterine infections.* Elsevier Excerpta Medica, North Holland, 135-149, 1973.

[37] GARN (S. M.), SHAW (H. E.), MCCABE (K. D.). — Effects of socioeconomic status and race on weight defined and gestational prematurity in the United States. *Epidemiology of prematurity.* URBAN and

SCHWARZENBERG. Baltimore, Munich, 127-144, 1977.

[38] GIBBS (C. E.). — Diagnosis and treatment of uterine conditions that may cause prematurity. *Clin. Obstet. Gynecol.*, *16*, 159-160, 1973.

[39] GLUCK (L.), RICHARDSON (C. J.). — Acceleration of the fœtal lung maturation following prolonged rupture of the membranes. *Am. J. Obstet. Gynecol.*, *119*, 11-15, 1974.

[40] GOLSTEIN (H.). — *Survey editorial team. Perinatal problems.* Livingstone, Edinburgh, 1969, 42-56.

[41] GOODWIN (J. M.), DUNN (J. T.), THOMAS (B. W.). — Antepartum identification of the fœtus at risk. *Can. Med. Assoc. J.*, *101*, 458-464, 1969.

[42] GORTMAKER (S. L.). — The effects of prenatal care upon the health of the newborn. *Am. J. Obstet. Public Health*, *69*, 653-660, 1979.

[43] GOUJARD (J.), HENNEQUIN (J. F.), KAMINSKI (M.), MARENDAS (R.), RUMEAU-ROUQUETTE (C.). — Prévision de la prématurité et du poids de naissance en début de grossesse. *J. Gynécol. Obstét. Biol. Reprod.*, *3*, 45-59, 1974.

[44] GREEN (L. K)., HARRIS (R. E.). — Uterine anomalies: frequency of diagnosis and associated obstetric complications. *Obstet. and Gynecol.*, *47*, 427-429, 1976.

[45] GRICE (A. C.). — Vaginal infection causing spontaneous rupture of the membrane and premature delivery. *Aust. N. Z. J. Obstet. Gynecol.*, *14*, 156-159, 1974.

[46] HAWKINSON (J. A.), SCHULMAN (H.). — Prematurity associated with cervicitis and vaginitis during pregnancy. *Am. J. Obstet. Gynecol.*, *94*, 898-902, 1966.

[47] HELVIN (G.), LAVIGNE (F.), PAPIERNIK (E.). — Twin delivery spontaneous labor or induction. *3rd international congress on twin studies*, Jerusalem, 16-20 June 1980.

[48] HOBEL (C. J.). — *Prevention of prematurity.* Privileged communication.

[49] HOFMEISTER (F. J.), SCHWARTZ (W. R.), VONDRAK (B. F.), MARTENS (W.). — Suture reinforcement of the incompetent cervix: experience at the Lutheran Hospital of Milwaukee. *Am. J. Obstet. Gynecol.*, *101*, 58-65, 1968.

[50] HUTCHINS (F. L.), RUBINO (J.), KENDALL (N.). — Experience with teenage pregnancy. *Obstet. Gynecol.*, *54*, 1-5, 1979.

[51] HENRY-SUCHET (J.), PEZ (J. P.). — Prévention de la prématurité grâce à l'auto-C. R. A. P. (modification du C. R. A. P. de Papiernik). Société Nationale de Gynécologie et d'Obstétrique. Réunion nationale de Bordeaux, 20 septembre 1975. *J. Gyn. Obstét. Biol.*, *5*, 843-845, 1976.

[52] JANSSON (I.). — Aetiological factors in prematurity. *Acta Obstet. Gynecol. Scand.*, *45*, 279-301, 1966.

[53] JEFFREY (R. L.), BOWES (W. A.), DELANEY (J. J.). — Role of bed rest in twin gestation. *Obstet. Gynecol.*, *43*, 822-826, 1974.

[54] JONES (J. M.), SWEETNAM (P.), HIBBARD (B. M.). — The outcome of pregnancy after cone biopsy of the cervix: a case control study. *Brit. J. Obstet. Gynecol.*, *86*, 913-916, 1979.

[55] JOHNSTON (J. W. C.), DUBIN (N. H.). — Prevention of preterm labor. *Clin. Obstet. Gynecol.*, *23*, 51-73, 1980.

[56] JOHNSTON (J. W. C.), AUSTIN (K. L.), JONES (C. S.), DAVIS (G. H.), KING (T. M.). — Efficacy of 17 α hydroxyprogesterone caproate in the prevention of premature labor. *The New Engl. J. Med.*, *293*, 675-680, 1975.

[57] JOHNSTON (J. W. C.). — Obstetric aspects of preterm delivery. *Clin. Obstet. Gynecol.*, *23*, 15-16, 1980.

[58] KAMINSKI (M.), GOUJARD (J.), RUMEAU-ROUQUETTE (C.). — Prediction of low birthweight and prematurity by a multiple regression analysis with maternal characteristics known since the beginning of the pregnancy. *Int. J. Epidem.*, *2*, 195-204, 1973.

[59] KAMINSKI (M.), PAPIERNIK (E.). — Multifactorial study of the risk of prematurity at 32 weeks of gestation. II. Comparison between an empirical prediction and a discriminant analysis. *J. Perin. Med.*, *2*, 37-44, 1974.

[60] KAMINSKI (M.), BLONDEL (B.), BREART (G.), FRANC (M.), DU MAZAUBRUN (C.). — Issue de la grossesse et surveillance prénatale chez les femmes migrantes. *Rev. Épidém. Santé publ.*, *26*, 29-46, 1978.

[61] KAMPER (J.), MOLLER (J.). — Long term prognosis of infants with idiopathic respiratory distress syndrome. Follow-up studies in infants surviving after the introduction of continuous positive airway pressure. *Acta Paediat. Scand.*, *68*, 149-154, 1979.

[62] KAUPPINEN (M. A.). — The correlation of maternal heart volume with the birth of the infant and prematurity. *Acta Obstet. Gynecol. Scand.*, Suppl. 6, 1967.

[63] KEIRSE (M. J. N. C.), RUSH (R. W.), ANDERSON (A. B. M.), TURNBULL (A. C.). — Risk of preterm delivery in patients with previous preterm delivery and/or abortion. *Brit. J. Obstet. Gynecol.*, *85*, 81-85, 1978.

[64] KIDESS (E.), PROBST (V.), FIECHTNER (E.). — Indikationstellung und Erfolg der Zervixcerclage (Shirodkar McDonald) in der Schwangerschaft. *Geburtsh. U. Frauenheilk*, *33*, 196-202, 1973.

[65] KLOOSTERMAN (G. J.). — Prevention of prematurity. In: *Séminaire sur la prématurité et l'insuffisance pondérale du nouveau-né.* Centre International de l'enfance, 9-11 juin 1969, Paris.

[66] KRUGER (P. S.). — Risk factors and pregnancy outcome among air force women. *Milit. Med.*, *144*, 788-791, 1979.

[67] KUBLI (F.). — In: *Preterm labor.* Proceeding of the fifth congress of the Royal College of Obstetricians and Gynaecologists. ANDERSON (A.), BEARD (R.), BRUDENELL (J. M.), DUNN (P. M.), London, 1978.

[68] KUCERA (H.), PAVELKA (R.), FUDELSTORFER (B.), REINOLD (E.). — The influence of socio-economic factors on the results of a prematurity dysmaturity prevention programme. *Wien Lin Wochenschr.*, *89*, 307-311, 1977.

[69] LAMBOTTE (R.). — In: *Preterm Labor.* Proceedings of the fifth study group of the Royal College of Obstetricians and Gynaecologists, 5-6 October 1977, Londres.

[70] LAUKARAN (V. H.), VAN DEN BERG (B. J.). — The relationship of maternal attitude to pregnancy outcomes and obstetric complications: a cohort study of unwanted pregnancy. *Am. J. Obstet. Gynecol.*, *136*, 374-379, 1980.

[71] LAZAR (P.), GUEGUEN (S.), DREYFUS (J.), PAPIERNIK (E.), RENAUD (R.), PONTONNIER (G.). — Multicentrered controlled trial of cervical cerclage

in women at moderate risk of preterm delivery. *Brit. J. Obst. Gyn.*, *91*, 731-735, 1984.

[72] LEHMANN (W. D.). — Die reisende Schwangere. *Munchen Med. Wschr.*, *118*, 1079-1082, 1976.

[73] LEES (D. H.), SUTHERST (J. R.). — The sequelae of cervical trauma. *Am. J. Obstet. Gynecol.*, *118*, 1050-1054, 1974.

[74] LEWIN (D.), SADOUL (G.), SYLVAIN LEROY (B.), MORY (I.). — Aspects échotomographiques de la béance isthmique pendant la grossesse. *La nouvelle presse médicale*, *7*, 2133-2136, 1978.

[75] LIGGINS (G. C.), HOWIE (R. N.). — A controlled trial of antepartum glucocorticoid treatment for prevention of the respiratory distress syndrome in premature infants. *Pediatrics*, *50*, 515-524, 1972.

[76] LIGGINS (G. C.), HOWIE (R. N.). — Clinical trial of antepartum betamethasone therapy for prevention of respiratory distress in preterm infants. *Preterm labor*, 1 vol. Proceeding of the 5th study group of the Royal College of Obstetricians and Gynaecologists. Ed. ANDERSON (A.), BEARD (R.), BRUDENELL (J. M.), DUNN (P. M.), London, 1978.

[77] LIPSHITZ (J.). — Cerclage in the treatment of incompetent cervix. *S. Afr. Med. J.*, *49*, 2013-2015, 1975.

[78] LORING (T. W.). — Pregnancy and uterine malformations. *Am. J. Obstet. Gynecol.*, *116*, 505-510, 1973.

[79] MAMELLE (N.), LAUMON (B.), LAZAR (P.). — Prematurity and occupational activity during pregnancy. *Am. J. Epidemiol.*, *119*, 309-322, 1984.

[80] MAYER (M.), MORIN (F.). — L'activité professionnelle de la femme enceinte, son influence sur la grossesse. *Rev. Hyg. Soc.*, *7*, 596-609, 1969.

[81] MARQUET (G.), MICHEL BRIAND (C.), QUICHON (R.), SCHIRRER (J.). — Influence de la situation professionnelle de la femme sur l'enfant à naître. *Arch. Mal. Prof.*, *37*, 329-346, 1976.

[82] McCORMACK (W. M.), BRAUN (P.), LEE (Y. H.), KLEIN (J. O.), KASS (E. H.). — The genital mycoplasma. *The New Engl. J. Med.*, *288*, 78-89, 1973.

[83] McCORMACK (W. M.). — Management of sexually transmissible infections during pregnancy. *Clin. Obstet. Gynecol.*, *1*, 5772, 1975.

[84] MEAD (P. B.), CLAPP (J. F.). — The use of betamethasone and timed delivery in management of premature rupture of the membranes in the preterm pregnancy. *J. Reprod. Med.*, *19*, 3-7, 1977.

[85] MELCHIOR (J.), BERNARD (N.). — *Prématurité et coefficient de risque calculé.* Séminaire « Usage de l'informatique en obstétrique ». Institut de Recherche Informatique et d'Automatique, 8-9 décembre 1975.

[86] NAEYE (R. L.), BLANC (W. A.). — Relation of poverty and race to antenatal infection. *New Engl. J. Med.*, *283*, 555-560, 1970.

[87] NAEYE (R. L.), DELLINGER (W. S.), BLANC (W. A.). — Fœtal and maternal features of antenatal bacterial infections. *Pediatrics*, *79*, 733-739, 1971.

[88] NESBITT (R. E. L.), AUBRY (R. H.). — High risk obstetrics. II. Value of semiobjective grading system in identifying the vulnerable group. *Am. J. Obstet. Gynecol.*, *103*, 972-985, 1969.

[89] NIEBYL (J. R.), BLAKE (D. A.), WHITE (R. D.), KUMOR (K. M.), DUBIN (N. H.), ROBINSON (J. C.), EGNER (P. G.). — The inhibition of premature labor with indomethacin. *Am. J. Obstet. Gynecol.*, *136*, 1014-1019, 1980.

[90] PANTEKALIS (S. N.), PAPADIMITRIOU (G. C.), DOXIADIS (S. A.). — Influence of induced and spontaneous abortions on the outcome of subsequent pregnancies. *Am. J. Obstet. Gynecol.*, *116*, 799-805, 1973.

[91] PAPAEVANGELOU (G.), VRETTOS (A. S.), PAPADATOS (C.), ALEXIOU (D.). — The effect of spontaneous and induced abortion on prematurity and birthweight. *J. Obstet. Gynecol. of the Brit. Commonwealth*, *80*, 418-422, 1973.

[92] PAPAGEORGIOU (A. N.), DESGRANGES (M. F.), MASSION (M.), COLLE (E.), SHATZ (R.), CELFANOL (M. M.). — Antenatal use of betamethasone in prevention of respiratory distress syndrome. A controlled double blind study. *Pediatrics*, *63*, 73-79, 1979.

[93] PAPIERNIK (E.). — Le coefficient de risque d'accouchement prématuré. *Presse Médicale*, *77*, 793-794, 1969.

[94] PAPIERNIK (E.). — Morts périnatales évitables par une action prénatale. *J. Gynécol. Obstét. Biol. Reprod.*, *7*, 605-610, 1978.

[95] PAPIERNIK (E.). — Prévention de la prématurité : résultats et limites en 1978. *Gynak. Rundschau.*, *18* (suppl.), 100-112, 1978.

[96] PAPIERNIK (E.). — *Preterm labor.* Royal College of Obstetricians and Gynaecologists, London, 1979.

[97] PAPIERNIK (E.), HULT (A. M.). — A prospective study of the prevention of prematurity and dysmaturity. *Perinat. Med.*, *IV*, 325-330, 1973.

[98] PAPIERNIK (E.), LEROY (B.), MASSE (N.), PAJSZCZYK-KIESZKIEWICZ (T.), SCHARTZ (D.), VIALA (J. L.). — *Vers une grossesse sans risque*, 1 vol., Nestlé Guigoz, Éd., Paris, 1973.

[99] PAPIERNIK (E.). — La grossesse et les déficiences intellectuelles de l'enfant. *Arch. Franç. Pédiat.*, *35*, 10-14, 1978.

[100] PAPIERNIK (E.), KAMINSKI (M.). — Multifactorial study of the risk of prematurity at 32 weeks of gestation. I. A study of the frequency of 30 predictive characteristics. *J. Perin. Med.*, *2*, 30-35, 1974.

[101] PAPIERNIK (E.). — Proposals for a programmed prevention policy of preterm birth. *Clinical Obstetrics and Gynecology*, *27*, 614-635, 1984.

[102] PAPIERNIK (E.), BOUYER (J.), DREYFUS (J.), COLLIN (D.), WINISDORFFER (G.), GUEGUEN (S.), LECOMTE (M.), LAZAR (P.). — Prevention of preterm births: a perinatal study in Haguenau, France. *Pediatrics*, *76*, 154-158, 1985.

[103] PETERSON (P. G.), KEIFER (W. S.). — Diagnosis of an incompetent internal cervical os. *Am. J. Obstet. Gynecol.*, *116*, 498-504, 1973.

[104] PEZ (J. P.). — Étude de 300 cerclages. *Thèse de médecine*, Paris, 1974.

[105] PINARD (A.). — Note pour servir à l'histoire de la puériculture. *Bull. Soc. Méd. Publ. et d'Hyg. Prof.*, *XVIII*, 326, 1895.

[106] POMERANCE (J. J.), UKRAINSKI (C. T.), UKRA (R.), HENDERSON (D. H.), NASH (A. H.), MEREDITH (J. L.). — Cost of living for infants weighing 1,000 g or less ar birth. *Pediatrics*, *61*, 908-910, 1978.

[107] RAIHA (C. E.). — Prematurity: its social consequences and our possibilities of decreasing the

number of premature babies. *Biol. Neonat. Basel,* *1,* 113, 1959.

[108] RANTAKALLIO (P.). — Group at risk in low birth weight infants and perinatal mortality. *Acta paediatr. Scand.,* Suppl. 193, 1969.

[109] REBELLO (R.), GREEN (F. H. Y.), FOX (H.). — A study of the secretory immune system of the femal genital trav. *Brit. H. Obstet. Gynecol.,* *82,* 812-816, 1975.

[110] ROBERSON (N. R. C.), TIZARD (J. P. M.). — Prognosis for infants with idiopathic respiratory distress syndrome. *Brit. Med. J.,* *3,* 271-274, 1975.

[111] ROOTH (F.). — Better perinatal health: Sweden. *Lancet,* December 1st, 1979.

[112] ROUVILLOIS (J. L.), PAPIERNIK (E.), AMIEL-TISON (C.). — Prophylaxie de l'infection en cas de rupture prématurée des membranes. A propos de 150 cas traités par antibiotiques et tocolytiques. *Gynéc. Obstét. Biol. Reprod.,* *2,* 271-281, 1973.

[113] RUBIN (R. A.), ROSENBLATT (C.), BALOW (B.). — Psychological and educational sequelae of prematurity. *Pediatrics,* *52,* 352-363, 1973.

[114] RYAN (G. M.), SCHNEIDER (J. M.). — Teenage obstetric complications. *Cl. Obstet. Gynecol.,* *21,* 1191-1197, 1978.

[115] RYAN (G. M.), SWEENEY (P. J.), SOLOLA (A. S.). — Prenatal care and pregnancy outcome. *Am. J. Obstet. Gynecol.,* *137,* 876-881, 1980.

[116] SALING (E.). — Prämaturitäts und Dysmaturitäts Präventions program (PDP Program). *Z. Geburtsh. U. Perinatol.,* 70-81, 1972.

[117] SARTI (D. A.), SAMPLE (W. F.), HOBEL (C. H.), STAISCH (K. J.). — Ultrasonic visualisation of a dilated cervix during pregnancy. *Radiology,* *130,* 417-420, 1979.

[118] SCHWARTZ (A.), BROOK (I.), INSLER (V.), KOHEN (F.), ZOR (U.), LINDNER (H. R.). — Effect of flufenamic acid on uterine contractions and plasma level of 15 keto 13,14 dihydroprostaglandin F2 in a preterm labor. *Gynec. Obstet. Investig.,* *9,* 139-149, 1978.

[119] SHIELDS (J. R.), RESNIK (R.). — Fœtal lung maturation and the antenatal use of glucocorticoids to prevent the respiratory distress syndrome. *Obstet. Gynec. Survey,* *34,* 343-363, 1979.

[120] SILVERMAN (W. A.). — In: *Duham's premature infants,* 1 vol., 3rd ed., 2nd printing, New York, Hoeber, 1964.

[121] SPEARING (G.). — Alcohol, indomethacin and salbutamo. A comparative trial of their use in preterm labor. *Obstet. Gynecol.,* *53,* 171-174, 1979.

[122] SPIRA (N.), COUCHARD (M.), PAPIERNIK (E.), LEFEBVRE (C.), JOURDAN (A.), BETHAMN (O.), MINKOWSKI (A.). — *Caractéristiques des mères des nouveau-nés hospitalisés dans un centre de réanimation néonatale.* 5es journées internationales de médecine périnatale (Le Touquet, 1975). Arnette, *Cahier médical,* 91-101, 1976.

[123] STEWART (A. L.). — A note on the obstetric effects of work. *Brit. J. Prev. Soc. Med.,* *9,* 159-161, 1955.

[124] STEWART (A. L.), REYNOLDS (O. R.). — Improved prognosis for infants of very low birthweight *Pediatrics,* *54,* 724-813, 1974.

[125] STEWART (A. L.), TURCAN (D.), RAWLINGS (C.),

HART (S.), GREGORY (S.). — *Outcome for infants at high risk of major handicap.* Ciba Found Symp., *59,* 151-171, 1978.

[126] STICKLE (G.), MA (P.). — Some social and medical correlates of pregnancy outcome. *Am. J. Obstet. Gynecol.,* *127,* 162-166, 1977.

[127] STOLTE (L.), ESKES (T.). — *Cervical incompetence.* 5th World Congress Gynaec. Butterworths, Sydney, WOOD and WALTES, 729, 1967.

[128] TERRIS (M.), GOLD (E. M.). — An epidemiologic study of prematurity. I. Relation to smoking, heart volume, employment and physique. *Am. J. Obstet. Gynecol.,* *103,* 358-370, 1969.

[129] TERRIS (M.), GOLD (E. M.). — An epidemiologic study of prematurity. II. Relationship to prenatal care, birth interval, residential history and outcome of previous pegnancies. *Am. J. Obstet. Gynecol.,* *103,* 371-379, 1969.

[130] TERRIS (M.), GLASSER (M.). — A life table analysis of the relation of prenatal care to prematurity. *A. J. P. H.,* *64,* 869-875, 1974.

[131] THALHAMMER (O.). — Verhütung von Frühgeburtlichkeit und pränataler Dystrophie I : ein einfaches System zur Vorausberechnung des Frühgeburts Risikos sowie des Aufwandes und Nutzens bei Ausschaltung von Risiko faktoren. *Z. Geburtsh. Perinat.,* *177,* 169-177, 1973.

[132] THIBEAULT (D. W.), EMMANOUILIDES (G. C.). — Prolonged rupture of fœtal membranes and decreased frequency of respiratory distress syndrome and patent ductus arteriosus in preterm infants. *Am. J. Obstet. Gynecol.,* *129,* 43-46, 1977.

[133] THORNFELDT (R. E.), FRANKLIN (R. W.), PICKERING (N. A.), THORNFELDT (C. R.), AMELL (G.). — The effect of glucocorticoids on the maturation of premature lung membranes: preventing the respiratory distress syndrome by glucocorticoids. *Am. J. Obstet. Gynecol.,* *131,* 143-148, 1978.

[134] TIMONEN (S.), UOTILA (U.), KUUSISTO (P.), VARA (P.), LOKKI (O.). — Effect of certain maternal, fœtal and geographical factors on the weight and length of the newborn and the duration of pregnancy. *Ann. Chir. Gynaec. Fenn.,* *55,* 196, 1966.

[135] TOAFF (R.), TOAFF (M. E.), BALLAS (S.), OPHIR (A..) — Cervical incompetence: diagnosis and therapeutic aspects. *Israel J. Med. Sci.,* *13,* 39-49, 1977.

[136] VIGNIER (B. I.), CHAPALAIN (M. T.), PAPIERNIK (E.). *La périnatalité, étude de rationalisation des choix budgétaires,* 3 vol. Pour une politique de santé. Documentation française, 1971.

[137] WEEKES (A. R. L.), MENZIES (D. N.), WEST (C. R.). — Spontaneous premature birth in twin pregnancy. *Brit. Med. J.,* *2,* 16-18, 1977.

[138] WEEKES (A. R. L.), FLYNN (M. S.). — Engagement of the fetal head in primigravida and its relationship to duration of gestation and time of onset of labour. *Brit. J. Obstet. Gynecol.,* *82,* 711, 1975.

[139] WEENER (W. J.), YOUNG (E. B.). — Non specific data at last menstrual period. An indication of poor reproductive outcome. *Am. J. Obstet. Gynecol.,* *82,* 711, 1975.

[140] WEIDINGER (H.), WIEST (W.). — A comparative study of the epidemiological data of pregnancies with and without tendencies to premature delivery. *J. Perinat. Med.,* *2,* 276-287, 1974.

[141] WIDMAIER (C.), REICHARDT (H. D.). — Erfahrungen mit einer erweiterten indikationsstellung zur Zervix-Cerclage in der Schwangerschaft. *Abl. Gynak.*, *95*, 16-21, 1973.

[142] WOOD (C.), BANNERMAN (R. H. O.), BOOTH (R. T.), PINKERTON (J. J. M.). — The prediction of premature labor by observation of the cervix and external tocography. *Am. J. Obstet. Gynecol.*, *91*, 396-402, 1965.

[143] ZACKLER (J.), ANDELMAN (S. L.), BAUER (F.). — The young adolescent as an obstetric risk. *Am. J. Obstet. Gynecol.*, *103*, 305-312, 1969.

[144] ZOLTRAN (I.). — The prognosis of twins and prematurity. *Acta Genet. Med. Gemellol.*, *22*, 7-9, 1974.

Intrauterine growth retardation

MALCOLM I. LEVENE, VICTOR DUBOWITZ

INTRODUCTION

Birth is an event which releases the fetus from its confined aquatic intrauterine environment into a breathing world which it must rapidly adapt to. The process of development is in part unrelated to the timing of birth and the rate of growth is unaffected by the change from fetal to neonatal life. Birth may liberate the fetus from a hostile environment in which poor nutrition and chronic hypoxia has caused the fetus to grow poorly and adequate postnatal nutrition may restore the infant to its full growth potential.

Knowledge of normal prenatal growth and intrauterine growth retardation are important and care of the poorly growing fetus must be shared by the perinatologist and the neonatologist. Gruenwald [35] in his original description of intrauterine growth retardation or as he described it, chronic fetal distress, found that the perinatal mortality and morbidity rates were very much higher in growth retarded fetuses. This is in contrast to the infant born prematurely who has a much higher risk of neonatal morbidity and mortality. An increased perinatal mortality rate of between four and eightfold compared with normally growing pregnancies has been reported throughout the world and close monitoring of these high risk pregnancies is necessary.

The mortality rate for any gestational age and birth weight can be predicted by studying large groups of infants. Figure I-38 illustrates such a graph derived from the late fetal and neonatal mortality rates from the British 1958 Perinatal Mortality Survey [33]. In general, the more severely growth retarded a fetus or infant is, the higher will be his chance of dying and in most cases this is more important as a risk factor than the degree of prematurity. Intrauterine growth retardation must not be considered to be only a neonatal problem. By identifying the at-risk pregnancy, and with careful monitoring and timely delivery, the infant may be given to the neonatologist in the best possible condition.

TERMINOLOGY

Increased mortality associated with early delivery and the identification of at-risk infants made necessary an international definition for prematurity. In 1948 the World Health Organisation decided that infants with birth weight less than or equal to 2,500 g should be designated "premature". Far from defining an homogeneous group of infants it became apparent that many so-called prematures behaved in a more

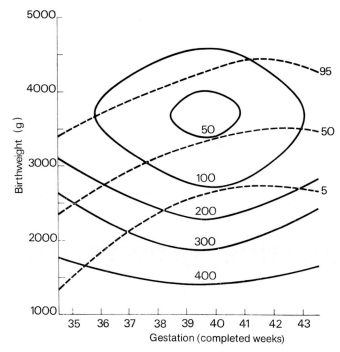

FIG. I-38. — *The late fetal and neonatal mortality rates by birthweight and gestation from the 1958 perinatal mortality survey* (GOLDSTEIN and PECKHAM) [33].

mature manner, and in 1961 the World Health Organisation decided that infants weighing less than 2,500 g at birth should be described as being "of low birthweight". Low birthweight could mean short gestation or poor intrauterine growth and in 1963 Gruenwald [35] and Lubchenco [46] almost simultaneously published papers that permitted differentiation of these two entities on a birth weight/gestational age basis. Gruenwald defined a group of infants whose birthweight was two standard deviations below the mean (third centile), and referred to these as "small for dates". These infants had much higher perinatal mortality and morbidity rates than infants with normal intra-uterine growth patterns. Lubchenco published data on 5,635 liveborn infants from 24 to 42 weeks post-menstrual age and produced the first birth weight for gestational age chart defining the tenth and ninetieth centiles. To avoid confusion the American Academy of Pediatrics in 1966 defined "small for gestational" age as those infants whose birth weight was below the tenth centile for post-menstrual age.

Unfortunately, confusion in nomenclature remains as some workers refer to the tenth centile, others to the fifth and yet others to the third as their criteria for diagnosing small for gestational age

(SGA) infants. In addition many terms have been coined to describe this condition. Light for dates, small for dates, dysmaturity and chronic fetal distress as well as SGA have all been used. In this discussion, SGA or intrauterine growth retardation (IUGR) will be used exclusively. It is important to describe newborn infants in terms of gestational age rather than birth weight and this is practical even in infants born to mothers with uncertain dates using schemes for assessment of gestational age [22]. Babies can then be referred to as preterm (below 38 weeks gestation [4]), small for gestational age, large for gestational age (above the 90th centile) or a combination of these. A definition of SGA dependent on weight is convenient as birth weight is an easy measurement to make; however, length, occipito-frontal head circumference and skin fold thickness also give important information on the state of growth and nutrition of the fetus and new-born infant.

GROWTH STANDARDS

Weight centiles for gestational age are useful only if the population from which they are derived

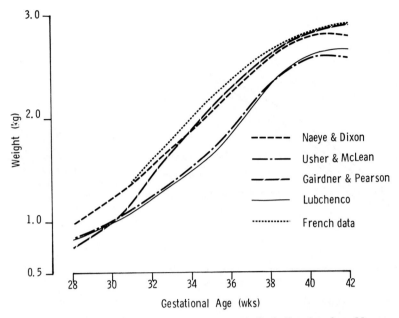

FIG. I-39. — *Composite chart for weight showing the 10th centile* (including data from NAEYE and DIXON [52]) *or the third centile* (USHER and MCLEAN [67]) *from different populations.*

is stated. There is considerable variation in birth weight dependent on sex, race, socio-economic class and many other factors. The most widely used weight centile charts are those devised by Lubchenco and her colleagues [46], from Denver, Colorado. The cohort studied were Caucasian live born infants derived from a population living at an altitude of 5,000 feet. The effect of this height on the fetus is to reduce the birth weight at term by an average of 400 g compared to an infant born at sea level [43]. Usher and MacLean [67] produced similar weight charts from infants born at sea level and Figure I-39 compares the Lubchenco tenth centile with the Usher and MacLean third centile. These lines are almost identical, emphasising the skew of the Denver data.

In Britain, Gairdner and Pearson's charts are most commonly used but this data is derived from multiple sources, from more than one country and in more mature infants only second or subsequently born babies have been included [31]. Figure I-39 also compares the tenth centile from the English chart to American and French [8] populations. There is a very close relationship between British and French birth weight centiles.

The weight of a newborn infant is of limited value unless compared to length and other body measurements. Growth charts of crown-heel length will suffer from the same bias as weight charts depending on the local population from which it is gathered. Figure I-40 shows length by gestational age from various sources comparing the tenth to the third centiles. Figure I-41 compares occipito-

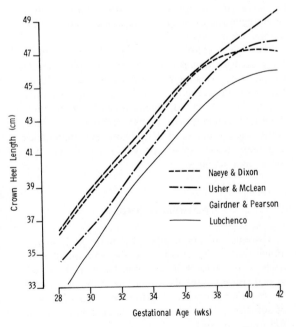

FIG. I-40. — *Composite chart for crown heel length showing the 10th centile* (USHER and MCLEAN [67]) *from different populations.*

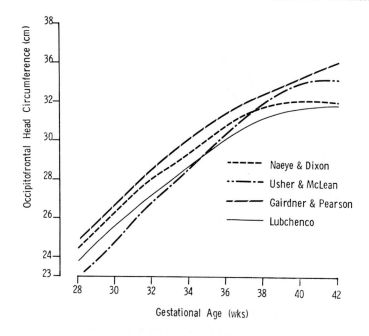

FIG. I-41. — *Composite chart for occipito-frontal head circumference showing the 10th centile or third centile (*USHER *and* MCLEAN [67]) *from different populations.*

frontal head circumference in a similar manner. Although measurements of length and head circumference are more difficult than an estimate of weight, regular practice will rapidly produce minimal interobservor error. Commercially produced neonatal crown-heel measuring devices are readily available, and a non-stretch flexible tape of steel or fibreglass is essential for accurate head circumference measurements.

The Denver charts consistently show tenth centile body measurements at or below the third centile for other American data in infants born at sea level. British (and presumably French) babies are generally slightly larger in all measurements than their American counterparts. Female infants are consistently slightly smaller in all measurements than males and most growth charts provide separate data for males and females.

PONDERAL INDEX

Absolute measurements of length and weight alone give no information on the amount of soft-tissue mass present in any one baby. Intrauterine growth retardation may leave an infant wasted of fat but of reasonable length. The relative amount of soft-tissue mass present can be calculated on the following formula:

$$\frac{\text{weight (g)}}{(\text{crown heel length (cm)})^3} \times 100$$

This is referred to as the ponderal index (PI). A low number represents a disproportionately long infant with little soft tissue mass. Miller and Hassanein [49] have calculated centiles for PI against gestational age in 1,692 infants (Fig. I-42). They conclude that infants with PIs below the third centile were considered to be malnourished either from failure to accumulate adequate soft-tissue mass or from excessive wasting of soft tissues.

SKIN FOLD THICKNESS

A more direct estimation of the amount of subcutaneous fat can be made by skin fold thickness. This measurement is made with a special spring loaded caliper and a double layer of skin is assessed at various sites, usually the triceps or subscapular region. Figure I-43 shows centile charts for triceps skinfold thickness from 37 to 42 weeks gestational age [54]. No data exists for infants below 37 weeks and the application of this technique is therefore limited to the more mature infant.

In conclusion, it is clearly important to consider various body measurements before concluding that an infant is normally grown. Two infants of identical weight and gestational age may have varying lengths, PIs and skin fold thickness but one may have suffered severe intrauterine growth retardation and have little soft tissue mass with low skinfold thickness, and the other may be shorter

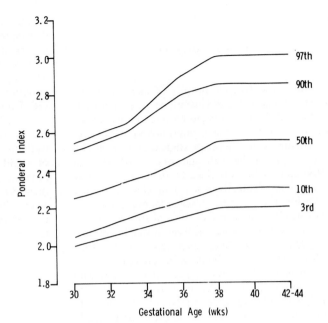

FIG. I-42. — *Range of ponderal index for gestational age* (from MILLER and HASSANEIN [49]).

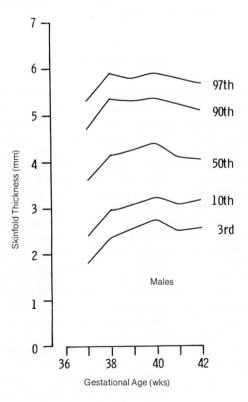

FIG. I-43. — *Range of skinfold thickness for gestational age* (from OAKLEY, PARSONS and WHITELAW [54]).

in length and well nourished. A variety of anthropometric measurements are available and all should be used in the investigation of intrauterine growth retardation.

INCIDENCE

Birth weight for a given maturity follows a Gaussian distribution and centile charts of birth weight by gestational age will identify the lower range of a *normal* population. Babies who are small for pathological reasons will be more likely found in the lower centile groups, but being placed below the tenth or third centile does not diagnose abnormality. 3 % of normal children will have a birth weight below the third centile.

If the tenth centile is used to identify SGA infants, then theoretically the incidence of this condition should be 10 % of a population. As discussed above the use of centile charts derived from a different population to the one sampled will invalidate the expected incidence and this will vary from population to population. Studies of large numbers of consecutive deliveries stating the frequency of diagnosis of SGA infants are rare. Using the Lubchenco charts for weight, the incidence of SGA (below the tenth centile) newborns was found variously as 0.8 % (Cap Bon, Tunisia), 1.6 % (Providence, Rhode Island), 4.3 % (New York State) and 7.6 % (Birmingham, Alabama).

FETAL GROWTH

Growth is a dynamic process of increase in the size of organs and consequently of the organism. Protein and lipid are integrated into cellular structure thus shaping organ morphology and size. Growth has been extensively studied by Winick [70] who has shown that cell numbers (based on total DNA) initially increase linearly, then begin to slow in rate, and eventually reach a maximum number well before the organ has reached its maximum size. To explain this he describes three phases of growth. The first is proportional increase in weight, protein and DNA content (increasing cell number), then a slower increase in DNA accretion than that of protein or weight (fewer number of new cells with simultaneous hypertrophy of existing ones), and finally no further increase in DNA content, but with continuing increase in net protein and weight (hypertrophy alone).

In the fetus, the rate of growth and maturation of organs vary widely but growth is influenced by placental function. In early pregnancy placental function far exceeds the growth requirements of the fetus and the growth rate depends largely on fetal or maternal factors. It is generally not until the last trimester that the fetal requirements may exceed placental function. The placenta continues to grow until 36 to 38 weeks of gestation before weight gain becomes static. This is about two to four weeks earlier than fetal weight increase significantly slows, and the ratio of fetal to placental weight changes in the third trimester from 5 : 1 to 7 : 1.

Hormonal growth control in fetal animals has been much studied [44]. Growth hormone, adrenal and probably thyroid hormones have little effect on prenatal linear growth. Insulin however appears to have the most potent effect on the regulation of fetal size. Differential organ growth is poorly understood but recently examination of the fetus by ultrasound has provided important information on normal growth of various organs. The conceptus is first detected by ultrasound in the third week after fertilisation and accurate measurement of embryonic crown-heel length is possible by 6 to 14 weeks. Linear growth is exponential up to 12 weeks and thereafter is linear. In the first trimester, length increases by about 10 mm per week [10].

Somatic growth may also be dependent on brain development and interference with cerebral development even for a short time at critical stages may significantly reduce eventual birth weight. The developing brain has two growth spurts. The first occurs at 10 to 18 weeks and is due to neuroblast multiplication to near adult numbers of neurones. The second occurs between 24 and 34 weeks of gestation due to a massive proliferation of glial cells from the germinal matix of the caudate nucleus. The cerebellum has a late growth spurt towards the end of the third trimester and continues until well after birth. At around term there is also a phase of rapid myelination and increasing numbers of synaptic connections. Organ growth and development does not stop at birth but continues for many years. The manner by which individual organs and the organism as a whole grows may be primed in the prenatal period.

CAUSES OF IUGR

The rate of prenatal growth is governed directly by three factors; maternal, fetal and placental. Table I lists the known cause of intrauterine growth retardation by these categories.

FETAL FACTORS

Chromosomally abnormal babies are often born small. In Down's Syndrome (Trisomy 21) gestation is often shortened, but growth retardation usually occurs despite this. Similarly in Trisomy 13 there is usually mild growth retardation whereas infants with Trisomy 18 are usually severely growth retarded with a mean birthweight of 2,200 g at 42 weeks. Trisomy syndromes are associated with intellectual retardation (often severe) and show characteristic dysmorphic features. The diagnosis is confirmed by chromosomal analysis. Apart from Down's syndrome survival beyond six months is unusual.

Turner's syndrome (X0) has a regular constellation of abnormal features including growth retardation but is often associated with normal intellect. There are a number of rare dysmorphic syndromes with normal chromosomes that are associated with intrauterine growth retardation. Table II lists these syndromes together with a brief description of each.

The commonest fetal cause of IUGR is prenatal viral infection and the commonest virus to cause this condition is rubella. Examination of the fetus may suggest this diagnosis if some of the charac-

TABLE I. — VARIOUS CAUSES OF INTRAUTERINE GROWTH RETARDATION

Fetal	*Placental*	*Maternal*
1. Chromosomal abnormalities: Trisomy 13 (Patau's syndrome), Trisomy 18 (Edward's syndrome), Trisomy 21 (Down's syndrome), Turner's syndrome (X0), Cri du chat syndrome.	1. Toxaemia of pregnancy. 2. "Placental vascular insufficiency". 3. Multiple pregnancy.	1. Maternal disease: Cyanotic heart disease, Anaemia, Hypertension, Structural uterine abnormality, Urinary tract infection [1], Arteritis.
2. Prenatal viral infection: Rubella, CMV, Toxoplasmosis.	4. Small placental size. 5. Site of implantation. 6. Vascular transfusion in monochorial twin placentas.	2. Toxins: Alcohol, Cigarette smoking, Narcotics.
3. Dysmorphogenesis (see Table II).	7. Chorioangioma.	3. Malnutrition.
4. Ionizing radiation.		4. Altitude.
5. Drugs [1].		5. Short stature [1].
		6. Low socio-economic class [1].
		7. Maternal age (young or old) [1].

[1] Evidence for this as a cause of IUGR is not good.

TABLE II. — SOME DYSMORPHIC SYNDROMES ASSOCIATED WITH INTRAUTERINE GROWTH RETARDATION.

Invariably associated with intrauterine growth retardation:

Silver's syndrome.	Prenatal dwarfism, body asymmetry.
Sekel's bird headed dwarfism.	Characteristic facies, microcephaly low IQ.
Bloom's syndrome.	Photosensitivity, high risk of malignancy.
Dubowitz's syndrome.	Eczema, characteristic facies.

Commonly associated with intrauterine growth retardation:

Progeria.	Dwarfism, alopecia, premature senility.
Kenny syndrome.	Dwarfism, dense tubular bones.
Prader-Willi syndrome.	Dwarfism, obesity, hypogonadism, hypotonia, low IQ.
Smith-Lemli-Opitz.	Reduced growth, characteristic facies, genital anomalies.
Cornelia de Lange syndrome.	Physical and intellectual retardation, abnormal facies.
Occulo-cerebro-renal syndrome.	Low IQ, cataracts and tubular abnormalities.
Asphyxiating thoracic dystrophy.	Thoracic constriction, dwarfism.

Sometimes associated with intrauterine growth retardation:

Treacher-Collins syndrome.	Malar and mandibular abnormalities, eye and ear involvement.
Menkes' syndrome.	Cerebral deterioration, abnormal hair.
Ataxia telangiectasia.	Ataxia, telangiectasia and immunological deficiency.
Rubenstein-Taybi syndrome.	Low IQ, broad thumbs, growth limitation.
Ellis-Van Creveld syndrome.	Dwarfism, ectodermal dysplasia, polydactyly.

teristic features such as cataracts, hepatospleno-megaly, skin rashes, microcephaly or prolonged jaundice are present. In addition, other viruses such as cytomegalovirus and parasitic infestations such as toxoplasmosis of prenatal origin may cause intrauterine growth retardation. Any process that will interfere with the early brain growth spurt will cause stunting of somatic growth. Excessive radiation may do this and certain drugs (e. g. steroids) have been implicated but not proven.

PLACENTAL FACTORS

Toxaemia of pregnancy together with essential hypertension are the commonest causes of IUGR in developed countries, and account for about one third of all SGA infants. The placenta of growth retarded infants often shows specific abnormalities, particularly if associated with toxaemia. The placental weight usually correlates more closely with the birth weight than with the length of gestation although in some growth retarded infants the placenta is disproportionately larger for their body weight. This may be associated with transplacental viral infection.

The pathological abnormalities usually affect primarily the blood vessels. Small infarcts of less than 3 cm are commonly seen with or without multiple micro-infarcts, associated with occlusion of small vessels, proliferation of the intima and much intervillous fibrin deposition. Ischaemic involution of chorionic villi and excessive overgrowth of the trophoblast with groups of avascular villi are also reported. The mechanism of placental dysfunction is probably a reactive vasculitis in response to hypertension which consequently retards utero-placental blood flow. This may be a patchy process and the severity of fetal growth retardation will depend on the extent of the placental involvement.

Partial placental abruption insufficient to cause fetal death, large or multiple haemangiomas and large vessel placental thrombosis may all cause in utero growth retardation. Rarely abnormalities of the placenta such as choriangioma or other tumours may affect its function. If the demands on placental function exceed its supply then growth failure will occur. This happens in multiple pregnancies but only occurs in the last trimester from about 34 weeks onwards. Not uncommonly, the placenta of one twin is smaller than the other, or the umbilical cord of the smaller monozygotic twin is inserted marginally into one edge of the placenta with vessels running to only a small proportion of the placental surface. Very rarely early twin to twin transfusion may cause discrepant size.

MATERNAL FACTORS

In world wide terms, maternal malnutrition is probably the commonest cause of IUGR. Limited food supply, parasites and poverty are common features in underdeveloped countries and infants born in this environment are significantly smaller than in developed countries. Studies in Guatemala [36] have shown that caloric supplementation in pregnancy increases the average weight of the baby at term by 50 g for every 10,000 kcal consumed by the mother. They showed that nutritional supplement caused the numbers of infants weighing more than 2.5 kg at birth to be increased by 40 % and suggested that by improving birth weight perinatal mortality rates may also fall. This has enormous implications in improving perinatal care in developing countries.

Periods of acute nutritional deprivation in developed countries such as during wartime also reduce the birthweight. Women who were pregnant during the siege of Leningrad or during the post war Dutch famine had smaller infants than those born before or after this time. Unfortunately poverty and poor nutrition exists in so-called affluent countries and this is an important cause of IUGR. Pre-pregnancy weight is important in predicting fetal malnutrition; those women who weigh less than 120 lbs (54 kg) at conception had a high incidence of low birthweight infants. Similarly, small weight gain during pregnancy of less than 11 lbs (5 kg) is also associated with poor fetal growth [25]. If these women can be identified and adequate nutrition given in the last trimester, improved fetal weight gain will occur. Conversely, abnormally large weight gain in pregnancy is associated with increased birth weight, and obese women give birth to infants who also have more subcutaneous fat than controls [69].

The evidence for short maternal stature causing IUGR in the same way as for low weight is not good. Ounsted suggests however that slow intrauterine growth is due in part to constraint exercised by a maternal regulator and if the mother herself was born small then her own babies were likely to be smaller than controls [55]. This is likely to be independent of paternal size. The socioeconomic class of the woman probably only acts on fetal size indirectly through the associated factors of nourishment, smoking, maternal size and antenatal care.

A maternal haemoglobin of less than 6.5 g/dl will on the average reduce the birth weight by 400 g compared to controls with a haemoglobin of 10.5g /dl or more [48]. Structural uterine abnormalities may inhibit growth by constraint and vasculitis as found in systemic lupus erythematosus or polyarteritis nodosa affecting uterine vessels will reduce placental blood flow. Most women however with systemic lupus erythematosus produce babies of normal size.

Excessive intake of alcohol in pregnancy is now well recognised as a potent cause of IUGR and congenital malformations. Almost all affected infants are severely growth retarded affecting length and head circumference as well as weight. Many have a characteristic facies with short palpebral fissures, epicanthic folds, maxillary hypoplasia, micrognathia, thin upper lip and occasionally cleft palate. Cardiac abnormalities are sometimes seen (usually septal defects) as well as joint, limb and genital abnormalities [42, 59]. Their later mental as well as physical development is often retarded. There is some evidence that lesser degrees of alcohol consumption if taken regularly through pregnancy are associated with less severe growth retardation. The fetal alcohol syndrome whilst common in the United States, is rarely seen in Britain.

Heroin addiction as well as other opiate abuse is associated with growth retardation [51] but this may in part be related to concurrent nutritional deficiencies. Cigarette smoking is the commonest agent producing IUGR. As little as five cigarettes a day may be associated with fetal growth impairment and mothers who smoke heavily have a three times higher chance of having growth retarded infants. In a study of all babies born in England and Wales in one week in 1958, smoking after the fourth month of pregnancy regardless of age, parity, social class, height or presence of severe pre-eclamptic toxaemia was found to significantly increase the risk of both fetal and neonatal death [9].

The relative importance of each of the above factors depends on the community studied. At an international symposium in 1974, a hypothetical distribution of causes of IUGR in the United Kingdom was compiled (Table III) [20]. If the tenth centile is again used as the definition of SGA infants then 10 % of the hypothetical total will be due to this normal variation. The commonest cause is utero-placental vascular disease of the mother which will largely be due to pre-eclamptic toxaemia and hypertension. With recent awareness of the potential hazards of smoking this as a cause of IUGR is a small proportion of the total. 32 % of infants have been allocated to miscellaneous

TABLE III. — SUGGESTED PERCENTAGE DISTRIBUTION OF CAUSES OF SMALL FOR GESTATIONAL AGE INFANTS IN THE UNITED KINGDOM (DAWES [20]).

Normal variation	10
Chromosomal and other congenital anomalies.	10
Infections (maternal and fetal). .	5 (perhaps <5?)
Poor uterus	1
Placenta and cord	2
Vascular disease in the mother. .	35
Drugs, medications and smoking.	5
Other.	32
	100

causes which includes many of the items listed the Table I.

ASSESSMENT OF FETAL WELL-BEING

The art of perinatology is to know when to intervene in a compromised pregnancy. In intrauterine growth retardation the fetus is considerably at risk and has a sixfold chance of dying in utero compared to a fetus of "optimal birth weight" [56]. The perinatologist needs to know in which pregnancy poor intrauterine growth is occurring, and should the fetus be left in utero or should he or she be removed prematurely from a hostile environment. The growth retarded infant tolerates the rigours of labour less well and the neonatologist should be forewarned and present at the birth in order to provide rapid and expert resuscitation to avoid the effects of birth asphyxia.

There is no precise way at present of determining these factors. In addition to physical examination of the mother, other techniques, such as ultrasound, aid the detection of IUGR. Function of the fetus is also important and many biochemical tests have been devised to follow the performance of the feto-placental unit. More recently the response of the fetus to external stimuli has been used as an index of fetal well-being and as a predictor of perinatal death.

CLINICAL EXAMINATION

The date of the last menstrual period is an aid to determining the age of the fetus as about 80 %

of pregnancies will terminate within two weeks on either side of this date. Unfortunately, many women are unsure of their dates, have irregular cycles or conceive within a short time of stopping the contraceptive pill and their uncertain dates are of little value in determining the estimated date of delivery of their progeny.

An early clinical examination during the first trimester is most likely to give an accurate estimate of duration of pregnancy. The height of the fundus however has often proven quite fallacious in estimating the duration of pregnancy particularly if the first assessment is delayed [21]. In a study of preterm SGA infants the diagnosis of intrauterine growth retardation was made in only 3 of 103 pregnancies, 75 of whom were high risk. In a British study only 29 % of infants whose birth weight was below the fifth centile were recognised clinically prior to birth [69]. Clinical examination is therefore a poor method of detecting IUGR.

ULTRASOUND

Over the last 20 years ultrasound has become the most widely used aid to assess fetal growth. Measurement of the biparietal diameter (BPD) has traditionally been used as an index of fetal size. A single measurement of the fetus before 20 weeks gestation (either BPD or crown-heel length) allows a prediction of fetal age which is better than clinical assessment or calculation from uncertain dates [10, 24]. As growth retardation often does not become apparent until the midle of the second trimester an early ultrasound measurement is an important yardstick by which to monitor an abnormal rate of fetal growth. Using serial BPD measurements made on ultrasound examination, 68 % of infants born small for gestational age (weight below the fifth centile for gestation in this study) were correctly identified antenatally, whilst only 30 % were detected clinically [11]. Campbell has described two patterns of abnormal fetal growth detected on ultrasound. The first shows normal head growth until the third trimester with a sudden reduction in the rate of growth from that time. This "late flattening" is usually associated with hypertensive disorder. The second type shows a persistent low growth rate usually from early in the second trimester without any tendency to cross centile lines in a downward direction. These infants at birth are usually symmetrically retarded in growth and the infant with chromosomal abnormalities often shows this growth pattern. The latter abnormal

growth curve is much less common than the late flattening type [10].

Ultrasound measurement of biparietal diameters has improved antenatal detection, but over 30 % of fetuses with IUGR will still be missed. In the more common asymmetric type of growth retardation, head growth is usually spared at the expense of impaired somatic growth. Measurement of abdominal circumference or diameter will reflect liver size which is usually reduced in this type of asymmetric growth retardation. A ratio of abdominal size to head size increases the detection rate of IUGR. The abdominal circumference is normally smaller than that of the head until 32 to 36 weeks of gestation, when the ratio approaches unity. If the abdominal circumference is measured at the level of the umbilical vein and its ratio to BPD used, then 87 % of babies whose birth weight was below the fifth centile for gestation could be detected before 32 weeks and 75 % at 36 weeks or more, provided that an early ultrasound scan had been performed so that gestational age was accurately known.

An estimate of fetal weight is the most useful measurement that could be used in diagnosing growth retardation. Multiple measurements of different fetal dimensions by ultrasound permits a mathematical model to be derived to calculate fetal weight. In one study this method produced a standard error in 20 patients of $\pm$ 106 g, but the process is time consuming and difficult and cannot be used as a routine test [50]. More recently a formula has been used to estimate fetal weight based on abdominal diameter, occipito-frontal head diameter and biparietal diameter measured on ultrasound. Close correlation between estimated weight and actual weight has been found in a small number of reported cases [6]. An estimate of total intrauterine volume including fetus, placenta and liquor predicted SGA infants (weight below the 10th centile for gestation) in 21 of 28 cases. No normally grown infant was thought to be growth retarded on ultrasound estimations in this study [32]. Ultrasound provides the best estimate of IUGR, but at present still does not routinely detect more than three quarters of SGA infants near term. Larger series using multiple measurements and volumetric or weight formulae may improve the detection rate of growth retarded fetuses.

Ultrasound also gives important information on placental maturity and the volume of liquor amnii. Placentas can be graded on the appearance of the basal and chorionic plates as well as the structure of the organ itself. Grade I is the least and Grade III the most mature, the latter showing the chorionic plate interrupted by indentations dividing the placental substance into compartments. Placentae showing the Grade III appearance correlated highly with lung maturity predicting that at delivery the infant was very unlikely to develop respiratory distress syndrome [34]. Oligohydramnios commonly accompanies IUGR due to hypertensive disorders. In the absence of an amniotic leak scanty liquor as assessed on ultrasound correlates very highly with the growth retarded fetus [40].

FETAL HEART RATE MONITORING

The responsiveness of the fetus to external stimuli such as uterine contraction has been found to be effective in assessing well-being. Fetal heart rate monitoring before or during labour may be performed with or without stressing the feto-placental unit with oxytocin. Non-stress testing relies on the regular painless contractions normally present in pregnancy and is non-invasive. In many cases useful information is obtained and the margin of reserve of the growth retarded infant may be assessed. To perform this test an external monitor is strapped to the maternal abdomen to detect fetal heart rate, and an external pressure transducer simultaneously measures uterine activity. The heart rate pattern in response to uterine contractions or fetal movements is observed. In the last trimester of pregnancy the normal fetus will show a stable heart rate (120 to 150 beats per minute), good variability (this is considered to be a heart rate changing by more than 10 but less than 25 beats per minute) and acceleration with fetal movement or uterine contraction. If these factors are present then the fetus is said to have a reactive pattern. Chronic hypoxia due to uteroplacental dysfunction will depress the fetal central nervous system and beat to beat variation is reduced or absent. The most omnious feature of the abnormal pattern is late heart rate deceleration with movement or contraction [61]. Fetal heart rate monitoring is reliable after 33 to 34 weeks, however interpretation in the less mature fetus is as yet not fully evaluated.

Observation over a sufficient period of time (10 minutes) is essential in obtaining a good tracing on which to base a diagnosis. If the non-stressed test is unreactive or shows late decelerations, an oxytocin stress test may be performed. An infusion of oxytocin is started if no contractions occur during an initial period of observation. The infusion rate is increased in a stepwise fashion until contractions lasting 50 to 60 seconds occur every 3 to 10 minutes. As for the non-stress test, it is positive if persistent

and repeated late decelerations occur in more than 50 % of uterine contractions. The stress test has a much higher risk to the fetus in that premature labour or even fetal death may be precipitated.

If the test is normal then the chance of perinatal death in a period of one week is very low (1.3 %). This gives confidence to the medical attendants that the fetus is in good condition and observations may be made regularly with sequential testing. If the non-stressed test is abnormal then the fetus is at risk. Confirmation of the presence of late decelerations on oxytocin stress testing indicates that the infant has a 22 to 50 % chance of death in the perinatal period and the conceptus is clearly at considerable risk. Infants with an abnormal non-stress test, but normal oxytocin stress test remain at relatively low risk as only 5 % will die in a similar period of time [61].

As mentioned earlier, the fetus who has suffered IUGR stands a much higher chance of death during labour than a normally grown infant. Monitoring of intrapartum fetal heart rate is necessary in order to expedite delivery if signs of fetal distress occur. Monitoring is performed in the same manner as described above; however, an electrode may be clipped to the fetal scalp to provide a better heart rate trace free from interference. The presence of persistent fetal tachycardia, bradycardia or more significantly, late deceleration associated with contractions, indicates a high risk of acute fetal hypoxia. Fetal scalp pH estimation may be helpful in deciding whether Caesarian section or other methods of termination of labour are necessary. If variable or delayed decelerations occur then 47 % of cases in one study had a fetal scalp pH of $\leqslant 7.25$ requiring rapid delivery [65]. Fetal cardiotochography in conjunction with scalp pH measurement during labour will identify many of those growth retarded fetuses who have exhausted their reserves during an adverse gestation and a difficult labour.

BIOCHEMICAL TESTS

The variety of biochemical tests available attest to the fact that none of them are particularly good at discriminating between the well and the compromised fetus. The two most commonly used assays are œstriol and human placental lactogen. Œstriol is produced by the feto-placental unit in the latter half of pregnancy and requires normal function of fetal adrenals and liver as well as placental sulphatase enzyme activity. Œstriol is also produced normally in the maternal liver even in the non-pregnant state and before 32 weeks of pregnancy, estimation of œstriols does not reflect feto-placental production. In intrauterine growth retardation the fetal liver and sometimes the adrenals are reduced in size and compromised in function. Hydroxylation of œstriol precursors in these organs may be impaired thus causing a reduction in its excretion. Abnormally low œstriols may be found in anencephaly (due to deficiency of fetal adrenal tissue), deficiency of placental sulphatase activity, adrenal hypoplasia or drug interference (ampicillin, steroids, heroin). Œstriols may be assayed in maternal urine or blood. A 24 hour collection of urine is required and the range of normal is wide thus limiting the value of the test. Diurnal variation of production and excretion will influence the level found in maternal blood at any time. For these reasons œstriol is an unreliable indicator of fetal growth retardation. However, if the urinary œstriol excretion is consistently below 2 standard deviations from the mean for uncomplicated deliveries, then most of the products of these pregnancies are growth retarded. IUGR may however occur even in the presence of normal œstriols.

Human placental lactogen is a polypeptide produced by the syncythiotrophoblast and has been used as a screening test between 30 and 32 weeks. However, in intrauterine growth retardation there may be a false negative rate of up to 33 %. The use of biochemical tests is therefore limited but if found to be consistently low, probably indicates some impairment of feto-placental function. There is however no evidence that the use of biochemical tests alone as an index of fetal well-being makes any difference to the perinatal mortality rate.

OTHER METHODS

Determination of gestational age may not be possible late in pregnancy by ultrasound alone if the woman has not previously been examined. The practice of X-raying the fetus to assess maturity by the presence of ossification centres has been used in the past. This is of very limited value in the growth retarded fetus because the X-ray appearance of epiphyseal centres at the knee and elsewhere are delayed by at least two weeks and great care must be taken if gestational age is to be established by this method [66].

The decision whether or not to prematurely terminate the pregnancy of a growth retarded fetus should be taken with consideration of the functional maturity of the infant's lungs. Amniocentesis and estimation of the lecithin to spingomyelin ratio of the liquor will enable a prediction of lung maturity to be made. If the ratio is more than 2 : 1 then the fetal lungs are capable of producing surfactant and the chance of hyaline membrane disease is very low.

MONITORING THE HIGH RISK PREGNANCY

It is often impracticable to monitor every pregnancy in an attempt to identify deviant growth. An attempt must be made to recognise those women whose fetuses will be more at risk of IUGR (Table IV) and who require an intensive monitoring plan. Early and regular antenatal visits with careful physical examination particularly noting poor weight gain or failure of the fundal height to increase at an expected rate should alert the clinician. All such women should have early ultrasound exami-

TABLE IV. — HIGH RISK WOMEN FOR INTRAUTERINE GROWTH RETARDATION.

Malnourished.
Previous growth retarded infant.
Maternal disease (see Table I).
Smoking.
Possibility of alcohol or drug abuse.
Short stature (less than 5 ft).
Hypertension.
Toxaemia.
Multiple pregnancy.
Drug ingestion in early pregnancy.
Extremes of reproductive age.
Poor weight gain in pregnancy.

nations repeated frequently and from 32 weeks regular oestriol assays. If growth failure is noted then regular non-stress testing should be performed and if abnormal, oxytocin stress testing considered. If abnormal then premature delivery may be advantageous, especially if the lecithin to sphingomyelin (L/S) ratio suggests pulmonary maturity. Table V summarises this protocol. Careful monitoring with multiple tests of fetal well-being has reduced the incidence of perinatal death due to intrauterine growth retardation by timely intervention in threatened pregnancies.

TABLE V. — PROTOCOL OF INVESTIGATIONS
IN A PREGNANCY THAT IS AT RISK
OF INTRAUTERINE GROWTH RETARDATION

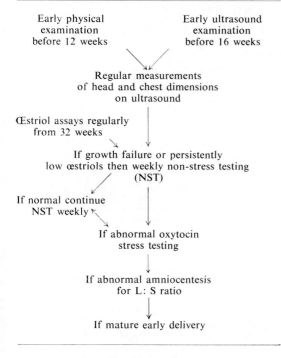

Early physical   Early ultrasound
examination   examination
before 12 weeks   before 16 weeks

Regular measurements
of head and chest dimensions
on ultrasound

Œstriol assays regularly
from 32 weeks

If growth failure or persistently
low œstriols then weekly non-stress testing
(NST)

If normal continue
NST weekly

If abnormal oxytocin
stress testing

If abnormal amniocentesis
for L: S ratio

If mature early delivery

CLINICAL DIAGNOSIS

Intrauterine growth retardation occurs through multiple aetiologies and the appearance of the poorly grown infant at birth will accordingly differ. About half of all SGA babies however will show loss of soft tissue mass and consequently a pattern of external appearances may be recognised. Usher [66] described the characteristic signs of intrauterine growth retardation most eloquently: "They have loose, thin skin, their ribs show through, the abdomen is scaphoid at birth to the point that diaphragmatic hernia may be suspected, and the wasting of muscle mass is very evident over cheeks, arms, buttocks and thighs. The flesh may be dry and cracked or even peeling over palms and soles. The hair is sparse; one almost never sees a fetal malnutrition infant with a heavy shock of hair. Skull sutures are often widened at birth but without any increase in fontanelle pressure. The umbilical cord is very thin, often discoloured yellow-brown at birth, and dries and hardens within hours."

The behaviour of the SGA infant at birth is more difficult to describe. Factors that will affect the way the neonate responds are the presence of asphyxia and hypoglycaemia, both of which are more common in the growth retarded infant. Most studies of newborn behaviour have not excluded the effects of these factors. Apathy, immature and sometimes abnormal reflexes, reduced passive movements of arms and legs and poorer rooting and sucking have all been described in term SGA infants. The work of Als et al. [1] suggests that these infants are less responsive resulting in diminished parent-infant interaction and consequently less stimulation to the detriment of later development.

Dubowitz and colleagues [23] studied a group of SGA infants who were likely to have suffered nutritional deprivation but little intrapartum asphyxia or obstetric interference (a Cape Town coloured population) and compared them with SGA Caucasian babies in whom no birth asphyxia had occured with little analgesia used in labour. The growth retarded infants of both races exhibited "hyperalert" behaviour with increase in visual and auditory orientation, heightened alertness, more frequent startles and increased tone. There was also some reduction in auditory and visual habituation. This study suggests that IUGR in some way affects the neonatal nervous system modifying newborn behaviour.

The fetal nervous system matures in an orderly and sequential manner through the course of gestation in parallel with other organ systems. It is possible to examine an infant at birth and assess accurately its gestational age on the basis of various items. The Dubowitz method of gestational assessment is the most widely used scheme for this purpose (see Fig. I-44). The method consists of 10 neurological items and 11 external criteria which are considered independently and the score for each item summated and gestational age calculated from a straight regression line [22]. Neurological items include mainly those of tone and have been selected to be relatively independent of neonatal illness. External items which overall give a better index of gestation than neurological criteria include appearance of skin, breast, nipple, ear and genitalia. The total score however using both external and neurological items gives a better result than either alone. The system is simple and relies on the comparison of appearance to simple diagrams and can be completed in less than 10 minutes. Accuracy of this method is ± 2 weeks (95 % confidence limits) of the actual gestational age and can be performed without loss of reliability up to five days from birth.

Comparison of neurological to external criteria

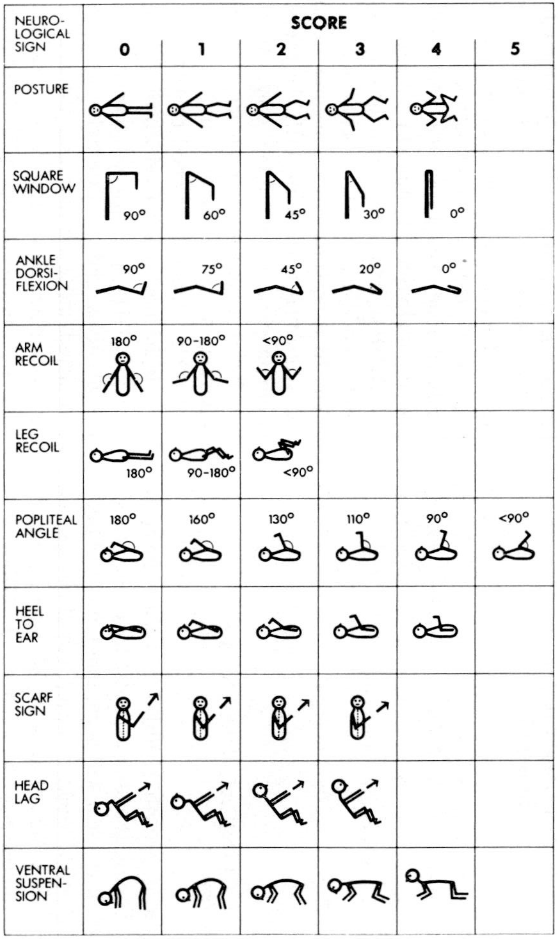

External (superficial) Criteria

EXTERNAL SIGN	SCORE 0	1	2	3	4
OEDEMA	Obvious oedema hands and feet; pitting over tibia	No obvious oedema hands and feet; pitting over tibia	No oedema		
SKIN TEXTURE	Very thin, gelatinous	Thin and smooth	Smooth; medium thickness. Rash or superficial peeling	Slight thickening Superficial cracking and peeling esp hands and feet	Thick and parchment-like; superficial or deep cracking
SKIN COLOUR (Infant not crying)	Dark red	Uniformly pink	Pale pink: variable over body	Pale Only pink over ears, lips, palms or soles	
SKIN OPACITY (trunk)	Numerous veins and venules clearly seen especially over abdomen	Veins and tributaries seen	A few large vessels clearly seen over abdomen	A few large vessels seen indistinctly over abdomen	No blood vessels seen
LANUGO (over back)	No lanugo	Abundant; long and thick over whole back	Hair thinning especially over lower back	Small amount of lanugo and bald areas	At least half of back devoid of lanugo
PLANTAR CREASES	No skin creases	Faint red marks over anterior half of sole	Definite red marks over more than anterior half; indentations over less than anterior third	Indentations over more than anterior third	Definite deep indentations over more than anterior third
NIPPLE FORMATION	Nipple barely visible; no areola	Nipple well defined; areola smooth and flat diameter <0.75 cm	Areola stippled, edge not raised diameter <0.75 cm	Areola stippled, edge raised diameter >0.75 cm	
BREAST SIZE	No breast tissue palpable	Breast tissue on one or both sides <0.5 cm diameter	Breast tissue both sides; one or both 0.5-1.0 cm	Breast tissue both sides; one or both >1 cm	
EAR FORM	Pinna flat and shapeless, little or no incurving of edge	Incurving of part of edge of pinna	Partial incurving whole of upper pinna	Well-defined incurving whole of upper pinna	
EAR FIRMNESS	Pinna soft, easily folded, no recoil	Pinna soft, easily folded, slow recoil	Cartilage to edge of pinna, but soft in places, ready recoil	Pinna firm, cartilage to edge; instant recoil	
GENITALIA MALE	Neither testis in scrotum	At least one testis high in scrotum	At least one testis right down		
FEMALES (With hips half abducted)	Labia majora widely separated, labia minora protruding	Labia majora almost cover labia minora	Labia majora completely cover labia minora		

(Adapted from Farr et al Develop Med Child Neurol 1966, **8**, 507)

Neurological Criteria

NEUROLOGICAL SIGN	SCORE 0	1	2	3	4	5
POSTURE						
SQUARE WINDOW	90°	60°	45°	30°	0°	
ANKLE DORSIFLEXION	90°	75°	45°	20°	0°	
ARM RECOIL	180°	90-180°	<90°			
LEG RECOIL	180°	90-180°	<90°			
POPLITEAL ANGLE	180°	160°	130°	110°	90°	<90°
HEEL TO EAR						
SCARF SIGN						
HEAD LAG						
VENTRAL SUSPENSION						

GESTATIONAL AGE CHART

(Dubowitz Score)

Name

Hospital No.

Sex   Race

Date/time of birth

Date/time of examination

Age

Weight

Length

Head circumference

Score   Neurological
         Superficial
         Total

FDD (certain/uncertain)

Gest by dates

Gest by Assessment

Comments

FIG. 1-44.

has been made in SGA infants. This has shown that stress in utero such as poor placental perfusion significantly accelerates the neurological score by up to four weeks in preterm infants of gestational age $\leqslant 32$ weeks compared to the overall score for external criteria [2]. This raises the intriguing possibility that in utero stress such as that producing IUGR may accelerate neurological maturation in much the same way as functional lung maturation is enhanced. In contrast to the central nervous system peripheral nerve myelination appears to proceed despite fetal malnourishment. Motor nerve conduction velocities are clearly related to gestational age ($\pm$ 2 weeks) in normal infants and IUGR does not appear to affect this [62]. Motor nerve conduction velocities can therefore be used as an estimate of gestational age if confusion exists and are useful in cases with conflicting results on other grounds.

NEWBORN COMPLICATIONS

Hypoglycaemia. — The blood glucose in the newborn is generally lower than the older child or adult. Significant hypoglycaemia is considered to be present with a blood glucose of 20 mg/100 ml or less in preterm and 30 mg/100 ml or below in term and post term-infants. The association between hypoglycaemia and IUGR is well recognised and commonly occurs. Its overall incidence is 12 to 25 % in SGA infants. It appears to be much more common in the preterm infant. 40 % of preterm SGA infants developed hypoglycaemia in one study compared to 3 % of similar appropriate for gestational age infants [45]. Boys are more commonly affected than girls, only a proportion of cases however are symptomatic.

The asymetrically growth retarded infant is most at risk of neonatal hypoglycaemia. These infants tend to be thinner and longer and have a low ponderal index. In a prospective study, 23 out of 62 of such growth retarded infants had hypoglycaemia within 12 hours of birth compared to only 8 % of proportionately growth retarded neonates [41]. Infants with the lowest PIs probably represent a syndrome of late under-nutrition due either to placental dysfunction or maternal nutritional deprivation. These infants, who have previously grown normally, lose soft tissue mass in the last trimester. The severely growth retarded but symmetrically small infant is more likely to have had long term nutritional deprivation and be uniformly stunted.

These infants have not acutely exhausted their glycogen stores as have the former group and are less prone to hypoglycaemia. The risk of hypoglycaemia is directly related to tissue glycogen. In SGA infants the glycogen content per gram of tissue is the same as normally grown infants however the total glycogen content was substantially lower in neonates born with growth retardation [57].

Neonatal hypoglycaemia in intrauterine growth retarded pregnancies usually occurs within the first 24 hours of life and may continue for several days. The hypoglycaemia may be symptomatic and the infant presents with convulsions, jitteriness or apathy but more commonly may be completely asymptomatic. It is important for this reason to regularly monitor the blood sugar in SGA infants and try and prevent hypoglycaemia by early and regular feeding and when needed I. V. glucose administration. Screening for hypoglycaemia is most conveniently performed by stick tests utilising an enzymatic colour change reaction. Those infants with asymptomatic hypoglycaemia do well in follow-up studies, however the same is not true for hypoglycaemia associated with convulsions. Almost half of all infants who have hypoglycaemic seizures in the neonatal period suffer some neurologic deficit and its importance is underlined since it is one of the few truely preventable causes of neurological handicap occuring in the neonatal period.

Hyperglycaemia. — A syndrome of transient diabetes mellitus may on rare occasions occur in the severly SGA infant. These children are usually born at term and are symmetrically growth retarded. Hyperglycaemia develops in the first few days of life and if successfully treated is a transient condition resolving by six months of age. High blood glucose is found in the absence of ketonuria and insulin therapy is required. Some infants have been weaned from insulin to chlorpropramide before recovery occured. Transient diabetes mellitus is associated with immaturity of the insulin releasing mechanism and endogenous insulin levels are low. Interestingly, when insulin treatment is started rapid catch up growth, particularly in length, often occurs. One case report describes an infant born below the third centile for length who increased in crown-heel measurement to above the 97th centile by one year of age [60].

Birth asphyxia. — The small for gestational age fetus embarks on the voyage of labour already depleted of energy stores and having to rely in many cases on a poorly functioning placental supply. Episodes of acute hypoxia and under-perfusion are likely and intrapartum asphyxia is a common complication. The risks of asphyxia are well recognised but the precise incidence is difficult to determine due to differing criteria used in its diagnosis. Generally asphyxia at birth appears to be about four times more common in the SGA infant than in the appropriately grown neonate. In a study of 38,405 consecutive deliveries, 1.2 % of babies overall had birth asphyxia (defined as requiring positive pressure ventilation for more than one minute before sustained respiration occured). 4 % of SGA infants (< 3rd centile for weight) born after 36 weeks were asphyxiated as were 34 % of SGA infants of 36 weeks of less. The presence of asphyxia in the growth retarded infant significantly increases the risk of the infant dying [47]. It is generally agreed that the preterm SGA infant is most at risk of asphyxia and this is found to be a highly significant association with later neurological handicap. Almost 50 % of asphyxiated infants (five minute Apgar score of < 6 or a need for positive pressure resusitation for > 2 minutes) born at 37 weeks post-menstrual age or less had significant neurological handicap at two years of age. The degree of handicap was unrelated to severity of the growth retardation [16].

The aim of the perinatologist is to identify the poorly grown fetus and closely monitor his well-being in pregnancy and labour. If signs of distress are detected then expedited delivery is essential in order to avoid the harmful effects of asphyxia. The treatment of birth asphyxia is somewhat controversial and is discussed in detail elsewhere. The aim must be in prevention rather than cure.

Polycythemia. — There is no generally accepted definition for polycythemia in the neonate but a haematocrit of above 60 or 65 % on venous blood or a haemoglobin of over 20 mg/dl is usually considered to be the minimal requirement for this diagnosis. The incidence of this condition in SGA infants is increased compared to the appropriately grown neonate and various reports of a frequency of 12 to 50 % are cited. In 23 full term SGA infants, haemoglobin, haematocrit, total erythrocyte count and HbF concentrations were all significantly raised compared to the term or pre-term well nourished neonate. Intrauterine hypoxia associated with placental dysfunction stimulates erythropoietin production and this is the stimulating factor for red blood cell production in the latter months of fetal life.

Polycythemia is associated with hyperviscosity and a small increase in haematocrit may cause a considerable increase in blood viscosity with the consequent risk of sludging in small blood vessels and infarction. An incidence of hyperviscosity of 18 % was found in SGA infants and a venous haematocrit of more than 64 % was predictive for this condition [37]. Over twice as many infants in the hyperviscous group exhibited symptoms either in the cardiorespiratory or neurological systems. Treatment of severe polycythemia by partial exchange transfusion (venous haematocrit of < 70 %) may be necessary in some SGA infants to prevent further complications.

Neurological complications. — The interpretation of abnormal neurological behaviour and intracerebral pathology in the neonatal period is influenced by birth asphyxia, hypoglycaemia, drugs and other insults which will exert their own abnormal effect on performance. Separating these various factors is not easy and relatively little attention has been paid to their modifying effect.

The electroencephalogram changes in a consistent pattern with advancing gestational age and variations from this may be detected. Several studies have shown a higher incidence of abnormal EEG's in small for gestational age infants but most of these studies have not controlled for the perinatal neurological insults discussed above. Schulte and colleagues reported a study of 22 SGA infants of toxaemic mothers ranging in gestation from 36 to 45 weeks and a similar number of normal newborn controls. They found that the SGA infants had significantly more immature EEG patterns both in active and quiet sleep than the controls. In addition many of the tracings were considered to be frankly abnormal for an infant of any age, even in those who had no known hypoxia or hypoglycaemia [63]. Abnormal sleep cycles have also been reported in infants of undernourished mothers causing the total duration of sleep to be significantly shortened [5].

Dreyfus-Brisac has also recognised a variety of unusual EEG patterns as well as bioelectric developmental retardation and patterns of different maturity in small-for-gestational age infants compared to normally grown babies of similar gestation [21 b].

Intraventricular haemorrhage (IVH) is an important cause of death and handicap in severely preterm infants. Whether this condition is more or less common in the infant with intrauterine growth retardation is not clear. Post-mortem data suggests that IVH was more common in the small for gestational age infant. In one study infants with IVH had a mean reduction in body weight for gestational age of 14 % compared with infants who died without haemorrhage [39]. Unfortunately, post mortem studies are severely limited in that only a highly selected group of babies with IVH are included. The suggestion that intraventricular haemorrhage is less common in growth retarded infants has been made on the basis of a retrospective study with matched controls [58]. The incidence of hyaline membrane disease and IVH was 74 and 42 % respectively in the appropriately grown group and 5 and 11 % in the small for gestational age infants. Diagnosis was made initially on clinical criteria and confirmed by computerised tomography or necropsy, however, as most intraventricular haemorrhages are "asymptomatic" this study will again not be representative of the entire spectrum of this condition. The growth retarded neonate has a lower incidence of hyaline membrane disease due to prenatal "stress" and the absence of extreme haemodynamic changes associated with severe respiratory disease may account for the apparently reduced incidence of IVH in this study. Careful scrutiny of the figures show that the relative proportion of IVH to hyaline membrane disease is in fact higher in the growth retarded group suggesting that the frequency of haemorrhage in this group is partially independent of hyaline membrane disease and its incidence is therefore higher than expected.

Pulmonary haemorrhage. — Massive pulmonary haemorrhage is a well described complication of intrauterine growth retardation. In the 1958 survey of all the births in Britain in one week, massive pulmonary haemorrhage accounted for 46 of the 832 first week deaths (6 %) and was the third commonest cause of mortality in small for gestational age infants. Infants were usually well until the second or third day of life, and most deaths occured on the fourth or fifth day. In many infants, cerebral irritation was noted and in some, convulsions occured shortly before the haemorrhage. This condition appears to be more common in the products of multiple pregnancy. Lung pathology shows massive diapedesis of red cells into the alveoli but there is usually no evidence of pneumonia.

The incidence of massive pulmonary haemorrhage has been reported as occuring in about 15 % of small for gestational age infants, however, it appears to be much less common in the last few years than hitherto. The reason for this is not clear but the pulmonary haemorrhage may have been related to hypoglycaemia or hypothermia which with present management occurs much less frequently.

Meconium aspiration. — Fetal distress in labour is associated with the passage of meconium and if hypoxia or asphyxia persist, gasping during labour may occur with aspiration of meconium laden liquor. Oligohydramnios frequently accompanies fetal growth retardation and the inhaled meconium will be more concentrated and more likely to affect pulmonary function. Meconium aspiration occured in one series in 18 % of SGA infants and causes a patchy pneumonic process with much inflammation and considerable ventilation perfusion inequalities. The infants are usually at or near term and rapidly develop symptoms and signs of respiratory distress. Suctioning of the naso-pharynx prior to delivery of the thorax may reduce the chance of meconium being aspirated into the lower bronchial tree.

Fluid balance. — In the full term neonate complicated homeostatic mechanisms exist to conserve body water. In more immature infants these controls are less reliable and the infant is more prone to abnormalities of fluid balance. The SGA infant behaves differently to the appropriately grown neonate in the way in which water is distributed in his body. Growth retarded infants commonly lose little or no weight in the first few days of life and significantly less so than infants appropriate for gestation. This weight loss is largely due to changes of water in body compartments and excretion from the organism.

Cassady [12] has studied water composition in growth retarded infants in considerable detail and has shown that SGA infants have an elevated plasma volume at birth, as well as an expanded extracellular compartment compared to normally grown infants. This means that although the infant is small for gestational age, his intravascular and extracellular water is proportionately much less depleted. The most striking and significant expansion of the extracellular fluid space occurs in the most length retarded infants suggesting a more chronic and severe insult to fetal growth. The odema seen in some growth retarded infants is related to these findings.

Conservation of water is mediated through the kidneys, bowel and skin. Little is known about the renal function of growth retarded neonates, however evaporative losses through the skin have been recently studied [38]. The rate of evaporation of water from the skin of full-term SGA infants is lower than that of normally grown term infants at corresponding relative humidity. Transepidermal water loss is consistently lower in growth retarded infants than appropriately grown infants over varying gestational ages. The precise mechanism for this is multifactorial but in the immediate neonatal period, SGA infants probably require less fluid than normal infants of the same gestational age.

Temperature control. — There is conflicting evidence as to whether small for gestational age infants are better at conserving heat than an AGA infant of the same birth weight. Measurements of metabolic rate have been shown to be related to gestational age by one group of investigators and others have found that changes in metabolic rate in response to cold stress were related to birth weight irrespective of gestation.

Another factor in promoting heat loss is the relatively large skin surface area to body weight ratio in disproportionately growth retarded neonates. Heat loss is liable to occur over a larger surface area in those infants particularly from the head and dressing the infant and the use of scalp caps are important in reducing the heat loss. Whether the infant is pre-term, SGA or both, careful attention to ways of avoiding cold stress and consequent raised metabolic rate is important.

Infection. — Infection is commoner in growth retarded infants and immunological function of these children has been investigated in some detail. Humoral immunity and the levels of immunoglobins have been studied by Chandra [14] and consistently low IgG measurements have been found in the SGA infants. This is probably related to placental dysfunction and impaired transfer of this protein. There was no catch-up in IgG levels by three to five months and this was associated with frequent bacterial infections during this time. Measurements of IgM and IgA did not show the same abnormality.

In addition to impaired humoral immunity, Ferguson showed considerable abnormalities in cellular immunity in growth retarded neonates [27]. There was a reduction in the number of circulating lymphocytes and this was due to reduction in the number of T-lymphocytes whereas B-cells were of normal number. Opsonisation, chemotactic activity, bactericidal and phagocytic cellular activity were all reduced. Follow-up studies of SGA infants show that in later life the numbers of T-lymphocytes increase to normal levels but their function is considerably impaired. These abnormalities of cellular immunity in general and thymus related lymphocytes in particular, are probably related to the marked thymic hypoplasia seen in growth retarded babies at birth.

Careful observation for infection is essential in the care of the SGA infant, particularly if he is also pre-term. Prophylactic antibiotics are not recommended but scrupulous hand washing technique and isolation of infected cases will reduce the incidence of infection in these children.

Metabolic disorders. — In addition to abnormalities in glucose metabolism, alteration in calcium homeostasis may be found. Plasma venous calcium has been shown to be significantly lower and inorganic phosphorus higher in growth retarded neonates, compared with normally grown controls. No differences in magnesium levels were found in the two groups [15]. Hypocalcaemia may be associated with jitteriness and convulsions.

Neonatal jaundice does not seem to differ in incidence very much from normally grown infants of the same gestational age. The very pre-term SGA baby or those with polycythemia may become more jaundiced than others although this is not usually a problem.

CONGENITAL ABNORMALITIES

The incidence of congenital abnormalities has been reported to be high in some studies. Certain chromosomal and dysmorphic syndromes are associated with degrees of intrauterine growth retardation but these babies are usually excluded from studies of SGA children. It is possible that some insult has occured early in gestation which has caused the developmental abnormality as well as impairing growth. Usher states that congenital anomalies occur 10 to 20 times more commonly in these infants and are usually not of sufficient severity to account for the growth retardation.

In the older literature, cataracts were seen more frequently in SGA infants, particularly when pregnancy was associated with toxaemia. This no longer appears to be a recognised association, and is probably related to prenatal rubella infection.

LONG TERM OUTCOME

Intrauterine growth retardation may permanently affect the child's physical and intellectual development. Which infants are most likely to be affected is an important question but few answers are forthcoming at this time. Follow-up studies are fraught with difficulties. The severity of IUGR must be considered—some studies include only infants born below the fifth or third centiles, and others consider any infant below the 10th centile for gestational age. The onset of growth retardation and the maturity at birth must also be considered.

The older literature cannot be reliably interpreted as feeding regimes were insufficient to provide adequate calories and temperature control was poor; these factors may have effects on later development. Feeding methods in the newborn period should be stated in any description of long term outcome. Environment is an important criterion as to whether the child is likely to do well or not, particularly in consideration of later intelligence. Sibling or twin studies give a certain amount of information which is independent of environment assuming the children are brought up in roughly similar circumstances. Attention to these considerations allow trends to be recognised and prediction of future growth and development may be made from factors observable at birth.

In discussing long term outcome, growth, intelligence and physical handicap will be considered separately.

GROWTH

Growth, unlike brain function, can be accurately measured and compared to controls. Much work on post natal growth patterns has been published and some generalisations can be made.

In SGA infants born at or near term, complete catch-up growth may occur. Growth velocity measurements plot the rate of increase in growth per unit time. For catch-up to occur the growth velocity must exceed that of normal infants of similar age. A growth retarded child at birth will remain small if his growth velocity subsequently follows a normal pattern. Children with mild "growth retardation" (which may reflect the lower end of an entirely normal population) may be found, not surprisingly, to be of normal stature, weight and head size some years later.

In a group of SGA infants of varying maturity at birth and followed until nearly two years of age, their mean weights remained below a random sample of normal babies. They had however moved closer to the mean of the controls over the two year period and had clearly increased their growth velocity. Some of the children had increased their weight rapidly compared to others and by two years were indistinguishable from the controls [13]. The head size and length remained in proportion to their weight. Severely growth retarded infants (weight below the fifth percentile) were significantly smaller

in weight and height at five years than infants born preterm but not growth retarded. Head circumference however did not differ from the premature group indicating that there had been some catch-up growth [53]. A group of mildly growth retarded infants (birth weight below the 10th but above the 5th percentile) also grew less well but did better than the severely growth retarded group of infants.

Fitzhardinge and Steven [28] reported a careful prospective study of 96 SGA full term singleton infants followed for at least four years. All were below the third weight percentile at birth. The average weight and height of these infants increased rapidly over the first six months from a point below the third percentile to between the 10th and 25th percentiles. Thereafter, until they reached six years of age, the average weight and height continued to grow along a constant percentile line. By six years the height was above the 50th percentile in only 8 % of the total group. 35 % were still at or below the third percentile. Increase in head size followed the increase in length. Thirty-three of these infants were paired with siblings of the same sex and in 24 of the sibling pairs, the normal birth weight child was taller than his or her brother or sister of low birth weight. 45 % of the control siblings were at or over the 50th percentile while only 12 % of the study children reached the same level in height. Particular attention was paid to the most severely growth retarded infants in this study (the lightest 20 %) but these children grew as well as those less severely growth retarded and all remained on average well below the mean for normal children.

Those infants who eventually reached normal height had a significantly greater growth velocity in the first year of life, but if catch-up had not occured by this time, no child eventually reached normal height or weight. This study ensured that no changes in feeding regimen occured during its course, parental height was normal, and only singleton births with no evidence of congenital abnormalities were included. The authors felt that many of the infants who failed to show catch-up growth came from a deprived home environment.

Davies et al. [17] have questioned whether late intrauterine growth retardation or continuous poor fetal growth throughout pregnancy affects the catch-up potential. Wasting as determined by a very low ponderal index suggests late undernutrition, and a normal or slightly low PI suggests mainly uniform growth retardation. All growth retarded infants were allocated to one or other group and the infants followed for six months. Babies in both groups showed average growth velocities greater than the mean for normally grown infants, however, the "wasted" babies with the lowest PIs had a considerably more rapid growth velocity over the first two to three months of life, after which time their growth rates slowed and normalised with no further catch-up occuring.

The severely preterm SGA infant has a double burden to overcome before realising full growth potential. Little reliable information is available on the growth patterns of these infants. Seventy-one babies born below 37 weeks who were more than two standard deviations below the mean were studied [16]. On comparison with intrauterine growth rates (which is probably not valid in prematurely born infants) linear growth was poor for the first few weeks after birth and this was most marked in those infants of gestation less than 33 weeks but was unrelated to the degree of growth retardation at birth. A spurt in linear growth velocity occured at about the time of the expected date of delivery and remained increased for six months compared with the standard for North American children. Their growth velocity overall from birth to six months was however, almost identical to the standard, largely due to the delay in the first weeks from birth. Head circumference velocity rates showed no deviation from the standards. These infants although showing a limited catch-up potential fell well below the mean at two years, and this pattern of poor catch-up was particularly seen in males. Only six of 71 infants were above the 50th percentile for weight and length at two years of age and 24 were below the third percentile.

Infants of very low birth weight ($\leqslant 1,500$ g) born or admitted to Hammersmith Hospital have been reviewed over a 10 year period [18]. One third were SGA (below the 10th percentile). The differences between the retarded and appropriately grown groups were small although the SGA infants were lighter at four years of age, and proportionately more were shorter and had smaller heads at the same age. Those infants poorly grown *in utero* and born very prematurely grow less well than infants normally grown but born severely preterm.

Head size is closely related to brain size in infants and careful studies of head growth give important information on brain growth. Brandt [7] has followed up two groups of poorly grown infants over an 8 year period whose birth weights were below the 10th centile of Lubchenco. One group showed catch-up of head growth by six months from birth with favourable neurological development (21 infants) and the other group entirely failed to show satisfactory catch-up head growth (22 infants). There was no difference in the degree

of IUGR in these two groups, and both showed normal head growth on ultrasound measurements until the beginning of the third trimester. Brandt examined changes in management of the infants over the eight year period of this study and most of the infants with good catch-up were born after introduction of early feeding (3 to 6 hours after birth), whereas most of those whose head growth remained poor were born before the early feeding regime was introduced. This illustrates how important it is to establish adequate feeding in infants growth retarded at birth.

To summarise our present understanding on expected growth of an infant who has suffered IUGR:

i. Adequate and early feeding is essential if full growth potential is to be realised.

ii. On the whole, the severity of intrauterine growth retardation does not seem to strongly influence the growth potential, although evidence remains conflicting.

iii. Catch-up growth if it is going to occur does so usually by six months. Catch-up growth for head circumference follows linear growth.

iv. Full term growth retarded infants stand a good chance of catch-up particularly if growth retardation is due to maternal factors.

v. Severely preterm SGA infants are much less likely to reach average size than infants of the same degree of prematurity but normally grown.

vi. Environmental factors probably play a large part in subsequent growth potential.

NEUROLOGIC HANDICAP

Intelligence. — It is necessary to again consider separately full term and preterm SGA infants. There have been two good studies comparing intelligence in term growth retarded infants from Newcastle [53] and Montreal [29]. Neligan and colleagues from Newcastle (England) studied a selected proportion of all births occuring during a 3 year period from 1960 to 1962. These were categorised into three groups: those born too soon (before 255 days of gestation), those born too small (below the 10th centile for local population distribution) providing they were 255 days of gestation or more, and this group was further considered as severe SGA if their weights fell below the fifth centile for gestational age. Group III consisted of 187 normal term infants born in the same year and of similar social class. Many children were followed for seven years. Overall they found that with a wide range of psychometric testing between the ages of five and seven years the effects of being born too small at term were more severe in degree (although similar in kind) to the effects of being born prematurely. Those infants born more severely growth retarded consistently scored worse at 5 or 7 years than the more mildly growth retarded infant. Males tended to be more severely affected than females. They also found that social class had a modifying effect on the child's performance.

Fitzhardinge and Steven [29] studied 96 full term SGA infants (below the third centile) from Montreal, and examined them at ages between four and eight years. Intelligence testing produced figures lower than the controls but the mean was well in the normal range. Generally boys scored worse than girls and 25 % of boys had an IQ of 80 or less. The degree of IUGR did not relate to subsequent intelligence scores.

Intelligence testing generally shows no difference in SGA infants born at term but one study found the mean IQ to be 10 points lower in a group of infants born SGA whose OFC remained below the 10th centile compared to a similar SGA group who showed effective catch-up in head growth [3].

Preterm infants are more likely to have complications during the neonatal period which may affect subsequent neurological performance. One hundred and nine preterm SGA infants (below the third percentile) were born between 1974 and 1975 of which 71 were followed up for two years [16]. The method of feeding did not alter over this period of time. Bayley mental and psychomotor developmental indices were performed at 18 months of age from expected full term delivery date. An average score of $\leqslant 80$ was found in 35 of 71 infants (49 %) and when SGA infants with gestation below 33 weeks were considered separately 12 of 47 (26 %) had Bayley scores $\leqslant 80$.

Data from Hammersmith Hospital over an eight year period found a significant difference between distributions of IQ score for SGA infants weighing 1,500 g at birth and normally grown prematures of the same birth weight [30]. The mean full-scale IQ of the former was 92 and of the latter 99. One fifth of the children showed a performance score significantly below their verbal ability and this was evenly distributed between the 2 groups of children. Those infants whose heads exhibited catch-up growth to lie above the 50th percentile had a mean IQ of 102 and this was significantly different from infants whose heads had failed to reach this percentile line. Stewart and Reynolds [64] report a follow up study of 95 infants with birth weight below 1,500 g born between the years 1966 and 1970. Infants were

followed to a mean age of five years, and 90.5 % had no detectable handicap. Twenty of the 95 were below the tenth percentile for gestational age and no difference in IQ could be found between them and the normally grown infants.

Major neurological handicap. — It has been discussed earlier that EEGs often show abnormalities suggesting a diffuse disorder related to poor intrauterine growth. More specific neurological handicap may also arise in such infants. In a retrospective study of seven year old children with cerebral palsy, many tended to be preterm and poorly grown at birth [26]. Preterm SGA infants are likely to suffer from neurological problems related to their prematurity as well as their poor growth and separation of the two may be difficult. Commey and Fitzhardinge [16] found hydrocephaly, cerebral palsy and recurrent nonfebrile convulsions amongst 71 infants who were SGA (below the third centile) and preterm. Spastic diplegia was the commonest form of cerebral palsy, and 75 % of them had an IQ below 80. Major neurological handicap or an IQ of $\leqslant 80$ was found in 49 % of those infants. There was however a very strong correlation between later handicap and the presence of cerebral depression (usually due to birth asphyxia) recorded on admission to the neonatal intensive care unit. The very high incidence of severe neurological handicap found in this study is in excess of that seen in full term SGA infants, and may reflect the preselection of the more critically ill infants who were outborn and transferred in.

If significant neurological handicap is defined as one or a combination of the following; an IQ of less than 70, neurological abnormality (major or minor) and moderate to severe hearing or visual deficit then 24 % of SGA infants weighing less than 1,500 g at birth were significantly handicapped. Only 16 % of normally grown infants of the same birthweight cared for over the same 10 year period at Hammersmith Hospital in the 1960s had similar problems [19].

A study of full term infants with growth retardation [29] revealed seven of 96 children (7.3 %) with cerebral palsy, 6 % had repeated convulsions and 15 % had signs of "minimal brain damage". In addition, 32 % of infants had severe speech defects, 16 % had ocular defects requiring correction and 43 % of those children in whom school performance could be obtained were considered to have learning problems despite in many cases, an adequate IQ. The difference in school performance between the study and control children was highly significant.

Similarly the disparity between the SGA and a control appropriate for gestational age group of similar maturity was statistically significant for "minimal brain damage". There appeared to be no association between neurological handicap and severity of growth retardation. In contrast to the preterm SGA study described above giving an incidence of major neurological handicap of 49 %, only 25 % of the term SGA infants had major neurological handicap or an IQ of ⩽ 80. Again neonatal asphyxia was found in a number of infants with the most severe handicap.

In the previously mentioned Newcastle study comparing term SGA with normally grown preterm infants the severely SGA infants (below the fifth centile) had more behaviour and temperament abnormalities than controls and more behaviour difficulties than the preterm infants. The severely SGA also exhibited more hyperactive behaviour. The number of abnormal physical neurological signs were also higher in the poorly grown infants than controls.

To summarise these studies and present knowledge:

i. Infants born SGA at term have more developmental, behavioural and learning problems than infants born mildly preterm.

ii. Males are more vulnerable to the neurological effects of intrauterine growth retardation than females.

iii. The severity of IUGR probably affects brain development but this in some cases does not relate to the severity of neurological problems.

iv. Effective catch-up head growth is associated with higher IQ scores than infants whose heads remain small.

v. Small for gestational age preterm infants have a high incidence of serious neurological abnormalities in some reports, but this is probably largely related to the effects of perinatal asphyxia rather than pure growth retardation.

vi. Environmental factors play a large part in subsequent neurological outcome.

REFERENCES

[1] ALS (H.), TRONICK (E.), ADAMSON (L.), BRAZELTON (T. B.). — The behaviour of the full-term but underweight newborn infant. *Develop. Med. Child. Neurol.*, *18*, 590-602, 1976.

[2] AMIEL-TISON (C.). — Possible acceleration of neurological maturation following high-risk pregnancy. *Am. J. Obstet. Gynecol.*, *138*, 303-306, 1980.

[3] BABSON (S. G.), HENDERSON (N. B.). — Fetal undergrowth: Relation of head growth to later intellectual performance. *Pediatrics*, *53*, 890-893, 1974.

[4] BATTAGLIA (F.), LUBCHENCO (L.). — A practical classification of newborn infants by weight and gestational age. *J. Pediatr.*, *71*, 159-163, 1967.

[5] BHATIA (V. P.), KATIYAR (G. P.), AGARWAL (K. N.), DAS (T. K.), DEY (P. K.). — Sleep cycle studies in babies of undernourished mothers. *Arch. Dis. Child.*, *55*, 134-138, 1980.

[6] BIRNHOLZ (J. C.). — Ultrasound characterization of fetal growth. *Ultrason Imaging*, *2*, 135-149, 1980.

[7] BRANDT (I.). — *The Biology of Human Fetal Growth*. ROBERTS D. F., THOMPSON A. M. (Eds). Taylor and Francis Ltd., London, 1976.

[8] BRÉART (G.), HENNEQUIN (J.-F.), CROST-DENIEL (M.), RUMEAU-ROUQUETTE (C.). — Étude de l'insuffisance pondérale à la naissance. *Arch. Franç. Péd.*, *34*, 221-232, 1977.

[9] BUTLER (N. R.). — ALBERMAN (E. D.) (Eds). *Perinatal Problems*, Livingstone, Edinburgh, 1969.

[10] CAMPBELL (S.). — The antenatal assessment of fetal growth and development. In: *Biology of Human Fetal Growth*. ROBERTS D. F., THOMPSON A. M. (Eds), Taylor and Francis Ltd., London, 1976.

[11] CAMPBELL (S.), DEWHURST (C. J.). — Diagnosis of the small for dates fetus by serial ultrasound cephalometry. *Lancet*, *2*, 1002-1006, 1971.

[12] CASSADY (G.). — Body composition in intrauterine growth retardation. *Ped. Clin. N. Amer.*, *17*, 79-99, 1970.

[13] CHAMBERLAIN (R.), DAVEY (A.). — Physical growth in twins, postmature and small for dates children. *Arch. Dis. Child.*, *50*, 437-442, 1975.

[14] CHANDRA (R. K.). — Fetal malnutrition and postnatal immunocompetence. *Am. J. Dis. Child.*, *129*, 450-454, 1975.

[15] COCKBURN (F.). — Some biochemical aspects of intrauterine growth retardation. *Arch. Dis. Child.*, *44*, 136, 1969.

[16] COMMEY (J.), FITZHARDINGE (P. M.). — Handicap in the preterm small-for-gestational age infant. *J. Pediatr.*, *94*, 779-786, 1979.

[17] DAVIES (D. P.), PLATTS (P.), PRITCHARD (J. M.), WILKINSON (P. M.). — Nutritional status of light for dates infants at birth and its influence on early postnatal growth. *Arch. Dis. Child.*, *54*, 703-706, 1979.

[18] DAVIES (P. A.). — In *Nutrition, Growth and Development*. FALKNER F., KRETCHMER N., ROSSI E. (Eds). Modern Problems in Paediatrics, vol. 14, 119-133, Karger S., Basel, 1975.

[19] DAVIES (P. A.). — Infants of very low birth weight: An appraisal of their present neonatal care and later prognosis. In *Recent Advances in Paediatrics*. HULL D. (Ed.). Churchill Livingstone, Edinburgh, 1976.

[20] DAWES (S.). — *Size at birth*. ELLIOTT K., KNIGHT J. (Eds). Elsevier, Amsterdam, 1976.

[21a] DEWHURST (C. J.), BEAZLEY (J. M.), CAMPBELL (S.). — Assessment of fetal maturity and dysmaturity. *Am. J. Obstet. Gynecol.*, *113*, 141-149, 1972.

[21b] DREYFUS-BRISAC (C.). — The electroencephalogram of the premature infant and the fullterm newborn: normal and abnormal development of waking and sleeping patterns. *In:* KELLAWAY P., PETERSEN J. (Eds): *Neurological and electroence-*

phalographic correlative studies in infancy. Grunner and Stratton, New York, 186-207, 1964.

[22] DUBOWITZ (L. M. S.), DUBOWITZ (V.), GOLDBERG (C.). — Clinical assessment of gestational age in the newborn infant. *J. Pediatr.*, 77, 1-10, 1970.

[23] DUBOWITZ (L. M. S.), DUBOWITZ (V.). — Neurological assessment of the newborn. *Neuropaediatrie*, 8, 505-506, 1977.

[24] DUBOWITZ (L. M. S.), GOLDBERG (C.). — Assessment of gestation by ultrasound in various stages of pregnancy in infants differing in size and ethnic origin. *Br. J. Obstet. Gynaecol.*, 88, 255-259, 1981.

[25] EASTMAN (N. J.), JACKSON (E.). — Weight relationships in pregnancy. *Obstet. Gynecol. Surg.*, 23, 1003-1025, 1968.

[26] ELLENBERG (J. H.), NELSON (K. B.). — Birth weight and gestational age in children with cerebral palsy or seizure disorders. *Am. J. Dis. Child.*, 133, 1044-1048, 1979.

[27] FERGUSON (A. C.). — Prolonged impairment of cellular immunity in children with intrauterine growth retardation. *J. Pediatr.*, 93, 52-56, 1978.

[28] FITZHARDINGE (P. M.), STEVEN (E. M.). — The small for dates infant. 1. Later growth patterns. *Pediatrics*, 49, 671-681, 1972.

[29] FITZHARDINGE (P. M.), STEVEN (E. M.). — The small for dates infant II. Neurological and intellectual performance. *Pediatrics*, 50, 50-57, 1972.

[30] FRANCIS-WILLIAMS (J.), DAVIES (P. A.). — Very low birth weight and later intelligence. *Develop. Med. Child. Neurol.*, 16, 709-728, 1974.

[31] GAIRDNER (D.), PEARSON (J.). — A growth chart for premature and other infants. *Arch. Dis. Child.*, 46, 783-787, 1971.

[32] GOHARI (P.), BERKOWITZ (R. L.), HOBBINS (J. C.). — Prediction of intrauterine growth retardation by determination of total intrauterine volume. *Am. J. Obstet. Gynecol.*, 127, 255-260, 1977.

[33] GOLDSTEIN (H.), PECKHAM (C.). — *The Biology of Human Fetal Growth*. ROBERTS D. F., THOMPSON A. M. (Eds). Taylor and Francis Ltd., London, 1976.

[34] GRANNUM (P.), BERKOWITZ (R. L.), HOBBINS (J. C.). — The ultrasonic changes in the maturing placenta and their relation to fetal pulmonic maturity. *Am. J. Obstet. Gynecol.*, 133, 915-922, 1979.

[35] GRUENWALD (P.). — Chronic fetal distress and placental insufficiency. *Biol. Neonate*, 5, 215-265, 1963.

[36] HABICT (J. P.), LECHTIG (A.), YARBROUGH (C.), KLEIN (R. E.). — Maternal nutrition, birth weight and infant mortality. In *Size at birth*. ELLIOT K., KNIGHT J. (Eds). Elsevier, Amsterdam, 1976.

[37] HAKANSON (D. O.), OH (W.). — Hyperviscosity in the small for gestational age infant. *Biol. Neonate*, 37, 109-112, 1980.

[38] HAMMARLUND (K.), SEDIN (G.). — Transepidermal water loss in newborn infants. *Acta Paediatr. Scand.*, 69, 377-383, 1980.

[39] HARCKE (H. T.), NAEYE (R. L.), STORCH (A.), BLANC (W. A.). — Perinatal cerebral intraventricular haemorrhage. *J. Pediatr.*, 80, 37-42, 1972.

[40] HOBBINS (J. C.). — Use of ultrasound in complicated pregnancies. *Clin. Perinatol.*, 7, 397-411, 1980.

[41] JARAI (I.), MESTYAN (J.), SCHULTZ (K.), LAZAR (A.), HALASZ (M.), KRASSY (I.). — Body size and neonatal hypoglycaemia in intrauterine growth retardation. *Early Hum. Develop.*, 1, 25-38, 1977.

[42] JONES (K. L.), SMITH (D. W.). — Recognition of the fetal alcohol syndrome in early infancy. *Lancet*, 2, 999-1001, 1973.

[43] LICHTY (J. A.), TING (R. Y.), BRUNS (P. D.), DYER (E.). — Studies of babies born at high altitudes. I. Relation of altitude to birthweight. *Am. J. Dis. Child.*, 93, 666-669, 1957.

[44] LIGGINS (G. C.). — The influence of the fetal hypothalamus and pituitary on growth. In *Size at birth*. ELLIOT K., KNIGHT J. (Eds). Elsevier, Amsterdam, 1976.

[45] LUBCHENCO (L. O.), BARD (H.). — Incidence of hypoglycaemia in newborn infants classified by birthweight and gestational age. *Pediatrics*, 47, 831-838, 1971.

[46] LUBCHENCO (L. O.), HANSMAN (C.), DRESSLER (M.), BOYD (E.). — Intrauterine growth as estimated from live-born birth weight data at 24-42 weeks of gestation. *Pediatrics*, 32, 793-800, 1963.

[47] MACDONALD (H. M.), MULLIGAN (J. C.), ALLEN (A. C.), TAYLOR (P. M.). — Neonatal asphyxia. I. Relationship of obstetric and neonatal complications to neonatal mortality in 38,405 consecutive deliveries. *J. Pediatr.*, 96, 898-902, 1980.

[48] MENON (M. K. K.). — *Obstetrics in India*. KELLAN R. J. (Ed). Butterworth, London, 1969.

[49] MILLER (H. C.), HASSANEIN (K.). — Diagnosis of impaired fetal growth in newborn infants. *Pediatrics*, 48, 511-522, 1971.

[50] MORRISON (J.), McLENNON (M. J.). — The theory, feasibility and accuracy of an ultrasonic method of estimating fetal weight. *Br. J. Obstet. Gynecol.*, 83, 833-837, 1976.

[51] NAEYE (R. L.), BLANC (W.), LEBLANC (W.), KHATAMEE (M. A.). — Fetal complications of maternal heroin addiction: Abnormal growth, infections and episodes of stress. *J. Pediatr.*, 83, 1055-1061, 1973.

[52] NAEYE (R. L.), DIXON (J. B.). — Distortions in fetal growth standards. *Pediatr. Res.*, 12, 987-991, 1978.

[53] NELIGAN (G. A.), KOLVIN (I.), SCOTT (D. M.), GARSIDE (R. F.). — Born too soon or born too small. *Clinics in Developmental Medicine 61*. Spastics International Medical Press, 1976.

[54] OAKLEY (J. R.), PARSONS (R. J.), WHITELAW (A. G. L.). — Standards for skinfold thickness in British newborn infants. *Arch. Dis. Child.*, 52, 287-290, 1977.

[55] OUNSTED (M.). — Fetal growth. In *Recent Advances in Paediatrics 4*. GAIRDNER D., HULL D. (Eds). Churchill Livingstone, Edinburgh, 1971.

[56] OUNSTED (M.), OUNSTED (C.). — On fetal growth rate. *Clinics in Developmental Medicine 46*. Spastics International Medical Press, 1973.

[57] PRIBYLOVA (H.), RAZOVA (M.), VONDRACEK (J.). — Glycogen content in subcutaneous adipose tissue of newborns of different birthweights in the first week of life. *Biol. Neonate*, 38, 154-160, 1980.

[58] PROCIANOY (R. S.), GARCIA-PRATS (J. A.), ADAMS (J. M.), SILVERS (A.), RUDOLPH (A. J.). — Hyaline membrane disease and intraventricular haemorrhage in small for gestational age infants. *Arch. Dis. Child.*, 55, 502-505, 1980.

[59] PYTKOWICZ-STREISSGUTH (A.), HERMAN (C. S.), SMITH (D. W.). — Intelligence, behaviour and dysmorphogenesis in the fetal alcohol syndrome: A report of 20 patients. *J. Pediatr.*, 92, 363-367, 1978.

[60] SCHIFF (D.), COLLE (E.), STERN (L.). — Metabolic and growth patterns in transient neonatal diabetes mellitus. *N. Engl. J. Med.*, *287*, 119-122, 1972.

[61] SCHIFRIN (B. S.). — In *Intrauterine asphyxia and the developing fetal brain*. GLUCK L. (Ed), Year Book Medical Publishers, Chicago, 1977.

[62] SCHULTE (F. J.). — Fetal malnutrition and brain development. In *Size at birth*. ELLIOT K., KNIGHT J. (Eds), Elsevier, Amsterdam, 1976.

[63] SCHULTE (F. J.), HINZE (G.), SCHREMPF (G.). — Maternal toxaemia, fetal malnutrition and bio-electric brain activity of the newborn. *Neuropae-diatrie*, *2*, 439-460, 1971.

[64] STEWART (A. L.), REYNOLDS (E. O. R.). — Improved prognosis for infants of very low birth weight. *Pediatrics*, *54*, 724-735, 1974.

[65] TEJANI (N.), MANN (L. J.), BHAHTHAVATHASA-

LAN (A.). — Correlation of fetal heart rate-uterine contraction patterns with fetal scalp *p*H. *Obstet. Gynecol.*, *46*, 392-396, 1975.

[66] USHER (R. H.). — Clinical and therapeutic aspects of fetal malnutrition. *Ped. Clin. N. Amer.*, *17*, 169-183, 1970.

[67] USHER (R.), MCLEAN (F.). — Intrauterine growth of live-born Caucasian infants at sea level. *J. Pediatr.*, *74*, 901-910, 1969.

[68] WALLIS (S. M.), HARVEY (D. R.). — In *Topics in Perinatal Medicine*. WHARTON B. (Ed.), Pitman Medical, England, 1980.

[69] WHITELAW (A. G. L.). — Influence of maternal, obesity on subcutaneous fat in the newborn. *Br. Med. J.*, *1*, 985-986, 1976.

[70] WINICK (M.). — Cellular growth in intrauterine malnutrition. *Ped. Clin. N. Amer.*, *17*, 69-78, 1970.

Perinatal asphyxia

G. PONTONNIER and H. GRANDJEAN

INTRODUCTION

Perinatal mortality is estimated to be about 15 $\%_{oo}$ in industrially developed countries. A third, or 5 $\%_{oo}$, is due to birth complications. Morbidity following peripartum asphyxia is less well established. We must in fact judge it at school age, that is to say long after the initial event. The after-effects are essentially neurological, and one can roughly distinguish two main types, psychomotor infirmity and mental retardation. In developed countries the frequency of cerebral palsy at school age is approximately 2.5 $\%_{oo}$ according to the "Collaborative Perinatal Study". One can estimate that about a third, or 0.8 $\%_{oo}$ cases, are linked to complications at birth. The frequency of severe mental retardation has, moreover, been estimated at 3.6 $\%_{oo}$, while that of less severe mental retardation, at 30 $\%_{oo}$. Between 1976 and 1978, several studies concluded that 10 % of severe mental retardation cases were provoked by complications at birth. It is more difficult to estimate the responsibility of birth complications in mild cases of mental retardation, since these after-effects are greatly modified by the child's environment and some of them were perhaps not clinically evident at the time of birth, as shown by Myers' study in the monkey [24].

Many perinatal complications due to peripartum asphyxia could be avoided by the application of our knowledge of the physiology and physiopathology of *in utero* fetal respiration. In addition, the early detection of high risk cases, the correct use of electronic monitoring and finally, properly adapted obstetrical management would enable us to prevent, or at least limit, the risk of death and after-effects.

The study of fetal asphyxia will therefore include several sections:

— the placenta,
— transplacental exchange of gases,
— fetal circulation,
— physiopathology of fetal asphyxia,
— acute fetal distress.

THE PLACENTA

The fetus does not have a functional lung before birth. Blood oxygenation takes place through contact with the maternal blood in the placenta. It is therefore indispensable to know the structure of this organ and its hemodynamic function, in order to understand the mechanism and pathology of fetal oxygenation *in utero*.

THE STRUCTURE OF THE PLACENTA

At term, the placenta is a fleshy mass of roughly circular shape. Its diameter varies from 16 to 20 cm and its weight represents about one sixth that of the fetus. It is located on the fundus of the uterus and has two sides. The fetal side is shiny and lined with the amnion. The umbilical cord is attached to the centre of this side. The maternal side is fleshy and is subdivided by grooves of varying depths which form 15 to 30 anatomical elements called maternal cotyledons. The placenta, which has a life cycle of 9 months, is a structure which is modified with its age. We can however consider that from the fifth month onwards, the general structure of the placenta varies very little. On microscopic anatomy one can distinguish (Fig. I-45):

The chorion plate. — This is located on the fetal side of the placenta. It is made up of the amniotic epithelium and of the chorion through which run the allanto-chorionic vessels which originate from the division of the two umbilical arteries and the umbilical vein. They subdivide to form the intravillous vessels.

The basal plate. — This corresponds to the zone of adherence of the placenta to the uterine mucosa. It is essentially composed of the decidua basalis which is evacuated with the placenta at delivery. It is into this area that the maternal vessels drain.

The intervillous space (I. V. S.). — This is the space in which the maternal blood, brought by the spiral arteries, circulates freely. In this blood are bathed the villous stems which become chorionic villi. The villous stems are projections of the chorionic plate. They contain arterial and venous branches from the allanto-chorionic vessels. According to the studies of the Brussels School [39], the main villous stems are 30 to 40 in number and hang perpendicularily from the chorionic plate. Each main primary stem divides into smaller secondary branches which descend to the basal plate onto which some of them anchor themselves, forming anchoring villi. They then form a loop and, following a recurrent path, make their way back towards the chorionic plate without actually reaching it. It is from these tertiary stems that the terminal villi are formed. They number approximately one million. According to the classical description, the villous stems formed from a primary villous stem make up a "drum system" which is the functional unit of the placenta; there are about 30 to 40 drum systems per placenta; they correspond to the maternal cotyledons, each drum system being separated from its neighbour by a septum which is a prolongation of the basal plate into the intervillous space; the theory of location of the orifices of this anatomical scheme is currently under criticism as it would seem that the maternal arteries do not open out into the center of the drum system. Gruenwald [16] ascertains that there is no correspondence between the maternal arteries and the drum system. Together with Ramsay [32], he describes a haphazard distribution of the arterial orifices in the basal plate. The majority of them open onto the zones separating

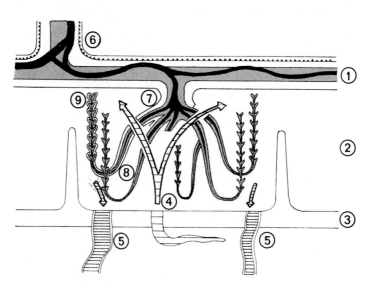

FIG. 1-45. — *Microscopic anatomy of the placenta: chorionic plate* (1), *intervillous space* (2), *basal plate* (3), *maternal artery* (4) *and vein* (5), *umbilical cord* (6), *primary* (7), *secondary* (8) *and tertiary* (9), *villous stems.*

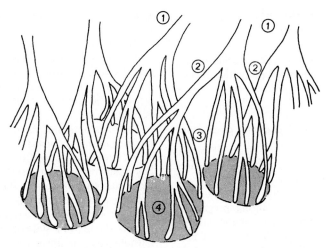

FIG. I-46. — *Scheme of the placental lobe from* GRUENWALD.
Primary (1), *secondary* (2) *and tertiary* (3) *villous stems; placental lobe* (4).

the drum system rather than onto the zone corresponding to the axis of this system. For Gruenwald the drum system, still called the placental lobe, is not formed from one main villous stem alone; it is made up by a ring of tertiary villous stems formed from several adjoining main villous stems. These lobes constitute the fetal cotyledons, and do not correspond anatomically to the maternal cotyledons (Fig. I-46).

This description takes into account the anatomical relationship between the fetal and maternal circulations. As in all mammals, the two circulations are separated. In the human placenta, and in that of primates in general, the fetal capillaries bathe in maternal blood. Fetal blood is simply separated from maternal blood by vascular endothelium and by the villous chorion which constitutes the placental membrane. This characteristic anatomical feature, called hemochorial structure, optimises feto-maternal exchanges.

PLACENTAL HEMODYNAMICS

Maternal circulation

This has been studied by radioangiography, by measurement of blood pressure, and by injection of tracers either into the maternal circulation, or into the intervillous space. The maternal blood runs through the arterial openings in the basal plate into the I. V. S. Under systolic pressure, which is about 80 mm Hg in the region of the uterine arteries, the blood flows in spurts, without lateral dispersion,

as far as the chorionic plate. These intermittent spurts correspond to the systolic output. It would seem that not all of the arterial orifices open at each systole. The utero-placental arteries probably do not all function simultaneously, either because of their own contractility or because of the contraction of the myometrium. The blood then mixes in the intervillous space where there is a pressure of 10 mm Hg. It is finally led off by the utero-placental veins where the pressure is about 8 mm Hg. The orifices of these veins open, as do those of the arteries, into the region of the basal plate.

The total volume of the intervillous space has been estimated by several authors at 250 ml. The maternal blood flow in the intervillous space can only be measured approximately after the injection of tracers directly into the intervillous space. Using 24 Na, Browne and Veall [7], thus estimated the rate of this flow at 600 ml/min. Pontonnier and Grandjean have had similar results with a method using 133 Xe injected into the intervillous space [27].

Fetal circulation

This is difficult to study in humans as there is no direct access to the villous stem. Only the umbilical cord is accessible at the moment of birth, but this cannot be considered as giving an accurate representation of the physiological conditions existing during pregnancy. The umbilical flow of a fetus at term can be estimated at approximately 200 ml/min. The pressure has been estimated at 70 mm Hg in the umbilical artery, at 35 mm Hg in the villous vessels, and at about 25 mm Hg in the umbilical vein.

Factors influencing placental hemodynamics

A number of factors, physiologic, pharmacologic and pathologic, can influence placental hemodynamics, and can cause repercussions on feto-maternal exchanges.

Factors influencing maternal placental circulation.

Arterial pressure. — The utero-placental blood flow is directly dependent on the perfusion pressure. Maternal hypotension of under 100 mm Hg can reduce the efficiency of placental perfusion. The causes of maternal hypotension during pregnancy can be pathological (hemorrhage, septic shock) or pharmacological, mainly during anesthesia and particularly peridural anesthesia. Acute or chronic arterial hypertension is also accompanied by a decrease in utero-placental blood flow; there is usually peripheral vasoconstriction, often with placental lesions. Treatment in these cases must try to prevent vasoconstriction while avoiding a too sudden drop in arterial pressure in order to preserve an efficient perfusion pressure.

Uterine contraction. — Many experimental studies have shown the existence of a reduction, and even an interruption, in the utero-placental blood flow during uterine contractions. Pose and Caldeyro-Barcia, recording the tissue pO_2 in the buttock of the fetus, showed that during uterine contractions there is a transitory and progressive drop in the fetal pO_2, the minimum of which occurs 30 or 40 seconds after the height of the contraction [30]. Uterine contraction reduces the utero-placental blood flow in two ways: by compression of the intra-myometrial vessels and by compression of the aorta and the iliac arteries by the contracted uterus. Uterine contraction brings about a rise in pressure in the intramyometrial vessels, and interrupts venous return, while the arteries, where the pressure is higher, continue to supply the intervillous space where the blood accumulates. When the intra-amniotic pressure reaches 30 to 55 mm Hg, the blood supply to the intervillous space is also interrupted and gas exchange takes place with maternal blood which becomes increasingly poor in oxygen. To this is added the fact that when a woman in labor is in a supine position, there is a decrease in the arterial circulation by compression of the aorta, or of one of its terminal branches, usually the right common iliac artery. This effect can be shown clinically by the temporary disappearance of the femoral pulse on the corresponding side and has been well demonstrated by the angiographic studies of Poseiro [31]. Arterial compression by the contracted uterus can lead to almost complete interruption of blood flow, with a sharp drop in arterial femoral systolic pressure and a slight rise in aortic systolic and diastolic pressure. This effect disappears when the patient is placed in the lateral decubitus position in which the uterus can no longer compress the great vessels.

The interruption of the utero-placental circulation during uterine contraction is usually for 10 to 20 seconds, and is well tolerated by a fetus which has a normal oxygen reserve. However there may be acute fetal distress if the contractions are too prolonged, or too close together, or if uterine relaxation is not sufficient between contractions, or if the fetus is already in a state of hypoxia due to different pathological circumstances.

Posture. — Compression of the inferior vena cava and of the pelvic venous system by the gravid uterus, together with the arterio-venous fistula constituted by the placenta, leads to hypertension in the veins of the lower limbs. In an upright position, there is venous stasis which short-circuits part of the blood mass. The supine position aggravates these effects and venous stasis can, in some cases, represent as much as a third of the volume of circulating blood and bring about a reduction in venous return to the heart, hypotension, and a state of shock. This syndrome of postural hypotension is frequently observed. It is promoted by the existence of a tonic uterus in the primipara, of hydramnios, a twin pregnancy or of venous abnormality in the lower limbs. This appears only in the last 3 months of gestation, and most often, near term. It is furthermore aggravated by blockade of the sympathetic nervous system, in particular during peridural anesthesia, or by the muscular relaxation provoked by a general anesthetic. Its treatment is simple, and consists of putting the patient into lateral decubitus. In the case of anesthesia, a slightly left lateral decubitus is a good preventive measure.

Muscular exercise. — Muscular exercise, which diverts blood from the splanchnic areas to that of the striated muscles, tends to diminish the blood supply to the placenta. This underlines the importance of rest in the treatment of all conditions likely to affect placental hemodynamics. Because of the effects of vascular compression due to posture, the resting position should be a left lateral one.

Stress. — Many animal experiments have shown that maternal stress provokes a decrease in utero-placental blood flow, due to the liberation of endogenous catecholamines. If this is prolonged, it can lead to fetal distress. Anesthesia can, in this case, be an efficient therapeutic measure during labor.

Pharmacologic modifications. — We know very little about the direct effects of drugs on the utero-placental blood flow. Vasopressive substances generally bring about a decrease in utero-placental blood flow, usually proportional to the increase in systemic arterial pressure, and to the degree of vasoconstriction of the uterine vessels. Local anesthetics also reduce the utero-placental flow. Their action seems to be directly on the uterine vessels and is not hindered by sympathetic block. The action of prostaglandins on utero-placental flow is difficult to estimate as it is combined with that of the uterine contractions which they produce. There is no known substance capable of increasing utero-placental flow. In fact it seems that the vessels already function at maximum vasodilatation. Thus, if one experimentally reduces the uterine flow for several minutes by compression of the aorta, it then goes back to its original state, but reactional hyperemia, which can be seen in other areas, has never been seen here.

Factors influencing fetal placental circulation. — The study of the factors affecting fetal circulation can only be indirect. The correlation existing between fetal arterial pressure, and umbilical blood flow has been studied experimentally by in vitro perfusion of the placenta. It appears that at physiological pO_2 and pCO_2 there is a close relationship between perfusion pressure and blood flow. Most research carried out on the vasomotricity of the umbilical cord vessels is difficult to interpret, as it was carried out under conditions too far from the physiological state. The umbilical cord vessels do not seem to be very sensitive to the biochemical elements in the blood, in particular the catecholamines. Only serotonin and bradykinin can trigger vasoconstriction. As Goodin [15] remarks, it seems that the main factor regulating the fetal placental flow is the pressure gradient between the umbilical arteries and vein. In the case of severe anoxia, the redistribution of fetal blood initially comprises an increase in umbilical flow. The experimental studies quoted above would lead one to believe that this increase in flow is linked to the fetal arterial hypertension triggered by the asphyxia.

During labor a compression of the umbilical cord may take place in the case of a prolapse or coiling around the fetal neck and may bring about a decrease and even an interruption of the oxygenated blood supply to the fetus.

TRANSPLACENTAL GAS EXCHANGE

TRANSPLACENTAL OXYGEN EXCHANGE

Oxygen consumption in the human fetus has been estimated at approximately 16 ml/min/kg. The quantity of oxygen present in the fetal organism is about 36 ml, which represents, at most, two minutes of survival for a fetus of 3 kg. Therefore, in order to survive and develop, the fetus needs an uninterrupted oxygen supply even though anaerobic glycolysis is, for the fetus, a more important source of energy than for the adult.

Oxygen is brought to the intervillous space by the maternal blood contained in the uterine artery. It crosses the placenta and passes into the fetal blood contained in the umbilical vein. The fetal circulation takes it to the tissues where it penetrates into the cells and is finally used by the fetal mitochondria.

Fetal oxygenation presents two specific characteristics: on the one hand the partial pressure of oxygen (pO_2) is very low in the arterial blood; it is 15 mm Hg; a partial pressure of oxygen at which the adult would be in anoxic coma; on the other hand the fetus uses, relatively speaking, twice as much oxygen as the adult. This is due to the immaturity of its enzyme systems, to the impossibility of oxidation of its fatty acids—a major source of ATP—and to the reduced number of mitochondria in its cells. In order to understand the origins of asphyxia in utero, and to try to prevent it, it is essential to understand how a fetus can live and develop in such a poor oxygen environment especially without any reserves. We must therefore study the nature and relative importance of the regulating mechanisms of transplacental oxygen exchange.

Among the many factors playing a part in this transfer, the main ones are:

(1) The progressive drop in oxygen partial pressure from the atmospheric air to the fetal mitochondria.

(2) The thickness and surface area of the placental membrane.

(3) The oxygen binding capacity of hemoglobin.

(4) The maternal placental blood flow.

(5) The fetal placental blood flow.

(6) The spatial relationship of the maternal and fetal circulatory currents and shunts.

The relative importance and role of these factors

are better known today thanks to research carried out in women during pregnancy and labor, chronic animal preparations (essentially monkeys and ewes) and lastly the mathematical models of placental gas exchange.

Oxygen pressure gradients

Oxygen moves from zones of high pressure to zones of low pressure (Fig. I-47). The partial pressure of oxygen is about 150 mm Hg in the air, 90 mm Hg in the uterine artery, 40 mm Hg in the intervillous space (the partial pressure equivalent to that of mount Everest), 27 mm Hg in the umbilical vein and only a few mm Hg in the fetal cell. The pressure gradient between the intervillous space and the intravillous capillaries is therefore about 13 mm Hg. This figure is too high to be explained by the simple fact of diffusion and is probably due to the hemodynamic factors limiting exchange and to the oxygen consumption of the placenta. This consumption is very high as it represents about a third of that of the fetus.

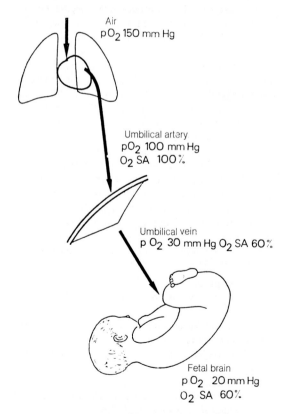

Air
pO_2 150 mm Hg

Umbilical artery
pO_2 100 mm Hg
O_2 SA 100%

Umbilical vein
pO_2 30 mm Hg O_2 SA 60%

Fetal brain
pO_2 20 mm Hg
O_2 SA 60%

FIG. I-47. — *Oxygen pressure gradients from mother to fetus.*

Longo, using a mathematical model, and the perfusion of a ewe's cotyledon in situ, studied the oxygen pressure gradients. A slight reduction of the maternal pO_2 to 70 mm Hg does not modify oxygen supply. If the maternal pO_2 falls to 50 mm Hg the oxygen transfer rate decreases from 24.8 ml/min to 20 ml/min, and the pO_2 in the villous capillaries decreases from 31.8 mm Hg to 25.9 mm Hg. This still allows the fetus to have a normal oxygen consumption. Fetal anoxia only appears if the maternal pO_2 falls below 50 mm Hg. This experimental observation is corroborated by measurements carried out in human fetuses in mothers living at high altitudes. These measurements show that the fetal pO_2 is normal although that of the mother only reaches 60 mm Hg. Furthermore, an increase of maternal pO_2 above normal has very little influence on the transplacental passage of oxygen. Indeed in hyperbaric oxygenation the fetal pO_2 only goes up by 10 % while the maternal pO_2 reaches 600 mm Hg.

Physiological variations in maternal pO_2 being small, it would seem probable that they play only a secondary role in the regulation of oxygen transfer to the fetus. It is obviously not the same in pathological circumstances where the decrease in maternal pO_2 will have a rapid effect on fetal oxygenation as soon as it falls below a certain level.

On the other hand, physiological variations in fetal pO_2 play an important role in the regulation of oxygen transfer. Longo has shown that variations of 1 mm Hg in the pO_2 in the umbilical artery bring about a variation of 6 % in placental oxygen transfer. He concluded from his experiments that, in physiological conditions, the rate of placental oxygen transfer is more influenced by a variation in the umbilical vein pO_2 than by a variation in any other factor.

The thickness and surface area of the placental membrane

Aherne and Dunill, using morphometry, estimated the distribution of the different placental compartments in women [1]. 21 % of the placental mass is made up of a non-parenchymal part, the basal plate and the chorionic plate. The parenchymal part is that which is concerned with gas exchange. It is made up of the intervillous space (36 %), the villi (58 %) and fibrin (4 %). The fetal capillaries occupy about 12 % of the parenchyma. The total surface area of the villi is about 11 m² but only a part of this is concerned in gas exchange. The zone of exchange was estimated by Aherne and Dunill at 1.8 m² at term. The thickness of the *placental membrane* is greater in the young placenta than in the term placenta. At the end of pregnancy it is about 3.5 microns to which one must add about 1 micron for the villi and 2 microns for the plasmic layer on each side of the villi walls. The thickness of the *alveolar membrane* is 2.5 microns in the newborn and 0.5 micron in the adult. However, the placental capacity is not very different from that of the lung as regards oxygenation, since, if the thickness of the membrane to be crossed is greater in the placenta, the surface area of exchange is also greater.

The capacity of oxygen binding by hemoglobin

The binding capacity of fetal blood is about 25 ml of oxygen per 100 ml of blood—that of adult blood is only 15 ml/100 ml. This capacity depends essentially on 3 factors: hemoglobin's affinity for oxygen, the concentration of hemoglobin in the blood, and the blood pH (Bohr effect). A study of the dissociation curves of oxygen showing the hemoglobin oxygen saturation percentage (O_2 Sa) related to the pO_2, demonstrates that in identical pH conditions, fetal hemoglobin has a higher affinity for oxygen than adult hemoglobin. In fact the fetal hemoglobin curve for a given pH is shifted to the left of the adult curve (Fig. I-48). However, in vivo fetal pH being lower than that of the mother, the gap between the two tends to be reduced, as acidosis shifts the curve towards the right. Analysis of the slopes of these dissociation curves shows that in the mother the pO_2, in the region of 100 mm Hg, can

vary greatly without significantly modifying the O_2 Sa, while, in the fetus, any variation of the pO_2, which is usually about 30 mm Hg, brings about a large modification of the O_2 Sa. The greater affinity of fetal hemoglobin for oxygen promotes oxygen binding by the fetal blood in the placenta. However this factor is probably not very important for survival as, on the one hand certain animals—cats, rabbits and rhesus monkeys—have a fetal hemoglobin affinity identical to that of the adult, and on the other hand, in severe Rhesus immunisation, fetal transfusion in utero with adult erythrocytes maintains oxygen exchange. It is interesting to note that the difference in the affinity of hemoglobin for oxygen only exists when the erythrocyte is intact, and disappears if the hemoglobin is extracted from the erythrocyte by hemolysis. This difference is due to the binding of 2.3-diphosphoglycerol to the β-chain of adult hemoglobin. This link does not exist with the α-chain of fetal hemoglobin which is free to bind with oxygen. The β-chain is mainly synthesised after birth.

The concentration of hemoglobin also influences the transfer capacity of oxygen. It is 16 g/100 ml in the fetus and only 12 g/100 ml in the adult. This helps the fetal blood in the placenta to bind oxygen. Alkalosis, whether it be gaseous or metabolic, increase the blood's affinity for oxygen. This leads to a shift to the left in the dissociation curve. Acidosis, on the contrary, shifts the curve to the right. This is the Bohr effect. In the placenta the transfer of the CO_2 and acid ions of the fetal blood to the maternal blood brings about an increase in fetal pH and helps oxygen binding by the fetal hemoglobin. On the maternal side, the arrival of the CO_2 from the fetus decreases the pH facilitating liberation of oxygen from the maternal hemoglobin. The Bohr effect is therefore doubly beneficial. It can, however, be harmful in certain cases of extreme maternal hypocapnia. Maternal hyperventilation during labour can bring about severe maternal respiratory alkalosis, which reduces the liberation of oxygen from the maternal blood.

Maternal placental blood flow

The transfer of O_2 is closely linked to the maternal blood flow. Proof of this link has been established in the gravid ewe by Assali [3]. If the ewe is submitted to experimental hypotension there is a drop in fetal pO_2, although the maternal arterial pO_2 is maintained at normal levels by assisted ventilation. This fall is due to a reduction in the transplacental

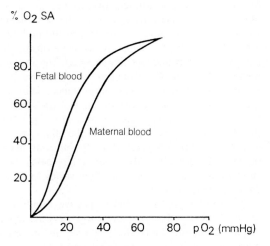

FIG. I-48. — *Dissociation curves of oxygen for maternal and fetal blood.*

passage of oxygen, which is itself related to a decrease in placental flow due to hypotension.

A number of other experimental studies have shown the harmful effects of a decrease in utero-placental flow on fetal oxygenation whether this be pharmacological or physiopathological, linked to hypotension, stress, or to uterine hyperactivity. The harmful effect on the fetus is greater when the decrease in flow is prolonged or when the fetus is already acidotic.

Fetal placental blood flow

The existence of sufficient umbilical blood flow is essential for the passage of oxygen from the mother to the fetus. However it would seem that the fetus has little control over the flow through the umbilical vessels. We know that the existence of an innervation of the umbilical cord and placental vessels has not been irrefutably demonstrated. Studies on the placental cotyledons perfused in vitro show that an increase in pO_2 could bring about vasoconstriction of the fetal vessels; yet Dawes has shown experimentally in vivo that the umbilical flow does not vary despite large variations in the fetal pO_2 and pCO_2 [12]. It would also seem that in the case of severe anoxia the umbilical flow is, at least at first, preserved due to an increase in fetal arterial pressure.

The spatial relationship between the maternal and fetal circulation currents and shunts

The spatial relationship between the maternal and fetal circulation currents in the placenta are not well understood and several theories have been proposed.

The existence of parallel flows in the same or opposite directions seems improbable. It is rather more plausible to think that the maternal circulation creates a blood pool, or several blood flows which each meet several villi during their crossing of the intervillous space. The hypothesis of a maternal blood pool supposes that the blood penetrates in sufficient quantities and in a large enough space, for the mixture in which the villi float to be homogeneous. The pO_2 would be identical throughout the space and comparable conditions of exchange would thus exist in all of the fetal villi. On the contrary, in the hypothesis of several flows, each of their pO_2's would decrease as it crossed the intervillous space. Thus the villi, according to the place they

were at, would float in more or less oxygenated blood, and the conditions of exchange would differ. The mixture of blood of different pO_2's would take place in the umbilical vein.

Furthermore, it is known that the utero-placental arteries do not function simultaneously. It is thus thought that certain zones of the intervillous space are not so well irrigated as others. This leads to the equivalent of a shunt.

Conclusion

It has been noted that oxygen transfer across the placenta depends on many different factors, which are still the subject of discussion. Their relative importance has only just begun to be suspected and they should therefore be the object of further research. We can however consider briefly that oxygen transfer depends on the existence of contrary forces.

The main element in the exchange is made up by the oxygen pressure gradient existing between the maternal circulation and the fetal circulation. The relative thickness of the placental membrane, the inequality of placental perfusion and the placental consumption of O_2 constitute a hindrance to exchange. These negative forces are counterbalanced by the greater capacity of the fetal blood to bind oxygen.

The use of mathematical models of placental exchange enabled Longo to appreciate the relative importance of the different factors influencing fetal oxygenation. He concluded that, under physiological circumstances, few of the factors play a part in the regulation of transplacental exchange. The transfer of oxygen is above all sensitive to the prevailing pO_2 in the umbilical artery and to the fetal hemoglobin affinity for oxygen. The pO_2 in the umbilical artery being linked to fetal tissue metabolism, this parameter forms a direct link between the requirements and the supply of oxygen. Other factors play a part but they are of lesser importance. Thus, for example, the consequences of physiological variations in the maternal arterial pO_2 are slight and the changes in concentration or in the affinity of the hemoglobin takes several days to have an effect on fetal oxygenation. Moreover it has never been shown that placental maternal flow varies in accordance with fetal needs.

In pathological cases, the respective importance of the factors influencing placental oxygenation is totally different. Thus the decrease in maternal placental flow plays a predominant role as it is at the origin of most fetal anoxia during labor.

Insufficient oxygenation of the maternal blood is, on the other hand, a less frequent cause of fetal distress. A decrease of blood flow in the umbilical cord and a reduction of the surface area of placental exchange can also disturb fetal-maternal oxygen exchange.

THE TRANSPLACENTAL EXCHANGE OF CO_2

At physiological partial pressure, only 10 % of the carbon dioxide produced by tissue metabolism can be transported in its dissolved form. The rest must be transformed and becomes mainly bicarbonate (70 %) and to a lesser extent (20 %) combined with hemoglobin forming carboxyhemoglobin. The liberation of fetal carbon dioxide in the placenta depends on the same factors as those regulating the transplacental passage of oxygen. We shall only examine four of them in detail: the fetal-maternal pCO_2 gradient, hemoglobinemia, blood carbon dioxide affinity, and the Haldane effect.

In the mother, at the end of pregnancy, there is a physiological gaseous alkalosis. The pCO_2 is at that moment about 32 mm Hg. During normal labor the maternal pCO_2 decreases to 23 mm Hg. In the fetus the pCO_2 is higher. It is 35 to 40 mm Hg in the scalp during labor and 40 mm Hg in the umbilical artery at birth. There is therefore a gradient of 15 to 20 mm Hg between the maternal and fetal blood during labor. Some authors estimate this gradient at only 5 mm Hg during pregnancy. However as carbon dioxide is a very diffusible gas, this low gradient suffices to establish exchange. The greater hemoglobin concentration of the fetal blood allows it to transport more carbon dioxide for a given increase of partial pressure with smaller modifications of the pH, when compared to adult blood.

For a given pCO_2, carbon dioxide saturation of the fetal blood is less than that of the mother. This can be seen in the dissociation curve of carbon dioxide in the blood, which gives the relationship between the quantity of total blood carbon dioxide, dissolved and combined, and the pCO_2. The dissociation curve of the fetus is to the right of the mother's (Fig. I-49). The lesser affinity of the fetal blood constitutes a factor helping the transfer of fetal CO_2 towards the mother.

The binding capacity of CO_2 by the blood depends directly on the quantity of hemoglobin which is not linked to oxygen. Thus, at the same pCO_2, blood which gives up oxygen can accept more CO_2. This is the Haldane effect. In the placenta the transfer

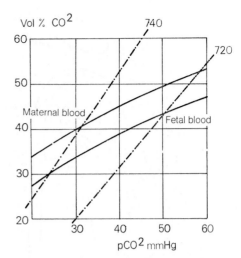

Fig. I-49. — *Dissociation curves of carbon dioxide for maternal and fetal blood.*

of CO_2 from the fetus to the mother is thus facilitated by the simultaneous transfer of oxygen from the mother to the fetus. On the maternal side, in contrast, the release of oxygen will favor carbon dioxide binding to hemoglobin. As with the Bohr effect, the Haldane effect is doubly beneficial in placental exchange.

FETAL CIRCULATION

The distribution of oxygen to the fetal tissues depends on two main factors. The oxygen saturation of the fetal blood, and blood flow in the tissues. We have already seen that the fetal arterial blood has an oxygen transport capacity which is greater than that of an adult due to its higher concentration of hemoglobin. The fact that the fetal hemoglobin has a greater affinity for oxygen is an advantage for oxygen binding in the placenta, but becomes a disadvantage in the tissues. Arterial blood flow is probably the most important factor in tissue oxygenation. In order to study this, we must first look at the anatomical characteristics of the fetal circulatory system, then at the heart and peripheral circulatory regulation.

ANATOMY

The fetal circulation includes three elements which disappear after birth. The ductus venosus,

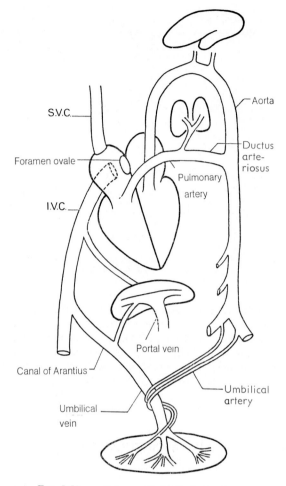

of the deoxygenated blood coming from the superior vena cava (S. V. C.) and the coronary veins, and 75 % of the oxygenated blood coming from the I. V. C. Only half of the blood from the right atrium goes into the right ventricle. The rest of it passes into the left atrium through the foramen ovale. The fact that the foramen ovale is adjacent to the orifice opening into the I. V. C. means that the blood crossing the foramen ovale is oxygenated blood coming directly from the I. V. C. This blood merges, in the left atrium, with a small quantity of deoxygenated blood coming from the pulmonary veins, and flows into the left ventricle, enters the ascending aorta and flows towards the cerebral circulation. 10 % of the merged blood contained in the right ventricle goes towards the lungs and 90 % of it joins the ductus arteriosus and flows into the descending aorta below the source of the carotid arteries. This anatomical arrangement explains how the blood destined to the brain has the highest oxygen saturation of the entire fetal organism, 62 %, whereas that of the femoral artery and the pulmonary artery are only 58 % and 52 % respectively. In cases of hypoxia, or under different pharmacologic influences, the ductus arteriosus is susceptible to vasoconstriction. This closure greatly reduces the circulation in the pulmonary artery, bringing about intracardiac modifications of pressure, and orienting the blood preferentially towards the left of the heart, which results indirectly in an increase in cerebral flow. Among the drugs likely to produce this vasoconstriction of the ductus arteriosus, are acetylcholine, cathecholamines, histamine and prostaglandin inhibitors. Severe anoxia and the prostaglandins can, on the contrary, keep the ductus arteriosus open after birth. The existence of the foramen ovale, and of the ductus arteriosus leads to parallel functioning of the right and left sides of the fetal heart, while in the adult the two sides function in series.

FIG. I-50. — *Scheme of the fetal circulation.*

the ductus arteriosus and the foramen ovale (Fig. I-50).

Umbilical vein blood flows in two directions, 60 % joins the ductus venosus and flows directly into the inferior vena cava (I. V. C.), by-passing the liver, and 40 % goes into the portal vein and crosses the liver. Two thirds of the I. V. C. blood flows through the right atrium and directly into the left atrium due to the presence of the foramen ovale, a third remains in the right atrium. A pressure gradient of about 3 mm Hg between the I. V. C. and the left atrium helps this opting of the oxygenated blood for the left atrium. Any compression of the umbilical cord can modify this pressure gradient altering the intracardiac distribution of oxygenated blood. The same thing happens during respiratory movements of the fetus in utero. Under normal conditions, the right atrium receives 25 %

REGULATION

The heart

In order to understand the cardiac response to hypoxia better, it is necessary to know the mechanical and chemical characteristics differentiating the fetal heart from that of the adult. Friedmann et al. [14] have shown that the proportion of contractile heart tissue is only about 30 % in the fetus, while in the adult it reaches as much as 60 %. They conclude that under physiological circumstances the fetal heart functions at a maximum rate in order to satisfy the needs of the tissues.

The degree to which the parasympathetic innervation of the myocardium is developed is an important factor in cardiac regulation. The cardiac concentration of noradrenaline, the principal neurotransmitter of the sympathetic nervous system, indicates the degree of development of this system. Friedmann et al. [14] in their histochemical studies have shown that this concentration is much lower in the fetal myocardium than in that of the adult. On the other hand, the parasympathetic innervation is the same. Furthermore, the immaturity of the sympathetic system renders the fetal heart hypersensitive to noradrenaline, because the sympathetic nerves play a part in the complex system of the inactivation of noradrenaline. This lack of balance in the autonomic innervation of the heart explains why the myocardial response to asphyxia is usually predominantly vagal. Moreover, the fetal adrenal glands contain a large quantity of catecholamines which, in the event of asphyxia, are liberated into the circulation, and to which the myocardium is very sensitive. This, plus the fact of adrenal circulatory conservation, in cases of stress, leads us to a better understanding of the fetal heart's response to asphyxia.

Study of the role of the autonomic nervous system in the regulation of cardiac function has been carried out by two methods: injection of adrenergic or cholinergic transmitters, or, on the contrary, administration of sympathetic or parasympathetic system blocking agents. The injection of a beta-stimulating drug soon brings about fetal tachycardia. This becomes extremely marked during the last third of the gestation period in the fetus of the ewe. Injection of acetylcholine during the second half of gestation causes bradycardia and hypotension. Atropine obviously has the opposite effect on the heart rate. The injection of beta-blocking drugs causes slight bradycardia during the last third of gestation. Numerous experiments on animals have taught us that the autonomic nervous system has an increasing influence on the heart from the second half of gestation onwards and also that there are differences in the development of the different regulatory systems, the parasympathetic system predominating.

The systemic circulation

In animals the fetal cardiac flow, expressed per kg weight, is estimated at three times that of the adult. According to studies carried out on animals, under normal conditions, the placenta receives about 50 % of the cardiac flow, the heart receives 4 %, the lungs 5 %, the brain 3 % and the adrenal glands 2 %. If one looks at the blood flow of each organ, not as a percentage of the total flow but in relation to weight, the myocardium receives twice as much blood per minute and per gram, as the brain, the lungs and the placenta, which receive approximately the same amount of blood. The regulation of the systemic circulation is of nervous and humoral origin. In the majority of mammals the autonomic nervous system develops rapidly near term and continues to develop after birth. Contrary to the nervous control of the heart, that of the vessels is, in the fetus, essentially sympathetic. The sympathetic system is mediated by baroreceptors and peripheral chemoreceptors. These develop during the second half of gestation in the aorta, the main blood vessels and the carotid sinus. The sensitivity of the α- and β-noradrenergic receptors increases with the age of the fetus. The contribution of sympathetic control of the vessels can be estimated by blockade with the sulfonium derivative of trimetophan. This produces only minimal hypotension. In fact, the regulation of the fetal circulation is essentially humoral. Animal experimentation has shown that the levels of circulating catecholamines are very high in the fetus —much more so than in the adult. It is the same in the adrenal glands. The fetal circulation responds in a violent manner to stimulation by catecholamines in comparison to the slight changes brought about by blockade of the nervous control of the circulatory vessels. The injection of adrenalin and the consequent beta-stimulation leads to tachycardia, with an increase in cardiac output, and hypotension caused by a decrease in peripheral resistance. Noradrenalin, by alpha stimulation, produces moderate bradycardia with a decrease in cardiac output and hypertension, indicating an increase in peripheral resistance. Other substances can also be made to act on fetal vasomotricity. The renin-angiotensin system, serotonin, histamine, bradykinin, vasopressin, and the E_2 prostaglandins modify vascular and systemic resistance. These substances probably play an important part in the cardiovascular adaptation to anoxia.

PHYSIOPATHOLOGY
OF FETAL ASPHYXIA

The fetus is more resistant to asphyxia than the adult. This has been shown experimentally many times. Moreover, fetal resistance to a lack of oxygen is evident, since the conditions of oxygenation of the fetal tissues during human pregnancy are incompatible with the survival of an adult. Myers has observed that the length of time necessary for asphyxia to cause cerebral lesions decreases with the time of gestation in the monkey. Faced with anoxia, the fetal organism reacts by a modification of its acid-base balance, and by cardiovascular adjustment. This is seen in a modification of the fetal heart rate curves (F. H. R.) the observation of which can help in the diagnosis of acute fetal distress. After having discussed the influence of asphyxia on acid-base balance and cardio-vascular adjustment, we will examine the physiopathological mechanisms which are basic to the different aspects of fetal heart rate observed in labour.

MODIFICATION
OF THE ACID-BASE BALANCE AND GASES
IN THE BLOOD

Whatever the cause, acute fetal distress can be considered, from a physiopathological point of view, to be the consequence of an abnormal decrease in transplacental gas exchange. This leads to a decrease in oxygen transfer from the mother to the fetus and therefore to fetal hypoxemia which itself leads to hypoxia or anoxia. Furthermore, there is carbon dioxide retention in the fetus which leads to an increase in the concentration of bicarbonate and therefore to respiratory acidosis.

The first signs of fetal asphyxia are a drop in the pO_2, hypercapnia and a fall in the pH due to respiratory acidosis. The decrease in oxygen supply to the tissues in the case of severe hypoxemia rapidly modifies their metabolism. Although other elements have been shown to play a specific energy role, such as the amino-acids and fatty acids, the main source of energy in the fetal organism is still glucose which is normally catabolised in the presence of oxygen. When this is lacking the fetus produces the energy necessary for the survival of the cells by anaerobiosis. In normal circumstances, anaerobic glycolysis is already used much more easily by the fetus than by the adult. Villee has shown that if one incubates fetal and adult tissue with a given quantity of glucose in the absence of oxygen, fetal tissue produces three times more pyruvate than does the adult tissue. This could be attributed to the nature of glycolytic enzymes which are different in the fetus and the adult. In the event of hypoxia, anaerobic glycolysis becomes important.

At first it only occurs in areas of vaso-constriction, but if the hypoxia continues all areas are progressively involved. However anaerobic glycolysis can only be a short-term solution, since it has three serious consequences: a decrease in energy production, draining of glycogen reserves, and metabolic acidosis.

Decrease in energy production. — Anaerobic glycolysis is a weak energy producing process. Aerobic oxidation of a molecule of glucose gives 36 molecules of ATP. Anaerobic catabolism of the same molecule gives only 2 ATP molecules. Thus when oxygen is lacking, the tissues must increase catabolism in order to generate enough energy.

The wastage of glycogen reserves. — The fetal glycogen reserves are primarily in the liver, heart and kidneys. In physiological conditions, it would seem that gluconeogenesis is relatively unimportant in the maintenance of normoglycemia. Glucose needs in the muscles and brain are in fact largely met by maternal glucose which diffuses easily across the placenta. It is only when maternal supplies become insufficient that the fetus is obliged to use its reserves. In pathological conditions, two mechanisms combine to drain the reserves: the decrease in maternal glucose supply and the increase in glycogen catabolism. Maternal supply can decrease chronically which sometimes happens in certain fetal hypotrophies; in these cases the fetus becomes unable to withstand anoxia for any length of time. Any acute alteration in feto-maternal exchange is also unfavourable, since an insufficient maternal glucose supply adds to the massive consumption of the glycogen reserves produced by the fetal anoxia.

Metabolic acidosis. — Glucose is normally catabolised into pyruvic acid following the Emden and Meyerhof pathway which is completely anaerobic; pyruvic acid is then decarboxylated in the presence of oxygen; this constitutes the Krebs cycle which occurs inside the mitochondria. This catabolism results in the formation of CO_2 and H_2O and produces the energy necessary for the regeneration of ATP which is essential for cell synthesis, the active transport of ions and molecules across the membranes and the transformation of liberated energy into mechanical energy for the contractile systems of the cell. During anoxia, the lack of oxygen prevents the decarboxylation of pyruvic acid, which is therefore metabolized into lactic acid. This accumulates in the fetal tissues and brings about metabolic acidosis with a fall in blood pH. In the resistance to acidosis the fetal organism cannot, as with the adult, use the pulmonary elimination of CO_2. As the passage of acid ions across the placenta towards the mother does not allow sufficient elimination, the buffer systems of the fetal blood, and in particular reduced hemoglobin, are fully utilized. Acidosis, as previously noted, decreases hemoglobin affinity for oxygen (Bohr effect); leading to a fall in oxygen saturation for a given pO_2. This has a doubly beneficial effect: the quantity of reduced hemoglobin available as a buffer is increased and oxygen is more easily liberated into the tissues. But this relief is obviously only temporary as, if acidosis increases, the cell cannot carry out anaerobic glycolysis. The pH incompatible with survival is estimated at about 6.90.

CARDIOVASCULAR ADJUSTMENT

Cardiac adjustment

The fetal heart's response to anoxia results in metabolic adjustment and a modification in its hemodynamic function. From a metabolic point of view the fetal heart uses glucose as the sole source of energy, and its relatively good resistance to anoxia can be explained by its enzyme system which is particularly adapted to anaerobic glycolysis. Friedman et al. compared the effects of asphyxia on fragments of adult and fetal cardiac muscle. The spontaneous contractions of the fetal myocardium last much longer than those of the adult, in a poor oxygen environment. All authors agree that fetal cardiac resistance is due to the fact that anaerobic glycolysis is greater than in the adult. Friedman et al. showed that oxidation blockade by dinitrophenol arrests myocardial contraction in the adult much more rapidly than in the fetus. In contrast, the blockade of anaerobic glycolysis by iodoacetate stops the fetal heart even when oxygen is present whereas it has no effect on adult muscle. If one considers the force of the contractions rather than their frequency, the results are much the same. Oxidation blockade produces a decrease in the force of cardiac contractions in the fetus and in the adult; the blockade of anaerobic glycolysis only affects fetal muscle. Mott [23] and then Dawes et al. [13] have also shown that there is a correlation between the glycogen concentration in the myocardium and resistance to asphyxia. Therefore a lack of glycogen due to undernutrition could decrease the time of survival. In the same way, the fetus resists asphyxia all the better for being

young and it is known that the glycogen content of the myocardium diminishes during gestation. The importance of glycogen is all the greater in that the fetus cannot use the oxidation of fatty acids, due to a lack of carnitine which transports them to the mitochondria. The oxidation of fatty acids represents 70 % of the myocardium's source of energy in the adult at rest and 20 % in the active adult, the remainder being supplied by glucose. The predominance of anaerobic metabolism of glucose could be due to the paucity of mitochondria in the fetal heart cells, which are, moreover, immature.

The hemodynamic function of the fetal heart is modified by anoxia. The majority of experiments done on animals show that hypoxia, whether it is associated or not with acidosis, brings about bradycardia in the fetus. This is the opposite of the reaction in the adult animal where the first reaction to hypoxia is tachycardia. In fact tachycardia does not seem to be a direct reaction of the myocardium. At first there is an alveolar reflex which is generated by hyperventilation appearing after hypoxia. If this hyperventilation is experimentally suppressed in animals, hypoxemia leads to bradycardia in the adult. The fetus does not respond to hypoxemia by hyperventilation, so it is normal that there is bradycardia. This would seem to be a specific response of cardiac muscle to anoxia. This is proven by the fact that the fetal or adult heart in experimental isolation, responds to anoxia with a decrease in the force and frequency of its contractions. On the other hand certain observations made in humans suggest that the initial fetal response to hypoxemia is tachycardia and that bradycardia only appears at a more advanced stage. These contradictions can only be explained by differences in the production mechanisms of hypoxia, or by a difference in maturity of the autonomic nervous systems, the adrenal glands, or the vasoreceptors. In fact it is interesting to note that in the ewe's fetus, the cardiac response to hypoxia varies with age. During the first two thirds of gestation, hypoxia brings about tachycardia. It is only later that the response is bradycardia, that is more marked as term approaches, perhaps because of a relationship to vagal activity.

The influence of fetal bradycardia induced by hypoxia on the cardiac flow is of current interest. In theory bradycardia increases the length of diastole and therefore permits a better filling of the left ventricle which in turn leads to stretching of the myocardial fibres. These two factors, a better filling and stretching, should allow for an increase in the volume of ventricular ejection and therefore a conservation of cardiac output. Cohn and Rudolph, in fact, found that in the fetus of the ewe, there is a decrease in cardiac flow which is slight and not significant in the case of isolated hypoxemia, but significant in the case of hypoxemia associated with acidosis [11]. Although this decrease in cardiac output has not been proven in the case of hypoxia in the human fetus, it is possible that it exists, since the fibres of the fetal myocardium have a contractile speed and force lower than that of the adult. This means that in physiological conditions the fetal heart already works maximally. The absence of an increase in cardiac output, in the event of anoxia, explains the necessity for a redistribution of the blood mass. This takes place in the peripheral circulation and also in the cardiac cavities. Animal experimentation has shown that asphyxia and more particularly acidosis triggers vasoconstriction of the pulmonary circulation and of the ductus arteriosus. This results in a decrease in right ventricular flow and in a drainage of part of the blood of the SVC by the foramen ovale. This redistribution maintains, and sometimes increases, the left ventricular output to the detriment of the right ventricle.

Adjustment
of the systemic circulation

In 1959 Schollender suggested that the fetal reaction to anoxia could be compared to that of certain mammals submitted to long periods of immersion [36]. During these phases of asphyxia it has been observed that there is a redistribution of the blood towards the organs which are indispensable for survival, such as the heart and the brain, and that this occurs to the detriment of other less important areas (the skin, kidneys, etc.). Since this hypothesis was advanced, many experimental studies have tried to analyse the fetus' circulatory adjustment to anoxia. This adjustment is characterised by variations in blood pressure and by a redistribution of visceral blood flow. In the case of blood pressure, hypoxia brings about hypertension in the fetus near term; it has no effect prior to then. The redistribution of visceral blood in hypoxia has been proven by chronic animal preparations. Rudolph and co-workers [11] measured visceral blood flow by using marked microspheres. Anoxia was induced in a ewe's fetus by making the mother breathe a mixture poor in oxygen. Although the experimental conditions were identical, half the fetuses showed symptoms of pure hypoxia, and the others, hypoxia associated with acidosis. In both groups hypoxia led to bradycardia, with conserva-

tion of cardiac output in cases of hypoxia associated with acidosis. Umbilical blood flow is not modified in absolute terms, but represents, on the other hand, a more important part of the cardiac output. The blood flow to the lungs, intestines, spleen and skeleton is decreased while the flow to the brain, myocardium and adrenals is increased. These changes in flow in the different areas also exist in absolute terms as well as in percentage of cardiac output. They appear in the two groups of fetuses but are more marked in the acidosis group. These results have been confirmed in primates by Behrman et al. who have shown that, in cases of hypoxia, the percentage of cardiac flow destined to the brain doubles and that in this organ there is a redistribution of blood giving preference to noncortical zones [5]. Moreover it must be noted that apart from an increase in cerebral flow, they observed that there is also a modification in the composition of the blood going to the brain. In physiological conditions deoxygenated blood from the SVC only represents 1 % of the blood irrigating the brain, in the event of hypoxia it represents 26 %. Although the brain blood flow increases in the event of hypoxia, with or without acidosis, the oxygen saturation decreases and finally, depending on the degree of hypoxia, the oxygenation of the brain is only just maintained or even decreased.

The experiments quoted above have studied the redistribution of visceral blood flow in fetal hypoxia produced by insufficient oxygen supply to the mother. This has not been studied in cases of acute fetal distress from other causes, such as maternal hypotension or cord compression. It is however probable that the same hemodynamic changes would take place.

Redistribution of cardiac flow in the case of hypoxemia is a safeguard mechanism which preserves oxygenation of the viscera indispensable for survival, to the detriment of other areas. There are many factors concerned in this response, and their relative importance is not well known. Research has given us a better knowledge of fetal circulatory physiology and the results given above allow us to make certain hypotheses. The effects observed are probably the direct result of (1) hypoxemia and acidosis on the heart and blood vessels, (2) secretion of catecholamines and other vasomotor substances and (3) of an excitation of the autonomic nervous system. The different responses to hypoxemia according to the age of the fetus can be explained by the greater or lesser maturity of the systems involved. The adrenals, an important source of catecholamines, play an essential role in circulatory readjustment following hypoxemia.

PHYSIOPATHOLOGICAL MECHANISMS RESPONSIBLE FOR CHANGES IN FETAL HEART RATE (FHR) CURVES

Baseline FHR and rapid oscillations

Regulation of the FHR takes place on two levels, that of the heart where the sino-auricular node controls automatic heart activity, and that of the central nervous system where the vagal cardio-inhibiting centre and sympathetic cardioaccelerating centre are found. At all times these different systems can adapt the FHR to fetal hemodynamic needs. Their action is mainly modulated by the chemical and hemodynamic variations of the circulating blood. These can act directly on nodal tissue or on nervous centres. They can also act indirectly by means of baroreceptors and chemoreceptors. Mendez-Bauer showed the consistent role of the vagus. By injection of atropine into a normal human fetus he obtained an acceleration of 30 beats/minute. Renou et al. injecting a beta blocker into the mother, noticed a slowing of the FHR by 10 beats/min. The FHR would therefore seem to be the result of accelerating and slowing effects of the sympathetic and parasympathetic systems. In normal conditions, these effects result in a rhythm of 120 to 140 beats/min with additional temporary fluctuations of 5 to 20 beats/min. On top of these rapid oscillations, the tracings of FHR show waves with a cycle of about 1 minute. According to Dawes, these variations are related to breathing movements in utero.

The disappearance of rapid oscillations of the FHR results in a flat tracing. This can be produced by several mechanisms: (1) a depression of the nervous centres under the effects of hypoxia, hypercapnia and their resulting metabolic changes, (2) a resting state similar to that of sleep where exterior excitation makes normal oscillations reappear; (3) the action of drugs such as atropine, which are central depressants. One can also see a flat tracing in certain fetal abnormalities: anencephaly, cardiac malformations and immaturity.

The accelerations

The baseline heart rate can show accelerations related to uterine contraction or fetal movements. These are due to several mechanism: (1) sympathetic excitation triggered by pressure on the trunk or fetal limbs, by sound waves or ultra-sound: (2) brief excitation of the chemoreceptors: (3) temporary compression of the umbilical vein which triggers hypotension and stimulates the baroreceptors: lastly (4) periods of breathing movement in utero. In the human fetus, these accelerations have an average amplitude of 20 beats per minute and last from 20 to 60 seconds. All authors agree that these accelerations are the sign of a healthy fetus.

Periodic decelerations

These are decelerations of the FHR due to uterine contraction. They have been widely studied in the human fetus and classified in several ways; we will refer only to the two main classifications by Caldeyro-Barcia and Hon since they permit a simple description of all observed periodic decelerations. According to Hon [18] there are 3 types of deceleration, defined in relationship to the onset of uterine contraction. Early decelerations start at the beginning of the contractions and have a regular shape. Late decelerations start afterwards and have an irregular shape. Variable decelerations start at various moments of the contractions and their shape varies.

According to Caldeyro-Barcia [8], the decelerations are not defined in relationship to the start of contractions, but rather in relationship to the time lapse between the lowest point of bradycardia and the peak of uterine contractions. Type 1 DIP is a transitory bradycardia and there is a time lapse of 3 to 20 seconds between its lowest point and the highest point of uterine contraction. This corresponds to Hon's early deceleration. Type 2 DIPS are characterised by a time lapse of 20 to 60 seconds and correspond to Hon's late deceleration. Types 1 and 2 DIPS can also be associated and partly correspond to Hon's variable decelerations.

The physiopathology of periodic decelerations is well known. It has been mostly studied by Hon and above all Caldeyro-Barcia more than a decade ago. Since then, experimental work has confirmed their hypotheses. The correlation between the clinical and biological condition of the newborn child and periodic decelerations have shown the practical importance of these physiopathological studies.

Early decelerations. — Early decelerations are due to a compression of the fetal head by means of a reflex mechanism. Caldeyro-Barcia showed that the rate of contraction with DIP 1 is practically zero at the beginning of labour and progressively increases by 50 % till the moment of expulsion.

In the same way, membrane rupture increases the type 1 DIP rate. Conditions enhancing the appearance of type 1 DIPS at the end of labor, that is with membranes ruptured and the head engaged, also help fetal head compression. Schwarcz has shown that the pressure exerted on the head is twice as strong under these conditions as the intra-amniotic pressure. Mendez-Bauer observed decelerations comparable to type 1 DIPS when he manually compressed the head of the fetus [21]. Moscary et al. have shown that if one experimentally produces an intracranial pressure of more than 55 mm Hg, a bradycardia reflex appears [22]. Compression of the head seems to be the main cause of type 1 DIP. This compression provokes stimulation of the cardio-moderator vagal centre by means of a mechanism similar to that of the oculo-cardiac reflex, or by intracranial hypertension leading to temporary ischemia of the vagal centre. The role of the vagus in the reflex mechanism is proved by the disappearance of the type 1 DIPS after injection of atropine into the fetus. Some investigators believe that early bradycardia could be the result of moderate temporary hypoxemia. According to them, the decrease in pO_2 noticed during uterine contractions could stimulate the chemoreceptors and trigger a temporary bradycardia.

Late decelerations. — Late decelerations are related to fetal hypoxia provoked by uterine contractions in certain pathological circumstances. Caldeyro-Barcia showed, by means of a polarographic electrode placed in the buttock of the fetus in utero, that there is a fall in fetal pO_2 during type 2 DIPS. He estimates the critical pO_2 at 18 mm Hg, under which type 2 DIPS appear. He also showed that oxygen given to the mother decreases the amplitude of the type 2 DIPS. Myers' studies also showed that fetal hypoxia is accompanied by late decelerations and that the time-lapse between the two is inversely proportional to the degree of hypoxia. Uterine contraction can alter fetal oxygenation either by compressing the umbilical cord, or by reducing the arterial blood supply to the intervillous space. This drop in circulatory flow is due to a compression of the intramyometrial vessels and occasionally to the compression of the retrouterine part of the aorta. Type 2 DIPS can be seen in the case of hyperactivity, but also with normal contractions added to chronic fetal distress and insufficient placental circulation. Fetal hypoxia induced by uterine contraction produces type 2 DIPS in different ways: firstly the lack of oxygen and acidosis can act directly on the nodal tissue. Secondly a fall in the pO_2 below a critical level can stimulate the cardio-

regulatory nervous centers. This takes place either directly in the medullary center of the vagus or via the chemoreceptors. The action of the chemoreceptors on the nervous centers seems to be indirect, their stimulation brings about hypertension. This has an effect on the baroreceptors and bradycardia is thus induced. Fetal hypoxia, which is the cause of type 2 DIPS, reaches its maximum point towards the end of uterine contraction, when the oxygen reserve of the intervillous space is drained. The fetal blood, poor in oxygen, must make its way towards the cardiomotor centres in order to trigger cardiac deceleration. This explains the time-lapse between the bradycardia and uterine contraction.

Variable decelerations. — Experimental compression of the cord during cesarean sections, in the human fetus or that of the ewe, triggers similar decelerations to those described by Hon as variable decelerations. For him, these decelerations are the results of vagal excitation due to cord compression. The prognostic significance depends on the duration, amplitude and rate of these decelerations. However, a certain amount of recent research shows that variable decelerations can have other causes than cord compression, in particular compression of the aorta, and the inferior vena cava.

ACUTE FETAL DISTRESS

ETIOLOGY

Schematically, acute fetal distress during labor appears either when there is abnormal uterine contraction, or when an intercurrent cause renders the fetus incapable of tolerating even normal uterine contractions.

Acute fetal distress due to hyperactivity

Dynamic dystocia may be primary but is more often secondary and is the result of the struggle of the uterus against an obstruction, as in the case of fetal pelvic disproportion.

Three abnormalities of uterine dynamics can disturb fetal maternal exchange, (1) hypersystole, which can be defined as an average intensity of contractions greater than 60 mm Hg, (2) tachysystole, which is characterised by an average rate of contractions greater than 5 per 10 minutes and (3) hypertonia, which corresponds to an average basal tone greater than 20 mm Hg. In these three cases, there is a disturbance of uterine placental hemodynamics. The oxygen reserve of the IVS is altered by prolonged circulatory arrest and by insufficient resting time between contractions. Abnormal contractions have a more rapid effect on fetal oxygen when maternal pathology restricts the placental reserves of oxygen.

Acute fetal distress in the absence of dynamic dystocia

If the fetal maternal exchanges are disturbed by intercurrent causes, uterine contraction, even when it is normal, can trigger acute fetal distress. These causes can be maternal, fetal or adnexial.

Maternal causes. — Maternal disease can bring about a lack of oxygenation of the fetal blood due to an insufficient quality or quantity of oxygenated blood.

Insufficiency in the quantity of oxygenated blood to the placenta can be chronic. Diseases such as diabetes, prolonged pregnancy and vascular-renal syndromes present on the one hand circulatory problems responsible for a fall in uterine blood flow, and on the other hand placental alterations which decrease exchange across the placental membranes. An acute decrease in utero-placental flow can be caused by a compression of the iliac arteries by a gravid uterus during contractions, or by general circulatory difficulties during states of shock, iatrogenic hypotension, or the hypotensive decubitus syndrome.

Insufficiency of maternal blood oxygenation can be the result of a respiratory problem (bronchitis, asthma, emphysema, etc.), of a general anesthetic complication, or of deficiency in oxygen transport by the maternal blood (severe anemia, decompensated cardiopathy).

Adnexial causes. — Certain placental lesions are accompanied by a reduction in surface exchange. One can see this in the case of an abruptio placentae, or of placenta praevia which causes a partial interruption in feto-maternal exchange due to detachement of the villi. Other placental alterations, such as chorio-angioma (benign vascular tumor leading to an arterio-venous shunt) also bring about a decrease in the transplacental passage of oxygen.

Several different abnormalities can moreover produce a decrease or stoppage of circulatory currents in the umbilical cord: prolapse and less frequently lateral prolapse, tight coiling, knotting, abnormal length and more rarely anatomical abnormalities of the cord. These funicular complications represent a major cause of fetal distress during labour.

Fetal causes. — These are numerous and we shall only mention the main ones. Because of their intrinsic fragility, certain infants risk distress during labor. This is the case with premature, dysmature, and infected fetuses. What is more, certain circumstances enhance fetal distress by exaggerating oxygen needs; this is the case, for example, in twins. Finally, hemolytic anemia and congenital heart disease can disturb oxygen transport.

DIAGNOSIS

Clinical diagnosis

During labor, acute fetal distress (A. F. D.) usually results in two clinical signs: meconium stained amniotic fluid, and modification of the heart beat. Other than in breech presentation, meconium in the amniotic fluid is considered to be a symptom of fetal distress. The passage of meconium into the amniotic fluid results in an adjustment of fetal circulation to anoxia: e. g. vasoconstriction in the blood supply to the digestive apparatus. This stimulates the parasympathetic system which relaxes the anal sphincter while stimulating intestinal peristalsis.

The diagnostic significance of stained amniotic fluid is, in fact, rather controversial. Many studies have shown that it is possible to have stained fluid without anoxia, and on the contrary, that A. F. D. may be accompanied by clear amniotic fluid. Saling, for example, only found 3 cases of acidosis out of 176 in which an amnioscopy revealed stained amniotic fluid where the pH was measured immediately. Pontonnier et al. found only 37 stained fluids out of 70 deliveries accompanied by fetal acidosis. These findings have been verified by numerous researchers, and have led to the abandonment of routine amnioscopy at the beginning of labor. However, this policy would only seem to be justified if all deliveries are monitored. In contrast, a stained amniotic fluid does have a certain value since, in the majority of published statistics, the risk of A. F. D. is greater when the amniotic fluid is stained, than when it is clear.

The value of cardiac auscultation is also questioned as being too subjective and not able to locate bradycardia in relation to uterine contractions. In fact the greatest disadvantage of auscultation, is that it is not continuous. Benson calculated that it only takes into account 5 % of the labour period [6]. Moreover, in contrast to monitoring tracings, it cannot be reviewed at a later date.

The clinical signs of A. F. D. therefore appear to be incomplete. Depending on the credence that one accords them, in conjunction with other obstetrical findings, two risks occur: either to act too early, at the first sign of abnormality, and to practise unnecessary intervention, or, on the other hand, to wait until the signs are very clear by which time there is a state of A. F. D. which could have been avoided. These are the reasons which explain the success of the paraclinical surveillance of labor.

Paraclinical diagnosis

Study of fetal heart rate. — The baseline fetal heart rate is defined as the average F. H. R. between contractions; a normal baseline F. H. R. is between 120 and 160 beats per minute. When the F. H. R. is below or above these limits, for at least 10 minutes, one speaks of bradycardia or of tachycardia. Although experiment has proven that anoxia can be the origin of these two abnormal states, their prognostic significance is still questioned. When there are no other modifications of the F. H. R. they can be accompanied by the birth of healthy infants. However we can see in Table I that they are more often present in births complicated by fetal distress, than in normal births. From a practical

TABLE I. — BASAL FETAL HEART RATE DURING NORMAL LABOR AND LABOR COMPLICATED BY FETAL ACIDOSIS.

Basal fetal heart rate	Fetal acidosis 79 cases	Normal labor 30 cases
Continuous bradycardia *	4 %	0 %
Continuous tachycardia *	19 %	0 %
Normal basal heart rate plus sustained bradycardia **	19 %	7 %
Normal basal heart rate plus sustained tachycardia **	28 %	13 %
Normal basal heart rate	30 %	80 %

* Continuous: during the entire time of recording.
** Sustained: during at least 10 minutes.

point of view it is more worrying when these abnormal states are prolonged and intense (bradycardia below 100 or tachycardia above 180) and, above all, when they are accompanied by late decelerations. Lastly, in the presence of fetal tachycardia one must be able to exclude causes which have no relation to anoxia, such as prematurity, maternal hyperthermia, or pharmacological effect (atropine, betamimetics).

Even though the pathological significance of a flat tracing is now accepted during pregnancy, its significance during labor is more controversial. However, our study, in accordance with that of Hammacher, shows that T0 patterns, a flat tracing with oscillations < 5 beats/min, are never present in absolutely normal births whereas they predominate in births complicated by acidosis, associated sometimes with T1 patterns: e. g. a fetal heart tracing with oscillations between 5-10 beats/min.

As regards accelerations of the F. H. R., produced by contractions or fetal movements, it is generally agreed that they are the sign of a healthy fetus.

The different interpretations of periodic decelerations, regardless of the classification adopted, can be summarized as follows. Early decelerations, or type 1 DIPS, are not the direct consequence of fetal anoxia and are not usually associated with neonatal depression. However, the decrease in cerebral flow experimentally shown in the case of head compression, makes one think that frequent repetition of early decelerations, especially when they are of high amplitude and are prolonged, are signs of trauma which can lead to fetal distress. Late decelerations, or type 2 DIPS, are, on the contrary, a direct sign of fetal anoxia. However, they are only the sign of a momentary fall in fetal pO_2 below a critical level and when few in number, should not necessitate urgent extraction.

To sum up, one can say that although a normal F. H. R. during labor usually corresponds to a healthy vigourous infant, the analysis of pathological tracings must be very carefully examined. This analysis must be not only qualitative but also quantitative, and take into account the number and intensity of the abnormalities. In addition, apart from a few very serious cases in which the diagnosis of distress is evident, the pathological F. H. R. curve must be accompanied by an analysis of blood pH in order to evaluate the degree of anoxia, and therefore to adapt obstetrical management.

Measurement of pH in the fetal scalp. — The acid-base equilibrium of the mother and of the fetus is by now well known. Tables II and III give the results of a study carried out by our group on 70 selected normal deliveries. The mother's pH varies

TABLE II. — FETAL ACID-BASE EQUILIBRIUM AND pO_2 DURING NORMAL LABOR

	3-4 cm	*5-6 cm*	*7-8 cm*	*9-10 cm*	*Second stage*	*U. A.*	*U. V.*
Number of measurements	28	35	32	29	17	103	103
pH	7.37 ± 0.05	7.36 ± 0.05	7.37 ± 0.07	7.37 ± 0.05	7.31 ± 0.07	7.27 ± 0.06	7.35 ± 0.06
pCO_2 mm Hg	36 ± 9	34 ± 9	34 ± 8	31 ± 9	36 ± 14	40 ± 7	32 ± 7
B. D. mEq/l	−4 ± 3	−6 ± 4	−5 ± 3	−6 ± 5	−8 ± 4	−8 ± 4	−7 ± 3
pO_2 mm Hg	19 ± 7	19 ± 6	21 ± 8	18 ± 5	14 ± 3	15 ± 5	25 ± 6
O_2 sat. %	41 ± 17	42 ± 16	47 ± 18	40 ± 15	22 ± 11	23 ± 14	57 ± 16

TABLE III. — MATERNAL ACID-BASE EQUILIBRIUM AND pO_2 DURING NORMAL LABOR

	3-4 cm	*5-6 cm*	*7-8 cm*	*9-10 cm*	*Second stage*	*Birth*
Number of measurements	28	35	32	29	17	103
pH	7.47 ± 0.07	7.47 ± 0.05	7.49 ± 0.07	7.47 ± 0.06	7.46 ± 0.05	7.40 ± 0.06
pCO_2 mm Hg	24 ± 7	22 ± 6	21 ± 6	21 ± 6	20 ± 5	22 ± 4
B. D. mEq/l	−5 ± 4	−6 ± 3	−5 ± 3	−6 ± 3	−7 ± 3	−10 ± 3
pO_2 mm Hg	80 ± 20	84 ± 18	88 ± 24	84 ± 17	87 ± 21	87 ± 20
O_2 sat. %	96 ± 1	97 ± 2	97 ± 2	97 ± 2	97 ± 2	96 ± 2

very little; during dilatation, it increases very slightly due to hypocapnia linked to hyperventilation and is partly compensated for by an increase in the base deficit. At the moment of delivery, a moderate metabolic acidosis linked to muscular work brings the pH down slightly. The picture of maternal acid-base equilibrium can vary according to different authors. This probably depends on the manner in which labor is managed. The pH of the fetus remains practically unchanged during dilatation and falls at the moment of delivery, due to moderate hypercapnia and slight metabolic acidosis, probably transmitted by the mother. Oxygen saturation falls from 44 % to 28 % but the absence of marked metabolic acidosis suggests that there is no oxygen deficit.

In 1962, Saling proposed measuring scalp pH in order to diagnose A. F. D. The physiopathology of anoxia explains the appearance of fetal acidosis which is firstly respiratory and then mixed. Total anoxia experimentally induced in the animal fetus results in a pO_2 of zero within 2.5 minutes, an increase in pCO_2 by 10 mm Hg/min and a decrease in pH of 0.1 U/min. But these experimental conditions are far removed from clinical reality where asphyxia never happens so abruptly or so totally. The normal limits of the pH of the scalp were established from the relationship between the pH and the clinical state of the newborn. In agreement with Saling it can be considered that pH 7.25 indicates the onset of anoxia; if the pH falls to 7.20, anoxia is established. However one must eliminate any transmitted maternal acidosis before taking such a decision

In spite of numerous publications confirming Saling's experiments, the usefulness of pH measurement on the scalp is still questioned for theoretical and practical reasons. Some authors have again recently cast doubts on the fact that scalp blood constitutes an indication of general fetal circulation. Animal experimentation has, however, demonstrated beyond doubt that the values of the parameters of the acid-base equilibrium and of the gases of the arterial blood are comparable to those measured in the scalp of ewe, and monkey fetuses. Several authors have compared pH values just prior to birth to those of the cord blood vessels. The coefficient of correlation is significant. Table IV reports the results obtained by our team from 36 samples taken from the scalp within 3 minutes preceding birth, then on the cord vessels before the first breath. The comparison of results shows that the capillary blood taken from the scalp resembles very closely that of the umbilical artery.

TABLE IV. — ACID-BASE EQUILIBRIUM AND pO_2 ON FETAL SCALP AND UMBILICAL VESSEL BLOOD

	pH	pCO_2 mm Hg	B. D. mEq/l	pO_2 mm Hg
Scalp . . .	7.28 ± 0.08	40 ± 6	8 ± 2	14 ± 5
U. A.. . .	7.26 ± 0.08	42 ± 6	8 ± 2	13 ± 4
U. V.. . .	7.33 ± 0.08	33 ± 6	8 ± 2	23 ± 5
Scalp/U. A. .	$r = 0.91$	$r = 0.62$	$r = 0.91$	$r = 0.57$
Correlation .	$p < 0.001$	$p < 0.01$	$p < 0.001$	$p < 0.01$

Experimental asphyxia induced in animals has shown that the pH measured in the scalp is a good indicator of anoxia. This cannot be proven so irrefutably in the human fetus since it would be necessary to examine it at the moment of measurement of the scalp pH, which tends to be compared to the state of the infant at birth. However, this is liable to error, as there can be a certain number of complications between the moment of blood

sampling *in utero* and the evaluation of the Apgar score; in these cases the pH cannot be an indicator since it is evaluated before the complications. The only moment when one is able to judge the clinical and biochemical state together, is at birth, by comparing the pH of the umbilical artery to the Apgar score before the first breath. We carried out these measurements in 503 births in which we had these two parameters as well as that of the maternal pH at birth. In 92 % of the cases, there was a concordance between the pH and the Apgar score. In 41 cases (8 %) there was a clear discordance. In 10 cases the pH of the umbilical artery was lower than 7.10 while the Apgar score was greater than 6; in 31 cases the Apgar score was less than 6 while the pH was normal. Analysis of these cases showed that the majority of false negatives was due to anesthetic depression, and the majority of the false positives was explained by the transmission of maternal acidosis.

The difficulty of taking blood samples from the fetal scalp is inversely proportional to the experience of the person doing the sampling. It is the same for the errors. The majority of errors and difficulties are due to incorrect sampling or malfunctioning of the pH meter. These technical problems are even more striking when pH measurements are not performed every day. Numerous authors have, however, reduced these difficulties in a satisfactory manner. Saling [34] for example, estimates at only 1 % the frequency of a gap between two successive samples greater than 0.06 which are unexplainable and therefore due to errors of measurement. In our study the gap between two measurements immediately repeated was always less than 0.05 and less than or equal to 0.02, in 91 % of cases.

Apart from very rare scalp abcesses, the only complication of blood sampling from the scalp is hemorrhage. This occurred in less than 1 in 1,000 cases. Out of 20,000 samples over 10 years, we have had only 2 serious hemorrhages in Toulouse. One was due to a technical error, and was fatal; the other allowed us to discover that the fetus was a hemophiliac.

The surveillance of the pH must be carried out systematically in all high-risk labors—hypotrophy, prematurity, diabetes, prolonged pregnancy—and in any normal labour as soon as the F. H. R. is disturbed.

TREATMENT

Until the last few years, the golden rule in the treatment of acute fetal distress was immediate extraction of the infant, either by the vaginal route, or by cesarean section, according to the clinical case at hand. Nowadays diagnosis and treatment of acute fetal distress has been transformed by breakthroughs in the physiology and physiopathology of fetal oxygenation, and by the discovery of modern means of detecting anoxia. Today, the basic principle of treatment is prevention rather than emergency extraction. Apart from the few cases in which there are unforeseeable complications such as cord prolapse or abruptio placentae, fetal anoxia should no longer be seen during labor. The systematic use of monitoring, the detection of high-risk pregnancies, and the surveillance of fetal pH in cases of dystocia permit us, in general, to anticipate it and to take preventive measures.

The position of the mother

Lateral decubitus is the recommended position during labor. This is a simple, safe and economic precaution and much local or general hypotension due to compression of the I. V. C. or aorta can thus be avoided. Changing from the dorsal decubitus to lateral decubitus can also cause the disappearance of certain late fetal bradycardia. In addition, a change in the mother's position can free a cord compressed by the fetus.

Management of labour

This constitutes the most essential element in the prevention of acute fetal distress. Prevention of fetal anoxia must, above all, consist of the detection of all high-risk cases (contracted pelvis, abnormal presentation, fragile fetus) before the onset of labour. In certain cases elective cesarean section should be performed, but once spontaneous labor has begun, the golden rule should be to obtain birth in the shortest possible time with the minimum of force. This is why ineffective contractions, which are a cause of anxiety and strain, should be treated particularly early by oxytocin infusion, by membrane rupture and analgesics, as soon as possible.

Hyperactivity is not always due to feto-pelvic disproportion or to a therapeutic error. It can be primary, in which case there is a "precipitate" birth and the infant runs the risk of anoxia. A correctly calculated infusion of beta-mimetic drugs should bring the different parameters of uterine contraction back into normal bounds, thus limiting fetal trauma.

Following the work of Caldeyro-Barcia we had recommended, some ten years ago, fetal reanimation

in utero by the use of I. V. beta-mimetics in the case of confirmed anoxia. This method suppresses uterine contraction and allows the normalization of fetal pH and heart rate in cases of hyperactivity. However reanimation in utero has lost its interest since the development of modern methods of labor management which allow us to foresee the onset of anoxia. It is now used only during the time it takes to prepare an emergency extraction in the case of unforeseeable acute fetal distress.

Uterine hyperactivity can be induced by an incorrectly dosed infusion of oxytocin. This error can be avoided by using an electronic pump and by placing an intra-amniotic catheter to keep a close eye on uterine contractions.

Adjuvant medical treatment

A whole series of adjuvant medical treatments for anoxia have been proposed, infusion of alkaline substances, infusion of glucose, and oxygen administration. In fact the influence of these adjuvants can only be secondary since the basic physiopathological characteristic of acute fetal distress is the difficulty in transplacental gas exchange. If oxygen, a highly diffusible substance, crosses the placenta with difficulty, it is probable that any substances given to the mother will reach the fetus too slowly and in too low a quantity compared to the speed of events. This is particularly true in the case of bicarbonate and T. H. A. M. A 10 % glucose infusion is, however, indirectly beneficial to the fetus since it prevents maternal acidosis due to fasting during labor. As for the administration of oxygen, its effects are still questioned. Some authors have obtained an improvement in fetal heart rate disturbance and an increase in fetal pO_2 using this method, others, on the contrary, have found no significant effect. Maternal oxygenation does not, however, present a danger and is undoubtedly useful in cases of maternal anoxia. Hyperventilation is, on the contrary, more dangerous as it is a factor in hypocapnia and sometimes in maternal hypoxemia. Hyperventilation can be either spontaneous or induced. Pain and anxiety often produce an exaggeration of the rapid superficial respiration recommended during the psychoprophylactic preparation of labor, and this results in spontaneous hyperventilation. In this case analgesia is an effective measure. Hyperventilation can also be induced during general anesthesia with curarization. In exceptional cases the result would be fetal anoxia by vasoconstriction secondary to hypocapnia in the placental vessels.

REFERENCES

[1] AHERNE (W.), DUNHILL (M. S.). — Quantitative aspect of placental structure. *J. Path. Bact.*, *91*, 123, 1966.

[2] ANTENATAL DIAGNOSIS. — V Department of health, education, and welfare. NIH Publication n° 79, 1973, III, 18, 1979.

[3] ASSALI (N. S.), BRINKMAN (C. R.), NUWAYHID (B.). — Uteroplacental circulation and respiratory gas exchange. *In* GLUCK L.: *Modern Perinatal Medicine*, Year Book Medical Publishers, Chicago, p. 67, 1974.

[4] BATTAGLIA (F. C.), WILKENING (R. B.). — Soins aux nouveau-nés de très faible poids de naissance. *Rev. Prat.*, *31*, 353-363, 1981.

[5] BEHRMAN (R. E.), LEES (M. H.), PETERSON (E. N.), DE LANNOY (C. W.), SEEDS (A. E.). — Distribution of the circulation in the normal and asphyxiated fetal primate. *Am. J. Obstet. Gynecol.*, *108*, 956, 1970.

[6] BENSON (R. C.), SHUBECK (F.), DEUTSCHBERGER (J.), WEISS (W.), BERENDES (H.). — Fetal heart rate as a predictor of fetal distress. A report from the collaborative project. *Obstet. Gynecol.*, *32*, 259, 1968.

[7] BROWNE (J. C.), VEALL (N.). — The maternal placental blood flow in normotensive and hypertensive women. *J. Obstet. Gynaecol. Brit. Emp.*, *60*, 141, 1953.

[8] CALDEYRO-BARCIA (R.), MENDEZ-BAUER (C.), POSEIRO (J. J.), ESCARCENA (L.), POSE (S. V.). BIENIARZ (J.), ARNT (I.), GULIN (L.), ALTHABE (O.). — Control of human fetal heart rate during labor. *In* D. E. CASSELS: *The heart and circulation in the newborn and infant*. New York, Grune Stratton, Inc., 7-36, 1966.

[9] CALDEYRO-BARCIA (R.), CASACUBERTA (C.), BUSTOS (R.), GIUSSI (G.), GULIN (L.), ESCARCENA (L.), MENDEZ-BAUER (C.). — Correlation of intrapartum changes in fetal heart rate with fetal blood oxygen and acid-base state. *In* ADAMSONS K. Edit.: *Diagnosis and treatment of fetal disorders*. Springer Verlag, Berlin, p. 205, 1968.

[10] CALDEYRO-BARCIA (R.), POSE (S. V.), POSEIRO (J. J.), MENDEZ-BAUER (C.), ESCARCENA (L.), BEHRMAN (R.). — Effects of several factors on fetal pO_2 recorded continuously in the fetal monkey. *In* GLUCK L.: *Intrauterine asphyxia and the developing brain*. Year Book Medical Publishers, Chicago, p. 237, 1977.

[11] COHN (H. E.), SACKS (E. J.), HEYMANN (M. A.), RUDOLPH (A. M.). — Cardiovascular responses to hypoxemia and acidemia in fetal lambs. *Am. J. Obstet. Gynecol.*, *128*, 817, 1974.

[12] DAWES (G. S.). — *Fœtal and neonatal physiology*. Year Book Medical Publishers, Chicago, p. 66, 1968.

[13] DAWES (G. S.), MOTT (J. C.), SHELLEY (H. J.). — The importance of cardiac glycogen for the maintenance of life in fetal lambs in newborn animals during anoxia. *J. Physiol.*, *146*, 516, 1959.

[14] FRIEDMAN (W. F.), KIRPATRICK (S. E.). — Fetal cardiovascular adaptation to asphyxia. *In* GLUCK L.: *Intrauterine asphyxia and the developing fetal brain*. Year Book Medical Publishers, Chicago, p. 149, 1977.

[15] GOODWIN (J. W.). — The fetal circulation. *In* GOODWIN J. W., GODDEN J. O., CHANCE G. W.: *Perinatal Medicine*. The Williams and Wilkins Co., Baltimore, p. 143, 1976.

[16] GRUENWALD (P.). — Maternal blood supply to the conceptons. *Europ. J. Obstet. Gynec. Reprod. Biol.*, *5*, 23, 1975.

[17] HAMMACHER (K.). — The clinical significance of cardiotocography. *In* HUNTINGFORD P. J. et al.: *Perinatal Medicine*. Georg Thiem Verlag, Stuttgart, 80-93, 1969.

[18] HON (E. H.), QUILLIGAN (E. J.). — The classification of fetal heart rate. II. A revised working classification. *Com. Med.*, *31*, 779, 1967.

[19] HON (E. H.), QUILLIGAN (E. J.). — Electronic evaluation of fetal heart rate. *Clin. Obstet. Gynec.*, *II*, 145-167, 1968.

[20] LONGO (L. D.). — Disorders of placental transfer. *In* ASSALI N. S.: *Pathophysiology of gestation*. Academic Press, New York, vol. 2, 1, 1972.

[21] MENDEZ-BAUER (C.), POSEIRO (J. J.), ARELLANO-HERNANDEZ (G.), ZAMBRANA (M. A.), CALDEYRO-BARCIA (R.). — Effects of atropine on the heart rate of the human fetus during labor. *Am. J. Obstet. Gynecol.*, *85*, 1033,1963.

[22] MOSCARY (P.), GAAL (J.), KOMAROMY (B.), MIHALY (G.), POHANKA (O.), SURANYI (S.). — Relationship between fetal intracranial pressure and fetal heart rate during labor. *Am. J. Obstet. Gynecol.*, *106*, 407-411, 1970.

[23] MOTT (J. C.). — The ability of young mammals to withstand a total oxygen lack. *Br. Med. Bull.*, *17*, 144, 1961.

[24] MYERS (R. E.). — Two patterns of perinatal brain damage and their conditions of occurrence. *Am. J. Obstet. Gynecol.*, *112*, 246-276, 1972.

[25] MYERS (R. E.). — Brain damage induced by umbilical cord compression at different gestational ages in monkeys. *In* GELDSMITH E. T., MOORJANOWSKI J. Edit.: *Medical Primatology*, Karger, Basel, 394, 1970.

[26] MYERS (R. E.). — Predictability of the state of fetal oxygenation from a qualitative analysis of the components of late decelerations. *Am. J. Obstet. Gynecol.*, *115*, 1083, 1973.

[27] PONTONNIER (G.), GRANDJEAN (H.), SARRAMON (M. F.), DEGOY (J.), GUIRAUD (R.), FAVRETTO (R.). — Chronic fetal distress. Research on placental blood flow and therapy. *In* B. SALVADORI: *Therapy of Feto-Placental Insufficiency*. Springer Verlag, Berlin, 251, 1975.

[28] PONTONNIER (G.), GRANDJEAN (H.), DELMASLATOUR (E.), ROLLAND (M.), LELOUP (M.), REME (J. M.). — Le rythme cardiaque fœtal au cours de l'accouchement compliqué d'acidose fœtale. Kontron Edit., vol. 1, p. 227, Paris, 1976.

[29] PONTONNIER (G.), TOURNIER (C.), DAT (S.), DELMAS (H.), MONROZIES (M.), PONTONNIER (A.). — Premiers essais de réanimation du fœtus humain *in utero* pendant l'accouchement. *Rev. Franç. Gynec.*, *66*, 517, 1971.

[30] POSE (C. V.), ESCARCENA (L.), CALDEYRO-BARCIA (R.). — La pression parcial d'oxygeno en el feto durante el parto. *N. Congr. Mexico Ginec. Obstet.*, *2*, 41, 1963.

[31] POSEIRO (J. J.), CALDEYRO-BARCIA (R.), BIENIARZ (J.), CURUCHET (E.), ARAMBURU (G.), CROTTOGINI (J. J.). — Utero placental circulation in late human pregnancy. V. — Effects of uterine contraction. *Scientific Exhibition IV World Congr. Int. Fed. Gynec. and Obst. Mar del Plata*, Argentina, 1964.

[32] RAMSEY (E. M.). — Circulation in the intervillous

space of the primate placenta. *Am. J. Obstet. Gynec.*, *84*, 1649, 1962.

[33] RENOU (P.), NEWMAN (W.), WOOD (C.). — Automatic control of fetal heart rate. *Am. J. Obstet. Gynec.*, *105*, 949, 1969.

[34] SALING (E.). — Possible errors in fetal blood analysis and their prevention. *In* GLUCK L.: *Modern Perinatal Medicine.* Year Book Medical Publishers, Chicago, p. 169, 1974.

[35] SALING (E.). — Comments on optical evaluation of the amniotic fluid by amnioscopy. *In* HUNTINGFORD P. J., HUTER K. A., SALING E.: *Perinatal Medicine*, George Thieme Verlag, Stuttgart, 17, 1969.

[36] SCHOLANDER (P. F.). — Experimental studies on asphyxia in animals. *In* WALKER W., TURNBULL A. C. Edit.: *Oxygen supply to the human fetus.* Charles Thomas, Springfield, 267, 1959.

[37] SCHWARCZ (R. L.) et coll. — Pressure exerted by uterine contractions on the head of the human fetus during labor. *Obstet. Gynecol.*, *13*, 115-126, 1959.

[38] SNOECK (J.). — *Le placenta humain.* Masson Paris, 1958.

[39] VILLEE (C. A.). — Bioenergetic consideration in fetal and mature tissues. In: *Brain damage in the fetus and newborn from hypoxia and asphyxia.* Report of the Fifty Seventh Ross Conference of Pediatric Research. Ross Laboratory, 1967.

8

Perinatal anesthesia

Geneviève BARRIER

THE INDICATIONS

If one considers obstetrical development in the last decade, it can be noted that the gap between the progress achieved in monitoring labor and drug management in analgesia and anesthesia has disappeared. The progress achieved has undoubtely contributed to the reduction in perinatal death and morbidity which could be observed. Such progress might have made one believe, probably incautiously, that anesthesia had become a usual and non hazardous medical act. However, more recent statistics show that maternal death under anesthesia has not decreased over the last 10 years and still remains around 13/100,000 in the last decade [65]. The percentage of maternal deaths due to anesthesia has increased during this period from 10.4 % to 13.2 % [72]. Therefore one may wonder whether anesthesia in maternity units has followed scientific progress in all hospitals. Apparently this is not the case. Efforts must be made so that all parturients can benefit from anesthesia in the most secure conditions. This task is urgent since the number of obstetric anesthesia cases is increasing at a rate which requires consideration:

— the indications for obstetrical anesthesia have risen during the last few years;

— the average number of cesarean sections has increased threefold during the last ten years [15, 28];

— breech presentations, dystocias, diabetes have become almost automatic indications for cesarean sections to save the fetus, as have intra-uterine growth retardation and late pregnancies.

In large hospitals the number of cesarean sections has been known to generally increase quickly [32]. Present obstetrical management will undoubtely lead to the closing of small clinics. The decrease in the rate of fecundity and fear of law suits against obstetricians for neonatal damage after vaginal delivery may also play a role in the increasing number of cesarean sections.

The parallel increase in uterine cervix cerclage at the beginning of pregnancy is an important part of anesthesia, as is the rapid diagnosis of acute fetal distress during labor, requiring either a cesarean section or an instrumental delivery, with anesthesia in both cases. A previous cesarean section will influence the obstetrical decision in subsequent pregnancies. Finally, pain relief requested by more and more parturients is now added to indications required by doctors for obstetrical pathology.

Women want to benefit from obstetrical analgesia for their delivery. As it is a common phenomenon, one must search for the deep and true reasons. The average increase in the standard of living may account for it, as noted in a recent prospective enquiry, showing that the socio-cultural level of women requesting epidural anesthesia is higher than a comparative group of non requesters but corresponds often to psychological and family difficulties [35]. In the group with peridural analgesia more obstetric pathology requiring hospital care during pregnancy is noted.

Similarly, it must be noted in France that today's parturients belong to the first generation born to mothers who have been trained for the Lamaze method. If their mothers have successfully experienced their parturitions, the daughters will benefit from the experience. Nevertheless if the mothers have born the cost of the myth of painless parturition and exceeding naturalism of some obstetricians, their daughters will have learnt to dissociate pain and parturition, and will not claim more than the preparation can provide. These elements are found in the two groups of the survey, who have attended training in comparative proportions. This shows that the request for analgesia is not related to a lack of training.

On the contrary, training plays a great part in analgesia, since trained parturients require smaller doses of general analgesics, and less locoregional anesthesia [74]. This clearly shows that the Lamaze method and obstetrical analgesia are not antagonistic but complementary methods. This is especially true as we now use technics which relieve parturients without affecting consciousness. In this way, psychological difficulties remain untouched with or without epidural anesthesia, and in the case of difficulties, the request for anesthesia was probably a call for help, which will not be satisfied with only a medical, analgesic or anesthetic response. Lastly, the present parturients belong to the first generation which was able to control fecundity and dissociate sexuality and reproduction. Nowadays couples willing to have a well defined number of children, want a quality of life which is evident in their choice to determine the moment of pregnancy, to fully experience parturition and be rewarded when a healthy and wanted child is born. In this respect, obstetric analgesia has a significant social role to play, especially in the lower classes of society.

THE ROLE OF BACKGROUND

Obstetrical anesthesia can be classified into two large groups: emergency anesthesia and planned anesthesia. In all cases, the anesthesiologist should never give priority to the parturient's comfort instead of her security. If anesthesia should be performed in an emergency, general anesthesia should be undertaken, its quick induction will permit any surgical procedure within a few minutes. In other cases, in agreement with the obstetrician and the parturient, one can choose between locoregional anesthesia and general anesthesia. Finally, for labor analgesia, various locoregional, or systemic or inhalatory methods can be selected.

Before enumerating the different possibilities, one must recall some anatomics and physiological particularities of parturients, and the consequences of anesthesia on labor and the fetal condition.

The parturient's stomach is always full. — The gastric emptying time of pregnant women decreases from the 34th week of pregnancy. Labor equally delays gastric evacuation, and the patient often goes into labor after a meal; in such a way that inhaling stomach contents is one of the main causes of anesthetic maternal death. That is why premedication associating an anticholinergic substance with an antacid is a measure of prevention against this terrible complication [80, 31, 38]. Some prefer glycopyrrolate which does not cross the placenta to atropine which can have undesirable fetal and neonatal secondary effects [1, 8, 10]. Tracheal intubation, with compression of the cricoid cartilage should quickly follow general anesthesia induction in the case of pregnant women.

Parturients should not lie in supine position. — During pregnancy, the cardiac output increases by 30 or 40 %. The relative decrease in the last trimester accounts for the compression of the inferior vena cava and of the aorta by the supine position of the uterus. This decrease is not recorded in the left lateral position [22].

The decrease in the uterine blood flow provoked by the supine position may be enough to cause fetal distress (Fig. I-51). This can cause neonatal distress which might be wrongly attributed to anesthesia. When such anomalies of Fetal Heart Rate (F. H. R.) are observed, it is sufficient to place the parturient in the left lateral position, while putting a small cushion under her right hip, maintaining a left uterine displacement (L. U. D.) manually during the maneuver. This should be systematically done when a parturient is placed on the operating table for a cesarean section.

Those symptoms of fetal distress may be aggraved by maternal hypotension as is the case for some anesthetics with vasodilatation effects such as halogenated agents or locoregional anesthesia. In these cases, one should not only move the uterus and do L. U. D. as seen previously, but also drastically prevent hypotension by I. V. infusion of fluids, or the injection of ephedrine.

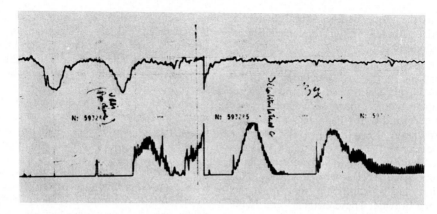

FIF. I-51. — *Normalized fetal heart rate with left uterine displacement of the parturient* (G. BARRIER, 1981).

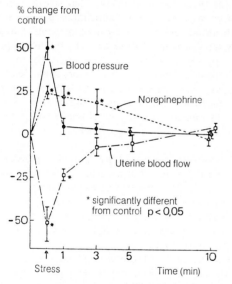

FIG. I-52. — *Pain effect on the blood level of catechol-amines, maternal arterial pressure and utero-placental blood flow.* Sol M. SHNIDER, University of California, Department of Anesthesia, Mofitt Hospital, San Francisco, California. *Anesthesiology, 50, 6, 526, 1979.*

The pain caused by uterine contractions implies an increasing maternal blood level of catechol-amines. However there is a correlation between blood levels of catecholamines and the utero-placental blood flow (Fig. I-52). In addition, Myers [64, 65] and Morishima [58, 59] have experimentally produced in the animal fetal hypoxia and acidosis by maternal stress only. Similarly Shni-der [78] noted that maternal stress reduced the uterine blood flow. These important studies justify obstetrical analgesia in the case of hyperalgic parturitions. As proof of their value we may consider cases of

fetal distress which can be reduced by anesthesia.

Thus, each indication for obstetrical analgesia or anesthesia must be considered and for each treatment to a pregnant woman a possible subsequent anesthesic must be considered, so it is that we know how labor begins, but not how and when the delivery could happen. No medication should be administered without thinking about this possibility of anesthesia in an emergency. Nevertheless, some commonly administered medications during pregnancy and labor increase the anesthesia risk by drug interaction. For example, in the case of drugs which are administered to prevent or treat premature labor, especially betamimetics.

Betamimetics drugs are used in obstetrics as tocolytics, that is to stop uterine contractions in case of premature labor. All except the effect of uterine relaxation, could be considered as side effects in obstetrics [45].

The betamimetics, most commonly use in France in obstetrics, have a prevaling β 2 effect (Ritodrine and Salbutamol). However, they unquestionably preserve a β 1 effect, from which their side effects derive:

— cardiovascular: tachycardia, increasing cardiac output, arterial pressure variability (most often hypotension, seldom hypertension) increasing fetal heart rate (F. H. R.);

— metabolic: maternal and fetal hyperinsulinemia, hypoglycemia, lipolysis.

The counterindications to the use of betamimetics are therefore maternal hemorrhage and hypotension, and cardiovascular disease. They should be cautiously used for diabetic and toxemic parturients, all the more as anesthesia is more usually needed for those patients than in the rest of population of pregnant women. But noxious drug interactions of betamimetics with some anesthetics drugs are observed:

— halogenated agents are also positive bathmotropes. Their cardiac effects may be potentiated with resulting arrhythmia;

— the tachycardic effect of theses agents are potentiated by acetylcholinomimetics and curare like substances;

— epidural anesthesia provokes vasodilatation. Associated with betamimetics, it can produce collapse resulting in severe fetal distress.

Antihypertensive drugs should be continued prior to any obstetrical anesthesia. The anesthesia should be deep enough to avoid the sharp hypertensive attacks caused by pain during parturition or nociceptive stimuli during cesarean section. Any anesthesia involving vasoplegia may, for the patients under treatment, cause hypotension especially as some of them are hypovolemic. Thus, it is only after a careful pre-anesthetic check up, including the evaluation of the mother's state, fetal condition and uterine contraction evaluation, that the drug or method which is best adapted to the anesthesia must be chosen while considering the planned intervention and the obstetrician's and parturient's desires.

ANESTHESIA AND ANALGESIA

(A) In case of emergency, general anesthesia is usually chosen. All the drugs available for I. V. general anesthesia cross the placenta and will be found in the placental circulation.

Penthiobarbital has been used in obstetrics since 1936, and is the most commonly used anesthetic in obstetrics. Its success is partly due to its quick induction, its efficiency and easy use. Its effects on labor, which have been studied by the Toulouse Medical School [69] show that it does not change uterine activity which always remains within physiological limits. Because of its rapid placental transfer [35], there is much illusory hope that the fetus may be delivered before being affected by thiopental, but the transfer involves no fetal acidosis nor change in the F. H. R. If used in a single dose for induction, no fetal depression is observed. In case of higher doses, neonatal consciousness may be affected, and hypotonia seen in the first minutes of life. They will disappear in few

minutes if birth care and especially the neonate's warming have been correctly performed.

Propanidid (or Epontol) may be selected for brief operations because of its short term effects (3 or 4 minutes). It should be used by infusion for cesarean sections. Its effects on uterine activity are controversial. It has no neonatal depression effect, but its noxious side effects (hypotension, allergic reactions) restrict its use.

Althesin (or Alfatesine) a steroid anesthetic was used in obstetrics on account of its low toxicity, its high therapeutic index and its quick action. Repeated doses are not cumulative since it is metabolized instantaneously. After a slow induction, Althesin should be administered in regular supply. It does not change labor; some authors have noted neonatal acidosis in the case of high doses [33], which contrasts with the remarks of most authors, noticing the excellent birth state of neonates born after maternal administration of Althesin, and their normal development during the first week of life [25, 41]. However severe allergic incidents and accidents have been described while using Althesin, with collapse which may induce a severe fetal distress. For this reason, its use must be avoided in emergency cases, and in the case of a patient known to be allergic.

Ketamine has been used in obstetrics since 1968 [46, 23]. It is a short acting anesthetic. It is useful in obstetrics because it provides a "dissociative anesthesia" including certain analgesia and slight sleep. The psychodysleptic effect which is often observed when no premedication is given, is avoided by benzodiazepine administration. No respiratory or cardiovascular depression is noted. Ketamine is one of the rare anesthetics well known for its oxytocic effects [32]. It increases the basic uterine tone, and uterine contraction frequency.

Ketamine does not only depress neonates, but it can provoke muscular hypertonicity at birth and hyperexcitability.

It can be used as an induction agent for general anesthesia at a dose of 2 mg/kg, or as an analgesic (0.25 mg/kg) at small doses. It must be avoided for patients suffering from psychiatric diseases.

Hydroxybutyrate (Gamma OH in France) has been used in obstetrics since 1961 [26]. This is an anesthetic of long duration which is used in cesarean sections and dystocias, with hypotonic uterus, in vaginal deliveries.

It has no maternal respiratory or cardiovascular maternal depressive effect, and is even slightly hypertensive. As in the case of ketamine, it has an oxytocic effect: it increases the basic uterine tone, and decreases the active phase of labor without any other oxytocic. Its lack of analgesic effect is a drawback in obstetrics, but because of its fetal benefit in the case of anesthesia indicated by fetal distress (Fig. I-58), it has proven to be a first quality anesthetic in case of a maternal emergency involving fetal distress. The work in progress concerning the treatment of post-anoxia brain damage [43, 74] emphasizes the studies related to the use of barbiturates and hydroxybutyrate in obstetrics in the indication of anesthesia for fetal distress, and will probably allow us to understand the benefits of hydroxybutyrate on fetal distress, which are not now elucidated. Preeclampsia and eclampsia are counterindications for it.

All these methods of anesthesia can be completed after birth by adding inhalation anesthetics (nitrous oxide, halogenated agents), and curare-like agents which will permit muscular relaxation needed for the performance of surgical proceedures.

(B) If there is no emergency, one may use different analgesic and anesthetic methods which will obtain pain relief without change of consciousness.

When a simple additional analgesic is requested by the mother, the simplest methods must be chosen first for adequate psychoprophylactic preparation.

Transcutaneous electric stimulation can be selected rather than acupuncture, on account of the latter's disappointing results in this matter.

It is a very simple method with no maternal or fetal side effects, providing a possible analgesia for the parturients who were deprived from other drug analgesia due to fetal distress or counterindication, and can be complemented by very low doses of analgesic drugs to be completely efficient in normal deliveries. It is the case for multiparas and primiparas until 5 or 6 cm of dilatation, when traditional analgesia can be started, with an important saving of drugs.

Narcotics have been used in obstetrics for a long time, since morphine associated with scopolamine was used by Sertuner in 1902. It was rejected after meperidine had reached the market (1940), and then aroused a new keen interest when used by epidural injection [47, 12, 88]. Contingent on further studies, it can be stated that this method permits the same analgesia as systemic administration, with fewer doses.

In obstetrics, the interest of narcotics is not only their central analgesic effect, but also their oxytocic effect [40] although there is controversy about it. Simple use, and this double efficacy with very little

side effects for moderate doses accounts for their constant success and their incessant use in obstetrics in spite of certain shortcomings. Indeed, they have desagreable maternal side effects: lethargy, nausea. With small doses, certain analgesia is obtained without considerable side effects, but the pain relief is not much improved by increasing the doses, on the contrary the side effects increase, except when they are minimized by adding a neuroleptic drug [39].

All narcotics cross the placenta and therefore can cause neonatal respiratory depression if used at high doses. This trouble is less dangerous since naloxone (Narcan), a strong and selective antimorphinic drug can be used for adults and the neonate. For the adult, a dose of 0.4 mg should be used, renewable, IV or IM. For the neonate, the advised dose is 10 µg/kg IM, with when necessary concomitant ventilatory assistance [13, 48].

Meperidine (Dolosal, Pethidine) is the most common narcotic drug used in obstetrics. It can be administered IV or IM. The usual dose for labor is 50 to 100 mg of meperidine IM or 12.5 to 50 mg IV. At this dose, adverse neonatal effects are not to be anticipated, except for lack of suck, which could be antagonized by naloxone.

Above this dose, neonatal respiratory depression may occur. These adverse effects are related to the dose, and time between administration of meperidine and birth.

Fentanyl: its rapid action allows immediate analgesia, but its rapidity of effect (30 to 60 minutes) requires repeated doses.

Phenoperidine is a strong narcotic, belonging to the phenylpiperidines like meperidine.

Its effect is rather long (30 to 45 minutes), and like other narcotics it has a respiratory depressive effect. In obstetrics, its interest lies in the fact that it is the only narcotic devoid of vomiting action. Phenoperidine, with rapid effect, is used like fentanyl especially in neuroleptanalgesia [39, 40].

Inhalation analgesia is traditionally used in obstetrics, since the use of ether by Simpson in 1847.

Replacing of ether by chloroform in November 1847 was the beginning of a long use of *halogenated agents* in obstetrics since chloroform was followed by halothane, methoxyflurane and now ethrane. They provide quick induction and awakening, are easy to administer, but have two effects which restrict their obstetrical use: the drugs have cardio-circulatory depressive effects, and are highly tocolytic, except in the case of slight anesthesia. Therefore, they are used as a complementary anesthetic in small concentration, or in the treatment of uterine hypertonia with higher concentrations. They have no neonatal adverse effects.

Nitrous oxide has been constantly used in obstetrics since 1890. This is one of the strongest elements in obstetrical analgesia. It can be continuously or intermittently administered by the parturient herself or the midwife. A clinical study performed in a large number of cases in Great Britain [73] has shown that 90 % of the users were relieved. Pain relief is obtained from a concentration of 50 % of nitrous oxide/oxygen. These concentrations involve no maternal or fetal risk, causing no cardiovascular depression, and no change in uterine contractility. The sale of an equimolecular mixture of nitrous oxide/oxygen (Entonox), eliminating all anoxic risks permits self-administration by the parturient herself when requested. Placental transfer, which is now demonstrated, involves no neonatal adverse effects.

Local and regional anesthesia has proven to be a success for several years, especially lumbar epidural block.

For cesarean section, it is used to avoid general anesthesia and its risks of inhalation of gastric contents. Except in an emergency, it can be performed in most cases without accident when counterindications are observed.

Concerning parturition, it provides not only good analgesia, but also maternal comfort in normal deliveries; in addition it can treat uterine dystocias and avoid fetal consequences of maternal pain. It has been clearly demonstrated [80] that lumbar epidural anesthesia decreases the epinephrine level in maternal blood by 46 % and the norepinephrine level by 20 %. This decrease is all the greater as the mother's blood level was higher before anesthesia. The other reason for its success lies in the maintenance of consciousness, which avoids the occurence of Mendelson's syndrome, and enables the mother to fully attend the delivery. But, these methods also have adverse effects:

— Hypotension is usual in the absence of systematic prevention. It can be aggravated by aorto-vena cava compression by the gravid uterus which is more frequent in epidural anesthesia. It requires a preliminary IV perfusion of Ringers Lactate, left lateral position of the parturient or L. U. D. [71] and, according to some authors, previous IM administration of ephedrine IM before block.

— Headaches due to cerebro-spinal fluid loss by

dural puncture are sharp and unpleasant, but are stopped, most often, when using common antalgesic drugs, and do not produce any sequellae.

— Decreasing uterine efficiency which was sometimes controversial is now admitted. A prospective study [44] comparing epidural analgesia during labor with bupivacaine, and the Lamaze method has clearly shown that for the same length of labor, the population that received epidural analgesia needed twice as many oxytocic drugs.

— An increasing number of forceps deliveries has been demonstrated in the same studies. This may be minimized by good training in the Lamaze method, teaching parturients to push under epidural analgesia.

The other severe complications described are exceptional and avoided by respecting the counterindications to the method (clotting troubles, neurologic disease, infected back pustules, allergy to local anesthetics).

In these circumstances, neonatal consequences of epidural anesthesia are small [44, 71]. The neurobehavioural scores of babies born after epidural anesthesia are similar to the control group. Scanlon [75, 76] noted no signs of neonatal central depression after epidural anesthesia, but in a previous study muscular hypotonicity especially that related to the tests evaluating passive tone (recoil of the head, trunk tone) was present. This passive hypotonicity has not been noted either on further study [73] or in the french study [44]. The apparent contradiction is probably due to the fact that in the population under study by Scanlon, the anesthetics used were lidocaine and mepivacaine now abandonned for this indication, whereas in the latter studies by Scanlon and ourselves, bupivacaine was used. This local anesthetic is especially well adapted to obstetrics, since it provides good analgesia but only involves very moderate myoresolution. This is consequently the local anesthetic which best facilitates pushing efforts. It is used in concentrations from 0.125 to 0.375 % in obstetrical analgesia and 0.5 % for cesarean section.

NEONATAL CONSEQUENCES
OF OBSTETRICAL ANESTHESIA

As most of the drugs administered to the mother during pregnancy and parturition cross the placenta, they can involve fetal and neonatal symptomatology secondary to their administration. These symptoms should be known even if they are not severe, simply to perform a differential diagnosis at birth among facts implying different treatments.

The study of the neonatal fate of drugs given to mothers now developing, related to the study of fetal physiology and noenatal neurobehaviour will undoubtely enable us to better understand some problems of neonatal adaptation to extra-uterine life. Placental transfer of drugs has been presumed, and now, during labor, it can be proved by modifications of F. H. R. subsequent to their maternal administration, and at birth by the study of maternal and fetal pharmacokinetics of drugs, and systematic clinical examination of the newborn, in the search for neonatal secondary effects of drugs. The rules for placental transfer of drugs and their fetal and neonatal metabolism will not be described here in, as they are included in the chapter devoted to perinatal pharmacology.

Fetal evaluation during labor should include the study of F. H. R. (amplitude and frequency), fetal acid-base balance by scalp blood samples which measure the pH and lactic acid.

Fetal Heart Rate is obtained externally by Doppler signal and recorded on a cardiotachograph. A rapid baseline (from 120 to 160 beats/minute), is indicative of a good prognosis (Fig. I-53). An apparently decreased variability or flat line, or decelerations may be negatively significant and indicate fetal distress (Figs. I-54 and I-55).

The F. H. R. should be studied for a fairly long time prior to any obstetrical analgesia in order to eliminate fetal distress which could be previously present and attributed to analgesia by mistake. We also must know the modifications of F. H. R. induced by placental transfer of drugs, so as not to confuse them with symptoms of very different significance.

F. H. R. regulation is dependant on many factors: control of the adrenergic nervous system and vagal tone, baro and chemo-receptor reflexes. The variations are linked with the interferences between the activity of the sinus node and the beta-adrenergic and vagal nervous system. Consequently, it is easy to understand that all the drugs with central or peripheral action modifying vagal tone or adrenergic responses will change F. H. R. For example, as in the case of chlorpromazine, atropine and betamimetic drugs.

Chlorpromazine (Fig. I-56) eliminates physiological variability beat to beat, by showing a flat drawing of the baseline, which could involve fetal distress if maternal administration of this drug is unknown. This is equally the case, to a lesser degree, with hydroxyzine and meperidine [84, 85].

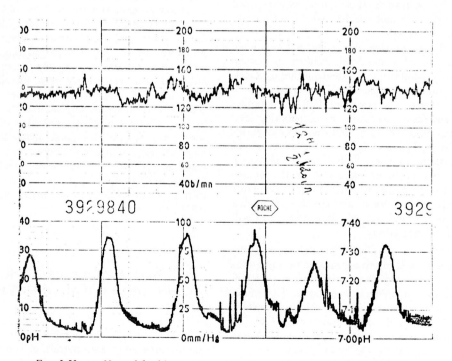

Fig. I-53. — *Normal fetal heart rate and uterine contractions* (G. Barrier, 1981).

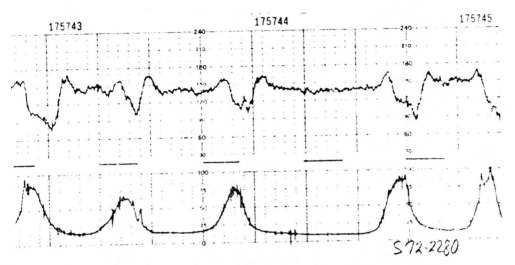

FIG. I-54. — *Early decelerations of uterine contractions* (G. BARRIER, 1981).

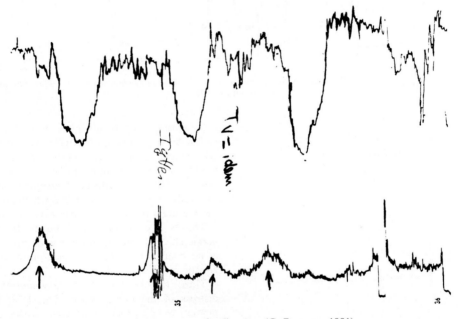

FIG. I-55. — *Late decelerations* (G. BARRIER, 1981).

Conversely, *Betamimetic drugs* [84] increase the basic rate and variability.

The feto-neonatal pharmacokinetics of *Atropine* [8] have shown that placental transfer of this drug is easily accomplished, but also that individual large variations could be observed in maternal and fetal blood concentrations after administration of the same dose to the mother (12.5 μg/kg IV). This suggests that placental transfer of atropine varies from one patient to the other in the absence of any pathology. On the other hand, the increase in F. H. R. by atropine on which the "atropine test" used by some authors to detect chronic fetal distress was based, occurs after an apparent delay. If maternal-fetal blood equilibrium is obtained within five minutes, atropinic fetal tachycardia, following a short period of bradycardia gradually rises to reach its maximum level in a mean time of 25.7 ± 8.5 minutes [66]. This may lead to errors in the interpretation of the test (Fig. I-57).

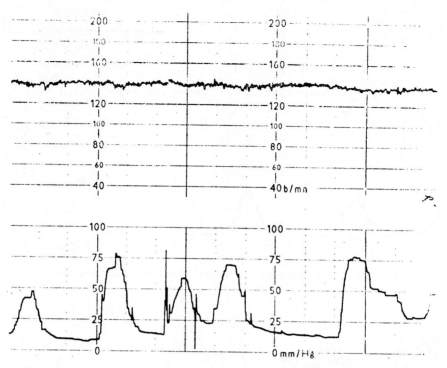

FIG. I-56. — *Silent fetal heart rate following maternal administration of chlorpromazine "Flat drawing"*
(G. BARRIER, 1981).

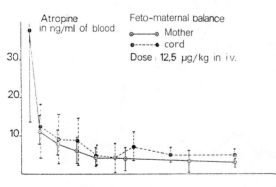

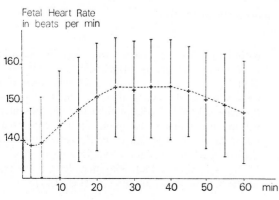

In contrast, use of atropinic drugs for premedication before maternal anesthesia is still valid, but the changes of F. H. R. induced by atropine and modifying fetal symptomatology, as well undesirable neonatal side effects of atropine have led to the study of atropinic substances which do not cross the placental barrier: i. e. glycopyrrolate [1, 10, 70].

This is a quaternary ammonium. Its anticholinergic effect is similiar to the one of atropine. There is no change in F. H. R. which preserves its diagnostic value in fetal distress.

Thus, the benefit of hydroxybutyrate in fetal distress of metabolic origin (Fig. I-58) has been proven, whereas there is no effect if this distress is due to a nuchal cord (Fig. I-59). This effect has been partly ascribed to atropine used as a vagolytic agent in hydroxybutyrate anesthesia. But it has been recently demonstrated that it persists when atropine is replaced by glycopyrrolate which does not cross

FIG. I-57. — *Level of atropine in maternal venous blood and in the umbilical cord.* There is an increase in F. H. R. after IV Atropine (12.5 µg/kg). Studies in 45 women in labour (From ONNEN *et al.* Placental transfer of atropine at the end of pregnancy. *Europ. J. Clin. Pharm.*, *15*, 443-446, 1979).

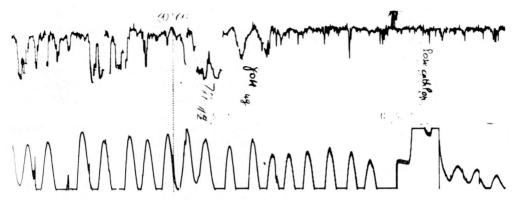

FIG. I-58. — *Benefits of hydroxybutyrate in fetal distress of metabolic origin* (G. BARRIER, 1981).

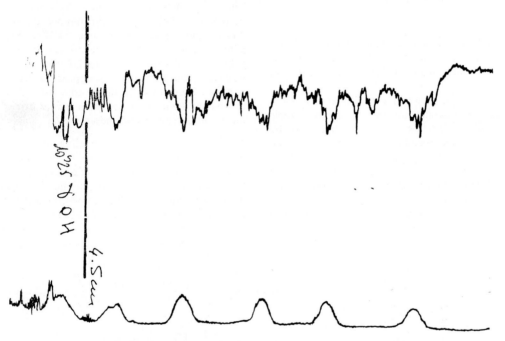

FIG. I-59. — *Persistant decelerations under hydroxybutyrate with nuchal cord (loop around the neck)*
(G. BARRIER, 1981).

the placenta in hydroxybutyrate anesthesia for acute fetal distress.

Finally, without considering in detail the placental transfer of drugs and their fetal and neonatal metabolism, we can illustrate by some examples the fetal and neonatal consequences involved in placental transfer of anesthetics and analgesics, and the role played by the prior fetal condition in the metabolism of drugs.

The study of acid-base fetal balance is necessary to be able to choose the most suitable drug, whose secondary effects would not add to the previous fetal

pathology. The neonatal side effects of drugs should be as short as possible, in order to be independant of neonatal symptomatology.

Fetal absorption of drugs is known to be influenced by the pH gradient between the maternal and fetal blood; it has been demonstrated that in the presence of fetal acidosis and a constant injection of a local anesthetic, lidocaine, the level in blood is higher [14] than with a normal pH before infusion (Fig. I-60). Similarly, the neonatal decrease of the blood level of local anesthetic agents is quicker for a normothermic neonate than for an hypothermic one [60].

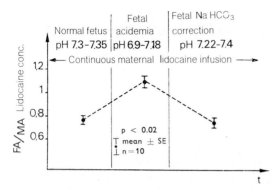

FIG. I-60. — *Influence of acidosis on lidocaine metabolism.*

The study of fetal and neonatal pharmacokinetics of drugs administered to the mother is important in understanding fetal physiology and neonatal pathology.

In the neonatal period, the clinical status of the infant may be modified not only by drugs or their metabolites via placental transfer, but also by changes of their metabolism secondary to the clinical status (temperature, acidosis) and by drug interactions between drugs administered to the mother during delivery and some others administered to the newborn at birth.

The increasing number of drugs administered to pregnant women, either by doctors or by self-medication [7] does not facilitate the understanding

of neonatal pathology. A neonate is not a "mini adult". His anatomical and physiological characteristics (high hematocrit, high percentage of water in the organism, small plasma protein concentration) cannot be applied to the data of adult pharmacology. At birth, the interruption of the umbilical circulation forces the neonate to metabolize and eliminate by himself the drugs he has received during the end of pregnancy and parturition with his own biochemical potential, since they cannot any longer be eliminated by the mother.

This adaptation to extra-uterine life will be exposed to large variations caused by gravidic or obstetrical fetal pathology, as well as to the secondary effects of some drugs received via placental transfer. Thus it is necessary to study the pharmacology of drugs administered to the mother during pregnancy and labor, and correlate the data obtained with the clinical status of the neonate, to perform a behavioural diagnosis of pathological symptoms observed at birth, and then give appropriate treatment.

As an illustration of drugs administered during pregnancy, we shall consider the studies carried out on benzodiazepines and indomethacin.

Benzodiazepines are usually given to anxious or insomniac parturients, especially at the end of the pregnancy. The neonatal side effects of these drugs have been described [5]: hypotonia, hypothermia with no response to cold, acidosis, neurologic and respiratory depression were observed for apparent moderate doses. However, the study of placental transfer of drugs emphasizing the conditions for the

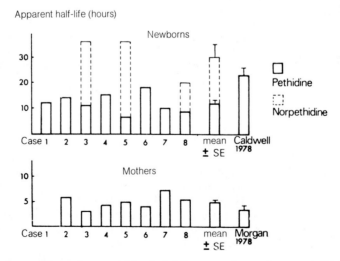

FIG. I-61. — *Half-life of meperidine and normepiridine in 8 full-term newborns. Apparent half-life of meperidine in full-term mothers during delivery.* From: TALAFRÉ M. L., ROVEI V., BARRIER G., LASSNER J., SAN JUAN M., MORSELLI P. L., SUREAU C.: Pharmacocinétique de la péthidine chez le nouveau-né et la mère pendant le travail. INSERM, *Pharmacologie du développement,* vol. 89, 287-296, 1979.

transfer [42] and the study of neonatal pharmaco-kinetics have shown that these side effects could be more related to the blood level of a metabolite (nordiazepam) than to the initial drug. Prior to these studies, some pediatricians would have surely tried to ascribe this neonatal symptomatology to the obstetrician, even one skillfully manipulating a forceps, or to the anesthesiologists who cautiously manipulate drugs. In addition because benzodiaze-pine absorption during the end of pregnancy can result from either self-medication or medical pres-cription from a family doctor it may consequently be unknown to the obstetrician or midwife.

It is known that treatments recommended in premature labor use drugs with antiprostaglandin effects especially *Indomethacin*. The study of its neo-natal secondary effects associated with the pharmaco-kinetics of indomethacin have demonstrated an important oligo-anuria [52] and a transient ileus, and above all neonatal cyanosis [51, 14], which could be related to a constriction of the ductus arteriosus implying the presence of pulmonary hypertension.

The placental transfer of indomethacin [16] is known, and in the animal model, anatomic and functional changes occuring in the fetus by placental transfer have been reproduced [49]. At present, such neonatal effects can be related to their true causes, whereas previously, the observation of such events in neonates whose mothers had received indomethacin and obstetrical analgesia would have probably allowed some pediatricians to ascribe the difficulties to analgesia.

The study of neonatal pharmacology is equally of importance to evaluate the effects of drugs administered to the mother during labor; parti-cularly analgesics. Meperidine which has been used since 1940 is the most commonly used agent. Its side effects are well known. Recently the study of meperidine metabolism in parturients and the neonate explains some surprising and controversial facts. Central depressive effects of meperidine like those of all narcotics are known. They have been described for the neonate [17], but the relationships between effect-dose and effect-time from fetal expo-sure at birth have been controversial. For some [61], the noxious side effects on the neonate are all the more significant as the length of time between admi-nistration of meperidine to mother and birth is important. In recent studies [24, 82], it has been demonstrated that there was a correlation between the time of meperidine administration and birth, and meperidine $\dfrac{\text{umbilical vein}}{\text{maternal vein}}$ ratio. This ratio tends to increase with time, and 3 or 4 hours are

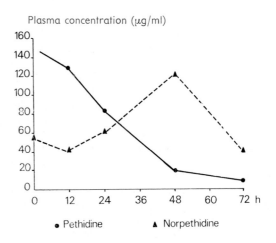

Plasma concentration (µg/ml)

● Pethidine   ▲ Norpethidine

Fig. I-62. — *Plasma levels of pethidine and norpethidine in a term newborn-1st 72 hours of life.*

required to obtain equilibrium. Therefore, the diffe-rences of appreciation of various authors can be explained by different times when neonates where examined after birth following administration of meperidine to the mother. On the other hand, the half-life of meperidine is 3 hours. In parturients it is 3.1 to 7.1 hours which assumes a slower meta-bolism of drugs. For neonates, the half-life is 6.5 to 18 hours [24, 82] (Fig. I-61). In addition, normoperi-dine with its convulsive effects is apparently more pre-judicial to the neonate than meperidine itself [53], and increases in the 24 to 48 hours after birth corro-borating preliminary studies carried out on diazepam and mepivacaine which suggest moderately reduced demethylation by the neonate. In contrast, hydroxyla-tion and binding capacities are very much reduced. The fact that normeperidine tends to accumulate in the neonate for 24 to 48 hours after birth, that its half-life is twice or three times as long as mepe-ridine which is metabolized 5 or 8 times more slowly by the neonate than the adult, can, in the case of fetal distress and acidosis, have obvious noxious neonatal effects, and increases neonatal pathology with obstetrical causes (Fig. I-62). This may explain some late distress in neonates born after obstetrical dystocias, whose mothers were given high doses of meperidine, i. e. greater than 100 mg.

Naloxone is the antagonistic drug of narcotics. But as its effect lasts only 90 to 120 minutes [13], one can appreciate some late depression after admi-nistration of naloxone to the newborn. One pharma-cokinetic approach to neonatal metabolism of the drug allowed us to adjust the dose and time of antagonist administration in order to avoid late neonatal side effects of narcotics (10 µg/kg of naloxone IM, renewed if necessary after 2 hours).

Studies of placental transfer of *local anesthetics* have demonstrated that local anesthetics with long term effects (bupivacaine, etidocaine) have a high maternal-fetal ratio, as they are preferentially bound to maternal rather than fetal proteins [86, 50], which explains their low concentration in fetal blood. It was thought that this was the explanation of good fetal and neonatal tolerance to these substances. However several authors [86, 56] have shown in man and animal experiments that the strong binding to maternal proteins did not eliminate placental transfer. The plasma concentration of free drug, which is most important for the transfer, may be low without preventing the materno-fetal equilibrium and similar tissue ratios are reached. For example, fetal tissue concentration of etidocaine or lidocaine are similar, whereas the protein binding of etidocaine is more higher than for lidocaine (Fig. I-63). Therefore this implies that other factors influence placental transfer, such as liposolubility, or the rate of drug-protein dissociation. It can be dependant of the fetal condition and acid-base balance, as Morishima et al. have demonstrated for the ewe [57]. They have demonstrated that fetal tolerance to lidocaine is higher than the neonate's, and the tolerance is decreased by anoxia and acidosis.

In healthy neonates, they have noted that high levels of local anesthetics, can involve no side effects as long as the umbilical circulation was normal. But in case of acidosis and asphyxia, the excretion of the drug toward the mother is modified as studied by comparing normal lambs and asphyxiated lambs. In the latter group within 10 minutes, blood levels of lidocaine were higher than in the control group and within 15 minutes, umbilical arterial concentration of the studied group was higher than venous concentration, resulting in fetal uptake.

As for meperidine and benzodiazepines, this work has allowed us to understand some contradictory facts which have previously raised controversies. It can be assumed that healthy human fetuses can sustain high concentrations of local anesthetics provided that they are well oxygenated, their acid-base balance normal, and placental and umbilical flow normal. But with the same blood concentration anoxic and acidotic fetuses will have a higher tissue concentration, which can have severe hemodynamic consequences, as demonstrated in man [20, 21]. Consequently, it is of great importance that the diagnosis of fetal distress be established *prior to any obstetrical analgesia* for want of aggravating distress by noxious side effects of a drug overdose. This is one of the reasons for which we recommend the systematic recording of the F. H. R., complemented when necessary by the study of fetal acidosis on samples of fetal scalp blood before any significant or long duration planned obstetrical analgesia. In particular one should refuse to perform epidural

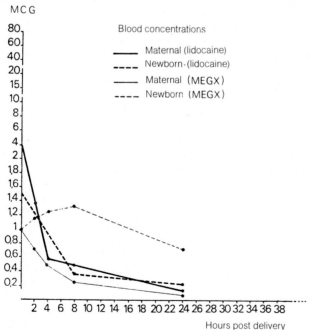

MCG

Blood concentrations

——— Maternal (lidocaine)
- - - - Newborn (lidocaine)
——— Maternal (MEGX)
- - - - Newborn (MEGX)

80, 60, 40, 20, 15, 10, 8, 6, 4, 2, 1,8, 1,6, 1,4, 1,2, 1, 0,8, 0,6, 0,4, 0,2

2 4 6 8 10 12 14 16 18 20 22 24 26 28 30 32 34 36 38

Hours post delivery

FIG. I-63. — *Maternal and neonatal lidocaine concentrations in the first 24 hours of life.* From: OSTHEIMER G. W., DATTA S., SCANLON J. W., CORKE B. C., BROWN W. U., CROCKER J. S., WEISS D. B., ALPER M. H.: Abstract S. O. A. P. Meeting, Boston) 1980.

analgesia if a persistant abnormality of F. H. R. is observed, and not modified by L. U. D. or left lying position of the mother, or without excluding fetal acidosis by the measurement of pH or lactate.

Neurobehavioural evaluation of the neonate is the third type of the study which, in the last decade has allowed us to extend, understand and improve neonatal security concurrently with maternal security in obstetrical anesthesia. If the study of fetal heart rate allowed us to detect before analgesia fetal distress which could be a counterindication to its administration and the study of perinatal pharmacokinetics enabled us to understand some unpredicted neonatal side effects of anesthetics or analgesics, and then treat them properly; systematic studies of neonatal neurobehaviour following obstetrical analgesia may demonstrate additional neonatal effects of drugs used during labor. These studies will need to be long term since side-effects may be slight and may be only perceived under careful examination. The proper detection of these phenomena at first in healthy infants, then after fetal distress, will allow us to finally know what is related to pathology and what to anesthesia in the state of a neonate.

Although the **Apgar score** is still the predominant instrument for evaluating the neonatal state at birth, and appreciating care or resuscitation performed in the first minutes of life, it should not be used for estimating neonatal behavioural modifications occuring after administration of maternal analgesia. These modifications are too slight to be easily observed except in case of overdoses, drug interactions or underlying fetal pathology.

By 1961, Brazelton [18] noted that neonates whose mothers had received a large amount of drugs during labor feed less than the others. He continued his work and published the "Brazelton Neonatal Neurobehavioral Assessment Scale" in 1973 [79], from which the subsequent work concerning neurosensorial behaviour in neonates in the days following normal delivery is derived. Brazelton's credit was to call attention to neonatal behaviour. His test allowed us to evaluate the capacity of the neonate to adapt himself to his environment, to eliminate inappropriate sensorial stimuli and modulate his response in relation to external events. Unfortunately, this examination is time consuming and requires experienced observers.

Utilizing the same principle, the test subsequently published by Scanlon [75] was especially designed to study the effects on the neonate of anesthetics administered to the mother. The Early Neonatal Neurobehavioural Scale (ENNS) which is simpler and quicker than the Brazelton test, has selected neonatal effects of epidural anesthesia [75, 76].

More recently, following the work of Amiel-Tison about neurologic behaviour of the newborn in the first days of life [3], Amiel-Tison, Barrier and Shnider have described a new neurosensory assessment of the full-term infant [79]. This test is based on the study of passive tone, active tone, primary reflexes, state of consciousness, adaptative capacity to light and sound, and response to consolability. We have included a total of 20 objective tests or criteria within these categories. Each criterion is rated 0,1 or 2 based on whether the response to testing is absent or grossly abnormal: score 0; mediocre or slightly abnormal: score 1; or normal: score 2 with a maximum score of 40.

The items in the score can be performed in any order but we have listed them in a sequence which we have found to be most conducive and logical to follow. The examiner determines the neonate's best performance and if, in an individual item the neonate scores 1 or 0, the test should be repeated later in the examination to confirm this low score.

Evaluation of adaptive capacity (items 1 to 5). — The interaction of the infant with his environment is tested with 5 criteria composed of sensory stimuli (light and sound) observing consolability when the baby is agitated.

The equipment needed for the behavioural capacity score are a bell and a flashlight. The infant must be in a state of quiet alertness and tested in a quiet environment preferably prior to being unwrapped or undressed to minimize distracting stimuli.

If the infant is too sleepy or fussy, the maximal response may not be easily elicited. In such cases it is advisable to complete the neurological portion of the examination initially and retest adaptive responses afterward. This affords the infant the opportunity to score optimally.

(1) *Response to sound.* — Ring the bell sharply but briefly a few inches behind the infant's head in the midline out of visual range. We suggest a bell similar to the one used in a standard Gesell Test. Evaluate the response on movements, activity, startle, blinking and respiratory changes. If there is no response to the first ring, awaken the infant by gentle stimulation then repeat the test again up to three times before giving a score of zero. Ring the bell three times and use the maximum response.

0. No reaction.
1. Moderate reaction.
2. Vigorous reaction with startle and possible searching for the bell.

(2) *Habituation to sound.* — Repeat the sound stimulus after the previous response has ended. Observe

and describe the sequential responses as similar, diminished or altered, or absent. Repeat the stimulus until
obtaining a modified or absent response to the stimulus.
Discontinue the test after 12 stimuli if there is no modification of the response. If the response to sound had
been scored 0, the habituation or response decrement
is also scored 0.

0. No decrement or alteration observed after 12 stimuli.
1. Decrement or alteration of the response after 7 to
12 stimuli.
2. Decrement of the response before or at the 6th stimulus.

(3) *Response to light.* — Briefly shine a bright light
from a pocket flashlight into the infant's eyes three
times. Evaluate the best response on blink, startle, or eye-
widening reflex, general motor activity or respiratory
changes. It is best to perform this test in a quiet darkened
room. If no response, awaken the infant by gentle stimulation then repeat the test again up to three times
before giving a score of 0.

0. No reaction.
1. Sluggish or delayed reaction.
2. Brisk blink or startle.

(4) *Habituation to light.* — Repeat the stimulation
after the infant's best response has been observed and
each sequential reaction up to 12 is observed. If the
response to light has been scored 0 the habituation is
score 0.

0. No decrement or alteration.
1. Decrement or alteration of the response after 7 to
12 stimuli.
2. Decrement or alteration of the response before or
at the 6th stimulus.

(5) *Consolability.* — This is measured in an infant
actively fussing or crying for 15 seconds or more. Usually
crying accompanies part of the neurologic examination,
especially the Moro maneuver. Absence of crying or
fussiness during the examination or with mild stimulation
would be distinctly abnormal and scored 0. Consolability is first tested with the infant lying on the examination table. Apply soothing stimuli, such as placing of
the examiner's hand on the infant's abdomen and res-
training the activity of the infant's arms. If necessary,
hold or rock the infant in the supine, or even better,
the prone position. Consolability is demonstrated when
the infant quiets for at least 5 seconds.

0. No consoling even with caressing, holding, rocking and finger sucking for 60 seconds.
1. Difficult but obtainable on the examination table
by the preceding maneuvers.
2. Easily obtainable by examiner's voice and face or
by the preceding maneuvers.

Neurological assessment. — This portion of the examination requires no equipment and can always be
completed even if the infant is lethargic, irritable or
almost inconsolable. The only major prerequisite is
that the general condition of the infant allows testing
in the upright position. This is necessary to assess accurately the supporting reaction (a test of active tone,
item 14) and automatic walking (a primary reflex,
item 15). The technique for testing each of the 15 criteria is listed below.

Evaluation of passive tone (items 6 to 9):

(6) *Scarf sign.* — A positive scarf sign means that the
arm encircles the neck like a scarf. Sustain the infant
in a semireclining position using the palm of the hand
as a support; then take the infant's hand and try to
pull the arm across his chest towards the opposite
shoulder, continuing as far posteriorly as possible.
Observe the position assumed by the elbow in relation
to the umbilicus. Both sides are tested successively.
Three positions are described:

0. Very ample movement, the arm encircles the neck
without resistance.
1. Elbow passes midline.
2. Elbow does not reach midline.

(7) *Recoil of elbows.* — This can be checked only when
the infant is in a spontaneously flexed posture. Both
sides are tested simultaneously. With the infant supine
fully extend the arms by pulling on the hand and release;
observe how quickly the forearms return to a position of
flexion.

0. Absent or not able to test if initial position is in
extension.
1. Recoil sluggish or weak.
2. Brisk, reproducible.

(8) *Popliteal angle.* — While maintaining the pelvis
flat on the table, flex each thigh at the hip and fix the
knees on either side of the abdomen. Then, simultaneously
lift the lower segment of the legs and observe the angle
between the leg and the thigh, that is, the popliteal angle.

0. The angle formed is more than 110°.
1. The angle formed is 100° to 110°.
2. The angle formed is a right angle or less.

(9) *Recoil of lower limbs.* — With the infant supine
the hips and knees are usually flexed. Simultaneously
extend both legs by pushing the knees downward and then
release them.

0. Absent or not able to test if initial position is in
extension.
1. Recoil sluggish or weak.
2. Brisk, reproducible.

Remarks on testing passive tone:

(*a*) The examiner can evaluate *passive tone* by observing
and manipulating the infant while he is quiet but not
asleep. The resistance of an extremity to these manipulations is measured by noting the angle formed by the
movement or the amplitude of the movement or a recoil.
During these maneuvers keep the infant's head in the
midline position to avoid eliciting the asymmetric
tonic reflex. The maneuvers must be performed slowly
and gently and to the point of meeting resistance.

(*b*) In case of an asymmetrical response, code the best
side, as the hypotonic side is very likely abnormal from
a peripheral nerve injury.

(*c*) In the case of breech delivery, the passive tone in
the lower limbs will be modified transiently by the intrauterine posture. The resulting apparent hypotonia in the
lower limbs will therefore result in an abnormal popliteal
angle and recoil of the lower extremities unrelated to
central nervous system dysfunction. With breech presentation these two criteria should not be tested but to
complete the scoring of passive tone the same scores
as obtained for scarf and for recoil of elbows should

be used. We believe that this is legitimate since mild central nervous system dysfunction will cause hypotonicity only in the upper limbs. Thus in the breech infant if the tone is normal in the upper limbs, the assumption can be made that it would have been normal as well in the lower limbs had the baby been born in the vertex position.

Evaluation of active tone and primary reflexes (items 10 to 17). — The quality of most *primary reflexes* is dependent on the quality of the active tone. Since poor primary reflexes signify more profound central nervous system depression than poor tone, it is important to dissociate as much as possible the two kinds of abnormalities.

(10) *Active contraction of the neck flexors.* — Grasp the shoulders and pull the supine infant to the sitting position while noting the position of the head in relation to the trunk. In the oblique position, just before the vertical position is reached, one can observe that the flexor muscles contract to raise the head. In the full-term infant extensor and flexor tone is balanced and the head is maintained for about 3 to 5 seconds in the axis of the trunk.

0. Absent if the head, which is pendulent at first, passively passes the midline and immediately drops forward, or abnormal if permanent hypertonicity of neck extensors maintains the head backward and keeps the head from falling downward with gravity at the end of the maneuver.
1. Mediocre—head maintained in the axis but only for 1 to 2 seconds; difficult to obtain, not reproducible.
2. Perfect—head is maintained a few seconds in the axis of the trunk; reproducible.

(11) *Active contraction of the neck extensors.* — With the infant sitting and leaning forward and the head hanging down on the chest, move the trunk backward and observe the reaction of the head. In the oblique position, just before the vertical position is reached, a reaction of the extensors will raise the head of the term infant and maintain this position for 3 to 5 seconds.

0. *Absent* if the head, which is pendulent at first, passively passes the midline and drops backward, or *abnormal*, if the head is unable to hang, on the chest at the beginning of the movement, being maintained strongly by the extensors. The head then passes backward too quickly in such a way that the reaction appears too good.
1. Mediocre, head maintained in the axis but only for 1 to 2 seconds; difficult to obtain, not reproducible.
2. Perfect, reproducible, the head is maintained a few seconds in the axis of the body.

(12) *Palmar grasp.* — Although this is primarily a reflex, palmar grasp is inserted in the active tone tests as a necessary prerequisite to testing response to traction (item 13). Failure to elicit a palmar grasp does not allow testing of traction as a parameter of active tone.

With the infant lying in the supine position the arms are extended and the fists unclenched by the examiner. The examiner inserts his index fingers into the hands of the infant from the ulnar side and gently presses against the palmar surface; this palmar stimulation produces a flexion of the infant's fingers onto the examiner's index fingers.

0. If no grasp of the fingers is observed.
1. If mediocre.
2. Perfect.

(13) *Response to traction.* — At the very moment that a strong grasp of the fingers is obtained, the observer then raises his index fingers approximately 12 inches (keeping his thumbs ready to hold the infant's hand if necessary).

The normal term infant will respond to this maneuver by flexing his upper extremities and literally lifting himself from the bed completely. The observer should not grasp the infant's hands and lift the baby as this maneuver will not evaluate active tone. It is important that the baby's hands are clean and dry.

0. Absent when no active flexion of the upper extremities is noted or not able to test when there is no palmar grasp.
1. When the strength of the contraction only allows part of the body weight to be lifted before the palmar grasp is released or if the knees are not flexed when both feet are off the table.
2. Excellent, when the infant is able to lift his body weight completely and the maneuver is halted when both feet are off the table. When the reaction is perfect the head usually moves forward and the infant maintains itself for a few seconds in an active semiflexed position.

(14) *Supporting reaction.* — The infant is held in the standing position with the examiner placing his hand on the infant's anterior chest with thumb and fingers in the axillae. Observe if the legs straighten and the trunk muscles contract to allow the infant to support some of his own weight. Ascertain that the infant's soles are firmly on the table. If the infant's feet are cold or traumatized by heel sticks, the reaction might be difficult to obtain.

0. Absent, no tendency to contract the extensor muscles of the legs and trunk, the entire body weight is in the hands of the observer.
1. The contraction is incomplete and transitory.
2. The contraction is strong, maintained a few seconds and the infant supports all his body weight.

It is important to note that when the posture in flexion is very strong in a full term newborn, full extension of the legs may not occur during the first few days. Likewise, in breech deliveries the standing position cannot always be achieved because of the abnormal position of the lower limbs. If the trunk muscles contract in a visible and perceptible way, a score of 2 can be given even if the legs are not fully extended or are abnormally postured during the testing of the supporting reaction.

(15) *Automatic walking.* — When the supporting reaction is obtained automatic walking occurs spontaneously or is helped by tilting the infant slightly backward or forward.

0. Absent, no steps are observed.
1. A few steps but mediocre and repetitive.
2. Perfect, brisk, reproducible.

Note that walking can usually be obtained even if the infant's lower extremities are not in full extension. If automatic walking cannot be demonstrated due to excessive flexion or abnormal posture of the lower extremities (breech), the placing reaction should be substituted as a primary reflex.

Placing reaction. — With the infant suspended in the upright position, the body is raised until the dorsum of the foot touches a protruding bassinet edge. Scoring is based on flexion, then extension, of the stimulated leg until placement of the ipsilateral foot on the edge is accomplished.

0. No response.
1. Weak flexion and extension with poor placement of ipsilateral foot.
2. Brisk, reproducible.

(16) *Sucking*. — The examiner evaluates the sucking reflex by introducing a finger into the mouth and noting the strength, rhythmicity of sucking and the synchrony of swallowing.

0. Absent.
1. Weak, discontinuous, asynchronous with swallowing.
2. Perfect, continuous, rhythmic, synchronous with swallowing.

(17) *Moro reflex*. — Holding both hands of the infant in abduction while keeping the back of the head on the bed, lift the infant's shoulders a few centimeters off the bed. Then release the hands briskly at the point of maximum abduction. The normal reflex is a brisk abduction of the arms at the shoulder and extension of the forearms at the elbow followed by abduction of the arms at the shoulder (an embrace) and flexion of the forearms at the elbow. Complete opening of the hands occurs during the first part. In the normal newborn crying is consistently provoked.

0. Absent.
1. Weak, incomplete, no crying, no opening of the hand.
2. Perfect with full extension, abduction of the arms, opening of the hands and crying.

Because the Moro appears to be a frightening experience for the infant, if a spontaneous Moro response has been observed during the course of the evaluation, this reflex can be scored without actually performing the maneuver described above.

Remarks on testing active tone and primary reflexes. The examiner studies *active tone* when the infant moves spontaneously in response to a given stimulus. The infant must be well enough to allow manipulation of his head and trunk.

Defer testing of neck extensors if the child is crying. A crying normal infant demonstrates a mild hypertonicity of the neck extensors probably due to transitory elevation of intracranial pressure. It is best to postpone this test until the infant is consoled. The primary reflexes may also be transiently inhibited by excessive crying and testing of reflexes should be deferred until the infant is consoled.

General assessment (items 18 to 20):

(18) *Alertness*. — The judgement of alertness takes into account the predominant state of consciousness during the entire examination.

0. Comatose state, no response to stimuli.
1. Lethargy with poor contact, short periods of attention, sluggish response to stimulation.
2. Quiet alertness with occular contact; immediate responsivity to most stimuli.

(19) *Crying*. — The quality of the cry is evaluated. Normal babies usually cry at some point during the examination. Mild additional stimulation may be necessary to elicit crying.

0. Absent.
1. Abnormal (high-pitched, weak, monotonous, moaning, discontinuous, resulting in cyanosis or vasomotor changes, difficult to elicit).
2. Normal in quality and quantity.

(20) *Motor activity*. — Spontaneous motor activity is best evaluated by inspection of the infant while he lies undisturbed. The speed, intensity and amount of movement vary a great deal in the normal infant and only the most obvious alterations should be considered abnormal.

0. Absent, the infant lies motionless even when strongly stimulated or shows excessive motor agitation, incessant tremors or bursts of clonic movements.
1. Diminished or excessive motor activity with intermittent jitteriness.
2. Normal in quantity, harmonious in quality.

Remarks on alertness. — Scoring of infant alertness corresponds to the state of consciousness S_2, S_1, A_1, A_2, A_3, A_4, used in the Scanlon ENNS. A score of zero (0) designates the S_2 state with either no arousability or extremely poor arousability. A baby that is lethargic but able to be stimulated for the purposes of testing scores one (1) and corresponds to S_1 or A_1 infants. A_2, A_3, (A_4) state infants would be vigorous and in an awake state through most of the testing and score two (2). Arousal of the infant for testing may bring the infant to an artificially high state of consciousness and may not be a measure of the predominant state.

This is not an invasive score. It avoids the repeated Moro, pin-prick and therefore can be done many times in front of mothers. In addition it is designed to score each examination between 0 and 40 (maximum scoring is 40), and do a follow up of fetal behaviour during the first days of life.

However emphasizing more muscular tone than is noted in ENNS, there is a correlation between the test described by Amiel-Tison, Barrier and Shnider and the one illustrated by Scanlon. As it is quicker and only requires simple experience, it can be repeated without provoking hypothermia. It is apparently a good instrument for anesthesiologists willing to know the consequences of drugs administered to parturients. The first results published on the study of neonates following a normal delivery under obstetrical anesthesia or analgesia allow us to question the preliminary conclusions of Conway and Brackbill [28].

If the administration of a dose of 50 mg of meperidine may decrease habituation to sound [17], and a dose of 100 mg results in decreased sucking during 30 to 60 minutes after birth, with complete recovery at 2 hours of life, the study of neonatal behaviour after a dose less than 100 mg of meperidine [48] or its narcotic equivalent has shown that the global evaluation of our scoring system was normal. Similarly Scanlon has described decreasing passive tone of neonates whose mothers had received epidural anesthesia with lidocaine or mepivacaine but notes that the tone becomes normal at the 8th hour of life [76]. As a matter of interest, this symptomatology is not found after epidural analgesia with bupivacaine which is the drug most often used now.

Recently, a prospective study [44] comparing the results of two obstetrical analgesic methods (Lamaze method and epidural with bupivacaine) during labor and delivery of full-term primiparas found no differences between the neonates born from both groups.

Contrary to local anesthetics the neonatal effects of which are peripheral, general anesthetics may have a transitory depressive effect on the items reflecting consciousness. Preliminary results suggest the assumption that if obstetrical anesthesia or analgesia does result in slight, and transitory neonatal symptomatology, it does not by itself cause neonatal distress. No long term effect of obstetrical anesthesia or analgesia can as yet be ascertained [87].

This analysis does not justify the incautious use of drugs in anesthetic technics during delivery, but it tends to reconsider certain suggestions judging neonatal effects of obstetrical analgesia on a group of mixed neonates in which some of them were healthy infants whose mothers had received analgesia, and others infants from deliveries during which fetal distress was the indication for emergency anesthesia.

LAWSUITS AND OBSTETRICAL ANESTHESIA

These may be very serious since prosecutions following delivery are most often due to catastrophic accidents, jeopardizing the health or the life not of only one patient as usual in medicine, but the lives of two persons: mother and infant.

Obstetrical anesthesia is a difficult and very special medical act. It is one of the rare medical cases in which two patients should be cared for at the same time and whose requirements may be contradictory. This peculiar relationship gives the obstetrician and anesthesiologist the frightening honour of being the doctors most often prosecuted, and to have the most expensive insurance rates. This is aggravated by the special practice of anesthetists and obstetricians: in case of accidents, they cannot themselves correct their errors. If a pediatrician makes a wrong diagnosis and consequently there is erroneous treatment (which is permissible by the law which imposes obligation of means and not of

results, and acknowledges them, the right to error, provided that it occured in spite of accurate, steady and constant care corresponding to acquired scientific data), he is often able to acknowledge and correct it. He alone is responsible for it. If an anesthesiologist or an obstetrician makes an error in the diagnosis of fetal distress, prejudicial to the newborn, the latter will be sent to a neonatal resuscitation department where some physicians might be tempted to become prosecutors. This is all the more regretable, as the risk is always prevalent in anesthesia and obstetrics. Maternal or fetal accidents are not always due to a fault in the management of labor or delivery. Fetal distress during labor is often the first clinical symptom of a previous problem which has then been uncovered by labor acting as an effort test [64]. According to the accidental circumstances, the anesthesist's responsibility should be differently evaluated.

During an emergency for maternal or fetal safety, he does not know his patient. There is no relationship between the anesthesist and his parturient in danger. It is the obstetrician who concluded an agreement with the patient. He must briefly face actual risks implied by various interests. If he is called for acute fetal distress in order to quickly deliver the newborn, he must perform emergency anesthesia on a healthy young mother who runs no risk without anesthesia, and for which there is no time to empty the stomach or for premedication. Anesthesia represents for her a major risk by itself.

In contrast, if the anesthesist is urgently called for a parturient with sudden hemorrhage for example for abruptio placentae, he must administer drugs to the mother which could provoke or aggravate neonatal distress caused by shock and or prematurity secondary to what has happened in the pregnancy. If the fetal distress was the indication for anesthesia which required an operation, in case of a maternal accident, or newborn brain damage, the anesthesist may be prosecuted in a lawsuit initially engaged against the obstetrician, because it is sometimes difficult to claim if maternal anesthesia, by its own effects has created or aggravated the damage or is independant of it. Sometimes the true cause of accident will be demonstrated subsequently by experts during a lawsuit.

This fear should not prevent the anesthetist from being responsible and accept the indication proposed by the obstetrician, while permanently keeping in mind the idea of lawyers or pediatricians. If he has treated his patient to the best of his ability, and conscience while keeping up with present scientific data, and has shown no evidence of awkwardness, imprudence, carelessness, negligence or ignorance of the law and the rules [1], he can justify his action, having done his duty which was in any case to bring help to a mother or infant in jeopardy.

In such cases, the anesthesist's task is difficult, rapidly making decisions which can be so highly significant in the future. Requests for analgesia by parturients are very different. More and more parturients try to be delivered in hospitals where obstetrical analgesia is performed. Thus, it is asserted that in this case, the anesthesiologist is the performer, but he or she is not the director of the Institution. The anesthetist who is so asked should obviously, when accepting the request, send the patient to an obstetrician, but in this case, it is he who concluded the agreement with the parturient. He knows her, and has duties to her. If in an emergency, the anesthetist can benefit from extenuating circumstances, in the case of planned analgesia, he must insist upon safety and good organisation of his work.

In this case, where the request is made by the parturient herself, and not by a doctor for a medical indication, nothing can eliminate the obligation of the doctor to obtain from the parturient *clear consent* to anesthesia.

If the request is made to the obstetrician during pregnancy, he should send the parturient to an anesthetist, who is the one able to take responsibility for possible anesthesia during an out-patient pre-anesthetic consultation. During this consultation, the parturient should express her demand to the anesthetist, who should listen to her and consider as carefully as possible her desires and anxiety. If the patient requires it, he must answer all the questions concerning the incidental and accidental risks of each technique, not only as regards the mother's health, but also the labor and fetal consequences. There is no use explaining all possible complications of anesthesia, but the anesthetist should answer cautiously and honestly if it is not a necessary medically needed anesthesia. He should examine the patient, considering each method and demand a pre-anesthesia biological balance-sheet if necessary. At the end of the examination, he should inform the patient about his conclusions, especially if there is a counterindication to a method or a drug. If the patient's requirements are inconsistent with her security, the anesthesiologist can refuse the demand in the shortest possible time so that she can seek other medical advice.

The reports of consultation should be included in the file. In all cases, analgesia should be chosen in strict agreement with the obstetrician, who will perform the delivery, should be informed about the selected techniques, and can provide the obstetrical elements of the case necessary for the anesthetist. This will ensure a qualified team which will work in harmony. Finally, it is necessary to write an anesthesia report in which concurrently with labor, time, doses, administration of all drugs administered to mother or newborn are carefully noted. It may be an element of reference in case of further complications. But more often, this report is designed to find elements used in rapid and adequate treatment of the consequences of anesthesia on mother or infant, which, if added to previous pathology can raise problems concerning diagnosis and therapy following parturition.

CONCLUSION

It can be said that obstetrical anesthesia and analgesia which are administered cautiously and efficiently, do not entail noxious consequences on the state of the newborn who was a healthy fetus. Conversely, they can improve fetal distress during labor, either by effect of a drug, or by the pertinent selection of anesthesia which permits, without any delay and supplementary trauma, the delivery of a newborn who will be delivered after an optimal labor.

The time has come to judge quietly but carefully the side effects of the therapeutics we have, to use them properly by administering them to the parturient without prejudice to the newborn, an event that may be a positive factor in the binding with her child and her subsequent pregnancies. One may also ask whether the present way of life in large cities and Maternity hospitals does not result in increasing useage of obstetrical anesthesia and analgesia. Perhaps, mutual consideration of physicians, Administration and parturients would bring them each the security and comfort they desire, while preserving for valid indication only drugs and techniques which, in spite of their efficiency, nevertheless have their own limits.

REFERENCES

[1] ABBOUD (Th.), CHEN (T.), READ (J.), MILLER (F.), VALLE (R.), HENRIKSEN (E.). — Effects of placental transfer of glycopyrrolate. *Anesthesiology*, 53, 3S, 316, 1980.
[2] ALSAT (E.), HAUGUEL (S.), CEDARD (L.). — Action des bêta-mimétiques et des catécholamines sur

---

[1] Text of French Law.

le métabolisme du glycogène placentaire. *INSERM*, 89, 245-254, 1979.

[3] AMIEL-TISON (Cl.). — Neurologic evaluation of the small neonate. The importance of head-straightening reactions. *Modern Perinatal Medicine.* Louis Gluck edit., Year Book, 1974.

[4] AMIEL-TISON (Cl.), BARRIER (G.), SHNIDER (S. M.), HUGHES (S. C.), STEFANI (S. J.). — A new neurologic and adaptative capacity scoring system for medications in full-term newborns. *Anesthesiology*, 56, 340-350, 1982.

[5] ANDRÉ (M.), SIBOUT (M.), PETRY (J. M.), VERT (P.). — Dépression respiratoire et neurologique chez le prématuré de mère traitée par le diazépam. *J. Gyn. Obst. Biol. Reprod.*, 2, 357-366, 1973.

[6] APGAR (V. A.). — A proposal for a new method of evaluation of the newborn infant. *Anesth. Analg. Cur. Res.*, 32, 260-267, 1953.

[7] BARRIER (G.), BADIN (N.), BOUCHAMA (S.). — La consultation d'anesthésie périnatale. *Agressologie*, 17, 3, 155-158, 1976.

[8] BARRIER (G.), OLIVE (G.), OHNEN (I.), DAILHE-DUPONT (D.), MERCERON (L.). — La pharmacocinétique de l'atropine chez la femme enceinte et le fœtus en fin de grossesse. *Anesth. Analg. Réan.*, 33, 795-800, 1976.

[9] BARRIER (G.), TALAFRÉ (M. L.), LASSNER (J.). — Neonatal pharmakokinetics of pethidine administered to mothers during labour. *European Academy of Anaesthesiology.* 1st Scientific Meeting, London, 1979.

[10] BARRIER (G.), DURUPTY (D.), MERCERON (L.), VALTER (P.), VIGÉ (P.). — Étude du passage transplacentaire d'une substance atropinique : le glycopyrrolate. *X^es Journées de la Soc. Fr. de Méd. Périnat.*, Abstract. Arnette édit., Paris, 1980.

[11] BARRIER (G.), DURUPTY (D.), LASSNER (J.). — L'analgésie électrique en obstétrique. *Analg. Anesth. Réan.*, 1980.

[12] BEHAR (M.), OLSHWANG (D.), MAGORA (F.), DAVIDSON (J. T.). — Epidural morphine in treatment of pain. *Lancet*, I, 527, 1979.

[13] BERG (E.). — Effets sur le nouveau-né de la péthidine administrée à la mère. Évaluation neurologique, action de la naloxone. *Thèse DAR Cochin-Port-Royal*, Paris, 1979.

[14] BIEHL (D.), SHNIDER (S. M.), LEVINSON (G.) et coll. — Placental transfer of lidocaine: effects of fetal acidosis. *Anesthesiology*, 48, 409, 1978.

[15] BOTTOMS (S. F.), ROSEN (M. G.), SOKOL (R. J.). — The increase in the cesarean birth rate. *New Engl. J. Med.*, 302, 10, 559-563, 1980.

[16] BOULLEY (A. M.), DEHAN (M.), VIAL (M.), HERNANDORENA (X.), ROPERT (J. C.), LAUDIGNON (N.), LHERMITTE (C.), GABILAN (J. C.). — Grossesse gémellaire, indométacine et cyanose néonatale. *Arch. Fr. Péd.*, 37, 317-319, 1980.

[17] BRACKBILL (Y.), KANE (J.), MANIELLO (R. L.), ABRAMSON (D.). — Obstetric meperidine usage and assessment of neonatal status. *Anesthesiology*, 40, 116-120, 1974.

[18] BRAZELTON (T. B.). — Psychophysiologic reactions in the neonate. Effect of maternal medication on the neonate and his behaviour. *J. Pediatr.*, 58, 513, 1961.

[19] BRAZELTON (T. B.). — *Neonatal behavioral assessment scale.* J. B. Lippincott, Philadelphia, 1973.

[20] BROWN (W. U.), BELL (G. C.), ALPERT (M. H.). — Acidosis, local anesthetics and the newborn. *Obst. Gynec.*, 48, 27-30, 1976.

[21] BROWN (W. U.), BELL (G. C.), LURIE (A. O.), WEISS (J. B.), SCANLON (J. W.), ALPER (M. H.). — Newborn blood levels of lidocaine and mepivacaine in the first post-natal day following maternal epidural anaesthesia. *Anesthesiology*, 42, 698-707, 1975.

[22] BULEY (R. J. R.), DOWNING (J. W.), BROCK-UTNE (J. G.), CUERDEN (C.). — Right versus left fateral tilt for cesarean section. *Br. J. Anaesth.*, 49, 1009, 1977.

[23] BUNODIÈRE (M.), DELIGNE (P.). — Le chlorhydrate de kétamine (kétalar) en anesthésie obstétricale (césariennes et forceps). *Ann. Anesth. Fr.*, 12, 2, 227-241, 1971.

[24] CALDWELL (J.), WAKILE (L. A.), NOTARIANNI (J. J.), SMITH (R. L.), CORREY (G.) et coll. — Maternal and neonatal disposition of pethidine in child birth. *Life Sci.*, 22, 589-596, 1978.

[25] CHADENSON (O.), BENOIT (M. P.). — Effets de l'anesthésie générale par l'alfatésine sur le nouveau-né en pratique obstétricale. *Ann. Anesth. Fr.*, 17, 1, 9-17, 1976.

[26] CHARTIER (M.), BARRIER (G.), HIDDEN (J.). — Première utilisation du 4-hydroxybutyrate de Na en obstétrique. *Bull. Gyn. Obst.*, 14, 5, 649, 1962.

[27] *Compte rendu des VIIIes Journées de la Soc. Fr. de Mé. Périnat.*, La Baule. Arnette édit., 1978.

[28] CONWAY (E.), BRACKBILL (Y.). — Delivery medication and infant outcome. An empirical study. *Monograph. Soc. Res. Child Der.*, 35, 24, 1970.

[29] DATTA (S.), ALPER (M. H.). — Anesthesia for cesarean section. *Anesthesiology*, 53, 142-160, 1980.

[30] *Décret n° 79-506 du 28 juin 1979 portant le Code de Déontologie médicale.*

[31] DEWAN (D. M.), WHEELER (A. S.), JAMES (F. M.) III, FLOYD (H. M.). — Antacid anticholinergic premedication in the parturient. *Anesthesiology*, 53, 3S, 308, 1980.

[32] DICK (W.), BORST (R.), FODOR (H.) et coll. — Ketamine in obstetrical anesthesia: clinical and experimental results. *J. Perinat. Med.*, 1, 252-262, 1973.

[33] DOWNING (D. W.), COLEMAN (A. J.), MEER (F. M.). — An intravenous method of anesthesia for cesarean section. Part III. Althesin. *Brit. J. Anaesth.*, 45, 381-387, 1973.

[34] EVRARD (J. R.), GOLD (E. M.). — Cesarean section: risk/benefit. *Perinatal Care*, 2, 4-10, 1978.

[35] FINSTER (M.), MARK (L. C.), MORISHIMA (H. O.) et coll. — Plasma thiopental concentrations in the newborn following delivery under thiopental nitrous oxide anesthesia. *Am. J. Obst. Gynecol.*, 95, 621, 1966.

[36] GALLOON (S.). — Ketamine for obstetric delivery. *Anesthesiology*, 44, 522-524, 1976.

[37] GAREL (M.), CROST (M.). — Quelques aspects psychologiques de l'analgésie péridurale. *X^es Journées de la Soc. Fr. de Méd. Périnat.* Deauville. Arnette édit., Paris, 1980.

[38] GIBBS (C. P.), KUCK (E. J.), HOOD (I. C.), RUIZ (B. C.). — Antacid plus foodstuff aspiration. *SOAP Annual meeting*, Boston, Abstract, 1980.

[39] GRANDJEAN (H.), BERTRAND (J. C.), GRANDJEAN (B.), REME (J. M.), DEGOY (J.), PONTONNIER (G.). — La neuroleptanalgésie dans la direction majeure du travail. *J. Gyn. Obst. Biol. Reprod.*, 6, 563-577, 1977.

[40] GRANDJEAN (H.), DE MOUZON (J.), CABOT (J. A.), DESPRATS (R.), PONTONNIER (G.). — Comparaison des effets fœtaux de deux méthodes d'analgésie utilisées au cours de l'accouchement normal. *INSERM*, 89, 271-278, 1979.

[41] GRENOM (A.), ECHINARD (K.), MERCIER (C.), LEROY (G.), SOUTOUL (J. H.). — Anesthésie à l'alfatésine utilisée comme agent unique de narcose. *Cah. Anesth.*, 23, 5, 513-520, 1975.

[42] GUERRE-MILLO (M.), CHALLIER (J.), REY (E.), RICHARD (M. O.), OLIVE (G.). — Protein binding and placental transfer of benzodiazepines. *INSERM*, 89, 447-454, 1979.

[43] HOSSMANN (A.). — Prevention and treatment of ischemia of the brain. *Communication au VIIe Congrès Mondial d'Anesthésiologie*, Hambourg, Abstract, 1980.

[44] JASSON (J.). — Étude comparative des conséquences maternelles et néonatales de deux méthodes utilisées en analgésie obstétricale. *Compte rendu des X^es Journées de la Soc. Fr. de Méd. Périnat.*, Deauville. Arnette édit., Paris, 1980.

[45] JOUHET (Ph.). — Effets secondaires des bêta-mimétiques prescrits en obstétrique. *Conférence aux X^es Journées de la Soc. Fr. de Méd. Périnat.*, Deauville. Arnette édit., Paris, 1980.

[46] LANGREHR (D.), STOLP (W.). — Ketamine anesthesia for obstetrical-gynecological interventions. *Z. Prakt. Anaesth. Wiederbel*, 5, 3, 145-156, 1970.

[47] LASSNER (J.), BARRIER (G.), TALAFRÉ (M. L.), DURUPTY (D.). — Utilisation of extradural morphine to provide pain relief in labour. European Academy of Anaesthesiology. *2nd Scientific Meeting, Nijmegen*, 1980.

[48] LASSNER (J.), BARRIER (G.), LOOSE (J. P.), BERG (A.). — L'analgésie obstétricale médicamenteuse : étude de la dépression respiratoire néonatale liée à la péthidine. *Cah. Anesth.*, 26, 5, 595-608, 1978.

[49] LEVIN (D. L.), MILLS (L. J.), PARKEY (M.), GARRIOT (J.), CAMPBELL (W.). — Constriction of the fetal ductus arteriosus after administration of indomethacin to the pregnant ewe. *J. Pediat.*, 94, 647, 1979.

[50] LEVINSON (G.), SHNIDER (S. M.). — Placental transfer of local anesthetics: clinical implications. In *Parturition and Perinatology*. G. F. MARX ed. F. A. Davis, Philadelphia, p. 173, 1973.

[51] MANCHESTER (D.), MARGOLIS (H. S.), SHELDON (R. E.). — Possible association between maternal Indomethacin therapy and primary pulmonary hypertension of the newborn. *Amer. J. Obst. Gynecol.*, 126, 467, 1976.

[52] MARCHAL (F.), BIANCHETTI (G.), MONIN (P.), DUBRUCQ (C.), MORSELLI (P.), BOUTROY (M. J.), VERT (P.). — Pharmacocinétique et effets pharmacodynamiques de l'indométacine chez le nouveau-né. *INSERM*, 89, 499-508, 1979.

[53] MATHER (L. E.), MEFFIN (P. J.). — Clinical pharmacokinetics of pethidine. *Clin. Pharmacok.*, 3, 352-365, 1978.

[54] MERKOW (A. J.), MCGUINNESS (G. A.), ERENBER (A.), KENNEDY (R. A.). — The neonatal neurobehavioural effects of bupivacaine, mepivacaine and 2-chloroprocaine used for pudental block. *Anesthesiology*, 52, 309-312, 1980.

[55] MORGAN (D.), MOORE (G.), THOMAS (J.), TRIGGS (E.). — The disposition of meperidine in pregnancy. *Clin. Pharm. Ther.*, 23, 288-295, 1978.

[56] MORISHIMA (H. O.), FINSTER (M.), PEDERSEN (H.) et coll. — Placental transfer and tissue distribution of etidocaine and lidocaine in guinea pigs. Abstracts of Scientific papers. *Annual meeting ASA*, Chicago, 1975.

[57] MORISHIMA (H. O.), HEYMANN (M. A.), RUDOLPH (A. M.), BARRETT (C. T.), JAMES (L. S.). — Transfer of lidocaine across the sheep placenta to the fetus. *Am. J. Obst. Gynec.*, 122, 581-588, 1975.

[58] MORISHIMA (H. O.), GUTSCHE (B. G.), STARK (R. I.), MILLIEZ (J.), JAMES (L. S.), KEENAGHAN (J. B.), COVINO (G. G.). — The mecanism of fetal bradycardia following regional anaesthesia in obstetrics. *Am. J. Obst. Gynecol.*, 134, 3, 289-296, 1979.

[59] MORISHIMA (H. O.), PEDERSEN (H.), FINSTER (M.). — The influence of maternal psychological stress on the fetus. *Am. J. Obst. Gynecol.*, 131, 286, 1978.

[60] MORISHIMA (H. O.), MULLER-HEUBACH (E.). — Body temperature and disappearance of lidocaine in newborn puppies. *Anesth. Analg.*, 50, 941, 1971.

[61] MORRISSON (J. C.), WISER (W. L.), ROSSER (J. J.), GAYDEN (J. O.), BUCOVAZ (E. J.), WHYBREW (W. D.), FISH (S. A.). — Metabolites of meperidine related to fetal depression. *Am. J. Obst. Gynecol.*, 115, 1132-1137, 1973.

[62] MORSELLI (P. L.). — Clinical pharmacokinetics in the neonate. *Clin. Pharmacok.*, 1, 87-98, 1976.

[63] MORSELLI (P. L.). — Problems of drugs administration in the neonatal period. *Clin. Pharmacol.*, 6, 57-66, 1978.

[64] MYERS (R. E.), WILLIAMS (M. V.). — Lost opportunities for the prevention of fetal asphyxia: sedation, analgesia, and general anaesthesia. *Clin. Obstetr. Gynaecol.*, 9, 2, 369-414, 1982.

[65] MYERS (R. E.). — Maternal psychological stress and fetal asphyxia: a study in the monkey. *Am. J. Obst. Gynecol.*, 122, 47, 1975.

[66] ONNEN (I.), BARRIER (G.), D'ATHIS (P.), SUREAU (C.), OLIVE (G.). — Placental transfer of atropine at the end of pregnancy. *Europ. J. Clin. Pharmacol.*, 15, 443-446, 1979.

[67] OSTHEIMER (G. W.), DATTA (S.), SCANLON (J. W.), CORKE (B. C.), BROWN (W. U.), CROCKER (J. S.), WEISS (D. B.), ALPER (M. H.). — Epidural anesthesia in obstetrics: clinical implications for mother and newborn. *SOAP Meeting, Boston*, Abstract, 1980.

[68] PAKTER (J.), SCHIFFER (M. A.), NELSON (F.). — Maternal and perinatal mortality. In *Clinical management of mother and newborn*, G. F. MARX edit. Springer-Verlag, New York, 1979.

[69] PONTONNIER (G.), TOURNIER (C.), LAGORCE (J. C.), DELMAS (H.), JOSSERAND (P.), DJIAN (P.), BABANI (E.), FAVRETTO (D.). — Pression amniotique, fréquence cardiaque et pH fœtaux au cours de l'accouchement sous perfusion intraveineuse de syntocinon associée à l'anesthésie générale au Penthotal. *Rev. Franç. Gynecol.*, 65, 10, 537-560, 1970.

[70] PROAKIS (A. G.), HARRIS (G. B.). — Comparative penetration of glycopyrrolate and atropine across the blood, the brain barrier and placental barrier in anesthized dogs. *Anesthesiology*, 48, 339-344, 1978.

[71] RALSTON (D. H.), SHNIDER (S. M.). — The fetal and neonatal effects of regional anesthesia in obstetrics. *Anesthesiology*, 48, 34-64, 1978.

[72] Report on confidential enquiries into maternal deaths in England and Wales. Her Majesty's Stationery Office. London, 1978.

[73] Report by MRC Committees Sir Dugald Biard. Clinical trials of different concentrations of oxygen and nitrous oxide for obstetric analgesia. *Br. Med. J., 1,* 709, 1970.

[74] SAFAR (P.). — Brain resuscitation after cardiac arrest and head injury. *Communication VIIe Congrès Mondial d'Anesthésiologie, Hambourg,* Abstract, 1980.

[75] SCANLON (J. W.), BROWN (W. U.) Jr., WEISS (J. B.), ALPER (M. H.). — Neurobehavioral response of newborn infants after maternal epidural anesthesia. *Anesthesiology, 40,* 121-128, 1974.

[76] SCANLON (J. W.), OSTHEIMER (G. W.), LURIE (A. O.) et coll. — Neurobehavioral responses and drug concentrations in newborns after maternal epidural anesthesia with bupivacaine. *Anesthesiology, 45,* 400, 1976.

[77] SCOTT (J. R.), ROSE (N. B.). — Effect of psychoprophylaxis (Lamaze preparation) on labour and delivery in primiparas. *N. Engl. J. Med., 294,* 22, 1205-1235, 1976.

[78] SHNIDER (S. M.), WRIGHT (R. C.), LEVINSON (G.) et coll. — Uterine blood flow and plasma norepinephrine changes during maternal stress in the pregnant ewe. *Anesthesiology, 50,* 524, 1979.

[79] BARRIER (G.), SUREAU (Cl.). — Effects of anaesthetic and analgesic drugs on labour, fetus and neonate. *Clin. Obstet. Gynaecol., 9,* 2, 351-367, 1982.

[80] SHNIDER (S. M.), ABBOUD (T.), ARTAL (R.), HENRIKSEN (E.), STEFANI (S. J.), LEVINSON (G.). — Maternal endogenous catecholamines decrease during labour after lumbar epidural anesthesia. *Annual meeting of SOAP, Boston,* Abstract, 1980.

[81] STEFANI (S. J.), HUGHES (S. C.), SHNIDER (S. M.). — Neonatal neurobehavioral effects of inhalation analgesia for delivery. *Anesthesiology* (à paraître).

[82] TALAFRE (M. L.), ROVEI (V.), BARRIER (G.), LASSNER (J.), SAN JUAN (M.), MORSELLI (P. L.), SUREAU (C.). — Pharmacocinétique de la péthidine chez le nouveau-né et la mère pendant le travail. *INSERM, 89,* 287-296, 1979.

[83] TAYLOR (G.), PRYCE-DAVIES (J.). — The prophylactic use of antacids in the prevention of the acid-pulmonary aspiration syndrome (Mendelson's syndrome). *Lancet, 1,* 288, 1966.

[84] THOULON (J. M.), SELIGMANN (G.). — Médications antispasmodiques et utéro-relaxantes. Leur influence sur le rythme cardiaque fœtal. *INSERM, 89,* 365-370, 1979.

[85] THOULON (J. M.), SELIGMANN (G.). — Influence des médicaments sur le rythme cardiaque fœtal. *Rev. Franç. Gynécol., 73,* 4, 309-313, 1978.

[86] TUCKER (T. T.), BOYES (R. N.), BRIDENBAUGH (P. O.), MOORE (D. C.). — Binding of anilide-type local anaesthetics in human placenta. II. Implications *in vivo* with special reference to transplacental distribution. *Anesthesiology, 33,* 304-314, 1970.

[87] VAN DEN BERG (B. J.), LEVINSON (G.), SHNIDER (S. M.), HUGHES (S. C.), STEFANI (S. J.). — Evaluation of long-term effects of obstetric medication and child development. *SOAP meeting, Boston,* Abstract, 1980.

[88] WRITER (W. D. R.), JAMES (F. M.), WHEELER (A. F.). — A double blind comparison of morphine/dextrose with bupivacaine in continuous lumbar epidural analgesia in labour. *12th Annual meeting SOAP, Boston,* Abstract, 1980.

9

Birth injury

M ANDRE and P. VERT

THE EVALUATION
OF CONDITION AT BIRTH

THE APGAR SCORE

Definition. — To the vague notions of "apparent death", infant coma, asphyxia or apnea at birth, delay of the first cry: Virginia Apgar, an anesthesiologist, in 1953 proposed [3] the substitution of a scoring system which was both simple and clear and could be used both for the interpretation of the results of obstetrical practice, of anesthesia and analgesia as well as of resuscitation techniques.

Universally used, the Apgar score assesses, 60 seconds after birth, five criteria which are easily appreciable without interfering with any care the child might need (Table I).

Of these five criteria, each one being rated 0, 1 or 2, Apgar considered the cardiac rhythm to be the most useful; absent beats, rate under 100 or over 100. The appreciation of the respiratory condition must only take account of the respiration truly recorded after 60 seconds and not of any possible previous breaths. The response to stimulation—irritability reflex—as well as the muscle tonicity are simple to

TABLE I. — The Apgar score

Criteria	0	1	2
Heart rate.	Absent.	Below 100.	Over 100.
Breathing.	Absent.	Slow, irregular.	Good.
Muscle tone.	Massive hypotonia.	Slight flexion of the extremities.	Bent position Active movements.
Reaction to stimulation.	Nil.	Weak cry.	Strong cry.
Colour.	Blue or pale.	Bluish extremities.	Completely pink.

score provided that two is given only to perfect states, nil to major abnormalities and one to all the intermediate states. All three assess the neurological condition. From her first publication, she noted that color was the least satisfactory sign; cyanosis, often assessed subjectively, can fail to reveal a pathological condition.

Significance. — The natural history of perinatal asphyxia is well known in rhesus monkeys [25]. One can suppose that it is the same in man, being divided into four periods: the first of primary hyperpnea, from 1 to 2 minutes, the second of primary apnea of about one minute, during which the organism remains capable of reacting to stimulation, the third of secondary hyperpnea, which comprises a succession of gasps for 5 or 6 minutes, then the fourth period of secondary apnea when all respiratory movement ceases, and respiratory stimulation is of no use.

Death takes place 13 to 14 minutes after the beginning of asphyxia. During these different stages, the arterial pressure and the cardiac rhythm decline progressively; the oxygen content becomes zero in 3 minutes, the PCO_2 rises by 10 mm Hg/minute until it exceeds 100 mm Hg, pH falls by 0.1 unit per minute. The level of blood lactic acid increases to more than 10 mEq/l (900 mg/l).

Clinical differentiation between these stages is difficult in the newborn child, all the more since the infant is more often liable to partial than to total asphyxia.

Drage (1966) considers that an Apgar score less than or equal to 3 corresponds to stage 4, a score between 3 and 6 to stage 3 whilst a score of seven and over corresponds to stages 1 or 2. Survival prognosis is in close correlation to the one minute score: 14 % mortality for a score of 1 or 2, 1.1 % for 3 to 7, 0.13 % for 8, 9 and 10.

The determination of the score at 5 or even 10 minutes adds a useful measure of evolution. For Naeye [62], moreover, the score after 5 minutes is the one which has the best correlation with the mortality rate: death rates 3-4 times greater than in children with a normal score (> 7) if the Apgar score is less than 4 at one minute, and 10 times if it is less than 4 at five minutes.

The later observations of Apgar [4] and of Drage [28] made the predictive value of this score on neonatal morbidity more accurate: more Hyaline Membrane Disease in premature infants if the score is low. They showed its importance in neurological prognosis. 7.4 % of neurological anomalies at one year for a score $\leqslant 3$, 1.7 % for a score > 7.

Some criticisms of the Apgar score have been expressed. Its variability according to the observers sometimes seems to be linked to the fact that the criteria for scoring are not adhered to, and especially to the lack of precision concerning the time elapsed since the birth. In situations of serious distress, its assessment is often retrospective. A simplified scoring system, such as the ABC system (Activity, Breathing, Circulation) of Morrow [61] could be useful. Apgar predictive value for morbidity and especially for prognosis is not always valid, especially in the long term (1969). Above all, contrary to these statistical data, the Apgar score has only a limited value as regards individual prognosis. A very low score can be linked to a very short period of distress; complete and speedy recovery is usual if the resuscitation is well carried out. On the other hand, a nearly normal score does not exclude a cerebral complication, especially after severe chronic fetal distress, or during severe circulatory difficulties caused by prolonged compression of the head in posterior deliveries.

OTHER SIGNS
OF PERINATAL ASPHYXIA

The antenatal and perinatal signs of asphyxia: clinical, cardiotocographic, biochemical are dealt with in other chapters of this work. At birth, apart from the criteria of the Apgar score, the clinical signs are elements of the post-asphyxial syndrome: amniotic fluid inhalation, neurological complications, visceral impairment... Several biochemical disturbances reflect previous perinatal distress.

The modification of the acid-base status. — Fetal asphyxia always brings about metabolic acidosis, notably by the accumulation of lactic acid found in the newborn infant. The pH is often much less than 7.20 (normal $\geqslant 7.25$). Low [54] defined post-asphyxial acidosis by the fall of base in umbilical arterial blood; from 41.2 ± 2.5 mEq/l in healthy cases, it falls to less than 34 mEq/l in full-term infants who have suffered from asphyxia.

Statistically, this acidosis is significantly related to a low Apgar score at one and five minutes, as well as to the need for intermittent positive pressure ventilation. Modanlou [60] found in 150 high risk deliveries that the acidosis during labour and birth was all the more noticeable when there was a low Apgar score ($\leqslant 6$). For Huisjes [43], the low umbilical venous pH (< 7.19) is associated with a poor Apgar score; the correlations are not as good with umbilical arterial pH.

On the other hand, in children who had intra-uterine growth retardation, Lin [50] found no correlation between acidosis and Apgar score. Similarly, Tooley [83] found no link between Apgar score at one and five minutes and the concentration of H+ ions in arterial blood in premature babies weighing less than 1,750 g.

Lactic and pyruvic acids. — In 1966, Daniel [24] showed that the increase in lactates and pyruvates in the newborn was a sign of ante-natal asphyxia, due to the increase of anaerobic glycolysis, secondary to tissue hypoxemia.

Matthieu (1971) in 106 newborns, confirmed, the importance of the amount of lactacidemia in the evaluation of the severity of asphyxia. There is no difference in lactacidemia between premature babies and full-term healthy babies, nor between the arterial and venous levels. The lactates are 2.6 ± 0.4 mEq/l (234 ± 36 mg/l), the pyruvates 0.09 ± 0.01 mEq/l (7.9 ± 0.88 mg/l). The amount of pyruvates does not seem to supply any useful additional information in practice.

The critical level for lactates is 3.9 mEq/l (350 mg/l). The lactacidemia may have some prog-nostic significance: normalisation of the level is desirable within the first 24 hours of life; the combi-nations of lactacidemia greater than 8.5 mEq/l (766 mg/l) within 3 hours and a cumulative Apgar score (at 1, 5 and 10 minutes) of less than 10 and/or lactacidemia greater than 12 mEq/l (1,080 mg/l) within 96 hours are always followed by the child's death.

Svenningsen and Siesjö (1972) showed an increase of lactate and of the lactate/pyruvate ratio in the CSF in the period immediately following as-phyxia. Mathew et al. (1980) verified the normal values for CSF lactate in healthy cases: 21.51 and 23.45 mg/100 ml (at full term with or without O_2 for respiratory distress without hypoxia), 16.53 and 17.97 mg/100 ml in premature babies. They point to a significant increase in the lactate level in the 8 hours following fetal asphyxia (defined by a low Apgar score). The levels are all the more increased (>60 mg/ 100 ml) when the other criteria of asphyxia are severe. The level returns to normal in less than 8 hours in the absence of persistant hypoxemia. These authors consider that this early increase constitutes a reflection of cerebral hypoxemia and may have some prognostic significance. However, their work does not include any follow-up of the children.

Enzymes. — The anoxemia and tissue damage at birth may be responsible for the rise in the level of serum enzymes.

Lending [49] found an increase in lactate dehydro-genase activity (LDH) in newborns who had suffered from asphyxia. The average plasma activity is 11 % higher than normal, it is 309 % in the CSF. This work does not include the quantification of the various enzymatic fractions.

The same author has made similar observations for glutamo-oxaloacetic transaminases. The increase seems related to the neurological prognosis.

Hall [38] tried to define the degree and the mecha-nism of the increase in LDH in CSF following perinatal asphyxia, during the first week of life. The increase in the level in CSF is significant, without any connection with the increase in the blood level. Death occured 9 times out of 10 during the post-asphyxial syndrome when the LDH was greater than 100 mU/ml. This same level separates normal survivors and those who survive with neurological sequelae. The study of isoenzymes has not allowed the pinpointing of the origin of LDH, the hypothesis of an increase in the permeability of the hemocerebral barrier is feasible. The increase in fraction 3 (neu-rons) is not sufficient to indicate an abnormal neural break-down.

The increase of serum creatine phosphokinase (CPK) is often due to the release of enzymes by the muscles. Thus Rudolph finds an activity 2 to 5 times higher after vaginal delivery than after cesarean section. On the other hand, it is specifically the isoenzyme BB, almost exclusively of cerebral origin, which is markedly higher after major peri-natal distress (more than 4 %, normal < 0.5 %) (Cao; Becker). Its increase allows a retrospective diagnosis of hypoxia (Lavaud); when it is short, a return to normal comes about between 24 and 48 hours.

Meberg [59] considers that a high level of the CPK isoenzyme BB in the CSF is a better indicator of post-asphyxial cerebral damage. He finds values of 5 to 25 U. I./l in children born with an Apgar score below 2 (normal < 5 U. I./l).

Lipids. — Sabata [72] showed, in newly born children with hypoxemia, an increase in free fatty acids and even more of glycerol in the umbilical arterial blood. Gärdmark [34] also found an increase in glycerol in fetal blood during episodes of severe or prolonged bradycardia.

For Tsang [86] as for Andersen and Friis-Hansen [2], the cord blood hypertriglyceridemia (> 70 mg/100 ml) correlates with fetal distress (fetal bradycardia, meconium stained amniotic fluid, low Apgar score). This increase is not of maternal origin.

It is likely that the catecholamines which increase

during asphyxia (Holden [42]) favour the lipolysis of the triglycerides of the fatty tissue. This causes the increase in free fatty acids and glycerol. The free fatty acids which are not oxidised and resynthesized locally are metabolized by the placenta, or processed by the fetal liver for endogenous synthesis of the triglycerides; the latter appear in the fetal serum. When maternal degradation ceases at birth, the serum level increases even more. Triglyceride determination can have some significance, together with the Apgar score in the evaluation of perinatal asphyxia.

Other biochemical disturbances. — Engel (1970) showed a hypermagnesemia, associated with hyperkalemia, which he attributes to a passage of intracellular ions to the plasma.

The plasma arterial hypoxanthine is significantly increased after fetal asphyxia: the maximum is noted 10-20 minutes after birth (33.7 μmole/l, 11.9 μmole/l in controls). A significant correlation is noted with the level of lactate and the base deficit. The increase in hypoxanthine is briefer [14, 79].

RESUSCITATION
IN THE DELIVERY ROOM

Most newborns whose Apgar score does not exceed 7 at 60 seconds or at 5 minutes show poor adaptation. They should be given help to limit the short and long term effects of the asphyxia.

TECHNIQUES

Preparations. — Some difficulties at birth follow high risk obstetric situations and are forseeable. But unforseen complications can always occur. The resuscitation equipment must always be ready near the labour room, and should be checked before each delivery by the person in charge (Table II).

An individual experienced in resuscitation of newborn infants should be available. For serious situations, a well prepared team must be able to be assembled at any time. All treatment should be carried out under the strictest aseptic conditions; a newborn child with hypoxemia is particularly vulnerable to infections. To combat hypothermia the child must be dried quickly with a warm cloth and kept under a radiant heater of at least 400 watts throughout the resuscitation.

TABLE II. — EQUIPMENT FOR RESUSCITATION
OF A BABY AT BIRTH

— Sterile, radiantly heated resuscitation platform.
— Sterile polyethylene catheters, for aspiration, sizes 6, 8 and 10.
— Source of vacuum (−20, −30 cm H_2O).
— Source of oxygen and air, with if possible, oxygen-air proportioner and heated nebulizer.
— Bag for manual ventilation (type Penlon) which cannot exceed 30 cm H_2O pressure and masks.
— Sterile endotracheal tubes, sizes 2.5 to 4 mm with appropriate connections.
— Laryngoscope, with blades for full term newborns and premature children.
— Stethoscope.
— Stopwatch.
— Material for injection of solutions: sterile gloves, sheets, syringes, catheters.

Suction. — This allows the airways to be cleared of liquids or foreign material which may be obstructing them. Firstly one carries out suction of the pharynx, gently and carefully done in order to avoid any irritation of the posterior wall of the pharynx, a cause of laryngospasm and of bradycardia, or even of cardiac arrest (Cordero, 1971), so as to check any possible leakage of the liquid at the larynx; then an aspiration of the nostrils.

Aspiration of the stomach avoids secondary inhalation of intragastric liquid during vomiting.

An endotracheal aspiration after intubation is needed whenever there is any suspicion of inhalation of amniotic fluid and prior to any ventilation using an endotracheal tube.

Ventilation. — This is used to insufflate and ventilate the lungs and to stimulate spontaneous breathing. It is carried out, at a rate of 15-30/minute, using a manual bag attached to a face mask or to a tracheal tube, with a flow of gas of 3 to 8 l/min. If ventilation with air does not cause the child to turn pink, one uses a mixture with an increasing concentration of oxygen. Great care must be taken in using oxygen with premature babies because of the risk of retinopathy. The positive pressure applied must not exceed 30 cm H_2O (2.94 KPa). This pressure is often sufficient to induce gasps followed soon afterwards by normal respiratory movements. The initial response to intratracheal insufflation is normally an expiratory effort and more rarely a paradoxal Head inspiration reflex (Boon, 1979). Whilst in newborn babies breathing spontaneously, delivered normally, there is no raised "opening pressure", Boon [13] showed, in asphyxiated babies

delivered by caesarian section, the existence of an opening pressure of 13 to 32 cm H_2O. In the course of the first insufflations with intermittent positive pressure (IPP) he noted a progressive increase in tidal volume. The functional residual capacity was established during the first 30 seconds, whether spontaneous respiratory movements appeared or not. An interruption of ventilation for approximately 15 seconds every 3 minutes allows the evaluation of the quality of the spontaneous respiratory movements. Too efficient ventilation risks bringing about alkalosis and convulsions. It encourages the occurence of interstitial emphysema and pneumothorax. Ventilation using a mask may also be inadequate and hinder the movements of the child.

External cardiac massage. — Whenever the circulation is insufficient, cardiac massage may become essential to deliver the necessary oxygen to the tissues. It is carried out at a rate of 100-120/min. It is only used with efficient ventilation. During the insufflation of the lungs, cardiac massage must be stopped: this coordination is imperative to avoid the occurrence of pneumothorax or pneumomediastinum.

The treatment of acidosis. — The consequences of acidosis in the newborn are well known: increase in pulmonary resistance, decrease in myocardial efficiency, destruction of surfactant, change in glucose metabolism, impairment of oxygen transport by hemoglobin. The re-establishment of efficient ventilation corrects the ventilatory aspect of its production.

Dawes and Co-workers (1963) showed, in the lamb and the rhesus monkey, that the infusion of a hypertonic solution of bicarbonate improved cardio-respiratory tolerance during perinatal asphyxia and decreased the recuperation time during resuscitation [26].

In 1963, Usher [27] and in 1972, Hobel [41] noted less severe respiratory distress and an improved survival rate in premature babies whose acidosis had previously been corrected by injection of sodium bicarbonate at the rate of 0.4 × base deficit mmol/kg or even 5 mmol/kg.

It is imperative that only babies with good ventilation are given sodium bicarbonate. Ostrea [65] showed *in vitro* that the injection of bicarbonate in a closed system brought about an increase in PCO_2 and could even, in the case of rapid injection of a hypertonic solution, result in a drop in pH, because of the giving off of intracellular protons as a response to the hypertonicity of the extracellular fluid.

Steichen and Kleinman [76] confirmed, with hypoventilated dogs, that the injection of 2 mmol/kg of bicarbonate brought about a decrease of PaO_2 and an increase of PCO_2. The blood pH decreases considerably, more in dogs who received the bicarbonate than those who only received glucose serum. In newborn babies the changes in the blood gases are linked to the rapidity of the injection (> 1 mmol/min) [7]. Even when the ventilation is efficient, the injection of hypertonic bicarbonate solution can be dangerous. A slow correction (0.3 mmol/kg/min) following the classic formula [1/3 base deficit mmol/kg] of metabolic acidosis modifies the natremia and the osmolarity without any major changes in the PaO_2 (Rhodes [70]).

These changes in osmolarity and $PaCO_2$, factors of variation of the cerebral vascular bed, together with loss of autoregulation of the cerebral flow in the distressed newborn (Lou [53]), considerably increase the risk of cerebral haemorrhage and particularly of intraventricular haemorrhage in the very premature baby (Papile). The administration of bicarbonate at birth must therefore be used very sparingly (Eidelman). It is only when resuscitation proves inadequate and the ventilation is good (pH < 7.25 despite a PCO_2 ⩽ 30 mm Hg, Tooley), that the injection of sodium bicarbonate is necessary. One injects 1 to 2 mmol/kg at the rate of 0.5 mmol/min, of semimolar bicarbonate solution, or better, half diluted with 5 % glucose serum. This can be injected into the umbilical vein after catheterization under conditions of the utmost cleanliness and security, or into a peripheral vein. Ideally, this alkalinisation should not be carried out without having previously determined the pH and the PCO_2, the quantity administered corresponding to the correction of half of the base deficit.

Drugs. — The use of respiratory analeptics is not indicated. The injection of cardio-circulatory analeptics into the umbilical vessels has been responsible for sciatic palsy. In newborns with cardio-circulatory collapse Lindemann [50 *bis*] proposes to give Epinephrine intratracheally: 0.25 ml (0.1 mg/ml solution) under 1,500 g body weight, 0.50 ml between 1,500 g and 2,500 g, and 1 ml above 2,500 g.

If the mother has received pethidine shortly before birth, or morphine or other opiates, the child may be given an antagonist. The one used at present is naloxone *(Narcan)* at the rate of 0.01 mg/kg by intravenous or intramuscular injection. The drug also appears able, in the newborn rabbit, to reduce the period of post asphyxial primary apnea, most likely by the inhibition of endorphins and enkephalins [19].

POSSIBLE SITUATIONS

The Apgar score is at least equal to 7.
— Only a clearing of the pharynx and the nose, and gastric aspiration are necessary.

Apgar score less than 6.
— The majority of asphyxiated newly born babies are in the period of primary apnea, so that cleaning of the nasopharynx and brief ventilation with a mask are usually sufficient to induce efficient respiration and a return to normal cardiac rhythm. Otherwise, tracheal intubation is indicated. Endotracheal aspiration must be performed before any insufflation. Gregory [36] showed that meconium was present in the tracheas of 56 % of newly born infants with meconium staining of the amniotic fluid.

Ventilation with an inflatable bag must be continued until the child has spontaneous and efficient respiratory movements. When cardiac massage is required, it is performed by a second person. If the condition remains poor (Apgar < 3), sodium bicarbonate may be used.

Exceptional cases.
— Two surgical emergencies are of clinical importance: atresia of the esophagus and diaphragmatic hernia; ventilation must be carried out using a tracheal tube in conjunction with continuous gastric aspiration.

Pneumothorax, which may require urgent thoracocentesis is rare. The diagnosis must be confirmed by X-rays beforehand.

Hypovolemic shock, after fetal haemorrhage, should be corrected immediately by infusion of 20 % albumin or plasma, while waiting for the blood for transfusion. On the other hand vascular overfilling in the absence of certain loss carries a risk of pulmonary edema.

Infants of less than 1,000 g: For some years now, the proportions of long term survival of children without cerebral sequelae have been improving. The use of intensive care: intubation and ventilation carried out when respiratory effort is ineffective has contributed to this. It is justifiable to abandon the reanimation attempts, if the cardiac condition and the asphyxia are immediately very severe in a child who appears very immature. Any intermediary position rapidly increases the chances of survival with a seriously damaged brain. In these children, it is important to emphasize the need for technical perfection of the mechanical aspects of the resuscitation. It may be useful in a case with good spontaneous ventilation but with a cardiac rhythm of less than 100, to begin respiratory assistance at an early stage by continuous positive pressure since the very small premature baby seems unable to maintain good expansion without adequate opening pressure. The use of oxygen makes the measurement of PaO_2 (transcutaneously) indispensable as soon as possible. The administration of bicarbonate must be even more sparing than in larger infants. Lactic acidosis, the result of tissue hypoxia improves tissue perfusion. When the tissue oxygenation returns to normal the lactic acid is metabolised.

The outcome of the resuscitation.
— If the immediate results are satisfactory, with a return to efficient, spontaneous ventilation, and good hemodynamics, the infant should be watched closely for at least several hours, including in particular a neurological and general examination, an assessment, with correction if necessary, of pH, glycemia, calcaemia and a chest X-ray.

When the results are not satisfactory, with the reappearance of signs of vitality in the circulation but with the persistence of respiratory difficulties, the infant must be moved to an intensive care unit.

Failure. — This is death with irreversible cardiorespiratory failure. It is usually stated that the absence of the reappearance of signs of life after 20-30 minutes of a well carried-out reanimation justifies the abandonment of such measures. The situation is more difficult to define where there is cardiac, but not respiratory recovery. Steiner and Neligan [77] have shown that when spontaneous breathing does not resume 30 minutes after the resumption of a normal cardiac rhythm there is death or serious sequelae. The prognosis is good on the other hand when there is cardiac recovery in less than 5 minutes with normal breathing in less than 30 minutes.

A systematically negative or active attitude appears also to be unjustified. Each case must be considered individually. Apart from the undeniable failures of reanimation, it should not be the person responsible for the initial resuscitation in the labour room to make the decision alone as to whether or not it is appropriate to continue. Resuscitation must be started in the best possible conditions, without a continual questioning of whether it is fully justified, which leads to half measures, dangerous in that they are likely to allow the survival of the child with increased damage. The diagnosis of failure of reanimation and of cerebral death is often easier after a short period of intensive care than at the very moment of birth. Whatever the moment decided to discontinue resuscitation it is essential that it be strictly adhered to.

HEAD INJURIES

Lesions are most often secondary to compression (2/1,000 newborn children—Brown, 1976) or distension. They are dangerous by themselves and also indirectly through alterations of the cerebral circulation and/or cerebral edema.

OSSEOUS LESIONS

Cephalhematoma. — Seen in 0.2 to 2.5 % of newborn babies, it is usually harmless. It may be associated with more important osseous lesions: 25 % with linear fractures out of 64 cases for Kendall and Woloshin [44]. Zelson [91] found 111 cases of cephalhematomas in 7,250 newborn babies (1.5 %), only 6 (5.4 %) being associated with a fracture. In 4 of these 6 cases, forceps had been used. However, cesarean section does not completely eliminate the risk: as there were 3 cases of cephalhematoma, one with fracture. The fractures are more frequent when the cephalhematoma is bilateral (18 %). None of the children studied by Zelson showed any neurological problem. Young [90] has shown the association between occipital cephalhematoma and subdural hematoma of the posterior fossa. When it is voluminous, it can bring about anemia and jaundice. A secondary osteomyelitis is possible especially if an attempt is made to aspirate it. Spontaneous regression is usual.

Fractures of the skull. — Natelson and Sayers (1973) in a report of 42 observations of neonatal injuries of the skull noted one fracture of the base, two linear fractures and 15 depressed or "ping-pong ball" fractures. The prognosis for linear fractures is often poor because of underlying cerebral lesions or "growing fracture" associated with leptomeningeal cyst development; the prognosis of depressed skull fractures seems, in general, to be good. The latter, often attributed to obstetric intervention (1 case/1,000 in Europe, almost always after forceps) can come about spontaneously. They were noted by Axton and Levy in Africa and Tan in Singapore, in 1/4,000 spontaneous births, who considered them to be the result of the compression of the baby's head against the mother's pelvis.

Spontaneous resolution may be expected (Loeser). Surgery is necessary if there are any reasons for fearing cerebral complications (softening or hematoma): bone fragments in the brain tissue, neurological deficiency, signs of increased intracranial pressure, anomalies of the CSF or again in the event of failure of conservative management: e. g. observation or elevation by aspiration using an obstetrical vacuum extractor (Saunders).

Wigglesworth (1977) has emphasized the severity of certain occipital injuries in babies in breech presentation born vaginally. In 2/3 of these babies, weighing more than 3,000 g, who died during or after delivery, there existed an occipital osteodiastasis, that is to say a separation between the bones of the occiput and the lateral parts.

Facial fractures. — There may be fracture or subluxation of the bones or the septal cartilage of the nose, especially first born babies with a long labour. Some dental malocclusions seems secondary to hypoplasia of the mandible due to traumatic neonatal epiphysial lesions.

INTRACRANIAL LESIONS

Known for a long time only to anatomo-pathologists, looked upon with a fatalistic attitude by clinicians, they have only recently become lesions whose diagnosis can be made while the patient is alive thanks to radiology and ultrasound, and which are sometimes within the scope of effective neurosurgical treatment.

Subdural and subtentorial hemorrhages. — Cephalic moulding which is too accentuated causes a distortion of the dural structures, and in particular an excessive traction on the tentorium and falx cerebri which exceeds their elasticity. It causes a tear of the veins and of the other dural structures (Towbin [84]), at the origin of subdural haemorrhages.

In the full term baby, hematoma of the convexity of the brain, often small and of good prognosis, results from a tear of the superficial veins. When the vertical moulding is very marked, more severe trauma with fracture is frequently observed. A lesser degree of vertical moulding, on the other hand, combined with lateral compression, causes considerable parietal overlapping; this may damage the sagittal sinus or the veins leading into it, which may result in subarachnoid haemorrhage and subsequent hydrocephaly.

Posterior fossa hematomas occur in the full term as well as in the premature baby; they are secondary to the rupture of the junction of the falx cerebri and tentorium near the confluence of the vein of Galen. The rupture may be secondary to considerable antero-posterior elongation as in forehead and face presentation, or when forceps are used. When the haemorrhage is massive, the accumulation of blood in the posterior fossa may cause compression of the brain-stem with severe neurologic problems. More uncommonly (Blank) one finds subdural hematoma following milder lesions, especially in full-term babies, born by normal delivery without any apparent complications who, after a time lag of a few hours to days develop signs of intracranial hypertension with hydrocephalus, combined with signs of subtentorial impairment: respiratory difficulty, nystagmus, 6th nerve paresis. There is usually no 3rd nerve paresis or convulsions. The diagnosis can be made with computed tomography. Recovery can be expected following emergency surgical treatment. Tank has described tearing of the tentorium cerebelli with intracranial haemorrhage after breech delivery [82].

In 15,000 births (1968-1970), Brown found lesions in 82 babies following cephalic compression, of which 29 had subarachnoid hemorrhages, 26 cerebral edema, 13 contusions with unilateral symptomatology, 7 subdural hematoma and 5 hydrocephalus [16, 17].

Extra-dural hematoma. — This is more exceptional, following a difficult breech delivery, the use of forceps or vacuum extractor. It results from an injury to the branches of the middle meningeal artery or to the lateral venous sinuses (Takagi). It is not necessarily combined with a fracture since phenomena of compression are just as important in its determination. If it is diagnosed at a sufficiently early stage by angiography or C. T. Scan, it is treated surgically.

Lesions following application of a vacuum extractor are not very common. A swelling is observed in all babies which recedes after a few hours. In a review of the literature in 1979, Plauche [68] found 18 subaponeurotic haemorrhages out of 14,276 cases, an average of 12.6 %, (variation from 0.8 to 37.6 %) of abrasions or lacerations of the scalp, 6 % (1 to 25 %) of cephalematoma and 0.35 % of intracranial haemorrhages. Retinal heamorrhages are often found in up to 100 % of cases if extraction takes more than 15 minutes. If one considers that retinal vascularization is the reflection

of vascularization of other areas dependent on the internal carotid, one might well wonder about the possible occurrence of "minimal cerebral lesions". However the early or delayed signs of neurological lesions do not seem to be much different from those following spontaneous deliveries (5.3 % with motor handicaps or delayed development after vacuum extraction, 5.9 % in controls).

FACIAL PARALYSIS

The facial nerve is particularly vulnerable in the newborn baby owing to its superficial position after its emergence from the stylomastoid foramen, the mastoid not being well developed at this age. Facial paralysis is most often unilateral following compression by forceps or by the maternal promontory. The impairment is peripheral varying according to the case and according to the muscles involved. Spontaneous recuperation is noted usually in less than a month. If occlusion of the eye is insufficient, the cornea must be protected by the frequent instillation of eye drops and occlusion of the eyelids. Surgical exploration of the nerve is justifiable only in the case of signs of complete persistant denervation.

*
* *

The consequences of these post-traumatic lesions are all the more severe since they are frequently combined with post-asphyxial lesions. However obstetric manipulations alone seem rarely to be responsible for serious trauma by themselves. The need to avoid post-asphyxial lesions must always be a priority.

SPINAL INJURY

During delivery, whatever the method, the neck undergoes considerable strain. Since the observations of Kennedy (1836) and then Parrot (1870) great emphasis has been placed on spinal cord injuries during breech deliveries. Yates (1959) studied the neck of 60 infants who were stillborn or who died very early. Among them, 8 were breech-births and 8 were delivered by cesarean section. Marked signs of cervical trauma were apparent in 27 cases: extra and sub-dural haemorrhages, often extensive, haemorrhages into joint capsules and synovial villi, tearing of ligaments and dura. These lesions, particularly severe after breech delivery were also noted after cephalic delivery or cesarean section. Only two cases of extensive destruction of the cord itself were reported which followed breech delivery. Bruising and tearing of spinal nerve roots were found in 9 cases, especially the anterior roots. The author emphasizes above all the great frequency of damage to the vertebral arteries.

DAMAGE TO THE VERTEBRAL ARTERIES

These have been well described in Yates' work, most authors having limited their study to the spinal cord.

In 24 cases (out of 27 cervical trauma cases) there was an intramural hematoma of one or both vertebral arteries, most frequently at the transverse processes of vertebrae; it was frequently combined with a rupture of the neighbouring venous sinuses. These hematomas are usually caused by a tear at the junction of the principal stem of the vertebral artery and of its branches. They are most likely brought about during delivery when, under the influence of uterine contractions, the intravascular pressure often rises to 250 mm Hg. Any small rupture could be the source of a hematoma whose pressure is high and which will remain localised since the wall of the vertebral artery is resistant. After the baby has been delivered the intravascular pressure again becomes identical to the aortic pressure; because of the hematoma, for a period of a few minutes to a few hours, this pressure is not sufficient to maintain an effective perfusion. Adventitial lesions can also be the cause of arterial spasm through lesions of autonomic innervation.

Ischemic lesions in areas dependant on the vertebrals and on the basilar truncus can result from vertebral arterial damage: e. g. brain-stem, cerebellum, occipito-temporal area. They can be fatal from the outset or be the cause of sequelae: anomalies of the cranial nerves, hypotonia through cerebellar lesions; cerebral palsy is likely when the disorder is symetrical and/or combined with cortical blindness. However, most authors believe that this situation is not the consequence of vertebral arterial damage but represents associated lesions following the same initial insult.

SPINAL CORD INJURY

The lesions are varied: laceration, edema, congestion, softening which is more or less localised, haemorrhage (Towbin).

Clinical manifestations. — These almost always occur after breech delivery, but have also been described with cephalic delivery. Dystocia is frequent, the obstetrician has sometimes been aware of a muffled cracking sound while traction is exerted on the trunk in order to extract the head.

Hellström and Sallmander (1968) have shown the frequent combination of hyperextension of the head in utero and spinal trauma. During intra-uterine hyperextension of the head in breech presentations, diagnosed through X-rays, cesarean section protects against cord trauma: 14 cord section out of 56 by vaginal delivery, none out of 26 cesarean sections (Bresnan and Abroms, 1974). In these cases, the cervical angulation is at maximum at the 8th cervical vertebra and can persist for a long time, 14 days to 25 months. However, Maekawa and co-workers observed quadriplegia despite a cesarean section [55], due perhaps to a particularly marked hyperextension; the fact that there was a decrease in fetal movement during the last third of pregnancy suggests that the cord lesion had originated in utero.

At birth. — There is practically always a period of shock with difficulty in initiating respiration. The motor signs vary with the site of the lesion. Above C3 and C4, the lesions are rapidly fatal. If the lesion is a low cervical one, there is flaccid paralysis of the upper limbs; occasionally the "Thorburn posture" can be seen, which must be distinguished from the decerebrate position, with the hand in the shape of a pistol and which occurs particularly in hyperextension of the neck. Breathing is shallow and at times paradoxical. In dorsal lesions there is defect of the intercostal and abdominal muscles. A flaccid, isolated paraplegia follows the more rare lumbosacral trauma.

An accurate assessment of the loss of sensation is not possible, but one can usually demonstrate a lack of response to pinpricks over a wide area. Sphincter disorders are usual; automatic micturition is quickly established (except in cases of lumbosacral lesions). The presence of blood in the CSF is not specific and may be lacking. X-rays of the spine are usually normal; sometimes a dislocation can be seen.

Evolution. — The initial phase of "spinal shock" lasts a few weeks, a time which is necessary for the resorption of the edema and the haemorrhage. An assessment of the neurological status can then be made: motor and sensory lesional syndrome, rapidly spasmodic sub-lesional syndrome. The study of evoked somato-sensitive potentials can be useful in specifying the level of the lesion. Spasticity produces few retractions; these are prevented by physiotherapy. Vesical rehabilitation is indispensable. The lack of sweating below the lesion can bring about bouts of fever. Cutaneous trophic disorders are rare. There is sometimes exclusively motor impairment (isolated lesion of the anterior horn?). The long term evolution varies, a deterioration of the neurological condition can be an expression of the healing process, or sometimes the beginning of hydromyelia justifying surgical intervention. The picture can be complicated by combined cerebral lesions.

Treatment. — If a blockage is shown by myelography, a laminectomy is debatable but, bearing in mind the lesions, it is of little practical use and risks affecting the subsequent stability of the spine. In view of the surprising recuperation of some children a conservative attitude is justified. Orthopedic treatment is indicated if there is vertebral dislocation. The essential part of the treatment is symptomatic.

LESIONS OF THE SPINAL NERVES (BRACHIAL PLEXUS)

The lesions. — Whatever the movement in question, the tension exerted on the brachial plexus during relative lowering of the shoulder related to the spine can cause lesions of the roots of the brachial plexus.

If the traction is moderate, as is most often the case, the axons are either shattered or broken within sheaths which always remain intact. This allows them to regrow. There is complete recovery in 2 to 3 months.

During stronger traction, one can see radicular rupture with a gap reaching the extraspinal segment of the root. The root loses all contact with the central nervous system. In the case of tearing, the gap affects the intraspinal portion of the root where, not being covered by a sheath, it divides into radicles which are very fragile systems. The rupture takes place at the junction between the radicles and the cord. In these two situations there is no chance of a spontaneous recovery.

The type of lesion differs according to the level of emergence of the affected roots. In C5 and C6 it is most often a radicular rupture. In C7, C8, D1, tears are almost the rule. C5 and C6 are always the first affected then possibly C7, C8 and occasionally D1.

One can also add to or mingle with this, ischaemic disorders from lesions of the small arteries vascularizing the roots.

Clinical picture. — There is always flaccid paralysis of the peripheral type, of which three topographic varieties are usually described.

Upper palsy (Erb-Duchenne) corresponds to an injury limited to C5 and C6. The shoulder is affected with loss of abduction, external rotation and flexion of the elbow. This creates a muscular maladjustement so that the arm is in an incorrect position of adduction, internal rotation and extension of the elbow. The hand is normal. If there is C3, C4 injury, there may be phrenic palsy. In rare cases the diaphragmatic paralysis is isolated [74] or bilateral [1]. The clinical picture is respiratory distress of varying severity, sometimes requiring assisted ventilation with intermittent positive pressure. The X-rays show an elevation of the diaphragm, with displacement of the mediastinum towards the opposite side. The paradoxical movements of Kienboeck can be seen with radioscopy.

There is much debate about the existence of *"lower isolated injury"* (Dejerine-Klumpke). This almost always is part of a combined injury with complete paralysis of the entire upper limb. It is, however, unusual that not a single innervated muscle remains and that the limb is completely slack. Most frequently it is in adduction and internal rotation. The elbow is often not completely extended. The forearm is in pronation and the hand in cubital inclination. The fingers remain capable of some movement, not sufficient for a good grip. A Claude Bernard-Horner syndrome or phrenic paralysis are possible. Intermediate forms between these types are common.

Evolution. — It is impossible to decide with any certainty on a prognosis in the initial phase. In upper lesions, only regular supervision can note any improvement, or even frequently, spontaneous recovery (50-90 % of cases).

Complete paralyses have little chance of full spontaneous recovery. The coexistence of paralyzed muscles opposed to healthy muscles which have kept their tone causes the imbalance of peri-articular muscular tension. The articulation is, then, in an incorrect position set by the secondary muscular and capsulo-ligamentary retractions. In time, this imbalance changes the articular surfaces themselves.

Complementary examinations

Electromyography: in the initial stage this provides information about the extent of the damage without judging what its evolution might be. It is especially worthwhile in the supervision of recovery and the decision about surgical treatment and possibly during the operation as well.

Myelography: this shows up certain intraspinal lesions: absence of one or several roots from their dural sheath; meningocele showing an avulsion and the rupture of the meningeal covering of a root. Although it is difficult to carry out and to interpret, it is especially useful in secondary therapeutic surgical indications.

Treatment

(1) The initial period corresponds to the three first months during which 50 to 90 % of obstetric paralyses recover spontaneously.

Incorrect positions must be guarded against by physiotherapy because spontaneous re-innervation or surgical reattachment can only be effective if each articulation has retained its normal mobility.

(2) Early surgery on the plexus allows direct exploration of the lesions. Radicular ruptures, the most usual case, are reparable with the possibility of the interposition of a nerve graft; avulsions, on the other hand, are not. Phrenic paralyses are treated by plication of the diaphragm.

The decision to operate can be taken about the 3rd month if there has been no sign of re-innervation, possibly earlier in the diaphragm in the event of the necessity for prolonged assisted ventilation.

(3) When sequelae have begun, muscle transfers are the only possibility for functional salvage of the limb. It is then a matter of a redistribution of unaffected muscles whose aim is to re-establish essential function at the expense of a less important movement.

TRAUMA TO THE LIMBS

FRACTURES

The clavicle is the bone most often fractured, especially during delivery of large babies and during shoulder dystocia. Recovery is rapid and always of good quality. If there is displacement it is worthwhile immobilising the limb with a figure of eight bandage to prevent injury to the brachial plexus or

to the apex of the pleural cavity. It may be that the fracture can be recognised only at the callus stage. The latter is always resorbed without any aesthetic ill-effects.

Fractures of the long bones almost exclusively involve the femur and the humerus; usually, 4 cases out of 5, following breech-delivery. Fractures of the humerus are located in the middle third and are transverse or spiral. A transient paresis of the radial nerve is possible.

Fractures of the femur are also located in the middle third and are transverse. Their prognosis is excellent if the diagnosis is made early and the treatment carried out in good circumstances.

EPIPHYSIAL SEPARATION

This is the tearing of an epiphysis from a long bone at the growth plate. It occurs especially at the upper end of the femur. The usual mechanism is an hyperextension with abduction and rotation combined with strong traction on the lower limb during breech delivery [51, 85].

The clinical presentation is typical: the baby's limb remains in flexion, abduction and external rotation. He or she avoids all motion, passive mobilization is very painful. Edema of the inguinal crease and of the gluteal area occurs rapidly. Thigh shortening of the limb can be discerned.

The X-rays show a displacement of the upper epiphysis of the femur upwards and outwards. This can mimic a congenital dislocation of the hip.

Arthrography pinpoints the lesions and allows differentiation from septic neonatal arthritis. If possible the treatment should be conservative. Surgical reduction must be reserved for very serious forms. The failure to utilize appropriate operative treatment can bring about serious sequelae such as coxa vara, aseptic necrosis, premature fusion of the epiphysis, nonunion, etc.

Similar lesions have been noted in the knee and in the upper end of the humerus. Differential diagnosis from paralysis of the brachial plexus is not always easy [48].

MUSCULAR TRAUMA

These are particularly frequent during breech deliveries, especially if methods of extraction of the baby are used (Ralis [69]). Widespread lesions can cause a "crush syndrome" with its general consequences.

Less serious lesions of the sternocleidomastoid muscle brought on by poor intra-uterine position with retraction of the muscle, is shown by a firm lump joined to the muscle and wrongly called "hematoma". In fact this nodule is made up of torn, retracted muscle fibres. The physiotherapist must set about limiting the retraction of the muscle in order to prevent the occurrence of torticollis. Only rarely is surgery necessary.

VISCERAL LESIONS

For a long time these had been discovered mainly during autopsy. Recent methods of diagnosis particularly using ultra-sound allow for earlier diagnosis and thus improve the prognosis.

SUBCAPSULAR HEMATOMA OF THE LIVER

Not unusual, since it is found in 2 to 3.5 % of neonatal autopsies, this constitutes one of the principal causes of serious internal haemorrhage in the newborn [37].

Pathogenesis. — Some complementary factors should be mentionned: obstetric trauma (breech-delivery), hepatic fragility, coagulation disorders. Difficult labours, and macrosomia are sometimes involved in direct trauma to the right side; one can most frequently observe excessive traction on the support ligaments of the liver (coronary ligament and round ligament) which constitute superficial lacerations. This progressive haemorrhage distends the capsule which ruptures into the peritoneal cavity after a period of time becoming shorter the heavier the bleeding becomes. The haemorrhage which until then has been limited by the tension of the hematoma, resumes freely at a volume of 50 to 500 ml.

The fragile nature of the liver of the newborn baby, especially the premature, can be increased because of venous congestion following anoxia. Postnatal injuries (umbilical catheter, handling) may be predisposing factors. Very occasionally a vascular hepatic anomaly is discovered: hemangiomatosis, hemangioendothelioma.

Coagulation disorders constitute the major predisposing factor: haemorrhagic disease of the newborn, side-effects of drugs taken by the mother (salicylic acid, anticonvulsants) and rarely constitutional defects (hemophilia). Consumptive coagulopathy following considerable blood loss, which aggravates the haemorrhagic disorders, quickly follows.

The clinical history is in two stages. The first phase of unbroken hematoma is marked by the progressive increase of a tumefaction of the right side which is joined to the liver. After an interval of 1 to 7 days the general signs become serious: haemorrhagic shock and collapse, whereas the local signs decrease and the liver is extended by a very vague mass. A bluish peri-umbilical patch or hematinic intra-scrotal effusion, signs of hemoperitoneum, are usually observed.

X-rays of the abdomen show an opacity of the right side pushing back the intestinal loops towards the left. The echotomogram which is easier to carry out than a CT Scan confirms its localisation and its liquid nature. Following rupture, visualization shows a peritoneal effusion with the intestinal loops framed like stained glass-windows.

Management is first and foremost medical: correction of the anemia and the disorders of hemostasis. In the event of failure, hemostasis is to be obtained by surgery. If the bleeding is controlled, the evolution of the hemoperitoneum is favorable as the peritoneum resorbs red cells well.

ADRENAL HAEMORRHAGE

Described by Corcoran and Strauss (1924), this represents a cause of mortality which cannot be overlooked (1.7 per 1,000 autopsies). Its actual frequency is certainly much higher than is usually admitted since it can give few or no symptoms.

The factors which bring it about, are the same as in hepatic hematoma. It is 3 to 4 times more common on the right, the gland being even more compressed between the spine and the liver. In 8 to 10 % of cases it is bilateral.

The signs appear during the first week, they are often atypical: digestive disorders (anorexia, vomiting, diarrhoea, pseudo-occlusive signs), poor behavior, dyspnea, hematuria. The characteristic situation is a combination of a variable reduction of hemoglobin, prolonged jaundice and a lumbo-abdominal tumefaction, which is often difficult to investigate because of considerable bloating of the abdomen. It is located in the lumbar fossa and is dull, firm and homogenous.

Intravenous pyelography shows a homogenous mass displacing the kidney downwards and outwards, flattening its upper pole. The ipsilateral kidney can be non visible. The cystic nature of the mass is confirmed by echotomography and possibly by a CT Scan [64].

The immediate evolution depends on the degree of the haemorrhage and on its possible bilaterality.

Rupture, whether it be in the peritoneum or rather in the retroperitoneal space, is often fatal. In favourable cases, the volume of the tumor decreases slowly. From the third week calcifications may appear. During the acute phase there is no adrenal insufficiency. The long term prognosis is good although a risk of delayed hormonal insufficiency cannot be categorically excluded. This fact justifies attentive supervision of these children.

The combination of thrombosis of the renal vein and adrenal haemorrhage has been described. Haemorrhage must be differentiated from other abdominal hematomas and neuroblastoma, particularly necrotic and haemorrhagic tumors [46].

Management is medical. Surgical treatment is to be used only for massive uncontrolled haemorrhages and for possible suppurative forms.

HEMATOMA OF THE SPLEEN

This is five times less common than that of the liver. Initially it is characterized by a subcapsular hematoma which is susceptible to rupture. These hematomas often affect abnormal spleens (during erythroblastosis for instance) but this is not always the case [20, 39].

The clinical picture is of a splenic tumour with anemia, which is liable to be complicated by hemoperitoneum. The latency period can be longer, approaching 11 days. Surgery is the usual treatment.

The risk of serious infection following splenectomy in a child of less than 4 years (OPSI syndrome: overwhelming post splenectomy infection) seems to be less than following splenectomy for other causes. It does occur in 4.25 % of cases, pneumococcus being especially common [6].

OTHER LESIONS

Other injuries are rare, and found mainly after breech deliveries: rupture of the kidney (Eraklis, Conner and Curran), of the bladder (Tank) or of the esophagus.

REFERENCES

[1] ALDRICH (T. K.), HERMAN (J. H.), ROCHESTER (D. F.). — Bilateral diaphragmatic paralysis in the newborn infant. J. Pediatr., 97, 988-991, 1980.

[2] ANDERSEN (G. E.), FRIIS-HANSEN (B.). — Neonatal hypertriglyceridemia. A new index of antepartum-intrapartum fetal stress? Acta Paediatr. Scand., 65, 369-374, 1976.

[2 bis] ANGELL (L. K.), ROBB (R. M.), BERSON (F. G.). — Visual prognosis in patients with ruptures in Descemet's membrane due to forceps injuries. Arch. Ophthalmol., 99, 2137-2139, 1981.

[3] APGAR (V.). — A proposal for a new method of evaluation of the newborn infant. Current Res. Anaesth., 32, 260-267, 1953.

[4] APGAR (V.), JAMES (L. S.). — Further observations on the newborn scoring system. Am. J. Dis. Child., 104, 419-428, 1962.

[5] AXTON (J. H. M.), LEVY (L. F.). — Congenital moulding depressions of the skull. Br. Med. J., 1, 1644-1647, 1965.

[6] BALFANZ (J. R.), NESBIT (M. E.), JARVIS (C.), KRIVIT (W.). — Overhelming sepsis following splenectomy for trauma. J. Pediatr., 88, 458-460, 1976.

[7] BAUM (J. D.), ROBERTSON (N. R. C.). — Immediate effects of alkaline infusion in infants with respiratory distress syndrome. J. Pediatr., 87, 255-261, 1975.

[8] BECKER (M.), MENZEL (K.). — Brain typical creatine kinase in the serum of newborn infants with perinatal brain damage. Acta Paediatr. Scand., 67, 177-180, 1978.

[9] BERGEN (R.), MARGOLIS (S.). — Retinal hemorrhages in the newborn. Ann. Ophthalmol., 8, 53-56, 1976.

[9 bis] BERGER (S. S.), STEWART (R. E.). — Mandibula‧ hypoplasia secondary to perinatal trauma: report of a case. J. Oral Surg., 35, 578-582, 1977.

[10] BESIO (R.), CABALLERO (C.), MEERHOFF (E.). — Neonatal retinal hemorrhage and influence of perinatal factors. Am. J. Ophthalmol., 87, 74-78, 1979.

[11] BLANK (N. K.), STRAND (R.), GILLES (F. H.), PALAKSHAPPA (A.). — Posterior fossa subdural hematomas in neonates. Arch. Neurol., 35, 108-111, 1978.

[12] BOON (A. W.), MILNER (A. D.), HOPKIN (I. E.). — Physiological responses of the newborn infant to resuscitation. Arch. Dis. Child., 54, 492-498, 1979.

[13] BOON (A. W.), MILNER (A. D.), HOPKIN (I. E.). — Lung expansion, tidal exchange and formation of the functional residual capacity during resuscitation of asphyxiated neonates. J. Pediat., 95, 1031-1036, 1979.

[14] BRATTEBY (L. E.), SWANSTRÖM (S.). — Hypoxanthine concentration in plasma during the first two hours after birth in normal and asphyxiated infants. Pediatr. Res., 16, 152-155, 1982.

[15] BRESNAM (M. J.), ABROMS (I. F.). — Neonatal spinal cord transection secondary to intrauterine hyperextension of the neck in breech presentation. J. Pediatr., 84, 734-737, 1974.

[16] BROWN (J. K.). — Infants damaged during birth, Pathology, In D. HULL: Recent advances in paediatrics, Churchill Livingstone ed., Edinburgh, 35-56, 1976.

[17] BROWN (J. K.). — Infants damaged during birth. Perinatal asphyxia, In D. HULL: Recent advances

in paediatrics, Churchill Livingstone ed., Edinburgh, 57-88, 1976.

[18] CAO (A.), TRABALZA (N.), DE VIRGILIS (S.), FURBETTA (M.), COPPA (G.). — Serum creatine kinase activity and serum kinase isoenzymes in newborn infants. *Biol. Neonate*, *17*, 126-134, 1971.

[19] CHERNICK (V.), MADANSKY (D. L.), LAWSON (E. E.). — Naloxone decreases the duration of primary apnea with neonatal asphyxia. *Pediatr. Res.*, *14*, 357-359, 1980.

[20] CHRYSS (C.), AARON (W. S.). — Successful treatment of rupture of normal spleen in newborn. *Am. J. Dis. Child.*, *134*, 418-419, 1980.

[21] CONNER (E.), CURRAN (J.). — *In utero* traumatic intra-abdominal deceleration injury to the fetus, a case report. *Am. J. Obstet. Gynecol.*, *125*, 567-569, 1976.

[22] CORCORAN (W. J.), STRAUSS (A. A.). — Suprarenal hemorrhage in newborn. *JAMA*, *82*, 626-628, 1924.

[23] CORDERO (L.), HON (E. H.). — Neonatal bradycardia following nasopharyngeal stimulation. *J. Pediatr.*, *78*, 441-447, 1971.

[24] DANIEL (S. S.), ADAMSONS (K.), JAMES (L. S.). — Lactate and pyruvate as an index of prenatal oxygen deprivation. *Pediatrics*, *37*, 942-953, 1966.

[25] DAWES (G. S.). — Fetal and neonatal physiology, Chicago, Year Book Medical Pub., 1968.

[26] DAWES (G. S.), JACOBSON (H. N.), MOTT (J. C.), SHELLEY (H. J.), STAFFORD (A.). — The treatment of asphyxiated mature fetal lambs and rhesus monkeys with intravenous glucose and sodium bicarbonate. *J. Physiol.*, *169*, 167-184, 1963.

[27] DRAGE (J. S.), KENNEDY (C.), BERENDES (S.), SCHWARZ (B. K.), WEISS (W.). — The Apgar score as an index of infant mortality. *Dev. Med. Child Neurol.*, *8*, 141-148, 1966.

[28] DRAGE (J. S.), BERENDES (H. W.), FISCHER (P. D.) — The Apgar scores and four year psychological examination performance. In *Perinatal Factors affecting human development*, Scientific Publication n° 185, Washington, D. C., Pan American Health Organization, 222, 1969.

[29] EIDELMAN (A. I.), HOBBS (J. F.). — Bicarbonate therapy revisited. A study in therapeutic revisionism. *Am. J. Dis. Child.*, *132*, 847-848, 1978.

[30] ELLIS (S. S.), MONTGOMERY (J. R.), WAGNER (M.). — Osteomyelitis complicating neonatal cephalhematoma. *Am. J. Dis. Child.*, *127*, 100-103, 1974.

[31] ENGEL (R. R.), ELIN (R. J.). — Hypermagnesemia from birth asphyxia. *J. Pediatr.*, *77*, 631-637, 1970.

[32] ERAKLIS (A. L.). — Abdominal injury related to the trauma of birth. *Pediatrics*, *39*, 421-424, 1967.

[32 bis] FRASER (G. R.). — *The causes of profound deafness in childhood*, Baltimore Johns Hopkins University Press, 1976.

[33] FRENCH (C. E.), WALDSTEIN (G.). — Subcapsular hemorrhage of the liver in the newborn. *Pediatrics*, *69*, 204-208, 1982.

[34] GÅRDMARK (S.). — Studies on acid-base balance, carbohydrate and lipid metabolism in human fetal and maternal blood in clinical and experimental conditions during labor, Student literature Lund, 1974.

[35] GREENE (W.), L'HEUREUX (P.), HUNT (C. E.). — Paralysis of the diaphragm. *Am. J. Dis. Child.*, *129*, 1402-1404, 1975.

[36] GREGORY (G. A.), GOODING (C. A.), PHIBBS (R. H.), TOOLEY (W. H.). — Meconium aspiration in infants,

prospective study. *J. Pediatr.*, *85*, 848-852, 1974.

[37] GRUENWALD (P.). — Rupture of liver and spleen in the newborn infant. *J. Pediatr.*, *33*, 195-201, 1948.

[38] HALL (R. T.), KULKARNI (P. B.), SHEEHAN (M. B.), RHODES (P. G.). — Cerebrospinal fluid lactate dehydrogenase in infants with perinatal asphyxia. *Dev. Med. Child Neurol.*, *22*, 300-307, 1980.

[39] HALVORSEN (J. F.). — Rupture of the normal spleen occurring as a birth injury. *Acta Obstet. Gynecol. Scand.*, *50*, 95, 1971.

[40] HELLSTRÖM (B.), SALLMANDER (U.). — Prevention of spinal cord injury in hyperextension of the fetal head. *JAMA*, *204*, 1041-1044, 1968.

[41] HOBEL (C. J.), OH (W.), HYVARINEN (M. A.), EMMANOUILIDES (G. C.), ERENBERG (A.). — Early versus late treatment of neonatal acidosis in low-birth-weight infants: relation to respiratory distress syndrome. *J. Pediatr.*, *81*, 1178-1187, 1972.

[42] HOLDEN (K. R.), YONG (R. B.), PILAND (J. H.), HURT (W. G.). — Plasma pressors in the normal and stressed newborn infant. *Pediatrics*, *49*, 495-503, 1972.

[43] HUISJES (H. J.), AARNOUDSE (J. G.). — Arterial or venous umbilical *p*H as a mesure of neonatal morbidity. *Early Hum. Dev.*, *3*, 155-161, 1979.

[44] KENDALL (N.), WOLOSHIN (H.). — Cephalhematoma associated with fracture of the skull. *J. Pediatr.*, *41*, 125-132, 1952.

[45] KENNEDY (E.). — Observations on cerebral and spinal apoplexy, paralysis and convulsions of newborn infants. *Dublin J. Med. Sci.*, *10*, 419, 1836.

[46] KHURI (F. J.), ALTON (D. J.), HARDY (B. E.), COOK (G. T.), CHURCHILL (B. M.). — Adrenal hemorrhage in neonates: report of 5 cases and review of literature. *J. Urol.*, *124*, 684-687, 1980.

[47] LAVAUD (J.), CHOPIN (N.), JEQUECE (S.), BESSON-LEAUD (M.), CHASSEVENT (J.), MSELATI (J. C.). — Isoenzyme BB de la créatine kinase sérique témoin de la souffrance cérébrale néonatale. *Nouv. Presse Méd.*, *8*, 3821-3824, 1979.

[48] LEMPERG (R.), LILIEQUIST (B.). — Dislocation of the proximal epiphysis of the humerus in newborns. *Acta Paediatr. Scand.*, *59*, 377-380, 1970.

[49] LENDING (M.), SLOBODY (L. B.), STONE (M.), HOSBACH (R. E.), MESTERN (J.). — Activity of glutamic-oxalacetic transaminase and lactic deshydrogenase in cerebrospinal fluid and plasma of newborn and abnormal newborn infants. *Pediatrics*, *24*, 378-388, 1959.

[50] LIN (C. C.), MOAWAD (A. H.), ROSENOW (P. J.), RIVER (P.). — Acid-base characteristics of fetuses with intrauterine growth retardation during labor and delivery. *Am. J. Obstet. Gynecol.*, *137*, 553-559, 1980.

[50 bis] LINDEMANN (R.). — Resuscitation of the newborn. *Acta Paediatr. Scand.*, *73*, 210-212, 1984.

[51] LINDSETH (R. E.), ROSENE (H. A.). — Traumatic separation of the upper femoral epiphysis in a newborn infant. *J. Bone Jt. Surg.*, *53 A*, 1641-1644, 1971.

[52] LOESER (J. D.), KILBURN (H. L.), TOLLEY (T.). — Management of depressed skull fracture in the newborn. *J. Neurosurg.*, *44*, 62-64, 1976.

[53] LOU (H. C.), LASSEN (N. A.), FRIIS-HANSEN (B.). — Impaired autoregulation of cerebral blood flow in the distressed newborn infant. *J. Pediatr.*, *94*, 118-121, 1979.

[54] Low (J. A.), Galbraith (R. S.), Muir (D.), Killen (H.), Karchmar (J.), Campbell (D.). — Intrapartum fetal asphyxia: a preliminary report in regard to long-term morbidity. *Am. J. Obstet. Gynecol.*, *130*, 525-533, 1978.

[55] Maekawa (K.), Masaki (T.), Kokubun (Y.). — Fetal spinal cord injury secondary to hyperextension of the neck: no effect of caesarean section. *Dev. Med. Child Neurol.*, *18*, 229-232, 1976.

[56] Mathew (O. P.), Bland (H.), Boxerman (S. B.), James (E.). — CSF lactate levels in high risk neonates with and without asphyxia. *Pediatrics*, *66*, 224-227, 1980.

[57] Matthieu (J. M.), Gautier (E.), Prod'Hom (L. S.), Frei (J.). — Lactate sanguin dans l'asphyxie périnatale et les syndromes de détresse respiratoire. *Helv. Paediatr. Acta*, Suppl. *26*, 3-27, 1971.

[58] Matthieu (J. M.), Gautier (E.), Prod'Hom (L. S.). — Relation entre l'équilibre acidobasique, le degré d'oxygénation artérielle et la lactacidémie au cours des 96 premières heures de vie. *Helv. Paediatr. Acta*, Suppl. *26*, 29-37, 1971.

[59] Meberg (A.), Hetland (O.), Sommer (F.), Pervaagenes. — Creatine kinase in cerebrospinal fluid in newborn infants. *Clin. Chim. Acta*, *85*, 95-97, 1978.

[60] Modanlou (H.), Yeh (S. Y.), Hon (E. H.), Forsythe (A.). — Fetal and neonatal biochemistry and Apgar scores. *Am. J. Obstet. Gynecol.*, *117*, 942-951, 1973.

[60 bis] Monks (F. T.). — A fractured mandible in the newborn. *Br. J. Oral Surg.*, *14*, 270-272, 1977.

[61] Morrow (W. F. W.), Myles (T. J. M.). — Simplified scoring system for newborn. *Br. Med. J.*, *2*, 820-821, 1969.

[62] Naeye (R. L.). — Underlying disorders responsible for the neonatal deaths associated with low Apgar scores. *Biol. Neonate*, *35*, 150-155, 1979.

[63] Natelson (S. E.), Sayers (M. P.). — The fate of children sustaining severe head trauma during birth. *Pediatrics*, *51*, 169-174, 1973.

[64] Nordshus (T.), Monn (E.). — Ultrasonography in the diagnosis of neonatal adrenal haemorrhage. *Acta Paediatr. Scand.*, *69*, 695-698, 1980.

[65] Ostrea (E. M.), Odell (G. B.). — The influence of bicarbonate administration on blood *p*H in a closed system: clinical implications. *J. Pediatr.*, *80*, 671-680, 1972.

[66] Papile (L. A.), Burstein (J.), Burstein (R.), Koffler (H.), Koops (B.). — Relationship of intravenous sodium bicarbonate infusions and cerebral intraventricular hemorrhage. *J. Pediatr.*, *93*, 834-836, 1978.

[67] Parrot (J.). — Note sur un cas de rupture de la moelle chez un nouveau-né par suite des manœuvres pendant l'accouchement. *Bull. Mém. Soc. Méd. Paris*, *6*, 38-45, 1869.

[68] Plauche (W. C.). — Fetal cranial injuries related to delivery with the Malmström vacuum extractor. *Obstet. Gynecol.*, *53*, 750-757, 1979.

[68 bis] Radecki (L. L.), Tomatis (L. A.). — Continuous bilateral electrophrenic pacing in an infant with total diaphragmatic paralysis. *J. Pediatr.*, *88*, 969-971, 1976.

[69] Ralis (Z. A.). — Birth trauma to muscles in babies born by breech delivery and its possible fatal consequences. *Arch. Dis. Child.*, *50*, 4-13, 1975.

[70] Rhodes (P. G.), Hall (R. T.), Hellerstein (S.). — The effects of single infusions of hypertonic sodium bicarbonate on body composition in neonates with acidosis. *J. Pediatr.*, *90*, 789-795, 1977.

[71] Rudolph (N.), Gross (R. T.). — Creatine phosphokinase activity in serum of newborn infants as an indicator of fetal trauma during birth. *Pediatrics*, *38*, 1039-1046, 1966.

[72] Sabata (V.), Wolf (H.), Lausmann (S.). — Glycerol levels in the maternal and umbilical cord blood under various conditions. *Biol. Neonate*, *15*, 123, 1970.

[73] Saunders (B. S.), Lazoritz (S.), McArtor (R. D.), Marshall (P.), Bason (W. M.). — Depressed skull fracture in the neonate. Report of three cases. *J. Neurosurg.*, *50*, 512-514, 1979.

[74] Smith (B. T.). — Isolated phrenic nerve palsy in the newborn. *Pediatrics*, *49*, 449-451, 1972.

[75] Sokol (D. M.), Tompkins (D.), Izant (R. J.). — Rupture of the spleen and liver in the newborn: a report of the first survivor and a review of the literature. *J. Pediatr. Surg.*, *9*, 227, 1974.

[76] Steichen (J. J.), Kleinman (L. I.). — Studies in acid-base balance. I. Effect of alkali therapy in newborn dogs with mechanically fixed ventilation. *J. Pediatr.*, *91*, 287-291, 1977.

[77] Steiner (H.), Neligan (G.). — Perinatal cardiac arrest, quality of the survivors. *Arch. Dis. Child.*, *50*, 696-702, 1975.

[77 bis] Stocksted (P.), Schonsted-Madsen (U.). — Traumatology of the newborn's nose. *Rhinology*, *17*, 77-82, 1979.

[78] Svenningsen (N. W.), Siesjo (B. K.). — Cerebrospinal fluid lactate/pyruvate ratio in normal and asphyxiated neonates. *Acta Paediatr. Scand.*, *61*, 117-124, 1972.

[79] Swanström (S.), Bratteby (L. E.). — Hypoxanthine as a test of perinatal hypoxia as compared to lactate, base deficit and pH. *Pediatr. Res.*, *16*, 156-160, 1982.

[80] Takagi (T.), Nagai (R.), Wakabayashi (S.), Mizawa (I.), Hayashi (K.). — Extradural hemorrhage in the newborn as a result of birth trauma. *Child's Brain*, *4*, 306-318, 1978.

[81] Tan (K. L.). — Cephalhematoma. *Aust. NZJ Obstet. Gynecol.*, *10*, 101, 1970.

[82] Tank (E. S.), Davis (R.), Holt (J. F.), Morley (G. W.). — Mechanisms of trauma during breech delivery. *Obstet. Gynec.*, *38*, 761, 1971.

[83] Tooley (W. H.), Phibbs (R. H.), Schlueter (M. A.). — Delivery room diagnosis and immediate management of asphyxia, In *Intrauterine asphyxia and the developing fetal brain*. L. Glück ed., Year Book Medical Pub., Chicago-London, 251-261, 1977.

[84] Towbin (A.). — Central nervous system damage in the human fetus and newborn infant. Mechanical and hypoxic injury incurred in the fetal-neonatal period. *Am. J. Dis. Child.*, *119*, 529-542, 1970.

[85] Towbin (R.), Crawford (A. H.). — Neonatal traumatic proximal femoral epiphysiolysis. *Pediatrics*, *63*, 456-459, 1979.

[86] Tsang (R. C.), Glueck (C. J.), Evans (G.), Steiner (P. M.). — Cord blood hypertriglyceridemia. *Am. J. Dis. Child.*, *127*, 78-84, 1974.

[87] Usher (R.). — Reduction of mortality from respiratory distress syndrome of prematurity with early administration of intravenous glucose and sodium bicarbonate. *Pediatrics*, *32*, 966-975, 1963.

[88] WIGGLESWORTH (J. S.), HUSEMEYER (R. P.). — Intracranial birth trauma in vaginal breech delivery: the continued importance of injury to the occipital bone. *Br. J. Obstet. Gynaecol.*, *84*, 684-691, 1977.

[89] YATES (P. O.). — Birth trauma to the vertebral arteries. *Arch. Dis. Child.*, *34*, 436-441, 1959.

[90] YOUNG (R. S. K.), ZALNERAITIS (E. L.). — Retro-auricular cephalhematoma as a sign of posterior fossa subdural hematoma. Diagnosis in the newborn by tomography. *Clin. Pediatr.*, *19*, 631-632, 1980.

[91] ZELSON (C.), LEE (S. J.), PEARL (M.). — The incidence of skull fractures underlying cephalhematomas in newborn infants. *J. Pediatr.*, *85*, 371-373, 1974.

10

Perinatal pharmacology

P. L. MORSELLI and J. F. THIERCELIN

INTRODUCTION

IMPORTANCE AND NEED
OF INFORMATION ON DRUG DISPOSITION
IN THE PERINATAL PERIOD

Increasing concerns about the toxic effects of drugs in newborns and infants have underlined the need for a better knowledge of drug kinetics and effects in the early period of life. Such a need has been mainly conditioned by the fact that at the adult level thanks to a better understanding of the physiological variables regulating drug disposition, drug safety has been greatly improved. Furthermore, the identification of therapeutic and toxic plasma level thresholds for various classes of drugs as well as an improved understanding of possible modifications of the kinetic variables in several physiological or pathological conditions has led in many instances to a more rational use of therapeutic agents with the consequent optimization of their therapeutic potential and reduction of the incidence of adverse reactions.

More recently the development of the concept of "Therapeutic Drug Monitoring" has permitted us to illustrate the importance not only of defining the kinetic profile of any given drug, but also the necessity for regular monitoring of plasma concentrations of drugs because of possible modifications (within a given individual) of the variables conditioning drug disposition due to environmental factors and/or physiopathological conditions. On the other hand, numerous examples do illustrate that "steady" plasma drug concentrations within the therapeutic range, are the correct "premise" for an optimal therapeutic response.

Among the various factors capable of modifying drug kinetics and hence drug effects *age* is a very important one. For several years, despite a consistent body of information at the animal level indicating that drug kinetics and effects do change substantially with age, our knowledge of drug disposition in the human newborn has been rather scanty if not completely absent. More recently, the situation has substantially changed: the information on drug disposition in the perinatal period has considerably increased. Today, for several classes of therapeutic agents, the kinetic profiles in the perinatal period are known and the possible therapeutic and toxic effects are better understood. Furthermore, thanks to this development, important differences in drug disposition have been observed between premature newborns, full-term neonates and young infants. An increased awareness of the necessity of taking into consideration, when prescribing, variables such as gestational age and/or postnatal age has developed. However the relative bearing of other factors such as: *in utero* exposure to drugs, hypoxic conditions, haemodynamic alterations, and the presence of cardiorenal pathology are not fully understood at the clinical level and only very seldom taken into account when prescribing a therapeutic regimen for a neonate. Evidence indicates that all these factors may further modify drug disposition and effects. Furthermore, because the maturational process is not fully predictable and because all the above mentioned factors may interact to a varying extent, depending on the clinical situation, it has become evident that therapeutic drug monitoring may be necessary at the perinatal level as well. By applying the concept of therapeutic drug monitoring we have acquired more insight about the relative weight and importance of the different factors as well as about the maturation rates of the various physiological functions conditioning drug disposition.

However for several therapeutic classes, currently used in the perinatal period, we still lack systematic data, and in the absence of data defining the risk/benefit ratios, drugs are still used in a rather uncontrolled and empirical manner. In such a situation, "assignation of meaningful dosages is a practically impossible task" (Stern L., 1975). On the basis of the information acquired up to now we should continue the efforts to better understand drug disposition and effects in the perinatal period with the aim of making the "task" mentioned above no more "impossible" but on the contrary "rational and logical".

In the following pages we have tried to summarize the available information on drug disposition in the perinatal period. Because of the necessary space limitation some points will not be discussed in detail. For more detailed information the reader is referred to specific articles and reviews indicated for each subchapter.

GENERAL PRINCIPLES OF PHARMACOKINETICS AND PHARMACODYNAMICS

A drug is not a mysterious entity, but a well defined molecular chemical entity which exerts its action by interacting with protein structures of the body (or of the host in the case of bacteria) modifying the function of the structures with which it interacts. The effect of such an interaction can be either an inhibition or an enhancement of function conditioned by the interacting "receptor" proteins.

For many compounds these actions are reversible and the intensity and/or duration of the effects are directly related to the *quantity* of drug which reaches the "site of action", "the receptors" and to the *time* a given "active" concentration is maintained.

If this applies to an acute situation (as in the case of a single dose), in the course of repeated administration we may have compensatory and adaptative mechanisms leading to a modification of either the number of receptors at the site of action or of the affinity of these proteins for the administered compound. For these reasons relationships between drug concentrations in biological fluids and effects observed after a single dose cannot always be extrapolated to repeated dosages and vice versa. Each situation should hence be considered separately.

In a living organism, an exogenous compound (as a drug can be considered in most instances) in order to reach the "sites of action" has to go through a series of complex steps, schematically illustrated in Figure I-64. Most of these steps consist of dissolution in biological fluids, passage of biological membranes, reversible binding to proteins and distribution (according to its physicochemical properties) in extracellular and/or intracellular fluids. Liposolubility is an important factor since the ease of membrane penetration is proportional to this physicochemical characteristic. Similarly the rate of elimination will depend on processes such as metabolization to more polar compounds and/or biliary and renal excretion intended to dispose of the exogenous agent.

ABSORPTION

With this word we define a process by which drugs are delivered from their site of administration into the blood stream or into the body area in which we wish them to act.

Considering the first step, the rate of entry into the blood stream depends on the *route* by which the drug is given and on the physico-chemical properties of the compound. In any case however, whatever may be the route (oral, rectal, intramuscular, subcutaneous, topical), in order to reach the circulation drugs have to cross barriers such as lipoidal membranes and/or endothelial walls.

Such passage generally takes place by "passive diffusion" according to a non saturable process in which the transfer is directly proportional to: (*a*) the concentration gradient, (*b*) the lipid/water partition coefficient of the drug and (*c*) the absorbing surface area.

When in solution, drugs exist in ionized and nonionized form and according to their pKa and the pH

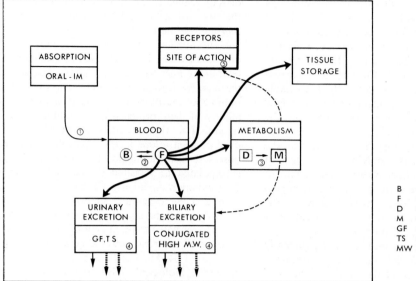

FIG. I-64. — *Schematic representation of the fate of drugs in the body.* The passage in each compartment implies the passage across lipoidic membranes. Its rate is regulated by factors such as the drug's concentration-gradients, polarity of the molecules, binding to plasma and tissue proteins, haemodynamic conditions, etc. The drug concentration in blood can be taken as an expression of this dynamic situation and in "steady state" conditions the concentration in blood may be considered as "representative" of the drug concentrations at the sites of action.

of the medium one or the other form prevails. However, even if the two forms are in dynamic equilibrium it is only the unionized form which can cross the membrane walls. The degree of ionization is hence an important variable.

Other mechanisms such as active transport, filtration through pores and pynocytosis play a small role for most of the therapeutic agents, with the exception of vitamins and a few very polar compounds.

Gastrointestinal absorption. — After oral administration most absorption occurs in the small intestine which provides a very large surface area and a wide range of pHs ($\sim$ 4.00-8.00) which may favour the absorption of several non-ionized compounds. As previously noted in order to be absorbed a drug must be present in solution at the surface of the cell membranes preferably in a non-ionized form. This implies that the physicochemical properties of the drug, the characteristics of the formulation, the gastric and the intestinal pH, the gastric emptying time, the status of the intestinal mucosa and the presence of food are all factors which may play an important role. Among these, the dissolution rate of the formulation, gastric emptying time and gastrointestinal motility appear to be the most important factors in determining the rate of gastrointestinal absorption,

together with the degree of liposolubility of the drug. Presence or absence of bile salts and modification of gastrointestinal blood flow may also influence intestinal transit time and rate of drug removal.

Rectal absorption. — The basic mechanisms regulating rectal absorption of drugs are identical to those described for gastrointestinal absorption. Even if the absorbing surface is considerably reduced, the high vascularization permits an efficient absorption of several compounds, provided that these are administered in a suitable form. *Solutions* or *enemas* are usually well absorbed, while in the case of *suppositories* the absorption may be quite variable depending on the speed of dissolution. Presence of fecal material may of course limit the amount absorbed.

Intramuscular and subcutaneous absorption. — The main factors conditioning the rate of absorption of a drug administered in aqueous solution either *subcutaneously* or *intramuscularly* are:

— the ease of penetration through the endothelial capillary walls;

— the surface area over which the solution has spread;

— the rate of blood flow through the area.

Evidence indicates that the absorption rate and

the total amount absorbed may vary significantly by injecting into different muscles. Such a difference may, on given occasions, be very important since as in the case of lidocaine or insulin the rates of absorption are not without significance for the effectiveness of the drug.

Percutaneous absorption. — Skin is designed to prevent absorption. However given certain conditions the skin may be used to administer drugs. The thickness of the stratum corneum, the status of the skin and its hydration, the vehicle in which the drug is dissolved and the degree of liposolubility are the important variables. Increased hydration of the skin and a rise in skin temperature (increased blood flow) usually enhance skin permeability.

PLASMA PROTEIN BINDING AND DISTRIBUTION

Once entered into the blood stream drugs are usually distributed to the rest of the body. The degree and rate of distribution depend on several factors such as:

— physicochemical properties of the drug (liposolubility, pKa, ionization constant);
— pH of body fluids;
— blood flow to individual organs and tissues;
— extent of drug binding to plasma and tissue proteins;
— size and mass of the patient;
— proportion of extracellular body water;
— amount of adipose tissue.

The time of onset of action and the intensity and duration of the effects of drugs depend not only on their absorption and elimination rates but also on their kinetics of distribution in various tissues and body compartments.

Drugs are distributed between extracellular water and fat depots according to their lipid/water partition coefficient. Alterations in acid-base balance or of tissue pH may influence the amount of drug present as the unionized fraction or modify the degree of binding to plasma and tissue proteins. Furthermore, the penetration into tissues is also a function of blood flow. It follows that the size of the body water compartment and of adipose tissue depots, cardiac output, regional blood flow, organ perfusion pressures, acid-base balance and degree of binding are all physical variables capable of significantly modifying the distribution of many drugs in the body and hence their effects.

A kinetic parameter which gives an idea of the extravascular distribution of drug is the Apparent Volume of Distribution (AVD). AVD is a mathematical expression calculated by dividing the total amount of drug in the body by the theoretical plasma concentration that would exist at zero time, (assuming an instant equilibration) following an intravenous bolus injection. In practice it is computed extrapolating to zero time the slope of the concentrations observed during the terminal exponential phase (Fig. I-65). AVD can also be defined as the

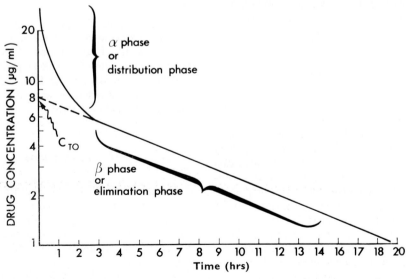

FIG. I-65. — *Schematic representation of the decrease of drug blood concentrations as a function of time, after either i. v. administration or rapid oral absorption, and of the extrapolation for obtaining the value of drug concentration at time 0* (C_{TO}).

volume that must be filled before the desired plasma concentration can be achieved.

In general, acidic drugs bind mostly to albumin, while in the case of basic drugs other proteins such as γ globulins, lipoproteins and α1-acid glyco-protein (α1-AGP) may play an important role in the "binding" phenomenon.

Drug binding to plasma proteins can be described as a reversible interaction between a small molecule (the drug) and a macromolecule (the protein) where the extent and the degree of interaction depends on several variables such as the type and the amount of binding protein, the affinity constant of the drug for the protein, the blood pH and the eventual pre-sence of other substances (endogenous and exoge-nous) capable of modifying the drug/protein interaction.

It should also be recalled that: only the unbound fraction of any given drug can cross biological membranes and interact with the receptor sites; and only the unbound fraction is available to metabolizing enzymes and can be filtered at the glomerular level.

METABOLISM

The majority of compounds used as therapeutic agents are highly liposoluble and because of this they cannot be excreted via the kidney. In order to be excreted via the kidney or via the bile they need to be transformed into more polar compounds, into compounds with higher water solubility. This process of biotransformation occurs primarily, but not necessarily, in the liver.

Metabolic reactions are usually divided into two groups: (*a*) Phase I reactions or non synthetic reactions and (*b*) Phase II reactions or synthetic reactions.

Phase I reactions include processes of oxi-dation, reduction and hydrolysis and in most instances they lead to a modification of the activity of the compound. The activity of *oxidation* and *reduction* processes are dependent on cyto-chrome P-450 and NAPH-cytochrome-c-reductase enzymatic systems, present in the membranes of the hepatic microsomal endoplasmic reticulum. The capability of these systems can be depressed (inhi-bition) or enhanced (induction) by concomitant or previous treatment with other drugs and can also be modified in several pathological conditions.

The process of *hydrolysis*, very important for many endogenous substances, is linked to both enzymatic systems present in the liver (as for instance deaminases) and to enzyme systems present in blood and in several tissues (as the esterases).

It should be recalled that the "product" of a phase I reaction is not always a "non-active meta-bolite". In several instances the derivative may be equally or more active than the parent compound.

In contrast, conjugation processes *(Phase II reactions)* do lead in general to the complete inac-tivation of the molecule, which is transformed to a very polar derivative and so more easily excreted at the biliary or renal level. These processes are endothermic reactions and require the presence of ATP. The enzyme systems catalyzing these processes are present in the liver but also in other organs, in smooth microsomes, in mitochondria and also in solution within the cell cytoplasm.

Most common conjugation reactions include conjugation with glucuronic acid, with glycine, and the formation of sulphates.

Glucuronoconjugation consists in the trans-fer (via transferases) of a molecule of glucuronic acid from UDGPA to an acceptor group (phenol, alcohol, aromatic amine, carboxylic acid). The compound so formed may be excreted via the kidney or the bile. In the latter case in the intestine it may be hydrolized by a glucuronidase system and so be reabsorbed and return into the systemic circulation via the portal system.

The formation of *glycine* conjugates usually occurs for acidic compounds which first form a CoA derivative and subsequently conjugate with glycine.

The formation of *sulphates* occurs mainly in the case of aromatic and aliphatic hydroxyl groups reacting with activated forms of sulphates thanks to the intervention of specific sulphokinases.

Other reactions of phase II include processes of acetylation, methylation and the formation of mercapturic acid derivatives.

EXCRETION

Renal excretion. — The primary pathway of drug elimination from the body is that of renal excretion. In general, parent drugs and metabolites can be removed from the body via the kidney by two major mechanisms: glomerular filtration and tubular secretion.

At the *glomerular* level only drugs present in plasma water are *filtered*. This means that only the free fraction of any given drug can be filtered while the plasma protein bound fraction cannot pass. Depending on its physicochemical properties, on the pH of the filtrate and on the concentration gradient between filtrate and plasma, part of the drug filtered at glomerular level with plasma water, is *reabsorbed at the tubular level* by a passive process. It follows that in most cases only a fraction of the drug filtered at the glomerular level may be found in the final urine. This is the case with most liposoluble substances.

Another mechanism of renal elimination is represented by *tubular secretion*. This is a process predominantly occuring at the level of the proximal tubule. The process is an active one involving the participation of a carrier protein. Up to now two carrier systems have been identified: one for anions and one for cations. It is interesting to recall that drugs transported by the same mechanism may compete with each other (one example is represented by probenecid and penicillin).

DEVELOPMENT
OF PHYSIOLOGICAL VARIABLES
IMPORTANT FOR DRUG DISPOSITION
IN THE HUMAN NEONATE

Most of the physiological variables conditioning drug absorption, distribution and elimination are at birth (both in premature and full term neonates), rather immature thus leading to important modifications in drug kinetics. Such a situation can be further altered by the presence of severe pathological states.

We will first describe the basic conditions in a "normal" or "not severely ill" newborn and then discuss the possible effects of severe disease.

NORMAL PHYSIOLOGICAL CONDITIONS

Gastrointestinal absorption

As noted before *gastric emptying time* and *pH dependent diffusion* are two main factors modulating the gastrointestinal absorption of drugs. In the newborn these two variables are remarkably different from those present in infants, children or adults. Most important is the fact that they undergo continuous maturational change for several months after birth.

Gastric emptying time is considerably prolonged at birth. Recent studies have indicated that it is a function of both gestational maturity and postnatal age as well as the nature of the feeding. The gastric emptying time is not affected by posture and is characterized by a biphasic pattern with an initial rapid phase followed by a slower exponential phase. Such a biphasic pattern is apparently not present in the premature newborn where the gastric emptying rate is linear and considerably slower. In the newborn the rate of gastric emptying is highly irregular and normally associated with an unpredictable peristalsis which may be further modified by diet and feeding habits.

At birth gastric pH is about 6.0 to 8.0 but it falls to 1.5-3.0 within a few hours and returns to about 6.0-7.0 within 24 hours. Such a drop is not observed in the preterm newborn because of immaturity of secretory mechanisms. The acid secretion is closely related to the development and maturity of the gastric mucosa; it is thus understandable that the amount of acid produced in the first 24 hours by the preterm neonate is less than that observed in the full term neonate. The gastric pH then persists close to neutrality for about 8-10 days after birth when a gradual lowering of pH together with an increased secretion of acids can be observed. Adult values are reached only at about 2 years of age.

It may be interesting to recall that concomitant with this relative achlorhydria there is a consistent hypergastrinemia. The relative achlorhydria may partially account for the higher bioavailability reported in the newborn for several penicillins as well as for the reduced absorption of acid compounds such as phenobarbitone, phenytoin and nalidixic acid.

Other factors which may play a variable role are: the relative immaturity of the intestinal mucosa, the gradual maturation of biliary function, a factor which may influence both the absorption of drugs as well as their disposition in those cases where enterohepatic recycling is implicated; the high level of β-glucuronidase activity present in the neonatal intestine; the variable colonization rate of the intestine by the microbial flora. In connection with the latter it may be worthwhile to remember that diet and developmental age may greatly influence both the nature of the micro-organisms as well as the colonization rate.

Because of the immaturity of all the above variables, it is understandable that in either the preterm or full term neonate drug bioavailability may be substantially modified.

The few data available on *rectal* absorption

indicate that in contrast with the to route, if a proper formulation is used, this route of administration may lead to a better bioavailability with highly reproducible results. Examples are diazepam and theophylline where by the use of rectal *solutions* peak plasma concentrations higher than the oral ones can be obtained within 15-30 minutes with minimal intersubject variability.

Intramuscular absorption

The absorption rate and efficiency of intramuscularly administered drugs are very variable in the neonate. Reasons for such variability are several.

As, previously mentioned the blood flow through the area where the drug is applied is an important factor. In the newborn there are progressive changes in the blood flow of various muscles due to maturation. Furthermore the muscle mass contains a higher percentage of water and the muscular concentrations useful in spreading the injected solution over a larger absorptive area may be relatively inefficient. In addition, the extreme peripheral vasomotor instability, the exaggerated vasoconstrictive response to exposure to an unduly cold environment, and the frequent presence of relative hypoxic conditions may be important modifiers.

Because of these factors intramuscular absorption in both the preterm and full term neonate is rather erratic depending on both physicochemical characteristics of the drug and on the maturational stage. It may be excellent as in the case of phenobarbital, delayed as in the case of diazepam or reduced as in the case of gentamicin and digoxin.

Percutaneous absorption

As previously noted percutaneous absorption is inversely related to the thickness of the stratum corneum and directly related to the degree of hydration. In the newborn, the stratum corneum is reduced and the degree of hydration is increased resulting in an increased percutaneous absorption which may be further augmented by the use of abrasive tapes frequently used for monitoring or therapeutic devices.

The reported toxicity of boric acid powders, hexachlorophene soaps and emulsions, salicylic acid ointments and napthaline stored clothes are good examples of increased percutaneous absorption.

Drug plasma protein binding and drug distribution

In the preterm neonate as well as in the full term newborn reduced drug binding to plasma proteins is well documented.

The decrease in drug plasma protein binding is due to the concurrence of several factors such as: a reduced total plasma protein concentration associated with qualitative differences in plasma protein content (there is a reduced albumin concentration together with persistance of fetal albumin showing lower affinity for drugs); a significantly lower concentration of gamma-globulins and lipoproteins; a high plasma concentration of unconjugated bilirubin and FFA which compete with highly bound acidic drugs at albumin binding sites; a relatively acidic blood pH (7.20-7.35) associated with a condition of relative hypoxemia (two factors which tend to reduce drug binding to proteins); and finally the possible presence of substances of maternal origin, capable of "competing" at the plasma protein binding sites. Another factor which may play an important role is the relative or total absence of protein Y, the major anion binding protein in the liver.

All the above factors may potentiate each other. For example, an undue exposure to a cold environment may condition an increase in plasma FFA and a slight decrease in blood pH, thus influencing the plasma levels of free, unconjugated, bilirubin which may rise because of displacement by FFA. High FFA levels, high unconjugated bilirubin and lower blood pH may lead to a further increase in the free fraction of highly albumin bound acidic drugs.

The importance of gamma-globulins for binding of non acidic compounds is now well accepted. In premature and full term newborns the already low level of gamma-globulins may be further decreased by insufficient dietary intake.

The reduced plasma protein binding of drugs together with the fact that in the newborn the various body compartments have different absolute and relative sizes as compared to adults may have a variable effect on drug distribution in various organs and tissues as well as on the apparent volume of distribution of drugs.

In the newborn, the total body water content is larger and the ratio of extracellular water to intracellular water is higher. The adipose tissue is scarce (about 15 % of b. w.) and contains less fat and more water. The skeletal muscle mass is also considerably reduced ($\sim$ 20-25 % of b. w.). The brain is much larger in relation to body weight. Its myelin content is lower. The cerebral blood flow is higher than in adults while other regional blood flows may be lower. Since it has been shown that for various lipophylic drugs, brain concentrations are flow dependent, it is not unlikely that the brain of neonates may be exposed to higher amount of liposoluble drugs.

Depending on the physicochemical properties of the drug, on the maturational stage, and on the physiological status of each given individual, the drug distribution to various tissues and organs may be rather variable with an increase or decrease in the apparent volume of distribution (AVD).

Drugs are in fact distributed between extracellular water and fat depots according to their lipid/water partition coefficient and to the relative perfusion of the various areas. The continuous modification of variables such as protein content and body compartment, together with the progressive haemodynamic changes with constant increase in organ perfusion and regional blood flow do strongly influence the distribution of therapeutic agents as well as their therapeutic effects.

From a practical point of view, we should remember that, because of the possibility of an altered AVD, a given drug plasma concentration in the preterm or full term neonate may be associated with a tissue/plasma ratio different from those normally encountered in adults.

For these reasons, the simple measurement of blood or plasma concentrations of drugs without information about variables such as blood pH, FFA and bilirubin level and protein content, etc., may be of little value in the course of therapeutic drug monitoring in neonates.

In such a situation, we cannot in fact extrapolate to neonates the values of therapeutic and/or toxic thresholds observed in either adults or children, because the observed plasma drug concentrations do not reflect the same amount of drug present at the site of action assumed from data in children and/or adults.

Drug metabolism

Most of the enzymatic activity responsible for drug metabolic degradation associated or not with the hepatic microsomal system is either depressed or reduced in the neonate.

Esterase activity. — Esterases are deficient at birth. Their activity is closely related to the developmental stage. In the premature newborn their rate is usually lower than in the full term neonate.

Reduced activity of acetylcholinesterases, acetylesterases and pseudocholinesterases have been described by several authors and their low levels may explain the relative long-lasting cardiorespiratory depression observed in newborns when drugs containing "ester-bonds" (*i. e.* local anaesthetics) are given to the mother during delivery. The increase in plasma esterase activity parallels that of the plasma proteins and full activity is reached only at 10-12 months of age.

Hepatic microsomal activity. — *In vitro* studies showing that "at term" cytochrome P.450 and NADPH-cytochrome C-reductase activities are about one-half of adult values are in good agreement with *in vivo* observations indicating that both in preterm and full term newborns the enzymatic activities catalyzing phase I biotransformation reactions may be significantly reduced. However, recent evidence indicates that the various metabolic activities do not reach maturation at the same time and that they may be differently influenced by the maturational process.

This may explain some of the "discrepancies" present in the literature when comparing data obtained with different drugs.

While hydroxylation rates appear in general as greatly depressed, dealkylation reactions appear to be less impaired. Compounds for which an impaired metabolic degradation has been documented include: acetanilid, amobarbital, phenobarbital, phenytoin, diazepam, mepivacaine, lidocaine, nortriptyline, phenylbutazone, salicylates, indomethacin, tolbutamide, nalidixic acid, furosemide and several sulpha drugs.

As discussed in more detail below, the situation may be completely different in the case of *in-utero* exposure to "inducing" agents, capable of increasing hepatic metabolic activity.

Considering phase II synthetic reactions, they also are unevenly reduced. In fact, while sulphate conjugation and glycine conjugation are present at titres comparable to those found in adults, the conjugations with glucuronic acid are considerably depressed and reach adult values only at 24-30 months of age.

The mechanisms regulating the development of metabolic activities in man are still unknown. Several hypotheses have been put forward in the last ten years. However, up to now none has been totally proven and it is most likely that several factors are implicated at the same time. Whatever may be the cause, it should be kept in mind that a reduced capability to metabolize drugs is constantly observed in prematures and full term newborns during the first 2 weeks of extra-uterine life. Such a stage is then followed in most cases by a dramatic increase in the metabolic rate of phase I reactions.

This very rapid switch from a situation where the metabolic rates are 1/5-1/3 of the adult one to a situation where metabolic rates are 2-6 times faster than in adults may have important therapeutic implication. We pass in fact from a clinical situation where the risk is that of *overdosing* to a situation where the risk is that of *underdosing*.

One exception to such a rapid switch is theophylline and the related xanthines for which the metabolic rates increase gradually and progressively up to 10-12 months of age.

RENAL DRUG EXCRETION

In the newborn, the kidney is anatomically and functionally immature and renal function is reduced. Furthermore, we encounter a situation of glomerular/tubular imbalance due to the more advanced maturational stage of glomerular function. Such an imbalance may persist up to 6 months of age.

The development and maturation of renal function depends essentially on two main factors: gestational age and the sequential changes in haemodynamics which take place in the first days of life.

A sudden increase in glomerular function is generally observed at about 34 weeks (2,000 g) and corresponds to the cessation of formation of new glomeruli. At birth, the glomerular filtration rate (GFR) is between 2-4 ml/min in full term neonates, but it may be as low as 0.6-0.8 ml/min in preterm newborns. The adaptive increase in GFR in the first days of life is greater in full term than in preterm babies and is due to several factors resulting in an increased renal blood flow and probable changes in the permeability of the glomerular membrane.

It has been shown that after 48-72 hours of extra-uterine life, GFR may be from 8-12 ml/min in full term newborns against 2-3 ml/min in the preterm infant.

Such a reduced GFR is not without effect on the excretion of drugs which depend on GFR for their elimination. Clearance values 10-30 times lower than those observed in adults have been described for several compounds (e. g. aminoglycosides, antibiotics, digoxin, indomethacin, furosemide, etc.).

The reduced GFR may be partially compensated in selected cases by a reduction in tubular resorption conditioned by either the low urinary pH or the "physiological" presence of proteins in the urinary filtrate which has been shown to exist in about 20-30 % of full and preterm newborns.

Tubular secretory function is even further reduced: low tubular functional capacities have been described for the transport of bicarbonate, glucose, phosphates and PAH. Such a low capacity of tubular transport does affect drugs too as documented by the very low clearance values usually observed in the newborn of drugs whose excretion depends upon tubular secretion (e. g. penicillins and several sulphonamides).

EFFECT OF VARIOUS PATHOLOGICAL STATES ON DRUG KINETICS IN THE NEWBORN

It is evident from the data reported in the previous pages that drug disposition in the preterm and full term newborn is significantly different from what may be observed in older children and adults. This is due mainly to the immaturity of most of the physiological variables conditioning drug kinetics. This situation can be further aggravated by the presence of severe pathological states.

Hypoxemic conditions, acute renal and gastrointestinal pathology, cardiac insufficiency, respiratory distress syndrome and modifications of normal haemodynamic development may have a considerable impact on drug kinetics and effects in the neonate.

Furthermore, all these clinical situations not only modify drug kinetics in a manner similar to that observed in adults in comparable conditions, but in addition they can interfere with the maturational processes of the different physiological variables conditioning drug kinetics.

In the following section, we will attempt to describe the possible impact on drug disposition of some of the more common and severe pathological situations encountered in the neonate. The available material on this topic is still rather poor or totally nonexistant. For these reasons, some of the assumptions described below are derived more from physiopathological considerations than from live concrete examples.

Absorption

Gastroenteritis, stetorrheas of preterm and full term newborns, insufficient dietary intake, cardiac insufficiency and hypoxic conditions are all situations where the absorptive process can be further reduced.

In the first three situations, causes for reduced absorption can be identified in an accelerated gastrointestinal transit time, an altered bile acid concentration with ileal dysfunction and bile acid loss.

In the case of hypoxemia and/or cardiac insufficiency it has been shown that intestinal motility may be markedly decreased. In addition, because of reduced arterial blood pressure and reduced cardiac output, the perfusion rate of the splanchnic area may be significantly decreased. This can lead to an œdematous state of the gastrointestinal mucosa resulting in reduced and/or delayed drug absorption.

Considering intramuscular administration any situation leading to vasoconstriction or to a reduction in systemic blood flow (as in the case of cardiocirculatory insufficiency, respiratory distress, etc.) may impair the absorptive process.

Drug protein binding and distribution

In situations such as respiratory distress syndrome, PDA, congenital cardiac defects, all characterized by reduced arterial blood pressure and modified tissue perfusion, drug distribution may be further modified and drug plasma protein binding further reduced because of a trend towards acidosis and the association with a lower dietary protein intake with a consequent further drop in plasma proteins. It should also be mentioned that "small for date" newborns may present excess of extracellular water, even lower protein levels and reduced gastrointestinal motility. This last factor may lead to stagnation of conjugated bilirubin in the intestinal lumen. Because of the elevated beta-glucuronidase activity in the newborn increased hydrolysis may occur with subsequent resorption and high plasma levels of unconjugated bilirubin competing with acidic drugs for plasma protein binding.

Blood pH variation of 0.20-0.25 which can be frequently observed in post-anoxic convulsive states may lead to important redistribution phenomena for compounds whose pKa (as in the case of phenobarbital) is close to the blood pH.

Another point which should be underlined is the fact that the threshold of response of the cerebral vasculature to ambient gases is much lower in the preterm and full term newborn. As a consequence, in the case of CNS acting drugs, higher concentrations may be attained in brain stem structures in situations of relative hypoxia or perinatal asphyxia. This is due to the fact that concomitantly with systemic hypotension preferential perfusion of brain stem structures occurs together with the reduction of total cerebral blood flow.

Drug biotransformation

All metabolic activities related to the microsomal enzymes may be significantly reduced in pathological states such as respiratory distress, cardiac insufficiency, hyperbilirubinemia and insufficient dietary intake. In these situations the clinical picture is accompanied by a more or less severe hypoxemia, a trend towards acidosis and a diminished hepatic perfusion, factors which all condition reduced liver enzyme activity.

Furthermore, the same factors may condition an increased free fraction of the drug with consequent higher drug concentration in the tissues. This may further complicate a situation characterized by a very reduced elimination rate.

Renal drug excretion

Any pathological state capable of reducing or altering renal haemodynamics may lead to a delay in the maturation of a function which, as described above, is already very poorly developed.

Situations such as perinatal anoxia, hypotensive states secondary to respiratory distress, diarrhea and dehydration may all lead to renal failure with a strong influence on drug renal elimination rates.

The newborn kidney is very sensitive to oxygen deprivation: depending on the duration of the hypoxic condition different effects may be observed. While a short lasting mild hypoxic episode may be followed (in hypocapnoeic conditions) by an increased diuresis and decreased tubular drug resorption and/or secretion, a longer lasting episode with persistant reduction in renal blood flow may involve glomerular function resulting in oliguria.

In all the above situations a further reduction in renal clearance should be expected for those drugs which are mainly eliminated via the kidney.

EFFECT OF "IN UTERO EXPOSURE TO DRUGS" ON THE MATURATION OF PHYSIOLOGICAL VARIABLES IMPORTANT FOR DRUG KINETICS

A consistent body of evidence indicates that drugs administered chronically to the mother during the last month of pregnancy may have several effects on the fetus and the newborn. Among these effects we wish to comment on the important variations in hepatic microsomal activity and in renal function which can be observed in cases of *in utero* exposure to certain therapeutic agents.

EFFECT OF "INDUCING AGENTS" ON NEONATAL DRUG METABOLISM

As previously noted "induction" may take place *in-utero* resulting in metabolic rates at birth similar to those which can be observed in 2-3 month old infants.

Barbiturates and anticonvulsant drugs are the most common example of inducing agents, but the effect can be observed with a large number of compounds and with "social" drugs as well (e. g. high consumption of caffeine and/or tobacco).

It may be interesting to recall that the various metabolic pathways may be stimulated and/or increased to different extents. This could partially explain some of the discrepancies that can be found in the literature on this topic. The basis for the difference in responses to inducing agents in the newborn, could be on the one hand the presence of different enzymes with a substrate specificity higher than currently thought; or on the other the presence of endogenous competitive inhibitors. The enzymatic systems responsible for drug metabolism do in fact catalyze the biotransformation of free fatty acids, bile acids and steroid hormones.

EFFECT OF KIDNEY FUNCTION

Recent studies indicate that at the renal level the transport system for weak organic acids and weak organic bases may increase its capacity in response to either a load or to repeated administration.

Several reports have shown that stimulation of renal tubular transport processes for xenobiotics as well as stimulation of water and electrolyte renal excretion is possible in the newborn following *in utero* exposure to the specific agent.

As in the case of drugs cleared by hepatic mechanisms prenatal drug administration may influence the rate of development of kidney function in the newborn. In selected cases unexpectedly high renal drug clearances may be encountered. Drugs for which such a phenomenon has been described include: oxacillin, sulphonamides, phenobarbital, ethachrynic acid, and several diuretics.

CONCLUSIONS

It is evident that any "standardized" approach to therapeutic regimens in the neonatal period may very easily lead to either under or overdosing in a large part of the treated population. Due to the unpredictable development of those physiological variables important for drug kinetics and to the superimposed pathological conditions, any meaningful prediction of doses and regimens becomes a very difficult task. In adult patients we can sometimes base our reasoning for correcting the dose on the presence of more or less severe side effects or on the delay of the therapeutic responses. In newborns we cannot have such an approach for practical and ethical reasons.

For each individual patient variables such as gestational and conceptional ages, days of extra-uterine life, previous exposure to drugs (*in utero* or during the first days of life), haemodynamic conditions, blood pH, etc., should be considered very carefully together with the actual developmental stage of the excretory organs. The knowledge and consideration of these parameters should be coupled with therapeutic drug monitoring in any situation at risk.

Therapeutic drug monitoring is currently the only safe and rational approach to the correct individualization of doses and dose regimens taking into consideration the variables mentioned above. For these reasons we believe that services of therapeutic drug monitoring should be available in each perinatal unit. This should not be regarded as experimentation but as an integral part of a rational individualized therapeutic approach to patients at high risk.

REFERENCES

I. — *General Reading on*
"Importance and Need of Information
on Drug Disposition in the Perinatal Period".

DANCIS (J.), HWANG (J. C.). — *Perinatal pharmacology Problems and priorities.* Raven Press Publ., New York, 1975.

MIRKIN (B. I.). — *Clinical pharmacology and therapeutics. A paediatric perspective.* Year Book Medical Publ. Inc., Chicago, 1978.

MORSELLI (P. L.). — Paediatric clinical pharmacology: routine monitoring or clinical trials? *In* GOUVEIA, TOGNONI and VAN DER KLEIJN (Eds). *Clinical Pharmacy and Clinical Pharmacology*, 277-287, Elsevier-North-Holland, Amsterdam, 1976 *b*.

SERENI (F.), PRINCIPI (N.). — Developmental pharmacology. *Annual Review of Pharmacology*, *8*, 453-466, 1968.

SHIRKEY (H.). — Therapeutic orphans. *J. Pediatr.*, *72*, 119-120, 1968.

SHIRKEY (H. C.). — Paediatric clinical pharmacology and therapeutics. *In* AVERY (Ed.). *Drug Treatment*, 2nd Ed., 100, Adis Press, Sydney and New York, Churchill Livingstone, Edinburgh, 1980.

STERN (L.). — Drug therapy in the perinatal period. *In* MORSELLI, GARATTINI and SERENI (Eds). *Basic Aspect of Perinatal Pharmacology*. Raven Press Publ., New York, 7-12, 1975.

YAFFE (S.), STERN (L.). — Clinical implication of perinatal pharmacology. *In* MARTIN B. L. (Ed.). *Perinatal Pharmacology and Therapeutics*. Academic Press, New York, 355-428, 1976.

WILSON (J. J.). — Pragmatic assessment of medicine available for young children and pregnant or breastfeeding women. *In* MORSELLI, GARATTINI, SERENI (Eds). *Basic Aspect of Perinatal Pharmacology*. Raven Press, New York, 411-421, 1975.

II. — *General Reading on Pharmacokinetics and Pharmacodynamics.*

ARIENS (E. J.). — *Molecular pharmacology:* the mode of action of biologically active compounds. Vol. 1. Academic Press Inc., New York, 1964.

BRODIE (B. B.), GILLETTE (J. R.). — *Handbook of experimental pharmacology. Concepts in biochemical pharmacology.* Vol. XXVIII. Parts I and II. Springer-Verlag, Berlin, 1971.

GARATTINI (S.), MORSELLI (P. L.). — *Interazioni tra farmaci.* 2nd Ed. Ferro, Ed., Milano, 1974.

GIBALDI (M.). — *Biopharmaceutics and clinical pharmacokinetics.* Lea and Febiger, Philadelphia, 1971.

GILLETTE (J. R.), MITCHELL (J. R.). — *Handbook of experimental pharmacology. Concepts in biochemical pharmacology.* Vol. XXVIII. Part III. Springer-Verlag, Berlin, 1975.

GOLDSTEIN (A.), ARONOW (L.), KALMAN (S. M.). — *Principles of drug action. The basis of pharmacology.* 2nd Ed. John Wiley and Sons Inc., New York, 1974.

LA-DU (B. N.), MANDEL (H. G.), WAY (E. L.). — *Fundamental of drug metabolism and disposition.* Williams and Wilkins, Baltimore, 1971.

MELMON (K. L.), MORELLI (H. F.). — *Clinical pharmacology. Basic Principles in Therapeutics.* 2nd Ed. MacMillan Publishing Co. Inc., New York, 1978.

ROWLAND (M.), TOZER (T. N.). — *Clinical pharmacokinetics. Concepts and applications.* Lea and Febiger, Philadelphia, 1980.

III. — *Selected Reading on Development of Physiological Variables Important for Drug Disposition in the Human Neonate.*

a) *General.*

DAVIS (J. A.), DOBBING (J.). — *The scientific foundation of paediatrics.* Heinemann, London, 1974.

MORSELLI (P. L.). — *Drug Disposition During Development.* Spectrum Inc., New York, 1977.

MORSELLI (P. L.). — Cinétique de distribution des médicaments chez le nouveau-né et l'enfant normal et pathologique. *Le Colloque de l'INSERM. Pharmacologie Périnatale.* Vol. 73, 92-128, INSERM, 1978.

MORSELLI (P. L.), FRANCO-MORSELLI (R.), BOSSI (L.). — Clinical pharmacokinetics in newborns and infants. Age-related differences and therapeutic implications. *Clin. Pharmacokinet.*, *8*, 485-527, 1980.

YAFFE (S. J.), JUCHAU (M. R.). — Perinatal pharmacology. *Ann. Rev. Pharmacol.*, *14*, 219-238, 1974.

WEBER (W. W.), COHEN (S. N.). — Aging effects and drugs in man. *In* GILLETTE, MITCHELL (Eds). *Concepts in Biochemical Pharmacology.* Vol. 28, 213-233, Springer, Berlin, 1975.

b) *Drug Absorption.*

BLUMENTHAL (I.), EBEL (V.), PILDES (R. S.). — Effect of posture on the pattern of stomach emptying in the newborn. *Paediatrics*, *63*, 532-536, 1979.

CAVELL (B.). — Gastric emptying in preterm infant. *Acta Paediatr. Scandin.*, *68*, 725-730, 1979.

GUPTA (M.), BRANS (Y. W.). — Gastric retention in neonates. *Paediatrics*, *62*, 26-29, 1978.

JANICK (J. S.), AKBAR (A. K.), BURRINGTON (J. D.), BURKE (G.). — Serum gastrin levels in infants and children. *Paediatrics*, *60*, 60-65, 1977.

HEIMANN (G.). — Enteral absorption and bioavailability in children in relation to age. *Europ. J. Clin. Pharm.*, *18*, 43-50, 1981.

LONG (S. S.), SWENSON (R. M.). — Development of anaerobic fecal flora in healthy newborn infant. *J. Pediatr.*, *91*, 298-301, 1977.

MURPHY (G. M.), SINGER (E.). — Bile acid metabolism in infants and children. *Gut*, *15*, 151-163, 1974.

SCHELINE (R. R.). — Drug metabolism by intestinal microorganism. *J. Pharmac. Sc.*, *57*, 2021-2028, 1968.

SMITH (C. A.). — *The physiology of the newborn infant.* And. Ed., 180-198, Thomas, Springfield, 1951.

TYRALA (F. F.), HILLMAN (L. S.), HILLMAN (R. F.), DODSON (W. E.). — Clinical pharmacology of hexachlorophene in newborn infants. *J. Pediatr.*, *91*, 481-486, 1977.

c) *Drug Plasma Protein Binding and Drug Distribution.*

EHRNEBO (M.), AGURELL (S.), JALLING (F.), BOREUS (I. O.). — Age differences in drug binding by plasma binding proteins: studies on human fœtuses, neonates and adults. *Europ. J. Clin. Pharmacol.*, *3*, 189-193, 1971.

FRIIS-HANSEN (B.). — Body water compartment in children: changes during growth and related changes in body composition. *Paediatrics*, *28*, 169-181, 1961.

KRASNER (J.), GIACOIA (G. P.), YAFFE (S. J.). — Drug-protein binding in the newborn infant. *Ann. New York Academy of Sciences*, *226*, 101-114, 1973.

KURZ, (H.), MAUSER-GASNBORN (A.), STICKEL (H. H.). — Differences in the binding of drugs to plasma proteins from newborn and adult man. I. *European Journal of Clinical Pharmacology*, *11*, 463-467, 1977.

KURZ (H.), MITCHELS (H.), STICKEL (H. H.). — Differences in the binding of drugs to plasma proteins from newborn and adult man. II. *European Journal of Clinical Pharmacology*, *11*, 469-472, 1977.

ØIE (S.), LEVY (G.). — Interindividual differences in the effect of drugs on bilirubin plasma binding in newborn infants and in adults. *Clin. Pharmacol. Therapeut.*, *21*, 627-632, 1977.

SETTERGREN (G.), LINDBLAD (B. S.), PERSSON (H. B.). — Cerebral blood flow and exchange of oxygen, glucose ketone bodies, lactate, pyruvate and aminoacids in infants. *Acta Paediatrica Scandinavica*, *65*, 343-353, 1976.

WALLACE (S.). — Altered plasma albumine in the newborn infant. *Brit. J. Clinical Pharmacol.*, *4*, 82-85, 1977.

WIDDOWSON (E. M.). — Changes in body proportions and composition during growth. In: *Scientific Foundations of Pediatrics*, Heineman, London, 153, 1974.

ZOPPI (G.), ZAMBONI (G.), SIVIERO (M.), BELLINI (P.), LANZONI CANCELLIERI (M.). — γ-globulin level and dietary protein intake during the first year of life. *Paediatrics*, 62, 1010-1018, 1978.

d) *Drug Metabolism.*

ARANDA (J. V.), MACLEOD (S. M.), RENTON (K. W.), EADE (N. R.). — Hepatic microsomal drug oxidation and electron transport in newborn infants. *Journal of Pediatrics*, 85, 534-542, 1974.

BOREUS (L. O.), JALLING (B.), KALLBERG (N.). — Clinical pharmacology of phenobarbital in the neonatal period. In MORSELLI, GARRATTINI, SERENI (Eds). *Basic and Therapeutic Aspects of the Perinatal Pharmacology*, 331-340, Raven Press, New York, 1975.

COOK (D. R.), WINGARD (I. B.), TAYLOR (F. H.). — Pharmacokinetics of succinylcholine in infants, children and adults. *Clinical Pharmacology and Therapeutics*, 20, 493-498, 1976.

DUTTON (G. J.). — Developmental aspects of drug conjugation with special reference to glucuronidation. *Annual Review of Pharmacology and Toxicology*, 18, 17-35, 1978.

ECOBICHON (D. J.), STEPHENS (D. S.). — Perinatal development of human blood esterases. *Clinical Pharmacology and Therapeutics*, 14, 11-17, 1973.

LEVY (G.), KHANNA (N. N.), SODA (D. M.), TSUZUKI (O.), STERN (L.). — Pharmacokinetics of acetaminophen in the human neonate: formation of acetaminophen glucuronide and sulfate in relation to plasma bilirubin concentration and D-glucaric acid excretion. *Pediatrics*, 55, 818-825, 1975.

MIHALY (G. W.), MOORE (R. G.), THOMAS (J.), TRIGGS (G. J.), THOMAS (D.), SHANKS (C. A.). — The pharmacokinetics and metabolism of the anilide local anaesthetics in neonates. 1. Lignocaine. *European Journal of Clinical Pharmacology*, 13, 143-152, 1978.

MILLER (R. P.), ROBERTS (R. J.), FISCHER (C. J.). — Acetaminophen elimination in neonates, children and adults. *Clinical Pharmacology and Therapeutics*, 19, 284-294, 1976.

MORSELLI (P. L.), PRINCIPI (N.), TOGNONI (G.), REALI (E.) et al. — Diazepam elimination in premature and full term infants. *J. of Perinatal Medicine*, 1, 133-141, 1973.

MORSELLI (P. L.). — Clinical pharmacokinetics in the neonate. *Clinical Pharmacokinetics*, 1, 81-98, 1976.

NEIMS (A. H.), MANCHESTER (D. K.). — Drug disposition in the developing human. In Mirkin (Ed.) *Clinical Pharmacology and Therapeutics. A pediatric perspective*, 35-48 (Year Book Medical Publishers, Chicago and London, 1978).

ZSIGMOND (E. K.), DOWNS (J. R.). — Plasma cholinesterase activity in newborns and infants. *Canadian Anaesthesists' Society Journal*, 18, 278-285, 1971.

e) *Renal Drug Excretion.*

ARANT (B. S.). — Developmental patterns of renal functional maturation compared in the human neonate. *Journal of Pediatrics*, 92, 705-712, 1978.

BARNETT (H. I.), HARE (W. K.), McNAMARA (N.), HARE (R. S.). — Influence of postnatal age on kidney function of premature infants. *Proceedings of the Society for Experimental Biology and Medicine*, 69, 55-67, 1948.

BRAUNLICH (H.). — Kidney development-drug elimination mechanisms. *In* MORSELLI (Ed.). *Drug Disposition During Development*, 89-100, Spectrum, New York, 1977.

GLADTKE (F.), HEIMANN (G.). — The rate of development of elimination functions in kidney and liver of young infants. In MORSELLI, GARATTINI, SERENI. *Basic and Therapeutic Aspects of Perinatal Pharmacology*, 393, Raven Press, New York, 1975.

GUIGNARD (J. P.), TORRADO (A.), DA CUNHA (O.), GAUTIER (F.). — Glomerular filtration rate in the first three weeks of life. *Journal of Pediatrics*, 87, 268-272, 1975.

HOUSTON (I. B.), ŒTLIKER (O.). — The growth and the development of the kidneys. *In* DAVIS, DOBBING (Eds.). *Scientific Foundations of Paediatrics*, 297-307, Heinemann, London, 1974.

LEAKE (R. D.), TRYGSTAD (C. W.). — Glomerular filtration rate during the period of adaptation to extra-uterine life. *Paediatric Research*, 11, 959-962, 1975.

IV. — *Selected Reading on Effect of Pathological conditions on drug kinetics in the neonate.*

ARANT (B. S.). — Developmental patterns of renal functional maturation compared in the human neonate. *Journal of Pediatrics*, 92, 705-712, 1978.

BARBARA (L.), LAZZARI, RODA (A.) et al. — Serum bile acids in newborns and children. *Paediatric Research*, 14, 1222-1225, 1980.

BELL (M. J.), SHACKELFORD (P. G.), FEIGIN (R. D.), TERNBERB (J. Y.), BROTHERTON (T.). — Alterations in gastrointestinal microflora during antimicrobial therapy for necrotizing enterocolitis. *Paediatrics*, 63, 425-428, 1979.

COHEN (M. D.), RAEBURN (J. A.), DEVINE (J.) et al. — Pharmacology of some oral penicillins in the newborn infant. *Arch. Dis. Child.*, 50, 230-234, 1975.

DAUBER (I. M.), KRAUS (A. N.), SYMCHYCH (P. S.), AULT (P. A. M.). — Renal failure following perinatal anaxia. *Journal of Pediatrics*, 88, 851-855, 1976.

DU SUICH (P.), McLEAN (A. J.), LALKA (D.), ERILL (S.), GIBALDI (M.). — Pulmonary diseases and drug kinetics. *Clin. Pharmacokin.*, 3, 257-266, 1978.

JONES (A. S.), JAMES (F.), BLAND (H.), CROSHONG (T.). — Renal failure in the newborn. *Clinical Paediatrics*, 18, 286-291, 1979.

KRISHNASWAMY (K.). — Drug metabolism and pharmacokinetics in malnutrition. *Clinical pharmacokinetics*, 3, 216-240, 1978.

LOU (H. C.), LASSEN (N. A.), FRIIS-HANSEN (B.). — Low cerebral blood flow in hypotensive perinatal distress. *Acta Neurologica Scandinavica*, 56, 343-352, 1977.

MORSELLI (P. L.), VIBERT (M.), MONIN (P.), ANDRE (M.), SANJUAN (M.), ROVEI (V.). — Surveillance du taux plasmatique du phénobarbital chez le nouveau-né. In *Les Colloques de l'INSERM du Développement*. INSERM juin 1979. Vol. 89, 509-518, 1980.

MORSELLI (P. L.). — Effects of various pathological states on drug pharmacokinetics in the newborn. In *1st European Congress of Biopharmaceutics and Pharmacokinetics*. Vol. III, *Pharmacocinétique Clinique*, 34-42, 1981.

RAHILLY (P. M.). — Effects of 2 % carbon doxide, 0.5 % carbon dioxide and 100 % oxygen on cranial blood flow of the human neonate. *Paediatrics*, 66, 685-689, 1980.

SONDHEIMER (J. M.), HAMILTON (J. R.). — Intestinal function in infants with severe congenital heart disease. *Journal of Pediatrics*, *92*, 572-578, 1978.

VOLPE (J. J.). — Cerebral blood flow in the newborn infant: relation to hypoxic-ischemic brain injury and periventricular hemorrhage. *J. Ped.*, *94*, 170-173, 1979.

VERT (P.), BROQUAIRE (M.), LEGAGNEUR (M.), MORSELLI (P. L.). — Pharmacokinetics of furosemide in the neonatal period. *Eur. J. Clin. Pharmacol.*, *22*, 39-45, 1982.

V. — *Selected Reading on Effect of* in utero *exposure to drugs on the maturation of physiological variables important for drug kinetics.*

BRAUNLICH (H.). — Excretion of drugs during postnatal development. *Pharmac. Ther.*, *12*, 229-320, 1981.

FRENZEL (J.), BRAUNLICH (H.), SCHRAMM (D.) et al. — Effect on maturation of kidney function in newborn infants of repeated administration of water and electrolytes. *Europ. J. Clin. Pharm.*, *11*, 317-320, 1977.

HOOK (J. B.), HEWITT (W. R.). — Development of mechanisms for drug excretion. *Amer. J. Med.*, *62*, 497-505, 1977.

MORSELLI (P. L.), MANDELLI (M.), TOGNONI (G.) et al. — Drug interaction in the human fœtus and in the newborn infant. *In* MORSELLI, GARRATTINI, COHEN (Eds). *Drug Interactions*, 259-270, Raven Press, New York, 1974.

MORSELLI (P. L.). — Clinical pharmacokinetics in neonates. *Clin. Pharmacokin.*, *1*, 81-96, 1976.

SERENI (F.), MANDELLI (M.), PRINCIPI (M.) et al. — Induction of drug monitoring metabolizing enzymes activities in the human fetus and in the newborn infant. *Enzyme*, *15*, 318-329, 1973.

SCHWARTZ (G. J.), HEGGY (T.), SPITZER (A.). — Subtherapeutic dicloxacillin levels in a neonate possible mechanisms. *Journal of Pediatrics*, *89*, 310-312, 1976.

11

Infants of chronically ill mothers

Paul VERT and Monique ANDRE

Therapeutic progress has permitted pregnancy in women who formerly were very ill and who sometimes died as a result of it. The first example described of fetal repercussions of a chronic maternal disease was that of the infant of a diabetic mother. Numerous other diseases as well as drug addiction, which remained little known for a long time can now be added. The experience of neonatal units reveals that infants of chronically ill mothers make up an important group of neonates exposed to multiple risks. Long term studies of the development of these infants frequently show a poor prognosis.

MODALITIES AND PERIODS OF RISK

Although some studies show a possible risk of teratogenesis when the father is exposed to certain chemical substances (anesthesiologists, dentists...) [130 *bis*] this chapter will be limited to the relationship between maternal disease and development.

The embryo and fetus are theoretically exposed to the effects of both the maternal disease and the drugs used in its treatment. They thus unwillingly receive drugs or poisons which almost always cross the placenta to a large degree, leading to a kind of pollution of the developing organism. The abnormalities of development during organogenesis cause embryopathies during the first three months of pregnancy and particularly from the 20th to the 60th day. During the last two trimesters, fetopathy can take place by inducing growth retardation, homogenous or limited to specific organs [132].

The birth of an infant of a sick mother presents all the risks of a possible handicap induced by anomalous development (fetal distress) and by the effect of drugs on neonatal adaptation. There is increasing data showing that these infants can suffer from long term developmental disorders due, at least in part, to the alterations in intra-uterine environment. However, it is sometimes difficult in these long term assessments to differentiate the effects of a disturbed post-natal environment: starvation, child neglect, deleterious effects of an unbalanced psychosocial environment.

VULNERABLE FUNCTIONS
IN NEONATES

Birth suddenly deprives the infant of the means of eliminating drugs and their metabolites into the maternal circulation by way of the placenta. The infant must face its physiological adaptation overloaded with inherited drugs and handicapped by its own immature metabolic and excretory functions.

Cerebral function can be depressed by neurosedatives, giving disorders of respiratory drive and swallowing which may lead to apnea and aspiration. Some such infants show delayed weight gain because of poor sucking. These drugs often act as muscle relaxants inducing hypotonia (benzodiazepines) and disorders of visceral motility such as urine retention and transient ileus.

The neonatal haemodynamic pattern following the changes in pulmonary and systemic vascular tone can be disturbed by vasodilator and hypotensive drugs, such as procaine derivatives and beta-blockers [20]. Renal function is also affected by these vasomotor alterations, as well as by diuretics [145] and certain nephrotoxic drugs (aminoglycosides, indomethacin).

Thermoregulation is a result of the operation of very fragile energy mechanisms. Hypothermia may be due to neuro-sedatives and ganglioplegics such as chlorpromazine and pethidine, which are used to induce hypothermia in adults.

The positive or negative effects of drugs on the **transport, metabolism and excretion of bilirubin** are detailed elsewhere in this volume (chapter 36).

Coagulation defects may cause serious hemorrhages through a deficiency of vitamin K dependant clotting factors (antiepileptics, dicoumarins, moxalactam) or through platelet disturbances, e. g. thrombocytopenia due to thiazides, or an alteration of platelet aggregability by prostaglandin inhibitors (acetylsalicylic acid, indomethacin).

Antibiotics, which alter the physiological process of bacterial colonization, select out resistant pathogenic bacterial strains, exposing the neonate to the risk of infection.

In practice, one finds situations complicated by the simultaneous effects of several drugs—for example, arterial hypotension and respiratory depression... The wide range of chronic maternal diseases capable of affecting the development or adaptation of the infant are suggested in Table I. Only the most common situations, which are not described in other chapters, are presented here.

TABLE I. — MATERIAL CONDITIONS AND INTOXICATIONS WHICH AFFECT THE CHILD

Endocrine disorders — Diabetes mellitus. — Thyroid disorders. — Hyper and hypoparathyroid states.	*Drug abuse* — Heroin and other narcotics. — Alcohol. — Tobacco.
Neuropsychological states — Epilepsy. — Psychological instability (lithium).	*Cardiopulmonary diseases* — Cardiopathy. — Hypertension. — Asthma.
Muscle defects — Steinert's disease. — Myasthenia	
Immunological conditions Systemic Lupus Erythematosus. Thrombocytopenia. Immune depression: kidney transplant.	*Gastro-intestinal conditions* — Cholestasis.
Maternal infections	
Intoxications Carbon monoxide.	

INFANTS OF EPILEPTIC MOTHERS

About 3 out of 1,000 pregnant women are epileptic. Attention was first drawn to their infants by hemorrhagic problems [2], and then by the increased incidence of malformations [89, 131]. Numerous studies have confirmed these risks and reported anomalies of post-natal development [33, 66]. An entire volume devoted to the problems of pregnancy and of infants of epileptic mothers has been published [74].

Intra-uterine growth seems normal if assessed by weight and size, but the head circumference (HC) is often small. Some cases of microcephaly had been reported, but, in our experience 30 % of cases had a head circumference $\leqslant -2$ standard deviations compared with standard growth charts. This was accompanied by an enlarged fontanelle and morphological signs of a small skull which can be measured on X-ray. Table II [9]. All mothers of infants with HC < -2 SD had been treated with phenobarbitone alone or together with other drugs. The blood level of phenobarbitone at birth in a group of infants with small HC was

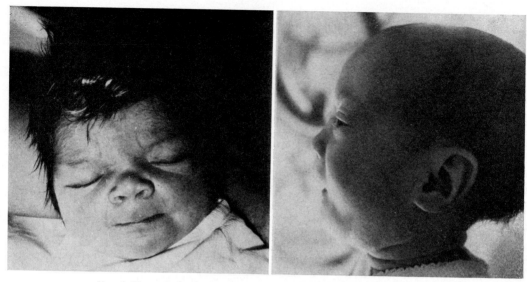

Fig. I-66. — *Left: the facial features of the child of an epileptic mother.*
Right: typical profile of fetal alcohol syndrome.

TABLE II. — Cephalic morphology.
CEM: child of epileptic mother

	CEM	Controls	P
Fontanelle area mm² ± SD [31] . . .	560 ± 360	336 ± 141	< 0.02
Intercaruncular space mm ± SD . . .	23.6 ± 2.5	21.5 ± 2.2	< 0.001
Austin's and Gooding's Index [9] . . .	395 ± 13.5	312 ± 16.5	< 0.001

significantly higher than for those with HC ⩾ −2 SD. The phenobarbitone carbamazepine association seems to induce an even greater proportion of retarded cephalic growth. The increased frequency of retarded head circumferential growth has been confirmed by other groups [19, 52]. Echographic measurements have shown that in some cases, the evolution of the biparietal diameter is already retarded at 21 weeks of gestation. These findings could be correlated with alterations in cerebral protein synthesis observed in rats treated with hydantoins and barbiturates [77, 135].

The incidence of congenital malformations is controversial, depending on the epidemiological methods used. For some, it is about two to three times higher that in control populations (6 to 7 % instead of 2 %) [68, 73, 148], for others, whilst certainly existing, the increase is no greater

than 0.26 %. Both Janz and Bossi confirm the increased risk by putting together the data from 25, and 48 studies respectively concerning several thousand infants of epileptic mothers [19] Table III.

TABLE III. — Congenital malformations found in 9,540 neonates of treated epileptic mothers. Review of 48 studies published between 1964 and 1981 (L. Bossi) [19].

Malformations	Number	⁰/₀₀ Live births
Facial or auricular abnormalities .	168	17.6
Cleft lip and/or palate. . .	155	16.2
Cardiac malformations	169	17.7
Ventricular septal defect. . .	51	5.3
Skeletal abnormalities	217	22.7
Digit or nail hypoplasia. . .	68	7.1
Clubbed foot	60	6.3
Congenital hip dislocation . .	51	5.3
CNS abnormalities	74	7.8
Microcephaly	30	3.1
Hydrocephaly	11	1.1
Meningomyelocele	14	1.5
Gastro-intestinal malformations .	86	9.0
Inguinal Herniae	37	3.9
Genito-urinary abnormalities . .	88	9.2

Hill found up to 19 % major congenital defects in infants of epileptic mother. The most frequent malformations were cleft lip and palate which could increase to 2 % (risk multiplied by 9 to 16) and congenital heart defects such as ventricular septal defect, Fallot's tetralogy, hypoplasia of the left heart, with an incidence ranging from 2 to 3,5 %. Dislocated hip, club foot and anomalies of the neural tube are also more frequent. For neural tube defects attention has recently been focused on sodium valproate as a possible cause [117 *bis*]. Malformations of the extremities with hypoplasia of the distal phalanges and nails have been described as the "Fetal hydantoin syndrome" [61].

This syndrome also includes more or less marked facial anomalies: hypertelorism, epicanthal folds, palpebral ptosis, flat nasal bridge sometimes associated with a short nose (Fig. I-66). The scalp may be extended in front and behind the low-set ears and there may be a hypoplasic mandible with retrognathism [128]. These signs are found alone or associated in about 12 % of cases; they are also described in infants of mothers treated with phenobarbitone [17]. Measurements show a significant widening of intercaruncular and interorbital spaces (Table II).

The debate is still open concerning the responsibility of drugs in malformative or other alterations of prenatal development. It is difficult to separate the genetic and environmental factors also associated with epilepsy, and particularly the socio-economic level. However, more and more experimental data confirm the possible teratogenic role of various anti-epileptic agents in animals: phenytoin, phenobarbitone, trimethadione. Amongst the arguments incriminating anti-epileptics, there are:

— the greater incidence of malformations in infants of treated epileptics compared with non-treated epileptic mothers [73],
— the higher blood levels of drugs in mothers giving birth to malformed infants [30],
— the increased risk in cases of polychemotherapy.

The hemorrhagic risk reported as early as 1942 [49] is due to a deficit in vitamin K dependant clotting factors (prothrombin, II, proconvertin, VII, anti-hemophilic factor B, IX, and Stuart factor, X). Phenobarbitone and diphenylhydantoin can both be responsible for this occurrence which has been experimentally reproduced in cats. This "hemorrhagic disease" induced by anticonvulsants can also be a source of hematomas and other forms of neonatal hemorrhage [146]. In our study, 27 % of children born to epileptic mothers had a prothrombin level below 20 % with control findings of 42 ± 18 % (± 1 SD) at birth. Out of 115 infants

there were 8 cases of serious hemorrhage, 5 hepatic hematomas, one intracranial hemorrhage with mild cerebral palsy, and two gastro-intestinal hemorrhages. The prevention of this risk by giving 20 mg of vitamin K_1 orally every day, during the last two weeks of pregnancy led to a mean prothrombin level of 90 % in 14 children of epileptic mothers at birth.

Neonatal neurological abnormalities comprise the depressive effects of drugs followed by the effects of their withdrawal. The drepressive effects are characterized by apnea, hypotonia and poor sucking. These are explained by blood levels of anti-epileptic drugs in the child similar to those of the mother at the time of birth which remain steady for several days. The withdrawal syndrome is comparable to that of infants of drug addicted mothers, although less severe. The infants present with signs of irritability, fine tremors, myoclonia and muscular hypertonia, crying, voracity, vomiting, and delay in weight gain. The EEG shows a somewhat poor basal activity with small fast spikes, in short fits. The sleep pattern is normal. In our experience, the withdrawal syndrome is more frequent in infants with a HC < — 2 DS (12 out of 22) than in those with HC ⩾ to — 1 SD (11 out of 52). If one compares infants of 39 and 40 weeks gestational age, the mean head circumference is 32.6 ± 1.4 cm in the presence of withdrawal symptoms, and 33.9 ± 1.32 cm in their absence (p < 0.01). The association of withdrawal symptoms, small head circumference and electro-encephalographic anomalies suggests the presence of brain damage.

Postnatal development.

Somatic growth. — In our study, 80 infants were followed for 6 months to 6 years. The measurements, compared with those of normal French children, showed retarded growth ⩽ — 2 SD, more often in their weight (18 cases) and head circumference (20 cases) than in their height (10 cases): see Table IV. Hypotrophy appears during the first three months of life, the growth patterns then remaining in the same growth percentile range. The small head circumference at birth is a risk criterion for development, as out of 18 hypotrophic infants over 6 months of age, 14 had HC ⩽ — 2 SD, and among 27 infants with a small head circumference reexamined 6 months or more later, 13 were still severely growth retarded.

Psychomotor development, evaluated according to the criteria of Brunet-Lezine and of the Denver

TABLE IV. — Postnatal development of children born of epileptic mothers. Head circumference at birth and subsequent risk for growth retardation in 80 children followed up at 6 months to 6 years of age.

Birth HC	N=80	Growth		
		Weight ≤ −2 SD	HC ≤ −2 SD	Height ≤ −2 SD
> −2 SD	52	4 7.6 %	7 13.4 %	5 9.6 %
≤ −2 SD	27	14 51.8 %	13 48.1 %	5 18.5 %

Developmental Test, shows a development quotient (DQ) below 90 in 33 % of cases (< 80 in 7 %). Although it is difficult to know what is due to antenatal drug exposure and what is due to the post-natal environment, this proportion of more or less retarded infants warrants appropriate screening measures and guidance. Here again, the small head circumference at birth (< − 2 SD) indicates a risk as it involves almost half the infants with a DQ below 90 (Table V). Similar findings concerning the retarded skull development (13 %) of children with DQ < 90 (26 %) have been reported by Hill et al. These authors report that infants of epileptic mothers present with learning difficulties in particular those of language, two or three times greater than in control groups. Finally, 35 % of the children of this series needed special education, versus 8 % in the control group [67].

Hill studied the risk factors of these learning problems and identified intra-uterine growth retardation, growth deficiency in the first months, the presence of a major malformation, 9 or more minor malformations, and polychemotherapy associating hydantoins and phenobarbitone.

Experimental data concerning the long term development of animals exposed to antiepileptics in utero are still scarce. Gupta and Yaffe have shown anomalies in pubertal development and in fertility in rats exposed to phenobarbitone in utero [56, 57].

Despite the uncertainty and arguments about the mechanism of the observed problems, the infant of an epileptic mother is a matter of concern to the physician before, as well as after birth.

INFANTS OF ALCOHOLIC MOTHERS

Idiocy due to parental alcoholism was part of the classic descriptions of the end of the 19th century. Authors at the time attributed the deleterious effects of alcohol to damage of genetic inheritance affecting either the father or the mother. However in 1888, Combemale wrote his thesis at Montpellier on the effects of "absinthe", given to pregnant bitches, on the antenatal development of the puppies. In 1900 Nicloux showed that blood alcohol levels were identical in the mother and the neonate. In 1957, Rouquette and in 1968 Lemoine, described the major symptoms of infants of alcoholic mothers. In 1973, Jones gave the name "fetal alcohol syndrome" to the alcoholic embryo-fetopathy.

In addition to the severe alteration of development resulting from alcoholic intoxication, we must

TABLE V. — Head circumference at birth, risk for growth retardation and mental retardation during development

Psychomotor Level	N	Birth HC < −2 SD	Growth	
			Weight ≤ −2 SD	HC ≤ −2 SD
DQ ≥ 90	53	8 15.1 %	2 3.7 %	5 9.4 %
DQ < 90	27	12 44.4 %	14 51.8 %	16 59.2 %
P		< 0.01	< 0.001	< 0.001

consider the difficulties due to episodic or moderate intoxication, in particular malformations and behavioural anomalies. The incidence of female alcoholism is difficult to evaluate and certainly varies with geography and social habits [78]. For the fetal alcohol syndrome, the published incidence varies between 1.3 to 5 per 1,000 births [34]. It usually involves poor mothers living in economically deprived conditions, poly-intoxicated (wine, beer, tobacco, coffee). Many already have neurological or major hepatic symptoms from alcoholism. These women have numerous pregnancies and often neglect prenatal care. Blood tests show hypochromic anemia, alterations of hepatic function, a rise in gamma-glutamyl-transferase, and alcohol levels more than or equal to 1.5 g/litre. Poor weight gain during pregnancy and even weight loss, are suggestive signs. Premature delivery occurs in nearly one third of cases. The premature or full term infants are often growth retarded, their weight diminishing with parity [34].

The fetal alcohol syndrome comprises intra-uterine growth retardation affecting all measurements [104]. In the presence of unexplained microcephaly in a neonate this etiology must be considered. Cranio-facial dysmorphia is comprised of shrinking of palpebral fissures, hypoplasia of the middle part of the face, flat nasal bridge, shortening of the nose, lengthening of the upper lip with a long and badly designed philtrum (Fig. I-66). The mouth is large with falling commissures, the line of Cupid's bow is effaced, and the lips are thin. Micro-retrognathism can also be present. More rarely one finds frontal hirsutism, synophrism, anti-mongoloid obliqueness of the eyelids, ptosis, and epicanthal folds. The ears can be badly rimmed and low-set. These features have been compared with the anti-convulsant dysmorphia, although in the latter case, the signs are more discreet and rarer. The associated malformations include cardiac defects, particularly septal defects, anomalies of the skeleton, dislocated hip, joint ankyloses, thoracic deformation, and hypoplasia of the fingers and nails. Cleft palate, spina bifida, multiple tuberous hemangiomas and anomalies of the external genital organs are also possible. Amongst the visceral anomalies are diaphragmatic herniae, renal malformations and pyloric stenosis. The possibility of ocular anomalies, and particularly of the retinal vessels, are not rare [134].

Neonatal adaptation is often abnormal, with a high frequency of low Apgar scores; withdrawal symptoms appear at 6 to 12 hours of life [114, 133]. Tremors, muscular hypertonia, hyperacusis, apnea and convulsions are possible. As alcohol is a good inducer of hepatic enzymes, there is no hyperbilirubinemia.

Infants presenting with this syndrome have a poor prognosis, as much for growth as for mental development. Physical development often shows a deficiency of -2 to -3 standard deviations compared with normal infants. Retarded weight gain is obvious from the first days of life.

Mental retardation is often impressive with a very low intellectual quotient, averaging 65 according to Dehaene and Streissguth. The extremely perturbed environment makes it difficult to evaluate what is due to alcohol itself.

Pathological analysis of the brains of these infants shows major alterations of morphogenesis with heterotopia (abnormal cellular migration) constituting an aberrant neuroglial layer on the surface of the cortex [26].

The possible effects of regular consumption of alcohol by pregnant women who are not chronic alcoholics has been studied prospectively [105]. The studies distinguish between "heavy" drinkers, who absorb 30 to 48 g of pure alcohol a day, and moderate or occasional drinkers. These studies tend to show that heavy drinkers expose their infants to a degree of growth retardation, and a significantly high incidence of stillbirths (25 $^o/_{oo}$ versus 9 $^o/_{oo}$ in the control population). In a study in Boston, Ouellette found a 32 % incidence of congenital anomalies (major and minor) in the infants of heavy drinkers as opposed to 14 % in moderate drinkers and 9 % in occasional drinkers. This suggests a relationship between the dose of alcohol and the response. In a study in Seattle, the behaviour of infants was compared, according to the alcohol consumption of the mothers, using the Brazelton score [133]. The infants of heavy drinkers scored badly in habituation and had weak alertness responses. Landesman and Dwyer found that neonates exposed to alcohol showed: (1) increased body tremors, (2) eyes opened for longer periods, (3) increased head turning to the left (an atypical position in neonates), (4) increased hand-to-mouth behavior, (5) body activity of diminished vigor. In the longer term, mental and motor development can be significantly altered [133].

Experimentation has reproduced the mechanism of fetal alcoholism on development and malformations [43] and has shown an alteration in the placental transfer of amino-acids such as valine, alanine, leucine, lysine, etc. [65].

It is important to note that a woman whose infant has suffered from an intra-uterine exposure to alcohol, can have a perfectly normal infant in another pregnancy if removed from all intoxication.

THE SMOKING HABIT

The smoking habit has become more and more common in women; in Western countries, about a quarter of unborn children are exposed to the effects of tobacco *in utero*. Amongst the numerous substances coming from tobacco, likely to affect the fetus, the best studied are carbon monoxide, nicotine, hydrocyanic acid which is transformed into thiocyanate, enzyme inducers such as 3 methyl-cholanthrene and benzopyrene, and the carcinogens.

Studies show that the incidence of **prematurity** rises with the quantity of cigarettes smoked [4, 32, 47, 112]. The risk increases from 50 to over 100 %. In a study of 5,000 pregnancies in the city of Nancy in 1972, the prematurity rate ranged from 5.1 % in non smokers to 13.2 % when the mothers smoked 20 or more cigarettes a day. Naeye has shown a rise in the incidence of placenta praevia (+ 143 %), of abruptio placentae (+ 72 %) and large placental infarcts (+ 37 %), all complications capable of having serious effects on the fetus and neonate. The frequency of these complications, mainly due to poor placental perfusion, was influenced both by the length and the degree of the addiction during pregnancy.

Fetal growth retardation affects weight, length and head circumference [90, 92, 112]. In a series of 55 infants born to mothers smoking 20 or more cigarettes a day, we found a mean deficit of 440 g for weight, 2.8 cm for length and 1.6 cm for head circumference compared to standard growth charts. The association of smoking with toxemia is known to induce severe growth retardation. There is no data in the literature on the bone development of these infants; however, in our study, we found bone growth to be significantly retarded [32].

Naye showed that women who smoked during a first pregnancy and then stopped during a second one, had smaller infants when they had smoked, which would seem to incriminate tobacco. This could be the effect of a chronic relative hypoxia from carbon monoxide which alters maternal and fetal oxygen transport. The level of carboxyhemoglobin at birth in the infants of mothers who smoke can reach 10 % [11]. It is in reaction to this chronic hypoxemia that the infants of mothers who smoke are born with a significantly higher hematocrit, similar to infants of mothers living at high altitudes [40]. Nicotine, by its powerful vaso-constrictive action reduces the utero-placental blood flow,

and could, by this mechanism, also be the cause of growth retardation.

The role of thiocyanate produced by the detoxification of cyanide has been implicated because its metabolism interferes with vitamin B_{12}, which is low in the blood of mothers who smoke. The blood level of thiocyanate, which is identical at birth in the infant and mother, is a good indicator of the severity of the smoking habit [91].

The risk of malformation is controversial. Some authors have found an increased incidence of cleft lip and palate [46], of cardiac defects [81, 98], anencephaly or malformations in general. The interlocking with other toxic or nutritional factors makes the interpretation of these facts uncertain and sometimes questionable [122, 152], deserving further investigation.

The early neonatal adaptation of these infants is related above all to their state of prematurity or hypotrophy, or both. The importance of hyperbilirubinemia is reduced by the effect of the enzyme inducers of tobacco smoke, such as 3-methyl-cholanthrene [103]. Although no withdrawal syndrome has been described for the infants or mothers who smoke, we have noticed hyperexcitability with tremors, crying and feeding difficulties in a quarter of these children with no other explanation.

Mothers who smoke and breastfeed can transmit derivates of tobacco in this way to their infants. Rare cases of digestive difficulties such as feeding problems, vomiting or diarrhea, attributed to nicotine ingestion, have been reported.

The long term effects of antenatal exposure to the risks of tobacco are difficult to evaluate, because these infants remain "passive smokers" after their birth. However, an increase in the incidence of sudden death has been noted [15, 97], and later in childhood, a greater frequency of behavioural problems such as hyperactivity or learning difficulties with dyslexia, has been observed.

The troubling question of the risk of malignancies occuring as a result of the numerous carcinogens present in tobacco crossing the placenta, has been raised. Animal experiments have given a positive reply, but the substantiality of this danger has not yet been established in man [46].

INFANTS OF MOTHERS
TREATED WITH LITHIUM

The teratogenic effects of lithium in mammals have been well demonstrated by Szabo [136].

From the beginning of the use of this product in the treatment of manic-depressive psychosis, the question of its harmlessness was raised. The register of "Lithium babies" opened by Schou showed a moderate increase in the incidence of malformations in infants whose mothers had been treated with lithium during the first trimester of pregnancy. Placental transfer of lithium has been documented. The levels in the mother and infant are identical [116]. These infants are exposed to two kinds of risks: malformations and neonatal effects.

Malformations. — Thirteen of the 143 infants on the register had malformations. In 11 cases, the malformations were cardiovascular: patent ductus arteriosus, mitral atresia, aortic coarctation, ventricular septal defect, and Ebstein's anomaly (4 cases). Other observations of cardiac defects and in particular Ebstein's anomaly were reported afterwards [101, 108]. The usual frequency of Ebstein's anomaly is 1/20,000 live births, which would indicate that lithium plays a role in its occurrence.

Difficulties of neonatal adaptation [141, 150]. — These are primarily neurological: hypotonia, difficulties in sucking and swallowing, hypoventilation. Also noted are episodes of hypothermia and hypoglycemia. The critical level of lithium is 1.6 mEq/l, easily reached because of the frequent increase in blood lithium level during pregnancy (reduced excretion).

Lithium passes easily into the maternal milk, the blood level in the infant then being 1/4-1/3 of that of the mother [121]. A single case of goitre has been reported. Tseng has suggested the occurence of interstitial myocarditis. This would seem to account for cardiomegaly, cardiac arrhythmias, atrial flutter, bundle branch block, and possibly transient tricuspid incompetence [8].

These disorders regress when the infant's blood lithium level falls below 1 mEq/l (half life 68 H). The long term prognosis is good.

MYASTHENIA GRAVIS

This is a rare disorder of the neuro-muscular junction and particularly of the post-synaptic region, characterized by muscle weakness, increased by effort, helped by rest and anticholinesterase drugs. In the neonate, this sometimes produces serious hypotonia with severe respiratory problems.

Transient neonatal myasthenia. — Infants whose mothers have myasthenia, even in clinical remission [42], are particularly at risk (10 to 20 % of infants of sick mothers). A maternal immunological factor, anti-acetylcholine receptor (Ac Ch R) antibody, responsible for the disease, can cross the placenta and bind to acetylcholine receptor protein [37, 80]. To explain why many children are not affected, Brenner suggested that alpha feto-protein could inhibit the binding of anti-Ac Ch R antibodies on the receptor protein. However maternal anti Ac Ch R antibodies differ from those of children with neonatal myasthenia; it seems more likely therefore that the fetus produces its own antibodies even before birth. Antibody production in the child may be due to transfer of a cellular clone from the mother [85].

If the effect occurs antenatally, contractures linked to immobility, occasionnally even arthrogryposis can be seen at birth [69, 127].

As early as the first hours of life, and always before the fourth day, muscle weakness appears, the cry is weak, the face is unexpressive, but ptosis is rare. Sucking and swallowing are inefficient requiring tube feeding. Respiratory distress is of variable intensity.

After 2 to 3 weeks, the disorder improves spontaneously. Its severity and duration do not seem to be related to the titer of anti-Ac Ch R antibodies. The Tensilon test (1 mg subcutaneously) brings about spectacular improvement in 10 to 20 minutes, confirming the diagnosis.

The EMG is not essential. Treatment is indicated if the functional repercussions are harmful. Neostigmine is used: 0.1 mg as an intramuscular injection or 1 mg orally. An exchange transfusion can hasten recovery by removing the transmitted antibodies; this is indicated in cases of severe respiratory distress [38, 109].

Congenital myasthenic syndromes appearing neonatally differ from the preceeding by the absence of maternal myasthenia, and the absence of anti-acetylcholine receptor antibodies. Three clinical forms are classically recognised, but intermediate forms exist which makes the distinction arguable [48].

(1) In congenital myasthenia, the symptoms which do not regress appear at birth or soon after, predominantly affecting the extrinsic ocular muscles. Hypotonia is moderate. It is transmitted as a recessive autosomal trait.

(2) Hereditary infantile myasthenia, which is very rare, begins in the neonatal period with respiratory

and feeding difficulties, often severe. There is no ophtalmoplegia. Spontaneous remission is frequent, but later recurrence with apnea and risk of sudden death has been observed in infants [28]. It is transmitted as an autosomal recessive trait. In both these forms, anticholinesterase drugs are effective.

(3) Newer forms of neonatal myasthenia [44]. Three types of anomalies have been pinpointed in patients suffering from early infantile or neonatal myasthenia:

— an enzymatic deficiency in the resynthesis of acetylcholine;

— a form associating small nerve endings, a decrease in the release of acetylcholine and of end plate acetylcholinesterase;

— a decreased conductance or opening time of the ionic channels induced by acetylcholine. This is seen later, apparently transmitted as a dominant autosomal trait.

STEINERT'S MYOTONIC DYSTROPHY

Steinert's myotonic dystrophy is a disease transmitted as a dominant autosomal trait. The clinical signs usually begin in late childhood or early adulthood; they include facial and distal limb muscle weakness, cataract, multiple endocrinopathies, baldness and myotonia.

The problems can sometimes begin in fetal life (myotonica dysembryoplasia of Pruzanski). The mother is then the parent affected in 94 % of cases, which would seem to show that the antenatal origin of the disease is the result of the influence of the maternal disease on a genetically predisposed fetus.

Worsening maternal muscular weakness and myotonia during pregnancy is often seen, but the diagnosis of myotonic dystrophy is often not yet suspected. However, the diagnosis of the neonatal form of Steinert's disease will be almost exclusively based on the family history. Miscarriages, sometimes repeated, are frequent. Polyhydramnios is common, the fetus moves little, delivery is often difficult because of the poor quality of uterine contractions.

The appearance of the infant is characteristic: hypotrophy, facial diplegia, odd-shaped mouth (upper lip like an inverted V "shark mouth") high-arched palate, articular deformations ranging from bilateral clubbed feet to a generalised arthrogryposis, difficulties in sucking, swallowing and breathing, testicular ectopia. On X-ray, the ribs are thin,

atelectasis is frequent. Muscular deficiency is mostly proximal, deep tendon reflexes are present. Its potential severity is due to respiratory failure [110, 126].

Serum enzymes are normal. Muscle biopsy, often normal, can show an aspect of arrested maturation, particularly in the neighbourhood of the affected joints. The fibres are small and round, with a central nucleus and few myofibrils. Where there is evidence of differentiation, type II fibers predominate, corresponding to a fetal maturity of 20 weeks of pregnancy [6]. Retarded maturation has been shown in other organs: kidney, pancreas [153].

Neonatal death is frequent, due to respiratory failure. In those cases that do survive, mental deficiency and motor retardation occur and the degree of involvement is worsened.

In some cases, antenatal assessment of the risk can be made on amniocentesis, by examining the fetal ABH secretor state [50, 63].

INFANTS OF CARDIAC MOTHERS

Although pregnancy in women suffering from various cardiac conditions is not rare, no proper studies exist dealing with the ante- and post-natal development of the child. In maternal cyanotic heart disease, the incidence of prematurity and hypotrophy is increased. The use of drugs in cardiac mothers is all the more frequent as analgesics are given to avoid pain, which may lead to hypertension and tachycardia [144]. The cardiac glycosides, digoxin in particular, cross the placenta, and fetal blood levels, measured in cord blood, are identical to those of the mother [118]. Digoxin myocardial affinity is directly related to the immaturity of the child [82]. Although digoxin half-life is in the range of 25-96 hours in the neonate, cases of fetal overdoses of maternal origin are rare [54]. Diuretics, furosemide and especially thiazides, also give fetal blood levels similar to the maternal ones [14, 145]. They can therefore have a pharmacodynamic effect both in utero and in the first few hours of life, with a loss of water and electrolytes, and even a risk of dehydration [111, 145]. The half-life of furosemide acquired transplacentally is about 33 hours. This is inversely proportional to the gestational age, and individual variations range from 6 to 96 hours. Chlorothiazide has been considered as a cause of some rare cases of leucopenia and neonatal thrombocytopenia.

Amongst the drugs which are used, the risks of

oral anticoagulants have been well demonstrated, and their use is contra-indicated during pregnancy.

The risk of serious, often lethal, hemorrhage, during labour or at birth is due to hypoprothrombinemia induced in the neonate by the transplacental passage of vitamin K antagonists [18]. In several reported cases maternal overdose was also noted. The time necessary for the fetal prothrombin time to return to normal limits after maternal treatment has been stopped is unknown but is likely greater than 7 days.

"Warfarin embryopathy" has in fact been seen with all oral anticoagulants [60]. The exposure of the embryo to vitamin K antagonists during the first trimester of pregnancy can lead to a malformation syndrome associating nasal hypoplasia and stippled epiphyses [13]. The nose is very flat, sometimes appearing to have been squashed, with a pronounced bridge and a deep groove between the alae and the tip of the nose. The airways are reduced in size which explains the frequency of respiratory distress from upper airway obstruction at birth [113]. True choanal stenosis has been reported on four occasions.

Small epiphyseal calcifications, "Stippled epiphyses" which are only visible during the first year, have been seen in the long bones (proximal end of the femur), the calcanea and the spine. The distribution of the anomalies makes it easy to distinguish this syndrome from Conradi-Hunermann's disease which is asymmetric, and from rhizomelic chondrodysplasia punctata, where the lesions are most prominent in the knees, elbows and wrists.

This embryopathy does not seem due to secondarily calcified fetal microhemorrhages but rather to an inhibition by vitamin K antagonists of the vitamin K dependant oesteocalcins, whose role in embryonic calcification is well known. The affected infants will be small.

Central nervous system anomalies. — A small proportion of infants exposed to vitamin K antagonists in utero have various anomalies of the central nervous system (3 %); hydrocephalus, perhaps secondary to an intra-uterine cerebral hemorrhage, but also callosal agenesis, Dandy-Walker syndrome and cerebellar atrophy. Some ocular anomalies, in particular optic atrophy, have also been described. In such cases, the dangerous time of exposure to these drugs appears to be the second and third trimesters. There are always some sequellae: mental retardation, blindness (half the cases), convulsions, spasticity. Taking into account the period of exposure, the cerebral anomalies seem to be due to a growth disorder (perhaps secondary to an early fetal hemorrhage), rather than a real malformation occuring during organogenesis.

ARTERIAL HYPERTENSION

Arterial hypertension complicates 6 % of pregnancies. Whether it exists before pregnancy, or whether it appears in the 3rd trimester as a sign of toxemia, it often causes intra-uterine growth retardation secondary to placental dysfunction. The decision to induce the birth of the infant prematurely is taken by the obstetricians when there are signs of serious fetal distress and arrested intra-uterine growth confirmed by echography.

Antihypertensive drugs have various effects on the fetus and the neonate which justify singling out this category of high-risk infants. The transplacental passage and the unwanted effects of these drugs in the perinatal period have however been poorly studied.

The peripheral vasodilators are essentially represented by hydralazine and dihydralazine. Cases of fetal bradycardia have been reported for the latter. Experimentally, hydralazine diminishes uterine arterial blood flow, and induces a fall of PO_2 in the lamb [83]. Diazoxide, rarely used for prolonged periods as an antihypertensive can induce alopecia and hypertrichosis as well as deficient fetal bone maturation [102].

Alpha-methyldopa is a commonly used antihypertensive drug. Its placental transfer gives fetal blood levels, measured in cord blood, equivalent to those of maternal venous blood [75]. The possibility of arterial hypotension in the newborn has been reported [149]. The half-life of alpha-methyldopa in neonates is 9 to 20 hours. Moar in comparing the infants of non treated hypertensive mothers and mothers treated with alpha-methyldopa, found a significant reduction in mean head circumference in the latter. This difference was no longer seen at one year of age, and the developmental prognosis at 4 years was identical for both groups of infants [94].

It is above all the beta-blockers which have been incriminated in deaths in utero and in difficulties at birth. Not only propanolol, but all the beta-blockers (metoprolol, oxprenolol, atenolol, etc.) cross the placenta, and are found in the infant, with their metabolites, at similar blood levels as in the mother, *i. e.* in a high enough concentration for a pharmacodynamic effect to be present [20, 41].

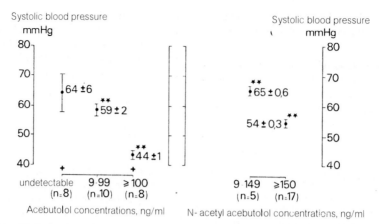

Fig. I-67. — *Relationship between acebutolol and its metabolite, N-acetyl acebutolol, and neonatal blood pressure on the first day of life* (mean ± SE). Statistical significance according to Student's *t* test. The mean of systolic pressures is significantly lower (* < 0.01, ** < 0.001) when the concentrations of beta-blockers are high. BOUTROY et al. [20].

Among the effects seen are prolonged episodes of bradycardia of less than 100 b. p. m. before, during and after birth; a loss of physiological oscillations of fetal heart rate giving a "flat" line on the recording. This effect is comparable to observations made in lambs whose blood pressure adaptation and post-anoxic tachycardia were abolished after having been given propanolol [72].

In a study carried out on 31 neonates exposed to acebutolol in utero compared to neonates of similar gestational age and mode of delivery, arterial hypotension was present in 30 cases for the 3 days of observation. This low pressure was proportional to the plasma concentration of acebutolol and its principal metabolite, N-acetyl-acebutolol (Fig. I-67). Unexpected cardiogenic shock occurred in two cases; this compares well with identical accidents described with propanolol and atenolol [58, 87, 137].

Transient tachypnea in 6 cases corresponded to mean blood levels (± 1 SD) of acebutolol higher than those found in infants without respiratory disorders (260 ± 124 as opposed to 87 ± 23 ng/ml, $p < 0.05$). This is probably connected to the beta-adrenergic inhibition of the secretion of lung liquid at birth, as shown in the lamb. Experimental propanolol adrenergic block maintains this secretion despite the administration of isoproterenol [147]. Finally the possibility of episodes of hypothermia and hypoglycemia, also due to the adrenergic block, has been reported [58].

All the beta-blockers are found in maternal milk at concentrations several times higher than in plasma. This is due to their great solubility in fat and their physical characteristics (weak bases). However, the quantity of beta-blockers which is in fact absorbed by the infant of a treated mother is not sufficient to reach pharmacodynamic levels.

The use of magnesium sulfate in the preventive treatment of eclampsia exposes the neonate to the risk of hypermagnesemia, even more so as the excretion of magnesium is low at this age [88]. Respiratory depression with a low Apgar score and the risk of apnea can occur. Neuro-muscular hypotonia and defects of myocardial conduction (lengthening of the PQ interval and widening of the QRS complex) are seen in serious overdoses. Finally, hypocalcemia can result from hypermagnesemia, probably by the inhibition of parathyroid hormone secretion [120].

The administration of calcium is indicated in cases of severe overdose. Exchange transfusion may also be performed.

As a result of these risks, the cardiovascular and respiratory functions of infants of treated hypertensive mothers must be carefully monitored for the first 2 or 3 days of life. Data is however lacking on the long term effects of antenatal exposure to these antihypertensive agents.

ASTHMA

Asthma is seen in 0.4-1.3 % of all pregnancies [93, 142], but there is little data concerning the infants of asthmatic mothers. There appears to be an increased risk of complicated pregnancies, prematurity, and perinatal mortality [10]. The mean weight at birth would seem to be slightly smaller than in the general population [36]. During status asthmaticus hypoxia and maternal alkalosis are likely to affect the fetus with a greater risk of perinatal death, hypotrophy and neurological sequellae [53]. The effects of the drugs used in the treatment of asthma must be taken into account. Theophylline gives limb abnormalities when given to the pregnant mouse [140]; nothing similar has been described in man. It is difficult to know the human clinical significance of the experimental evidence for the undesirable effects of methylxanthine derivatives on cholesterol synthesis in glial cells [3]. Both theophylline and aminophylline given during pregnancy have a possibly beneficial effect on surfactant synthesis and maturation in the rabbit [79, 125], as well as on the rate of idiopathic respiratory distress in the premature newborn [59]. Although theophylline appears in vitro to favor opening of the ductus arteriosus, no clinical cases have yet been reported to confirm this risk in the neonate. When the mother has been given large doses of theophylline during the delivery, the child can show signs of overdose with tachycardia, polyuria, irritability, feeding difficulty and vomiting [7, 151]. In one such case, we have seen neonatal status epilepticus. Methylxanthine derivatives lower the epileptic threshold in the mouse [55]. The fetal half-life of the drug is very long, being about 32 hours, *i. e.* 5-6 times longer than in the adult [5, 21]. Moreover, the fetus and neonate metabolise a significant proportion of theophylline into caffeine, which has a half-life of about 100 hours [5, 21]. It has been suggested that weaning from theophylline may be a possible cause of apnea.

Steroids, which are often prescribed during asthma, have no confirmed teratogenic effect in man. They may speed up surfactant maturation.

Some beta-mimetic drugs such as isoxuprine and ritodrine increase fetal insulin secretion [138], growth rate, and may be responsible for a transient increase in the thickness of the interventricular septum [29]. This does not seem to have been studied for salbutamol, the beta-mimetic given to asthmatic patients.

Although only rarely given in asthma, iodine containing drugs such as potassium iodide, can lead to fetal goiter with a risk of asphyxia in the first few days of life.

INFANTS OF MOTHERS
WITH SYSTEMIC LUPUS ERYTHEMATOSUS

The possibility of the placental passage of the "LE factor" was described by Bridge and Foley (1954). This transfer only concerns the IgG which disappears from the infant's serum at 15 weeks [12]. Transmission may be asymptomatic. Nevertheless, in some cases, there is neonatal lupus with various manifestations [62].

Maternal lupus is accompanied by a high level of miscarriages (30 %). 60 % of the neonates are hypotrophic. Amongst 54 infants affected, 34 were girls, 19 boys. Some (41 %) showed cutaneous lupus: facial skin rash, sometimes associated with hepatosplenomegaly (22 %). Also described is haemolytic anemia with leucopenia and thrombocytopenia. These lesions are transient, disappearing during the first months of life [99, 124].

More serious (30 % mortality) but rare, is a possible congenital complete heart block [16, 71]. It can be diagnosed in utero if the fetal heart rate is slow and regular, occasionally with heart failure and anasarca. This bradycardia must not be confused with that of fetal distress. The electrocardiogram shows atrio-ventricular dissociation with normal atrial rhythm, and normal ventricular complexes at 40-60/min. Although the bradycardia is often well tolerated, it can be treated with isoproterenol, and if necessary by electrosystolic pacing. The atrio-ventricular block is permanent. There is no other cardiac malformation.

Endocardial fibroelastosis is frequently found at autopsy of dead infants. The nodal tissue seems to be interrupted by a process of connective tissue degeneration, probably because of transmitted specific antibodies.

Pericarditis has also been described [39].

Occasionally, maternal lupus may remain undiagnosed. It is therefore necessary to consider this possibility in all infants with isolated congenital atrio-ventricular block.

CARBON MONOXIDE POISONING

Acute or chronic carbon monoxide poisoning can occur during pregnancy. It is usually serious for the fetus, particularly because of maternal hypoxia, which does not allow sufficient placental exchange. On the other hand, carbon monoxide diffuses only slowly from the mother to the fetus [51].

Out of 45 observations collected by Turpin in 1978, there were 19 fetal deaths (with 11 maternal deaths), 8 neonatal deaths with neurological disorders, invariably severe, ressembling those observed in the post-asphyxial syndrome. Among the 14 survivors most had severe neurological sequellae:

microcephaly, convulsions, Little's syndrome (spastic diplegia)...

The neuro-pathological alterations are represented by necrotic lesions of anoxic appearance, of variable intensity, involving the lenticular nucleus and the cerebral cortex.

OTHER DISEASES

Among the other risks of pathological pregnancies likely to affect the fetus and the neonate, there is the risk of hypotrophy in infants of mothers who, following a kidney transplant, remain on immunosuppressive drugs [123]. The child is also at risk for infection, in particular from cytomegalovirus [45]; the infant may however also have apparently normal humoral immunity [25].

Recurring cholestasis of pregnancy, occasionally familial [95], increases the risk of death in utero, prematurity and fetal distress [117]. The mechanisms involved are not known.

REFERENCES

[1] AICARDI (J.), CONTI (D.), GOUTIERES (F.). — Neonatal forms of Steinert's myotonic dystrophy. J. Neurol. Sciences, 22, 149-164, 1974.

[2] ALAGILLE (D.), ODIEVRE (M.), HOULLEMARE (L.). — Avitaminose K néonatale sévère chez deux enfants de mère traitée par anti-épileptiques. Arch. Fr. Pédiatr., 25, 31-41, 1968.

[3] ALLEN (W. C.), VOLPE (J. J.). — Reduction of cholesterol synthesis by Methylxanthines in cultured glial cells. Pediatr. Res., 13, 1121-1124, 1979.

[4] ANDREWS (J.), McGARRY (J. H.). — A community study of smoking in pregnancy. J. Obstet. Gynecol. Br. Commonw., 79, 1057-1073, 1972.

[5] ARANDA (J. V.), TORMEN (T.), SASYNIUK (B. I.). — Pharmacokinetics of diuretics and methylxanthines in the neonate. Eur. J. Clin. Pharmacol., 18, 55-63, 1980.

[6] ARGOU (Z.), GARDNER-MEDWIN (D.), JOHNSON (M. A.), MASTAGLIA (F. L.). — Congenital myotonic dystrophy. Fiber type abnormalities in 2 cases. Arch. Neurol., 37, 693-696, 1980.

[7] ARWOOD (L. L.), DASTA (J. F.), FRIEDMAN (C.). — Placental transfer of theophylline: two case reports. Pediatrics, 63, 844-846, 1979.

[8] ARNON (R. G.), MARIN-GARCIA (J.), PEEDEN (J. N.). — Tricuspid valve regurgitation and lithium carbonate toxicity in a newborn infant. Am. J. Dis. Child., 135, 941-943, 1981.

[9] AUSTIN (J. H.), GOODING (C. A.). — Roentgenographic measurement of skull size in children. Radiology, 99, 641-646, 1971.

[10] BAHNA (S. L.), BJERKEDAL (T.). — The course and outcome of pregnancy in women with bronchial asthma. Acta Allergol., 27, 397-406, 1972.

[11] BARIBAUD (L.), YACOUB (M.), FAURE (J.), MALINASY CAU (G.). — L'oxycarbonémie de l'enfant né de mère fumeuse. Méd. Lég. Dom. Corp., 3, 272-274, 1970.

[12] BECK (J. S.), OAKLEY (C. L.), ROWELL (N. R.). — Transplacental passage of antinuclear antibody. Study in infants of mothers with systemic lupus erythematosus. Arch. Dermatol., 93, 656-663, 1966.

[13] BECKER (M. H.), GENIESER (N. B.), FINEFOLD (M.), MIRANDA (D.), SPACKMAN (T.). — Chondrodysplasia punctata. Is maternal warfarin therapy a factor? Am. J. Dis. Child., 129, 356-359, 1975.

[14] BEERMAN (B.), GROSCHINSKY-GRIND (M.), FANREUS (L.), LINDSTRÖM (B.). — Placental transfer of furosemide. Clin. Pharmacol. Ther., 24, 560-562, 1978.

[15] BERGMAN (A. B.), WILSNER (L. A.). — Relationship of passive cigarette smoking to sudden infant death syndrome. Pediatrics, 58, 665-668, 1976.

[16] BERUBE (S.), LISTER (G.), TOEWS (W. H.), CREASY (R. K.), HEYMANN (M. A.). — Congenital heart block and maternal systemic lupus erythematosus. Am. J. Obstet. Gynecol., 130, 595-596, 1978.

[17] BETHENOD (M.), FREDERICH (A.). — Les enfants des anti-épileptiques. Pédiat. Lyon, 30, 227-248, 1975.

[18] BLOOMFIELD (D. K.). — Fetal deaths and malformations associated with the use of coumarin derivatives in pregnancy. A critical review. Am. J. Obstet. Gynecol., 107, 883-888, 1970.

[19] BOSSI (L.). — Fetal effect of anticonvulsants. In: Antiepileptic drug therapy, P. L. MORSELLI, C. E. PIPPENGER, J. KIFFIN PENRY Edit. Raven Press, New York, 37-64, 1983.

[20] BOUTROY (M. J.), VERT (P.), BIANCHETTI (G.), DUBRUCQ (C.), MORSELLI (P. L.). — Infants born to hypertensive mothers treated by Acebutolol. Pharmacological studies in the perinatal period. Dev. Pharmacol. Ther., 4, suppl. 1, 109-115, 1982.

[21] BOUTROY (M. J.), VERT (P.), ROYER (R. J.), MONIN (P.), ROYER-MORROT (M. J.). — Caffeine a metabolite of theophylline during the treatment of apnea in the premature infant. J. Pediatr., 94, 996-998, 1979.

[22] BRENNER (T.), ABRAMSKY (O.). — Suppression of clinical and experimental myasthenia gravis by alpha-fetoprotein. Neurology, 30, 380-381, 1980.

[23] BRIDGE (R. G.), FOLEY (F. E.). — Placental transmission of the lupus erythematosus factor. Amer. J. Med. Sci., 227, 1-8, 1954.

[24] BUTLER (N. R.), GOLDSTEIN (H.). — Smoking in pregnancy and subsequent child development. Brit. Med. J., 4, 573-575, 1973.

[25] CEDERQVIST (L. L.), MERKATZ (I. R.), LITWIN (S. D.). — Fetal immunoglobulin synthesis following maternal immunosuppression. Am. J. Obstet. Gynecol., 129, 687-690, 1977.

[26] CLARREN (S. K.), ALVORD (E. C.), SUMI (S. M.), STREISSGUTH (A. P.), SMITH (D. W.). — Brain malformations related to prenatal exposure to ethanol. J. Pediatr., 92, 64-67, 1978.

[27] COMBEMALE (F.). — La descendance des alcooliques. Thèse Méd., Montpellier, 1888.

[28] CONOMY (J. P.), LEVINSOHN (M.), FARANOFF (A.). — Familial infantile myasthenia gravis: a cause of sudden death in young children. J. Pediatr., 87, 428-429, 1975.

[29] CRAWFORD (C. S.), HALL (M. L.), OTIS (C.). — Echocardiographic effects of intrauterine Rito-

drine exposure. Abstract 270. *Pediatr. Res., 16,* 123 A, 1982.

[30] DANSKY (L.), ANDERMANN (E.), ANDERMANN (F.), SHERWIN (A. L.), KINCH (R. A.). — Maternal epilepsy and congenital malformations: correlations with maternal plasma anticonvulsant levels during pregnancy. In: *Epilepsy, Pregnancy and the child.* D. JANZ Edit. Raven Press, New York, 251-258, 1982.

[31] DAVIES (D. P.), ANSARI (B. M.), COOKE (T. J. H.). — Anterior fontanelle size in the neonate. *Arch. Dis. Child., 50,* 81-83, 1975.

[32] DEBLAY (M. F.), VERT (P.). — Le tabac et le développement de l'enfant. In : *Médecine Périnatale.* G. BARRIER, J. M. THOULON Édit., Arnette, Paris, 215-228, 1981.

[33] DEBLAY (M. F.), VERT (P.), ANDRE (M.). — L'enfant de mère épileptique. *Nouv. Presse Méd., 11,* 173-176, 1982.

[34] DEHAENE (P.), CREPIN (G.), DELAHOUSSE (G.), QUERLEU (D.), WALBAUM (R.), TITRAN (M.), SAMAILLE-VILLETTE (C.). — Aspects épidémiologiques du syndrome d'alcoolisme fœtal. *Nouv. Presse Méd., 10,* 2639-2643, 1981.

[35] DENSON (R.), NANSON (J. L.), MCWATTERS (M. A.). — Hyperkinesis and maternal smoking. *Can. Psychiatr. Assoc. J., 20,* 183-187, 1975.

[36] DE SWIET (M.). — Diseases of the respiratory system. *Clin. Obstet. Gynaecol., 4,* 287-296, 1977.

[37] DONALDSON (J. O.), PENN (A. S.), LISAK (R. P.), ABRAMSKY (O.), BRENNER (T.), SCHOTLAND (D. L.). — Antiacetylcholine receptor antibody in neonatal myasthenia gravis. *Am. J. Dis. Child., 135,* 222-226, 1981.

[38] DONAT (J. F. G.), DONAT (J. R.), LENWON (V. A.). — Exchange transfusion in neonatal myasthenia gravis. *Neurology, 31,* 911-912, 1981.

[39] DOSHI (N.), SMITH (B.), KLIONSKY (B.). — Congenital pericarditis due to maternal lupus erythematosus. *J. Pediatr., 96,* 699-701, 1980.

[40] D'SOUZA (S. W.), BLACK (P. M.), WILLIAMS (N.), JENNISON (R. F.). — Effect of smoking during pregnancy upon the haematological values of cord blood. *Br. J. Obstet. Gynaecol., 85,* 495-499, 1978.

[41] DUMEZ (Y.), TCHOBROUTSKY (C.), HORNYCH (H.), AMIEL-TISON (C.). — Neonatal effects of maternal administration of acebutolol. *Brit. Med. J., 283,* 1077-1079, 1981.

[42] ELIAS (S. B.), BUTLER (I.), APPEL (S. H.). — Neonatal myasthenia gravis in the infant of a myasthenic mother in remission. *Ann. Neurol., 6,* 72-75, 1979.

[43] ELLIS (F. W.), PICK (J. R.). — An animal model of the fetal alcohol syndrome in Beagles, Alcoholism. *Clin. Exper. Research, 4,* 123-134, 1980.

[44] ENGEL (A. G.). — Morphologic and immunopathologic findings in myasthenia gravis and in congenital myasthenic syndrome. *J. Neurol. Neurosurg. Psychiat., 43,* 577-579, 1980.

[45] EVANS (T. J.), MCCOLLUM (J. P. K.), VALDIMARSSON (H.). — Congenital cytomegalovirus infection after maternal renal transplantation. *Lancet, 1,* 1359, 1975.

[46] EVERSON (R. B.). — Individuals transplacentally exposed to maternal smoking may be at increased cancer risk in adult life. *Lancet, 2,* 123-127, 1980.

[47] FAVIA (J.). — Cigarettes pendant la grossesse,

poids de naissance et mortalité périnatale. *Can. Med. Assoc. J., 109,* 1104-1107, 1973.

[48] FENICHEL (G. M.). — Clinical syndromes of myasthenia in infancy and childhood. *Arch. Neurol. 35,* 97, 1978.

[49] FITZGERALD (J. E.), WEBSTER (A.). — Obstetric significance of barbiturates and vitamin K. *JAMA, 119,* 1082-1085, 1942.

[50] GIBSON (S. L. M.), FERGUSON-SMITH (M. A.). — The use of genetic linkage in counselling families with dystrophia myotonica. *Clin. Genet., 17,* 443, 1980.

[51] GINSBERG (M. D.), MYERS (R. E.). — Fetal brain injury after maternal carbon monoxide intoxication. Clinical and neuropathologic aspects. *Neurology, 26,* 15-23, 1976.

[52] GÖPFERT-GEYER (I.), KOCH (S.), RATING (D.), JÄGER-ROMAN (E.), HARTMANN (L.), JACOB (S.), OFFERMANN (G.), HELGE (H.). — Delivery, gestation, data at birth, and neonatal period in children of epileptic mothers. In: *Epilepsy, pregnancy and the child,* D. JANZ et al. Edit. Raven Press, New York, 179-187, 1982.

[53] GORDON (M.), NISWANDER (K. R.), BERENDES (H.), KANTOR (A. G.). — Fetal morbidity following potentially anoxigenic obstetric conditions. VII. Bronchial asthma. *Am. J. Obstet. Gynecol., 106,* 421-429, 1970.

[54] GORODISHER (R.). — Cardiac drugs. In: *Pediatric Pharmacology,* S. J. YAFFE Edit. Grune and Stratton Pub., New York, 281-304, 1980.

[55] GROSS (R. A.), FERRENDELLI (J. A.). — Effects of reserpine, propanolol and aminophylline on seizure activity on CNS cyclic nucleotides. *Ann. Neurol., 6,* 296-301, 1979.

[56] GUPTA (C.), SHAPIRO (B. H.), YAFFE (S. J.). — Reproductive dysfunction in male rats following prenatal exposure to phenobarbital. *Pediatr. Pharmacol., 1,* 55-62, 1980.

[57] GUPTA (C.), YAFFE (S. J.). — Reproductive dysfunction in female offspring after prenatal exposure to phenobarbital: critical period action. *Pediatr. Res., 15,* 1488-1491, 1981.

[58] HABIB (A.), MCCARTHY (J. S.). — Effects on the neonate of propanolol administered during pregnancy. *J. Pediatr., 91,* 808-811, 1977.

[59] HADJIGEORGIOU (R.), KITSIOU (S.), PSAROUDAKIS (A.), SEGOS (C.), NICOLOPOULOS (D.), KASKARELIS (D.). — Antepartum aminophylline treatment for prevention of the respiratory distress syndrome in premature infants. *Am. J. Obstet. Gynecol., 135,* 257-260, 1979.

[60] HALL (J. G.), PAULI (R. M.), WILSON (K. M.). — Maternal and fetal sequelae of anticoagulation during pregnancy. *Am. J. Med., 68,* 122-140, 1980.

[61] HANSON (J. W.), SMITH (D. W.). — The fetal hydantoin syndrome. *J. Pediatr., 87,* 285-290, 1975.

[62] HARDY (J. D.), SOLOMON (S.), BANWELL (G. S.), BEACH (R.), WRIGHT (V.), HOWARD (F. M.). — Congenital complete heart block in the newborn associated with maternal systemic lupus erythematosus and other connective tissue disorders. *Arch. Dis. Child., 54,* 7-13, 1979.

[63] HARPER (P. S.). — Congenital myotonic dystrophy in Britain. I. Clinical aspects. II. Genetic basis. *Arch. Dis. Child., 50,* I: 505-513, II: 514-521, 1975.

[64] HASSEL (T. M.), JOHNSTON (M. C.), DUDLEY (K. H.).

— *Phenytoin-induced teratology and gingival pathology.* Raven Press, New York, 1980.

[65] HENDERSON (G. I.). — Maternal ethanol consumption and fetal development: two potential mechanisms. *Dev. Pharmacol. Ther.*, 4, suppl. 1, 66-78, 1982.

[66] HILL (R. M.), VERNIAUD (W. M.), HORNING (M. G.), MACCULLEY (L. B.), MORGAN (N. F.). — Infants exposed *in utero* to epileptic drugs. A prospective study. *Amer. J. Dis. Child.*, 127, 647-653, 1974.

[67] HILL (R. M.), VERNIAUD (W. M.), RETTIG (G. M.), TENNYSON (L. M.), CRAIG (J. P.). — Relationship between antiepileptic drug exposure of the infant and developmental potential. In: *Epilepsy, Pregnancy and the child*, D. JANZ et al. Edit. Raven Press, New York, 409-417, 1982.

[68] HILL (R. M.). — Fetal malformations and antiepileptic drugs. *Am. J. Dis. Child.*, 130, 923-925, 1976.

[69] HOLMES (L. B.), DRISCOLL (S. G.), BRADLEY (W. G.). — Contractures in a newborn infants of a mother with myasthenia gravis. *J. Pediatr.*, 96, 1067-1068, 1980.

[70] HOROWITZ (D. A.), JABLONSKI (W.), MEHTA (K. A.). — Apnea associated with theophylline withdrawal in a term neonate. *Am. J. Dis. Child.*, 136, 73-74, 1982.

[71] HULL (D.), BINNS (B. A. O.), JOYCE (D.). — Congenital heart block and widespread fibrosis due to maternal lupus erythematosus. *Arch. Dis. Child.*, 41, 688-690, 1966.

[72] HYMAN (A. I.), HAWORTH (G.), BOWE (E. T.), DANIEL (S. S.), JAMES (L. S.). — Effects of sympathetic blokade on fetal responses to asphyxia. *Biol. Neonat.*, 21, 1-8, 1972.

[73] JANZ (D.). — On major malformations and minor anomalies in the offspring of parents with epilepsy: review of the litterature. In: *Epilepsy, Pregnancy and the child*, D. JANZ et al. Edit. Raven Press, New York, 211-222, 1982.

[74] JANZ (D.), DAM (M.), RICHENS (A.), BOSSI (L.), HELGE (H.), SCHMIDT (D.). — *Epilepsy, Pregnancy and the child.* Raven Press, New York, 1 vol., 552, 1982.

[75] JONES (H. M. R.), CUMMINGS (A. J.), SETCHELL (K. D. R.), LAWSON (A. M.). — A study of the disposition of α-methyldopa in newborn infants following its administration to the mother for the treatment of hypertension during pregnancy. *Br. J. Clin. Pharmacol.*, 8, 433-440, 1979.

[76] JONES (K. L.), SMITH (D. W.), ULLELAND (C. N.), STREISSGUTH (A. P.). — Pattern of malformation in offspring of chronic alcoholic mothers. *Lancet*, 1, 1267-1277, 1973.

[77] JONES (G. L.), WOODBURY (D. M.). — Effects of diphenylhydantoin and phenobarbital on protein metabolism in the rat cerebral cortex. *Biochem. Pharmacol.*, 2, 53-61, 1976.

[78] KAMINSKI (M.), RUMEAU-ROUQUETTE (C.), SCHWARTZ (D.). — Consommation d'alcool chez les femmes enceintes et issue de la grossesse. *Rev. Épidémiol. Sant. Publ.*, 24, 27-40, 1976.

[79] KAROTKIN (E. H.), KIDO (M.), CASHORE (W. J.), REDDING (R. A.), DOUGLAS (W. J.), STERN (L.), OH (W.). — Acceleration of fetal lung maturation by aminophylline in pregnant rabbits. *Pediatr. Res.*, 10, 722-724, 1976.

[80] KEESEY (J.), LINDSTROM (J.), COKELY (H.), HERRMAN (C.). — Antiacetylcholine receptor antibody in neonatal myasthenia gravis. *N. Engl. J. Med.*, 296, 55, 1977.

[81] KELSEY (J. L.), DWYER (T.), HOLFORD (T. R.), BRACKEN (M. B.). — Maternal smoking and congenital malformations: an epidemiological study. *J. Epidem. Com. Health*, 32, 102-107, 1978.

[82] KIM (P. W.), KRASULA (R. W.), SOYKA (L. F.), HASTREITER (A. R.). — Post-mortem tissue digoxin concentrations in infants and children. *Circulation*, 52, 1128-1131, 1975.

[83] LADNER (C. N.), WESTON (P. V.), BRINKMAN (C. R.), ASSALI (N. S.). — Effects of hydralazine on uteroplacental and fetal circulations. *Am. J. Obstet. Gynecol.*, 108, 375-381, 1970.

[84] LANDESMAN-DWYER (S.), KELLER (L. S.), STEISSGUTH (A. P.). — Naturalistic observations of newborns: effects of maternal alcohol intake. *Alc. Clin. Exp. Res.*, 2, 171-177, 1978.

[85] LEFVERT (A. K.), OSTERMAN (P. O.). — Newborn infants to myasthenic mothers: a clinical study and an investigation of acetylcholine receptor antibodies in 17 children. *Neurology*, 33, 133-138, 1983.

[86] LEMOINE (P.), HARROUSSEAU (H.), BORTEYRU (J. P.), MENUET (J. C.). — Les enfants de parents alcooliques. Anomalies observées à propos de 127 cas. *Ouest Méd.*, 25, 476-482, 1968.

[87] LIEBERMAN (B. A.), STIRRAT (G. M.), COHEN (S. L.), BEARD (R. W.), PINKER (G. D.). — The possible adverse effect of propanolol on the fetus in pregnancies complicated by severe hypertension. *Brit. J. Obstet. Gynaecol.*, 85, 678-683, 1968.

[88] LIPSITZ (P. J.). — The clinical and biochemical effects of excess magnesium in the newborn. *Pediatrics*, 47, 501-509, 1971.

[89] MEADOW (S. R.). — Anticonvulsant drugs and congenital abnormalities. *Lancet*, 2, 1296, 1968.

[90] MEBERG (A.), HAGA (P.), SANDE (H.), FOSS (O. P.). — Smoking during pregnancy: hematological observations in the newborn. *Acta Paediatr. Scand.*, 68, 371-374, 1979.

[91] MEBERG (A.), SANDE (H.), FOSS (O. P.), STENWIG (J. T.). — Smoking during pregnancy. Effects on the fetus and on thiocyanate levels in mother and baby. *Acta Paediatr. Scand.*, 68, 547-552, 1979.

[92] MEYER (M. B.), JONAS (B. S.), TONASCIA (J. A.). — Perinatal events associated with maternal smoking during pregnancy. *Am. J. Epidemiol.*, 103, 464-476, 1976.

[93] MINTZ (S.). — Pregnancy and asthma in WEISS (E. B.), SEGAL (M. S.) Eds. *Bronchial Asthma, Mechanisms and Therapeutics.* Little Brown, Boston, 971-982, 1976.

[94] MOAR (V. A.), JEFFERIES (M. A.), MUTCH (L. M. M.), OUNSTED (M. K.), REDMAN (C. W. G.). — Neonatal head circumference and the treatment of maternal hypertension. *Brit. J. Obstet. Gynaecol.*, 85, 933-937, 1978.

[95] MONIN (P.), VERT (P.), PETRY (J. M.). — Cholostase récidivante de la grossesse. Maladie autosomique dominante. *Nouv. Presse Méd.*, 9, 1779, 1980.

[96] NAEYE (R. L.). — Effect of maternal cigarette smoking on the fetus and placenta. *Brit. J. Obstet. Gynaecol.*, 85, 732-737, 1978.

[97] NAEYE (R. L.). — Sudden infant death syndrome: a prospective study. *Am. J. Dis. Child.*, 130, 1207-1210, 1976.

[98] NAEYE (R. L.). — The duration of maternal ciga-

rette smoking, fetal and placental disorders. *Early Hum. Dev.*, *3*, 229-237, 1979.

[99] NATHAN (D. J.), SNAPPER (I.). — Simultaneous placental transfer of factors responsible for LE cell formation and thrombocytopenia. *Am. J. Med.*, *25*, 647-653, 1958.

[100] NICLOUX (M.). — Recherches expérimentales sur l'élimination de l'alcool dans l'organisme. Détermination d'un alcoolisme congénital. *Thèse Méd.*, *Paris*, 1900.

[101] NORA (J. J.), NORA (A. H.), TOEWS (W. H.). — Lithium, Ebstein's anomaly and other congenital heart defects. *Lancet*, *2*, 594-595, 1974.

[102] NUWAYHID (B.), BRINKMAN (C. R.), KATCHEN (B.), SYMCHOWICZ (S.), MARTINEK (H.), ASSALI (S.). — Maternal and fetal hemodynamic effects of diazoxide. *Obstet. Gynecol.*, *46*, 197-203, 1975.

[103] NYMAND (G.). — Maternal smoking and neonatal hyperbilirubinemia. *Lancet*, *2*, 173, 1974.

[104] OLEGARD (R.), SABEL (K. G.), ARONSSON et coll. — Effects on the child of alcohol abuse during pregnancy. *Acta Paediatr. Scand.*, suppl. *275*, 112-121, 1979.

[105] OUELETTE (E. M.), ROSETT (H. L.). — A pilot prospective study of the fetal alcohol syndrome at the Boston city hospital. II. The infant. *Ann. N. Y. Acad. Sci.*, *273*, 123-129, 1976.

[106] OUELLETTE (E. M.), ROSETT (H. L.), ROSMAN (N. P.), WEINER (L.). — Adverse effects on offspring of maternal alcohol abuse during pregnancy. *N. Engl. J. Med.*, *297*, 528-530, 1977.

[107] OUNSTED (M. K.), MOAR (V. A.), GOOD (F. J.), REDMAN (C. W. G.). — Hypertension during pregnancy with and without specific treatment; the development of the children at the age of four years. *Br. J. Obstet. Gynaecol.*, *87*, 19-24, 1980.

[108] PARK (J. M.), SRIDAROMET (S.), LEDBETTER (E. O.). — Ebstein's anomaly of the tricuspid valve associated with prenatal exposure to lithium carbonate. *Am. J. Dis. Child.*, *134*, 703-704, 1980.

[109] PASTERNAK (J. F.), HAGEMAN (J.), ADAMS (M. A.), PHILIP (A. G. S.), GARDNER (T. H.). — Exchange transfusion in neonatal myasthenia. *J. Pediatr.*, *99*, 644-646, 1981.

[110] PEARSE (R. G.), HÖWELER (C. J.). — Neonatal form of dystrophia myotonica. Five cases in preterm babies and a review of earlier reports. *Arch. Dis. Child.*, *54*, 331-338, 1979.

[111] PECORARI (D.), RAGNI (N.), AUTERA (C.). — Effetti sul neonato della somministrazione di furosemide alla madre durante il travaglio di parto. *Ateneo Parmense*, *40*, 89-97, 1969.

[112] PERSSON (P. H.), GRENNERT (L.), GENNSER (G.). — A study of smoking and pregnancy with special reference to fetal growth. *Acta Paediatr. Scand.*, suppl. *78*, 33-39, 1978.

[113] PETTIFOR (J. M.), BENSON (R.). — Congenital malformations associated with the administration of oral anticoagulants during pregnancy. *J. Pediatr.*, *86*, 459-462, 1975.

[114] PIEROG (S.), CHANDAVASU (O.), WEXLERI. — Withdrawal symptoms in infants with the fetal alcohol syndrome. *J. Pediatr.*, *90*, 630-633, 1977.

[115] PRUZANSKI (W.). — Variants of myotonic dystrophy in preadolescent life. *Brain*, *89*, 563-568, 1966.

[116] RANE (A.), TOMSON (G.), BJARKE (B.). — Effects of maternal lithium therapy in a newborn infant. *J. Pediatr.*, *93*, 296-297, 1978.

[117] REID (R.), IVEK (K. J.), RENCORET (R. H.), STOREY (B.). — Fetal complications of obstetric cholestasis. *Brit. Med. J.*, *1*, 870, 1976.

[117 bis] ROBERT (E.), GUIBAUD (P.). — Maternal valproic acid and congenital neural tube defects. *Lancet*, *II*, 937, 1982.

[118] ROGERS (M. C.), WILLERSON (J. T.), GOLDBLATT (A.), SMITH (T. W.). — Serum digoxin concentrations in the human fetus, neonate and infant. *N. Engl. J. Med.*, *287*, 1010-1013, 1972.

[119] ROUQUETTE (J.). — Influence de la toxicomanie alcoolique parentale sur le développement physique et psychique des jeunes enfants. *Thèse*, *Paris*, 1957.

[120] SAVORY (J.), MONIF (G. R. G.). — Serum calcium levels in cord sera of the progeny of mothers treated with magnesium sulfate for toxemia of pregnancy. *Amer. J. Obstet. Gynecol.*, *110*, 556-559, 1971.

[121] SCHOU (M.), GOLDFIELD (M. D.), WEINSTEIN (M. R.), VILLENEUVE (A.). — Lithium and pregnancy. I. Report from the register of lithium basis. *Brit. Med. J.*, *2*, 135-136, 1973.

[122] SCHWARTZ (D.), GOUJARD (J.), KAMINSKI (M.), RUMEAU-ROUQUETTE (C.). — Smoking and pregnancy: results of a prospective study of 6,989 women. *Rev. Eur. Et. Clin. Biol.*, *17*, 867-879, 1972.

[123] SCIARRA (J. J.), TOLEDO-PEREYRA (L. H.), BENDEL (R. P.), SIMMONS (R. L.). — Pregnancy following renal transplantation. *Am. J. Obstet. Gynecol.*, *123*, 411-425, 1975.

[124] SEIP (M.). — Systemic lupus erythematosus in pregnancy with haemolytic anaemia, leucopenia and thrombocytopenia in the mother and her newborn infant. *Arch. Dis. Child.*, *35*, 364-366, 1959.

[125] SEVANIAN (A.), GILDEN (C.), KAPLAN (S. A.), BARRETT (C. T.). — Enhancement of fetal lung surfactant production by aminophylline. *Pediatr. Res.*, *13*, 1336-1340, 1979.

[126] SIMPSON (K.). — Neonatal respiratory failure due to myotonic dystrophy. *Arch. Dis. Child.*, *50*, 569-571, 1975.

[127] SMIT (L. M. E.), BARTH (P. G.). — Arthrogryposis multiplex congenita due to congenital myasthenia. *Dev. Med. Child Neurol.*, *22*, 371-374, 1980.

[128] SMITH (D. W.). — Hydantoin effects on the fetus. In: *Phenytoin-induced teratology and gingival pathology*, T. M. HASSEL, M. C. JOHNSTON, K. H. DUDLEY Edit. Raven Press, New York, 1980, 35-40.

[129] SOLOMON (G. E.), HILGARTNER (M. D.). — Coagulation defects caused by diphenylhydantoin. *Neurology*, *22*, 1165-1171, 1972.

[130] SOLOMON (G. E.), HILGARTNER (M. D.), KUTT (H.). — Phenobarbital induced coagulation defects in cats. *Neurology*, *24*, 920-924, 1974.

[130 bis] SOYKA (L. F.), JOFFE (J. M.). — *Male mediated drug effects on offspring in drug and chemical risks to the fetus and newborn*; SCHWARZ R. H., YAFFE S. J. Edit. Alan R. Liss Pub., New York, 49-66, 1980.

[131] SPEIDEL (B. D.), MEADOW (S. R.). — Maternal epilepsy and abnormalities of the fetus and newborn. *Lancet*, *2*, 839-843, 1972.

[132] STERN (L.). — *In vivo* assessment of the teratogenic potential of drugs in man. *Dev. Pharmacol. Ther.*, *4*, suppl. *1*, 10-18, 1982.

[133] STREISSGUTH (A. P.), LANDESMAN-DWYER (S.), MARTIN (J. C.), SMITH (D. W.). — Teratogenic effect of alcohol in humans and laboratory animals. *Science, 209*, 353-361, 1980.

[134] STRÖMLAND (K.). — Eyeground malformations in the fetal alcohol syndrome. *Neuropediatrics, 12*, 97-98, 1981.

[135] SWAIMAN (K. F.), KENNETH (F.), STRIGHT (P. L.). — The effect of anticonvulsants on *in vitro* protein synthesis in immature brain. *Brain Res., 58*, 515-518, 1973.

[136] SZABO (K. R.). — Teratogenic effect of lithium carbonate in the fetal mouse. *Nature, 225*, 73-75, 1970.

[137] TCHOBROUTSKI (C.). — Les bêtabloquants au cours de la grossesse. *Arch. Fr. Pédiatr., 35*, 571-577, 1978.

[138] TENENBAUM (D.), COWETT (R. M.). — The mechanism of ritodrine effects on neonatal glucose kinetics. *Pediatr. Res., 17*, 157 A, 1983.

[139] TSENG (H. L.). — Interstitial myocarditis probably related to lithium carbonate intoxication. *Arch. Pathol. Lab. Med., 92*, 444-448, 1971.

[140] TUCCI (S. M.), SBELKO (R. G.). — The teratogenic effects of theophylline in mice. *Toxicol. Let., 1*, 33, 341, 1978.

[141] TUNNESSEN (W. W.), HERTZ (C. G.). — Toxic effects of lithium in newborn infants: a commentary. *J. Pediatr., 81*, 804-807, 1972.

[142] TURNER (E. S.), GREENBERGER (P. A.), PATTERSON (R.). — Management of the pregnant asthmatic patient. *Ann. Int. Med., 93*, 905-918, 1980.

[143] TURPIN (J. C.), ESCOUROLLE (R.), GRAY (F.), FOURNET (J. P.), CASTAING (H.), DUPARD (M. C.). — Intoxication oxycarbonée chez le fœtus. A propos d'une observation anatomo-clinique. *Rev. Neurol., 134*, 485-495, 1978.

[144] UELAND (K.), METCALFE (J.). — Heart disease in pregnancy. *Clin. Perinatol., 1*, 349-367, 1974.

[145] VERT (P.), BROQUAIRE (M.), LEGAGNEUR (M.), MORSELLI (P. L.). — Pharmacokinetics of furosemide in neonates. *Eur. J. Clin. Pharmacol., 22*, 39-45, 1982.

[146] VERT (P.), DEBLAY (M. F.). — Hemorrhagic disorders in infants of epileptic mothers. In: *Epilepsy, Pregnancy and the Child*, JANZ D. *et al.* Edit. Raven Press, New York, 387-388, 1982.

[147] WALTERS (D. W.), OLVER (R. E.). — The role of catecholamines in lung liquid absorption at birth. *Pediatr. Res., 12*, 239-242, 1978.

[148] WEBER (M.), SCHWEITZER (M.), MUR (J. M.), TRIDON (P.), VERT (P.). — Épilepsie, médicaments antiépileptiques et grossesse. *Arch. Fr. Pédiatr., 34*, 374-383, 1977.

[149] WHITELAW (A.). — Maternal methyldopa treatment and neonatal blood pressure. *Brit. Med. J., 283*, 471, 1981.

[150] WILBANKS (G. D.), BRESSLER (B.), PEETE (C. H.), CHERNY (W. B.), LONDON (W. L.). — Toxic effects of lithium carbonate in a mother and newborn infant. *JAMA, 213*, 865-867, 1970.

[151] YEH (T. F.), PILDES (R. S.). — Transplacental aminophylline toxicity in a neonate. *Lancet, I*, 910 (letter), 1977.

[152] YERUSHALMY (J.). — Congenital heart disease and maternal smoking habits. *Nature, 242*, 262-263, 1973.

[153] YOUNG (R. S. K.), GANG (D. L.), ZALNERAITIS (E. L.), KRISHNAMOORTHY (K. S.). — Dysmaturation in infants of mothers with myotonic dystrophy. *Arch. Neurol., 38*, 716-719, 1981.

12

Infants of drug-addicted mothers

Cynthia T. BARRETT and J. Stephen ROBINSON

INTRODUCTION

During the last two decades, drug abuse has reached epidemic proportions in the United States. It has been estimated that there are 400,000 opiate drug users in the United States, of whom 100,000 are thought to be of child-bearing age. In addition, there are large but undocumented numbers addicted to other psychotropic agents including barbiturates, diazepam, propoxyphene and pentazacine, among others. Alcohol addiction is a major social and medical problem world-wide. In addition to the above pharmacologic agents, a majority of opiate addicts are polydrug users and most smoke cigarettes. Aside from alcohol, drug abuse, particularly opiate abuse, has been a far greater problem in the United States than it has been in Europe. Almost all pharmacologic agents administered to a pregnant woman are transferred across the placenta and appear in the fetal circulation. Exceptions are highly protein bound agents such as thyroxin and large molecules such as insulin. Some have major effects on fetal growth; all of them affect neonatal behavior and some even affect infant behavior beyond the first year of life.

HEROIN AND METHADONE

In addition to the direct effects upon the fetus, there are multiple indirect effects which may relate to the lifestyle and socio-economic status of the pregnant addict, particularly the opiate addict who is not in a methadone maintenance program. Malnutrition is frequently observed in opiate addicts, both because narcotics depress the appetite, and also because food has a lower priority than drugs in the budget of the addict; poor health care in conjunction with poor general health compound this problem. Venereal diseases occur with increased frequency in women addicted to opiates because they often resort to prostitution to obtain money to buy their drugs. Hepatitis is thought to occur in approximately three-quarters of addicts who administer their drugs intravenously, since sterility of needles, syringes, diluent and drug is not maintained. Thrombophlebitis can also result from unsterile equipment and lead to sepsis or pulmonary emboli. In addition, foreign bodies such as talc and cornstarch are frequently present in street drugs and may cause foreign body granulomata following venous injection. Pulmonary fibrosis and hypertension can be long-term complications. Quinine, an agent used to dilute the concentration of heroin, is highly sclerotic and responsible for much of the superficial scarring and abscesses which occur in opiate addicts.

During the last decade, methadone has become a widely utilized pharmacologic agent used in the place of heroin. It has been administered in controlled fashion by numerous methadone maintenance treatment programs in the United States and is also available as an illicit drug. Its advantages over heroin include: (1) longer half-life so that it need be administered only once daily, (2) availability as an oral preparation which obviates the risks of intravenous administration, (3) low cost or no charge when it is administered through a licensed methadone maintenance program, and (4) a very low street price compared with heroin. Many methadone users also abuse other psychotropic agents, and may also indulge heavily in alcohol and cigarette smoking.

COMPLICATIONS OF PREGNANCY, LABOR AND DELIVERY

Although for many years the woman addicted to heroin was thought to have decreased fertility, recent studies suggest that this is not true, and that, indeed, the parity of heroin addicts may be greater than that of a control population of both comparable and lower maternal age [26, 27]. A study from Vancouver, B. C., covering a span of 20 years, reported a lower mean age of heroin addicted mothers than in the general population with more women delivering in the 15-19 year age group [10]. Ability to maintain a pregnancy through embryogenesis is probably not impaired by opiate addiction, and teratogenesis is not thought to be related to opiates in humans. The incidence of stillbirths is increased in women who are detoxified late in pregnancy [14], and thus third trimester detoxification is not recommended. Approximately one-third of opiate addicted mothers have evidence of meconium in the amniotic fluid at the time of rupture [2], and three-fourths of the heroin addicts receive no antenatal care [5]. In one study, pregnancy was complicated in 27 % of opiate addicts by syphilis and in 18 % by hepatitis [14].

Pre-term delivery occurs with increased frequency in women addicted to heroin, possibly secondary to increased uterine irritability during times of relative withdrawal [5]. In one large series, premature labor occurred in 24 % of patients [10]. Methadone maintenance is associated with a pre-term delivery rate of approximately 18 % [14].

Disturbance of fetal growth is a major side effect of heroin addicts. Incidence of infants who are small for gestational age ranges from 30-40 % [7], compared to only 11-14 % for pregnancies of women in methadone maintenance programs [14, 35]. Poor intrauterine growth of fetuses of heroin addicts has often been attributed to poor maternal nutrition, but Naeye and his co-investigators have evidence

from autopsy specimens that heroin has a more direct effect on antenatal cell growth and number [24]. In addition, they noted a very high incidence of intrauterine infection which contributes to poor fetal growth as well as to an increased risk of preterm delivery. Mean birth weights of infants of mothers in methadone maintenance programs are less than those of a control population, but greater than those of heroin addicts [20, 26, 27, 28]. In contrast, Rajegowda et al. reported lower birthweights in 15 infants of methadone dependent mothers compared with 38 infants of heroin addicts [31]. The majority of women who are in methadone maintenance programs smoke cigarettes, which likely contributes to the relatively low birth weight of their fetuses [14, 15]. A dose relationship for methadone in the first trimester of pregnancy and birth weight has been observed [20], with higher birth weights of newly born infants being directly correlated with the maternal dose of methadone [20]. Several theories to support this observation have been suggested relating to alteration of carbohydrate metabolism by this agent, but none has been proved [20]. Animal studies have confirmed that heroin has a direct inhibitory effect on fetal growth unrelated to maternal nutrition [39, 42]. Similar effects have been noted with methadone administration; in particular, adverse effects have been described in brain growth with decreased concentrations of protein and DNA in fetal brains [8].

Complications of labor occur with increased frequency in women addicted to heroin and include fetal distress in approximately 20 % [10], prolonged rupture of the fetal membranes in 11 % and preeclampsia in 10 % [6]. All of these complications are significantly elevated when compared with a control population. In a population in a methadone maintenance program, prolonged rupture of the fetal membranes occurred in 7 % of the population and pre-eclampsia in 8 %.

PHARMACOKINETICS OF METHADONE

Studies of pharmacokinetics of opiates are few in the pregnant human, but include determinations of methadone concentrations in maternal plasma and urine, amniotic fluid, cord blood and neonatal blood and human milk [1, 2, 21]. Blinick et al. reported concentrations of methadone in maternal plasma ranging from 0.14-0.40 µg/ml and in amniotic fluid from 0.07-0.39 µg/ml with a mean ratio of 0.73 of amniotic fluid/maternal plasma concentrations.

Umbilical cord concentrations ranged from 0.04-0.25 µg/ml with a mean ratio of 0.57 (cord blood/maternal plasma). Breast milk in the first 10 days of life had a range of 0.05-0.57 µg/ml with a mean ratio of 0.83 compared with maternal plasma. Neonatal urine concentration of methadone averaged 37 % of maternal urine on day 1 and 16 % on day 3, with the baby receiving no methadone after delivery [1]. Harper and her associates reported a methadone concentration in cord blood that was usually less than 50 % of the concentration in maternal plasma obtained intrapartally and postulated this might be due either to protein binding preventing transport across the placenta or to enhanced excretion in the fetal urine [15]. Methadone can be detected in the first urine of almost all infants at risk and is undetectable in the plasma by day 5 of life. In one study of a mother-infant pair, two months after birth, analysis of tissue fluids (bloods, urines and breast milk) revealed methadone levels within the ranges noted above and a mean breast milk/maternal plasma ratio of 0.45-0.75. Following the oral administration of methadone, each of the body fluids (maternal and infant) showed an increase in concentration peaking at approximately 4 hours and gradually declining during the remainder of the day. Although the dose of methadone ingested by this infant with the mother receiving 45 mg daily was estimated to be 50-100 µg/day, the baby was completely free of symptoms [33].

Methadone is extensively metabolized in the liver utilizing enzyme systems thought not to be mature at the time of birth. It is excreted in the urine both as pure methadone and as metabolites. In addition, methadone is highly tissue-bound, tending to prolong its half-life. Thus the newly born infant, with considerable tissue-bound methadone and a decreased capability to metabolize drugs, may sequester significant amounts of methadone for weeks, resulting in a prolonged course of withdrawal or a late onset of symptoms of methadone abstinence.

NEONATAL ABSTINENCE SYNDROME

A neonatal abstinence syndrome has been described in infants with antenatal exposure both to heroin and to methadone. In most respects the syndromes are similar, but they may appear disparate. In general, neonatal signs of the abstinence syndrome include central nervous system, gastrointestinal and respiratory dysfunction [7, 11]. The most frequent signs in the central nervous system are coarse tremors at rest, hyperactivity, hypertonicity and irritability [15, 35]. Hyperphagia is frequently described and associated with excessive fist sucking [27, 28, 33]. In addition, neonatal patients with narcotic abstinence syndrome have deficits in habituation to light stimuli during Brazelton examinations [37, 38]. Even in the absence of other signs of opiate abstinence, sleep patterns are abnormal in infants of drug-dependent women [3]. Despite excessive fist-sucking, nutritive sucking is impaired in infants undergoing narcotic withdrawal [9] which leads to excessive weight loss and poor weight gain, especially for methadone addiction [20].

The incidence of signs of the narcotic abstinence syndrome varies widely in different series and may reflect quantitative differences of both heroin and methadone doses. It has been estimated that whereas a bag (capsule in Canada) of heroin contained 45 mg of the agent in 1960, the same bag in 1977 contained only 3-5 mg [10]. The smaller doses in recent years would tend to produce a lower percentage of babies with symptoms of heroin abstinence and to make the neonatal course of those infants with signs of withdrawal more mild. Most investigators report a lower incidence of neonatal heroin abstinence than of methadone abstinence. Investigators have found that 40-100 % of infants of heroin addicts have signs of withdrawal [2, 10, 20, 25, 31, 41] while the incidence is 58-94 % for infants of women who are methadone dependent [2, 14, 20, 26, 31, 34, 35]. Withdrawal from methadone seems to be more severe and more prolonged than withdrawal from heroin [31, 43]. In addition, there are reports of an increased incidence of seizures occurring during withdrawal from methadone compared with heroin [14, 15]. In one study the incidence of seizures was 7.8 % in infants of mothers maintained on methadone, 1.2 % in infants of heroin addicts and 5.1 % in infants of mothers maintained on methadone who also had evidence of heroin abuse [16]. The incidence of seizures appeared to correlate with the pharmacologic agent used to treat the abstinence syndrome, occurring in 4 % of infants treated with paregoric and 42 % of infants treated with diazepam. The mean onset of seizures was 10.1 days of age with a range of 3-34 days [16]. Seizure incidence in a mixed population of infants withdrawing from heroin and methadone indicated an incidence of seizures less than 1 % with treatment of the abstinence syndrome by paregoric [12]. Severity of signs of methadone abstinence has been reported to be unrelated to the maternal dose of methadone [16], to occur less frequently and with less severity in women on low doses of methadone [5, 23], and to occur more frequently in women on moderate to high doses of methadone [15, 26, 27, 28]. Age of onset of signs of the narcotic abstinence syndrome is earlier in infants of heroin addicts than those of methadone-maintained women. Whereas signs of heroin withdrawal usually appear within 24-48 hours, in one study 21 % of infants of women maintained on methadone first evidenced withdrawal between 6 and 8 days of age [35]. This was influenced by the proximity of the mother's last administered dose. If her last dose of methadone was more than 20 hours prior to delivery, most infants had signs of withdrawal in 3-24 hours after delivery; if, however, the last dose of methadone was administered less than 20 hours before delivery, the onset of symptoms was generally delayed to 30-52 hours after delivery [35].

DIFFERENTIAL DIAGNOSIS OF NEONATAL OPIATE ABSTINENCE SYNDROME

The differential diagnosis of an infant who is hyperactive and hyperirritable must include, in addition to the narcotic abstinence syndrome, hypoglycemia, hypocalcemia, hypomagnesemia and hyperthyroidism. In the presence of hyperthermia, sepsis must be considered, and with seizures, hyponatremia, pyridoxine dependency, polycythemia, meningitis, encephalitis, and intracranial trauma deserve consideration. The gastrointestinal symptoms of the narcotic abstinence syndrome must be differentiated from those of gastroenteritis. Even in the presence of the narcotic abstinence syndrome, any of the above abnormalities may also be present, and laboratory studies should be obtained to exclude them. In particular, the incidence of hypoglycemia and hypocalcemia is increased because of the increased incidence of poor intrauterine growth and pre-term delivery. The risk of neonatal sepsis is increased because of the increased incidence of prolonged rupture of the fetal membranes in a narcotic-addicted population. In addition, whenever maternal narcotic dependency or addiction is suspected, maternal urine and the first voided neonatal urine should undergo toxicologic examination. Serum should be obtained for determination of the presence of hepatitis-associated antigen (HAA) and cord blood should have a serologic test for syphilis and IgM.

MANAGEMENT OF NEONATAL NARCOTIC ABSTINENCE SYNDROME

Medical management of an infant with signs of the narcotic abstinence syndrome includes pharmacologic and non-pharmacologic aspects. Although an environment with decreased sound, light and physical stimuli is frequently recommended for infants withdrawing from narcotics, one study has reported that control of light and noise in the nursery setting did not alleviate the severity of the opiate abstinence syndrome [27, 28]. Often, however, by simple measures such as holding and rocking a baby, giving it a pacifier and feeding it on demand, one can alleviate much of the hyperactivity and hyperirritability of a baby during withdrawal and obviate the need for pharmacologic intervention. Assuring adequate intake, by use of gavage feeding if necessary, will help maintain normal fluid balance and by providing calories, diminish the excessive weight loss experienced by these babies. In the presence of significant vomiting or diarrhea, intravenous fluids may be necessary.

Scoring systems have been devised to assess the need for pharmacologic intervention in an infant with the narcotic abstinence syndrome [9]. If symptoms are mild, do not interfere with nutrition, and if the baby can be quieted for a large part of time, pharmacologic intervention is not indicated. In mothers using only heroin, 55-70 % of infants require pharmacologic intervention. With heroin and methadone 77 % of infants require pharmacologic treatment, and this increases to 97 % if methadone is the only maternal opiate [6, 20]. The need for pharmacologic intervention is also thought to be increased in infants born at term with weights less than 2,500 grams [7]. Pre-term infants have less severe signs and symptoms of the narcotic abstinence syndrome, presumably because their muscle tone is not yet fully developed [4, 7]; this may account in part for the differences in incidence of the narcotic abstinence syndrome in infants of mothers with heroin addiction who have a high rate of pre-term deliveries and those of mothers with methadone dependency who have a much lower rate of pre-term deliveries.

Three categories of agents have been used to treat babies with the narcotic abstinence syndrome. These are: (1) opiates, (2) tranquilizers and (3) barbiturates.

Opiates

In general, this is the most logical approach to management of an infant with narcotic abstinence syndrome, but it has been the least widely used of the three approaches.

Paregoric. — The most widely utilized opiate for treatment of infants with neonatal abstinence syndrome is paregoric, a camphorated tincture of opium [10, 16, 22, 41, 43]. The recommended dose is 0.15-0.8 ml every three to four hours as necessary to control the signs and symptoms. It has been reported to be more effective than sedatives and tranquilizers in reversal of the impairment of nutritive sucking [22] and in improving adaptive functioning [18]. It is particularly effective in infants with diarrhea because of the effect of opium to decrease motility of the gastrointestinal tract [42]. Potential concerns with the use of paregoric are related to its non-opiate components. Camphor, 4 grams/liter, is present in paregoric and as a central nervous system stimulant might augment the signs of hyperirritability. In addition, paregoric contains 4 grams/liter benzoic acid which can displace bilirubin from albumin and presents a potential risk to the infant with a high serum bilirubin.

Tincture of opium. — Tincture of opium, on the other hand, is a concentrated solution and must be diluted to 1/25 of its original concentration to provide morphine in the same concentrations as paregoric. The necessary dilution increases the risk of errors of medication and for this reason, this agent is not more frequently used [30].

Methadone. — Methadone has been administered in doses of 0.25-0.50 mg every six hours. Methadone has also been administered by means of breast feeding to a very few infants who never showed significant signs or symptoms of narcotic abstinence [33]. One tendency not to use either opium or methadone to treat neonatal narcotic abstinence is related to major concerns about prolonging the period of addiction to a narcotic agent. Breast-feeding is only rarely permitted in methadone dependent mothers and babies because of the very high frequency of maternal abuse of other agents which would also be secreted into milk and ingested by the baby [2, 33].

It has been reported, however, to be a highly effective means to avoid symptoms of methadone withdrawal in a small series of patients [33]. This form of management requires very close medical supervision, daily in the first week of life, to ascer-tain that the baby is receiving adequate nutrition for growth and is not undergoing narcotic abstinence. Mild symptoms are managed non-pharmacologically just as they are managed in the hospital setting. It is imperative that the methadone-maintained woman not miss any breast feedings as the infant receives methadone with each feeding throughout the day, the greatest amount coming within the first 4-6 hours after the mother has received her methadone.

Detoxification can be achieved in one of two ways:

(1) The mother may decide to wean the baby while continuing her own methadone dependence. In this instance she should eliminate one breast feeding every 3-5 days, beginning with the night feedings initially followed by the first feedings after her methadone administration and, finally, by the remaining daytime and evening feedings. This will usually accomplish withdrawal in 3-4 weeks.

(2) The mother may undergo detoxification over a 3-4 week period and continue all breast feedings until detoxification has been completed for 1-2 weeks. In the reported series, both methods were used with success, and the infants so treated did not undergo any signs of narcotic abstinence and had no noted behavioral disturbances in the first year of life [33].

Tranquilizers

Diazepam and chlorpromazine are the most widely-used tranquilizers to alleviate the signs and symptoms of neonatal narcotic abstinence syndrome.

Diazepam. — Diazepam has been utilized in many studies to treat the narcotic abstinence syndrome [12, 16, 23, 43]. Recommended doses range from 0.5-2.0 mg every 6-8 hours depending upon the severity of the symptoms. It was noted, however, in one study, to be associated with a greater incidence of seizures during withdrawal from methadone than was paregoric, and subsequently its use has been curtailed by that group [16]. Other investigators have noted that, when used to treat methadone withdrawal, it impairs nutritive sucking more than does methadone alone [9, 22]. Diazepam may produce apnea when used in conjunction with barbiturates; it also contains 5 % sodium benzoate and, therefore, could result in dissociation of bilirubin from albumin [25, 43].

Chlorpromazine. — Chlorpromazine is administered in a dose of 2.2 mg/kg/day divided into four doses. This agent has sedative, hypnotic, anticonvulsant and antiemetic properties and has been used with success in several large series [18, 43]. It has also been reported to correct the abnormal sleep patterns that occur during opiate withdrawal.

Sedatives

Phenobarbital. — Phenobarbital has been administered extensively in the management of infants during opiate withdrawal [10, 14, 23, 43]. Recommended doses range from 5-8 mg/kg/day divided into three doses [23, 43]. Phenobarbital may cause respiratory depression, particularly in combination with diazepam, but is an effective anticonvulsant [18, 43].

Regardless of the pharmacologic agent used to treat infants with symptomatic opiate abstinence, the usual duration of treatment is 1 and ½-3 weeks, and some infants require treatment for several months. It is important that the dosage of pharmacologic agents should be decreased as the symptoms of withdrawal improve.

OTHER NEONATAL EFFECTS OF OPIATES

Other neonatal observations include decreased jaundice, accelerated maturation of surfactant production, and thrombocytosis in babies with antenatal exposure to opiates [3, 25, 27, 28].

Significantly higher serum bilirubin concentrations were reported in a control neonatal population on days 1, 2 and 3 of life, compared with a population of infants with heroin and methadone exposure [25]. In this report glucuronyl transferase activity was also enhanced in mice that had been habituated to morphine sulfate for 12 weeks. Electron microscopy revealed an increase of smooth endoplasmic reticulum in the livers of these animals [25].

A decreased incidence of neonatal respiratory distress syndrome has been observed in infants of heroin addicts [11]. This observation was confirmed in fetal rabbits in which some aspects of lung maturation were accelerated after administration of heroin to the pregnant doe [39].

Thrombocytosis has recently been described in a number of infants of methadone-dependent women with a history of polydrug abuse [3]. The thrombocytosis developed in the second week of life and persisted for several months.

SOCIAL EVALUATION

An important aspect of the management of the infant of a heroin or methadone dependent woman is a careful evaluation of the environment into which the baby will be discharged. This involves a close liaison with a social worker who is, in general, best able to initiate this investigation, usually performed in conjunction with community social service organizations and the police department. Some hospitals have a SCAN (Suspected Child Abuse and Neglect) team to perform the evaluation and decide whether the baby can safely be discharged to its mother's care. A large proportion of infants of heroin addicts are discharged to foster placement, whereas the majority of infants of methadone-dependent women are discharged to the care of their mothers.

LATE NEONATAL EFFECTS OF OPIATES

Later neonatal effects of methadone include a delayed onset of signs of the abstinence syndrome. Kandall and his co-investigators reported a series of infants who first developed signs and symptoms between 12 and 30 days of age [19]. One baby in this report died. In many infants, however, agitation, colic, vomiting, tremors, hyperphagia, incessant sucking, increased sweating, hyperacusis and poor sleep patterns persist for several months [7, 41], and there is a well-described phenomenon of worsening of these symptoms at the time of discharge from the hospital which may last for 3-6 months [41].

NEONATAL AND INFANT MORTALITY

Neonatal mortality in infants of opiate dependent women is primarily related to complications of prematurity and infection. The narcotic abstinence syndrome should not cause death if an infant is in a nursery setting. Infants who have been discharged from the nursery and developed signs of narcotic abstinence have died secondary to dehydration in consequence of their withdrawal. An unexplained phenomenon is an apparent increase of sudden infant death in children of opiate-dependent women.

In one recent report, 2.4 % of infants of methadone dependent women died with the diagnosis of sudden infant death syndrome. In infants with moderate-to-severe signs of withdrawal, this rose to 6.7 %, and in infants with mild to minor symptoms it was 1.9 %. Sudden, unexplained infant death occurred in 0.5% of infants of non-drug-dependent women [4].

GROWTH AND DEVELOPMENT
IN INFANCY

Development of infants of methadone dependent women is abnormal through the first year of life. In general, they perform appropriately for age on Gesell testing [41], but at 12 months of age have decreased psychomotor performance on Brazelton evaluation [37, 38]. More than 50 % have behavior dysfunction with poor fine motor skills compared with gross motor skills. Beyond one year of age, they continue to have disturbances of activity level, short attention span, temper tantrums, low frustration tolerance, sleep disturbances and poor somatic growth [41].

AGENTS OTHER THAN HEROIN
AND METHADONE

Scattered reports have appeared describing an abstinence syndrome similar to the opiate abstinence syndrome in infants of mothers habituated to barbiturates [6, 17], pentazocine [13], diazepam [32], ethchlorvynol [36], propoxyphene [40] and alcohol [28].

In general, the signs and symptoms are similar to those of opiate abstinence and occur within the first one to two days of life. Propoxyphene *(Darvon)* and diazepam *(Valium)* are probably two of the most frequently prescribed pharmacologic agents in the United States; neither agent is recommended for treatment during pregnancy. Both have early onset of neonatal withdrawal symptoms.

Barbiturates, in contrast with the other agents, are associated with a delayed onset of symptoms of withdrawal, usually from four to seven days of age, although they have begun as late as two weeks of age. Barbiturate abstinence syndrome occurs not only following barbiturate abuse, but also in infants whose mothers are receiving prescribed barbiturates for seizure control or other indications [6, 17].

The clinical features associated with the fetal alcohol syndrome are well recognized and include intrauterine growth retardation, microcephaly, mid-face hypoplasia, short palpebral fissures, micrognathia, a low, convex upper lip with a narrow vermilion border. In addition, these babies have signs and symptoms of an abstinent state beginning in the first day of life and accompanied by seizures in approximately 50 % of affected babies [29].

Management of infants with signs and symptoms of abstinence from pharmacologic agents other than heroin and methadone is identical to the management described for those agents. In general, the agent chosen to treat the withdrawal state should be as similar as possible to the agent to which the fetus was habituated, with the exception of alcohol withdrawal. Treatment of the withdrawal state may be necessary for several months.

REFERENCES

[1] BLINICK (G.), INTURRISI (C. E.), JEREZ (E.), WALLACH (R. C.). — Methadone assays in pregnant women and progeny. *Am. J. Obstet. Gynecol.*, *121*, 617-621, 1975.

[2] BLINICK (G.), WALLACH (R. C.), JEREZ (E.), ACKERMAN (B. D.). — Drug addiction in pregnancy and the neonate. *Am. J. Obstet. Gynecol.*, *125*, 135-142, 1976.

[3] BURSTEIN (Y.), GIARDINA (P. J.), RAUSEN (A. R.), KANDALL (S. R.), SILJESTROM (K.), PETERSON (C. M.). — Thrombocytosis and increased circulating platelet aggregates in newborn infants of polydrug users. *J. Pediat.*, *94*, 895-899, 1979.

[4] CHAVEZ (C. J.), OSTREA (E. M.), STRYKER (J. C.), SMIALEK (Z.). — Sudden infant death syndrome among infants of drug-dependent mothers. *J. Pediat.*, *95*, 407-409, 1979.

[5] CONNAUGHTON (J. F.), REESER (D.), SCHUT (J.), FINNEGAN (L. P.). — Perinatal addiction: outcome and management. *Am. J. Obstet. Gynecol.*, *129*, 679-686, 1977.

[6] DESMOND (M. M.), SCHWANECKE (R. P.), WILSON (G. S.), YASUNAGA (S.), BURGDORFF (I.). — Maternal barbiturate utilization and neonatal withdrawal symptomatology. *J. Pediat.*, *80*, 190-197, 1972.

[7] DESMOND (M. M.), WILSON (G. S.). — Neonatal abstinence syndrome: recognition and diagnosis. *Addictive Dis.*, *2*, 113-121, 1975.

[8] FIELD (T.), MCNELLY (A.), SADAVA (D.). — Effect of maternal methadone addiction on offspring in rats. *Arch. Internat. Pharmacodyn. Ther.*, *228*, 300-303, 1977.

[9] FINNEGAN (L. P.), CONNAUGHTON (J. F.), KRON (R. E.), EMICH (J. P.). — Neonatal abstinence syndrome: assessment and management. *Addictive Dis.*, *2*, 141-158, 1975.

[10] FRICKER (H. S.), SEGAL (S.). — Narcotic addiction, pregnancy and the newborn. *Am. J. Dis. Child.*, *132*, 360-366, 1978.

[11] GLASS (L.), EVANS (H. E.), RAJEGOWDA (B. K.), KAHN (E. J.). — Effect of heroin on perinatal respiration. *Addictive Dis.*, 2, 375-368, 1975.

[12] GODDARD (J.), WILSON (G. S.). — Management of neonatal drug withdrawal. *J. Pediat.*, 92, 861-862, 1978 (letter).

[13] GOETZ (R. L.), BAIN (R. V.). — Neonatal withdrawal symptoms associated with maternal use of pentazocine. *J. Pediat.*, 84, 887-888, 1974.

[14] HARPER (R. G.), SOLISH (G. I.), PUROW (H. M.), SANG (E.), PANEPINTO (W. C.). — The effect of a methadone treatment program upon pregnant heroin addicts and their newborn infants. *Pediatrics*, 54, 300-305, 1974.

[15] HARPER (R. G.), SOLISH (G.), FEINGOLD (E.), GERSTEN (W. N. B.), SOKAL (M. M.). — Maternal ingested methadone, body fluid methadone and the neonatal withdrawal syndrome. *Am. J. Obstet. Gynecol.*, 129, 417-424, 1977.

[16] HERZLINGER (R. A.), KANDALL (S. R.), VAUGHAN (H. G.). — Neonatal seizures associated with narcotic withdrawal. *J. Pediat.*, 91, 638-641, 1977.

[17] HILL (R. M.), VERNIAUD (W. M.), MORGAN (N. F.), NOWLIN (J.), GLAZENER (L. J.), HORNING (M. G.). — Urinary excretion of phenobarbital in a neonate having withdrawal symptoms. *Am. J. Dis. Child.*, 131, 546-550, 1977.

[18] KAHN (E. J.). — Paregoric in management of narcotic withdrawal syndrome. *J. Pediat.*, 89, 520-521, 1976 (letter).

[19] KANDALL (S. R.), GARTNER (L. M.). — Late presentation of drug withdrawal symptoms in newborns. *Am. J. Dis. Child.*, 127, 58-61, 1974.

[20] KANDALL (S. R.), ALBIN (S.), DREYER (E.), COMSTOCK (M.), LOWINSON (J.). — Differential effects of heroin and methadone on birth weights. *Addictive Dis.*, 2, 347-355, 1975.

[21] KREEK (M. J.), SCHECTER (A.), GUTJAHR (C. L.), BOWEN (D.), FIELD (F.), QUEENAN (J.), MERKATZ (I.). — Analyses of methadone and other drugs in maternal and neonatal body fluids: use in evaluation of symptoms in a neonate of mother maintained on methadone. *Am. J. Drug-Alcohol Abuse*, 1, 409, 1974.

[22] KRON (R. E.), LITT (M.), ENG (D.), PHOENIX (M. D.), FINNEGAN (L. P.). — Neonatal narcotic abstinence: effects of pharmacotherapeutic agents and maternal drug usage on nutritive sucking behavior. *J. Pediat.*, 88, 637-641, 1976.

[23] MADDEN (J. D.), CHAPPEL (J. W.), ZUSPAN (F.), GUMPEL (J.), MEJIA (A.), DAVIS (R.). — Observation and treatment of neonatal narcotic withdrawal. *Am. J. Obstet. Gynecol.*, 127, 199-201, 1977.

[24] NAEYE (R. L.), BLANC (W. A.), LEBLANC (W.). — Heroin and the fetus. *Pediat. Res.*, 7, 321, 1973.

[25] NATHENSON (G.), COHEN (M. I.), LITT (I. F.), McNAMARA (H.). — The effect of maternal heroin addiction on neonatal jaundice. *J. Pediat.*, 81, 899-903, 1972.

[26] NEWMAN (R. G.), BASHKOW (S.), CALKO (D.). — Results of 313 consecutive live births of infants delivered to patients in the New York City Methadone Maintenance Treatment Program. *Am. J. Obstet. Gynecol.*, 121, 233-237, 1975.

[27] OSTREA (E. M.), CHAVEZ (C. J.), STRAUSS (M. E.). — A study of factors that influence the severity of neonatal narcotic withdrawal. *Addictive Dis.*, 2, 187-199, 1975.

[28] OSTREA (E. M.), CHAVEZ (C. J.), STRAUSS (M. E.). — A study of factors that influence the severity of neonatal narcotic withdrawal. *J. Pediat.*, 88, 642-645, 1976.

[29] PIEROG (S.), CHANDAVASU (O.), WEXLER (I.). — Withdrawal symptoms in infants with the fetal alcohol syndrome. *J. Pediat.*, 90, 630-633, 1977.

[30] PUROHIT (D. M.). — Management of narcotic withdrawal in neonates. *J. Pediat.*, 92, 1031-1032, 1978.

[31] RAJEGOWDA (B. K.), GLASS (L.), EVANS (H. E.), MASO (G.), SWARTZ (D. P.), LEBLANC (W.). — Methadone withdrawal in newborn infants. *J. Pediat.*, 81, 532-534, 1972.

[32] REMENTERIA (J. L.), BHATT (K.). — Withdrawal symptoms in neonates from intrauterine exposure to diazepam. *J. Pediat.*, 90, 123-126, 1977.

[33] ROBINSON (J. S.), CATLIN (D. H.), BARRETT (C. T.). — Withdrawal from methadone by breast feeding. In *Intensive Care of the Newborn*, III. STERN (L.), OH (W.), FRIIS-HANSEN, eds. Masson Publ., New York, pp. 213-218, 1981.

[34] ROSEN (T. S.), PIPPENGER. — Disposition of methadone and its relationship to severity of withdrawal in the newborn. *Addictive Dis.*, 2, 169-178, 1975.

[35] ROSEN (T. S.), PIPPENGER (C. E.). — Pharmacologic observations on the neonatal withdrawal syndrome. *J. Pediat.* 88, 1044-1048, 1976.

[36] RUMACK (B. H.), WALRAVENS (P. A.). — Neonatal withdrawal following maternal ingestion of ethchlorvynol (Placidyl). *Pediatrics*, 52, 714-716, 1973.

[37] STRAUSS (M. E.), LESSEN-FIRESTONE (J. K.), STARR (R. H.), OSTREA (E. M.). — Behavior of narcotics-addicted newborns. *Child. Dev.*, 46, 887-893, 1975.

[38] STRAUSS (M. E.), STARR (R. H.), OSTREA (E. M.), CHAVEZ (C. J.), STRYKER (J. C.). — Behavior concomitants of prenatal addiction to narcotics. *J. Pediat.*, 89, 842-846, 1976.

[39] TAEUSCH (H. W.), CARSON (S.), WANG (N. S.), AVERY (M. E.). — The effects of heroin on lung maturation and growth in fetal rabbits. *Pediat. Res.*, 6, 335, 1972.

[40] TYSON (H. K.). — Neonatal withdrawal symptoms associated with maternal use of propoxyphene hydrochloride (Darvon). *Pediat. Pharm. Ther.*, 85, 684-685.

[41] WILSON (G. S.), DESMOND (M. M.), VERNIAUD (W. M.). — Early development of infants of heroin-addicted mothers. *Am. J. Dis. Child.*, 126, 457-462, 1973.

[42] ZAGON (I. S.), McLAUGHLIN (P. J.). — Effects of chronic morphine administration on pregnant rats and their offspring. *Pharmacol.*, 15, 302-310, 1977.

[43] ZELSON (C.). — Acute management of neonatal addiction. *Addictive Dis.*, 2, 159-168, 1975.

13

Structure and function of the neonatal intensive care unit

Paul R. SWYER

Introduction. — The Neonatal ICU's major function is to serve as a tertiary care referral unit for a geographic region in regard to the high risk newborn. There are other aspects of reproductive medical care for which the unit may also assume responsibility. These are regional administration, education and research, basic and applied. Staffing levels must reflect these additional responsibilities to clinical service.

It is also implicit that the neonatal special care nursery should be closely associated with the obstetrical special care unit, both functionally and geographically. The content of this chapter will, however, be confined to the paediatric neonatal component of perinatal intensive care except insofar as descriptions of the other components are necessary for orientation.

Regional administration. — The tertiary care centre should take a leading role in developing a network system for support of primary and secondary care institutions in the region. Essential to this function is a mechanism for the gathering of maternal and perinatal morbidity and mortality data for the region as a whole and for the individual hospitals in the region. These data provide the basis for the operational statistics of the region on which the development of personnel and material can be planned in relation to need. They will also provide, together with costing, a measure of the effectiveness of the program and will identify areas of deficiency for attention.

Follow-up program. — An integral part of a Perinatal Intensive Care Unit is an organised follow-up program adequately staffed by physicians skilled in developmental assessment and with the ability to call upon consulting services in psychology, psychometrics, neurology, audiology, ophthalmology and rehabilitation services. Such a follow-up program provides an essential check on the performance of the tertiary care neonatal unit in terms of mortality, morbidity and appropriateness and safety of treatment procedures [1].

Professional education. — The tertiary care neonatal unit will usually be associated with a University Health Sciences Centre and will therefore have a major responsibility in undergraduate and graduate professional education, including nursing and the paramedical disciplines such as Respiratory Technology.

The unit should also adopt the responsibility for developing an outreach educational program for the secondary and primary units in the region. This should consist of formal sessions both at the centre and at individual regional hospitals and should include medical, nursing and paramedical personal at all levels. New and imaginative programs need to be developed, such as properly funded educational exchange attachments of personnel between the tertiary care unit and other institutions in the region.

Probably the greatest potential for further reduction in perinatal mortality and morbidity resides not in still further refining treatment in the tertiary care referral unit, but in educating health care providers at the primary and secondary levels in preventive management techniques which will either avoid the necessity for tertiary care, or will ensure its prompt application when required (e. g., by maternal antenatal identification of risk and prenatal referral to a combined obstetric/paediatric perinatal intensive care unit).

Public education. — An important part of this preventive strategy should be programs aimed at public education regarding appropriate conduct and lifestyle in relation to human reproduction. A recent publication of the U. S. Surgeon General [2] rightly lays particular emphasis on these aspects and on personal responsibility for appropriate conduct.

Thus, particular attention should be paid by the regional administration and educators in the tertiary care unit to the provision of appropriate counselling services, premarital, marital, antenatal, genetic, dietetic, and public health in the community. Emphasis should be placed on promoting an appropriate life style before and during pregnancy with proper nutrition, effective antenatal care, the identification of risk factors in pregnancy, referral for consultation and their appropriate management, and the avoidance of potentially harmful drugs in pregnancy, including smoking [3] and alcohol abuse [4].

Research. — The staff of the NICU should be involved in basic, developmental and operational research in reproductive medicine in the region. Research is essential not only to develop new knowledge, but also as a means of maintaining a critical attitude toward standards of care; and for developing a cadre of knowledgeable individuals able critically to evaluate recent advances in the field from other jurisdictions and to abstract them for current application locally as indicated.

Operation of unit. — Numbers and types of patient admitted. — The tertiary care centre should take an active role in collating data on risk pregnancies for the region, using one of the antenatal risk scoring systems or formal pregnancy documentation in common use in many countries or jurisdictions as part of the antenatal care system [5, 6, 7]. The obstetric/paediatric staff provide an antenatal consultation service for women with pregnancies assessed as high risk who should then be booked for delivery in the centre.

Figure I-68 shows the outcome of 1,000 unselected pregnancies as an approximate experience in developed countries. 150 pregnant women in 1,000 will have some definable risk factor in pregnancy. In about 30/1,000 this risk will be sufficiently severe to mandate referral for delivery to a level III perinatal intensive care unit; the remainder could appropriately be delivered in a special care unit at intermediate level II.

27/1,000 infants require special care at level III of whom 5 will die and at least 4 will survive with major handicaps. About 2/3 of this 27 will arise from high risk pregnancies delivered in the associated perinatal intensive care unit, but up to 1/3 will be referred from other institutions as a result of unpredicted or undetected problems occurring in newborns delivered of women with pregnancies at lower or no risk. These proportions will obviously vary with the regional morbidity experience.

Definition of perinatal intensive care units (PICU) (level III and level II). — A PICU usually functions within a University Health Sciences Centre. It has intrapartum and neonatal intensive care areas in geographic continuity and is operationally integrated under co-directors of obstetrics and perinatal paediatrics. Associated should be a unit for normal obstetrics serving the immediate surrounding area. For each 1,000 annual pregnancies in the population the total obstetric bed requirements are:

19 beds for normals (level I);
3 beds for moderate risk (level II);
1.5 bed for high risk (level III). Obviously the referral area for level III would be much larger and there would be a concentration of level III beds in the PICU [8].

The antepartum area has short and long term beds for serious pregnancy problems (e. g., diabetes mellitus, antepartum bleeding, hypertension, intrauterine growth retardation). This component, staffed by specially trained nurses, should have a 24-hour service of laboratories: biochemical; ultrasound;

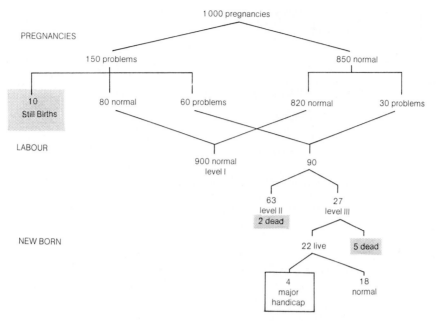

FIG. I-68. — *Schematic on the outcome of 1,000 unselected pregnancies.*

radiological; and consultation from: genetics; medical and surgical specialities; nutrition; anaesthesia; social services; and physiotherapy.

The intrapartum component consists of a labour and delivery unit with appropriate specialised staff and facilities for monitoring the condition of the mother and fetus during delivery and for providing skilled resuscitation to the newborn at delivery. The facilities should include the ability to perform immediate Caesarean section as indicated by monitoring of the maternofetal condition.

The neonatal component should be adjacent to the high risk delivery suite and resuscitation area. It provides for continuous surveillance by skilled staff and appropriate instrumentation for support of the infant for life and brain threatening disease. There should be provision for intermediate and convalescent care in separate but associated areas, with an open option to transfer the infants for convalescence to a hospital closer to the patient's home as soon as condition permits.

Indications for admission to a PICU.

Maternal. — Prior to the onset of labour: These include clinical fetal distress, abnormal maturity (pre- or post-term), significant medical complications (diabetes, cardiac, renal); obstetric complications (toxaemia, antepartum haemorrhage); gestational complications (intrauterine growth retarda-

tion, blood group iso-immunization, multiple pregnancy) other maternal or fetal and/or social factors (extremes of maternal age, parity and nutrition); conditions associated with labour include induction and trial of labour, disorders of uterine action, prolonged labour, lack of progress, clinical fetal distress, malpresentation, prior uterine surgery.

Neonatal. — Indications for admission to NICU: These include:

— severe respiratory distress (R. D. S., meconium aspiration, diaphragmatic hernia, pneumothorax, pneumonia);

— low birth weight, especially < 1,500 g whether due to prematurity or intra-uterine growth retardation;

— severe neonatal infection, septicaemia, meningitis, viral conditions;

— birth asphyxia;

— convulsions or other neurological disorders;

— metabolic disturbances, hypoglycaemia, electrolyte disorders, inborn errors of metabolism, hyperammonaemia;

— significant congenital anomalies including cardiac, gastrointestinal, central nervous system and genitourinary malformations.

Size of unit and number of beds-newborns. — Figure I-69 summarizes the numbers of newborns requiring care at levels I, II

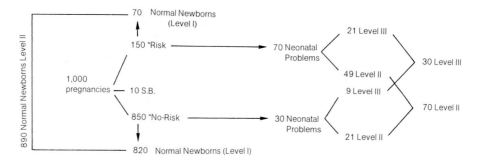

A. Schematic Showing the Derivation of the Numbers of Infants Requiring Levels I, II and III
   Facilities for Every 1,000 Live Births.

B. Summary of Distribution of 1,000 Live Births According of the Level of Care Required.

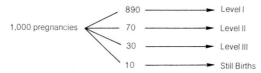

FIG. I-69. — *Summary of numbers of newborns requiring care at each level in a regionalized system.*

and III in a regional system. Specifically, for every 1,000 births, approximately 30 will require admission to the NICU each year.

Taking into account an occupancy factor of 80-85 % and an average stay of 7-10 days, 1.5-1.0 level III neonatal intensive care bassinets per 1,000 live births are needed.

The desirable size of a unit represents a compromise between administrative compactness and the need for a sufficient patient volume. This volume is necessary to maintain expertise in staff and to provide for full use of expensive facilities and equipment. Additional factors in determining bed capacity are the size of the population of the region, its geography and travel times, the birth rate and the rate of low birth weight deliveries. Table I gives the relevant numbers of beds and medical staff required for regional populations from 0.25 million to 1.5 million. Most would agree that 12-20 beds at level III is the desirable size for an NICU. Such a unit should be associated with ∼ 2/3 this number of intermediate care bassinets (level II) to care for infants with less severe illness and convalescents from level III who cannot be transferred back to local hospitals.

Structure. — The NICU should be adjacent to the high risk pregnancy unit with direct communication between the delivery/resuscitation area and the NICU.

Space allocation in the intensive care unit should be generous, 7.45-11 m² per bassinet, depending on the amount of monitoring and life support equipment necessary in a given case. Appropriate H type shelving is necessary to support the array of equipment and to provide local working and storage space [9].

Storage areas should be generous within the ICU itself, at least 11 m² per bassinet. Replenishable mobile cart supplies are useful.

There should be at least 4 oxygen, 4 compressed air, 4 suction and 16 electrical outlets provided per bassinet from a central system. Easily accessible high voltage supplies should be available in each patient area for radiographic apparatus.

Patient rooms should be temperature controlled and the relative humidity maintained between 50 and 60 %. Air circulation should be through High Efficaciency Particulate filters and provide for at least 12 changes per hour.

Hand washing facilities operated by foot taps should be generously provided in all patient care areas.

The size and numbers of patient rooms will depend on the size and organization of the unit but an open plan is to be preferred with some provision for isolation in the form of movable panel walls or separate rooms to contain a possible outbreak of infection.

TABLE I. — NUMERICAL CONSIDERATIONS DETERMINING STAFFING BY PAEDIATRIC PERINATOLOGISTS OF A LEVEL III FACILITY.

	Level III				
Population base (millions)	.25	.5	.75	1	1.5
No. live births (15/1,000 popn)	3,750	7,500	11,250	15,000	22,500
Incidence LBW/ 1,000 l. b.	70	70	70	70	70
Needing level III/ 1,000 l. b.	30	30	30	30	30
Patients/year	112	225	338	450	675
Length of stay (average) days	10	10	10	10	10
Patients days/year	1,125	2,250	3,375	4,500	6,750
Occupancy rate (%)	85	85	85	85	85
No. of beds	4	8	11	15	22
Neonatologists (equivalents)	1 *	1.5 *	2	3	4

* Single handed operation not possible unless part-time comparably skilled help available, or level II neonatologist associated.

Also required will be the following:

Components:

(*a*) patient rooms of appropriate size and number depending on the size and organization of the unit;

(*b*) each unit will require:
— nurses' station/control desk;
— chart storage and work room;
— clean supply room, can include medications and linens;
— soiled utility;
— examination and treatment room;
— instrument area, for maintenance and storage of electronic/respiratory equipment;
— admission room for outborn referrals;
— parents' room, near intermediate care area for parent contact and limited rooming-in (holding, feeding and bathing of infants).

Other requirements which may be shared with the adjacent obstetric care unit include:

— offices for medical and principal nursing staff;
— library/conference room;
— laboratory (micro blood gas and ultramicro-biochemical);
— X-ray (mobile, with image intensifier and viewing room);
— ultrasound;
— sleeping accommodation for medical staff;
— follow-up clinic for high risk infants (need not be in the same area);
— change rooms, lounges, washrooms;
— waiting room;
— in-house or other living accommodation for parents who must stay with a sick neonate.

Lighting. — General lighting should be provided by ceiling mounted fluorescent fixtures at lighting levels in accordance with those recommended in the Illuminating Engineering Society Handbook [10]. Lamps should be colour corrected to provide good colour rendition, especially for the detection of jaundice and cyanosis. Dimming facility is also recommended.

There should be a high intensity light fixture, preferably movable arm type to each patient station. This fixture should be grounded to the same "Capital Equipment Grounding bus" as all receptacles in the patient's vicinity [11].

Equipment. — Neonatal Care: The kinds of equipment required for neonatal care may be summarized under the following headings:

(1) Diagnostic. Individual stethoscopes, auriscopes, ophthalmoscopes, etc.; portable ECG, EEG, X-ray, fibreoptic lamps for transillumination; portable ultrasonographic machines; Doppler principle blood pressure apparatus.

(2) Life Support. Intubation and resuscitation equipment, ventilators, apparatus for paracentesis thoracic and abdominial drainage, cardiac pacemakers.

(3) Monitoring. Devices for direct and indirect measurement of blood pressure; micro blood gas apparatus; heart rate monitors, respiration monitors; apparatus for continuous display of patient and environmental temperature; oxygen monitoring equipment (paramagnetic, polarographic electrode and fuel cell types); transcutaneous oxygen and carbon dioxide electrodes. All monitoring apparatus should incorporate fail-safe and adjustable limit alarms.

(4) Thermal Protection. Incubators: standard, servo-controlled and transport, equipped with double walls or internal heat shields; warmers for infused

blood; radiant heaters. The thermal environment of the newborn is of extreme importance to successful outcome and has implications both for immediate care, in providing the least stressful environment for a sick infant whose thermoregulatory mechanisms are impaired, and for outcome in terms of minimizing the nutritional energy requirement for adequate growth and development (see chapter on, thermoregulation).

Medical staffing. — The three major specialties concerned are obstetrics, paediatrics and anaesthesia. The Director will usually be drawn from one of these with section heads from the other two. The Director may be aided by a management committee.

Administration of the unit. — Administrative responsibility for the unit must be clearly outlined and roles of the director(s) and unit advisory committee defined. The policy statements on administration should include the following:

(*a*) composition of advisory committee;
(*b*) relationship of committee to the board of the hospital and to the medical staff;
(*c*) responsibilities of the Director of the unit; nursing staff of the unit.

Paediatric perinatologists. — The Paediatric perinatologist should have had two years special training in the sub-specialty following certification as a specialist in Paediatrics. Skills will have been acquired with:

(*a*) critical care and life support;
(*b*) obstetric/paediatric bridge:
— growth and development of the fetus;
— perinatal resuscitation;
— adaptation to extrauterine life;
(*c*) cardiopulmonary function;
(*d*) ventilatory support;
(*e*) nutrition;
(*f*) i. v. alimentation;
(*g*) infection;
(*h*) thermoregulation;
(*i*) pharmacology of the newborn;
(*j*) administrative skills for level III unit:
— regionalization principles;
— transport;
(*k*) electronics:
monitoring and safety;
(*l*) research:
— ability to evaluate and incorporate new knowledge into practice,
— epidemiology,

— controlled trials,
— physiology.
(*m*) Follow-up program:
— assessment of growth and development,
— assessment of neurological state and behaviour.
(*n*) Education:
(*o*) Personnel management:
— ability to work with nurses, parents and technicians;
— ability to cope with tensions and emotions of all those connected with the unit.

Categories of care in a level III unit.

(1) Full life support including invasive type monitoring and ventilatory support (all modalities).

(2) Intensive care including full monitoring (invasive and noninvasive), oxygen administration, i. v. therapy, no ventilatory support.

(3) Intermediate care:
— oxygen administration,
— noninvasive monitoring,
— gavage feeding.

As part of a University Health Sciences Centre and teaching institution, the unit would have the services of residents and more importantly fellows-in training. These form a legitimate service component associated with training. There should be approximately 1 junior medical staff person to each 4 patients [16] in order to provide 24-hour medical coverage on a shift system at a level III intensity defined as (1) above.

This level of junior staffing designed to satisfy the service needs of the NICU may result in some over representation of this aspect of Paediatrics in the postgraduate curriculum, particularly as (even with this complement) work weeks of 70 hours are common. In order to partly overcome this problem, it is possible to train nurses to perform many of the technical procedures. In fact, because of their longer term commitment, nurses usually become very skilled, to the patient's advantage.

On the other hand, there are many medical judgemental decisions which need to be taken in intensive care situations which may, in the absence of junior medical staff, call for an increased time commitment by senior medical staff. The phenomenon of "burn out" has been much discussed and the current long hours and stressful nature of the work in the NICU documented [12, 13, 14]. If senior staff, already frequently overworked, and with additional academic and research commitments, are to be called upon to provide shift coverage, including night work, then new staffing schedules will be required. A 35-40-hour work week which is currently the norm in most hospitals for ICU nurses may equally need to be applied to medical staff at all levels, bearing in mind that to cover one post for 24 hours a day requires 5 persons to be employed. The budgetary implications are serious but it is contended that money expended in neonatal intensive care is more effective in saving life and function than in most other areas of special care. Moreover, it results in an offsetting saving in the direct and indirect costs of subsequent perinatally determined handicap which may last a lifetime [8].

Nursing staff. — The clinical nursing care of infants in an ICU requires a nurse-patient ratio of exceptionally 2/1; 1/1 or 1/2 more usually. A 1/3 ratio will usually classify the patient at level II rather than level III.

A shift system of about a 35-40-hour week is common, necessitating 5 persons employed for each 24 hours staffed post. For a 20-bedded ICU, therefore, a minimum of 50 nurses would be needed exclusive of administrative, teaching, clerical and domestic staff.

The most frequently mentioned problems in a recent nursing survey of ICU's [8] were the lack of sufficient competent relief staff for peak periods, and the difficulty in providing adequate in-service education in a rapidly changing sub-specialty. This difficulty consisted in insufficient available time free of patient care responsibilities and the lack of financial support for education. Solution of these difficulties is a matter of commitment to the concept of neonatal intensive care and the provision of adequate funds by the responsible authorities.

Providing the educational hurdle can be cleared there would seem to be a major scope for expansion of the nurses' care taking and therapeutic role in the ICU. The following is a list of procedures which have been authorized to be performed by specially trained nurses in some jurisdictions.

(1) Intubation of the trachea.
(2) Umbilical arterial and umbilical venous catheterization and/or blood sampling therefrom.
(3) Needling and/or drainage of the pleural space in an emergency to relieve tension pneumothorax.
(4) Radial artery puncture for blood sampling.
(5) Venepuncture.
(6) Setting up scalp or other peripheral venous infusion.

In order to avoid the phenomenon of "burn out" there should be adequate specialised back up staff available, senior medical, psychiatric and social, to cope with the many personal stresses, ethical and family problems impinging on both parents of seriously ill or dying infants and the caring staff of the unit. The individual bedside nurse should be closely involved in the decision making concerning her patient and should have representation in the administrative and policy decisions of the NICU.

Consulting and support services. — A detailed compendium of consulting and support services for reproductive medicine is available in several recent publications [9, 11, 15, 16, 24]. However it is useful to set out a listing of the consulting and special services required for a level III centre which must be available on an emergency basis 7 days a week, 24 hours a day.

An annotated listing of consultative and support services relating primarily to level III follows.

Medical and surgical consulting services. — There will need to be a full range of consulting services in general and paediatric medicine and surgery as well as their sub-specialties for the mother and the newborn respectively:

(a)	Mother	Infant
	General medicine	*Paediatric medicine*
	Cardiology	Paediatric Cardiology
	Nephrology	Paediatric Nephrology
	Endocrinology	Paediatric Endocrinology
	Pharmacology	Paediatric Pharmacology
	Dermatology	Paediatric Dermatology
	Infectious disease	Paediatric infectious disease
	Neurology	Paediatric Neurology
	Ophthalmology	Paediatric Ophthalmology
	Haematology	Paediatric Haematology
	Immunology	Paediatric Immunology

(b)	Mother	Infant
	General surgery	*Paediatric general surgery*
	Cardiovascular	Paediatric Cardiovascular
	Thoracic	Paediatric Thoracic
	Urological	Paediatric Urological
		Paediatric Neurosurgery
		Paediatric Orthopaedic
		Paediatric Plastic
		Paediatric E. N. T.

(c)	*Anaesthesia*	*Paediatric anaesthesia*
(d)	*Psychiatry*	*Child psychiatry*

mother/infant interaction and attachment, stresses surrounding serious illness and intensive care for patients, parents and staff.

Diagnostic and laboratory services. —

In the planning of Regional Perinatal Centres, attention is always given to the problems of staffing of such units, particularly with regard to health professional staff. However, little consideration is given to the fact that a Regional Perinatal Centre, like any other intensive care unit, places a considerable demand on the laboratory * and radiologic support facilities of the hospital in which they are located. Special financial arrangements need to be made for the support services that assist the perinatal unit.

Radiology. —

Continuously available consulting radiological services for both mother and infant are mandatory and are widely used. Services under this heading will include conventional diagnostic radiology; computerized tomography (level III), of major importance in the diagnosis of newborn intracranial lesions; and ultrasound (level II and level III) for materno-fetal and neonatal diagnosis. Table II estimates capital costs for conventional radiology for a neonatal unit, and table III estimates operating costs. In a recent analysis each bassinet in a Neonatal Intensive Care nursery generated 208 radiological examinations annually [8]. Infant ultrasound imaging, can be expected to play an increasing role.

TABLE II. — Estimate of capital costs for conventional radiology for a perinatal unit (1982 costs).

Capital Equipment	
Radiography unit with 105 mm spot film	$ 300,000
Radiography mobile unit	$ 30,000
Accessories	
Cassettes (various sizes) with I. screens .	$ 2,250
Protective lead aprons, gloves . . .	$ 750
Film Processor	
Kodak Automatic X-O-Mat Model M8. OR Dupont daylight system (no dark room needed)	$ 30,000
Film Viewer	
Single row five panel	$ 1,125
Shelves	
For film storage	$ 4,500
Total:	$ 368,625

* 60 % of all urgent biochemical tests performed at The Hospital for Sick Children (615 beds) originate in the 60-bedded Neonatal Unit.

TABLE III. — Operating costs for diagnostic radiology for a 30-bed (20 level III, 10 level II) neonatal unit, based on experience of the Hospital for Sick Children (courtesy Mr. Vartainen, HSC) for the year 1978.

Operating cost:	
Technologists for 8 a. m.-4 p. m. 4 p. m.-12 midnight .	$ 17,960
Standby duty Midnight to 8 a. m. & 24 hours weekends; $ 110 per week	2,860
Call back pay Average two calls per night minimum two hours per call; time and a half, 1,092 hours per year	7,776
Part-time stenographer	2,000
Radiologist	?
	$ 30,596
Supplies:	
X-Ray film. 2 films per examination based on average 10 examinations per day .	$ 2,000
Chemicals; 15 % cost of film . . .	300
X-Ray envelopes (individual)	150
X-Ray envelopes (master bags) . . .	300
Contrast media (barium, hypaque, etc.) .	150
	$ 2,900
Service and maintenance:	
X-Ray equipment; 5 % of cost of equipment per year	$ 10,000
	$ 43,496

N. B. Special equipment and its operation would be additional, e. g. ultrasound and CT scan.

Laboratory. —

A perinatal unit places considerable strain on the resources of the laboratory, particularly on the Clinical Chemistry Service. The strains affect both fiscal and staffing considerations since a 24-hour service is provided and many of the tests need to be performed manually. In a recent analysis [17] the cost of laboratory investigations (excluding any accounting for the professional component or depreciation of capital equipment) was $ 38.09 per neonatal intensive patient per day in 1977; similarly calculated laboratory investigation costs for all other in-patients in the Medical Centre averaged $ 5.74 per patient per day.

The cost figures used should be advanced by about 10 % annually (the prevailing inflation rate).

Table IV gives the laboratory units for a 25-bed tertiary care unit for one month and provides an indication of the usual monthly volume.

TABLE IV. — LABORATORY UNITS (LMS) FOR THE NEO-
NATAL INTENSIVE CARE UNIT AT MCMASTER UNIVER-
SITY MEDICAL CENTRE, FOR THE MONTH OF APRIL 1977.
EACH UNIT = $ 40.8 (1982).

	Neonatal unit
Anatomical pathology	1,589.0
Clinical chemistry	52,578.0
Biochemical genetics.	572.0
Cytogenetics	1,675.0
Haematology	28,551.0
Immunology	324.0
Microbiology	26,104.0
Other	—
Total	111,393.0
Beds	25 (list)

(*i*) Clinical chemistry. — Conventional clinical
chemistry should be continuously available for the
mother. For the newborn there should be ultra-
microchemical analyses immediately available, of
which the most important are: pH, pO_2, pCO_2,
HCO_3^-, Na^+, K^+, Cl^-, Ca^{++}, blood glucose, serum
bilirubin, BUN and creatinine. Laboratory diagnostic facilities for more esoteric metabolic biochemical
problems would be confined to level III.

(*ii*) Bacteriology (level III). — Facilities for rapid
identification of organisms and antibiotic sensitivities.

(*iii*) Virology (level III, available by consultation
at level II). — Facilities for virus isolation and
identification by culture, electron microscopy and
serological testing.

(*iv*) Haematology (level III). — Routine haemo-
grams, bone marrows, clotting profiles, blood
grouping and cross-matching.

(*v*) Genetic services (level III). — Cell culture,
karyotyping.

(*vi*) Pathology (level III). — It is essential to
maintain a high necropsy rate for diagnostic,
quality control, academic and research purposes.

Other support services.

(*a*) Respiratory technology (level III). — This
service performs an essential function in managing
and servicing life support equipment both within
the ICU and for transport. 24-hour service is
required.

(*b*) Medical engineering (level III). — This
service exercises advisory functions regarding selection of monitoring and life support equipment,
safety, maintenance and research.

(*c*) Pharmacy (level III). — A clinical pharma-
cologist (level III) with supporting pharmaceutical
services is necessary.

(*d*) Nutritional and dietetic (level III). — Maternal malnutrition is a recognized factor in compromising maternal and fetal well being in pregnancy,
while the nutrition of the neonate, particularly of
the high risk neonate, continues to present important
problems, including that of total parenteral nutrition.

(*e*) Social services (level III). — Social problems
tend to be over-represented in perinatal intensive
care units, comprising such problems as single
parents, teenage pregnancies, poor socioeconomic
circumstances. Social workers perform an essential
service in such conditions and also provide an important liaison between parents and professional staff
in the often highly stressful atmosphere of an intensive care unit.

(*f*) Physiotherapy (level III). — This service is
necessary for the care and rehabilitation of infants
with neurological and orthopaedic problems resulting from perinatal disease including that of genetic
origin.

(*g*) Occupational therapy (level III). — This
service can be extremely useful for the developmental
assessment of compromised infants and provision
of infant stimulation programs.

(*h*) Chaplaincy services (level III).

Transportation of the newborn and/or the expectant mother.

— Although approxi-
mately 70 % of risk pregnancies can be identified
antenatally, there remains still a substantial number
(30 %) of problems which are not identifiable and
which present during or immediately after delivery.
Thus, it is necessary that all levels of care (I, II
and III) be organised to deal with unforeseen
emergencies and that operational plans for support
of the lower levels by the higher, particularly by
the level III NICU be organised.

An integral part of a regional organisation is
a transportation system for mother and infant and
to a limited extent for staff, between the various
level institutions. This will mainly be by road but
there is a definite limited need for air transportation
where distance and geography, e. g., an alpine
terrain or heavy traffic make rapid road communications too time consuming.

Many transfers are for sick newborns but a significant and probably increasing number of transports are for in utero referrals of high risk mothers for delivery in level III units, from level II or level I units respectively. Because of the special medical requirements for providing care and dealing with problems in transit, a limited number of special purpose transport vehicles would ideally be desirable. These could be strategically located in depots throughout the region for maximum availability [18]. As an alternative, providing specially trained personnel and specialised equipment are available, standard ambulances may be used.

The Air Transport Service should be based centrally as fixed wing aircraft. Helicopters [19] have been found to be extremely valuable to transfer neonatal transport teams rapidly for emergency care and stabilisation prior to return by helicopter [20].

Table V indicates the advantages of transfer of the neonate by a specially trained team [21, 22].

TABLE V. — TRANSPORT OF THE NEWBORN < 1,500 G COMPARING VARIOUS MORBIDITY INDICES FOR INFANTS TRANSPORTED BY THE SPECIALLY TRAINED HOSPITAL FOR SICK CHILDREN TEAM AND BY STAFF OF REFERRING HOSPITALS (CHANCE et al., 1978) [21].

On admission	H. S. C. team	Outside team
Temp. (° C)	36.5	35.0
Arterial pressure (mm Hg) . .	58.2	46.0
pH	7.31	7.23
Duration of stay in NICU (days).	19.1	28.6
Duration of hospitalization (days)	37.9	62.4
Survival (%)	86	58

A recognized need in a regionalized system is the ability to transport the risk mother prior to delivery from a level I to a level II or III facility. For example, an increasing number (75 %) of the newborn infants in the level III facility at McMaster University Medical Centre are admitted following in-house delivery of high risk referred mothers [8]. This compares with less than 40 % referred at the initiation of the facility in 1973. Increasing in utero referral can be expected to reduce the need for difficult neonatal transport, as has been the experience at this Centre [8, 20].

There is a necessity for personnel especially trained in the transport of mothers prior to labour

and of sick infants [19]. There will be a limited requirement for skilled medical coverage of both types of medical personnel who will also need special background knowledge of transportation procedures. Specially trained nurses with physician back up in special circumstances, provide the care during transit. Such nurses have: (a) at least one year's experience of NICU nursing; (b) taken a 3-6 month course in neonatal nursing; (c) undergone a 3-month course in infant stabilisation and transport procedures; and (d) served an apprenticeship with a qualified transport nurse prior to receiving full certification as a transport nurse. Such transport nurses operate under the authority of the referral centre ICU physician and are in touch with the centre by special priority telephone or radio telephone at all times before and during transit.

Conclusion. — The complex functions, structure and operation of a Neonatal Intensive Care Unit has been described in its context as an integral part of a total patient care system for Reproductive Medical Care. The requirements for successful operation as described are very stringent if the best results are to be achieved. Less than optimal operation of such a unit will not produce the desired improvement in patient outcome.

Follow-up studies are establishing that treatment in Perinatal Intensive Care Units has:

(a) improved perinatal and neonatal mortality rates;

(b) resulted in a reduction in serious perinatal and neonatal asphyxia;

(c) improved both the mortality and outcome of very low birth weight infants weighing < 1,500 grams;

(d) despite much improved survival of newborns at risk, morbidity has not increased, but has probably somewhat decreased the total burden of perinatally determined handicap in the community;

(e) accomplished this improved outcome at significant expense to the community offset by as yet imperfectly assessed and appreciated cost savings as a result of avoidance of otherwise inevitable perinatally determined handicap.

REFERENCES

[1] FITZHARDINGE (P. M.), PAPE (K. E.). — Follow-up studies of the high risk newborn. In: *Neonatology*, Avery G. B. (ed.), third edition. J. B. Lippincott Co., Philadelphia, Toronto, 350-367, 1986.
[2] U. S. Surgeon General's Report on Health Promotion and Disease Prevention, Healthy People, 1979.

[3] MILLER (H. C.), MERRITT (T. A.). — *Fetal Growth in Humans*. Year Book Medical Publishers, Chicago and London, p. 103, 1979.

[4] MORRISON (A. B.), MAYKUT (M. O.). — Potential adverse effects of maternal alcohol ingestion on the developing fetus and their sequelae in the infant and child. *Can. Med. Assoc. J.*, *120*, 826-828, 1979.

[5] GOODWIN (J. W.), CHANCE (G. W.). — New system for managing high risk pregnancies. *Ontario Medical Review*, *46*, 563, 1979.

[6] GOODWIN (J. W.), DUNNE (J. T.), THOMAS (B. W.). — Antepartum identification of the fetus at risk. *Can. Med. Assoc. J.*, *101*, 458, 1969.

[7] AUBRY (R. H.), NESBITT (R. E. L.). — High risk obstetrics, Part I, Perinatal outcome in relation to a broadened approach to obstetric care for patients at special risk. *Am. J. Obstet. Gynecol.*, *105*, 241, 1969.

[8] *A Regionalised System for Reproductive Medical Care*. — Ed., Swyer P. R., Effer S., p. 61 et sq. Ministry of Health, Ontario, 1979.

[9] ROSS LABORATORIES. — *Planning and Design for Perinatal and Pediatric Facilities*. Columbus, Ross Labs., Division of Abbott Labs., 1972.

[10] *I. E. S. Lighting Handbook* (The Standard Lighting Guide) published by the Illuminating Engineering Society, 1860. Broadway, New York 23, N. Y. U. S. A. Refer to chapter Institutions and Public Buildings, Hospitals of current edition.

[11] *Recommended Standards for Maternity, and Newborn Care*, p. 90. Health & Welfare, Canada, 1975.

[12] MARSHALL (R. E.), KASMAN (C.). — Burnout in the Neonatal Intensive Care Unit. *Pediatr.*, *65*, 1161-1165, 1980.

[13] ASTBURY (J.), YU (V. Y. H.). — Determinants of stress for staff in a neonatal intensive care unit. *Arch. Dis. Child.*, *57*, 108-111, 1982.

[14] WALKER (C. H. M.). — Neonatal intensive care and stress. *Arch. Dis. Child.*, *57*, 85-88, 1982.

[15] *Special Care Units in Hospitals*, p. 35-49. Perinatal intensive care units. Health & Welfare Canada, 1975.

[16] *Standards and Recommendations for Hospital Care of Newborn Infants*. Amer. Acad. Pediatr., 6th ed., p. 36, 1977.

[17] *Op. cit.*, reference 8, appendix K.

[18] LALONDE (C.). — L'urgence : thème du congrès de l'Association des médecins de langue française du Canada. *Can. Med. Assoc. J.*, *117*, 1081, 1977.

[19] *Report of the Project Team on Neonatal Transportation*, Ministry of Health Ontario, 1978.

[20] MERENSTEIN (G. B.), PETTETT (G.), WOODALL (J.), HILL (J. M.). — An analysis of air transport results in the sick newborn. II. Antenatal and neonatal referrals. *Am. J. Obstet. Gynecol.*, *117*, 1081, 1977.

[21] CHANCE (G. W.), MATTHEWS (J. D.), GASH (J.), WILLIAMS (G.), CUNNINGHAM (K.). — Neonatal transport. A controlled study of skilled assistance. Mortality and morbidity of infants less than 1.5 kg birthweight. *J. Pediatr.*, *93*, 662-666, 1978.

[22] GUNN (T.), OUTERBRIDGE (E. W.). — Effectiveness of Neonatal Transport. *Can. Med. Assoc. J.*, *118*, 646, 1978.

[23] SWYER (P. R.), GOODWIN (J. W.) (eds). — *Regional Services in Reproductive Medicine*. Joint Committee of the Soc. of Obst. & Gyn. Can., Can. Paed. Society, 1973.

[24] SWYER (P. R.). — The organization of perinatal care with particular reference to the newborn. In: *Neonatology*, 3rd ed., Gordon B. AVERY, 17-47, 1986.

2

Neonatal neurology

Brain development and neurological survey during the neonatal period

C. AMIEL-TISON and J. Cl. LARROCHE

Introduction

Two fundamental remarks should be made as an introduction to these chapters, dedicated to the Central Nervous System. First, brain development is a continuous process and the stages chosen for defining the normal and abnormal appearance during growth and maturation are selected arbitrarily. Secondly, the part played by gestational age in determining brain pathology and its clinical and bioelectric expression make neonatal neurology a peculiar and fascinating subject for study.

Anatomical study

Following formation of the neural tube it is usual to recognise certain chronological stages in the cytological development of the Central Nervous System, such as cell proliferation by successive mitoses, migration, differentiation, growth and death of certain cell types. In fact, although this sequence of development remains valid as a whole, the heterogenous character of the Central Nervous System is such that both mature systems and those which are as yet undifferentiated, for example the subependymal matrix and cerebellar external granular layer co-exist at certain stages. Cellular differentiation begins while cells are still undergoing migration, well before each component has reached its predetermined destination. For example, synapses, already exist in the molecular layer of the embryonic brain at 60 days [28], at a time when the cortical plate is hardly formed. Furthermore, myelinisation, which begins in the brain stem of the fœtus at 22-24 weeks, is practically non-existent in the cerebral hemispheres of the newborn at term. Each of these processes, studied separately for convenience, is perfectly programmed and closely integrated with the others. In recent years there has been a wish to emphasize critical periods of Central Nervous System development, particularly in pathological circumstances such as malnutrition. In fact, the heterogenous character of the structures we have just considered and the extraordinary variation in the tempo of their maturation create a state of constant vulnerability throughout intrauterine life. Depending on their timing, adverse factors such as antimitotic drugs, viral infection, anoxia, ischaemia or maternal nutrition, might affect neuronal and glial cell multiplication, might interrupt their migration, curtail the branching process, or impair spine development; finally myelin may be manufactured in insufficient quantities. In the neonate the morphological appearance of lesions is very varied and depends both on the timing of the insult and on the elapse of time between the insult and examination of the brain.

The definition of morphological criteria for cerebral maturation has proved to be indispensable, both for the study of prenatal pathology, such as fœtal growth retardation or malformations, and for the understanding of neonatal cerebral pathology, because this is almost specific for a given gestational age (G. A.). Finally, the recent introduction of investigative techniques, such as the computerized tomographies (C. T.) and ultrasound (U. S.), have brought together two distinct disciplines of morphological study. Using these newer techniques the anatomist finds, in vivo, normal cerebral structures and pathological features, which are already familiar to him.

A number of parameters have been studied to define a norm for the level of maturity; some are coarse variables, e. g. weight, size and gross morphology, whilst others depend on histological and cytological criteria. Finally, the electron microscope allows the study of detailed intracytoplasmic cell structure, of neuropile and of synapses.

BRAIN WEIGHT
AND GROSS MORPHOLOGY

The structural development of the brain and its increase in weight are progressive and regular. In the embryo and fœtus the cranium is enormous in comparison to the rest of the body. During the final period of gestation the brain represents about 1/7th to 1/10th of the weight of the fœtus, whereas in the adult it represents only 1/50th of the total body weight. In contrast, in the newborn, the cerebellum represents only 1/25th of the weight of the brain, whereas, in the adult it represents 1/10th to 1/15th of the total brain weight.

The size of the hemispheres and more precisely the occipito-frontal diameter provides an indicator of maturation, notably from the 28th week. For example, at 28 weeks it is 80 mm, at 32 weeks: 90 mm, at 34 weeks: 100 mm, at 36 weeks: 110 mm, at 40 weeks: 120 mm [27]. But it is the change in the configuration of the surface of the hemispheres that is the spectacular and characteristic feature of gestational age (Fig. II-3). Up to the 18th week, the external surface of the hemispheres is smooth and the occipital pole hardly covers the cerebellum. On the interhemispheric surface the supracallosal sulcus is visible and the parieto-occipital and calcarine sulci form their characteristic Y-shaped figure. From the 20th week what was previously only a small dimple progressively hollows out to form the central sulcus or fissure of Rolando. By the 28th week the first temporal sulcus is visible in both hemispheres (Fig. II-1), and the precentral sulcus begins to appear. The so-called primary sulci, Rolandic, calcarine, supra-callosal, superior temporal and the beginning of deepenning of the Sylvian fissure are very reliable morphological criteria at this gestational age. From this moment on, the formation of gyri becomes complicated, as secondary sulci appear. Progressively and due to development of the frontal, parietal and temporal lobe, the Sylvian fissure closes, covering the insula or island of Reil. In horizontal plane sections as well as on the C. T. scan the closure can be followed week by week.

As the 34th week is approached, the arachnoid membrane appears immature, and a large volume of cerebrospinal fluid is present, filling the still rudimentary sulci and presenting as a wide peripheral space of low density on C. T. scan. The branches of the cortical meningeal arteries which derive from the primordial vascular plexus form, in the fœtus, large loops or convolutions mostly on the surface of the hemispheres. During the last months of intrauterine life, when the sulci are increasing in number some segments of arterial branches disappear and the number of anastomoses is reduced until only those between the three main arterial systems as in the adult brain remain [51]. At the same time the arteries become embedded in the depth of the sulci and the branches of the perforating arteries increase.

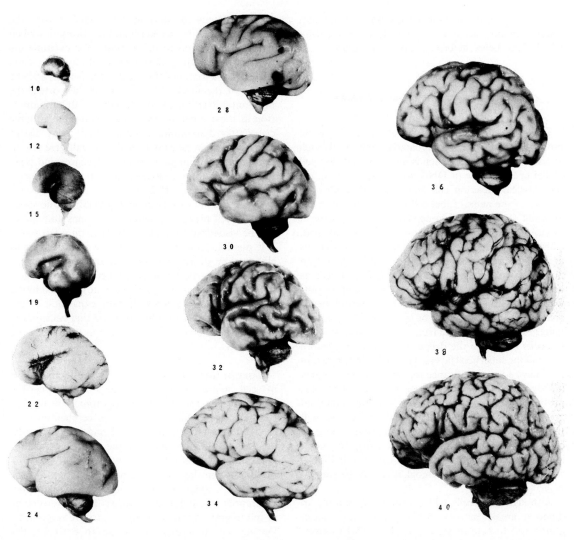

Fig. II-1. — *Morphologic aspects of external surface of the brain during intrauterine development* (from Larroche J. Cl.: *Developmental pathology of the neonate*, Amsterdam, 1977, excerpta medica. Elsevier/North-Holland Biomedical Press).

From the 12th week, all the cerebral structures are in place with the exception of the corpus callosum which develops from the rostral wall of the embryonal telencephalon, backwards, during the following weeks. This antero-posterior progression in development may explain why in partial agenesis it is generally the splenium which is absent. Furthermore, there exist constantly in the fœtus large cavities in the midline which are limited above by the corpus callosum and laterally by the leaves of the septum and the columns of the fornix. These cavities, cavum septi pellucidi in front, and cavum vergae behind, regress at the end of gestation and disappear progres-

sively after birth [27] in about 85 % of the population.

Until the 30th week, and more especially before the 20th week, the ventricles are enormous and large choroïd plexuses float in abundant cerebro-spinal fluid. This physiological hydrocephalus persists for a long time at the level of the occipital horns. The constituents and consistency of the fœtal brain are different from those of the infant and from those of the adult. During the course of development as the amounts of lipid and cell volume increase, the water content diminishes but still represents 90-91 % of the fresh brain weight between 10 and 34 weeks. The absence of myelin in the hemispheres, and the high water content, account for the low radiodensity which has been described on C. T. scan.

CYTOARCHITECTONIC DEVELOPMENT

Cerebral cortex. — Experimental work, mostly in rodents, using radioactive compounds such as tritiated thymidine which is incorporated into cell nuclei in the course of DNA synthesis, has modified the classical ideas on cell migration [7]. Following closure of the neural tube, cell divisions begin in the adjacent "ventricular" zone. Here starting from a monolayered epithelium millions of cells are formed. This cell population, at first, appears homogenous and we do not know what controls cell proliferation nor what is responsible for specialisation of cells as neurones and glia. The daughter cells migrate outwards to form, at the level of the cerebral hemispheres, the marginal layer or layer I and the cortical plate; the latter is formed from an inside-out process; the cells that form the deeper layers arriving before those of the superficial layers. This order of formation may have some significance for establishing contacts and synapses. The area between the zone of cellular proliferation or germinal layer and the marginal zone is known as the intermediate zone and will therefore be crossed by immature neurones and glial cells. Neuronal migration seems to take place along an elongated cell process, the so-called radial fibre, stretching from an ependymoglial cell to the subpial layer [43].

Although glial cells will continue to multiply in different areas, mitoses in the ventricular region, giving rise to neurones cease at about 15-16 weeks; however, daughter cells continue to migrate from the ventricular region after this period until the germinal matrix has been exhausted. At 26-28 weeks there is still a well marked germinal zone in the region of the thalamo-striate sulcus, partially covering the caudate nucleus; in this zone the density of immature cells is considerable and quite comparable to that of the cortex. In the earliest C. T. scans of premature babies it is probable that certain mistaken diagnoses of germinal layer haemorrhage were due to the high radiodensity of this region [40]. Similarly the diagnosis of subarachnoid haemorrhage was without doubt sometimes erroneously made, due to misinterpretation of the significance of the very dense narrow band of the highly cellular cortex.

Neuronal migration is not entirely synchronous in all parts of the brain, and the appearance of the cortical plate is not uniform; from the 28th week the major types of cortex, hetero- and isocortex, described in the adult, begin to differentiate, for example the motor cortex in the prefrontal convolution, the visual cortex in the margins of the calcarine fissure, and the cortex of the insula. The height of the cortex, the horizontal striation and the degree of cellular maturation at these different levels, can be used as reliable criteria for determining gestational age. Any distortion or delay in neuronal migration will give rise to topographical anomalies of varying degree and type, such as heterotopia, lissencephaly, and certain forms of microgyria (Fig. II-2).

By the use of Golgi impregnations [32] the development of cell processes, dendrites, axones and spines can be visualized (Fig. II-3). By electron microscopy it is possible to precisely follow the appearance and elaboration of the neuropile and of the synapses necessary for passing messages between cells. Since the total number of neurones is already defined in the foetus of less than 20 weeks it is the expansion of the cell surfaces and the proliferation of glial cells that is largely responsible for the increase in the volume of the brain.

Cerebellar cortex. — A better understanding of cell migration in the cerebellum is possible thanks to the use of autoradiographic histological techniques [34]. Maturation of the cerebellum proceeds by alternating divisions and migrations of cells, a process still incomplete at the end of gestation. Although the cerebral cortex (with the exception of the plexiform layer) is formed by migration of cells from inside-outwards, the cerebellar lamellae differentiate from outside inwards. The various steps of cell migration can be grouped into five stages [25]. During the embryonic period up to 8 weeks, the cerebellum is represented by a rhombencephalic outgrowth of bilaminar structure: an external layer of low cellularity and an internal layer in which Purkinje cells differentiate. During the foetal period an external granular layer forms, the cells of which, like a matrix, migrate inward to form the internal granular layer, which still persists in the newborn at term. Successive migrations of these cells and their differentiation give the appearance characteristic of different gestational ages. At first 3 layers, later 5 layers and still 4 at full term are recognised (Fig. II-4). During the first 6 to 8 months after birth the external granular layer gradually disappears via an inside migration of cells and the cerebellar lamellae acquire the adult configuration of three layers.

Anomalies or delay in migration of cells may lead to the appearance of dysplastic islands of cells of various types [27].

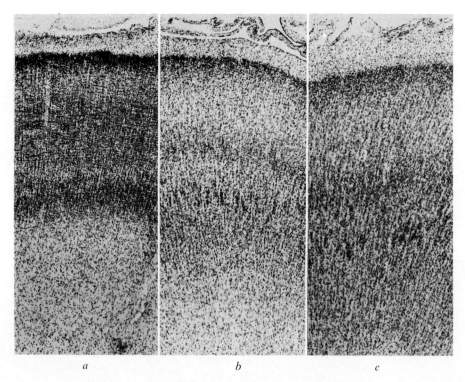

FIG. II-2. — *Motor cortex at 28 weeks*, (*a*) 34 weeks, (*b*) 40 weeks, (*c*) (cresyl violet stain)

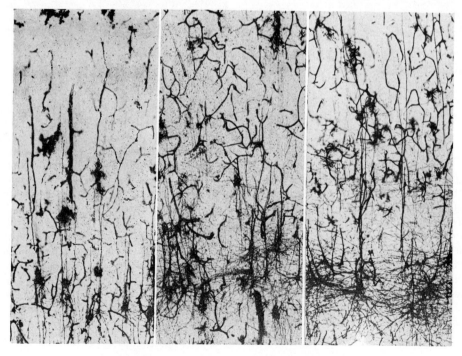

FIG. II-3. — *Same area at identical age as* (fig. II-2). (*Golgi cox.* preparation)

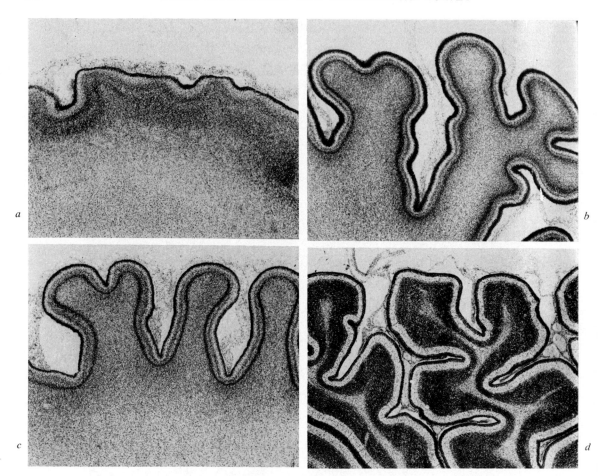

FIG. II-4. — *Development of cerebellar lamellae.*
(*a*) 16 weeks, (*b*) 24 weeks, (*c*) 32 weeks, (*d*) 40 weeks.

MYELOGENESIS

Various methods can be used to demonstrate myelinated fibres, such as the Loyez method or luxol fast blue stain. The number and the thickness of myelinated fibres is measured by the intensity of staining. This method is obviously subjective but is reliable in the hands of an experienced observer. In this way it is possible to map out the progress of myelinisation [26], though the asynchrony of the process in the different tracts and systems makes this study difficult. The regularity with which myelinisation occurs at any given level allows the anatomist to use each one of the stages as a reliable indication of maturation or gestational age. Myelinization begins in the second half of fœtal life. It develops in a caudocephalic direction. Spinal roots and ascending tracts are myelinated first, then follow brain stem, the statoacoustic, vestibular and extrapyramidal systems. Thalamocortical fibers and the optic system begin to myelinate around 36 weeks. The first myelinated fibers of the pyramidal tract are visible in the pons at about the same period. Myelination will continue well into infancy and after the first year of life, and even beyond the third decade. This is true notably of cortical association fibers. The duration of myelinization is specific for a given system. These myelogenetic "cycles" [55] reflect, reasonably accurately, the degree of specialisation and elaboration of each system.

Exploring cerebral function

NEUROLOGICAL EXAMINATION OF THE NEONATE AT TERM

The normality of the central nervous system in the neonate born at term can be verified very rapidly by routine systematic examination. A lively look, a vigorous cry, efficient sucking and swallowing, grasping, an active response to forward traction, can suffice within 30 seconds for investigation of conscious state, reflexes and active muscle tone. The ill neonate presents a different problem; neurological examination must be very detailed, repeated and interpreted as part of the general examination.

Clinical examination must be flexible enough to adapt itself to each individual neonate. An observation period will precede manipulations which will of necessity be very limited in ill neonates. If the infant has just had a feed, or on the contrary is too agitated or too hungry, the examination must be postponed.

Cranial and spinal examination

Cranial examination. — Cranial morphology is observed first: deformation of the skull may be very obvious in the first days of life and then disappear. The caput succedaneum at the site of the presenting part, often ecchymotic, changes its location with the position of the infant in the cot. Anomalies of the skin and hair are also looked for.

Abnormal cranial shapes suggest craniostenosis: the head being narrow and lengthened in the case of synostosis of the sagittal suture; or wide with a flat forehead in cases of synostosis of the coronal suture. A wide cranium, anteriorly, with a convex forehead suggests hydrocephalus. A large head with a very prominent occiput, suggests a Dandy-Walker malformation. Palpation is used to check for the presence of cephalhematomas, which are fluctant pools of blood lifting the periosteal membrane. The examiner's fingers should follow the suture line searching for disjunction, overlap or premature closure, the size of the anterior and posterior fontanelles is noted. Uneven ossification, craniotabes and cranial lacunae are looked for, by palpating the cranial bones.

Measurement of the cranium relies on the use of a tape-measure, to determine the largest occipito-frontal circumference. This is a simple and reproducible method, and it has been shown, that the values obtained closely parallel the results of more sophisticated radiological methods for measurement of cranial volume.

This measurement is entered on an intra-uterine growth curve and compared to the size and weight at birth. Head circumference should be measured several times during the first week, because the presence of a caput succedaneum and modelling of the cranium affect the initial figure.

Cranial auscultation should be undertaken in cases of cardiac insufficiency, as it may reveal a loud murmur due to arterio-venous malformation, most frequently an aneurysm of the vein of Galen.

If the neurological examination is abnormal or if the head circumference is unusually large or small the head is transilluminated. This should be a routine procedure on initial examination. A simple torch with a soft rim, or a more sophisticated cold light source (see below), will show abnormal light diffusion in cases of abnormal fluid accumulation, whether it is peripheral or intraventricular. It will demonstrate a subdural collection cerebral atrophy, porencephaly or hydrocephalus. The permissible size of the halo obtained, depends on the light source used. With an ordinary electric light, less than 1 cm is considered normal. Norms for successive gestational ages have been established with the chun-gun, thus avoiding many diagnostic errors [53].

Measurement of intracranial pressure should also enter into the routine examination because it is simple, reliable and informative. Non-invasive methods for measurement of pressure through the anterior fontanelle, using fibreoptics or tocography have recently been developed [39]. The results are expressed in cm of water. The norm, for an infant at rest, lies between 8 and 10 cm. A figure greater than 15 cm for a newborn, while lying still, is a sign of intracranial hypertension.

Examination of the vertebral column. — The vertebral column must be inspected and palpated during the course of routine examination to search, in particular, for congenital abnormalities, dimples, fistulae, angiomata, and tufts of hair. If any of these are present the examination should be completed with X-rays of the vertebral column.

State of alertness

Alertness of the neonate is judged by looking at spontaneous and stimulated motor responses: opening of the eyes, facial mimicry, breathing movements, and crying. A normal newborn infant can be easily woken by moderate stimulation, where upon he or she makes spontaneous movements and opens his eyes. A quiet awake state is easily achieved and maintained for some time. This represents the optimal state for neurological examination. The definition of the state of wakefulness in the neonate, has been shown to be so important in the interpretation of all the clinical examinations in the newborn that a classification of sleep or waking states, proposed by Prechtl, has been widely adopted [50].

Stage 1: Closed eyes, regular breathing, no movements.

Stage 2: Closed eyes, irregular breathing, a few movements.

Stage 3: Open eyes, a few movements.

Stage 4: Open eyes, highly active, no crying.

Stage 5: Open or closed eyes, crying.

This is a coarse assessment but sufficient for many neurological investigations. During the course of the examination as a whole, it is important to notice the state which predominates and also, sometimes, the precise stage at the time of each manœuvre. More refined observations of neonatal behaviour and potential interactions with the environment have been developed by Brazelton [11-12]. These observations have led to the establishment of "scores" allowing evaluation of qualitative differences and seeking to extract information of value in prognosis.

Examination of cranial nerves

This is performed simultaneously with initial evaluation of the level of consciousness, making contact with the neonate and observing its responses to stimulation. The 2nd and 7th cranial nerves can be explored by the response to bright light, which causes blinking and a facial grimace. Contraction of the pupils in response to light is a test for the 2nd and 3rd nerves. The neonate at term can fix on an object or face within an angle of some 60° and if the object or face is brought close enough, between 20 to 30 cm, he is able to focus on it. To complete the examination,

the retina is examined with an ophthalmoscope. A pale, greyish appearance of the optic disc is normal in the neonatal period; nystagmus due to an absence of fixation is without significance in the first weeks; on the other hand, blinking in response to a bright light can be obtained even if blindness is later shown to be present.

Discovery of chorioretinitis suggests toxoplasmosis or a cytomegaloviral infection. The oculomotor responses dependent on the 3rd, 4th and 6th cranial nerves are tested by observing spontaneous motor responses and by the permanence of visual fixation on a face or object when the head is moved from side to side. The integrity of the 7th nerve is more readily analysed when the infant is crying, than when he is quiet. Deviation of the mouth to the unaffected side is the most characteristic sign of lower motor neuron facial palsy. However, facial paralysis is too frequently diagnosed in the neonate due to confusion with a congenital, and sometimes genetic, defect of the peribuccal muscles. Diagnosis of bilateral facial paralysis is difficult; it is suggested by an absence of facial expressions and impaired sucking ability. Evaluation of the response to noise, allowing evaluation of the 8th nerve, is made by observations of its effect on the face, on breathing, and on spontaneous movements. Sucking brings into play the 5th, 7th and 12th nerves, swallowing the 9th and 10th. The tongue should be examined for atrophy, fasciculation, hypertrophy or hemihypertrophy.

Examination of motor function

Examination of the motor system is based on evaluating spontaneous movements and analysing muscle tone.

Spontaneous motor activity. — The frequency and symmetry of spontaneous limb movements are observed before disturbing the infant. This gives a rough guide to clinical status, spontaneous movements being qualified as normal, excessive or insufficient.

Passive tone. — Although in the past 30 years neurophysiological studies have added many new elements to the better understanding of tone, the different aspects of clinical examination of tone, as described by André Thomas, remain indispensable for clinical evaluation. The terminology is, therefore that of Thomas and his school [46, 48, 49].

Analysis of passive muscle tone involves study of extensibility and flapping.

Extensibility is judged, region by region, by means of a certain number of manœuvres, which assess the amplitude of a slow movement made by the observer, the infant remaining passive. The result can most often be expressed as an angle, estimated, but not measured; at other times it is expressed in relation to anatomical reference points (the scarf sign, lateral rotation of the head) or, by rough assessment of a curve, for example of the trunk. In all these manœuvres the examiner must control his own strength and look for the limit at which discomfort in the infant becomes perceptible.

The evaluation of flapping investigates the amplitude of a movement created by a rapid, but passive, movement of a distal segment and therefore looks at the extent of resistance in antagonist muscle groups.

During examination of passive muscle tone the infant's head must be maintained in the axis of the trunk, in order to avoid interference by the asymmetric tonic neck reflex. All the manœuvres used for assessment of passive muscle tone are described in several recent publications [5, 41, 46, 50]. Some of the most frequently used will be described here. The normal results of these manœuvres, in the neonate at term, are shown in tables (I-III) summarising the clinical stages of maturation.

Posture. — Before disturbing the newborn, observation of posture is important, as reflecting passive tone. The posture of the lower and upper limbs is observed: complete extension, intermittent flexion or very pronounced permanent flexion. However, the position *in utero*, and the fixation of the limbs, inevitably modify spontaneous posture during the first days of life.

The trunk posture is also observed, opisthotonos is obvious if present. It is due to permanent hypertonicity in the spinal extensor muscles, which keeps the trunk arched. The infant cannot stay flat on the back and the resting position is in the lateral decubitus position, in hyperextension. The wakeful state is optimal (stage 3) for judging a normal trunk posture. In fact, sleep causes a general relaxation of muscle tone, whereas wakefulness increases opisthotonos.

Heel to ear manœuvre. — With the infant lying on his back, the lower limbs, held together are lifted

TABLE I. — POSTURE AND PASSIVE TONE FROM 28 TO 40 WEEKS OF GESTATION, INDICATING INCREASING MUSCLE TONE IN UPPER AND LOWER EXTREMITIES, WHICH DEVELOP WITH INCREASING GESTATIONAL AGE. (From AMIEL-TISON, C. In: RUDOLPH A. M., BARNETT H. L. and EINHORN A. H., editors: Pediatrics, ed. 16 [Appleton-Century-Crofts book], Englewood Cliffs, N. J. 1977, Prentice Hall, Inc.).

Gestational age (weeks)	28	30	32	34	36	38	40
Posture	Completely hypotonic	Beginning of flexion of thigh at hip	Stronger flexion	Froglike attitude	Flexion of four limbs	Hypertonic	Very hypertonic
Heel-to-ear maneuver	150°			130°	100°		90°
Popliteal angle	150°		110°	100°	100°	90°	80°
Dorsiflexion angle of foot			40-50°		20-30°	Premature reached weeks 40° / Full term 0°	
Scarf sign	Scarf sign complete with no resistance		Scarf sign more limited		Elbow slightly passes the midline		Elbow does not reach midline
Return to flexion of forearm	Absent (upper limbs very hypotonic lying in extension)			Absent (flexion of forearms begins to appear when awake)	Present but weak, inhibited	Present, brisk, inhibited	Present, very strong, not inhibited

TABLE II. — ACTIVE TONE FROM 32 TO 40 WEEKS GESTATIONAL AGE
(ref. as for Table I).

Gestational age (weeks)	32	34	36	38	40
Lower extremity	Brief support	Excellent straightening of legs when upright			
Trunk	–	± Transitory straightening	Good straightening of trunk when upright		
Neck flexors	No movement of head	(face view) Head rolls on shoulder	Brisk movement, head passes in axis of trunk	Head maintained for a few seconds	Maintained in axis for more than a few seconds
Neck extensors	Head begins to lift but falls down	(profile view) Brisk movement head passes in axis of trunk	Good straightening but not maintained	Head maintained for a few seconds	Maintained in axis for more than a few seconds

up and moved as far as possible towards the ears. The amplitude of the arc traversed by the legs is evaluated. The pelvis must not be raised during examination. During this manœuvre, when the muscle tone in flexion is very strong, the popliteal angle is not completely open. Therefore, the angle formed by the thigh and table is not the one measured, but the angle formed by the line joining the heel to the pelvis and the table. Normal values are between 80° and 100°.

Popliteal angle. — The thighs are abducted and flexed on either side of the abdomen whilst the pelvis rests on the table; while maintaining this thigh position, the leg is maximally extended on the thigh. The angle formed by the thigh and calf is the popliteal angle. The right and left angles are measured simultaneously. Their normal value lies between 80° and 100°.

Dorsi-flexion angle of the foot. — While leg extension is maintained by a hand placed on the infant's knee, the examiner flexes the foot onto the leg, by applying thumb pressure on the sole of the foot. The angle formed by the back of the foot and the anterior surface of the leg, is the angle of dorsi-flexion of the foot. The manœuvre is carried out successively on the two sides. The normal value lies between 0° to 10°.

Recoil of lower limbs. — This can only be investigated if the spontaneous posture is in flexion. The two legs are simultaneously extended, by pushing the knees downward and then releasing them. The lower limbs rapidly return to their initial position.

Scarf sign. — The infant is supported in a half sitting position by a hand placed behind the back and neck: The examiner places his elbow on the table for support. One of the infant's hands is held and pulled in front of the chest, as far as possible towards the opposite shoulder. The position of the elbow in relation to the median line is noted. The result is expressed according to the position of the elbow. Both arms should be tested successively.

Position 1: The elbow fails to reach the median line.
Position 2: The elbow passes the median line.
Position 3: Movement very ample; the arm encircles the neck (like a scarf), very little resistance is detectable in the shoulder muscles.
Normal result in the fullterm = position 1.

Return to flexion of forearm. — This can only be investigated if the spontaneous posture of the infant is in flexion. The two sides are tested simultaneously. The arms are extended by pulling on the hand or lower forearm.

When released, the forearms return rapidly to the initial position of flexion, in a brisk and reproducible manner. When the response is active, it is not inhibited by maintaining the forearm in extension for ten seconds; in this case the response is described as "springy".

Active tone. — Anything that brings into play the motor or postural activity of the newborn should come under the heading of active tone. It is therefore impossible to describe it completely. A few manipulations will be described, where the examiner alters the posture of the newborn to obtain a directed motor response. Here again, only the most commonly used manœuvres will be described briefly.

Righting reactions of the lower limbs and of the trunk. — The infant is maintained in a vertical position (supporting reaction); the observer encloses the anterior surface of the thorax in his palm. The thumb and middle finger lie in each armpit and the index finger supports the chin. The lower limbs react by a righting movement. This is followed by contraction of spinal muscles, such that the infant supports a large part of his own weight for several seconds. The righting reaction is considered present even if the knees stay in semi-flexion, due to hypertonicity of the lower limbs flexor muscles.

Active contraction of the neck flexors. — The test known as "pulling to a sitting position" assesses the flexor muscles of the neck.

The infant is laid on his back. The observer takes the shoulders in the palm of his hand and raises the infant to a sitting position. The movement exerted on the trunk must neither be too quick nor too slow. The position of the head during the course of this movement, which induces a reaction from the neck flexor muscles, is observed. At first the head may or may not be bent back. Then the flexor muscles contract and bring the head forward, an active

"passage" occurs even though the trunk has not reached a vertical position (Fig. II-5).

In the normal infant at term, the tone of the extensor and flexor neck muscles is almost equal and the infant can keep his head in the axis of the trunk for several seconds, before letting it fall forward (Fig. II-5 *a*).

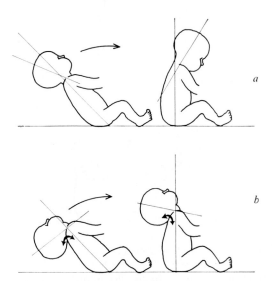

FIG. II-5. — *Head straightening with neck flexors in a full-term newborn.*

a) Normal reaction: before the full vertical position is reached, the flexor muscles are stimulated to raise the head.

b) Abnormal reaction: permanent hypertonia of the neck extensors maintains the head backward. The head remains extended and active forward "passage" is impossible.

(From AMIEL-TISON C. *et al.*: in neck extensor hypertonia. Early human development. *1*, 181-190, 1977 (with permission)).

The "passage" of the head is considered abnormal in the following instances :

If it is difficult to demonstrate, not maintained or not reproducible, it is classified as difficult.

If the head, hanging back passively at the beginning of the movement, passes the mid-line passively, by the action of gravity alone, and then falls immediately forward, the "passage" is classified as passive.

When there is permanent hypertonicity in the extensor muscles of the neck, the head remains extended and active forward "passage" is impossible. The contraction may be so strong that even passive forward movement of the head is prevented (Fig. II-5 *b*). The most easily recognised phenomenon is "forward fall impossible" in the leaning forward position.

Active contraction of the neck extensors. — Movement in the opposite direction assesses the neck extensor muscles (Fig. II-6).

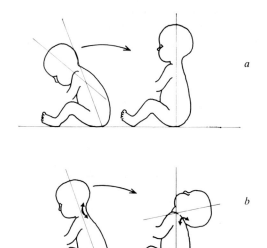

FIG. II-6. — *Head straightening with neck extensors in a full-term newborn.*

a) Normal reaction: before the vertical position is reached, the extensor muscles are stimulated to raise the head.

b) Abnormal reaction: the head, unable to fall forward on the chest at the beginning of the movement, passes backward too quickly in such a way that the reaction appears "too good".

(From AMIEL-TISON C. *et al.*: in neck extensor hypertonia. Early human development. *1*, 181-190, 1977 (with permission)).

The infant is sitting, leaning forward, head bent on chest; the observer takes him by the shoulders and moves him backwards. Observation is made of active head movement, provoked by this manipulation which must be neither too quick nor too slow. These movements in a vertical plane (forwards-backwards, and backwards-forwards) demonstrate the alternate contractions of extensors and flexors with symmetrical "braking" of the movement. This is normally observed in the neonate at term from the first days of life (Fig. II-6). The passage of the head is abnormal in the following cases:

— If it is difficult to demonstrate, not maintained or not reproducible, it is classified as difficult.

— If the head, hanging forward passively at the beginning of the movement, passes the midline, passively, by the action of gravity alone, and falls immediately backward, the passage is classified as passive, *i. e.* absent.

— When there is a permanent hypertonicity in the extensor muscles of the neck, the head is unable to hang on the chest at the beginning of the movement, being maintained strongly by the extensors. The head then passes backward too quickly, in such a way that the reaction appears too strong (Fig. II-6). Symmetrical "braking" of the movements of the head are not obtained when oscillations of the trunk around a vertical plane are applied.

The main difficulty in analysing these actions is linked to the impossibility to separately test these 2 sets of muscles. However, the addition of "foreward fall impossible" and "too good" passage backwards allows one to recognise neck extensor hypertonicity, often suspected on the basis of postural opisthotonos. A different situation can be recognised by the addition of "too good" passage backwards but a normal drop forwards of the head; this is the association observed in the case of poor active tone in the neck flexors, usually suspected because of an abnormally ample scarf sign.

Conclusion of the motor examination. — To conclude an examination of muscle tone, the upper and lower limbs and the right and left side must be compared. The quality of muscular contraction must be assessed. Its normality is evaluated from the strength of the righting reflexes and the response to traction.

Reflex activity

Primary vestigial reflexes. — These reflexes are stereotyped responses shown by the newborn in the first months of life. Thus they are one element of the neonatal neurological investigation. They must be present, symmetrical and reproducible. They retain their interest in the months following birth because of their progressive disappearance in the course of normal development or their abnormal persistence. Only those which are currently looked for will be described here.

Sucking-swallowing. — These two reflexes are tested with the teat or finger. In the neonate at term, sucking is vigorous, rhythmic and associated with synchronous swallowing movements.

Finger grasping. — The examiner places his index fingers in the palms of the infant. This stimulates strong finger flexion. The grasping response is very vigorous in the neonate at term.

Response to traction of the flexor muscles of the upper limb. — Having elicited the grasp reflex, the examiner raises his hands, putting traction on all the flexor muscles of the upper limb. The infant is raised up and can support all or part of his weight. This tonic flexor response depends on the quality of the infant's active tone.

Most often in the course of this manœuvre, the head raises in the axis of the trunk and the lower limbs are strongly flexed. This entirely active response is very spectacular.

Moro reflex. — The infant in dorsal decubitus is raised up several centimetres, by applying light traction to the two hands. The upper limbs are extended. When the hands are sharply released the infant falls back on the examining bench and the reflex appears.

Initially, the arms are abducted and extended (first stage), then adducted and flexed (the embracing movement of the second stage). The hands open completely during the first stage. Then the infant cries. Note whether the reflex is absent, asymmetrical or obtained after only slight excitation (low threshold).

In this case a series of clonic movements are often observed.

Crossed extension. — One foot is stimulated by rubbing the sole, whilst the lower limb is held in extension. The response is observed in the opposite lower limb.

(1) Extension, after a rapid movement of flexion.
(2) The toes fan-out.
(3) Adduction bringing the free foot onto the stimulated foot.

The first two elements of the response are constant. Adduction depends on the stage of maturity. It only becomes obvious at 39-40 weeks.

Automatic walking. — The infant is kept in a vertical position to obtain righting of the trunk and gently bent forward. If the feet are brought into contact with the examination table, the infant will take a few steps.

Tendon reflexes. — Several of these are systematically investigated, the biceps jerk, the knee jerk, and the ankle jerk. They are normally brisk.

TABLE III. — STRENGTH OF SIX REFLEXES FOR INFANTS BETWEEN 28 AND 40 WEEKS OF GESTATIONAL AGE *

Gestational age	28 weeks 30 weeks	32 weeks	34 weeks	36 weeks	38 weeks	40 weeks
Sucking reflex	Weak and not really synchronized with deglutition	Stronger and better synchronized with deglutition	Perfect — — — — → — — — — — — → — — — — →			
Grasp reflex	Present but weak	Stronger		Excellent		
Response to traction	Absent	Begins to appear	Strong enough to lift part of the body weight		Strong enough to lift all of the body weight	
Moro reflex	Weak, obtained just once, incomplete	Complete reflex — — — → — — — → — — — → — — — →				
Crossed extension	Flexion and extension in random pattern, purposeless reaction	Good extension but no tendency to adduction		Tendency to adduction but imperfect	Complete response with • Extension • Adduction • Fanning of the toes	
Automatic walking		Begins tip-toeing with good support on the sole and a righting reaction of the legs for a few seconds	Pretty good, very fast tiptoeing		A premature who has reached 40 weeks walks in a toe-heel progression or on tip-toes. A full-term newborn of 40 weeks walks in a heel-toe progression on the whole sole of the foot.	

* From Amiel-Tison, C.: In Rudolph, A. M., Barnett, H. L. and Einhorn, A. H., editors: Pediatrics, ed. 16 (Appleton-Century-Crofts book), Englewood Cliffs, N. J., 1977, Prentice-Hall, Inc.

Cutaneous plantar reflex. — This has been the subject of a considerable literature. However, it is little used because the response is very variable and dependent on the mode of stimulation. One can agree with Hogan that it is normally flexor when the lateral surface of the heel is stimulated [22]. An extensor response is usually related to a lesion in the brain stem or spinal cord.

NEUROLOGICAL EXAMINATION IN THE PREMATURE NEONATE

Clinical examination allows a schematic analysis of the different stages of cerebral maturation. Saint-Anne Dargassies described the stages by analysis of tone and reflexes [45, 46]. This examination can be simplified by choosing the most reliable tests. These have been illustrated on schemes, which can be included in every clinical record [1, 2].

The evolution of posture and passive tone is represented in table I. Flexion first appears in the lower limbs, then the upper limbs. It is this caudocephalic progression which defines the different stages. The evolution of active tone is shown in table II, this is the area most often neglected in examination, yet it is the most reliable. The different reactions show on the one hand the caudocephalic progression, and on the other, the predominance of axial extensor muscles over flexor muscles until their equalisation at about 40 weeks. Finally, the primary reflexes are illustrated in table III. They are present at 28 weeks but the quality of the response improves with gestational age and the progression of muscle tone changes their expression. The appearance of adduction and crossed extension is particularly significant because it is never observed before 35-36 weeks.

The stages of this evolution are described in two week periods; it is considered that to reach a conclusion, the responses must be clustered on a given maturational pattern. If the responses are too dispersed it may not be possible to reach a conclusion concerning gestational age. The examination gives an estimate and not a "score". It can only be carried out if the child's condition allows mobilisation of the head and trunk; it therefore has obvious limitations and other methods have been described that can give a "score" under all circumstances. Neurological examination is then restricted to evaluating the passive tone of the limbs; the addition of external criteria is claimed to improve the correlation with gestational age.

The most widely used scoring method is that of Dubowitz [17]. It has been followed by others which

are more simple [9]. Despite the difficulties, and limitations of this assessment of maturity, it remains necessary for paediatricians to know the stages of maturation; only from this starting point can neurological symptoms be assessed: Since a given tonic state, considered normal at 28 weeks, is abnormal at 40 weeks.

ELECTROENCEPHALOGRAPHIC FINDINGS

The bioelectrical phenomena recorded from the cranial surface undergo rapid changes during infant development. They have been the subject of numerous publications [14, 18, 24, 35, 38].

Maturation of cerebral electrical activity is not a continuous phenomenon. Study of the distribution of the major bioelectric phenomena over a period of time, leads to the recognition of groupings which correspond to stages of developmental maturation.

Between 24 and 32 weeks of gestational age, the speed of bioelectric development allows dating of the tracing to within 15 days. The features typical of this period are a discontinuous type of electrical activity, the low reactivity hardly appreciable without applying integrating techniques, and the difficulty in distinguishing clinically between waking and sleeping states.

At 24 weeks the tracing is disordered and polymorphous. It contains rhythms of delta, theta and alpha frequency and some high voltage spikes which are grouped together in bursts of several seconds separated by periods of electrical silence (lasting from 10 seconds to 2 or 3 minutes).

At 28 weeks (Fig. II-7) the dominant activity consists of brief bursts of theta rhythm at 5 c/s, synchronous over the whole of one hemisphere, alternating with slow, high amplitude waves.

At 30 weeks (Fig. II-7), associated with the theta rhythms, there appear bursts of slow fronto-occipital waves on which rapid rhythms are superimposed. These are characteristic of the tracing in the premature infant after 32 weeks.

At 32 weeks (Fig. II-7) the absence of differentiation between tracings of sleep and waking states persists. E. E. G. activity remaining discontinuous during deep sleep and becoming more continuous during active sleep and the waking state.

At 35 weeks (Fig. II-7) the first tracings of sharp frontal transient activity appear.

At 36-37 weeks, the difference between sleep and waking states can be detected in the tracing for the first time. This constitutes the first step in maturation. The tracing of the waking state will persist until one

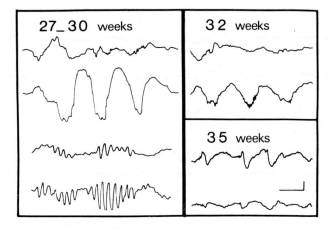

FIG. II-7. — *E. E. G. pattern at 27-30 weeks, 32 weeks and 35 weeks.*

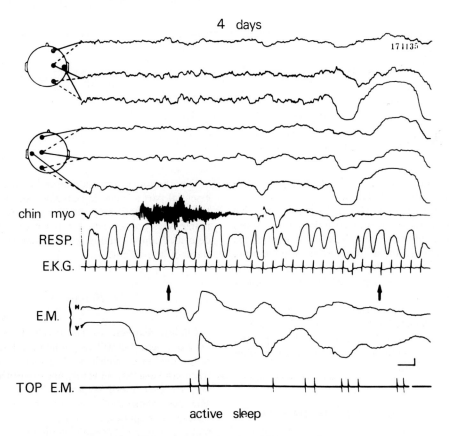

FIG. II-8. — *Active sleep in a full-term newborn.*

Polygraphic recording includes 6 scalp electrodes, electromyogram (E. M. G.), respiration (resp.), electrocardiogram (E. K. G.). Recorded eye movements (E. M.) and observed eye movements (TOP E. M.). Calibration = 1 sec. 50 μV. During active sleep, there is a continuous slow wave pattern, with respiratory irregularities; REMs are present and the E. M. G. disappears.

3 days

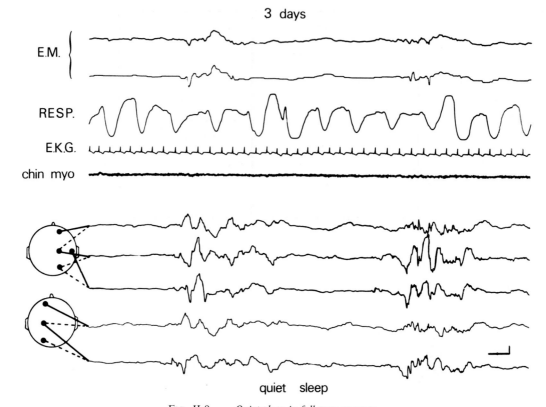

E.M.

RESP.

E.K.G.

chin myo

quiet sleep

FIG. II-9. — *Quiet sleep in full-term neonate.*
Idem as in fig. 8). The E. E. G. pattern is discontinuous, respiration is regular, eye movements absent; the activity on E. E. G. reflects brain activity; continuous E. M. G. activity.

month after normal term, remaining slightly rhythmical and uniform in all areas.

At 40-41 weeks (Figs. II-8, II-9) deep and active sleep are well differentiated. Active sleep is associated with a tracing of low amplitude, which is continuous and polyrhythmic, similar to that of the waking state. Quiet sleep shows an "alternating" pattern consisting of bursts of slow waves separated by intervals of low voltage activity.

Three months after normal term a second essential stage is reached: for the first time in the infant an organised occipital waking state rhythm appears, which can be interrupted by external stimulation (stopping reaction).

CLINICAL SIGNS OF BRAIN DAMAGE

Signs of brain damage can be obvious, they can also be very discret, for example, the finding of a head circumference on a percentile below that of the infant's length.

Observation of the neonate in his incubator is an essential part of neurological assessment. The rest of the examination may be carried out using the manœuvres appropriate for the neonatal period as described above, taking full account of the clinical state of the infant.

Seizures

Clinical features. — The cerebral cortex in the neonatal period is still very immature but is capable of producing convulsions. The clinical features of these convulsions, however, are often disconcerting and are even more atypical in the very ill infant. The development of tonic spasms is unusual. In certain cases apnoea, chewing movements and abnormal eye movements enable clonic movements in the limbs to be characterised as a convulsion. Prolonged observation is, therefore, indispensable. A clinical classification is necessary; that proposed by Volpe [52] is simple; it distinguishes five different types of convulsions, described in the order of decreasing frequency.

"Minimal" signs which are very discrete and therefore often missed: abnormal posture of a limb such as extension and internal rotation of an arm, lateral eyeball deviation, clonic movements of the eyelids or chin or diaphragm, blinking episodes and excessive salivation. Each of these episodes is accompanied by apnoea and a change in colour. These signs are all associated with a persistent disturbance of consciousness. Recording abnormal electrical activity simultaneously with these signs, will confirm the clinical suspicion of a convulsion.

Tonic convulsions produce an opisthotonic posture, accompanied by apnoea or stertorous breathing, ocular signs and tonic extension of all limbs.

Clonic seizures, arising from multiple foci (multifocal), are characterised by clonic movements migrating from one limb to another in a random manner, sometimes becoming generalized and spreading to the four limbs.

Focal seizures only affect one extremity and are not accompanied by a disturbance of consciousness. They have no value in localisation.

Myoclonic convulsions are usually located in one or several extremities. They consist of regular trembling lasting for a variable length of time. They are rare and particularly associated with metabolic disorders. They indicate a severe cerebral defect.

The diagnosis of seizures is often wrongly made when the infant displays bursts of clonic movements. An episode of such movements, affecting the four limbs, can look like a multifocal convulsion; however these incidents are usually induced by stimulation. They occur after stimulation in an alert infant and are accompanied neither by respiratory signs nor disturbances of consciousness. Prolonged observation by an experienced clinician is needed to recognize this activity as being of no special significance in the first days of life.

The diagnosis of status epilepticus deserves special attention.

It can be defined as the repetition of seizure activity at short intervals without a return to normal alertness and normal muscle tone in the intervals. Status epilepticus can be so designated when it continues for 30 minutes or more. The prognosis, for cerebral function, usually unfavourable, justifies making this distinction; the prognosis is based more on the characteristics of the tracing between convulsions than on their frequency.

Investigations. — These are designed to rapidly confirm or eliminate the principle causes of convulsions.

The electroencephalogram is an indispensable source of diagnostic and prognostic information. The recording should be made in the 24 hours following the convulsive episode and repeated 5 days later. Obviously treatment must begin immediately, without waiting for the recording.

Lumbar puncture is necessary to confirm or eliminate the diagnosis of meningitis. A series of bacteriological investigations will complete the evidence for or against the presence of infection.

Blood glucose and blood calcium must be measured immediately. Plasma electrolytes and acid-base status should also be measured immediately. The use of Dextrostix methods allows immediate evaluation of the blood glucose level and is of obvious importance.

Etiology. — Clinical and laboratory studies often establish the cause of the convulsions, i. e. perinatal anoxia, meningitis, hypoglycaemia or hypocalcaemia. In the absence of any of these, the search for a cause is longer and more complex. It begins by eliminating rare metabolic disorders. All these investigations may be negative and the convulsions remain unexplained [30]. "Delayed" status epilepticus (occurring late in the neonatal period) appears to be clinically different, showing particular features on the EEG and a benign clinical course [13]. Familial cases have been described [42].

Anticonvulsant treatment. — The convulsions must be stopped by eliminating the cause whenever possible but also by symptomatic treatment. The basis of treatment of neonatal convulsions remains phenobarbital. The intravenous route is used initially, so that a high blood level is rapidly obtained. The dose is 15-20 mg/kg. Injected slowly over a period of about five minutes, into a peripheral vein [20, 52]. The maintenance dose is 5-7 mg/kg/24 hours. Dosage is modified according to blood levels, effective concentrations are between 15 and 20 mg/l. In status epilepticus this treatment rarely suffices, and various other anticonvulsants are also used, the choice depending on local custom. This can be intravenous diazepam, given repeatedly in doses of approximately 2 mg/kg. Its action is rapid but often transient. Intravenous diphenylhydantoin, in a priming dose of 15-20 mg/kg and maintenance dose of 5-7 mg/kg/ 24 hours, is also used. As with phenobarbital the effective blood level for diphenylhydantoin is approximately 15-20 mg/kg. Alternatively a 4 % solution of paraldehyde (3 to 4 ml/kg) can be injected intravenously over a period of 10-15 minutes.

Since all these drugs depress respiration, a means of intubation must be readily available. The accumulation of these drugs in infants, who are often oliguric or anuric is a substantial risk and their blood levels must be monitored throughout.

Other signs of cerebral damage

The classification of all the possible deviations from normal, in the neurological examination, would be tedious. In current practice it is most useful to recognise combinations of typical signs.

Signs of central nervous system depression. — The waking state is difficult or impossible to obtain. The cry is weak or absent, visual perception and all the primary reflexes are diminished or absent. Feeding is made dangerous or impossible by inadequate sucking and incoordinate swallowing; spontaneous mobility is diminished or absent, passive and active tone is reduced, hypotonia is generalised. Coma and depressed breathing are signs of the severest form of depressed cerebral function. Convulsions, if they occur, will not be very evident and are difficult to recognise in the comatose infant.

Signs of hyperexcitability. — The reverse situation is represented by signs of hyperexcitability. The cry is sharp and excessive; the state of quiet sleep is difficult to obtain, primary and deep tendon reflexes are exaggerated with a low threshold of stimulation. Hyperactivity is present, with clonic movements of the limbs (large, slow movements) or with fine tremors of the extremities (very rapid, small movements). Passive tone is exaggerated and there is generalized hypertonia. These signs of irritability can precede the appearance of convulsions.

Signs of intracranial hypertension. — The signs found on examination of the head and the neurological signs of intracranial hypertension, are inversely proportional to each other because they both depend on the ability of the sutures to separate, in response to an increase in intracranial pressure.

Cranial signs. — The fullness of anterior and posterior fontanelles is increased; they are sometimes bulging and tense. The sutures are separated: at first the sagittal, then the coronal, the metopic and parieto-occipital; finally and therefore of most significance, the squamous or temporo-parietal sutures separate. Systematic examination by palpation of all the sutures, is necessary to evaluate their separation in millimetres. Excessive increase in head circumference is due to separation of the skull bones. The

maximum tolerable rate of increase, during the first weeks, is about 1 cm/week. A change in skull shape is only seen in very severe or long lasting intracranial hypertension.

Neurological signs. — Disturbances in level of consciousness, ocular signs, and respiratory signs, are the same as at other periods of life. Lethargy, downward deviation of the eyes, and apnoea are signs of severe intracranial hypertension since initially, the cranial bones are able to separate relieving pressure on the brain. On the other hand, disorders of tone should be investigated using techniques appropriate to the neonatal period [3]. Posture is abnormal, and the head is thrown back even during sleep. Examination of active tone in the anterior and posterior neck muscles and of the trunk shows a permanently increased extensor tone. Thus, when the infant is in a sitting position the head is held back and the drop forward no longer takes place when the infant is leaning forward (Fig. II-5). With movement in the opposite direction, from sitting to lying, the starting position is abnormal (the head is behind the axis of the trunk) (Fig. II-6) and this posture becomes more pronounced when the backward movement of the trunk is initiated. In extreme cases it is not possible to put the infant in a sitting position, he arches backwards in opisthotonos, and contraction of the axial muscles cannot be overcome. On the other hand, papilloedema is not part of the symptomatology in the newborn.

Fontanometry confirms the presence of intracranial hypertension when the values obtained are greater than 15 cm of water. It is also a usefull method of following the clinical course and assessing the effect of treatment.

There are many causes of intracranial hypertension in the neonate and treatment will obviously depend on the cause and whether the hypertension is acute or chronic. However, it is important not to neglect intracranial hypertension; it must be recognized, investigated and rapidly treated.

The acute hypertension of ischaemic-anoxic encephalopathy, for example, is usually treated by a combination of osmotically active agents and corticosteroids. Mannitol in a 10% or 20% solution is given at once, by the intravenous route for its rapid action.

A dose of 0.50 g/kg by rapid injection is sufficient and can be repeated every 6 hours during the first 24 hours. At the same time fluid intake is restricted. Dexamethazone may be started simultaneously but will only act after 12 to 24 hours, when it takes over as the important therapeutic agent. It can be administered either intravenously or intramuscularly every

6 hours in a total daily dose of 0.25-0.5 mg/kg following a priming dose of 0.5 mg/kg. The treatment is continued for 5 to 7 days.

In chronic intracranial hypertension repeated lumbar punctures or acetazolamide are at present considered the best expectant treatment, in the period preceding possible surgery. Acetazolamide is used in a dose of 10 mg/kg/24 hours, given by mouth, in two daily doses [6]. Treatment can be continued, without problems, for several weeks, with monitoring of potassium levels and of the acid-base state. It is not specific for one type of intracranial hypertension because it probably acts generally on secretion and re-absorption of cerebro-spinal fluid.

Localised signs. — They are infrequent during the neonatal period, however investigation must always be made on any differences between right and left throughout neurological examination, in inspecting body movements and the facial grimace and in evaluating tone and reflexes. The term hemisyndrome describes asymmetry between the right and left side of the entire body: it is not rare to find left sided hypotonia in the normal neonate at term. Perhaps it represents an early manifestation of laterality. Paralysis of one upper limb usually has an obstetric origin. A careful search for associated signs such as Horner's syndrome or phrenic paralysis must be made. Localised signs can be related to localised lesions such as a subdural haemorrhage, an abscess, or a vascular accident. However, frequently, localised signs, as in the case of focal convulsions, have no precise relationship to the site of the lesion.

In conclusion, various symptom complexes are commonly encountered, which may be transitory or may persist and become aggravated. Repeat examination is always necessary when any anomaly is detected.

Classification in the neonatal period. — Follow-up of full-term neonates and correlation with the long term prognosis has shown that neurological symptoms, during the first week of life [4], can usefully be classified into 3 grades of severity.

Minor signs (Stage 1). — Hyperexcitability and anomalies of tone are present without disturbance of consciousness. Primary reflexes are elicited and there are no convulsions.

Moderate signs (Stage 2). — A combination of signs suggesting depression of the nervous system is present. In particular consciousness is affected and the primary reflexes are diminished or absent. One or several isolated convulsions can appear.

Severe signs (Stage 3). — Status epilepticus, defined by repeated seizures on a background of altered consciousness and muscle tone.

The presence or absence of blood in the cerebrospinal fluid does not affect this symptomatic classification. By the end of the first week, half the Stage 1 cases return to normal. This is exceptional in Stage 2 cases and never occurs in Stage 3 cases.

The combination of these signs is interpreted in the total clinical context. Gestational age, the circumstances of pregnancy and labour, drugs administered to the mother and the possibility of infection are taken into account.

According to the suspected diagnosis, various further investigations will be necessary.

FURTHER INVESTIGATIONS

Cerebrospinal fluid

Lumbar puncture is mostly always necessary in the face of neurological problems. If the dura appears to be under tension during passage of the needle, this is an abnormal sign and suggests intracranial hypertension.

Meningitis must always be considered whenever there is the slightest sign of cerebral involvement, during the neonatal period. The normal limits for cerebrospinal fluid are wider during the neonatal period and especially in the premature than in later life: 10 to 25 white cells is an acceptable figure and likewise are several hundred red blood cells. The albumin concentration in C. S. F. is also raised, it can reach 1 g/l or more in the premature. Above 3,000 red blood cells the liquid is turbid, slightly pink, and intracranial haemorrhage can be diagnosed with certainty, although without any implication as to its site or severity. The difficulty is, in fact, to eliminate a traumatic puncture. The 3 tube test or the presence of xanthochromia do not always resolve the uncertainty, given that the C. S. F. albumin is often raised in the neonatal period. Culture is performed routinely even on haemorrhagic fluid.

Subdural puncture is, at present, rarely carried out. However, when severe neurological signs are present from birth after such traumatic events as a high forceps or difficult breech delivery, the possibility of bilateral subdural haemorrhage must be investigated. Subdural taps are done only if the anterior fontanelle is sufficiently wide to allow puncture at a good distance from the sagittal sinus.

Ventricular puncture is only performed in exceptional circumstances.

Retina

Ophthalmoscopy of the fundi will reveal retinal haemorrhage in cases of perinatal distress, but can be especially useful in diagnosing rare disease.

Electroencephalography

When and how should an E. E. G. tracing be performed to obtain the optimal information? The E. E. G. should be made within the first 2 or 3 days in the fullterm newborn and within the first 5 or 6 days of life in the preterm infant. The E. E. G. should be repeated in the course of the illness, especially in case of clinical worsening. A single tracing performed after the acute stage of the disease, 2 or 3 weeks after birth, has no prognostic value. Therefore, appropriate equipment should be available at the bedside in an intensive care unit. What kind of information can be obtained from the E. E. G.?

Evaluation of maturation. — The gestational age can be evaluated accurately to within 2 weeks. The E. E. G. will confirm the foetal age or indicate it when gestational data are lacking or in the small-for-dates infant. This is not possible, however, if there are too many abnormal figures on the tracing. Concordance between "electrical" and "clinical" age is a good prognostic sign. Absence of electrical criteria of maturation indicates a poor prognosis [15]. An E. E. G. tracing that appears too young for foetal age is abnormal but may be a transient finding without pronostic value.

Evaluation of sleep organisation from various polygraphic criteria (Figs. II-8 and II-9). — For this evaluation, it is necessary to record various parameters, eye movements, respiration, chin electromyogram, and to observe the infant carefully for at least 60 to 90 minutes. Good sleep organisation within the first 2 days of life in the fullterm infant is associated with a good prognosis in 70 % of cases, whereas the prognosis is poor in 70 % of cases in the absence of sleep organisation lasting longer than 3-4 days [16].

Abnormal patterns. — Three of these will be described.

Presence or absence of electrical discharges (electro-clinical or sub-clinical) such as rhythmical discharges of slow or rapid frequency: delta (0.5 to 3 cycles per second), theta (4 to 7 cycles per second), alpha (8 to 12 cycles per second), beta (over 12 cycles per second), or repetitive spikes of different frequencies, more or less high and sharp or complex patterns associating spikes and slow waves (Fig. II-10).

These discharges last from 10 seconds to several minutes; they usually start from a focus in one hemisphere and migrate from one region to another in the same hemisphere or from one hemisphere to the other (Fig. II-10) or diffuse to the whole scalp. Generalized discharges not preceded by a focal discharge are rarely seen. Electrical discharges without any clinical manifestation are more frequent in the preterm than in the fullterm baby. Electrical discharges with simultaneous complex symptomatology are seen both in premature and in fullterm babies. Continuous recording lasting several hours in a neonate who has had convulsions is a means of evaluating the efficacity of anticonvulsant therapy. Presence of electrical discharges on the E. E. G. of a premature infant is a disquieting prognostic sign. However, as in the fullterm newborn, prognosis cannot be based solely on the presence of electrical discharges but depends also on the quality of the background activity, recorded between the discharges.

Prognosis relies mainly on the *modifications of background activity*: the evolution is always severe with inactive tracings, that is to say absence of activity under good conditions of recording, lasting at least 2 hours; in a neonate of 9 hours or more (drugs given to the mother during or before delivery can modify the background activity of the E. E. G. of the neonate during the first 6-8 hours of life), paroxysmal tracings in the fullterm newborn and a permanent discontinuous tracing in the premature also have a poor prognosis (Fig. II-11). In these cases the E. E. G. has lost all physiologic pattern; activity consists of bursts lasting 1-10 seconds, of spikes, slow waves, theta rhythms or rarely beta rhythms occurring on an inactive background. In a fullterm newborn, during its first 24 hours of life, inter-burst intervals lasting 40 seconds or more indicate a poor prognosis. These paroxysmal or permanent discontinuous tracings show no reactivity and no sleep organisation. To affirm the severe prognosis the recording must be continued for at least 2 hours and the possibility of drug intoxication by phenobarbital, clomipramine, and/or diazepam must be eliminated.

Presence of pathologic patterns. — These are usually spikes, rapid rhythms without physiologic characteristics or focal slow waves. Positive spikes or sharp waves have a particular pathological value in the premature baby until 36 weeks gestational age.

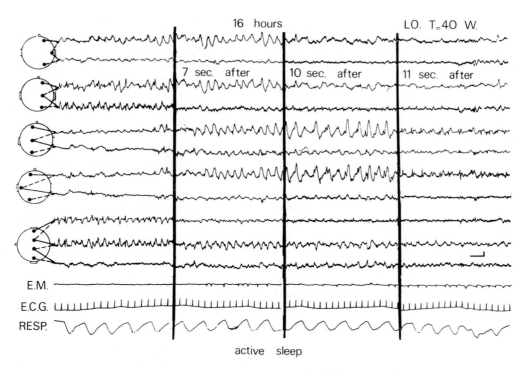

FIG. II-10. — *Alternative right and left electrical seizures in a full-term newborn at 16 hours of life = rhythmic activity of various types, slow waves, sharp waves and complex pattern associating spikes and slow waves.* The interseizure E. E. G. is moderately abnormal; late outcome has been good.

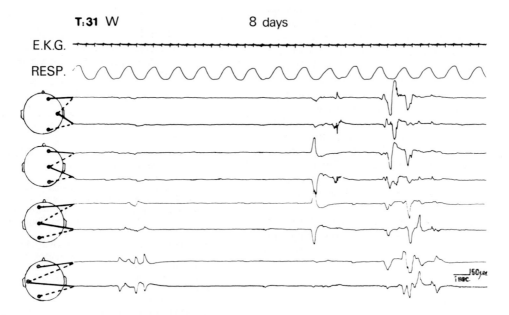

FIG. II-11. — *Permanent discontinuous recording in a 31 week old premature.* Absence of maturation of E. E. G. No physiological E. E. G. activity; Rolandic slow positive spikes. Death at day 14. At autopsy diffuse multicystic leuco-malacia and necrosis of the basal ganglia.

Correlations between E. E. G. and anatomical lesions. — Inactive and paroxysmal E. E. G.'s are mainly seen in neonates suffering from ischaemic-anoxic encephalopathy with cortical and/or subcortical neuronal necrosis.

Positive Rolandic spikes are often seen in premature babies with intraventricular haemorrhage or extensive leucomalacia.

Electrical discharges may be seen in various cerebral lesions. In the premature baby they often indicate intraventricular haemorrhage or extensive parenchymal lesions such as leucomalacia, meningo-encephalitis or intracerebral haemorrhage.

Electrical discharges are often focal in the neonate without indicating focal anatomical lesion. However, persistence of focal discharges on a prolonged recording or on several successive E. E. G.'s may be seen in cases of intracerebral haemorrhage or arterial occlusion. Arachnoid haemorrhage and subdural hematoma have no specific pattern on the neonatal E. E. G.; if E. E. G. abnormalities are seen with such haemorrhage, they indicate lesions of the subjacent cerebral parenchyma.

Radiographic and radio-isotopic investigations

Since 1976 the C.T. scan has revolutionised cerebral investigation during the neonatal period. The quality of the pictures obtained and the apparent harmlessness of the method have led to the almost complete disappearance of pneumoencephalography, angiography, and scintillation scanning. Normal appearances in the neonate have been described [40]. Studies of radiological anatomy have improved the interpretation of the pictures obtained, and therefore allow clinico-radiological correlations of improved accuracy in cases of survival [29]; by confirming the existence of ischemic or haemorrhagic lesions, and by making the chronology and sequential development of lesions more accurate [19]. More recently, however, the indications for C. T. scanning have been reduced and repeat examinations avoided because of fears that the immature brain and lens are particularly sensitive to X-rays.

Measurement of isotopic transit time still has certain rare indications in the investigation of intracranial hypertension, since it gives dynamic information on C. S. F. circulation, not provided by other methods.

Ultrasonography

This method has been rapidly replacing the C. T. scan for several indisputable reasons: the investi-gation is done without removing the child from its cot; it is innocuous, therefore repetition is possible, and it shows dynamic features—in particular, vascular pulsations [10, 23, 37, 47]. These non-invasive methods, have renewed interest in anatomico-clinical correlations in neonatal neurology, and put into question many of the physiopathological hypotheses of recent years.

Other investigations

Clinical examinations and radiological investigations require wide experience for interpretation of the evidence, and the results are expressed qualitatively. Quantitative methods for the newborn are at present under review. The study of visual or auditory potentials has again become profitable with recent technological progress, both in the study of maturation and for the detection of cerebral lesions [33].

Transcephalic impedance [44] is another method of study. It measures the resistance of the head to an alternating current. This resistance regularly increases with gestational age. It varies according to the cranial contents, and has been used to follow hydrocephalus and ischaemic-necrosis. Measurements of blood flow, using the Doppler effect [8] or xenon clearance [31], have not yet entered clinical practice. It is likely that C. T. scans using labelled glucose (positrion emission tomography) will be of considerable importance as will be functional studies utilizing the principles of nuclear magnetic resonance (N. M. R.).

Changes in C. S. F. enzymes, after asphyxia, reflect cerebral cellular destruction. However, the practical value of such measurements has not yet been established [21, 54].

References

[1] AMIEL-TISON (C.). — Neurological evaluation of the maturity of newborn infants. *Arch. Dis. Childh.*, *43*, 89-93, 1968.

[2] AMIEL-TISON (C.). — Neurological evaluation of the small neonate: The importance of head straightening reactions. In *Modern Perinatal Medicine.* L. GLUCK, Ed., Year Book Medical Publ., 347-357, 1974.

[3] AMIEL-TISON (C.), KOROBKIN (R.), ESQUE-VAU-COULOUX (M. T.). — Neck extensor hypertonia: a clinical sign of insult to the Central Nervous System of the newborn. *Early Hum. Dev., 1*, 181-190, 1977.

[4] AMIEL-TISON (C.). — A method for neurological evaluation within the first year of life. In *Major Mental Handicap.* Ciba Symposium n° 59. Elsevier, North-Holland, 107-126, 1978.

[5] AMIEL-TISON (C.), GRENIER (A.), Eds. — *Evaluation*

neurologique du nouveau-né et du nourrisson. Masson, Paris, 1980, 120.

[6] AMIEL-TISON (C.), KOROBKIN (R.), HORNYCH (H.) et al. — Delayed intracranial hypertension, in the premature neonate following chronic fetal distress. In *Newborn Intensive Care,* III. L. STERN and B. FRIIS-HANSEN, Eds., Masson Publ., New York, 1981, 239-252.

[7] ANGEVINE (J. B. Jr), SIDMAN (R. L.). — Autoradiographic study of cell migration during histogenesis of cerebral cortex in the mouse. *Nature,* 192, 766-768, 1961.

[8] BADA (H. S.), HAJJAR (W.), CHUA (C.) et al. — Non invasive diagnosis of neonatal asphyxia and intraventricular hemorrhage by Doppler ultrasound. *J. Pediatr.,* 95, 775-779, 1979.

[9] BALLARD (J.L.), KAZMAIERNOVAK (K.), DRIVER (M.). — A simplified score for assessment of fetal maturation of newly born infants. *J. Pediatr.,* 95, 769-774, 1979.

[10] BEJAR (R.), CURBELO (V.), COEN (R. N.) et al. — Diagnosis and follow-up of intraventricular and intracerebral hemorrhages by ultrasound studies of infant's brain through the fontanelles and sutures. *Pediatrics,* 66, 661-672, 1980.

[11] BRAZELTON (T. B.), Ed. — Neonatal behavioral assessment scale. *Clinics in Developmental Medicine,* n° 50, Philadelphia, Lippincott, 1973, 60.

[12] BRAZELTON (T. B.). — Behavioral competence of the newborn infant. *Seminars in Perinatology,* 3, 35-43, 1979.

[13] DEHAN (M.), QUILLERON (D.), NAVELET (Y.) et coll. — Les convulsions du cinquième jour de vie. *Arch. Fr. Péd.,* 34, 730-742, 1977.

[14] DREYFUS-BRISAC (C.), MONOD (N.). — The electroencephalogram of fullterm newborns and premature infants. In A. REMOND Ed., *Handbook of Electroencephalography and clinical neurology-physiology.* Amsterdam, Elsevier Publ. Co., 1975. vol. 6B, 6-29.

[15] DREYFUS-BRISAC (C.). — Neonatal electroencephalogram. In E. M. SCARPELLI, E. V. COSMI, Eds., *Reviews in perinatal medicine,* vol. 3. Raven Press, N. Y., 1979, 397-472.

[16] DREYFUS-BRISAC (C.), PESCHANSKI (N.), RADVANYI (M. F.) et coll. — Convulsions du nouveau-né: aspects cliniques, électrographiques, étiopathogéniques et pronostiques. *Rev. EEG Clin. Neurophysiol.,* 11, 367-378, 1981.

[17] DUBOWITZ (L. M. S.), GOLDBERG (C.). — Clinical assessment of gestational age in the newborn infant. *J. Pediatr.,* 77, 1-10, 1970.

[18] ENGEL (R. C.), Ed. — *Abnormal electroencephalograms in the neonatal period.* Springfield (Ill.), 1975, Charles C. Thomas Publ., 128.

[19] FERRY (P. C.). — Computed cranial tomography in children. *J. Pediatr.,* 96, 961-967, 1980.

[20] GOLD (F.), BOURIN (M.), GRANHY (J. C.) et coll. — Intérêt de la voie intraveineuse pour l'utilisation du phénobarbital chez le nouveau-né à terme asphyxié. *Arch. Fr. Péd.,* 36, 610-616, 1979.

[21] HALL (R. T.), KULKARNI (P. B.), SHEEHAN (M. B.) et al. — Cerebrospinal fluid lactate dehydrogenase in infants with perinatal asphyxia. *Develop. Med. Child. Neurol.,* 22, 300-307, 1980.

[22] HOGAN (G. R.), MILLIGAN (J. E.). — The plantar reflex in the newborn. *New Engl. J. Med.,* 285, 502-506, 1971.

[23] JOHNSON (M. L.), MACK (L. A.), RUMACK (C. M.) et al. — B-mode echoencephalography in the normal and high risk infant. *Am. J. Roentgen.,* 133, 375-381, 1979.

[24] KELLAWAY (P.). — Ontogenic evolution of the electrical activity of the brain in man and animals. In G. RADERMECKER Ed., *Fourth International Meeting of EEG and Clinical Neurophysiology.* Acta Med. Belg., 1957, 141-153.

[25] LARROCHE (J. Cl.). — Quelques aspects anatomiques du développement cérébral. *Biol. Néonat.,* 4, 126-153, 1962.

[26] LARROCHE (J. Cl.). — The development of the Central Nervous System during intra uterine life. In *Human Development.* F. FALKNER Ed., W. B. Saunders Company, Philadelphia, 257-276, 1966.

[27] LARROCHE (J. Cl.), Ed. — Developmental pathology of the neonate. Elsevier Excerpta Medica, 1977, 525.

[28] LARROCHE (J. Cl.). — Marginal layer in the neocortex of a 7 week old human embryo. *J. Anat. Embryol.,* 162, 301-312, 1981.

[29] LARROCHE (J. Cl.). — Critères morphologiques du développement du système nerveux central du fœtus humain. *J. Neuroradiology,* 8, 93-108, 1981.

[30] LOMBROSO (C. T.). — Convulsive disorders in newborns. In *Pediatric Neurology and Neurosurgery.* R. A. THOMPSON and J. R. GREEN Eds., New York, 1978. Spectrum Press Publ., 205-239.

[31] LOU (H. C.), LASSEN (L. A.), FRIIS-HANSEN (B.). — Low cerebral blood flow in hypotensive perinatal distress. *Acta Neurol. Scand.,* 56, 343-352, 1977.

[32] MARIN-PADILLA (M.). — Prenatal and early post natal ontogenesis of the human motor cortex: a Golgi study. The sequential development of the cortical layers. *Brain Research,* 23, 167-183, 1970.

[33] MARSHALL (R. D.), REICHERT (T. J.), KERLEY (S. M.) et al. — Auditory function in NICU patients revealed by auditory brain-stem potentials. *J. Pediat.,* 96, 731-735, 1980.

[34] MIALE (I. L.), SIDMAN (R. L.). — An autoradiographic analysis of histogenesis in the mouse cerebellum. *Exp. Neurol.,* 4, 277-296, 1961.

[35] MONOD (N.), THARP (B.). — Activité électroencéphalographique normale du nouveau-né au cours des états de veille et de sommeil. *Rev. Electroencephalogr. Neurophysiol. Clin.* (Paris), 7, 302-315, 1977.

[36] MONOD (N.), PEZZANI (C.), LARROCHE (J. Cl.) et al. — Prognostic value of the neonatal EEG of the fulterm newborn during the first 24 hours of life. In *Fetal and Neonatal Physiological Measurements.* P. ROLFE Ed., Pitman Med. Ltd. Publ., 1980, 327-330.

[37] PAPE (K. E.), CUSIK (G.), HOUANG (M. T. W.) et al. — Ultrasound detection of brain damage in preterm infants. *Lancet,* 2, 1261-1264, 1979.

[38] PARMELEE (A. H.), SCHULTE (F. J.), AKIYAMA (Y.) et al. — Maturation of EEG activity during sleep in premature infants. *Electroencephalogr. Clin. Neurophysiol.,* 24, 319-329, 1968.

[39] PHILIP (A. G. S.). — Non invasive monitoring of intracranial pressure. *Clinics in Perinatology,* 6, 123-137, 1979.

[40] PICARD (L.), CLAUDON (M.), ROLAND (J.) et al. — Cerebral computed tomography in premature infants, with an attempt at staging developmental features. *J. Comput. Assist. Tomogr.,* 4, 435-444, 1980.

[41] PRECHTL (H. F. R.), BEINTEMA (D.). — The neurological examination of fullterm newborn infant.

Clinics in Dev. Med., n° 12. Spastics International Medical Publ., Londres, 1964, 74.

[42] QUATTLEBAUM (T. G.). — Benign familial convulsions in the neonatal period and early infancy. *J. Pédiatr.*, 95, 257-259, 1979.

[43] RAKIC (P.). — Mode of cell migration to the superficial layers of fetal monkey neocortex. *J. Comp. Neurol.*, 145, 61-83, 1972.

[44] REIGEL (D. H.), DALLMAN (D. E.), SCARFF (T. B.), et al. (J.). — Transcephalic impedance measurement during infancy. *Develop. Med. Child. Neurol.*, 19, 295-304, 1977.

[45] SAINT-ANNE DARGASSIES (S.). — La maturation neurologique du prématuré. *Études Néonat.*, 4, 71-116, 1955.

[46] SAINT-ANNE DARGASSIES (S.), Ed. — Le développement neurologique du nouveau-né à terme et prématuré. Masson, Paris, 1974, 337.

[47] SILVERBOARD (G.), HORDER (M. H.), AHMANN (P. A.) et al. — Reliability of ultrasound in diagnosis of intracerebral hemorrhage and post hemorrhagic hydrocephalus: comparison with computed tomography. *Pediatrics*, 66, 507-514, 1980.

[48] THOMAS (A.), DE AJURIAGUERRA (J.), Eds. — *Étude sémiologique du tonus musculaire.* Éditions Médicales Flammarion, Paris, 1949, 420.

[49] THOMAS (A.), SAINT-ANNE DARGASSIES (S.), Eds. — *Études neurologiques sur le nouveau-né et le jeune nourrisson.* Masson, Paris, 1952, 434.

[50] TOUWEN (B.). — Neurological development in infancy. *Clinics in developmental medicine*, n° 58. Spastics International Medical Publ., Londres, 1976, 150.

[51] VANDER EECKEN (H.), Ed. — *Anastomoses between the leptomeningeal arteries of the brain. Their morphological pathological and clinical significance.* Thomas Publ., Springfield, 1959, 160.

[52] VOLPE (J. J.). Ed. — *Neurology of the newborn.* W. B. Saunders Company, 1981, 648.

[53] VYHMEISTER (N.), SCHNEIDER (S.), CHUL CHA. — Cranial transillumination norms of the premature infant. *J. Pediat.*, 91, 980-982, 1977.

[54] WARBURTON (D.), SINGER (D. B.), OH (W.). — Dose response relationship of creatine phosphokinase (CPK) isoenzymes in stressed newborn infants. *Clinical Research*, 28, 1980 (Abstracts of western society for pediatric research).

[55] YAKOVLEV (P. I.), LECOURS (A. R.), Eds. — The myelogenetic cycles of regional maturation of the brain. In *Regional development of the brain in early life.* BLACKWELL Ed., 1967. 1 vol. Oxford, Edimbourg, 3-70.

15

Brain damage: clinical and anatomical correlations

J. Cl. LARROCHE and Cl. AMIEL-TISON

Introduction

During the past twenty years, by careful clinical observations in conjunction with anatomical studies, it has been possible to distinguish a certain number of pathological entities during the neonatal period. It has become apparent that the stage of cerebral maturation is a factor determining both the morphological aspect of the cerebral lesions and their clinical expression.

Recently, newer methods of studying the brain during life have indicated the possibility of examining neurological abnormalities in terms of anatomical lesions, from the first days of life.

Hypoxic-ischaemic encephalopathy

The terminology of hypoxic-ischaemic encephalopathy was recently introduced into the literature and in fact, covers almost the total perinatal cerebral pathology. Various clinical signs as well as morphological features are described under the same label. We shall limit our discussion to the form which is observed in fullterm neonates; leucomalacia, a form of hypoxic-ischaemic cerebral damage occurring in the premature infant will be discussed separately.

CLINICAL DESCRIPTION

Fœtal asphyxia can cause cerebral dysfunction of diverse severity. In the severe form, manifesting as status epilepticus, the causes, neonatal course, and long-term consequences, have been well recognised for many years [22]. Signs of central nervous depression appear within hours of birth. Frequently, the infant presents with severe respiratory distress necessitating immediate mechanical ventilation.

Hypertonia and hyperexcitability follow an initial period of hypotonia. The child becomes lethargic and hyporeactive and convulsions develop. These are often difficult to recognise and may even be subclinical. Consciousness is progressively lost, often to deep coma. Status epilepticus has been defined as repeated convulsions separated by short intervals, without recovery of consciousness between the convulsive episodes. The diagnosis should be confirmed by E. E. G. The cerebrospinal fluid is generally normal; it may be xanthochromic due to an increased protein content, often greater than 1 g/l, and it is sometimes haemorrhagic. In comatose neonates a search should be made for clinical signs suggesting cerebral œdema. Separation of sutures is not a constant feature. Often œdema is suggested by the inability to obtain even a few drops of cerebrospinal fluid at lumbar puncture. Ultrasonography or the C. T. scan will demonstrate the markedly narrowed ventricles. Anticonvulsive therapy should be started at once, without waiting for E. E. G. confirmation. The development of a convulsive state within hours of birth and the associated gestational or obstetric problems leave the clinician in no doubt as to the urgency of the situation.

Measures to combat cerebral œdema may be started together with the anticonvulsive treatment, even though there is no certain proof of their effectiveness. If the respiratory centres are depressed, the child will need ventilatory assistance. Blood pressure and metabolic homeostasis must be maintained by appropriate fluid therapy.

The initial phase, characterised by coma and convulsions, lasts approximately 48 hours and is followed by a period of lethargy, hypotonia and hypoactivity which can last for several weeks; the sucking reflex reappears, the upper part of the body remains hypotonic while the extensor muscles of the neck and lower limbs become hypertonic. At about three weeks of age the infant can be bottle-fed; he develops eye contact and responds to his mother. Phenobarbital or sodium valproate should be continued in maintenance doses.

This period of clinical improvement is unfortunately often misleading. Head circumference should be measured weekly to detect microcephaly which may ensue. If spontaneous respiration is not established during the first days of life, episodes of bradycardia are frequent and the child generally dies in the course of the first week, often with pulmonary complications. The neonatal death rate is evidently also dependent on the ethical viewpoint of the intensive care unit.

Besides this major form, cerebral lesions of different degrees can be produced, according to the intensity and duration of acute fœtal distress. Clinical classification (previous chapter) into moderate and minor degrees, gives a rough, early indication of prognosis.

AETIOLOGY AND FREQUENCY

Various kinds of mechanical or asphyxial accidents may lead to acute cerebral dysfunction. The severity of cerebral lesions depends on the intensity and duration of the insult. Certain obstetric complications have long been known to cause fœtal death or severe cerebral damage. The British Perinatal Mortality Survey [16] and the Collaborative American Project [57] show correlations between mortality and cerebral damage on the one hand, and the position of the fœtus, the course of labour and mode of delivery on the other hand; thus, occipito-posterior and occipito-transverse positions are less favourable than occipito-anterior positions. All breech positions are potentially unfavourable. If labour is too short, less than 3 hours in a primipara, or too long, more than 15 hours, or if the second stage is prolonged, over two hours, there is an increased risk of cerebral damage. Obstetric problems known to be associated with damage include difficult forceps delivery, antepartum haemorrhage due to placenta previa, abruptio placentae, prolapse of the umbilical cord, and a tight cord round the neck. These classical problems have not disappeared, but the risk of serious accidents has been much reduced by improved prenatal diagnosis and the general use of fœtal heart rate monitoring. Inevitably, the aim of preventing acute fœtal distress during birth has led to an increase in the number of Caesarean sections performed at term. In fact, in many cases Caesarean section extraction was necessary but was performed too late, when fœtal asphyxia persisting for several hours had already damaged the brain; similarly, forceps extraction was often wrongly blamed for cerebral damage which was already present, caused by the asphyxia.

In contrast to the present day rarity of accidents at birth, cerebral lesions established before the onset of labour are becoming relatively more frequent. The clinical presentation during the first days of life is often identical; in the absence of obstetric complications C. T. scan or ultrasound examination (U. S.) performed at an early date, may help to identify lesions which have been present for some time before delivery (see below).

In assessing the results of modern obstetric care, cases of hypoxic ischaemic encephalopathy may usefully be divided into three groups according to severity [5]: In major maternity hospitals the incidence of the severe form has been reduced to about 1 in 1,000 births, and is still improving, though recent figures are not statistically significant (see table I). The incidence of the moderate form, has diminished significantly from 1 % to 1 °/$_{oo}$ with the widespread use of electronic monitoring of fœtal heart rate. The incidence of minor forms has decreased less dramatically; these are related to minor obstetric complications which cannot be eliminated completely without unduly increasing the number of Caesarean sections.

TABLE I. — INCIDENCE OF STATUS EPILEPTICUS IN TWO MATERNITY HOSPITALS, FROM 1962 TO 1984

Years	Maternities	N. of deliveries at term	N. of cases	°/$_{oo}$
1962 1963 1964	Baudelocque	6,200	10	1.6
1968 1969	Port-Royal	3,257	6	1.8
1974	Port-Royal	1,578	2	1.3
1976 1977 1978	Port-Royal	5,825	5	0.9
1979-80	Baudelocque	2,870	2	0.7
1981-82	Baudelocque	2,364	0	0
1983-84	Baudelocque	3,170	2	0.6

ANIMAL EXPERIMENTS

Since the classic work of Ranck and Windle [64], Myers and colleagues [56] have developed various methods of inducing ischaemic-hypoxic cerebral lesions in newborn monkeys designed to imitate pathological conditions in humans. The authors have established four different experimental models in the fœtal monkey causing distinct types of cerebral lesions.

— Total asphyxia by clamping the umbilical cord and preventing the onset of respiration leads to brainstem damage with a particularly high frequency of involvement of the inferior colliculi.

— Partial asphyxia by reducing placental per-

fusion leads to cerebral œdema and cortical necrosis.

— Partial asphyxia without acidosis leads to lesions involving mainly the white matter.

— Partial asphyxia followed by total asphyxia leads to necrosis of the basal ganglia and sometimes the cortex.

The authors recently emphasized the deleterious role of lactate accumulation in the brain, the production of which is related not only to the amount of oxygen delivery but also to the quantity of blood glucose and glycogen storage in the different areas of the brain.

ANATOMICAL FEATURES

Damage to nerve cells is the out standing hypoxic-ischaemic lesion in the fullterm neonate [43, 26, 67]. Corresponding to the range of clinical signs already described, cerebral lesions of varying degrees of severity are encountered. They may be focal or diffuse. In the severe form with status epilepticus, the infant often dies during the first week of life with associated cardiopulmonary lesions.

At autopsy, cerebral œdema is found in almost all cases; it presents the same characteristics as in the adult: absence of free cerebrospinal fluid in the arachnoid meshwork, flattening of gyri, narrowing of sulci, herniation of the uncus; in the posterior fossa, herniation of the cerebellar tonsils, and formation of a pressure cone at the level of the vermis may be present, all features explaining the frequent absence of cerebrospinal fluid at lumbar puncture. On section, the brain is pale, the ventricles are collapsed, and there may be herniation of the infundibulum. At times, the cortex, the deep gray matter and brainstem nuclei, especially the inferior colliculi may be greyish brown. Curiously, the basal part of the temporal lobe is usually spared.

The microscopic features of the damaged neuron are pycnosis or karyorrhexis (fragmented nucleus); vacuolated cytoplasm, when Nissl bodies are present, they are displaced to the periphery; finally the cell membrane disintegrates and the cell disappears. A microglial reaction develops within several days. If the infant survives long enough, areas of softening are found similar to those in the adult brain, with a polymorphic glial reaction, macrophages and prominent capillary endothelium (Fig. II-12 *a*). The cortical necrosis may be focal or diffuse, patchy or columnar in distribution. It is often more pronounced in the depth of the sulci (Fig. II-12 *a*) than on the crest of the gyri or it may be laminar (Fig. II-12 *b*). Necrosis of the basal ganglia is characterised by

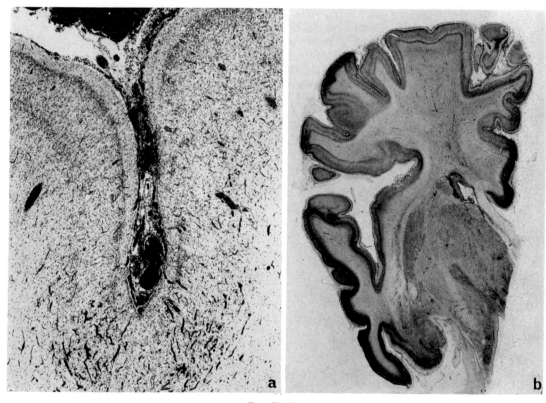

FIG. II-12.

a) Cortical necrosis, more severe in the borders and depth of the sulcus.   *b*) Cortical laminar necrosis.

the presence of spindle-shaped neurons with acidophilic cytoplasm and pycnotic nuclei, of areas of softening with neuronal loss, polymorphic glial cells and macrophages and prominent capillaries. Necrosis of the brainstem which can involve all the structures was for long ignored or wrongly interpreted. The inferior colliculi are often affected, as are the cranial nerve nuclei and the reticular formation; the large neurons of the pons often show karyorrhexis. In the cerebellum, the dentate nucleus is highly vulnerable; there is necrosis of Purkinje cells and internal granular layer cells particularly in the archicerebellum where many nuclei are karyorrhectic. The cerebellar tonsils are often the site of severe necrosis aggravated by œdema and herniation. The medulla and spinal cord are not spared. When the brainstem is preferentially involved, bioelectric anomalies appear during sleep.

The few tracts in the hemispheres already myelinated at birth may also be injured; the fibers are swollen, vacuolated, appearing as a string of beads or fragmented. In the neonatal period the breakdown of the brain tissue is often rapid, because even at term, the hemispheres have a high water

content and are almost devoid of myelin.

Unlike the lesions produced in the monkey by various anoxic or ischaemic insults, cerebral damage in the human infant is rarely of a pure type. However three dominant topographic patterns are observed:

— diffuse necrosis involves cortex, deep grey matter, brainstem and cerebellum in the majority of cases;

— necrosis is predominant in the basal ganglia and thalamus in about one third of cases;

— necrosis involves the cortex alone in about 10 % of cases.

The vulnerability of the cortex, either alone or in association with other structures may depend, to some extent, on the stage of maturation. The superficial network of arteries in particular [78], becomes modified towards the end of intrauterine life and anastomoses, as in the adult are rare. The blood supply to the brain thus comprises certain well defined arterial territories and the border zones between these territories are particularly vulnerable to alterations in blood pressure and anoxia. Parasagittal cerebral necrosis has been demonstrated in living infants [80, 81] with radionuclide brain scanning and parasagittal impairment of cerebral blood flow was also demonstrated with positron emission tomography in asphyxiated term infants [82]. The inferior colliculi and the visual cortex, are apparently at risk because of their dependence on an unusually rich blood supply. The vulnerability of a region depends also on the level of its metabolic activity, particularly on its oxygen consumption. In the human neonate at term, oxidative enzyme activity is detectable only in certain cortical layers (III and V); this might explain the laminar necrosis [36] observed in some cases of neonatal asphyxia and the damage so often located in archaic structures such as the archicerebellum. The neuropile itself, dendrites, spines and synapses undergoes considerable development close to term and vulnerability of nervous tissue increases with its increasing complexity.

SEQUELLÆ
OF HYPOXIC-ISCHAEMIC ENCEPHALOPATHY

After apparent clinical improvement and restoration of vital functions, the infant who survives develops severe neurological disorders such as spastic paraplegia or quadriplegia with or without choreoathetosis, seizures, severe mental retardation, sensory deficits and microcephaly.

In addition to clinical follow up, EEG and sensorial studies, the morphogical appearance of the brain contributes to the prognosis: a normal US or CT scan does not exclude sequellæ, but abnormal images are the best predictor for further handicaps [25]. Some of these may be transient as the brain develops and later on become fixed. CT scan and US show cerebral atrophy with enlarged ventricles (ex vacuo hydrocephalus), and/or porencephalic destructions. The structural sequellæ vary from case to case. The brain may undergo extensive disintegration and liquefaction (multicystic encephalomalacia). When necrosis is predominent in the cortex with neuronal loss and poor myelination the convolutions become shrunken or atrophic, the sulci widen (cortical atrophy); laminar necrosis and nodular atrophy are best seen on sections stained for myelin or by Holzer's method for fibrillary astrocytes. Similar scars or "plaques fibromyéliniques" in the basal ganglia are described as status marmoratus or "état marbré".

Intraventricular haemorrhage in premature infants

ANATOMICAL FINDINGS

Intraventricular haemorrhage (IVH) is generally secondary to bleeding in the subependymal germinal matrix, which is not completely involuted in premature infants of 26-34 weeks (see previous chapter). At this stage, the matrix consists of packed immature neurons and of glial cells. Electron microscopic studies have shown that in the matrix, capillaries and small venules cannot be differentiated on morphological grounds; their endothelial cells, basal membrane and glial coverings are already mature by 20 weeks but the number of capillaries tends to decrease, while increasing in the cortex [46].

Although the most frequent site of bleeding is the matrix near the head and the anterior part of the body of the caudate nucleus (Fig. II-13 a), haemorrhage may also occur in the germinal layer of the roof of the temporal horn (Fig. II-13 b) and in the external wall of the occipital horn. IVH results from rupture of the ependyma, previously necrosed and distended.

As well as in the matrix, haemorrhage occurs in the choroid plexuses in 15 % of IVH cases, found at autopsy, either as an isolated finding or in association with haemorrhage in the matrix. Whatever the primary site of bleeding, the blood fills the lateral ventricles, the 3rd and 4th ventricles and then collects in the arachnoid spaces around the brainstem and cerebellum (Fig. II-13 c), extending anteriorly to the basal cisterns and posteriorly to the spinal cord.

THE EVOLUTION OF IDEAS

Already known to pediatricians in the late nineteenth century, IVH aroused the interest of only a few obstetricians and pathologists until 1976, when CT scan [27] and soon after Ultrasound [17, 50] led clinicians and radiologists to define the morphology and pathology of the brain in the living infant.

For decades, premature infants were merely

rewarmed, often belatedly, then oxygen was given, at times too generously, while feeding was not initiated before the second day of life. "Idiopathic respiratory distress" or hyaline membrane disease (HMD) was the same disease as today, but, anoxia, acidosis and hypotension were not properly corrected; deterioration of the infant's state was rapid and death within a few days was the usual

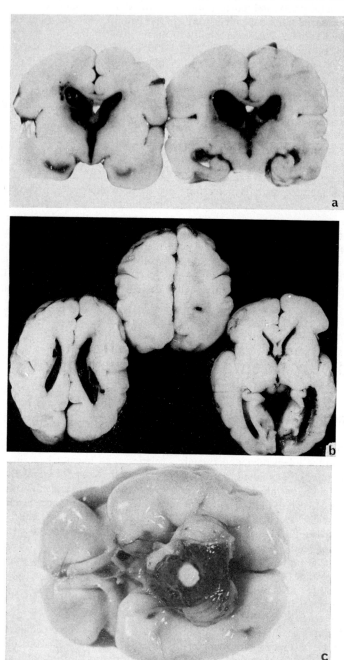

FIG. II-13. — *Various sites of intracerebral hemorrhages.*

a) Subependymal hemorrhage over the anterior part of the caudate nucleus and hemorrhagic ventricular cast.
b) Hemorrhage over the anterior, medial and inferior (temporal) part of the caudate nucleus.
c) Hemorrhage in the arachnoid space around the brain stem.

result. At autopsy, HMD was associated with IVH in 80 % of cases [3, 42]. More recently, Leech and Kohnen [49] found the association in 95 % of cases. Lungs with HMD were atelectatic and reddish purple; there was severe stasis in the right atrium, superior vena cava and brain, mainly in the deep venous system of Galen. Thromboses, secondary to venous stasis, impairment of coagulation factors and endothelial damage can only be assessed on microscopic examination, and the frequency of occurrence can only be established on serial sections of all specimens; this time-consuming procedure is rarely done; in such material, mural deposits of fibrin or true lamellated thrombi, are found in small vessels of the matrix or in the large veins of the system of Galen in 10 to 12 % of cases presenting with haemorrhage in the matrix and in the ventricles [45]. In addition, the thin walled veins of this region [32] can disrupt easily when submitted to increased pressure. In addition, in the matrix, ischaemic infarcts which predate or accompany the haemorrhage have been observed [67, 75]. Moreover, studies on semi thin and ultra thin sections of the subependymal zone of asphyxiated premature infants have shown swollen perivascular glial end feet, damage to the basal lamina, and dislocation of the endothelial cells with extravasation of blood [46]. Finally, the high fibrinolytic activity of the matrix [29] might explain the rapid and massive spread of an initially minimal haemorrhage.

For the last fifteen years or so, better care of the neonate in the delivery room and newer techniques for the treatment of HMD have lead to radical changes in cardiopulmonary haemodynamics and consequently in the circulation of the brain. Hence, other mechanisms have been proposed to explain the IVH. Some are iatrogenic such as hypernatremia secondary to infusion of bicarbonate; this hypothesis is controversial and it seems that only massive doses of hyperosmolar solutions, infused too rapidly, might be deleterious, and indeed not only to the central nervous system. For Hambleton and Wigglesworth (1976) [34], bleeding occurs in the capillary bed of the Heubner's artery, a branch of the anterior cerebral artery, when systemic pressure rises; however, this mechanism does not explain haemorrhages in the roof of the temporal horn and in the external wall of the occipital horn. More recently, microangiographic studies [72] have shown that in the premature neonate, the precaudate matrix is a terminal arterial territory with few capillaries, while the deep venous system undergoes rapid development in order to drain the growing hemispheres; in addition, in the newborn beagle pup, the matrix is

a low blood flow structure [61], hence vulnerable in the case of anoxia-ischaemia and hypotension. Other studies [52, 53] have shown that in asphyxiated newborn infants the autoregulation of cerebral blood flow is impaired; if there is no vascular mechanism to compensate for fluctuations in the systemic blood pressure, the vulnerability of the CNS is increased; when vascular walls have been damaged by hypoxia, they can easily be disrupted as a result of hypertensive episodes. All situations which impair cerebral blood flow such as HMD with hypoxia, hypothermia [54], hypercapnia and acidosis, blood pressure instability or low blood pressure during the first hours of life [28], occurrence of a pneumothorax, are common findings preceding or concomitant with an IVH. In addition, particular situations such as intubation, tracheal aspiration, blood sampling, noise, etc. [51] lead to significant variations in blood pressure with increased heart and respiration rate and fall in transcutaneous PaO_2. These aggressive manœuvers should be avoided as much as possible in sick premature infants.

Finally, experimental studies in fetal sheep [65] and newborn puppies [31] show that intermittent variations in intravascular pressure (arterial or venous), when associated with asphyxia, can produce haemorrhages in the germinal zone and the choroid plexus similar to those observed in premature infants. All this evidence is still fragmentary and is often derived from a small number of experiments or observations. We must modestly recognize that, while technology has revolutionized our diagnostic methods, there is still a long way to go before the physiopathology of these lesions is precisely known.

As far as *prevention of IVH* is concerned, phenobarbital and vitamin E have been proposed, the data are contradictory at the moment. Elimination of fluctuating cerebral blood flow velocity in preterm infants with RDS seems to reduce the incidence of IVH [63].

DIAGNOSIS

All infants born prematurely and presenting with respiratory distress which justifies admission to an intensive care center must be suspected of IVH. During the first 24/48 hours of life respiratory signs dominate. However, haemorrhage may silently be taking place in the germinal zone, most often during the first 24 hours [76]; only when the ependyma ruptures and the ventricles are flooded, will neurological signs appear with general deterioration in the state of the infant. The neurological signs are varied, including generalised hypertonia, or hypertonia in the posterior muscles of the trunk, abnormal eye movements, clonic movements of one limb or convulsions, sometimes difficult to recognize if the infant is in coma. If the haemorrhage is abundant and especially when there are parenchymal lesions, the EEG shows positive Rolandic spikes in a significant number of cases. Episodes of bradycardia or repeated apnoeic episodes, in an infant whose respiratory syndrome seems well controlled are warning signs. Neurological signs are rarely apparent in the very low birth weight infant who is intubated, and often immobilised. A drop in haematocrit [13] should raise suspicion of internal haemorrhage. Lumbar puncture does not always reveal the haemorrhage, and it is often traumatic; the glucose level in the CSF is reduced. In large haemorrhages, the anterior fontanelle may be abnormally tense and the head circumference rapidly increases. In summary, the warning signs are: prematurity, hypothermia on admission, respiratory distress with acidosis or blood pressure instability in the first 24 hours of life.

The CT scan (Fig. II-14 *a*, *b*) has modified the attitude of the neonatologist and allowed us to make the diagnosis with confidence [14, 40, 60]. However, it must be remembered that the premature brain contains zones of immature cells, with high mitotic potential (the subependymal germinal matrix and the external granular layer of the cerebellum), and this should limit the indications for CT scanning or for repeating the scan. It may be replaced by ultrasonography (Fig. II-15) using high resolution probes, which gives an excellent picture of cerebral structures in real time and in various planes [17, 38, 59]. The ease with which the apparatus can be handled makes it a precious diagnostic tool. The importance of early examination is to confirm clinical suspicion, to assess the size and the site of hemorrhage, whether unilateral or bilateral and to detect any associated hemorrhage in the surrounding matter. The classification of IVH into 4 stages, initially based on CT scan examination [60], is also valid for US: stage I: haemorrhage in the matrix; stage II: IVH without ventricular dilatation; stage III: IVH with enlarged ventricles; stage IV: IVH with parenchymal haemorrhage.

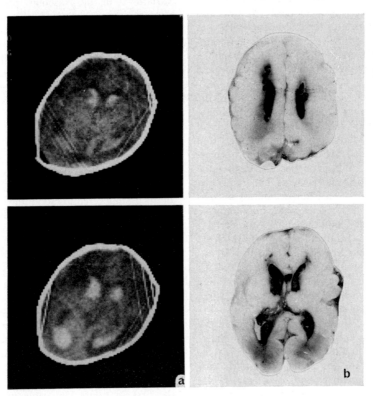

FIG. II-14.

a) CT scan; hemorrhage of the anterior matrices and in the ventricles (courtesy of Dr. VIGNAUD).
b) Horizontal sections of the brain of the infant who died 2 days after the ET.

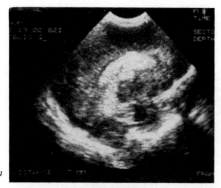

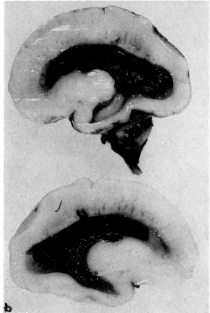

FIG. II-15.

a) Ultrasound; sagittal view: hemorrhage in the matrix and in the ventricles; slight erosion of the roof (courtesy of Dr. M. COUCHARD).

b) Section of the corresponding hemisphere through the same plane.

EPIDEMIOLOGY

Until recent years, diagnosis of IVH was made by careful clinical and paraclinical examinations and generally confirmed at autopsy. In the University Hospital Baudelocque in Paris, about 30 % of infants born at 28-32 weeks gestation had IVH at autopsy; an additional 10 % had haemorrhage in the matrix without rupture of the ependyma. Fedrick and Butler [24], based on the British Perinatal Mortality Survey, estimated the incidence to be

45 $^\circ/_{oo}$ live births at less than 32 weeks. With improved resuscitation and supportive measures for RDS, a large number of infants have overcome their lung problems which may have been associated with IVH and survived. It has therefore, been difficult to evaluate the incidence of IVH for many years. Systematic use of CT scan [10], has increased the figures, but the high cell density in the subependymal matrix has sometimes been mistaken for haemorrhage. Nowadays, with US, the rate of IVH is estimated to be 40 to 50 % of infants with a birth weight of less than 1,500 g, with a prevalence of stages I and II.

IMMEDIATE COURSE AND LATE CONSEQUENCES

The pathologist's point of view. — Minor haemorrhages may remain localized in the germinal zone and be clinically silent. They represent an incidental finding at autopsy but can be detected by CT scan and US in living infants. Ultimately, macrophages laden with iron pigments and pseudocysts [74, 45], will be the only remaining evidence of haemorrhage. The consequence to the ultimate development of the brain, of the massive loss of neurons is difficult to estimate.

In the past, massive ventricular haemorrhage was always rapidly fatal. With the use of mechanical ventilation, a large number of infants survive longer and this has modified the range of appearances now found in cerebral pathology. Thus, an increasing incidence of posthaemorrhagic hydrocephalus is observed in infants coming to autopsy: the incidence was less than 1 % of cases of IVH prior to 1967, the opening of our intensive care unit, and has since then increased progressively from 5 to 25 %. In fact, the incidence of severe sequelæ reflects the type of population at risk admitted into the ICU and the general policy concerning mechanical ventilation. Independently of the size of the initial haemorrhage, the cellular reaction in the arachnoid can obstruct the foramina of Magendi and Luschka and result in hydrocephalus by blocking the circulation of CSF [20, 44]. Dilatation of the ventricular system often precedes an increase in head circumference [39, 81] and can now be detected by US (Fig. II-16 *ab*) and CT scan (Fig. II-17 *ab*) [37, 17, 50]. In cases of severe bleeding, the ventricles are rapidly distended, the clotted blood forming a cast of the cavities or "haemocephalus". Blood clots persisting within the cavities during the development of hydrocephaly may be described as "haemohydro-

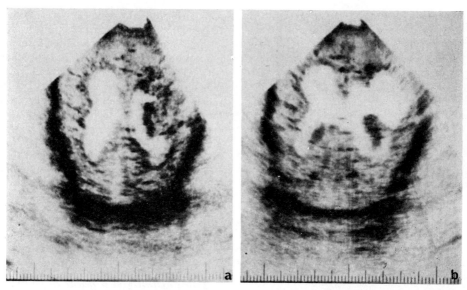

FIG. II-16. — *Ultra-sound.*
a) Post hemorrhagic hydrocephalus.
b) Evolution toward communicating porencephaly or diverticulum (courtesy of Dr. COUTURE).

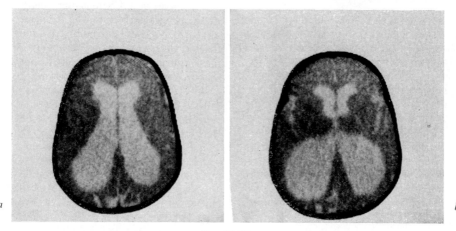

FIG. II-17.
a) and *b*) CT scan: posthemorragic hydrocephalus (courtesy of Dr. VIGNAUD).

cephalus". Severe IVH is often associated with ischaemic or haemorrhagic damage to the cerebral parenchyma leading to porencephaly or diverticula.

The clinician's point of view. — The immediate outcome depends on the size of the haemorrhage and on associated parenchymal damage: a high proportion of infants with stages III and IV IVH die in the neonatal period. Obstructive hydrocephalus begins early within weeks or months. The initial stage can be detected clinically from signs of intracranial hypertension (rapid increase of head circumference, distended sutures, opisthotonos, sunset sign, apnoeic spells and bradycardia) and confirmed by repeated ultrasound measurements of ventricular size.

This hydrocephalus with increased pressure needs to be differentiated from the hydrocephalus with normal pressure, *i. e.* hydrocephalus ex vacuo due to cerebral atrophy. This differentiation between the two forms is easy in typical cases, but mild and transient posthaemorrhagic hydrocephalus may be observed, and may be associated with some degree of ex vacuo hydrocephalus. Therefore a ventricular shunt is not usually immediately indicated: Repeated lumbar punctures are performed and/or acetazolamide is given in order to avoid the adverse effects of intracranial hypertension while waiting for a surgical decision.

Within the first year of life, motor function, psychological, sensorial and behavioral development should be tested. US studies show the stabilization of lesions if any; EEG studies are performed.

At one year of age, most of the severe sequelæ are diagnosed, with a global incidence which varies from one publication to another, but with an average rate of 10 %. Moderate and mild sequelæ obviously need longer follow-up studies to be evaluated and there are more conflicting views. However, in the VLBW groups, most of the publications agree on about 50 % of infants being completely normal at school age.

In fact, as shown by Stewart [70] 2 major groups emerge in the survivors, based on repeated US within the first month of life: *non complicated IVH* (grades 1 and 2 without any parenchymal complication grossly apparent at US) carries a good prognosis, just as good as a group of VLBW without IVH. *Complicated IVH* (grades 3 and 4 with hydrocephalus, cerebral atrophy, porencephaly already obvious on the one month US), results in a high incidence of major sequelæ from 30 to 60 % depending on the extent of the lesions.

Intraventricular haemorrhage in the fullterm infant. — There are few data concerning its frequency [12, 15, 35]. The source of the bleeding is usually the choroid plexus, a vascular malformation, extension of a parenchymal haemorrhage into the ventricle or blood dyscrasia. When IVH is an isolated finding, surgical removal of the haematoma may be attempted with a fairly good prognosis.

Other intracranial haemorrhages

SUBDURAL HAEMORRHAGE

By definition this is a collection of blood in the potential space between the dura and the arachnoid. Subdural haemorrhage can be uni- or bilateral; it may be several millimetres thick (true haematoma), or it may form only a thin surface layer over one or more lobes of one or both hemispheres (Fig. II-18). Subdural haemorrhage generally results from rupture of a superficial cerebral vein, either the great vein of Trolard which empties into the sagittal sinus, or the vein of Labbé which empties posteriorly into the transverse sinus, or of smaller accessory veins. These vascular tears are the result of opposing forces applied to the fœtal head during passage through the birth canal. In the neonate at term where the cranial bones are well ossified, there is often a history of difficult birth with cephalo-pelvic disproportion, a high forceps delivery, or a breech presentation with difficult extraction of the after-coming head; these complications are most often encountered in primiparae. In addition to the mechanical problems resulting in haemorrhage, there is an asphyxial component causing neuronal necrosis. It is essential to recognize these two types of lesions [47], since the clinical course and prognosis will be quite different

according to whether trauma occurs alone or in combination with asphyxia and nerve cell necrosis.

In the mixed form (haemorrhage and necrosis), which is unfortunately the more frequent, the clinical picture is dominated by signs of hypoxic-ischaemic

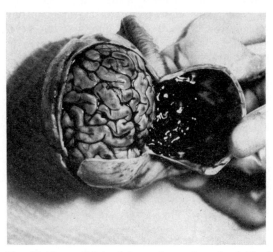

FIG. II-18. — *Subdural hemorrhage. Coagulated blood adherent to the parietal bone. There is no associated arachnoid hemorrhage.*

encephalopathy, as described above in fullterm neonates such as: acute fœtal distress, convulsions and coma developing during the first hours of life; focal signs are rare; the anterior fontanelle is tense, the sutures rapidly separate, and head circumference may increase significantly in 48 hours with signs of raised intracranial pressure and, possibly, retinal haemorrhages. The EEG findings are compatible with cellular necrosis.

In the pure form, with isolated haemorrhage, the clinical picture is less dramatic; there are focal signs such as unilateral convulsions, ocular signs, or a hemisyndrome. The clinical history should be scrutinised for revelant obstetric problems. In rare cases, the EEG shows contra-lateral focal changes [2].

At lumbar puncture, the cerebro-spinal fluid may be normal or slightly hemorrhagic. In cases with cerebral œdema no cerebro-spinal fluid is obtained. Subdural taps may be attempted if, on CT scan, the haemorrhage is abundant, collected and accessible; otherwise this procedure may be dangerous and it may provide no information. Ultrasonography through the anterior fontanelle does not detect the effusion when it is located close to the sagittal sinus or when it is very small.

Until recently the diagnosis of subdural haemorrhage was seldom made clinically, and the incidence was established from autopsy reports. In an intensive care unit [45] subdural haemorrhage was found in 15 to 18 % of autopsies. Even since the widespread use of the CT scan and ultrasonography, data on the frequency of these haemorrhages remains incomplete. Recognition of dystocia early in labour has practically eliminated the mechanical complications. Mention must be made of the special form of subdural haemorrhage, occurring in premature infants, found in 10 % of autopsies, but never suspected clinically. It is due apparently to the extraordinary malleability of the cranium, which permits distortion and sometimes considerable overlap of the parietal bones leading to venous tears. There is often associated arachnoid haemorrhage. Whatever the gestational age of the infant, although a large haemorrhage may be detected by CT scan or US, it remains difficult to distinguish subdural from arachnoid haematoma, or even from peripheral cerebral haemorrhage. Subdural haematoma have also been reported in hemophilic newborn infants [47, 81] and in cases of thrombocytopenia.

ARACHNOID HAEMORRHAGE

Haemorrhage in the arachnoid membrane is fairly common; as an isolated phenomenon it is of little significance. It may be traumatic, in cases of forceps or vacuum extraction, when distorsion or compression of the cranial bones leads to rupture of vessels; or it may result from extreme vasodilatation with diffuse extravasation of blood under conditions of asphyxia.

The condition is encountered most often in the baby of a primiparous mother who has experienced difficulties during the first and second stages of labour. Hyperexcitability, an abnormal cry, vasomotor instability, cyanosis and alterations of muscle tone, are the typical signs. The sutures and anterior fontanelle are often normal. The state of alertness and primary reflexes are unaffected. The cerebrospinal fluid is pink and under pressure. In the majority of cases these signs disappear within several days with symptomatic treatment, such as phenobarbital. Laboratory diagnosis is not always simple. Arachnoid haemorrhage is usually defined as a count of more than 3,000 red cells/mm³ in the CSF. Even under normal conditions the CSF of a premature infant may contain several hundred red cells/mm³; the liquid is then opalescent. The CSF, when pink, contains 8,000 to 10,000 red blood cells/mm³. Frankly bloody CSF contains several hundred thousand red blood cells/mm³. The real difficulty is to distinguish true arachnoid haemorrhage from a traumatic tap. If the CSF is very haemorrhagic when the needle enters the canal and then clears progressively, or if the liquid coagulates, the tap was traumatic. In true arachnoid haemorrhage the liquid is obtained very easily, it is pink or red, identical in the 3 tubes, and does not coagulate. A xanthochromic supernatant, or the presence of crenated red blood cells, favours true haemorrhage. Lumbar puncture is a simple procedure, but it demands experience. The operator must state in writing whether or not, in his opinion, the puncture was traumatic.

Before the advent of CT and US it was difficult, on the basis of clinical signs and lumbar puncture alone, to define accurately the site of intracranial bleeding. For instance IVH could be eliminated only because the gestational age of the infant, and the obstetric circumstances made the diagnosis unlikely. If, in addition to arachnoid haemorrhage, there are intracerebral lesions such as intracerebral haematoma and/or cortical necrosis, the clinical picture primarily reflects these lesions. In this case the infant is lethargic from birth, the primary reflexes are depressed, and there are alterations in muscle tone; the condition worsens progressively, apnoeic episodes and convulsions may develop, sometimes the sutures separate. Prognosis depends on the extent of the associated lesions and not on the size of the arachnoid haemorrhage [4]. Occasionally, however, hydrocephalus may develop, secondary to arachnoid thickening and occlusion of the foramina of Magendi and Luschka.

The incidence of arachnoid haemorrhage varies from one set of statistics to another because the figures rely essentially on the presence of blood in the CSF and therefore also on the number of lumbar punctures carried out in the neonatal unit concerned. Figures based on CT scan and US data are not known.

A special form of arachnoid haemorrhage is presented by haematoma covering one or several lobes, more or less completely (Fig. II-19) [45]. In many cases the underlying brain tissue is the site of ischaemic and/or haemorrhagic infarction. The distinction between subdural and arachnoid haematoma is difficult on CT scan and US. The pathogenesis is poorly understood but arterial emboli cannot be excluded.

CEREBELLAR HAEMORRHAGE

Cerebellar haemorrhages are frequent in the neonate but until recently were essentially an autopsy finding in about 15 % of cases [45]. They are either isolated or associated with IVH and appear as multiple haematomas several mm to several cm in diameter. Larger haematomas are easily recognized macroscopically (Fig. II-20) and these forms should be detectable by CT [66] or US [62]. Much more often there are disseminated petechial haemorrhages that only a systematic histological examination can reveal.

The mechanism of these haemorrhages is not known. However any rough manipulation or prolonged fixation of the head which tends to alter blood flow (arterial or venous) can be prejudicial to an infant in a state of hypoxia. In addition the frequency of haemorrhage in the immature cerebellar cortex may be related to the poorly formed capillary bed in this region [59].

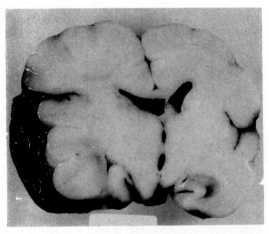

FIG. II-19. — *Hematoma in the arachnoid over the left temporal lobe; oedema and displacement of the left hemisphere.*

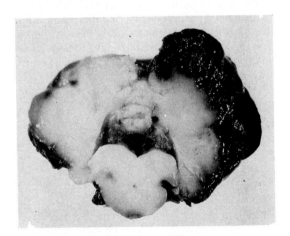

FIG. II-20. — *Left cerebellar hematoma in the arachnoid and the parenchyma.*

Leucomalacia

ANATOMY AND PATHOGENESIS

Periventricular leucomalacia (PVL) or necrosis of the white matter, generally occurs in patchy distribution throughout the centrum semiovale

(Fig. II-21), predominantly near the external angle of the lateral ventricles, in the corona radiata, in the temporal acoustic radiations and, posteriorly in the stratum sagittale or optic radiations. Sections of fixed brain show small whitish or pearly-white plaques, which stand out against the surrounding normal tissue, hence their name "white spots". Macroscopically the lesions are discrete and often overlooked. In histological preparations, acute lesions or coagulation necrosis (Fig. II-22 *a*) stain easily with PAS or luxol fast blue. Silver impregnation shows the disrupted axons, the proximal part retracted and swollen and the distal part degenerating (Fig. II-22 *b*). A polymorphous cellular reaction rapidly appears consisting of microglial cells, macrophages and astrocytes. The ultimate outcome, unpredictable in the individual lesion, may be scar formation with fibrillary gliosis, focal absence of myelin and calcium deposits. This sclerosis of the centrum semiovale is frequently associated with hydrocephalus ex vacuo (Fig. II-23 *a, b*). In other cases, tissue lysis with formation of multiple cavities (Fig. II-24), will develop [18].

The lesions of leucomalacia, already known in the last century, were described in details by Banker and Larroche in 1962 [8]. These authors considered the lesions to be a form of neonatal anoxic encephalopathy and to be the morphological basis for the spastic mono and diplegia reported by Little in 1861. The morphological attributes of the lesions, typical of ischemic necrosis, and their localisation in the boundary zone between ventriculopedal and ventriculofugal arterial system [77] favour an ischemic-hypoxic origin. Combining histological techniques and radioangiographs, Takashima and Tanaka, 1978 [73] demonstrated leucomalacia in these poorly vascularised zones. However, the fact that these lesions are characteristic of a limited stage of brain development, suggests that an additional factor in their pathogenesis is the extreme vulnerability of non-myelinated white matter or tissue in the process of myelinization.

CLINICAL DIAGNOSIS

In the early stages of leucomalacia, the clinical picture is non specific. Infants with these lesions generally have a history of long periods of hypoxia and/or acidosis, repeated apnoeic episodes with bradycardia and cardiac arrest, hypotension and eventually respiratory distress. In the premature baby, leucomalacia is at most, only a presumptive diagnosis, once IVH has been eliminated. In some cases of extensive leucomalacia verified at autopsy, the EEG shows positive Rolandic spikes. CT scan is of no use in diagnosis; areas of low density in the white matter have been interpreted, at times, wrongly as leucomalacia. The poor cellularity of the white matter, its high water content and lack of myelin are responsible for these hypodensities, which must be considered physiological even if they are not found in all infants of a given gesta-

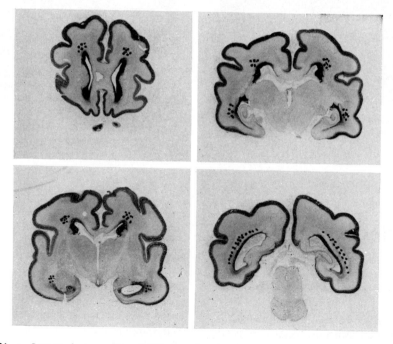

FIG. II-21. — *Leucomalacia: preferential topography of ischemic-anoxic necrosis of the white matter.*

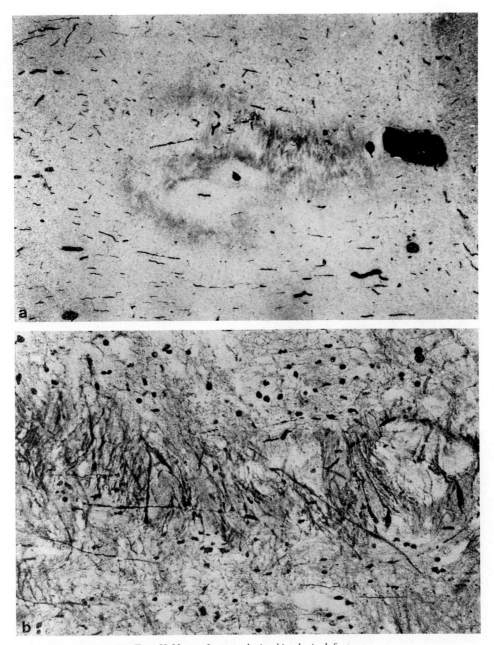

FIG. II-22. — *Leucomalacia, histological features.*

a) Coagulation necrosis on H and E stain.
b) Axonal damage, swelling and fragmentation on silver stain.

tional age. Recently, paradoxical hyperechogenic zones have been demonstrated by US, in the periventricular white matter and leucomalacia was confirmed at autopsy [19, 58, 68].

In the following weeks as the lesions progress, either to sclerosis or to multicystic encephalopathy, the clinical diagnosis is still uncertain. CT scan and US may show ventricular dilatation, with or without multiple cavities around the ventricles: poor myelination can be assessed by nuclear magnetic resonance imaging [23]. Psychomotor development of the infant is unsatisfactory but there are

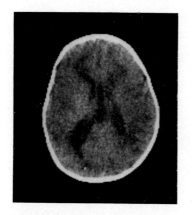

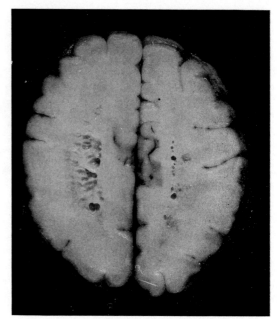

Fig. II-24. — *Bilateral multicystic leucomalacia (horizontal section).*

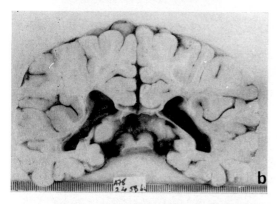

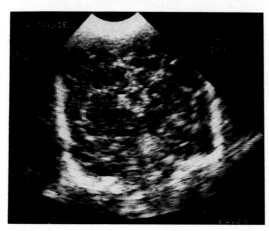

Fig. II-23. — *Sequelae of leucomalacia.*

a) On CT scan, sclerosis (?) and atrophy of the centrum semi-ovale with ex vacuo hydrocephalus.

b) Coronal section of the brain of the same infant who died at 4 months; atrophy of the white matter and dilatation of the ventricles.

c) Multicystic encephalomalacia (courtesy of Dr. M. COU-CHARD).

no specific neurological signs. Motor defects, in every possible combination become apparent only when the infant is several months old.

EPIDEMIOLOGY

The incidence of early lesions can only be established at autopsy. Twenty five years ago, leucomalacia was described in about 20 % of brains of premature infants. In many cases the lesions occurred alone, whithout other significant gross pathology, or with discrete neuronal necrosis in the striatum and dentate nucleus. In the full-term neonate, similar lesions were found in about 15 % of examined brains, but they were associated with diffuse neuronal necrosis. These infants died of various pathological conditions such as IUGR with hypoglycemia, congenital heart malformatiors or septicemia with meningo-encephalitis (see below). This probably explains why, in survivors, fullterm infants were more likely to suffer from diffuse encephalopathy with motor defects and mental handicap, rather than isolated mono or diplegia.

Today, improved antenatal and perinatal care has reduced neonatal mortality and babies who die have survived longer. Twenty five years ago, only 8 % of infants coming to autopsy had survived longer than 10 days, the comparative figure today is over

30 %, and the pathology of the brain has accordingly changed. Prolonging the survival of these children, often very ill, brings with it an increase in the risk of nosocomial infections. At autopsy the association of leucomalacia with meningo-encephalitis has increased from 8 % to 20 %. In addition, a longer survival in infants, allows the evolution of the lesions to be followed. At autopsy, the incidence of sclerosis of the centrum semiovale and multicystic encephalomalacia has increased from 2.2 % in 1956-1966, to 7.2 % in 1967-1973, then to 14.4 % in recent years. These figures reflect the pessimistic experience of the pathologist in contrast to the more encouraging data obtained in studies on surviving children.

Various types of leucomalacia:

— Leucomalacia is often associated with meningo-encephalitis. After fixation, the white matter is yellowish, may be firm or liquefied and contrasts with the surrounding cortex and deep grey nuclei. Histological studies show intense proliferation of large GFA positive glial cells in association with other features of severe softening. Similar reactions have been described in newborn rabbits after intra-abdominal injections of *Escherichia coli* endotoxin in pregnant animals [30].

— Haemorrhagic leucomalacia: although the primary lesion is usually ischaemic [7], secondary haemorrhage occurs in 7 to 25 % of cases when vascular walls and the surrounding white matter are severely damaged. This form is often associated with IVH; these two lesions may subsequently communicate and, on anatomical grounds, it is difficult to know if rupture was caused by pressure from within out or vice versa. In some cases, however, the occurrence of haemorrhagic infarction in the white matter as the initial event cannot be ruled out. The system of thin-walled veins arranged in a radial pattern without anastomoses or valves predisposes to diapedesis and rupture.

— Subcortical leucomalacia is seen more frequently in mature newborn infants, and at autopsy is often associated with œdema. This lesion is located in a poorly vascularized triangular arterial territory [71] and, in survivors may become cystic [69].

Arterial occlusions

Arterial occlusions were said to be rare in the neonatal period and until recently the diagnosis was made with certainty only at autopsy [9] or later in life after neurological deficits had developed. It is generally the middle cerebral artery, more frequently the left or one of its branches, that is occluded. Cerebral lesions correspond to the areas irrigated by the affected artery. However, in the neonate, haemorrhagic lesions often extend within and beyond the ischaemic areas. Microscopically, the lesions closely resemble those observed in the brain of older children and adults. The cortex and the subcortical white matter are totaly disorganised with pyknosis of nerve cell nuclei and, after several days, glial and macrophagic reactions, followed by capillary proliferation with prominence of endothelial cell nuclei. The causes of arterial occlusion in the neonate are not well understood. In some cases, emboli arising during umbilical venous catheterisation and exchange transfusion have been incriminated [45]. The late consequences with multicystic formations, glial and macrophage reactions, atrophy of the corresponding cerebral hemisphere and homolateral hydrocephalus, are not different from those observed in older infants. If the injury occurs early in fœtal life, anomalies of cell archi-

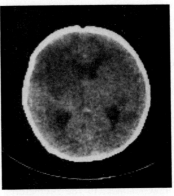

Fig. II-25. — *CT scan: softening in the territory of the middle cerebral artery in a 3 day old infant; he developed status epilepticus and subsequently a right hemiplegia.*

tecture comparable to forms of microgyria may develop (see below).

In the neonatal period, unilateral symptomatology is unusual and often submerged in a clinical picture dominated by major respiratory and neurological distress. However, when there are asymmetrical neurological signs, usually hypotonia with contralateral electrical abnormal tracings, arterial thrombosis must be considered in the differential diagnosis.

Nowadays, CT scan und US, allow for early diagnosis (Fig. II-25) and arteriography can be avoided. If these studies are performed soon after birth, the lesions can be diagnosed and dated; it is sometimes possible to state that the vascular accident must have occurred in utero and hence, "difficult birth" as a cause can be excluded. Whether the damage is antenatal or perinatal, motor defects become apparent only during the months that follow [41].

The brain and intrauterine growth retardation

Animal experiments have given much information on the development of the central nervous system in intrauterine growth retardation, whether this is secondary to maternal malnutrition or to reduced uterine blood flow. A reduction in the number of mitoses, alterations in cell migration, or defects of myelinization occur to a variable degree, according to the timing of the insult. Less is known about the hypotrophic small for dates human infant.

In the case of maternal hypertension with placental insufficiency, fœtal growth retardation generally occurs in the second half of gestation, and the central nervous system is relatively unaffected. The brain is much larger than would be predicted from the weight of the infant, but it is small in relation to gestational age. There is no significant modification in the external morphology of the cerebral hemispheres (Fig. II-26 a, b, c) and the number of nerve cells is apparently undiminished. On the other hand, the number of glial cells and the degree of myelinization may be altered and, in the cerebellum the final stages of cell migration may be affected (cf. chapter 14).

None of these anomalies can be considered by the neuropathologist as a lesion in the sense of tissue damage or destruction. Cerebral lesions, in the usual sense of the term, may, however be present in addition, in the hypotrophic infant. They are generally caused by obstetric or postnatal problems and are characteristic of the gestational age of the infant as described above in the eutrophic infant: IVH and leucomalacia in the premature, neuronal necrosis in the full-term infant. They result from diverse haemodynamic problems and in addition from hypoglycaemia.

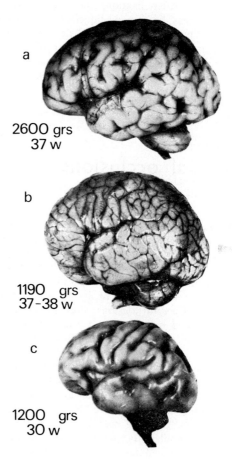

a

2600 grs
37 w

b

1190 grs
37-38 w

c

1200 grs
30 w

Fig. II-26. — *External morphological aspect of the brain.*

a) Eutrophic neonate of 37 weeks of gestation.

b) Hypotrophic infant.

c) Premature infant of same birth weight as b.

Fetal vascular encephalopathies

The generalized utilization of ultrasonography for prenatal diagnosis has lead, recently, to an increased number of reports of cerebral lesions that occur in utero. Although the mechanism of these lesions is not always well understood, they may be related to maternal, fœtal or placental abnormal conditions. Once identified, these lesions can no longer be attributed to difficult labor and birth (Fig. II-27).

Maternal pathological conditions. — In the past, toxaemia with hypertension, recurrent urinary tract infections, severe anemia or hypoxia, have been incriminated in the pathogenesis of fœtal brain damage. However, the lesions were described long after birth and their time of occurrence could not be proven with certainty. Nowadays, with the use of US, antenatal lesions have been diagnosed following maternal bee sting anaphylaxis and severe hypoxia for example.

Maternal trauma during pregnancy with subsequent cephalhematoma of the fœtus [33], subdural hematoma following a fall of the mother [6], multicystic encephalopathy, or hydranencephaly after an aircraft accident have been repeatedly reported. Car accidents without trauma to the mother were also thought to be a cause of intraventricular hemorrhage and multicystic encephalopathy and posed a difficult medico-legal problem [47]. In the pregnant rhesus monkey [55], maternal psychological stress can indeed cause catecholamine elaboration, leading to uterine vasoconstriction and impaired intervillous perfusion with fœtal brain damage similar to that observed in human fœtuses.

Inhalation of carbon monoxide during pregnancy is known to lead to fœtal cerebral damage and to neurological disorders in survivors. Inhalation of butane gas which is in itself non-toxic, utilized in an attempted suicide, can induce a state of pure anoxia, followed by severe maternal cardiovascular collapse with subsequent fœtal brain damage [48]. In these situations, the extent of the lesions is a function of the duration and severity of the maternal accident; in extreme cases death of the fœtus in utero results; in case of a surviving damaged fœtus, therapeutic abortion should be considered.

Fœtal pathological conditions. — In some monozygotic, multiple pregnancies, with placental anastomoses [11] it is not rare for one twin to be born dead and macerated, and for the survivor to present with cerebral lesions which are either isolated or associated with visceral lesions. The pathogenesis of these lesions is not well known: haemodynamic alterations in the case of twin-to-twin transfusion, multiple embolizations from the placenta of the macerated twin or production of thrombokinase are possible explanations. The cerebral lesions are most often described as multicystic leucomalacia, sometimes associated with extensive cortical damage. Faced with a pathological neurological picture not explained by the circumstances of birth, the clinician should have resort to an early US which may well show very extensive lesions, established long before birth (Fig. II-28 a and b). In infants who survive, a wide range of psychomotor handicaps develops, depending on the extent of the lesions and on their localization [1].

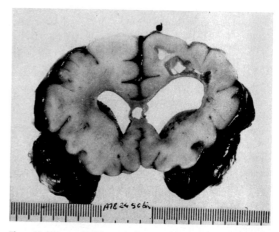

Fig. II-27. — *Stillborn infant at 38 weeks of gestation; posthemorrhagic hydrocephalus and multicystic leucomalacia that have developed* in utero (courtesy of Dr. NESSMANN).

Fœtal blood dyscrasia in the setting of isoimmune thrombocytopenia, haemolytic disease, hydrops fœtalis with or without blood group incompatibility, congenital rubella or ill defined intrauterine thrombopathy can lead to intracerebral haemorrhage and subsequent porencephaly.

Fœtal arterial occlusion, rarely described by

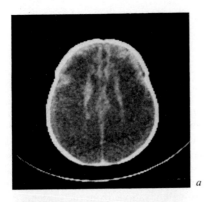

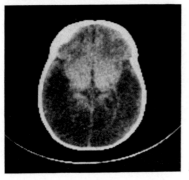

Fig. II-28. — *CT scan in a surviving twin*. The other infant was macerated and stillborn; diffuse hypodensity; basal ganglia and frontal poles are spared (hydranencephaly?) (courtesy of Dr. Vignaud).

pathologists in stillborn infants is probably more frequent than was once thought. In infants born alive, use of CT scan and US allows early diagnosis, measurement of the extent of the lesion and assessment of its age (Fig. II-25). The lesions are located in the arterial territory corresponding to the occluded vessel, and, are morphologically similar to those observed postnatally or in older infants. However, early occlusion can lead to anomalies of morphogenesis and cytoarchitecture or even to hydranencephaly.

Placental and cord anomalies. — Although we have little information on the relations between placental and cord anomalies and specific brain damage, the placenta and cord should be systematically and carefully examined, at least when the infant presents difficulties at birth, in order to search for pathological conditions which may impair fœtal circulation. A case of severe placental calcification has been reported [48], associated with diffuse brain hypodensities on CT scan compatible with the diagnosis of hydranencephaly. At autopsy of the

3 day old infant, the brain was œdematous and histological studies revealed a near total loss of neurons.

Finally an increasing number of cases of fœtal intracranial haemorrhages without apparent cause have been diagnosed by US [21] with or without autopsy control and reported in the literature.

REFERENCES

[1] Aicardi (J.), Goutieres (F.), Hodebourg-de-Verbois (A.). — Multicystic encephalomalacia in infants and its relation to abnormal gestation and hydranencephaly. *J. Neurol. Sc.*, *15*, 357-373, 1972.

[2] Allemand (F.), Monod (N.), Larroche (J. Cl.). — L'électroencéphalogramme dans les hémorragies sous-durales du nouveau-né. *Rev. EEG Neurophysiol.*, *7*, 365, 1977.

[3] Amiel (Cl.). — Hémorragies cérébrales intraventriculaires chez le prématuré. 2ᵉ partie : Les éléments du diagnostic clinique. *Biol. Neonat.*, *7*, 57-75, 1964.

[4] Amiel-Tison (Cl.). — Neurologic disorders in neonates associated with abnormalities of pregnancy and birth. *Curr. Probl. Pediatr.*, *3*, 3-50, 1973.

[5] Amiel-Tison (Cl.), Dalisson (C.), Henrion (R.). — Évolution de la pathologie cérébrale du nouveau-né à terme au cours des cinq dernières années de la maternité de Port-Royal. *Arch. Fr. Pédiatr.*, *37*, 87-92, 1980.

[6] Amiel-Tison (Cl.), Grenier (A.), Eds. — *La surveillance neurologique au cours de la première année de la vie*. Masson, publ., Paris, 1985.

[7] Armstrong (D.), Norman (H. G.). — Periventricular leucomalacia in neonates. Complications and sequelæ. *Arch. Dis. Child.*, *49*, 367-375, 1974.

[8] Banker (B. Q.), Larroche (J. Cl.). — Periventricular leukomalacia of infancy. A form of neonatal anoxic encephalopathy. *Arch. Neurol.*, *7*, 386-410, 1962.

[9] Barmada (M. A.), Moosy (J.), Shuman (R. M.). — Cerebral infarcts with arterial occlusion in neonates. *Ann. Neurol.*, *6*, 495-502, 1979.

[10] Bejar (R.), Curbelo (V.), Coen (R. W.) et al. — Diagnosis and follow-up of intraventricular and intracerebral hemorrhages by ultrasound studies of infant's brain through the fontanelles and sutures. *Pediatrics*, *66*, 661-673, 1980.

[11] Benirschke (K.), Driscoll (S. G.), Eds. — *The pathology of the human placenta*. Springer Verlag, Berlin, 1967.

[12] Bergman (I.), Bauer (R. E.), Barmada (M. A.) et al. — Intracerebral hemorrhage in the full-term neonatal infant. *Pediatrics*, *75*, 498-496, 1985.

[13] Blanc (W. A.), Rapmund (G.), Silverman (W. A.). — Falling hematocrit value in the premature infant as a sign of intraventricular haemorrhage. *Am. J. Dis. Child.*, *94*, 430, 1957.

[14] Burstein (J.), Papile (L.), Burstein (R.). — Subependymal germinal matrix and intraventricular hemorrhage in premature infants: diagnosis by CT. *Am. J. Roentgenol.*, *128*, 971-976, 1977.

[15] Cartwright (G. W.), Culbertson (K.), Schreiner (R. L.) et al. — Changes in clinical presen-

tation of term infants with intracranial hemorrhage. *Dev. Med. Child. Neurol.*, 21, 730-737, 1979.

[16] CHAMBERLAIN (R.), CHAMBERLAIN (G.), HOW-
LETT (B.), CLAIREAUX (A.), Eds. — *British births
1970.* London, William Heinemann Medical Book
Ltd., 1975, 278.

[17] COUTURE (A.), CADIER (L.). — *Échographie cérébrale par voie transfontanellaire.* Vigot Éditeur,
Paris, 1983.

[18] CROME (L.). — Multilocular cystic encephalopathy
of infants. *J. Neurosurg. Psychiat. (London),*
21, 146-152, 1958.

[19] DELAPORTE (B.), CHERINAT (C.), SIDIBE (M.) et al. —
Aspect échographique des lésions ischémiques et/ou
anoxiques non hémorragiques du nouveau-né
prématuré. *Arch. Fr. Pédiat.*, 41, 222, 1984.

[20] DEONNA (T.), PAYOT (M.), PROBST (A.) et al. —
Neonatal intracranial hemorrhage in premature
infants. *Pediatrics*, 56, 1056-1064, 1975.

[21] DONN (S. M.), BARR (M.), MCLEARY (R. D.). —
Massive intracerebral hemorrhage in utero: sono-
graphic appearance and pathologic correlation.
Obst. and Gyn., 63, N° 3 suppl., 28S-30S, 1984.

[22] DREYFUS-BRISAC (C.), MONOD (N.). — Electro-
clinical studies of status epilepticus and convulsions in the newborn. In *Neurologic and electro-
encephalographic correlative studies in infancy.*
KELLAWAY (P.), PETERSON (I.) Eds. Grune and
Stratton, Inc., New York, 1964, 250-272.

[23] DUBOWITZ (N. M. R.), BYDDER (G. M.), MUSHIN (J.).
— Developmental sequence of periventricular
leukomalacia. *Arch. Dis. Child.*, 60, 349-355, 1985.

[24] FEDRICK (J.), BUTLER (N. R.). — Certain causes of
neonatal death: II. Intraventricular hemorrhage.
Biol. Neonat., 15, 257-290, 1970.

[25] FITZHARDINGE (P. M.), FLODMARK (O.), FITZ
(C. R.) et al. — The pronostic value of computed tomography as an adjunct to assessment of
the term infant with post-asphyxial encephalopathy.
J. Pediat., 99, 777-781, 1981.

[26] FRIEDE (R. L.) Ed. — *Developmental neuropathology.*
Springer Verlag, 1975, Vienne, p. 524.

[27] FLODMARK (O.). — *Diagnosis by computed tomography of intracranial hemorrhage and hypoxic/
ischemic brain damage in neonates.* ISBN 91-7222-
420-7. Sweden Studentlitteratur, Stockholm, 1981.

[28] FUJIMURA (M.), SALISBURY (D. M.), ROBINSON
(R. O.) et al. — Clinical events relating tointra-
ventricular haemorrhage in the newborn. *Arch.
Dis. Childh.*, 54, 409-414, 1979.

[29] GILLES (F. H.), PRICE (R. A.), KEVY (S. V.),
et al. — Fibrinolytic activity in the ganglionic
eminence of the premature human brain. *Biol.
Neonat.*, 18, 426-432, 1971.

[30] GILLES (F. H.), AVERILL (D. R.), KERR (C. S.).
— Neonatal endotoxin encephalopathy. *Ann.
Neurol.*, 2, 49-56, 1977.

[31] GODDARD (J.), LEWIS (R. M.), ALCALA (H.) et al.
— Intraventricular hemorrhage. An animal model.
Biol. Neonat., 37, 39-52, 1980.

[32] GRUENWALD (P.). — Subependymal cerebral
hemorrhage in premature infants, and its relation
to various injurious influences at birth. *Am. J. Obst.
Gynecol.*, 61, 1285-1292, 1951.

[33] GRYLACK (L.). — Prenatal sonographic diagnosis
of cephalohematoma due to pre labor trauma.
Pediatric Path., 12, 145-147, 1982.

[34] HAMBLETON (G.), WIGGLESWORTH (J. S.). — Origin

of intraventricular haemorrhage in the preterm
infant. *Arch. Dis. Childh.*, 51, 651-659, 1976.

[35] HAYDEN (C. K.), SHATTUCK (K. E.), RICHARDSON
(C. J.) et al. — Subependymal germinal matrix
hemorrhage in full-term neonates. *Pediatrics*,
75, 714-718, 1985.

[36] HOPKINS (I. J.), FARKAS-BARGETON (E.), LAR-
ROCHE (J. Cl.). — Neonatal neuronal necrosis:
its relationship to the distribution and maturation
of oxidative enzymes of newborn cerebral and cerebellar cortex. *Early Human Develop.*, 4, 51-60, 1980.

[37] HORBAR (J. D.), WALTERS (C. L.), PHILIP (A. G.)
et al. — Ultrasound detection of changing ventricular size in posthemorrhagic hydrocephalus.
Pediatrics, 66, 674-678, 1980.

[38] JOHNSON (M. L.), RUMACK (C. M.). — Ultrasonic
evaluation of the neonatal brain. *Radiol. Clin.
North. Am.*, 18, 117-131, 1980.

[39] KOROBKIN (R.). — The relationship between head
circumference and the development of communicating hydrocephalus following intraventricular
hemorrhage. *Pediatrics*, 56, 74-77, 1975.

[40] KRISHNAMOORTHY (K. S.), FERNANDEZ (R. A.),
MOMOSE (K. J.) et al. — Evaluation of neonatal
intracranial hemorrhage by computerized tomography. *Pediatrics*, 59, 165-172, 1977.

[41] KULAKOWSKI (S.), LARROCHE (J. Cl.). — Cranial
computerized tomography in cerebral palsy. An
attempt at anatomo-clinical and radiological correlations. *Neuropediatrics*, 11, 339-353, 1980.

[42] LARROCHE (J. Cl.). — Les hémorragies cérébrales
intraventriculaires chez le prématuré. Anatomie
et physiopathogénie. *Biol. Neonat.*, 7, 26-56, 1964.

[43] LARROCHE (J. Cl.). — Nécrose cérébrale massive
chez le nouveau-né. Ses rapports avec la maturation,
son expression clinique et bio-électrique. *Biol.
Neonat.*, 13, 340-360, 1968.

[44] LARROCHE (J. Cl.). — Posthaemorrhagic hydrocephalus in infancy. Anatomical study. *Biol. Neonat.*,
20, 287-299, 1972.

[45] LARROCHE (J. Cl.), Ed. — *Developmental pathology
of the neonate.* Excerpta Medica, Amsterdam, 1977,
545.

[46] LARROCHE (J. Cl). — *The fine structure of matrix
capillaries in human embryos and young fetuses.*
The second Ross conference on intraventricular
hemorrhage, Washington, 1982.

[47] LARROCHE (J. Cl.). — *Perinatal brain damage in
Greenfield's Neuropathology.* J. HUME ADAMS,
J. A. N. CORSELLICS and L. W. DUCHEN, Eds.,
Edward Arnold, 1984, 4th Edition.

[48] LARROCHE (J. Cl.). — *Fetal brain damage of circu-
latory origin in the at-risk infant.* S. HAREL and
N. ANASTASIOW, Eds., Brookes Publ. and Co.,
Baltimore, 1985.

[49] LEECH (R. W.), KOHNEN (P.). — Subependymal
and intraventricular hemorrages in the newborn.
Am. J. Pathol., 77, 465-476, 1974.

[50] LEVENE (M. I.), WILLIAMS (J. L.), FAWER (C. L.),
Eds. — Ultrasound of the infant brain. *Clinics in
Developmental Medicine*, N° 92, London, SIMP,
Blackwell Scientific Publications Ltd., 1985.

[51] LONG (J. G.), LUCEY (J. F.), PHILIP (A. G.). — Noise
and hypoxemia in the intensive care unit. *Pediatrics*,
65, 143-145, 1980.

[52] LOU (C. H.), LASSEN (N. A.), FRIIS-HANSEN (B.).
— Low cerebral blood flow in hypotensive perinatal distress. *Acta. Neurol. Scand.*, 56, 343-352,
1977.

[53] LOU (C. H.), LASSEN (N. A.), FRIIS-HANSEN (B.). — Impaired autoregulation of cerebral blood flow in the distressed newborn infant. *J. Pediatr.*, *94,* 118-121, 1979.

[54] MORIETTE (G.), RELIER (J. P.), LARROCHE (J. Cl.). — Les hémorragies intraventriculaires au cours de la maladie des membranes hyalines. *Arch. Franç. Péd.*, *34*, 492-504, 1977.

[55] MYERS (R. E.). — Maternal psychological stress and fetal asphyxia: a study in the monkey. *Am. J. Obstet. Gyn.*, *122*, 47-59, 1975.

[56] MYERS (R. E.), DECOURTEN-MYERS (G. M.), WAGNER (K. R.). — Effect of hypoxia on fetal brain in *Fetal physiology and medicine*, 2ᵉ ed. BEARD and NATANIELSZ Eds., Bekker, 1983.

[57] NISWANDER (K. R.), GORDON (M.), Eds. — *The women and their pregnancies*. Philadelphia, 1972, W. B. Saunders Co., p. 540.

[58] NWAESSI (C. G.), PAPE (K. E.), MARTIN (D. J.), BECKER (L. E.) et al. — Periventricular infarction diagnosed by ultrasound. A post mortem correlation. *J. Pediat.*, *105*, 106-110, 1984.

[59] PAPE (K. E.), WIGGLESWORTH (J. S.), Eds. — *Hemorrhage, ischemia and the perinatal brain*, 1979, W. Heinemann Medical Books, London.

[60] PAPILE (L.), BURNSTEIN (J.), BURNSTEIN (R.) et al. — Incidence and evolution of sub-ependymal and intraventricular hemorrhage. A study of infants with birth weight less than 1,500 g. *J. Pediat.*, *92*, 529-534, 1978.

[61] PASTERNAK (J. F.), GROOTHUIS (D. R.), FISCHER (J. M.) et al. — Regional cerebral blood flow in the newborn beagle pup: the germinal matrix is a "low-flow" structure. *Ped. Research*, *16*, 499-503, 1982.

[62] PERLMAN (J. M.), NELSON (J. S.), MCALISTER (W. H.) et al. — Intracerebellar hemorrhage in a premature newborn: diagnosis by real time. Ultrasound and correlations with autopsy findings. *Pediatrics*, *71*, 159-162, 1983.

[63] PERLMAN (J. M.), GOODMAN (S.), KREUSSER (L.) et al. — Reduction in intraventricular hemorrhage by elimination of fluctuating cerebral blood flow velocity in preterm infants with respiratory distress syndrome. *New Engl. J. Med.*, *312*, 1353-1357, 1985.

[64] RANCK (J. B.), WINDLE (W. F.). — Brain damage in the monkey, *Macaca mulatta*, by asphyxia neonatorum. *Exp. Neurol.*, *1*, 130-154, 1959.

[65] REYNOLDS (M. L.), EVANS (C. A.), REYNOLDS (E. O.), SAUNDERS (N. R.) et al. — Intracranial haemorrhage in the preterm sheep fetus. *Early Human Develop.*, *32*, 163-186, 1979.

[66] ROM (S.), SERFONTEIN (G. L.), HUMPHRYS (R. P.). — Intracerebellar hematoma in the neonate. *J. Pediatr.*, *93*, 486-488, 1978.

[67] RORKE (L. B.), Ed. — *Pathology of perinatal brain injury*. Raven Press, New York, 1982.

[68] RUSHTON (D. I.), PRESTON (P. R.), DURBIN (G. M.). — Structure and evolution of echo dense lesions in the neonatal brain. *Arch. Dis. Child.*, *60*, 798-808, 1985.

[69] SMITH (J. F.), Ed. — *Pediatric neuropathology*. McGraw-Hill Book Cie, 1974.

[70] STEWART (A. L.). — Early prediction of neurological outcome when the very preterm infant is discharged from the intensive care unit. *Ann. Pediat.*, *32*, 27-38, 1985.

[71] TAKASHIMA (S.), ARMSTRONG (D.), BECKER (L. E.). — Subcortical leucomalacia; relationship to development of the cerebral sulcus and its vascular supply. *Arch. Neurol.*, *35*, 470-472, 1978.

[72] TAKASHIMA (S.), TANAKA (K.). — Microangiography and vascular permeability of the subependymal matrix in the premature infant. *J. Can. Sciences Neurol.*, *5*, 45-50, 1978.

[73] TAKASHIMA (S.), TANAKA (K.). — Development of cerebrovascular architecture and its relationship to periventricular leucomalacia. *Arch. Neurol.*, *35*, 11-15, 1978.

[74] TAKASHIMA (S.), ARMSTRONG (D.), BECKER (L. E.). — Old subependymal necrosis and hemorrhage in the prematurely born infant. *Brain Develop.*, *1*, 299-304, 1979.

[75] TOWBIN (A.). — Cerebral intraventricular hemorrhage and subependymal matrix infarction in the fetus and premature newborn. *Am. J. Path.*, *52*, 121-140, 1968.

[76] TSIANTOS (A.), VICTORIN (L.), RELIER (J. P.) et al. — Intracranial hemorrhage in the prematurely born infant: timing of clots and evaluation of clinical signs and symptoms. *J. Pediatr.*, *85*, 854-859, 1974.

[77] VAN DEN BERGH (R.). — The periventricular intracerebral blood supply. In *Research on the cerebral circulation*. J. MEYER, H. LECHNER, O. EICHHORN, Eds., Ch. Thomas, Publ., 1969, 52-65.

[78] VAN DER EECKEN (H. M.), Ed. — *The anastomoses between the leptomeningeal arteries of the brain*. Ch. Thomas, Publ., 1959, 160.

[79] VOLPE (J. J.), PASTERNAK (J. F.). — Parasagittal cerebral injury in neonatal hypoxic-ischemic encephalopathy. Clinical and neuroradiologic features. *J. Pediatr.*, *91*, 472-476, 1977.

[80] VOLPE (J. J.), PASTERNAK (J. F.), ALLAN (W. C.). — Ventricular dilation preceding rapid head growth following neonatal intracranial hemorrhage. *Am. J. Dis. Child.*, *131*, 1212-1215, 1977.

[81] VOLPE (J. J.), Ed. — *Neurology of the newborn*. W. B. Saunders Company, Philadelphia, 1981, 468.

[82] VOLPE (J. J.), HERSCOVITCH (P.), PERLMAN (J. M.) et al. — Positron emission tomography in the asphyxiated term infant: parasagittal impairment of cerebral blood flow. *Ann. Neur.*, *17*, 287-296, 1985.

16

Follow-up studies

Claudine AMIEL-TISON

Introduction

The difficulties in evaluating the consequences of different forms of cerebral pathology in the neonate are numerous. Apart from very severe forms of asphyxial encephalopathy, or post-haemorrhagic hydrocephalus, the parents should not be unduly alarmed because the long term prognosis is so uncertain. Anxiety must not be needlessly transmitted; an explanation of the perinatal history and the reasons for close surveillance should be given. Regular consultation during the first year gives a better approximation of the effects [2]. Indeed some children have shown normal development during the first year. This is very reassuring for the infant born at term but less clearly so, for the infant of low birthweight. In other cases early detection of cerebral anomalies, in particular motor anomalies, has been possible; if they persist at one year, they will be definitive. Finally there is an intermediate group of transient motor deficiencies, these children, despite their apparent normality at one year, will still be at risk of showing further moderate consequences at school age. This method of surveillance allows classification of the infants at one year, into three groups, a classification which has no value in accurate diagnosis of the individual infant, but is of overall importance for the obstetrician and paediatrician. The interest lies in obtaining statistics for prognostic evaluation, before school age, as the results at 7 years depend so much on education, social and cultural factors.

Unfortunately differences in methodology and definition of terms make comparisons between studies difficult. In general, classification of a handicap as major results if the child is unable to pursue a normal school life. This occurs for diverse reasons; cerebro-motor deficits, an IQ less than 70, auditory or visual handicaps. Major handicaps because of their severity are usually diagnosed before the infant is 1 year old. On the other hand, the definition of minor handicap remains extremely vague and varies with the age of the infant at the time of evaluation. The same infant may be classified as having minor handicaps during the first year of life due to motor anomalies, between 1 and 4 years as normal and then again as having minor handicaps interfering with his or her intellectual performance or behaviour at school. However, recently a good correlation has been shown [8] between a score of 85 using the Bayley psychomotor scale at 18 months, and a score of less than 90 on the Wechsler scale at 6 years. This is thus an acceptable method from the statistical point of view even if it is not in evaluation of the individual infant.

The importance of social and cultural conditions is very great at all ages. Socially disadvantaged children will suffer not only from poorer prenatal care, but also from poor social conditions after birth. It has been clearly demonstrated in the category of minor handicaps, grouped under the term "Minimal Brain Dysfunction" (MBD), that cultural conditions are as important as perinatal lesions. This considerable bias in interpretation is insurmountable in local studies in which the numbers involved are too small to be subdivided. It can probably only be avoided by very detailed evalua-tion of neuromotor anomalies during the first year.

In spite of all these difficulties to which one must often add a percentage of infants whose development is not followed, it is possible to predict the risk of consequences in different categories of infants.

Results in certain groups of infants at risk

The characteristics of lesions, as we have already seen, are directly linked with the degree of cerebral maturation at birth. It is therefore obvious that the long term neurological consequences will also depend on gestational age.

Neonates of very low birthweight

The group designated under the heading of "very low birth-weight" represents premature or small for dates infants of birthweight between 501 and 1,500 gm. This definition has only recently come into current use, since the neonate of less than 1,000 gm for a long time at the lower limits of all mortality and especially morbidity statistics, had been included with infants of greater weight. In addition to the weight at birth another factor needs to be considered in the interpretation of results, the place of birth, whether "inborn"—born in the hospital containing the intensive care unit—or "outborn"—born elsewhere and transported to the unit. The prognosis is different in the two cases.

The degree of foetal malnutrition in this group must also be analysed. A brief history of this subject is necessary before analysis of the most recent results. Three periods can be roughly distinguished, marked by different progress in the techniques of perinatal medicine. Each new technique brought with it changes in the attitude of the obstetric and neonatal team.

1965-1970. — Intensive postnatal care was at a hesitant stage. Mortality was considerable in artificially ventilated neonates weighing less than 1,500 gm to the extent that many teams refused to use artificial ventilation. In fact, this required a huge effort for little gain in survival, and there was always the fear of seeing an increase in cerebral damage. It was a period of doubt and little success.

1970-1975. — An improvement in intensive care, particularly in ventilation techniques, brought with it an increase in survival year by year. The results of

long term enquiries demonstrate a parallel improvement in mortality and neurological sequelae. It was, therefore, an encouraging period in paediatrics, driving the therapeutic effort to its maximum. It is a period when all the statistics local and national show a dramatic decrease of cerebro-motor disability with the prevention of apnoeic episodes in this group of prematures.

1975-1980. — This period is marked by considerable progress in the methods of evaluating the foetal state. The development of techniques for recording foetal heart rate and progress in physio-logical knowledge now allow a better understanding of distress in the very small foetus, and a better definition of the moment when prolonging intra-uterine life places the cerebral integrity of the foetus at risk. Because postnatal care was now of better quality it became logical to carry out very early delivery when the foetus is in danger. It represents a period of obstetric courage.

However, everyone questions their conscience about what limits to respect in this intervention. Fitzhardinge has recently drawn attention to repeatedly poor results obtained for the newborn weighing less than 800 gm [3]. In fact, the general feeling is against establishing general policies.

The results from several centres [7, 9, 14] dealing with large numbers of infants who have a well organised long term follow-up arrangement, provide indispensable reference points, as shown in Table I. These results give the percentage of major handicaps in relation to the survivors. They show important divergences; thus the percentage of major handicap varies from 8 to 30 %. The percentage for major handicap is a little higher in infants of less than 1,000 gm than for the group as a whole, but this is insignificant.

Other data [4] has shown, separately, the cerebral prognosis of small-for-dates neonates of less than 37 weeks with a weight less than two standard deviations below the average curve (all except 7 weighed less than 1,500 gm). The figure for the

TABLE I. — The percentage of major handicap observed amongst survivors
weighing 501 g to 1,500 g at birth

		501-1,500 g	501-1,000 g	1,001-1,500 g
Toronto [7]	Admissions to the ICU	250		
	Deaths	86		
FITZHARDINGE et al. (1978)	Lost to follow-up	15		
	Followed	149	44	105
Results at 2 years (mostly	Major handicap	44	16	28
"outborn")		44/149 = 30 %	16/44 = 36 %	28/105 = 27 %
Cleveland [9]	Admissions to the ICU	291		
	Deaths	79		
HACK et al. (1978)	Lost to follow-up	29		
	Followed	160	32	128
Results at 2 years	Major handicap	27	7	20
		27/160 = 17 %	7/32 = 22 %	20/128 = 16 %
London [14]	Admissions to the ICU	589		
	Deaths	269		
STEWART et al. (1978)	Lost to follow-up	2		
	Too young	59		
	Followed	259	39	220
Results at 18 months or	Major handicap	22	5	17
later		22/259 = 8 %	5/39 = 13 %	17/220 = 8 %
(mostly "inborn")				
	Assessment at 8 years	50		
	Attending normal schools	38 (76 %)		
	Help in normal schools or special schools	12 (24 %)		

total number of children having a major handicap reached 49 % in the work cited above. For the group from Toronto the premature small-for-dates infant has a cerebral prognosis less favourable than the small-for-dates infant born at term [6] or than the premature infants of appropriate birth weight [7]. Such figures may be biased by the conditions of transport and a possible selection as to suitability for transport. A similar increase in the risk, associated with intrauterine malnutrition has not in fact been found by Stewart or Hack [9, 14].

Neonates born at term

Cerebral pathology of the neonate at term has its origin at the time of birth. Whatever the respective proportions of ischaemia with anoxia, trauma, circulatory disturbance and œdema, the severity of symptoms observed during the first week allows a good evaluation of the long-term prognosis.

The prognosis of *severe forms* (Stage 3), *i. e.* status epilepticus, is poor [1, 13]. Associations of cerebro-motor defects of variable degree, often quadriplegia with mental retardation and poor

social adaptation, are usual. A more favourable development is however not impossible. The best prognostic sign during the first months is the head circumference growth curve because severe cerebral atrophy soon becomes associated with microcephaly and early closure of the fontanelles and sutures.

It is almost impossible to predict outcome in *moderate forms* (Stage 2) during the first months. Many of these children become apparently normal during the first year, but later problems of mental retardation and behaviour disturbance cannot be excluded.

The prognosis in *minor forms* (Stage 1 cases show neither convulsions, nor alertness or reflex disturbances) is excellent, because there is probably no cellular damage in these cases.

From a practical point of view the following points must be emphasized.

— Obstetric trauma has become a rare pathological condition, 1 in 1,000 fullterm births for Stage 3, 1 in 1,000 for Stage 2 (see ch. 14). It therefore occupies a modest place amongst cerebral problems, compared to malformations, metabolic defects and infections.

— Lesions arising in the antenatal period are often wrongly attributed to the conditions of birth. In fact, Sylvian softenings, or destruction of the hemispheres by multicystic leucomalacia can develop *in utero* and present at birth in the same way as recent and acute brain damage. The temptation for the paediatrician is to attempt to explain the neurological state as the result of difficulties at birth, sometimes against all the evidence.

The outcome in the small-for-dates infants at term has a special pattern. Cerebro-motor defects are very rare; psychomotor disturbance is often the only worrying sign during the first year; but the percentage of infants classed in the Minimal Brain Damage (MBD) group has been estimated as 25 % [6]. This, therefore, represents a far from negligible risk.

Neonates of diabetic mothers

The neonate of a diabetic mother is nowadays most often born at term and the improved control of maternal diabetes tends to equalise his or her chances with those of the general population. The results obtained from the Wechsler scale show a normal distribution for intelligence in these infants [5].

*
* *

IN SUMMARY the epidemiological picture has changed greatly over the last 20 years. It depends on a number of factors, and varies from country to country and within each country with the general health of the mother, the level of antenatal care, the incidence of prematurity, and the level of organization of obstetric and postnatal care. The long-term study of Hagberg in Sweden [10, 11, 12] which uses cerebro-motor handicaps as an indicator of damage has demonstrated the trends taking place in the county of Göteborg, over the last 30 years. The number of cerebro-motor defects has diminished in a very significant manner in the group of infants of birth weight less than 2,500 g. On the other hand, in the group with a birth weight greater than 2,500 g the number has remained unchanged in the last 20 years. In this group it is becoming more and more apparent that a number of unfavourable prenatal factors, including fœtal growth retardation and other abnormal factors add up in the course of gestation and can be grouped together under the heading "Fœtal deprivation of supply". To this, the addition of even a minor degree of intrapartum asphyxia can lead to cerebral pathology. The

multifactorial nature of causation thus appears in this group.

The epidemiological evidence agrees with the anatomical evidence, in particular the evolution in the distribution of leucomalacia during the last 20 years into different groups of neonates at risk (see ch. 15).

REFERENCES

[1] AMIEL-TISON (C.). — Cerebral damage in fullterm newborn. Aetiological factors, neonatal status and longterm follow-up. *Biol. Neonat.*, *14*, 234-250, 1969.
[2] AMIEL-TISON (C.). — A method for neurological evaluation within the first year of life. In *Major Mental Handicap*. Ciba Symposium n° 59. Elsevier, 1978, North-Holland, 107-126.
[3] BENNET-BRITTON (S.), FITZHARDINGE (P. M.). — Is intensive care justified for infants weighing less than 801 g at birth? *Pediatr. Res.*, *14*, abstract 989, 1980.
[4] COMMERY (J. O.), FITZHARDINGE (P. M.). — Handicap in the preterm small for gestational age infant. *J. Pediatr.*, *94*, 779-786, 1979.
[5] CUMMINS (M.), NORRISH (M.). — Follow-up of children of diabetic mothers. *Arch. Dis. Childh.*, *55*, 259-264, 1980.
[6] FITZHARDINGE (P. M.), STEVEN (E.). — The small for date infant. II. Neurological and intellectual sequelae. *Pediatrics*, *50*, 50-57, 1972.
[7] FITZHARDINGE (P. M.), KALMAN (E.), ASHBY (S.), PAPE (K. E.). — Present status of the infant of very low birth weight treated in a referral neonatal intensive care unit in 1974. In *Major Mental Handicap*. Ciba Symposium n° 59. Elsevier, 1978, North-Holland, 139-144.
[8] FITZSIMONS (R. B.), ASHBY (S. A.), FITZHARDINGE (P. M.). — The prediction of school age IQ during infancy in the premature child. *Pediatr. Res.*, *12*, abstract 41, 1978.
[9] HACK (M.), FANAROFF (A. A.), MERKATZ (I. R.). — The low-birth weight infant evolution of a changing outlook. *New Engl. J. Med.*, *301*, 1162-1165, 1979.
[10] HAGBERG (B.), HAGBERG (G.), OLOW (I.). — The changing panorama of cerebral palsy in Sweden 1954-1970. I. Analysis of the general changes. *Acta Paediatr. Scand.*, *64*, 187-192, 1975.
[11] HAGBERG (G.), HAGBERG (B.), OLOW (I.). — The changing panorama of cerebral palsy in Swenden 1954-1970. III. The importance of fœtal deprivation supply. *Acta Paediatr. Scand.*, *65*, 403-408, 1976.
[12] HAGBERG (B.), HAGBERG (G.), OLOW (I.). — The changing panorama of cerebral palsy. XVI International Congress of Pediatrics. Barcelone, 1980, 281.
[13] MONOD (N.), PAJOT (N.), GUIDASCI (S.). — The neonatal EEG. Statistical studies and pronostic value in fullterm and preterm babies. *Electroenceph. Clin. Neurophysiol.*, *32*, 529-544, 1972.
[14] STEWART (A.), TURCAN (D.), RAWLINGS (G.), HART (S.), GREGORY (S.). — Outcome for infants at high risk of Major Mental Handicap. In *Major Mental Handicap*. Ciba Symposium n° 59, Elsevier, 1978, North-Holland, 151-164.

3

Cardiocirculatory
and respiratory diseases

17

Circulatory adaptation to extrauterine life

C. Göran WALLGREN

Our concepts regarding the prenatal circulatory pattern are based mainly on studies in animals with pioneer contributions by Barcroft and Dawes in England. The species under study has usually been the sheep and the circulatory pattern of the lamb has been investigated in utero, after implantation of flow and pressure detectors and reclosing the uterine wall, as well as in the exteriorized animal.

Although caution has been exercised to alter as little as possible of the environmental conditions prevailing in utero, artifacts due to the experimental procedures per se are difficult to rule out. This dilemma is exemplified by the reactivity of the umbilical circulation where the vessels rapidly constrict in response to a variety of external stimuli and accordingly have to be handled with the utmost gentleness to avoid changes in the circulatory pattern existing in utero.

A second potential error is induced by the fact that species differences are known to occur which may make the relevance of data obtained in animal models not directly transferable to the situation in the human fetus at term.

With these precautions in mind, there should, however, be little reason to question the validity of the basic pattern of the fetal circulation derived from animal experiments. A limited number of observations in the human fetus in situ during cesarean section procedures further corroborate this assumption.

Whereas thus most of our knowledge of the prenatal circulation is for obvious reasons based on animal studies, the circulatory characteristics of the postnatal period have been extensively documented in the newborn infant. There is today a substantial pool of information available on this subject, gathered by direct invasive as well as indirect observations in the neonatal period. Extensive experimental studies in animals regarding the circulatory consequences of the initiation of breathing have enriched our concept of the dramatic changes occurring in the central circulation in relation to aeration of the lungs.

Our general notion of the circulatory adaptation to extrauterine life is built largely by inference from data obtained from pre- and postnatal animal studies, but is in part also based on retrograde extrapolations from studies of the human circulation in the immediate postnatal period.

Characteristics of the prenatal circulation

The metabolic needs of the fetus are satisfied through exchange with the maternal circulation, and the placenta also handles the excretory load that fetal metabolism gives rise to. Placental blood flow accounts for approximately 50 % of the combined (right and left) ventricular output (Fig. III-1), arising from the abdominal aorta through the paired umbilical arteries. In the human fetus at term this amounts to 125 ml/kg/min. The placental circulation is a relatively low resistance circuit, where, after exchange has taken place in the intervillous spaces between maternal and fetal circulation, the post-

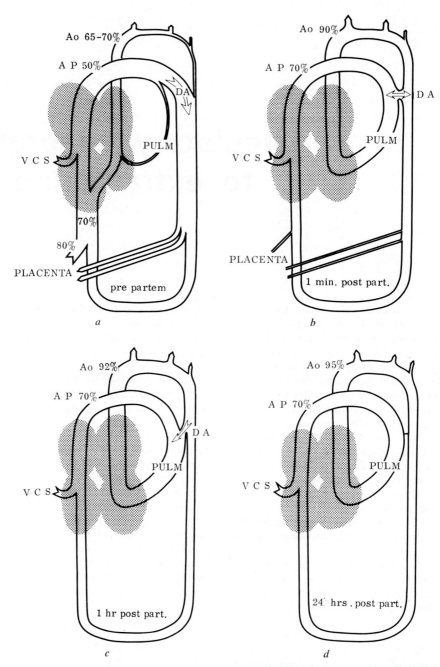

FIG. III-1 *a, b, c* and *d*. — *Perinatal changes in the central circulatory pattern.* AP, Ao, DA and VCS stand for pulmonary artery, ascending aorta, ductus arteriosus and superior caval vein respectively. Numbers indicate oxygen saturation and arrow direction of the ductal shunt. Shaded areas depict the four heart cavities. For details see text.

capillary blood is transported back to the fetus by way of the single umbilical vein connecting with the fetal portal sinuses. Umbilical venous blood with approximately 80 % saturation is the oxygen richest blood of the fetal circulation. It is shunted from the portal sinuses past the hepatic parenchyma to the inferior caval vein by way of the ductus venosus, with only a small fraction entering the portal circulation. Inferior caval venous blood which comprises approximately 2/3 of the systemic venous return to the heart, enters the fetal heart with an oxygen content that has dropped to some 70 % due to the admixture of umbilical venous blood with oxygen poor systemic venous blood. The inferior caval blood empties partly (2/3) into the right atrium and partly into the left (1/3) by way of the foramen ovale (via sinistra), which remains patent due to the prevailing left atrial hypotension. It mixes within the left atrium with the small amount of pulmonary venous blood draining the fetal lungs. Left ventricular ejection delivers blood to the ascending aorta with an oxygen saturation of 65-70 %, which is the highest oxygen content of blood leaving the fetal heart, providing an optimal oxygen supply to the upper part of the fetal body, notably the myocardial and cerebral circulations.

IVC blood entering the right atrium mixes with superior caval blood and small amounts of coronary sinus blood which reduces the oxygen saturation of blood expelled from the right ventricle to about 50 %. In contrast to IVC blood, SVC blood drains almost entirely into the right atrium with only very small amounts traversing the foramen ovale. Right ventricular output which, as a consequence of the prevailing volume load, is approximately twice that of the left ventricle, is mainly directed to the descending aorta through the patent ductus arteriosus and only a small fraction perfuses the high resistance pulmonary circulation. Right ventricular contribution reduces the aortic oxygen saturation to some 60 %. Descending aortic blood perfuses the lower part of the fetal body and the placental circulation. Under prevailing conditions the A-V oxygen difference across the placenta amounts to 35-40 ml/l.

With both ventricles emptying into the systemic circulation, their pressure loads are identical with the need to overcome an aortic systolic pressure of 60-70 mm Hg in the human fetus at term. As a consequence, the myocardial thickness of the ventricles is equal, whereas, due to the difference in volume load, the right ventricular cavity is approximately twice that of the left ventricle. The combined ventricular output of the fetus at term is roughly twice the univentricular output of the newborn (200 ml/kg in the newborn infant), indicating that a considerable extra volume load is put on the left ventricle at birth. The fetal heart rate usually aproximates 140 b.p.m. and cardiac output is mainly governed by changes in heart rate. The fetal heart rate and cardiac output are affected by a variety of stimuli, notably hypoxia, which is reflected in the fetal heart rate "dips" of prepartal fetal monitoring.

The high pulmonary vascular resistance in the fetus is mediated mainly by the low oxygen tension of the pulmonary tissue, which maintains a high tonus in the pulmonary arterioles. Various other factors have been identified as pulmonary vasoconstrictors, but it is reasonable to assume that oxygen tension is the main regulator of pulmonary resistance in the fetal lung. The peripheral systemic circulation also responds to hypoxia with increased vascular resistance in most vascular compartments. The most vital fetal organs, however, are less sensitive to fetal hypoxemia and there is experimental evidence for a redistribution of perfusion to the heart and the brain at the expence of perfusion during hypoxia to less vital parts of the body. Such "preferential" circulation serves the purpose of securing oxygen economy in the presence of impaired oxygen uptake from the placenta. In response to various vasoactive pharmacological substances, the fetal circulation does not seem to be substantially different from that in the newborn and the vascular reflex pattern is well developed.

THE IMMEDIATE CIRCULATORY CONSEQUENCES OF BIRTH

The birth process is accompanied by depressed placental function, due to the circulatory effects of the forceful uterine contractions during parturition. These impede gas exchange and the newborn infant enters the world with an oxygen debt and an accumulation of acid metabolites. The fact that placental perfusion usually continues, although at a falling rate, allows for some gas exchange during the first minute of extrauterine life, until separation occurs. With a basal metabolic need of 5 ml O_2/kg BW/min., hypoxia and respiratory acidosis can henceforth rapidly occur. Rapid institution of adequate ventilation and perfusion of the lungs are thus requisites for survival. At the time of the first respiratory movements, pO_2 is down to near 2-3 kPa (15-25 mm Hg) with a corresponding increase in

pCO_2 usually near 10 kPa (70 mm Hg) and a pH near 7.10.

Pulmonary vascular resistance (PVR), effect of aeration

The characteristically high pulmonary vascular resistance in the fetus is effected by vascular constriction in response to the relative tissue hypoxia and acidosis that exist in the unventilated lung. There is also a mechanical effect of the liquid-filled air spaces that promotes vascular compression, and the vascular geometry of the unexpanded lung further adds to the resistance to blood flow.

With the first few respiratory movements that usually occur within 20 seconds following delivery of the trunk, oxygen rich air enters the lungs and, as ventilation becomes effective, accumulated carbon dioxide is removed. The step-up in oxygen tension mediates an immediate relaxation of the pulmonary vessels, an effect which is further promoted by lowering of the carbon dioxide tension and acid-base correction (Fig. III-2). There is also good experimental support for the existence of a direct mechanical effect of aeration, which operates over surface tension forces in the liquid/air interface within the alveoli and small airways on one side, and negative inspiratory pressure on the other side, promoting vascular patency within the lungs. Local release of specific vasodilating material *i. e.* brady-

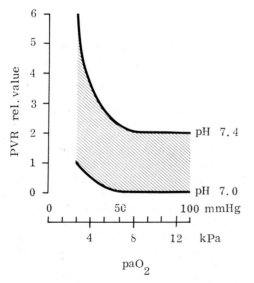

Fig. III-2. — *Effect of pH and paO_2 on pulmonary vascular resistance* (modified from RUDOLPH et al., 1966). Note vasoconstrictive response to increasing acidity with synergistic effect of hypoxemia.

kinin may further contribute to pulmonary vascular relaxation at the time of postnatal breathing. It is of particular importance that the pulmonary vascular resistance does not drop to the low adult levels immediately when breathing starts. The tone release, promoted by pulmonary ventilation, lowers the PVR down from the late fetal level of 1.5-2.0 mm Hg/ml/kg/min to a level only slightly below that of the systemic circulation 0.20-0.25 mm Hg/ml/kg/min. The persistent patency of the fetal communications between the pulmonary and systemic circuits during these hemodynamic conditions permits the dramatic changes of the neonatal central circulatory pattern, characterized by redistribution of the cardiac output. The ductal shunt, instead of routing right ventricular output past the lungs, now shifts to a left-to-right direction and actively contributes to the perfusion of the pulmonary parenchyma (Fig. III-1).

Functional closure of the "via sinistra"

The inflow of inferior caval blood through the foramen ovale to the left atrium presupposes a right atrial pressure in excess of that in the left atrium. This condition is fulfilled during fetal life, due to the very limited inflow to the left atrium of pulmonary venous blood and the relative volume overload of the right side. With the sudden drop in PVR during the first respiratory movements, pulmonary perfusion and consequently left atrial inflow are dramatically increased. The filling pressure of the left atrium exceeds that of the right side and the flap over the foramen ovale closes. With the intracardiac shunt closed, the systemic venous return to the heart drains to the right ventricle, whereas the left ventricle conveys arterialized blood. The pulmonary circulation is now being arranged in series with the systemic circuit.

The closure of the atrial shunt is purely a consequence of prevailing hydrostatic conditions. As a consequence of the small differences in vascular resistance between the pulmonary and systemic circulations, the central circulatory pattern of the newborn is labile, and relatively small changes in PVR will provoke relapses into the fetal circulatory pattern with ductal and/or atrial right-to-left shunting and arterial desaturation. This may be the case during crying, when the Valsalva manœuvre increases PVR to an extent, where the ductal shunt shifts to a right-to-left direction and the ensuing pulmonary hypoperfusion reduces left atrial pressures to levels below that of the right atrium, reopening the atrial shunt. Sudden and often pronounced alterations in arterial oxygen saturation is consequently a common experience in the newborn infant. Catheter studies in older children have revealed that the flap over the foramen ovale is not always fused to the septum, i. e. foramen ovale anatomically closed, but can be opened by a catheter tip in approximately 1/3 of studied children. With increasing postnatal age, the left-sided filling pressures will create a more stable pressure difference between the atria. Consequently functional patency of the foramen ovale may then not be provoked under "physiological" cardiorespiratory conditions, although the foramen ovale has not been anatomically sealed.

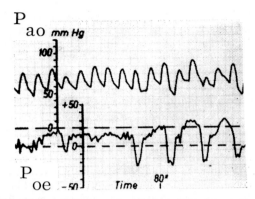

FIG. III-3. — *Pressure tracings from abdominal aorta* (Pao) *and œsophagus* (Poe) *demonstrating well maintained systemic blood pressure in the presence of forceful respiratory movements associated with the first breaths.*

The ductal shunt

With postnatal respiration, a pulmonary vascular resistance of subsystemic level is created and the shunt flow through the ductus arteriosus consequently is mainly left-to-right. The internal diameter of the fetal ductus at term is of the same size as that of the aortic arch and it may consequently accommodate a considerable flow. In the immediate postnatal period, the direction and rate of ductal flow is governed solely by the resistance ratio of the systemic and pulmonary circulations. There is good support for the view that early in neonatal life, there may exist a bidirectional shunt through the ductus arteriosus, suggesting that PVR is near that of the systemic circulation and that the ductus remains open for at least the first few hours of life. Whereas an increase in PVR to levels in excess of the SVR results in a right-to-left shunt and systemic desaturation below the level of the ductus, a too rapid fall in PVR will be associated with an oversized left-to-right shunt with pulmonary hyperperfusion and left sided overload of the heart. In view of the fact that the left ventricle during late fetal life accounts for only 1/3 of the combined ventricular ouput, it would seem reasonable to assume that a left-to-right ductal shunt may easily be associated with overtaxation of the myocardial resources. Successful coping with this situation requires an elaborate balance between forces that control PVR, SVR and the ductal calibre. The well maintained systemic pressure level in the neonate (Fig. III-3) suggests that the newborn infant is expertly equipped to control the size of the ductal shunt. There are two major factors that interact here. One is the already mentioned phenomenon that PVR does not immediately fall to low adult levels with aeration of the lungs, which prevents pulmonary overperfu-

sion. The other is the ductal constriction, which operates during the first days of extrauterine life.

In contrast to its effect on the pulmonary circulation, elevation of the partial pressure of oxygen increases the tone of the muscular wall of the duct. When oxygen enriched blood starts to perfuse the ductus arteriosus as a consequence of effective gas exchange in the newborn lung and a left-to-right ductal shunt direction, there is a prompt constrictive effect on the ductal musculature, with a reduction in ductal diameter. The effect is reversible and should paO_2 fall again, there is an immediate relaxation of the ductal wall muscles, and the diameter increases again.

Considerable effort has been devoted to elucidate the mechanism of ductal constriction, with studies performed both in animals and in the human neonate. Apart from the powerful vasoconstrictive response to the pO_2 increase in the aortic blood, the ductal muscles constrict when exposed to various other stimuli, e. g. vasoactive kinins, adrenalin-noradrenalin and prostaglandin inhibitors, such as indomethacin and salicyclic acid. Usually the constrictive effect of these agents is less pronounced, or sometimes even blocked during arterial hypoxemia. In the normal newborn infant, the initial constriction of the ductus arteriosus is followed by a slower caliber reduction in the first day of extrauterine life. Functional closure has usually occurred after 24 hours (see below).

Placental transfusion and neonatal blood volume

Effective umbilical circulation, i. e. perfusion participating in gas exchange within the placenta, usually ceases within the first minutes after birth, when separation from the uterine wall begins. A net shift of blood, however, occurs from the placenta to the newborn, due to uterine contractions, as long as the umbilical cord is left intact and the infant is kept well below the level of the placenta. It has been estimated that from the fetal part of the placenta, a total of 75-150 ml blood is transfused to the newborn at a falling rate during the first two minutes of postnatal life. Early clamping of the cord, as well as the common habit of placing the newborn infant above the level of the placenta, interferes with this transfusion. The infant may be handling a blood volume less than half of that provided by a full shift of placental blood. Thus whereas the newborn infant, deprived of the placental transfusion, circulates a blood volume of approximately 65 ml/kg BW, which also corresponds to the estimated blood volume of the fetus in utero, the newborn with a full placental transfusion has a circulating blood volume in the vicinity of 110 ml/kg BW.

The effects of early and late clamping of the umbilical cord, one of the variables in the birth process that is relatively easily controlled, have been the subject of intense studies with the ultimate purpose of seeking an answer to the question of an optimal time for ligation of the cord. There is ample documentation regarding the circulatory effects of early versus late clamping of the umbilical cord. It is evident that the additional blood volume, provided by the placental transfusion, creates a state of relative hypervolemia, which affects most studied variables. It is also obvious that this hypervolemic state is combatted by the infant through extravasation of plasma (Fig. III-4). It stands to reason that the increased blood volume is associated with increased circulatory work in the newborn. Right and left ventricular pre- and afterload are increased, as well as stroke volume and cardiac output. There does not seem to be an apparent beneficial effect of the placental transfusion, apart from the larger iron store provided by the initial blood volume increase. Infants delivered by cesarean section exhibit a smaller initial blood volume than vaginal deliveries, which is probably related to the hydrostatic conditions prevailing, but may also be a reflection of impaired uterine squeezing of the placenta. A significantly higher blood volume is found in infants who are developing perinatal distress and it is likely that this shift already takes place in utero.

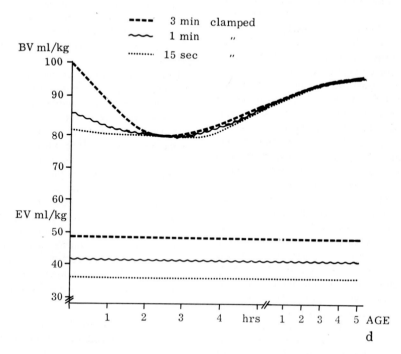

FIG. III-4. — *Effect of cord clamping on infant blood volume.* BV = blood volume. EV = erythrocyte volume. Note hemoconcentration during the first hours in the late clamped (hypervolemic) infants (Modified from YAO and LIND 1974).

THE INTERMEDIATE (TRANSITIONAL) CIRCULATORY PATTERN

The postnatal circulation is characterized by less dramatic hemodynamic changes than those occurring in immediate relationship to the initiation of breathing. The intermediate or transitional period lasts from approximately 5 minutes to 5 days of extrauterine life. The circulatory changes during this time are characterized by an initial labile balance between the pulmonary and systemic circulations, with potential relapses into the fetal circulatory pattern. There is a gentle stabilization of the circulation into an adult pattern, and the period is terminated, when both fetal channels are functionally closed and the pulmonary circulation has achieved definite low resistance, compared to the systemic circuit.

Neonatal blood volume changes

In proportion to the size of the placental blood transfusion, the initial blood volume is affected by plasma transudation during the first few hours. A high initial blood volume is followed by a subsequent withdrawal of plasma from the circulation, resulting in hemoconcentration. This extravasation of plasma is not seen in the newborn deprived of the placental transfusion, which suggests that there is indeed a state of hypervolemia in the late-clamped infants, who can sense the situation and are fully capable of effectively coping with it. Figure III-4 illustrates the changes in initial blood volume, related to the time of cord clamping and the subsequent plasma shift. It is evident that by the first 2-3 hours after birth, the average circulating blood volume of the newborn amounts to 75-80 ml/kg, irrespective of the size of the initial volume. The late-clamped infants, however, have a considerably higher erythrocyte volume fraction as a consequence of plasma extravasation. Although the reduction of circulating blood volume in these infants reduces the volume load of the heart, hyperviscosity due to hemoconcentration again adds to the myocardial work load. This is reflected in the presence of increased pre- and afterload levels for both ventricles and the common finding of a prolonged period of pulmonary hypertension in infants with an initial high blood volume.

Longitudinal studies of the blood volume in the transitional period indicate that, irrespective of the initial volume, there is during the first day of life an increase in the circulating blood volume, probably as a reflection of activation of new vascular compartments within the body. This volume increase is induced solely by hemodilution and there is nothing to suggest an increase in erythrocyte volume during this period.

The ductal shunt

It has earlier been emphasized that constriction of the ductus arteriosus is vital in avoiding volume overload of the left heart in the presence of a gradual lowering of the pulmonary vascular resistance. It is evident from studies by dye dilution in the newborn infant that there is a decreasing left-to-right shunt through the duct in the first day of life. In the presence of a falling PVR and an increasing pressure gradient between the aorta and the pulmonary artery, this denotes decreasing ductal diameter. Figure III-5 illustrates these findings, and it is clear that in most instances there is no more evidence of a ductal shunt after the first day of life, indicating functional closure of the duct. The pulmonary and systemic circulations are now separated from each other and arranged in series. Resistance and pressure may now vary independently, while perfusion

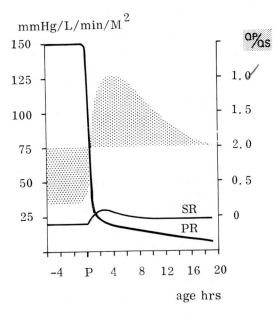

Fig. III-5. — *Pulmonary (PR) and systemic (SR) vascular resistance in the transitional period related to the size and direction of the ductal shunt (shaded areas). For details see text.*

remains equal in the two circuits. The establishment of an adult circulatory pattern signals the end of the transitional period, but it should always be kept in mind that the ductal constriction is highly dependent on "normal" oxygen and carbon dioxide tensions in the systemic circulation. During this period the ductal shunt may reopen instantly in response to the proper stimuli. The response of the ductal constrictors is related to the maturity of the newborn, and persistent patency of the duct is not an uncommon finding in the premature infant, where it may upset the transition to extrauterine life. This matter will be discussed later in the text.

Characteristics of the transitional pulmonary circulation

The steep fall in pulmonary vascular resistance, associated with the aeration of the lungs, is followed by a slower decline in resistance that takes PVR down to 1/2-1/3 of the systemic level within the first days of life (Fig. III-5). This slower phase may be regarded more as a process of maturation of the precapillary pulmonary arterioles, where the muscular wall thickness is subject to a continuous reduction during the first postnatal weeks. With the ductus arteriosus closed, pulmonary perfusion is equal to that of the systemic circulation, and amounts to some 200 ml/kg/min. Pulmonary vascular resistance during this period is very sensitive to changes in oxygen tension, carbon dioxide tension and pH of the perfusing blood. Hypoxemia and/or acidosis provoke immediate vasoconstriction in the neonatal lung, i. e. an effect opposite to the ductal response, where these stimuli provoke relaxation of the ductal constrictors. In association with a reopened ductal shunt, hypoxia and acidosis consequently may reinstitute a fetal circulatory pattern with right-to-left ductal shunting, leading to a vicious circle. These aspects of the central circulatory regulation have important bearings on the therapeutic approach to hypoxemia and acidosis in the neonate and will be further commented upon when the pathophysiology of the circulatory adaptation is discussed.

Ventilation/perfusion inequalities

Optimal gas exchange within the lungs requires that alveolar ventilation is matched by adequate perfusion to secure a balance between the gas tension of alveolar air and the perfusing capillary blood. An optimal ventilation/perfusion ratio (V/P) in usually not reached in the first days of life,

mostly due to poor airway stability, which creates areas with low V/P ratios that serve as physiologic intrapulmonary right-to-left shunts. This phenomenon is reflected in an increased alveolar/arterial oxygen gradient and in a failure to reach the expected high paO_2 levels during oxygen breathing. Although this shortcoming hardly exerts any negative effects on the adaptation to extrauterine life in the normal child, where the practical consequences are negligible, and only result in slight desaturation of the arterial blood (Fig. III-6), the degree of V/P imbalance in the pathologic lung may provoke massive life threatening right-to-left shunts. The V/P ratio in the normal child has usually reached adult standards by the end of the first week, when effective pulmonary perfusion, i. e. perfusion participating in gas exchange, becomes almost identical with total pulmonary perfusion.

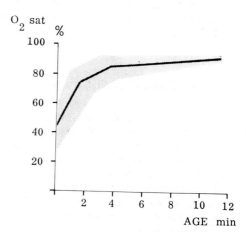

Fig. III-6. — *Systemic oxygen saturation in the immediate neonatal period* (HANSON and WALLGREN, 1970, unpublished observations).

Characteristics of the transitional systemic circulation

Peripheral circulation in the neonatal period has been investigated by means of various types of plethysmographic techniques, where as a rule the arterial inflow to a section of an extremity has been quantitated during various experimental conditions. The neonatal systemic circulation is characterized by low resistance and relatively higher peripheral blood flow than in adult man. With a systemic output near 2.5-3.5 l/min/m² BSA and a mean perfusing pressure of 50 mm Hg, the newborn infant has a peripheral vascular resistance half of that found in the adult. With peripheral blood flow related to kg BW, the neonatal systemic resistance will only amount to 1/3 of adult values. The previous statement that systemic pressure homeostasis is remarkably well maintained in the presence of the dramatic circulatory changes occurring at birth, with the sudden appearance of systemic run-off through the ductal shunt, denotes an efficient control of peripheral vascular tone. In this respect, the newborn is not different from the older child and adult man. It has been demonstrated that the newborn infant can handle acute depletion of blood volume up to 15 % of estimated total blood volume without any systemic pressure fall, although cardiac output decreases as a consequence of hypovolemia and lower filling pressures. The resting peripheral blood flow, as recorded in the segmental perfusion of the lower extremity, amounts to 5-10 ml/100 ml tissue, and vasomotor activity is capable of both reducing the flow to zero, as well as increasing 10-fold the peripheral perfusion in response to the proper stimuli. Peripheral vasoconstriction is elicited through chemoreceptors responding to hypoxia and acidosis, and baroreceptors that respond to hypotension. The cutaneous vessels react to thermal stimuli with vasoconstriction in response to cold exposure. Constriction is mediated through the adrenergic nervous system, but local release of vasodilating material is a likely mechanism, just as in adult man. The renal secretion of vasoactive material is well developed in the newborn and a fall in systemic blood pressure is followed by angiotension release. Peripheral vascular tone and the systemic perfusion pressures are directly related to the maturity of the infant, with significantly lower levels in the premature newborn.

MONITORING THE TRANSITIONAL CIRCULATORY PATTERN

Pulmonary vascular resistance

Physical findings. — The characteristic single heart sounds of the fetal circulation persist during the first days of life, but careful auscultation during quiet resting conditions may identify a splitting of the second heart sound near the end of the first postnatal week. The splitting is due to the established pressure difference between the systemic and pulmonary circulations, where the later closure of the pulmonary valves signals the pressure drop in the lung vessels.

Laboratory findings. — The fall in PVR may also be traced in the typical electrocardiographic pattern

of the neonatal period. The initial direction of the precordial T vector is to the right with positive T_1 and a flat or isoelectric T_6. After a usually short-lasting further shift to the right with negative T_6, which possibly reflects the temporary volume overload of the left ventricle before ductal constriction has occurred, the T vector swings over to the left during the first days of extrauterine life (Fig. III-7). T_1 becomes negative and T_6 distinctly positive. This electrocardiographic feature of the transitional circulation signals the normal right ventricular work reduction, as PVR is falling and right ventricular ejection pressure diminishes. This ECG finding is appreciated as a most sensitive index of a normal circulatory adaptation to extrauterine life. Persistence of a positive T_1 after the first week of life is highly suggestive of persistent right ventricular hypertension.

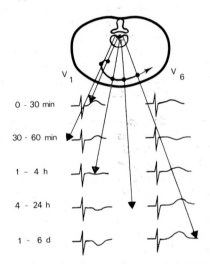

FIG. III-7. — *Evolution of the neonatal ECG.* Note the initial right- and then leftward shift of the horizontal T vector indicating diminishing right ventricular pressure load.

The use of ultrasound in cardiovascular diagnostic work has repeatedly been proven to be of great value and echocardiographic analysis of the neonatal circulatory pattern has contributed considerably to our concept of the central circulatory pattern. Through the use of the echo-signal, it has been possible to determine the systolic time intervals of the right ventricle non-invasively. This technique has shown that the ratio pre-ejection period (PEP), *i. e.* time from initial ventricular deflection in the ECG to beginning of ventricular emptying, as measured at the pulmonary valve opening, over right ventricular ejection (RVET), measured from opening to closing of the pulmonary valves, is directly related to right ventricular pressure. A decrease in this PEP/RVET/ratio from 0.4 to near 0.3 during the second day of life suggests a normal decrease in right ventricular afterload, *i. e.* PVR.

Left-to-right ductal shunt

Physical findings. — Frequent auscultation of the heart in the newborn detects constriction of the ductus arteriosus as the appearance of a ductal murmur usually within the first 48 hours. The murmur is localized along the left sternal border and over the pulmonic area and is usually not of the classical continuous type, but rather systolic with a protodiastolic tail. The disappearance of the murmur in the healthy child signals complete closure of the duct, and reappearance of the murmur in the cyanotic infants suggests reopening of the duct in response to impaired oxygenation. It is indeed possible to have the ductal murmur come and go in the infant in respiratory distress especially with respirator usage, merely by changing the oxygen fraction of the inspired air.

Laboratory findings. — Electrocardiography is less apt to identify the presence of a left-to-right ductal shunt, but an R/S ratio less than one in V_1 is highly suggestive of the presence of pulmonary hyperperfusion. The presence of a left-to-right ductal shunt is considerably easier to assess by echocardiography, where the increased pulmonary blood flow results in a volume increase of the left atrium, which may be indexed in the ratio left atrial diameter/aortic root diameter. Near or in excess of 1.3, this ratio is highly diagnostic of left-to-right shunting. The ratio falls to 1.0 or less, when the shunt disappears during the first days of life.

The radiological examination of the heart in the newborn does usually not provide a sensitive index of pulmonary overperfusion, and both cardiomegaly and the increase in vascular marking of the lungs that in the older child suggests left-to-right shunt, are often absent in the transitional period. It should in this context be pointed out that the radiological appearance of the heart in the immediate postnatal and transitional periods is characterized by an initial enlargement during the first hour of extrauterine life, followed by a reduction in heart size with the smallest dimension recorded after 3-4 days. It is likely that the initial enlargement of the heart is a reflection of volume overload, due to left-to-right ductal shunting, and that the presence of a persistent patency of the duct may be associated

with an absence of the normal heart volume reduction. With the notoriously wide scatter in cardiac volume between individuals, it is more rewarding to use the patient as his or her own control and compare repeated examinations. An absent volume reduction would suggest persistent left-to-right shunting.

Right-to-left shunts

The degree of arterial desaturation in the newborn reflects the overall effect of right-to-left shunts that may be intra- or extra-pulmonary. Usually there is a very rapid increase in arterial oxygen saturation after birth, when saturation increases from somewhere near 40 % immediately post partum to 90 % after the first 5-10 minutes (Fig. III-6), indicating a rapid reduction of overall right-left shunting.

Physical findings. — Visual observation of the infant with right-to-left shunting may identify cyanosis, if desaturation is marked. It should, however, be kept in mind that acrocyanosis, *i. e.* cyanosis of the most peripheral parts of the body, is a common finding, in normal newborn infants during the first days of life, reflecting impaired vascular tone in the periphery, rather than central right-to-left shunting. It is also clear that the polycythemic infant may often be mistaken for a cyanotic one, and erythrocyte volume fraction should always be determined when cyanosis is suspected. From these comments it is easily deduced that visual observation of cyanosis as an index of right-to-left shunting is full of pitfalls and should regularly be supplemented by laboratory means of assessing desaturation.

Laboratory findings. — The direct method for recording arterial oxygen saturation, oximetry, may be used externally by transillumination of the skin, e. g. ear-piece oximetry, or by oximetry on arterial blood samples. Arterial oxygen saturation may also be assessed via the oxygen tension value (paO_2), recorded by transcutaneous electrodes or on arterial and capillary samples. The corresponding saturation figures are then read from the oxygen dissociation curve for the prevailing pH (Fig. III-8).

The degree of arterial desaturation reflects the size of the venous admixture, *i. e.* blood added to the systemic circulation without having passed through aerated alveoli, and may consequently be due to intrapulmonary factors, *i. e.* uneven ventilation/perfusion ratios, or to extrapulmonary shunts through the fetal channels. The aim of such analyses

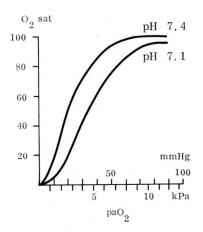

FIG. III-8. — *Oxygen dissociation curve at various pH.* Note higher oxygen affinity at higher pH.

should be to evaluate not only the size, but also the site of the venous admixture.

Quantitating the right-to-left shunt. — Calculation of the relative size of the overall right-to-left shunt may be done from the formula

$$Q_s/Q_t = \frac{C_{pv} - C_{ao}}{C_{pv} - \bar{C_v}}$$

where Q_s is the shunt flow, Q_t is total aortic blood flow, C_{pv} is the pulmonary venous oxygen content assumed to be equalized with and to correspond to the alveolar oxygen tension prevailing. C_{ao} is the aortic oxygen content and $\bar{C_v}$ is mixed venous oxygen content. With the further assumption of an oxygen content difference between aortic and mixed venous blood of 4 vol %, the equation may be solved if the oxygen fraction of the inspired air and the arterial oxygen saturation or tension are known. The graph in Fig. III-9 is constructed from the formula and allows the estimation of the overall right-to-left shunt from the arterial oxygen tension and alveolar oxygen tension, i. e. the alveolo/arterial oxygen gradient.

Localization of right-to-left shunts. — Intrapulmonary shunting may be due to the perfusion of inadequately ventilated or atelectatic non-ventilated areas, or to the presence of alveolo-capillary block, where the gas exchange between alveoli and perfusing blood is impeded. Respiratory physiology has since long recognized that increased oxygen tension of the alveolar air overrides the effect of alveolo-capillary block and inadequately ventilated areas on oxygen exchange. Oxygen breathing accordingly reduces or abolishes the effect of these factors

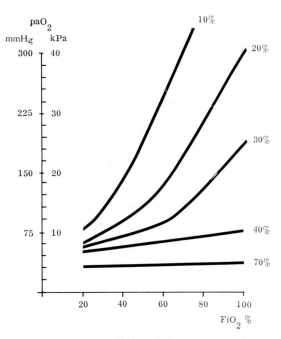

FIG. III-9. — *Nomogram for assessing overall right-to-left shunt from systemic oxygen saturation and alveolar oxygen content (FiO_2).*

on the overall venous admixture. This is the background for the *hyperoxia test*, where the infant is left to breathe 100 % oxygen for 10 minutes, which results in hyperoxia even in poorly ventilated areas of the lung. If the arterial oxygen tension reaches levels near 50 kPa (400 mm Hg), venous admixture should be due mostly to alveolo-capillary block or insufficiently ventilated areas. If, on the other hand, paO_2 remains lower than 25 kPa (200 mm Hg), this indicates the presence of sizeable non-ventilated areas of the lung and/or extrapulmonary shunt sites. Venous admixture from non-ventilated areas in the neonatal lung is, however, usually considered to be small, due to local tissue hypoxia and subsequent arteriolar constriction and hypoperfusion. An arterial oxygen tension at hyperoxia of less than 25 kPa consequently must reflect gross pulmonary pathology with extensive atelectasis. Absence of radiological evidence of such pathology certainly suggests extrapulmonary sites for the right-to-left shunt.

Extrapulmonary shunt sites. — Disregarding the possibility of cyanotic congenital heart disease, extrapulmonary channels of desaturation are the foramen ovale and the ductus arteriosus. The relative contribution of these two shunts may be assessed from recordings of arterial oxygen saturation (or tension) above and below the level of the ductus arteriosus. The presence of lower levels distal to the ductus arteriosus indicates right-to-left ductal shunting, whereas identical levels denote the presence of more "central" shunts, i. e. foramen ovale and/or intrapulmonary admixture. The fraction of the ductal right-to-left shunt may be estimated from the formula

$$Q_s/Q_t = \frac{A_{Aao} - C_{Dao}}{C_{Dao} - C_{\bar{v}}}$$

where Q_s is the ductal right-to-left shunt, Q_t is total aortic blood flow, C_{Aao}, C_{Dao} and $C_{\bar{v}}$ are oxygen content of ascending aortic blood, oxygen content of descending aortic blood distal to the duct, and oxygen content of mixed venous blood (assumed to be 4 vol % less than distal aortic blood), respectively.

It is clear that monitoring various parameters in the newborn may contribute substantially to our knowledge regarding the circulatory pattern of the transitional period. Although based on a number of assumptions and hence only a rough estimate of the circulatory pattern, this information has a bearing on therapeutic approaches, and as such is of great value to the neonatologist.

THE STABILIZED CIRCULATORY PATTERN AND NORMAL CIRCULATORY STANDARDS IN THE NEWBORN

The transitional (intermediate) phase of the circulatory adaptation to extrauterine life ends in the second half of the first week. The immediate circulatory consequences of birth are then usually ended and the circulatory pattern has stabilized in a form, which is a close reflection of the circulation in the older individual. Although there remains a potential hazard in the fact that fetal pathways may reopen at this age in response to proper stimuli and jeopardize the circulatory balance, this risk becomes less the older the infant gets. The characteristic finding in this period is the relative hyperkinetic type of circulation encountered in the newborn. This is further emphasized in the premature infant, where cardiac output may be 2-4 times that of the adult, whether body weight or surface area are used as references. The following circulatory standards are characteristic of the full term newborn infant at the end of the first week of life:

Blood volume: 90 ml/kg BW.

Heart volume: 45 ml.
Heart rate: 140 b. p. m.
Stroke volume: 6 ml.
Cardiac output: 250 ml/kg/min (4 l/min/BSA).
Pulmonary vascular resistance: 0.7 mm Hg/ml/kg/min.
Systemic vascular resistance: 1.4 mm Hg/ml/kg/min.
Aortic pressures: 70/45.
Pulmonary pressures: 35/15.

The fate of other fetal circulatory pathways. — Whereas the umbilical arteries obliterate along their entire length soon after birth, the umbilical vein, except for its most distal obliterated end, may remain open for a long period of time and may be cannulated in adult man.

The ductus venosus is usually functionally closed within the first week of life and the portal sinuses drain through the liver parenchyma. The ductus venosus may be penetrated by catheters during the first days of life and thus presents an alternative route for diagnostic heart catheterization in the newborn.

PATHOPHYSIOLOGY OF THE CIRCULATORY ADAPTATION TO EXTRAUTERINE LIFE

In view of the fact that the physiological consequences of birth are associated with a dramatic change of the working conditions for the heart and circulation, it stands to reason that various pathological conditions that affect the capacity of the cardiovascular system, may be hazardous to the neonatal adaptation to extrauterine life.

Hypovolemia and anemia of the newborn

Sudden uncontrolled bleeding from the fetal circulation may occur during labour or accidentally post partum from the umbilical vessels. If the blood loss is large enough to overtax the capacity of the cardiovascular system of the newborn, the condition will result in hypovolemic shock, with a failure to maintain systemic pressure homeostasis. The situation is life threatening and should be treated by immediate restitution of the circulating blood volume, preferably with whole-blood transfusion. Hypovolemic shock is likely to occur when the blood loss exceeds 15-25 % of total circulating blood volume.

Repeated smaller intrauterine hemorrhages may occur as a leak from the fetal part of the placenta in late gestation, or as an occult phenomenon in twin pregnancies, where one twin bleeds into the other's circulation, and may result in various degrees of anemia. A relatively common cause of anemia in the newborn are the various hemolytic conditions that may occur as a consequence of blood group incompatibilities between mother and child.

Anemia is, by definition, associated with hemodilution and impaired oxygen-carrying capacity, which provoke compensatory hyperkinetic circulation in the fetus and newborn. The high cardiac output, in association with ensuing myocardial hypoxemia, may cause cardiac failure already in utero. The newborn infant in anemic failure is pale, tachypnoeic with edematous tissues and hepatomegaly. Radiography indicates the presence of cardiomegaly and pulmonary vascular congestion. The condition must be attended to immediately with indicated therapeutic measures, such as exchange transfusion with packed red cells and removal of infant plasma, together with appropriate anticongestive treatment.

Polycythemia and the hyperviscosity syndrome

Hematocrit values in excess of 65 % are associated with a marked increase in blood viscosity. A clinical entity, named symptomatic neonatal plethora, or hyperviscosity syndrome, with symptoms related to impaired peripheral circulation, may ensue. The pathogenicity of the condition may be intrauterine, as a response to prolonged fetal anoxia, maternal-to-fetal or twin-to-twin bleeding, or it may be related to an excessive placental transfusion in the immediate neonatal period. Small for date infants and infants of diabetic mothers are particularly prone to be affected. From a circulatory point of view, the work of the heart is increased with elevated perfusion pressure, due to a viscosity-related increase in the peripheral resistance to blood flow (Fig. III-10). It is of particular interest in this context that there is good experimental evidence, suggesting that the pulmonary vascular resistance is relatively more affected by hyperviscosity. Hematocrit levels in excess of 70 % may thus in the neonate provoke a right-to-left ductal shunt, by reversing the pressure gradient between the aorta and the pulmonary artery (see p. 306).

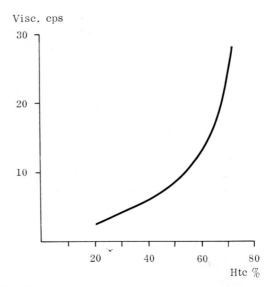

Visc. cps

Htc %

FIG. III-10. — *Hematocrit/blood viscosity relationship. Marked increase in blood viscosity occurs with htc (central venous sample) values in excess of 60 %.*

In the newborn infant, the clinical picture of hyperviscosity is characterized by a plethoric appearance, which, in the presence of the commonly pronounced tachypnea, may be mistaken for a cyanotic heart lesion. The diagnosis is established in the presence of high hematocrit levels and normal oxygen saturation. The newborn is likely to show neurological symptoms with lethargy, jitterness, and sometimes seizures, as a consequence of impaired perfusion of the central nervous system. Neurological sequelae may persist and therapy should be instituted promptly, when neurological symptoms are present. Adequate treatment comprises phlebotomy, with 10-20 % of the estimated blood volume, which eventually will result in blood volume expansion and hemodilution. A choice of more active treatment includes exchange transfusion, with addition of erythrocyte-free plasma. The latter procedure should be the therapy of choice in the presence of a subnormal blood volume in the patient. In the less severe cases, no treatment is necessary and symptoms usually subside within 48 hours, as a result of endogenous plasma expansion and vascular adaptation to the larger circulating blood volume.

Myocardial disease

Apart from gross congenital malformations of the cardiovascular system, some of which are capable of upsetting the normal adaptation (see below), myocardial dysfunction, due to infectious, degenerative or storage disease, may impair cardiac function to an extent, where survival of the newborn may be in question.

Infectious myocardial disease is usually of viral origin, and, as in the case of degenerative, i. e. endocardial fibroelastosis and various storage diseases, treatment is usually limited to symptomatic anticongestive measures. In the case of viral myocarditis, survival in the neonatal period is usually followed by spontaneous healing. This may also be the case in fibroelastosis, if gross cardiac defects are not present.

Perinatal arrhythmia

Among arrhythmias with life threatening neonatal consequences, sustained supraventricular tachycardia and third degree A-V block should be mentioned here. These conditions may be diagnosed antenatally by fetal heart sound monitoring. A heart rate in excess of 200 should suggest supraventricular tachycardia, and a fetal heart rate below 75 the presence of a congenital complete heart block. Whereas a ventricular rate below 40 b. p. m. usually is accompanied by a reduced cardiac output, severe enough to cause neonatal symptoms, tachycardia in excess of 250 is not compatible with adequate filling of the ventricles, and usually provokes cardiac failure, due to the falling stroke volume.

Digitalis has little effect on A-V block, where pacemaker treatment should be instituted, when symptoms of impaired cardiac output are present, i. e. circulatory failure or neurological symptoms, due to inadequate cerebral perfusion, but the drug should be used immediately in the presence of failure, due to supra-ventricular tachycardia. This treatment may indeed be started before birth, by digitalis administration to the mother.

Cardiovascular malformations

Whereas most congenital heart defects seem to affect the circulatory adaptation of the neonate relatively little, some lesions may, by virtue of their specific effect on the central circulatory pattern, and particularly on the pulmonary circulation, affect the normal pattern of the intermediate circulation. In relation to their effect on the pulmonary circulation, these congenital defects may be divided into three groups.

Increased pulmonary blood flow with pulmonary hypertension. — This is the common finding, when large communications exist between the pulmonary and systemic circulations, i. e. ventricular septal defects, and septation defects between the great arteries. In these instances, the left-to-right shunt that is initiated by the fall in PVR when breathing commences, persists irrespective of ductal constriction. The moderate pulmonary hyperperfusion that ensues is accompanied by marked pulmonary hypertension, due to the still relatively elevated PVR, which interferes with the normal decline in right ventricular work load, characteristic of the transitional period. The hemodynamic characteristics are usually those of right ventricular pressure overload. Signs of left ventricular volume overload, due to the persistance of the left-to-right shunt, are usually a later finding, due to a slower decline in PVR in these infants. Histologically, the precapillary pulmonary arterioles show hypertrophy of the media and muscular layer of the wall.

Decreased pulmonary blood flow with pulmonary hypertension. — This is the typical situation in backward failure, due to severe left sided obstruction. These lesions, mitral or aortic stenosis, hypoplastic left heart syndrome or severe coarctation of the aorta will, like pulmonary venous obstruction, by virtue of the pulmonary venous hypertension, result in increased PVR and obstruction to pulmonary blood flow. The clinical picture is one of pulmonary congestion and impaired pulmonary and systemic circulation, with hypoxia and acidosis further adding to the elevated PVR. These lesions almost invariably give severe symptoms during the transitional period and should be actively treated for survival.

Decreased pulmonary blood flow and pulmonary hypotension. — These are typical findings in right ventricular outflow obstruction in conjunction with restrictive arterio-venous communications. Examples of this entity are Tetralogy of Fallot and various hypoplastic right-sided lesions, where right ventricular outflow bypasses the obstruction by way of shunts. There is usually little interference with the early circulatory adaptation, as the pulmonary perfusion is maintained through a right-to-left intracardiac shunt and a left-to-right ductal shunt. Difficulties, however, arise, when ductal constriction occurs in spite of the persisting arterial desaturation, and primary treatment must be directed towards securing patency of the duct (see below).

Common to all cyanotic heart lesions is the metabolic effect of hypoxia and acidosis, which in the severe cases, e. g. transposition of the great arteries with intact ventricular septum (see chapter 18), may jeopardize the outcome of the neonatal period.

Circulation in severe respiratory insufficiency

Impaired gas exchange, due to pulmonary pathology, is a common clinical problem in the neonatal period. Whatever the primary cause, the pathophysiological mechanism is initially one of increased venous admixture, as a consequence of perfusion of non-ventilated areas of the lung. The ensuing metabolic effect is arterial desaturation and carbon dioxide retention, both of which affect the systemic and pulmonary circulation in the newborn. The pulmonary vessels of the neonate, by virtue of their great sensitivity to hypoxemia and acidosis, constrict in response to the metabolic disorder, and PVR very rapidly may reach systemic levels, which affects right ventricular working conditions. If severe enough, RV pressure overload may result in elevation of right atrial pressures as well. This may reopen the foramen ovale, and the right-to-left atrial shunt adds to the venous admixture. This may easily become a vicious circle with more constriction of the pulmonary vessels promoting further extrapulmonary venous admixture. This situation is found in severe cases of idiophatic respiratory distress (IRDS) of the newborn, where the overall right-to-left shunt may be as high as 80-90 % of the systemic output. The extrapulmonary shunt is mainly at the atrial level and relatively little is contributed by any right-to-left ductal shunt. Figure III-11 illustrates the findings in a group of premature infants with moderate IRDS at the height of their symptoms.

Severe hypoxia is usually associated with accumulation of acid metabolites, due to anaerobic metabolism. With decreasing pH values, the acid-base imbalance further adds to the pulmonary vascular constriction and reduction of effective pulmonary blood flow. It is easy to understand that a central part of therapy must include efforts to relax the pulmonary vascular constriction (see below).

The systemic circulation is also affected by the metabolic consequences of respiratory insufficiency in the neonatal period. Arterial desaturation in the newborn is associated with an increase in the peripheral vascular resistance and of systemic pressures, and is usually accompanied by bradycardia, just as in the fetus, where hypoxemia is signalled by deceleration of the fetal heart sounds. There is also experimental support for the presence of "preferential" circulation, i. e. circulation to more vital parts of the body, i. e. CNS and the coronary circulation, being increased at the expense of circulation to other regions. A similar redistribution of systemic output is seen during CO_2 retention, which is one of the most powerful dilators of the cerebral circulation.

Whereas there are thus closely similar vascular effects of hypoxemia and hypercapnia, the presence of metabolic acidosis with low blood pH values is considered as a circulatory depressant, which causes a drop in cardiac output possibly as a direct myocardial effect. As the typical metabolic consequence of respiratory insufficiency is hypoxia, with combined respiratory and metabolic acidosis, it is difficult to predict the overall effect on the systemic circulation of these partly opposed factors. The characteristic pattern of systemic perfusion in severe respiratory distress in the newborn, is, however, a decreased peripheral perfusion, due to increased SVR, with a relative increase to vital vascular compartments, e. g. the central nervous system. There are some indications of a reduced cardiac output and systemic hypotension in this condition.

It is of practical importance that the decreased peripheral perfusion tends to accumulate acid metabolites in the presence of severe hypoxia, which, when therapy is effective, may be released into the circulation and increase the buffer load of the system. From what has been said, it is evident that respiratory insufficiency, if severe enough, may interact profoundly with the normal circulatory pattern of the transitional period, with the presence of often massive intra- and extrapulmonary right-to-left shunts and reduced peripheral perfusion, blood pressure and cardiac output, and, ultimately, cardiac failure.

Other circulatory characteristics of severe IRDS include significantly lower hematocrit values, unrelated to the size of placental transfusion, and the

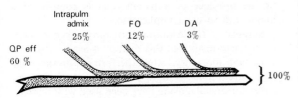

Fig. III-11. — *Fractional contribution to distal aortic blood flow in moderately sick premature infants with IRDS.* QP eff signifies pulmonary blood flow participating in gaseous exchange. Intrapulm admix indicates pulmonary blood flow not participating in gaseous exchange (intrapulmonary right-to-left shunt). FO and DA denote additional right-to-left shunts through foramen ovale and ductus arteriosus.

presence of a relative bradycardia. The heart rate is often particularly stable with very small beat-to-beat interval variations in infants with severe forms of IRDS, where this phenomenon indicates the presence of neurological damage, and, accordingly, is considered a poor prognostic sign.

In view of the central place of pulmonary vascular resistance in the pathophysiology of severe respiratory insufficiency in the neonate, effective treatment of the condition must include efforts to relax the pulmonary vascular constriction. These include administration of oxygen and correction of acid-base imbalance, without which measures ventilatory support remains useless. These matters will be discussed under other headings.

Persistent patency of the ductus arteriosus

Delayed closure of the ductus arteriosus means the presence of a usually left-to-right ductal shunt, in infants more than 1-2 days old. Theoretically, an open duct at this age may reflect a reopening after an initial constriction, or a primary failure to respond to the usual constrictive principles in the immediate postnatal period. The latter mechanism is usually held to be responsible for the presence of an open duct in this age group. From a pathogenetic point of view, an impaired constrictive response may be related to the gestational age of the infant, the more immature, the less effective the constrictive response. The incidence of persistent ductal patency in premature infants is as high as 25-30 %, and the incidence in premature infants with respiratory distress syndrome amounts to twice this figure. This is clearly a reflection of the fact that persistent patency may also be provoked by factors such as persistent arterial desaturation. Low environmental oxygen, *i. e.* at high altitudes, is also associated with a considerably higher incidence of delayed closure, which further corroborates an effect of lower arterial oxygen tension. The presence of persistent patency of the ductus arteriosus in a number of mature infants without associated cardio-pulmonary disease, suggests the presence of an "idiopathic" form of delayed closure as well.

Immediately post partum, the open duct may not be a great problem for the newborn, but as PVR falls to levels considerably below the systemic side during the first day of life, the left-to-right shunt increases and may provoke leftsided volume overload and failure. This development may be hazardous, especially to the infant who is already struggling with pulmonary pathology.

The presence of delayed closure of the duct is clinically reflected in the appearance of a ductal murmur, a hyperactive precordium and lively peripheral pulses, due to the connection between a high and a low pressure circuit. In the presence of left sided volume overload, an apical gallop sound is usually present, together with increased respiratory rate, tachycardia and hepatomegaly. Although radiology usually reveals pulmonary vascular congestion, cardiomegaly, which in the older individual is suggestive of cardiac overload and failure, is not always present in the newborn with volume overload.

Ultrasonographic studies indicate that in infants with large left-to-right ductal shunts there is a retrograde diastolic blood flow in the carotid arteries suggesting a hampered cerebral perfusion.

In association with IRDS, the presence of a patent duct may be reflected in a deterioration of the clinical situation, with distress out of proportion to the pulmonary pathology. The pulmonary disease does not follow the expected course, with spontaneous recovery in the first week. Weaning the child with ventilatory support from the respirator may be impossible in the presence of a patent duct.

In the very immature infant, persistent patency of the ductus arteriosus may be associated with considerably different symptomatology and an open duct may here be suspected in the presence of repeated periods of apnea.

The natural history of delayed closure of the ductus arteriosus in the newborn infant is often one of spontaneous closure, notably when the associated respiratory pathology has cleared. If closure occurs spontaneously, it usually takes place within the first month of life. Persistent patency beyond this period usually implies a permanent condition.

Anticongestive therapy is indicated whenever there are signs of cardiac overload, and acute measures aimed at closing the duct should always be considered when intractable failure is present, or the presence of a patent duct is considered a major and severe complication.

Surgery is the traditional therapy for persistent ductus arteriosus, but this therapy is associated with a certain mortality, when performed in the very immature infant in failure. Pharmacological principles for ductal closure have been used with increasing frequency in recent years. Since it was established in the mid 1970's that prostaglandin, present in the fetal circulation, promotes patency of the duct, an intense interest has been devoted to methods of pharmacological manipulation of the ductal caliber. Whereas adrenergic receptors in the ductal wall have been shown to play some, but not an essential role in ductal constriction, the use of prostaglandin inhibitors has been followed by successful ductal closure in an increasing number of infants, as well as in animal experiments. Examples of prostaglandin inhibitors are indomethacin and salicylic acid, and therapy with indomethacin in particular has been successful in the newborn infant.

Indomethacin is given by the oral or rectal route in a dose of 0.1-0.3 mg/kg BW or by the usually more effective i. v. route. Ductal constriction usually occurs within 24 hours. Restricted fluid intake (less than 120 ml/kg BW) seems to favour ductal closure. When therapy fails to close the duct or it re-opens, a second dose may be successful. It should be kept in mind however, that indomethacin is known to be nephrotoxic and particularly when repeated administration is needed, close observation of renal function is advocated. The drug seems to be less effective in the very premature infant (GA less than 28 w) as well as in newborns after the first few weeks of postnatal life. Surgical closure is indicated when pharmacologic therapy has failed.

The life supporting PDA. — Postnatal patency of the ductus arteriosus, although unwanted in most instances, may be a life saving "complication" in newborn infants with various types of cardiovascular malformations. Heart lesions, where the effective pulmonary circulation is inadequate, due to right-sided outflow obstruction at various levels, may be compatible with life, if the obstruction can be bypassed via the ductus arteriosus. Examples of this type of malformation are tricuspid atresia, pulmonary atresia and other varieties of the hypoplastic right heart syndrome. The obstruction is bypassed via an intracardiac right-to-left shunt and a ductal left-to-right shunt, and the patient may thus be provided with a sufficient pulmonary blood flow, as long as the duct remains open. In the presence of aortic anomalies, patency of the ductus arteriosus may be essential for survival. This is the case in severe preductal coarctation or aortic arch interruption, as well as in aortic atresia, in which conditions perfusion of the systemic side, or parts of it, is maintained through a right-to-left ductal shunt.

In these usually severe cardiovascular anomalies, some of which are amenable to surgery, patency of the ductus arteriosus is needed for survival, until surgery may be performed. In these instances, infusion of prostaglandin (PGE$_1$), preferably proximal to, or within, the duct, in doses of 0.05-0.1 μg/kg/min, may delay ductal constriction, or even reopen a constricting duct, making survival during the transitional period possible.

The syndrome of persistent fetal circulation (PFC)

This condition, which has synonymously been called abnormal pulmonary vasoconstriction, persistent pulmonary hypertension, and persistent pulmonary vascular obstruction, was first recognized 10 years ago as a neonatal syndrome, characterized by severe arterial desaturation, persistent pulmonary hypertension, and often minor or no pulmonary pathology. It has in previous paragraphs been stated that the fetal circulatory pattern may resume, as a consequence of impaired ventilation in severe respiratory distress. In PFC, however, pulmonary pathology is not a prerequisite, and most reported cases cannot be explained on the basis of primary respiratory insufficiency. Whereas the respiratory distress syndrome and its secondary circulatory changes, due to impaired gas exchange, predominantly occur in the premature infant, the PFC syndrome usually affects the newborn at term.

The infant is usually not noted to be cyanotic immediately post partum, but cyanosis appears within the first hours of life, and is often accompanied by tachypnea. A history of perinatal asphyxia is not uncommon, and the radiological examination usually reveals normal heart size and little pulmonary pathology. In association with the often severe hypoxemia, these findings make it difficult to rule out a congenital cyanotic heart lesion. Cardiac catheterization studies reveal the presence of pulmonary hypertension, with right-to-left shunts at the atrial and ductal levels, but no indications of gross cardiovascular malformations. The few reports available suggest normal gas exchange with blood that perfuses the lungs. Due to the presence of massive extrapulmonary right-to-left shunts, a hyperoxia test usually yields only a minor increase in paO$_2$, which further emphasizes the difficulty in separating this syndrome from cyanotic heart lesions.

From a pathogenetic point of view, it seems likely that the primary cause of the condition is an altered reactivity of the pulmonary vessels in the neonatal period. A deficient response to aeration and oxygen tension increase may maintain PVR at fetal levels at birth, and increased reactivity to hypoxia and acidemia may recall the fetal circulatory pattern in response to early respiratory dysfunction. Histologic studies have suggested the presence of vascular pathology with medial hyperplasia and an abnormal distribution of the muscular coat of the small vessels, which may lend some support to the idea of abnormal vascular reactivity.

As more reports have accumulated, it has become clear that PFC may be associated with a number of other findings in the newborn, none of which, however, seems to be pathognomonic for the disease. These include hyperviscosity, hypercalcemia, and hypoglycemia, as well as the association with perinatal distress. As some of these conditions are well known promotors of elevated PVR, there may be more than a coincidental relationship to PFC. Persistent fetal circulatory pattern has also been reported in infants with various types of atypical respiratory diseases, e. g. transient tachypnea of the newborn, or atypical respiratory distress syndrome in the term newborn. It has been speculated as to whether hyperinflation, commonly occurring in these conditions, may play a role in the pathogenesis of pulmonary hypertension. This line of thought has a bearing on the choice of therapeutic measures, and in particular the common use of continuous, positive airway pressure (CPAP) in respiratory distress may be contraindicated, when PFC is related to the presence of hyperinflation.

Whereas elevated PVR is the central mechanism behind most of the reported instances of PFC, a more complex variety has been identified, where myocardial dysfunction and heart failure with systemic hypotension may constitute the pathogenetic factor. It would seem as if this entity, which is dominated by cyanosis, by clinical signs of cardiac failure and by the presence of murmurs suggesting A-V valve dysfunction, exemplifies a different disease. Invasive studies in this complex form have identified A-V valve incompetence, possibly related to myocardial ischemia and papillary muscle dysfunction. Systemic hypotension and moderately elevated pulmonary vascular resistance, usually at levels close to systemic, are characteristic findings at cardiac catheterization. The central circulatory pattern is one of extrapulmonary right-to-left, or bidirectional, shunts.

The natural history of the simple form of PFC is usually one of spontaneous recovery within the first few weeks of life, but the condition may also be fatal. It is not uncommon that the cyanosis lessens, following diagnostic angiocardiography. Indeed, this happens often enough to suggest that the contrast medium may have a beneficial effect on pulmonary vascular resistance.

Therapeutic considerations. — Oxygen therapy and correction of acid-base imbalance are the cornerstones of the therapeutic approach. Whenever cardiac failure is present or suggested, anticongestive treatment should be started promptly.

Ever since pulmonary vascular constriction was recognized as a major mechanism behind the syndrome, efforts have not been spared to find a way of pharmacologically relaxing the pulmonary arterioles. There are mainly two different drugs that have been used; Tolazoline (Priscoline), an alpha-adrenergic blocker, chemically related to the histamines, and Prostacyclin (PG I_2). Whereas Tolazoline is both a pulmonary and a systemic vasodilator, Prostacyclin is selectively a pulmonary relaxant. Tolazoline is given by the intravenous route, in doses of 0.5-1 mg/kg/hour, and Prostacyclin in doses of 0.05-0.1 µg/kg/min. The effect of Tolazoline has been well studied, and it appears from a number of reports that this drug is highly effective in reducing PVR in this syndrome. Its effectiveness is however abolished if the pH is below 7.20 [16 bis]. The clinical effect is best monitored by serial determination of systemic oxygen saturation or tension, and the dose should be adjusted according to the individual response. Care should be exercised to monitor systemic pressures during the infusion of Tolazoline, as systemic hypotension is a potential hazard with this drug. Such systemic hypotension may jeopardize the beneficial effect of a falling PVR on the size of the right-to-left shunt.

Particularly in the complex variety of the disease with associated myocardial dysfunction and pre-existing systemic hypotension, the use of Tolazoline may be questioned. Treatment with Prostacyclin may be a better alternative in these cases, due to its selective (but less effective) pulmonary vasodilatation.

Infants, who recover from the PFC syndrome and are recatheterized at a later age, usually show normal circulatory conditions. There are, however, reports of instances where pulmonary hypertension has been irreversible and the circulatory pattern in the older child inseparable from that of primary pulmonary hypertension.

Electrolytes and the neonatal circulation

It is a well recognized phenomenon that cardiac function is susceptible to changes in the electrolyte pattern, due to effects on the membrane potentials and conductivity of the Purkinje system. The neonatal period is characterized by rather more pronounced changes in electrolyte balance, possibly as a combined effect of a less efficient control mechanism and the pronounced metabolic changes that burden this period.

Electrolytes of particular interest for circulatory hemeostasis are potassium and calcium, both of which are highly sensitive to changes in the acid-base balance; calcium, by virtue of its higher ion dissociation in acid media, and potassium, due to the risk of depletion in conditions of acidosis, when the potassium ion is shifted from the intra-to-extra-cellular space.

In particular the presence in neonatal life of hypocalcemia may be associated with severe circulatory dysfunction. From a neuromuscular point of view, the fraction of ionized calcium is the more important, and a low Ca^{++} level may be reflected in early electrocardiographic characteristics, *i. e.* prolongation of the Q-T interval. A more reliable diagnosis is, however, made by indirect or direct assessment of the Ca^{++} plasma level.

Neonatal cardiovascular symptoms reported with hypocalcemia include cardiac failure and peripheral edema without apparent gross cardiac defects. The condition may be fatal to the infant, but in cases where the connection with hypocalcemia has been recognized, calcium infusion has been beneficial.

Neonatal circulatory crises in endocrine dysfunction and fulminating sepsis

Most hormones can directly or indirectly influence the circulatory system. Life threatening circulatory crises are known to occur in the athyreotic newborn, and the circulatory insufficiency in acute adrenal dysfunction is a dreaded complication. Septic conditions may also jeopardize systemic circulatory homeostasis, due to endotoxic paralysis of the peripheral vasomotor response, which affects the venous return to the heart. Whereas adrenal dysfunction should be controlled by substitution therapy with adrenal hormones; septic shock, due to peripheral vascular paralysis, usually requires transfusions or plasma expanders. In these instances, a central venous catheter, which allows monitoring of the systemic venous filling pressures, facilitates adequate hydration.

Cardiovascular therapy in the newborn period. General remarks

Heart failure. — Cardiac decompensation, as evidenced by respiratory distress with tachypnea, tachycardia and auscultatory gallop sound, and hepato-cardiomegaly with or without cyanosis, should be treated by digitalis, diuretics and increased FiO_2. The drugs should be administered by the intravenous route whenever the condition is critical or the circulation deranged, to an extent where absorption of orally given treatment may be in doubt. In instances of neonatal failure, where the response to digitalis is inadequate, the administration of adrenalin has been reported as an effective alternative. This drug is effective through its positive ionotropic and vasotonic effects. Correction of metabolic derangement with buffer solution is essential for the outcome of severe failure, where the acid-base balance often is markedly upset. When gas exchange is impaired and is not enhanced by anticongestive treatment, ventilatory support is indicated.

Cyanosis. — Arterial desaturation should be treated by increased FiO_2, by mask or tube, acid-base correction and possibly respirator support. Whenever persisting pulmonary vascular constriction is suspected, trials with one of the pharmacological vasodilators Tolazoline or Prostacyclin may be indicated. When cyanosis is ductus related, due to the presence of a congenital heart defect, ductal patency may be enhanced by prostaglandin E_1.

Cardiovascular resuscitation. — Pronounced bradycardia with ventricular rates less than 30-40 b. p. m. does not provide adequate cardiac output, and failure with arterial hypotension results. The condition, like ventricular asystole, calls for mechanical circulatory support, which should be given promptly. While ventilation is being supported by mask or intratracheal tube, external cardiac massage is administered by rhythmic compression of the thoracic cage over the precordial area, at a rate of 100/min. Care should be exercised to secure a stiff dorsal support with a good response to compressions. The ECG should be continuously monitored and buffer should be given, either in relation to the level of base deficit, or, whenever laboratory data are not available, in a "predicted" dose, corresponding to at least 1 mmol HCO_3 per kg BW and minute of circulatory arrest.

The recovery capacity of the neonatal myocardium is very impressive, a phenomenon most likely related to the relatively high content of glycogen. If, however, electrocardiographic and mechanical signs of ventricular contractions fail to appear in response to the above procedures, an intracardiac injection of adrenalin 1-2 ml 1/10,000 and Ca gluconate should be given. If the various therapeutic measures have not resulted in myocardial activity after 20-30 minutes, chances for revival are improbable and further resuscitation efforts should be withheld.

TABLE

Digoxin: Term infant maintenance		0.01-0.015 mg/kg BW orally
	Premature maintenance	0.005-0.01 mg/kg BW orally
	Initial priming	3-4 times maintenance dose
	Intravenous dose	3/4 of oral dose
	Check plasma concentration levels 1-2 ng/ml	

Adrenalin: 0.1-0.3 µg/kg/min i. v.

Isoproterenol: 0.2-0.3 µg/kg/min i. v.

Furosemide: 1-2 mg/kg

Indomethacin: 0.1-0.3 mg/kg p. o. or i. v.

Alpha-blockers and prostaglandins: see p. 313, 314.

Acid-base correction: HCO_3^- dose (mmol) = base deficit (mmol/L) $\times$ 1/3 of BW (kg).

REFERENCES

General references

BARCROFT (J.). — *Researches on Prenatal Life.* Blackwell Scientific, Oxford, 1946.
CASSELS (D. E.) Ed. — *The Heart and Circulation in the Newborn and Infant.* Grune and Stratton, 1966.
DAWES (G. S.). — *Foetal and Neonatal Physiology.* Year Book Medical Publ. Chicago (Ill.), 1968.
HEYMANN (M. A.), RUDOLPH (A. M.) Eds. — *The Ductus Arteriosus.* Report of the 75th Ross Conference on Pediatric Research. Columbus (Ohio), 1979.
LIND (J.), STERN (L.), WEGELIUS (C.). — *Human Foetal and Neonatal Circulation,* Ed. J. ANDERSON. Ch. Thomas, Springfield (Ill.), 1964.
SALING (E.). — *Das Kind im Bereich der Geburtshilfe.* G. Thieme Verlag, Stuttgart, 1966.
WALLGREN (G.) Ed.— *Quantitative Studies of the Human Neonatal Circulation. Acta Paediat Scand.,* suppl. *179,* 1967.
WALSH (Z.), MEYER (W.), LIND (J.). — *The Human Fetal and Neonatal Circulation. Function and Structure,* Ed. Ch. SWINYARD. Ch. Thomas, Springfield (Ill.), 1974.

* *

[1] ASSALI (N. S.), MORRIS (J. A.), BECK (R.). — Cardiovascular hemodynamics in the fetal lamb before and after lung expansion. *Amer. J. Physiol., 208,* 122-129, 1965.
[2] CELANDER (O.). — Blood flow in the foot and calf of the newborn. *Acta Paediat. Scand.,* 49, 488-496, 1960.

[3] CHU (J.), CLEMENTS (J. A.), COTTON (E. K.), KLAUS (M. H.), SWEET (A. Y.), TOOLEY (W. H.). — Neonatal pulmonary ischemia. *Pediatrics, 40,* 709-712, 1967.
[4] COLLETTI (R. B.), PAN (M. W.), SMITH (E. W.), GENEL (M.). — Detection of hypocalcemia in susceptible neonates. *N. Engl. J. Med., 290,* 931-935, 1974.
[5] COOK (C. D.), DRINKER (P. A.), JACOBSON (H. N.), LEVISON (H.), STRANG (L.). — Control of pulmonary blood flow in the fœtal and newly born lamb. *J. Physiol., 169,* 10-29, 1963.
[6] ELDRIDGE (F.), HULTGREN (H. N.). — The physiological closure of the ductus arteriosus in the newborn infant. *J. Clin. Invest., 34,* 987-996, 1955.
[7] EMMANOULIDES (G. C.), MOSS (A. J.), DUFFIE (E. R.), ADAMS (F. H.). — Pulmonary arterial pressure changes in human newborn infants from birth to 3 days of age. *J. Pediatr., 65,* 327-333, 1964.
[8] FOURON (J. C.), HÉBERT (F.). — The circulatory effects of hematocrite variations in normovolemic lambs. *J. Pediatr., 82,* 995-1003, 1973.
[9] GERSONY (W. M.), DUC (G. V.), SINCLAIR (J. C.). — « PFC » syndrome (persistence of fetal circulation). *Circulation, 40,* suppl. III, 87-90, 1969.
[10] GOETZMAN (B. W.), SUNSHINE (P.), JOHNSON (J. D.), WENNEBERG (R. P.), HACKEL (A.), MERTEN (D. F.), BARTOLETTI (A. L.), SILVERMAN (N. H.). — Neonatal hypoxemia and pulmonary vasospasm. Response to tolazoline. *J. Pediatr., 89,* 617-621, 1976.
[11] HERSHKO (C.), CARMELI (D.). — The effect of packed red cell volume, hemoglobin content and red cell count on whole blood viscosity. *Acta Haemat., 44,* 142-154, 1970.
[12] HEYMANN (M. A.), RUDOLPH (A. M.), SILVERMAN (N. H.). — Closure of the ductus arteriosus in premature infants by inhibition of prostaglandin synthesis. *N. Engl. J. Med., 295,* 530-533, 1976.
[13] HIRSCHFELD (S. S.), GRIGGS (T.). — Neonatal circulatory changes: An echocardiographic study. *Pediatrics, 59,* 338-344, 1977.
[14] JAMES (S. L.), WEISBROT (I. M.), PRINCE (C. E.), HOLADAY (D. A.), APGAR (V.). — The acid-base status of human infants in relation to birth asphyxia and the onset of respiration. *J. Pediatr., 52,* 379-394, 1958.
[15] LINDERKAMP (O.), STROHHACKER (I.), VERSMOLD (H. T.), KLOSE (H. R.), RIEGEL (K. P.), BETKE (K.). — Peripheral circulation in the newborn. Interaction of peripheral blood flow, blood pressure, blood volume and blood viscosity. *Eur. J. Pediat., 129,* 73-81, 1978.
[16] LOCK (J. E.), OLLEY (P. M.), COCEANI (F.), SWYER (P. R.), ROWE (R. D.). — Use of prostacyclin in persistent fetal circulation. *The Lancet, 1,* 1343, 1979.
[16 bis] MONIN (P.), VERT (P.), MORSELLI (P. L.). — A pharmacodynamic and pharmacokinetic study of Tolazine in the neonate. *Dep. Pharmacol. Ther., 4,* suppl. I, 124-128.
[17] MURDOCK (A. I.), SWYER (P. R.). — The contribution to venous admixture by shunting through the ductus arteriosus in infants with respiratory distress syndrome of the newborn. *Biol. Neonat., 13,* 194-210, 1968.
[18] OLLEY (P. M.). — Nonsurgical palliation of congenital heart malformations. *N. Engl. J. Med., 292,* 1292-1294, 1975.

[19] REEVES (J. T.), LEATHERS (J. E.). — Circulatory changes following birth of the calf and the effect of hypoxia. *Circul. Res.*, *15*, 343-354, 1964.

[20] RIEMENSCHNEIDER (T. A.), NIELSEN (H. C.), RUTTENBERG (H. D.), JAFFE (R. B.). — Disturbance of the transitional circulation: Spectrum of pulmonary hypertension and myocardial dysfunction. *J. Pediatr.*, *89*, 622-625, 1976.

[21] ROWE (R. D.). — Clinical observations of transitional circulation. In *Adaptation to Extrauterine Life*. Report of the 31st Ross Conference on Pediatric Research, T. K. OLIVER, Ed. Columbus, Ohio, 1959.

[22] ROWE (R. D.), HOFFMAN (T.). — Transient myocardial ischemia of the newborn infant. A form of severe cardiorespiratory distress in full term infants. *J. Pediatr.*, *81*, 243-250, 1972.

[23] RUDOLPH (A. M.), YUAN (S.). — Response of the pulmonary vasculature to hypoxia and H+ ion concentration changes. *J. Clin. Invest.*, *45*, 399-411, 1966.

[24] RUDOLPH (A. M.), HEYMANN (M. A.). — Circulatory changes with growth in the fetal lamb. *Circ. Res.*, *26*, 298-306, 1970.

[25] SAIGAL (S.), USHER (R. H.). — Symptomatic neonatal plethora. *Biol. Neonat.*, *32*, 62-72, 1977.

[26] SHELLEY (H. J.). — Carbohydrate reserves in the newborn infant. *Brit. Med. J.*, *1*, 273-275, 1964.

[27] STARLING (M. B.), ELLIOTT (R. B.). — The effects of prostaglandins, prostaglandin inhibitors and oxygen on the closure of the ductus arteriosus, pulmonary arteries and umbilical vessels *in vitro*. *Prostaglandins*, *8*, 187-203, 1976.

[28] STRANG (L. B.), MCLEISH (H. M.). — Ventilatory failure and right-to-left shunt in newborn infants with respiratory distress. *Pediatrics*, *28*, 17-27, 1961.

[29] TROUGHTON (O.), SINGH (S. P.). — Heart failure and neonatal hypocalcemia. *Brit. Med. J.*, *4*, 76-79, 1972.

[30] YAO (A. C.), LIND (J.). — Placental transfusion. *Amer. J. Dis. Child.*, *127*, 128-141, 1974.

18

Congenital heart disease

Claude PERNOT

with the contribution of Cl. DUPUIS, J. KACHANER and A. J. MOULAERT

Introduction

The incidence of congenital heart disease at birth is estimated at about 7 to 8 $°/_{oo}$.

Most often, it is consistent with normal or slightly perturbed cardiovascular fœto-placental physiology. Only certain major malformations, incompatible with development and survival in utero, are responsible for abortions. In some cases cardiac failure appears at the end of the pregnancy, this being responsible for hydrops fetalis and often for the occurence of stillbirths. Conversely, the malformation often passes undetected during the neo-natal period, the diagnosis being made only later. The cardiopathies which are symptomatic during the neo-natal period are those that result from an incompatibility between the malformation and the new circulatory conditions (Table I). In order to understand the physiopathology and evolution of these cardiopathies, it is indispensable to understand the mechanisms of circulatory adaptation at birth.

The border-line between cardio-vascular malfor-mations *(organic)* and difficulties of neo-natal circulatory adaptation *(functional)* is sometimes indecisive. Thus, the persistence of the ductus arteriorus of the premature—and sometimes of the term newborn—is most often the consequence —and not the cause—of poor circulatory adaptation, just as is the syndrome of persistence of fœtal circulation.

As well as these real malformations, we will include cardiac *arrhythmias* and the *myocardiopathies* of the newborn.

After a revision of the principal *methods of investigation* useful for the diagnosis, we will identify two cardiopathic groups, following their principal mode of clinical translation: *cyanotic* cardiopathies; cardiopathies responsible for *cardiac failure*, and or for collapse or cardiogenic shock. *Rhythm difficulties* and various other problems will be considered. Some *therapeutic* considerations will conclude this chapter.

TABLE I. — MAJOR SERIES OF HEART DEFECTS IN THE NEWBORN. FREQUENCY OF THE FIVE PRINCIPAL TYPES OF EARLY SYMPTOMATIC CARDIAC DEFECTS, ACCORDING TO AUTOPSY STATISTICS, CATHETERIZATIONS STATISTICS, OR BOTH TOGETHER.

Studied series			Complete transposition of the great arteries	Hypoplastic left heart complex	Pulmonary stenosis or atresia with intact ventricular septum	Coarctation of aorta	Tetralogy of Fallot	Total of these defects
Age	Material	Authors						
0 to 1 month	Autopsies	ROWE and CLEARY 1960	10 %	27 %	8 %	13 %	5 %	63 %
		MEHRIZI 1964	11 %	13 %	7 %	21 %	7 %	59 %
		LAMBERT and coll. 1966	15 %	22 %	7 %	10 %	7 %	61 %
		GAUTIER 1969	30 %	12 %	15 %	10 %	2 %	69 %
		PERNOT and coll. 1972	19 %	20 %	10 %	10 %	6 %	65 %
	Catheterizations	VARGHESE and coll. 1969	20 %	9 %	12 %	9 %	5 %	55 %
		NEIMANN and PERNOT 1969	28 %	4 %	8 %	10 %	2 %	52 %
0 to 8 days	Together	LAMBERT and coll. 1969	22 %	21 %	7 %	6 %	2 %	68 %
0 to 10 days	Autopsies	GAUTIER 1969	28 %	18 %	18 %	8 %	2 %	74 %
	Together	KACHANER and CASASOPRANA 1972	29 %	13 %	12 %	9 %	8 %	71 %

Methods of investigation

CLINICAL EXAMINATION

The data collected at the physical examination of the newborn infant suspected of a cardiopathy form the basis of the initial diagnostic orientation.

Inspection is an important aspect as it permits the detection of functional respiratory troubles (tachypnea and dyspnea) which are constant in cases of cardiac failure; and the evaluation of a generalised cyanosis, often intense and immutable under oxygen-therapy, sometimes less evident, sensitive to oxygen and mixed with a palor to give a grey-cinder tint. This is sometimes associated with an erythrosis which gives a "berry" colouring to the lips and extremities. Difficult cases can benefit from oxymetric measurements.

Palpation serves to detect hepatomegaly and to compare the pulsation of the femoral, humeral, radial or carotid arteries: their abolition, exaggeration or asymmetry has considerable diagnostic value. The measurement of blood pressure of the superior and inferior limbs, using the flush technique or Doppler sensors, is mandatory. Finally, the state of the peripheral perfusion and the time needed for recoloration aids in the recognition of collapse.

Auscultation of the heart serves to count the cardiac frequency; determine the regularity of the rhythm; qualify the sounds (normal, bursting, dulled or diminished) detect abnormal sounds (gallop) and murmurs for which one can specify the time (systolic, systolo-diastolic or continuous), the intensity, the

timbre and the maximal site not omitting auscultation of the back or the skull.

RADIOLOGY

A frontal plain film roentgenogram is of great
value in diagnostic cardiology in the newborn.

The technique must be fautless and one should
not report on a film unless the following five criteria
have been met: an exact frontal view, demonstrated
by symmetry of the clavicles about the vertical axis;
thoracic focus on the nipple line; left/right orientation using a contrast index X-rayed with the child;
considerable lowering of the diaphragmatic arches
by deep inspiration; appropriate penetration of
the X-rays: not so strong that only the skeleton
appears and not so weak that the lung field is among
the soft tissues.

Analysis of the film requires the following procedures: exact determination of the cardiac position
in the thorax *i. e.*: apex on the left (levocardia),
on the right (dextrocardia), or in the middle (mesocardia); determination of the thoracic situs (solitus,
inversus, ambiguus) according to the bronchial
morphology and to the liver position; measurement
of the cardio-thoracic ratio (Fig. III-13), a ratio
greater than 0.60 may be defined as cardiomegaly;
appreciation of the cardiovascular shadow about
the position of the apex, protrusion or recession of
the arches of the left border, a possible right border

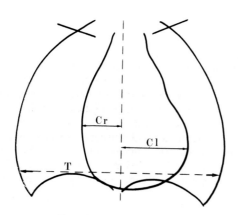

Fig. III-13. — *Measurement
of cardiothoracic ratio (CTR).*

T : Maximal transverse diameter of the thorax.
Cr : Maximal right hemidiameter of the heart.
Cl : Maximal left hemidiameter of the heart.
$$CTR = \frac{Cr + Cl}{T}$$

bulging, position of the aortic arch in relation to the
trachea; evaluation of the pulmonary vasculature:
decreased when the lungs appear clear without
any vascular pattern, or increased by an overload,
either of arterial origin, with hilifugian trabeculae,
or of venous origin via horizontal networks and
interstitial seeping.

ELECTROCARDIOGRAPHY

Pathophysiology

The appearance of the electrocardiogram is
dependant on the myocardial mass of the two ventricles and on the electrical activity of each one.
This activity depends firstly on the degree of volumetric distension, secondly on the resistance offered
to the flow from the vascular bed. This explains why
the neonatal period, a period of transition between
two very different hemodynamic situations, is
characterized by important and rapid variations
in the electrocardiographic patterns.

During foetal life, the activity of the right ventricle
is greater than that of the left ventricle; pulmonary
resistance is high, placental resistance low. At birth
the parietal thickness of the right ventricle exceeds
by one third that of the left ventricle. After ligation
of the cord, systemic resistance rises sharply,
pulmonary resistance falling with the first respiration.
Very quickly, systemic resistance become equal to
pulmonary resistance and then exceeds it. At the
end of the first day, pulmonary resistance has
fallen by half; by the fourteenth day they hardly differ
from those of the adult. After the first month,
the left ventricle becomes thicker than the right
ventricle.

In the newborn baby there is a physiological right
ventricular hypertrophy which evolves towards a
reduction with the progressive diminishing of
pulmonary resistance, a transient overloading of the
left ventricle related to the rapid increase of systemic
resistance. The ventricular depolarization (QRS
complex) is influenced above all by the myocardial
mass activated, that is to say the thickness of the
ventricular walls, whereas repolarization (essentially
T wave) depends on intraventricular pressures. This
is the reason why, during the neonatal period,
variations of the T wave are the most rapid and
demonstrative indicators of a normal or pathologic
hemodynamic evolution. The atriogram (P wave) is
influenced to a lesser degree by the hemodynamic
overloading of the right or left cavities.

In the physiological state the evolution of the

tracing is subject to individual variations which depend on several factors such as the degree of pulmonary vaso-constriction or the amount of the placental transfusion: thus a late clamping of the cord is followed by a slow recession of the electrocardiographic signs of the overloaded right ventricle.

In the premature infant, numerous factors intervene, sometimes in opposition, to modify the electrophysiology of the heart of the newborn. This explains why it is difficult to schematize the particularities of the electrocardiogram. We can retain the fact that right ventricular hypertrophy is less marked than that of the full term infant, voltages lower, the intervals (P, PR, QRS) shorter, modifications of repolarization more variable and less well systematised.

Analysis of the electrocardiogram

The frequency is extremely variable. Apart from pathological arrhythmias (see below) it oscillates generally between 200 (210 for the premature infant) and 70-80. At rest, it is on average at 130 per minute (slightly higher for the premature child). Sinus arrhythmias are frequent, a bradycardia (sometimes junctional) is not infrequent during the normal state, sleep or during breast feeding.

The P wave has a duration of between 0.03 and 0.06 sec. Its amplitude can vary in the neonatal period but does not exceed, in the normal state, 0.25 to 0.30 mV. A $+ -$ biphasic P wave in V1-V4R can often be noted during the first hours of life. The ample, and peaked P waves of right atrial hypertrophy are indicative of an obstruction on the right side of the heart (tricuspid atresia, pulmonary atresia with intact ventricular septum); the narrower the foramen ovale the more ample the waves.

The P-R Interval reaches between 0,07 and 0,12 sec, being slightly shorter in the premature baby. In Ebstein malformation of the tricuspid valve there can be a precocious elongation.

The QRS Complex varies little during the neonatal period but its morphology is subject to considerable individual variations; hence the interest of a statistical analysis for the interpretation of doubtful cases.

The QRS axis normally ranges between $+ 120°$ and $\pm 180°$. Only extremes have a definite pathological significance ($+ 30°$ to $- 150°$). During the first weeks of life, axial modifications are minimal and of little interest except where there is a case of extreme variation which would suggest a conduction problem in relation to major hemodynamic overload

(for example left axis deviation in a poorly tolerated coarctation of the aorta).

The duration of the QRS is between 0.04 and 0.06 sec (slightly less in the premature baby). Widening of the QRS is rare at birth but can appear progressively (as in Ebstein malformation for example): Right bundle branch block is more frequent than left bundle branch block whose prognosis is ominous at this age (cardiomyopathy, severe aortic stenosis). The Wolff-Parkinson-White syndrome is not infrequent and can be noted either after an episode of neonatal or fœtal paroxysmal tachycardia or in association with some congenital cardiopathies (Ebstein's anomaly or corrected transposition of the great vessels).

A low voltage Q wave (2-3 mm) is common in DII-DIII, more rare in DI. It is not frequent in V5 or V6 but has no pathological significance except if it exceeds 3 mm (left ventricular hypertrophy) or if it contrasts with signs of right ventricular hypertrophy brought into evidence in V1-V2 (combined ventricular hypertrophy). There is not normally a Q wave in V1 (except in cases of septal inversion or in definite patterns of right ventricular hypertrophy).

The amplitude of RS in V1-V2-V4R and in V6 varies considerably, but the progression—normal in the adult—of the relation R/S from V1 to V6 is never found in the normal state and always signifies left ventricular hypertrophy. A single R wave in V1 is rare but possible in the normal state, a notched R wave is frequent in V1. An R/S ratio less than 1 in V1-V4R is rare; below 0.7 it is always pathologic. The amplitude of R never normally exceeds 25 mm in V1, 15 mm in V6, that of S should not exceed 10 mm in V6.

The T wave can be subject to rapid variations. In standard derivations it is normally positive and not very prominent in DIII; the angle QRS-T becomes quickly accentuated during the first week: from 60° to 95°. In the premature baby, or during the first day the QT interval can often be longer (exclusive of electrolyte balance disturbances).

The most important variations to be considered are in V1-V4R. T is normally positive in these derivations in the first four days, then becomes negative. *If by the seventh day, the T wave has not become negative, one can conclude that there is pathological hypertension in the right ventricle* (unless there is a right bundle branch block with a large QRS).

In V5-V6 the T wave can be flat or even negative during the first two days; beyond this limit such negativity is *always pathological* (particularly in myocardial anoxia).

Pathological patterns

It is wise not to take into account doubtful tracings, particularly if the context does not favour a cardiopathy. *Arrhythmias* and *ischemia* will be described separately. *Atrial hypertrophy* (pure or associated with ventricular hypertrophy) can be confirmed in the presence of a P wave with an amplitude greater than 3 mm (in DII, V1-V4R) sometimes considerably larger. The diagnosis of right ventricular overload is difficult, occasionally necessitating the comparaison of successive tracings during the first month. It is rarely of the *diastolic* type with large QRS, qR on V1, notched complexes (agenesis of pulmonary valves, large left-to-right shunts, particularly at the atrial level, or total anomalous pulmonary venous drainage) but rather of the *systolic* type, sometimes associated with *left ventricular hypertrophy* (large left-to-right shunts): the diagnosis of *combined ventricular hypertrophy* is difficult, except in the case of an overall increase in the QRS voltage.

The criteria of overloading can be schematized as follows:

Right ventricular hypertrophy

TV1 positive beyond the fifth day.
qR in V1.
RV1 superior to 28 mm, RV4R superior to 19 mm.
SV6 superior to 11 mm.

Left ventricular hypertrophy

SV1 greater than 21 mm (26 for the premature baby).
R/S on V1 less than 1 (after the second day in the premature baby).
RV6 greater than 16 mm, QV6 superior to 3 mm.
$\overline{A}$QRS less than + 30° (+ 30° to − 150°).

Combined ventricular hypertrophy

Signs associated with RVH and LVH, in particular in the case of ample diphasic RS.
Signs of RVH with:
    Q greater than 1 mm on V6.
    R less than 5 mm on V6.
    T negative on V6.
Signs of LVH with:
    R greater than 5 mm on V1.

ECHOCARDIOGRAPHY

Echocardiography, M mode and, above all, real time two dimensional sector scan, is a non invasive technique whose applications have proved so useful in neonatal cardiology *that it is now the basic method to determine the management of distressed neonates with congenital heart disease.* Thus, in recent years, the indications for cardiac catheterization, especially in emergency conditions, have become less and less common. It is possible: to see and analyse cardiac *structures* (atrio-ventricular valves, semi-lunar valves, ventricular and atrial cavities, interventricular and interatrial septa); to study the inter-relations of the great vessels and their relations and connections with the ventricles; in complex congenital heart disease, to determine atriovisceral situs; finally to permit assessment of the cardiac *dynamics* and measures of some hemodynamic parameters (pulmonary pressure, for instance); to evaluate the follow-up of cardiopathies.

Subxiphoid cross-sectional echocardiography is the most useful in the newborn, allowing for multiple longitudinal, transverse or sagittal views of the cardiac chambers and the origin of the great vessels. Apical and classical parasternal approaches are of little interest at this age. On the other hand, the suprasternal approach is used to study the aortic arch and the bifurcation of the main pulmonary artery.

Contrast echocardiography is a complementary technique which is especially useful in the newborn and young infant, using the M-mode (chronologic study) and cross-sectional technique (morphologic study). The injection of 1 to 3 cm³ of physiological solution or of the patient's own blood into a peripheral vein (for example the umbilical vein) produces echoes which appear initially across the tricuspid valve, then in the right ventricle and finally in the pulmonary artery. In the normal newborn, abnormal echoes in the left sided cavities do not exist. If the right-to-left shunt is at the atrial level, abnormal echoes can be registered in the left atrium, then across the mitral valve and finally in the left ventricle and the aorta. If the right-to-left shunt is ventricular, abnormal echoes appear in the right ventricle then at the following systole in the left ventricle. Left-to-right shunts are more difficult to discern using this method and their identification relies on "wash out" contrast images.

Pulsed Doppler echocardiography provides very useful data on intracardiac or vascular flows, their accurate locations throughout the cardiac structures (identified by a "sample volume" on cross-sectional views), their directions, their "laminar" or "turbulent" patterns; it can identify more certainly some structures (ductus arteriosus for example) and may help to understand physiopathology; its use for indirect evaluation of hemodynamic parameters (output, pressure gradients) is now under study.

At the present time, two-dimensional echocardiography allows for an accurate diagnosis in most neonatal cardiopathies. *It is now possible to delay or avoid cardiac catheterization in a neonate in poor condition.* It is thus possible to restrict emergency intracardiac explorations to patients requiring therapeutic procedures (*i. e.* balloon septostomy).

The echocardiogram should be interpreted in the light of the clinical, electrical and radiological examination. Thus, several eventualities can be observed according to the degree of cyanosis and pulmonary vascularization.

The newborn is cyanosed; the pulmonary vasculature is increased

Transposition of the great vessels is easily detected by bidimensional echography: the anterior vessel arises vertically and corresponds to the aorta, the posterior vessel has a route parallel to the anterior one or slightly oblique towards the back and corresponds to the pulmonary artery. An upper transverse cross-section indicates if the aorta is to the right or to the left of the pulmonary artery. Unidimensional echography permits one, in the majority of cases, to localize the aorta in relation to the pulmonary artery by the angulation of the transducer and to study the systolic intervals. Contrast echography coupled with supra-sternal recordings shows abnormal echoes in the anterior aorta which is a continuation of the right ventricle.

In the case of total anomalous pulmonary venous return, the vessels are in place and the anterior pulmonary artery is dilated. The right ventricle is extremely dilated and the movement of the interventricular septum is most often abnormal. The abnormal venous collector is visible if there is a question of a return flow in the left ventricular vein or a sub-diaphragmatic venous return.

A common arterial trunk is suspected when one records one vessel which is large straddling the interventricular septum. The left atrium and left ventricle are dilated. If a pulmonary sigmoid valve is recorded a common trunk is out of the question. Echography permits one therefore to differentiate easily a common trunk from an interventricular communication with pulmonary hypertension.

The newborn is cyanosed; the pulmonary vasculature is diminished

Extreme tetralogy of Fallot or pulmonary atresia with ventricular septal defect can be suspected if one records the aorta straddling the interventricular septum. The contrast echography thus shows a right-to-left ventricular shunt.

Pulmonary atresia with intact ventricular septum is characterised by right ventricular hypoplasia, a small tricuspid valve, the absence of echoes of the pulmonary valve and a dilated left side of the heart. In contrast to the tetralogy of Fallot, a septo-aortic continuity exists and the contrast echography shows a right-to-left shunt, but there also exists a passage from the right atrium to the right ventricle.

Tricuspid atresia is suggested if the tricuspid valve echo is absent, the right ventricle small and the left side of the heart dilated. Contrast echography can estimate atrial right-to-left shunts. The opacification of the right ventricle is later than that of the left ventricle.

In some cases, the echocardiogram is qualitatively normal, the newborn is cyanosed and the pulmonary vasculature is normal or diminished. The vessels are in place and all the cardiac structures are recorded. This may be due to transient pulmonary hypertension or a persistence of the fetal circulation. The relationship between the pulmonary pre-ejection period and the pulmonary ejection-time is greater than 0.50. In addition, echography permits one to follow the evolution under the effect of treatment of the systolic intervals. There may also be a question of neonatal cyanosis without cardiopathy and the echocardiogram is then qualitatively and quantitatively normal.

The newborn is little or not at all cyanosed; the pulmonary vasculature is increased

Hypoplastic left heart syndrome is easily diagnosed: either hypoplasia of the mitral valve with a small left ventricle and small aorta; or mitral atresia with an absence of the mitral valve recording, small left ventricle and small aorta; or aortic atresia with a small aorta and an absence of the aortic valve.

The coarctation syndrome can be recognised above all by clinical diagnosis. Echography permits one to eliminate a hypoplastic left heart, to study the contractility of the left ventricle and sometimes to see the coarctation.

Amongst other left-to-right shunts, an atrio-ventricular canal is usually easy to detect: appearance of a single atrio-ventricular valve or the appearance of the mitral valve which crosses the interventricular septum to join the tricuspid valve. Ductus arteriosus of the newborn is visible only when using bidimensional techniques but its presence does not eliminate an associated ventricular septal defect which is difficult to discern using this method.

Single ventricle can be confirmed if one records two atrio-ventricular valves in the same ventricular cavity in front of, or behind which can be found an opacified accessory chamber by using the contrast, later than in the ventricular cavity which receives the mitral and tricuspid valves.

The newborn is not cyanosed; the pulmonary vasculature is normal

Bidimensional echography can detect a narrowing of the aortic orifice by showing a dome shaped aspect to the aortic valve or a sub-valvar membrane. The left ventricle is dilated.

An intramyocardial or intraventricular tumour can also be discovered by bidimensional echography; this should lead to a search for other signs of Bourneville's tuberous sclerosis. Finally, cardiomegaly can be due to a neonatal pericardiac discharge which is responsable for the free space tracing of the echo in front of the right ventricle and/or behind the left ventricle.

In summary, echocardiography now occupies the lead place in the evaluation of a newborn child suspected of congenital heart disease. Performed after the clinical, electrical and radiological examinations, it can confirm or exclude a cardiopathy. It always gives morphological and dynamic information which is very useful for the diagnosis.

CARDIAC CATHETERISATION AND ANGIOCARDIOGRAPHY

The aim of intracardiac catheterisation is to obtain, from pressure tracings, the measurement of

oxygen saturation in the different cavities, the localization of abnormal trajectories of the catheter and above all from the anatomic information furnished by selective cineangiography, a diagnosis of the malformation which is as precise and as complete as possible. The neonatal period is the period during which the risks involved in using this technique are the highest. However, during the last decade these risks have become far less. At the same time, the increasing precision of non-invasive techniques, in particular echocardiography, permits a limitation of indications and a reduction in their duration.

Indications

They should be established with considerable prudence, following a careful study of the clinical and paraclinical facts and above all after a rigorous standard echocardiographic exploration, possibly with contrast; this will not only serve to guide the plan of the catheterization and to specify for the operator the points on which he should focus attention, but equally will determine the degree of urgency of the intracardiac investigations. This can avoid certain long explorations which are not without risk and can simplify the technique compared to classical methods used in the older child.

The most urgent type of indication is complete transposition of the great vessels, for which catheterization has not only a diagnostic but also a therapeutic aim, permitting balloon atrial septostomy (for which this anomaly remains the best indication).

Catheterization is equally indicated in all cases of refractory cyanosis when it is likely to lead to immediate surgical treatment (pulmonary atresia with ventricular septum intact or open, tricuspid atresia). In the case of heart failure, its indications during the neonatal period are less urgent. In coarctation of the aorta, it is wise not to catheterize before having reduced the failure by medical treatment without however letting the optimal time go by.

When the data from simpler examinations has led to the suspicion of hypoplastic left heart syndrome, and the echocardiogram has confirmed this diagnosis, catheterization is not indicated because of the absence of any real possibility of surgery. It is equally unnecessary when the echocardiogram permits the confirmation of Ebstein's anomaly which should be treated medically except where there is a suspicion of pulmonary atresia. Similarly, when echocardiography confirms the presence of pulmonary arterial hypertension with normal cardiac structures, indicative of the syndrome of persistence of the fœtal circulation, catheterization is not justifiable.

Finally, cardiopathies discovered during the neonatal period which are well compensated do *not* call for immediate catheterization.

Technique

The approach is essentially *venous*: usually via the *percutaneous femoral route*. Venous dissection is rarely necessary if the team is well trained, and should be used only in cases of puncture failure, in children of very low birth weight and some premature babies. During the first week of life, the *umbilical vein* can be used but this has limitations since it leads to false routes, presents difficulties in manipulation of the catheter and does not easily permit performance of a Rashkind septostomy. The technique permits an approach to the left side of the heart through the foramen ovale: the left atrium is easily reached, the left ventricle sometimes with a little more difficulty. The use of a Swan-Ganz balloon catheter facilitates passage through the mitral orifice. *The retrograde arterial route;* difficult at this age using the percutaneous technique, often necessitates dissection not without risk of thrombosis and is little used. On the other hand, the *umbilical arterial route* which is rapid and of low risk, has specific indications: The exploration of the aorta or a common arterial trunk, the ductus arteriosus, the left ventricle, and arterio-venous fistulae.

Important progress has recently been made in **the materials** used thus rendering the technique more certain and less dangerous. One uses only very supple catheters of 4F or 5F, which are to be manipulated with prudence. For the injection of the contrast medium, one needs to avoid certain positions of the catheter which predispose to intra-myocardial breakage, particularly in the ventricular cavities.

Ventilatory support should be available during the examination, which requires no medication, the puncture or dissection being done under local anaesthesia. Assisted respiration, thermoregulation by a mattrass with water circulation, frequent control of blood parameters and rectal temperature, the use of bicarbonate, and avoiding fluid overload all permit the avoidance of hypoxemia, hypothermia and acidosis which are always to be feared at this age.

One needs also to carefully measure any blood loss and to correct it as indicated. In all cases where there is significant respiratory difficulty with hypercapnia, the procedure should be conducted under assisted ventilation.

Risks and complications

The risks of catheterization during the neonatal period are relatively high. The mortality rate is estimated at 5 %. However, given the often precarious state of these infants, it is difficult to distinguish between the part played by the procedure and that of the spontaneous evolution of the cardiopathy. With the improvement in materials and the experience of the teams, certain accidents *linked directly with the procedure* (myocardial perforations, persistent arrhythmias, accidents due to an excess of the contrast product or to fluid excess) have become less frequent. On the other hand, some "high risk" situations such as the hypoplastic left heart syndrome no longer necessitate catheterization and therefore do not augment the mortality rate.

Hypoxemia, acidosis, hypothermia and *hemorrhagic anemia* can be treated all the more efficiently if they have been rapidly detected. *Myocardial perforations and severe extravasations* caused by the contrast product were, until several years ago, a major concern. In the case of a perforation by the catheter, it is preferable to leave it in place and it is generally necessary to intervene surgically. *Acidents due to the contrast product* are mainly related to osmolar disturbances and the amelioration now obtained is indicative principally of the use of new products. Generally, one needs to avoid going beyond a total of 3 ml/kg and 1.5 ml/kg for each injection and to wait 15 minutes between injections. It is necessary to be even more prudent in the case of renal insufficiency, confirmed or suspected, as for example in the coarctation syndrome.

Results

The route of the catheter gives rapid information about certain malformations. *By the venous route* one can note the passage through the ductus arteriosus which remains largely permeable and from there is directed towards the descending aorta; the crossing of a perimembranous ventricular septal defect which leads to the ascending aorta from the right ventricle; more rarely a trajectory more complex and indicative of total anomalous venous drainage, systemic (azygos continuation, double superior vena cava) or pulmonary (supracardiac collector). *The retrograde umbilical arterial route* is useful for obtaining precise information about the anterior situation of the ascending aorta from which the catheter descends into the right ventricle in cases of complete transposition of the great vessels.

Oximetry leads to the diagnosis and localisation of left-to-right shunting: to an enrichement of oxygen in the superior vena cava in the case of arterio-venous cerebral fistula; a hightened level of saturation in the case of total anomalous pulmonary venous return; enrichement in the right ventricle in the case of ventricular septal defect, in the pulmonary artery in the case of patent ductus arteriosus or aorto-pulmonary window. In cases of severe obstruction of the left heart outlet (coarctation of the aorta or valvar aortic stenosis) the enrichement of the right auricle is due to a "forced" foramen ovale sometimes also observed in cases of "lower" large shunts hence the difficulties of diagnosis of a double or triple shunt. In the case of newborn infants in poor condition, oximetry can be difficult to interpret or even impossible particularly if it has been necessary to maintain the child in a high FiO_2 during the examination.

Pressures should be measured in stable conditions outside of shock. Hypertension in the right cavities indicates an obstruction in the lower part of the cavity in question; atrial hypertension in tricuspid atresia is more marked when the foramen ovale is less permeable; systolic ventricular hypertension may sometimes be very high, considerably above the aortic level in the case of pulmonary atresia with intact ventricular septum, with a pointed pressure curve. In pulmonary atresia with open ventricular septum and tetralogy, the systolic pressure in the right ventricle is the same as that of the aorta and the summit of the curve does not have a pointed aspect. Pulmonary arterial hypertension (above 30 or 35 mm of mercury end systolic) is the principle finding in right-to-left shunt cardiopathies, total anomalous pulmonary venous return. In complete transposition of the great vessels, it is prudent not to catheterize the pulmonary artery, a manœuvre

which is complex and delicate all the more so since the pulmonary arterial pressure, an important element in the prognosis, is subject to considerable variation during the first weeks of life. It is necessary however to obtain it at the repeat studies made around the third month. Recording of the *pressure gradients* permits the diagnosis of stenosis of the orifices. In the case of aortic stenosis, the gradient measurement is most often indirect. Finally, the pressure gradient between the two atria gives information on the size of the foramen ovale and permits an assessment of the results of atrial septostomy.

Angiocardiography gives the most precise information. Certain *indirect signs* are sometimes very revealing and can lead to, a particular orientation for the other studies. Massive and rapid reopacification of the superior vena cava suggests a cerebral arteriovenous fistula. The opacification, even feeble, of the descending aorta from the pulmonary artery, indicates a "systemic" ductus arteriosus; that of the ascending aorta after an injection into the right ventricle indicates a ventricular septal defect which is all the more important where there is an obstruction at the outflow tract of the right ventricle or major pulmonary arterial hypertension. Reopacification of the pulmonary artery indicates a ventricular septal defect. In the case of an important right-to-left shunt, the dilution is often such that is it difficult to obtain good opacification which may demonstrate lesions such as the aortic coarctation of the "coarctation syndrome". The different malformations of the right side of the heart, of the pulmonary outflow tract, of the left side of the heart, of the subaortic region and of the aorta, and of anomalous pulmonary venous drainage can usually be studied via a frontal and lateral view. Identification of the interventricular septum necessitates a doubly oblique angle, that of the mitral valve, a right anterior oblique angle.

Catheterization and angiocardiography should be reserved for severe cardiopathies susceptible to benefit from immediate therapy. If these indications are followed and if the procedure is conducted by an experienced team under the cover of good ventilatory assitance, it is an invaluable technique for diagnosis in the newborn infant.

Cyanotic cardiac disease

DIAGNOSIS OF NEONATAL CYANOSIS OF CARDIAC ORIGIN

Many types of heart disease reveal themselves in the first few hours or days by cyanosis of a particular type. This can be labelled as the *isolated refractory hypoxemia syndrome*, and its identification ofen serves as a first point of orientation in the diagnosis.

DEFINITION. FIRST APPROACH

The definition of this syndrome resides in one word: *cyanosis*. The cyanosis has often been noted in the first minutes and lowers the Apgar score. In some cases, it is noticed some hours later, sometimes in the form of an attack. It ends always by being intense, generalised, permanent, and accentuated by crying. Two of its characteristics are extremely important: it is *not sensitive* to any form of oxygenation; it is generally *isolated*: there is little or no respiratory difficulty, good neurological condition, central and peripheral blood flow is normal. Thus, it is a question of a newborn infant who is blue, extremely blue whatever one does, and who tolerates this state rather well, not giving the impression of being ill. Nothing is more erroneous than to be lead astray by this apparent tranquility: *far from being reassuring, this situation should immediately cause one to suspect a serious cardiac malformation and to initiate the investigative process.*

One should, without delay, obtain a thoracic radiograph, an electrocardiogram, an analysis of the acid base balance, and in doubtful cases an oxymetric measurement (PaO_2 or SaO_2) on samples of arterial blood collected under basal conditions and again after 15 to 20 minutes of intensive oxygenation of the child. One can thus confirm the hypoxemia and its refractory character.

If local conditions do not permit one to obtain this simple information immediately, it is necessary to transfer the newborn to a specialised unit.

ETIOLOGIC DIAGNOSIS

Diagnosis of cardiac origin

It is of course necessary to begin by confirming that the organ affected is the heart. Many respiratory infections are cyanotic in the newborn but almost all show functional respiratory problems or specific changes which are visible radiologically in the lung parenchyma or the pleura. Neurological disturbances, with or without convulsions, are often cyanotic too but the history and neurological evolution are specific. Attacks of cyanosis due to hypoglycemia or hypocalcemia result from a particular context (diabetic mother, post-maturity, dysmaturity) leading to conclusive biological examinations.

In addition, three disease can readily give rise to confusion:

Congenital methemoglobinemia is rare and gives a slate-coloured tint rather than cyanosis; the PaO_2 is normal, the blood is of chocolate colour when exposed; the measurement of methemoglobin proves the diagnosis.

Polycythemia is frequent and can be recognized by the tint which is erythrocytic rather than cyanotic, particularly in the lips, ears and nails with carmine coloured mucosa and bloodshot conjunctiva; oxymetry is usually normal and the hemogram leads to the diagnosis: more than 6,000,000 rbc/mm^3, greater than 20 g % of hemoglobin, hematocrit above 65 %.

The persistent fetal circulation syndrome usually affects term infants with prenatal distress. The cyanosis is usually associated with respiratory difficulties and sometimes with tricuspid insufficiency: a systolic murmur, cardiomegaly, and a clear pulmonary film. The diagnosis should only be made after an echocardiogram, that is to say by the identification of all cardiac structures in the normal position with pulmonary arterial dilation and signs of pulmonary hypertension. In cases of doubt, one can have recourse to tolazoline or to endocavitary

TABLE II

Syndrome	Major elements of orientation		Likely diagnosis	Other suggestive signs
Isolated refractory hypoxemia	Increased pulmonary vasculature		Complete transposition of the great arteries	Normal heart size, "egg-shaped" heart shadow
	Decreased pulmonary vasculature	Normal heart size	Tetralogy of Fallot	Heart shadow "en sabot" right aortic arch
			Pulmonary atresia + VSD (or + complex heart defect)	Continuous murmur
			Tricuspid atresia	QRS axis = − 30°
			Agenesis of the pulmonary valve	Systolo-diastolic murmur
		Moderate cardiomegaly	Pulmonary stenosis or atresia with intact ventricular septum	"ace of spades" heart shadow left atrial and ventricular enlargement
			Tricuspid insufficiency	Xiphoid systolic murmur
		Huge cardiomegaly	Ebstein's disease	Right atrial enlargement Right bundle branch block

investigation which shows pulmonary arterial hypertension and a right-to-left shunt in a normal heart, via the ductus arteriosus and the foramen ovale.

Specific diagnosis

It is in fact easy to attribute the responsibility for isolated refractory hypoxemia to the heart. The quality of the pulmonary vasculature and the volume of the heart on the thoracic film permit a precise diagnosis. The principal steps are summarized in Table II. The following simple rules can be utilized.

If the pulmonary vasculature is increased, the only diagnosis is that of transposition of the great vessels. Suspicion of this implies immediate transfer of the newborn to a specialised unit for confirmation of the diagnosis and urgent treatment by balloon atrial septostomy.

If the pulmonary vasculature is reduced, it suggests that there is a reduction of pulmonary output: either by severe obstruction of the pulmonary pathway with ventricular septal defect or with normal heart size (tetralogy of Fallot, tricuspid

atresia); or by tricuspid insufficiency, secondary to an obstruction at the pulmonary orifice with intact ventricular septum, or to structural anomalies of the right ventricle or the tricuspid valve. The heart is as a general rule large and sometimes even massively dilated as in the Ebstein malformation. All these malformations should be urgently identified by echocardiography and later endocavity exploration since certain ones can benefit from specific medical or surgical treatment.

COMPLETE TRANSPOSITION OF THE GREAT ARTERIES

Complete transposition of the great arteries in the newborn has merited great interest in the last decade not only because of its frequency, but, because enormous progress has been made in its treatment. In effect, before the therapeutic era, 95 % of the children suffering from this disease died early whereas now, with correct treatment, 70 to 80 % can survive.

PATHOLOGY

The malformation is characterised by a ventricular-atrial discordance *i. e.* the aorta rises from the right ventricle, the pulmonary artery from the left ventricle. Usually, the aorta is anterior and the pulmonary artery posterior. In the majority of cases the transposition is of the D type (dextro-transposition) with the aortic valve to the right of the pulmonary valve. In the L type transposition (rare in the case of complete transposition) the aortic valve lies to the left of the pulmonary valve. In the majority of cases, transposition of the great arteries is *isolated* (50 to 60 % of cases) or associated with simple intracardiac anomalies such as ventricular septal defect (30 %) or pulmonary stenosis (10 %). *Ventricular septal defect* is most often of the perimembranous type. *Pulmonary stenosis* is rarely valvar; it is more often related to a diffuse septal hypertrophy or a mitro-aortic malalignement with an excess of mitral valvular tissue. It is sometimes represented by a fibro-muscular tunnel. It often becomes more serious during the first months of life. In more than one third of the cases, it is associated with a ventricular septal defect. Amongst other associated anomalies, the persistance of a large ductus arteriosus or coarctation of aorta merit mention even though they are rare.

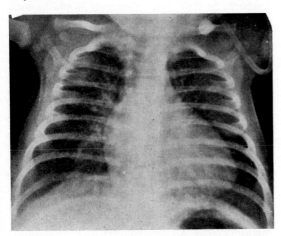

FIG. III-14. — *Complete transposition of the great arteries with intact ventricular septum.* "Egg-shaped" cardiac shadow, thin heart-pedicle, increased lung vasculature.

PATHOPHYSIOLOGY

In the form with intact interventricular septum, there is marked peripheral arterial desaturation and an overload of the two ventricles. In effect, pulmonary and systemic circulatory function is parallel and not in series as in the normal subject. During fetal life this abnormal circulation has no serious consequences. On the other hand, after birth it is incompatible with prolonged survival. Non-oxygenated blood which enters the right side of the heart via the vena cava returns to the periphery by the aorta. The oxygenated blood entering the lungs from the pulmonary veins returns to the lungs via the pulmonary artery. Survival depends on the mixing of the bloods. This can be done by the ductus and the foramen ovale as long as they are more or less open. Peripheral arterial desaturation is rapid and intense (the PaO_2 is often around 25 mm Hg or less). It provokes tissue anaerobic glycolysis and a severe metabolic acidosis. Hypoxemia, acidosis and hypoglycemia rapidly alter myocardial metabolism. The only system of defense that the organism has to raise the level of the mixing of the bloods is to increase the cardiac output; but owing to metabolic myocardial difficulties this results rapidly in cardiac insufficiency. Hypoxemia, acidosis, hypoglycemia and their habitual corollary in the newborn, hypothermia, are thus rapid and frequent complications of the isolated complete transposition. The subsequent cardiac failure further complicates this and often in the absence of treatment results in death within a few days.

In the form with large ventricular septal defect, the mixing of bloods is more effective and the peripheral arterial desaturation far less serious; however this compensation is at the price of a raised output and pulmonary arterial pressures and an important bi-ventricular overload. In this form, the two risks are therefore cardiac failure and the development of an obstructive pulmonary vascular disease. To these two important causes of pulmonary vascular disease which are high pulmonary output and hypertension can be added other causes: hypoxemia and systemic acidosis; the bronchial blood hypoxemia contrasting with the pulmonary arterial hyperoxemia, the polycythemia with blood hyperviscosity which generates pulmonary vascular micro-thrombosis. The initial good tolerance of this form is thus not sustained.

In the form with ventricular septal defect and pulmonary stenosis, if the ventricular septal defect is large enough to permit a good mixing of the bloods, and the pulmonary stenosis not too tight, the initial tolerance is good. There is neither risk of cardiac failure, nor secondary risks of obstructive pulmonary vascular disease. It was these forms which, before the therapeutic era, allowed the longest survival.

In the forms with a large ductus arteriosus or coarctation of aorta, the risk of early congestive cardiac failure is greater: in the first case because of the shunt, and in the second case owing to an obstruction at the exit of the right ventricle.

ETIOLOGY

Complete transposition represents about 9 % of child heart disease and about 25 % of newborn heart disease. It is more frequent in boys than in girls, the ratio in the majority of studies being 2 to 1. The masculine predominance is more marked in the forms with ventricular septal defect. Transposition appears rare in first born children. Initial studies showed that newborns suffering from transposition had a birthweight which was higher than normal. As this also characterizes children of diabetic mothers, it was concluded that glycemic perturbations in the mother were a possible etiological factor in transposition. This etiological factor has not been confirmed and more recent studies have not found evidence of increased birthweight in cases of transposition. Additional extracardiac malformations are rare in transposition, particularly in isolated transposition.

PRINCIPAL CLINICAL PATTERNS

Complete transposition with intact ventricular septum

The disease is symptomatic from birth. On inspection, the infant appears of normal size, cyanosed, tachycardic and polypneic. The pulses are strong, arterial pressure normal and the neurological examination without significant findings. The apex of the heart is in its normal place. At auscultation, the first sound is normal, there is a bursting second sound which is single or whose splitting is very close. One can usually hear a small systolic ejection murmur which is of low intensity, but there is generally no murmur. Blood gas study shows a lowered pH level with normal PCO_2 and a low PO_2. After 100 % oxygen for 10 minutes, the PO_2 remains unchanged or rises only a little.

These children being hypoxemic, hypothermic, acidotic and often hypoglycemic, they should be rapidly transported to a specialised center under oxygen therapy and an infusion designed to correct biological perturbations. In the absence of treatment, the state of the infant rapidly deteriorates. Signs of cardiac failure, particularly hepatomegaly, are noted. Respiratory distress, acidosis and hypoxemia become greater, the neurological state deteriorates and death follows. It is possible that the closing of the ductus arteriosus is the cause of many rapid deteriorations.

Chest radiography is an important element in the diagnosis of isolated transposition. Classically there is pulmonary hypervascularisation contrasting with the absence of the main pulmonary artery segment of the left border, a narrow pedicle, an oval-shaped heart and a rapid augmentation of cardiac volume, but the first three signs are not constant and the fourth should no longer be seen. The pulmonary vascularization and the absence of the main pulmonary artery segment are the most characteristic. However one cannot entirely exclude a diagnosis of transposition if the cardiac silhouette and the pulmonary vascularization appear normal.

The electrocardiogram has little value. The rhythm is a sinus one, the PR interval is normal, the QRS axis deviates to the right between + 90° and + 120° and there is atrial hypertrophy analogous to that which one can observe in a normal newborn. In time, this appearance would be more characteristic since right ventricular hypertrophy accentuates in transposition whereas it regresses in the normal newborn.

An echocardiogram associating uni- and bi-dimensional techniques along with ultrasonic contrast permit one practically always, to confirm or to refute the diagnosis of transposition. The mitral and tricuspid valves are easily localized and have normal motions. The interventricular septum and the right and left ventricular cavities are normal; the continuities are normal *i. e.* the anterior mitral valve is in continuity with the posterior wall of the posterior vessel (here the pulmonary artery). The septum is in continuity with the anterior border of this same vessel. All the signs permit one to eliminate the majority of the other cyanotic heart diseases of the newborn. The transposition is confirmed by the study of the position of the great arteries. The D transposition is the easiest to recognise since the anterior vessel is to the right of the posterior vessel, the inverse of that which can be observed in the normal subject. Often one records both great arteries at the same time owing to their parallel tract whereas in the normal subject this is rare. Finally the study of systolic intervals shows that the anterior valve (aortic valve) opens later and closes earlier than the posterior valve. As these signs are not absolute, it is preferable to use certain other techniques *i. e.*, bidimensional echocardiography, or multi-scan which shows that the anterior vessel has a vertical direction—it is therefore the aorta—whereas the posterior vessel has a horizontal direction corresponding therefore to the pulmonary artery; or a sector-scan which permits one to identify the division between the pulmonary artery and the posterior vessel. Contrast echocardiography shows the rapid passage of the contrast injected into a peripheral vein of the right side of the heart towards the aorta; this is easily identifiable in its suprasternal occurrence: it is always above the pulmonary artery, whatever the malformation.

Catheterization and angiocardiography should be done urgently since, even if the state of the newborn appears relatively good, a sudden and irreversible aggravation is always possible. The umbilical route can sometimes be used. The femoral percutaneous venous approach or catheterization of the femoral vein or its branches is more usual. One begins by recording the pressures and the saturation in the right atrium, superior vena-cava, right ventricle and left atrium. There is uniform desaturation in the right side of the heart, with normal saturation in the left atrium. The right ventricular pressures are at systemic level and there is usually an average left atrial pressure 3 to 6 mm Hg greater than the average right atrial pressure. Right ventriculography which, showing that the aorta is anterior and above all takes origin in the right ventricle, confirms the diagnosis of transposition, gives precisions on the anatomy of the isthmus and shows the aspect of the duct, still patent or closed on the pulmonary side. The Rashkind balloon septostomy should now be used. A catheter of 5F calibre is generally sufficient; however in an infant of low birth weight, it is possible to use a 4F catheter. The catheter should pass across the foramen ovale into the left ventricle or a pulmonary vein. If the tip of the catheter is located in a pulmonary vein, it is sufficient to pull it a little so that it will be in the left atrium. If one is not able to pass the catheter into a pulmonary vein, one needs to verify if it is well to the back. One can then inflate the balloon with a diluted contrast medium. The balloon is inflated firstly to 1 cm³ then to 2.5-3 cm³, thus assuring a diameter of 10 to 15 mm. It is withdrawn brusquely from the left atrium towards the right atrium in the direction of the inferior vena-cava to tear the valve of

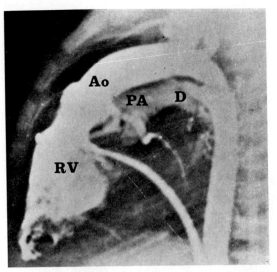

FIG. III-15. — *Complete transposition of the great vessels with intact ventricular septum.* Selective angiocardiogram in the right ventricle (RV), lateral view. Aorta (Ao) is anterior, pulmonary artery (PA) posterior, the latter injected from the aorta through the ductus (D), still slightly patent. Note the thin jet of contrast medium at the pulmonary end of the ductus.

the foramen ovale, then repassed towards the orifice of the inferior vena-cava towards the right atrium and then deflated. This operation should be repeated several times, increasing the volume of the balloon each time. It is necessary to avoid a slow withdrawal which can dilate the foramen ovale without really tearing it, and a too rapid withdrawal and the introduction of air bubbles when one inflates the balloon in order to avoid all risks of air embolism in case of rupture. The risks of this procedure: perforation of the left atrial wall by the catheter, uprooting of the inferior vena-cava, splitting of the balloon with a clot of rubber in a systemic artery, inability to deflate the balloon, have almost disappeared with improvement in the materials. Levoposition of the right atrium is rare but may constitute a trap which an experienced observer can avoid by noting the impossibility to enter a pulmonary vein and the less posterior position of the catheter.

The Rashkind balloon septostomy usually permits a tear of 10-15 mm in diameter and an immediate improvement in metabolic acidemia and arterial oxygen saturation. One can confirm its efficacy by noting the disappearance of the interatrial pressure gradient. The newborn being improved by this process, one can now, using a Swan-Ganz balloon catheter, easily pass the left atrium towards the left ventricle, measure the left ventricular pressure and perform left ventriculography. The left ventricular

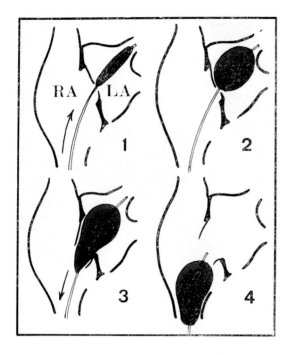

FIG. III-16. — *Rashkind balloon septostomy*. 1 : The catheter is introduced from right atrium (RA) into left atrium (LA), pushing the valve of the fossa ovalis. 2 : The balloon is inflated in the left atrium. 3, 4 : A vigorous traction of the catheter results in a large laceration of the valve.

pressure can be low (around 30 mm Hg); it is sometimes raised during the first week of life, even in the absence of pulmonary stenosis, by persistence of pulmonary arterial hypertension of the fetal type. Left ventriculography allows the evaluation of any associated pulmonary stenosis. Catheterization of the pulmonary artery has no merit at this stage only prolonging the examination unnecessarily.

Evolution. — *The majority of newborns* are improved for several months by balloon septostomy. It establishes good mixing of bloods between the atria, the cyanosis remains moderate, the PaO$_2$ is above 30 mm Hg, the cardiac failure disappears, the cardiac volume remains normal and growth continues relatively well. But these children remain fragile and, after a few months, the cyanosis intensifies, anorexia and hypotrophy appear, and there is a risk of cerebral vascular thrombosis. Until recently, the tendancy was to do a surgical Blalock-Hanlon septectomy between three and six months which enabled one to wait and to achieve the venous

transposition at the atrial level, using the Mustard procedure, at the age of between eighteen months and two years. However the mortality rate for the Blalock-Hanlon procedure is not negligible; the procedure favours the occurence of supra-ventricular arrhythmias; it does not prevent either the hypotrophy nor the risk of cerebro-vascular thrombosis. This explains why currently one tends to intervene early, between three and six months, with a venous transposition at the atrial level without a palliative intermediate procedure. The Mustard procedure, which uses a baffle of pericardium to bring the caval blood towards the tricuspid, the pulmonary venous blood being thus diverted gives good results; it may however lead to pulmonary venous or caval stenosis and to supraventricular arrhythmias. The Senning procedure, whose aim is identical, uses the wall of the atria and the atrial septum to achieve an analogous partitioning. It predisposes less to pulmonary or caval stenosis, but seems to result in the same supra-ventricular arrhythmias. The risk of the Mustard and Senning interventions is low after the age of three months. Practiced early, it puts the child out of danger of cerebro-vascular thrombosis and can in the majority of cases avoid the development of obstructive pulmonary vascular disease. The results are certainly acceptable. On the other hand, the Jatene procedure, or transposition at the arterial level, carries a high mortality in isolated transposition.

In some cases, Rashkind balloon septostomy improves the childs condition only a little or transiently. It may be a question of a poor mixing of bloods across the atrial septal defect or a persistence of fetal circulation. These failures do not appear rarely to be of technical origin since a second atrioseptostomy rarely proves successful. Prostaglandin used to reopen and dilate the ductus, or Tolazoline, used to reduce the vascular pulmonary resistance, have not proven efficacious. Early Blalock-Hanlon intervention or a Senning procedure are encumbered with a heavy mortality rate. Careful medical treatment can sometimes succeed and permit gaining time but the problem of the early failure of the Rashkind procedure has not yet been solved.

Transposition
with large ventricular septal defect

In this group, cyanosis and acidemia are less important. Tolerance is better and the onset of difficulties is less early than in an isolated transposition. The appearance is that of a large shunt with moderate cyanosis, polypnea, tachycardia and early appearance of global cardiac failure with hepatomegaly and pulmonary edema. The peripheral pulses are usually good, the precordium is hyperactive with a right parasternal impulse. At auscultation, one can generally hear a holosystolic murmur, intense and maximal low on the precordium. The measurement of blood gases shows a moderate peripheral arterial desaturation (PaO₂ between 30 and 40 mm Hg), PCO₂ and pH are usually normal. In the absence of treatment, cyanosis and acidemia become more severe and growth is interrupted.

Chest radiography is characteristic, with a large oval heart, a narrow pedicle and above all an important and diffuse pulmonary hypervascularisation which contrasts with a concave pulmonary arch. Images of pulmonary edema are not infrequent.

The electrocardiogram shows a biventricular enlargement.

The echocardiogram is interesting in these children since the appearance of the large shunt and the moderate cyanosis can mimic a truncus arteriosus, a single ventricle, or a large isolated ventricular septal defect. It reveals an anormal position of the great vessels and the dilatation of the pulmonary artery which is all the more marked when the shunt is larger.

Catheterization and angiocardiography confirm the diagnosis of transposition. A balloon septostomy is recommended in all cases to improve the blood mixing and to reduce the left atrial pressure which is usually high and obstructs pulmonary venous return. Systolic pressures are identical in the two ventricles, aorta and pulmonary artery. Oxymetry confirms the shunt at the ventricular level and estimates its importance. The angiography should be done in the right ventricle then in the left one. It gives precisions on the origin and size of the septal defect. There it is important to measure the pulmonary arterial pressure in order to note whether or not there exists a systolic gradient between the left ventricle and the pulmonary artery. The passage into the pulmonary artery can be performed either from the right ventricle via the septal defect, or from the left ventricle using a Swan-Ganz balloon catheter. In these children the risk of cardiac failure and obstructive pulmonary vascular disease of rapid evolution is such that medical management is

insufficient and they must in any case undergo early—before the age of 6 months—surgical treatment. One has therefore the choice of two procedures: either an early intervention of the Senning or Mustard, type at the same time closing the ventricular septal defect, or, at the latest at 3 months, undertake a banding of the pulmonary artery and subsequently, after the age of one year, an arterial switching using the Jatene procedure. At the moment it is impossible to say which approach will be of greatest value in the future.

Transposition with ventricular septal defect and pulmonary stenosis

Because of the stenosis of the pulmonary tract, there is no risk of obstructive pulmonary vascular disease, and no cardiac failure. The blood mixing is relatively good and cyanosis can be initially moderate. These forms resemble somewhat a tetralogy of Fallot. Cyanosis is variable, increasing during crying. On examination the pulses beat well, there is no cardiomegaly. At auscultation, the first sound is normal, the second sound pure, without splitting. There is usually a loud ejection murmur at the second left intercostal space. If pulmonary stenosis is severe, cyanosis, hypoxemia and acidemia can appear from the first days on and can suddenly become more severe due to the closing of the ductus.

Chest radiography differs little from that for the tetralogy of Fallot: the heart size is small and there is pulmonary hypovascularization; one can at most note that the middle part of the left border is more convex than in the tetralogy of Fallot.

The electrocardiogram rarely shows the signs of left ventricular enlargement that one might expect; vectorcardiogram permits one to evaluate the left ventricular overload.

The echocardiogram confirms the transposition and permits the study of pulmonary stenosis more easily than in the case of tetralogy of Fallot since the pulmonary orifice is behind. The aorta is dilated and the main pulmonary artery is small. The valvular, sub-valvular or diffuse muscular origin of the stenosis can be generally suspected.

Catheterization and angiocardiography confirm the diagnosis. Atrioseptostomy should be done in order to improve the blood mixing but the results are far less dramatic than for the isolated transposition. The left and right ventriculographies show the situation and the size of the ventricular septal defect, the site and degree of the pulmonary stenosis. Axial views are more useful than those in simple profile or the frontal plane. The right and left ventricular pressures are at the same level. It is important to catheterize the pulmonary artery and to measure the systolic pressure gradient between the pulmonary artery and the left ventricle. One can frequently note, in the absence of anatomic pulmonary stenosis, a gradient of between 5 and 20 mm Hg in all the different types of transpositions, but the left ventricle outlet is still normal at angiography. Some pulmonary stenoses are evolutive and can appear or become accentuated between two examinations performed some months apart.

The evolution can be marked by rapid aggravation of cyanosis and anoxic spells. It is legitimate to propose a Blalock-Taussig shunt or a Waterston shunt if the first proves impossible. Complete repair is difficult sincet he stenosis is rarely localized, valvular or sub-valvular and the surgical approach at the outlet of the left ventricle is particularly difficult. One can operate early in the forms where the pulmonary stenosis is moderate or negligeable. In other cases it is preferable to wait until at least the age of three or four years since one will probably need to use a ventriculo-arterial conduit.

Unusual and complex transpositions

Transpositions with pulmonary stenosis and intact ventricular septum are rare. If the stenosis is moderate, it resembles isolated transpositions. If the stenosis is severe it resembles forms with ventricular septal defect and pulmonary stenosis. Evolution and treatment vary according to the severity of the stenosis. It is preferable to ignore moderate stenosis and to operate early on these children. In severe stenosis, the treatment is as that for forms with ventricular septal defect and pulmonary stenosis.

Transpositions with large ductus arteriosus differ little from the form with large ventricular septal defect. There is generally a left sub-clavicular systolic murmur. As the shunt is essentially left-to-right, it is exceptional that one observes a differential cyanosis, more marked in the lower limbs. The diagnosis is generally made at angiography. Medical treatment is rarely sufficient and one is

often lead to an early ligation of the canal. One can associate with it a Blalock-Hanlon septectomy or an early Senning procedure depending on the type of the lesion and the preference of the surgical team.

Transpositions with coarctation of the aorta can be suspected if the femoral pulses are feeble, or if there is a clear gradient of pressures between the lower and the upper limbs. As there is often an associated ductus arteriosus, a bi-directional shunt can be produced between the aorta and pulmonary artery. It is in these forms that one can observe a differential cyanosis predominant in the upper limbs. Comparative oxymetry by a percutaneous approach can improve the accuracy of this sign. Angiography gives precisions on the severity of the coarctation and above all permits one to distinguish an interruption in the aortic arch, which has a more severe prognostic implication. When the coarctation is associated with a large ventricular septal defect, surgical treatment necessitates, in addition to the removal of the coarctation, a banding of the pulmonary artery.

Complex forms are very often the result of L transposition and of a variety of more or less complex Ivemark Syndromes (congenital heart disease and asplenia). Dextrocardia is frequent. It associates with the transposition, a single ventricle, atrioventricular valve anomalies, subaortic and above all subpulmonary obstructions. The anatomic and physiological account of the malformations can best be determined by echocardiogram and angiography. The usefulness of the Rashkind atrial septostomy is doubtful. One may be tempted to propose palliative interventions: banding of the pulmonary artery in the forms with large pulmonary flow, shunt in the forms with clear lungs. One should however keep in mind that if these interventions can be of a temporary benefit, they often lead within a few months or a few years to therapeutic dead-ends.

TOTAL ANOMALOUS PULMONARY VENOUS DRAINAGE

Total anomalous pulmonary venous drainage constitutes, in order of frequency, the fourth commonest cyanotic heart lesion in the newborn infant. It is usually symptomatic before the age of three months.

PATHOLOGY

The anomaly is due to an absence of the incorporation of the common pulmonary vein into the left atrium. According to the modalities of drainage in the fœtal venous system, one can distinguish: supracardiac venous drainage (50 % of the cases) which occurs in 4/5 of the cases into the left superior vena cava and in 1/5 into the right superior vena cava; cardiac venous drainage (25 % of the cases) which occurs in 4/5 of the cases into the coronary sinus and in 1/5 into the right atrium; infracardiac venous drainage (20 % of the cases) which goes into the portal vein or its afferent vessels; and mixed venous drainage (5 % of cases). In about 10 % of cases the venous return is one of the elements of Ivemark's syndrome previousely described.

PATHOPHYSIOLOGY

Total anomalous pulmonary venous return results in: a massive left-to-right atrial shunt since all the pulmonary blood returns to the right atrium; a right-to-left shunt between the atria via a persistent foramen ovale or an atrial septal defect. This shunt, which explains the cyanosis, is obligatory and conditions survival. In addition, there is *stenosis*, between the pulmonary veins and the right atrium, notably in the collector trunk of the pulmonary veins, which results in an obstruction to the pulmonary venous return and plays an important role in the aggravation of this condition. This obstruction is severe and constant in infradiaphragmatic pulmonary venous return since the pulmonary venous blood, in order to return to the right atrium, has to cross the hepatic parenchyma; it is frequent but less severe in supracardiac venous drainage and the exception in cardiac drainage.

CLINICAL PATTERNS

Forms with severe pulmonary venous obstruction and pulmonary hypertension. — Infra-diaphragmatic pulmonary venous drainage is the most characteristic. Functional impairment is early, with tachypnea, severe cyanosis with peripheral arterial desaturation resistant to oxygen therapy. There is always important hepatomegaly. There is no murmur but the second sound is accentuated.

Chest radiography shows a diffuse edema of the pulmonary fields which obscures the cardiac contours and gives a "foggy appearance" to the lungs. This appearance can be confused with that given by hyaline membrane disease. The heart is small: Total anomalous sub-diaphragmatic venous drainage is the only variety of cardiac failure which accompanies a small heart.

The electrocardiogram shows a right diastolic ventricular hypertrophy (right axial deviation of QRS, deep S waves in V5 and V6).

The echocardiogram shows signs of pulmonary hypertension, the left atrium is small, there is no abnormal motion of the septum. The most characteristic sign is the echo-free space behind the left atrium and the left ventricle which corresponds to a venous collector.

Catheterization and angiocardiography reveal severe pulmonary arterial hypertension which can make the injection of contrast material dangerous. Angiocardiography visualises the four pulmonary veins converging behind the heart in a unique vertical collector which crosses the diaphragm.

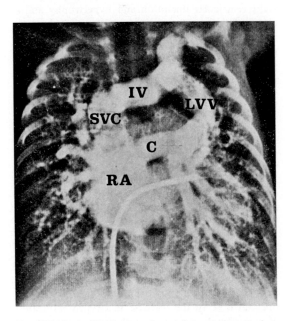

Fig. III-17. — *Total anomalous pulmonary venous drainage into the right atrium, of the supracardiac type. C : retrocardiac collector of the right pulmonary veins, draining into the left vertical vein (LVV). This later is drained to the innominate vein (IV), then to the superior vena cava (SVC) and finally to the right atrium (RA).*

Surgical treatment should be immediately undertaken since the evolution is always fatal in one to three weeks. Under by-pass and profound hypothermia a large anastomosis between the collector trunk and the left atrium is performed. The surgical mortality rate is high.

Forms with severe pulmonary arterial hypertension and moderate or absent venous obstruction.

— Pulmonary vascular resistances are slightly raised but, the pulmonary blood flow being extremely high, the pulmonary arterial pressure is often close to that of the systemic pressure.

Functional signs appear later but before the third month. In the absence of treatment, one can observe a rapid evolution towards congestive cardiac failure with hepatomegaly and pulmonary edema. There is usually no murmur and the second sound is accentuated in the pulmonary area.

The electrocardiogram shows right atrial and ventricular enlargement with a qR or rSR' in V3R and V1.

Chest radiography shows cardiomegaly with right ventricular dilatation and hypertrophy and a clear dilatation of the right atrium and the pulmonary artery; the pulmonary vasculature is definitely accentuated. More specific appearance of some varieties of venous drainage such as supracardiac opacity or figure of eight in the left superior vena cava drainage form are sometimes observed but are less evident when the infant is very young.

The echocardiogram shows indirect signs: diastolic overload of the right ventricle, dilatation of the cavity and abnormal motion of the septum: small left atrium. The direct signs: visibility of the venous collector or the coronary sinus behind the left atrium are less constant and highly debatable.

Catheterization and angiocardiography show greatly increased right heart pressures. On the other hand, it is the only heart disease where oxymetry of the left atrium is recorded below that found in the right atrium and pulmonary artery. The site where one can observe the increase in oxygen saturation of peripheral venous blood (innominate vein, superior vena-cava, right atrium) helps to establish the site of entry of the venous drainage but the most precise examination is selective angiography in the pulmonary arterial trunk. It shows the site of entry and can reveal stenosis of the collector.

Medical management is necessary but not sufficient. *Balloon atrioseptostomy* whilst permitting improved blood mixing between the atria is only transiently effective. It is preferable to undertake a *corrective procedure.* Effectively, the mortality rate is not greater when one operates early on the infant and the risk of rapid development of obstructive pulmonary vascular disease is great. One can carry out, under by-pass and profound hypothermia, an anastomosis between the collector and the left atrium. The surgical mortality rate is still high, at least 30 %; but, on the other hand the long term prognosis for operated cases is excellent.

PULMONARY OBSTRUCTION
WITH VENTRICULAR SEPTAL DEFECT

Lesions in this group have in common a severe obstruction of the pulmonary tract and a ventricular septal defect. The obstruction can extend to complete atresia (pulmonary atresia, tricuspid atresia) and the septal defect to the absence of the septum (single ventricle).

TETRALOGY OF FALLOT

Only the most severe forms of this disease are symptomatic in the neonatal period. The frequency is less than that for complete transposition and atresia or severe pulmonary stenosis with intact ventricular septum. There is no predominance of sex, the weight at birth is usually normal.

Pathology

The essential feature is the marked hypoplasia of the pulmonary tract: infundibular stenosis, valvar stenosis often with bicuspid valve, short main pulmonary artery parting from the annulus to the bifurcation, which is often of good size. The two branches may or may not be of adequate size: the most severe forms are those where the branches are narrow, thus preventing the early establishment of an aorto-pulmonary shunt. The ventricular septal defect is large. The aorta, which is always large, is more or less dextraposed above the ventricular septal defect. The aortic arch is to the right in 1/3 of cases.

Clinical features

Cyanosis is not always prominent. Anoxic spells can often be observed in forms of tetralogy which are only mildly cyanotic, but they are rare before the end of the first month. The systolic murmur is generally ejectional, of 2 to 3/6 intensity, located maximally at the second and third left intercostal space. Sometimes, it is of low intensity or even absent. In this case it is always a question of a very severe form. The second sound is pure and not split. In the forms with anoxic spells the murmur is extremely muffled or absent during the spell, which is also characterised by severe tachycardia. The intravenous injection of propranolol immediately improves the situation and causes the murmur to reappear. There are usually no signs of congestive cardiac failure.

Initial investigation

Chest radiography shows the heart to be rather small, sometimes slightly larger but never beyond a CTR of 0.55. The apex is lifted, the left border is concave or rectilinear. When the pedicle is not masked by the thymus one can see a large aorta overlapping to the right. In one out of three instances, the aortic arch is to the right: this can be suspected on the standard film and confirmed by œsophagal opacification. The lungs are clear with hilums pitted or not clearly defined, the periphery more or less empty.

The electrocardiogram shows a marked right axial deviation with a moderate right ventricular hypertrophy in the precordial leads: R wave is ample, sometimes not followed by an S wave on V1; from V2 or V3, the complex is of the RS type, with a relatively low voltage in V5-V6, an R/S ratio less than 1. In the first weeks the diagnosis of pathological right ventricular enlargement can be difficult: it is therefore necessary to give full attention to the absence of negative conversion of T waves in V1-V2 after the end of the first week.

The echocardiogram shows evidence of one septum and two ventricles. The right ventricle is dilated, the left rather small, the tricuspid echo being ample and easy to record. The recording of the pulmonary valve is difficult if not impossible, whereas the aortic orifice is large. Sweeping permits the recognition of a mitro-aortic continuity but there is not the usual septo-aortic continuity and the aorta straddles the two ventricles. Contrast injection via a venous approach causes echos to appear in the right ventricle, then simultaneously in the aorta and right pulmonary artery.

Catheterization and angiocardiography

These are required during the neonatal period only where there is severe cyanosis which is not improved by oxygen therapy, or which is complicated by acidemia, nursing difficulties, failure in weight gain or, if the cyanosis is moderate, in the case of anoxic spells. The catheter is easily placed in the aorta from the right ventricle. It is generally impossible—and not recommended—to catheterize the pulmonary tract. One confirms the equality of the systolic pressures of the aorta and the right ventricle. Good ventriculography in the frontal and profile view is generally sufficient (Fig. III-18). The ventricular cavity is dilated and the muscular outline is very marked. The infundibular hypertrophy, clearly visible in profile, can appear as a very close filiform stenosis. Above, can be seen a small sub-valvar chamber, then the annulus, most often of reduced size (one third of the aortic size), then the seat of a stenotic dome preceeding a short pulmonary trunk visible only in profile (or in the sitting-up position). In the newborn, the most important point to determine is the size of the branches of the pulmonary artery, which govern the possibilities for a surgical anastomosis. These depend in addition on other factors: i. e. the side of the aortic arch and the length of the innominate trunk and the sub-clavian artery of the opposite side, and the possible existence of an aberrant retro-œsophagal sub-clavian artery.

Treatment

Beta-blocking drugs are usefull in cases with anoxic spells. Often, it is a question of instances which are only mildly cyanotic, with moderate aortic dextroposition, and a particularly tight infundibular stenosis, with a true obliteration by infundibular spasm. At the time of the spells, the intravenous injection of one milligram of propranolol has an immediate effect. Orally, as initial treatment, the dose is from 2 to 5 mg per kg each day. Right heart failure may appear, particularly if one has to use a dose greater than 4 mg/kg, and it therefore can be useful to add small doses of Digoxin.

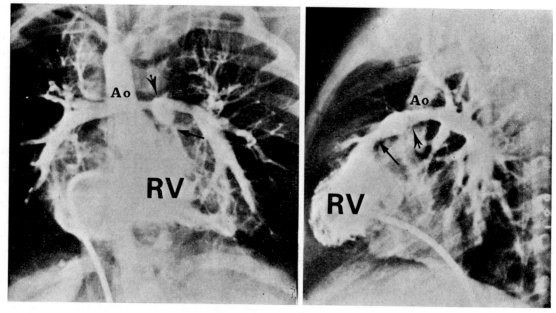

FIG. III-18. — *Tetralogy of Fallot*, severe form in a newborn. Right ventriculogram, frontal and lateral views. The right ventricle (RV) is dilated, pulmonary valve is stenosed, on a very tight annulus, the main pulmonary artery and its branches are small. Early opacification of a large aorta (Ao) straddling both the ventricles.

Surgical treatment is still most often a palliative anastomosis. The *Blalock-Taussig* technique, using the sub-clavian artery, can be used in the newborn thanks to micro-surgical techniques but the anastomosis is of very small calibre and may be either inefficient or become thrombosed. *The Waterston aorto-pulmonary shunt* (between the ascending aorta and the right pulmonary artery) was proposed for the newborn in order to overcome these problems: apart from the fact that it is difficult to calibrate, with a severe risk of pulmonary arterial hypertension, it has the feature of creating a kinking of the pulmonary artery, which compromise future surgical correction. Because of this, other palliative methods are preferred, with some advising recourse even at this age to complete correction.

Recent palliative techniques are: the placing of a small prosthetic aorto-pulmonary conduit, which will be left in place only for a limited time owing to the risk of obstructive pulmonary arterial hypertension; or the enlarging of the pulmonary tract under by-pass by a patch going from the infundibulum to the pulmonary bifurcation, without closure of the ventricular septal defect.

Complete correction is advocated by some in the neonatal period. It necessitates the enlarging of

the pulmonary tract and the closing of the ventricular septal defect. The mortality is still high, but in carefully selected groups has been reported to be not more than 10 % in children operated upon before six months. It is not recommended if the angiocardiography indicates diverse associated anomalies such as an abnormal coronary distribution, double ventricular septal defect, marked hypoplasia or aplasia of one of the two branches of the pulmonary artery.

PULMONARY ATRESIA
WITH OPEN INTERVENTRICULAR SEPTUM

This malformation is most often classed amongst the severe forms of tetralogy of Fallot in the newborn, and represents about one third of the cases.

Pathology

There is total atresia of the pulmonary orifice and sometimes the pulmonary arterial trunk. The right and left pulmonary arteries are often confluent. The pulmonary bifurcation can be fed by a ductus arteriosus either normal (issuing from the sixth distal arch on the same side from the aortic arch which itself issues from the fourth arch and whose concavity gives rise to a short route which rejoins the bifurcation) or aberrant (issuing from the sixth distal arch opposed to the aortic arch and uniting the sub-clavian to the corresponding pulmonary artery by a winding pathway). Most often however, it is the systemic arteries arising from the ascending aorta which assure pulmonary perfusion. They anastomose in the hila with the normal pulmonary arteries whose pathway they often follow. Sometimes, one or several of them vascularize a lobe or pulmonary segment in an autonomous fashion and without connection to the normal arterial tree. These arteries are of irregular calibre, and are twisted with stenosis, above their origin on the aorta, thus protecting the lung from an excess of pressure. The pulmonary infundibulum is reduced to a narrow cul-de-sac or is totally absent, the ventricular septal defect is large and the aorta strongly dextraposed.

Clinical features

The cyanosis is almost always intense, complicated sometimes by anoxic crises and there is no cardiac failure. But there exist forms with a moderate cyanosis, susceptible to develop, as a result of a particularly important pulmonary circulation from systemic arteries, cardiac failure like that of the common arterial trunk. In this case one can hear throughout the thorax, and particularly in the back, continuous, intense and diffuse murmurs. In the usual forms, it is the continuous murmur which, associated with severe cyanosis, suggests the diagnosis. There is often a ductus arteriosus murmur heard under the left clavicle or to the right. This may also be a dorsal murmur, whose confirmation is more difficult.

Complementary examinations

The results are highly comparable to those obtained in the tetralogy of Fallot.

The radiological silhouette is more "caricatural", with a marked concavity in place of the region of the pulmonary artery. Careful examination of the pulmonary zones and the hila show the abnormal vascularization: It is not unusual to find opacities due to large abnormal systemic arteries, twisting or appearing sliced in the form of rounded parahilar opacities.

The electrocardiogram does not differ from that of the tetralogy of Fallot. Sometimes, however, there is a combined ventricular enlargement.

The echocardiogram does not show evidence of a pulmonary orifice but this does not eliminate tetralogy; the aorta straddles the two ventricles. With a suprasternal approach, the appearance of the contrast injected via the venous tract in the right pulmonary artery, when one can record it under the aorta where there is a ductus arteriosus, is always second to its appearance in the aortic arch; Here it is continuous *i. e.* non pulsed.

Catheterization and angiocardiography

The aim of the technique is to show the likelihood of a pulmonary arterial bifurcation, in the case of severe precocious anoxia, to permit an anastomosis or to allow the placing of an aorto-pulmonary tube. The aorta is reached from the right ventricle and its injection gives the most useful information. In one out of two cases it is the ductus arteriosus which, clearly visible in the concavity of the aorta, permits this opacification. In the more favourable forms, the atresia involves only the sigmoid orifice and the retrograde opacification of the trunk reaches the adjacent region at the extremity of the narrow infundibulum. In less favourable cases aortography shows the twisted abnormal arterial trunks arising from the descending aorta and going into the lungs. It permits one often to see, via the intermediary of the anastomosis, that a pulmonary bifurcation exists. If one can not see it in this way, one can try a retrograde pulmonary venous injection which at this age is not without risk.

TREATMENT

Medical treatment is directed firstly to forms with voluminous systemic arteries, which are slightly cyanotic and often necessitate digitalization. In the highly anoxic forms, beta-blocking treatment, although illogical since there is no infundibular spasm, can however be useful.

Surgical treatment remains unsatisfactory. A Blalock shunt can be performed if the size of the branches permits it. The most interesting possibility consists, in the case of the bringing to light of a pulmonary arterial bifurcation of acceptable calibre (2 or 3 mm at least), of the placing of an aorto-pulmonary tube. The result can be spectacular as concerns the improvement of the anoxia and the subsequent growth of the pulmonary artery, permitting one to prepare for a more complete correction by a right ventricle to pulmonary artery valved tube and closing of the ventricular septal defect. In the case of pure valvar atresia, the opening and enlarging by a patch of the pulmonary infundibular tract without an associated closing of the interventricular communication is the most logical solution.

ABSENCE OF THE PULMONARY VALVE WITH VENTRICULAR SEPTAL DEFECT

This rare malformation was once considered as a special form of tetralogy of Fallot. In fact, its physiology is very different from that of the tetralogy, particularly in the newborn, where its gravity is caused more by the respiratory difficulty than by the consequence of the right-to-left shunt.

Pathology

The pulmonary ring is avalvar and most often stenosed. The ventricular septal defect is large, of the same type as in a tetralogy. *The aneurysmal dilatation of the pulmonary artery* is constant and large, giving an appearance of a large swollen bag to the arterial trunk and its bifurcated branches.

Clinical features

There is primarily respiratory distress: tachypnea, wheezing, episodes of dyspnea. Cyanosis is of lesser order, cardiac failure is rare. A liver lowered by emphysematous thoracic distension should not be mistaken for true hepatomegaly. The double meso-cardiac murmur, systolo-diastolic, intense and sometimes rough, is suggestive of the malformation but it is not entirely constant as the diastolic murmur can be missing. The phonocardiogram can show the absence of the second pulmonary sound.

Complementary examinations

On X ray, the pulmonary artery is salient and expansive. The dilatation of the main pulmonary artery sometimes shows as a transverse opacity which runs into the hila but this can be hidden by the thymus, and thus is more easily observed in profile. Beyond the very dilated hila the pulmonary zones are only slightly vascularised which is the basis of the atelectatic zones and obstructive emphysema.

The electrocardiogram reveals a right ventricular diastolic overload with large and crotcheted complexes in the right precordial leads.

The echocardiogram shows signs of a right ventricular diastolic overload with paradoxical septal movement. It is not possible to record the echo of the pulmonary valve.

Catheterization and angiocardiography

The right ventricular hypertension is usually at the systemic level and there is almost always a notable systolic gradient between the right ventricle and the pulmonary artery. The characteristic feature is the lowering of the diastolic pressure of the pulmonary artery, with the absence of dicrotic notching. The shunt is not exclusively left-to-right as in tetralogy, but bi-directional, via the ventricular septal defect. Selective angiography in the main pulmonary artery shows the aneurysm, but it is to be avoided during the neonatal period, it being preferable to undertake a right ventriculography and, if possible, a retrograde aortography, in order to eliminate the other two heart defects which present a double murmur during the neonatal period: e. g. truncus arteriosus and aorto-left ventricular tunnel.

Treatment

In forms which are poorly tolerated from birth, treatment remains highly unsatisfactory and the mortality rate exceeds 75 %.

Medical treatment involves pulmonary therapy and antibiotics. Digitalis like drugs have few indications. Artificial respiration should be avoided, except for the cases amenable to surgical treatment, since these children risk becoming machine dependent.

Surgical treatment, which is useful for older children, has not for the moment permitted success during the neonatal period. Aneurysmorraphy, early banding of the pulmonary artery and sometimes lobectomy have been proposed. Complet correction, the closing of the ventricular septal defect and the insertion of a valvar prosthesis, is only possible in older children. The most logical solution is perhaps simple closing of the communication, with or without aneurysmorraphy.

TRICUSPID ATRESIA

Pathology

This malformation can be defined by the absence of a right atrio-ventricular connection. In fact, with the exception of the rare cases where an imperforated tricuspid valve separates the right atrium from a patent but hypoplastic right ventricular sinus, tricuspid atresia is always associated with *the absence of the inlet chamber of the right ventricle.* The right ventricle is reduced to a trabeculated area and to an outflow tract communicating with the left ventricle via a ventricular septal defect. The ventricular morphology is the same as that for the single ventricle of the type A of Van Praagh (double inlet left ventricle and an outlet chamber giving rise to one of the great vessels). Only the absence of a right atrio-ventricular connection distinguishes tricuspid atresia from this type of single ventricle. The modern classification puts tricuspid atresia in the *univentricular heart* group (univentricular heart of the left type with absence of the right atrio-ventricular connection and outlet chamber).

There are some anatomic forms which comprise an increased pulmonary vasculature, a large heart, cardiac failure and mild cyanosis or its absence: its appearance is therefore identical to that of a large ventricular septal defect or single ventricle without pulmonary stenosis and the treatment is the same: digoxin and diuretics with palliative banding of the pulmonary artery, except where the ventricular septal defect becomes rapidly symptomatic.

The most frequent forms (75 % of cases) have decreased pulmonary vasculature. Occasionally it is a question of pulmonary atresia and the vasculature is assured by the ductus arteriosus. Most often there is either valvar or subvalvar pulmonary stenosis or a ventricular septal defect.

The evacuation of blood reaching the right atrium from the venae cavae can be made only towards the left atrium, more or less easily, by a real atrial septal defect, sometimes large, or by a "forced" foramen ovale, which can be narrow with a dilatation or hypertrophy of the right atrium.

Clinical features

The appearance is very close to that of severe tetralogy. Cyanosis is marked, a loud systolic murmur (3 to 4/6) harsh and holosystolic, of the ventricular septal defect type is generally heard. In the case of pulmonary atresia a continuous murmur is generally heard, as in other malformations with pulmonary atresia and patent ductus arteriosus. In the case of associated transposition of the great vessels, the second sound is particularly loud. Hepatomegaly is usual and there can be venous distension in the neck.

Complementary examinations

The X ray does not reveal a truly pathognomic silhouette. However, the prolongation of the left inferior arch which is convex and elongated, is suggestive of this defect. Sometimes, it shows a bulging in the upper part, in relation to the outlet chamber. The enlargement of the right border depends on the size of the atrial septal defect: it can be missing if the latter is large. The aortic arch is always on the left.

The electrocardiogram generally suggests the diagnosis: a marked left axis (— 30° to — 90°) is constant in the form with clear lungs and is associated with a left ventricular enlargement in the precordial leads: pattern rS with S deep in V1, qR in V6 with an RV6 which is not necessarily very ample. The T wave can be negative in V5 and V6. The P wave is generally ample and peaked in II-III-VF: in the case of a large atrial septal defect, it can even be gigantic.

The echocardiogram does not record a tricuspid valve in the M-mode and does not show a tricuspid orifice in the bidimensional mode. The left atrium and the left ventricle are dilated, the mitral valve is of great amplitude. The interventricular septum is easily visible, and hyperkinetic. The right ventricle and the main pulmonary artery appear to be small. Mitro-aortic and septo-aortic continuity is present.

Catheterization and angiocardiography

It is not possible to pass the catheter into the right ventricle: the only passage obtainable goes from the right atrium towards the left atrium and the left ventricle. In the neonatal period, it is not possible to enter the sub-pulmonary outlet chamber, nor the pulmonary artery. The right atrial hypertension and the systolic gradient between right atrium and left atrium are greater when the atrial septal defect is narrow. The frontal and lateral angio-cardiography with an injection into the right atrium gives the characteristic image of absence of the tricuspid valve and a right ventricular sinus: the contrast opacifies a large right atrium and flows into the supra-hepatic veins, then opacifies the left atrium and the dilated left ventricle. Frontal view shows an empty triangular area with the superior summit between the right atrium and the left ventricle. The ventricular septal defect and the sub-pulmonary outlet chamber are clearly visible and signify stenosis of the pulmonary tract. The main pulmonary artery is often narrow, but the branches are generally of good calibre, permitting palliative surgery. In the regular form, the great vessels are found in the normal position. In the forms with transposition, this is generally of the D-type: the aorta is prominent and to the right, arising from the accessory chamber, with a stenosed pulmonary artery emerging from the principal chamber. Forms with pulmonary atresia and opacification of the pulmonary artery via the ductus arteriosus are rare. Forms with increased pulmonary vasculature show a different picture; most often the aorta is transposed.

Treatment

The early mortality rate is extremely high (more than two thirds of the cases). The results of palliative procedures are still very poor. Some authors discuss the expediency of these measures. Waterston anastomosis before one month and Blalock-Taussig shunt beyond one month are logical, but hold a high surgical mortality (at least 30 %) and a secondary risk of distorsion of the pulmonary artery in the case of a Waterston anastomosis. If the child survives, it should generally undergo a second palliative procedure. Beyond the age of two, this can be a Glenn cavo-pulmonary shunt. Later the "ortho-terminal" physiological correction by the Fontan procedure (the insertion of a valvar tube between right atrium and main pulmonary artery) could be proposed. When right atrial stasis is very marked, catheterization during the neonatal period should be completed with balloon atrial septostomy, using the Rashkind technique. This should not however be done routinely. In cases of survival, it is important, in view of a possible future Fontan procedure, to assure good right atrial musculature, which is not the case if the atrial septal defect is too large.

COMPLEX CYANOTIC HEART DISEASES

This group of heart defects represents about 3 % of cardiac disease in the newborn. They fall principally into the category of the *syndrome of Ivemark*, with splenic abnormalities and anomalies of visceral situs. Indications for surgery are difficult to establish and the results of surgery particularly poor.

Pathology

Stenosis or atresia of the pulmonary tract is a feature common to these malformations. A *sequential approach* permits their classification. It is helpful to review successively: atrio-visceral situs, patterns of venous drainage into the atria, atrio-ventricular connections, ventricular morphology and ventriculo-arterial connections. The most common ventricular type is the *single ventricle*. Ventricular morphology permits us to definite a "left" type, the most frequent, or "right" type and an "ambiguous" type. There may or may not be an accessory chamber communicating with the main ventricular chamber. This accessory chamber can be blind (trabecular pouch) or lead to one of the two great vessels (outlet chamber). The position of the great vessels is variable. They are often *transposed* (aorta anterior and to the right of the pulmonary artery, or anterior and to the left). Each can originate from one of the ventricles or, in the case of a single ventricle, from each of the two chambers, the main one and the accessory one. Thus, in a frequent variety of single ventricle, the left type with sub-aortic outlet chamber, the aorta is anterior and to the left. Types with very varied morphology and connections can also be seen. The atrio-ventricular connections can be *"discordant"* with a heart in atrio-visceral situs solitus, the right atrium opens into a ventricle of the left type situated to the right, the left atrium into a ventricle of the right type, situated to the left. Atrio-ventricular connections can also be of the *atrio-ventricular canal* type, sometimes with a *single atrium*. The ventriculo-arterial connections are sometimes of the *double outlet type (right or left)*. There often exists straddling, as much in the atrio-ventricular connections (straddling of the tricuspid valve above the two ventricles, whereas the mitral valve only hangs over one part of the left ventricle) as in the ventriculo-arterial connections (overriding aorta or pulmonary artery). Finally, there may be associated *abnormal pulmonary or systemic venous returns*.

A complex heart defect is easily suspected when an anomaly of the visceral situs is found. Effectively in the presence of severe cyanosis and of ambiguus situs, one should think of the *Ivemark or asplenia syndrome*. Situs ambiguus, which is opposed to situs solitus or inversus, manifests itself in the form of a "double right side" or "dextro-isomerism". There is absence of the spleen, the liver is median and symetrical, with symetrical lungs both with three lobes. The stomach is to the left or the right, the heart in levocardia (apex to the left) or more rarely in dextrocardia, sometimes in mesocardia. Apart from stenosis or pulmonary atresia, there is most often an anomalous pulmonary venous drainage, an atrio-ventricular canal, a single ventricle or a double outlet right ventricle, or a transposition of the great vessels. *In the polysplenia syndrome* ("double left side" or "levo-isomerism", bi-lobed symmetric lungs, anomalous systemic venous drainage), stenosis or atresia of the pulmonary tract is less constant and it is the left-to-right shunt with pulmonary hypervasculature and a large heart which predominates.

Clinical features and diagnosis

The determination of the position of the thoraco-abdominal viscera is the initial procedure which will orientate one, in the presence of severe cyanosis and minimal enlargement of the heart, towards complex heart disease. Dextrocardia is sometimes noted but levocardia is more common. On the other hand, the medial and symetric liver is easy to diagnose both clinically and radiologically. The location of the gastric fundus is highly suggestive if it appears on the opposite side to the apex of the heart. The tracheal bifurcation, on a high penetration film is the best indicator of the visceral situs. Splenic scintigraphy, the presence or absence of the splenic artery on the aortogram, the search for Howell-Jolly and Heinz bodies in the blood can help the diagnosis but are not entirely without error.

The electrocardiogram is often useful, particularly if it shows a negative PI wave (inversed atrial situs), a positive PI (situs atrial solitus), sometimes a dual sinus rhythm (dextro-isomerism) or a junctionnal rhythm (levo-isomerism).

Echocardiography permits one to assess the complexity of the malformation and to attempt to analyse it with contrast injection. It is sometimes more reliable than the angiocardiogram for confirming certain findings: for example the absence of one of the atrio-ventricular orifices.

Catheterization and angiocardiography yield a complete and precise account of the lesions: abnormal pulmonary or systemic venous drainage, anomalies of the cavities, malpositions of the great vessels, stenosis or atresia of the pulmonary tract.

Evolution and treatment

The natural history is studded with complications related to the heart disease (anoxic spells), to the immunologic defect due to the splenic anomalies (severe infectious episodes) or to both (cerebral vascular accidents). It is most often quickly fatal.

Medical treatment rests on oxygen therapy, the prophylaxis of infections and sometimes digitalis.

Surgical treatment can only in exceptional cases result in a complete correction. If it is generally possible to envisage a palliative surgical intervention which will permit the child to survive, this is of high risk and generally leads after a few months to a therapeutic impasse.

PULMONARY OBSTRUCTION
WITH INTACT VENTRICULAR SEPTUM

Atresia or severe stenosis of the pulmonary valve with intact ventricular septum is quite common in the newborn. It is the degree of hypoplasia of the right heart structures (the right ventricular cavity ring and tricuspid valve) which determine their gravity.

Pathology

The basic lesion involves the pulmonary ring: It is always hypoplastic and, if accompanied either by a valvar dome pierced by a punctiform orifice, or an unperforated diaphragm, sometimes doubled with a layer of myocardium on its ventricular face, one can speak of severe stenosis or true atresia. The main pulmonary artery is generally hypoplastic but its calibre may be normal. Associated lesions are frequent and affect the right ventricle and tricuspid valve. The ventricular cavity is almost always underdeveloped and, in 80 % of the cases, this reduction is considerable: the infundibulum is often atretic and the inlet chamber is a small sphere communicating with the coronary arteries and the aorta by sinusoids whose development across the very thick right ventricular wall sometimes encompasses true coronary fistulas. The tricuspid ring is also small, all the more so where right ventricular underdevelopment is severe, and the tricuspid valve is often thick and dysplastic; it is not unusual that it indicates an Ebstein's anomaly. In a minority of cases, the ventricular cavity is less underdeveloped and allows for a complete but blind infundibulum: the tricuspid ring is thus less small but still insufficient. In all forms, the foramen ovale and the ductus arteriosus are the only paths permitting pulmonary perfusion.

Clinical features

Cyanosis is the major sign. It is generalised, intense and present from birth or within the first few hours of life. It is not responsive to any form of oxygenation and is accompanied by a deep and refractory hypoxemia. Rarely, cyanosis is considerably more discrete because the ductus arteriosus assures a large aorto-pulmonary shunt. In half of the cases, this cyanosis is the only visible anomaly in a newborn in apparently good health. But in the other half, it is associated with respiratory difficulties which reflect heart failure, acidemia or both. At examination, hepatomegaly is inconstant and modest: the peripheral pulses are variable; a jugular pulse is visible in the case of an associated massive tricuspid regurgitation. A significant murmur can be heard two out of three times: systolic, ejectional, maximal in the pulmonary area; pansystolic, low at the xiphoid; or continuous left sub-clavicular.

Complementary examinations

On X-ray, the most evident feature is the clarity of the two pulmonary areas. The size of the heart is slightly augmented in two thirds of the cases; it can be massively increased such that the cardio-thoracic ratio is greater than 0.75. In this case an associated

Ebstein anomaly may be suspected. In all cases, the silhouette associates a bulging right atrium on the right border and a large left ventricle on the left border with a blunt apex detached from the diaphragm and the absence of a pulmonary artery arch. The aortic arch is always to the left of the trachea.

The electrocardiogram almost always records right atrial enlargement, a QRS axis between $+ 150°$ and $0°$ (loop in the anti-clockwise direction) and a left ventricular overload or enlargment. Right ventricular overload is much more rare.

With this preliminary analysis, the association of a refractory hypoxemia with decreased pulmonary vasculature strongly suggests an obstruction at the right side of the heart. A distinct or moderate cardiomegaly suggests the integrity of the ventricular septum. One can hope that the right heart underdevelopment will not be too severe when the following signs are present: ejectional systolic murmur of tricuspid insufficiency, enlarged heart, right ventricular overload. Inversely one fears a severe right ventricular and tricuspid valve underdevelopment when there is no murmur or only a continuous murmur, the cardiomegaly is minimal or absent and the left ventricular overload distinct. When the size of the heart is only increased a little, it suggests severe pulmonary obstruction with open ventricular septum, tricuspid atresia, transposition of the great vessels with ventricular septal defect and pulmonary stenosis. When there is cardiomegaly and tricuspid insufficiency, it suggests all the other causes of right atrio-ventricular regurgitation ranging from Ebstein's anomaly to a normally structured heart with the syndrome of persistence of the fetal circulation.

The echocardiogram is of considerable value. It permits one to identify a normal or dilated posterior ventricular cavity and a large posterior vessel whose walls are in normal continuity with the ventricular septum in front and the posterior atrio-ventricular valve behind. The bi-dimensional study furnishes very clear images: distinct hypoplasia of the anterior ventricle and the anterior atrio-ventricular valve, impossibility to record the pulmonary valves, small pulmonary artery, identification of the posterior vessel as the aorta.

Catheterization and angiocardiography

Introduced by the venous route, the catheter easily reaches the left atrium from the right one

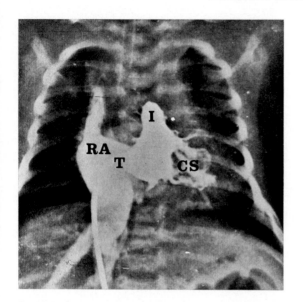

FIG. III-19. — *Pulmonary atresia with intact ventricular septum.* Right ventriculogram. Small right ventricle, blind infundibulum (I), large intramyocardial coronary sinusoids (CS), small tricuspid valve (T) which is insufficient, resulting in a large regurgitation into the right atrium (RA).

and can also lead to the left ventricle. Penetration into the right ventricle is often difficult owing to the small dimensions of the tricuspid ring and the ventricular cavity. One can record, on right atrial pressure curves, a very ample "*a*" wave, a mean pressure superior to that of the left atrium and, sometimes, a large regurgitation "*v*" wave. The right ventricular pressure is very high, being equal or superior to that of the left ventricle, with a sharp pointed aspect to the curve. A major right-to-left shunt at the atrial level is usually noted, reflecting the profound desaturation of the blood in the left heart. The angiocardiography should be done selectively in the right ventricle in the right anterior oblique view and in the lateral with a small quantity of contrast (0.5 ml/kg) pushed by hand. One can thus see a small blind ventricular cavity with infundibular atresia without any direct passage towards the pulmonary artery: it is in the most severe variety, "drop-shaped"; unfortunately, this is the most frequent appearance (70 % of cases). Less frequently the inlet chamber continues via a contractile infundibulum which frays like a "radish tail" or, in more favourable cases, ends under a well formed valvar roof which is atretic or slightly permeable. The following four anomalies can be commonly observed: a variable number of dilated and twisted sinusoids, sometimes opacifying the

coronary arteries and the aorta in the manner of ventriculo-coronary fistulae, running in the thickness of the right ventricular muscle; an underdevelopment of the tricuspid ring; a tricuspid regurgitation towards a dilated right atrium, then to the left side of the heart; pulmonary arterial filling from the aorta by the ductus arteriosus. This last point is identified by an oblique and left anterior ventriculography which in addition confirms the integrity of the ventricular septum, or by isthmic retrograde aortography in respect to the ductus arteriosus. In both cases, one can opacify the pulmonary trunk to the orificial diaphragm, principally visible in the lateral view, and eliminate any possibility of "functional" pulmonary atresia.

Natural history and management

The spontaneous evolution is extremely severe and the majority of newborns die in a few hours to a few days with a picture of anoxemia, acidosis and intractable cardiac failure. Some infants can survive for a few months after the neonatal period, thanks to the maintenance of the patency of a large ductus arteriosus.

Medical treatment is very limited: the digitalis like drugs are not very efficient and even dangerous; oxygen therapy is ineffective and can even contribute to the closing of the ductus arteriosus; the buffering of the acidemia has only transient and partial effects. Diuretics and artificial ventilation are the most useful of the temporizing methods. In the case of urgency, the only real effective treatment is the continuous infusion of prostaglandin E_1, if possible via an umbilical catheter at the level of the ductus arteriosus. The effect is immediate and dramatic: the canal dilates, the pulmonary output increases, the cyanosis and hypoxemia diminish or disappear, the hemodynamic condition normalizes and the acidemia corrects itself. To the extent that the effect of this treatment ceases immediately when one stops, but where its prolongation can lead to vascular alterations giving rise to fear of rupture, it should only, initially, be considered a palliative measure to be followed mandatorily by surgical intervention.

Surgical treatment in the newborn calls upon several surgical methods of unequal therapeutic value. Favourable forms, without extreme underdevelopment of the tricuspid ring and right ventricle, are potentially curable during the neonatal period with open heart surgery and should benefit from a pulmonary valvotomy by a pulmonary arterial or transventricular approach, associated with an aorto-pulmonary shunt. One can thus assure good pulmonary arterial output and hope that the size of the right ventricle will improve in time. In the light of this, the Rashkind atrioseptostomy is not advisable, as it promotes an atrial right-to-left shunt to the detriment of the direction of the right tract. Unfavourable forms are those where the tricuspid and right ventricular underdevelopment is very severe. One can choose between the former treatment mentioned, or a Rashkind atrioseptostomy followed by an aorto-pulmonary shunt, with a pulmonary valvotomy of "decompression" and a view to an ultimate procedure of the Fontan type. In fact, the results are poor, and even if the immediate mortality rate has declined, the long term future of these children is highly uncertain and the appropriateness of undertaking a major medico-surgical approach in these truly hypoplastic right heart syndromes should be seriously considered.

RIGHT-TO-LEFT ATRIAL SHUNTS

Some cases of refractory cyanosis in neonates are due to the entry of low-oxygenated blood into the left atrium, either from the right atrium by an organic or functional obstruction to any part of the right heart, or directly from the venous system resulting from an anomalous caval drainage.

OBSTRUCTIVE LESIONS OF THE RIGHT HEART

Abnormalities of very diverse types (malformations, tumours, degenerations, vaso-constrictive reactions) can affect the different segments of the right heart or its valves, causing an obstruction to the pulmonary outflow. In addition to the right-to-left shunt which results, there is tricuspid regurgitation, whose severity regulates the degree of cardiac failure and cardiomegaly with clear lungs which accompanies the cyanosis.

Anomalies of the right atrium

Specific tumours either develop in the atrial cavity from the septum or the tricuspid ring (rhabdomyomas) or compress the atrium from the pericardial cavity (teratomas). In all cases, they restrict the tricuspid flow and are easily recognisable on bidimensional echocardiography. Some are removable by a relatively simple procedure which should be curative.

Persistence of the valve of the sinus venosus can, occasionally, play a severely obstructive role. Echocardiography reveals the diagnosis. It is a lesion curable by surgery.

Anomalies of the tricuspid valve

The most severe form of tricuspid obstruction, atresia, has been discussed previously. Some other anomalies may also produce an obstruction: they constitute the group of *congenital tricuspid insufficiencies*.

Ebstein's anomaly. — Here there is a question of the attachment of the proximal part of the septal and posterior leaflets onto the corresponding walls of the right ventricle, hence a displacement towards the apparent point of insertion of these valves around a new orifice. Between the fibrous tricuspid ring and this distal orifice, the ventricular walls are very thin, *i. e.* "atrialised". This is the "intermediary chamber" between the right atrium and the outlet part of the right ventricle. The asynchronicity of the contractions between the right atrium and this intermediary chamber leads to a defect in the filling of the right ventricle, a reduction in pulmonary flow, tricuspid regurgitation and a right-to-left atrial shunt. These are all the more marked in the newborn where the pulmonary vascular resistence high and one can speak of true "functional pulmonary atresia". The most serious forms of this malformation are those which reveal themselves at birth and it is not uncommon for them to be associated with other anomalies, particularly atresia or stenosis of the pulmonary valve. Cyanosis is constant, sometimes accompanied by tachypnea and hepatomegaly. A soft systolic murmur low on the left sternal border or the xiphoid, suggestive of tricuspid regurgitation, is very common but additional sounds (3rd or 4th) are more rare than in the older child. The cardiomegaly, often massive, with a cardio-thoracic ratio greater than 0.75 and decreased pulmonary vasculature, are highly suggestive. On the electrocardiogram, right atrial enlargement and right bundle branch block are very common; not uncommonly one can observe arrhythmias (supra-ventricular tachycardia), disturbances of conduction or pre-excitation (Wolff-

Parkinson-White syndrome). Echocardiography is specific in diagnosis because it can easily record the anterior valve of the tricuspid, at the left border of the sternum which opens and above all closes distinctly later than the mitral valve. Only in doubtful cases is it necessary to have recourse to catheterization. The displacement of the true right ventricle to the left side, a right ventricular systolic pressure below 40 mm Hg and the recording of a peculiar endocavitary electrocardiogram are sufficient for the diagnosis. Angiocardiography is dangerous and should be reserved only for atypical cases or when one feels uncertain about pulmonary stenosis. It is then done in the distal right ventricle preferably in the right anterior oblique view so that one can see the succession of the three chambers (right atrium, intermediary chamber, outflow chamber) separated by two notches; the true tricuspid ring and the distal functional ring.

The prognosis is serious and death occurs in over half of the cases during the first month of life, particularly if there is massive cardiomegaly, severe cyanosis or an associated malformation. Beyond that, the decrease in pulmonary resistance permits one to hope for a more favourable evolution but three dangers still threaten these children: arrhythmias, cardiac failure and persistent hypoxemia causing polycythemia.

No surgical treatment is possible during the neonatal period. It is preferable above all to avoid any intervention likely to increase pulmonary vascular resistance. Some have even suggested using Tolazoline to diminish the resistance and to thus increase pulmonary flow.

Congenital tricuspid dysplasia. — In some cases the tricuspid tensor apparatus is badly formed: the free side of the valves are attached to the ventricular walls by cords which are much too short, rudimentary, or almost absent. The clinical picture is close to that of the Ebstein's anomaly: *i. e.* constant refractory cyanosis, frequent cardiac failure, murmur of tricuspid regurgitation, massive cardiomegaly, right atrial enlargement. The diagnosis is difficult to make precisely, even after angiography which above all shows the tricuspid regurgitation. Many of these newborns die but symptomatic treatment can be effective.

Transient tricuspid insufficiency. — This syndrome affects newborns who have generally had fetal compromise. Refractory cyanosis, respiratory difficulties, hepatomegaly, a systolic murmur maximal at the xiphoid, a sometimes massive radiological

cardiomegaly with clear lungs, and right and left ventricular overload are the principal features of it but are not specific. Diffuse alterations of repolarisation and high levels of creatine-phospho-kinase MB bear witness to the myocardial ischemia, which is probably the cause of this syndrome.

Echocardiography and hemodynamic studies show that the heart is structurally normal: the pressures in the right ventricle and the pulmonary artery are normal, the tricuspid is incontinent and there is a massive right-to-left shunt at the atrial level. A transient tricuspid insufficiency can complicate the syndrome of persistence of fetal circulation: the pulmonary pressures are then raised and treatment with Tolazoline may be tried.

Anomalies
of the right ventricle

Anomalies which change the compliance of the right ventricle to the point of favouring tricuspid regurgitation and a right-to-left shunt via the foramen ovale are rare in the newborn. They present with refractory cyanosis, cardiac failure and cardiomegaly of variable degree, clear lungs, right atrial enlargement, and sometimes electrical signs of left ventricular predominance.

Isolated hypoplasia of the right ventricle can be recognized on angiography by a marked reduction in volume of the right ventricular filling chamber with a proportional reduction of the tricuspid ring and dilatation of the right atrium. The prognosis is variable.

Uhl's anomaly consists of an absence of the myocardial fibres of the wall of the right ventricle wall, leading to a failure in its contractility. The forms in the newborn are generally associated with pulmonary valve atresia, and/or agenesis of the tricuspid apparatus. The evolution is rapidly fatal and diagnosis usually made at autopsy.

Tumours of the right ventricle, particularly rhabdomyomas, can obstruct the right tract. They can be easily recognised on echocardiography and are operable. Partial removal can suffice to free the obstruction and cure the child. There are in addition rare cases where the right ventricular cavity is encumbered by hypertrophic bundles which hamper pulmonary ejection. This *"proliferative myocardiopathy"*, *i. e.* pseudotumor, is capable of spontaneous remission.

Anomalies of the pulmonary valve

Stenosis and atresia of the pulmonary valve have been discussed separately. It suffices here to indicate that they constitute the essential diagnostic differential in all other right-to-left shunts at the atrial level which can mimic it, even on angiography, when the raised pulmonary arterial resistance forms an obstruction to ejection from the right ventricle.

Syndrome of persistence of foetal circulation

Already described elsewhere, this syndrome should be mentioned here since it raises problems of diagnostic possibilities with numerous organic or functional heart diseases.

It generally follows perinatal stress in a term infant. The persistence of the raised pulmonary arterial resistance is the cause of right ventricular and pulmonary arterial hypertension, of right-to-left shunt via the ductus arteriosus and sometimes with resultant tricuspid insufficiency via the foramen ovale. The refractory cyanosis is always associated with respiratory distress of variable degree and often with a large liver, a xiphoid systolic murmur and cardiomegaly with clear lungs. Echocardiography may identify a normal heart suggesting pulmonary hypertension. In case of doubt, an endocavitary investigation proves the pulmonary hypertension and the ductal and atrial right-to-left shunts, without any malformations. A trial of treatment with Tolazoline is often effective but demands strict hemodynamic control.

ANOMALIES OF CAVAL DRAINAGE

It can happen that part or all of the systemic venous drainage flows abnormally into the left atrium. This situation is exceptional, rarely isolated and commonly associated with complex malformations. In order that such a malformation be cyanotic, it is necessary that the abnormally connected vena cava carry the drainage from a large area. The cyanosis is isolated, in a child in apparently perfect health: the clinical and complementary examinations are normal and it is the angiography and contrast echocardiography via the veins of the left arm, the right arm or the inferior vena cava which will enable a diagnosis of abnormal drainage at the left atrium of a left superior vena cava (directly or by the coronary sinus), of an inferior vena cava, or of all the venae cavae. Only the very cyanotic forms are justifiable re surgery to avoid pulmonary infections or thrombotic accidents.

Neonatal heart failure, collapse and cardiogenic shock

DIAGNOSIS OF NEONATAL HEART FAILURE

Heart disease which presents at birth as serious cardiac failure is common and, often requires urgent diagnosis and treatment.

Definition. Initial signs

The newborns in this group quickly show themselves to be ill and sometimes even in danger of dying. Respiratory function is always perturbed: tachypnea, constant or post-prandial, or respiratory distress, leading to the child's exhaustion. On examination, hepatomegaly is always palpable and the cardiac sounds are rapid, dull, sometimes with a gallop rhythm. Two other non-specific signs can be observed: cyanosis, often mild and above all sensitive to the oxygenation of the child; collapse with a greyish face, a generalized marbled skin, with a lengthy time for recolouration; a weak or absent pulse; oligo-enuresis.

It is important to obtain the initial measures of diagnostic importance, that is a radiograph of the thorax and an electrocardiogram. It is also necessary to collect certain biological information in order to evaluate the gravity of the illness and to guide the initial therapeutic measures: acid base balance, electrolytes, glucose and calcium. Initiation of symptomatic treatment, possibly prior to any transfer of the child, is sometimes mandated by the severity of the lesion. One can resort to the administration of a strong diuretic (furosemide), to a digitalis preparation with rapid action (digoxin), to the correction of the principal biological disorders, principally acidemia and/or hypoglycemia and, in the most menacing cases, to artificial respiration with intermittent or continuous positive pressure.

Etiologic diagnosis

Diagnosis of the cardiac origin. — It is not always easy to see that serious illness in a child is due to heart disease since other diseases can express themselves by secondary cardiac involvement or can simulate cardiac failure.

Newborns of diabetic mothers often have large viscera, particularly the liver and the heart. It is easy to recognise these children by their cushingoid appearance, even if the maternal antecedent is not known. However, they are sometimes authentically subject to hypertrophic cardiomyopathies, which formally counterindicate digitalization: the echocardiograph confirms the diagnosis and should avoid catheterization.

Transient myocardial ischaemia is a syndrome affecting newborn-babies born at term after a perinatal insult, with cardiac failure, collapse and biological electrocardiographic and scintillographic signs of myocardial ischaemia. It is the echocardiograph which gives the most aid in the diagnosis: the heart is normally formed but shows hypokinetic movements and left ventricular enlargement.

Other diseases without cardiovascular defects can impair cardiac function: chronic or acute anaemias, hypoglycemia, hypocalcemia, hypo- and hyperthyroidism. All of these are rare but need to be considered by history or clinical context.

Neonatal infection may pose a most difficult problem since its signs and symptoms may resemble that of cardiac failure. The absence of cardiomegaly, the splenomegaly, the hematological impairments all should indicate an infection. Occasionally left obstructive heart diseases can reveal themselves by

TABLE III

Syndrome	Major elements of orientation	Likely diagnosis	Other suggestive signs
Severe heart failure	Heart of normal size	Total anomalous pulmonary venous drainage	Cyanosis. Pulmonary œdema
	Cardiomegaly-moderate	Hypoplastic left heart syndrome Valvar aortic stenosis Syndrome of coarctation of aorta	Severe collapse Systolic murmur. Left ventricular overload Difference of arterial pulses
		Single ventricle Double outlet right ventricle Atrio-ventricular canal Truncus arteriosus	Peculiar silhouette QRS axis = − 90° Systolo-diastolic murmur. Bounding pulses
		Transposition of the great vessels + large ductus arteriosus	Egg-shaped silhouette
		Ductus arteriosus	Prematurity. Bounding pulses
		Heterotopic tachycardia Atrio-ventricular block	Heart rate > 200/min. Heart rate < 80/min.
	Cardiomegaly-huge	Cerebral arterio-venous fistula Other systemic fistulae Purulent pericarditis (or other) Cardiomyopathies, tumours	Bounding carotid pulse, cranial murmur Examination of placenta, liver., context of septicemia None

an associated infection: the diagnostic distinction can usually be made by specialised investigation, essentially via the echocardiograph.

Lesional diagnosis. — The volume of the heart can aid in directing the diagnosis according to the schema represented in Table III. One can retain from it the following principal rules:

If the heart is of normal size, it is not true congestive failure which is in question but a clinical and radiological picture of pulmonary edema with a more or less intense cyanosis: the first diagnosis to be considered is total anomalous pulmonary venous drainage. Hemodynamic confirmation is urgently required since surgery may cure these children.

If the heart size is huge (cardio-thoracic ratio greater than 0.75) one should think first of a systemic arterio-venous fistula, principally intracranial, not failing to recognize a pericarditis, most frequently purulent at this age; or look for a cardiomyopathy or a tumour of the heart.

If the cardiomegaly is moderate, as is most often the case, one should consider the possibility of a severe left sided obstruction, of a large septal defect or, in the premature infant, a left-to-right shunt via the ductus arteriosus. A transposition of the great vessels with ventricular septal defect or ductus arteriosus may also be observed. All of these anomalies can be formally recognized or suggested by the echocardiograph.

Rhythm or conduction disturbances can in some cases cause congestive cardiac failure. Auscultation and the electrocardiogram can detect a heterotopic junctional tachycardia or, more rarely, atrial tachycardia. Conversely there may be an atrio-ventricular block whose poor tolerance may justify the urgent insertion of a pacemaker.

OBSTRUCTIVE LESIONS
OF THE LEFT HEART

The obstructions of the left heart are due to malformations: of the left atrium and the inlet chamber of the left ventricle (stenosis of the pulmonary veins, cor triatriatum, mitral and supra-mitral stenosis, mitral atresia); of the outlet chamber of the left ventricle (hypoplastic left heart syndrome, aortic stenosis and aortic atresia); and of the aortic arch, such as coarctation, tubular hypoplasia and

interruption. Each of these anomalies can appear as an isolated lesion. However it is much more common to find them associated. Thus "hypoplastic left heart syndrome" generally comprises mitral stenosis or atresia, hypoplasia of the left ventricle, aortic atresia, hypoplasia of the ascending aorta and often coarctation of aorta. As a result of the progress made in intracardiac investigations and above all in echocardiography, it is now possible to define with greater precision the complexity of the different anatomic lesions and, in some cases, to propose surgical intervention.

HYPOPLASTIC LEFT HEART SYNDROME

This term serves to designate failures of development of the aortic valve, left ventricle, mitral valve and ascending aorta. The degree and the location of the lesions vary notably from case to case. But there is one physiopathological common feature: the left ventricle is unable of assuming the systemic output which is taken over by the right ventricle, the pulmonary artery and the ductus arteriosus.

Pathology

The left ventricle is generally very hypoplastic, reduced to a vestigial slit, sometimes difficult to find in the thickness of the left wall of a ventricular cavity which seems initially to be single. *The aortic valve* is generally atretic, a diaphragm totally closing a ring of very small calibre. It may simply be hypoplastic and stenosed. *The mitral valve* is always underdeveloped: the ring is extremely hypoplastic and often completely obstructed by a diaphragm or a blind crater (mitral atresia). Sometimes the valvar apparatus has a normal architecture but is miniscule (mitral hypoplasia) and highly obstructive. *The ascending aorta* is generally underdeveloped, reduced to a cord posteriorly in relation to the voluminous pulmonary artery. It gives off the coronary arteries normally and reaches a satisfactory size at the horizontal segment and the origin of the first collaterals. The isthmus is often withdrawn above the ductus arteriosus.

Most of the lesions associated with these basic abnormalities have characteristics indispensible to minimal hemodynamic functioning. The left atrium is often small but above all heavily musculated. An atrial septal defect, of the foramen ovale or ostium secundum type, can be observed

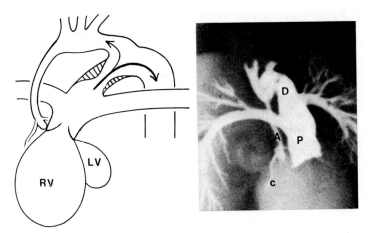

FIG. III 20. — *Hypoplastic let heart syndrome:* diagram and postmortem angiography.
P = pulmonary artery; A = hypoplastic aorta; D = ductus ateriosus; c = coronary artery; RV = right ventricle; LV = left ventricle.

in 80 % of cases. The interatrial septum can be totally closed by early and complete joining of the valve of the fossa ovalis. This can lead to an aneurysmal projection into the right atrium. In this case, survival can be assured by abnormal connections: *i. e.* intra-myocardial sinusoids, anomalous pulmonary venous drainage. The right sided structures (atrium, tricuspid valve, ventricle and pulmonary artery) are dilated and hypertrophied. The ductus arteriosus is naturally patent and continues without a reduction in calibre by the descending aorta. Generally there is no ventricular septal defect.

The different anatomical forms are sometimes classified in relation to the site of obstruction: mitral atresia, aortic atresia, mitro-aortic atresia. It is more in keeping with the anatomo-clinical features to describe three groups, according to the degree of hypoplastic left ventricle: *the major forms* associate aortic atresia, slit-like left ventricle, mitral atresia or extreme hypoplasia, with major underdevelopment of the ascending aorta. One almost always finds an atrial septal defect but the ventricular septum is intact and there is no endocardial fibro-elastosis. These are the most frequent forms. *The intermediary forms* are those where the left ventricular cavity remains highly hypoplastic but exists; there is complete aortic atresia. *The mild forms* are much less common; they have in common a left ventricular cavity of reduced dimensions but able to reach one third that of the right ventricular cavity. All the left sided structures can be patent but on a very reduced scale; it is here that the atrial septum can be intact. There can be mitral atresia with a normal aortic orifice and ventricular septal

defect, or an aortic atresia with a patent mitral valve and ventricular septal defect. These mild forms are at the nosological limit of the hypoplastic left heart syndrome but should be included to the extent that the right heart and the ductus participate considerably, if not exclusively, in the systemic outflow. The ascending aorta is less hypoplastic where the aortic ring is more functional.

Etiology

The different varieties of hypoplastic left heart represent a little more than 1 % of congenital heart disease. They are the principal cause of heart failure and death from cardiac distress in the newborn: 10 to 25 % of the cardiac malformations which reveal themselves in the first few days of life are hypoplastic left heart syndromes. There is a clear masculine predominance (sex-ratio: 2/1 to 3/1). Familial cases are not uncommon. The role of the early closing of the foramen ovale (excluding the left heart from the fetal circulation) has often been advanced as an explanation for the genesis of hypoplastic left heart but this has been verified only in a minority of cases. It is more probable that the primitive defect obstructs one of the valves of the left heart and that the exclusion of the above or underlying structures by the new drainage circuit leads to their involution.

Pathophysiology

The upstream consequences are: above all a syndrome of pulmonary venous obstruction, analogous for example to a tight mitral stenosis, all the more severe where the atrial septal defect is less permeable; a right-to-left total atrial shunt leading all the pulmonary drainage to the tricuspid valve and the right ventricle; a considerable diastolic overload of the right ventricle which becomes exhausted in assuring not only the pulmonary output, but also the systemic one, by the pulmonary artery: Right ventricular and pulmonary hypertension are constant; an obligatory right-to-left shunt through the ductus for aortic perfusion leading to peripheral desaturation and, subsequently, rapid death on closure of the ductus: hypoplastic left heart is a form of "ducto-dependant" heart disease.

The downstream consequences are those resulting from a systemic perfusion which is inadequate because it is often hampered in the ductus and badly pulsatile: whence a situation of collapse with renal failure and sometimes hepatic failure with centro-lobular necrosis and perturbations of acid-base balance occurs. In addition the perfusion of the superior half of the body, *i. e.* the brain and the heart, is achieved in a retrograde manner and in conditions which are even more difficult in the case of associated pre-ductal isthmic stenosis.

Clinical features

Functional impairment always appears very early but after an interval which varies from a few hours to a few days. It occurs in the newborn who until that moment was considered to be well as a sudden collapse, accompanied by respiratory distress, cyanosis, hypothermia and hypotonia. Occasionally it is the appearance and rapid accentuation of cyanosis which attracts attention.

On examination, dyspnea is severe; there is often severe respiratory distress which requires artificial ventilation. The colour may reflect a mixture of cyanosis and palour, thus giving a greyish cinder colour which is characteristic. Hepatomegaly and tachycardia with forceful heart sounds and sometimes a gallop rhythm while the murmurs are frequently non intense and of little significance, are the features which complete the picture of severe cardiac failure. Associated are more or less intense signs of collapse: symmetrical arterial pulses which are weak or totally abolished, general mottling of the skin and prolongation of the time of recolouration.

Complementary procedures

The chest X ray generally shows a distinct but never massive cardiomegaly: the cardio-thoracic ratio is generally between 0.60 and 0.65, with a constant right prominence and salient left border. Whence a cardiac silhouette circular or piriform with a raised apex, like a "rugby-ball". The pulmonary vasculature can appear normal but it is most often increased: with arterial overload and venous stasis parallel to the degree of obstruction to the pulmonary venous drainage leading to the fuzzy characteristic of lung edema.

On the electrocardiogram, the most specific abnormalities are right atrial and ventricular enlargement, which is significant and isolated. Associated with it sometimes are disturbances of atrio-ventricular conduction and diffuse alterations of repolarisation. There are also atypical forms with the appearance of left ventricular overload, probably in

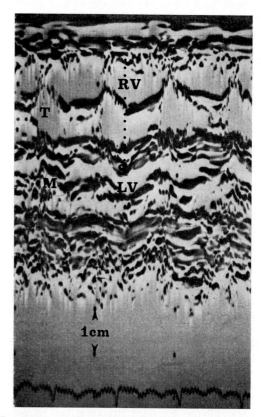

FIG. III-21. — *Hypoplastic left heart syndrome.* M-mode echocardiogram, showing the small diameter of the left ventricle (LV) and mitral valve (M), contrasted with the large right ventricle (RV) and tricuspid valve (T).

relation to a rotation of the heart which directs the hypertrophy of the right ventricle towards the left.

The echocardiogram is essential for the diagnosis. TM recording permits not only the recognition of the syndrome but the specification of the variety with remarkable reliability. The size of the ascending aorta does not exceed 5 mm. The left ventricular cavity cannot be identified or does not measure more than 11 mm, with a ratio of the size of the left ventricle to the right ventricle less than 0.6. The mitral valve is not identified or appears very small and of abnormal morphology. There is overload with multiple echos. When these criteria are present, diagnosis of a major form can be made with certainty.

Catheterization and angiocardiography

Umbilical arterial catheterization consists of pushing the catheter up to the aortic isthmus with an angiogram in the left anterior oblique position. Two findings give support for the diagnosis: retrograde opacification of the entire aortic arch and the vessels of the neck without the slightest washing out by non-opacified blood coming from the left ventricle, thus giving very dense images; and the extreme underdevelopment of the ascending aorta seen as a fine cord which ends as a swelling from which the coronary arteries emerge.

A right sided venous catheter permits one to reach the left atrium via the foramen ovale (except in the case of an intact atrial septum). The right heart is explored up to the pulmonary branches and one can penetrate into the ascending aorta through the ductus arteriosus: this latter manoeuvre is often poorly tolerated since it obstructs the only source of systemic outflow and should therefore be very brief. The principal oxymetric findings are a left-to-right shunt at the atrial level, with homogenous saturations up to the pulmonary and aortic branches. The pressures are considerably raised in the atria, particularly the left one; they are often at the systemic level (even supra-systemic in the first days of life, in the right ventricle and pulmonary artery). The aortic pressure is poorly pulsatile. Angiocardiography with injection in the trunk of the pulmonary artery or the ductus, may show the characteristic aspect of the retrograde aortography; in the left atrium in the left anterior oblique position with a strong cranio-caudal inclination, which will permit one to see the small atrial cavity, the mitral atresia with massive reflux towards the

right atrium through the atrial septal defect; or the crater of a severe mitral valve hypoplasia, which allows the injection of a blind left ventricular cavity.

Prognosis and management

The prognosis of hypoplastic left heart syndrome is poor: whatever the measures taken, death usually occurs from a few hours to a few days in the major forms; from a few weeks to a few months for the less severe varieties, particularly those with a ventricular septal defect.

Medical management is generally only a means of permitting the organisation and execution of diagnostic procedures: artificial respiration, diuretics, digitalis and possibly even perfusion with prostaglandins to delay the closing of the ductus arteriosus in preparation for surgery.

Surgical measures are usually palliative gestures such as the enlargening of the atrial septal defect with banding of the two pulmonary branches: or a major open heart procedure aimed at the division of the right atrium into one caval part, anastomosed at the bifurcation of the pulmonary artery, and one pulmonary part, following via the tricuspid valve, the right ventricle and the main pulmonary artery, anastomosed by a conduit at the horizontal aorta: few of the newborns who have undergone surgery have survived.

AORTIC VALVAR STENOSIS

Aortic valvar stenosis represents 6 % of congenital heart disease but less than 10 % of these stenoses are sufficiently severe to be symptomatic in the neonatal period, with a picture of intractable cardiac failure, mimicking that of the hypoplastic left heart syndrome. It is important to recognize this malformation, since it is amenable to surgery. There is a distinct male predominance.

Pathology

The aortic valve is stenosed, often bicuspid, with the valves thick and rigid and a punctiform orifice more or less off-center. The left ventricle is dilated and sometimes the seat of endocardial fibroelastosis. Some forms with a small ventricle represent a transition to the hypoplastic left heart syndrome.

Pathophysiology

At birth, the establishment of the pulmonary circulation involves an increase of about 25 % of the left ventricular output. In valvar aortic stenosis, the left ventricle cannot assure a sufficient output, heart failure appears more or less quickly. Intracardiac shunts can appear at the level of the foramen ovale and ductus arteriosus. The "forced" foramen ovale permits the passage of blood from the left atrium to the right atrium, which leads to an overloading of the right heart and can explain the right ventricular enlargement sometimes observed. At the level of the ductus, which remains open, the shunt is from the pulmonary artery towards the aorta, as in the fetal circulation. In more serious forms, whose hemodynamics approach those of the hypoplastic left heart, there is a rapid lethal evolution towards death with features of intractable cardiac failure and irreducible metabolic acidemia, the perfusion of the organs remains insufficient and the deficit becomes greater with the progressive reduction of the calibre of the ductus. The delayed closing of the ductus explains some later worsening when the total blood flow of right ventricular origin has to pass through the lungs and return to the left heart, whose work is thus increased. The progressive diminution of the pulmonary resistance also intervenes in the hemodynamic modifications of this period.

Clinical features

Critical aortic stenosis causes intractable cardiac failure that sets in abruptly between the first few days and the end of the first month. Clinically, it resembles the hypoplastic left ventricle syndrome: irritability, pallor and weak arterial pulses, suggesting a low cardiac output. When left heart failure appears, the infant may show tachypnea, dyspnea and diffuse rales may be heard over the lungs. Slight cyanosis may result from the pulmonary congestion. Failure of the right ventricle may occur. The intensity of the cardiac murmur depends on the cardiac output. It is often soft and may even be absent.

Complementary procedures

The chest X-ray shows global cardiomegaly with left predominance and pulmonary congestion.

The electrocardiogram is usually compatible with severe left ventricular hypertrophy. This finding is important in the differential diagnosis with hypoplastic left ventricle syndrome. Pre- and afterload of the right ventricle is augmented when a left-to-right shunt at the atrial level and pulmonary hypertension develop, secondary to left heart failure; which may also induce right heart failure.

The echocardiogram is usually sufficient for the diagnosis, giving precision to the anatomic characteristics of the malformation: thick aortic valve, nearly immobile with an eccentric opening, hypoplasia of the aortic ring and post-stenotic dilatation of the ascending aorta. The size of the left ventricle, the degree of hypertrophy of its walls and also the absence of signs suggesting endocardial fibroelastosis are important in regard to the prognosis.

Catheterization and angiocardiography

The left ventricle is reached through the foramen ovale and one can, by in addition puncturing the femoral or axillary artery, determine the systolic pressure gradient. Pulmonary arterial pressure is most often raised and one can demonstrate a left-to-right shunt at the atrial level, sometimes a right-to-left shunt via the ductus arteriosus, occasionally with retrograde filling of the aortic arch at the start of the injection.

Angiocardiography in the left ventricle shows a dome-shaped image, the jet-lesion with dilation of the ascending aorta, and sometimes an associated coarctation. It is important to specify the dimensions of the left ventricular chamber, whose contractability is weak. An injection in the left atrium may sometimes discover an associated mitral stenosis.

Natural history and management

Medical treatment is ineffective Digitalis may be dangerous and is poorly tolerated. Reanimation and the correction of metabolic disorders can however lead to improvement from which one should profit to make a decision concerning surgery if conditions are favourable (left chamber of sufficient dimension, absence of associated malformation). Emergency valvotomy, performed under cardiopulmonary by-pass, may save the patient's life. The efficacy of a valvulotomy depends on the dimension of the aortic ring. If it is too small the anomaly is inoperable. The surgical mortality rate remains high and the postoperative results depend on the degree of myocardial failure due to subendocardial ischemia, the presence of endocardial fibroelastosis, hypoplasia of the left ventricule, residual aortic stenosis, and secondary aortic regurgitation. If the immediate results are favourable, the long-term results are also often good, despite an aortic insufficiency, more or less severe, and the necessity of valve replacement later.

The clinical picture of critical aortic stenosis in the neonate resembles that of a coarctation. Compared with coarctation, there usually is no marked pressure difference between the upper and lower limbs. Left ventricular preponderance on the electrocardiogram excludes the hypoplastic left ventricular syndrome. The non-invasive 2-dimensional echocardiogram is extremely valuable for an immediate and accurate diagnosis. The images obtained from the various cross-sections are usually pathognomonic for this particular anomaly.

COARCTATION OF THE AORTA

Pathology and morphogenesis

Coarctation is a stenosis situated in the aorta, at the juncture of the horizontal and descending segment, just upstream or downstream from the ductus arteriosus. The classical lesion is a localised plication, diaphragm-shaped, of the media, which results in a reduction of the calibre of the vessel. At the level of this diaphragm the aorta displays a localised kinking. In longitudinal section this exterior appearance faces the arterial ligament. The coarctation, defined in this way, is thus to be distinguished from *tubular hypoplasia* of the aorta, characterised by an aortic segment which is too long and too narrow.

During fetal life, the quantity of blood passing via the pulmonary artery→ductus arteriosus→ descending aorta, is about 60 % of the total outflow, with a percentage of 10 % across the aortic isthmus, the segment of the aortic arch situated between the left sub-clavian artery and the insertion of the ductus.

Any modification of the fetal circulation resulting in preferential flow towards the pulmonary artery and the ductus, to the prejudice of flow across the ascending aorta and aortic arch, can result in aortic underdevelopment or malformations of the aortic arch, such as tubular hypoplasia, atresia or interruption of the aortic arch. It is observed in some ventricular septal defects, caused by malalignement of the septa, and in partial obstructions of the left

ventricular outflow tract; in some cases of double outlet right ventricle with subaortic obstruction (Taussig-Bing complex).

Frequently, tubular hypoplasia of the aortic arch is accompanied by a localised diaphragm. This association is all the more frequent where the child is young (60-90 % of tubular hypoplasias presenting under six months). Coarctation can in these cases be explained by the same process which is responsible for the appearance of the tubular hypoplasia; where a reduction of the blood flow across the preductal aorta results in raising of the blood flow in the pulmonary arterial trunk and ductus. This latter structure has a tendance to prolong itself, to insert itself into the descending aorta. The exterior kinking of the coarctation can be explained solely by the hemodynamics: it is simply the exaggeration of the physiological indentation of the aortic arch at the level of the junction of the ductus arteriosus with the descending aorta. The coarctation also has a histological substratum: it is the tissue of the ductus arteriosus which is responsible for the localized stenosis. The tubular hypoplasia, which often preceeds the coarctation in the newborn, can disappear later as the aortic flow becomes normal: only the localised stenosis, which is fixed and inextensible, remains. The relationships which exist between the ductal tissue and the coarctation of the aorta have been identified by microscopic studies. Normally there is always a certain invasion of ductal tissue in the aortic wall at the level of the junction of the ductus. Generally this does not surpass one third of the circumference of the aorta. In localised coarctation, there is a prolongation of the ductus such that the ductal tissue almost entirely surrounds the circumference of the aorta. The closing, followed by fibrosis, of the ductus is then an important factor in the secondary appearance of the coarctation, since it results in a fibrosis of the media at the level of the diaphragm of ductal tissue in the aortic wall. The process of sclerosis can exaggerate the effect of the coarctation by traction exerted on the two arms of the stenosing sling coming from the ductus. It is also probable that the pulse wave in the aorta is interrupted at the level of the fibrous tissue coming from the ductus, which results in a dilation upstream from the coarctation. The closing of the ductus arteriosus is not mandatory for the creation of a coarctation.

Isolated coarctation and coarctation associated with obstructive malformations of the left heart have the same histological appearance and can be explained by the same process of downstream sliding of the ductal tissue in the aorta, the consequence of a preferential circulation via the pulmo-

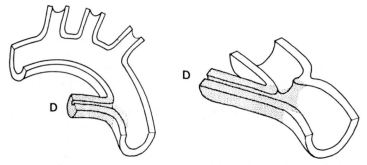

F IG. III-22. — *Extension of ductal tissue into the aorta in a normal neonate* (a) *and in coarctation* (b).
D = ductus arteriosus.

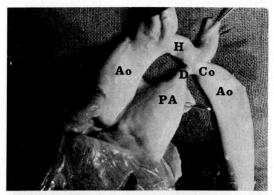

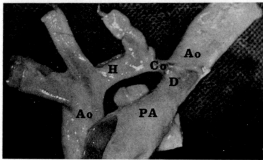

F IG. III-23. — *Coarctation of aorta.* Top : post-ductal coarctation; the stenosis is discrete, after the origin of the left subclavian artery and the opening of a small ductus arteriosus (D). The horizontal aorta (H) is slightly hypoplastic. Bottom: preductal coarctation; the main pulmonary artery (PA) from which one can see both the branches emerging, continues itself without transition by the ductus (D) and descending aorta (Ao); the stenosis is very tight and the horizontal aorta (H) hypoplastic.

nary trunk→ductus arteriosus→descending aorta, to the prejudice of the flow across the ascending aorta. The frequency of forms associating tubular hypoplasia and localised coarctation in the two groups, the transformation of tubular hypoplasia into localised coarctation with increasing of the flow through the aorta, the high percentage of bicuspid aortic valve in the two groups and the possibility of spontaneous closing, fetal or postnatal, of an associated ventricular septal defect, are arguments in favour of a common pathogenesis for tubular hypoplasia and localised coarctation.

When the ductus is patent, it can open above the stenosed area: this *preductal* coarctation comprises the fetal type, with persistance of continuity of pulmonary artery trunk→ductus→descending aorta, onto which the retracted aortic isthmus opens laterally. This anatomic form is observed in association with obstructive malformations of the left heart, or with ventricular septal defect: it is the *"coarctation syndrome"*.

At its most severe, fetal hemodynamic problems which result in both aortic tubular hypoplasia and coarctation can lead to *complete interruption of the aortic arch*.

A ductus of small calibre can be open at the level of the stenosis or below it (juxta or postductal coarctation); it terminates often by closing itself and its presence does not involve the same serious hemodynamic disturbances as those in preductal coarctation, but only a left-to-right shunt in addition. The clinical consequences are those of an isolated coarctation.

Clinical features

Coarctation is third amongst heart disease which is symptomatic in the neonatal period after complete transposition and hypoplastic left heart syndrome. It is more frequent in boys and appears sometimes in a familial context or associated with a polymalformative syndrome of ovarian dysgenesis or its male "Turner" counterpart (Bonnevie-Ulrich syndrome). Less than 10 % of the coarctations reveal themselves during the neonatal period as serious cardiac failure.

Isolated coarctation, or coarctation associated with a small juxta or prestrictural ductus, is generally latent but can, during the first weeks, suddenly become symptomatic. In this case, cardiac failure is usually moderate and responds well to digitalis and diuretic drugs. Often, these children have an elevated blood pressure in the upper limbs.

With or without failure, isolated coarctation is disclosed by palpation of the femoral pulses, which are weak or absent. In contrast, in the absence of heart failure, humeral and radial pulses are abnormally ample. The absence or weakness of the femoral pulses is often difficult to detect in the newborn. It is therefore necessary to simultaneously measure the arterial blood pressure in the upper limb and the homolateral inferior limb with a double cuff and single manometer, by flush or Doppler technique: a gradient of at least 20 mm of mercury is needed to confirm the diagnosis; this examination, sometimes difficult to interpret, should be repeated. Auscultation reveals a soft systolic murmur at the base, sometimes more easily perceived in the back, and sometimes a continuous murmur of a ductus arteriosus.

The "coarctation syndrome" is the malformative association which corresponds, from a clinical point of view, to early and serious distress, all the more serious when it manifests itself early, leaving no hope for lasting improvement by medical treatment and justifying an early surgical approach. The coarctation is preductal, associated with hypoplasia of the horizontal aorta and most often with one or several intracardiac malformations: commonly ventricular septal defect, mitral stenosis or insufficiency, sometimes complex heart disease such as transposition or double outlet right ventricle.

The symptoms are the same as those for hypoplastic left heart syndrome; but the latency period is longer and it is towards the end of the first week that they begin to appear in a baby who until that moment presented only signs of good health: feeding difficulties, dyspnea, an abnormal weight gain due to fluid retention, then rapidly the features of severe cardiac failure with collapse, respiratory distress, greyish apperance, and hepatomegaly.

Auscultation may reveal a systolic murmur (in one third of the cases), sometimes a gallop rhythm. Cyanosis is evident only in cases of associated transposition. In the usual case one should observe a differential cyanosis, in respect to the head and upper limbs, because the right ventricle empties into the descending aorta. However, this sign is almost always lacking because of intracardiac shunts. However, the measure of the percutaneous PO_2 can show a gradient (which is accentuated by the hyperoxia test) between the sub-clavian area and the lower limbs. The most definitive sign is the lack of femoral pulses and measures of blood pressure: providing that these measures are repeated, particularly after the reestablishment of improved myocardial function, one can notice a significant difference in two out of three cases. Weak pulses in the four limbs (particularly at the first examination) or noticed equally in the four limbs, will not eliminate the diagnosis. Moreover, a good perception of radial pulses in a newborn with heart failure is always unusual. After the improvement in cardiac function, pulsatile carotids and a vibrant aorta perceived at the sternal notch are also important signs.

Complementary procedures

The chest X-ray is not characteristic in isolated coarctation. The inferior left border can appear abnormally rounded and overlap the diaphragm. In the coarctation syndrome, a global and severe cardiomegaly is associated with marked pulmonary hypervascularity. When it is huge, it is sometimes indicative of an accompagning pericardial effusion.

The electrocardiogram is of little help. One can sometimes identify atrial enlargement. A left ventricular enlargement is possible but rarely isolated, except in uncomplicated forms, which are most often well tolerated. Rarely one observes impressive right ventricular enlargement or sometimes a combined ventricular enlargement. A strain pattern is common: flat or negative T wave, depressed ST segments. One can attribute these either to coronary or myocardial impairment of sometimes to an associated pericardial effusion.

The echocardiogram, as a simple bidimensional procedure, shows the coarctation via a suprasternal approach. TM mode is helpful since it permits one to eliminate hypoplastic left heart syndrome, to suspect associated malformations, to appreciate the left ventricular function, to show a possible pericardial effusion and appreciate the effects of cardiac drugs.

Catheterization
and angiocardiography

These are used only for those forms which show early poor tolerance, principally the coarctation syndrome, since an early surgical decision is necessary and it requires a complete account of the malformations. The degree of urgency varies according to the case but, most often, despite previous medical treatment, the child remains in a precarious state which makes the procedure difficult and dangerous. It should be performed rapidly, little contrast medium should be used because of the risk of renal failure, but it should nevertheless be precise and complete. The route of the catheter gives information on the existence of a ductus arteriosus, a ventricular or atrial septal defect, or any other abnormal route. Oxymetry, can be a useful indicator for detecting shunts. The recording of pressures is important. It is necessary to pay particular attention to: the level of the pulmonary arterial pressures, the existence of pressure gradients: between the aorta and pulmonary artery via the ductus; above and below the coarctation; between aorta

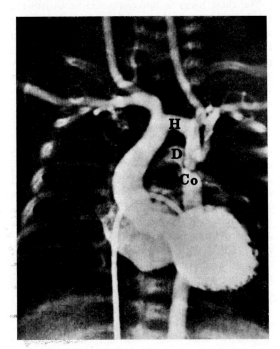

FIG. III-24. — *Coarctation of aorta.* Left ventriculogram; slight regurgitation to the left atrium; very tight stenosis (Co), small patent ductus (D), allowing slight opacification of the main pulmonary artery; the ascending aorta is "too long", the horizontal aorta (H) is hypoplastic.

and left ventricle; between the diastolic pressure of the left ventricle and the pressure of the left atrium; between the mean pressures of the left atrium and right atrium.

The choice of selective injections and angiographic views should be carefully established for each case, the most useful being the aortogram, in frontal and lateral or left oblique anterior views, left ventriculography in a long axial oblique view (ventricular septum, left outlet chamber) or in a right anterior oblique view (mitral valve); the injection in the main pulmonary artery in frontal and lateral views.

Isolated coarctation appears as a localised stenosis of the aortic isthmus preceded by a moderately hypoplastic horizontal aorta an ascending aorta which often appears "too long" and is abnormally curved. A small ductus is sometimes visible.

Coarctations with large shunts involve one or other or sometimes several of the following associations: large substrictural ductus, emptying directly into the descending aorta from the pulmonary artery and without a notable pressure gradient between these two vessels; perimembranous ventricular septal defect, sometimes associated with a subvalvar aortic stenosis, sometimes with one or several other defects in the trabeculated septum; atrial septal defect with left-to-right shunt, most often a "forced" foramen ovale; sometimes an atrio-ventricular canal ("goose-neck" pattern on the ventriculogram); aorto-pulmonary window, revealed only by aortography.

Coarctations with left heart anomalies represent 25 % of the cases. They involve: mitral malformations, stenosis and sometimes severe insufficiency; valvar or subvalvar aortic anomalies (*the Shone syndrome* associates: parachute mitral valve, mitral supravalvar ring, sub-valvar aortic stenosis, and coarctation).

Coarctations with complex malformations are principally associated with a double outlet right ventricle, with transposition of the great vessels and a univentricular heart.

Natural history. Management

Isolated coarctation complicated by early cardiac failure responds favourably to digitalis and diuretic drugs. In the case of significant hypertension, it is not usual to institute antihypertensive drugs: the most effective are the beta-blocking drugs, less desirable because of their depressant effect on the myocardium. The use of diuretics is thus preferable for this purpose.

Coarctation syndrome, in contrast to hypoplastic left heart syndrome, usually responds to medical treatment. Digoxin should however be used with prudence taking into account the renal failure which may occur in this malformation. If this occurs, it is necessary to move to intracardiac investigations without delay and to determine the indications for surgery. Improvement on medical management is temporary and a downhill course is usually observed, except in rare cases which involve delayed closing of the ductus or even of a ventricular septal defect.

Surgical intervention consists of a resection of the coarctation followed by resuturing of the aorta. The difficulties arise above all from the hypoplastic horizontal aorta: diverse techniques of aortoplasty have been proposed, using, for example, the left sub-clavian artery to enlarge the aorta. The ductus is ligated. In the case of a large ventricular septal defect, a banding of the pulmonary artery may be considered but its real value is questionable. The mortality rate is still high (at least 15-20 %). It is above all the associated lesions which lessen the surgical prognosis.

COMPLETE INTERRUPTION OF THE AORTIC ARCH

This malformation is rare and usually isolated. Clinically it resembles a severe form of the coarctation syndrome, but it poses more complex surgical problems.

Pathology

The continuity between ascending and descending aorta is completely interrupted. Sometimes, a fibrous cord joins the two segments. The ductus is practically always patent. According to the point of interruption, one can distinguish three types: *in type A* (44 % of the cases) the interruption is between the left sub-clavian artery and the ductus; *in type B* (52 % of the cases), it is between the left carotid and the left sub-clavian; *in type C* (4 % of the cases), the interruption is situated between the innominate arterial trunk and the left carotid. Each of these types is divided into two groups, according

to whether the right sub-clavian artery has a normal origin and course or whether it originates from the descending aorta and has an aberrant retro-œsophagal course (types A1, B1, C1). Type B1 is encountered in 17 % of cases.

There is almost always a ventricular septal defect. More complex malformations are found in 40 % of cases (truncus arteriosus type I or aorto-pulmonary window, transposition, double outlet right ventricle).

Clinical features

The malformation behaves like a preductal coarctation; the cardiac failure is early and severe. One should think of this above all when the pressure in the left arm is lower than that in the right arm and equal to that of the lower limbs: In findings of this kind, an interruption of type B is the most frequent, whereas in coarctation the obstruction is rarely situated above the origin of the left sub-clavian artery. In type B1 the four limbs are under the same pressure condition, depending on the right ventricle by way of a ductus which, according to whether it starts to close or remains widely dilated, more or less dampens the systolic wave of the right ventricle. Differential cyanosis should be observed in this malformation (on the feet and one hand, for example); in actual fact, for the same reasons as in coarctation, this sign is evident only in some instances but can be demonstrated by comparative measurement of the percutaneous PO_2.

The X-ray, electrocardiogram, echocardiogram and catheterization findings are as in the coarctation syndrome.

Angiocardiography

This is the procedure which confirms the diagnosis. Right ventriculography opacifies the ductus then the descending aorta. Left ventriculography fills the ascending aorta and the arteries that emerge from it. However, the superimposition of the dilated pulmonary vessels hampers the interpretation considerably and only the selective opacification of the ascending aorta, reached via the ventricular septal defect or, if it is not possible, by retrograde arterial catheterization allows an exact diagnosis.

Evolution and management

Medical management alone is ineffective, but surgery permits some limited successes. Prostaglandins may maintain the open ductus and permit surgery in more optimal conditions. Different proceedures are used to reestablish aortic continuity. In the neonatal period, some authors have proposed banding of the pulmonary artery associated with injection of formalin in the wall of the ductus in order to keep it open; the reestablishment of continuity will only then, be performed secondarily with or without a prothesis or graft.

MITRAL STENOSIS

Obstructive anomalies of the mitral apparatus (the ring, the area immediately supravalvar, the valves, cords and papillary muscles) are rare and almost always associated with other malformations. The left ventricle usually has a dimension large enough to permit adequate cardiac output.

Pathology

Isolated forms comprise: *valvar lesions* (thickening and shrinking of the leaflets, fusion of the commissures, funnel or diaphragm-shaped mitral valve); *subvalvar lesions* (chordae tendinae short or basal, papillary muscles thick and short, more or less fusioned, or absent, "parachute mitral valve", with the chordae converging towards a single large papillary muscle); sometimes there is a supravalvar stenosis ring.

Associated forms represent 60-90 % of the cases, according to different series, and consist of complex left sided obstructions (coarctation syndrome, Shone syndrome or associated left-to-right shunts).

Clinical features

The most severe obstructions become symptomatic within the first weeks of life as respiratory distress, sudden attacks of dyspnea, of coughing or, sometimes of pulmonary œdema; the "white" anoxic spells or convulsive seizures may appear later.

The baby is pale and sweating, signs of congestive cardiac failure are common. Auscultation is dominated by rales of pulmonary edema and by the murmurs due to the associated heart defects. A diastolic apical murmur can be detected in some cases and has the advantage of drawing one's attention to the mitral valve.

Complementary procedures

The heart generally shows an increased volume on the X-ray, but the classical "mitral silhouette" is not observed at this age. The pulmonary vascular anomalies are more significant: venous congestion, predominant at the apices, Kerley's septal lines.

Signs of atrial enlargement are constant (left or combined) as are those or right ventricular enlargement. A left ventricular enlargement is not infrequent and orients one towards an associated aortic stenosis or coarctation.

The echocardiogram contributes in a major way to the diagnosis but does not permit a diagnosis of the anatomical form of the stenosis. The mitral valve echo is of reduced amplitude, the posterior leaflet has a systolic movement towards the front and the anterior leaflet has a rapid closing (accentuated EF slope).

Catheterization and angiocardiography

The level of pulmonary arterial and wedge pressure is very high, as is the pressure in the left atrium reached via the foramen ovale. The injection of contrast should be made in this latter cavity and clearly shows, in a right anterior oblique view, the lesions of the mitral apparatus. Failing this, an injection in the pulmonary artery will also show them, but this may be dangerous owing to the degree of hypertension.

Prognosis and treatment

Prognosis is particularly poor. Death usually follows from severe lung edema. Medical treatment is supportive at best. There is little hope of surgical correction, except possibly if stability can be obtained for several months. A simple mitral commissurotomy is sometimes sufficient and it is even possible, in the case of a supravalvar diaphragm, to undertake a complete correction; In other cases the only solution consists of a valve replacement; a procedure which is highly risky in the newborn.

PULMONARY VENOUS OBSTRUCTION. COR TRIATRIATUM

These lesions are: obstructed anomalous pulmonary venous drainage, already described; pulmonary venous stenosis and atresia of the common pulmonary vein; triatrial heart (cor triatriatum).

All of these have a similar *embryological origin*: abnormalities in the connection of the pulmonary venous plexus and the common pulmonary vein, difficulty in the incorporation of the common pulmonary vein into the wall of the left atrium.

Their pathophysiology is identical. The pulmonary venous hypertension leads to interstitial edema and sometimes to lymphangiectasis, then to pulmonary edema from alveolar exudation. Cyanosis can appear because an impairment of hemoglobin status or more rarely as a result of a right-to-left shunt through the foramen ovale, when it is situated below the obstruction (as in some forms of cor triatriatum). The heart remains of normal size and the malformation presents as a pulmonary condition.

Multiple stenoses of the pulmonary veins are rare and rarely reveal themselves at birth. *Atresia of the common pulmonary vein* is rare. *Cor triatriatum*, on the other hand, is not a rare malformation and can be symptomatic within the first few weeks of life.

Pathology of cor triatriatum

The basic lesion is a muscular membrane, covered with endocardium on the two sides, which divides the left atrium into two chambers; one, dorsal or proximal, receives the pulmonary veins: it is in fact the common pulmonary vein not incorporated into the left atrium; the other, ventral or distal, carries the left appendage, communicates with the left ventricle through the mitral valve and is in fact the real left atrium. The membrane is perforated with one or several openings, which bring the two chambers into communication. In one out of three cases, a foramen ovale makes the right atrium communicate with the distal chamber or, rarely, with the proximal chamber. In one out of four cases, a partial anomalous pulmonary venous drainage is associated.

Clinical features and routine examinations

Intolerance is all the more precocious where the opening of the membrane is smaller. It manifests itself by dyspnea, coughing, sometimes a suffocating attack of severe lung edema. Auscultation reveals little: there is sometimes a latero-sternal systolic murmur or, more rarely, a systolo-diastolic apical murmur. On the X-ray the heart is of normal size

but the images of venous and lymphatic pulmonary congestion are suggestive. The electrocardiogram shows an enlargement of the right cavities.

The echocardiogram is a key examination, since it shows the linear echo corresponding to the membrane in the left atrium.

Catheterization and angiocardiography

Catheterization can exclude total anomalous pulmonary venous drainage. Severe pulmonary arterial hypertension may make angiography dangerous; it should be undertaken in a highly prudent manner, or avoided if the echocardiogram is sufficiently clear. It shows the presence of pulmonary venous congestion and opacifies the two left atrial chambers separated by the membrane. It thus permits a differential diagnosis between the triatrial heart and the rarer pulmonary venous stenosis or atresia.

Prognosis and treatment

The prognosis is usually poor. Even worse is that of atresia of the common pulmonary vein, whereas that for stenosis of the pulmonary veins is variable, according to their degree. However the triatrial heart is potentially surgically curable.

The treatment should initially be medical and include measures which are all the more urgent and drastic when the edema is particularly menacing; diuretic drugs, fluid restriction, artificial respiration with positive pressure for the most serious cases. In cor triatriatum, surgical intervention is simple and consists of excising the membrane under cardiopulmonary by-pass. It is not the same for venous stenosis, and especially not for atresia of the common pulmonary vein, where it is necessary to anastomose the cul-de-sac into which the pulmonary veins enter at the left atrium. This procedure has to date not been performed with much success.

LEFT-TO-RIGHT CARDIAC SHUNTS

Large left-to-right shunts are rarely symptomatic in the neonatal period since the pulmonary vascular resistances, which are still high, prevent the establishment of the shunt. In addition, a wide communication between the two circulations results in delaying the maturation of the resistances. It is from six weeks to two months that the intolerance usually appears. However, it can be earlier, particularly if another hemodynamic disturbance is added to that of the shunt, for example valvar regurgitation, as in the atrio-ventricular canal.

The symptoms common to this group are: dyspnea with tachypnea and intercostal retractions, related to the considerable augmentation of the intrapulmonary blood volume and often complicated by bronchial hypersecretion and airways obstruction, repeated attacks of pulmonary infections and failure to thrive; precordial hyperactivity with an abnormal thrust palpable over the apex and the subxiphoid area, thoracic bulging due to cardiomegaly and hyperinflation of the lungs; congestive heart failure with tachycardia, liver enlargement, excessive sweating, rapid exhaustion during feeding. The X-ray shows global cardiomegaly and an increased vasculature, predominant at the apices; the electrocardiogram shows a biventricular enlargement predominant in the left ventricle, with high voltages; the echocardiogram suggests dilated right and left chambers with features of pulmonary hypertension, which can be ascertained by the measurement of systolic time intervals.

DUCTUS ARTERIOSUS

Ductal closure is completed in two stages. It consists of a first stage of contraction of the muscular cells of the media. This contraction results in a thickening of the wall of the vessel, with protrusion of the media and the intima into the lumen of the ductus, and its functional closure 10-15 hours after birth. The rise in the PaO_2, related to the onset of respiration, is considered to be the principal factor in this functional constriction. The second stage, or definitive anatomical closure, usually lasts from one to three weeks. It can happen that the ductus remains open as a result of a congenital anomaly of its wall. There may be also a delay of up to three months in the closing of the ductus. Different factors can cause this delay: chronic hypoxemia due to pulmonary or cardiac disease; imbalance between the vasodilatator and vasoconstrictor factors which affect the prostaglandin system, for example in prematurely born children suffering from the respiratory distress syndrome; special hemodynamic conditions occuring in "ducto-dependant" cardiac malformations; finally,

physiological or histological immaturity of the ductus, in the premature. It is therefore difficult, and often impossible, for the clinician, to distinguish, during the first three months of life, the difference between a delay in closure and true persistence of the ductus arteriosus.

Nevertheless, histological study of the evolution of the ductus permits us to establish the difference between a ductus whose maturity is simply delayed, but which is still susceptible to closure, and true persistence of the ductus. Without going into details, it appears that the maturation takes place in four phases: at the third phase, all the elements necessary for the closure of the duct are present, particularly thickening of the intima, and fragmentation of the elastic internal membrane. If a deviation appears (phase IIIA, characterised by the appearance of another internal elastic membrane) the duct will no longer be susceptible to closure. Certain lesions of the wall of the duct, which appear early (in rubella syndrome, for example), prevent its further maturation and consequently its closure.

Patent ductus arteriosus in the preterm infant

The degree of constriction of the ductus arteriosus under the effect of oxygen is directly related to the gestational age, and it is not surprising therefore that the incidence of delayed ductal closure in the preterm baby suffering from respiratory distress syndrome is increased with the degree of prematurity. Thus it can occur in 70 to 80 % of the small prematures born aged 28-30 weeks and in infants having a birth weight of less than 1,200 g. The overall incidence for children whose gestational age is less than 36 weeks is about 30 %.

Pathophysiology. — The first signs indicating a patent ductus arteriosus in the preterm baby are generally noted during the phase of improvement of the initial respiratory distress, often when artificial respiration is discontinued. The ductus remains patent at birth; the pulmonary resistance, remaining high because of the hypoxemia caused by the respiratory distress, prevents the establishment of a left-to-right shunt. When improvement in the pulmonary condition appears, the PaO_2 rises. This produces a vasodilatation of the small pulmonary arteries and a decreasing pulmonary arterial pressure, and stimulates the constriction of ductus media. However, efficient constriction does not always take place, owing to the immaturity of the ductus. Thus, the left-to-right shunt begins and the condition of the baby deteriorates again. The stroke volume of the left ventricle increases in relation to the increase in the left-to-right shunt through the ductus. There is an enlargement of the left ventricle with an increase in the end diastolic ventricular pressure and the left atrial pressure. It needs little therefore to result in left cardiac failure, with dilatation of the left atrium and pulmonary edema. The latter is favoured by the increased pulmonary outflow. The weakness of the compensatory mechanisms in the newborn, and more so in the preterm baby, explains the precociousness and severity of the cardiac failure. Several factors make the preterm baby particularly sensitive to the slightest change in circulatory volume: (1) The sympathetic innervation of the myocardium is complete only after full gestation; it is often even absent in the preterm baby; (2) The myocardium of the preterm born contains more water and connective tissue and less contractile elements; it is therefore not surprising that the Frank-Starling mechanism may be less efficient; (3) The increase in the left ventricular diastolic pressure and the fall in the aortic diastolic pressure, caused by the runoff through the ductus, can impair the perfusion of the myocardium, thus producing a degree of myocardial ischemia and even further depressing ventricular function. Hypocalcemia, hypoglycemia and physiological or iatrogenic anaemia can also reduce myocardial performance.

Clinical features. — Findings depend on the severity of the primary pulmonary distress, the magnitude of the left-to-right shunt through the ductus and the possibility of the initiation of compensatory mechanisms for the volumetric overload of the ventricles. The usual appearance is that of a preterm baby of several days of age suffering from respiratory distress syndrome, whose conditions of artificial respiration improve and who develops the following signs: a precordial murmur, excessive pulses palpable at the tips of the fingers, a hyperactive precordium and spells of apnea and bradycardia. On the X-ray, the enlarged heart becomes evident and the pulmonary image suggests vascular congestion. The echocardiogram permits one to evaluate the magnitude of the left-to-right shunt: a left atrium/aorta ratio greater than 1.2 is pathological. Respiratory difficulties become more serious again and necessitate an increase in the concentration of oxygen with a readaptation of the frequency and the pressures of the ventilator. When the left-to-right shunt increases considerably, the perfusion of the descending aorta can become insufficient. As a result of this, there can be intestinal

ischemia with distension and ileus, and a reduction in the renal flow with oliguria. The metabolic acidemia results from the ischemia of the region drained by the descending aorta and from the perturbation of the hepatic metabolism of lactic acid.

Treatment consists of restriction of the fluid intake, if necessary to 60 to 70 ml/kg daily, the correction of hypoglycemia and hypocalcemia, the use of diuretic drugs and digitalisation adapted to the premature infant. The hematocrit should be maintained above 40 to 45 %. If, after such treatment for two to three days, the respiratory condition deteriorates, if the cardiac failure remains intractable and if the clinical and echocardiographic signs of a left-to-right shunt persist, surgical closure of the ductus is called for. To wait too long risks the creation of pulmonary and cardiac lesions. The mortality rate and complications resulting from surgical intervention have become negligible in those centers where there is good cooperation between the surgical and pediatric groups.

Studies in vitro and animal experimentation had shown that *Indomethacin* was capable of producing a constriction of the ductus by inhibition of the synthesis of the type E prostaglandins, which dilate the ductus. This has been used by different groups to stimulate the constriction of the ductus, thus provoking in the premature closure that until then would have had to be performed surgically. The results appear within 24 hours: the constriction of the ductus is accompanied by a spectacular change in the clinical status with an improvement in the blood gases, permitting a rapid cessation of artificial respiration; the murmur becomes less loud and disappears, the pulses are no longer bounding, the cardiac rhythm becomes normal and the signs of cardiac failure disappear; on the X-ray, the pulmonary congestion improves and the size of the heart diminishes rapidly; on the echocardiogram, there is a reduction of the left atrium/aorta ratio of at least 30 %. The recommended dose is 0.2 mg/kg, administered intravenously. It can be repeated, at the maximum twice, with an interval of 24 hours. A second attempt can be considered if necessary but one can, in that case, pose the question of the benefit of surgery. The contra-indications are a suspicion of necrotizing enterocolitis, coagulation disturbances and bleeding problems, hyperbilirubinemia, alterations in renal function and presence of an infection. The early results in the literature were highly encouraging. However, there have been an increasing number of failures of Indomethacin treatment, or of recurrences, which necessitate a new attempt or perhaps surgical ligature of the duct. It is possible that, while the ductus is immature, it is unable to achieve definitive anatomical closure, because it does not yet have the thickness of the intima, which is essential for its closure. When a preterm infant has a ductus with an histological structure typical of that of persistence of the ductus, it is evident that its spontaneous or pharmacologic closure will not take place. The clinician cannot distinguish these different groups and this uncertainty is, among others, one of the reasons why there is a tendency towards a return to surgical ligation of the canal.

Patent ductus arteriosus in the full-term infant

Cardiac failure secondary to a wide persistent ductus arteriosus rarely appears in the neonatal period, since the high pulmonary vascular resistance prevents the establishment of a left-to-right shunt. Such an eventuality can however appear, either in the event of fetal distress or dysmaturity towards the end of the first week, or, rarely, from birth or in the first twelve hours following. In the first instance, the appearance is that of a large left-to-right shunt with ample pulses, a left sub-clavian continuous murmur, and there is no notable difference with that observed in a premature baby suffering from respiratory distress. In the second case, the picture becomes rapidly dramatic. It consists of *cyanosis*, the auscultation and the pulse are not characteristic, the increase in size of the heart is huge, death follows within a few hours due to irreversible failure. The autopsy shows only a voluminous ductus arteriosus, of a size equal or superior to that of the aorta. The causes of "functional" neonatal heart failure now being more clear, one can ask whether this "malignant ductus arteriosus" merits continued inclusion in the nosology.

Whatever the age of the child born at term, patent ductus arteriosus which becomes precociously complicated by cardiac failure poorly controlled by medical treatment should lead to ligation or to division of the duct. Indomethacin is of no use. If the digitalo-diuretic drugs are effective, it is better to wait, since it is indeed possible to observe a delayed closure.

VENTRICULAR SEPTAL DEFECT

It is rare that an isolated ventricular septal defect is poorly tolerated from the first weeks, for the reasons already indicated. Most often, this malformation is discovered towards the end of the first week, a date which corresponds to the lowering of pulmonary resistance to such a level as to allow the shunt to become established, allowing the detection of a more or less rough mesocardiac pansystolic murmur, in a newborn who apart from that is perfectly well. This eventuality is quite frequent, since the malformation is encountered in two out of 1,000 newborns. In at least half of the cases, *the septal defect will close spontaneously* in the months that follow, particularly if it occurs in children of low birth weight or in preterm babies: the murmur becomes brief, proto-mesosystolic, then disappears completely or persists in the form of a soft and brief murmur. It is necessary to know, however, that some of these ventricular septal defects of the newborn, if they are large, will deteriorate towards the end of the second month. However, the criteria of a large septal defect are not evident before this period: it is therefore necessary to attentively observe the feeding pattern, the growth curve and the cardio-pulmonary condition. On the other hand, in the newborn who is well and in whom one can auscultate a systolic murmur, certain elements should lead one to suspect a *more complex* malformation and to attentively follow its evolution. Thus, the absence of negative conversion of the T wave in lead V1 at the end of the first week may cause one to suspect tetralogy of Fallot, as yet non-cyanotic; an electrocardiographic image of septal inversion and an unusual silhouette on the radiograph (high angulation on the left border) suggests a corrected transposition; left ventricular enlargement can correspond to a double outlet right ventricle with a limiting septal defect. In all of these cases, the *echocardiogram* is irreplaceable and intracardiac procedures should only be considered afterwards. Finally, ventricular septal defect is a congenital heart defect that one must think of when confronted by a newborn child suffering from a polymalformative syndrome and a cardiac murmur.

Ventricular septal defects which decompensate precociously are *large defects*, which are perimembranous or trabecular, sometimes there is a *multiperforated* septum ("swiss-cheese" defects).

The early appearance of heart failure in preterm infants may be explained by myocardial immaturity and by the insufficiently developed media of the pulmonary muscular arteries, which causes a rapid decrease of the pulmonary resistance and consequently the early onset of a large left-to-right shunt. The heart failure in full-term infants with a large ventricular septal defect however appears later, between the 4th and 12th week of life. This is caused by a slower regression of the media of the pulmonary muscular arteries, due to the stress of the increased pulmonary flow. The pulmonary vascular resistance remains elevated for a longer period which diminishes the magnitude of the left-to-right shunt and explains the delayed appearance of heart failure. The signs are rarely dramatic: tachypnea, fatigue, feeding difficulties, hepatomegaly. Auscultation reveals a rough pansystolic murmur with maximal intensity at the 4th left intercostal space, along the sternal border. The intensity of the systolic murmur depends on the pressure difference between the two ventricles. If the pressures are equal, the shape of the murmur may loose its pansystolic pattern, and even disappear. If the left-to-right shunt is very large, a mid-diastolic flow murmur due to the rapid inflow from left atrium to left ventricle will also be heard. A cardiac thrill is palpable in about 25 % of the cases.

The electrocardiogram of a large ventricular septal defect is compatible with biventricular hypertrophy and often atrial dilatation. Isolated right ventricular hypertrophy suggests the development of pulmonary vascular obstruction (Fig III-26).

The echocardiogram visualizes the left atrial and left ventricular volume overload, which provides a

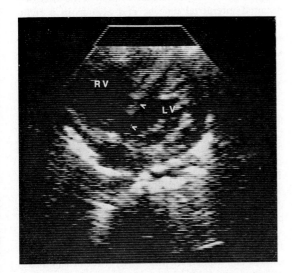

FIG. III-25. — *Ventricular septal defect*. Echocardiogram of a short axis view of the heart made with a two-dimensional real time sector scan: the arrows show the localization of the two ventricular septal defects: a posterior one and one situated at the junction of the inlet septum and the trabecular septum. RV = right ventricle; LV = left ventricle.

rough estimation of the magnitude of the left-to-right shunt. Right ventricular hypertrophy and the delayed closure of the pulmonary valve may indicate the presence of pulmonary hypertension. With the two-dimensional sector scan echocardiogram the size and the exact localization of the ventricular septal defect can be determined. It may also reveal associated lesions such as mitral stenosis, subaortic obstruction, anomalies of the aortic arch. All of this information is important, particularly when surgery is contemplated.

Cardiac catheterization is necessary to determine the exact magnitude of the left-to-right shunt and the degree of the pulmonary vascular resistance. Left ventricular angiocardiography can reveal the exact localization of the ventricular septal defect, provided the correct projection is used to outline the appropriate part of the interventricular septum. It remains important to exclude associated malformations.

Medical therapy should be directed at the control of the heart failure and any pulmonary infection if present. Intractable cardiac failure requires *early surgical closure* of the defect despite the age of the child. This happens in approximately 5 % of these infants. The surgical mortality rate varies between 0 and 5 %. At present, banding of the pulmonary artery is only justifiable for multiple ventricular septal defects and possibly in preterm infants with severe cardiopulmonary distress. In the latter case it is advisable to also close the ductus at the same time. Re-operation, in order to complete the correction with removal of the band, should be carried out within 18 months, because of the risk of secondary lesions.

COMMON ATRIOVENTRICULAR CANAL

The complete form of this defect is sometimes symptomatic, and poorly tolerated, from the early neonatal period. It is due to an *endocardial cushion defect*: lack of fusion of the anterior and posterior endocardial cushions of the primitive atrioventricular canal, and comprises: A large low atrial septal defect, in direct continuity with a high posterior ventricular septal defect, at the level of the inlets of the ventricles. The differentiation of the atrioventricular valve is incomplete, resulting in a common anterior and posterior atrioventricular valve for the two ventricles.

The partial forms, principally represented by a low atrial septal defect of the ostium primum type with a cleft in the mitral valve, are well tolerated and can only be detected by a *characteristic electrocardiographic pattern, which is common to all the forms of endocardial cushion defect*: left upper QRS axis (between − 60° and − 140°), deep SI SII SIII waves, frequently with an increased PR interval. This pattern is not absolutely specific for this defect and can be sometimes observed in other malformations. Nevertheless, it is of great value in the presence of a systolic murmur and morphologic features of *Down syndrome* or, more rarely, of other polymalformative syndromes.

The common atrioventricular canal represents about 2 % of congenital cardiac malformations. Its incidence in Down syndrome is about 20 %.

The findings in the poorly tolerated forms is the same as that of any large left-to-right shunt and commonly appear in the first weeks of life. Sometimes there is a blowing pansystolic murmur at the apex, radiating to the left axilla, which is caused by the associated mitral incompetence.

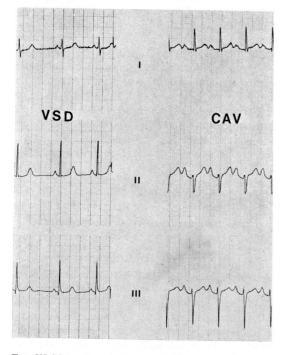

FIG. III-26. — *Ventricular septal defect and atrio-ventricular canal.* Electrocardiograms to show the mean QRS electrical axis of + 90 degrees in a ventricular septal defect (VSD) and of −60 degrees in a common atrioventricular canal (CAV). In the CAV the PR interval is increased and a P-pulmonale is present.

The electrocardiogram, in addition to the characteristic features described above, shows right or biventricular hypertrophy on the precordial leads, depending on the degree of pulmonary hypertension and overload of the ventricles.

The chest X-ray often shows marked cardiomegaly, suggesting a dilatation of the four chambers. The cardiomegaly is often greater than in the other malformations with a large left-to-right shunt.

The echocardiogram visualizes the typical interatrial and interventricular defects of this malformation. Compared with angiocardiography, the two-dimensional sector scan echocardiogram provides more information about the anomaly. It clearly visualizes the lesions on the atrioventricular valve and the place of insertion of its chordae tendinae. The dimensions of the various cardiac chambers can be determined and easily outlined.

Anatomical details, essential for surgical intervention, can be analysed. In most of the cases cardiac catheterization confirms the presence of pulmonary hypertension and sometimes the early development of increased pulmonary resistance. 50 % have a slight arterial desaturation that may result from pulmonary venous desaturation due to pulmonary congestion, from the presence of some left-to-right shunt, as frequently seen in the inferiorly situated interatrial defects, and also from a right-to-left shunt when pulmonary vascular obstruction is present. The left ventricular angiocardiogram shows a typical "goose-neck" deformity of the outflow tract and can estimate the degree of atrioventricular regurgitation.

Medical treatment is usually disappointing without surgical intervention. About 50 % of these infants die before the age of 6 months, 80 % before 5 years. The technical problems of *surgery* for this complex malformation have improved considerably. The surgical mortality rate is about 20 % in infants between 6 and 12 months. Before the age of 3 months, the mortality rate is still higher, due to cardiac immaturity, hyperreactivity of the pulmonary arteriolar bed and severity of the heart failure. Pulmonary artery banding gives poor results and should be reserved for the forms without significant mitral regurgitation. The current tendency is to perform an early complete correction. Beyond the age of two years the surgical mortality rate increases, depending primarily on the presence of associated malformations and the severity of the acquired obstructive lesions of the pulmonary arterial tree.

TRUNCUS ARTERIOSUS

The common arterial trunk, or persistent truncus arteriosus, is a single vessel arising from the heart, above a high ventricular septal defect, and leading to the ascending aorta, the pulmonary arteries and the coronary arteries. Several anatomical types have been described: the most frequent is type I, the trunk of the pulmonary artery detaching itself from the common trunk before dividing; in types II and III, the right and left pulmonary arteries arise separately from the common trunk; one of these may also be missing. Finally, an appearance very close, from a physiopathological point of view, occurs with a large aorto-pulmonary window, which differs from type I only by the existence of two valvar rings—aortic and pulmonary—but whose surgical correction is much simpler. In truncus arteriosus, the single valvar ring straddles a high, anterior and generally wide ventricular septal defect and is most often situated in frank dextroposition, for the most part above the right ventricle; levo-position is much rarer. The truncal valve consists of 2 to 6 cusps; they are thick, abnormal, resulting in stenosis or regurgitation in more than 50 % of the cases. The aortic arch is to the right in one third of the cases. Associated malformations are common: interruption of the aortic arch, coarctation, double aortic arch, anomalies of distribution of the coronary arteries, absence of one of the two pulmonary arteries.

The malformation is frequently symptomatic during the neonatal period (75 % of the cases are symptomatic before one month) manifested by respiratory distress and congestive cardiac failure due to a large left-to-right shunt. Cyanosis is usually present: It is almost inapparent demanding confirmation by measurement of the SaO_2. It can be more marked to the extent that a diagnosis of transposition is sometimes suggested. The systolic murmur resembles a ventricular septal defect murmur but is sometimes associated with a protosystolic click; the second sound is a single, non-split sound, sometimes followed by a diastolic murmur of truncal valve insufficiency. In two out of three cases there is arterial hyperpulsatility. Only a few characteristic findings can be listed at this age; *the X-ray*, which sometimes shows an egg-shaped heart as in transposition, an arch of the left pulmonary artery too high ("comma" sign); an aortic arch to the right, whose diagnostic value is considerable when it is observed with a

picture of cyanosis and hypervascularised lungs; or *the electrocardiogram* which shows combined ventricular enlargement rather than an exclusively right or left one; on the other hand, the *echocardiogram* shows the single vessel straddling the two ventricles, as in pulmonary atresia with open interventricular septum; there is also a mitro-truncal valve continuity; indirect features of a large left-to-right shunt (right atrium/aorta ratio increased), truncal semi-lunar valves which are sometimes thick, mitral and tricuspid diastolic fluttering which resembles an insufficiency of the truncal valve may also be present.

Cardiac catheterization shows an equality of ventricular pressures and a bidirectional ventricular shunt, and the angiography permits one to diagnose the anatomical type and associated lesions: Usually stenosis of the pulmonary arteries or the absence of one of them, insufficiency or stenosis of the truncal valve.

The prognosis is poor in the short term: in the case of failure of digitalo-diuretic treatment, since the banding of the main pulmonary artery (or of each one of its branches in types II or III) entails a heavy mortality rate; on a long term basis, in the case of successful stabilisation from the first months, since obstructive vascular pulmonary disease is common and gives deceiving results for complete correction, which consists of the placing of a valved conduit between the right ventricle and the pulmonary artery detached from the common trunk. The surgical mortality rate varies between 20 and 30 %.

COMPLEX DEFECTS:
UNIVENTRICULAR HEART,
DOUBLE OUTLET RIGHT VENTRICLE

When these defects are not complicated by stenosis or atresia of the pulmonary tract, their serious nature is not necessarily evident from the neonatal period. A polymalformative syndrome is frequently noted, a systolic murmur is usually heard, pulmonary hypervascularity and cardiac failure rarely appear before the end of the first month. They are often confused with a trivial ventricular septal defect, more so where cyanosis is not evident. This is why it is necessary to measure the PaO_2, which shows a moderate hypoxemia, and to attentively examine the electrocardiogram, which occasionally reveals unusual signs: monotonous precordial recordings with rS on all the precordial leads in the single ventricle, for example; these unusual signs are however not constant. In fact, only the echocardiogram is able to show the characteristic anomalies; single ventricular chamber, absence of mitro-aortic continuity, malposition of the great vessels. Cardiac catheterization and angiocardiography can give precision as to the anatomic diagnosis but are performed only in the case of early cardiac failure which is poorly controlled by medical treatment.

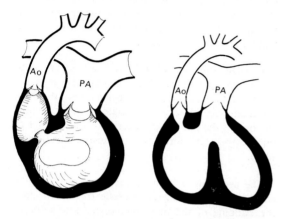

FIG. III-27. — *Single ventricle and double outlet right ventricle.* Diagram of the usual pattern of univentricular heart (*a*) and a double outlet right ventricle with a subpulmonary ventricular septal defect (*b*).

Ao = aorta; AP = pulmonary artery.

Banding for the pulmonary artery is the initial choice procedure in surgical management, the possibilities for ultimate complete correction are poor in univentricular heart, to such an extent that the indications for banding can be questioned.

MYOCARDIAL ISCHEMIA IN THE NEWBORN

Ischemic myocardial disease is a condition whose frequency is increasingly recognized in neonatal pathology. It is responsible for congestive cardiomyopathy of variable gravity and results from diverse causes: sometimes congenital heart disease, but also iatrogenic accidents, systemic disease and, primarily, functional disturbances of a heart which is structurally normal.

Clinical features

The majority of the functional and physical signs are not specific: they simply explain the ventricular hypocontractility, particularly the left side, which results from the myocardial ischemia. Similarly, their gravity varies considerably in relation to the extent of the ischemia. On the other hand electrocardiogram, laboratory findings and scintilography are useful adjunct tools in diagnosis.

Non specific signs.

Functional findings are usually serious. Even though the ischemia can be detected by chance on the electrocardiogram of a newborn, the most common instance is that of respiratory distress, occuring shortly after birth and accompanied by tachypnea and moderate cyanosis. The situation can be even more serious, reflecting true asphyxia, with or without collapse.

Physical findings can be minimal but it is usual to discover signs of *cardiac failure*: hepatomegaly,

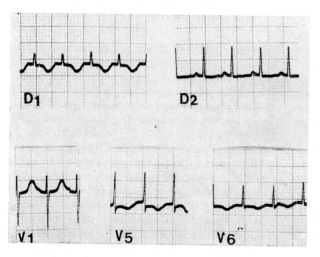

FIG. III-28. — *Transient myocardial ischemia in a newborn.* Electrocardiogram at twelve hours of life, after severe fetal compromise. Inverse T waves, prolonged QT interval, in DI V5 V6.

tachycardia, dull heart sounds with a gallop rhythm. In half of the cases one can hear a xiphoid systolic murmur from tricuspid insufficiency or, more rarely, an apical one from mitral insufficiency. Most severe cases eventuate in *collapse*, with a greyish tint and generalised arterial pulse weakness.

The radiological data can be summarized as *cardiomegaly* of varying degree and an increased density of the pulmonary area by images of interstitial and venous congestion; thus the term "humid lung", or, in more serious cases, frank lung edema.

Routine laboratory findings add little: mixed acidemia of varying degrees, moderate hypoxemia, partially responsive to oxygenation, sometimes hypoglycemia, and in the case of prolonged collapse, hyperazotemia and hyperkalemia.

The echocardiogram has the principal merit of excluding the possibility of hypoplasic left heart syndrome, whose clinical features are identical and affirming that the heart is structurally normal. It may show hypokinetic activity of the left ventricular myocardium and can also suggest pulmonary arterial hypertension.

Invasive explorations are of little use, since they do not reveal any more information than utrasound.

Specific signs.

The electrocardiogram is always pathological and provides the most important criteria for the diagnosis. Apart from the right ventricular predominance, normal at this age, one can observe at least a flattening or inversion of the T-wave in several leads. Associated with it there can be an ST-segment depression or elevation, and even some Q waves of necrosis, which permit one to describe four degrees of increasing severity. The classical tracing of a transmural infarction is rare in the newborn.

Myocardial enzyme findings may also help in the diagnosis since it is usual to observe a significant rise in the amount of the MB fraction of creatine phosphokinase (CPK).

Perfusion scintilography with Thalium 201 clearly shows a defect in myocardial fixation, which is all the more marked when myocardial ischemia is severe. This defect is usually diffuse throughout the left ventricle.

Etiological diagnosis

Malformative causes. — Several of the congenital malformations can cause myocardial ischemia; principally *severe obstructions of the left outlet*, as in critical aortic stenosis and coarctation syndromes, poorly tolerated from birth on. It is, in fact, often because of myocardial ischemia that the tolerance is precociously poor. These are anomalies which should be recognized immediately, as their early surgical treatment is the key to therapy. It is to be noted that *anomalous pulmonary origin of the left coronary artery*, which is the principal cause of myocardial infarction in children is *rarely detected in the neonatal period*. This fact is probably related to the persistence of high pulmonary resistance, maintaining, in the anomalous left coronary artery, high pressures to preserve satisfactory left myocardial perfusion. It is usually towards the age of two to six months that the infantile forms of this defect become symptomatic. *Atresia of a coronary ostium* can, on the other hand, become symptomatic early: supravalvar aortography can detect the lesion.

Non malformative causes. — These are by far the most common in the newborn.

Coronary thrombosis can result from an embolus originating from the umbilical vein. The traumatic role of catheterization of this vein, particularly during exchange-transfusion, is highly probable. The myocardial infarction is usually massive and detected at autopsy.

Infantile idiopathic calcifying arteriopathy can reveal itself within the first days of life as severe cardiac failure, with cardiogenic shock and myocardial ischemia. If the child survives, arterial hypertension appears and periscapsular calcifications can be seen on the X-ray. The evolution is rapidly fatal and histological examination shows an obliterative intimal fibroelastic proliferation of small muscular, renal and all coronary arteries, with calcification of the media and the internal elastic membrane. It is often a familial defect. Early treatment with diphosphonate seems promising of being curative.

Congenital rubella can include a severe ischemic myocardiopathy which often evolves towards death, in a picture of septicemia with necrotic lesions at autopsy.

Transient myocardial ischemia syndrome generally occurs in infants born at term, having had fetal distress or birth difficulties, with an Apgar score often below 6. The degree of coronary ischemia is variable: from simple transitory tachypnea to severe collapse. There is often a *tricuspid insufficiency*, due to ischemia of the papillary muscles, or, more rarely, *mitral insufficiency*. Histological lesions in fatal cases vary from myocardial cellular edema, in the case of rapid evolution, to areas of necrosis, eventually calcified, in cases of death at a later stage. Clinically, the evolution can be favourable within a few days; This is more so the case where the clinical attack has been less severe but the electrocardiogram may take several months to normalize.

Treatment

The less serious cases require only simple symptomatic measures: oxygen therapy, correction of acidemia and hypoglycemia. In the case of confirmed cardiac failure, artificial ventilation is indicated for a difficult period of several days, as is treatment with furosemide. Digoxin can be more dangerous than useful. The use of vasoactive drugs should be seriously considered in the case of severe collapse; nitrates, such as sodium nitroprusside, to lower the systemic afterload, or beta-mimetic drugs such as dopamine. Close hemodynamic surveillance (pulmonary arterial and wedge pressures) is necessary.

NEONATAL CARDIOMYOPATHIES

The term "cardiomyopathy" is used, in a specific way, to designate primary myocardial disease which affect a normally formed cardiovascular system. The development of echographic methods of investigation has contributed to the detection of these diseases in the newborn and to the recognition of their pathophysiologic and anatomic types: At this age, they can be divided into "hypertrophic", "concentric", "asymmetric" and possibly "obstructive" varieties; the so-called "congestive" or hypokinetic forms are more rare. The prognosis and treatment depend considerably on a possible etiology but on the whole they are serious illnesses.

General symptoms and diagnosis

Neonatal cardiomyopathies are generally detected as a severe functional syndrome associating *congestive cardiac failure and peripheral collapse*: respiratory distress, cyanosis, liver enlargement, weak peripheral pulses, tachycardia, dull cardiac sounds with a gallop rhythm and sometimes a systolic murmur due to mitral insufficiency. The routine complementary examinations are not speci-

fic: cardiomegaly and pulmonary venous congestion on the X-ray; right, left or combined ventricular enlargement with frequent repolarization disturbances on the electrocardiogram; acidemia with hypobasemia, hyperkalemia and hyperazotemia in the case of associated renal function failure.

Given such a situation the diagnostic procedure is based on the *echocardiogram*.

One can begin by excluding the diagnosis of *pericardial effusion*, which should be considered if the cardiomegaly evolves rapidly.

One should next try to recognise the *cardiovascular malformations* which are often accompanied by *secondary cardiomyopathies*, and which are more frequent at this age that the primary varieties. In the case of concentric myocardial hypertrophy with hypokinesis, one can look for a left sided obstruction such as critical aortic stenosis, coarctation syndrome or aortic arch interruption. This last diagnosis can be difficult to exclude without endocardial exploration. In the case of dilatation and severe diastolic overload of the ventricles, one should direct attention towards a systemic arterio-venous fistula, above all an intracranial one which can reflect hypervolemia as hydrops fetalis (rhesus illness; prolonged fetal paroxysmal tachycardia).

One can recognize, finally, *ischemic myocardial disease* when the dilatation and hypokinesis of the left ventricle seen on the echocardiogram, is associated with electrocardiographic, biochemical and scintilographic anomalies suggestive of ischemic cardiomyopathy: at this age, this syndrome most often follows fetal or obstetrical distress and has a good chance of being cured.

When all of these possibilities have been excluded, and the myocardial dysfunction remains unexplained, one can speak of a *primary cardiomyopathy*.

Etiological diagnosis of primary cardiomyopathies

Cardiomyopathies of known causes.

The infant of a diabetic mother is often affected by an hypertrophic cardiomyopathy. It is generally sub-clinical and can be detected by routine echocardiogram study. However it can be much more severe, concentric or obstructive, leading to serious cardiovascular difficulties. The characteristic appearance of these newborns is an aid in the diagnosis, when the maternal antecedent is not known. The disease is relatively self limited but symptomatic treatment may help through a difficult period. One should avoid the administration of all inotropic drugs, particularly digitalis, which will aggravate the sub-aortic obstruction. Some have even suggested using beta-blockers: one should reserve these for the most severe cases.

Neonatal hypoglycemia (other than in the context of maternal diabetes mellitus) has also been incriminated in the explanation of associated cardiomyopathy. One can ask if, in many cases, the myocardial dysfunction is not the ischemic consequence of perinatal distress, responsible in addition for the hypoglycemia.

Serious hypocalcemia can, on the other hand, be the cause of severe cardiac failure with considerable dilatation of the heart. The systematic measurement of calcemia in all seriously ill newborns permits its recognition and treatment with calcium preparations.

Type II glycogen storage disease due to the absence of acid maltase (Pompe's disease) sometimes reveals itself in the neonatal period as severe cardiac failure with hypertrophic cardiomyopathy. The lethargy and generalised hypotonia of this disease in the older infant is absent in the first few days. The electrocardiogram is more specific: short PR-interval, left axis QRS, repolarization changes and above all very high voltages of the ventriculograms in all leads. The appearance of the glycogen storage of the myofibrils on the muscle biopsy and the lack of acid maltase in the muscle, liver and even leucocytes of the peripheral blood, leads to the diagnosis. The disease evolves inevitably towards death within a few weeks to a few months. The interest to identify it lies in the possibility of prenatal detection by specific enzymatic activity in the amniotic cells of future pregnancies. The disease is inherited and transmitted as an autosomal recessive.

Lipid storage diseases, secondary to difficulties in the metabolism of carnitine, only rarely begin at birth. They can be confirmed by the lipid storage in the cells at muscle biopsy, and proven by biolochemical evidence of generalised or muscular deficiency of carnitine, or lack of palmityl-carnitine transferase. Its importance lies in the sensitivity of some forms to substitutive treatment with carnitine chloride, associated with a specific diet.

Cardiomyopathies of unknown cause. — This is essentially a question of early forms of *idiopathic hypertrophic subaortic stenosis* or "asymmetric septal hypertrophy" in the newborn. It should be clearly distinguished from the physiologic asymmetric septal hypertrophy of the newborn, whose natural evolution is towards its disappearance: It is generally asymptomatic. But, when the septal hypertrophy becomes huge and shows no tendency towards involution, it has pathologic importance. It is then very serious, poorly tolerated and leads to death in a few weeks or a few months despite all medical (beta-blockers) or surgical (subaortic myotomy) treatment. It is often familial and is transmitted as a dominant trait. More rarely, the characteristic disarray of the septal fibres relates to an embryopathy, for example, rubella or alcohol.

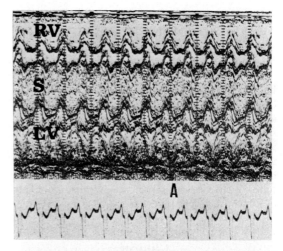

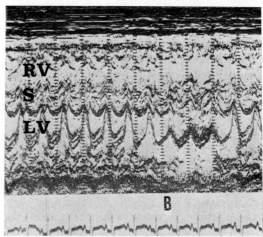

FIG. III-29. — *Hypertrophic cardiomyopathy in a newborn of a diabetic mother.*

A : M-mode echocardiogram at 6 hours of life; significant hypertrophy of the ventricular septum (S) and posterior wall of the left ventricle (LV). The mitral valve is "cramped for room" in a small ventricular cavity.

B : Same patient, after 20 days: clear decrease in septal hypertrophy. The mitral valve has "plenty of room" in the cavity.

Together with the cardiomyopathies one needs to consider *primary endocardial fibro-elastosis* which becomes symptomatic occasionally right from the neonatal period, in the form of rapidly dramatic cardiac failure often in a familial pattern. Its pathogenesis is debatable but the primordial element is myocardial: the thickening endocardium is probably not the cause, but rather the consequence of the hemodynamic disturbances.

ARTERIOVENOUS FISTULAE

Three types of systemic arteriovenous fistulae can be symptomatic in the newborn. They are, in order of frequency: cerebral, hepatic and peripheral arteriovenous fistulae. They can create a considerable shunt. The left heart has to compensate for this with tachycardia and an increase in the stroke volume. The increase in the systemic venous drainage overloads the right heart. This leads therefore to congestive heart failure, which consists initially of a high cardiac output.

Clinical and paraclinical signs

Heart failure appears early, it is global and severe. The newborn is tachycardic, tachypneic, sometimes cyanotic, with liver enlargement. A systolic murmur is heard, which may be due to tricuspid insufficiency but which is most often the radiation of a cervico-cephalic or hepatic murmur due to the fistula. A gallop rhythm is rare. There is almost always huge cardiomegaly, the pulmonary vasculature is normal or increased due to pulmonary venous congestion. The electrocardiogram can show right ventricular enlargement, biventricular enlargement and quite often negative T waves in the left precordial leads.

Often, the extracardiac origin of the cardiac failure is not detected before catheterization and angiography or even before the autopsy. However, certain signs should attract attention, suggest a fistula and give precision to its site.

Topographic diagnosis

Cerebral arteriovenous fistulae can be suspected if neurological signs exist: convulsions, tone changes,

rapid augmentation of the volume of the skull, but these signs are rare and appear late. If one thinks of auscultating the skull, one can usually discover a loud continuous murmur. Unfortunately, this murmur is not constant nor pathognomonic, since one can hear it in some cardiac diseases, such as truncus arteriosus. The peripheral pulses are ample and bounding, at least at the beginning, with a hyper-pulsatility of the neck vessels, suggesting a coarctation. The veins of the neck and the scalp are dilated: this sign is characteristic, but not constant. The echocardiogram is of interest for differential diagnosis. It shows the vessels in normal place, dilated cardiac chambers and absence of valvar anomalies. On catheterization, the right sided pressures are raised to the systemic level, and there is above all a notable increase of the oxygen level in the superior vena cava in contrast to the inferior vena cava. When cardiac failure is severe, there is sometimes a desaturation of left atrial blood from a right-to-left shunt across the foramen ovale. Left ventriculography permits one to confirm the diagnosis by showing a massive rapid return of the contrast via the jugular veins and superior vena cava. In addition, it illustrates the dilatation and tortuosity of the carotid arteries and jugular veins. An aortogram via the umbilical route can yield the same information: it is the best method in the first few days of life because of its simplicity. When one suspects a cerebral arteriovenous fistula before catheterization, or as soon as this method has demonstrated some indirect signs of this, the angiogram, with the skull in the field of the X-rays, will show the site and size of the fistula.

Hepatic arteriovenous fistulae. — Hepatomegaly is constant. At auscultation of the hepatic area, a systolic murmur or a continuous murmur is heard, radiating into the precordium. At catheterization, the oxygen content of the inferior vena cava is extremely high, in contrast to that of superior vena cava. The left ventriculogram and aortogram indirectly confirm the diagnosis by showing a precocious and torrential venous return of the contrast via the inferior vena cava, and direct visualization if the liver is included into the field of the X-rays. They are essential in establishing the sites and sizes of the fistulae.

Peripheral arteriovenous fistulae are the easiest to diagnose, since those associated cutaneous angiomas are frequent, as is a sometimes huge enlargement of the affected limb. On the other hand, a localised thrill is often noticeable before the appearance of cardiac failure.

Natural history and management

Cardiac failure due to arteriovenous fistulae is often difficult to control by tonicardiac therapy, which is indispensable whatever the origin of the fistulae.

Cerebral arteriovenous fistulae have a severe prognosis and many newborns die from heart failure or neurological complications (convulsions, intracranial haemorrhages). At this age, neurosurgical treatment and embolisation seem at the moment to be difficult. In the patients who survive the neonatal period: mental retardation, intracranial haemorrhages or hydrocephaly can remain. Even after the age of one year treatment by ligation of the afferent arteries is difficult and despite repeated interventions the result is hazardous. It can however be good.

Hepatic arteriovenous fistulae have a slightly better but less forseeable prognosis. The hemangiomas can become complicated with profuse intratumoural haemorrhages, provoking a consumptive coagulopathy. Corticoids have sometimes given excellent results as has radiotherapy. Surgery is possible only when the fistulae are localised. It has had some successes.

Peripheral arteriovenous fistulae have a variable evolution sometimes severe and rapidly malignant. In very extensive forms, ligation of the afferent artery can save the patient, particularly where an excision of the angiomatic mass is difficult or dangerous.

Other types of arteriovenous fistulae

Placental arteriovenous fistulae can be at the origin of precocious neonatal cardiac failure, or even in utero, with hydrops fetalis. Cardiac failure disappears after delivery and the diagnosis is made only upon examination of the placenta which shows a hemangiopericytoma, whose size can be of some importance.

Pulmonary arteriovenous fistulae are rarely symptomatic in the newborn but they can be the cause of neonatal cyanosis.

Fistulae between a systemic artery and pulmonary vessels can be observed in the "Scimitar syndrome", whose neonatal forms are precociously severe. This syndrome is associated, with a right anomalous pulmonary venous drainage in the inferior vena cava, dextrocardia and a hypoplastic right lung. There is almost always a decrease in the arterial vasculature of the right lung and a systemic vascularization of varying importance, generally coming from the abdominal aorta. If this systemic vasculature is highly developed, the defect is symptomatic right from the neonatal period. The systemic arterial blood is drained by the pulmonary veins towards the right atrium; pulmonary hypertension results from it at the systemic level, provoking cardiac failure with respiratory distress. This diagnosis should always be suspected in a newborn with congestive cardiac failure or with respiratory distress, when there is dextrocardia and a right lung

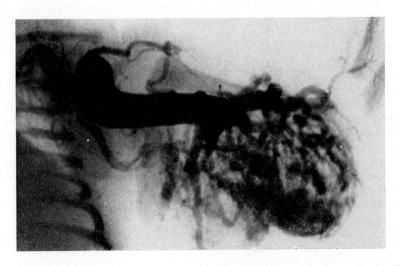

Fig. III-30. — *Malignant arteriovenous fistulas* in a newborn; early view of an arteriogram: huge axillary and humeral arteries, angiomatous network very dilated, resulting in brachial hypertrophy. Note the cardiomegaly, the left border of the heart comes in contact with the axillary thoracic wall.

which is clearly hypoplastic. The angiocardiogram confirms the diagnosis: the right ventriculogram shows a right anomalous pulmonary venous drainage in the inferior vena cava and the left ventri-culogram or aortography shows the abnorma systemic arteries. In the case of failure of tonicardiac medical therapy, ligation of the abnormal systemic vessels is the only efficient surgical procedure.

Special problems

CARDIAC ARRHYTHMIAS

Cardiac rhythm disorders observed in the new-born are congenital or acquired. When congenital they are sometimes detected in utero. Where acquired the rhythmic disorders are most often the consequence of serious hemodynamic disturbances in relation to congenital heart disease, myocardial ischemia, serious perturbations of electrolyte balance or iatrogenic factors (digitalis intoxication, cardiac catheterization or neonatal surgery).

Anatomical and physiological review

The conduction system of the heart comprises: a centre of production of the stimulus, the sino-atrial node; internodal pathways which link the sinoatrial node to the atrioventricular node; atrio-ventricular junction from whence arise; atrionodal fibres, then the atrioventricular node, finally the bundle of His which penetrates into the central fibrous body from where it emerges to divide itself into two branches; the right and left bundle-branches, which continue in the terminal Purkinje network to the contractile myocardial fibres.

The fundamental property of these cells of nodal tissue is their automaticity, which permits them to depolarize slowly, but spontaneously, just to the threshold level, which produces the rapid depola-rization and the impulse. The common myocardial cells do not possess this property and can only be depolarized under the effect of an impulse. Normally it is the sinoatrial node which has the preponderant automatism and which regularly emits impulses which cross the sino-atrial junction and depolarize the atria. This activity is marked on the electrocardio-gram by a P wave, whose axis and morphology depend upon the origin of the centre of production, or pacemaker. The impulse thus reaching the auriculo-ventricular junction, its propagating speed is considerably reduced in the atrio-ventricular node before increasing again in the bundle of His and its branches through which it reaches and depolarizes the ventricles. The ventricular activity appears on the electrocardiogram as the QRS complex. This is separated from the P wave by a space going from the beginning of P to the beginning of QRS and which is the sum of three conduction times: P-A interval, the sino-nodal conduction time between the moment of production of the impulse and that of its entry into the atrio-ventricular node; A-H interval, intra-nodal conduction time measuring the delay of the crossing of the atrio-ventricular node; H-V interval, conduction time of the His-Purkinje system between the entry of the impulse in the bundle of His and it's arrival at the distal myocardial cells. This timing can be measured by endocavitary recording. This autonomous centre of production and conduction is connected to the rest of the organism by sympathetic and parasympathetic systems. The latter selectively influences the sino-atrial node, whose emission frequency it slows and the atrio-ventricular node, whose conduction-power it limits.

The mechanisms responsible for arrhythmias are; the anomalies of the formation of the impulse, depression of the sinus node or abnormal hyper-excitability of a focus situated elsewhere (hetero-topic or ectopic focus); the anomalies of con-duction of the impulse, propagation blocked, slowed down or non-homogenous; a frequent combination of these two mechanisms leading to desynchronization (fibrillation), and a circuit said to be of "reentrance" (reciprocal rhythms).

Anomalies of sinus rhythm

Sinus tachycardia can reach a frequency of 220/m. It is a response to different stimuli. It is characterised by a P wave with an axis between 0º and +90º, and a PR interval at least equal to 80 ms.

Sinus bradycardia is characterised by a frequency below 90/m. It can be due to a lesion of the sinus node, but is then rarely isolated and alternates with other disorders, resulting in the "sick sinus syndrome". Most often it is due to vagal stimuli and disappears with atropine. A marked sinus bradycardia can cause escape coming from the bringing into play of a pacemaker situated lower, generally junctional: This is a common phenomenon in the newborn. At a more marked degree, a junctional rhythm can appear transiently, each time that the sinus rhythm slows down: this "displacement of the pacemaker" has no pathological significance.

Sinus arrhythmia is most often of respiratory origin in the child, but is rarely observed in the newborn.

Premature beats

These are frequent in the newborn and even in the fetus and occur most often in a healthy heart. This "extrasystolic disorder" remits spontaneously within a few days to a few weeks. It is a reflection of a hyperexcitability of a centre of automatism or a re-entrance phenomenon ("echo" premature beats). If the centre is atrial or junctional, the ventricular complex is not enlarged. If it is ventricular, the ventricular complex is wide, but a wide complex may also be due to functional intraventricular blocking of a supra-ventricular premature beat. The place of the P′ atriogram depends on the position of the ectopic centre. P′ may not be followed by QRS (blocked supraventricular premature beat). A premature beat is generally followed by a compensatory pause. The premature beats arise isolated, in short bursts or coupled with sinus complexes following fixed rhythms or allorhythmias, such as bigeminism. This latter, when it arises in utero, can mimic a severe bradycardia, leading to a caesarian section; in fact, each normal beat is audible whereas the extrasystole is not, thus giving a false bradycardia on auscultation of the maternal abdomen.

In the presence of premature beats, it is essential to assure their isolated nature, since it can also reveal organic cardiac disease. Occasionally, frequent and precocious ventricular premature beats, appearing on a record with prolongation of the QT interval, can have an ominous character: This is the "long QT syndrome" which is generally genetically determined and may be responsible for sudden death.

Heterotopic tachycardias

Supraventricular tachycardia. — These occur with a predilection for boys during the first three months, and in half of the cases in the first month. Some are detected in utero. They are only rarely associated with a congenital heart lesion (Ebstein's disease) or with a cardiac tumor (rhabdomyoma). Most often, the prognosis, after their control, is good. However, the high frequency (300/m and more) can be responsible for severe cardiac failure, sometimes initiating in-utero hydrops fetalis. The frequency is extremely high, not countable without the electrocardiogram, it is regular and remarkably fixed. Signs of cardiac failure (tachypnea, hepatomegaly, edema) are coupled with signs of low cardiac output (collapse, convulsions). The cardiomegaly is evident and accompanied by pulmonary edema.

QRS complexes are not enlarged, with some exceptions (functional bundle branch block, or reciprocal rhythm with anterograde conduction in an accessory pathway and retrograde in the bundle of His). The study of the atriogram and its relationship to the ventriculogram permits one to approach the mechanism of the crisis. If the surface electrocardiogram is not sufficiently explicit, one can have recourse to œsophagal recordings and—rarely in the newborn—to intracardiac recordings.

Junctional tachycardias with reciprocal rhythm are due to a mechanism of "reentry", coupling in two ways, one anterograde, the other retrograde. This circuit can be situated in the junction itself, whose fibres are dissociated in two tracts whose electrophysiological properties differ; (at the moment of the arrival of the stimulus, one is excitable in the anterograde direction, the other is in the refractory period and will be excitable, a little later, only in the retrograde sense, thus the initiation of the "reentry" circuit. It is most often constituted by the normal nodohisian tract (travelled through generally in the anterograde direction) and by an accessory atrio-ventricular connection, constituted by an aberrant bundle, which is excitable in the retrograde direction. Such bundles, such as the bundle of Kent, can be due to an immaturity of the central fibrous body which allows persistent myocardial fibres permitting this by-pass: if maturation is delayed, these fibres can involute and the tachycardia, which appeared during the neonatal period, will never reappear. In fact, it is more often a question of a simple latency of the accessory connection, which has become non-functional beyond the first few months of life by the diminution of its excitability; in this case, a "concealed" connection permits that which may, much later, be at the origin of another attack of reentrant tachycardia.

The presence of a bundle of Kent has as a consequence a ventricular pre-excitation when there is a return to sinus rhythm: when taken in the anterograde direction (like the nodo-hisian tract, which it by-passes), the accessory path permits an early activation of a part of one of the ventricles, which is connected to the atrial myocardium. A rather particular recording is the result, with a short PR, and a wave of pre-excitation at the foot of the rapid wave of ventricular depolarization, thus the enlargement of QRS. This is the *Wolff-Parkinson-White syndrome*. This syndrome can be detected in at least 50 % of the cases of the reciprocal tachycardias in the newborn, at the time of the sinus rhythm return, but the "concealed" bundles of pre-excitation are also almost as numerous. The surface recording differs according to the localization of the aberrant bundle. Schematically one can distinguish A-type (left ventricular bundle of pre-excitation) and B-type (right ventricular bundle). During the neonatal period, the incidence of the two types is about equal; later the B-type is more frequent; it is also this B-type that one encounters in association with congenital heart disease (Ebstein's disease, corrected transposition of the great vessels). It is

possible that A-type bundles of Kent are more often subject to post-natal involution or to latency than those of the B-type.

During the course of the attack of tachycardia, the heart rate is around 300, QRS complexes are usually not enlarged, the atriogram P' is more or less drowned in the ventricular repolarisation wave, there is a P' wave for every QRS complex, the P' axis is directed upwards, that is to say that P' is negative in DII-DIII-aVF. Other criteria, when present, are characteristic of reciprocal rhythms.

A particular variant form of reciprocal tachycardia should to be mentioned: considerably slower (200 at birth) it rarely entails decompensation but, on the other hand, it is particularly refractory to all therapeutic measures and generally persists in a "repetitive" form, that is characterised by strips of reciprocal rhythm separated each time by a few sinus complexes: This should be termed *chronic reciprocal tachycardia*, as opposed to the common paroxysmal tachycardias, which can usually be stopped by therapy.

Atrial tachycardias are due to a taking over by an ectopic focus whose rate can reach 400: above 300, there is generally an atrio-ventricular functional dissociation, therefore more P' waves than QRS complexes. This block can also be pro-

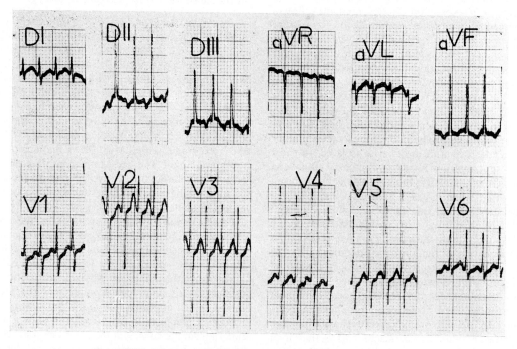

FIG. III-31. — *Paroxysmal supraventricular tachycardia in a newborn.*
Heart frequency: 300/m. P wave is inverted in DII-DIII.

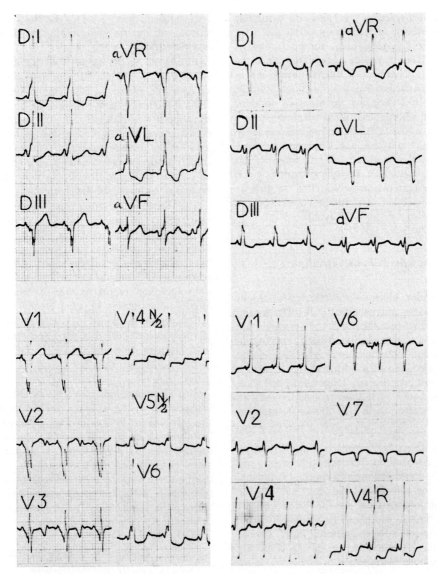

FIG. III-32. — *Wolff Parkinson White syndrome.* On the left, B-type: the "delta" wave (enlarged, at the beginning of the R wave) is positive in DI DII *a*VL and V4 V5 V6. On the right, A-type: the "delta" wave, less enlarged, is at the beginning of the R wave in V1 and V4R.

voked by vagal stimulation, which aids in the diagnosis.

Atrial flutter is due to an intra-atrial circular depolarization at 300 per min., with a ventricular response of 1/1, also susceptible to control by treatment: the atriogram is a succession of "saw teeth".

Atrial fibrillation is rare in the newborn: the basal line is irregular, animated by more or less regular quivering, going up to 700 per min., there is always a ventricular tachyarrhythmia.

Chaotic atrial tachycardias, sometimes called "polymorphic", "multifocal", are peculiar to the newborn; when they are not associated with organic heart disease, their prognosis is favourable. The atriogram has an unstable morphology with the appearances of atrial tachycardia corresponding to several different foci, strips of flutter, of fibrillation, of sinus rhythm. The ventricular rhythm is irregular, the complexes not enlarged, but one can often observe some large complexes with functional blocking of intraventricular conduction.

Ventricular tachycardias. — These are extremely rare in the newborn and are most often tied to a specific etiology (myocarditis, tumour, digitalis intoxication). The complexes are large and the principal problem consists of differentiating supraventricular tachycardias from a functional bundle branch block. It is necessary, in order to do that, to identify the ventriculo-atrial dissociation (there are fewer P waves than QRS waves) and the existence of "fusion beats". An œsophagal and endocavitary exploration is often necessary. *Ventricular fibrillation* is characterised by a desynchronisation which corresponds to a circulatory arrest. The "torsade de pointe" is a brief burst of fibrillation which can be seen specifically in the "long QT syndrome".

Non sinus bradycardias

Atrio-ventricular block. — *First degree* blocks are characterised by a lengthening of the PR, beyond 140 ms; although rare in the newborn, it is sometimes observed in some congenital heart conditions (atrio-ventricular canal, Ebstein's disease). *Second degree* blocks are most often of the Mobitz type I, that is the PR becomes progressively longer until a P wave is blocked and the period starts again; one can sometimes observe these in digitalis intoxication.

Complete or third degree block is characterised by a complete dissociation between the atrial and ventricular rhythms. The atrial frequency is normal for the age, the ventricular frequency slowed, the severity being proportional to the extent of the bradycardia. Such a block can be acquired, in the terminal stage of severe cyanotic heart disease with acidemia, hypothermia, or during a poorly tolerated cardiac catheterisation.

Complete congenital heart block is a rare disease (1 in 20,000 births). In 30 % of cases, it is associated with congenital heart disease (corrected transposition, complex heart defects) and increases the severity of the prognosis. When it is isolated, its morbidity depends on the degree of the bradycardia. Often it is detected in utero, in the form of a stable bradycardia, under 100/m, not influenced by uterine contractions. Sometimes, there is a familial pattern. It has been observed in children whose mothers suffer from connective tissue disorders, specifically systemic lupus erythematous, for which it is necessary to look for maternal clinical manifestations and biological signs, since it may be a presentation which is clinically latent. The lesions of the nodo-hisian sys-

tem which are responsible for the block are the consequence of the transplacental passage of immune complexes.

Intolerance in the neonatal period, and sometimes in utero, is the case for 10 % of these blocks and can be observed where the frequency is less than 60/m. Even though very slow rhythms can be accompanied by a poor neurological comportement, sometimes coma, apnea (due to sudden slowing of the rhythm, asystole or "torsade de pointe"), they are rare under three months of age and the presentation is usually as cardiac failure with collapse and cardiomegaly, related to a slowing of the rhythm.

The factors favouring poor prognosis are: a rate below 50/m; a progressive slowing from the first days; an infrahisian block with enlarged ventricular complexes; ventricular premature beats (which cause one to suspect ventricular fibrillation); prolonged QT interval and any important disorders of ventricular repolarisation. A familial pattern augurs unfavourably in heart block.

The prognosis for a block with a slow frequency in the neonatal period is poor and treatment, even with electrosystolic pacing yields poor results, the mortality rate being 50 %.

Sick sinus syndrome. — This is a rare cause of bradycardia in the neonatal period. It is generally the response to severe myocardial disease but can be observed as part of complex congenital heart lesions (Ivemark's syndrome). It associates a non-sinus bradycardia, usually junctional, with polymorphous supraventricular arrhythmias, junctional tachycardia, atrial flutter or fibrillation (bradycardia-tachycardia syndrome). The prognosis is poor.

Emergency treatment of arrhythmias

General management aims to reestablish the vital functions compromised by the rhythmic disorder: oxygenation, artificial respiration, or in case of serious heart failure with collapse, correction of the acidemia, and fluid depletion by furosemide. When the arrhythmia is discovered in utero, caesarian section may be indicated. Fetal echography and echocardiography can give information i.e. the severity of the cardiac failure. The administration of Digoxin to the mother has been recommended. Antiarrhythmic drugs which cross the placental barrier, such as propranolol, have shown some short term success in the treatment of heterotopic tachycardia.

Supraventricular tachycardias should be initially treated with digoxin, preferably administered from the beginning intravenously in the usual doses for the treatment of acute cardiac failure in the newborn. The techniques of vagal stimulation are not efficient or stop the tachycardia only for a few seconds. Digoxin is effictive in 80 % of tachycardias of the reciprocal type and in more than half of the atrial tachycardias. Treatment should be undertaken for one year. Relapses can be observed in 25 % of the cases, being more frequent in the case of reciprocal tachycardia. It is difficult to predict the natural history, some children, after a neonatal attack, may, several months later, be seen to suffer from a chronic form. There is no difference in prognosis between children showing the pattern of a Wolff-Parkinson-White syndrome and those who do not have it; the disappearance of the syndrome on the recording after several weeks or months adds nothing to the prediction. In the case of ineffectiveness of digoxin after 48 hours, one should add either beta-blockers (propranolol, 1 to 3 mg.kg/24 h) or preferably amiodarone (500 mg/m²/24 h as an initial dose, 250 mg/m²/24 h for ongoing treatment); this should be continued for 6 months. With atrial tachycardia or flutter, one can deliver an electric shock, if the situation is critical, or use an endo-atrial overdrive pacer. In the case of chaotic tachycardia, amiodarone is often effictive, one can also use isopyramide (250 mg/m²/24 h).

Ventricular tachycardias justify electric shock or, if the situation is not critical, amiodarone. Treatment of the "torsades de pointe" is more delicate and depends on the etiology (pacing, beta-blockers in genetic forms). That of ventricular fibrillation consists of cardiac massage, artificial respiration, the correction of the acidemia and immediate external electric shock (100 joules/m²).

Complete heart block justifies urgent treatment only in the case of a slow ventricular rate. Infusion of isoprenaline is sometimes sufficient but it is usually necessary to resort to endocavitary pacing. According t o the evolution (return or not of spontaneous rhythm greater than to 60/m, regression or not of the cardiomegaly) and to the type of block (enlarged or narrow ventricular complexes, isolated or associated with curable congenital heart disease) one can decide for or against pacemaker implantation. The miniaturization of lithium generators permits one to consider an implantation even in the newborn, under conditions which have become technically acceptable.

Sick sinus syndrome is extremely difficult to manage. Often it is necessary to couple pacing with substantial antiarrhythmic treatment, principally using amiodarone.

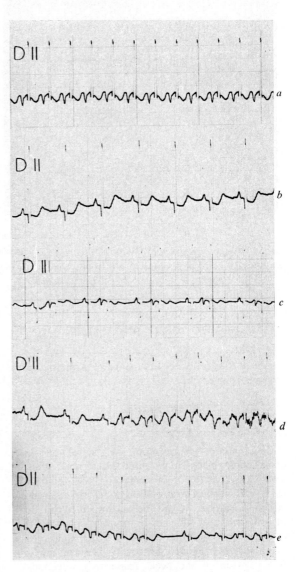

FIG. III-33. — *Chronic supraventricular tachycardia.* Heart frequency: 180/m.

a : Heterotopic rhythm present from birth, P wave inverted in DII.

b : After digoxin, return to a normal sinus rhythm.

c : Reapparence of a reciprocal rhythm, in the form of "echoes"; resulting in an extrasystolic bigeminism (an extrasystolic echo after each sinus complex).

d, e : Repetitive form of the heterotopic rhythm, with a few short phases of sinus rhythm.

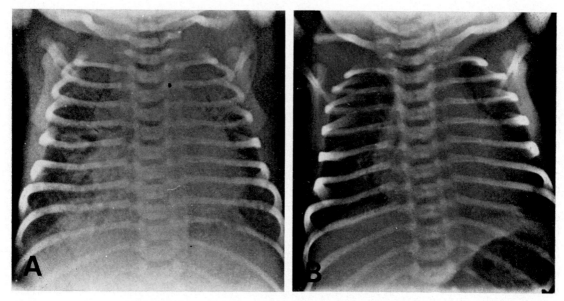

Fig. III-34. — *Complete congenital heart block in a newborn.*

A) At birth, ventricular rate: 50/m, cardiomegaly, pulmonary edema, cardiac failure.

B) After 24 hours with infusion of Isoprenalin, ventricular rate: 100/m, normal heart size, disappearance of pulmonary edema.

AORTIC ARCH ANOMALIES

Few of the aortic arch anomalies are symptomatic in the newborn.

Anomalies compressing the tracheo-œsophagal axis

The findings depend on the degree of the constriction being more precocious and severe where the constriction is significant; the dominant element is tracheal compression. Stridor is the most common feature; it can be accompanied by fits of suffocation, episodes of respiratory distress with cyanosis and sometimes attacks of reflex apnea. All of these are magnified by crying, the passage of food, flexion of the neck, respiratory infections, and the accumulation of tracheobronchial secretions. Rest and hyper-extension of the neck can reduce the distress. Dysphagia and false passages for alimentation are of a secondary nature. The frontal X-ray with high voltage gives information on the topography of the aorta and the morphology of the trachea. The most useful examinations are the barium-oesophagogram and angiocardiography. The study of œsophagal notches, which is facilated by cineradiography, often permits a diagnosis. Tracheo-

bronchography should be avoided because of the risk. The localization of the œsophagal notches and the angiocardiographic findings reveal the origin of the compression. Four principal malformations are encountered.

Retro-œsophagal sub-clavian artery. — This anomaly occurs frequently but is rarely symptomatic. It is often associated with some congenital heart lesions and may be found in chromosomal aberrations. Most often the right sub-clavian artery is involved, but, in the case of a right aortic arch, a left retro-œsophagal sub-clavian artery can occur. Diagnosis is made by barium-œsophagogram. It shows a posterior notch with an oblique "bayonet" trajectory from below to above and left to right. The notch is not very wide, except in the case of a left retro-œsophagal sub-clavian artery, since at the origin of the sub-clavian there is often an aortic diverticulum (Komerell's diverticulum). This disorder rarely justifies an operation. Frequent small feedings, treatment of bronchial infections and attentive nursing are indicated in the rare symptomatic cases which regress and progressively disappear during the first year of life.

Abnormal origin of the innominate arterial trunk. — The term "abnormal origin" can be criticized since, in the normal newborn, the innominate artery always originates to the left of the trachea and crosses its anterior face, on which it leaves a notch which is clearly visible in a lateral view under high voltage. In fact, the disorders are due to a tracheo-malacia and perhaps a shortness of the innominate artery, the two elements combining to accentuate the tracheal physiological constriction. This anomaly does not cause any œsophagal notch. Angiography has a negative value: it eliminates the other anomalies of the aortic arch. Surgery is rarely required.

Double aortic arch (vascular ring). — This anomaly constitues a vascular ring, surrounding the tracheo-œsophagal axis. Symptoms are precocious and may be severe. The œsophagogram shows on lateral view, a large posterior notch, which is due to the aorta; in a frontal view, a double notch on the right and left borders of œsophagus, the right one being often at a higher level. Left ventriculogram or aortogram shows the topography of the two arches, the type of the ring, complete or incomplete (with an intermediate fibrous part). This opacification also permits one to determine the preferred site of sectioning: fibrous part or the more narrow part of the complete ring. It is necessary to operate early, only if the symptoms are precociously severe. The surgeon usually performs a left thoracotomy, because the left arch is the smaller one in 95 % of cases, and therefore easier to resect.

Abnormal origin and course of the left pulmonary artery (vascular sling). — The left pulmonary artery is directed to the right above the right main bronchus, then turns to the right, passes between the trachea (in front) and œsophagus (behind) to reach the left hilum. It thus forms a vascular sling around the trachea. In addition to the stridor, usually expiratory, and to the attacks of respiratory distress, there may be associated disorders related to the compression of the right main bronchus: emphysema of the right lung or more rarely atelectasis. When compression exists from birth, one can observe an opacity of the right lung owing to a retention of alveolar fluid. Œsophagogram shows, in the lateral and left anterior oblique view, a notch which compresses the trachea in front and œsophagus behind. Angiography in the "sitting up" position shows the abnormal course of the left pulmonary artery. Surgical treatment is indicated in severe forms: with sectioning of the left pulmonary artery, which is rejoined in front of the trachea under circulatory by-pass.

Right pulmonary artery originating from the aorta

In this malformation, the right pulmonary artery arises from the aorta mid-way between the aortic valve and the aortic arch. There is often an associated ductus arteriosus. The clinical feature is that of a large left-to-right shunt with a rapid evolution towards heart failure. One can hear a systolic or systolo-diastolic murmur and palpate bounding pulses. The electrocardiogram shows biventricular enlargement and the X-ray a global cardiomegaly. A close examination of the pulmonary fields can show a differential vasculature with hypervasculature of the right lung, the left lung being of smaller size. If the diagnosis is suspected, a pulmonary scan will indicate that only the left pulmonary artery is vascularized from the right ventricle. Cardiac catheterization and angiocardiography confirm the diagnosis. The right ventriculogram opacifies the left pulmonary artery whereas the left ventriculogram opacifies the right pulmonary artery from the ascending aorta. The pressures in the right ventricle and pulmonary artery are at systemic level. Surgery is imperative before the age of 6 months in order to avoid persistent alterations of the pulmonary vascular bed. The surgical results are good.

Therapy

MEDICAL THERAPY

Congenital heart disease which become symptomatic during the neonatal period justifies the rea-nimation procedures used in other forms of neonatal distress: the correction of metabolic disorders, particularly acid-base imbalance; artificial respiration; prevention against thermal loss. Rehydration, the re-establishment of an appropriate hemoglobin pool. The administration of sodium ions (bicarbonate) should be carefully monitored as volumetric overload is sometimes poorly tolerated, particularly in obstructive left heart syndromes.

Cyanotic heart diseases require oxygen therapy with high FiO_2. The therapeutic means which are particularly relevant to heart disease are: digitalis and diuretic drugs, antiarrhythmic drugs; vaso-active drugs, which consists of: the prostaglandins of the E-type, the prostaglandin-inhibitors (indo-methacin, see p. 364) the catecholamines and the vasodilating drugs.

Digitalis

This is a highly active drug owing to its strong inotropic action, but also dangerous because of its electrophysiological properties, which should lead to very strict regulation concerning prescription. In neonatal heart failure, the goal to be reached is the obtaining as quickly as possible of an active tissue concentration without going beyond the toxic level.

The choice of medication depends on its metabolic characteristics: *Digoxin* is the preferred form for the newborn: Its digestive absorbtion is less than that of digitoxin, but its action and its renal elimina-tion are quicker and it is easier to control via all routes of administration. Lanatoside-C is reserved for intravenous use.

In the majority of cases the drug is administered orally: digoxin solution at 0.05 $^o/_{oo}$ is the most easy to prescribe since it contains 5 micrograms per 0.1 ml. In the case of vomiting, or in severe cases, the venous route is chosen (ampules of 2 ml = 500 micrograms of digoxin or of 2 ml = 400 micrograms of Lanatoside-C).

The dosage depends on weight and the renal status. In the newborn of more than 3 kg with normal renal function, typical treatment demands a "loading" oral dose of 20 micrograms/kg of digoxin followed, eight hours later, by one third of that dose, to be repeated every eight hours. The main-tenance dose is thus 20 micrograms/kg/24 h. Below 3 kg, the "loading" dose is only 15 micro-grams/kg and the maintenance dose 15 micro-grams/kg/24 h. If the child is suffering from renal failure, one reduces the dose by multiplying the standard doses by 0.6 if the azotemia is between 8 to 17 mmol/l; by 0.3 for azotemia between 17 and 25 mmol/l; by 0.15 below that. Finally, all of these dosages are reduced by one third if one choses digoxin or Lanatoside-C by the parenteral route or digitoxin by any route.

The control of therapy should be rigourous and constantly alert to signs of overdosage. The clinical symptoms (vomiting) and electrical signs prolong-ed PR interval, bundle branch block, premature beats, heterotopic tachycardias) show themselves later. Progress in our knowledge of pharmaco-kinetics and in the techniques of measurement of the digitalis drugs in the plasma permit more precise observation; in the newborn, the therapeutic level of digoxin in plasma is of the order of 3 ± 0.5 ng/ml and the toxic level is generally above 5 ng/ml.

Diuretic drugs

Diuretic therapy occupies a principal place in neonatal cardiac therapy because the congestive manifestations related to congenital cardiac lesions are widespread and menacing at this age.

Emergency treatment calls for *furosemide* which has an extremely rapid action whatever the method of administration and has little real toxicity. In the case of significant peripheral fluid overload, parti-cularly pulmonary, one administers 2 mg/kg by the parenteral route to be repeated several times during the first 24 hours. If the renal response is clear, the hydro-electrolyte losses need to be surveyed and compensated for, and the plasma and urinary ionic constants observed. *Ethacrynic acid*, prescribed in the same doses, is equally efficient, but its adminis-tration to the newborn may risk interference with bilirubin metabolism.

Long-term management makes use of furosemide at a dose of 2 mg/kg/24 h three times a week admi-nistred orally.

In the case of hyperaldosteronism, proven by urinary ionogram, some children can benefit from treatment by the oral administration of *spirono-lactone* starting with 3 mg/kg/24 h and, if needed, raising it progressively to 15 mg/kg/24 h while following the urinary elimination of sodium and potassium.

E-prostaglandins

Prostaglandins E_1 and E_2 play a major role in the relaxation of the ductus arteriosus and are probably important mediators in the maintenance of its patency during the fetal period. This property has lead to their use as infusions for children suffering from cardiac malformations in whom life depends on the patency of the ductus arteriosus (ducto-dependant heart diseases).

The indications fall into two principal groups:

Malformations in which pulmonary circulation and oxygenation depend on a left-to-right shunt across the ductus: pulmonary atresia, with or above all without ventricular septal defect, tricuspid atresia and tetralogy of Fallot.

Malformations whose distal systemic circulation depends on the persistence of a right-to-left shunt across the ductus: interruption of the aortic arch and severe preductal coarctation, generally accompanied by serious intracardiac defects, such as ventricular septal defect with obstruction of the left heart outflow, double outlet right ventricle with subaortic stenosis, some forms of single ventricle and aorto-pulmonary window.

On the other hand, prostaglandins can be used in *specific circumstances*. Particularly in emergencies when the newborn presents in a poor condition and it is difficult to make a diagnosis: some coarctations of the aorta cannot be differentiated from a hypoplastic left heart syndrome, without an improvement in the condition of the circulation. The administration of prostaglandin in the catheterization room can also permit one to more clearly visualize the pulmonary arteries and the pulmonary venous drainage in complex malformations.

In transposition of the great vessels, a prostaglandin infusion can be valuable where a Rashkind atrio-septostomy has proven insufficient. Not only does it dilate the ductus, but its action as a vasodilator of the pulmonary arterioles can reduce the pulmonary hypertension, thus improving the pulmonary circulation. Finally, in *Ebstein's anomaly* with a low right ventricular output and a large right-to-left interatrial shunt provoking severe hypoxemia, prostaglandin can help in a crisis period by increasing the pulmonary circulation via the ductus and by producing a fall in pulmonary resistance.

The vasodilating effect of the prostaglandins on the pulmonary vessels is under study and could justify their use in the treatment of the syndrome of persistence of the fetal circulation.

The administration should begin in the catheterization room. The catheter is placed as near as possible to the ductus, at the level of the aortic isthmus just downstream from the left sub-clavian artery when there is a left-to-right shunt, in the main pulmonary artery when the circulation in the descending aorta depends on the patency of the ductus. Prostaglandins being very rapidly metabolised, their effect may depend on the site of the catheter. However, at the present time, a simple intravenous infusion is performed in most instances and appears to be as effective as the intraductal route.

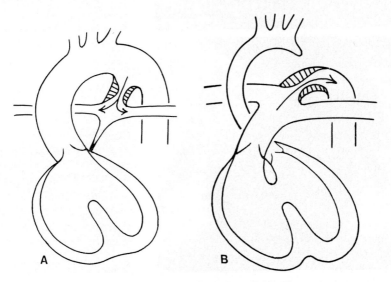

FIG. III-35. — *Ductus-dependent malformations.*

A) Pulmonary artery with a ventricular septal defect: prototype of ductal dependent cardiac anomalies with a left-to-right shunt through the ductus.

B) Interruption of the aortic arch with a ventricular septal defect: prototype of ductal dependent cardiac anomalies with a right-to-left shunt through the ductus.

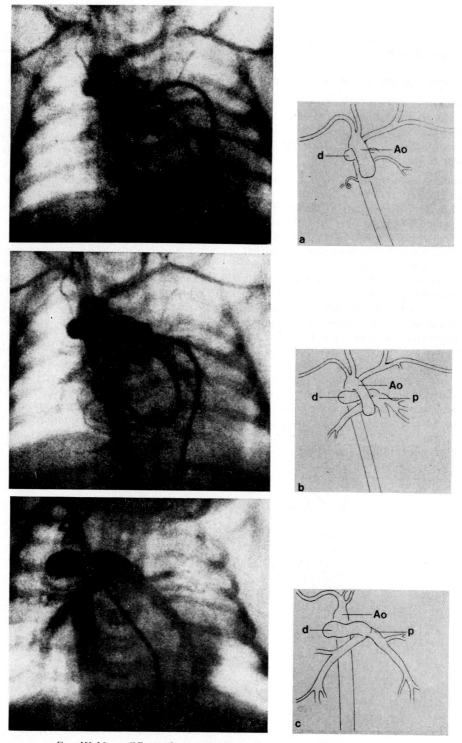

FIG. III-36. — *Effects of prostaglandin:* aortograms in pulmonary atresia.

a) Before prostaglandin administration: absence of filling of pulmonary arteries.
b) After 10 minutes prostaglandin trial; visualization of the ductus and beginning pulmonary circulation.
c) After 3 days of prostaglandin infusion: impressive dilatation of the ductus with considerable improvement of the pulmonary circulation.
Ao = aorta; *d* = ductus arteriosus; *p* = pulmonary artery.

The dosage is initially 0.1 µg/kg/mn for 10 minutes. The response is generally apparent in the first few minutes; it is characterized by an improvement in the general condition and can be confirmed by angiocardiography, which shows the dilatation of the ductus. In the cyanotic group with an obligatory left-to-right shunt, PaO_2 should show an increase of at least 10 mm Hg. The group with an obligatory right-to-left shunt should show an increase in the distal systemic pressures, with a reduction of the pressure gradient between the descending aorta and the pulmonary artery at the level of the ductus: the femoral arteries become palpable again and a diuresis may occur. If the response is positive, the dosage can be reduced by half and the improvement can sometimes be maintained even with doses of only 0.01 µg/kg/mn. The infusion should be continued intravenously within the intensive care unit. The period of infusion should be short and followed by emergency surgical treatment. It is sometimes necessary during the post-operative period. Infusions of longer duration have been advised for children who are not immediately operable. The cessation of the infusion is accompanied by constriction of the ductus with an aggravation of the circulatory condition, even if the perfusion has been of long duration Fig. III-36.

The side effects are not negligible. When the catheter is correctly placed, they are rarer and less severe. Peripheral vasodilation can produce systemic hypotension. A cutaneous flush of the drainage region of the perfused artery can be seen in about 10 % of the cases. It is then advisable to withdraw the tip of the catheter from the sub-clavian or carotid artery and to replace it in the aortic isthmus. A temporary elevation in temperature can be attributed to the direct action of prostaglandin on the thermoregulatory centres. The most severe complication is apnea followed by bradycardia, which may necessitate artificial respiration; it generally appears at the beginning of treatment and its mechanism is not yet clearly elucidated; it occurs in about 10 % of cases. Convulsions have been reported. The side effects are not more frequent in the case of venous infusion than by intraductal administration.

Catecholamines, vasodilators

The catecholamines are indicated for serious heart failure which does not respond to digitalis therapy and in states of cardiogenic shock and collapse. They are also used in the post-operative phase of heart surgery. Dopamine is infused at an initial dose of 2 to 5 micrograms/kg/mn, this being increased until an effect is obtained, up to 10 micrograms/kg/mn maximum. Isoprenalin is preferable in the case of bradycardia (0.2 to 2 micrograms/kg/mn). Adrenalin (0.05 to 0.3 microgram/kg/mn) is sometimes more efficient but may risk dangerous renal vasoconstriction.

The vasodilating drugs have two types of use depending on whether one wants to obtain pulmonary or systemic vasodilation. Apart from oxygen, there is no selective vasodilator of the pulmonary arterioles, but *tolazoline* is used to reduce pulmonary arterial hypertension, by infusion at a dose of 2 mg/kg/hour following a ten minute initial dose of 2 mg/kg. The indications are principally the syndrome of persistence of the fetal circulation, transposition of the great vessels where a Rashkind atrioseptostomy correctly undertaken has not permitted the rapid establishment of an interatrial left-to-right shunt, or the Ebstein's anomaly.

The use of systemic vasodilators has been proposed in cases of severe cardiac failure, to relieve the myocardium by reducing the afterload. The indications and dosage for the neonatal period are still poorly defined. *Nitroglycerin* seems preferable to sodium nitroprusside, used in the older child, but more toxic (0.2 to 2 micrograms/kg/minute). *Prazosine* has been used in the infant at a dosage 0.1 to 0.4 microgram/kg/minute.

CARDIOVASCULAR SURGERY

Only heart disease where medical management has not improved matters and where there is hope of improving the condition justify early surgical intervention. Pulmonary atresia with intact ventricular septum, coarctation of aorta syndrome, critical aortic valvar stenosis and total anomalous pulmonary venous drainage are neonatal surgical emergencies. Hypoplastic left heart syndrome remains beyond reasonable surgical possibilities. Tetralogy of Fallot and pulmonary atresia with open ventricular septum can necessitate an early surgical approach in cases of severe anoxia.

Closed heart surgical correction is limited to ligation of a ductus arteriosus (isolated in the premature born, or more often associated) and to the resection of a coarctation. *The direct approach* to an intracardiac lesion is sometimes undertaken with the aid of a brief circulatory arrest which permits, for example, a transarterial pulmonary or aortic valvulotomy. The pulmonary or aortic transventricular instrumental valvulotomies may be useful in the neonate.

Open heart surgery is indispensable either for surgery with direct vision of the intracardiac lesions (open aortic valvotomy) or to allow a great vessel conduit (anastomosis of a pulmonary venous collector into the left atrium).

The majority of procedures undertaken during the neonatal period are *palliative*. They are primarily *pulmonary systemic anastomoses*, and *banding of the pulmonary artery*. The Blalock-Taussig shunt between the sub-clavian artery and the homolateral pulmonary artery is technically difficult or impossible in the newborn, even with micro-surgical techniques. The Waterston shunt, between ascending aorta and right pulmonary artery, allows for more severe lesions and for pulmonary arterial kinking. *Blalock-Hanlon septectomy* is now rarely used and it is now preferred, in transposition, to wait a little and to undertake a Mustard or Senning open heart procedure.

The procedures cannot be decided upon without hemodynamic investigation and an angiocardiogram.

Neonatal cardiac surgery obeys the same rules as for all thoracic surgery in the newborn. Amongst other things, it presupposes a specific delineation of myocardial function and the cardiac rhythm. The restoration of good myocardial function demands that one improves, in specific circumstances the "preload" (filling), the contractility (catecholamines), or the "afterload" (vasodilators). Rhythm disorders due to hyperexcitability are often provoked by aggressive pre-surgical digitalisation. It is thus preferable to reduce the dosage pre-operatively. They are difficult to treat because of the myocardial depressant effect of the majority of the anti-arrhythmic drugs. In the case of bradycardia with heart block, a pacemaker may be necessary.

REFERENCES

[1] AUJARD (Y.), BEAUFILS (F.), BOURRILLON (A.). — La persistance de la circulation fœtale. *Arch. franç. Pédiat.*, *35*, 681-690, 1978.

[2] BARR (P. A.), CELERMAJER (J. M.), BOWDLER (J. D.), CARTMILL (T. B.). — Severe congenital tricuspid incompetence in the neonate. *Circulation*, *49*, 962-967, 1974.

[3] BATISSE (A.), CARON (M.). — Les tumeurs du cœur du nouveau-né. Journées paris. Pédiat. Paris, Flammarion, 297-307, 1978.

[4] BATISSE (A.), DUBAUX (P.), FERMONT (J.), KACHANER (J.). — Blocs auriculo-ventriculaires complets congénitaux. *Arch. Mal. Cœur*, *73*, 455-462, 1980.

[5] BATISSE (A.), PETIT (J.), FERMONT (L.), KACHANER (J.). — Les tachycardies supraventriculaires du nouveau-né et du nourrisson. *Arch. franç. Pédiat.*, *36*, 551-562, 1979.

[6] BERDEAUX (A.), BATISSE (A.), RICHER (C.), KACHANER (J.), GIUDICELLI (J. F.). — Le dosage de la digoxine plasmatique chez le nouveau-né. Applications pratiques. *Nouv. Presse méd.*, *6*, 2142-2144, 1977.

[7] BOZIO (A.), PAYOT (M.), ESPELTA-VELA (F.), KRATZ (C.), NORMAND (J.), DAVIGNON (A.). — Le syndrome d'hypoplasie du cœur gauche. Corrélations anatomo-échocardiographiques. *Arch. Mal. Cœur*, *71*, 1-8, 1978.

[8] BUCCIARELLI (R. L.), NELSON (R. M.), EGAN (E. A.), EITZMAN (D. V.), GESSNER (I. H.). — Transient tricuspid insufficiency of the newborn: a form of myocardial dysfunction in stressed newborns. *Pediatrics*, *59*, 330-337, 1977.

[9] CHÉTOCHINE (F. L.), WORMS (A. M.), REY (C.), MARTELLI (H.), THIBERT (M.). — Fistules artério-veineuses thoraco-brachiales malignes du nouveau-né. *Arch. Mal. Cœur*, *71*, 496-501, 1978.

[10] CLARKE (D. R.), STARK (J.), DE LEVAL (M.), PINCOTT (J. R.), TAYLOR (J. F. N.). — Total anomalous pulmonary venous drainage in infancy. *Br. Heart J.*, *39*, 436-444, 1977.

[11] DE GEETER (B.), MESSER (J.), BENOIT (M.), WILLARD (D.). — Interruption de la crosse aortique et PO₂ cutanée. *Arch. franç. Pédiat.*, *36*, 144-148, 1979.

[12] DIDIER (F.), HOEFFEL (J. C.), WORMS (A. M.), HENRY (M.), LERBIER (N.), PERNOT (C.). — Étude anatomoradiologique du syndrome d'hypoplasie du cœur gauche, à propos de 72 observations. *Ann. Radiol.*, *19*, 673-686, 1976.

[13] FAROOKI (Z. Q.), GREEN (E. W.). — Multifocal tachycardia in two neonates. *Br. Heart J.*, *39*, 872-874, 1977.

[14] FERMONT (L.), BATISSE (A.), PIÉCHAUD (J. F.), KACHANER (J.). — Myocardiopathie hypertrophique transitoire du nouveau-né de mère diabétique. *Arch. franç. Pédiat.*, *37*, 113-115, 1980.

[15] FERMONT (L.), KACHANER (J.), BATISSE (A.), LUCET (P.), NEVEUX (J. Y.), LEMOINE (G.). — Le cœur triatrial chez le nourrisson. A propos de quatre cas dont deux opérés avec succès. *Arch. franç. Pédiat.*, *34*, 825-843, 1977.

[16] FINLEY (J. P.), HOWMAN-GILES (R. B.), GILDAY (D. R.), BLOOM (K. R.), ROWE (R. D.). — Transient myocardial ischaemia of the newborn infant demonstrated by thallium myocardial imaging. *J. Pediatr.*, *94*, 263-270, 1979.

[17] FINLEY (J. P.), RADFORD (D. J.), FREEDOM (R. M.). — « Torsades de pointe » ventricular tachycardia in a newborn infant. *Br. Heart J.*, *40*, 421-424, 1978.

[18] FREED (M. D.), ROSENTHAL (A.), CASTANEDA (A. R.), NADAS (A. S.). — Use of prostaglandin El in an infant with interruption of aortic arch. *J. Pediatr.*, *91*, 805-807, 1977.

[19] FRIEDMAN (W. F.), HIRSCHKLAU (M. J.), PRINTZ (M. P.), PITLICK (P. T.), KIRKPATRICK (S. E.). — Pharmacological closure of patent ductus arteriosus in premature infants. *New Engl. J. Med.*, *295*, 526-529, 1976.

[20] GARSON (A.), GILLETTE (P. C.), McNAMARA (D. G.). — Propranolol: the preferred palliation for tetralogy of Fallot (abstr.). *Circulation*, *59-60*, Suppl. II, 250, 1979.

[21] GITTENBERGER-DE GROOT (A. C.), MOULAERT (A. J.), HARINCK (E.), BECKER (A. E.). — Histopathology of the ductus arteriosus after prostaglandin E1 administration in ductus dependant cardiac anomalies. *Br. Heart J.*, *40*, 215-220, 1978.

[22] GODMAN (M. J.), MARQUIS (R. M.). — Heart disease in the newborn. Paediatric Cardiology, vol. 2, Churchill-Livingstone. Edinburgh-London-New York, 1979.

[23] GODMAN (M. J.), THAM (P.), KIDD (B. S. L.). — Echocardiography in the evaluation of the cyanotic newborn infant. *Br. Heart J.*, *36*, 154-166, 1974.

[24] GRAHAM (T. P.), ATWOOD (G. F.), BOUCEK (R. J.). — Use of prostaglandin E1 for emergency palliation of symptomatic coarctation of the aorta. *Cathet. cardiovasc. Diagn.*, *4*, 97-102, 1978.

[25] GUTGESELL (H. P.), SPEER (M. E.), ROSENBERG (H. S.). — Characterization of the cardiomyopathy in infants of diabetic mothers. *Circulation*, *61*, 441-450, 1980.

[26] HAGAN (A. D.), DEELY (W. J.), SAHN (D.), FRIEDMAN (W. F.). — Echocardiography criteria for normal newborn infants. *Circulation*, *48*, 1221-1226, 1973.

[27] HALLIDAY (H.), HIRSHFELD (S.), RIGGS (T.), LIEBMAN (J.), FANAROFF (A.). — Echographic ventricular systolic time intervals in normal term and preterm neonates. *Pediatrics*, *62*, 317-321, 1978.

[28] HALLIDIE-SMITH (K. A.), FOX (K. M.), ANDERSON (R. H.). — Fetal tachycardia. *Br. Heart J.*, *43*, 106-107, 1980.

[29] HARDY (J. D.), SOLOMON (S.), BANWELL (G. S.), BEACH (R.), WRIGHT (V.), HOWARD (F. M.). — Congenital complete heart block in the newborn associated with maternal systemic lupus erythematous and connective tissue disorders. *Arch. Dis. Child.*, *54*, 7-13, 1979.

[30] HEYMAN (M. A.), RUDOLPH (A. M.), SILVERMAN (N. H.). — Closure of the ductus arteriosus by prostaglandin inhibition. *New Engl. J. Med.*, *295*, 530-533, 1976.

[31] KACHANER (J.), CASASOPRANA (A.). — Cardiopathies congénitales néonatales. XXIIIᵉ Congr. Assoc. Pédiat. Langue franç., Allier, Grenoble II, 37-172, 1972.

[32] KACHANER (J.), GAUTIER (M.), CASASOPRANA (A.), TRAN VAN DUC. — Principaux types de l'insuffisance tricuspidienne néo-natale. *Arch. franç. Pédiat.*, *31*, 359-389, 1974.

[33] KACHANER (J.), NOUAILLE (J. M.), BATISSE (A.). — Les cardiomégalies massives du nouveau-né. *Arch. franç. Pédiat.*, *34*, 297-322, 1977.

[34] KLEINMAN (C. S.), HOBBINS (J. C.), JAFFE (C. C.), LYNCH (D. C.), TALNER (N. S.). — Echocardiographic studies of the human fetus: prenatal diagnosis. *Pediatrics*, *65*, 1059-1067, 1980.

[35] LAMBERT (E. C.), CANENT (R. V.), HOHN (A. R.). — Congenital cardiac anomalies in the neonatal period. A review of conditions causing death or severe distress in the first month of life. *Pediatrics*, *37*, 343-351, 1966.

[36] LANDRIEU (P.), CHAUMONT (P.). — Hémangiome solitaire du foie révélé par une insuffisance cardiaque néo-natale. Guérison par radiothérapie. *Arch. franç. Pédiat.*, *34*, 763-768, 1977.

[37] LANG (P.), FREED (M. D.), BIERMAN (F. Z.), NORWOOD (W. I.), NADAS (A. S.). — Use of prostaglandin E1 in infants with *d*-transposition of the great arteries and intact ventricular septum. *Am. J. Cardiol.*, *44*, 76-81, 1979.

[38] LEWIS (A. B.), LURIE (P. R.). — Prolonged prostaglandin E1 infusion in an infant with cyanotic congenital heart disease. *Pediatrics*, *61*, 534-536, 1978.

[39] McCARTY (J. S.), ZIES (L. G.), GELBAND (H.). — Age dependant closure of the patent ductus arteriosus by indomethacin. *Pediatrics*, *62*, 706-712, 1978.

[40] McMANUS (Q.), STARRR (A.), LAMBERT (L. E.), GRUNKEMEIER (G.). — Correction of aortic coarctation in neonates: mortality and late results. *Ann. thorac. Surg.*, *24*, 544-549, 1977.

[41] McREID (M.), REILLYB (J.), MURDOCK (A. I.), SWYER (P. R.). — Cardiomegaly in association with neonatal hypoglycemia. *Acta Paediat. Scand.*, *60*, 295-301, 1970.

[42] MADISON (J. P.), SUKHUM (P.), WILLIAMSON (D. P.), CAMPION (B. C.) — Echocardiography and fœtal heart sounds in the diagnosis of fetal heart block. *Am. Heart J.*, *98*, 505-509, 1979.

[43] MANTAKAS (M. E.), McCUE (C. M.), MILLER (W. W.). — Natural history of Wolff-Parkinson-White syndrome discovered in infancy. *Am. J. Cardiol.*, *41*, 1097-1103, 1978.

[44] MESSER (J.), VORS (J.), KRUG (J. P.), PHILIPPE (E.), WILLARD (D.). — Pathologie fœtale et néo-natale en rapport avec le chorio-angiome du placenta. *Ann. Pédiat.*, *21*, 891-897, 1974.

[45] MONIN (P.), DIDIER (F.), VIBERT (M.), ANDRÉ (M.), VERT (P.). — Diagnostic des cardiopathies congénitales dans la période néonatale. Intérêt de la mesure transcutanée de la PO₂. *Nouv. Presse méd.*, *7*, 289, 1978.

[46] MOODIE (D. S.), KLEINBERG (F.), RELANDER (R. L.), KAYE (M. P.), FELDT (R. H.). — Tolazolin as adjuvant therapy for ill neonates with pulmonary hypoperfusion. *Chest*, *74*, 604-605, 1978.

[47] MOULAERT (A.), ENDERS (R.), VAN ERTBRUGGEN (J.), HUYSMANS (H.), HARINCK (E.). — Effect of E1 type prostaglandins on hypoxaemia in cyanotic congenital cardiac malformations. *Europ. J. Cardiol.*, *5*, 321-325, 1977.

[48] MOULAERT (A.), GITTENBERGER-DE GROOT (A.), HARINCK (E.). — Effets de la prostaglandine dans les malformations cardiaques avec canal artériel obligatoire. Étude clinique et histologique. *Arch. franç. Pédiat.*, *35*, 717-725, 1978.

[49] NEIMANN (N.), PERNOT (C.), GENTIN (G.), VERT (P.), WORMS (A. M.). — Le syndrome d'Ivemark : cardiopathie congénitale cyanogène sévère, hétérotaxie thoraco-abdominale complexe et asplénie ou polysplénie. *Pédiatrie*, *21*, 511-532, 1966.

[50] NEIMANN (N.), PERNOT (C.), PRÉVOT (J.). — Aspects chirurgicaux des détresses néonatales. XXIIᵉ Congr. Assoc. Pédiat. Langue franç., Expansion scientifique, Paris II, 269-399, 1969.

[51] NEIMANN (N.), PERNOT (C.), RAUBER (G.). — Aplasie du myocarde du ventricule droit (ventricule droit papyracé congénital). *Arch. Mal. Cœur*, *58*, 421-430, 1965.

[52] PERNOT (C.), LOTH (P.), GAUTIER (M.). — Myocardiopathies des glycogénoses. *Arch. Mal. Cœur*, *71*, 428-436, 1978.

[53] PERNOT (C.), MARCHAL (C.), RAVAULT (M. C.), CLOEZ (J. L.), LAMBERT (A.). — La fermeture prématurée du foramen ovale. *Arch. franç. Pédiat.*, *36*, 949-958, 1979.

[54] PERNOT (C.), WORMS (A. M.), GRUN (G.). — Agénésie des valves pulmonaires révélée par des troubles

de la ventilation chez le nouveau-né. *Arch. franç. Pédiat.*, *32*, 637-646, 1975.

[55] PERNOT (C.), WORMS (A. M.), HENRY (M.), DIDIER (F.). — Les communications interventriculaires du nourrisson. Aspects actuels. XXIIIe Congr. Pédiat. Langue franç., Allier, Grenoble II, 259-329, 1972.

[56] PETIT (A.), NIVELON (L. J.), MICHIELS (R.), FOUCHERES (G.), NIVELON-CHEVALLIER (A.), SANDRE (D.). — Les cardiomyopathies obstructives du nouveau-né et du nourrisson. A propos d'une observation personnelle à révélation néonatale. *Pédiatrie, 33,* 733-738, 1978.

[57] PONTÉ (C.), DUPUIS (C.), REMY (J.), LEQUIEN (P.), REY (C.). — Le syndrome de Halasz néonatal. A propos de trois observations. *Arch. franç. Pédiat., 32,* 299-300, 1975.

[58] RASHKIND (W. J.), MILLER (W. W.). — Creation of an atrial septal defect without thoracotomy. *J. Am. Med. Assoc., 196,* 991-992, 1966.

[59] REY (C.), LABLANCHE (J. M.), DELOCHE (A.). — Apport de l'échocardiographie au diagnostic d'un retour veineux pulmonaire anormal total infradiaphragmatique. *Arch. Mal. Cœur, 70,* 997-1001, 1977.

[60] ROWE (R. D.), HOFFMAN (T.). — Transient myocardial ischaemia of the newborn infant. A form of severe cardio-respiratory distress in full-term infants. *J. Pediart., 81,* 243-250, 1972.

[61] ROWE (R. D.), IZUKAWA (T.), MULHOLLAND (H. C.), BLOOM (K. R.), COOK (D. H.), SWYER (P. R.). — Non structural heart disease in the newborn. Observations during one year in a perinatal service. *Arch. Dis. Child., 53,* 726-730, 1978.

[62] ROWE (R. D.), MEHRIZI (A.). — The neonate with congenital heart disease. Saunders, Philadelphia-London-Toronto, 1968.

[63] SARDET (A.), KACHANER (J.). — L'insuffisance tricuspide transitoire du nouveau-né. Journées paris. Pédiat. Paris, Flammarion, 275-283, 1979.

[64] SOLINGER (R. E.), ELBL (F.), MINHAS (K.). — Echocardiography in the normal neonate. *Circulation, 47,* 108-118, 1973.

[65] SOUTHALL (D. P.), ORREL (M. J.), TALBOT (J. F.) et coll. — Study of cardiac arrhythmias and other forms of conduction abnormality in newborn infants. *Br. med. J., 2,* 597-599, 1977.

[66] STERN (L.), RAMOS (A. D.), WIGGLESWORTH (F. W.). — Congestive heart failure secondary to cerebral arteriovenous aneurysm in the newborn infant. *Am. J. Dis. Child., 115,* 581-587, 1968.

[67] TEUSCHER (A.), BOSSI (E.), IMHOF (P.), ERB (E.), STOCKER (F. P.), WEBER (J. W.). — Effect of propranolol on fetal tachycardia in diabetic pregnancy. *Am. J. Cardiol., 42,* 304-307, 1978.

[68] THIBERT (M.), CHÉTOCHINE (F. L.). — Sténose et atrésie pulmonaire à septum interventriculaire intact. I : nouveau-né. *Cœur, 3,* 1-22, 1972.

[69] WALSH (S. Z.). — ECG changes during the first 5-6 days after birth. *Praxis, 64,* 747-753, 1975.

[70] WALSH (S. Z.). — Characteristic features of the ECG of premature infants during the first year of life. *Praxis, 64,* 754-759, 1975.

[71] WOLFF (G. S.), HAN (J.), CURRAN (J.). — Wolff-Parkinson-White syndrome in the neonate. *Am. J. Cardiol., 41,* 559-563, 1978.

[72] WORMS (A. M.), HENRY (M.), PERNOT (C.). — Cathétérisme cardiaque par voie percutanée chez le nourrisson et le nouveau-né. *Cœur, 8,* 75-81, 1977.

[73] WORMS (A. M.), STEHLIN (H.), DIDIER (F.), PLÉNAT (F.), NEVEUX (J. Y.), PERNOT (C.). — La sténose aortique valvulaire à expression néonatale. A propos de 8 observations. *Arch. Mal. Cœur, 70,* 329-336, 1977.

19

Respiratory diseases of the newborn

William OH and Leo STERN

Introduction

During adaptation to extrauterine life, the physiologic changes of the respiratory system are the most critical tasks which the newborn infant has to achieve for normal transition to the neonatal period. Adaptive phenomena relating to metabolic competence, thermoregulation, renal function, etc., all occur, but can be graded and spaced over a prolonged period of time. However, the adaptation of the lungs and cardiovascular system is crucial to the maintenance of life. Any abnormality relating to this adaptation can lead to conditions which may require neonatal intensive care.

In intrauterine life, the lungs are collapsed and the pulmonary resistance accordingly high. This resistance to pulmonary flow is the major determinant of the fetal circulation whereby the ventricles work in parallel and the output of the one is *not equal* to that of the other. With the onset of extrauterine life, there is immediate expansion of the lungs. Under normal circumstances this will occur with the first effective breath and can be demonstrated radiographically in as short a period of time as 1/3

of a second. The expansion of the lung results in an immediate fall in pulmonary resistance and a concomitant increase in pulmonary blood flow. The overall result is a fall in pulmonary artery pressure, which acts as the fulcrum around which the cardiovascular adaptive changes occur. These changes within a relatively short period of time will convert the fetal circulation with its parallel output of the right and left ventricles to the neonatal circulation in which the ventricles now work in series and where the *output* of one is totally equal to that of the other. In order for this to occur, a series of events resulting ultimately in the closure of both the ductus arteriosus and the foramen ovale are initiated.

Thus, while expansion of the lungs has as its immediate objective the initiation of extrauterine respiration, the physiologic changes will invariably involve an essential alteration in the normal cardiovascular system as well. Because of this interrelationship, diseases of the respiratory system are often associated with cardiovascular signs and symptoms.

TABLE I. — Embryology and functional maturation of the lung

| Time after conception | Developmental events | | |
	Pulmonary morphology	Pulmonary vascular and lymphatic system	Biochemical
24-26 days	Protrusion of lung bud from gut.	—	—
26-28 days	First branching of lung bud.	Appearance of anlage of pulmonary arteries and veins.	—
1-3 months	— Lung is glandular. — Dichotomus branching continues. — Epithelium columnar. — Muscle fiber for trachea, primary, secondary and tertiary bronchi appears. — Elastic tissue appears and develops in trachea and bronchi.	— Branching of pulmonary vessels along with bronchi. — Lymphatic vessels appear (60 days).	—
20-24 weeks	— Alveoli duct appear. — Epithelium lined by glycogen-rich cells.	— Capillaries appear.	— Surfactant synthesis via methylation pathway begins.
24-28 weeks	— Alveolai developed from alveolar duct. — Epithelium attenuates. — Cell predominantly, type I.	— Proliferation of vascular and lymphatic capillaries around the terminal alveoli.	— Above process continues.
28-32 weeks	— Type II cells increase.	— Closer approximation of capillaries to alveolar lining.	— Surfactant synthesis via choline incorporation pathway begins.
32-36 weeks	— Increasing number of type II cells with lamellar bodies.	— Increasing anastomosis of capillaries. — Collateral circulation through bronchial arteries appears.	— Increasing production of lecithin by choline incorporation.

EMBRYOLOGY AND BIOCHEMICAL DEVELOPMENT OF THE LUNG
(Table I)

During intrauterine life, the morphologic development and differentiation of the lung parenchyma, pulmonary vascular and lymphatic structures, and biochemical changes are closely interrelated. The endpoint of this development is to equip the fetus with a lung that is morphologically and functionally sufficiently well developed to sustain normal respiratory function in extrauterine life.

At 24 to 26 days of conceptual age, the lung bud protrudes from the foregut to form the primary structure of the lung. At 26 to 28 days, the first branching occurs along with the invasion of the anlage of the pulmonary arteries and veins. From here on, dichotomous branching of the bronchi into smaller bronchioles continues during the first three months of gestation. Muscle fibers and elastic tissue also begin to appear in the trachea, bronchi and bronchioles. In the meantime, the pulmonary vessels continue to branch out along with the bronchi and bronchioles and at about two months gestation, the lymphatic vessels also begin to appear. During this period of time, there is virtually no biochemical activity occurring in the primitive lung. At 20 to 24 weeks of gestational age, the alveolar ducts begin to appear. The epithelial lining of the alveolar ducts is cuboidal in nature and rich in glycogen content. The capillaries of the pulmonary vasculature also begin to appear. At 24 to 28 weeks of gestation, the alveoli begin to appear out of the alveolar ducts. The epithelium in the alveoli starts to attenuate. The cells will differentiate into the type I cells which are primary cellular structures for gas exchange and the centrally located type II cells which contain lamellar bodies—the highly specialized cellular structure for the synthesis and storage of surfactants. Meanwhile the pulmonary vessels and lymphatics continue to proliferate and anastomose around the terminal alveoli. Collateral circulation with bronchial vessels also appears at this time which rapidly enhances the blood supply to the alveoli. Biochemically, the synthesis of surfactant also begins, primarily via the methylation pathway for the formation of lecithin. This pathway for lecithin synthesis is extremely sensitive to hypoxia and acidosis, thus accounting for the marked severity of hyaline membrane disease in very immature infants with perinatal asphyxia. At 28 to 32 weeks of gestation, the number of specialized type II cells within the alveolar lining increases; at the same time, closer approximation of capillaries to the alveolar lining occurs. Surfactant synthesis continues to flourish with the shifting of the synthetic pathway from the methylation to the choline incorporation process. The latter is less susceptible to acidosis and hypoxemia. Between 32 and 36 weeks gestation, the morphologic maturation is established, particularly with increasing anastomosis of the capillaries for perfusion. There is an increasing predominance of the choline incorporation pathway for the synthesis of lecithin.

GENERAL CONSIDERATIONS OF NEONATAL PULMONARY FUNCTION

Lung compliance

Lung compliance measures the distensibility of the lung. It represents the change in tidal volume in relation to the change in trans-pulmonary pressure (lung compliance = tidal volume/Δ pressure), at the point of no flow. Lung compliance is dependent on the functional residual capacity (FRC) and the intrinsic elasticity of the lung itself. Therefore,

if a specific compliance value is desired, the lung compliance should be measured simultaneously with FRC.

In normal newborn infants, the lung compliance is low at the initiation of the first breath; hence accounting for the high pressure (frequently up to 25 to 30 cm H_2O) required for its initiation. With the establishment of respiration and with the gradual clearance of lung fluid during the first 3 to 6 hours of life, the FRC increases with concomitant improvement of the lung compliance. Since the improvement in lung compliance is due to the improvement in FRC, the specific compliance is unchanged. There is considerable variability of compliance values in the first 2 hours of life, and this accounts for the frequent observations of a higher respiratory rate in infants during this period of time. It is important that in interpreting the significance of higher respiratory rates during the first 2 hours of life, this physiologic variation be taken into account and the clinical signs interpreted accordingly. If a higher respiratory rate is associated with any form of retraction, grunting or cyanosis requiring oxygen supplementation, the infant must have a pathological condition accounting for the manifestations, until proven otherwise.

Ventilation-perfusion ratio (V_A/Q ratio)

For normal gas exchange, the ventilation perfusion ratio should be very close to 1.0, *i. e.*, for every ml of air ventilation, there should be a proportionate degree of perfusion. In healthy adults, this V_A/Q ratio is about 0.8. In the presence of cardiopulmonary disease, the V_A/Q ratio may be abnormal depending on the nature of the pulmonary pathology. In cases of intrinsic pulmonary disease associated with hypoventilation, the V_A/Q ratio will be less than 1.0. In cardiac anomalies with right to left shunt and in pulmonary disease where a large portion of the alveoli are ventilated but underperfused, a V_A/Q ratio greater than 1.0 can be observed.

Breathing pattern of newborn infant

It is well known that the pattern of breathing of newborn infants is frequently irregular and this irregularity in the control of respiration is even more pronounced in preterm, low birth weight infants. The so-called periodic breathing frequently observed in preterm infants is characterized by a period of apnea lasting for 10 to 20 seconds followed by a burst of rapid irregular respiration and again by a (10 to 20 second) pause of respiratory effort. This type of respiratory pattern is generally not associated with bradycardia during the apnea period. If apnea is associated with bradycardia secondary to significant myocardial hypoxemia, the condition is no longer physiologic and should be considered as a significant apneic episode requiring diagnostic and therapeutic interventions.

Scope and intent of this section

We will not attempt to cover all of the possible respiratory diseases in the neonate. Such coverage would be inappropriate in a general book on neonatology and may be found in more specialized volumes dealing exclusively with neonatal respiratory disorders. The present section is intended to highlight some of the major diseases and to present an approach which stresses specific aspects of the illnesses, their pathophysiology, and treatment.

Upper airway problems

Posterior choanal atresia. — This is a congenital malformation characterized by an obstruction either in the form of bone or membrane at the junction of the posterior nares and nasopharynx. The unilateral form is associated with difficulty in respiration when the patent side is obstructed by a mucus plug, mucosal congestion or foreign body. In the bilateral form, the infant is, by virtue of the fact that neonates are obligate nose breathers, in immediate respiratory difficulty and the diagnosis can be suspected in the delivery room. Under these circumstances, there is intense cyanosis with respiratory difficulty, which is relieved by forcing the infant's mouth open with an airway device.

Diagnosis can be made when an attempt to pass a catheter through the nostril is unsuccessful. Radiographic confirmation with instillation of radio-opaque material will outline both the nature and extent of the defect. If the defect is membranous, an attempt may be made early to surgically create an adequate aperture in the area. Immediate therapy consists of the maintenance of an oral airway either via intubation or the insertion of a small mouthpiece. The previously almost mandatory tracheotomy has now been replaced by insertion of plastic tubes and repeated dilations of the area, a method of treatment which seems preferable in that tracheotomies at this age are often associated with a high morbidity. If the defect is osseous and thick, the immediate treatment is supportive with maintenance of upper airway patency and the definitive surgical correction delayed.

Unfortunately, the condition is frequently associated with other midline defects in the area of the sphenoid bone, and along with it, of the central nervous system. The uncomplicated case, however, will be profoundly influenced as to outcome by the speed of diagnosis, since failure to accurately establish the cause of such unexplained cyanosis may result in permanent irreversible hypoxic central nervous system damage.

Laryngeal web. — This form of intrinsic laryngeal obstruction is usually located in the region of the vocal cords, but may occur in both the supraglottic and subglottic areas. The lesion develops as a result of an arrest in development at 7 to 10 weeks of gestation and is exceedingly rare. The complete form is obviously incompatible with any prolonged period of survival and requires immediate tracheotomy or opening from above if at all possible. Incomplete forms may present as stridor, predominantly inspiratory, and a hoarse cry if movement of the vocal cords is restricted. Laryngoscopic examination will usually reveal the nature of the problem and appropriate therapy can then be undertaken.

Extrinsic laryngeal compression. — A number of tumors and cysts can result in compression not only of the larynx but of the upper airways in general. These may include cystic hygromas, thyroid masses either aberrant or of a goitrous nature, and a number of primitive congenital cysts derived from the embryonic arch structures. Hemangiomas and teratomas have occasionally been located in the laryngeal and tracheal areas, as have some of the congenital fibromatous neoplasms. The therapy of this type of obstruction depends both on its nature and upon its surgical accessibility. Goiters may respond to appropriate thyroid therapy, and there have been recent encouraging results with the use of corticosteroids for the treatment of extensive obstructing hemangiomas. The degree of compression will clearly dictate the urgency of surgical intervention, and the anatomical disposition of the lesion will govern the nature of the surgical approach that can be undertaken. The rare but clinically impressive laryngocele which occurs as an outpouching in the area of the vocal cords may only appear as a lateral swelling in the neck upon crying but its compression effect on enlargement may occasionally give rise to laryngeal obstruction as well.

Laryngomalacia. — This condition which has been variously ascribed to as floppy epiglottis, redundant aryepiglottic folds, or loose arytenoids appears to represent a weakness of the structures of the upper respiratory tract which results in their lack of stability and collapse during inspiration, hence the presentation as inspiratory stridor. The condition can be diagnosed by direct laryngoscopy and also has a characteristic appearance on cineangiography of the upper respiratory tract. Although noisy and frightening to the observer and parents, the condition is generally benign and will disappear by six months to one year of age as the structures mature and strengthen. Diagnosis is important from the point of view of reassurance and conservative therapy should be maintained throughout.

Laryngeal nerve paralysis. — Paralysis of the vocal cords may be both the result of congenital malformation or birth injury. Under these circumstances, direct visualization can ascertain the movement of the cords themselves. If complete paralysis occurs, the vocal cords tend to be fixed in the mid-inspiratory position. In Moebius syndrome (motor neuron disease affecting the cranial nerves) the condition tends to be associated with other evidence of upper nuclear paralysis (immobile facies, drooping eyelids), which will afford a clue as to the underlying condition.

Tracheomalacia. — In contrast to laryngomalacia, the etiology of the inspiratory stridor is much more clearly defined at this level, being due to a weakness of the supporting cartilagenous tracheal rings. Diagnosis can be confirmed by cineradiography after having been suspected on ordinary inspiratory films. The condition is self limited, and treatment is expectant only.

Vascular ring compression. — A variety of aberrant vascular structures may compress the respiratory tract in its upper portion but the most common one found on X-ray (aberrant subclavian) is almost never if at all a cause of such compression. The condition is usually associated with inspiratory stridor, and in severe cases the infant may tend to lie in a position with the neck hyperextended and a form of vocalization which has been described as "the cough of a barking seal". When not diagnosed in the immediate neonatal period, the condition may present as recurrent attacks of croup in later infancy and early childhood. A double aortic arch would appear to be statistically the most common form of presentation, with the aberrant left pulmonary artery causing both respiratory and digestive tract obstructive signs presenting a peculiar type of knuckle indentation on radiographic study. Initial suspicion may be obtained from ordinary antero-posterior and lateral chest radiographs which show tracheal narrowing and compression but final anatomic delineation of the lesion is dependent upon angiographic demonstration.

Phrenic nerve palsy. — Although aplasia of the phrenic nerve has been reported, the condition is usually secondary to birth trauma and may be associated with other evidence of injury to the brachial plexus. Unilateral forms will result in evidence of paradoxical respiration on chest fluoroscopy, whereas its bilateral occurrence if complete, may impose serious limitations on respiratory excursion. Cineradiographic demonstration of the movement of the diaphragms will lead to diagnostic classification, but there is little effective form of active therapy other than the hope that the partially impaired pathways can recover. It should be remembered that the early lesion may result from edema in the area of a cervical root injury and will therefore to some extent be reversible. Efforts to artificially stimulate the diaphragm by a variety of electronic devices have so far not proven to be of any major therapeutic advantage. It must also be remembered that the presence of any severe type of birth injury may often be accompanied by other evidence of CNS impairment which may of itself influence both central and peripheral respiratory drive and function.

Tracheo-esophageal fistula. — This condition occurs in approximately 1 in 3,000 births and is often associated with other major abnormalities in other systems. In the most common form, there is atresia of the proximal end of the esophagus while the distal segment of the esophagus is connected and in continuation with the trachea.

Clinically, the condition may present as poly-hydramnios during pregnancy. The inability to pass a catheter through the esophagus into the stomach may establish the diagnosis in the delivery room. In this connection, it should be noted that a catheter may coil extensively in the upper segment (blind pouch) of the esophagus giving the false impression that the catheter is passing through the esophagus. A useful maneuver is to auscultate the gastric area with a stethoscope while air is being injected via a syringe into the catheter. The sound of air passage indicating the entry of air into the stomach will confirm the patency of the esophagus. Radiographic visualization with radio-opaque dye is often necessary for confirmation of the obstructed site. This maneuver is particularly useful to provide the surgeon with precise information on the type of anomaly and the distance between the blind proximal end and the distal segment of the esophagus. The latter is an important piece of information for the surgeon in deciding on the surgical procedure for definitive anastomosis of the esophagus.

The earliest suspicious sign of this condition is the presence of mucous requiring frequent excessive suctioning of the infant's oro-nasal cavity. This is due to the upper esophageal obstruction and the resultant inability of the infant to swallow his or her own secretions. The report of the nursing staff that a diaper placed at the head of the infant is continuously wet should lead to an index of suspicion by which the diagnosis may be readily suspected. Delay in this diagnostic procedure will result in aspiration pneumonia, as feeding attempts are undertaken. The diagnosis becomes more clearly and painfully obvious, with progressive cyanosis each time feeding is attempted. An additional radiographic clue can be adduced from the rapid and early distention of the abdomen with gas, an occurrence explained by the existence of a virtually direct communication between the trachea and the distal end of the esophagus so that air is forced into the lower GI tract with each successive respiration.

Radiographic diagnosis can be made from simple AP and lateral films showing the level of esophageal atresia; however, it is often necessary to resort to contrast filling of the upper segment of the esophagus (Fig. III-37).

Treatment is surgical. Division and anastomosis of the fistula is usually fairly simple, but a longer missing segment may necessitate either blind pouch suction and dilation in the hope of lengthening

the segment to be able to carry out a primary apposition or the interposition of some form of other intestinal tissue (colon has been used for this purpose) in an attempt to complete the esophageal continuity. Under such circumstances, a feeding gastrostomy will be necessary while awaiting the definitive surgical procedure and its outcome.

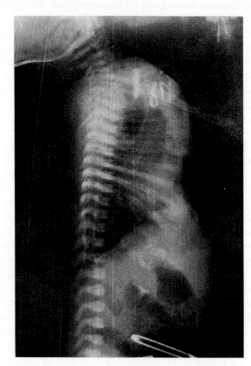

FIG. III-37. — *Tracheoesophageal fistula.*
The contrast medium outlines the proximal blind end of the esophagus.

The rarer H-type fistula which is not associated with esophageal atresia is rarely diagnosed at birth. It more commonly will result in repeated bouts of pneumonia which may only become recognized in older children or early adult life as being due to the presence of the condition. Demonstration of such a fistula usually requires distention of the esophagus with contrast medium under pressure for demonstration of the aberrant passage. A more complete form of this type of fistula in which there is virtual continuity between the posterior wall of the trachea and the anterior wall of the esophagus results in massive entry of food contents into the lung and is generally incompatible with any degree of prolonged survival.

Lower respiratory problems

HYALINE MEMBRANE DISEASE
OR RESPIRATORY DISTRESS SYNDROME

Hyaline membrane disease or respiratory distress syndrome is the most common pulmonary disorder in the newborn. It occurs almost exclusively in premature infants and the incidence is inversely proportional to gestational age. The precise incidence is not known; although, the best estimate shows that it occurs in 60 % of infants less than 28 weeks of gestation and 15-20 % in those between 32 and 36 weeks of gestation. Beyond 37 weeks of gestation, the incidence is approximately 5 %. Hyaline membrane disease is also a leading cause of neonatal death accounting for 25,000 neonatal deaths annually in the United States. It has been estimated that 50 % of all neonatal deaths are the result of hyaline membrane disease and its complications.

A large body of knowledge has accumulated in the last decade dealing with the etiology, pathogenesis, diagnosis and management of this disease. It appears likely that within the next decade, further breakthroughs in defining the etiology and prevention of this disease will continue to unfold, resulting in a reduction in incidence, morbidity, and mortality of this disease.

ETIOLOGY AND PATHOGENESIS

During the past three decades, numerous hypotheses have been advanced to account for the occurrence of hyaline membrane disease. The most recent and probably most plausible theory is based on the concept that hyaline membrane disease is primarily a result of the lack or reduction of surfactant in the pulmonary alveolar lining in an immature infant. With increasing degrees of maturation, increased amounts of phospholipids (primarily lecithin) are synthesized and stored in the type II cells of the alveoli. These surface active agents are released into the alveoli reducing the surface tension and helping to maintain alveolar stability during expiration. The Laplace law, $P \propto \dfrac{2T}{R}$

states that the pressure required to distend a sphere is directly proportional to the surface tension and inversely to the radius of the sphere. Therefore, with a lack of surfactant and high surface tension, it requires progressively higher pressures to maintain alveolar patency in expiration with resultant alveolar collapse. Hence, pulmonary atelactasis is the most prominent pathologic feature of infants with hyaline membrane disease. As shown in Figure III-38, a series of events will occur: the extensive atelectasis will result in hypoventilation resulting in both hypoxemia and hypercarbia; in other alveolar areas, the extensive atelectasis will produce a right to left intra-pulmonary shunt resulting in hypoxemia. The combined effect of hypoxemia and hypercarbia is one of respiratory and metabolic acidosis. It is known that hypoxemia and acidosis may cause pulmonary vasoconstriction resulting in pulmonary hypoperfusion and further diminution in surfactant synthesis. In the presence of hypoperfusion, increased endothelial permeability of the pulmonary capillaries with leakage of plasma into the interstitial space ensues. The conversion of fibrinogen present in the plasma into fibrin forms the hyaline-like material, from which the term hyaline membrane disease was derived. The presence of hyaline membranes in the interstitial space constitutes the other major pathological finding in infants who die of hyaline membrane disease. This hyaline membrane-like material also may reduce the diffusion capacity of gases across the alveolar capillary membrane resulting in further compromise in oxygen and carbon dioxide exchange.

Surfactant synthesis in the alveoli is a dynamic process and is dependent on an intact physiologic environment; i. e., normal pH, temperature, and perfusion. The presence of hypoxemia and hypoperfusion, particularly in the presence of hypovolemia, hypotension and cold stress, will compromise surfactant synthesis. Moreover, in the presence of ischemia, and other unfavorable factors, such as exposure to high oxygen concentration, poor drainage of the upper airway, and the effect of respirator management, the epithelial lining of the alveoli may be damaged, resulting in a further reduction of surfactant synthesis. Thus, it appears that the pathogenesis of the hyaline membrane disease is a sequence of events beginning with impair-

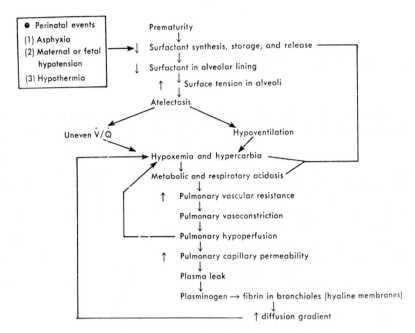

FIG. III-38. — *Pathogenesis of hyaline membrane disease.*

ment in surfactant synthesis followed by a series of events which leads to a vicious cycle accounting for the progressive increment in the severity of the disease during the first three days of life. The recovery phase of the disease is characterized by the regeneration of the alveolar tissue including the type II cells and the return of surfactant activity.

SIGNS AND SYMPTOMS

The majority of infants with respiratory distress syndrome will have signs of respiratory insufficiency starting immediately after birth. The signs of respiratory insufficiency include: tachypnea, intercostal retractions, subcostal retractions, expiratory grunting (grossly audible or by auscultation) and cyanosis with or without oxygen supplementation.

DIAGNOSIS

The diagnosis of respiratory distress syndrome is based on the following criteria:

1. Biochemical evidence of lung immaturity. The latter includes a low lecithin sphingomyelin (L/S) ratio ($< 2 : 1$) or negative foam stability tests in

amniotic fluid or other biological fluids, such as gastric aspirate, hypopharyngeal secretion, or tracheal fluid.

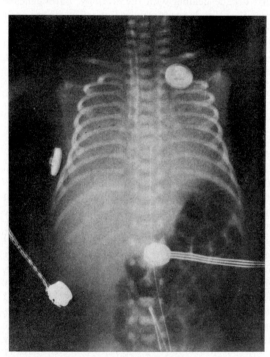

FIG. III-39. — *Hyaline membrane disease.*
Note the reticulogranular infiltrate and air bronchogram.

2. Physical signs of respiratory insufficiency as described previously.

3. Exclusion of other conditions that might account for the respiratory distress.

4. Radiographic evidence of hyaline membrane disease which includes a reticulo-granular infiltrate, enlarged heart, and the presence of an air bronchogram (Fig. III-39).

DIFFERENTIAL DIAGNOSIS

Table II lists conditions that might produce respiratory distress in the newborn infant. These conditions should be considered and excluded before a diagnosis of respiratory distress syndrome is entertained. In most cases, a carefully obtained history of the pregnancy and clinical course, a thorough physical examination in the first hour of life, an adequate anterior-posterior and lateral

TABLE II. — DIFFERENTIAL DIAGNOSIS
OF HYALINE MEMBRANE DISEASE

I. DISORDERS OF THE RESPIRATORY SYSTEM
CAUSING RESPIRATORY DISTRESS IN THE NEWBORN

1. Posterior choanal atresia.
2. Laryngeal webs or cysts: vocal cord paralysis.
3. Tracheal stenosis.
4. Laryngo-tracheal malacia.
5. Double aortic arch.
6. Congenital lung cyst.
7. Congenital lobar emphysema.
8. Congenital hypoplastic lung.
9. Congenital agenesis of the lung.
10. Congenital bacterial or viral pneumonia.
11. Perinatal aspiration syndrome:
    a) Meconium aspiration syndrome;
    b) Thick mucus aspiration;
    c) Blood aspiration.
12. Pneumothorax and pneumomediastinum.
13. Pulmonary lobar interstitial emphysema.
14. Transient tachypnea of the newborn.
15. Chylothorax.

II. EXTRA-PULMONARY DISORDERS
CAUSING RESPIRATORY DISTRESS IN THE NEWBORN

1. Tracheo-esophageal atresia.
2. Diaphragmatic hernia.
3. Muscular weakness:
    a) Amyotonia congenita;
    b) Myasthenia gravis.
4. Phrenic nerve injury or paralysis.
5. Depressant drugs, e. g. meperidine.
6. Central nervous system pathology, e. g. cerebral hemorrhage, meningoencephalitis, subdural hematoma.
7. Congenital heart disease with congestive heart failure or pulmonary edema.

chest roentgenogram, and in a few instances, an electrocardiogram will provide sufficient information to consider or exclude the various other diagnoses. Thus, a careful physical examination and chest roentgenogram will provide the basis for the diagnosis of such conditions as tracheo-esophageal fistula, posterior choanal atresia, laryngeal obstructions from various pathologies, diaphragmatic hernia, congenital pneumonia, pneumothorax, pneumomediastinum, pulmonary hypoplasia, meconium aspiration syndrome, and transient tachypnea of the newborn. In addition, chest roentgenograms and electrocardiographic data will provide useful information that will exclude or include the diagnosis of congenital heart disease as the cause of respiratory distress.

Recently, it has been shown that gastric aspirate obtained during the first few hours of life may be useful in establishing the diagnosis of respiratory distress syndrome. Foam stability tests performed on the gastric aspirate collected at birth may provide information reflecting the status of pulmonary maturation and surfactant activity.

MANAGEMENT

Antenatal treatment for the prevention of respiratory distress syndrome (RDS)

It has recently been shown that a number of pharmacologic agents can enhance fetal pulmonary maturation by the alteration of specific mechanisms in the synthesis and secretion of surfactants. Of the agents identified (thyroxine, aminophylline and corticosteroids), the corticosteroids have been studied most extensively in human subjects. The data of Liggins and Howie based on a large controlled study has shown that administration of a synthetic corticosteroid (betamethasone) to the mother 24-72 hours prior to the delivery of the fetus results in a significant reduction in the incidence of RDS, particularly in infants less than 32 weeks of gestational age. Since the publication of these results, several clinical trials including a large collaborative study in the United States have confirmed the beneficial effect of glucocorticoids in reducing the incidence of RDS. Based on these clinical findings, it seems reasonable to suggest that with appropriate consideration of risk/benefit, corticosteroid may be given to a pregnant woman who might deliver an infant at risk for RDS. With the exception of an observed increase in fetal death when corticosteroid is given to a severely affected toxemic mother, most of the known risks of corticosteroid treatment of the fetus are confined to animal observations. However, while additional follow-up data on children who were exposed to corticosteroid prior to birth are being collected, the use of corticosteroid should be confined only to cases where clear indications of immature fetal lung are present (amniotic fluid L/S ratio $\leqslant$ 2 : 1).

Acceleration of fetal lung maturity may also be accomplished by natural events. It has been shown that prolonged rupture of amniotic membranes ($\geqslant$ 24 hours) and high risk pregnancies resulting in placental insufficiency and chorionamniotis may result in the acceleration of fetal lung maturation probably on the basis of increased endogenous production of corticosteroid under stress conditions. Therefore, in situations where such risk factors are present, the use of corticosteroid treatment should be avoided since the natural event itself may be adequate to produce an acceleration of lung maturation without the additional use of an exogenous agent. Furthermore, the clinical events that might enhance lung maturation are also the conditions that might impose additional risks on the mother and the fetus when corticosteroids are used. For instance, in the presence of premature rupture of membranes with chorionamnionitis, corticosteroid may enhance the severity and complication of infection both in the mother and the fetus. Also, the risk of fetal death is higher when corticosteroid is administered to toxemic mothers with placental insufficiency. The latter is frequently associated with the enhancement of fetal lung maturation.

It is apparent that the largest group of subjects who are appropriate candidates for corticosteroid treatment for the acceleration of lung maturation are pregnant mothers of less than 32 weeks of gestation with evidence of fetal lung immaturity who are admitted for premature labor. In these instances, the success of corticosteroid therapy depends largely on the effectiveness of arresting labor by the use of uterine muscle inhibitors. Several pharmacologic agents are currently being evaluated, notably beta-mimetic drugs such as Ritodrine. If the premature labor can be stopped and the delivery of the fetus delayed for more than 24 hours, there is considerable chance that fetal exposure to corticosteroid may enhance lung maturation with a reduced incidence of RDS.

Intrapartum care of the fetus

It is well established that fetal and neonatal asphyxia could exaggerate the severity of hyaline membrane disease particularly in the presence of an inadequately developed lung. Therefore, an important component in the management of hyaline membrane disease is to minimize the insult to a premature fetus during labor. It is recommended that all fetuses in premature labor be monitored with a continuous fetal heart rate monitoring device; and that when appropriate, fetal scalp sampling should be done to assess the biochemical status of the fetus for appropriate management including interruption of pregnancy when indicated. It is of the utmost importance that the maternal complications, such as circulatory compromise, and acidosis, be treated promptly to avoid fetal jeopardy. The use of oxytocin for induction and augmentation of labor, heavy analgesic medication, and some forms of anesthesia, such as spinal anesthesia, should be avoided to reduce the risk of fetal depression and hypoxemia.

Immediate neonatal care

Attending a premature birth requires the concerted efforts of a perinatal team to insure the optimal outcome of the infant. The infant should be kept warm, the upper airway should be maintained and resuscitation appropriately carried out by the most experienced person on the team. The question of early versus late clamping of the umbilical cord in relation to the incidence of respiratory distress syndrome has been a matter of controversy for many years. However, the current consensus is that the effect of placental transfusion on the incidence and severity of respiratory distress syndrome is probably minimal and that the best approach in this regard is to clear the infant's airway during the first minutes after the delivery of the body allowing the placental transfusion to occur during this time period.

Neonatal care of infants with respiratory distress syndrome

Since hyaline membrane disease is a self-limiting disorder, the aim of neonatal therapy is to provide support to maintain the optimal physiologic conditions of the infant. These supports include temperature control, oxygen therapy, fluid and electrolyte as well as nutritional management, correction of metabolic acidosis when present, and assisted ventilation when the indications arise. Temperature control, fluid and electrolyte management, and nutritional support are discussed elsewhere in this textbook. Oxygen therapy, correction of acid base imbalance, and assisted ventilation will be discussed in detail below.

Oxygen therapy. — The goal of oxygen therapy in newborn infants with respiratory distress syndrome is to maintain normal tissue oxygenation by providing adequate oxygen with proper monitoring without subjecting the infants to the risk of oxygen toxicity to the eye and lung. To provide adequate tissue oxygenation, the infant must have normal oxygen tension, oxygen saturation, hemoglobin content, blood pressure, and tissue perfusion. From the clinical standpoint, it is virtually impossible to measure on a minute to minute basis the oxygen content, oxygen dissociation curve, blood pressure and tissue perfusion, therefore, the arterial oxygen tension has become the most commonly used parameter in monitoring oxygen therapy. Arterial blood samples can be obtained either by peripheral arterial punctures (temporal, radial, or brachial arteries) when intermittent arterial PO_2 monitoring is sufficient for the clinical management. When more frequent PO_2 monitoring is indicated, umbilical artery catheter placement is the most commonly used method of blood sampling. A polyethylene radiopaque lined catheter (French 3.5, 5 or 8) is generally used for the catheterization with the catheter retrogradely passed into the descending aorta and placed either above or below the diaphragm. There has been considerable discussion regarding the advantage of either above or below the diaphragm placement; the consensus of opinion is that the complication rate is probably similar in both locations of placement and that either location is probably satisfactory provided that the tip of the catheter is not placed directly above or adjacent to the bifurcation or branching of the renal or celiac arteries.

Warmed capillary blood has also been used for the measurement of PO_2 when arterial punctures or umbilical arterial placement are impossible. This is an undesirable blood sampling route since the correlation between warm capillary blood PO_2 and arterial blood PO_2 is poor particularly in instances where the peripheral tissue perfusion is reduced as a result of either immaturity, young age, or poor clinical condition. During the recovery phase, the capillary blood PO_2 at high levels is also very inaccurate. Venous blood PO_2 should not be used for the assessment of tissue oxygenation. Transcutaneous PO_2 measurements are now clinically available; in newborns the correlation between arterial and transcutaneous PO_2 is good and reliable particularly if the calibration and care of the instru-

ments for transcutaneous PO_2 measurement are well maintained. This method of oxygen monitoring is encouraged particularly in very sick infants where continuous assessment of oxygen therapy is indicated.

There is an absolute necessity to deliver oxygen at all times that is both warm and humidified. Oxygen as it emerges from the standard source in the wall or portable oxygen tank is both cold and dry. The dry property adds to evaporative heat loss and to the drying effect on the respiratory tract. The coldness of the oxygen delivered is particularly dangerous when given through a face mask over the trigeminal area of the nose and mouth. It is known that the peripheral receptors for cold stimulation are located over the forehead in the trigeminal area of the face in the newborn infants. The application of a cold stimulus to these areas will force a mandatory increase in oxygen consumption on the part of the infant irrespective of the rest of the environmental temperature. This fact tends to be forgotten when oxygen is used, via a face mask directly from a wall source, particularly in emergency situations for purposes of resuscitation from apneic spells.

Finally, it should be stressed again that the apparent recrudescence of the incidence of retrolental fibroplasia in small premature infants is only marginally related to the increase in the number of infants with severe respiratory distress syndrome. Since retrolental fibroplasia is a function of arterial oxygen tension, the infant with severe cardiopulmonary disease rarely reaches arterial PO_2 levels of sufficient magnitude to result in the retinopathy of prematurity. It is the infant with an *intact* cardiopulmonary system who is being resuscitated frequently from apneic spells with a bag and mask attached to a pure oxygen line who is subject to intermittent high peak PaO_2 exposure. Under these circumstances it is recommended that a self inflatable bag be kept within the incubator and that if and when resuscitation is necessary, it be carried out in the same inspired air concentration at which the infant has been kept throughout.

Assisted ventilation for the treatment of severe respiratory distress syndrome. — In the moderate to severe forms of respiratory distress syndrome, it is often necessary to utilize the various mechanical means of assisted ventilation in the management of this disease. In infants with severe hypoxemia but minimal or moderate hypercarbia, continuous positive airway pressure (CPAP) breathing is often utilized to combat the hypoxemia. This mode of treatment is based on the theory that by mechanically applying a certain amount of distending pressure during the end expiratory phase, in an infant with spontaneous breathing, pulmonary atelectasis due to surfactant deficiency can be minimized or avoided. During the initial phase of the development of this method of treatment, endotracheal intubation was required to apply the continuous positive airway pressure (CPAP) therapy; therefore, the criteria for instituting this treatment were rather rigid and included 1) arterial blood $PO_2 \leqslant 50$ mm Hg with an FIO_2 of 1.0, 2) $PCO_2 \leqslant 60$ mm Hg, and 3) pH $\geqslant 7.20$. More recently, with the introduction and use of non-invasive technique of applying CPAP by nasal prongs, more liberal criteria for early treatment of these infants by such means have been utilized. Criteria of $PO_2 \leqslant 50$ mm Hg at FIO_2 of 0.7 are now utilized as an indication for CPAP treatment. Data collected at various centers have shown that this approach may effectively reduce the severity of the disease, reduce the amount of O_2 needed, shorten the course of the disorder, lower the incidence of chronic lung disease, and improve the survival rate.

In infants with severe respiratory distress syndrome with respiratory failure, or those who develop complications resulting in persistent apnea, intermittent cycled respirator management is indicated. The criteria for placing an infant on a positive intermittent pressure respirator include 1) arterial blood pH$\leqslant 7.20$, 2) arterial blood $PCO_2 \geqslant 60$ mm Hg, 3) arterial blood $PO_2 \leqslant 50$ mm Hg at FIO_2 of 1.0, and 4) persistent apnea. There are two forms of positive pressure respirators: 1) pressure constant volume variable (e. g., Bird 8 Q Circle Respirators) and 2) volume constant and pressure variable respirators (e. g., Bourns respirator). The various types of the positive pressure respirators offer different kinds of mechanical or technological sophistication and economic advantage; however, the effectiveness of respirator management is much more dependent on the training, experience, and devotion of the neonatal intensive care team rather than on the type of respirator employed.

COMPLICATIONS

Patent ductus arteriosus (PDA)

In normal term infants, the ductus arteriosus normally closes within 24-48 hours after birth, partly in response to the rise in oxygen saturation following birth. In preterm infants with respiratory distress and hypoxemia, the ductus frequently remains patent for several days or weeks with significant shunting of blood from left to right leading to pulmonary edema. PDA with left to right shunt as a complication of RDS is often associated with low gestational age and low birth weight. The majority of these complications develop in infants below 32 weeks and $< 1,750$ g. The diagnosis can be made by clinical signs and symptoms as well as laboratory and other diagnostic aids. Typically, the infants begin with a classical course of RDS with increasing degree of severity which will start to improve by the third day of life. At this time, there may be worsening of the clinical status with: 1) occurrence of persistent apnea unaccountable by other causes, and 2) physical findings of a) heaving and active precordium, b) bounding peripheral pulses, c) presence of a systolic or diastolic murmur. The laboratory findings will include 1) CO_2 retention with metabolic and respiratory acidosis, 2) increasing requirement of ambient oxygen concentration to maintain a normal arterial PO_2. In addition, there may be 1) radiological evidence of cardiomegaly and increased pulmonary vascular markings, and 2) echocardiography will reveal a high left atrial to aortic root ratio ($\geqslant 1.3$).

The medical management of PDA with left to right shunt includes: 1) fluid restriction, 2) diuretics (furosemide, 1 mg/kg), 3) maintaining a normal hemoglobin and hematocrit level and 4) assisted ventilation when necessary. The evidence suggests that digitalis is of little value in treating this condition.

If conservative medical management is unsuccessful, and findings of a left to right shunt persist beyond 24 to 48 hours, a prostaglandin synthetase inhibitor (Indomethacin) may be used to hasten the closure of the ductus. The dose is 0.2 mg/kg intravenously every 12 hours. If more than 3 doses have been used and the clinical status is unchanged, surgical ligation should be considered.

The surgical management of PDA with left to right shunt consists of transthoracic ligation of the ductus. The success rate of the surgical intervention is dependent on the skill of the surgeon and the cohesive pre-operative and post-operative management of the infant by the perinatal team.

Bronchopulmonary dysplasia (chronic or respirator lung disease)

Bronchopulmonary dysplasia is a complication of RDS particularly in those infants who require assisted ventilation. Clinically, infants with bronchopulmonary dysplasia may have respiratory symptoms persisting up to 3 to 6 months of life. Many infants may require prolonged hospitalization with oxygen therapy. Pathologically, the condition is characterized by the presence of alveolar and bronchiolar epithelial damage followed by bronchiolar metaplasia, peribronchial and interstitial fibrosis. Radiologically, the progressive pulmonary changes are divided into four stages by Northway et al. Stage 1 are non-specific changes indistinguishable from those of hyaline membrane disease, stage 2 is characterized by the opacification of the lung with persistence of a bronchogram, stage 3 is characterized by the presence of cystic infiltrates, and stage 4 by the presence of hyperlucency and strandlike infiltrates, representing bronchiolar and interstitial fibrosis. The treatment for this complication is conservative and consists mostly of appropriate oxygen therapy and other supportive measures. Most infants with bronchopulmonary dysplasia gradually recover by 6-12 months of age in most cases with normal pulmonary function.

The etiology of bronchopulmonary dysplasia is probably multi-factorial; the combination of previous alveolar damage from hyaline membrane disease, exposure to high oxygen concentrations, the use of the respirator, the use of endotracheal intubation, and the prolonged duration of these therapies probably together account for the development of this complication. In this connection, one needs to clearly differentiate the assumption that the condition is synonymous with oxygen toxicity from the evidence which actually exists to support this contention. The condition has been reported both in newborn infants and in adults following prolonged assisted ventilation with positive pressure respirators utilizing both high oxygen concentrations and endotracheal or nasotracheal tubes. By contrast, there are essentially no reports of its occurrence in prolonged ventilation with negative pressure equipment in either newborn infants or adults despite the fact that high oxygen concentrations have been used under these circumstances for periods even longer than those suggested in the original reports of the condition. If this is correct, then it is unlikely that oxygen by itself is responsible for this form of chronic respirator lung disease but that it would indeed require both the co-existence of an endotracheal tube and/or a positive pressure respirator for the effect to occur. The current best estimate would suggest that the damage is primarily a function of both the intubation and the time that assisted ventilation is necessary, and that efforts to either avoid or shorten both of these would effect a reduction of the incidence and/or the severity of the disease.

Extrapulmonary extravasation of air

Pulmonary interstitial emphysema, pneumomediastinum, with pneumothorax are the results of accumulation of air in the pulmonary interstitial tissue, anterior mediastinum, and pleural cavity, respectively. Pulmonary interstitial emphysema (Fig. III-40) or pneumomediastinum (Fig. III-41) may occur with or without the use of positive pressure resuscitation or a respirator. The diagnosis is usually made radiologically. No active treatment is available. However, the presence of pulmonary interstitial emphysema in infants with respiratory distress syndrome should portend the occurrence of pneumothorax particularly if the infant is being treated with assisted ventilation using high inspiratory peak pressures.

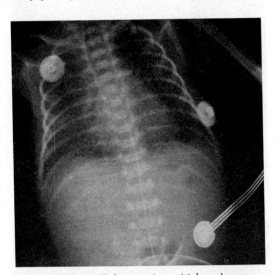

FIG. III-40. — *Pulmonary interstitial emphysema.*

Pneumothorax occurs in about 30 % of infants with severe hyaline membrane disease on respirator treatment. A direct correlation exists between the amount of inspiratory pressure used and the incidence of pneumothorax. This association should be taken into account in determining the pressure to be used in the respirator treatment of hyaline membrane disease. The diagnosis of pneumothorax is based on sudden deterioration, often accompanied by hypotension. Physical examination reveals reduction or absence of breath sounds on the affected side of the chest and shifting of heart sounds to the contralateral side. Chest roentgenogram provides definitive diagnosis (Fig. III-42). In emergency, and if delay in the radiological diagnosis is anticipated, one may use a high intensity lamp to demonstrate the presence of pneumothorax. However, it is clear that chest roentgenogram is the preferred method of diagnosis. Treatment consists of close observation, if the infant is asymptomatic or mildly symptomatic and the degree of pneumo-

thorax is small (e. g., less than 10 %); but in infants with significant chest retraction with a large pneumothorax, immediate evacuation of pleural air by insertion of a needle is mandatory to be followed by chest tube drainage of the pleural space.

In addition to the above three, two additional complications of extrapulmonary air accumulation have been reported in conjunction with respirator usage. Pneumopericardium may present as sudden shock and circulatory collapse during the course of respirator management, and its clinical appearance can occasionally be detected by hearing an extremely rapid heart rate indicative of cardiac tamponade. A prompt diagnosis should be made radiographically since this complication can be rapidly fatal unless it is immediately treated by evacuation of the entrapped air. Similarly, pneumoperitoneum (Fig. III-43), which occurs as air is forced down through the diaphragmatic apertures, may present a therapeutic dilemma in that it needs clearly to be differentiated from the pneumoperitoneum secondary to a perforated viscus. Given a desperately ill infant already under respirator care, one would prefer to avoid surgical exploration under these circumstances. The instillation of a small amount of contrast material into the stomach may afford a diagnostic maneuver of value in that the contrast medium can then be seen to either remain within the gastrointestinal tract excluding a perforated viscus or to be found outside it, suggesting that one

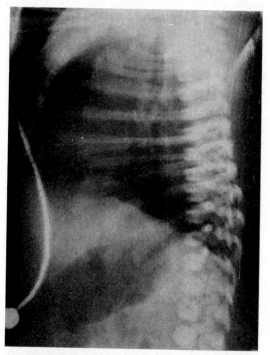

FIG. III-41. — *Pneumomediastinum.*

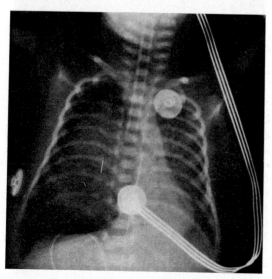

FIG. III-42. — *Pneumothorax, right.*
Note presence of pulmonary interstitial emphysema in both lung fields.

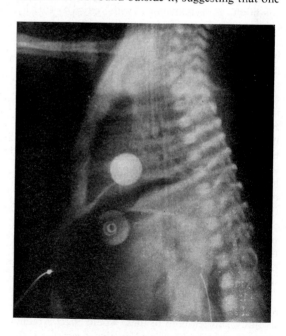

FIG. III-43. — *Pneumoperitoneum.*
Note presence of pneumomediastinum.

has indeed occurred and indicating the necessity for surgical intervention.

Intraventricular hemorrhage

Intraventricular bleeding is a common complication in infants with hyaline membrane disease. The usual causes of intraventricular hemorrhage include hypoxemia and acidosis, abnormalities in the mechanism responsible for coagulation, and the excessive use of large volumes of hypertonic solutions, such as sodium bicarbonate. Correction or avoidance of these abnormal clinical factors is the best means of preventing the complication of intracranial hemorrhage. Diagnosis of this condition is based on a sudden fall in hemoglobin, onset of apneic spells and/or seizures. Recently, ultrasonography has been found to be very useful in making a diagnosis of intraventricular hemorrhage. When intraventricular hemorrhage occurs, the prognosis of these infants is poor; a large number will die. In those who survive, hydrocephalus is a common sequelae. The long-term developmental outcomes are also poor, particularly if the hemorrhage is large and seizures occur during the neonatal period.

TRANSIENT TACHYPNEA OF THE NEWBORN

This condition is a poorly understood entity and difficult to define pathologically since it almost invariably results in recovery of the patient. It is thought to be due in most cases to a delay in absorption of lung fluid. Radiographically there is the appearance of a "wet lung" with fluid lines present in the fissures. It should be remembered that in adults pulmonary edema is not an uncommon result of central nervous system injury, and it may therefore be that a certain number of these cases are associated with birth asphyxia and a degree of pulmonary edema and pulmonary vasoconstriction. Treatment is purely supportive and similar to that outlined for the management of RDS. Fortunately, the prognosis for these infants is excellent and almost all infants will recover without significant sequelae.

ASPIRATION SYNDROMES (OTHER THAN MECONIUM)

Either blood or mucus may be aspirated by the newborn in the course of passage through the birth canal. Aspiration of blood (either the infant's own or that of the mother) may occur from a variety of causes associated with third trimester bleeding and particularly in situations where sudden bleeding occurs just as the delivery is being completed. Most of the blood under such circumstances usually enters the GI tract, where it can be differentiated as to fetal vs. maternal origin on the basis of its reaction with alkali. Aspirated blood in the lung is usually of a rapidly transient nature rarely requiring therapy beyond its recognition, and will tend to disappear rather quickly. Amniotic fluid does not persist to any great extent within the lung; the fluid being in relatively easy equilibrium with other body fluids across the alveoli. However, the debris associated with the amniotic fluid aspiration may well remain in the form of a variety of cellular fragments, mucus plugs, etc. Unless the material is known or assumed to be infected, therapy should be of a supportive nature.

MECONIUM ASPIRATION SYNDROME

The aspiration of meconium presents a characteristic picture which has in the past been primarily considered as essentially a pulmonary disease. To the extent, however, that such aspiration almost invariably accompanies an asphyxiating delivery or represents the end manifestation of peripartum asphyxia, it is more appropriate to consider the meconium aspiration syndrome as part and parcel of the peripartum asphyxia situation and its causes in the newborn.

Nevertheless, the aspiration itself may cause severe intrinsic pulmonary problems. If sufficiently massive, the meconium will result in not only alveolar but primarily bronchiolar obstruction with overdistention of the peripheral alveoli and massive arterial alveolar block in those alveoli in which meconium has managed to pass even the smaller bronchioles. The characteristic X-ray which has been described as "wet snow flakes on pavement" is usually diagnostic even when the distribution is widespread and diffuse.

The aspiration usually occurs in the terminal stages of the birth process, but has been demonstrated to occasionally occur earlier in utero as a result of gasping respiratory movements associated with the hypoxic release of meconium from the gastrointestinal tract in utero. Although little can be done to remove meconium from the distal portions of the respiratory tract, there is considerable advantage in attempting to clear as much meconium as possible

TABLE III. — Protocol
FOR COMBINED OBSTETRIC AND PEDIATRIC MANAGEMENT

1. As soon as the baby's head appears on the perineum, the obstetrician passes a DeLee suction catheter through the nares to the level of the nasopharynx and aspirates any mucus or meconium, then suctions the mouth and hypopharynx.
2. Immediately after delivery the pediatrician suctions the oropharynx with a bulb syringe and, if meconium is present, inspects the cords by direct laryngoscopy while an assistant monitors the heart rate.
3. If meconium is present at the cords, direct suctioning of the trachea with either a DeLee catheter or mouth-endotracheal tube is performed.
4. Usual measures of ventilation and resuscitation are carried out.

from the upper airways providing this can be done atraumatically. More recently, it has been shown that a combined obstetric and pediatric approach (Table III) to the removal of meconium from the upper airway will improve the outcome of these infants. The procedure is therefore encouraged as part of the regime in the management of the meconium aspiration syndrome. Respiratory supportive therapy with oxygen, intravenous fluids, and eventually respirator management is indicated in severe cases. The use of antibiotics under these circumstances is debatable. Where there is no evidence that infected material has been aspirated the meconium itself should be considered as being sterile. Nevertheless, experimental studies have suggested that meconium affords an enhanced medium for bacterial growth and the use of antibiotics to prevent "secondary" superinfection has been advocated. There is, however, little evidence to suggest that deaths from this condition are indeed of bacterial origin, and the use of antibiotics under such circumstances, therefore, remains of questionable value.

Functionally there may be a profound depression of arterial PO_2 as well as an enormous elevation in arterial PCO_2. The latter results from the broncho-obstructive features of the disease secondary to obstruction of the smaller bronchioles with the sticky meconium. Under these circumstances if assisted ventilation is necessary, the use of CPAP is probably contraindicated since the alveoli are already overdistended and adding a continuous distending pressure under these circumstances will only increase the dead space further raising the arterial carbon dioxide tension.

Finally, it must be recognized that the severe forms of meconium aspiration are almost invariably associated with severe central nervous system asphyxia. The frequent accompaniment of convulsive disorders and cerebral edema only attest to this point. Such evidence of CNS injury will need to be managed with anticonvulsant medication. To date there is no convincing evidence that osmotic diuretic agents such as mannitol are useful in the treatment of cerebral edema secondary to asphyxial or anoxic injury. The ultimate prognosis for infants with meconium aspiration syndrome may depend not so much upon the pulmonary disability but more on the central nervous system injury which is in turn a reflection of the underlying asphyxiating cause.

EARLY NEONATAL SEPSIS
WITH OR WITHOUT CONGENITAL
PNEUMONIA

Bacterial sepsis with or without pneumonia can be acquired by the infant from the mother through a variety of routes which include hematogenous and direct extension from infected uterine and genital sources. The degree of maternal illness often is not associated with that seen in the infant. Evidence for the spread can often be obtained by examination of the placenta, cord, and membranes which will show exudation and/or polymorphonuclear infiltration in the tissues as evidence of the route of transmission. The organisms involved are often group B Streptococcus, and gram negative organisms such as *E. coli* or *Klebsiella pneumoniae*.

Clinically, bacterial sepsis of early onset is a highly dangerous event. The symptoms appear soon after birth in the form of respiratory distress. Radiographically, all degrees of involvement from streaky infiltrations to lobar consolidation may be seen. A febrile response may or may not be present but is most often absent under these circumstances. In this connection, the failure to maintain a stable body temperature is a far better index of sepsis than fever itself in a newborn infant. Hypotension is also a frequent manifestation. Depression of the white blood cell count to levels below 5,000/mm³ with a reduced polymorphonuclear count is a particularly ominous sign and will usually indicate impending demise irrespective of the energetic use of antibacterial therapy (Fig. III-44). Culture of the organisms may be obtained either from tracheal aspirate or blood. Treatment consists of antibiotics, usually a combination of Ampicillin and one of the

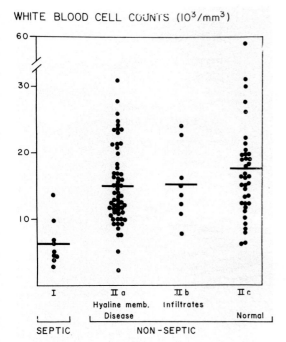

WHITE BLOOD CELL COUNTS (10³/mm³)

Fig. III-44. — *White blood cell counts in infants with neonatal sepsis.*

aminoglycosides such as Kanamycin or Gentamycin. In severe cases fresh whole blood exchange transfusion has been used with good results; but clear evidence for the effectiveness of this form of therapy is still lacking. Because of severe leukopenia, white blood cell transfusion has also been suggested as an adjunct in the treatment of neonatal sepsis; however, this therapy is still in the experimental stage.

A number of viruses have been implicated in transplacental pneumonias of maternal origin and isolation of viruses of the Coxsackie, Herpangina, Echo, and Myxovirus group have been reported from fatal cases. The history may often show evidence of a minor respiratory or gastrointestinal illness in the mother and in the case of the herpes hominus virus there may have been prior evidence of either vaginal or cervical herpes. The radiographic appearance tends to be more diffuse and streakier than in the well-organized bacterial variety but ante mortem differentiation between the two is often not possible unless specific bacterial cultures have been obtained. Viral isolation should be undertaken in suspicious cases, but it is difficult to avoid antibiotic therapy because of the similarity between the bacterial and viral presentations, particularly with respect to the systemic manifestations of generalized illness as well as the respiratory symptomatology.

As with congenital pneumonias of bacterial origin, there is a high mortality rate and a tendency towards rapid downhill progression. Failure to maintain thermal balance and the depression of the white blood cell count are grave prognostic signs.

Both bacterial and viral pneumonias can present in a neonatally acquired form with the transmission usually coming from other neonates, parents, or nursery personnel. In the bacterial category staphylococcal disease from a maternal breast abscess or streptococcal spread from the upper respiratory tract of either symptomatic or asymptomatic carriers may be implicated. A number of viruses of the adenovirus, parainfluenza, and respiratory syncytial virus groups have been implicated in nursery epidemics with severe respiratory impairment often necessitating respirator support in the first few weeks of life. Reports of upper respiratory viral disease in epidemic fashion in nurseries have also been described with the specific isolation of influenza virus of the Hong Kong type during the 1970 and 1971 epidemics in North America.

PNEUMOTHORAX

The two major causes of pneumothorax in the newborn are the meconium aspiration syndrome and hyaline membrane disease. In the former condition the sticky meconium tends to fix along the bronchus and results in a partial fixed obstruction. The rupture tends to occur early in the course of the disease and the relatively compliant overdistended lung is easily subject to massive tension displacement with serious major shifts of the cardiovascular structures resulting in the classical picture of tension pneumothorax (see p. 445 for additional discussion).

LOBAR EMPHYSEMA

A variety of congenital cysts of the lungs may occur either from de novo malformation of alveolar structures or as a result of bronchomalacia in one or more major subdivisions of the bronchial tree. In the condition associated with bronchomalacia, the alveoli may initially be normal but the progressive emphysema with collapse of the bronchus during expiration due to the intrinsic weakness of its cartilaginous rings results in a progressively enlarging cystic area which may necessitate total removal of the lung on that side as a life-saving procedure.

Less extensive degrees may be treated by attempted repair of the bronchus or removal of the affected portion of the lung.

DIAPHRAGMATIC HERNIA

Congenital diaphragmatic hernia is the result of failure of the pleuroperitoneal folds to fuse either completely or partially. The condition is more common on the left than on the right side. In the area where the pleuro-peritoneal folds do not develop, the peritoneum and pleura are absent and allow a communication between the thoracic and abdominal cavities. In the usual left-sided defect the intestine, stomach, and spleen may all be elevated into the thorax. By contrast a right-sided defect especially if an incomplete one may have the liver as a guard in that the organ may effectively block or minimize the entry of other organs into the thoracic cavity. If the defect is complete, however, it is possible to have the entire liver or certainly its right-sided portions displaced into the thorax as well.

The result of such displacement is both severe respiratory embarrassment as well as the impairment of development of the lung on the affected side. The impairment is, however, not permanent since even the most vestigial appearing lung has been shown to expand to normal size and function with postnatal growth of the alveoli by one to one and a half years of age if the infant survives the initial insult. Diagnosis depends on early recognition of a newborn infant in acute respiratory distress. The auscultation of bowel sounds in the thoracic cavity affords an obvious clue but the appearance of a scaphoid abdomen due to displacement of the intestinal contents in the thorax may afford the major diagnostic indication of the underlying pathology present. Radiographic confirmation of the defect showing displacement of the abdominal organs will lead to a more definitive diagnosis (Fig. III-45). Great care must be taken in resuscitating such an infant not to attempt oxygenation via a bag and mask apparatus over the face, since this will only result in the entry of more air into the intestinal tract and further compromise the respiratory system by the displaced intestinal organs. Immediate intubation with delivery of oxygen through an intratracheal source should be carried out and transport of the infant to a surgical center arranged for with this mode of resuscitation and oxygenation in place.

Surgical success depends heavily on the speed of diagnosis and the correction of underlying acidemia

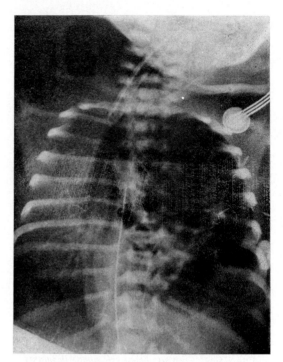

Fig. III-45. — *Diaphragmatic hernia.*
Note bowel in the left chest.

and hypoxia. Surgical repair of the defect where possible with replacement of the intestinal organs is the treatment of choice but both the size of the defect and the massiveness of the displaced organs may limit the technical ability to achieve this desired result. The vestigial underlying lung may pose problems in the immediate recovery period. In addition, persistent fetal circulation with a large right to left shunt is often associated with diaphragmatic hernia. Postnatal alveolar development, however, will occur and normal lung function can be anticipated with further growth of the infant.

WILSON-MIKITY SYNDROME

In 1959, Wilson and Mikity described a form of respiratory distress in premature infants associated with a radiographic appearance of cystic "soap-bubble like" changes in the lung on radiographic examination. This condition has been variously called cystic emphysema of prematurity or soap-bubble lung but is still most commonly referred to under its descriptive name.

The etiology of the condition is still unclear. It seems likely to be an associated phenomenon of extreme prematurity possibly due to the absence of sufficient pulmonary surface for gas exchange. Pathologically the disease is manifested by an almost classical type of compensatory emphysema with widely dilated alveolar spaces and fracture of the alveolar walls. Special elastic stains on lung specimens have demonstrated relatively heavy elastic reduplication in the emphysematous areas. The condition has been variously ascribed to oxygen toxicity but the occurrence of the disease in prematures who have both been in, and not been in, oxygen enriched environments prior to development of the disease tends to mediate against this as the sole etiologic agent. Symptoms of respiratory insufficiency together with the characteristic radiographic appearance have been noted as early as one week and as late as six weeks after birth. Other causes suggested include progressive injury from prolonged left to right shunting secondary to patent ductus arteriosus, viral infections, and even milk allergy. It would seem more appropriate to conceive of the disease as an affliction of extreme immaturity associated with a variety of potential compromising insults and eventuating in a final common pathway of compensatory overdistention of the alveoli in an effort to provide a greater respiratory surface.

Pathophysiologically the condition may lead to severe respiratory impairment and associated cor pulmonale with right-sided failure. Conservative management, however, has proven to be successful in most instances with regression of the changes over a protracted period of time as long as 1 to 2 years. Prolonged oxygen therapy represents a dangerous risk for the development of retrolental fibroplasia, particularly when one is obliged to administer added oxygen to infants of very low birth weight at times when easy access to arterial blood gases is not available. Management of cor pulmonale and congestive failure with digitalis has proven helpful in those circumstances where it occurs. Attempts to reverse the process with corticosteroids have not met with any documented success. Deaths which have occurred have been either from intercurrent pulmonary infection or cor pulmonale. Efforts to relate the disease to an inherited defect in lung structure possibly associated with alpha$_1$-antitrypsin deficiency while attractive have so far not been productive.

CHYLOTHORAX

In this rare situation a pleural effusion with milky fluid is present usually because of congenital malformation or traumatic injury to the thoracic duct. The milky nature of the fluid can be reversed by restricting the lipid intake and a formula of medium chain triglycerides will usually result in a change in the milky characteristics of the fluid removed. Drainage of the fluid if it accumulates to a degree of respiratory embarrassment is indicated. The condition tends to improve or ameliorate with time.

PULMONARY HEMORRHAGE

Primary pulmonary hemorrhage is associated with a variety of hypoxic insults and is far more common in small premature infants than in older more mature babies. However, even full-term infants subject to profound asphyxia have demonstrated the condition often in association with hypoxic hemorrhages in the central nervous system and/or adrenals. The condition is serious and there is a high mortality not so much from the pulmonary impairment as from the accompanying asphyxic and anoxic insults. Occasionally hemorrhagic disorders may manifest primarily as pulmonary hemorrhage and the disease is a common although unexplained accompaniment of kernicterus particularly in premature infants.

Diagnosis can usually be made by the characteristic appearance of the X-ray with a coarser infiltrate than one would anticipate in hyaline membrane disease. Where the condition is primarily microscopic and alveolar, no specific respiratory symptoms may be seen and the diagnosis would only be made at autopsy examination of the lungs. With more massive hemorrhage there is profound respiratory embarrassment and blood may be seen either grossly coming from the respiratory tract or appearing in the form of a bloody foam at the mouth and upper pharynx. Treatment is supportive for the pulmonary involvement with oxygen and even respiratory support if indicated, but the determining factor in survival is far more likely to be that of the underlying anoxia than of the pulmonary lesion itself.

REFERENCES

[1] ARANDA (J. V.), STERN (L.), DUNBAR (J. S.). — Pneumothorax with pneumoperitoneum in a newborn infant. *Am. J. Dis. Child.*, **123**, 163, 1972.
[2] AVERY (M. E.), FLETCHER (B. D.). — *The lung and its disorders in the newborn infant*, 3rd Edition. W. B. Saunders Company, Philadelphia, 1974.

[3] AVERY (M. E.), MEAD (J.). — Surface properties in relation to atalectasis in hyaline membrane disease. *Am. J. Dis. Child*, 97, 517, 1959.

[4] BAUER (C. R.), COLLE (E.), STERN (L.). — Prolonged rupture of membranes associated with a decreased incidence of respiratory distress syndrome. *Pediatrics*, 53, 7, 1973.

[5] BAUER (C. R.), ELIE (K.), SPENCE (L.), STERN (L.). — Hong Kong influenza in a neonatal unit. *JAMA*, 223, 1233, 1973.

[6] BOYLE (R.), CHANDLER (B. D.), STONESTREET (B. S.), OH (W.). — Early identification of sepsis in infants with respiratory distress. *Pediatrics*, 62, 744-750, 1978.

[7] CHU (J.), CLEMENTS (J. A.), COTTON (E.), KLAUS (M. H.), SWEET (A. Y.) *et al.* — The pulmonary hypoperfusion syndrome. *Pediatrics*, 35, 733, 1965.

[8] CLEMENTS (J. A.), PLATZKER (A. C. G.), TIERNEY (D. F.), HOBEL (C. J.), CREASY (R. K.), MARGOLIS (A. J.), THIBEAULT (D. W.), TOOLEY (W. H.), OH (W.). — Assessment of the risk of the respiratory-distress syndrome by a rapid test for surfactant in amniotic fluid. *New Engl. J. Med.*, 286, 1077, 1972.

[9] COWETT (R. M.), UNSWORTH (E. J.), HAKANSON (D. O.), WILLIAMS (J. R.), OH (W.). — Foam stability test on gastric aspirate and the diagnosis of respiratory distress syndrome (RDS). *New Engl. J. Med.*, 293, 413, 1975.

[10] GLUCK (L.), KULOVICH (M.). — Lecithin-sphingomyelin ratios in amniotic fluid in normal and abnormal pregnancy. *Am. J. Obst. Gynecol.*, 115, 539, 1973.

[11] GLUCK (L.), KULOVICH (M.), BORER (R.) *et al.* — Diagnosis of the respiratory distress syndrome by amniocentesis. *Am. J. Obst. Gynecol.*, 109, 440, 1971.

[12] GREGORY (G.), KITTERMAN (J.), PHIBBS (R.), TOOLEY (W.) *et al.* — Treatment of the idiopathic respiratory distress syndrome with continuous positive airway pressure. *New Engl. J. Med.*, 284, 1333, 1971.

[13] HOBEL (C. J.), HYVARINEN (M. A.), OH (W.). — Abnormal fetal heart rate and fetal acid base balance with special reference to respiratory distress syndrome. *Obst. and Gynec.*, 39, 83, 1972.

[14] LIGGINS (G. C.), HOWIE (R. N.). — A controlled trial of antepartum glucocorticoid treatment for prevention of the respiratory distress syndrome in premature infants. *Pediatrics*, 50, 515, 1972.

[15] LIND (J.), STERN (L.), WEGELIUS (C.). — *Human Fœtal and Neonatal Circulation* (Amer. Monographs in Pediatric Series, John ANDERSON, ed.). Charles C. Thomas and Sons, Springfield, 1964.

[16] MURPHY (D. A.), OUTERBRIDGE (E. W.), STERN (L.), KARN (G. M.), JEGIER (W.), ROSALES (J.). — Management of premature infants with patent ductus arteriosus. *J. Thor. and C. V. Surg.*, 67, 221, 1974.

[17] NELSON (N. M.), PROD'HOM (L. S.), CHERRY (R.B.), LIPSITZ (P. J.), SMITH (C. A.). — Pulmonary function in the newborn infants; the alveolar-arterial gradient. *J. Appl. Physiol.*, 18, 534, 1963.

[18] NORTHWAY (W. H.), ROSAN (R. C.), PORTER (D. B.). — Pulmonary disease following respiratory therapy. *New Engl. J. Med.*, 276, 357, 1967.

[19] OH (W.), LIND (J.), GESSNER (I. H.). — Circulatory and respiratory adaptation to early and late cord clamping in newborn infants. *Acta Pediatr. Scand.*, 55, 17, 1966.

[20] OH (W.), WALLGEN (C.), HANSON (J. S.), LIND (J.). — The effects of placental transfusion on respiratory mechanics of normal term newborn infants. *Pediatrics*, 40, 7, 1967.

[21] PHELPS (D. L.), LACHMAN (R. S.), LEAKE (R. D.), OH (W.). — The radiologic localization of the major aortic tributaries in the newborn infant. *J. Pediatr.*, 81, 336, 1976.

[22] SINGH (K.), WIGGLESWORTH (F. W.), STERN (L.). — Pneumopericardium in a newborn: a complication of respiratory therapy. *Can. Med. Assoc. J.*, 106, 1195, 1972.

[23] STAHLMAN (M.), MALAN (A. F.), SHEPARD (F.) *et al.* — Negative pressure assisted ventilation in infants with hyaline membrane disease. *J. Pediatr.*, 76, 174, 1970.

[24] STERN (L.). — The use and misuse of oxygen in the newborn infant. In *Pediatric Clinics of North America*, Symposium on Respiratory Disorders in the newborn. GLUCK, L. (ed.), W. B. Saunders Company, 20, 447-464, 1973.

[25] STERN (L.), FLETCHER (B. D.), DUNBAR (J. S.), LEVANT (M. N.), FAWCETT (J. S.). — Pneumothorax and pneumomediastinum associated with renal malformations in newborn infants. *Amer. J. Roentgenol.*, Radium Therapy and Nuclear Medicine, 116, 785, 1972.

[26] THIBEAULT (D. W.), EMMANOUILIDES (G. C.), NELSON (R. J.), LACHMAN (R. S.), ROSENGART (R. M.), OH (W.). — Patent ductus arteriosus complicating the respiratory distress syndrome in preterm infants. *J. Pediatr.*, 86, 120, 1975.

[27] BELL (E. F.), WARBURTON (D.), STONESTREET (B. S.), OH (W.). — Effect of fluid administration on the development of symptomatic patent ductus-arteriosus and congestive heart failure in premature infants. *N. Engl. J. Med.*, 302, 598-604, 1980.

[28] CARSON (B. S.), LOSEY (R. W.), BOWES (W. A., Jr.), SIMMONS (M. A.). — Combined obstetric and pediatric approach to prevent meconium aspiration syndrome. *Am. J. Obst. Gynecol.*, 126, 712-715, 1976.

[29] THIBEAULT (D. W.), HOEBEL (C. J.), KWONG (M.). — Perinatal factors influencing the arterial oxygen tension in preterm infants with RDS while breathing 100 % oxygen. *J. Pediatr.*, 84, 898, 1974.

[30] WILSON (M. G.), MIKITY (V. G.). — A new form of respiratory disease in premature infants. *Am. J. Dis. Child.*, 99, 489, 1960.

20

Neonatal apnea

F. MARCHAL

INTRODUCTION

Recurrent protracted apnea is associated with neurologic sequelae in premature infants [123]. With impending definitive cardiorespiratory arrest, bag and mask resuscitation is sometimes required. When using high FIO_2 hyperoxic episodes may occur increasing the risk of retrolental fibroplasia. In most infants the apnea rate decreases with growth. However, respiratory instability may persist in some thus probably increasing the risk of sudden infant death.

Apnea may occur at any age of life. In normal adults, 10 to 20 second apneas can range from 10 to 20 a night [105]. In normal term infants, the rate of apnea longer than five seconds ranges from 20 to 30 per 100 minutes of sleep [57]. In the fetus, percentage time where breathing movements occur ranges from 55 to 90 [166]. The more premature the baby, the higher the apnea frequency: apnea occurs in 25 % of babies below 2,500 g [39], 30 % below 1,750 g [123], 84 % below 1,000 g [1]. The severity is related to the delay in or absence of spontaneous apnea offset rather than to apnea frequency associated with immaturity. Apnea occurs mainly during sleep. Its duration, type and organization varies with age. Percentage of sleep time is 30 % in adults and 70 % in newborns. There are also qualitative differences. In adults, quiet sleep repre-

sents 85 % of total sleep time and active sleep 15 %. In full term babies, both quiet and active sleep each represent 30 % of total sleep time, 40 % corresponding to a poorly differentiated state called transitional or indeterminate sleep. At 28 weeks gestation quiet sleep is almost absent, active sleep represents 20 to 30 % of sleep time and indeterminate sleep 80 to 70 %. The percentage time of active sleep progressively increases up to 50 % at 34 weeks gestational age [141].

Control of breathing is largely dependent upon the activity state which may account for some mechanisms promoting apnea.

The neonatologist is confronted with three practical problems; prevention and treatment of apnea, identification of neonates at risk for sudden infant death and long term follow up of neurologic development allowing for various forms of treatment.

CLINICAL PRESENTATION

In premature babies below 32 weeks gestation, apnea usually occurs by the end of the first week of life. Apneas longer than 20 seconds are usually associated with cyanosis, hypotonia and bradycardia below 100 beats per minute. Manual stimulation is required and usually brings about respiratory

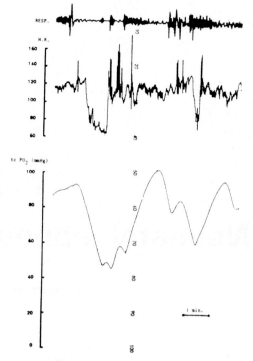

FIG. III-46. — *Central apnea.*

From top to bottom: respiratory impedance (resp.), heart rate (HR), transcutaneous PO_2 (TcPO$_2$).
Apnea is associated with bradycardia and with a drop in TcPO$_2$ from 90 to 45 mmHg. After P. J. MONIN et al.) [128].

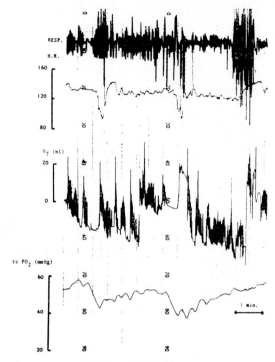

FIG. III-47. — *Obstructive apnea* *(middle part of the recording).*

From top to bottom: respiratory impedance (resp.), heart rate (HR), tidal volume (VT), transcutaneous PO_2 (tcPO$_2$).
Ventilatory arrest with ongoing thoracic movements, bradycardia and a drop of tcPO$_2$ from 50 to 40 mmHg. Note a mixed apnea at the left part of the recording: obstruction following central apnea. After P. J. MONIN et al. [128].

recovery. The infant may be placed on an apnea and heart rate monitor. The respiratory signal is usually recorded through thoracic impedance electrodes. Central or diaphragmatic apnea is related to primary cessation of diaphragmatic movements. Figure III-46 illustrates this type of apnea and its effects on heart rate and transcutaneous PO_2. When ventilatory arrest is secondary to upper airway obstruction no apnea is detectable on the thoracic impedance signal and bradycardia may occur. Figure III-47 shows a typical obstructive apnea on the middle part of the recording. Ventilation has ceased although thoracic movements are still present. There is a concomittent drop in heart rate and transcutaneous PO_2. Mixed apnea is a combination of diaphragmatic and obstructive apnea. Periodic breathing consists of regular alternance of short apnea (usually less than 10 seconds duration) with breathing movements (Fig. III-48).

Apnea of prematurity may be secondary to various underlying diseases such as sepsis, meningitis, intracranial hemorrhage, hypoglycemia and abnor-

mal temperature control. Frequently no aetiology is to be found. However, there are many physiologic and pathophysiologic factors whose association may determine apnea.

PATHOGENESIS

DIAPHRAGMATIC APNEA

Fetal breathing movements

In the human fetus, intermittent breathing movements may be detected as early as eleven weeks of gestation. However they become continuous only near term. They are irregular with a frequency of 30 to 70 breaths per minute. In the sheep fetus,

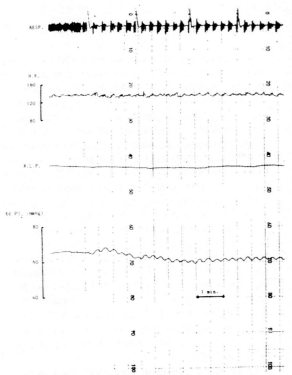

FIG. III-48. — *Periodic breathing*. From top to bottom: respiratory impedance (resp.), heart rate (HR), relative blood flow (RLP), transcutaneous PO₂ (tcPO₂). Note the absence of bradycardia and sinusoidal variations in tcPO₂. After P. J. MONIN et al. [128].

they occur during periods of electroencephalographic desynchronisation and rapid eye movement. This state corresponds to active sleep in newborns and adults. Large movements called gasps occur at a frequency of 1 to 4 per minute during 5 % of the time. With maturation, the duration of periods of thoracic inactivity decreases and a cycle appears with an increase in periods of breathing movements during daytime. These variations are detectable by 80 days (mid-gestation) in the sheep fetus. Breathing movements vary according to maternal glycemia. Maternal hypoglycemia is associated with a decrease in breathing movements [166]. Maternal smoking is also responsible for a decrease in fetal breathing movements. This effect is thought to be related to nicotine rather than to an increased carboxyhemoglobin level [60, 115].

Fetal breathing movements play an important role in fetal lung maturation [108, 109]. However, little is known about their initiating mechanisms. The fetal chemoreceptor function has extensively

been reviewed by Purves [150]. Aortic chemoreceptor activity may be recorded in utero [148] and its stimulation by hypoxemia results in cardiac output redistribution toward the placenta [44, 45, 154, 164]. In contrast carotid chemoreceptors are silent and insensitive to hypoxemia [14] which leads to cessation of breathing movements in the immature fetus [16]. In the near term fetus, carotid chemoreceptor activity may occasionally be recorded [87] and asphyxia promotes gasping [16 b]. These gasps still occur in the carotid body denervated fetus [201]. Experimental umbilical artery occlusion or uterine contraction promoting mild hypoxemia during active sleep, induces cessation of breathing activity associated with the onset of quiet sleep [74]. From a teleologic point of view this change in activity state appears to be an appropriate response since, in the newborn, oxygen consumption is lower in quiet sleep than in active sleep [179].

It is likely that central chemoreceptors do not play an important role in the onset of fetal breathing. Although fetal breathing increases during hypercapnia [16], this activity is not modified by acidic cerebrospinal fluid application on the ventral surface of the medulla [80].

Stretch receptor activity may be recorded in the fetus in utero [148]. However respiratory center activity is not modified by bilateral cervical vagotomy [35, 46]. Central mechanisms inhibiting respiration have been shown in adult animals. Stimulation of the amygdaloid area abolishes the respiratory center response to alteration of blood gases and pH [151]. In newborn piglets, central respiratory inhibition has been advocated as explaining the prolonged apnea following electrical stimulation of the superior laryngeal nerve [105 b]. Recent experiments of mid brain transection in fetal lambs suggest that chemoreceptor activity is suppressed by a central inhibitory pathway [47].

Prostaglandins may play a role in the regulation of fetal breathing. Prostaglandin injection into fetal lambs causes a reduction of fetal breathing [97] and injection of prostaglandin synthesis inhibitors increases fetal breathing movements and promotes their apparance during quiet sleep [96].

Prolonged periods of fetal apnea are thus probably related to a number of mechanisms: "immaturity" of respiratory centers, insensitivity of peripheral chemoreceptors, central inhibition of vagal afferents and perhaps of the respiratory centers themselves. Furthermore, fetal breathing occurs during active sleep which is associated in adults with a relative loss of metabolic drive [145]. Thus fetal breathing movements appear to depend on behavioral rather than on metabolic factors.

Respiratory depression with hypoxemia

It may be surprising that continuous respiratory movements may appear after birth in a 28 week fetus formerly apneic for about 50 % of the time of its intrauterine life. Indeed, breathing movements are of trivial consequence for gas exchange in utero and become of the utmost importance after birth. Carotid body activity appears soon after birth [87] and undergoes functional maturation during the first days of life in lambs [12, 29]. However, its importance in the onset of respiration at birth is variously appreciated [75, 149, 201]. In adult cats, carotid body stimulation has a facilitatory effect on respiration which may last for hours beyond the stimulation period [124] and may play a role in the neonate in the maintenance of continuous breathing movements beyond the first inspiration. A progressive increase in the respiratory response to hypoxemia occurs during the first days of life in term neonates [23] and during the first weeks for preterm babies [157]. This response is intermediary between that of the fetus and of the adult; an initial hyperventilation is followed by hypoventilation. The latter part of the response seems to be related to a central depressant effect of hypoxemia overwhelming the carotid body stimulus [158]. Dopamine and noradrenaline carotid body concentration increases with gestational age in the fetus [150] and this may explain their functionnal immaturity in prematures.

The respiratory response to hypercapnea increases with gestational and postnatal age in prematures [17]. By about 4 weeks postnatal age, the response is identical to that of the adult [159]. The decreased ventilatory response to CO_2 may be related either to immature central drive or to high total lung resistances. Indeed, during hypercapneic challenge tests premature neonates may increase the work of breathing with little change in ventilation [103]. Oxygen concentration in the inspired gas affects the response to CO_2 tremendously: the lower the FIO_2, the less the response [159]. These findings have important clinical implications. Firstly, during apnea, asphyxia may depress respiratory center activity thus increasing apnea duration. Secondly, any situation resulting in alveolar hypoventilation will be associated with an increased incidence of apnea. Such situations frequently occur in low birth weight babies with high chest wall compliance [56], low functional residual capacity [188] and a relatively high closing volume [133].

Vagal pulmonary inputs

Sighing reflects Head's paradoxical reflex and plays an important role in the maintenance of lung volume in the neonate [186]. Sigh frequency increases during experimental hypoxia [10]. Hypoxia has a facilitatory effect on the discharge of irritant receptors, probably related to stimulation of peripheral chemoreceptors [63]. Sighs are responsible for the recruitment of atelectatic alveolar units and for the reopening of terminal airways [122], thereby increasing lung compliance and oxygen stores. The increased expiratory pause following a sigh has therefore a distinctly different significance from that of apnea occuring during alveolar hypoventilation. The increased expiratory period is related to stretch receptors whose tonic activity regulates expiratory time [119, 172] and whose phasic activity regulates inspiratory time [137, 172, 192]. In other words, a decrease in lung volume increases inspiratory duration and an increase in functionnal residual capacity increases expiratory duration. The magnitude of Hering-Breuer's reflex seems to decrease with gestational age [95].

In adults, chemical or mecanical stimulation of irritant receptors promotes cough, increases respiratory rate and decreases tidal volume. In premature babies below 35 weeks gestation it frequently induces apnea [55]. The signal is transmitted through myelinated fibers and it is possible that a lack of myelinization related to immaturity is responsible for distortion of the transmitted signal leading to erroneous responses [27]. Likewise other irritant receptor reflexes, such as increased inspiratory effort related to decreased lung volume in adults might induce an abnormal response leading to apnea in premature babies.

J receptor stimulation induces apnea and bradycardia in adult animals [139] but their role in the pathogenesis of apnea associated with patent ductus arteriosus has not been established.

The intercostal inspiratory inhibitory reflex

A high chest wall compliance is responsible for paradoxical breathing with inspiratory inward motion of the lower part of the thorax called chest distortion which increases with decreasing gestational age [43] and which may induce stimulation of intercostal muscle gamma afferents leading to the inhibition of phrenic discharge [98]. The decreased apnea frequency observed with positive airway pressure [91] may be explained through chest wall stabilization and suppression of this intercostal reflex.

Upper airway receptors

Different reflex apneas may originate from chemical or mechanical stimulation of upper airway receptors. Such reflexes are particularly powerful in the neonate. For instance pharyngeal mechanoreceptor stimulation may result from pharyngeal suction or orogastric feeding [36, 136]. Small amounts of gastric content regurgitation lead to upper airway obstruction and also to reflex apnea related to stimulation of laryngeal chemoreceptors. In newborn animals such stimulation leads to profound apnea [51, 88, 101, 113, 116, 183].

Similarly, reflex apnea may result from the stimulation of thermoreceptors located in the trigeminal area. Such apnea may result from cold oxygen blown over the face [25].

Sleep state influences

Irregular breathing [18, 54] with frequent pauses [65, 84] represents a characteristic manifestation of active sleep as well as rapid eye movements [72, 145]. Metabolic drive plays a trivial role during this sleep state. Indeed, in animals, irregularity of breathing movements is not influenced by hypercapnea [144], metabolic alkalosis [180], hypoxia [147], pulmonary inflation [143] or vagotomy [46, 143]. This breathing pattern may be regarded as a caricature of phasic wakefulness where cortical influences adapt breathing to activity such as phonation or swallowing, involving laryngeal reflexes which may also be triggered during active sleep [116, 181]. The pattern of the ventilatory response to hypercapnea and hypoxia during active sleep is still controversial in animal or human newborns. They have been reported to be decreased [26, 78, 161] or identical [43, 52, 78] compared to quiet sleep. The lack of reproducibility of these responses during active sleep is not surprising. Indeed, there is a high variability of tidal volume; and chest distortion may vary according to maturation [43] or animal species [78]. Identification of sleep states is difficult in immature babies and active sleep may correspond to different types of paradoxical sleep; tonic and phasic [145]. An important aspect of the neonatal response to respiratory stimuli during active sleep consists of the arousal reaction which has unfortunately frequently been overlooked.

In animals the arousal reaction to stimuli such as hypercapnea [144], hypoxia [147], bronchopulmonary [182] and laryngeal stimulation [181] and airway occlusion [77] is regularly depressed compared to quiet sleep.

Finally there are important modifications of chest and lung mechanics during active sleep. Intercostal muscle hypotonia and loss of laryngeal expiratory adduction [73] lead to a decreased lung volume and oxygen stores [79]. Despite an usual increase in minute ventilation [18, 54, 72] there is a fall in PaO_2 [24] and chest wall distortion [38] may trigger the intercostal inspiratory inhibitory reflex [98]. However, the protective effect of active sleep during chronic hypoxemia has been demonstrated. In kittens, after several days of hypoxemia, apnea occuring during quiet sleep disappears with the onset of active sleep [9].

It is possible that these modifications of lung mechanics may have consequences during the following quiet sleep period, when the respiratory drive "specific" for active sleep is suppressed. Indeed, during quiet sleep, the appropriate transmission and integration of various mechanical and chemical, peripheral or central stimuli is of the utmost importance for the maintenance of gas exchange.

In the overall there are many mechanisms leading to diaphragmatic apnea in premature babies, whether of reflex origin with the possibility of abnormal transmitted signals promoting an erroneous response, or resulting from instability or immaturity of metabolic drive during transitional or quiet sleep or related to the "mandatory" irregular breathing of active sleep.

PERIODIC BREATHING

The definition of periodic breathing unfortunately differs with authors. It may be defined as the regular repetition of breathing pauses of less than 10 seconds duration alternating with breathing movements of regularly increasing and then decreasing amplitude for 10 to 15 seconds. During such episodes, there is no bradycardia or cyanosis. The incidence of periodic breathing is inversely related to gestational age, and may be seen in 95 % of prematures below 1,500 g [53]. Its significance is differently appreciated. For some authors it is a common phenomenon related to respiratory immaturity [53] for others, it is related to hypoxic respiratory depression [155]. Indeed periodic breathing can be induced by administration of a hypoxic gas mixture [156] and suppressed by administration of an oxygen [53] or gas mixture containing 2 to 4 % CO_2 [53, 160]. It may occur during active sleep [57, 84], quiet sleep particularly in full term newborns [196] and also during transitional sleep [57, 84]. It is tempting to compare the latter to stages I and II of sleep in adults which are a transition between quiet wakefulness and deep quiet sleep and during which periodic breathing may normally occur [28].

Under normoxic conditions, $PaCO_2$ is the main metabolic stimulus. Drowsiness is characterized by a succession of light sleep and periods of wakefulness. With the onset of sleep, there is a progressive withdrawal of reticular substance activity and an increase in $PaCO_2$ set point with subsequent hypoventilation. With sudden awakening, the sleep $PaCO_2$ set point becomes an error signal promoting hyperventilation. The greater the difference between sleep and waking ventilatory level or in other words the more unstable the $PaCO_2$ set point during drowsiness, the more important the periodic breathing [28, 156].

During hypoxemia, such as that resulting from acclimatation to high altitude in adults, PaO_2 becomes the main metabolic stimulus. During drowsiness when ventilation decreases, PaO_2 decreases and becomes an error signal on awakening. Such a stimulus is suppressed with oxygen administration as is periodic breathing [145].

It is likely that in premature babies both mechanisms play a role during transitional sleep which probably corresponds to different levels of reticular activating substance tone resulting in an instability of $PaCO_2$ and PaO_2 set points respectively during normoxemia and hypoxemia. Indeed, different mechanisms may lead to periodic breathing since both hyper [33, 53] and hypoventilation [155] have been reported during such breathing patterns.

MIXED AND OBSTRUCTIVE APNEA

With thoracic impedance monitors obstructive apneas are frequently overlooked [197] although they commonly occur in prematures [67, 126].

The newborn is an obligate nose breather [37, 185] and is therefore vulnerable to obstruction of this part of the airway. Such an obstruction may result from secretions produced by the inflamed nasopharyngeal mucosa, occuring frequently after prolonged nasotracheal intubation.

A recent study has shown that most obstructive apnea of premature babies occurs at the oropharyngeal level [121] in a similar fashion as in adults [76,

152]. Hyperflexion of the head on the chest is an important mechanism promoting obstruction through backward motion of the tongue [171, 187, 200] and folding of the highly compliant cervical trachea. It is important to bear in mind that the phasic activity of pharyngeal muscles during breathing is, like diaphragmatic activity, dependant upon metabolic drive. During a hypoxic or hypercapneic challenge test there is a progressive decrease in upper airway resistance concomittent with the increase in diaphragmatic activity [142]. When metabolic drive is unstable during quiet or transitional sleep, a modification of pharyngeal muscle phasic activity may occur resulting in airway obstruction. In fact, adults with obstructive sleep apnea may also present an impaired ventilatory response to hypoxemia [203]. During active sleep, pharyngeal muscle tone is suppressed and obstruction may result from either passive reduction of airway calibre or active contraction of pharyngeal or laryngeal muscles occuring analogous to rapid eye movements. Therefore, it is clear that many obstructive apneas are of central origin.

Mixed apnea may correspond to two combinations of diaphragmatic and obstructive apnea. With primary obstruction, during which oxygen content decreases more rapidly than during central apnea [90], probably because of ongoing breathing movements and higher oxygen consumption, the resulting asphyxia is responsible for ventilatory depression and cessation of diaphragmatic activity. A reflex mechanism has also been advocated. In prematures below 31 weeks gestation apnea may result from upper airway occlusion [135]. During central apnea, cessation of pharyngeal muscle activity may lead to pharyngeal occlusion. In adult dogs, the thresholds of the response to hypercapnia and hypoxemia of the hypoglossal and recurrent laryngeal nerves are respectively higher (CO_2) and lower (O_2) than the phrenic's [199]. This could explain the dissociation between the reoccurrence of diaphragmatic movements and the disappearance of pharyngeal obstruction.

APNEA OFFSET

The main factor in delaying the turning off of apnea is related to the ventilatory depressant effect of hypoxemia. On the one hand, premature babies present no sign of struggle or arousal reaction during apnea. However, it is well demonstrated in adult animals that hypoxemia is a potent stimulant of the reticular activating substance, this effect being potentiated by hypercapnea [86]. With the reoccurrence of wakefulness, there is an increase in metabolic drive [146]. The study of events occurring at the offset of apnea in adults [105] and infants [69] has shown the regular occurrence of an arousal reaction. In premature babies most apnea can be turned off by gentle manual stimulation which induces reoccurrence of breathing movements and behavioral modifications reflecting arousal.

When pharyngeal occlusions occurs, the more potent the inspiratory effort, the more negative the pressure below the obstructed airway, thus tending to perpetrate pharyngeal collapse rather than to restablish ventilation. The mechanism indispensable for the disappearance of pharyngeal obstruction and the reappearance of efficient ventilation is the return of pharyngeal muscle tone related to awakening [153].

Premature babies in intensive care units are submitted to frequent stimuli leading to perturbation of an already poorly organized sleep. In adult animals, sleep fragmentation alters arousal metabolic thresholds to hypoxemia and hypercapnia [22]. Furthermore, in humans, sleep deprivation decreases the respiratory sensitivity to hypercapnea [34].

HEMODYNAMIC ADAPTATION
DURING APNEA

Bradycardia occurs frequently during apnea and results in a drop in cardiac output while an increase in systemic vascular resistance is responsible for maintenance or increase in arterial blood pressure [62, 178].

In newborn lambs, similar circulatory changes occur during apnea resulting from laryngeal chemoreflex stimulation, reflecting cardiac output redistribution toward the heart, brain and adrenals [66], in a similar fashion to the hemodynamic adaptation occurring in diving mammals [3, 82] and in the hypoxemic fetus [164] and neonate [176]. When stretch receptor activity is minimal with cessation of breathing movements usually occurring at end expiration [39, 133], the inflation reflex, promoting tachycardia and vasodilation, is abolished and replaced by a reflex vasoconstriction resulting from partial lung collapse [41] related to the decreased functional residual capacity during apnea [188]. Arterial chemoreceptor stimulation by hypoxemia and hypercapnea results in bradycardia and enhances vasoconstriction [5, 40]. The latter is related to an increase in sympathetic tone from vasomotor center

stimulation and is suppressed by α blockade; the increased parasympathetic tone accounts for bradycardia which is suppressed by atropine [66]. This reflex protecting high oxygen consumption areas might be inefficient in prematures: with prolonged apnea, systemic hypertension is replaced by hypotension [62]. This may be related to sympathetic system immaturity. Indeed, in fetal rabbits, catecholamine tissue concentration increases with gestational age and during the early neonatal period [138]. Furthermore, in apneic premature infants, there is a decreased urinary excretion of catecholamines [92].

During asphyxia, there is a loss of cerebral blood flow autoregulation [111, 112]. Arterial blood pressure plays a determinant role in the maintenance of cerebral oxygenation. The increase in cerebral perfusion with systemic hypertension compensates for the decreased arterial blood oxygen content. However, such sudden increases in cerebral perfusion pressure may induce an increase in periventricular capillary transmural pressure resulting in haemorrhage, while hemodynamic non-adaptation to apnea i. e. systemic hypotension, promotes cerebral ischemia leading to leucomalacia [140].

Finally, cardiac output redistribution away from mesenteric vessels is responsible for intestinal ischemia, a determining factor in necrotizing enterocolitis [191]. Indeed, recurrent apneas are particularly frequent in babies presenting with necrotizing enterocolitis [184].

In summary, bradycardia which is frequently thought to result from cardiorespiratory failure, reflects an adaptation to gas exchange alterations providing a temporary adaptation of arterial blood pressure and allowing for the maintenance of cerebral oxygenation at the cost of increased cerebral perfusion pressure and decreased systemic blood flow.

QUANTITATIVE ASPECTS

There is a little agreement in the literature as regards the incidence of apnea in the neonatal period according to activity states. This may be related to large interindividual variations, to different criteria defining both apnea and sleep states, to different methods of recording physiologic parameters and to the relatively small number of infants in each study.

The premature baby

Frequency of apnea longer than two seconds is higher during active than during quiet sleep, but its mean duration is similar [124]. For a given recording period, the apnea index is defined as the sum of all apnea durations divided by the corresponding sleep time and multiplied by 100. Index of apnea longer than 3 seconds is higher during active sleep at any gestational age [167]. A longitudinal study shows that in a given infant the frequency of apnea equal to or longer than 10 seconds may be higher during quiet than during active sleep and vice versa at different postnatal ages. However, the incidence of apnea equal to or longer than 10 seconds is higher during quiet sleep than active sleep between 30 and 33 weeks gestation (Table I).

TABLE I. — MAXIMAL VALUE OF FREQUENCY OF APNEA $\geqslant$ 10 s PER 100 MINUTES IN 24 PREMATURE BABIES STUDIED AT VARIOUS POST-CONCEPTIONAL AGES AND IN 4 TERM NEONATES (Recording duration: 90 minutes) (after A. N. KRAUSS et al. [104]).

N	G. A.	C. A.	Q. S.	A. S.	T. S.	W
8	26, 28	26-29	57	83	108	13
		30-33	23	13	20	17
		36	0	0	0	0
16	30, 32, 33	30-33	50	36	55	0
		34-37	43	13	40	0
		38	0	0	0	0
4	34, 35	34-37	8	9	0	0
		41	0	0	0	0
4	39, 40	39-40	0	10	0	0

G. A.: gestational age; C. A.: conceptional age; Q. S.: quiet sleep; A. S.: active sleep; T. S.: transitional sleep; W: wakefulness; N: number of infants.

In 11 prematures below 2,000 g studied between 3 and 9 weeks of age, 68 % of apnea 10 seconds or longer occurred during quiet or transitional sleep, the longer apneas always occurring during quiet sleep. In 4 infants weighing between 2,400 and 3,500 g and studied between 6 and 14 weeks of age, 54 % of 130, 3 to 9 second apneas occurred during active sleep while 61 % of 18 apneas equal to or longer than 10 seconds occurred during quiet or transitional sleep, 2/3 being central and 1/3 obstructive or mixed [67]. These data are consistent with Deuel's in an infant population of more heterogeneous age where 80 % of apnea occurring during active sleep lasts 2 to 5 seconds and 54 % of apnea occuring during quiet sleep lasts 5 to 20 seconds [48].

On the other hand, in Gabriel's study, apneas were more frequent and also lasted longer in active sleep than in quiet or transitional sleep in 8 prematures between 28 and 34 weeks gestation, studied on several occasions between 31 and 35 weeks postconception [59].

Term neonates

The index of apnea equal to or longer than 2 seconds is higher during active than during quiet [57, 65] or transitional sleep [65]. Mean values range from 0.7 during quiet sleep to 5.9 during active sleep [65], with an extreme upper value of 25 [57].

The frequency of respiratory pauses (less than 5 seconds) (Table II a) and of apnea 6 to 9 seconds duration (Table II b) is high particularly during active sleep.

The frequency of apnea equal to or longer than 5 or 6 seconds is not significantly different among sleep states (Table II c) nor is the frequency of apnea equal to or longer than 10 seconds. The latter are infrequent whatever the sleep state, from 0.4 per 100 minutes of transitional sleep [65] (one apnea every four hours), to 8 per 100 minutes of active sleep [85] (one apnea every 15 minutes). The high incidence of apnea in Hoppenbrouwer's study [85] may be related to the duration of recording [85] and to the apnea detecting method [57] (Table II d).

Apneas equal to or longer than 15 seconds are exceptional. None is reported in Thoman's [190], Hoppenbrouwer's [85], Stein's [173] or Flores Guevarra's [57] studies. In Gould's [65] there is no apnea longer than 20 seconds. In a former study [84], Hoppenbrouwers reported 4 apneas longer than 20 seconds of the 640 recorded (0.6 %).

It appears that the high apnea index during active sleep is related to the high incidence of short respiratory pauses, while prolonged apnea is scarce as during quiet sleep. Occurrence of apnea shorter than 10 or 15 seconds seems to reflect a physiologic phenomenon in the newborn.

Mixed and obstructive apneas are scarce usually occurring during active sleep [57].

Percentage time of periodic breathing is highly variable in full term neonates. Waite showed that in infants studied at 2 days of age, periodic apneas are not found and by 2 weeks of age their frequencies are similar during quiet and active sleep ranging from 2 to 4 per hour of sleep [196]. Similarly, Flores Guevarra showed that during the first week of life, the percentage time of periodic breathing is similar during quiet, active and transitional sleep, 3.6,

TABLE II. — FREQUENCY OF APNEAS PER 100 MINUTES OF SLEEP IN TERM NEONATES [57, 84, 85] AND PREMATURES AT 40 WEEKS POST-CONCEPTION [65]

Apnea duration	Author	N	Q.S. $\bar{x}$	Q.S. S.D.	Q.S. range	A.S. $\bar{x}$	A.S. S.D.	A.S. range	T.S. $\bar{x}$	T.S. S.D.	T.S. range
a < 5 s	Flores-Guevarra [57]	16	23	27	0-100	60	46	0-148	40	33	0-104
	Hoppenbrouwers * [85]	25	100	—	—	200	—	—	140	—	—
	Gould [65]	26	7.3	6.7	—	76.5	48.6	—	55.1	30.2	—
b 5-9 s	Hoppenbrouwers * [85]	25	15	—	—	25	—	—	15	—	—
	Gould [65]	26	4.2	5.1	—	22.7	22.0	—	18.8	10.6	—
c ≥ 5 s	Flores-Guevarra [57]	16	20	25	0-172	30	46	0-148	30	49	0-189
≥ 6 s	Flores-Guevarra [57]	16	15	35	0-134	19	33	0-113	21	44	0-178
	Hoppenbrouwers * [84]	9	2.8	2.5	0-6.2	12.4	11.5	2.8-40.8	8.5	5.5	2.9-16.7
d ≥10 s	Flores-Guevarra [57]	16	1.1	2	0-7	0.8	1.7	0-5.7	0.5	1.8	0-7
	Hoppenbrouwers * [85]	25	4	—	—	8	—	—	5	—	—
	Gould [65]	26	0.4	1.2	—	0.9	2.3	—	1.5	2.2	—

N: number of infants; Q.S.: quiet sleep; A.S.: active sleep; T.S.: transitional sleep; $\bar{x}$: mean; S.D.: standard deviation.
* 12 hours recording.

4.8 and 2.6 % respectively with a range of 0 to 53 %; and that this percentage increases during the 2nd week particularly during active sleep [57].

Studies have been made on neonates of 38 to 42 weeks gestation. Flores-Guevarra's study shows that the apnea index and frequency are always higher in 38-39 week than in 40 to 42 week neonates and so is periodic breathing [57]. This factor probably accounts for the variation in apnea index and frequency from one study to another where the precise gestational age of each baby is not always reported.

Duration and time of recording may also influence apnea parameters. The longer the recording period, the higher the incidence of apnea. 24 hour recordings show that there frequently is a clustering of apneas during the second part of the night [175]. This is in agreement with Guilleminault's study in infants [69]. Finally, the infant's position during the recording session does not seem to influence apnea frequency [57].

In summary, a normal sleeping full term infant beyond 38 weeks gestation may present during the first week of life one to two pauses shorter than 5 seconds per minute, 9 to 15 apneas of 6 to 9 seconds duration per hour or 1 to 19 apneas equal to or longer than 10 seconds every 4 hours, but no apnea longer than 15 seconds. Obstructive apneas are scarce, less than 3 per 12 hours. Percentage of periodic breathing is highly variable, up to 50 % sleep time.

With growth, apnea frequency decreases and apnea equal to or longer than 10 seconds is practically nonexistent at one month.

ETIOLOGY

Various pathological conditions must be considered in babies presenting apneic episodes.

SEPSIS

Neonatal infection should always be considered particularly when apnea occurs during the first hours of life. After the 2nd week, apnea may also be secondary to nosocomial infection in low birth weight babies in intensive care units. When abdominal symptoms such as bowel distension are present, necrotizing enterocolitis should be considered.

Central nervous system disorders

Apnea may be the only expression of neonatal seizures. Electroencephalography may be necessary for the diagnosis. Intracranial haemorrhage should be considered in prematures below 1,500 g with perinatal asphyxia or severe respiratory distress and cerebral echography should be performed. When apnea is associated with other neurologic abnormalities and clinical or biological signs of infection, meningitis should be considered and a lumbar puncture performed.

Perinatal asphyxia may induce respiratory depression whether or not organic cerebral lesions are present. In such circumstances, the Apgar score is usually below 6 and apnea may occur during the first hours of life.

Respiratory depression may also result from transplacental transfer of drugs administered to the mother during labor such as anaesthetic agents or narcotics.

Cardiorespiratory causes

Neonatal respiratory distress may cause apnea resulting from a number of mechanisms: respiratory depression with hypoxemia, decreased lung compliance and increased chest distorsion and the incapacity of the premature infant to compensate by an increase in the work of breathing.

By the 3rd or 4th day of life, apnea may reflect the occurrence of a large left to right ductal shunt.

Some hemodynamic situations may lead to decreased cerebral oxygenation even though arterial PO_2 is normal. For example, in hypotensive babies with asphyxia or respiratory distress, the decreased cerebral blood flow may promote respiratory depression. Such depressant effects may also be related to the decreased oxygen content of arterial blood due to anemia [93]. Furthermore, anemia may be associated with metabolic acidosis which induces respiratory depression in newborn lambs [30].

Infants born to β blocker treated hypertensive mothers may present with apnea during the first days of life [21].

Other causes of apnea

Hypo- or hyperthermia is frequently associated with apnea. Furthermore, even though the rectal temperature is normal, an elevated environmental temperature may induce apnea [39].

Metabolic causes such as hypoglycemia, hypocalcemia or hyponatremia are managed by appropriate intravenous infusions.

When apnea occurs in the neonate, an underlying disease must be ruled out. The history should be examined for maternal drug administration and for signs of neonatal infection such as maternal fever,

prolonged rupture of membranes and fetal distress. One should measure rectal and environmental temperature of the baby and inquire for the possible association of apnea with nursing manœuvres such as gastric feeding or pharyngeal suction. On physical examination, one should look for respiratory distress symptoms, decreased blood pressure, ensure the patency of upper airways and look for abnormal muscle tone or abnormal movements indicative of a central nervous system disorder. The abdomen should be examined for bowel distention, hepato- or splenomegaly suggesting sepsis.

Blood samples should be taken for measurement of arterial blood gases and pH, glycemia, calcemia, hematocrit, white blood cell count and for blood culture. Spinal tap should be considered according to the clinical presentation. In low birth weight babies or in babies with perinatal asphyxia the work up should be completed by cerebral ultrasound examination and sometimes with an electroencephalogram.

MANAGEMENT

Symptomatic treatment may be instituted when possible underlying disease requiring specific treatment has been ruled out.

Monitoring

Careful clinical monitoring is required for all sick neonates. Infants weighting less than 1,800 g at birth should ideally be placed on an apnea and heart monitor for the first two weeks of life. Such monitoring is mandatory when an infant has shown an episode of prolonged apnea. The respiration alarm delay is usually set at 20 seconds and the heart rate alarm at 100 beats per minute. When the alarm sounds, the infant should be looked at before the monitor. One should look for cutaneous coloration and evidence of breathing movements. If the infant stops breathing with pallor or cyanosis, cutaneous stimulation is required and usually effective. With prolonged apnea, bag mask ventilation using the same FIO_2 received by the patient should be started and rapid pharyngeal suction should be performed to ensure upper airway patency. Prematures presenting several apnea attacks per 24 hours should also be placed on a transcutaneous PO_2 monitor for prolonged periods of time in order to determine the gravity of the apnea and to avoid hyperoxic episodes during resuscitation manœuvres.

Care of the infant

Careful nursing is mandatory in preventing apnea and reducing apnea frequency.

Infant's position. — With hypotonic neck muscles, hyperflexion of the neck can easily occur and should be prevented. Whenever possible, particularly when moderate respiratory distress related to bronchopulmonary dysplasia is present, the infant should be nursed in the prone position which is associated with better oxygenation [50, 120, 194] and lung compliance [194], shorter gastric emptying time [83, 202] and a decreased incidence of regurgitation [15] and gastric content aspiration [81].

Thermal environment. — The thermal environment should be set, to obtain a central temperature between 36.5 and 37° C, in the lower zone of thermal comfort.

Nursing manœuvers. — The duration and rate of pharyngeal suction should be minimal. During gavage, the orogastric tube should be carefully placed and sudden gastric distension should be avoided. Continuous gastric feeding should be considered when apnea occurs regularly with gavage.

Air and oxygen administered via a head box should be warmed to incubator temperature.

Cardiorespiratory monitoring. — Frequent measurement of blood gases is required although a single PaO_2 value obtained after arterial puncture is of little interest whenever the baby has been struggling or crying during the sampling procedure. Prolonged transcutaneous PO_2 monitoring gives a better evaluation of oxygenation. In apneic neonates, PO_2 should be maintained between 65 and 75 mm Hg although there is little data showing that these values are safe as regards the risk of retrolental fibroplasia, particularly in infants of less than 28 weeks gestation.

Arterial blood pressure should be measured frequently and hypotension with oliguria below 2 ml/kg/h should be treated according to cause: dehydration, hypovolemia, cardiac failure or anemia. Hematocrit should be maintained above 45 %.

Treatment

When despite the above mentioned precautions the infant continues to present more than 3 apneas longer than 20 seconds per day [89], symptomatic therapy should be started.

Stimulation. — It is assumed that prematures have a decreased number of afferent signals toward respiratory centers. This can be compensated for by increasing the number of external stimuli. Cutaneous stimulation decreases apnea frequency [91]. Placing the infant on a water or rocking bed results in labyrinthine stimulation and is an effective method of reducing apnea frequency [99, 193].

Continuous positive airway pressure. — The effectiveness of continuous positive airway pressure (CPAP) in preventing apnea [91] is related to different mechanisms: increased PaO_2 with increased lung volume and lung compliance and decreased venous admixture [189] and work of breathing; as well as the elimination of the intercostal inspiratory inhibitory reflex. Nasal or pharyngeal CPAP may be effective even in infants with a normal PO_2 [118] and is always worth a trial. Its disadvantages are related to abdominal distension and feeding difficulties and to irritation of the nose.

Respiratory stimulants.

METHYLXANTHINES.

Pharmacodynamic effects. — Methylxanthines (theophylline and caffeine) are effective in treating apnea of prematurity [6, 11, 166]. They promote stimulation of metabolic drive with a decreased threshold [61] and increased sensitivity to CO_2 [7, 42]. Other effects may contribute to the reduction of apnea. Increased skeletal muscle tone and contraction [7] and decreased diaphragmatic fatigue [110]. At a dose of 2 mg/kg/d, theophylline decreases apnea frequency without altering CO_2 sensitivity [130]. This effect may be related to an alteration of sleep organization [49, 100]. The bronchodilatory effect of theophylline in prematures has not been established.

The inhibitory effect of methylxanthines on phosphodiesterase, increasing cyclic AMP explains their action on a number of systems. The increased CAMP in the medullary respiratory centers may be responsible for an increase in neurotransmitters [93]. They also induce smooth muscle relaxation and systemic vasodilatation; and influence metabolic homeostasis, increasing blood glucose [106, 109], the basal metabolic rate and oxygen consumption [61, 127].

Methylxanthines may alter cerebral blood flow, although there are conflicting reports in the litterature: cerebral vasoconstriction [162, 198], vasodilation [64] and no significant changes in cerebral blood flow [177] have all been reported. These apparent contradictions may be explained by the presence or absence of hypocapneic alkalosis and by different mechanisms of action related to different dosages. In vitro, millimolar concentrations of theophylline increase the diameter of pial arteries, this effect is thought to be related to an increased CAMP concentration. However, at micromolar concentrations, there is an inhibition of the vaso-dilatory effect of adenosine [195] which is an important local regulating factor in the cerebral circulation. Therefore, it is possible that under normal conditions of oxygenation theophylline may not affect cerebral blood flow, but during cerebral hypoxia the reactive increase in local perfusion promoted by adenosine tissue release [163] could be blocked by theophylline. Respiratory alkalosis induces cerebral vasoconstriction and in newborn piglets cerebral blood flow is not modified by theophylline when $PaCO_2$ is kept normal [177]; however cerebral tissue acidosis may occur during hyperventilation in theophylline treated piglets [117].

Persistant apnea in theophylline treated babies may have more severe consequences in the face of the possible loss of hemodynamic adaptation of the brain to asphyxia. Other secondary effects may be observed: sinus tachycardia, vomiting, hyperexcitability or seizures and polyuria. Experimental data show that theophylline may also alter neuronal growth [2, 107]. However, follow-up studies show that the development of prematures treated with caffeine or theophylline is not different from population controls [70, 134] up to three years of age.

Indications for methylxanthine therapy should be carefully examined because of the lack of knowledge of its long term effects. Their use should be controlled with pharmacokinetic monitoring.

PRACTICAL UTILIZATION. — A number of pharmacokinetic studies have determined their therapeutic modality.

In newborns, theophylline half-life is longer than in adults, ranging from 12 to 57 hours [7]. Therapeutic levels range from 6 to 13 mg/l and are usually obtained after a loading intravenous dose of 6 mg/kg followed by a maintenance dose of 2 mg/kg every 12 hours. Plasma concentrations should be measured after 2 or 3 days of treatment, before drug administration to determine the trough level. Plasma clearance increases with postnatal age and dosage should be appropriately adapted. A special metabolic pathway of interconversion of theophylline to caffeine has been shown in premature infants. Therefore, caffeine levels should also be monitored

during theophylline treatment although the portion of the pharmacodynamic effect attributable to caffeine is difficult to evaluate [8, 19, 20].

Caffeine half-life is longer than theophylline, ranging from 70 to 150 hours. The recommended loading dose is 10 mg/kg followed by a single daily maintenance dose of 2.5 mg/kg [7]. Therapeutic levels range from 5 to 20 mg/l. A recent double blind study shows that caffeine is as efficient and has fewer secondary effects than theophylline. Further, plasma caffeine concentrations may be measured less frequently than theophylline, *i. e.* once a week instead of every second or third day (A. Bairam et al., *Progress in Neonatologie*, A. Minkowski, J. P. Relier ed., Karger, Basel, 5, 196-207, 1985). Caffeine citrate is prefered to the sodium benzoate preparation as the latter displaces bilirubin from its albumin binding sites [165].

DOXAPRAM. — Doxapram at a dosage of 2.5 mg/kg/h I. V., has been proposed in association with caffeine when the latter alone is not effective (Alpan, *J. Pediatr.*, 104, 634, 1984 and Eyal et al., *Pediatrics*, 75, 709, 1985). Recent observations from our institution suggest that in association with caffeine Doxapram may be effective at a dose of 0.25 mg/kg/h I. V. Thus the pharmacodynamics and kinetics of Doxapram alone requires further investigation.

Artificial ventilation. — When prolonged apnea persists in spite of previous therapeutic attempts artificial ventilation should be initiated using a constant flow respirator allowing for spontaneous breathing. Minimal peak inspiratory and end expiratory pressure together with a short inspiratory time should be used. Weaning from the respirator may be considered when the infant tolerates a rate lower than 5 per minute.

Neonatal apnea and the risk of sudden infant death syndrome (SIDS)

Some SIDS victims have presented with apnea for a variable period of time prior to death [13, 32, 68, 94, 114, 129, 174] and a higher risk for SIDS is reported in premature infants [58, 102, 135]. However, a recent cooperative study on 1,157 neonates below 37 weeks gestation and/or weighing less than 2,500 g at birth did not show any relationship between the occurrence of prolonged apnea on cardiorespiratory monitoring, performed one week prior to discharge from the NICU and the incidence of SIDS. Indeed in this study, none of the 5 SIDS cases had apnea equal to or longer than 20 seconds. These were

TABLE III. — APNEA PARAMETERS DURING THE FIRST WEEK OF LIFE IN 1,301 NEONATES; DATA OBTAINED DURING 24 HOUR RECORDINGS. REPORTED VALUES ARE PERCENTILE 84.1 (corresponding to the mean + 1 standard deviation) (After A. STEINSCHNEIDER et al. [175]).

	Index of apnea ≥ 2 s	Index of apnea ≥ 6 s	% periodic breathing (with pauses ≥ 2 s)	Longest apnea (s)	Apnea mean duration (s)
Q. S.	—	—	—	9.0	3.76
A. S.	—	—	—	9.7	3.84
T. S. T.	4.08	0.86	8.21	—	—

Q. S.: quiet sleep; A. S.: active sleep; T. S. T.: total sleep time.

present in 33 babies who survived of which 6 were however treated with theophylline or placed on a home monitoring system [168]. In a prospective study, respiration recorded during the first 24 hours of life in 1,301 infants was compared with the neonatal recordings of 10 infants who later died of SIDS. The 84.1 percentile value of the normative data (mean + 1 standard deviation) for different apnea parameters is reported in Table III. Apnea index during feeding, number of 15 second sleep episodes where at least one apnea occurred, index of central apnea equal to or longer than either 2 or 6 seconds and percentage time of periodic breathing were more frequently elevated in the SIDS group than in the control population. In 5 to 6 of 10 SIDS victims, the value of one or more of these parameters was greater than the 84.1 percentile's [175]. In other words, the risk for SIDS in infants with such values would be 24 to 29 %oo against 2 %oo in the general population. This study confirms that some SIDS victims may have neurologic abnormalities long before death, as has previously been reported [4, 131, 132, 170].

Unfortunately, a systematic SIDS identification programme based on neonatal pneumogram analyses would not be practical for two reasons [175]: firstly, there is a lack of specificity: only 3 % of infants with "apnea scores" greater than percentile 84.1 will eventually die and secondly there is a lack of sensitivity: 40 to 50 % of future SIDS victims would not be screened.

It appears likely that apnea plays a definite role in the terminal event of SIDS. However apnea is not always present long before death and when present it is not systematically associated with SIDS. Nonetheless high risk neonates should benefit from careful supervision which might depend on local possibilities: home visiting [31], cardiac or respiratory home monitoring [94] or hospital consulta-

tions. Improvement in infant surveillance techniques during the first weeks of life is associated with decreased SIDS and a reduced infant mortality [31].

CONCLUSION

Long term outcome of apneic premature infants should be particularly evaluated for neurologic and behavioral development. It is possible that the poor long term neurologic prognosis usually reported with apnea would be improved with early treatment. Systematic detection of intracranial hemorrhage in apneic prematures may show that this, rather than the apnea itself is responsible for the later development of neurologic sequellae.

REFERENCES

[1] ALDEN (E. R.), MANDELKORN (T.), WOODRUM (D. E.) *et al.* — Morbidity and mortality of infants weighing less than 1,000 grams in an intensive care nursery. *Pediatrics, 50,* 40, 1972.

[2] ALLAN (W. C.), VOLPE (J. J.). — Reduction of cholesterol synthesis by methylxanthines in cultured glial cells. *Pediatr. Res., 13,* 1121-1124, 1979.

[3] ANDERSEN (H. T.). — Cardiovascular adaptations in diving mammals. *Am. Heart. J., 74,* 295-298, 1967.

[4] ANDERSON (R. B.), ROSENBLITH (J. F.). — Sudden unexpected death syndrome. Early indicators. *Biol. Neonate, 18,* 395-406, 1971.

[5] ANGELL (James J. E.), DE BURGH DALY (M.). — Cardiovascular responses in apnoeic asphyxia: role of arterial chemoreceptors and the modification of their effects by a pulmonary vagal inflation reflex. *J. Physiol., 201,* 87-104, 1969.

[6] ARANDA (J. V.), TURMEN (T.). — Methylxanthines in apnea of prematurity. *Clin. Perinatol., 6,* 87-108, 1979.

[7] ARANDA (J. V.), GRONDIN (D.), SASYNIUK (B. I.). — Pharmacologic considerations in the therapy of neonatal apnea. Pediatr. Clin. North Amer., 28, 113-133, 1981.

[8] BADA (H. S.), KHANNA (N. N.), SOMANI (S. M.) et al. — Interconversion of theophylline and caffeine in newborn infants. J. Pediatr., 94, 993-995, 1979.

[9] BAKER (T. L.), McGINTY (D. J.). — Reversal of cardiopulmonary failure during active sleep in hypoxic kittens: implications for sudden infant death. Science, 198, 419-421, 1977.

[10] BARTLETT (D.). — Origin and regulation of spontaneous deep breaths. Resp. Physiol., 12, 230-238, 1971.

[11] BEDNAREK (F. J.), ROLOFF (D. W.). — Treatment of apnea of prematurity with aminophylline. Pediatrics, 58, 335-339, 1976.

[12] BELENKY (D. A.), STANDAERT (T. A.), WOODRUM (D. E.). — Maturation of hypoxic ventilatory response of the newborn lamb. J. Appl. Physiol.: Respirat. Environ. Exercise Physiol., 42, 630-635, 1977.

[13] BERGMAN (A. B.), RAY (C. G.), POMEROY (M. A.) et al. — Studies of the sudden infant death syndrome in King county, Washington. III. Epidemiology. Pediatrics, 49, 860-870, 1972.

[14] BISCOE (T. J.), PURVES (M. J.), SAMPSON (S. R.). — Types of nervous activity which may be recorded form the carotid sinus nerve in the sheep fœtus. J. Physiol., 202, 1-23, 1969.

[15] BLUMENTHAL (I.), LEALMAN (G. T.). — Effect of posture on gastro-œsophageal reflux in the newborn. Arch. Dis. Child., 57, 555, 1982.

[16] BODDY (K.), DAWES (G. S.), FISHER (R.) et al. — Fœtal respiratory movements, electrocortical and cardiovascular responses to hypoxaemia and hypercapnia in sheep. J. Physiol., 243, 599-618, 1974.

[16 bis] BODDY (K.), DAWES (G. S.). — Fetal breathing. Br. Med. Bull., 31, 3-7, 1975.

[17] BODEGARD (G.). — Control of respiration in newborn babies. III. Developmental changes of respiratory depth and rate responses to CO_2. Acta Paediatr. Scand., 64, 684-692, 1975.

[18] BOLTON (D. P. G.), HERMAN (S.). — Ventilation and sleep state in the newborn. J. Physiol., 240, 67-77, 1974.

[19] BORY (C.), BALTASSAT (P.), PORTHAULT (M.) et al. — Metabolism of theophylline to caffeine in premature newborn infants. J. Pediatr., 94, 988-993, 1979.

[20] BOUTROY (M. J.), VERT (P.), ROYER (R. J.) et al. — Caffeine, a metabolite of theophylline during the treatment of apnea in the premature infant. J. Pediatr., 94, 996-998, 1979.

[21] BOUTROY (M. J.), VERT (P.), BIANCHETTI (G.) et al. — Infants born to hypertensive mothers treated by acebutolol. Pharmacological studies in the perinatal period. Dev. Pharmacol. Ther., 4, 109-115, 1982.

[22] BOWES (G.), WOOLF (G. M.), SULLIVAN (C. E.) et al. — Effect of sleep fragmentation on ventilatory and arousal responses of sleeping dogs to respiratory stimuli. Am. Rev. Respir. Dis., 122, 899-908, 1981.

[23] BRADY (J. P.), CERUTI (E.). — Chemoreceptor reflexes in the newborn infant: Effect of varying degrees of hypoxia on heart rate and ventilation in a warm environment. J. Physiol., 184, 631-645, 1966.

[24] BROOKS (J. G.), SCHLUETER (M. A.), NAVELET (Y.) et al. — Sleep state and arterial blood gases and pH, in human newborn and young infants. J. Perinat. Med., 6, 280-286, 1978.

[25] BROWN (W. V.), OSTHEIMER (G. W.), BELL (G. C.) et al. — Newborn response to oxygen blown over the face. Anesthesiology, 44, 535, 1976.

[26] BRYAN (H. M.), HAGAN (R.), GULSTON (G.) et al. — CO_2 response and sleep state in infant. Clin. Res., 12, 689 A, 1976.

[27] BRYAN (A. C.), BRYAN (M. H.). — Control of respiration in the newborn. Clin. Perinatol., 5, 269-281, 1978.

[28] BÜLOW (K.). — Respiration and wakefulness in man. Acta Physiol. Scand., 59 (suppl.), 209, 1963.

[29] BUREAU (M. A.), BÉGIN (R.). — Postnatal maturation of the respiratory response to O_2 in awake newborn lambs. J. Appl. Physiol.: Respirat. Environ. Exercise Physiol., 52, 428-433, 1982.

[30] BUREAU (M. A.), BÉGIN (R.). — Depression of respiration induced by metabolic acidosis in newborn lambs. Biol. Neonate, 42, 279-283, 1982.

[31] CARPENTER (R. G.), EMERY (J. L.). — Final results of study of infants at risk of sudden death. Nature, 268, 724-725, 1977.

[32] CARPENTER (R. G.), GARDNER (A.), McWEENY (P. M.) et al. — Multistage scoring system for identifying infants at risk of unexpected death. Arch. Dis. Child., 52, 606-612, 1977.

[33] CHERNICK (V.), HELDRICH (F.), AVERY (M. E.). — Periodic breathing of premature infants. J. Pediatr., 64, 330, 1964.

[34] COOPER (K. R.), PHILLIPS (B. A.). — Effect of short-term sleep loss on breathing. J. Appl. Physiol.: Respirat. Environ. Exercise Physiol., 53, 855-858, 1982.

[35] CONDORELLI (S.), SCARPELLI (E. M.). — Fetal breathing: induction in utero and effects of vagotomy and barbiturates. J. Pediatr., 88, 94-101, 1976.

[36] CORDERO (L. J.), HON (E.). — Neonatal bradycardia following nasopharyngeal stimulation. J. Pediatr., 78, 441, 1971.

[37] CROSS (K. W.), LEWIS (S. R.). — Upper respiratory obstruction and cot death. Arch. Dis. Child., 46, 211-213, 1971.

[38] CURZI-DASCALOVA (L.). — Phase relationships between thoracic and abdominal respiratory movement during sleep in 31-38 weeks CA normal infants. Comparison with full-term (39-41 weeks) newborns. Neuropediatrics, 13, 15-20, 1982.

[39] DAILY (W. J. R.), KLAUS (M.), MEYER (H. B. P.). — Apnea in premature infants: monitoring, incidence, heart rate changes, and effect of environmental temperature. Pediatrics, 43, 510-518, 1969.

[40] DALY (M.), DE BURGH, SCOTT (M. J.). — An analysis of the primary cardiovascular reflex effects of stimulation of the carotid body chemoreceptors in the dog. J. Physiol., 162, 555-573, 1962.

[41] DALY (M.), DE BURGH, HAZZLEDINE (J. L.), UNGAR (A.). — The reflex effects of alterations in lung volume in systemic vascular resistance in the dog. J. Physiol., 188, 331-351, 1967.

[42] DAVI (M. J.), SANKARAN (K.), SIMONS (K. J.) et al. — Physiologic changes induced by theophylline in the treatment of apnea in preterm infants. J. Pediatr., 92, 91-95, 1978.

[43] DAVI (M.), SANKARAN (K.), McCALLUM (M.) et al. — Effect of sleep state on chest distorsion and on the ventilatory response to CO_2 in neonates. Pediatr. Res., 13, 982-986, 1979.

[44] DAWES (G. S.), DUNCAN (S. L. B.), LEWIS (B. V.) et al. — Hypoxaemia and aortic chemoreceptor function in fœtal lambs. J. Physiol., 201, 105-116, 1969.

[45] DAWES (G. S.), DUNCAN (S. L. B.), LEWIS (B. V.) et al. — Cyanide stimulation of the systemic arterial chemoreceptors in fœtal lambs. J. Physiol., 201, 117-128, 1969.

[46] DAWES (G. S.), FOX (H. E.), LEDUC (B. M.) et al. — Respiratory movements and rapid eye movement sleep in the fœtal lamb. J. Physiol., 220, 119-143, 1972.

[47] DAWES (G. S.), GARDNER (W. N.), JOHNSTON (B. M.) et al. — Breathing pattern in fetal lambs after mid brain transsection. J. Physiol., 208, 29 p., 1980.

[48] DEUEL (R. K.). — Polygraphic monitoring of apneic spells. Arch. Neurol., 28, 71-76, 1973.

[49] DIETRICH (J.), KRAUSS (A. N.), REIDENBERG (M.) et al. — Alterations in state in apneic pre-term infants receiving theophylline. Clin. Pharmacol. Ther., 24, 474-478, 1978.

[50] DOUGLAS (W. W.), REHDER (K.), BEYNEN (F. M.) et al. — Improved oxygenation in patients with acute respiratory failure: the prone position. Am. Rev. Respir. Dis., 115, 559-566, 1977.

[51] DOWNING (S. E.), LEE (J. C.). — Laryngeal chemosensitivity, a possible mechanism for sudden infant death. Pediatrics, 55, 640, 1975.

[52] FAGENHOLZ (S. A.), O'CONNELL (K.), SHANNON (D. C.). — Chemoreceptor function and sleep state in apnea. Pediatrics, 58, 31-36, 1976.

[53] FENNER (A.), SCHALK (U.), HOENICKE (H.) et al. — Periodic breathing in premature and neonatal babies: incidence, breathing pattern, respiratory gas tensions, response to changes in the composition of ambient air. Pediatr. Res., 7, 174-183, 1973.

[54] FINER (N. N.), ABROMS (I. F.), TAEUSCH (H. W.). — Ventilation and sleep states in newborn infants. J. Pediatr., 89, 100-108, 1976.

[55] FLEMING (P.), BRYAN (A. C.), BRYAN (M. H.). — Functional immaturity of pulmonary irritant receptors and apnea in newborn preterm infants. Pediatrics, 61, 515, 1978.

[56] FLEMING (P. J.), MULLER (N. L.), BRYAN (M. H.) et al. — The effects of abdominal loading on rib cage distortion in premature infants. Pediatrics, 64, 425-428, 1979.

[57] FLORES-GUEVARRA (R.), PLOUIN (P.), CURZI-DASCALOVA (L.) et al. — Sleep apneas in normal neonates and infants during the first 3 months of life. Neuropediatrics, 13, 21-28, 1982.

[58] FROGGATT (P.), LYNAS (M. A.), MARSHALL (T. K.). — Sudden death in babies: epidemiology. Am. J. Cardiol., 22, 457-468, 1968.

[59] GABRIEL (M.), ALBANI (M.), SCHULTE (F. J.). — Apneic spells and sleep states in preterm infants. Pediatrics, 57, 142-147, 1976.

[60] GENNSER (G.), MARSAL (K.), BRANTMARK (B.). — Maternal smoking and fetal breathing movements. Am. J. Obstet. Gynecol., 123, 861-867, 1975.

[61] GERHARDT (T.), McCARTHY (J.), BANCALARI (E.). — Effect of aminophylline on respiratory center activity and metabolic rate in premature infants with idiopathic apnea. Pediatrics, 63, 537-542, 1979.

[62] GIRLING (D. J.). — Changes in heart rate, blood pressure, and pulse pressure during apnoeic attacks in newborn babies. Arch. Dis. Child., 47, 405-410, 1972.

[63] GLOGOWSKA (M.), RICHARDSON (P. S.), WIDDICOMBE (J. G.) et al. — The role of vagus nerves, peripheral chemoreceptors and other afferent pathways in the genesis of augmented breaths in cats and rabbits. Resp. Physiol., 16, 179-196, 1972.

[64] GOTTSTEIN (U.), HELD (K.), SEBENING (H.) et al. — Is decrease of cerebral blood flow after intravenous injections of theophylline due to direct vasoconstrictive action of the drug? Europ. Neurol., 6, 153-157, 1971-1972.

[65] GOULD (J. B.), LEE (A. F. S.), JAMES (O.) et al. — The sleep state characteristics of apnea during infancy. Pediatrics, 59, 182-194, 1977.

[66] GROGAARD (J.), LINDSTROM (D. P.), STAHLMAN (M. T.) et al. — The cardiovascular response to laryngeal water administration in young lambs. J. Dev. Physiol., 4, 353-370, 1982.

[67] GUILLEMINAULT (C.), PERAITA (R.), SOUQUET (M.) et al. — Apneas during sleep in infants: possible relationship with sudden infant death syndrome. Science, 190, 677-679, 1975.

[68] GUILLEMINAULT (C.), ARIAGNO (R. L.), FORNO (L. S.) et al. — Obstructive sleep apnea and near miss for SIDS. I. Report of an infant with sudden death. Pediatrics, 63, 837-843, 1979.

[69] GUILLEMINAULT (C.), ARIAGNO (R.), KOROBKIN (R.) et al. — Sleep parameters and respiratory variables in Near miss sudden infant death syndrome infants. Pediatrics, 68, 354-360, 1981.

[70] GUNN (T. R.), METRAKOS (K.), RILEY (P.) et al. — Sequelae of caffeine treatment in preterm infants with apnea. J. Pediatr., 94, 106-109, 1979.

[71] HADDAD (G. G.), EPSTEIN (R. A.), EPSTEIN (M. A. F.) et al. — Maturation of ventilation and ventilatory pattern in normal sleeping infants. J. Appl. Physiol.: Respirat. Environ. Exercise Physiol., 46, 998-1002, 1979.

[72] HADDAD (G. G.), LAI (T. L.), MELLINS (R. B.). — Determination of ventilatory pattern in REM sleep in normal infants. J. Appl. Physiol.: Respirat. Environ. Exercise Physiol., 53, 52-56, 1982.

[73] HARDING (R.), JOHNSON (P.), McCLELLAND (M. E.). — Respiratory function of the larynx in developing sheep and the influence of sleep state. Resp. Physiol., 40, 165-179, 1980.

[74] HARDING (R.), POORE (E. R.), COHEN (G. L.). — The effect of brief episodes of diminished uterine blood flow on breathing movements, sleep states and heart rate in fetal sheep. J. Dev. Physiol., 3, 231-243, 1981.

[75] HARNED (H. S. J.), HERRINGTON (R. T.), GRIFFIN (C. A.) III et al. — Respiratory effects of division of the carotid sinus nerve in the lamb soon after the initiation of breathing. Pediatr. Res., 2, 264-270, 1968.

[76] HARPER (R. M.), SAUERLAND (E. K.) — The role of the tongue in sleep apnea, in Sleep Apnea Syndromes, C. GUILLEMINAULT, W. C. DEMENT ed. Alan R. Liss, Inc., New York, 1978, 219-234.

[77] HENDERSON-SMART (D. J.), READ (D. J. C.). — Depression of intercostal and abdominal muscle activity and vulnerability to asphyxia during active sleep in the newborn, in Sleep Apnea Syndromes, Alan R. Liss, Inc., New York, 1978, 93-117.

[78] HENDERSON-SMART (D. J.), READ (D. J. C.). — Ventilatory responses to hypoxaemia during sleep in the newborn. *J. Dev. Physiol.*, 1, 195-208, 1979.

[79] HENDERSON-SMART (D. J.), READ (D. J. C.). — Reduced lung volume during behavioral active sleep in the newborn. *J. Appl. Physiol.: Respirat. Environ. Exercise Physiol.*, 46, 1081-1085, 1979.

[80] HERRINGTON (R. T.), HARNED (H. S.), FERREIRO (J. I.) *et al.* — The role of the central nervous system in perinatal respiration: studies of chemoregulatory mechanisms in the term lamb. *Pediatrics*, 47, 857-864, 1971.

[81] HEWITT (V. M.). — Effect of posture on the presence of fat in tracheal aspirate in neonates. *Aust. Paediatr. J.*, 12, 267-271, 1976.

[82] HOCHACHKA (P. W.). — Brain, lung, and heart functions during diving and recovery. *Science*, 212, 509-514, 1981.

[83] HOOD (J. H.). — Effect of posture on the amount and distribution of gas in the intestinal tract of infants and young children. *Lancet*, July 18, 107-110, 1964.

[84] HOPPENBROUWERS (T.), HODGMAN (J. E.), HARPER (R. M.) *et al.* — Polygraphic studies of normal infants during the first six months of life. III. Incidence of apnea and periodic breathing. *Pediatrics*, 60, 418-425, 1977.

[85] HOPPENBROUWERS (T.), HODGMAN (J. E.), ARAKAWA (K.) *et al.* — Respiration during the first six months of life in normal infants. III. Computer identification of breathing pauses. *Pediatr. Res.*, 14, 1230-1233, 1980.

[86] HUGELIN (A.), BONVALLET (M.), DELL (P.). — Activation réticulaire et corticale d'origine chémoceptive au cours de l'hypoxie. *Électroencéphalogr. Clin. Neurophysiol.*, 11, 325-340, 1959.

[87] JANSEN (A. H.), PURVES (M. J.), TAN (E. D.). — The role of sympathetic nerves in the activation of the carotid body chemoreceptors at birth in the sheep. *J. Dev. Physiol.*, 2, 305-321, 1980.

[88] JOHNSON (P.), ROBINSON (J. S.), SALISBURY (D.). — The onset and control of breathing after birth, in R. S. COURLINE ed., *Fœtal and Neonatal Physiology*, Cambridge University Press, 1973, 217.

[89] JONES (R. A. K.). — Apnea of immaturity. I. A controlled trial of theophylline and face mask continuous positive airways pressure. *Arch. Dis. Child.*, 57, 761-765, 1982.

[90] KAHN (A.), BLUM (D.), WATERSCHOOT (P.) *et al.* — Effects of obstructive sleep apneas on transcutaneous oxygen pressure in control infants, siblings of sudden infant death syndrome victims, and near miss infants: comparison with the effects of central sleep apneas. *Pediatrics*, 70, 852-857, 1982.

[91] KATTWINKEL (J.), NEARMAN (H. S.), FANAROFF (A. A.) *et al.* — Apnea of prematurity. *J. Pediatr.*, 86, 588-592, 1975.

[92] KATTWINKEL (J.), MARS (H.), FANAROFF (A. A.) *et al.* — Urinary biogenic amines in idiopathic apnea of prematurity. *J. Pediatr.*, 88, 1003-1006, 1976.

[93] KATTWINKEL (J.). — Neonatal apnea: pathogenesis and therapy. *J. Pediatr.*, 90, 342-347, 1977.

[94] KELLY (D. H.), SHANNON (D. C.), O'CONNELL (K.). — Care of infants with near miss sudden infant death syndrome. *Pediatrics*, 61, 511-514, 1978.

[95] KIRKPATRICK (S. M. L.), OLINSKY (A.), BRYAN (M. H.) *et al.* — Effect of premature delivery on the maturation of the Hering-Breuer inspiratory inhibitory reflex in human infants. *J. Pediatr.*, 88, 1010-1014, 1976.

[96] KITTERMAN (J. A.), LIGGINS (G. C.), CLEMENTS (J. A.), TOLLEY (W. H.). — Stimulation of breathing movements in fetal sheep by inhibitors of prostaglandin synthesis. *J. Dev. Physiol.*, 1, 453-466, 1979.

[97] KITTERMAN (J. A.), LIGGINS (G. C.), FEWELL (J. E.) *et al.* — Inhibition of breathing movements in fetal sheep by prostaglandins. *J. Appl. Physiol.: Respirat. Environ. Exercise Physiol.*, 54, 687-692, 1983.

[98] KNILL (R.), BRYAN (A. C.). — An intercostal phrenic inhibitory reflex in human newborn infants. *J. Appl. Physiol.*, 40, 352-356, 1976.

[99] KORNER (A. F.), KRAEMER (H. C.), HAFFNER (M. E.) *et al.* — Effects of water bed flotation on premature infants: a pilot study. *Pediatrics*, 56, 361-367, 1975.

[100] KORNER (A. F.), RUPPEL (E. M.), RHO (J. M.). — Effects of water beds on the sleep and motility of theophylline-treated preterm infants. *Pediatrics*, 70, 864-869, 1982.

[101] KOVAR (I.), SELSTAM (U.), CATTERTON (W. Z.) *et al.* — Laryngeal chemoreflex in newborn lambs: respiratory and swallowing response to salts, acids and sugars. *Pediatr. Res.*, 13, 1144-1149, 1979.

[102] KRAUS (J. F.), BORHANI (N. O.). — Post-neonatal sudden unexplained death in California: a cohort study. *Am. J. Epidemiol.*, 95, 497-510, 1972.

[103] KRAUSS (A. N.), WALDMAN (S.), AULD (P. A. M.). — Diminished response to carbon dioxide in premature infants. *Biol. Neonate*, 30, 216-223, 1976.

[104] KRAUSS (A. N.), SOLOMON (G. E.), AULD (P. A. M.). — Sleep state, apnea and bradycardia in preterm infants. *Dev. Med. Child Neurol.*, 19, 160-168, 1977.

[105] KRIEGER (J.), KURTZ (D.). — EEG changes before and after apnea, in *Sleep Apnea Syndromes*, C. GUILLEMINAULT, W. C. DEMENT ed. Alan R. Liss, Inc., New York, 1978, 161-176.

[105 bis] LAWSON (E. E.). — Prolonged central respiratory inhibition following reflex induced apnea. *J. Appl. Physiol.*, 50, 1981, 874-879.

[106] LAZARO-LOPEZ (F.), COLLE (E.), DUPONT (C.) *et al.* — Metabolic effects of caffeine in the preterm neonate. *Pediatr. Res.*, 14, 468 (Abstract), 1980.

[107] LEHEUP (B.), GRIGNON (G.). — Croissance et théophylline : effet inhibiteur *in vivo* et *in vitro* chez le fœtus de rat. *Dev. Pharmacol. Ther.*, 4, 206, 1982.

[108] LIGGINS (G. C.), VILOS (G. A.), CAMPOS (G. A.), KITTERMAN (J. A.), LEE (C. H.). — The effect of spinal cord transection on lung development in fetal sheep. *J. Dev. Physiol.*, 3, 267-274, 1981.

[109] LIGGINS (G. C.), VILOS (G. A.), CAMPOS (G. A.), KITTERMAN (J. A.), LEE (C. H.). — The effect of bilateral thoracoplasty on lung development in fetal sheep. *J. Dev. Physiol.*, 3, 275-282, 1981.

[110] LOPES (J. M.), LESOUEF (P. N.), HEATHER (M.) *et al.* — The effects of theophylline on diaphragmatic fatigue in the newborn. *Pediatr. Res.*, 16, 355 A (Abstract), 1982.

[111] LOU (H. C.), LASSEN (N. A.), FRIIS-HANSEN (B.). — Impaired autoregulation of cerebral blood flow in the distressed newborn. *J. Pediatr.*, 94, 118, 1979.

[112] LOU (H. C.), LASSEN (N. A.), TWEED (W. A.) *et al.* — Pressure passive cerebral blood flow and breakdown of the blood brain barrier in experimental fetal asphyxia. *Acta Paediatr. Scand.*, 68, 57-63, 1979.

[113] LUCIER (G. E.), STOREY (A. T.), SESSLE (B. J.). — Effects of upper respiratory tract stimuli on neonatal respiration: reflex and single neuron analyses in kitten. *Biol. Neonate*, 35, 82, 1979.

[114] MANDELL (F.). — Cot death among children of nurses. Observations of breathing patterns. *Arch. Dis. Child.*, 56, 312-314, 1981.

[115] MANNING (F. A.), FEYERABEND (C.). — Cigarette smoking and fetal breathing movements. *Br. J. Obstet. Gynaecol.*, 83, 262-270, 1976.

[116] MARCHAL (F.), CORKE (B. C.), SUNDELL (H.). — Reflex apnea from laryngeal chemo-stimulation in the sleeping premature newborn lamb. *Pediatr. Res.*, 16, 621-627, 1982.

[117] MARCHAL (F.), MONIN (P.), VERT (P.). — Theophylline induced cerebral acidosis during hyperventilation in the newborn piglet. *Pediatr. Res.*, 16, 127 A (Abstract), 1982.

[118] MARSHALL (T. A.), KATTWINKEL (J.). — Functional residual capacity and oxygen tension in apnea of prematurity. *J. Pediatr.*, 98, 479-482, 1981.

[119] MARTIN (R. J.), OKKEN (A.), KATONA (P. G.), KLAUS (M. H.). — Effect of lung volume on expiratory time in the newborn infant. *J. Appl. Physiol.: Respirat. Environ. Exercise Physiol.*, 45, 18-23, 1978.

[120] MARTIN (R. J.), HERRELL (N.), RUBIN (D.) et al. — Effect of supine and prone positions on arterial oxygen tension in the preterm infant. *Pediatrics*, 63, 528-531, 1979.

[121] MATHEW (O. P.), ROBERTS (J. L.), THACH (B. T.). — Pharyngeal airway obstruction in infants with mixed and obstructive apnea. *Pediatr. Res.*, 15, 671 A (Abstract), 1981.

[122] MEAD (J.), COLLIER (C.). — Relation of volume history of lungs to respiratory mechanics in anesthetized dogs. *J. Appl. Physiol.*, 14, 669-678, 1959.

[123] MILLER (H. C.), BEHRLE (F. C.), SMULL (N. W.). — Severe apnea and irregular respiratory rhythms among premature infants. *Pediatrics*, 1959.

[124] MILLHORN (D. E.), ELDRIDGE (F. L.), WALDROP (T. G.). — Prolonged stimulation of respiration by a new central neural mechanism. *Resp. Physiol.*, 41, 87-103, 1980.

[125] MILNER (A. D.), SAUNDERS (R. A.), HOPKIN (I. E.). — Apnoea induced by airflow obstruction. *Arch. Dis. Child.*, 52, 379-382, 1977.

[126] MILNER (A. D.), BOON (A. W.), SAUNDERS (R. A.) et al. — Upper airways obstruction and apnoea in preterm babies. *Arch. Dis. Child.*, 55, 22-25, 1980.

[127] MILSAP (R. L.), KRAUSS (A. N.), AULD (P. A. M.). — Effect of theophylline on metabolic rate in premature infants. *Clin. Pharmacol. Ther.*, 27, 271-272, 1980.

[128] MONIN (P.), VERT (P.), ANDRÉ (M.) et al. — Transcutaneous PO_2 Monitoring ($tcPO_2$) in the newborn during apneic spells, convulsions, cardiac catheterizations and exchange transfusions. *Birth Defects*, 15, 469, 1979.

[129] MONOD (N.), CURZI-DASCALOVA (L.), GUIDASCI (S.). et al. — Pauses respiratoires et sommeil chez le nouveau-né et le nourrisson. *Rev. EEG Neurophysiol.*, 6, 105-110, 1976.

[130] MYERS (T. F.), MILSAP (R. L.), KRAUSS (A. N.) et al. — Low-dose theophylline therapy in idiopathic apnea of prematurity. *J. Pediatr.*, 96, 99-103, 1980.

[131] NAEYE (R. L.), LADIS (B.), DRAGE (J. S.). — Sudden infant death syndrome. *Am. J. Dis. Child.*, 130, 1207-1210, 1976.

[132] NAEYE (R. L.), MESSNER III (J.), SPECHT (T.) et al. — Sudden infant death syndrome temperament before death. *J. Pediatr.*, 88, 511-515, 1976.

[133] NELSON (N. M.). — Respiration and circulation after birth, in *The Physiology of the Newborn Infant*, C. A. SMITH and N. M. NELSON eds, C. C. Thomas, Springfield, 1976, 117.

[134] NELSON (R. M.), RESNICK (M. B.), HOLSTRUM (W. J.) et al. — Developmental outcome of premature infants treated with theophylline. *Dev. Pharmacol. Ther.*, 1, 274-280, 1980.

[135] OAKLEY (J. R.), TAVARE (C. J.), STANTON (A. N.). — Evaluation of the Sheffield system for identifying children at risk from unexpected death in infancy. *Arch. Dis. Child.*, 53, 649-652, 1978.

[136] ODELL (G.) in *Care of the High Neonates*, A. H. KLAUS and A. A. FANAROFF eds, Saunders Philadelphia, 147, 1973.

[137] OLINSKY (A.), BRYAN (M. H.), BRYAN (A. C.). — Influence of lung inflation on respiratory control of neonates. *J. Appl. Physiol.*, 36, 426-429, 1974.

[138] PADBURY (J. F.). — DIAKOMANOLIS (E. S.), LAM (R. W.) et al. — Ontogenesis of tissue catecholamines in fetal and neonatal rabbits. *J. Dev. Physiol.*, 3, 297-303, 1981.

[139] PAINTAL (A. S.). — Vagal sensory receptors and their reflex effects. *Physiol. Rev.*, 53, 159-227, 1973.

[140] PAPE (K. E.), WIGGLESWORTH (J. S.). — The clinico-pathological relationship and aetiological aspects of intraventricular haemorrhage. In *Haemorrhage, Ischemia and the Perinatal Brain, Clinics in Developmental Medicine*, 133, 69-70, 1979.

[141] PARMELEE (A. H.), STERN (E.). — Development of States in infants, in C. CLEMENTE, D. PURPURA, F. E. MAYER, *Sleep and the Maturing Nervous System*, Academic Press, New York, 199-228, 1972.

[142] PATRICK (G. B.), STROHL (K. P.), RUBIN (S. B.) et al. — Upper airways and diaphragm muscle responses to chemical stimulation and loading. *J. Appl. Physiol.: Respirat. Environ. Exercise Physiol.*, 53, 1133-1137, 1982.

[143] PHILLIPSON (E A.), MURPHY (E.), KOZAR (L. F.). — Regulation of respiration in sleeping dogs. *J. Appl. Physiol.*, 40, 688, 1976.

[144] PHILLIPSON (E. A.), KOZAR (L. F.), REBUCK (A. S.) et al. — Ventilatory and waking responses to CO_2 in sleeping dogs. *Am. Rev. Resp. Dis.*, 115, 251-259, 1977.

[145] PHILLIPSON (E. A.). — Control of breathing during sleep. *Am. Rev. Resp. Dis.*, 118, 909-939, 1978.

[146] PHILLIPSON (E. A.), SULLIVAN (C. E.). — Arousal: the forgotten response to respiratory stimuli. *Am. Rev. Resp. Dis.*, 118, 807-809, 1978.

[147] PHILLIPSON (E. A.), SULLIVAN (C. E.), HEAD (D. J. C.), MURPHY (E.), KOZAR (L. F.). — Ventilatory and waking responses to hypoxia in sleeping dogs. *J. Appl. Physiol.*, 44, 512-520, 1978.

[148] PONTE (J.), PURVES (M. J.). — Types of afferent nervous activity which may be measured in the vagus nerve of the sheep fœtus. *J. Physiol.*, 229, 51-76, 1973.

[149] PURVES (M. J.). — The effects of hypoxia in the newborn lamb before and after denervation of the carotid chemoreceptors. *J. Physiol.*, 185, 60-77, 1966.

[150] Purves (M. J.). — Chemoreceptors and their reflexes with special reference to the fetus and newborn. *J. Dev. Physiol.*, *3*, 21-57, 1981.

[151] Reis (D. J.), McHugh (P. R.). — Hypoxia as a cause of bradycardia during amygdala stimulation in monkey. *Am. J. Physiol.*, *214*, 601-610, 1968.

[152] Remmers (J. E.), de Groot (W. J.), Sauerland (E. K.) *et al.* — Neural and mechanical factors controlling pharyngeal occlusion during sleep. In *Sleep Apnea Syndromes*, C. Guilleminault, W. C. Dement ed. Alan R. Liss, Inc., New York, 211-217, 1978.

[153] Remmers (J. E.), de Groot (W. J.), Sauerland (E. K.) *et al.* — Pathogenesis of upper airway occlusion during sleep. *J. Appl. Physiol.: Respirat. Environ. Exercise Physiol.*, *44*, 931-938, 1978.

[154] Reuss (M. L.), Rudolph (A. M.). — Distribution and recirculation of umbilical and systemic venous blood flow in fetal lambs during hypoxia. *J. Dev. Physiol.*, *2*, 71-84, 1980.

[155] Rigatto (H.), Brady (J. P.). — Periodic breathing and apnea in preterm infants. I. Evidence for hypoventilation possibly due to central respiratory depression. *Pediatrics*, *50*, 202-218, 1972.

[156] Rigatto (H.), Brady (J. P.). — Periodic breathing and apnea in preterm infants. II. Hypoxia as a primary event. *Pediatrics*, *50*, 219-228, 1972.

[157] Rigatto (H.), Brady (J. P.), de La Torre Verduzco (R.). — Chemoreceptor reflexes in preterm infants: I. The effect of gestational and postnatal age on the ventilatory response to inhalation of 100 % and 15 % oxygen. *Pediatrics*, *55*, 604-613, 1975.

[158] Rigatto (H.). — Ventilatory response to hypoxia. *Sem. Perinatol.*, *1*, 357-362, 1977.

[159] Rigatto (H.). — Ventilatory response to hypercapnia. *Sem. Perinatol.*, *1*, 363-367, 1977.

[160] Rigatto (H.), Kalapesi (Z.), Leahy (F. N.) *et al.* — Chemical control of respiratory frequency and tidal volume during sleep in preterm infants. *Resp. Physiol.*, *41*, 117-125, 1980.

[161] Rigatto (H.), Kalapesi (Z.), Leahy (F. N.) *et al.* — Ventilatory response to 100 % and 15 % O_2 during wakefulness and sleep in preterm infants. *Early Hum. Dev.*, *7*, 1-10, 1982.

[162] Rosenkrantz (T. S.), Oh (W.). — Reduction of cerebral blood flow (CBF) in low birth weight (LBW) infants after aminophylline administration. *Pediatr. Res.*, *16*, 306 A (Abstract), 1982.

[163] Rubio (R.), Berne (R. M.), Bockman (E. L.), Curnish (R. R.). — Relationship between adenosine concentration and oxygen supply in rat brain. *Am. J. Physiol.*, *228*, 1896-1902, 1975.

[164] Rudolph (A. M.), Itskovitz (J.), Iwamoto (H.) *et al.* — Fetal cardiovascular responses to stress. *Sem. Perinatol.*, *5*, 109-121, 1981.

[165] Schiff (D.), Chan (G.), Stern (L.). — Fixed drug combinations and the displacement of bilirubin from albumin. *Pediatrics*, *48*, 139-141, 1971.

[166] Shannon (D. C.), Gotay (F.), Stein (M.) *et al.* — Prevention of apnea and bradycardia in low birth weight infants. *Pediatrics*, *55*, 589, 1975.

[167] Siassi (B.), Hodgman (J. E.), Cabal (L.) *et al.* — Cardiac and respiratory activity in relation to gestation and sleep states in newborn infants. *Pediatr. Res.*, *13*, 1163-1166, 1979.

[168] Southall (D. P.), Richards (J. M.), Rhoden (K. J.) *et al.* — Prolonged apnea and cardiac arrhythmias in infants discharged from neonatal intensive care units: failure to predict an increased risk for sudden infant death syndrome. *Pediatrics*, *70*, 844-851, 1982.

[169] Srinivasan (G.), Singh (J.), Pildes (R. S.) *et al.* — Plasma glucose changes during theophylline therapy. *Pediatr. Res.*, *16*, 132 A (Abstract), 1982.

[170] Stanton (A. N.), Downham (M. A. P. S.), Oakley (J. R.), Emery (J. L.). — Terminal symptoms in children dying suddenly and unexpectedly at home. *Br. Med. J.*, *2*, 1249-1251, 1978.

[171] Stark (A. R.), Thach (B. T.). — Mechanisms of airway obstruction leading to apnea in newborn infants. *J. Pediatr.*, *89*, 982-985, 1976.

[172] Stark (A. R.), Frantz (I. D.). — Prolonged expiratory duration with elevated lung volume in newborn infants. *Pediatr. Res.*, *13*, 261-264, 1979.

[173] Stein (I. M.), White (A.), Kennedy (J. L.). — Apnea recordings of healthy infants at 40, 44 and 52 weeks postconception. *Pediatrics*, *63*, 724-730, 1979.

[174] Steinschneider (A.). — Prolonged apnea and the sudden infant death syndrome: Clinical and laboratory observations. *Pediatrics*, *50*, 646-654, 1972.

[175] Steinschneider (A.), Weinstein (S. L.), Diamond (E.). — The sudden infant death syndrome and apnea/obstruction during neonatal sleep and feeding. *Pediatrics*, *70*, 858-863, 1982.

[176] Stonestreet (B. S.), Laptook (A.), Schanler (R.) *et al.* — Hemodynamic responses to asphyxia in spontaneously breathing newborn term and premature lambs. *Early Hum. Dev.*, *7*, 81-97, 1982.

[177] Stonestreet (B. S.), Nowicki (P. T.), Hansen (N. B.) *et al.* — The effect of aminophylline on brain blood flow in the piglet with controlled ventilation. *Pediatr. Res.*, *16*, 132 A, 1982.

[178] Storrs (C. N.). — Cardiovascular effects of apnoea in preterm infants. *Arch. Dis. Child.*, *52*, 534-540, 1977.

[179] Stothers (J. K.), Warner (R. M.). — Oxygen consumption and neonatal sleep states. *J. Physiol.*, *278*, 435-440, 1978.

[180] Sullivan (C. E.), Kozar (L. F.), Murphy (E.) *et al.* — Primary role of respiratory afferents in sustaining breathing rhythm. *J. Appl. Physiol.*, *45*, 11, 1978.

[181] Sullivan (C. E.), Murphy (E.), Kozar (L. F.) *et al.* — Waking and ventilatory responses to laryngeal stimulation in sleeping dogs. *J. Appl. Physiol.*, *45*, 681-689, 1978.

[182] Sullivan (C. E.), Kozar (L. F.), Murphy (E.) *et al.* — Arousal, ventilatory, and airway responses to bronchopulmonary stimulation in sleeping dogs. *J. Appl. Physiol.*, *47*, 17-25, 1979.

[183] Sutton (D.), Taylor (E. M.), Lindeman (R. C.). — Prolonged apnea in infant monkeys resulting from stimulation of superior laryngeal nerve. *Pediatrics*, *61*, 519, 1978.

[184] Sweet (A. Y.). — Epidemiology in neonatal necrotizing enterocolitis. E. G. Brown and A. Y. Sweet eds, Grune and Stratton, Inc., New York, 11 1980.

[185] Swift (P. G. F.), Emery (J. L.). — Clinical observations on response to nasal occlusion in infancy. *Arch. Dis. Child.*, *48*, 947-951, 1973.

[186] Thach (B. T.), Taeusch (H. W.). — Sighing in newborn human infants: role of inflation-augmenting reflex. *J. Appl. Physiol.*, *41*, 502-507, 1976.

[187] Thach (B. T.), Stark (A. R.). — Spontaneous neck flexion and airway obstruction during apneic spells in preterm infants. *J. Pediatr.*, *94*, 275-281, 1979.

[188] THIBEAULT (D. W.), WONG (M. M.), AULD (P. A. M.). — Thoracic gas volume changes in premature infants. *Pediatrics, 40*, 403-411, 1967.

[189] THIBEAULT (D. W.), POBLETE (E.), AULD (P. A. M.). — Alveolar-arterial O_2 and CO_2 differences and their relation to lung volume in the newborn. *Pediatrics, 41*, 574-587, 1968.

[190] THOMAN (E. B.), MIANO (V. N.), FREESE (M. P.). — The role of respiratory instability in the sudden infant death syndrome. *Dev. Med. Child Neurol., 19*, 729-738, 1977.

[191] TOULOUKIAN (J. T.). — *Etiologic role of the circulation in neonatal enterocolitis*, E. G. BROWN and A. Y. SWEET eds., Grune and Stratton Inc., New York, 41, 1980.

[192] TRIPPENBACH (T.). — Laryngeal, vagal and intercostal reflexes during the early postnatal period. *J. Dev. Physiol., 3*, 133-159, 1981.

[193] TUCK (S. J.), MONIN (P.), DUVIVIER (C.) *et al.* — Effect of a rocking bed on apnoea of prematurity. *Arch. Dis. Child., 57*, 475-477, 1982.

[194] WAGAMAN (M. J.), SHUTACK (J. G.), MOOMJIAN (A. S.) *et al.* — Improved oxygenation and lung compliance with prone positioning of neonates. *J. Pediatr., 94*, 787-791, 1979.

[195] WAHL (M.), KUSCHINSKY (W.). — The dilatatory action of adenosine on pial arteries of cats and its inhibition by theophylline. *Pflügers Arch., 362*, 55-59, 1976.

[196] WAITE (S. P.), THOMAN (E. B.). — Periodic apnea in the full-term infant: individual consistency, sex differences, and state specificity. *Pediatrics, 70*, 79-86, 1982.

[197] WARBURTON (D.), STARK (A. R.), TAEUSCH (H. W.). — Apnea monitor failure in infants with upper airway obstruction. *Pediatrics, 60*, 742-744, 1977.

[198] WECHSLER (R. L.), KLEISS (L. M.), KETY (S. S.). — The effect of intravenously administered aminophylline on cerebral circulation and metabolism in man. *J. Clin. Invest., 29*, 28-30, 1952.

[199] WEINER (D.), MITRA (J.), SALAMONE (J.) *et al.* — Effect of chemical stimuli on nerves supplying upper muscles. *J. Appl. Physiol.:* Respirat. Environ. Exercise Physiol., *52*, 530-536, 1982.

[200] WILSON (S. L.), THACH (B. T.), BROUILLETTE (R. T.) *et al.* — Upper airway patency in the human infant: influence of airway pressure and posture. *J. Appl. Physiol.:* Respirat. Environ. Exercise Physiol., *48*, 500-504, 1980.

[201] WOODRUM (D. E.), STANDAERT (T. A.), PARKS (C. R.) *et al.* — Ventilatory response in the fetal lamb following peripheral chemodenervation. *J. Appl. Physiol.:* Respirat. Environ. Exercise Physiol., *42*, 630-635. 1977.

[202] YU (V. Y. H.). — Effect of body position on gastric emptying in the neonate. *Arch. Dis. Child., 50*, 500, 1975.

[203] ZWILLICH (C. W.), SUTTON (F. D.), PIERSON (D. J.) *et al.* — Decreased hypoxic ventilatory drive in the obesity-hypoventilation syndrome. *Am. J. Med., 59*, 343, 1975.

21

Pulmonary infection in the newborn

J. P. RELIER and J. Cl. LARROCHE

Pulmonary infection has for a long time represented an important part of neonatal pathology. As early as 1884, Silberman [30] showed "Pneumonia" to be a possible cause of neonatal death. In 1939, McGregor in England [21] thought that "Pneumonia" was responsible for 20-25 % of neonatal mortality. For Fedrick and Butler in 1958 [7], the incidence of fatal pulmonary infection was 3.81 per 1,000 live births. This incidence has evolved parallel to that of materno-foetal infection, which swings between 1 to 4 % of live births in France [16]. It represents a large part of the admissions to a neonatal intensive care unit, as the gravity of the respiratory signs increasingly justify assisted ventilation.

The incidence of respiratory distress due to pulmonary infection seems to be on the increase, especially as there is a relative decrease in other causes of neonatal respiratory distress (NRD) such as hyaline membrane disease (HMD). Thus in the neonatal intensive care unit at Port-Royal, over a period of five years (1975-1980), out of 2,160 neonates, 200 were admitted for respiratory distress due to pulmonary infection (usually of maternal origin), an incidence of about 10 %.

Neonatal pulmonary infection as is much neonatal pulmonary pathology, is largely a feature of prematurity. In the Port Royal maternity hospital [2] the frequency of pulmonary infection is 5.7 % in neonates of less than 2,500 g as against only 0.7 % in neonates of more than 2,500 g. This proportion increases to 15 % in premature infants of less that 1,550 g (Fessard et al. [8]).

Neonatal pulmonary infection remains a serious disease. Mortality is at a mean of 50 %, attaining 88 % in some statistics of premature infants of less than 1,500 g [8]. From the autopsies of neonates dying during the first 15 days, whatever the cause of death, pulmonary infection was found in 36 % of cases in Fedrick and Butler's [7] series, but only in 22 % of the cases examined by Larroche [19].

ETIOLOGY
AND PATHOGENESIS

Neonatal pulmonary infection can be divided into two categories: bacterial and viral. As in all neonatal infections, pulmonary infection may occur at 3 different times; before birth, during labour and birth and after birth.

Before birth. — Three mechanisms are involved; from the mother's blood system via the placenta, per vaginam and via premature rupture of the membranes.

The route via the placenta is difficult to prove. It is rarely responsible for pulmonary infection. The most plausible examples are those of listeriosis and certain viral infections where the pulmonary infection is a localisation of a general foetal infection. Foetal infection often occurs after a maternal illness which may be neglected or pass unnoticed. The prognosis is extremely unfavourable. It is in such cases that death in utero may occur.

The route per vaginam is often involved even when the membranes are still intact. When there is a focus of infection in the endometrium or a severe vaginal infection, an amniotitis occurs. The foetus may be contaminated by swallowing or inhaling the amniotic fluid during foetal gasps.

Premature rupture of the membranes occuring well before labour, may be a source of pulmonary infection, either because this rupture is a symptom of a pre-existing amniotic infection, or because the rupture then opens the way for an amniotitis. The risk of neonatal pulmonary infection is clinically linked to the length of rupture [21].

Penner and McInnes [24] have shown at autopsy, that the incidence of pulmonary infection increases from 10 % when the rupture of the membranes is 6 hours or less, to 60 % for a rupture of 24 hours or more. The bacteria involved are those in the vagina, whose flora may be modified by the indiscriminant use of antibiotics prescribed prophylactically, sometimes creating bacterial resistance, despite their limited therapeutic spectrum.

During labour and birth. — A newborn infant may become contaminated by inhaling infected amniotic fluid or when passing through the genital tract. Gosselin in 1945 [13], showed that the longer the labour the greater the risk of infection, even when the membranes remain intact.

Infection is not inevitable: It would imply massive contamination while repeatedly gasping during acute foetal distress, or the presence of a major vaginal infection. The first clinical signs are often delayed but always appear before the 5th day of life. The infectious agents are most frequently bacterial.

After birth. — This is as a general rule "iatrogenic" infection, as it appears in neonates, more often admitted to an intensive care or special care unit for acute neonatal distress and/or gross prematurity.

It occurs from the 5th to 30th postnatal day. Although these "hospital" organisms are more often bacterial, they may also be viral.

MECHANISM

The mechanism of respiratory distress during bacterial or viral pulmonary infection remains debatable. It is in fact, complex and involves different elements:

In viral pneumonia. — Some [9, 34] believe that viral injury to type II cells may alter the production of surfactant, leading to alveolar instability and thereby to a functional right to left shunt secondary to the abnormality of the ventilation-perfusion relationship. These hypotheses are supported by microscopic and mechanical studies on extracts of lung matter.

In bacterial pneumonia. — The mechanism is sometimes evident when there is extensive bronchoalveolar injury. In some gram negative infections, such as Pseudomonas [19], it is impossible to recognise the normal structure of the pulmonary architecture. The necrosis of the pulmonary vessels and the microthrombi in the capillaries in specifically designated parenchymatous zones makes it easy to imagine the severity of the lung perfusion disorder. Such forms tend to envolve towards a picture of pulmonary haemorrhage.

The mechanism is less obvious in curable bacterial pulmonary infection. Scarpelli [28] and Strang [32] have reported abnormalities in the surface tension of infected lung samples.

Taylor and Abrams [33] have even suggested that fibrinogen could inactivate the surfactant locally at the level of the alveoli. However bacterial pulmonary infection does not modify the biochemical profile of the lung of the term neonate. This has been studied by Gluck's group using streptococcal pulmonary infections [27] as well as other organisms such as *E. coli* and *H. influenzae* [17].

These authors have shown that, during neonatal pulmonary infection, respiratory distress is not due to a deficit or alteration in the composition of the phospholipids in surfactant. It even seems that antenatal infection may be a factor encouraging pulmonary maturation. Our group has in fact shown [26] that 17 premature neonates (27 to 35 wks, mean GA = 30 wks) with pulmonary infection from birth, had phosphatidyl-glycerol

(PG), as early as the first 24 hours, in the pulmonary liquid aspirated from the trachea during assisted ventilation; whereas 16 neonates of the same gestational age (27 to 35 wks, mean GA = 30 wks) with HMD, had no PG before the 4th or 5th postnatal day.

Thus, the mechanism is far from clear; if one retains the possibility of abnormal surfactant, one must give as much importance to other causes of abnormal alveolar ventilation such as occlusion of bronchiolo-alveolar units by muco-purulent blockage, weakness of respiratory muscles, and abnormalities of the pulmonary circulation which lead to these complications.

Another factor which must not be neglected in the determination of infectious respiratory distress is an **abnormality of lung perfusion** following infectious shock during certain severe infections even without an obviously abnormal lung parenchyma.

Lastly the mechanism of respiratory distress is further complicated by the fact that frequently, especially in the preterm neonate, the infection is associated with other pulmonary pathology such as HMD, inhalation, problems with the reabsorption of lung liquid, or even pulmonary haemorrhage.

PATHOLOGY

General morphological characteristics

As in the child or the adult, the basic lesion is a leucocytic alveolitis with more or less altered polynuclei. This inflammatory cellular reaction may be focal or confluent, nodular or lobular, extending over one lobe or over the entire pulmonary parenchyma. In severe and prolonged forms, the necrosis of the alveolar epithelium can be seen under an optic microscope in the form of an amorphous eosinophil border. The fibrino-leucocytic alveolitis classically described in the adult is rarely observed in the neonate.

A peri-bronchial inflammatory reaction is equally unusual hence the English preference for the term "pneumonia" to the term broncho-pneumonia too often used in France. Only viral infections merit this term (see below).

Pleural involvement is frequent, initially in the form of a serous infiltration followed by cellular poly-

morphism. In severe and extensive forms and especially in intubated infants, the bronchial epithelium is also necrosed, flaking off in the lumen, with an inflammatory reaction.

All these findings are in fact those of inflammation. The pathologist can only, on a slide, speak of infection if he or she demonstrates the causative organism with a specific stain.

The pneumonia of "amniotic aspiration" is pathologically a rather special form as numerous horny squames and globules of meconium are generally mixed with inflammatory elements thus signifying the intra-uterine origins of the infection.

Secondary pneumonia due to inhalation is difficult to confirm from isolated morphologic criteria. In fact, a few drops of milk or glucose often cannot be discovered even by minute dissection of the bronchial tree or histological segmentation.

In contrast, true aspiration pneumonia is rare.

Morphological characteristics specific to certain pathogenic agents
(Fig. III-49)

"Listeria monocytogenes": the basic lesion is the granuloma that one finds in all the tissues. Sometimes difficult to isolate in an inflammatory pulmonary parenchyma, it is classically recognisable at the level of the bronchial epithelium, which it invades and destroys, overflowing into the neighbouring tissues (Fig. III-49 *a*).

Pseudomonas: these are ragged necro-haemorrhagic lesions which characterise the gram negative infections in general and more particularly pseudomonas infections. The inner walls of all types of vessels are necrosed. The organisms carried in the blood invade the perivascular spaces, "colonize" the endothelium, then the other constituents of the walls, thus facilitating mural thrombi. Pseudomonas in the lungs particularly invades the peri-bronchial cartilage (Fig. III-49 *c*).

"Candida albicans": the site of origin is generally bronchial by inhalation of Candida, during passage through the vagina. The mycelium travels through the bronchial mucosa which may sometimes appear intact (Fig. III-49). True granulomas composed of mycelian filaments, spores and inflammatory cells separate the parenchyma. The point of origin may also be oesophageal with ulceration of the mucosa and the direct passage of the mycelium into the

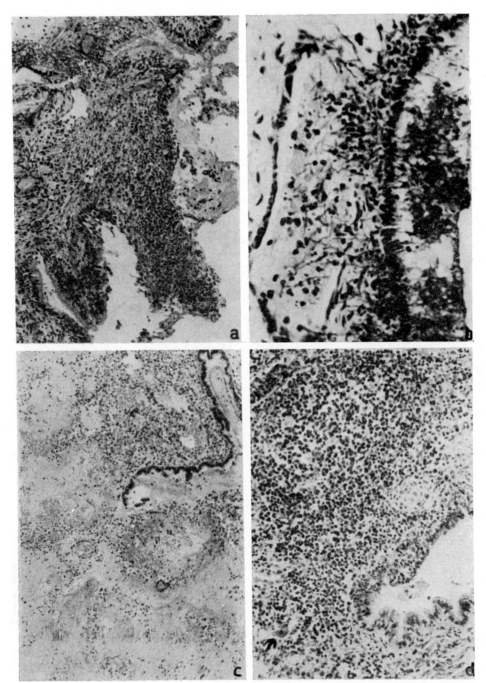

FIG. III-49.

(a) *Listeria monocytogenes* showing the basic "granuloma", lesion which invades and destroys the bronchial epithelium.

(b) *Candida albicans* with numerous spores and mycelian filaments, traveling through the bronchial mucosa.

(c) *Pseudomonas* with large necro-haemorrhagic lesions with total necrosis of the parenchyma and bronchus.

(d) *Cytomegalovirus* infection with severe interstitial pneumonia secondary to mononuclear type cells. The large characteristic cells in the bronchial epithelium are typical of CMV.

sub-mucosal vessel leading to a Candida septicaemia (Fig. III-49 *b*).

Viral infections

The inflammatory cellular reaction is generally of a mononuclear type. It invades the alveolar cavities, but, during the neonatal period, it mainly infiltrates the septa and the peri-bronchial spaces in particular giving rise to the term interstitial pneumonia and even bronchial-pneumonia. The necrosis of the alveolar lining leads to secretory abnormalities of the surfactant in the mucous membranes.

A particular form is seen in Cytomegalovirus infections in which one finds large characteristic cells either free in the lumen or more often than not in the bronchial epithelium (Fig. III-49 *d*).

CLINICAL SIGNS

As with all neonatal infection, the time of appearance of clinical signs of pulmonary infection is extremely variable according to the mode of contamination and the severity of the infection. All scenarios are possible from death in utero to an asymptomatic picture where one considers prescribing antibiotics only on the evidence of maternal signs indicating the possibility of foetal contamination [25]. These signs are described in detail elsewhere.

In pulmonary infection due to maternal contamination, early RD is the symptom that is most commonly found. It is often difficult during this period of adaptation to tell the difference between RD due to pulmonary infection, and RD of different origin, such as hyaline membrane disease, transient tachypnea or inhalation of amniotic fluid, especially as there are frequently several mechanisms involved. Certain serious forms are fairly suggestive, associating severe respiratory distress with an early mixed acidosis, without evidence of inhalation, a deterioration of the general state with early jaundice, disruption of thermal control and disturbances of glycaemic adjustment, lethargy and especially cardio-vascular collapse, which should all be measured and corrected. Such forms have a poor prognosis.

Certain clinical pictures are a function of the etiologic agent and will be reviewed in this chapter.

In fact, the large diversity of clinical pictures justify one's worry above other anomalies in the behaviour of the neonate and, as rapidly as possible, an attempt to assemble all the arguments in favour of infection in order to begin treatment before the return of the bacteriological results which often arrive too late. These cultures however allow information on the diagnosis and may possibly result in an alteration of antibiotic therapy.

In pulmonary infection contracted after birth by nosocomial contamination, the signs are difficult to interpret.

Sometimes they appear secondarily in a previously well neonate; and the diagnosis of infection should be suspected in view of the absence of any anomaly, particularly of respiratory origin.

Sometimes signs will appear following the initial respiratory illness and may be difficult to interpret posing the problem either of an aggravation of the initial pathology (a fact due either to the iatrogenesis of assisted ventilation or disruptions of lung perfusion due to a left-right shunt through the Ductus Arteriosus in the premature infant) or of a secondary infection.

The problem is not too difficult to resolve as long as the infant has not received any prophylactic antibiotics. It is far more worrying when the infant is already under antibiotic therapy due to a suspicion of materno-foetal infection unconfirmed by bacteriological studies. In all cases, the contribution of complementary investigations are indispensable.

BIOLOGICAL DATA

Amongst the bacteriological findings encountered during neonatal infection none are in fact specific for pulmonary infection. Acidosis, hypoxia and hypercapnia are the signs of all pulmonary pathology of the neonate.

Haematological abnormalities found during these infections are numerous and are described in another chapter. The most suggestive are:

— a leucocytosis greater than 25 or 30,000 per mm^3,

— a leucopenia of less than 4,000 or a neutropenia of less than 1,000 per mm^3,

— a thrombopenia of less than 100,000 per mm^3,

— an elevation in the levels of fibrinogen, orosomucoid and C reactive protein.

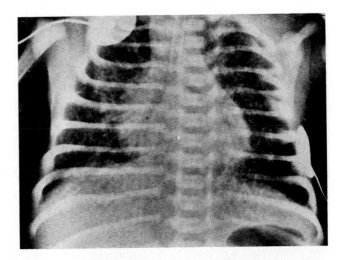

FIG. III-50. — *Listeria pulmonary infection in a 2 day old newborn.*

The initial aspect of alveolar opacities with bronchogram (HMD like) has been modified by the picture of converging alveoli of unequal irregular opacity, alternating with a picture of emphysema.

RADIOLOGICAL SIGNS

As in all respiratory pathology, the radiological pathology of the lungs constitutes the basic investigation for diagnosis, to follow its evolution and to appreciate the efficacy of treatment.

The initial radiological aspect depends particularly on the mode of contamination [3].

Infections "by maternal contamination"

Haematogenic dissemination transplacentally gives the particular appearance of rounded opaque alveoli with blured edges, of differing sizes going as far as coarse and granite-like, dense, bilateral, associated with a bronchogram with interstitial emphysema. This may be thought to be the typical aspect of hyaline membrane disease. However, the development is different. There may often appear after 24-48 hours, either the picture of converging alveoli of unequal opacity, irregular and alternating with a picture of emphysema (Fig. III-50), aggravated by intermittent positive pressure ventilation (IPPV) often mixed with continuous positive pressure ventilation (CPPV), or findings of pulmonary haemorrhage which imply that the broncho-pneumonia is of haematogenic origin. It may be a segmentary picture of ventilation disorders in which it is difficult to determine the exact origin: *i. e.* a complication of assisted ventilation and/or a manifestation of a broncho-pulmonary infection.

This type of image is particularly encountered in pulmonary infections of haematogenic ori-

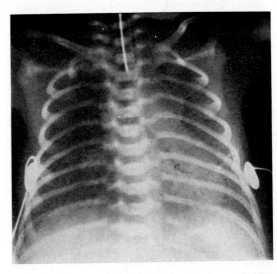

FIG. III-51. — *B Streptococcal-pulmonary infection.* The mixture of granite-like opacities and an air-bronchogram can be confused with HMD which can also be associated.

gin; Streptococci, Listeria and Colibacilli are most often the causal organism (Figs. III-50, III-51, III-52).

Pulmonary infections due to inhalation of infected amniotic fluid, ante or peri-natally show themselves at variable times according to the date of contamination. They are usually confined to pulmonary manifestations with a negative blood culture.

All forms may be encountered. The lungs may even appear normal during the first hours of life. A further stage is that of asymetrical abnormalities in different areas: linear opacities scattering out

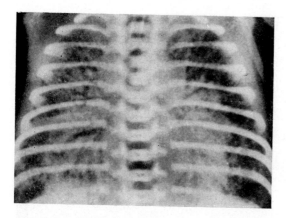

FIG. III-52. — *Gram negative pulmonary infection due to maternal contamination*. Initial granite-like opacity with air bronchogram is replaced, on the third day, by irregular opacities with interstitial emphysema, aggravated by assisted ventilation.

from the hilum, images of poorly defined lumps, small zones of atelectasis, sometimes lobular or segmentary atelectasis more often affecting the superior lobes.

In this case, a bacteriological study of the pulmonary liquid aspirated after physiotherapy allows for a diagnosis. Before receiving the results of the culture an argument that remains in favour of infection is that of a persistence of all the signs of "inhalation" after several effective sessions of respiratory physiotherapy. In these forms of infection there is frequently pleural involvement.

The diagnosis of purulent pleurisy is rarely made clinically. More often than not it is a matter of a border line between a pleural reaction which is difficult to distinguish from a problem of reabsorption of the lung liquid.

Other radiological aspects. — Certain forms of pulmonary infection due to maternal contamination reveal themselves as a pneumothorax uni- or even bilaterally. It is, difficult in such cases, to interpret the images of the interior of the lungs while collapsed or even after drainage. It is however important to suspect pulmonary infection with such a picture.

Certain forms show themselves from birth as a characteristic interstitial pneumonia with a homogenous and dense opacity of one lobe, of one segment, or even one entire lung. Lastly there are characteristic images according to the causal agent even though no single aspect is pathognomonic. They should be studied clinically, especially those of viral origin.

Infections
due to "postnatal contamination"

The clinical and radiological signs appear secondarily after the 5th day of life.

As a general rule these are iatrogenic secondary infections in an intubated and catheterized neonate admitted to an intensive care unit for what was initially non infective pulmonary pathology. After amelioration of the signs of the original pathology, one sees a new clinical and radiological deterioration, with more or less converging lumpy opacities difficult to differentiate with from pictures of an overperfused pulmonary vascular system (Fig. III-53). This could also be the picture of atelectasis reacting badly to physiotherapy and local aspiration.

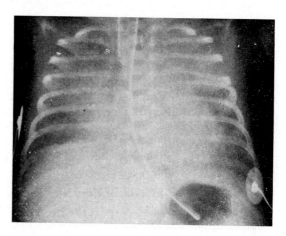

FIG. III-53. — *Acquired pulmonary infection due to* Candida albicans *after surgery for ductus arteriosus.*

Two days after surgery, converging lumpy opacities appeared, responding poorly to physiotherapy and tracheal suction. Diagnosis was made by the association of infectious clinical signs, high fibrinogen, leucocytosis greater than 30,000 p. mm³ and the presence of *Candida albicans* on tracheal aspirate.

The infant treated with Flucytosine recovered completely after 20 days.

It can also represent an aspiration bronchopneumonia, especially in low birth weight neonates, the neonate in a poor neurological state, or a neonate with a tracheo-oesophageal abnormality. The feature is one of aspiration, that is to say lumpy opacities associated with lobular or segmental atelectasis, coexisting with zones of emphysema. Classically this is predominant in the right lung, frequently with an atelectasis of the superior lobe or the inferior lobe whereas the middle lobe is full of emphysema. It is in these forms that one may rarely encounter a pulmonary abcess [23, 29].

BACTERIOLOGICAL TYPES

The organisms involved are generally different according to whether primary infection by maternal contamination or secondary infection acquired after birth is involved.

Infections due to maternal contamination

In our experience: infections by maternal contamination are due to 3 dominant organisms: Streptococcus, especially group B, Listeria and E. coli.

Although the clinical signs reveal themselves early on, they may vary from minor respiratory distress to the picture of major general distress with acute respiratory insufficiency, heart failure and cardio-vascular collapse irremediable despite all the mechanical and medicinal methods that it is at present possible to employ in intensive care units. Such a serious picture is classically described in certain streptococcus B infections but may also be seen with Listeria and E. coli in the neonate.

This is equally true for the radiological aspect. Indeed since Ablow et al.'s publication in 1976 [1], it is usual to suspect a streptococcal origin in a radiological alveolar syndrome. Apart from hyaline membrane disease which is often associated, this appearance may also be encountered in colibacillic or listeria infections (see above).

Due to the seriousness of certain streptococcal infections, many authors propose systematic treatment with penicillin G of all syndromes of "transient distress" and/or hyaline membrane disease. This prophylactic attitude is not entirely justified as penicillin G is not always active against organisms such as colibacillus and could cause a partial selection of digestive flora [12]. On the other hand there are neonatal pulmonary infections due to streptococcus B where the evolution is consistantly fatal despite early antibiotic therapy in which in vitro bacterial efficacy has been proven against the organism responsible.

Surprisingly however, in such rapidly evolving forms, the X-ray, is not necessarily dramatic. The diagnosis is not therefore established (until later) with the results of blood culture and culture of the bronchial fluid.

At present there are no studies to explain the severity of such infections in certain neonates so much so that it is impossible to define at birth the group of neonates at a high risk of infection. Other organisms can be the cause of primary neonatal pulmonary infection but merit only a rapid description due to their infrequent occurence.

These include Proteus, Enterobacter, occasionally Klebsiella pneumoniae, Pneumococcus, anaerobic organisms (Ristella fragilis) or even Pseudomonas.

Neonatal pulmonary infection by *Chlamydia trachomatis* is often suggested due to the frequent contamination of the female genital tract during pregnancy and the time of labour. The frequency of healthy carriers varies between 2 % [15] and 9 % [11]. Pulmonary manifestations at birth are relatively rare in comparison to the frequency of conjunctivitis. It is seen more often at 2 to 6 weeks after birth [11, 35]; appearing as a subacute or even chronic interstitial pneumonia. Recent progress in defining the organism by inoculation of cellular cultures or on serology by immunofluorescence should allow the diagnosis of these infections as a matter of routine [6]. The importance of early diagnosis is further reinforced by the ease of treatment since Chlamydia-Trachomatis is sensitive to sulfamethoxazole-trimethoprim and erythromycin. Tetracycline and Rifampin although active, should not be used in the neonate.

Primary pulmonary infection due to "*Mycobacteria*" are very rare, and are most frequently due to a secondary infection contracted in hospital from a humidifier or even from food [31].

Although of a different mechanism and etiology, one can compare the unusual pneumonias with *congenital tuberculosis*. In their publication of 5 cases in 1976, Couvreur et al. [4] indicated that even when maternal tuberculosis is active during pregnancy, diagnosed or not the first symptoms in general appear 15 days to 6 weeks after birth even if the neonate is immediatly separated from its mother. These authors however reported one case of a premature infant of 29 weeks gestational age, whose immediate respiratory distress was attributed to hyaline membrane disease and then to Wilson-Mikity syndrome. It was not until after the death of the infant on the 55th day, that the autopsy revealed diffuse tubercular lesions predominant in the lungs. The pulmonary infection shows itself as an interstitial or miliary pneumopathy (3/5).

The primitive pulmonary form most frequently corresponds to an inhalation of tubercular amniotic fluid followed by secondary general spread. Genital tuberculosis of the mother, a localization of a previous systemic infection, is without doubt the most frequent form of maternal infection. Diagnosis is difficult. The search for tubercular lesions in the placenta is not always interpretable: it may be negative even though the infant has been infected whereas, conversely, the existence of lesions does not necessairly signify the contamination of the infant (in Couvreur [4]).

Primary pneumonia due to *Candida albicans* is a rare complication of neonatal infection by Candida, acquired either at the time of passage through the birth canal or more often by ascending infection, or after birth. There is no specific clinical or radiological picture. More often the diagnosis is suspected due to the existence of a cutaneous and/or digestive mycosis (Fig. III-53). It is confirmed by the presence of the microorganism in different samples, and the examination of the placenta and membranes. In a series of 2,500 autopsies, Larroche [19] noted 10 cases of pulmonary infection due to Candida with a pure culture of monilia at the level of the respiratory tree and mycelial granulomata present in almost all the organs. The exact pathogenesis of these severe forms remains uncertain. In fact, it is remarkable to note the small number of pulmonary infections by Candida despite the frequency of neonatal carriers and the overextensive use of antibiotics.

Congenital syphilis has become a rare entity. The classical aspect of "Pneumonia alba" is only of real value when this clinical and radiological "Pneumonia" is associated with hepatosplenomegaly and the existence of the particular bony picture due to a periostial reaction in the long bones, which should lead to verification of the serological reactions of the mother.

Acquired bacterial pulmonary infection

Bacterial pulmonary infection acquired in the neonatal period is largely seen in sick neonates admitted to a neonatal centre for other pathology, frequently non-infectious pulmonary pathology.

It is most frequently a secondary iatrogenic pulmonary infection in neonates on assisted ventilation, undergoing frequent tracheo-bronchial suction, and who have had peripheral or especially central catheters. These secondary pulmonary infections may also be seen in non-intubated neonates, especially, premature infants, resulting from tracheo-pulmonary micro-aspirations, or as a pulmonary localization of an acquired septicaemia. The elements of clinical, biological and radiological diagnosis have been described previously. The bacteriological diagnosis rests entirely on the examination and culture of the bronchial secretions obtained after respiratory physiotherapy.

The organisms responsible for these acquired pulmonary infections are most often gram negative hospital organisms: Klebsiella, Enterobacter, Proteus, Pseudomonas. Secondary infection by anaerobic bacilli is more theoretical than real as is secondary infection by Enterococcus. Although rare at the moment in neonates, secondary pulmonary infection by Staphylococcus merits a separate description due to its radiological peculiarity. Dense segmental opacities co-exist with zones of emphysema. A pleural reaction is frequent. As in the infant, the illness may evolve into an abcess and sometimes a pyopneumothorax; and then under treatment into a pneumatocele. Such an evolution may also be seen during secondary infection by Klebsiella and Pseudomonas.

VIRAL PNEUMONIAS

Primary pneumonias. — Apart from a presentation implying maternal causes, viral pulmonary infections in the neonate are difficult to diagnose. More often than not it is a diagnosis by elimination. It is suggested after negative bacteriological findings and continuation of the radiological picture despite treatment with wide spectrum antibodies, established from the clinical and bacteriological features of infection. The prognosis is poor due to the extent of the lesions but it is in fact impossible to give exact figures, due to the difficulties involved in establishing a proven diagnosis of a viral infection (Fig. III-54).

Radiological aspect. — The *primary viral pneumonias* give a picture of reticular opacities of variable density found in the interstitial spaces beginning at the hilum. The association of a diffuse miliary appearance and cutaneous vesicles, sometimes haemorrhagic, may imply *varicella* or *congenital herpes*.

The predominance of an interstitial reticular aspect allied with hepatosplenomegaly, jaundice and intracranial calcification allows one to suspect

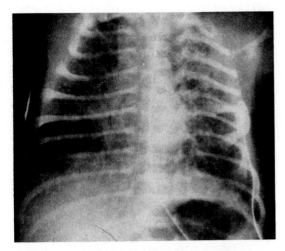

Fig. III-54. — *Viral pulmonary infection in a 900 g premature.*

The reticular interstitial image is rapidly altered by the appearance of emphysema. This picture shows the particular fragility of premature lungs exposed to infections.

cytomegalic viral infection, or even *rubella.* In order to establish rubella one must look for osseous striated bands with no periosteal reaction, and other ocular and/or cardiac findings.

The coexistence of severe cardiac failure with myocarditis suggests infection with *Coxsackie virus* which is frequently fatal.

A fatal interstitial pneumonia during neonatal *mumps transmitted by the mother* has also been described [10]. Neonatal pneumonias due to adenovirus occur and can be fatal. They show the classical aspect of an interstitial pneumonia, sometimes beginning with a predominance in one lung. Fatalities are due either to a secondary bacterial infection, to a deficient immune-response, or to the *type of adenovirus* [20]. Most of the fatal cases are due to adenovirus type 7, and more rarely to types 1, 3, 5 or 22. As in the majority of viral infections, it seems that the neonate is protected by the antibodies transmitted by the mother during pregnancy.

Although different from viral involvement, it must be noted that *congenital toxoplasmosis* may be accompanied by pulmonary localization in the form of an interstitial pneumopathy.

Secondary viral pneumonias are not unusual. They arise, as a general rule, during the course of an epidemic in a nursery and may be especially dramatic in the premature infant who already has pulmonary pathology from other causes. The initial contagion is usually due to an adult carrier of a minor upper respiratory tract infection. The causative viruses, most often reported, are Echovirus [5], Influenza [18], respiratory syncythial virus [14, 22] and adenovirus [7].

The onset is abrupt, with apnea, an episode of cyanosis, thermal imbalance and respiratory distress even with a cough which is a rare phenomenon in the neonate. The radiological aspect is that of non homogeneous infiltrations, irregularly distributed beginning at the hilum and often associated with an obstructive type of emphysema. The evolution is often severe, with cardiac failure especially in the premature infant, necessitating assisted ventilation.

Pneumonias due to *Pneumocystis carinii* should be compared. They are rarely seen before the first month and appear more often with a congenital or acquired deficient immune-response [36].

ELEMENTS OF PROGNOSIS

The general prognosis for neonatal pulmonary infection is poor. Certain factors determine this severity:

— The mechanism: with a more serious outcome in infections from maternal contamination.

— The organism responsible: a more serious outcome in viral pneumopathies.

— Gestational age and often therefore the association of another pathology. Pulmonary infections in premature infants of less than 35 weeks gestational age may be accompanied by hyaline membrane disease which further impairs lung function. The appearance of cerebral complications such as intra-ventricular haemorrhage and leucomalacia, is facilitated by the often severe haemodynamic and metabolic consequences of the pulmonary infection. It is moreover in this age group that the prognosis is worst, mortality according to some statistics [8] reaching 50 % or more.

In the long term the prognosis is made worse by the appearance of severe pulmonary sequellae, such as broncho-pulmonary dysplasia seen especially in the premature infant and occasionally with viral pneumopathies from maternal contamination.

TREATMENT

It is not intended to discuss here the details of the treatment of infection, acute respiratory insufficiency, collapse and of the general state, which are largely dealt with in other chapters of this book.

It is necessary however to underline certain points:

— Antibiotic therapy should be initiated as soon as a diagnosis of pulmonary infection is suspected; using broad spectrum antibiotic coverage and readily discontinued if a viral origin of the infection is certain (which is possible) or modified once the organism has been isolated and bacteriologically identified.

— Maintainance of vital function is all important at all times justifying transfer to an intensive care unit.

— Maintainance of pulmonary function, if necessary by intermittent positive pressure ventilation or with continuous positive pressure, adapted to the low weight neonate. With regard to this problem, the extreme bronchio-alveolar fragility of very premature lungs, especially during *viral infections* (Fig. III-54) should be underlined. It is therefore important to have at ones disposal equipment, allowing the very exact modification of the maximum inspiratory pressure, inspiration time, I/E relationship as well as the usual necessities such as frequency and the fraction of inspired oxygen.

Respiratory physiotherapy is desirable during the acute phase, during intubation, and following extubation; to avoid congestion and ventilatory problems, to prevent inequalities of lung perfusion and to aid as far as possible the ventilation-perfusion relationship.

— Maintainance of metabolic constancy, via a parenteral infusion with a constant turnover. The gravity of the general condition, especially in the premature infant, usually forbids enteral alimentation, often for several days, hence the necessity to resort to parenteral nutrition frequently adapted to cover any special metabolic problem, and varying according to the seriousness of the illness.

CONCLUSION

Neonatal pulmonary infection remains a frequent cause of neonatal illness. Although it is difficult to put an exact figure on the incidence of viral pulmonary infections, it represents an important part of this pathology. Bacterial infections either by maternal contamination, or by postnatal contamination, remain worrying despite therapeutic advances.

There is however the possibility of prevention, allowing for early detection and treatment of maternal infection during pregnancy while at the same time avoiding unnecessary prophylactic antibiotic therapy after birth. There should be adherence to strict hygiene in the vicinity of all neonates, but particularly premature infants and other neonates at risk.

REFERENCES

[1] ABLOW (R. C.), DRISCOLL (S. G.), EFFMAN (E. L.) et al. — A comparison of early-onset group B streptococcal neonatal infection and the respiratory distress syndrom of the newborn. *N. Engl. J. Med., 294*, 65-70, 1976.

[2] AMIEL-TISON (C.), PILLA GROSSI (S.), HENRION (R.). — Infection bactérienne néo-natale par contamination materno-fœtale, 67 cas. *J. Gynéc. Obstét. Biol. Reprod., 9*, 479-487, 1980.

[3] COUCHARD (M.), BOMSEL (F.). — Infection of the newborn lung. *Clinical Practice in Pediatric Radiology.* Vol. 2: The respiratory system. J. LEFEBVRE, J. KAUFMANN ed., Masson Publishing Inc. (USA), New York, 174-182, 1979.

[4] COUVREUR (J.), GRIMFELD (A.), LEMOING (G.) et al. — Une fœtopathie « oubliée » : la tuberculose congénitale cinq observations récentes. *Rev. Pédiat., 12*, 487-496, 1976.

[5] CRAMBLETT (H. G.), HAYNES (R. E.), AZIMI (P. H.) et al. — Nosocomial infection with ECHO virus type II in handicapped and premature infants. *Pediatrics, 51*, 603-607, 1973.

[6] EB (F.), ORFILA (J.). — État actuel du diagnostic biologique des chlamydiases. *Bull. Inst. Pasteur, 76*, 247, 1978.

[7] FEDRICK (J.), BUTLER (N. R.). — Certain causes of neonatal death. III. Pulmonary infection (a). Clinical factors. *Biologia neonat., 17*, 458-471, 1971.

[8] FESSARD (Cl.), LEROY (J. D.), MULLER (C.), JORAM (A.). — L'antibiothérapie de dissuasion : essai de limitation chez le nouveau-né de poids inférieur ou égal à 2 500 g. *Rev. Pédiat., 24*, 459-464, 1978.

[9] FINUCANE (K. E.), COLEBATCH (H. J. H.), ROBERTSON (M. R.), GANDEVIA (B. H.). — The mecanism of respiratory failure in a patient with viral pneumonia. *Am. Rev. Resp. Dis., 101*, 949-958, 1970.

[10] FRICKER (H.), MUHLETHALER (J. P.), KRECH (U.). — *Fatal prenataly acquired mumps infection in a newborn.* VIth Congress of European Perinatal Medicine. Vienne, 1978 (Abstract 293).

[11] FROMMEL (G. T.), ROTHENBERG (R.), WANG (S.) et al. — Chlamydial infection of mothers and their infants. *J. Pediatr., 95*, 28-32, 1979.

[12] GAMARRA (E. DE). — Communication personnelle.

[13] GOSSELIN (O.). — *Contribution à l'étude de l'invasion des organismes maternel et fœtal par les microbes des voies génitales inférieures au cours du travail.* Vaillant-Carmanni, S. A. Liège, 1945.

[14] HALL (C. B.), KOPELMAN (A. E.), DOUGLAS (R. G.) et al. — Neonatal respiratory syncitial viral infection. *N. Engl. J. Med., 300*, 393-396, 1979.

[15] HAMMERSCHLAG (M. R.), ANDERKA (M.), SEMINE (D. Z.) et al. — Prospective study of maternal and

infantile infection with *Chlamydia trachomatis*. *Pediatrics*, *64*, 142-148, 1979.

[16] HENRION (R.), RELIER (J. P.), PAUL (G.). — *Conduite à tenir devant une infection materno-fœtale. Mises à jour en gynécologie et obstétrique*. IIIes journées nationales du collège des gynécologues et obstétriciens français. Éd. Vigot, Paris, 47-82, 1979.

[17] JACOB (J.), EDWARDS (D.), GLUCK (L.). — Early onset sepsis and pneumonia observed as respiratory distress syndrom. *Am. J. Dis. Child.*, *134*, 766-768, 1980.

[18] JOSHI (U.), ESCOBAR (M.), STEWART (L.), BATES (R.). — Fatal influenza as viral pneumonia in a newborn. infant. *Am. J. Dis. Child.*, *126*, 829-840, 1973.

[19] LAROCHE (J. Cl). — *Developmental pathology of the neonate*. Excerpta Medica, Elsevier, Amsterdam, 525, 1977.

[20] LETAN VINH, LEBON (P.), ROUSSET, HUAULT (G.). — Pneumonie mortelle à adénovirus du nouveau-né. *Ann. Pédiat.*, *25*, 35-39, 1978.

[21] MACGREGOR (A. R.). — Pneumonia in the newborn. *Arch. Dis. Child.*, *14*, 323-335, 1939.

[22] MINTZ (L.), BALLARD (R.), SNIDERMAN (S.) *et al*. — Nosocomial respiratory syncytial virus infections in an intensive care nursery: rapid diagnostic by direct immunofluorescence. *Pediatrics*, *64*, 149-153, 1979.

[23] MOORE (T. C.), BATTERSBY (J. S.), STANLEY (J.). — Pulmonary abscess in infancy and childood: report of 18 cases. *Ann. Surg.*, *151*, 216-220, 1960.

[24] PENNER (D. W.), McINNES (A. L.). — Intra-uterine and neonatal pneumonia. *Am. J. Obstet. Gynecol.*, *69*, 147-168, 1955.

[25] RELIER (J. P.), HELFFER (L.), LARROCHE (J.-Cl). — Approach to materno-fetal contamination in a neonatal intensive care unit. *Paediatrician*, *5*, 278-291, 1976.

[26] RELIER (J. P.), DAVIT (N.), CORRÉA-FILHO (L.), JACQUOTOT (Ch.), TORDET (C.). — Maturation pulmonaire post-natale. VIIes Journées Nationales de néonatologie, Paris, 77-78, 20-22 mai 1977.

[27] SAUNDERS (B. S.), MERRITT (T. A.), KIRKPATRICK (E.), GLUCK (L.). — Group B streptococci in the newborn. *Lancet*, *1*, 1053, 1977.

[28] SCARPELLI (E. M.). — *The surfactant system of the lung*. Lea and Febiger, Philadelphia, 269, 1968.

[29] SIEGEL (J. D.), McCRACKEN (G. H.). — Neonatal lung abscess. A report of 6 cases. *Am. J. Dis. Child.*, *133*, 947-949, 1979.

[30] SILBERMAN (O.). — Über septische Pneumonie der Neugeboren und Säuglinge. *Deutsche Arch. Klin. Med.*, *34*, 334-351, 1884.

[31] SPEERT (D. S.), MUNSON (D.), MITCHELL (C.) *et al*. — *Mycobacterium chelonei* septicemia in a premature infant. *J. Pediatr.*, *96*, 681-683, 1980.

[32] STRANG (L. B.). — *Neonatal respiration. Physiological and clinical studies*. Blackwell Scientific Publications, Oxford, 316, 1977.

[33] TAYLOR (F. B.), ABRAMS (M. F.). — Effect of surface active lipoprotein on clotting and fibrinolysis and of fibrinogen on surface tension of surface active lipoprotein. *Am. J. Med.*, *40*, 346-350, 1966.

[34] THOMAS (S. A.), HARRIMAN (B. B.), KMIECIK (J. E.). — Pulmonary surfactant in lung of patients with desquamative interstitial pneumonia. *Am. Rev. Resp. Dis.*, *101*, 967-968, 1970.

[35] VASMANT (D.), BERGER (J. P.), LASFARGUES (G.). — Infection pulmonaire néo-natale à *Chlamydia trachomatis*. *Arch. Fr. Pédiatr.*, *37*, 193-195, 1980.

[36] VESSAL (K.), POST (C.), DUTZ (W.), BANDARIZADEH (B.). — Roentgenologic changes in infantile *Pneumocysti carinii* pneumonia. *Am. J. Roentgenol. Rad. Ther. Nucl. Med.*, *120*, 254-260, 1974.

22

Intrathoracic air-block syndromes

P. MONIN and F. PLENAT

INTRODUCTION

Intrathoracic air-block syndromes occur frequently in the neonate [2, 7, 54, 57]. They are complications of respiratory distress in the newborn and their severity is related to the induced disturbances of pulmonary mechanics and haemodynamics.

INCIDENCE. CLASSIFICATION

Among the intrathoracic air-block syndromes 4 types can be distinguished:

— interstitial emphysema; an extravasation originating in the connective tissue of the peribroncho-vascular sheaths, the interlobular septae and the visceral pleura;

— pneumothorax; air accumulated in one part or the totality of the space located between the parietal and visceral pleura;

— pneumomediastinum; a collection of air which dissects the mediastinal structures;

— pneumopericardium; an extravasation in the space between the two layers of the pericardium.

Interstitial emphysema and pneumothorax are the most frequently observed. When present, the other air block syndromes are generally associated with them [57]. Their frequency differs according to the selection of babies in newborn intensive care units, the quality of the radiographic equipment, the incidence of resuscitation maneuvers and the training of the personnel involved [2, 7, 32, 45, 58]. The importance of interstitial emphysema, initially described by Laennec [38] has been recognized since neonatal resuscitation began. Radiologically described since 1919 [6], the characteristics of the intrapulmonary air cavities were detailed a few years later by Miller [48]. In the neonate, the first description was given by Guillot [25]. The first pathological studies were reported in 1964 [60]. At present, several descriptive terms have been proposed for interstitial emphysema: intralobular emphysema [38], subpleural emphysema [40], alveolar rupture syndrome [16], air block syndrome [44].

To avoid any confusion with dystrophic emphysema of the adult, the term interstitial pulmonary pneumatosis has been proposed [57]. Two topographic types, sometimes associated, are described. In the first, interstitial intrapulmonary pneumatosis, the air is trapped in the interlobular septae and broncho-vascular sheaths (Fig. III-55). In the second, intrapleural pneumatosis, the air collections develop into the thickness of the visceral pleura (Fig. III-56). Intrapulmonary pneumatosis is observed in 6 %

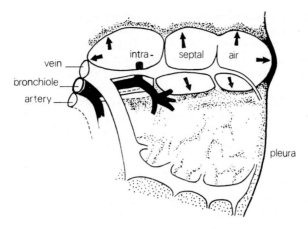

FIG. III-55. — *Schematic drawing of intrapulmonary pneumatosis* (PLENAT et al. [57]).

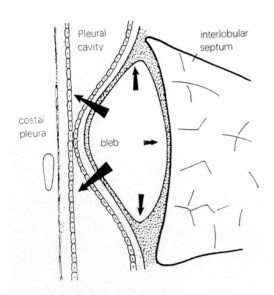

FIG. III-56. — *Schematic drawing of intrapleural pneumatosis.*

PATHOGENESIS

The development of intrathoracic air block syndromes is aided by perinatal events. The history often reveals prematurity which is an essential cause of the development of HMD, birth asphyxia associated with amniotic fluid or meconium aspiration, a delay in lung fluid resorption, resuscitation maneuvers in the delivery room and/or cesarean section [68]. To understand the mechanism involved in air space ruptures, and the development of air block syndromes, it is important to appreciate the physiology of the lungs during the perinatal period, and to correctly appreciate both the histologic structure of the lungs of the newborn, and the lesions observed in the course of HMD.

Mechanisms involved in air space rupture

of non malformative respiratory distress [57]. However this frequency is probably under-estimated. The intrapulmonary and intrapleural types occur with a similar incidence. The intrapulmonary form is more frequent in the premature and the intrapleural form occurs predominantly in full term neonates. Initially described by Ruge in 1878, pneumothorax in the neonate is usually a complication of interstitial emphysema. The frequency of pneumothorax reported in the literature is nearly 1 % of live births [18, 51, 68] and only 0.1 % for symptomatic forms. In some studies a greater incidence in boys is reported.

Except for very rare etiologies such as bronchial perforation by a nasotracheal tube, lung injury induced by rib fracture or Boerhave's syndrome (spontaneous rupture of the oesophagus) [1, 28, 73] the mechanism for air block syndrome is a single or multiple rupture of the terminal air spaces [57]. The rupture is secondary to a localized excess pressure in one or several terminal air spaces in one segment, lobe, or in both lungs. The risk of rupture is increased in case of focal or disseminated cell or tissue injuries, which are often associated. High pressure plays a role by inducing an overdistension of the lung parenchyma. These mechanisms occur in many different clinical situations. The occurence immediately at birth of numerous air block syndromes suggests a precocious rupture during the first inspiration [16]. During the first inspiration, the transpulmonary pressure reaches 40 cm H_2O and can sometimes be above 100 cm H_2O [34].

The compression of the thorax in the birth canal, enhances the development of these high pressures, the inspiratory muscles being thus placed in a favourable mechanical situation. Subsequently the establishment of the functional residual capacity avoids the necessity of the newborn developing transpulmonary pressures above 30 cm H_2O except in cases of lung disease with low lung compliance.

Lung aeration is often irregular. Ventilation inequalities may induce alveolar rupture. This risk is mainly related to an absence of collateral ventilation in the newborn. The anatomical structures involved are not yet developed (interalveolar and interbronchoalveolar pathways) [37, 44]. Therefore any focal or generalized excess pressure in the airways induces an overdistension of the parenchyma which increases the risk of rupture. The high pressure itself may have different origins. More often it is a partial bronchiolar obstruction secondary to pneumonia, amniotic fluid aspiration, persistance of lung liquid, etc. The risk of rupture is also increased by artificial ventilation [5, 7, 75]. The positive pressure techniques are the most dangerous especially if end expiratory pressure is also used. Assisted ventilation by pericorporeal depression does not significantly increase the risk of air block syndromes [50]. The major factor in the development of these disorders is the mean airways pressure value. It depends on insufflation pressure, end expiratory pressure and the inspiration/expiration ratio. The risk related to assisted ventilation increases when lung compliance improves during the course of the respiratory distress.

The air blocks are located on the right side in 2/3 of the cases. They occur bilaterally in 15 to 20 % of the cases [7, 31]. This distribution is related to the anatomical disposition of the bronchial tree. The right lung is more exposed to barotrauma, and the right main stem bronchus to the repeated trauma of endo-bronchial aspiration [1, 73].

Mechanisms for the development of air-block syndromes

As soon as the most distal air spaces of the secondary lobules are ruptured the air penetrates into the interstitium (interlobular septum, peribronchovascular sheaths) where there is negative pressure.

In the premature the interstitial tissue is thick and loose. A significant volume of gas can be collected inside without causing excessive pressure. In contrast, in full term infants, the interstitium is more dense. The air cannot accumulate inside and diffuses towards the pleura or the mediastinum. The relative lack of cohesion of the different layers of the conjunctive-adipose tissue of the mediastinum explains the facility and rapidity of the development of important air collections. The differences in histological structure of the interstitium according to its maturation explains the higher incidence of intrapulmonary pneumatosis in the premature and of pleural pneumatosis in full term infants.

Pneumothorax is only rarely related to the destruction of the most distal subpleural air spaces by infectious necrosis or the rupture of a malformative or acquired parenchymatous bubble, or of the peripheral air space of a distended subpleural lobule. Usually it is produced by the rupture of an intrapulmonary or pleural bubble directly into the pleural cavity. Three facts oppose the Macklin hypothesis [44] according to which the air penetrates in the mediastinum first before reaching the pleural cavity: the rare direct occurrence of pneumotosis bubbles bursting into the pleural cavity (Fig. III-57).

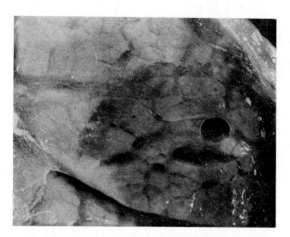

FIG. III-57. — *Rupture of a bubble of intrapulmonary pneumatosis in the pleural cavity.*

The low frequency of pneumomediastinum associated with pneumothoraces and its rarity at autopsies of infants dead from tension pneumothorax; the low incidence of bilateral pneumothorax despite the absence of anatomical delimitation of the pneumomediastinum. Although radiologically recognized in only 50 % of the cases, interstitial pneumatosis is probably a necessary intermediate step for pneumothorax [57]. The air in the peribroncho-vascular sheaths and in the interlobular septae may remain only for a very short period of time particularly in full term infants; bubbles of small volume are not consistently recognized.

Pneumomediastinum is usually related to the extension of an intrapulmonary pneumatosis, less frequently, to the rupture or perforation of the trachea, the main stem bronchi or the oesophagus. From the mediastinum the air may reach up into the subcutaneous spaces of the neck (subcutaneous emphysema) or down following the triangular ligaments and peri-œsophageal conjunctive sheaths, the retroperitoneal space and sometimes the intestinal wall [57]. Contrary to what is observed in the adult, cervical subcutaneous emphysema and pneumomediastinum are rarely associated.

The mechanism for the development of the pneumopericardium is not well established. In the most documented studies, pneumopericardium is constantly associated with interstitial emphysema or pneumomediastinum [46]. Some observations indicate that the air penetrates the pericardial serous membrane around the great vessels of the heart at the level of the reflection. This fact is inconstant [67]. Direct penetration of air into the pericardial cavity related to rupture of the membraneous part of the trachea has been reported in one case [42].

Gaseous embolism is rare. Its mechanism is not yet known. The eruption of interstitial air into the pulmonary lymphatic vessels could explain this embolism because these vessels drain towards the superior vena cava. However if this hypothesis is true, gaseous embolism should be much more frequently observed than it is [17, 40].

DIAGNOSIS

The diagnosis of the air block syndrome is assessed by anatomical, radiological and clinical findings. Different entities can be separated. To distinguish between them radiological techniques must be perfect. The equipment used must allow for very short exposures (1/100 of second). The thoracic films are taken during deep inspiration (with an automatic system) but in some cases, the contrast between abnormal air collections and the parenchyma can be increased during expiration [57]. Some films (lateral, lateral with horizontal beam, etc.) are useful to show images not visible on the antero-posterior films taken with vertical X-rays.

Interstitial pneumatosis.

Acute intrapulmonary interstitial pneumatosis (AIIP). — This is seen in prematures with hyaline membrane disease. It is characterized by circular or oval gaseous collections generally uniform and of a moderate size (3 to 8 mm) (Fig. III-58 *a*), developed in the interlobular septae and the peribronchovascular sheaths. These bubbles separate the interlobular planes and dissect the perilobular veins which remain in contact with the lobules only through their collateral branches (Fig. III-58 *b*). The extent of the lesions is variable, from the isolated micro bubble to the dissection of several segments of the lobes of one or two lungs. Frequently the bubbles are grouped together in chains along the bronchial tree from the hilum towards the peripheral areas. Their walls, often fragmented are composed of compressed collagen and connective tissue, coming from the interlobular septae or from the more dense connective tissue of the peribronchovascular sheaths. Pieces of endothelium or of lymphatic valves are also incorporated in their walls [12]. The interstitial gases are not exclusively or preferentially lymphatic and AIIP is not the equivalent of arterial or venous gaseous embolism. The parenchyma usually shows signs of HMD. AIIP occurs within the first hours of life; less frequently within the first days. It has no specific clinical signs other than that of the associated respiratory disorder [36, 57]. Isolated AIIP is generally not responsible for acute respiratory deterioration. In prolonged forms, it can be associated with thoracic overdistension.

Radiological recognition of interstitial air depends on the size of the gaseous collections and necessitates gradient opacity of X-rays between interstitial air and adjacent lung tissue. These conditions are achieved when the gaseous collection is voluminous and the lung tissue is compressed or presents signs of associated disease. One observes clear linear pictures, crossing each other and separating dense opacities with well defined limits and frequently irregular contours. The opacities are the secondary lobules dissected and compressed by the interstitial air. Clear circular pictures of greater size, pear shaped and oriented towards the hilum are sometimes observed when the air is collected in an intersegmentary fashion. To sum up, AIIP is a clear interstitial syndrome, a mirror image of the dense interstitial radiological syndrome observed in pulmonary fibrosis. The distribution of AIIP lesions is variable, they can be localized in only one segment, in one or several lobes or in the whole lung. The most severe localized forms induce a mediastinal shift. The

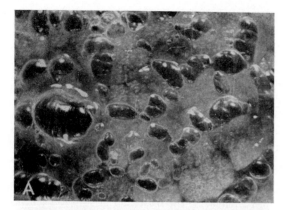

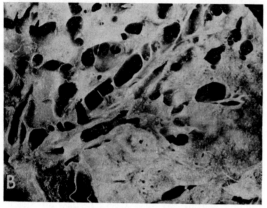

FIG. III-58. — *Intrapulmonary pneumatosis.*

a) Numerous air cavities bulging under the visceral pleura at the level of interlobular septae, *b*) note the dissection of the segmental venous sheaths.

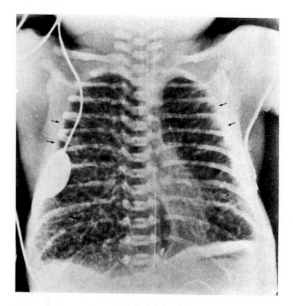

FIG. III-59. — *Bilateral intrapulmonary pneumatosis: note the mediastinal compression, the transmediastinal parenchymatous hernia, the horizontalization of the ribs and the widening of the intercostal spaces.*

bilateral diffuse forms are responsible for an intra-thoracic hyperpressure syndrome which is clinically characterized by a distension of the thorax and radiologically by a horizontalization of the ribs, an eversion of the diaphragm and a narrowing of the radiological pattern of the mediastinum (Fig. III-59). The diagnosis of AIIP is difficult in its moderate form when the linear clear pictures originating from the hilum can be confused with an air bronchogram or normal parenchyma, situated between 2 parallel vessels. In these cases the diagnosis is based on the discovery of clear linear peripheral pictures of areas where air bronchograms cannot exist and on the variations of images on exposures taken in rapid succession. The recognition of these limited forms makes it possible to anticipate the development, sooner or later, of other intrathoracic air block syndromes (pneumothorax, pneumo-mediastinum...) which are present in more than 60 % of the cases of acute interstitial intrapulmonary

pneumatosis. The evolution of AIIP is severe and its prognosis is poor. Among 19 cases of AIIP developing during the course of non malformative respiratory distress, 16 deaths occured mostly within the first 24 hours [57]. The improvement in resuscitation techniques has however reduced the mortality rate and when the infants survive, the air collections disappear. When study of the interstitial tissue is possible, it shows a normal anatomical aspect.

Persistent localized or diffuse interstitial pneumatosis. — These are characterized from a clinical point of view by a slow evolution and from a pathological point of view by the appearance, around the abnormal air cavities, of an inflammatory macrophagic reaction similar to that observed in the case of a foreign body resorption. The persistence of the pneumatosis and the inflammatory reaction are not explained. We distinguish localized and diffused forms.

The localized forms are the most frequent. About 20 cases have been reported since 1970. Pathological findings are abnormal gaseous cavities of different size often greater than in AIIP sometimes reaching 8 cm. These are surrounded by a more or less thick limit of collagenous fibrosis with irregular zones of hemosiderin, where macrophages and numerous giant multinuclear cells can be observed [8, 21, 76].

Bronchopulmonary dysplasia is rarely associated. The circumstances of the development of this form of pneumatosis are not significantly different from those leading to AIIP. The persistant localized forms are characterized by the duration of their course, the variable diameter, often large, of the very clear pulmonary pictures responsible for a multicystic aspect on X-rays and by poor clinical tolerance especially when the lesions induce intrathoracic compression with a mediastinal shift. The extrapulmonary intrathoracic air block syndrome is associated with persistent interstitial pneumatosis in more than 50 % of the cases. The improvement in the treatment (surgical or conservative) gives a survival rate in 70 % of the cases at the moment. This radiological and clinical pattern is sometimes difficult to distinguish from certain adenomatoid pulmonary malformations. The prolonged and diffuse forms where the two lungs in their totality are involved, are rarer ($\simeq$ 100 observations). In addition to the prolonged course and the presence of an inflammatory reaction around the abnormal gaseous cavities they are characterized by the small size of the interstitial gaseous collection and the high incidence of an associated bronchopulmonary dysplasia, which makes the radiological diagnosis between these two conditions difficult. Pneumothorax occurs in more than 75 % of the cases, however even when unilateral it rarely induces a mediastinal shift. The prognosis is very poor and in all the cases published, the infant died.

Pleural pneumatosis. — In this form, the pleura is dissociated over a more or less extended area by a gaseous collection which bulges into the pleural cavity (Fig. III-56). This lesion is described in the literature as a pneumatocele, pseudocyst, subpleural emphysema, bleb [48]. The diameter of the bubble varies from several mm to over 5 cm [24]. These gaseous collections are more frequent and more important at the level of the mediastinal pleura, in the hilum or along the segmentary or lobar veins (Fig. III-60). The adjacent parenchyma is not compressed; but the pleural pneumatosis can be associated with intrapulmonary pneumatosis. The etiologic circumstances are different. Pleural pneumatosis occurs specifically in full term infants with perinatal asphyxia. There is often an amniotic or meconium inhalation of variable intensity, less frequently a delay in pulmonary fluid resorption. In pleural pneumatosis, X-rays show clear pictures of various shapes and localizations. Their identification depends on the volume of the gaseous collection and on the radiological density of the adjacent parenchyma. If the parenchyma is properly

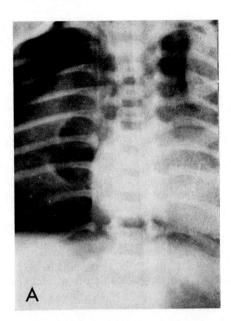

Fig. III-60. — *Intrapleural pneumatosis:* voluminous bleb located in the visceral pleura just next to the mediastinal pleura.

aerated (because it is normal) the very small bubbles are not visible. It is moreover difficult to detail the pleural topography of these lesions. However, the blebs are usually located in the visceral pleura of the mediastinal side of the lungs and appear radiologically in contact with the mediastinum. Without any other sign of pneumomediastinum, the observation of air collections in these areas implies a pleural localization. In the case of a significant associated pneumothorax, the internal surface of the displaced lung becomes oriented towards the front outer side and the abnormal air cavities are projected in the middle of the lung parenchyma (Fig. III-60). The development of a clear picture or its prolongation in an interlobar fissure also points to pleural localization. Pleural pneumatosis is by itself asymptomatic but it is often associated with other intrathoracic air blocks which are extrapulmonary and symptomatic. It can be a premonitory radiological sign. The mortality in this type of pneumatosis is low.

Pneumothorax. — The clinical signs of pneumothorax are variable. The physical signs usually occur after a more or less long period of functional disturbances. Grunting and tachypnea are frequent but not specific [2, 7, 29, 81].

In serious pneumothorax, the tachypnea turns into bradypnea. Persistent or intermittent cyanosis rapidly develops during crying or gavage feedings. The appearance of apnea and bradycardia during treatment are suspicious signs.

Physical signs are more easily found for more severe pneumothoraces. The thorax is distended and asymetric when, facing the incubator one looks at the baby placed in a strictly supine position [7, 29, 45]. The heart sounds are displaced as a result of mediastinal displacement. This shift is absent in the case of bilateral pneumothorax. On the side of the air block [24, 58], the vascular flow murmur is reduced or absent. When the air collection is important, there is right cardiac failure with hepato-megaly and a drop in systemic arterial pressure. In some cases the pneumothorax is revealed by acute clinical deterioration indicating the rapid development of a tension pneumothorax which can cause death through cardiac failure. Strict observation of these clinical parameters does not always allow for rapid and early diagnosis of pneu-mothorax [54]. The drop in systemic arterial pressure or the occurence of bradycardia in infants with interstitial emphysema seems particularly sug-gestive [9]. The great overlap of the clinical signs of pneumothorax, between the asymptomatic ones and those with cardiac arrest due to abrupt intra-thoracic hyperpressure, can be the origin of a dangerous delay in diagnosis.

Only X-ray can confirm the diagnosis. The presence of air in the pleural space separates the visceral and parietal layers of the pleura. The lung is away from the thoracic wall and more or less retracted towards the hilum. The limit of the lung is covered by the visceral pleura and is visible as a denser line. The absence of trabeculations between the thorax wall and the lung limit is not always clearly seen except in the case of pulmonary disease which is responsible for an increase in the density of the parenchyma. In some cases, a skinfold may be identical to the picture provided by the lung limit, however, in this case, the image formed usually cuts across the diaphragm. Often, a small gaseous collection which accumulates behind the anterior wall of the diaphragm only shows on X-rays as a difference in the density of the two lung fields [7, 56]. This situation observed in nearly 50 % of the pneu-mothoraces shows how imperative is the use of a lateral film with the baby in the supine position and a horizontal beam. This is the only way of showing a retrosternal collection. On these lateral films, it is possible to see the two separated layers of the pleura. In the case of serious pneumothorax, X-rays show the signs of high intrathoracic pressure, similar to those observed in the severe forms of interstitial emphysema: contralateral mediastinal shift, eversion

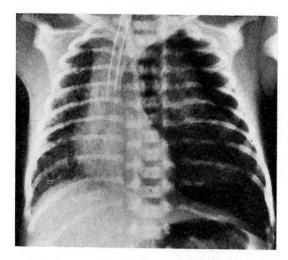

Fig. III-61. — *Left tension pneumothorax.* Note the mediastinal shift and the eversion of the diaphragm.

and lowering of the diaphragm, widening of the intercostal spaces, horizontalisation of the ribs (Fig. III-61). In the case of bilateral tension pneu-mothorax there is frequently a microcardia because of a compression of the heart without any mediastinal shift (Fig. III-62).

When it is difficult to obtain an X-ray rapidly [37], thoracic transillumination may permit the diagnosis. This technique gives positive results only for severe

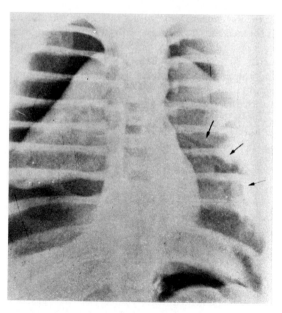

Fig. III-62. — *Bilateral tension pneumothorax.* Note the microcardia.

pneumothoraces and allows for rapid control of their disappearance following aspiration. The occurrence of acute changes in thoracic impedence also suggests the development of pneumothorax [47, 53]. Any unexplained change in the amplitude of the thoracic impedence should lead to a chest X-ray.

Pneumomediastinum. — A pneumomediastinum dissociates all the mediastinal structures. When it is serious (Fig. III-63) one or two thymic lobes can be separated and shifted upwards giving the characteristic aspect of a spinnaker sail [49].

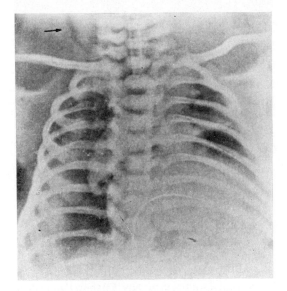

Fig. III-63. — *Pneumomediastinum.* "Spinnaker sail" appearance.

From the mediastinum, the air can diffuse into the adipose cellular spaces with the development of cervical subcutaneous emphysema. In some cases, a pneumomediastinum may induce dextrorotation of the heart [22]. When the pneumomediastinum is serious, signs of intrathoracic hyperpressure may occur with microcardia as in the case of tension pneumothorax.

Pneumopericardium. — Pneumopericardium may, if it is serious, be responsible for cardiac tamponade which associates cardiovascular shock, an increase in venous pressure and hepatomegaly. Radiologically, it is represented by a clear image (Fig. III-64) located in the pericardial sac. Major attention should be paid to the visualization of the inferior limit of the heart

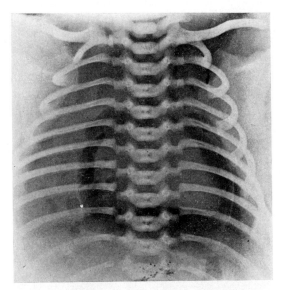

Fig. III-64. — *Pneumopericardium.* Note the translucent image surrounding the heart.

and the diaphragm and the line describing the air collection. The occurence of microvoltage on the EKG suggests the diagnosis.

PHYSIOPATHOLOGY

Interstitial pneumatosis

The pathophysiological consequences of pulmonary pneumatosis differ with the different types. In AIIP, pathological studies usually show important phenomena of lobular compression by the abnormal gaseous cavities. If the lesions are widespread it is logical to consider ventilatory consequences as demonstrated by Brook, using xenon scintigraphy, showing the absence of ventilation in abnormal areas [11].

The vascular consequences are important and the venous circulation is seriously involved. The areas involved with AIIP are not opacified by barium sulfate injection in the pulmonary veins. Areas of compression of perilobular veins or even larger veins are histologically patent. The arterial consequences are mainly a problem of microvascularization. There is no injection of peripheral divisions and rarely any evidence of cup shaped blockade (Fig. III-65) of the more proximal ramifications. However the compression is rarely strong enough to prevent arterial filling before the 6th to the 10th generation [57]. In the cases studied, the arterial

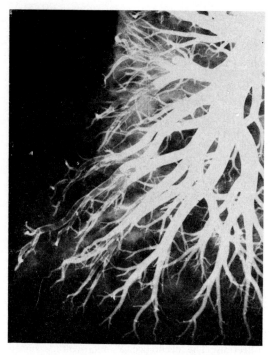
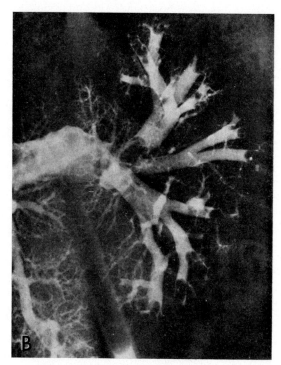

Fig. III-65. — *Arterial vascularisation in intrapulmonary pneumatosis.*
(*a*) Distal ramifications have disappeared.
(*b*) Aspects of cup shaped blockade (see text).

bronchial circulation was normal. Angiography and haemodynamic studies in experimental alveolar rupture syndromes carried out in animals show injuries too different from those observed in the newborn to allow a direct transfer to human pathology [55] without discussion. The occurrence of disturbances in the oxygen alveolar-arterial gradient before and after the development of interstitial pneumatosis during the course of hyaline membrane disease was not demonstrated [12]. This fact confirms the pathological findings which show an absence of vascularization in the areas where ventilation is excluded. Finally, it is realistic to consider the general effect of AIIP on vascular resistance and pulmonary blood flow. Prolonged pulmonary pneumatosis has not been studied. No intrapulmonary vascular consequences related to pleural pneumatosis have been demonstrated despite the existence of large blebs around the pulmonary veins of the mediastinal pleura [57].

Pneumothorax
and pneumomediastinum

The disturbances related to pneumothorax do not parallel its radiological appearance.

Tachypnea is always present [26]. It is the result of the inspiratory reflex of Hering and Breuer induced by lung deflation as demonstrated by its disappearance following vagatomy in the animal [10, 74]. Experimental studies in rabbits [52] show that tachypnea initially related directly to lung deflation is rapidly followed by bradypnea in more serious pneumothoraces as observed clinically in tension pneumothoraces. The tidal volume is reduced proportionnally to the importance of the air collection. The ventilation, initially slightly increased because of the tachypnea, decreases progressively. The intrapleural pressure rises with the gaseous collection and the difference between inspiratory and expiratory pleural pressures is reduced. When intrapleural pressure is above the barometric pressure, there is a tension pneumothorax.

The haemodynamic disturbances due to the pneumothorax and/or mediastinum are important (Fig. III-66). In animal studies, there is a close correlation between cardiac output, the size of the collection and the arterial systemic pressure; this is not significantly affected by collections of mild degree and drops only with the larger ones. The elevation of central venous pressure experimentally demonstrated is the origin of the fall in

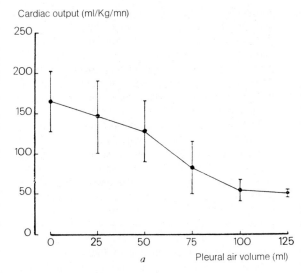

Cardiac output (ml/Kg/mn)

a Pleural air volume (ml)

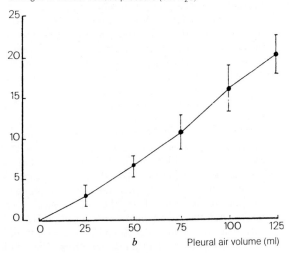

Changes in central venous pressure (cm H$_2$0)

b Pleural air volume (ml)

FIG. III-66. — *Hemodynamic changes during experimental pneumothorax in the rabbit.*

(*a*) Cardiac output (ml/kg/min);
(*b*) changes in central venous pressure (cm H$_2$O).

cardiac output through a reduction of the systemic venous return [52, 61, 63, 65]. The rise in pulmonary resistance, the displacement of the mediastinal structures and the elevation of intrapleural pressure act together to increase central venous pressure [13, 63, 64]. The changes in pulmonary resistance occurring with a pneumothorax are difficult to appreciate and depend largely on the associated lung disease. Thus slight improvement may occur when a pneumothorax develops from significant interstitial emphysema because of a reduction in the

interstitial abnormalities themselves. This supports the observed differences between the clinical and radiological signs of these air blocks. When the lung is stiff, a mediastinal shift may occur without any significant alveolar collapse and be responsible for severe haemodynamic disturbances. Moreover, the compression of the contralateral lung jeopardizes its ventilation and perfusion [16]. Finally, the reduction in cardiac output is the result of these events all of which are responsible for an increase in pulmonary vascular resistance [52].

Hypoxia, acidosis and hypercapnia resulting from ventilatory and haemodynamic disturbances also increase pulmonary resistance. When severe respiratory distress is present, the effect of the pneumothorax is greater than with a normal lung. The pneumomediastinum can also be responsible for an intrathoracic hyperpressure with pulmonary collapse and induce ventilatory and haemodynamic disturbances similar to those observed with a pneumothorax. These hemodynamic changes may alter cerebral blood flow [76].

Pneumopericardium

In pneumopericardium, the high pressure within the pericardial sac decreases the diastolic filling of the heart and reduces the systolic volume and the cardiac output. The venous return decreases and stasis occurs. These haemodynamic disturbances are not directly related to an elevation of pulmonary vascular resistance such as occurs in pneumothorax and pneumomediastinum.

TREATMENT

The therapy of air blocks depends on the type; the results are related to the rapidity of the diagnosis.

Treatment of interstitial emphysema

This is firstly based on prevention. In any infant presenting a risk of interstitial emphysema, any added resistance to air flow in the airways should be eliminated by adapted aspirations and physiotherapy. Any iatrogenic hyperpressure should be ruled out particularly by using preset bags with a security system for manual ventilation; as well as by limiting barotrauma and the risk of alveolar rupture by avoiding continuous positive pressure greater than 5 cm H$_2$O, peak pressure above 30 cm H$_2$O and high inspiratory/expiratory ratios. The infant should be adjusted to the respirator. The improvement in assisted ventilation techniques and particularly the introduction of intermittent mandatory ventilation allowing for low frequencies have considerably reduced the incidence of interstitial emphysema [3]. High frequencies also seem to reduce the occurrence of interstitial emphysema and its severity [8].

The position of the tip of the endotracheal tube should be regularly checked to avoid an accidental selective intubation of the right main stem bronchus, which is responsible for hyperpressure in the inferior lobe and exposes it to air space rupture [75].

Along with this preventative care, some curative therapeutics are possible in limited forms. Limited interstitial emphysema causing compression has in rare cases justified a lobectomy of the involved area [21]. Despite the apparent tolerance of this surgery in the newborn, it is important first to attempt conservative management because complete healing is always possible. In the case of limited interstitial emphysema, if signs of compression are present, Leonidas [43] recommends regular instillation of saline with thoracic percussion, drainage and aspiration. He suggests associating these maneuvers with 5 to 10 minutes of assisted ventilation at an FIO_2 of 1.0 to accelerate the resorption of extrabronchopulmonary air. The efficacy of this technique, despite the success reported by its author, remains questionable because, as reported above, the areas with interstitial emphysema are not correctly ventilated and perfused. Other authors have proposed a selective ventilation of the normal lung when only one lung is affected by interstitial emphysema [11]. This technique is effective and leads to healing within days. No treatment is effective in the diffuse bilateral forms. In practice the discovery of interstitial pneumatosis should give rise to an enhancement of the surveillance of the baby, with the setting up of the appropriate devices for an eventual pleural or pericardial drainage procedure. Assisted ventilation with a high frequency and a low tidal volume has been recently proposed [8].

Treatment
of other air block syndromes

Most of the pneumothoraces usually need only close surveillance in an intensive care unit [57]. The respiratory rate and the arterial systemic pressure should be monitored. The arterial pressure can be significantly reduced before pneumothorax or other air block syndrome occurs in infants having interstitial emphysema [9]. Nevertheless, it can also be tran-

sitionally increased when pneumothorax starts to develop. These opposed changes limit the value of this clinical parameter; in the absence of any cardiac output determinations, the central venous pressure could provide an evaluation of the haemodynamic status. The patency of the umbilical vein in the neonatal period makes this measurement theoretically possible.

The resolution of a pneumothorax can also be obtained by exposure to a high FIO_2 (0.8-1) [2, 16]. Oxygen enhances the elimination of nitrogen from blood and tissues by increasing the partial pressure gradient between the air collection and the blood. In animals, the disappearance of a pneumothorax is 6 times faster in pure oxygen. This technique is dangerous and exposes the baby to the risks of hyperoxia and retinopathy. The technique requires strict continuous monitoring of PaO_2.

It is reasonable in the case of pneumothorax, to decide on drainage if the following are present: sudden clinical and/or biological (pH, $PaCO_2$ and PaO_2) deterioration, significant drop in systemic arterial pressure, radiological signs of intrathoracic hyperpressure, rise in central venous pressure and clinical signs of right ventricular failure. The indication is imperative when the pneumothorax occurs during assisted ventilation.

Needle aspiration may give good results but exposes the lung to injury. It is better to use a chest tube with a lateral opening, allowing continuous aspiration. This is introduced through a tiny skin incision in the third or fourth intercostal space in the medial axillary line. It is then pushed towards the inferior third of the sternum with the purpose of placing its tip where the air collects anteriorly when the baby is in a supine position [19, 33]. The insertion of the tube should be technically perfect, performed by well trained operators. The rabbit has been proposed by Henderson as an animal teaching model [30]. The chest tube is then connected to an aspiration set, delivering a suction of -15 to -20 cm of water below barometric pressure. When the pleural air collection has disappeared suction is discontinued and replaced by a simple siphoning tube. After a variable period of time, the tube is clamped for 24 hours during which the possible reappearance of the pneumothorax is evaluated by X-rays. The tube is then removed.

The treatment of the mediastinum is not so easy. With conservative management, in the case of intrathoracic hyperpressure with important haemodynamic disturbance a decompression aspiration can be performed with prudence near the sternum in the 2nd or 3rd intercostal space. In the case of pneumopericardium a decompression aspiration can be performed through the retroxiphoid route or by an anterior route through the 5th intercostal space near the sternum.

Evolution

The evolution of intrathoracic air block syndrome differs with its type. The generalized forms of interstitial emphysema have a poor prognosis. The localized forms are more amenable to different treatments and have a better prognosis. When the evolution is favourable, a complete healing of the lung tissue occurs. However the occurence of interstitial emphysema may be involved in the development of broncho-pulmonary dysplasia.

The mortality related to the pneumothorax and pneumomediastinum depends largely on the nature of the lung disease. Sometimes when the pneumothorax progresses rapidly giving rise to intrathoracic hyperpressure, death may occur very suddenly. Rapidly drained, the pneumothorax is not by itself of poor prognosis.

The overall mortality of symptomatic air block syndromes is of the order of 47 % when interstitial emphysema is considered [54]. For all the air block syndromes observed in a population of neonates, the overall mortality was 0.04 % (5/1,110 live births) [75]. The prognosis of a pneumothorax well drained without any evident lung disease is excellent. In hyaline membrane disease, the pneumothorax significantly increases the mortality rate which rises from 14 % to 30 % [75].

The natural course of pneumopericardium is more difficult to analyse because of the rarity of this type of intrathoracic air block syndrome. Because of the risk of cardiac tamponade, only prompt and effective drainage can provide a favourable outcome

REFERENCES

[1] ANDERSON (K. D.), CHANDRA (R.). — Pneumothorax secondary to perforation of sequential bronchi by suction catheters. J. Pediatr. Surg., 11, 687-695, 1976.

[2] AVERY (M. E.). — The lung and its disorders in the newborn infant. Philadelphia W. B., Saunders Co., 1968.

[3] BARR (P. A.). — Weaning very low birth weight infants from mechanical ventilation using intermittent mandatory ventilation and theophylline. Arch. Dis. Child., 53, 598-600, 1978.

[4] BASHOUR (B. N.), BALFE (J. W.). — Urinary tract anomalies in neonates with spontaneous pneumothorax and/or pneumomediastinum. Pediatrics, Neonatology suppl., 1048-1049, 1977.

[5] BERG (T. J.), PAGTAKHAN (R. D.), REED (M. H.) et al. — Bronchopulmonary dysplasia and lung rupture in hyaline membrane disease. Pediatrics, 55, 51-54, 1975.

[6] BERKLEY (H. K.), COFFEN (T. H.). — Generalized interstitial emphysema and spontaneous pneumothorax. JAMA, 72, 535-538, 1919.

[7] BOCQUETIN (F.), LALLEMAND (D.), HUAULT (G.), TRAN VAN DUC (H.), ROSSIER (A.). — Le pneumothorax du nouveau-né : à propos de 66 observations. Arch. Fr. Pédiatr., 30, 319-339, 1973.

[8] BLAND (R.), KIM (M.), WOODSON (J. L.). — High frequency mechanical ventilation of low birth weight infants with respiratory failure from hyaline membrane disease. Pediat. Res., 11, 531, 1977.

[9] BRAZY (J. E.), BLACKMON (L. R.). — Hypotension and bradycardia associated with air block in the neonate. J. Pediatr., 90, 796-802, 1977.

[10] BREUER (J.). — Self steering of respiration through the nervus vagus. Sitzungbericht der akademie des Wissenschaften. In Wien, 57 part 2, 909-937, 1868. Translated by Ullmann in breathing Ciba Foundation. Hering. Breuer Centenary Symposium. Churchill, London, 365-391, 1970.

[11] BROOKS (J. G.), BUSTAMANTE (S. A.), KOOPS (B. L.) et al. — Selective bronchial intubation for the treatment of severe localized pulmonary interstitial emphysema in newborn infants. J. Pediatr., 91, 648-652, 1977.

[12] BURNARD (E. D.), GRATTAN-SMITH (P.), JOHN (E.). — A radiographic, pathologic and clinical study of interstitial emphysema complicating hyaline membrane disease. In STERN (L.) (ed.), Intensive care in the newborn. New York, Masson, 1976.

[13] BURTON (A. C.), PATEL (D. J.). — Effect on pulmonary vascular resistance of inflation of rabbit lungs. J. Appl. Physiol., 12, 239-246, 1958.

[14] CHABROLLE (J. P.), BRIOUDE (R.), GUÉRIN (J.) et al. — Pneumothorax néonatal et malformation de l'appareil urinaire. Discussion à propos de trois cas. Arch. Fr. Pédiat., 8, 771-782, 1976.

[15] CHASLER (C.). — Pneumothorax and pneumomediastinum in the newborn. Am. J. Roentgenol., 91, 550-559, 1964.

[16] CHERNICK (V.), AVERY (M. E.). — Spontaneous alveolar rupture in newborn infants. Pediatrics, 32, 816-824, 1963.

[17] CHIU (C. J.), GOLDING (M. R.), LINDER (J. B.). — Pulmonary atelectasis in subjects breathing oxygen at sea level or at simulated altitude. J. Appl. Physiol., 21, 828-836, 1966.

[18] DAVIS (C. H.), STEVENS (G. W.). — Value of routine radiographic examinations of the newborn based on a study of 702 consecutive babies. Am. J. Obstet. Gynecol., 20, 73-76, 1930.

[19] DUFFY (B. C.). — Neonatal pneumothorax. A simple drainage device. Anaesthesiology, 31, 403-405, 1976.

[20] EMERY (J. L.). — Interstitial emphysema, pneumothorax and « air-block » in the newborn. Lancet, 1, 405-409, 1956.

[21] FLECHTER (B.), OUTERBRIDGE (E.), YOUSSEFF (S.) et al. — Pulmonary interstitial emphysema in the newborn. J. Canad. Assoc. Radiol., 21, 273-279, 1970.

[22] FRANKEN (E. A.). — Pneumomediastinum in newborn with associated dextroposition of the heart. Am. J. Roentgenol. Radium Ther. Nucl. Med., 109, 252-255, 1970.

[23] GARDNER (M. D.), FERNET (P.). — Etiology of vaginitis emphysematosa. *Am. J. Obstet. Gynecol.*, *88*, 680-694, 1964.

[24] GERBEAUX (J.). — *Pathologie respiratoire de l'enfant.* Paris, Flammarion, 1975.

[25] GUILLOT (N.). Cited by EMERY (J. L.). — Interstitial emphysema, pneumothorax and « air-block » syndrome in the newborn. *Lancet*, *1*, 405-409, 1975.

[26] GUZ (A.), NOBLE (M. I. M.), EISELE (J. H.) *et al.* — The effect of lung deflation on breathing man. *Clin. Sci.*, *40*, 451-461, 1971.

[27] HALL (R.), RHODES (P.). — Pneumothorax and pneumomediastinum in infants with idiopathic respiratory distress syndrome receiving continuous positive airway pressure. *Pediatrics*, *55*, 493-495, 1975.

[28] HARRELL (G. S.), FRIEDLAND (G. W.), DAILY (W. J.) *et al.* — Neonatal Boerhaave's syndrome. *Radiology*, *95*, 665, 1970.

[29] HARRISON (V. C.), HESE (H.), KLEIN (M.). — The significance of grunting in hyaline membrane disease. *Pediatrics*, *41*, 549-559, 1968.

[30] HENDERSON (R.), ALDEN (E.), JENNINGS (P.) *et al.* — Tension pneumothorax: a teaching model. *Pediatrics*, *58*, 861-862, 1976.

[31] HIGH (R.). — Pneumothorax and pneumomediastinum. In KENDING (E. L.), *Disorders of the respiratory tract in children.* Philadelphia W. B., Saunders Co., 1972.

[32] HOWIE (V. M.), WEED (A. S.). — Spontaneous pneumothorax in the first ten days of life. *J. Pediatr.*, *50*, 6-9, 1957.

[33] JOLY (J. B.). — Drain pleural à usage pédiatrique. *Presse Méd.*, *76*, 18-20, 1968.

[34] KARLBERG (P.). — Respiratory studies in newborn infants. *Acta Paediatr. Scand.*, *51*, 121-136, 1962.

[35] KAUFMANN (M. J.), MAHOUBI (S.). — Unusual air distribution patterns in prematures on positive pressure ventilation. *Ann. Radiol.*, *18*, 431-438, 1975.

[36] KIRSCHNER (P. A.), STRAUSS (L.). — Pulmonary interstitial emphysema in the newborn. Precursors and sequelae. A clinical and pathological study. *Dis. Chest.*, *46*, 417-426, 1964.

[37] KUHNS (L. R.), BEDNAREK (F. J.), WYMAN (M. L.) *et al.* — Diagnosis of pneumothorax or pneumomediastinum in the neonate by transillumination. *Pediatrics*, *56*, 355-360, 1975.

[38] LAENNEC (R. T. H.). — *Traité de l'auscultation médiate.* Édition 4. J. S. CHAUDE (ed.), Paris, 1837.

[39] LAMBERT (H. W.), WANGH (H.). — Accessory, bronchioloalveolar communications. *J. Pathol. Bacteriol.*, *70*, 311-315, 1955.

[40] LENAGHAN (R.), SILVA (Y. J.), WALT (A. S.). — Hemodynamic alterations associated with expansion rupture of the lung. *Arch. Surg.*, *99*, 339-343, 1969.

[41] LEONIDAS (J. C.), HALL (R. T.), RHODES (P. G.). — Conservative management of unilateral pulmonary interstitial emphysema under tension. *J. Pediatr.*, *87*, 776-778, 1975.

[42] LOFTIS (J. W.), SUSSEN (A. F.), MARCH (J. H.) *et al.* — Pneumopericardium in infancy. *Am. J. Dis. Child.*, *103*, 61-65, 1962.

[43] LOHRER (A.). — Zur Pathogenese des pneumoperikard, beim neugeborenen. *Schweiz. Med. Wschenschr.*, *102*, 1248-1251, 1972.

[44] MACKLIN (M. T.), MACKLIN (C. C.). — Malignant interstitial emphysema of the lung and mediastinum as an important occult complication in many respiratory diseases and other conditions. An interpre-

tation of the clinical litterature in the light of laboratory. *Medicine (Baltimore)*, *23*, 281-358, 1944.

[45] MALAN (A. F.), HESSE (H. DE V.). — Spontaneous pneumothorax in the newborn. *Acta Paediatr. Scand.*, *55*, 224-228, 1966.

[46] MANSFIELD (P. D.), GRAHAM (C. M.), BECWITH (J. B.) *et al.* — Pneumopericardium and pneumomediastinum in infants and children. *J. Pediatr. Surg.*, *8*, 691-699, 1973.

[47] MERENSTEIN (G. B.), DOUGHERTY (K.), LEWIS (R. N.). — Early detection of pneumothorax by oscilloscope monitor in the newborn infant. *J. Pediatr.*, *80*, 98-101, 1972.

[48] MILLER (W. S.). — Study of the human pleura pulmonalis: its relation to the blebs and bullae of emphysema. *Am. J. Roentgenol. Radium Ther. Nucl. Med.*, *15*, 399-407, 1926.

[49] MOSELEY (J. E.). — Loculated pneumomediastinum in the newborn: a thymic « spinnaker sail » sign. *Radiology*, *75*, 780-783, 1960.

[50] MONIN (P.), CASHORE (W. J.), HAKANSON (D. O.) *et al.* — Assisted ventilation in the neonate. Comparison between positive and negative respirators. *Pediat. Res. Abstr.*, *10*, 483, 1975.

[51] MONIN (P.), VERT (P.). — Pneumothorax. *Clinics in Perinatol.*, *52*, 335-350, 1978.

[52] MONIN (P.), BOUGLE (D.), CRANCE (J. P.) *et al.* — Hemodynamics and ventilatory effects of tension pneumothorax in rabbits. In *Intensive care in the newborn.* L. STERN (ed.), Masson, New York, 37-49, 1978.

[53] NOACK (G.), FREYSCHUSS (U.). — The early detection of pneumothorax with transthoracic impedance in newborn infants. *Acta Paediat. Scand.*, *66*, 677-680, 1977.

[54] OGATA (E. S.), GREGORY (G. A.), KITTERMAN (J. A.) *et al.* — Pneumothorax in the respiratory distress syndrome: incidence and effects on vital signs. Blood gases and pH. *Pediatrics*, *58*, 177-183, 1976.

[55] OVENFORS (C.). — Pulmonary interstitial emphysema. An experimental roentgen diagnostic study. *Acta Radiol.* (Stockh.), *224* (suppl.), 1-131, 1964.

[56] OZONOFF (M. B.), RUDHE (U.). — Some theoretical aspects of pneumomediastinum in infants and children. *Ann. Radiol.*, *9*, 295-298, 1966.

[57] PLENAT (F.), VERT (P.), DIDIER (F.), ANDRÉ (M.). — Pulmonary interstitial emphysema. *Clinics in Perinatol.*, *5*, 351-375, 1978.

[58] PONTE (C.), REMY (J.), BONTE (C.), LEQUIEN (P.), LACOMBE (A.). — Pneumothorax et pneumomédiastins chez le nouveau-né. Étude clinique et radiologique de 80 observations. *Arch. Fr. Pédiatr.*, *28*, 817-836, 1971.

[59] POTTER (E. L.). — Bilateral renal agenesis. *J. Pediatr.*, *29*, 68, 1946.

[60] PROSSER (R.). — Interstitial emphysema in the newborn. *Arch. Dis. Child.*, *39*, 236-238, 1964.

[61] RICHARDS (D. W.), RILEY (C. B.), HISCOCK (H.). — Cardiac output following artificial pneumothorax. *Arch. Intern. Med.*, *49*, 964-1006, 1932.

[62] RUGE (C.). — Pneumothorax bei einem Neugeboren. *Zeitsch. Geburtsh. Gyn.*, *2*, 31-33, 1878.

[63] SIMMONS (D. H.), HEMINGWAY (A.), RICHIUTI (N.). — Acute circulatory effects of pneumothorax in dogs. *J. Appl. Physiol.*, *12*, 255-261, 1958.

[64] SIMMONS (D. H.), HEMINGWAY (A.). — The pulmonary circulation following pneumothorax and vagotomy in dogs. *Cir. Res.*, *7*, 93-100, 1959.

[65] SIMMONS (D. H.), LINDE (L. M.), MILLER (J. H.). — Relation between lung volume and pulmonary vascular resistances. *Cir. Res.*, *9*, 465-471, 1960.

[66] SMITH (B. M.), WELTER (L. H.). — Pneumatosis intestinalis. *Am. J. Clin. Pathol.*, *48*, 455-465, 1967.

[67] SHAWKER (T. H.), DENNIS (J. M.), GAREIS (J.). — Pneumopericardium in the newborn. *Am. J. Roentgenol. Radium Ther. Nucl. Med.*, *116*, 514-518, 1972.

[68] STEELE (R. W.), METZ (J. R.), BASS (J. W.) *et al.* — Pneumothorax and pneumomediastinum in newborn. *Pediat. Radiol.*, *98*, 629-632, 1971.

[69] STERN (L.), FLECHTER (B. D.), DUNBAR (J. S.), LEVANT (M. N.), FAWCETT (J. J.). — Pneumothorax and pneumomediastinum associated with renal malformation in newborn infants. *Am. J. Roentgenol.*, *116*, 785-788, 1972.

[70] STOCKER (J. T.), MADEWELL (J. E.). — Persistant interstitial emphysema: another complication of the respiratory distress syndrome. *Pediatrics*, *59*, 847-857, 1977.

[71] TODRES (I. D.), DE BROS (F.), KRAMER (S. S.), MOYLAN (F. M. B.), SCHANNON (D. C.). — Endotracheal tube displacement in the newborn infant. *J. Pediatr.*, *89*, 126, 1976.

[72] THIEBAULT (D. W.), LACHMAN (R. S.), LAUL (V. R.) *et al.* — Pulmonary interstitial emphysema, pneumomediastinum and pneumothorax: occurrence in the newborn. *Am. J. Dis. Child.*, *126*, 611-614, 1973.

[73] TRAN VAN DUC (H.). — Perforation of the lung by aspiration catheter. *Ann. Radiol.*, *16*, 69-70, 1973.

[74] WIDDICOMBE (J. G.). — Respiratory reflex in man and other mammalian species. *Clin. Sci.*, *21*, 163-170, 1961.

[75] YU (V. Y. H.), LIEW (S. W.), ROBERTON (N. R. C.). — Pneumothorax in the newborn: changing pattern. *Arch. Dis. Child.*, *50*, 449-453, 1975.

[76] BATTON (D. C.), HELLMAN (J.), NARDIS (E. E.). — Effect of pneumothorax induced systemic blood pressure alterations on the cerebral circulation in newborn dogs. *Pediatrics*, *74*, 350-353, 1984.

23

Chronic lung disease in the newborn infant*

Mildred T. STAHLMAN

Chronic respirator lung disease following hyaline membrane disease

INTRODUCTION

In the era before the successful development of mechanical ways to maintain ventilation artificially in small newborn infants with respiratory insufficiency, oxygen therapy (often used in low concentration because of the fear of inducing retrolental fibroplasia) intravenous glucose and buffers, and careful nursing care, constituted the therapeutic armamentarium. Immature infants with clinical hyaline membrane disease had high mortality rates, death almost always occurring in the first 3 days after birth, with the most immature usually dying

* This work was supported by Pulmonary SCOR Grant HL 14214.

Acknowledgement. The author wishes to acknowledge the valuable assistance of Dr. Mary E. Gray in taking and interpreting the light and electron microscopic illustrations, and of Mr. Fred Morris for technical assistance.

earliest. Survivors followed a predictable course of a period of progressive hypoxemia, often refractory to added inspired oxygen, increasing respiratory effort evidenced by severe infracostal and sternal retraction producing paradoxical respiration, loud grunting associated with reflex partial closure of the glottis on expiration, peripheral muscle hypotonia and central depression. If death had not ensued from ventilatory failure or intraventricular hemorrhage, on the 3rd or 4th day of life these infants underwent dramatic improvement, both clinically and metabolically. The oxygenation of their arterial blood began to improve, their respiratory rate and effort decreased, they ceased to grunt, gained in muscle tone, diuresed their edema fluid and became alert. They usually required no further supplemental oxygen by 5 or 6 days, and recovery was progressive and complete. The larger and more mature the infant, the more physically able to ventilate his damaged lung and stabilize successfully through the acute and reparative phases of this disease. Residual evidence of roentgenological or clinical pulmonary pathology was very rarely seen, and consisted of signs of increased hilar markings for some time on X-ray.

With the development of successful methods of assisting ventilation in the newborn infant and the liberalization of the use of increased inspired oxygen concentrations, infants began to survive their period of ventilatory failure in increasing numbers, and with lower birth weights. However, prolonged survival was frequently associated with prolonged use of increased supplemental oxygen and of assisted ventilation well beyond the natural history of uncomplicated hyaline membrane disease. Also, complications rarely seen before assisted ventilation, such as pneumothoraces, disseminated interstitial air, fluid overload, prolonged symptomatic patent ductus arteriosus with heart failure, secondary infection associated with chronic endotracheal intubation, recurrent bronchial obstruction necessitating suction and reintubation, and chronic malnutrition appeared in these infants. The natural history of the disease became distorted, and clinical, roentgenological and pathological changes reflected the degree of distortion. This chronic phase of hyaline membrane disease has variously been called "chronic respirator lung", "bronchopulmonary dysplasia" (BPD), and other descriptive terms. Its etiology is in dispute, primarily by those who favor one single pathogenic factor over all others, such as oxygen toxicity or barotrauma. Most, however, agree that its etiology is multifactorial, and that its prevention and management must take all of these complicating factors into account.

CLINICAL PICTURE

The symptom complex almost invariably begins with the birth of a preterm infant, usually below 2,000 g, who presents with the clinical signs and symptoms of severe hyaline membrane disease. These infants usually have progressive hypoxemia and acidosis, both metabolic and respiratory, and are frequently hypotensive, hypoglycemic, hypothermic and may be hypovolemic. They are usually vigorously treated for these derangements with warming, plasma expanders, buffers and glucose infusions. Increasing levels of inspired oxygen are used to compensate for the progressively increasing venous admixture. Lining cells of alveolar ducts and respiratory bronchioles slough into their lumen, type II alveolar cells undergo necrosis, and, as high protein containing fluid leaks into the terminal

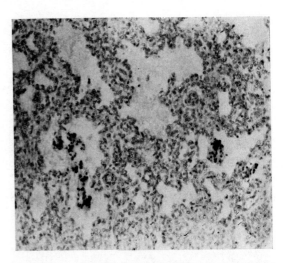

Fig. III-67. — Photomicrograph of lung from an infant of 30 weeks' gestation who died at 2 hours with hyaline membrane disease. The epithelium which lined terminal conducting airways has sloughed from its basement membrane and is aggregated in the air spaces. Pyknotic nuclei are present in the aggregates. Protein-rich fluid and a few erythrocytes fill some of the terminal airways. Arterioles are tightly constricted. Periodic acid-Schiff (original magnification: ×160).

conducting airways, compliance worsens with the progressive loss of surfactant necessary for stabilization of alveolar volume (Fig. III-67). As corrective measures are instituted for demonstratable pathophysiology, pulmonary vasoconstriction is replaced by pulmonary arterial vasodilatation and extensive capillary dilatation occurs (Fig. III-68). Sudden alveolar flooding may follow, as the ability of the lymphatics to remove interstitial fluid is overwhelmed, and an X-ray appearance of a "white-out" replaces the diffuse reticulogranular pattern of interstitial edema and decreased alveolar volume. If ventilatory assistance has not already been instituted, it becomes mandatory, or the patient will die with sudden or rapidly progressive respiratory failure. Infants are usually intubated and placed on mechanical ventilators with added positive endexpiratory pressure. The baby is now at the mercy of the machine. In the presence of fluid-filled terminal conducting airways, increasing mean added airway pressure frequently leads to air dissection, which may present as a sudden tension pneumothorax or pneumomediastinum, or as disseminated interstitial air in one or more lobes (Fig. III-69, III-70). Interstitial air is then forced directly into peribronchial, interstitial, subpleural and perivascular lymphatics (Fig. III-71). With tension pneumothoraces, one or more chest tubes are placed for unilateral, bilateral or reaccumulated pleural air. High mean added airway pressures are necessary for adequate ventilation and higher inspired oxygen levels are used in the face of increasing hypoxemia, despite evidence that the increased venous admixture

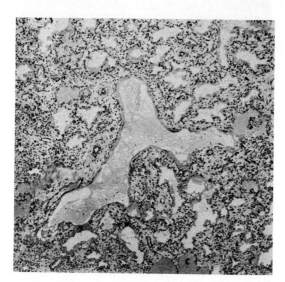

Fig. III-68. — Photomicrograph of lung from an infant of 28 weeks' gestation who died at 30 hours with severe hyaline membrane disease. Y-shaped alveolar duct system is denuded of epithelium, lined with an early membrane material, and filled with protein-rich fluid. Small arterioles are tightly constricted and some pulmonary capillaries are grossly overdistended with blood (C). Hematoxylin and eosin (original magnification: ×80).

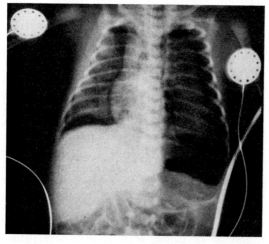

Fig. III-69. — Chest radiograph of a 3-day-old infant with hyaline membrane disease showing massive tension pneumothorax in the left side of the chest and interstitial air dissection in the right, with subpleural air collection and pneumomediastinum.

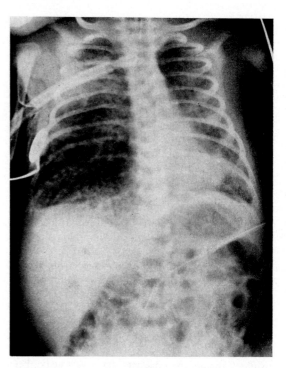

Fig. III-70. — Chest radiograph of a 13-day-old infant with severe hyaline membrane disease treated with positive pressure ventilation. Disseminated interstitial air is present in both lungs, most marked on the right; overdistention is prominent. A chest tube was placed for drainage of a right pneumothorax.

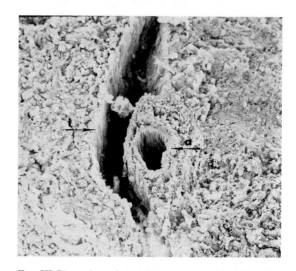

Fig. III-71. — Scanning electron micrograph of the lung of a 3-day-old, 26-week gestation, infant with severe hyaline membrane disease who had disseminated interstitial air dissection. A small muscular artery (arrow) is seen in the center of the field with an adjacent dilated, air-filled perivascular lymphatic channel (arrow 1) (original magnification: ×250).

and not a diffusion defect is the primary pathophysiological problem.

Edema formation resulting from the use of buffers and fluids for crises is exaggerated because the normal mechanism for clearance of lung fluid from the interstitium via the lymphatics has been disrupted by the dissection of air into these channels.

If these events have not occurred during the initial management of the disease, the appearance of a large left-to-right shunt through the ductus

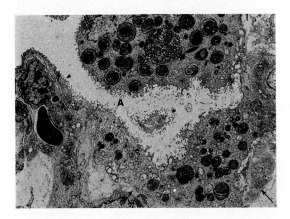

FIG. III-72. — Electron micrograph of lung from an infant born at 34-weeks' gestation who lived 7 days. Hyaline membrane disease is in a regenerating phase. The airway (A) has been relined with alveolar Type II cells filled with large lamellar bodies. Active capillary invasion has stretched the epithelium of a Type II cell over an epithelial and endothelial cells and between epithelium and interstitium (arrows). Uranyl acetate and lead citrate (original magnification: ×3.275).

arteriosus frequently accompanies the falling pulmonary vascular resistance on the 3rd to 5th day after birth. Recurrent pulmonary edema associated with congestive heart failure may necessitate the reinstitution of high inspired oxygen use and of high ventilatory pressures in a small infant previously improving from hyaline membrane disease.

With the passage of time, the oxygen dependence of these infants becomes sustained by the toxicity of oxygen itself, since prolonged high levels of inspired oxygen are toxic to type I epithelium and to capillary endothelium. Areas lined by type I epithelium and terminal conducting airways which have undergone slough of their lining cells are relined with proliferating type II pneumocytes, and large portions of the capillary bed which have been obliterated must repair and remodel the damaged lung (Fig. III-72). A diffusion barrier is now created, leading to further hypoxemia, and high inspired O_2 concentrations must be maintained. The presence of interstitial air, associated with non-ventilated false airspaces, and gross abnormalities in the matching of ventilation and perfusion leads to CO_2 retention. Pressure and distention damage may occur to conducting airways and alveolar junctional areas resulting in necrotizing bronchiolitis (Figs. III-73, III-74). Eventually, squamous metaplasia of epithelial lining of conducting airways and fibroblastic proliferation with excessive collagen production appears (Figs. III-75, III-76, III-77). The lung tissue becomes progressively stiff and overdistended as these changes occur.

The hyaline membranes, if extensive, may form

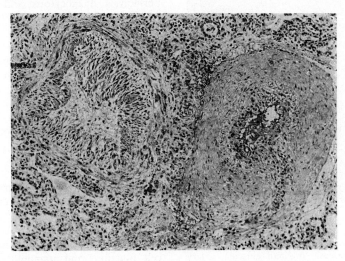

FIG. III-73. — Bronchiole of an infant with hyaline membrane disease who died after 10 days of intermittent positive pressure ventilation and high oxygen inhalation. Bronchiolar mucosa is proliferating in a highly abnormal fashion with necrosis of surface cells in many areas. Adjacent small muscular artery shows intimal thickening and medial hypertrophy. Hematoxylin and eosin (original magnification: ×160).

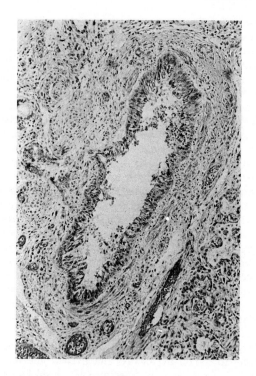

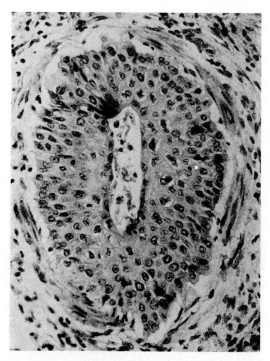

FIG. III-74. — Small intrapulmonary bronchus from same infant as Figure III-73 showing necrosis of surface cells and abnormal hyperplasia of basal cells. Hematoxylin and eosin (original magnification: ×160).

FIG. III-76. — Small intrapulmonary bronchiole of an infant with hyaline membrane disease who survived 14 days on IPPV and high oxygen inhalation which has undergone advanced squamous metaplasia. Hematoxylin and eosin (original magnification: ×520).

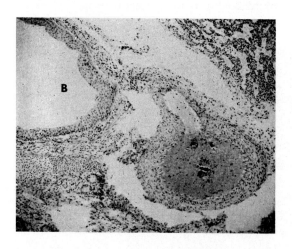

FIG. III-75. — Photomicrograph of lung from an 11-day-old infant who had disseminated interstitial air dissection following respirator treatment for severe hyaline membrane disease. A small muscular artery is surrounded by lymphatic channels dilated with air. Adjacent to this is a bronchiole (B) whose lining has undergone squamous metaplasia. Hematoxylin and eosin (original magnification : ×65).

casts of the distal conducting airways, and require fibrinolysis, phagocytosis, and mechanical removal by cough and suction (Fig. III-78). These membranes undergo invasion by the new population of lining cells, and with delayed resolution associated with adverse factors such as high inspired O_2, barotrauma, recurrent edema fluid, infection and loss of mechanical properties of cilia and mucous, membrane remnants act as an obstruction to normal air flow to the distal airways (Fig. III-79). Low grade infection of the airways is often seen, especially associated with *Pseudomonas aeruginosa, Staphylococcus epidermidis, Aerobacter klebsiella*, and other opportunistic organisms (Fig. III-80). Injury to the laryngeal and tracheal epithelium from repeated intubation and suctioning prepares the tissue for invasion of these organisms, which are especially difficult to eradicate in a chronically intubated infant. With the loss of cilia movement and goblet cell function, and immobilization of the infant, often in the supine position promoting pooling of secretions, pulmonary toilet becomes an increasing problem and occlusion of smaller conducting airways

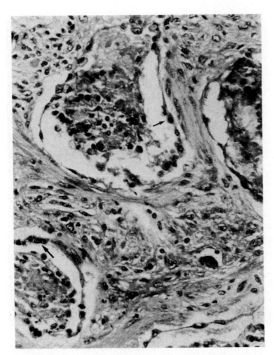

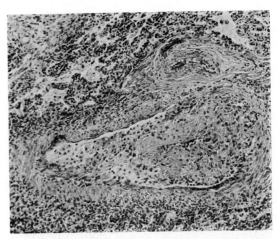

FIG. III-79. — Membrane cast fills a small bronchiole of an infant with hyaline membrane disease who survived 11 days on IPPV and high inspired oxygen showing necrosis and slough of epithelium with relining and invasion of cast by new cells. Hematoxylin and eosin (original magnification: ×400).

FIG. III-77. — Terminal airways of an infant with hyaline membrane disease who died after 64 days of IPPV and high O₂ inhalation. There is a new population of epithelial lining cells (arrow). Remnants of membrane casts are still present and are invaded by lining cells. Extensive dense connective tissue now makes up the alveolar walls and an air-blood interface is difficult to find. Hematoxylin and eosin (original magnification: ×640).

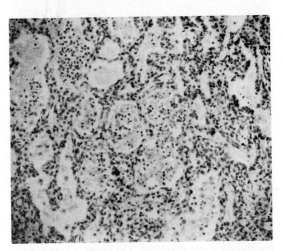

FIG. III-80. — Photomicrograph of the terminal airways of infant lung seen in Figure III-75, showing protein containing edema fluid, round cell and polymorphonuclear leukocyte accumulation associated with infection with *Pseudomonas aeruginosa*. Hematoxylin and eosin (original magnification: ×160).

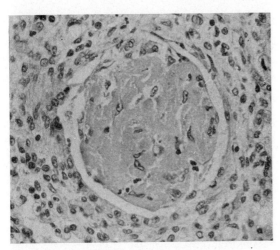

FIG. III-78. — Photomicrograph of the lung of an infant of 34 weeks' gestation who survived 7 days with severe hyaline membrane disease. A membrane cast still exists in the lumen of a terminal airway which is undergoing invasion by new cells, which are also relining the airway. Hematoxylin and eosin (original magnification: ×400).

may occur with ease. This may be complete, leading to areas of parenchymal collapse, or partial, leading to ball-valve overdistention of terminal airways. Chronic hypoxemia and hypercarbia lead to pulmonary hypertension and right heart hypertrophy, often exaggerated by a persistently open ductus, which now may shunt in both directions, and cor pulmonale appears with cardiomegaly and recurrent bouts of congestive heart failure (Fig. III-81).

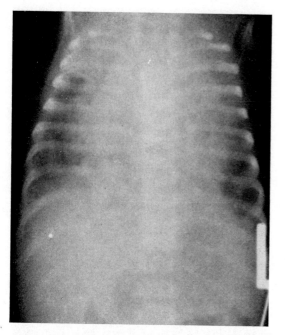

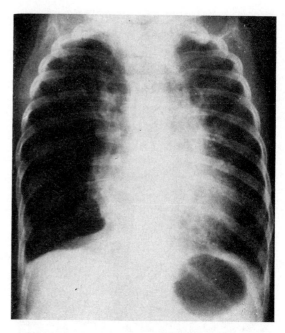

FIG. III-81. — Chest radiograph of same infant as in Figure III-69 now 7 weeks of age. Infant was still ventilator and oxygen dependent, with superimposed chronic *Pseudomonas aeruginosa* pneumonia. Cardiomegaly is also apparent.

FIG. III-82. — Chest radiograph of same infant as in Figures III-69 and III-81 now 6 months of age during terminal hospitalization. Right lung is grossly overdistended, with depression of the right diaphram, and is essentially functionless, except as dead space. Left lung is also distended. There are dense fibrotic scarred areas around the hilum. The heart is enlarged.

Digitalis and diuretics may improve symptoms temporarily, but often the heart failure is progressive and ductus closure at this stage is useless. Adequate nutrition is difficult to maintain in calories and in other nutrients, such as vitamins and minerals, and growth failure is common. Vitamin A deficiency in very low birth weight infants unable to sustain enteral feeding may contribute to conducting airway epithelial necrosis followed by squamous metaplasia described above. The infant is now oxygen and ventilator dependent, and chronic lung pathology is well established. Infants who die may succumb to progressive cardiopulmonary failure with hypoxemia and hypercarbia resistant to all therapeutic measures, or they may die with an acute, superimposed respiratory infection or sepsis (Fig. III-82). It has recently been shown that there are increased numbers of pulmonary paracrine cells in the conducting airways of infants dying with chronic lung disease following HMD. The peptide hormones, bombesin and calcitonin have been demonstrated in these cells (Figs. III-83, III-84). Since bombesin is capable of raising airway resistance in animals, the possibility exists that it's secretion into the interstitial space, either in response to hypoxia, hypercarbia or airway distortion with

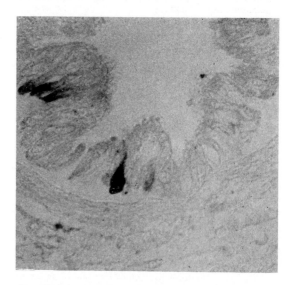

FIG. III-83. — Photomicrograph of bronchiole from the lung of an infant of 42 days postnatal age who died of bronchopulmonary dysplasia. Tissue was stained for IR bombesin. K-like cells and a cell cluster can be identified. Immunoperoxidase with no counterstain (original magnification: ×640).

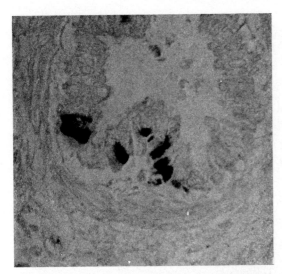

FIG. III-84. — Photomicrograph of a bronchiole from the lung of an infant of 55 days postnatal age who died of bronchopulmonary dysplasia. Tissue was stained for IR calcitonin. Many positively staining K-like cells can be identified. Immunoperoxidase with no counterstain (original magnification: ×640).

respirator use might contribute to the recurrent bouts of wheezing which occur. The role of calcitonin in the lung is, at present, unknown.

Infants who are not so severely affected may survive, especially if they can be successfully extubated early, if respirator pressures and inspired oxygen levels can be kept low, if ductus closure occurs early, either spontaneously or by surgical or pharmacological means, if secondary infection can be avoided, and if adequate nutrition can be maintained. Meticulous attention to the details of medical and nursing care throughout the course of the disease is essential. Even with a prolonged healing phase of HMD, many infants are salvageable. They may have recurrent bouts of wheezing and severe respiratory distress, often resembling bronchiolitis in the first 2 to 3 years of life. These sometimes respond to diuretic treatment. Frank pneumonia may occur, necessitating repeated hospitalization and acute care. These bouts of acute pulmonary insufficiency, which are superimposed on varying levels of chronic pulmonary impairment, usually gradually decrease in frequency and intensity with time, and by the 3rd or 4th year of life, the child may become essentially asymptomatic with good exercise tolerance. The originally involved areas of pulmonary damage scar around the hilum and newly developed airway units may compensate for impaired or non-functional ones, allowing relatively normal pulmonary function throughout

childhood. The eventual outcome of these children is not known.

In the original description of BPD, 4 stages could be separated according to the roentgenological picture of the lungs. Stage I consisted of the X-ray picture of acute uncomplicated HMD with a reticulogranular pattern and air bronchograms. Stage II appeared with a "white-out" and complete parenchymal opacification, which cleared into a bubbly appearance, stage III. This picture, if persistent for 30 days or more, was described as stage IV. Since the natural history of HMD is one of acute distress for 48 to 72 hours followed by prompt and complete resolution both clinically and roentgenologically within about a week, a pattern which is consistent with the uncomplicated regeneration of those portions of the lung originally affected, we must conclude that the prolonged healing process and its advancement into chronicity must occur as the result of either naturally occurring or iatrogenic complications associated with the treatment of severe disease.

The incidence of the secondary disease depends upon the strictness of the criteria for its diagnosis and that of the base population of HMD. It has been reported to vary between 3 % and 46 % of infants with HMD. Most definitions now rely only on those patients reaching stage IV, or roughly one month chronicity, since all earlier stages may be fairly readily reversible if death has not supervened. The criteria of Bancalari, which combine clinical history, pulmonary findings and radiographic outcome seem useful. They consist of the following: (1) The use of intermittent positive pressure ventilation during the first week of life and for a minimum of 3 days. (2) Clinical signs of chronic respiratory disease characterized by tachypnea, intercostal and subcostal retraction, and rales on auscultation, all persisting longer than 28 days. (3) Dependence on supplemental oxygen for more than 28 days to maintain a PaO_2 over 50 mm Hg. (4) Chest radiographic findings of persistent strands of densities in both lungs, alternating with areas of normal or increased lucency. In some infants, these areas become coalescent into larger structures resembling bullae.

Role of the underlying pathology of HMD

Pathology resembling chronic respirator lung disease, or BPD, has been described sporadically in the lungs of infants suffering from other types of initial problems than HMD, such as meconium aspiration pneumonia, tracheoesophageal fistula and

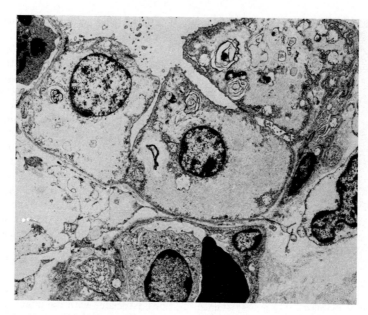

FIG. III-85. — Electron micrograph of terminal airway from an infant who survived for 15 days with hyaline membrane disease on IPPV and high oxygen inhalation showing severely damaged type II cells with disruption of organelles, and marked interstitial edema beneath the basement membrane. Uranyl acetate and lead citrate (original magnification: ×6,400).

congenital heart disease. For practical purposes, however, it is a sequal to complicated HMD. The baby who is susceptible to HMD has an immature lung, both anatomically and physiologically, and the areas which are damaged initially are remarkably constant. Alveolar duct and respiratory bronchiolar epithelium and developing alveolar type II cells appear to be exquisitely sensitive to the initiating injury, which in most cases apparently is perinatal ischemia and acute oxygen deprivation. These target cells line the budding, rapidly developing terminal conducting airways and, as in the case of type II cells, have high metabolic requirements for oxygen when compared with other parts of the lung. Likewise, vascular endothelial cells seem initially affected, with increased permeability and leakage of protein-rich fluid. Necrosis and cell slough of the injured epithelial cells is the result of the perinatal ischemic insult, followed by exudation of the protein-rich fluid into the terminal air spaces (Figs. III-85, III-86). With continued ventilation, the fibrinogen containing fluid clots in the presence of tissue thromboplastin, and an eschar is formed, lining the injured area (Fig. III-87). The low surface tension required for alveolar stability at end expiration increases, as available surfactant is utilized and not regenerated, and alveolar air volume diminishes. The more immature the lung, the greater the portion made up of these terminal budding units and the more imma-

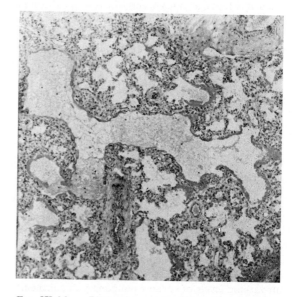

FIG. III-86. — Photomicrograph of lung from an infant of 28 weeks' gestation who died at 30 hours with severe hyaline membrane disease. Small tightly constricted arterioles lie adjacent to a respiratory bronchiolar-alveolar duct system, which has sloughed most of its lining epithelium and is now lined with early hyaline membrane material. The lumen contains protein-rich edema fluid. There is loss of volume of many terminal air sacs and thickening of alveolar septa. Hematoxylin and eosin (original magnification: ×80).

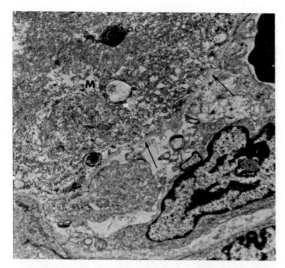

FIG. III-87. — Electron micrograph of hyaline membrane eschar (M) containing cellular remnants and lamellar bodies adherent to the basement membrane (arrows) of the pulmonary capillary bed from which the overlying epithelial cells have disappeared. Uranyl acetate and lead citrate (original magnification: ×8,000).

ture the surfactant system. Cell damage is more widespread and the physiological problems are exaggerated.

The lung has a limited number of ways in which it can undergo repair. Denuded epithelial surfaces are rapidly relined over a 2 to 3 day period with what appear to be migrating type II cells, presumably rapidly differentiated from a residual stem cell population. These cells not only line airways previously lined with type I cells, they appear to actively invade residual membrane material. Capillaries, which appear to have been damaged must now invade these newly lined terminal airways and induce differentiation of the new type II lining cells into type I membranous pneumocytes. This sequence of events seems to occur in the lung which has undergone a wide variety of insults, and accounts for the appearance of "hyaline membranes" in a wide variety of diseases and in mature lungs. However, the immature lung seems exquisitely susceptible to this type of injury, and the degree of immaturity must be taken into account when prolonged healing is considered.

Role of oxygen toxicity

All eukaryotic cells require oxygen for survival but their requirements for and their toxicity to oxygen vary widely. The fetus in utero develops under conditions which are considered oxygen poor, as compared with the adult, but thrives in this environment with a number of compensatory mechanisms. However, low PO_2 has been considered a growth factor for many fetal tissues, and even atmospheric oxygen tension may distort some cell growth patterns.

If a fetus is delivered prematurely, many of its organs are still undergoing rapid growth and differentiation, and the lung is no exception. Additionally, there is ample evidence that the normal adult lung can be altered in its physiology by prolonged exposure to an increased oxygen environment. In adult primates, continuous exposure to 100 % oxygen inhalation produces a sequence of events, some phases of which closely resemble the infant with HMD exposed to high oxygen therapy. The first evidence of pathology is in the vascular endothelium which becomes permeable to protein-rich fluid. Type I pneumocytes are selectively injured rather than terminal lining cells of conducting airways. The animal develops a protein-rich edema and a "white-out", and frequently dies in this acute stage. If it survives the first few days, the denuded terminal airways are relined by new type II pneumocytes, relatively resistant to oxygen effects. As capillaries begin to invade these areas, differentiation and remodeling begin. Fibroblastic activity is stimulated, and increased collagen may be laid down. The animal becomes oxygen dependent and, at the same time, oxygen tolerant.

The cellular mechanism thought to be responsible for oxygen toxicity is the formation of the free radical, superoxide anion (O_2^-). This free radical is formed in the cell during the course of many normal biological reactions, and can be handled rapidly and efficiently by means of the specific enzyme, superoxide dismutase (SOD). Hyperoxia is believed to promote the intracellular formation of O_2^-. If a deficiency of SOD should exist in the presence of hyperoxia, cell damage or cell death may occur as the result of O_2 promoting lipid peroxidation and the induction of denaturation of certain important enzymes and nucleoproteins. There is an age dependent relationship from the human fetus to infant to adult in the amount of pulmonary activity of SOD/mg of DNA. The amount of SOD activity in lungs or sera of infants dying with HMD has not been found to differ with that in lungs of other premature infants. However, studies suggest that HMD infants may be able to handle hyperoxia less effectively than non-HMD infants since HMD plasma is less effective in inducing SOD in lungs exposed to hyperoxia in vitro.

Selenium is a trace metal which is a necessary

part of certain antioxidant enzymes capable of preventing lipid peroxidation of both intra- and extracellular membranes. The possible role of selenium deficiency in chronic respirator lung disease in premature infants is not known at present.

Vitamin E has been shown to protect tissues from oxygen toxicity, and vitamin E deficient animals are said to have increased oxygen damage to the lung, the red cell and the central nervous system as compared to animals receiving a control diet. The vitamin E status of premature infants has been shown to be deficient by adult standards, and its role in the prevention of the changes of BPD, though still controversial, deserves further study under controlled conditions.

That oxygen toxicity alone is not the single etiological factor in the development of this complex patho-physiological picture is strongly suggested by the lack of correlation of its induction in HMD infants treated with prolonged and often high oxygen in conjunction with CPAP or negative pressure respirators, neither of which produces the direct barotrauma to the conducting airways caused by IPPV. The lack of satisfactory experimental animal evidence that BPD can be produced solely by high concentrations of oxygen or by its prolonged use, is also against a single factor role. Nevertheless, high inspired oxygen concentrations, and probably lower concentrations over a prolonged period, certainly, can produce injury to a wide variety of pulmonary tissues. Undoubtedly excessive oxygen use contributes to the ultimate picture of chronic respirator lung disease, and therefore should be avoided or minimized when possible.

Role of barotrauma and air dissection in chronic respiratory lung disease

Chronic respirator lung disease, either clinically or pathologically defined, has been a new phenomenon since the introduction of positive pressure ventilators in the treatment of HMD in premature infants. The observations from several centers that infants ventilated with negative pressure ventilators, infants treated with constant distending airway pressure, even when used with prolonged and/or high oxygen do not lead to the same picture, strongly implicates barotrauma as one of the etiological factors. There is extensive damage to the conducting airways, presenting in the initial healing phase of HMD as necrotizing bronchiolitis, followed by extensive proliferation of surrounding connective tissue and often followed by the appearance of squamous metaplasia (Figs. III-88, III-89, III-90). The use of

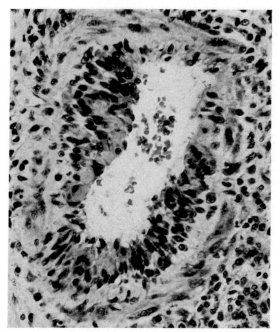

FIG. III-88. — Small bronchiole showing severe acute necrotizing broncholitis from an infant who survived hyaline membrane disease for 15 days on IPPV and high inspired oxygen. Basal cell proliferation is seen alternating with areas of epithelial necrosis and slough. Hematoxylin and eosin (original magnification: ×640).

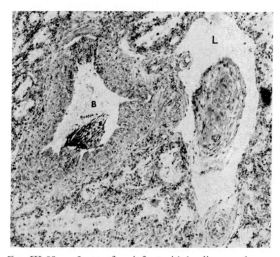

FIG. III-89. — Lung of an infant with hyaline membrane disease who survived 7 days on IPPV and high inspired oxygen showing bronchiole (B) with marked proliferation of epithelium developing into squamous metaplasia. The adjacent arteriole is surrounded by air dissected into the perivascular lymphatic channel (L). Terminal airways are open but contain polymorphonuclear leucocytes, macrophages and some edema fluid. Hematoxylin and eosin (original magnification: ×160).

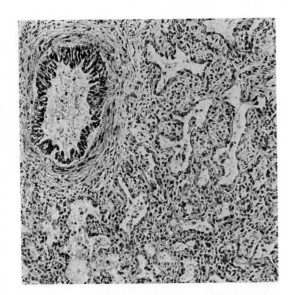

FIG. III-90. — Lung of an infant with hyaline membrane disease who survived 18 days on IPPV and high inspired oxygen. Marked proliferation of lining cells of bronchiole is occuring in a highly abnormal pattern. Terminal airways are open and relined with what appears to be a new cell population. Thickened interstitial areas show fibroblastic proliferation but also reflect underlying degree of lung immaturity. Hematoxylin and eosin (original magnification: ×400).

high inspiratory pressures is especially common when compliance of the lung is as its lowest. It is precisely when terminal airways are closing on end expiration and difficult to reopen, even on peak inspiration, and when terminal conducting airways are filled with fluid or membrane casts that the highest airway pressures are called on for ventilation and oxygenation. In these instances, dissection of air into the interstitial space and thence into the lymphatics is common. The prior occurrence of air dissection, either pneumothorax or disseminated interstitial air, is highly correlated with the incidence of residual pulmonary disease following HMD. Likewise, infants recovered from HMD who had received intermittent positive pressure ventilation during their acute disease have been shown to have a raised airway resistance when compared with non-ventilated infants, including those who had received up to 5 days of oxygen therapy over 80 %. Barotrauma probably plays a major role in the continued damage of an already injured lung and evidence of deranged regeneration and healing processes are evident pathologically. The development of systems which will avoid the need for high added airway pressures may dramatically decrease the incidence of chronic respirator lung in the future.

The human lung is richly laced with lymphatics, mainly following a peribronchial and perivascular distribution to the level of the alveolar ducts and the precapillary arterioles and small venules. The interstitial spaces of the terminal airways, which are widened and of greater capacity in the developing lung relative to the mature lung, are in direct communication with the pulmonary lymphatics, without intervening valves. The interstitial septa and visceral pleura are also richly endowed with lymphatic channels. A network for fluid exchange from intravascular to interstitial space to lymphatic space is readily possible. When fluid exchange from intravascular to interstitial space is very high, such as with increased Starling forces, lymphatic flow can increase several fold before alveolar flooding occurs, if endothelial permeability has not been increased or epithelial cell damage has not occurred. However, when fluid moves from the intravascular space into the distal conducting airways, as happens early in the course of HMD when lining epithelium sloughs, as high oxygen treatment alters microvascular permeability, when membrane casts fill terminal airways, or, later in the course of the disease when a left-to-right ductus shunt produces alveolar flooding, high transmural pressures are frequently used as life-saving efforts to maintain oxygenation and ventilation in the presence of a fluid-filled or membrane-filled airway or lung. The progressive loss of surfactant activity with worsening pulmonary compliance exaggerates the need for increased transmural pressure. The frequent result is air dissection into the interstitial spaces leading directly into the peribronchial and perivascular lymphatics, and into those of the septa and visceral pleura (Fig. III-91). Dissection into the mediastinum frequently occurs, as does rupture into the pleural space, producing a tension pneumothorax. Occasionally, dissection occurs into the pericardium or below the diaphragm into the abdominal lymphatics, or appears as free peritoneal air.

The pulmonary lymphatics dominate the fluid homeostatic mechanisms of the lung, and the imbalance created by interstitial air filling lymphatics leads to frequents bouts of pulmonary edema.

If air continues to be forced into the false air spaces created by air dissection into lymphatics, a large dead space needing ventilation is created, and a greatly overdistended "bubble lung" results (Fig. III-92). These spaces may become permanent, increasing in size with the passage of time. If only one lobe is involved, the picture of lobar emphysema may appear (Figs. III-93, III-94). These false air spaces frequently have new large cells invade and attempt to line them. These cells may be multi-

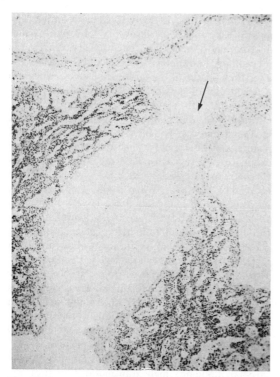

FIG. III-91. — Photomicrograph of lung from an 11-day-old infant who had disseminated interstitial air dissection following respirator treatment for severe hyaline membrane disease. Subpleural lymphatic vessel (arrow) which is overdistended with air extends into lymphatic channels in an interlobular septum. Pulmonary parenchyma is compressed. Hematoxylin and eosin (original magnification: ×65).

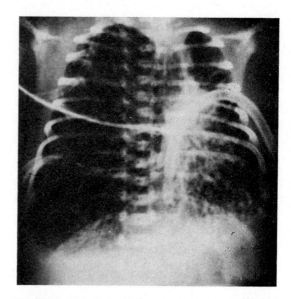

FIG. III-92. — Chest radiograph of a 9-day-old infant of 28 weeks' gestation with severe hyaline membrane disease. There is extensive dissection of air, both interstitial and into both pleural cavities, treated with chest tube drainage. There is gross overdistention of both lungs, especially on the right, and a bubble appearance typical of lymphatic distribution of dissected air.

nucleated and appear as giant cells, occasionally they have cilia, and often contain lammelar inclusions similar to those of alveolar type II cells (Fig. III-95). With the expansion of false channels, neighboring lung tissue is compressed leading to progressively less functional gas-diffusing surface area. This contributes to further hypoxemia, hypercapnea and respiratory acidosis and to the development of chronic pulmonary hypertension and cor pulmonale, ventilator dependence, and oxygen dependence. Any and all of the predisposing factors for the development of air dissection in the course of hyaline membrane disease should be avoided, especially factors which produce fluid-filled airways, such as high inspired oxygen use, aggressive fluid management of acidosis, persistent ductus left-to-right shunt, as well as other factors which demand high transmural airway pressures for management. The early and careful use of constant distending airway pressures before crises, and possibly the future development of effective ventilatory systems which do not demand high transmural pressures, or the effective use of artificial surfactant, may prevent this disastrous sequence of events in the future. Preliminary studies using human artificial surfactant suggest that chronic lung disease can be lessened in ventilated low birth-weight infants with HMD.

Other complicating factors in the development of chronic respirator lung disease

The problems resulting from recurrent pulmonary edema from any cause have already been alluded to. Most often this is associated with a persistent ductus patency and a large left-to-right shunt. However, acute fluid overload, especially early in the course of HMD, often associated with acute resuscitation maneuvers, injudicious rapid transfusions of blood or colloid, or simply overestimation of fluid requirements, may precipitate alveolar flooding and its secondary consequences relating to air dissection. Early ductus closure and the judicious use of fluid therapy may lessen these risks.

Infection of the airways is almost universally present in infants who are chronically intubated

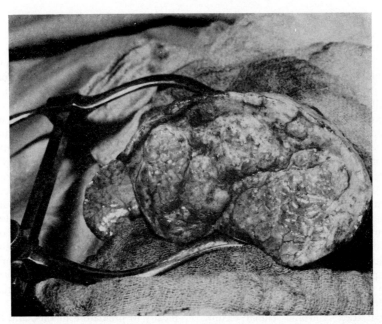

FIG. III-93. — Left lower lobe taken at lobectomy from the lung of a one-month-old infant who initially had hyaline membrane disease. Interstitial air dissection had progressed to lobar emphysema with herniation across the mediastinum. The left lower lobe was at least four times the normal volume of an infant of this age. Thin-walled, gas-filled vesicles can be seen on the external surface.

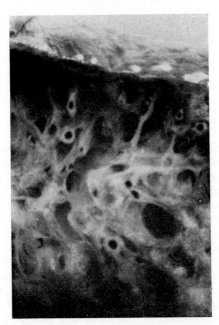

FIG. III-94. — Cut surface of lung from specimen seen in Figure III-91, viewed under a dissecting microscope. The lobe was inflated by bronchial injection of glutaraldehyde two days before sectioning. After fixation, serial sections revealed that the air-filled spaces seen exteriorly extended throughout the lobe. They occurred outside the respiratory passages and were found about arteries, veins, bronchi, in interlobular septa and subpleural tissue. The intervening alveolar tissue appeared collapsed.

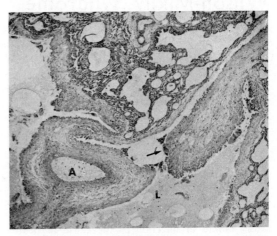

FIG. III-95. — Photomicrograph of lung seen in Figures III-91 and III-92. Large dilated lymphatic vessel (L) is seen surrounding a small muscular artery (A). Lymphatic endothelium in many areas is replaced with large epithelial-like cells, many of which are multinucleated (arrow). Hematoxylin and eosin (original magnification: ×65).

and ventilated. The types of organisms are those which typically produce low grade respiratory infection, but may induce fatal sepsis and other complications such as necrotizing enterocolitis. They are especially difficult to eradicate with antibiotic treatment as long as an endotracheal tube is in place, since mechanical trauma from the movement of the tube, and frequent suction of secretions continue to damage epithelium. The destruction of ciliated cell and goblet cell function, so necessary for adequate pulmonary toilet, is a serious loss, and infection usually lasts until the tube can be removed. Early extubation, whenever possible, is strongly recommended to prevent this spiral of events.

Proper nutrition is often difficult to achieve in small, sick pre-term infants for a wide variety of reasons. The problems associated with chronic gastric feeding in infants on mechanical ventilators or CPAP are often related to overflow of air into the gastrointestinal tract. Chronic jejunal feeding is not without risk, as frequent tube replacement is needed, and the potential hazards of perforation and dumping syndrome are present.

Parenteral alimentation, if given through a peripheral vein is low in calories, and if a central line is placed, runs a significant risk for clotting, emboli, superior caval syndrome, and infection. Additionally, the proper composition of parenteral alimentation in premature infants is unknown. Vitamin supplements, trace minerals, and total calories are frequently inadequate for optimal growth in the chronically ill premature, and growth failure is a common concomitant of chronic respirator lung disease. What role this plays in the prolonged and deranged healing phase of the lung is not known. However, the vitamins known to affect epithelial growth patterns, including that of the respiratory tract, such as Vitamin A, may modify lung regeneration. The possible role of Vitamin E in modifying the effects of O_2 produced lipid peroxidation on cell membranes has already been discussed. More needs to be known about the nutritional needs of chronically ill premature infants, and efforts to promote better nutrition may help prevent abnormal growth and development of the lung, especially during the healing phase.

Chronic respiratory disease in premature infants, Wilson-Mikity syndrome

In 1960, Wilson and Mikity described a form of respiratory distress occurring in small, premature infants which has certain similarities in clinical course and characteristic roentgenological findings. The clinical picture consisted of 1. premature infants in the first month of life; 2. insidious onset of hyperpnea and cyanosis; 3. later dyspnea, especially on effort; 4. frequently overexpanded chest, wheezing and coughing; 5. no rales, unless failure occurred; 6. no fever unless secondary infection occurred; 7. tendency to cor pulmonale; 8. variable effect on general growth; 9. cardiac failure, respiratory failure or infection as the cause of death; and 10. tendency for the pulmonary disease to resolve in surviving infants.

Laboratory results were summarized as follows: 1. radiographical course, streaky infiltration with small areas of emphysema, occasionally appearing cystic; 2. EKG showing progressive right ventricular hypertrophy; 3. failure to demonstrate bacteria, viruses, fungi or parasites; 4. no evidence of

fibrocystic disease; and 5. histological demonstration of emphysema in all, occasionally of interstitial fibrosis and interstitial mononuclear cellular infiltration.

Since that time, a number of reports have appeared describing similar clinical and roentgenological findings, and suggesting a number of patho-physiological antecedents to account for the clinical and radiological findings. These have included abnormal lung development in the extremely premature infant, pulmonary oxygen toxicity, undiagnosed viral disease, abnormal surfactant production, and unequal distribution of ventilation and airway obliteration associated with dyspnea from a wide variety of neonatal causes in the small premature.

There probably exists a spectrum of pulmonary dysfunction of the immature lung. Its time and mode of appearance, its degree of severity, its radiological appearance, and its outcome probably depend somewhat upon secondary factors, such as the chronic use of oxygen, ductus patency with left-to-right shunt, the use of a bag and mask for acute episodes or apnea, or CPAP with or without IPPV for frequently recurrent episodes of apnea or chronic respiratory insufficiency. Typical cases are below 1,500 g birth weight, are without significant respiratory distress in their first few days after birth, and have a gradual and insidious onset of respiratory distress beginning as early as 4 days after birth to several weeks later. The course of the illness is long, with gradual resolution. Apneic spells associated with cyanosis and collapse may be interspersed with more insidiously increasing dyspnea, hypoxia and hypercarbia. Oxygen dependence is common. By the second to third months, marked respiratory symptoms and radiographic changes are present. Gradual improvement usually begins between the fourth to sixth month after birth, and, unless the patient dies of cor pulmonale, improvement continues throughout the next six months.

The earliest radiological signs usually appear by one month of age and consist of a bilateral diffuse reticulonodular or retricular pattern with small, round lucent foci producing a bubbly appearance. Over many weeks, the densities become more defined, and later, coarse streaks radiate from the hilus. The lower zones are usually more radiolucent than the upper, and, along with flattened diaphragms, suggest overaeration.

Physiological studies have shown decreased dynamic lung compliance, gradual loss of lung volume, and the appearance of hypoxia and hypercarbia. Many patients also have elevated airway resistance. Resolution of physiological abnormalities accompanies clearing of clinical symptoms, and more gradually the X-ray becomes normal.

It is suggested that the lung of the very immature infant, with its small bore conducting airways, its shallow terminal air sacs, its immature surfactant system, and its widened interstitial space filled with loose connective tissue and lying between budding capillaries and incompletely differentiated epithelial lining cells, is capable of easy physical and physiological distortion. The increased volume which can be filled with interstitial edema fluid, combined with surfactant production which is not continuously regenerated commensurate with its requirements for terminal airway stability at low transmural pressures, leads to decreased lung compliance. The high incidence of persistent ductus patency with left-to-right shunts in these very low birth weight infants makes this more probable. In addition, the chest cage of these infants is abnormally compliant. During REM sleep, which occupies a large portion of these infants' time, intercostal muscle function is either absent or abnormal, the result of which is a collaps-

ing chest cage on inspiration producing paradoxical respiration. The ease with which complete collapse of pulmonary terminal airways can occur is further exaggerated by the infants' inability to cough vigorously and clear the small bore conducting airways. Recurrent apnea with collapse is common, and hypoxia and hypercarbia are seen, at first intermittently, and later, continuously. Additionally, the immature infant has active vagal reflexes which lead to apnea and bradycardia, including the laryngeal chemoreflex and the trigeminal dive reflex. Undoubtedly, other afferent pathways exist such as tactile reflexes in the upper airway activated by suctioning, producing the same result on stimulation. The infant may be resuscitated from such a collapse with a bag and mask, and often is left on low levels of inspired oxygen chronically. IPPV may be instituted to prevent such episodes.

Oxygen toxicity to the lung, air dissection associated with increased respiratory effort on inspiration in the face of poor compliance either self induced or iatrogenic and probably intermittent narrowing or even occlusion of terminal conducting airways on forced inspiration associated with poorly developed musculature surrounding these airways, all may contribute to inequalities of ventilation from one area of the lung to the next. Air trapping or over-distention of some terminal airways may destroy alveolar septa or chronically distort their

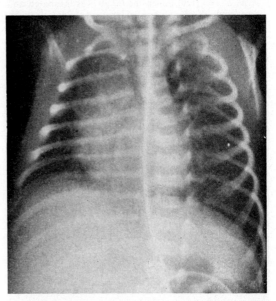

FIG. III-96. — PA chest radiograph on the 1st day of birth of baby C, a non-HMD infant who developed chronic respirator lung disease. Birth weight was 1,106 gms. at 28 weeks gestation. Infant was on F_1O_2 of .3 and CPAP on day 1. X-ray shows some hilar infiltrates compatible with interstitial edema.

growth. Other terminal airways may remain collapsed and distort neighbouring normal tissue. The physiological findings and the pathology seen at biopsy or autopsy suggest such a pattern of events. An example of the radiographic progression in such a situation is shown in Figs. III-96-100. Growth and maturation, both of the lungs and of the chest wall, would gradually overcome much of the patho-

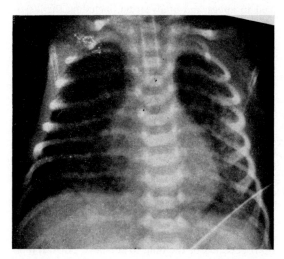

FIG. III-97. — PA chest radiograph of baby C on day 3. A ductus murmur had appeared on day 2. With the onset of recurrent apnea the infant was intubated and ventilated. X-ray shows widespread bilateral disseminated interstitial air dissection.

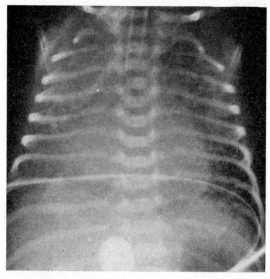

FIG. III-98. — Baby C's X-ray on day 6 shows increasing pulmonary infiltrates and interstitial air along with increasing heart size associated with a large ductus shunt.

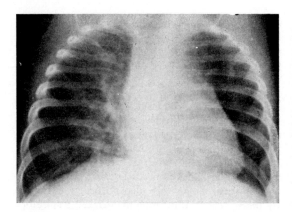

FIG. III-99. — At 6 months of age, baby C's chest x-ray shows residual increased hilar infiltrates on the right. Infant had a positive ET tube culture at 20 days, treated with antibiotics. Extubated at 41 days. Recurrent wheezing episodes post-hospitalization.

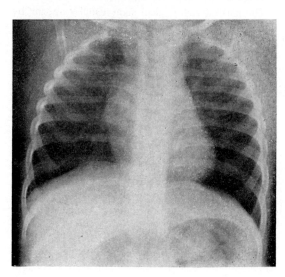

FIG. III-100. — Chest X-ray of baby C at 13 months shows essentially clear lung fields and a normal size heart. Slight hilar scarring on the right remains. Recurrent wheezing and infections persist.

physiology, as is suggested by the natural history of the condition and its resolution. It is not possible to mature all systems of the lung in a short time in the very low birth weight infant. However, the use of low pressure nasal CPAP with room air, or the lowest reasonable inspired oxygen concentration, might prevent some of these events. CPAP can stabilize a flail chest wall, prevent terminal airway collapse and loss of alveolar volume with apnea, lessen the mean transmural pressures needed for ventilation and thereby lessen the possibility of inspiratory closure of small bore respiratory bronchioles. This would tend to equalize ventilation and perfusion so that either oxygen toxicity or chronic hypoxia and hypercarbia may be avoided. Careful attention to the details of medical and nursing care including nutrition, may allow these very low birth weight infants to survive with minimal damage to their lungs.

Pulmonary pneumocystis carinii infection in the newborn

Interstitial plasma cell pneumonia due to *Pneumocystis carinii* has been described as prevalent in central Europe for the last 25 years. Its occurrence in newborns in the United States is much more rare and sporadic. A diffuse or focal pneumonia in the newborn first began to appear in institutional epidemics. This form occurs almost exclusively in premature or debilitated infants between 6 weeks and 4 months of age. The onset of symptoms is usually insidious, with failure to thrive, poor weight gain, and either irritability or lethargy. Pulmonary signs of tachyponea, cyanosis and cough productive of tenacious secretions increase gradually. Temperature elevation is not extreme. Physical findings may be few and misleading, and fine crepitant rales and bronchial breathing may be the only abnormalities. In contrast, the chest X-ray is often strikingly abnormal. Patchy, soft pulmonary infiltrates may spread from the apex to the middle and lower lung fields. Lower areas of focal emphysema may appear.

Laboratory data are non-specific with normal or slightly elevated white cell count with, on occasion, eosinophilia. High plasma calcium levels have been reported on occasion. Clinical diagnosis can be suspected from a fully developed clinical picture and typical chest X-ray. Lung biopsy may be necessary for confirmation. Organisms are more readily identified from tissue imprint smears studies or tissue emulsion than from tissue sections. The most characteristic form of the parasite is a cyst 7 to 10 μ in diameter which contains 8 bodies, each measuring about 1 to 2 by 1 μ surrounded by a mucoid, somewhat refractile capsule. Some cysts have a similar shape. The bodies within cysts may be round, oval or elongated, consisting of a nucleus and protoplasm. These bodies are sometimes present as free forms. Giemsa staining is especially useful in this identification.

At autopsy, lesions are confined to the lungs. With widespread infection, the lungs completely fill the chest. Septal markings are prominent on the surface and pleural reaction is absent. With massive consolidation the lungs are firm and the cut surface shows a prominent alveolar pattern with a gray or tan color. Evidence of air dissection may appear as parenchymal interstitial or mediastinal emphysema, or frank pneumothorax. The most prominent histological finding is the PAS-positive foamy material distending the alveoli. Exudation of granulocytes is absent. In many instances, there is marked thickening of septa and infiltration of mature plasma cells. The foamy alveolar material consists of innumerable pneumocystis organisms.

Treatment is non-specific and epidemics have suggested direct transmission from an infected infant, either by droplet or caretaker contact. Predisposition has been suggested to be related to an immature or suppressed immune reaction. The incubation period has been estimated as 1 to 2 months. Fortunately, this is a rare and sporadic disease in most parts of the world, and more basic information needs to be understood about its epidemiology and prevention.

REFERENCES

Chronic respirator lung disease following hyaline membrane disease.

[1] ANDERSON (R. W.), STRICKLAND (M. B.). — Pulmonary complications of oxygen therapy in the neonate. *Arch. Path., 91,* 506-514, 1971.
[2] ANDERSON (R. W.), STRICKLAND (M. B.), TSAID (S. H.), HAGLIN (J. J.). — Light microscopic and ultrastructural study of the adverse effects of oxygen therapy on the neonate lung. *Am. J. Pathol., 73,* 327-339, 1973.
[3] AULD (P. A. M.). — Oxygen therapy for premature infants. *Fetal and Neonatal Medicine, 78,* 705-709, 1971.
[4] AUTOR (A. P.), FRANK (L.), ROBERTS (R. J.). — Developmental characteristics of pulmonary super-

oxide dismutase: relationship to idiopathic respiratory distress syndrome. *Pediatr. Res., 10*, 154-158, 1976.

[5] BANCALARI (E.), ABDENOUR (G. E.), FELLER (R.), GANNON (J.). — Bronchopulmonary dysplasia, clinical presentation. *J. Pediatr., 85*, 819-823, 1979.

[6] BANERJEE (C. K.), GIRLINE (D. J.), WIGGLESWORTH (J. S.). — Pulmonary fibroplasia in newborn babies treated with oxygen and artificial ventilation. *Arch. Dis. Child., 47*, 509-518. 1972.

[7] BARNES (N. D.), HULL (D.), GLOVER (W. J.), MILNER (A. D.). — Effects of prolonged positive-pressure ventilation in infancy. *Lancet, 2*, 1096-1099, 1969.

[8] BARTLETT (D. Jr.). — Postnatal growth of the mammalian lung: influence of low and high oxygen tensions. *Resp. Phys., 9*, 58-64, 1970.

[9] BONIKOS (D. S.), BENSCH (K. G.), NORTHWAY (W. H. Jr.), EDWARDS (D. K.). — Bronchopulmonary dysplasia: the pulmonary pathologic sequel of necrotizing bronchiolitis and pulmonary fibrosis. *Hum. Pathol., 7*, 643-666, 1976.

[10] BOROS (S. J.), ORGILL (A. A.). — Mortality and morbidity associated with pressure—and volume—limited infant ventilators. *Am. J. Dis. Child., 132*, 865-869, 1978.

[11] BRYAN (H.). — Physiologic changes in bronchopulmonary dysplasia. *J. Pediatr., 85*, 844, 1979.

[12] BROWN (J. K.), COCKBURN (F.), FORFAR (M. R. L.), STEPHEN (G. W.). — Problems in the management of assisted ventilation in the newborn and follow-up of treated cases. *Br. J. Anaesth., 45*, 808-822, 1973.

[13] BROWN (E.). — Increased risk of bronchopulmonary dysplasia in infants with patent ductus arteriosus. *J. Pediatr., 85*, 865-866, 1979.

[14] BRYAN (M. H.), HARDIE (M. J.), REILLY (B. J.), SWYER (P. R.). — Pulmonary function studies during the first year of life in infants recovering from the respiratory distress syndrome. *Pediatrics, 52*, 169-178, 1973.

[15] COATES (A. L.), BERGSTEINSSON (H.), DESMOND (K.), OUTERBRIDGE (E. W.), BEAUDRY (P. H.). — Long-term pulmonary sequelae of premature birth with and without idiopathic respiratory distress syndrome. *J. Pediatr., 90*, 611-616, 1977.

[16] DINWIDDIE (R.), MILLOR (D. H.), DONALDSON (S. H. C.), TUNSTALL (M. E.), RUSSEL (G.). — Quality of survival after artificial ventilation of the newborn. *Arch. Dis. Child., 49*, 703-710, 1974.

[17] EDWARDS (D. K.), DYER (W. M.), NORTHWAY (W. H.). — Twelve years' experience with bronchopulmonary dysplasia. *Pediatrics, 59*, 839-846, 1977.

[18] EHRENKRANZ (R. A.), BONTA (B. W.), ALBOW (R. C.), WARSHAW (J. B.). — Amelioration of bronchopulmonary dysplasia after vitamin E administration. *N. Engl. J. Med., 11*, 564-569, 1978.

[19] FARREL (P. M.). — Vitamin E deficiency in premature infants. *J. Pediatr., 85*, 869-872, 1979.

[20] FITZHARDINGE (P. M.), PAPE (K.), ARSTIKAITIS (M.), BOYLE (M.), ASHBY (S.), ROWLEY (A.), NETLEY (C.), SWYER (P. R.). — *J. Pediatr., 88*, 531-541, 1976.

[21] FRANK (L.), AUTOR (A. P.), ROBERTS (R. J.). — Oxygen therapy and hyaline membrane disease: The effect of hyperoxia on pulmonary superoxide dismutase activity and the mediating role of plasma or serum. *J. Pediatr., 90*, 105-110, 1977.

[22] HARROD (J. R.), L'HEUREUX (P.), WAGENSTEEN (D.), HUNT (C. E.). — Long-term follow-up of severe respiratory distress syndrome treated with IPPB. *J. Pediatr., 84*, 277-286, 1974.

[23] IMPICCIATORE (M.), BERTACCINI (G.). — The bronchoconstrictor action of the tetradecapeptide bombesin in the guinea-pig. *J. Pharm. Pharmacol., 25*, 872, 1973.

[24] JOHNSON (D. E.), LOCK (J. E.), ELDE (R. P.), THOMPSON (T. R.). — Pulmonary neuroendocrine cells in hyaline membrane disease and bronchopulmonary dysplasia. *Pediat. Res., 16*, 446, 1982.

[25] JOHNSON (J. D.), MALACHOWSKI (N. C.), GROBSTEIN (R.), WELSH (D.), DAILY (W. J. R.), SUNSHINE (P.). — Prognosis of children surviving with the aid of mechanical ventilation in the newborn period. *Fetal and Neonatal Medicine, 84*, 272-276, 1974.

[26] JOSHI (V. V.), MANDAVIA (S. G.), SHAROD (G.), STERN (L.), WIGGLESWORTH (F. W.). — Acute lesions induced by endotracheal intubation. *Am. J. Dis. Child., 124*, 646-649, 1972.

[27] KAPANCI (Y.), WEIBEL (E. R.), KAPLAN (H. P.), ROBINSON (F. R.). — Pathogenesis and reversibility of the pulmonary lesions of oxygen toxicity in monkeys. II. Ultrastructural and morphometric studies. *Lab. Invest., 20*, 101-118, 1969.

[28] KAPLAN (H. P.), ROBINSON (F. R.), KAPANCI (Y.), WEIBEL (E. R.). — Pathogenesis and reversibility of the pulmonary lesions of oxygen toxicity in monkeys. I. Clinical and light microscopic studies. *Lab. Invest., 20*, 94-100, 1969.

[29] LAMARRE (A.), LINSAO (L.), REILLY (B. J.), SWYER (P. R.), LEVISION (H.). — Residual pulmonary abnormalities in survivors of idiopathic respiratory distress syndrome. *Am. Rev. Respir. Dis., 108*, 56-61, 1973.

[30] MERRITT (A.), HALLMAN (M.), GLUCK (L.), COCHRANE (C.). — Reduction of lung injury in RDS by surfactant therapy. *Pediat. Res., 17*, 383 A, 1983.

[31] MIKITY (V. G.), TABER (P.). — Complications in the treatment of the respiratory distress syndrome. *Pediat. Clin. North Am., 20*, 419-431, 1973.

[32] NORTHWAY (W. H.), ROSAN (R. C.), PORTER (D. Y.). — Pulmonary disease following respiratory therapy of hyaline membrane disease. *N. Engl. J. Med., 276*, 357-368, 1967.

[33] PHILLIP (A. G. S.). — Oxygen plus pressure plus time: The etiology of bronchopulmonary dysplasia. *Pediatrics, 55*, 44-50, 1975.

[34] PUSEY (V. A.), MacPHERSON (R. I.), CHERNICK (V.). — Pulmonary fibroplasia following prolonged artificial ventilation of newborn infants. *Can. Med. Assoc. J., 100*, 451-457, 1969.

[35] REYNOLDS (E. O. R.), TAGHIZADEH (A.). — Improved prognosis of infants mechanically ventilated for hyaline membrane disease. *Arch. Dis. Child., 49*, 505-514, 1974.

[36] SHENAI (J. P.), CHYTIL (F.), STAHLMAN (M. T.). — Liver vitamin A reserves of very-low-birth-weight (VLBW) neonates. *Pediat. Res., 16*, 177 A, 1982 (Abstract).

[37] STAHLMAN (M.), HEDVALL (G.), DOLANSKI (E.), FAXELIUS (G.), BURKO (H.), KIRK (V.). — A six-year follow-up of clinical hyaline membrane disease. *Pediat. Clin. North Am., 20*, 433-446, 1973.

[38] STAHLMAN (M. T.). — Clinical description of bronchopulmonary dysplasia. *J. Pediatr., 85*, 829-834, 1979.

[39] STAHLMAN (M. T.), CHEATHAM (W.), GRAY (M. E.). — The role of air dissection in bronchopulmonary dysplasia. *J. Pediatr., 85*, 878-882.

[40] STERN (L.), RAMOS (A.), OUTERBRIDGE (E. W.), BEAUDRY (P. H.).— Negative pressure artificial respiration: use in treatment of respiratory failure of the newborn. *Can. Med. Assoc., J.*, *102*, 595-601, 1970.

[41] STERN (L.). — The role of respirators in the etiology and pathogenesis of bronchopulmonary dysplasia. *J. Pediatr.*, *85*, 867-869, 1979.

[42] STEVENS (J. B.), AUTOR (A. P.). — Oxygen-induced synthesis of superoxide dismutase and catalase in pulmonary macrophages of neonatal rats. *International Academy of Pathology*, *37*, 470-478, 1977.

[43] STOCKS (J.), GODFREY (S.), REYNOLDS (E. O. R.). — Airway resistance in infants after various treatments for hyaline membrane disease: special emphasis on prolonged high levels of inspired oxygen. *Pediatrics*, *61*, 178-183, 1978.

[44] STOCKS (J.), GODFREY (S.). — The role of artificial ventilation, oxygen and CPAP in the pathogenesis of lung damage in neonates: Assessment by serial measurements of lung function. *Pediatrics*, *57*, 352-362, 1976.

[45] TAGHIZADEH (A.), REYNOLDS (E. O. R.). — Pathogenesis of bronchopulmonary dysplasia following hyaline membrane disease. *Am. J. Pathol.*, *82*, 241-258, 1976.

[46] TAPPEL (A. L.). — Free-radical lipid peroxidation damage and its inhibition by vitamin E and selenium. *Fed. Proc.*, *24*, 73-78, 1965.

[47] TRUOI (W. E.), PRUEITT (J. L.), WOODRUM (D. E.). — Unchanged incidence of bronchopulmonary dysplasia in survivors of hyaline membrane disease. *J. Pediatr.*, *92*, 261-264, 1978.

[48] WATTS (J. L.), ARIAGNO (R. L.), BRADY (J. P.). — Chronic pulmonary disease in neonates after artificial ventilation: Distribution of ventilation and pulmonary interstitial emphysema. *Pediatrics*, *60*, 273-281, 1977.

[49] WONG (Y. C.), BUCK (R. C.). — An electron microscopic study of metaplasia of the rat tracheal epithelium in vitamin A deficiency. *Lab. Invest.*, *24*, 55-66, 1971.

Chronic respiratory disease in premature infants, Wilson-Mikity syndrome.

[1] AVERY (M. E.). — *The lung and its Disorders*. Second edition, 210-212. Philadelphia, W. B. Saunders, 1968.

[2] BAGHDASSARIAN (O. M.), AVERY (M. E.), NEUHAUSER (E. D. B.). — A form of pulmonary insufficiency in premature infants. Pulmonary dysmaturity? *Am. J. Roentgenol.*, *89*, 1020, 1963.

[3] BURNARD (E. D.). — The pulmonary syndrome of Wilson and Mikity, and respiratory function in very small premature infants. *Pediat. Clin. North Am.*, *13*, 999-1016, 1974.

[4] MIKITY (V. G.), HODGMAN (J. E.), TATTER (D.). — The radiological findings in delayed pulmonary maturation in premature infants. *Progr. Pediat. Radiol.*, *1*, 149-159, 1967.

[5] KRAUSS (A. N.), KLAIN (D. B.), AULD (P. A. M.). — Chronic pulmonary insufficiency of prematurity (CPIP). *Pediatrics*, *55*, 55-58, 1975.

[6] THIBEAULT (D. W.), GROSSMAN (H.), HAGSTROM (J. W. C.), AULD (P. A.).— Radiologic findings in the lungs of premature infants. *Pediatrics*, *74*, 1-10, 1969.

[7] WILSON (M. G.), MIKITY (V. G.). — A new form of respiratory disease in premature infants. *Am. J. Dis. Child.*, *99*, 119-489, 1960.

Pneumocystis carinii.

[1] GAJDUSEK (D. C.). — *Pneumocystis carinii*. Etiologic Agent of Interstitial Plasma Cell Pneumonia of Premature and Young Infants. *Pediatrics*, *19*, 543-565, 1957.

[2] SHELDON (W. H.). — Pulmonary *Pneumocystis carinii* Infection. *J. Pediatr.*, *61*, 780-791, 1962.

[3] KRAMER (R. I)., CIRONE (V. C.), MOORE (H.). — Interstitial Pneumonia due to *Pneumocystis carinii*, Cytomegalic Inclusion Disease and Hypogamma Globulinemia Occurring Simultaneously in an Infant. *Pediatrics*, *29*, 816-827, 1962.

24

Mechanics of breathing and lung volumes in the newborn

F. GEUBELLE and C. MOSSAY

ABREVIATIONS

C_l dyn = dynamic lung compliance.
C_l stat = static lung compliance.
C_w dyn = dynamic compliance of the thoracic wall.
C_w stat = static compliance of the thoracic wall.
C_{lw} or C_{rs} = compliance of the respiratory system.
R_l = total pulmonary flow resistance.
R_{aw} = airway resistance.
R_{lt} = viscous resistance of the lung tissue.
P_l = pressure due to the elastic recoil of the lung.
P_w = pressure due to the elastic recoil of the thorax.
P_{rs} = P − P_w.
$P_{œs}$ = intraœsophageal (intrathoracic) pressure.
P_{alv} = alveolar pressure.
P_{ao} = pressure of the airway opening (mouth and/or nose).
P_{aw} = P_{alv} − P_{ao} = pressure gradient between the alveoli and the airway opening.
P_{pl} = pleural pressure.
P_{pl} − P_{ao} = $P_{œs}$ − P_{ao} = transpulmonary pressure.
$\overset{\circ}{\Delta V}$ = gasflow change ($\overset{\circ}{V}$ = flow).
ΔV = volume change (V = volume).
FRC = functional residual capacity.
V_l = lung volume.
TGV = total thoracic gas volume.
TG = trapped gas.
ELV = efficient lung volume.
CV = closing volume.
cpm = cycles per minute.

DEFINITIONS

The two most frequent values that are used to describe the mechanical behavior of the lung and the thoracic cage are the compliance and the resistance.

Compliances

Compliance (C) is the ratio between the volume change (ΔV) of a structure (lung, thorax...) and the pressure change (ΔP) required for this ΔV. The term "Elastance" (E) is also used: E = 1/C.

Strictly speaking, ΔV and ΔP should be measured in "static conditions" when there is no movement of gas in the lung, i. e. when the gas flow ($\Delta V/t$ or $\overset{\circ}{V}$) is zero. Theoretically ΔV and ΔP should be measured at the beginning and at the end of inspiration, the movement being interrupted by a voluntary apnea with the glottis open. If gas is flowing in any part of the bronchial tree, frictional forces influence the ΔP.

This type of voluntary apnea is unrealistic in

newborns, as well as in children or in dyspneic adults. For this reason, terms such as "dynamic compliance" of the lung (C_l dyn), of the thorax (C_w dyn) or of both structures (C_{lw} dyn or C_{rs} dyn) are used in order to define the $\Delta V/\Delta P$ between two points of zero flow, without apnea. Terms like "dynamic", "apparent", or "effective" are thus used instead of "static" (C_{stat}).

Lung compliance. — C_l dyn is the ratio between the lung volume change from the beginning to the end of inspiration—*i. e.* between two points of the breathing cycle when the flow is zero at *the mouth*—and the simultaneous transpulmonary pressure (P_l) change. P_l is the difference between the so called pleural pressure (P_{pl}) and the pressure simultaneously measured at the proximal end of the airways (P_{ao}, *ao*: airway opening).

ΔP_{pl} is similar to pressure changes in the œsophagus ($P_{œs}$) when technical conditions are respected.
$P_{pl} = P_l = P_{œs}$ when P_{ao} (at the mouth, at the nose or at the end of the tracheal tube...) is equal to the barometric pressure (P_{bar}).

C_l stat corresponds to the ratio $\Delta V/\Delta P_l$ when apnea is maintained for at least a few seconds at the end of the inspiration or the insufflation of air into the lung.

Thoracic wall compliance. — Thorax compliance and its elastic forces can be measured in "dynamic" (C_l dyn) or in "static" conditions (C_l stat) only if the muscular forces of the thorax are inhibited: the newborn must be curarized and artificially ventilated. C_w dyn is the ratio between ΔV during the insufflation and that of ΔP_l (or $\Delta P_{œs}$); C_w stat is the same ratio measured during a brief interruption—*i. e.*: a few seconds—of the gas flow at the end of the insufflation.

Compliance of the respiratory system. — The muscular force of the thorax being inhibited (curarization), the C_{lw} (or C_{rs}) is the ratio between ΔV and ΔP_{ao}. The equation being

$$C_{lw} = \frac{1}{C_l} + \frac{C}{C_w} \text{ (Fig. III-101).}$$

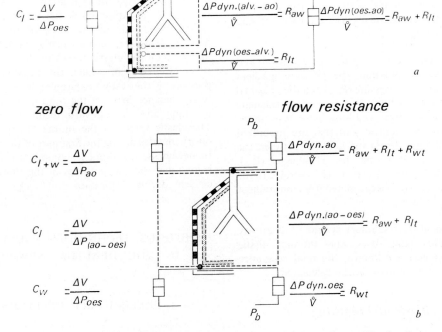

FIG. III-101. — *The required data for determination of the compliances (C_l, C_w, C_{lw}) and of the resistances (R_l, R_{aw}, R_{lt}, R_w) as defined in the text, during spontaneous ventilation and after curarization and artificial ventilation.*

(*a*) Intubated spontaneous breathing.
(*b*) Artificial breathing-relaxed.

Resistances

Pulmonary resistances. — The pulmonary resistances that oppose gas flow are expressed by the relation between the pressure gradient and air flow (Fig. III-101).

Some authors use the term "elastic resistance" or "visco-elastic resistance" in order to define the elastic or the visco-elastic forces of the lung. These terms are confusing. Elasticity or viscoelasticity of a structure is defined as the relation between its volume change and the pressure required to obtain this volume change under static conditions (zero flow).

This pressure gradient may be measured between two points at different levels of the bronchopulmonary system. If the gradient is measured between the nostril and the pharynx, the upper airway resistance can be calculated. If the pressure gradient is measured between the mouth (or: the nose) and the alveoli, the airway resistance (R_{aw}) is calculated expressing the frictional forces due to the movement of the gas molecules within the air stream and against the walls of the bronchial tree. The total pulmonary flow resistance of the lung (R_l) is calculated by measuring the gradient between the airway opening and the external surface of the lung. The difference between R_l and R_{aw} corresponds to the lung tissue viscous resistance (R_{lt}) due to the friction of the lung tissues against each other.

Thoracic resistances. — After curarization and during artificial ventilation, the pressure gradient between the ambient pressure (P_{bar}) and the proximal end of the tracheal tube (P_{ao}) is used to calculate total resistances: airway and lung tissue resistances, and those of the thoracic wall that are mobilized during insufflation. From the gradient between the airway opening (P_{ao}) and the œsophagus ($P_{œs}$), both R_{aw} and R_{lt} are calculated. The thoracic tissue viscous resistance (R_{wt}) is calculated from the gradient between P_{bar} and $P_{œs}$.

Resistances of the respiratory system. — If airway resistance plus lung tissue and thoracic tissue viscous resistances are known, the total resistance of the respiratory system can be calculated.

Work of breathing

Briefly and schematically, the work required for ventilation may be expressed by the product of the pressure change multiplied by the volume change (Fig. III-102).

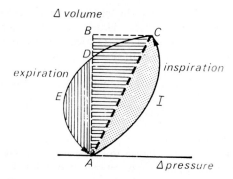

FIG. III-102. — *The ventilatory work calculated from the pressure-volume loop.*

On an X-Y diagram, the surface area of the loop described by the intrathoracic pressure change and the lung volume change may be analyzed in the following way.

The triangle ABC corresponds to the work required to overcome the elastic forces of the lung during inspiration. The semi-elliptical surface area AIC corresponds to the forces necessary to overcome the airway resistance (R_{aw}) and the lung tissue viscous resistance (R_{lt}). The potential energy of the elastic forces of the distended lung at the end of inspiration is used for expiration, as long as this is passive. If the expiration is active, the surface area DEA corresponds to the work of the expiratory muscles. However, such a calculation does not take into account the elastic forces of the thoracic wall. In children and in adults, the negative "pleural" pressure at the resting expiratory level corresponds to the balance between the inward elastic recoil of the lung and the outward recoil of the thorax. The elastic forces of the thorax "help" the inspiratory muscles during the first part of the movement. In newborns, the thoracic compliance is high (see below) and the elastic forces of the thorax are less efficient during inspiration.

METHODS, TECHNIQUES AND VALUES IN THE HEALTHY NEWBORN

PRELIMINARY REMARKS

In the newborn and the healthy infant, the lung mechanics have not been compared between awake and various stages of sleep. In the neonatal period, two types of sleep are identified: active sleep (or: "rapid eye movement sleep, REM sleep") and quiet sleep (or: "non-rapid eye movement sleep, NREM sleep"). Diagnostic features of REM sleep are the presence of body movements and rapid ocular movements, as well as irregular breathing. Those of NREM sleep are the absence of body movements and of rapid eye movements as well as regular breathing. The neuro-physiological criteria of REM sleep are of an irregular low voltage EEG tracing, absence of tone on EMG of chin area; those of NREM sleep are a slow large EEG tracing and tonic muscular activity of the chin. The periods of sleep which are difficult to classify are called indeterminate or transitional sleep. Neonatal sleep organization is periodic. Each sleep cycle has a duration of less than an hour, starting with REM followed by NREM with an equal proportion of REM and NREM. The newborn spends 50 % of his total sleep time in REM [86]. During the night, REM and NREM have no systematic distribution [87].

During wakefulness and NREM sleep, in the supine position, tonic activity of the diaphragm and intercostal muscles is recorded [88]. In REM sleep, the tonic activity of the diaphragm disappears [88] and the rib cage being then unstable, it will deform under the effect of phasic inspiratory diaphragmatic contraction which will cause the thorax to move inwards rather than to expand (so-called distortion or paradoxical breathing). Distortion is not invariably a feature of REM: it is also observed in NREM in premature and in full-term babies as well [17].

Distortion is one of the factors responsible for a decrease of the lung volume (see below). According to Lesoüef [89], when the rib cage is distorted the intraœsophageal pressure changes would not reflect mean pleural pressure.

Lung compliance

The lung volume change (ΔV) is usually measured with a pneumotachograph fixed to a mask. It measures the inspired and expired gas flow changes ($\Delta \overset{\circ}{V}$). The electrical integration of $\Delta \overset{\circ}{V}$ corresponds to ΔV. ΔV may also be measured with a mini-spirograph as long as its resistance and its inertance are negligible. In addition, if the spirograph is ventilated by a pump, the continuous positive pressure within the mask must also be minimal; if not, a pressure of more than a few mm of water could induce an increase in the lung volume (see: hyaline membrane disease).

The reliability of the **transpulmonary pressure** (P_l) must be analysed. First, it must be stressed that the intrathoracic ΔP, measured with an intra-œsophageal catheter, is only a "global" measurement of the transpulmonary pressures that exist on the outer surface of the lung. These forces are not identical everywhere: local differences have been observed in adults at different levels within the œsophagus [20], and local pleural pressure measurements in animals [1] demonstrate that these local differences are due to the density and the weight of the lungs (and are consequently modified by the body position). Secondly, it is assumed that the intra-œsophageal pressure ($P_{œs}$) corresponds to the pressure on the outer surface of the lung. Finally, the calculation of lung compliance and resistances is based upon the hypothesis that the lung is a mono-alveolar and homogenous model: flow changes ($\Delta \overset{\circ}{V}$), volume changes ($\Delta V$), and intra-alveolar ($P_{alv}$) as well as extra-alveolar (P_l or $P_{œs}$) pressure changes are assumed to be identical in all lung units during a breathing cycle. The value of the dynamic lung compliance (C_l dyn) depends on the elastic properties of the lung, but also on the distribution of the gas within the different lung units. From argon gas distribution curves at different expiratory levels in adults, Fowler et al. [24] suggested inequalities in gas distribution. Later, it was demonstrated that ventilatory asynchronism leads to a fall of C_l dyn [69].

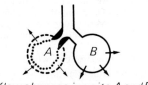

gas flow changes in units A and B

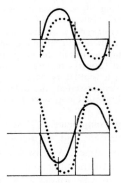

intraalveolar pressure changes
in units A and B

FIG. III-103. — *Schematic illustration of ventilatory asynchronism: flow and intra-alveolar pressure changes.*

Ventilatory asynchronism is observed when resistances opposing air flow in the air passages of different lung units, are different and unequally distributed within the entire lung: time constants calculated by analogy with those of an electrical circuit (resistance X capacitance, i. e.: resistance X compliance) are different from one lung unit to the other.

As indicated by the term "asynchronism", the ventilation of these lung units is not synchronized. The "global" intrathoracic ΔP does not necessarily correspond to the "local" ΔP: it is erroneously too high (the compliance being too low). In a heterogenous lung, P_{alv} and P_{ao} are not identical at the end of inspiration as long as the intraalveolar pressures are not similar in all the lung units. The transpulmonary pressure ($P_{pl} - P_{ao}$ or $P_{œs} - P_{ao}$) is erroneously too low [66, 67, 68] (Fig. III-103).

In children and in adults, ventilatory asynchronism is demonstrated by two methods: the interruption of air flow at the mouth and the comparison between the static and dynamic lung compliances.

Buccal pressure changes during brief and repeated interruptions of air flow are modified when the lung units are asynchronously ventilated: the equalization of the pressures between the alveoli and the mouth is incomplete during the brief time of air flow interruption when the small peripheral airway resistances are not similar in all lung units [69].

Simultaneously, with the modifications of the buccal pressure changes, a fall in C_l dyn is observed [69]. The static lung compliance is then measured during very slow and deep respiratory movements or by measuring the intrathoracic pressure at different levels of the inspiratory capacity [85]. From the difference between the static and the dynamic lung compliance, the severity of the ventilatory asynchronism may be estimated.

Finally, in some cases, when lung nitrogen is washed out by inhaling pure oxygen (see below), poorly ventilated lung units may be discovered.

In healthy or in respiratory distressed newborns, poorly ventilated lung units whose N_2 washout by O_2 is slow have not been observed [13, 63, 64]. However, during these measurements a sudden increase of the N_2 concentration at the mouth, after a deep inspiration, suggests the presence of totally or partially obstructed small airways and poorly or non ventilated lung units [63, 64]. Thus a ventilatory asynchronism may be suspected but not demonstrated, the difference between the static and the dynamic compliance not being known.

The static lung compliance (C_l stat) has been measured in curarized and artificially ventilated newborns or during apnea. A known volume of air is injected slowly into the lung and the pressure is measured at the airway opening (P_{ao})—i. e. the proximal end of the tracheal tube—and in the œsophagus ($P_{œs}$). The ratio between the ΔV and the pressure gradient ($P_{ao} - P_{œs}$) corresponds to the static lung compliance (C_l stat). Apnea may also be provoked in newborns by suddenly applying a positive pressure (a few cm of water) at the mouth and nose. A deep and rapid gasp is followed by an inspiration and apnea (Head reflex) [16]. However the C_l stat measured under these conditions is higher than the compliance measured during normal breathing. The sudden positive intra-alveolar pressure change and the large expansion of the lung during the gasp (before the apnea) may induce a recruitment of poorly or non ventilated lung units or a change in the visco-elastic properties of the lung. In healthy adults after a deep inspiration, the C_l dyn increases [70].

C_l stat has also been measured in vitro, the lung being insufflated or kept in an airtight box in which a progressively increasing negative pressure is applied to the outer surface of the lung. Under these experimental conditions, the distribution of the air in the lung is quite variable from one region to another, as demonstrated by the surface area of the lung units on histological slides. This distribution is mostly dependent upon the conditions of post mortem dissection [53]. The FRC values calculated in vitro [36] are lower than the values measured in vivo [13] in distressed newborns. In addition, the slope of the $\Delta V/\Delta P$ curves is different during the inflation and deflation of the lung, as well as from one inflation to the next [36]. Such variability is not observed in the curarized newborn during measurement of C_l stat.

Values of lung compliance in the healthy newborn. — Lung compliance increases with lung volume: during growth its value increases from birth (5 ml/cm H_2O) to the end of puberty (150-200 ml/cm H_2O). Therefore, it is necessary to express lung compliance by units of lung volume. Different methods have been used in order to measure the lung volume (see below). In some cases, the total volume of the intrathoracic gas (TGV) (including poorly or non ventilated lung units) is measured. In other cases, only the volume of well ventilated units is determined (functional residual capacity, or: FRC). During the first breaths, the *dynamic compliance* (C_l dyn) is very low (1.5 ml/cm H_2O): the volume of the ventilated alveoli is small and the FRC will progressively increase during the first hours of life.

In healthy term newborns, C_l dyn increases progressively [13, 28, 47, 48]. The FRC [26] and TGV [12] increase being less than that of C_l dyn, the increase of C_l/FRC and of C_l/TGV is mostly dependent upon the C_l increase. The C_l increase is not yet well defined and some hypotheses have been suggested.

For some authors, a progressively increasing resorption of the lung liquid would explain the change of the elastic properties of the lung [80]. For others, it is the consequence of repeated stretching of the lung parenchyma [3]. However, the C_l dyn increase could also be due to a more equal distribution of the inspired air into the different lung units. Assuming that the volume of the trapped gas (TG) decreases during the first days of life, one may also assume that in addition to non ventilated lung units (TG), other units may be poorly ventilated, their airways being partially obstructed. Such a situation leads to ventilatory asynchronism and explains the relatively low values of C_l dyn. These values must be carefully interpreted: the accuracy of the measured intrathoracic pressure change (P) might be reduced due to certain poorly or non ventilated lung units.

After the first few days of life, the C_l dyn value is about 5 ml/cm H_2O, in newborns whose weight is 3 to 3.5 kg. From the data collected in the literature, the following values may be suggested.

Birth weight kg	Intrathoracic gas volume (TGV) ml	C_l dyn ml/cm H_2O	Specific C_l dyn ml/cm H_2O ml^{-1} TGV
1-1.5	80	3.0	0.036
3-35.	110	5.8	0.054

The so called "specific" C_l dyn is expressed per unit of TGV. Indeed, both values—C_l dyn and TGV —are measured with the child breathing ambient air. The specific C_l dyn of the FRC might be higher in premature babies breathing a gas mixture enriched in oxygen during the measurement of FRC (see below: lung volumes).

Comparing dysmature newborns and premature babies with similar birth weight, Hutchinson et al. [42] observed that the FRC is smaller in premature babies, but the C_l dyn is similar (5-6 ml/cm H_2O) in both groups. The difference between the elastic properties of the lung in newborns with a low birth weight (dysmature or premature) and in at term healthy babies must be cautiously interpreted.

The C_l dyn observed by Reynolds et al. [73] has been measured during artificial ventilation and anesthesia with relatively low respiratory frequency (20 to 30 cpm): the distribution of the insufflated air may be more homogenous under these conditions and one has to assume that the data may be similar during spontaneous ventilation at a higher respiratory frequency.

The measurement of the *static lung compliance* (C_l stat) was performed in a few un-distressed newborns during anesthesia and curarization. The values are between 1.5 and 5 ml/cm H_2O [32, 73].

It must be stressed that the lung volume was not known during this measurement. It is now known that mechanical parameters are influenced by this volume (see below).

The difference between C_l stat and C_l dyn, which could demonstrate the presence and impor-

tance of ventilatory asynchronism, is poorly understood in the healthy newborn and has not been determined during respiratory distress.

Compliance of the thorax

C_l dyn and C_l stat have been measured in some curarized and ventilated newborns. The values vary from 20 to 24 ml/cm H_2O—*i. e.* 5 to 10 times the value of C_l dyn [32, 73]. In adults the C_l and C_w are similar. In addition, C_l dyn and C_l stat are similar in the artificially ventilated newborn.

Compliance of the respiratory system

The C_{rs} may be calculated from the previously cited equation (see p. 475): C_l being about 5 ml/cm H_2O and C_{wl} about 20 ml/cm H_2O; the C_{rs} is about 4 ml/cm H_2O.

This value has been observed by Olinsky et al. [65] during measurements of the so called "passive elastance". When the upper airways are suddenly obstructed at different levels and at the end of inspiration, apnea is observed in some newborns and in most premature babies as a consequence of the Hering-Breuer reflex. It may be assumed that the activity of the respiratory muscles is zero, and from the pressure measured at the nose and the mouth (P_{ao}) the C_{rs} is calculated ($\Delta V_{rs}/P_{ao} = C_{rs}$). The observed value is about 4.8 ml/cm H_2O in term newborns and 2.8 ml/cm H_2O in premature babies. The difference between these two values is essentially due to the relatively high rigidity of the lung and the high compliance of the thorax in premature infants.

It must be stressed that the so called "effective elastance" measured by these authors is the ratio between the lung volume and the ΔP_{ao} during an inspiratory effort immediately after the occlusion of the upper airways. Thus the values are also dependent upon the force of the respiratory muscles, and especially on the recruitment of fibers of the inspiratory intercostal muscles.

Total pulmonary flow resistance and airway resistance

It is assumed that the **lung is a mono-alveolar model**. In addition, the measured pressures are representative of the actual pressures if the air is equally distributed. Finally, one must also assume that resistances do not change according to the flow.

Indeed, turbulence is more important in the airways when the flow increases.

The airways resistance (R_{aw}) is defined by the pressure gradient (ΔP_{aw})—*i. e.* the gradient from the mouth (P_{ao}) to the alveoli (P_{alv})—divided by the flow ($\overset{\circ}{V}$): $R_{aw} = \Delta P_{aw}/\Delta \overset{\circ}{V}$.

According to Poiseuille's law, R_{aw} is directly related to the dimensions of a straight and rigid tube, and the viscosity and density of the gas flow, as long as the stream is laminar. However, most of the airways are not rigid and their calibers change during a breathing cycle by the application of intrathoracic pressure changes to their outer surface. In addition, the bronchial tree being branched, the stream may be more turbulent than laminar. In order to describe P_{aw} and owing to the turbulence, an equation was proposed:

$$P_{aw} = K_1 \overset{\circ}{V} + K_2 (\overset{\circ}{V})^2.$$

The first term takes into account the laminar flow, the second term the turbulent flow when the speed of the gas flow is high. R_{aw} would thus change during the breathing cycle and would also depend on the flow:

$$R_{aw} = P_{aw}/\overset{\circ}{V} = K_1 + K_2 \overset{\circ}{V}.$$

It is assumed that the second term of the equation ($K_2 \overset{\circ}{V}$) may be neglected, K_2 being small, at least in the bronchial airways. However, in the nose and in the pharynx the flow is turbulent and R depends on this flow.

For the first respiratory movements in term healthy newborns, only R_l has been calculated, the transpulmonary pressure being measured with an intra-œsophageal catheter. R_l may be as high as 100 cm $H_2O/l.sec^{-1}$ during the first hours of life. It then decreases to between 30 to 50 cm $H_2O/l.sec^{-1}$ during the first few days and weeks.

The range of the R_l values is large and may be explained by the lung volume changes, the position of the head [78] influencing the opening of the glottis.

R_l is also influenced by the position of the body of premature babies, it being larger in the prone than in the supine position [43]. Usually, R_l and R_{aw} are measured between two points of the respiratory cycle, where the lung volume is identical during inspiration and expiration. The ΔP between these two isovolume points depends only on the resistances to the gas flow, and it is assumed that the elastic forces of the lung which are increasing during inspiration are restored during expiration. Thus they are identical at isovolume inspiratory and expiratory points.

This hypothesis may be accepted if the lung compliance—*i. e.* the ratio between the volume and the pressure that describes the elastic forces of the lung—is identical during both the inspiratory and the expiratory phases of the breathing cycle. Actually, this assumption is confirmed in vivo in the curarized newborn. However, in vitro, C_l stat is different during inspiration and expi-

ration. It is likely that under dynamic conditions and during normal breathing, C_l is identical during both phases of the cycle.

R_l and R_{aw} thus express resistance between two phases of the respiratory cycle and not the resistance encountered during the entire cycle. Other methods of calculation have been described and take into account the force developed and the flow changes involved during the entire respiratory cycle [25, 40].

How are the different parts of the total pulmonary flow (R_l) distributed? The respective influence of R_{aw} and R_{lt} (airway and lung tissue viscous resistances) in newborns is not well known. According to an estimation of R_{lt} from successive measurements of R_l and R_{aw}, R_{lt} might be as high as 40 % of R_l (in adults R_{lt} is 5 to 10 % of R_l) [71]. This value must be cautiously accepted. Indeed, no argument is found from histological studies of the lung, except during the first hours of the life where a dilation of the lymphatics is observed during the resorption of the lung liquid [81].

The newborn is a "nose-breather" and one third of the total pulmonary resistance could be due to the upper airways (mostly the nose) [71].

A balance between the flow resistance by the nose on one hand and the whole lung on the other hand has been suggested from successive measurement of the resistances with the baby breathing through one and both nostrils [52]. However, it must be assumed that the resistance is still a simple and linear function of the flow even when one nostril is completely obstructed. This assumption is improbable and it is likely that the nasal resistance is overestimated [61].

The distribution of airway resistance between the so called "central" and "peripheral" airways has been investigated in vitro. The resistances opposing the peripheral airways, whose caliber is less than 2 mm, represent 50 % of R_{aw} (only 10 % in adults) [41]. Indeed, the diameter of the peripheral bronchi after the 18th generation is small in newborns and in infants. More studies of this subject are needed since it is known that the lung volume and the inflation of the pulmonary units may influence the caliber of some airways (see p. 485).

Thoracic resistances

Thoracic wall movement produces flow resistance that can only be measured in curarized and artificially ventilated newborns (see p. 476). This thoracic tissue viscous resistance is relatively high (up to 25 cm $H_2O/l.sec^{-1}$) and could be explained by the weight and the elasticity of the abdominal organs (liver, stomach...) [10].

Resistance of the respiratory system

This is the sum of the total flow resistance due to the upper airways (mainly the nose and the glottis), the large and the small bronchi, the lung parenchyma and the thoracic walls (including the abdominal viscera). This resistance is called R_{os} in the literature as it is measured by the so called oscillatory technique proposed by Dubois et al. in 1956 [26] and later modified [76].

The adult breathes ambient air against a low resistance (Zo) i. e. a small tube whose dead space is negligible. A pump introduces an oscillation gas flow into the mouth corresponding to a small volume change (2 ml) at a fixed frequency (10 cpm). This volume is distributed between the added resistance (Zo) and the resistance (Zx) of the total respiratory system (R_{os}). Volume changes induce pressure changes in the known added resistance (Zo) as well as in the unknown resistance (Zx or R_{os}).

These pressure changes are related to both resistances and are measured by transducers that produce electrical potentials, which are then related to both Zo and Zx resistances according to the equation: $\overset{\circ}{V} = \dfrac{U}{Zo} + \dfrac{U}{Zx}$, where $\overset{\circ}{V}$ is the flow of the pump, and U the difference between both potentials. Zo is the known impedance of the system and its mechanical equivalence is the resistance of the tube.

Zx is the unknown resistance of the subject:

$$Zx = \frac{ZoU}{\overset{\circ}{V}Zo - U} \quad (Zx \simeq R_{os})$$

As far as we know, no large investigation of R_{os} in newborns has been published.

Work of breathing

In the healthy newborn, the work of breathing is between 800 and 1,400 g.cm per minute. It is not higher than in adults if the volume ventilated per minute is taken into account [15]. This work corresponds to 1 % of the total metabolism and O_2 consumption.

In non distressed premature babies, the work of breathing is between 1,000 and 1,400 g.cm per minute [84] and corresponds to an energy expenditure of 0.9 ml O_2 per 0.5 l of ventilated air—i. e. a higher value than in adults (0.5 ml O_2 per 0.5 l of air). It is difficult to estimate the mechanical efficiency of the respiratory muscles—i. e. the ratio between the work and the O_2 consumption. At first it seems similar to the mechanical efficiency of other striated

muscles (about 20 %). Thus one has to assume that the mechanical efficiency is two times less in premature infants than in term newborns. The energy cost would be 0.3 to 0.4 ml O_2 per minute in a premature baby (2 kg)—i. e. about 5 % of the total metabolic cost (6 to 10 ml O_2). This percentage is 5 to 10 times higher than in adults. In adults, the respiratory frequency and tidal volume are balanced, thus the work of breathing is minimal, the alveolar ventilation being efficient. From the equation describing the relationship between the frequency, the tidal volume, the alveolar ventilation and the work of breathing, the respiratory frequency that corresponds to the lowest energy cost must be 37 cpm in healthy newborns—i. e. a value near to the actual figure: 40 cpm [15].

MECHANICS OF BREATHING AND LUNG VOLUMES

DEFINITION OF THE LUNG VOLUMES

The functional residual capacity (FRC) is the volume of gas in the alveoli at the end of a quiet and normal expiration (tidal volume). It is usually measured by the dilution of an inert gas (that is not significantly diffusing throughout the alveolo-capillary membrane) or by the dilution of the lung nitrogen by pure oxygen.

The efficient lung volume (ELV) describes the same volume but measured during a shorter time, the inert gas (helium) being rebreathed for 30 to 60 seconds. It is assumed that the volume of well ventilated (or "efficient") lung units is measured.

The intrathoracic gas volume (TGV) is the total volume of gas within the thorax, including the volume of the lung units, the airways being fully obstructed (mucus, œdema of the mucosa...). In addition, any pathological intrathoracic gas volume is measured by the body plethysmographic method (pneumothorax, gas in the mediastinum, intra- or extra-parenchymatous cyst...).

The trapped gas (TG) is the difference between the intrathoracic gas volume (TGV) and the functional residual capacity (FRC) or the efficient lung volume (ELV).

The closing volume (CV) measured during a deep expiration is the lung volume at which the inferior regions of the lung no longer empty themselves, while the superior regions still expell their gas.

METHODS, TECHNIQUES AND VALUES
OF THE LUNG VOLUMES AND CAPACITIES

In order *to measure FRC* by the usual method of helium dilution, the child is connected by nose plugs [28] or by a mask to a small bell spirograph. The gas mixture is pumped into the spirographic circuit and the helium is progressively diluted in the lung until a final and stable concentration is obtained which is identical in the newborn's lung and in the spirograph.

Some authors also use the term "efficient lung volume" owing to the relatively short time left for the dilution, the inert gas being distributed only to well ventilated lung units [42].

When the dilution time is longer, some airways may be obstructed during the measurement, the helium being trapped in certain lung units. However, other air ducts and alveoli may open up.

This is observed in older children when FRC is measured by another classical method—*i. e.* the washout of lung nitrogen by pure oxygen.

Two one-way valves distribute the inspired O_2 and the expired gas, which is collected in a bag or a spirograph. The F_{N_2} (nitrogen fraction) changes are continuously measured at the mouth and the F_{N_2} decreases to 1 %. The lung units are filled only with O_2 and the dissolved N_2 of the blood continuously diffuses throughout the alveolo-capillary membrane. The initial F_{N_2} in the lung (79.6 %), the volume of the expired gas and its known F_{N_2}, the volume of the alveoli and the bronchial tree in which N_2 is substituted by O_2, may be calculated. In some patients with obstructive lung disease, when F_{N_2} approaches 1 %, a sudden F_{N_2} increase is sometimes observed for a few respiratory cycles. This increase may correspond to an opening of some of the previously fully obstructed airways. During the measurement of FRC with the helium dilution technique in a closed spirograph circuit, F_{O_2} (oxygen fraction) is maintained at 20.8 % by continuously adding oxygen to the circuit, the CO_2 being absorbed by soda-lime. However at the end of the measurement using the washout method with pure O_2, the F_{O_2} in the alveoli progressively increases to 98 %: the consequences of such hyperoxia in unstable alveoli of certain newborns is discussed below.

Both methods (helium dilution and N_2 washout) require the use of much equipment for the newborn and this practical drawback explains the use of the rebreathing method.

A small bag of a known volume (100 to 200 ml) filled with O_2 (90 %) and helium (10 %) is connected through a mask to the newborn; after 30 to 60 seconds the F_{He} (helium fraction) is similar in the lung and in the bag. The lung volume may be calculated from the measured bag volume, F_{O_2} (or F_{CO_2}) and F_{He} [49, 50]. Using this rapid method, hyaline membrane disease

has been detected early before the appearance of clear cut clinical signs and the evolution of the disease can be easily followed. The FRC decrease is a typical sign of the unstable alveoli.

The concentration changes of F_{N_2}, F_{O_2} and F_{CO_2} during rebreathing are complex. Indeed the CO_2 partial pressure (P_{CO_2}) of the alveolar gas and the gas mixture of the bag tends to be progressively equilibrated. In addition, the alveolar P_{O_2} continuously increases and the alveolo-capillary P_{O_2} gradient gradually increases. The O_2 transfer and its consumption ($\overset{o}{V}_{O_2}$) increase while the volume of the bag decreases. The respiratory quotient ($\overset{o}{V}_{CO_2}/\overset{o}{V}_{O_2}$) changes during the measurement. The F_{N_2} in the bag and in the lung obviousely depends on the gaseous exchanges [75].

During rebreathing and N_2 washout, the O_2 transfer depends on the P_{AO_2} and on the lung perfusion: anesthesists have observed during a thoracotomy that lung units filled with insufflated O_2 easily collapse. More recently, the decrease in lung volume has been measured in adults breathing pure oxygen [82].

In premature infants and possibly in healthy newborns, where surfactant is insufficient in the alveolar film, a rapid transfer of oxygen may induce a decrease of the volume in unstable alveoli until a critical value is reached, at which point the surface tension forces will induce a collapse of the alveolar sac.

Some experimental data confirm this hypothesis:

(1) The values of FRC measured with the helium dilution method in a spirograph are usually higher than the data observed by Krauss et al. [49, 50], with the rebreathing method. Such a difference might be explained by an insufficient dilution time. However these authors observe that FRC did not change after a 3 minute rebreathing period [49, 50]. These values are similar to the values observed with the N_2 washout method [63, 64].

(2) FRC values measured using helium in a closed spirographic circuit in which the inert gas was mixed with air (F_{O_2}: 20.9 %) were higher than the FRC measured with the same method, but with an F_{O_2} of 90 %, in 10 to 40 day old non distressed newborns that had a normal or low birthweight [26].

The volume of some lung units decreases due to the significant O_2 alveolo-blood transfer.

A similar mechanism is suggested by intrathoracic gas values (TGV) measured by the body plethysmographic method. The newborn is placed in an airtight box with the head kept in a position which allows for the placement of a face mask with a valve. When the valve is closed, the infant attempts to inspire and expire against this infinite resistance.

The pressure changes during these static respiratory efforts are measured in the mask and are similar to the intraalveolar pressure changes, the glottis being open. The pressure changes are also recorded in the box and they depend on the volume changes of the intrathoracic gas during the inspiratory and expiratory efforts. If the buccal pressure is similar to the intraalveolar pressure [59], the TGV may be calculated.

TGV is usually higher than FRC. The difference between both volumes is greater in small than in large newborns [13, 63, 64] and corresponds to the volume of the trapped gas (TG), which could explain the relative hypoxemia observed even in healthy newborns. The trapped gas induces a right to left intrapulmonary shunt in the lung units whose airways are totally obstructed. However, in most cases, FRC was measured by N_2 washout with O_2 [63, 64] or by the rebreathing method with gas mixtures enriched with O_2 [13], the TGV being measured when the baby was breathing ambient air. It is probable that the inhalation of oxygen produces an FRC decrease and thus the value of the trapped gas is overestimated.

This fact might explain the following observations:
(1) the difference between TGV and FRC is larger in smaller newborns [63, 64], and
(2) FRC is significantly smaller in premature infants (27 ml/kg body weight) than in dysmature babies with similar body weights (35 ml/kg). In both cases, FRC was measured with O_2 enriched gas mixtures.

The decrease in the lung volume is probably due to the instability of the alveoli and the alveolar film, whose surface tension is high due to the lack of surfactant. The lung compliance is surprisingly similar (5 and 6 ml/cm H_2O) in both groups, premature babies and dysmature infants. The C_l dyn is measured with the child breathing ambient air [42].

Until now ventilatory parameters have been expressed in kg of body weight and the difference between dysmature and premature babies has seldom been considered.

(a) Body weight cannot be considered as a reliable biometric unit. Indeed, the lean body mass is relatively larger in small than in larger newborns [23] and the differences between light and/or small for date and premature babies are not well known.
(b) Height may be a reliable biometric unit. After birth a significant relationship is observed between lung volumes and ventilatory capacities on one hand, and height on the other hand. However, in dysmature infants organ size may vary from one organ to the next.
(c) Finally, it is currently known that the maturation of the lung tissue depends on several factors during gestation. For example, the alveolar film and its surfactant system influences the elastic properties of the lung parenchyma, and thus a premature baby cannot be compared with a dysmature infant of similar weight.

All these facts must be taken into account when appreciating the reliability of the data and of the predictive equations for lung volumes and capacities.

FRC measured with the helium dilution method,

without an O_2 enriched gas mixture, is about 25 to 30 ml/kg after the first hours of life in at term newborns. This value does not significantly increase during the first few days [28]. FRC is thus about 90 ml and TGV about 100 to 110 ml (when the child is breathing air) according to the equation TGV (ml) $= - 276 \times 7.85 \times$ height (cm) [50]. TGV decreases during the first week of life. This decrease may be as much as 45 % in newborns with a birth weight less than 1,750 g and as much as 25 % in larger babies [50, 84]. In newborns with a birth weight of less than 1,750 g, the TGV, after the 8th day of life, is 0.9 ml/cm ($\pm$ 0.2) and 1.5 ml/cm ($\pm$ 0.03) in larger newborns. But the gestational age has not been taken into account.

Inasmuch as future investigations concerning FRC measurement in ambient air confirm the stability of the lung volume in term newborns, a TGV decrease might correspond to the presence and the decrease of trapped gas (TG) in newborn non ventilated lung units. This gas trapping is not yet well explained. Obstruction of small airways has not been demonstrated by autopsy in premature babies with hyaline membrane disease, except in bronchodysplasia.

However it is possible that some airways collapse at the resting expiratory level as they would in older children and in adults at some expiratory reserve volume level—*i. e.* below the FRC level. This closing volume has been measured by different methods during deep expiration in older subjects.

It may be assumed that in newborns and most certainly in premature babies, the elastic forces of the lung which tend to decrease the alveolar bag are greater than the elastic forces of the thorax. Thus the volume of the alveoli of the lower regions might be smaller than those of the upper regions. The small peripheral airways of these lower regions not being pulled out by these reduced elastic lung forces (the alveolar volume being reduced) are collapsed and gas is trapped.

Intrathoracic pressure measurements at the resting expiratory level could allow a better understanding of the closing volume and the trapping of gas.

Maximal lung volume change is observed during the large inspiration that precedes a cry and the deep expiration during the cry. *The crying vital capacity (CVC)* is about 100 ml in term newborns (*i. e.* 1.9 to 2 ml/cm height) and 1.5 ml/cm in premature babies at 37 to 40 weeks of gestational age [51, 83]. The largest inspired volume is about 85 ml and the volume expelled during the cry is about 15 ml below the FRC level [2]. In anesthetized and curarized newborns, the maximal insufflated volume is between 100 and 150 ml, the P_{ao} being 35 cm H_2O [74].

The total lung capacity (TLC) is close to 200 ml in term newborns. The predictive equation has been described by Auld et al. [2]:

$$TLC \ (ml) = -381 + 11.68 \times height \ (cm).$$

The residual volume (RV) is thus relatively larger in newborns than in children and in adults. Indeed, it corresponds to 85 % of the FRC and 40 % of the TLC. The TLC being about 200 ml, the FRC/TLC ratio is about 50 to 55 %—*i. e.* a higher value than in children 5 to 6 years of age (40 %) or in adults (45 %) (Fig. III-104).

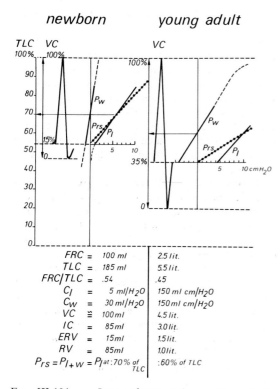

	FRC	=	100 ml	2.5 lit.
	TLC	=	185 ml	5.5 lit.
	FRC/TLC	=	.54	.45
	C_l	=	5 ml/H$_2$O	150 ml cm/H$_2$O
	C_w	=	30 ml/H$_2$O	150 ml cm/H$_2$O
	VC	≅	100 ml	4.5 lit.
	IC	=	85 ml	3.0 lit.
	ERV	=	15 ml	1.5 lit.
	RV	=	85 ml	1.0 lit.

$P_{rs} = P_{l+w} = P_l$ at : 70 % of TLC   :60 % of TLC

FIG. III-104. — *Lung volumes and capacities, elastic pressures (lung, thorax and respiratory system), and mechanics of breathing in newborns and in young adults* (VC = vital capacity; IC = inspiratory capacity; ERV = expiratory reserve volume; other abbreviations are described in the list of abreviations and the text).

RELATIONSHIPS BETWEEN LUNG VOLUMES, ELASTIC FORCES AND RESISTANCES TO GAS FLOW, WITH RESPECT TO ALERTNESS AND SLEEP

In 1965, Macklem et al. [56] demonstrated that in vitro R_l is high when lung volume (V_l) is lower than normal and that R_l decreases when the lung is inflated.

In adults, the airway resistance (R_{aw}) varies inversely with V_l. By increasing V_l, the intrathoracic pressure (P_l) becomes more negative. The elastic forces of the lung being greater, the negative pressure applied on the outer surface of the airways is also higher and the caliber of these airways increases while the R_{aw} decreases.

The relationship between R_{aw} and V_l (or: TGV) is complex. Indeed, R_{aw} depends on the opening of the glottis and of the upper airways [44, 45], as well as on the changes in the tone of the smooth muscles in the small airways and on any pathological change in the elastic properties of the lung parenchyma.

Irregular breathing and apnea have been observed in the premature baby. These phenomena have been recently quantified [79]. It is known that apnea is most often observed during active sleep with rapid eye movement. Breathing is irregular and accompanied by frequent movement of the eyes, the face muscles, and the extremities. Hypotonia and hyporeflexia are also observed. In some cases paradoxical breathing is observed: the volume of the thorax decreases during inspiration, while the volume of the abdomen increases [17, 18, 19, 22, 31]. With a reduction in the thoracic muscle tone, the volume of the thorax as well as that of the lung decreases: FRC [30, 62] and TGV [39] are smaller while the elastic forces which are a function of the lung volume also decrease.

The behavior of the thoracic muscles and of the diaphragm in newborns during active sleep is still disputed, but their decreased activity has been demonstrated. Diaphragmatic activity at the start of expiration is one of the possible mechanisms for limiting expiratory flow. A decrease in this "braking" activity might explain the fall in the lung volume [37]. In the newborn lamb, the activity of the glottis adductors is significantly reduced during active sleep [38]. The influence of the vagus nerve on the rhythm and amplitude of the breathing cycles through reflexes originating in the lung parenchyma and thoracic walls is still disputed.

Thus observations on proprioceptive and chemoceptive reflexes in newborns must be cautiously interpreted. An example is given by the measurement of the elastance of the respiratory system calculated by dividing the inspiratory pressure, at the mouth and nose after occlusion of these airway openings, by the tidal volume preceding this occlusion. The efficiency of the inspiratory muscles depends on their initial length, which itself depends on the volume and shape of the thorax. Volume and shape must be known during these measurements and not assumed to be "normal" [7].

Since the resistances to airflow are largely influenced by the caliber of the small peripheral airways in newborns and in infants [41], the R_l increases when FRC and TGV decrease. C_l dyn also decreases since partial obstruction of these small ducts is explained by a decrease in the elastic-stretching on their outer surface.

However, per unit of lung volume (FRC or TGV), C_l dyn may be relatively higher in active than in quiet sleep. This fact may be explained by a shift towards the lower part of the volume-pressure curve. This V_l/P_l ratio is assumed to be asymptotic and a larger P_l change is required for a similar V_l change when the lung volume is high, the lung being relatively overinflated and less compliant during quiet sleep. An argument for this assumption is given by the relatively high FRC/TLC ratio (0.50-0.55) in newborns compared to that in children and adults (0.40-0.45).

The obstruction of the small airways explains the increase in the work of breathing [11] and the intra-pulmonary veno-arterial blood shunting with a fall in PaO_2 [57, 58]. This hypoxemia is most likely due to gas trapping as well as to ventilatory asynchronism.

Similar changes have been observed when the newborn is breathing pure oxygen at barometric pressure. With an increase in the alveolar-capillary O_2 transfer (the P_AO_2 being high), the lung volume decreases. As the elastic forces decrease [26], the resistance of small airways to gas flow increases. These observations justify a small positive pressure when oxygen is administered to newborns. Thus, collapse of the lung and increase in the resistances are avoided.

The work of breathing has been studied in vitro when the lung volume is decreased [33]. In the deflating lung, small airways may be totally obstructed by a mucous plug: the surface tension of the liquid film on the mucosa of the small ducts being high when their calibers decrease. These ducts will re-open during the next inflation, but at a higher transmural pressure gradient than the one observed during the preceding deflation. The duct being open, the volume of the dependent lung units increases faster than if the duct had been closed at the start of the inflation. The pattern of the volume-pressure curve is thus dependent upon the successive opening and closing of these units, as well as on the elastic properties of the parenchyma. These mechanisms may be modified by collateral ventilation, which may be assumed to be less important in newborns than in adults. Indeed, Cohn's pores have not been observed in the fœtus and the newborn, but they appear later and their numbers rapidly increase with age [55]. Lambert's ducts have not been observed by Boyden before 7 years of age [8].

These changes in lung volumes according to the alertness and the state of sleep and the subsequent changes in the mechanics of breathing (R_l, R_{aw} and C_l dyn) might explain the relatively large range of values collected in the literature. Thus it must now be required to take into account the gestational and post-conceptional age of the newborn, its birth-weight and height, the state of alertness and the quality of the sleep, and the respective size of the thorax and of the abdomen.

AERATION OF THE LUNG AND MECHANICS OF BREATHING IN DISTRESSED NEWBORNS

Hyaline membrane disease (HMD) as well as aspiration syndrome (AS) are identified by similar clinical signs: high respiratory frequency, dyspnea and cyanosis. In most cases, the radiological signs are usefull in the differential diagnosis. Functional studies of both diseases have been performed by Hjalmarson [40].

HYALINE MEMBRANE DISEASE (HMD)

In this group of patients with HMD, the birth-weight was low ($\overline{m} = 2,070$ g) and the mean gestational age was 34 weeks. In order to keep the PaO_2 at 50-80 Torr, the mean O_2 concentration in the inspired gas (FIO_2) was about 52 % and the right to left shunt about 30 % (17 to 48 %). High FIO_2 was required for several days.

The C_l dyn decreased in all patients and even more when the venoarterial shunt increased. The physiological relationship between the tidal volume and the C_l dyn was not observed in these patients and their V_T (tidal volume) significantly decreased (from 14 ml to 7 ml). The decrease in C_l dyn was observed by several authors [13, 72].

The R_l increased but the range of values is large and the highest values were observed when the patient was grunting. However, grunting is not always accompanied by a severe obstruction and a high R_l. The R_l increase is more significant during inspiration than during expiration, as demonstrated by the increase in the negative inspiratory P_{pl}. The inspiratory flow ($\overset{\circ}{V}$) is similar in healthy and in distressed newborns. The higher the R_l, the higher the respiratory frequency and the lower the C_l dyn. The total ventilation per minute is similar or lower than in healthy subjects.

The TGV is significantly decreased: the mean value is 40 ml in distressed and 87 ml in non distressed newborns whose birthweights were similar. The decrease in the lung volume is due to the lack of surfactant and is facilitated by the high compliance of the thoracic wall and by an elevation of the diaphragm when the volume of the abdomen is increased.

It has been demonstrated that even when the abdomen is not distended, the tilting of the body to 45° does not significantly influence the lung volume: the increase of FRC is only 7 ml [3] in newborns, while in children [27] and in adults it can attain 600 ml. The shift of the diaphragm in newborns might depress the lower parts of the thorax.

This decrease in the lung volume was observed by measurements of the TGV [2] as well as of FRC while the patient breathed air [6] or an O_2 enriched gas mixture [49, 50]. The decrease in the FRC when breathing such mixtures is discussed elsewhere [26].

This may explain the decrease of C_l dyn. When the newborn is intubated, the C_l dyn decrease is more significant: The lung volume is probably reduced during expiration when the ventilatory obstruction (expressed by grunting) is abolished by the tube. Conversely, if the tube is partially obstructed, C_l dyn increases [34]. However, the relationship between C_l dyn and the lung volume must be cautiously interpreted.

It has been demonstrated that the volume of the trapped gas (TG = TGV − FRC) could be increased in these patients. However, the TGV is measured when the child is breathing air, and the FRC when he is breathing an O_2 enriched gas mixture [29].

If the TG is actually increased, the P_{oes} could not give an accurate value of the P_{pl}, the pressure at the outside surface of the lung (see p. 476). If the increase of the TG is less than that estimated from the difference between TGV and FRC (measured according to the conditions described here above), the C_l dyn decrease could correspond to changes in the lung parenchyma.

Proof of this assumption, could be given by a decrease of the C_l stat (static lung compliance) per unit of lung volume (FRC or TGV). But this measurement is not routinely performed, since curarization and artificial ventilation are required.

An increase in the elastic recoil has been described in newborns with HMD [3]. A relation between this increase and the lack of surfactant has been suggested [5, 12].

The so called "elastic resistance" opposed to the inspiratory flow via the alveoli, whose volume is markedly decreased at the end of expiration, might explain the high negative inspiratory pressure and the fall of C_l dyn.

Hjalmarson [40] observed that in some patients the pressure-volume loop is concave to the pressure axis, the C_l dyn being significantly decreased during the second part of the inspiration and the first part of the next expiration.

At the start of the inspiration, the C_l dyn would depend on the surface tension forces and the pressures required to open the fairly atelectatic alveoli. During the second part of the inspiration, P_{pl} would depend on the visco-elastic forces of the parenchyma in which the volume of the interstitial liquid is increased as is the volume of the lymphatic network [54].

This difference between the C_l dyn at the start and at the end of V_T is typical of HMD, and is not observed in patients whose respiratory syndrome is not due to a lack of surfactant [40]. Finally, ventilatory asynchronism could explain the fall of C_l dyn. With an increased respiratory frequency, the small differences between the time constants and the air flow resistance from one lung unit to an other might justify a decrease in the C_l dyn.

In some groups of patients, a negative correlation is first observed between the breathing frequency and the C_l dyn. However, from multiple regression analysis and taking into account all the factors influencing C_l dyn, this relationship is not statistically significant [40].

As far as we know, ventilatory asynchronism has not been demonstrated in these patients (namely by comparing the C_l stat and the C_l dyn). However, in the preterm baby with HMD, who is intubated and artificially ventilated, an increase in the C_l dyn has been observed when the breathing frequency is decreased. The distribution of the inspired air when slowly insufflated might be different. This has been demonstrated in adults. From regional differences between ventilated lung volumes and, consequently, between the mechanics of breathing, differences in "inspired" gas distribution may be assumed; but they have not been definitively proven. The V_T being decreased and the breathing frequency (f) being increased, the total ventilation per minute ($\overset{\circ}{V}$) is similar to the values observed in healthy newborns. However, the alveolar ventilation is most likely decreased (see below).

The decrease of V_T and the simultaneous increase of f are in agreement with the concept of adjusting the ventilation to do a minimal amount of work [60, 66]. This concept described in adults also seems applicable in healthy newborns [14].

However, the regulation and control of the respiratory centers in the distressed newborn, by hypoxemia and hypercapnia, is not well understood.

ASPIRATION SYNDROME (AS)

In newborns with an aspiration syndrome, the birthweight is usually higher and the gestational age longer than in babies with HMD. The FIO_2 required for a PaO_2 between 50 and 80 Torr is lower and the duration of oxygen therapy is shorter than in newborns with HMD [40].

C_l dyn is lower than in healthy babies, but the data are variable and this ventilatory parameter does not differentiate between aspiration syndrome and HMD. The C_l dyn decrease is transient, but the more marked the decrease, the higher the FIO_2 required.

The R_l is not always increased, but when such is the case, the obstruction occurs during expiration: the relationship between R_l and the maximal expiratory P_{pl} is statistically significant. However, the latter is not always increased and the maximal inspiratory P_{pl} is less negative than in newborns with HMD. The TGV values are very variable. As in patients with HMD, respiratory frequency (f) is increased and V_T is decreased, the total ventilation being larger than in healthy newborns. However, (f) being similar to that in HMD and V_T being less reduced, the total ventilation is larger in aspiration syndrome than in HMD: the decrease of TGV, when observed, might be due to atelectatic lung units that have been observed in vitro. This might explain the transient decrease of C_l dyn observed in some patients. However, the low C_l dyn might also be explained by transient changes in the lung parenchyma or by ventilatory asynchronism.

Generally speaking, the values of these ventilatory parameters are more variable in aspiration syndrome than in HMD: the quantity and the quality of the inhaled material and its distribution in the airways are more variable as demonstrated by X-ray examination.

The pattern of the pressure-volume curve is similar to the one observed in healthy children, and the concave pattern described in HMD has not been observed in patients with aspiration syndrome.

VENTILATORY WORK

This work was previously considered to be very high in distressed newborns [13, 15, 24, 46] and it was said that "these patients died exhausted and that therapy may help by decreasing the ventilatory work" [15]. But the compliance of the thoracic cage being 5 to 10 times higher than the lung compliance, the elastic forces of the thorax are far less involved in this ventilatory work (see p. 479 and p. 481) which has been estimated by Hjalmarson et al. [40].

These authors first demonstrated that, as in adults, the diaphragm is actually contracting, not only during inspiration but also during the first part (and not during the second half) of expiration, as shown by the EMG. The volume of the respiratory system at the end of expiration is thus a relaxation volume, if the muscular respiratory activity is near zero. This volume depends only on the respective elastic qualities of the lung and the thorax.

The relationship between $\overset{\circ}{W}$ (ventilatory work) and $\overset{\circ}{V}$ (ventilation) per minute is not linear in newborns (nor in children or adults): the logarithmic correlation between $\overset{\circ}{W}$ and $\overset{\circ}{V}$ is more accurate. In distressed newborns, the $\overset{\circ}{W}$ per liter of ventilated gas is actually higher than in healthy babies, but the difference is not large. However, the $\overset{\circ}{W}$ is much less than in a crying healthy newborn, whose $\overset{\circ}{W}$ is 25 to 50 times higher than during quiet breathing, and 4 to 9 times higher than in a distressed baby. During a cry, the resistance to expiratory flow is very high.

An adult is capable of performing maximal ventilatory work that is 500 times greater than that required during quiet breathing [66].

The energy cost of this ventilatory work is higher in the premature baby (0.9 ml O_2 per 0.5 l of ventilated gas) than in the adult (0.5 ml O_2) [84]—i. e. a few percent of the total metabolism and of the O_2 consumption—. O_2 consumption and CO_2 excretion should be similar in distressed and in healthy newborns [46, 77].

The increase of P_aCO_2 without a simultaneous increase in ventilation suggest exhaustion. However, the observations described above do not confirm this assumption. It is not known why the regulation of f and V_T for minimal ventilatory work is more efficient than the influence of P_aCO_2 increase on the respiratory centers.

REFERENCES

[1] AGOSTINI (E.), D'ANGELO (E.). — Comparative features of the transpulmonary pressure. *Res. Physiol.*, *11*, 76-83, 1971.
[2] AULD (P. A. M.), NELSON (N. M.), CHERRY (R. B.), RUDOLPH (A. J.), SMITH (C. A.). — Measurement of thoracic gas volume in the newborn infant. *J. Clin. Invest.*, *42*, 476-483, 1963.
[3] AVERY (M. E.). — *The lung and its disorders in the newborn infants.* Ed. W. B. Saunders, Philadelphia, 1968.
[4] AVERY (M. E.), COOK (C. D.). — Volume-pressure relationship of lungs and thorax in fetal newborn and adults goats. *J. Appl. Physiol.*, *16*, 1034-1038, 1961.
[5] AVERY (M. E.), MEAD (J.). — Surface properties in relation to atelectasis and hyaline membrane disease. *Amer. J. Dis. Child.*, *97*, 517, 1959.
[6] BERLUND (G.), KARLBERG (P.). — Determination of the functional residual capacity in the newborn infants. *Acta Paediat. Scand.*, *45*, 541-544, 1956.

[7] BOYCHUK (R. B.), SESHIA (M. M. K.), RIGATTO (H.). — The effects of gestational age on the effective elastance of the respiratory system in neonates. *Pediat. Res., 11*, 791-793, 1977.

[8] BOYDEN (E. A.). — Notes on the development of the lung in infancy and early childhood. *Am. J. Anat., 121*, 749-762, 1967.

[9] BRENDSTRUP (A.). — The effect of artificial respiration on the regional distribution of ventilation examined with 133 Xenon. *Acta anaesth. Scand., 10-2*, 180-186, 1966.

[10] BRODY (A. W.), CONNOLY (J. J. Jr), WANDER (H. I.). — Influence of abdominal muscles, mesenteric viscera and liver on respiratory mechanics. *J. Appl. Physiol., 14*, 121-128, 1959.

[11] BRYAN (M. H.). — The work of breathing during sleep in newborns. *Am. Rev. Resp. Dis., 119*, 137-138, 1979.

[12] BRYAN (M. H.), HARDIE (M. J.), REILLY (B. J.), SWYER (P. R.). — Pulmonary function studies during the first year of life in infants recovering from the respiratory distress syndrome. *Pediatrics, 52*, 169-178, 1973.

[13] CHU (J.), CLEMENTS (J. A.), COTTON (E. K.), KLAUS (M. H.), SWEAT (A. Y.), TOOLEY (W. H.). — Neonatal pulmonary ischemia. I. Clinical and physiological studies. *Pediatrics, 40*, 709-782, 1967.

[14] COOK (C. D.), CHERRY (R. B.), O'BRIEN (D.), KARLBERG (P.), SMITH (C. A.). — Studies of respiratory physiology in the newborn infant. I. Observation on normal premature and full-term infants. *J. Clin. Invest., 34*, 975-982, 1955.

[15] COOK (C. D.), SUTHERLAND (J. M.), SEGAL (S.), CHERRY (R.), MEAD (J.), MCILROY (M. B.), SMITH (C. A.). — Studies of respiratory physiology in the newborn infant. III. Measurements of mechanics of respiration. *J. Clin. Invest., 36*, 440-448, 1957.

[16] CROSS (K.), KLAUS (M.), TOOLEY (W. H.), WEISSER (K.). — The response of the newborn baby to inflation of the lungs. *J. Physiol. (Lond.), 151*, 551-565, 1960.

[17] CURZY-DASCALOVA (L.). — Thoracico-abdominal respiratory correlation in infants: constancy and variability in different sleep states. *Early Human Development, 2*, 25-38, 1978.

[18] CURZY-DASCALOVA (L.), PLASSART (E.). — Mouvements respiratoires au cours du sommeil du nouveau-né à terme : comparaison des enregistrements thoraciques et abdominaux. *Rev. EEG Neurophysiol., 6*, 97-104, 1976.

[19] CURZI-DASCALOVA (L.), PLASSART (E.). — Respiratory and motor events in sleeping infants: their correlation with thoracico-abdominal respiratory relationships. *Early Human Development, 2*, 39-50, 1978.

[20] DALY (W. J.), BONDURANT (S.). — Direct measurements of respiratory pleural pressure changes in normal man. *J. Appl. Physiol., 18*, 513-518, 1963.

[21] DU BOIS (A. B.), BRODY (A. W.), LEWIS (D. H.), BURGESS (B. F.). — Oscillation mechanics of lung and chest in man. *J. Appl. Physiol., 8*, 587-594, 1956.

[22] FLEMING (P. J.), MULLER (N. L.), BRYAN (M. H.), BRYAN (A. C.). — The effects of abdominal loading on rib cage distortion in premature infants. *Pediatrics, 64*, 425-428, 1979.

[23] FOMON (S. J.), JENSEN (R. L.), OWEN (G. M.). — Determination of body volume of infants by a method of helium displacement. *Ann. N. Y. Acad. Med., 110*, 80, 1963.

[24] FOWLER (K. T.). — Relative compliances of well and poorly ventilated spaces in the normal human lung. *J. Appl. Physiol., 19*, 937-945, 1964.

[25] GEUBELLE (F.), DEFECHEREUX (J.). — Calculateur analogique pour mécanique ventilatoire. *Bull. Scient. AIM Liège, 4*, 153-161, 1970.

[26] GEUBELLE (F.), FRANCOTTE (N.), BEYER (M.), LOUIS (I.), LOGVINOFF (M. M.). — Functional residual capacity and thoracic gas volume in normoxic and hyperoxic newborn infants. *Acta Paediat. Belg., 30*, 221-225, 1977.

[27] GEUBELLE (F.), GOFFIN (C.). — Respiratory studies in children. IV. Lung volume and body positions in healthy children. *Acta Paediat. Scand., 51*, 255-260, 1962.

[28] GEUBELLE (F.), KARLBERG (P.), KOCH (G.), LIND (J.), WALLGREN (G.), WEGELIUS (C.). — L'aération du poumon du nouveau-né. *Biol. Neonate, 1*, 169-210, 1959.

[29] GEUBELLE (F.), LAGNEAUX (D.). — *La fonction respiratoire du nouveau-né.* Ed. Nélissen, Liège, Belgique, 1977.

[30] GEUBELLE (F.), MOSSAY (C.). — Mécanique ventilatoire chez le nourrisson. Presented at the 7th Meeting of « Groupe de Pneumologie et Phtisiologie de Langue Française » (Paris, 21-22 septembre 1979).

[31] GEUBELLE (F.), MOSSAY (C.). — Lung volumes and mechanics of breathing in newborn. *In:* Physiological and Biochemical Basis for Perinatal Medecine. Samuel Z. Levine Conf., 1st Int. Meet., Paris 1979, pp. 13-19, Basel 1981, Karger.

[32] GEUBELLE (F.), SENTERRE (J.). — Methods of investigation of the mechanics of breathing in the artificially ventilated newborn. *Biol. Neonate, 16*, 35-46, 1970.

[33] GLAISTER (D. H.), SCHROTER (R. C.), SUDLOW (M. F.), MILIC-EMILI (J.). — Transpulmonary pressure gradient and ventilation distribution in excised lungs. *Resp. Physiol., 17*, 365-385, 1973.

[34] GRAFF (T. D.), SEWALL (K.), LIM (H. S.), KANT (O.), MORRIS (R. E.), BENSON (D. W.). — The ventilatory response of infants to airway resistance. *Anesthesiology, 27*, 168-175, 1966.

[35] GREGG (R. H.), BERNSTEIM (J.). — Pulmonary hyaline membranes and the respiratory distress syndrome. *Amer. J. Dis. Child., 102*, 871-890, 1961.

[36] GRIBETZ (I.), FRANK (N. R.), AVERY (M. E.). — Static volume-pressure relations of excised lungs of infants with hyaline membrane disease, newborn and stillborn infants. *J. Clin. Invest., 38*, 2168-2175, 1959.

[37] HAGAN (R.), BRYAN (A. C.), BRYAN (M. H.), GULSTON (G.). — Neonatal chest wall afferents and regulation of respiration. *J. Appl. Physiol., 42*, 362-367, 1977.

[38] HARDING (R.), JOHNSON (P.), MCCLELLAND (M. E.). — The expiratory role of the larynx during development and the influence of behavioural state. In *Proceedings of the Wenner Gren Symposium, 1978*, Oxford, Pergamon.

[39] HENDERSON-SMART (D. J.), READ (D. J. C.). — Reduced lung volume during behavioural active sleep in the newborn. *J. Appl. Physiol., 46*, 1081-1085, 1979.

[40] HJALMARSON (O.). — Mechanics of breathing in newborn infants with pulmonary disease. *Thèse, Göteborg*, 1974.

[41] HOGG (J. C.), WILLIAMS (J.), RICHARDSON (J. B.),

MACKLEM (P. T.), THURLBECK (W. M.), PATH (C. H.). — Age as a factor in the distribution of lower, airway conductance and the pathologic anatomy of obstructive lung disease. *New Engl. J. Med. 282*, 1283-1287, 1970.

[42] HUTCHINSON (A. A.), FORBES (A. M. W.), RUSSEL (G.). — Effective pulmonary blood flow in preterm and light for date infants. *Pediatrics, 57*, 187-190, 1976.

[43] HUTCHINSON (A. A.), ROSS (K. R.), RUSSEL (G.). — The effect of posture on ventilation and lung mechanics in preterm and light-for-date infants. *Pediatrics, 64*, 429-432, 1979.

[44] HYATT (R. E.), WILCOX (R. E.). — Extrathoracic airway resistance in man. *J. Appl. Physiol., 16*, 326-330, 1961.

[45] JAEGER (M. J.), BOUHUYS (A.). — Loop formation in pressure versus flow diagrams obtained by body plethysmographic techniques. *Prog. Resp. Res., 4*, 116, 1969.

[46] KARLBERG (P.), COOK (C. D.), O'BRIEN (D.), CHERRY (R. B.), SMITH (C. A.). — Studies of respiratory physiology in the newborn infant. Observations during and after respiratory distress. *Acta Paediat. Scand., 43* (suppl. 100), 397-411, 1954.

[47] KOCH (G.). — Alveolar ventilation, diffusing capacity and the A-*a* PO$_2$ difference in the newborn infant. *Respiration Physiol., 4*, 168-192, 1968.

[48] KOCH (G.). — Lung function and acid-base balance in the newborn infant. *Acta Paediat. Scand.*, suppl. *181*, 1968.

[49] KRAUSS (A. N.), AULD (P. A. M.). — Measurement of functional residual capacity in distressed neonates by helium rebreathing. *J. Pediatr., 77*, 228-232, 1970.

[50] KRAUSS (A. N.), AULD (P. A. M.). — Pulmonary gas trapping in premature infants. *Pediat. Res., 5*, 10-16, 1971.

[51] KRAUSS (A. N.), KLAIN (D. B.), DAHMS (B.), AULD (P. A. M.). — Vital capacity in premature infants. *Amer. Rev. Resp. Dis., 108*, 1361-1366, 1973.

[52] LACOURT (G.), POLGAR (G.). — Interactions between nasal and pulmonary resistance in newborn infants. *J. Appl. Physiol., 30*, 870-873, 1971.

[53] LAUWERIJNS (J. M.). — Hyaline membrane disease in newborn infants. *Hum. Path., 1*, 175, 1970.

[54] LAUWERIJNS (J. M.), CLAESSENS (S.), BOUSSAUW (L.). — Pulmonary lymphatics in neonatal hyaline membrane disease. *Pediatrics, 41*, 917-930, 1968.

[55] MACKLEM (P. T.). — Airway obstruction and collateral ventilation. *Physiol. Rev., 51*, 368-436, 1971.

[56] MACKLEM (P. A.), WILSON (N. J.). — Measurements of intrabronchial pressure in man. *J. Appl. Physiol., 20*, 653-663, 1965.

[57] MARTIN (R. J.), HERREL (N.), RUBIN (A.), FANAROFF (A.). — Effect of supine and prone positions on arterial oxygen tension in the preterm infant. *Pediatrics, 63*, 528-531, 1979.

[58] MARTIN (R. J.), OKKEN (A.), RUBIN (D.). — Arterial oxygen tension during active and quiet sleep in the normal neonate. *J. Pediatr., 94*, 271-274, 1979.

[59] MATTHYS (H.), HERZOG (H.). — Die Differentialdiagnose der obstruktiven Lungenkrankheiten mittels Ganzkörperplethysmographie. *Pneumologie, 144*, 1-9, 1971.

[60] MEAD (J.). — Volume displacement body plethysmograph for respiratory measurements in human subjects. *J. Appl. Physiol., 15*, 736-740, 1960.

[61] MEAD (J.). — Respiration: pulmonary mechanics. *Ann. Rev. Physiol., 35*, 169, 1973.

[62] MOSSAY (C.), GEUBELLE (F.). — Apnée et respiration périodique chez le prématuré. Apport des épreuves fonctionnelles respiratoires. In *Comptes rendus de la Soc. Belge de Pédiatrie*, n° *11*, 105-106, 1979.

[63] NELSON (N. M.), PROD'HOM (L. S.), CHERRY (R. B.), LIPSITZ (P. J.), SMITH (C. A.). — Pulmonary function in the newborn infant: the alveolar-arterial oxygen gradient. *J. Appl. Physiol., 18*, 534-538, 1963.

[64] NELSON (N. M.), PROD'HOM (L. S.), CHERRY (R. B.), LIPSITZ (P. J.), SMITH (C. A.). — Pulmonary function in the newborn infant. V. Trapped gas in the normal infant's lung. *J. Clin. Invest., 42*, 1850-1857, 1963.

[65] OLINSKY (A.), BRYAN (M. H.), BRYAN (A. C.). — Influence of lung inflation on respiratory control in neonates. *J. Appl. Physiol., 36*, 426-429, 1974.

[66] OTIS (A. B.), FENN (W. O.), RAHN (H.). — Mechanics of breathing in man. *J. Appl. Physiol., 2*, 592-607, 1950.

[67] OTIS (A. B.), McKERROW (C. B.), BARTLETT (R. A.), MEAD (J.), McILROY (M. B.), SELVERSTONE (N. J.), RADFORD (E. P.). — Mechanical factors in distribution of pulmonary ventilation. *J. Appl. Physiol., 8*, 427-443, 1956.

[68] PESLIN (R.). — Theoretical analysis of airway resistances in an inhomogenous lung. *J. Appl. Physiol., 24*, 761-767, 1968.

[69] PETIT (J. M.). — *Physiopathologie de la dyspnée chez l'asthmatique*. Ed. Arscia, Bruxelles, 1965.

[70] PETIT (J. M.), SENTERRE (J.), BOCCAR (M.), DELHEZ (L.), DAMOISEAU (J.), LAGNEAUX (D.), NAMUR (M.). — Variabilité de la compliance pulmonaire pendant la ventilation de repos chez l'adulte normal. *Path. et Biol., 10*, 1179-1185, 1962.

[71] POLGAR (G.), STRING (S. T.). — The viscous resistance of the lung tissues in newborn infants. *J. Pediatr., 60*, 787-792, 1966.

[72] PROD'HOM (L. S.), LEVISON (Y.), CHERRY (R. B.), SMITH (C. A.). — Adjustment of ventilation, intrapulmonary gas exchange and acid-base balance in early respiratory distress. *Pediatrics, 35*, 662-676, 1965.

[73] REYNOLDS (R. N.), ETSTEN (B. D.). — Mechanics of respiration in apneic anesthetized infants. *Anesthesiology, 27*, 13-19, 1966.

[74] RICHARDS (C. C.), BACHMAN (L.). — Lung and chest wall compliance of apneic paralyzed infants. *J. Clin. Invest., 40*, 273-278, 1961.

[75] RONCHETTI (R.), STOCKS (J.), KEITH (I.), GODFREY (S.). — An analysis of a rebreathing method for measuring lung volume in the premature infant. *Pediat. Res., 9*, 797-802, 1975.

[76] SCHMIDT (U.), LOLLGEN (H.), NIEDING (G.), FRANETZKI (M.), KORN (V.), PRESTELE (K.). — A new oscillation method for determining resistance to breathing. *Progr. Resp. Res., 6*, 402, 1976.

[77] SCOPES (J. W.), AHMED (I.). — Minimal rates of oxygen consumption in sick and premature newborn infants. *Arch. Dis. Child., 41*, 407-416, 1966.

[78] SPOELSTRA (A. J. G.), SRIKASIBHANDHA (S.). — Dynamic pressure-volume relationship of the lung and position in healthy neonates. *Acta Paediatr. Scand., 62*, 176-180, 1973.

[79] STEIN (I. M.), WHITE (A.), KENNEDY (J. L.), MERISALO (R. L.), CHERNOFF (H.), GOULD (J. B.). — Apnea recordings of healthy infants at 40, 44 and 52 weeks postconception. *Pediatrics, 63*, 724-730, 1979.

[80] STRANG (L. B.). — The pulmonary circulation in the respiratory distress syndrome. *Pediat. Clin. N. Amer.*, *3*, 693-701, 1966.

[81] STRANG (L. B.). — The permeability of lung capillary and alveolar walls as determinants of liquid movements in the lung. In *Ciba Foundation Symposium, Lungs liquids.* Ed. PORTER R. and O'CONNOR M. Amsterdam and New York, Elsevier, 1976.

[82] SUTER (P. M.), FAIRLEY (H. B.), SCHOLBOHM (R. M.). — Shunt, lung volume and perfusion during short periods of ventilation with oxygen. *Anesthesiology*, *43*, 617-627, 1975.

[83] SUTHERLAND (J. M.), RATCLIFF (J. W.). — Crying vital capacity. *Amer. J. Dis. Child.*, *101*, 67-75, 1961.

[84] THIBEAULT (D. W.), WONG (M. M.), AULD (P. A. M.). — Thoracic gas volume changes in premature infants. *Pediatrics*, *40*, 403-411, 1967.

[85] VON DER HARDT (H.), LOGVINOFF (M. M.), DICKREITER (J.), GEUBELLE (F.). — Static recoil of the lungs and static compliance in healthy children. *Respiration*, *32*, 325-339, 1975.

[86] ELLINGSON, R. J., PETERS, J. F. — Development of EEG and daytime sleep patterns in normal full-term infants during the first 3 months of life. *Electroencephalog. Clin. Neurophysiol.*, *49*, 112-124, 1980.

[87] HOPPENBROUWERS, T., HODGMAN, J. E., HARPER, R. M., STERMAN, M. B. — Temporal distribution of sleep states, somatic activity and autonomic activity during the first half year of life. *Sleep*, *5*, 131-144, 1982.

[88] PRECHTL, H. F., VAN EYKERN, L. A., O'BRIEN, M. J. — Respiratory muscle EMG in newborns: a nonintrusive method. *Early Hum. Dev.*, *1*, 265-283, 1977.

[89] CURZI-DASCALOVA (L.). — Thoracic-abdominal respiratory correlations in infants: constancy and variability in different sleep states. *Early Hum. Dev.*, *2*, 25-38, 1978.

[90] LESOÜEF, P. H., LOPES, J. M., ENGLAND, S. J., BRYAN, M. H., BRYAN, A. C. — Influence of chest wall distortion on œsophageal pressure. *J. Appl. Physiol. Respir. Environ. Exercise Physio.*, *55*, 353-358, 1983.

25

Oxygen transport in blood and tissues

Maria DELIVORIA-PAPADOPOULOS

INTRODUCTION

The oxygen transport system in man depends on a number of factors, including the fraction of oxygen in the inspired air, the partial pressure of oxygen in the inspired air, alveolar ventilation, the relation of ventilation to perfusion of the lungs, arterial pH and temperature (the Bohr effect), cardiac output, blood volume, hemoglobin concentration, and the affinity of hemoglobin for oxygen.

The major focus of clinical interest in oxygen transport has centered on factors governing oxygen uptake and little attention has been paid to the factors governing oxygen release, the unloading of oxygen to the tissues.

In normal subjects, this complex system is so adjusted to tissue requirements as to maintain an adequate end-capillary oxygen tension. The system has a reasonable reserve capacity, as well as an ability to respond rapidly to changes in oxygen need, but each of its components responds in a different manner.

The lungs, under basal conditions, load about 4 ml of oxygen per minute per kilogram of body mass on hemoglobin but are capable of increasing this about 15 times. Respiration is regulated by the carotid and aortic bodies (responsive to arterial oxygen content) and brainstem chemoreceptors.

The cardiovascular system affects oxygen supply through variation in the cardiac output and the distribution of blood flow. The major determinant of cardiac output is the metabolic activity [35] which acts by local vasodilatation to increase blood flow and venous return and, thereby, cardiac output. Cardiac output does not appear to be responsive to moderate changes in PaO_2 or oxygen content [20], presumably because other mechanisms are able to make an adequate adjustment. It is virtually unaffected by an increase in $PaCO_2$ to 50 mm Hg. Blood viscosity and volume are additional determinants. If volume is kept constant and viscosity altered by a change in hematocrit, a reciprocal change in cardiac output occurs [14]. Cardiac output changes are in the same direction as blood volume, presumably through the modification of venous return. These changes in cardiac output induced by both viscosity and volume manipulations are subsequently returned toward normal by changes in peripheral resistance [22]. Other neurohumeral factors affect cardiac output by their direct action on the heart, reflected in the strength and especially the rate of cardiac contraction.

The normal distribution of blood flow serves not only oxygen needs, but also other functions of blood flow. Consequently, different controls exist for different tissues [28]. Coronary flow reflects the metabolic activity of heart muscle; since oxygen extraction is normally high, changes in cardiac work must be closely paralleled by changes in coronary blood flow [23]. When oxygen supply becomes limited, flow is restricted in tissues with low oxygen extraction in favor of tissues with high extraction. The high-flow/low-extraction areas of circulation constitute an oxygen reserve system that may be deployed in times of oxygen deprivation.

Hemoglobin concentration is regulated by a renal sensing mechanism that seeks to maintain a balance between oxygen supply and oxygen requirement of renal tissues. Any decrease in concentration or arterial oxygen saturation of hemoglobin, or any increase in hemoglobin affinity for oxygen, causes increased erythropoietin production [21]. Although moderate changes in renal blood flow do affect oxygen delivery, they do not alter erythropoietin production, presumably because renal oxygen consumption is also decreased and the ratio between supply and demand remains unaffected. The effect of erythropoietin on the bone marrow is usually limited by available iron; the increase in red-cell production is about twice the basal value *i. e.*, from a daily rate of 1 %. Thus, changes in red-cell mass in response to hypoxia occur slowly [33]. Because of raised viscosity, a higher hemoglobin concentration at the same blood volume reduces blood flow, and normal cardiac output is regained by a re-establishment of normal plasma volume (increase in total blood volume) [32].

The affinity of hemoglobin for oxygen, in concert with flow distribution, translates oxygen flow into available oxygen. This behavior of hemoglobin is depicted by the oxygen dissociation curve (oxygen equilibrium curve) and is customarily expressed as the oxygen tension at which 50 % of hemoglobin is saturated with oxygen (P_{50}) under standard conditions of temperature and pH.

PHYSIOLOGIC FACTORS INFLUENCING THE OXYGEN-HEMOGLOBIN EQUILIBRIUM CURVE

The oxygen-hemoglobin equilibrium curve reflects the affinity of hemoglobin for oxygen (Fig. III-105). As blood circulates in the normal lung, the arterial oxygen tension rises from 40 mm Hg and reaches approximately 110 mm Hg, a sufficient pressure to ensure at least 95 % saturation of the arterial blood. The shape of the oxygen-hemoglobin equilibrium curve is such that the further increase in the oxygen tension in the lung results in only a very small

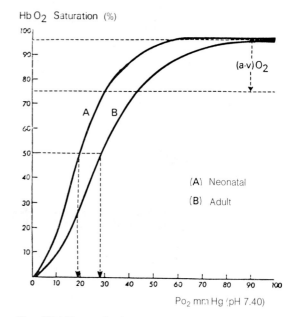

FIG. III-105. — *Oxyhemoglobin equilibrium curves of blood from term infants at birth and from adults*. The P_{50} is 19.4 mm Hg on day one in the term infant (curve A) and 20.8 mm Hg in the adult (curve B).

increase in the degree of saturation of the blood. The oxygen tension falls as blood travels away from the lungs and oxygen is released from the hemoglobin. In the normal adult, when oxygen tension has fallen to approximately 27 mm Hg, at a pH of 7.40 and a temperature of 37° C, 50 % of the oxygen bound to the hemoglobin has been released. The whole-blood oxygen tension at 50 % oxygen saturation (P_{50}), would thus be 27 mm Hg. When the affinity of hemoglobin for oxygen is reduced, more oxygen is released to the tissues at a given oxygen tension. In such situations, the oxygen-hemoglobin equilibrium curve is shifted to the right of normal. Alternatively, if the affinity of hemoglobin for oxygen is increased, the oxygen tension must drop lower than normal before the hemoglobin releases an equivalent amount of oxygen, causing the equilibrium curve to shift to the left.

The sigmoidal shape of the oxygen-hemoglobin equilibrium curve can be explained only if two assumptions are made: (*a*) that the heme groups react with oxygen in a definite order, and (*b*) that the oxygenation and deoxygenation of one profoundly affects the oxygenation and deoxygenation of the others. This phenomenon has been termed "heme-heme interaction" and is reflected in the shape of the curve, which indicates that as each heme group accepts oxygen it becomes progressively easier for the next heme group to pick up oxygen. X-ray crystallographic studies have confirmed the fact that oxygenated and deoxygenated hemoglobins differ in their conformation. These conformational changes are crucial for the interactions of hemoglobin with organic phosphates [27].

Physiological interpretations of the alteration of the position of the oxygen-hemoglobin equilibrium curve

The steep and flat parts of the curve facilitate the functions of oxygen release to the tissues and oxygen uptake in the lungs. The oxygen tensions in alveoli and capillaries of the normal lung lie within the high affinity area of the oxygen dissociation curve; however, in peripheral systemic capillaries, as oxygen is given off there is at first a rapid fall in oxygen tension until the steep part of the dissociation curve is reached, after which capillary PO_2 decreases very little, even though large amounts of oxygen are given off. Since the oxygen tension on the mitochondrial surface, the point of oxygen utilization, is always about 1.0 to 0.5 mm Hg [12], the driving potential for, and consequently the rate of oxygen delivery, is determined uniquely by the mean PO_2 in capillary blood which, in turn, is set by the position of the dissociation curve on the PO_2 axis, and by its steepness, which has the effect that relatively little change in driving potential takes place as the red cell progresses through the capillary.

A shift of the position of the oxyhemoglobin equilibrium curve to the left indicates that the affinity of hemoglobin for oxygen is increased. For example, while a PO_2 of 40 mm Hg results in an oxygen saturation of 75 % at 37° C and pH 7.40, a leftward shift of the curve would result in a higher saturation at the same PO_2. The lower P_{50} of the newborn noted above reflects the increased oxygen affinity of the predominantly fetal hemoglobin. A shift of the position of the oxyhemoglobin equilibrium curve to the right indicates reduced affinity of hemoglobin for oxygen.

Oxygen unloading is determined by the PO_2 gradient between blood and tissues. Thus, the shift of the oxyhemoglobin dissociation curve to the right, as CO_2 enters the blood from the tissues, tends to raise the oxygen tension and to increase this gradient for any given oxyhemoglobin saturation and thereby permits additional transfer of oxygen to the tissues. These movements occur by a process of diffusion. The rate of diffusion depends on several factors: (1) the oxygen pressure gradient existing between capillary and cell, (2) the distance between the closest perfusing capillary and the cell, and (3) the impedance to diffusion provided by the tissues, which is called the diffusion coefficient. As the partial pressure of oxygen decreases, tissue oxygenation may become impaired. The term "critical PO_2" was introduced to indicate the oxygen tension of blood below which diffusion is impaired and organ function is disturbed [25]. A critical PO_2 cannot be a well-defined value that applies to all tissues under all conditions. The oxygen requirements of tissues vary and in some tissues, such as striated muscles, oxygen requirements are determined by the level of activity. The critical PO_2 for the brain appears to be 20 mm Hg. With a shift to the left in the position of the oxygen hemoglobin equilibrium curve, oxygen is released at lower partial pressures and this could ultimately result in impaired diffusion.

pH, PCO₂ and temperature

The dissociation curve of both adult and fetal blood is shifted to the right by an increase in PCO_2, a decrease in pH, or an increase in temperature. The shift caused by a rise in PCO_2 or fall in pH is known as the Bohr effect. The P_{50} of the oxyhemoglobin curve in Figure III-105 is 27 mm Hg. A shift to the right, also referred to as a decrease of oxygen affinity (or rise in P_{50}), favors oxygen release from red cells in peripheral capillaries by increasing the driving potential for oxygen diffusion. The physiological importance of these shifts to the right is therefore clear. An increase in tissue metabolism causes a rise in local temperature and PCO_2, both of which cause a rise in P_{50} (reduced affinity), and a higher gradient of O_2 tension between capillary plasma and the mitochondria. The effect of PCO_2 and pH are, of course, interrelated; a rise in PCO_2 lowers pH and most of the Bohr shift can be explained in that way, given that there is also a small effect specific to CO_2.

The Bohr effect can be expressed as the change in log P_{50} per pH unit [Δ log P_{50}/Δ pH]. The value for adult human blood is 0.48 and that for the newborn human 0.44—which is not significantly different [3]. In mammals with a very high metabolic rate per unit mass, the value is higher.

ROLE OF ORGANIC PHOSPHATES

It has long been recognized that the oxygen affinity of adult hemoglobin in solution is considerably greater than that of the intact fresh erythrocyte. This difference suggests that the erythrocyte contains a substance or substances capable of interacting with hemoglobin and reducing its affinity for oxygen. In 1967, Benesch and Benesch [7] and Chanutin and Curnish [13] demonstrated that the affinity of a hemoglobin solution for oxygen could be decreased by interaction with a number of organic phosphates. Of the organic phosphates tested, 2,3-diphospho-glycerate (2,3-DPG) and adenosine triphosphate (ATP) were found to be most effective in lowering oxygen affinity for hemoglobin, and adenosine diphosphate, adenosine monophosphate, pyrophosphate, and inorganic phosphates had progressively decreasing degrees of effectiveness. Benesch and co-workers found that the highly charged anion 2,3-DPG binds to deoxyhemoglobin and that 1 mole of 2,3-DPG binds reversibly to 1 mole of deoxyhemoglobin tetramer under physiological conditions of solute concentrations and pH.

There are two mechanisms by which 2,3-DPG binds preferentially to deoxyhemoglobin and thereby alters the equilibrium between oxygen and hemoglobin. The preferential binding to deoxyhemoglobin is thought to be due to the change in quaternary structure of hemoglobin with oxygenation. The central cavity of deoxyhemoglobin can bind to 1 molecule of 2,3-DPG per molecule of hemoglobin, whereas the smaller central cavity of oxyhemoglobin cannot. Although it was initially thought that oxyhemoglobin did not bind 2,3-DPG, other studies demonstrated that oxyhemoglobin did bind small amounts of 2,3-DPG [10]. Since measurement of the amount of 2,3-DPG bound to oxygen varied, and because most studies of 2,3-DPG binding were performed with dilute solutions of hemoglobin rather than the higher concentration of hemoglobin found in the erythrocyte, precise quantitation of intracellular changes in 2,3-DPG binding that occur with oxygenation and deoxygenation of blood is not available. Nevertheless, preferential binding of 2,3-DPG to deoxyhemoglobin is generally accepted as a mechanism whereby 2,3-DPG affects the affinity of hemoglobin for oxygen. The second mechanism by which 2,3-DPG reduces oxygen affinity is by altering the intra-erythrocytic pH relative to plasma pH. In accordance with the Donnan equilibrium, increased erythrocytic 2,3-DPG reduces red cell pH. The reduction in pH decreases oxygen affinity by the Bohr effect. It has been shown that both mechanisms apply in the intact erythrocyte, and that at concentrations of 2,3-DPG above normal the latter predominates [33].

Of the organic phosphates normally found in the human erythrocyte, 2,3-DPG is found in largest concentrations and thus is quantitatively the most important with respect to modulation of hemoglobin-oxygen affinity. The content of 2,3-DPG in the erythrocyte (RBC) averages 4.5 μmole/ml RBC's (range 3.4-5.2 μmole/ml) and ATP 1.0 μmole/ml RBCs (range 0.8-1.4 μmole/ml), whereas the remainder of the organic phosphates generally totals less than 0.4 μmole/ml RBCs. Among the factors considered important for oxygen transfer from the maternal blood to the fetus is the position of the oxygen-hemoglobin dissociation curve in the maternal erythrocytes, and one of the most important regulators of the position of the curve in the maternal blood is the concentration of 2,3-DPG. Rorth and Brake concluded from their studies on pregnant women that the 2,3-DPG level is increased during normal human pregnancy [30]. However, whether this increase indicates the existence of a physiological mechanism operating in all pregnant women or merely reflects the effect of the anemia of pregnancy is not known.

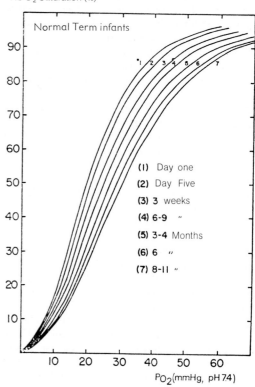

FIG. III-106. — *Oxygen equilibrium curves of blood from term infants at different postnatal ages;* each curve represents the mean value of the infants studied in each age group.

OXYGEN AFFINITY OF FETAL
AND ADULT HEMOGLOBIN

The observation that the oxygen affinity of human fetal blood is greater than that of maternal blood was first made in 1930 [1]. Subsequent studies in older children and adults showed a precise relationship between erythrocyte 2,3-DPG content and the position of the oxygen-hemoglobin equilibrium curve. Studies employing stripped fetal hemoglobin failed to demonstrate this interaction of 2,3-DPG, and both 2,3-DPG and ATP had little effect on lowering the oxygen affinity of fetal hemoglobin, although their effect on the oxygen affinity of adult hemoglobin was profound [8].

In 1971, the deoxygenation kinetics of isolated fetal and adult hemoglobin were studied and significant functional differences between their tetrameric hemoglobins were found [31]. It was observed that these functional differences closely paralleled the differences between beta and gamma chains. These studies first reconfirmed that 2,3-DPG had no significant effect on the deoxygenation rate of fetal hemoglobin. It had been shown that 2,3-DPG binds to fetal hemoglobin,

although the binding constant is lower than for adult hemoglobin [19]. As a result, 2,3-DPG in physiological concentrations was discovered to have no effect on the oxygen affinity of fetal hemoglobin in solution [11, 24]. Other experiments performed on whole blood demonstrated a significant fall in P_{50} when erythrocytes were depleted of 2,3-DPG, even in samples of blood having a very high percentage of fetal hemoglobin [9]. In vitro experiments using pure solutions of fetal and adult hemoglobin showed that the effect of 2,3-DPG on the P_{50} of fetal hemoglobin is approximately 40 % of 2,3-DPG's effect on the P_{50} of adult hemoglobin [29]. On the basis of these findings, one would expect the P_{50} of whole blood to be related to the 2,3-DPG level and to the relative concentration of adult and fetal hemoglobin. The results of the in vitro and in vivo experiments testing this hypothesis proved that even in whole blood the effect of 2,3-DPG on fetal hemoglobin is approximately 40 % of its effect on adult hemoglobin. Since the concentrations of adult hemoglobin and the 2,3-DPG level, and therefore the "functioning fraction of DPG" (FFDPG) (Fig. III-107), increase during gestation, it is not surprising that the P_{50} of whole blood correlates with gestational age. The correlation of P_{50} with gestational age is even closer than with the FFDPG, presenting the

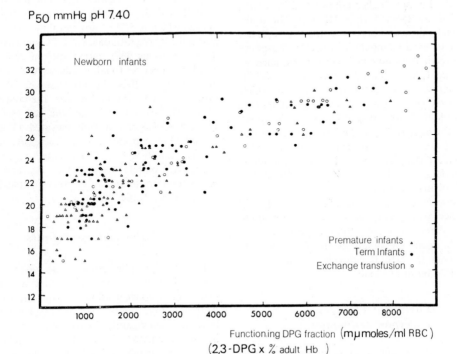

FIG. III-107. — The P_{50} and functioning DPG fraction of all infants studied.

possibility that other unknown factors contribute to the rise of P_{50} during gestation. The changes in oxygen affinity during postnatal life should be taken into account when the oxygen saturation or content of arterial blood in the neonate is derived from measurements of PO_2 and pH. In the absence of other measurements, gestational age can be utilized for a reasonably accurate estimation of the oxygen affinity of fetal blood. There is no satisfactory explanation for the rise in 2,3-DPG levels during gestation. Since it was shown in vitro that the reduced hemoglobin of adults is more effective than reduced hemoglobin in stimulating 2,3-DPG synthesis [5], it is attractive to speculate that the increase in 2.3-DPG with gestation is the result of increased synthesis of adult hemoglobin. This hypothesis is also supported by the significant correlation between the percentage of adult hemoglobin and 2,3-DPG content in the neonatal period (Fig. III-107). The relationship between the changes in 2,3-DPG and P_{50} in adult blood in vitro is almost identical to those calculated using results obtained in patients exhibiting changes in P_{50} and 2,3-DPG levels secondary to a variety of causes [26].

Oxygen dissociation curve of fetal blood

Fetal blood has a higher affinity and lower P_{50} than that of adult blood (Fig. III-105). The difference, which depends both on the hemoglobin molecule and on the amount of organic phosphate in the red cell, is greater in other species, such as the sheep, goat, and guinea pig, than in man [4]. In the placenta, because of the low PO_2's at which transfer of oxygen is achieved, the high affinity of fetal hemoglobin favors oxygen uptake in the fetus.

Indeed, the highest PO_2 in the fetus is in umbilical vein blood leaving the placenta, usually about 30 mm Hg. At that oxygen tension, the saturation of human fetal blood is 6-8 % higher than the saturation of maternal blood [6].

In addition to its high oxygen affinity, fetal blood has a higher hemoglobin concentration than adult blood and hence a higher total oxygen-carrying capacity. In man, the blood of the fetus at term contains about 18 g Hb/dl, equivalent to an oxygen capacity of 24 ml/dl of blood.

Postnatal changes in oxygen transport

The high oxygen affinity of fetal blood is well adapted to oxygen uptake in the placenta, but has disadvantages in postnatal life. Provided the lungs are functioning adequately, the blood flowing through them is exposed to an oxygen tension of 80 mm Hg or more, so that the high affinity at low oxygen tensions has no advantage for oxygen uptake in the newborn period. At tissue level, the low P_{50} decreases the driving potential for oxygen diffusion and therefore limits the rate at which oxygen can be supplied. The newborn needs more oxygen than the fetus; even in a neutral thermal environment and at rest, the oxygen consumption of most species increases by 100-150 % in the first few days of life [2]; colder environments and muscular activity further increase the demand. Hence, a P_{50} adequate for tissue supply in the fetus could provide an insufficient rate of net oxygen diffusion in the newborn.

In most species, postnatal changes take place in both oxygen affinity and oxygen-carrying capacity, but at different rates and by different amounts. During the first day of life, P_{50} in normal infants is 19.4 (plus or minus 1.8) mm Hg, as contrasted with a value of 27.0 (plus or minus 1.1) mm Hg for the normal adult. In the term infant, P_{50} rises during the first 5 days of life to 26.6 (plus or minus 1.7) mm Hg. From day 5, the P_{50} continues to gradually increase and reaches normal adult values by 4-6 months of life (Fig. III-106). The red cell 2,3-DPG on day one averages 5,433 (plus or minus 1,041) mµmol/ml red cells and thus does not differ significantly from that of adults which is 5,114 (plus or minus 418) mµmol/ml red cells. By the fifth day, 2,3-DPG increases to 6,580 (plus or minus 996) mµmol/ml red cells and then gradually declines to adult values. At 8 to 11 months of age, P_{50} in these infants averages 30.3 mm Hg which exceeds the value for the normal adult (Fig. III-106). At this age, the red cell 2,3-DPG content is also considerably elevated while the fetal hemoglobin concentration is decreased to that of normal adult levels. The average values for the percentage of fetal hemoglobin, P_{50}, and 2,3-DPG levels for term infants of various postnatal ages are shown in the Table.

Premature infants

In general, smaller infants have lower erythrocyte 2,3-DPG content, lower P_{50}, and a higher fetal hemoglobin concentration. During the first several weeks of life, these small infants have FFDPG's that are significantly lower than those of term infants. Premature infants have a smaller oxygen unloading capacity initially than do term infants, and do not catch up during the first three months of

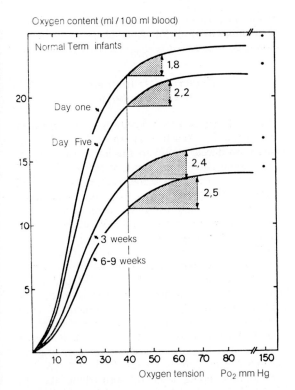

Oxygen content (ml / 100 ml blood)

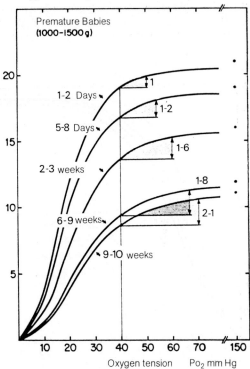

Oxygen content (ml / 100 ml blood)

FIG. III-108. — *Oxygen equilibrium curves of blood from term infants at different postnatal ages.* Double arrows represent the oxygen unloading capacity between a given "arterial" and "venous" PO₂. Points corresponding to 150 mm Hg on the abscissa are the O₂ capacities; each curve represents the mean value of the infants studied in each age group.

FIG. III-109. — *Oxygen equilibrium curves of blood from all weight groups of premature infants at different postnatal ages.* Double arrows represent the oxygen-unloading capacity between a given "arterial" and "venous" PO₂. Points corresponding to 150 mm Hg on the abscissa are the O₂ capacities; each curve represents the mean value of the infants studied in each age group.

life [20] (Fig. III-108, III-109). For various weight groups of infants, the mean oxygen unloading capacities are different.

After birth, oxygen-carrying parameters of blood are profoundly changed. Fetal hemoglobin is replaced by adult hemoglobin within 6 months of birth. Oxygen-carrying capacity is high in the newborn infant but falls within 6 months when hemoglobin levels decline to values that would be called anemic in the adult. Oxygen affinity, also high in the newborn, falls during the first 4 months of extrauterine life to subnormal values. These facts have been known for some time, but it was not possible to explain changes and interaction of relevant parameters completely. A significant correlation between fetal hemoglobin and P_{50} was first reported in 1958 [29] but was not as convincing as had been expected for several reasons: (*a*) In cord blood, identical P_{50} values at different fetal hemoglobin levels were observed, and vice versa; (*b*) blood of adults with persistently

high fetal hemoglobin shows the same oxygen affinity as normal adult blood [32]; (*c*) the blood of infants 3 months of age has a lower oxygen affinity than adult blood, despite a significant amount of fetal hemoglobin. A typical fetal blood oxygen affinity has been demonstrated in several mammals with no apparent fetal hemoglobin [3]. More recently, such studies were extended to the first year of life, which noted a more differentiated postnatal course of erythrocyte 2,3-DPG. This has physiologically meaningful implications with regard to transport mechanisms which concern tissue oxygen supply.

Acute changes in the position of the oxygen-hemoglobin equilibrium curve

An acute shift of the oxyhemoglobin dissociation curve to the right in the newborn infant can be achieved by performing an exchange transfusion with fresh adult blood of low oxygen affinity [16] (Fig. III-110). Acute shifts of the oxyhemoglobin dissociation curve to the left can be achieved in newborn animals by increasing their blood carboxy-hemoglobin to 15 % following inhalation of carbon monoxide in a closed rebreathing system [18].

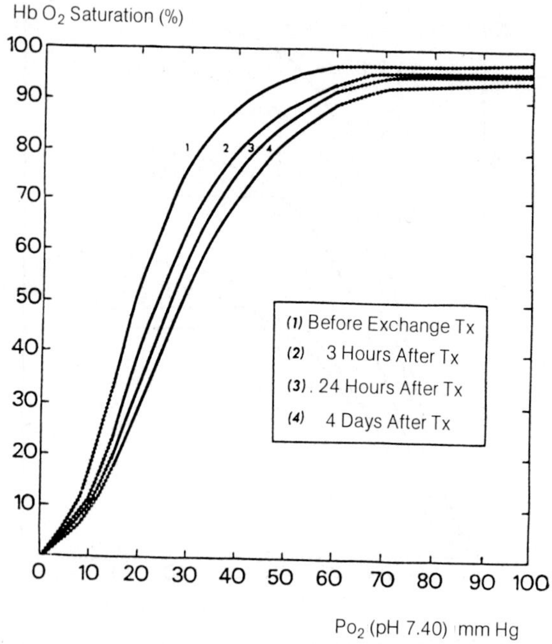

Exchange transfusion in the newborn

In 1954, Valtis and Kennedy first demonstrated that blood for transfusions stored for 7 days or longer produced a shift to the left in the oxygen-hemoglobin equilibrium curve of the recipient [34] and that the recipient's blood retained the increased affinity for oxygen for as long as several days. In 1969, Bunn and associates demonstrated that the increase in oxygen affinity which occurs with blood storage correlated with the fall of 2,3-DPG occurring simultaneously. The consequences of exchange transfusions with fresh versus stored blood were examined in 1971 [17] and it was found that prior to exchange transfusion the P_{50} and erythrocyte 2,3-DPG were similar in each group of infants; in those infants who received blood that had been stored for 4-5 days, the P_{50} value 2 hours after transfusion declined from its original mean value of 20.6 ± 1.7 to 17.1 ± 1.8 mm Hg. Twenty-four hours after the procedure, the P_{50} averaged 23.0 ± 1.1 and by 5 days it reached 27.9 ± 1.0 mm Hg, a value comparable to that of normal adults. The change in 2,3-DPG paralleled the change in P_{50} values (Fig. III-111).

Hb O_2 Saturation (%)

(1) Before Exchange Tx

(2)   3 Hours After Tx

(3) . 24 Hours After Tx

(4)   4 Days After Tx

Po_2 (pH 7.40) mm Hg

FIG. III-110. — *The effect of exchange transfusion on the oxyhemoglobin dissociation curve of newborn infants.*

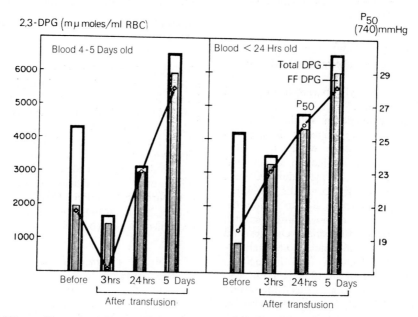

FIG. III-111. — *Comparison of P_{50}, total 2,3-DPG, and "functioning DPG fraction" in two groups of infants receiving 4- to 5-day-old blood, and blood less than 24 hours old for an exchange transfusion.*

In contrast, the infants who received blood that had been stored for less than 24 hours demonstrated a rise in the mean P_{50} only 2 hours after the exchange transfusion, when P_{50} values averaged 23.1 $\pm$ 1.5 mm Hg, compared with the pre-exchange transfusion value of 19.5 $\pm$ 1.3 mm Hg. At 2 hours of age, the P_{50} value was 25.9 $\pm$ 0.6 mm Hg and by the fifth day it was 28.1 $\pm$ 0.9 mm Hg. Again, the change in 2,3-DPG paralleled the change in the P_{50} values. The P_{50} values before and after the exchange transfusion correlated precisely ($r = 0.939$) with the FFDPG (Fig. III-111).

The calculated oxygen-unloading capacity appears decreased in infants receiving transfusions with 5-day-old blood, while in those receiving fresh blood it appears increased [17]. These studies demonstrated that during the immediate post-transfusion period the infant's blood reflects the storage characteristics

Oxygen content (ml / 100 ml blood)

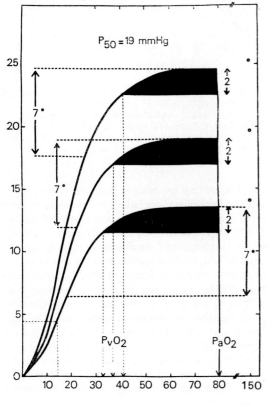

FIG. III-112. — *The effect of altered hematocrit at a constant P_{50} of 19.0 mm Hg on the tissue oxygen unloading of newborn infants.* The asterisk (*) represents the calculated myocardial extraction of oxygen. In this study the P_{50} equals 19.0 mm Hg at a pH of 7.40 and temperature of 37° C.

Oxygen content (ml / 100 ml blood)

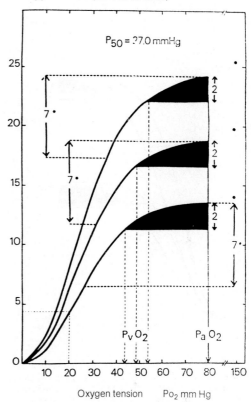

FIG. III-113. — *The effect of exchange transfusion of adult blood of varying hematocrit on the tissue oxygen unloading of newborn infants.* The asterisk (*) represents the calculated myocardial extraction of oxygen. In this study P_{50} equals 27.0 mm Hg at a pH of 7.40 and temperature of 37° C.

of the blood received. Blood stored in acid-citrate-dextrose (ACD) changes its oxygen affinity rapidly because of the prompt fall in 2,3-DPG; thus, blood less than 5 days old is quite dissimilar since blood stored for only 1 day has a lower oxygen affinity than does blood stored for 5 days (Figs. III-116 and III-117). When blood is stored in citrate-phosphate-dextrose, its oxygen affinity and 2,3-DPG content remain essentially unchanged during the storage period [17]. When blood with a lower P_{50} is used for exchange transfusion, the amount of oxygen unloaded between two arbitrarily selected points can be shown to decrease. In the infants exchanged with "old blood", the amount of oxygen unloaded at a venous PO_2 of 40 mm Hg declined from a pretransfusion value of 1.9 ml to a post-exchange transfusion value of 1.0 ml. If oxygen consumption during this interval is to remain

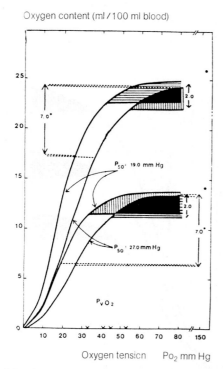

Oxygen content (ml / 100 ml blood)

Oxygen tension   Po₂ mm Hg

FIG. III-114. — *The effect of altering the oxygen affinity and hematocrit in comparing tissue oxygen unloading of the newborn infant.* The asterisk (*) represents the calculated myocardial extraction of oxygen. The P_{50} measurements were made at pH of 7.40 and temperature of 37° C.

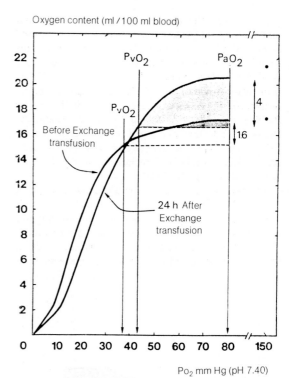

Oxygen content (ml / 100 ml blood)

Po₂ mm Hg (pH 7.40)

FIG. III-115. — *Effect of exchange transfusion with settled red blood cells on tissue oxygen unloading of newborn infants.* Oxygen unloading capacity after exchange transfusion increased from 1.6-4.0 ml/O₂/100 ml blood, while at the same time O₂ affinity decreased from a P_{50} of 17 mm Hg to 28 mm Hg.

unchanged, the infant must either increase its cardiac output while maintaining a narrower arteriovenous oxygen difference, or must increase the arteriovenous oxygen difference while keeping the cardiac output unchanged. The latter situation would produce a lowering of the venous oxygen tension. Such a decrease in the pressure gradient could then result in impairment of oxygen diffusion from the capillaries to the tissues.

In contrast, when blood of a higher P_{50} is used for exchange transfusion, the amount of oxygen unloaded between two arbitrarily selected points is increased. In the infants exchanged with "fresh blood", the amount of oxygen unloaded at a venous PO₂ of 40 mm Hg increased from 1.6 to 2.5 mm Hg. Again, if oxygen consumption remains constant and cardiac output could decrease, or if cardiac output remains unchanged, the central venous oxygen tension will rise. These studies showed that blood stored in ACD more than 5 days old should not be used for exchange transfusion. Blood less than 24 hours old appears to be preferable

for sick infants in whom impaired blood flow, decreased peripheral perfusion, and maximal cardiac effort may already exist. An abrupt and still further shift to the left of the position of the curve in infants whose compensatory mechanisms may be inadequate would lead to further tissue hypoxemia. In subsequent studies in infants where, in addition to their arterial indwelling catheter a catheter was inserted in the inferior vena cava, it was demonstrated that the venous oxygen tension where oxygen appeared to unload was never "fixed". Following alteration of the oxygen affinity with either old blood or fresh blood, the venous PO₂ either decreased or increased respectively, maintaining a constant unloading capacity of the exchanged blood.

Later studies performed on piglets indicate that exchange transfusion with maternal pig blood produces a shift to the right in the position of the oxygen-hemoglobin equilibrium curve with no change in oxygen consumption, but an increase in central venous tension [15] (Fig. III-118).

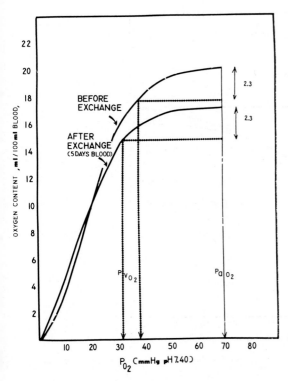

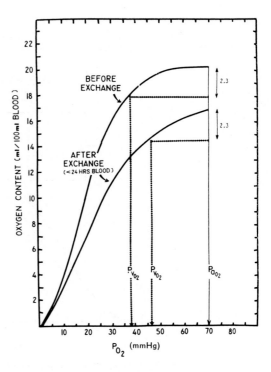

FIG. III-116. — *Oxygen equilibrium curve of infants receiving an exchange transfusion with 4- to 5-day-old blood.* The double arrows represent the oxygen unloading capacity at a given "arterial" and "venous" PO_2; each curve represents the mean value of the infants studied.

FIG. III-117. — *Oxygen equilibrium curve of infants receiving an exchange transfusion with blood less than 24 hours old.* The double arrows represent the oxygen unloading capacity at a given "arterial" and "venous" PO_2; each curve represents the mean value of the infants studied.

Relative effect of oxygen capacity and affinity on oxygen delivery to the tissues

Anemia is a common clinical problem in the premature infant. The hemoglobin level and the other red cell characteristics which influence oxygen transport are frequently altered by exchange transfusion. Thus, a series of measurements relating the effects of oxygen-carrying capacity and oxygen affinity in premature infants was made. Assuming that an infant is healthy and has no evidence of cardiac disease, pulmonary disease, or increased metabolic needs, the oxygen-carrying capacity should be a source of concern only if oxygen delivery to the tissues approaches the limit of oxygen stores. Infants at birth with significant differences in total oxygen capacity but similar oxygen affinity have the same arterial-venous oxygen content differences. It is worth noting that when oxygen capacity decreases significantly due to anemia, sufficient oxygen unloading occurs without lowering the venous

oxygen tension below 30 mm Hg. However, the myocardial extraction of oxygen in the anemic infant requires a blood PO_2 that approaches the critical PO_2 of the tissue.

Anemia infrequently occurs after exchange transfusion due to improper exchange transfusion technique. The reduced oxygen-carrying capacity which results from such anemia is shown in Figure III-113. The arterial-venous content difference can still be maintained due to the change in oxygen affinity resulting from the administration of red cells containing hemoglobin A. However, in this group of anemic infants with an increased P_{50} and decreased oxygen affinity after exchange transfusion, adequate myocardial oxygen extraction requires a PO_2 approaching the critical level. These data illustrate the need to avoid anemia resulting from exchange transfusion.

A comparison of oxygen-carrying capacities and oxygen affinities shows the relative significance of hematocrit level in infants before and after exchange transfusion (Fig. III-114). In the two groups of

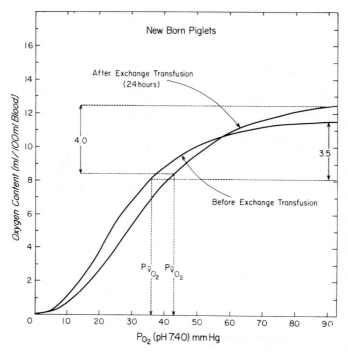

Fig. III-118. — *The effect of exchange transfusion on the oxyhemoglobin dissociation curve of newborn piglets.*

TABLE I. — Oxygen transport in term infants

No. of infants	Age	Total Hb, g/100 ml blood	Hct %	MCHC %	O₂ capacity ml/100 ml blood	P₅₀ at pH 7.40 mm Hg	2,3-DPG μmoles/ml RBC	Fetal Hb, % of total	FFDPG [1] μmoles/ml RBC	Reticulocyte count %
19	1 d	17.8 ±2.0 [2]	52.7 ±7.1	34.2 ±1.9	24.7 ±2.8	19.4 ±1.8	5,433 ±1,041	77.0 ±7.3	1,246 ±570	4.7 ±1.74
18	5 ds	16.2 ±1.2	46.9 ±6.0	34.1 ±0.8	22.6 ±2.2	20.6 ±1.7	6,580 ±996	76.8 ±5.8	1,516 ±495	2.15 ±1.64
14	3 wks	12.0 ±1.3	33.5 ±4.3	35.9 ±1.2	16.7 ±1.9	22.7 ±1.0	5,378 ±732	70.0 ±7.33	1,614 ±252	0.88 ±0.71
10	6-9 wks	10.5 ±1.2	30.2 ±3.9	34.9 ±0.6	14.7 ±1.6	24.4 ±1.4	5,560 ±747	52.1 ±11.0	2,670 ±550	1.63 ±0.65
14	3-4 ms	10.2 ±0.8	30.3 ±2.4	33.8 ±1.7	14.3 ±1.2	26.5 ±2.0	5,819 ±1,240	23.2 ±16.0	4,470 ±1,380	1.36 ±0.45
8	6 ms	11.3 ±0.9	34.0 ±3.6	33.4 ±0.7	14.7 ±0.6	27.8 ±1.0	5,086 ±1,570	4.7 ±2.2	4,840 ±1,500	1.42 ±1.15
8	8-11 ms	11.4 ±0.6	34.8 ±1.9	32.8 ±0.9	15.9 ±0.8	30.3 ±0.7	7,381 ±485	1.6 ±1.0	7,260 ±544	0.82 ±0.27

[1] Functioning fraction of 3,2-diphosphoglycerate.
[2] All values are given as mean ± 1 SD.

anemic infants, those of higher oxygen affinity are definitely compromised in extracting oxygen at the limit of oxygen stores. Those patients with lower oxygen affinity, but the same degree of anemia, appear to be unloading at oxygen tensions further away from the critical PO_2, assuming the infants are at rest. The moment an increased demand for oxygen exists, those infants with either high or low oxygen affinity but with low oxygen capacity, will be at the limit of oxygen stores. The fact that the infants are compensated at rest does not insure that there will be adequate oxygen unloading when body activity is increased.

CONCLUSIONS

From studies to date, some general conclusions can be drawn. In vivo oxygen unloading of hemoglobin is restricted by the oxygen tension at the end of the capillary which cannot fall below a critical level without jeopardizing tissue oxygen supply. Hemoglobin desaturation and thus oxygen delivery to the tissues is limited in blood with low P_{50} values. This deficiency can be balanced by an increase in hemoglobin concentration or by an increase in cardiac output when the hemoglobin concentration is low.

At rest, changes in cardiac output parallel those in oxygen consumption so that oxygen extraction is relatively constant. The decline in hemoglobin concentration in normal infants could be offset by the decreasing oxyhemoglobin affinity. An increase in oxygen need, or a limitation of one of the determinants of oxygen delivery, may rapidly exceed the adaptive capacity in the newborn and cause tissue hypoxia. In our studies of lambs, oxygen delivery has been found to be limited when hemoglobin concentration decreases below 5.0 g/dl at rest, when arterial oxygen saturation is less than 50 %, or when a cardiac shunt is greater than 35 % of the cardiac output.

As seen in Figure III-115, the oxygen unloading capacity in the newborn can be raised considerably by replacing the newborn's blood (P_{50} 17 mm Hg) by blood from an adult (P_{50} 28 mm Hg) with settled cells (hematocrit 50-55 %). However, below an arterial PO_2 of 45 torr, oxygen delivery to the tissues depends more on the blood's oxygen-carrying capacity than on the oxygen affinity. Especially in such cases, it is advisable to keep the hemoglobin concentration above 13 g/100 ml of blood during the first days after birth. By transfusion with adult red cells,

the infant will benefit not only from the higher oxygen-carrying capacity, but also from the lower oxygen affinity of this blood.

REFERENCES

[1] ANSELMINO (K. Y.), HOFFMAN (F.). — Die Ursachen des Icterus Neonatorum. *Arch. Gynaekol.*, *143*, 477, 1930.

[2] AVERY (M. E.). — *The Lung and Its Disorders.* 3rd ed., Saunders, Philadelphia, 1974.

[3] BARTELS (H.). — *Prenatal Respiration.* Amsterdam, North-Holland Publ. Co.

[4] BARTELS (H.), HILPERT (P.), REIGEL (K.). — Die O_2-Transportfunktion des Blutes während der ersten Lebensmonate von Mensch, Ziege und Schaf. *Pfluegers Arch. Ges. Physiol.*, *271*, 169-184, 1960.

[5] BAUER (C.), LUDWIG (L.), LUDWIG (M.). — Different effect of 2,3-diphosphoglycerate and adenosine triphosphate on the oxygen affinity of human and adult fetal hemoglobin. *Life Sci.*, *7*, 1339, 1968.

[6] BEER (R.), DOLL (E.), WENNER (J.). — Die Verschiebung der O_2-Dissoziationskurve des Blutes von Säuglingen während der ersten Lebensmonate. *Pfluegers Arch.*, *265*, 526-540, 1958.

[7] BENESCH (R.), BENESCH (R. E.). — The effect of organic phosphates from the human erythrocyte on the allosteric properties of hemoglobin. *Biochem. Biophys. Res. Commun.*, *26*, 162, 1967.

[8] BENESCH (R.), BENESCH (R. E.), RENTHAL (R.), GRATZER (W. B.). — Cofactor binding and oxygen equilibria in haemogoblin. *Nature (New Biol.)*, *234*, 174-176, 1971.

[9] BREWER (G. J.), EATON (J. W.). — Erythrocyte metabolism; interactin with oxygen transport. *Science*, *171*, 1205-1211, 1971.

[10] BUNN (H. F.), BRIEHL (R. W.). — The interaction of 2,3-DPG with various human hemoglobins. *J. Clin. Invest.*, *49*, 1088, 1970.

[11] BUNN (H. F.), MAY (M. H.), KOCHAOLATY (W. F.), SHIELDS (C. R.). — Hemoglobin function in stored blood. *J. Clin. Invest.*, *48*, 311, 1969.

[12] CHANCE (B.), SCHOENER (B.), SCHINDLER (F.). — In *Oxygen in the Animal Organism*. p. 367-392, F. DICKENS and E. NEIL, eds., London, Pergamon Press, 1964.

[13] CHANUTIN (A.), CURNISH (R. R.). — Effect of organic and inorganic phosphates on the oxygen equilibrium of human erythrocytes. *Arch. Biochem. Biophys.* *121*, 96, 1967.

[14] CONWAY (J.). — Hemodynamic consequences of induced changes in blood volume. *Circ. Res.*, *18*, 190-198, 1966.

[15] DELIVORIA-PAPADOPOULOS (M.), MARTENS (R. J.), FORSTER (R. E.), OSKI (F. A.). — Postnatal changes in oxygen hemoglobin affinity and erythrocyte 2,3-diphosphoglycerate in piglets. *Pediat. Res.*, *8*, 64-66, 1974.

[16] DELIVORIA-PAPADOPOULOS (M.), MILLER (L. D.), FORSTER (R. E. III), OSKI (F. A.). — The role of exchange transfusion in the management of low birth weight infants with and without severe respiratory distress syndrome. I. Initial observations. *J. Pediatr.*, *89*, 273, 1976.

[17] DELIVORIA-PAPADOPOULOS (M.), MORROW (G. III), OSKI (F. A.), COHEN (R.), O'NEAL (P.). — Exchange

transfusion in the newborn infant with fresh and « old » blood: The role of storage in 2,3-diphosphoglycerate, hemoglobin-oxygen affinity and oxygen release. *J. Pediatr.*, 79, 898, 1971.

[18] DELIVORIA-PAPADOPOULOS (M.), PARK (C. R.), CHEN (J. H.) *et al.* — Effect of increased cardiac tissue unloading of lambs following inhalation of carbon monoxide. *Pediat. Res.*, 8, 348, 1974.

[19] DELIVORIA-PAPADOPOULOS (M.), RONCEVIC (N. P.), OSKI (F. A.). — Postnatal changes in oxygen transport of term, premature, and sick infants; the role of red cell 2,3-diphosphoglycerate and adult hemoglobin. *Pediat. Res.*, 5, 235-245, 1971.

[20] GUYTON (A. C.). — Regulation of cardiac output. *Anesthesiology*, 29, 314-326, 1968.

[21] KRANTZ (S. B.), JACOBSON (L. O.). — *Erythropoietin and the Regulation of Erythropoiesis.* Chicago, University of Chicago Press, 1970.

[22] MELLANDER (S.). — Contribution of small vessel tone to the regulation of blood volume and formation of œdema. *Proc. R. Soc. Med.*, 61, 66, 1968.

[23] NAKAMURA (Y.), TAKAHASI (M.), TAKEI (F.) *et al.* — The change in coronary vascular resistance during acute induced hypoxemia with special reference to coronary vascular reserve. *Cardiologia*, 54, 91-103, 1969.

[24] NECHTMAN (C. M.), HUISMAN (T. H. J.). — Comparative studies of oxygen equilibria of human adult and cord blood red cell hemolysates and suspensions. *Clin. Chim. Acta*, 10, 165, 1964.

[25] OPIZ (E.), SCHNEIDER (M.). — Über die Sauerstoffversorgung des Gehirns und der Mechanisms von Mangeliverkungen. *Ergebn. Physiol.*, 46, 126, 1950.

[26] OSKI (F. A.), GOTTLIEB (A. J.), MILLER (L. D.), DELIVORIA-PAPADOPOULOS (M.). — The effects of deoxygenation of adult and fetal hemoglobin on the synthesis of red cell 2,3-diphosphoglycerate and its *in vivo* consequences. *J. Clin. Invest.*, 49, 400, 1970.

[27] PERUTZ (M. F.). — Stereochemistry of cooperative effects of hemoglobin. *Nature*, 228, 726-733, 1970.

[28] WEISSE (A. B.), REGAN (T. J.), NADIMI (M.). *et al.* — Late circulatory adjustments to acute normovolemic polycythemia. *Am. J. Physiol.*, 211, 1413-1418, 1966.

[29] RIEGEL (K. P.). — Respiratory gas transport characteristics of blood and hemoglobin. I. *Physiology of Neonatal Period*, edited by U. STAVE, Appleton-Century-Crofts, New York, 1970.

[30] RORTH (M.), BRAKE (N. E. B.). — 2,3-Diphosphoglycerate and creatinine in the red cell during human pregnancy. *Scand. J. Clin. Lab. Invest.*, 28, 271, 1971.

[31] SALHANY (J. M.), MIZUKAMI (H.), ELIOT (R. S.). — The deoxygenation of kinetic properties of human fetal hemoglobin: Effect of 2,3-diphosphoglycerate. *Biochem. Biophys. Res. Commun.*, 45, 1350, 1971.

[32] SCHRUEFER (J. J. P.), HELLER (C. J.), BATTAGLIA (F. C.), HELLEGERS (A. E.). — Interdependence of whole blood and hemoglobin oxygen dissociation curves from hemoglobin type. *Nature (Lond.)*, 196, 550, 1962.

[33] THORLING (E. B.), ERSLEV (A. J.). — The « tissue » tension of oxygen and its relation to hematocrit and erythropoiesis. *Blood*, 31, 332-343, 1968.

[34] VALTIS (D. J.), KENNEDY (A. C.). — Defective gas-transport function of stored red blood cells. *Lancet*, 1, 119, 1954.

[35] WADE (O. L.), BISHOP (J. M.). — *Cardiac Output and Regional Blood Flow.* Oxford, Blackwell Scientific Publications, 1962.

26

Oxygen therapy

G. DUC

Increasing the oxygen concentration in inspired air remains the most widely used method of treatment for neonatal hypoxemia. The indications for supplemental oxygen, its dangers, and methods of control to minimize hazard, cannot be understood without a grasp of the physiological principles governing oxygen transfer from the gaseous environment to the mitochondria. Thus, we will first devote a large part of this chapter to the pathophysiological mechanisms of hypoxia. This will be followed by a discussion of techniques for controlling oxygen administration according to clinical conditions. A glossary of terms used most often in this chapter and the chapter dedicated to the transfer of the oxygen in the blood, appears in the appendix (p. 531).

HISTORICAL CONSIDERATIONS

The history of oxygen use in neonatal care is highlighted by numerous dilemmas that have arisen since this supportive measure was first used widely in the 1930s. Liberal administration of oxygen, as well as curtailment of its use have been associated with tragic complications. In 1900, Budin recommended the utilization of oxygen for therapy in "cyanosis" [26]. Increased use of oxygen admi-nistered by a funnel [26], gastric tube [183], sub-cutaneous injections (noted but not recommended by Hess [70]), or in incubators [71], was the factor credited with an increase in survival among premature babies according to Hess [71]. Confidence in the benefits of oxygen therapy was reinforced by the 1942 observation that periodic breathing in small premature infants was regularized in a high oxygen environment [178].

The description of the first case of retrolental fibroplasia (RLF), during the same year [166] had no effect on the widespread belief concerning the important benefit of therapeutic oxygen. The international RLF epidemic occured during the decade 1942-1952. The clinical observations of Crosse [42] and Campbell [27] and the experimental studies of Ashton in Britain [6, 7] and those of Patz in the U. S. A. [129, 130, 131, 132] raised the suspicion that supplemental oxygen was implicated as the cause of RLF. That suspicion was confirmed in 1964 by the results of the first collaborative study [89] demonstrating that the risks of RLF were significantly increased by placing premature infants who had survived more than 48 hours and weighed less than 1,500 grams in an oxygen-enriched (over 50 % concentration) environment, for a period of 28 days (the program of care that had been routine since the early 1940s). In the hope that the risk of RLF could be eliminated it was recommended [67, 182] (without a critical test), that oxygen in concentrations greater than 40 % be used only under exceptional circumstances. These recommendations were made in spite of Gordon's concern [62] regarding the effect of such a recommendation on the survival of premature infants in the first 48 hours of life. A retrospective study [10] later demonstrated that the concern was well founded: during the five years (1954 to 1958), a period of oxygen curtailment, the mortality as well as the incidence of hyaline membrane disease increased compared to the years 1944-1948 when oxygen was administered quite liberally. In addition, MacDonald [110] demonstrated that in premature infants, less than 31 weeks gestation, followed for 2 to 8 years, an inverse relationship existed between the incidence of spastic diplegia and the duration of oxygen therapy. It was this very concern (*i. e.* neurological risks following curtailment of oxygen therapy) as well as the experimental observations [29] suggesting a beneficial effect of oxygen in postnatal adaptation that provided the rationale for the increased use of oxygen in the 60's. However, new side-effects attributed to oxygen were noted (bronchopulmonary dysplasia [123] and pulmonary hemorrhage [21, 154]).

During the midsixties, it became practical to measure arterial oxygen tension in samples obtained from umbilical artery catheters or from puncture of peripheral arteries. The problem of the critical fractional concentration of oxygen in inspired air (FIO_2), though unsolved, was rendered obsolete and replaced by the question: what is the critical PaO_2?

A second collaborative study (employing an observational format, rather than experimental methodology) was conducted between the years 1969-1972. The report of this effort published in 1977 [90] did not help define safe limits of PaO_2 or levels at which risks of RLF increase significantly. The risk of RLF appeared to be related to the birth weight and the duration of oxygen therapy; these findings were similar to the ex post facto associations found by re-examining the data from the first collaborative study [89].

The use of the transcutaneous oxygen monitoring [51, 76] in the 70's where continuous measurement of the PaO_2 was achieved, showed that in any baby this parameter is highly variable, particularly during the respiratory distress syndrome. Measurements of PaO_2 in samples obtained intermittently do not detect all states of hyperoxemia; it is conceivable that this may explain the absence of correlation between PaO_2 and the risk of RLF observed in the second collaborative study [90]. Thus, the history of oxygen use in newborn care tells us only that "too much" oxygen is associated with an increase

in the frequency of RLF and "too little" is associated with an increase in mortality and in neurological problems among survivers; the precise limits of the ill defined states of "too much" and "too little" continue to elude us (Table I).

TABLE I. — HISTORY OF O_2 USE
IN NEONATAL MEDICINE

Beneficial effects:

    Cyanotic spells (Budin, 1900) [26]
    Mortality (Hess, 1934) [71]
    Periodic breathing (Wilson, 1942) [178]
    Adaptation of the pulmonary circulation (Cassin, 1964) [29]

Deleterious effects:

    Hyperoxia:
        Retrolental fibroplasia (1942-1954) [89]
        Bronchopulmonary dysplasia (Northway, 1967) [123]
        Pulmonary hemorrhage (Shanklin, 1967) [154]
    Hypoxia:
        Mortality in "HMD" (Avery, 1960) [10]
        Spastic diplegia (McDonald, 1962) [110, 112 *a*]

PHYSIOLOGICAL CONSIDERATIONS

The role of oxygen in cellular metabolism. — Molecular oxygen participates in numerous types of oxidative reactions necessary for cellular metabolism: (*a*) As a terminal acceptor of electrons in the respiratory (cytochrome) chain, (*b*) As an oxidant in the reaction of monoxygenases with cytochrome P450. These monoxygenases are responsible, for example, for the hydroxylation of certain pharmacological substances, e. g. amino acids, steroids and catecholamines, (*c*) As an oxidant in deoxygenase reactions responsible, for example, for the production of prostaglandins (cyclogenases). Given the fact that the respiratory chain (oxidative phosphorylation) accounts for more than 90 % of an organism's total oxygen consumption, we will focus the discussion on this particular aspect of cellular oxygen metabolism.

OXIDATIVE PHOSPHORYLATION
(RESPIRATORY CHAIN)

The major portion of the energy consumed by an organism is derived from the degradation on oxidation of glucose in the glycolytic and citric acid cycles according to the general reaction indicated in the Figure III-119.

$$C_6H_{12}O_6 + 6 O_2 \longrightarrow 6 CO_2 + 6 H_2O$$
GLUCOSE
2863 KJ

FIG. III-119. — *Oxidation of glucose (glycolysis).*

This available energy is not consumed instantaneously, but is stored in the form of ATP. Furthermore, this energy is not liberated in blocks during the degradation of glucose, but in small steps, thus gaining optimal efficiency in the production of ATP. The transformation from ATP to ADP (and partly to AMP) liberates energy from the second and third phosphate bond (Fig. III-120).

As the reserves of ATP are small, the constant synthesis of the product is necessary in all cells in order to ensure adequate energy reserves. ATP can be synthesized from both aerobic and anaerobic glycolysis. The differences between these two types

of transformation are indicated in Figure III-121. Aerobic transformation produces 19 times more energy than the anaerobic process.

LOCALIZATION OF OXYGEN CONSUMPTION IN THE CELL

The oxygen consumption takes place in the mitochondria where oxygen combines with electrons to produce water (Fig. III-121). Glycolytic enzymes are present in the cytoplasm: those of the respiratory chain are localized in the inner membrane of mitochondria. Pyruvic acid and NADH formed during glycolysis diffuse from the cytoplasm into the mitochondria where they are oxidized. Hydrogen is liberated in the form of NADH. The latter substance is oxidized in the respiratory chain (flavine, quinone, cytochrome *b*, *c*, *a*, *a₃*, and its electrons finally bind to oxygen forming water (Fig. III-121). The binding reaction takes place only when the partial pressure of oxygen in the mitochondria in greater than 2 mm Hg.

ADENOSINE -(P)~(P) + (P) ⟶ ADENOSINE -(P)~(P)~(P)

A D P   A T P

FIG. III-120. — *Energy reserve coming from glycolysis* ~ *represents energy-rich bindings.*

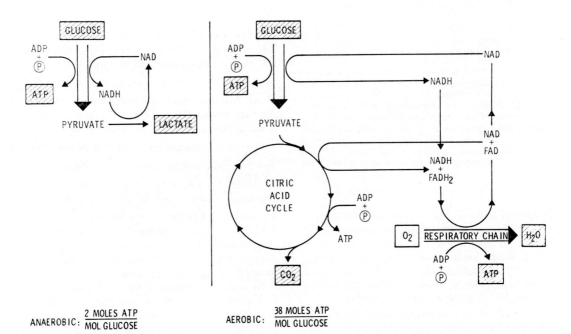

FIG. III-121. — *Differences between aerobic and anaerobic glycolysis.*

TRANSFER OF THE OXYGEN
FROM AIR
INTO THE MITOCHONDRIA

An understanding of the mechanisms regulating transfer of oxygen from environmental air to the mitochondria is necessary in order to rationalize the indications, dosage and control of oxygen therapy. The three principal levels of this transfer are represented in Figure III-122; inspired air, alveolar air and arterial blood. Each of these steps may be characterized by the composition of vital gases: concentration and partial pressure of O_2 and CO_2.

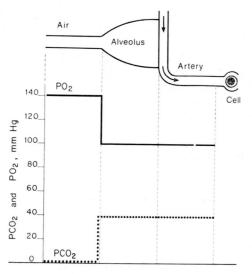

FIG. III-122. — *The lung is represented as a single alveolus perfused by a single vessel. The PO_2 and PCO_2 in three considered environments (inspired air, alveolar air, and arterial blood) are represented in the lower part of the figure. This lung is called "ideal" because it is functionally homogeneous (the same PAO_2 and $PACO_2$ in all the alveoli) and exhibits perfect equilibrium between the alveolar air and arterial blood, and also because all the pulmonary perfusion goes through the alveoli.*

Inspired air. — The oxygen concentration in the inspired air is expressed by the fraction (F) of that gas in the ambient gaseous environment, ignoring water vapor. Note that such classical instruments as Haldane, Scholander measure that fraction directly. In the atmospheric air, the fraction (concentration of oxygen (FIO_2)) is 0.2094.

The partial pressure of oxygen in the inspired air (PIO_2) takes into account temperature and humidity conditions of the body. The PIO_2 may be calculated when the FIO_2 and barometric pressure (PB) of dry gas are known.

$$PIO_2 = FIO_2 \cdot (PB - PH_2O) \text{ (Equation 1)}$$

where PB is the environmental barometric pressure, PH_2O is the pressure of the water vapor saturated at body temperature. At 37° C PH_2O is equal to 47 mm Hg or 6.3 kPa.

Example: The PIO_2 at sea level (BP = 760 mm Hg or 101.3 kPa) at a temperature of 37° C is equal to:

$$PIO_2 = 0.2094 \times (760 - 47)$$
$$= 149 \text{ mm Hg or } 19.9 \text{ kPa}$$

Note that PIO_2 but not FIO_2 decreases progressively with altitude (Table II).

TABLE II. — ALTITUDE AND PARTIAL PRESSURE OF O_2 IN INSPIRED AIR (PIO_2)

Altitude in meters	Barometric pressure in mm Hg	PIO_2 in mm Hg
sea level	760	149
1,000	674	131
2,000	596	115
3,000	526	100
4,000	462	87
5,000	495	75

Alveolar air. — Alveolar air is the gas contained within alveoli. Its composition depends partially on the consumption and/or production of gas exchanged ($\dot{V}O_2$, $\dot{V}CO_2$) and on alveolar ventilation ($\dot{V}A$). Alveolar ventilation is the volume of inspired air that renews the alveolar air every minute. The alveolar partial pressure of CO_2 ($PACO_2$) is proportional to the production of carbon dioxide ($\dot{V}CO_2$) and inversely proportional to $\dot{V}A$. When the ratio of $\dot{V}CO_2$ to $\dot{V}A$ is less than normal, $PACO_2$ is decreased. This state is called *hyperventilation.* Conversely, when the ratio of $\dot{V}CO_2$ to $\dot{V}A$ increases, $PACO_2$ rises and we define this state as *hypoventilation.* Reciprocally, the alveolar partial pressure of oxygen (PAO_2) is raised during hyperventilation and lowered during hypoventilation.

In research settings, PAO_2 and $PACO_2$ can be measured continuously at the mouth during end-expiration with instruments having rapid response times (e. g. mass spectrometer). Ordinarily, $PACO_2$ is estimated, and PAO_2 is calculated.

Estimation of alveolar PCO₂. — It is generally accepted that PACO₂ differs very little from the partial pressure of CO_2 in the arterial blood (PaCO₂) because the pulmonary diffusing capacity for CO_2 is large (3 to 6 times that of oxygen) [34, 56]. Since the arterial venous difference for PCO₂ is small, the pressure in the capillary blood (PcCO₂) is very close to that of the arterial blood (PaCO₂). This is why, in practice, the PcCO₂ or the PaCO₂ are accepted as accurate indicators of states of hyper- and hypo-ventilation.

Calculation of PAO₂. — The PAO₂ may be calculated by a simplified form of the alveolar gas equation:

$$PAO_2 = PIO_2 - \frac{PaCO_2}{R} \qquad \text{(eq. 2)}$$

R = Respiratory Gas Exchange Ratio, varies between 0.8 and 1.0

The relationship that exists between $\dot{V}A$, PAO₂ and the PACO₂ is represented in Figure III-123. This illustration permits the visualization of some principals that are important in everyday practice.

The relationship between $\dot{V}A$ and the alveolar gases is that of a hyperbola. When $\dot{V}A$ increases PAO₂ rises and approaches the value of PIO₂ asymptotically. The effect of hyperventilation on PAO₂ is not the same as that of hypoventilation. For instance, when $\dot{V}A$ doubles the PAO₂ increases by only 20 mm Hg (100-120 mm Hg) (and when $\dot{V}A$ is halved PAO₂ decreases by 40 mm Hg (100 to 60 mm Hg)). It appears, thus, that at the same variation, hypoventilation has a greater effect on PAO₂ than does hyperventilation. The asymmetry as seen in Figure III-123, is enhanced in arterial blood when one considers oxygen saturation, because of the sigmoidal form of the hemoglobin dissociation curve.

An inverse relationship is observed for CO_2: when $\dot{V}A$ is halved the PACO₂ doubles and when $\dot{V}A$ is doubled PACO₂ decreases by half. As in the case of oxygen in relatively equal variations of ventilation, PACO₂ increases disproportionately in hypoventilation as compared with the decrease observed when there is hyperventilation.

The effect on PAO₂ of increasing FIO₂ from 20.9 % to 30 % is displayed graphically in Figure III-123. When $\dot{V}A$ is lowered by one-fourth from the normal value, the augmentation of FIO₂ from 20.9 to 30 % is sufficient to maintain the PAO₂ at about 130 mm Hg. However, note that this hypoventilation is followed by a parallel increase of

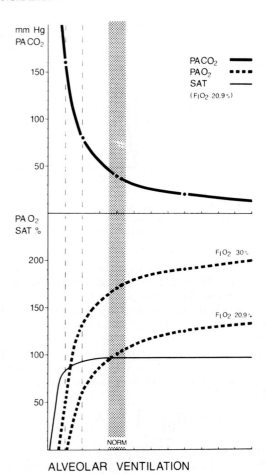

FIG. III-123. — *The relationship between alveolar ventilation* ($\dot{V}A$), *PACO₂ and PAO₂ for FIO₂ of 20.9 % and 30 % are represented in this figure.* The relationship that exists between $\dot{V}A$ and O₂ saturation of the Hb (in the terminal pulmonary capillary blood of a subject breathing 20.9 % O₂) is also represented. $\dot{V}A$ size is only qualitative here. This figure illustrates the difference between effects of hyperventilation and hypoventilation on PACO₂, PAO₂ and Hb saturation (see also Fig. III-125).

PACO₂ to 160 mm Hg, an abnormal state which is not corrected by the increase in FIO₂.

Arterial blood. — Arterial blood transports oxygen from the pulmonary capillaries to the tissues where it is utilized. The properties of the circulatory transport of oxygen can be described in terms of concentration and partial pressure, on the one hand, and cardiac output on the other. The situation is, however, more complicated than that in the transport of O₂ in air because blood, unlike

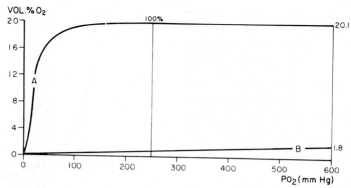

FIG. III-124. — *Comparison between the dissociation curve of Hb* (line A) *and the quantity of O_2 dissolved in plasma* (line B) *for PO_2 from 0 to 600 mm Hg.* Here the dissociation curve of Hb has been determined for a blood sample of 100 ml with 15 g Hb at pH of 7.40 and 38° C.

air, is not a homogeneous carrier. Oxygen is transported both bound to hemoglobin (HbO_2) and dissolved in plasma (dissociated O_2).

There is a linear relationship between PO_2 and oxygen concentration in plasma (also called oxygen content). The association is described by Henry's law: the quantity of oxygen dissolved in a liquid (expressed as volume %) is directly proportional to the partial pressure of oxygen (see Fig. III-124, line B),

$$O_2 \text{ dissolved} \left(\frac{ml}{100 \ ml} \right) = PaO_2 \text{ (mm Hg)} . \alpha.$$

Where α is the solubility coefficient for oxygen which is .003 ml at 37° C (For a PaO_2 of 100 mm Hg 0.3 ml of O_2 are dissolved in 100 ml of plasma.)

The relationship between PO_2 and the quantity of oxygen transported by the hemoglobin is expressed by a sigmoidal curve for the oxygen dissociation curve of hemoglobin (Fig. III-124, line A). When the PO_2 increases to 250 mm Hg or more, the curve becomes horizontal and the number of molecules of oxygen that can be bound to hemoglobin has reached a maximum. This maximal quantity is called the oxygen capacity of Hb.

One gram of hemoglobin (adult or fetal) has the capacity of carrying 1.30 ml of oxygen. The capacity of 100 ml of blood that contains 15 grams of hemoglobin is 19.5 ml of oxygen (15 × 1.30).

The term oxygen saturation expresses the relationship between the quantity of oxygen bound to hemoglobin (concentration) for a given PO_2 and oxygen capacity. The facility with which hemoglobin binds to oxygen is expressed in terms of its affinity. Affinity varies with conditions in the internal and external environment of the erythrocyte. The PO_2 necessary to saturate half of the hemoglobin is a measure of affinity, termed P_{50}.

Note the quantitative difference between oxygen transported by hemoglobin and that dissolved in the plasma (Compare lines A and B in Fig. III-124.)

Delivery of oxygen to the tissues. — The delivery of oxygen from the capillary blood to the cells depends on the PaO_2, the arterial oxygen content, the oxygen affinity for hemoglobin, the local perfusion, and the tissue diffusion capacity. The PaO_2 (head pressure, "driving force") must be high enough to permit diffusion of the oxygen molecules from the capillaries to the mitochondria. The oxygen content of the arterial blood (concentration) is usually high enough to supply the cellular oxygen needs adequately. When PaO_2 or oxygen content are low, increased local perfusion and lessened oxygen affinity for hemoglobin (increase in P_{50}), are compensatory mechanisms to avoid tissue hypoxia.

The extraction of oxygen from the arterial blood is measured by the arterial venous difference. This difference varies for every organ. It is greatest for the heart and working skeletal muscles, moderate for the brain and liver and relatively small for the kidneys and skin.

MECHANISMS OF HYPOXIA AND OXYGEN THERAPY

Among the pathologic mechanisms which influence the quantity of oxygen delivered to the tissues, the following deserve special mention because of their importance in neonatal care [48].

1. Alveolar hypoventilation.
2. Alveolar capillary diffusion disturbances.

3. Right-to-left shunts.

4. Ventilation perfusion abnormalities.

5. Diminution of the oxygen capacity for the transport of oxygen.

6. Abnormalities of tissue perfusion.

7. Increased relative affinity of hemoglobin for oxygen.

To explain the end consequences of these different mechanisms with respect to decreased oxygen transfer from air to tissues, we will use a graphic scheme that describes PO_2 and PCO_2 in the three media described above: inspired air, alveolar air, and arterial blood (Fig. III-122).

Alveolar hypoventilation
(Fig. III-125)

Alveolar hypoventilation is characterized by an elevated $PACO_2$ with secondarily elevated $PaCO_2$. Since $PACO_2$ is proportional to CO_2 production ($\dot{V}CO_2$) and inversely to alveolar ventilation ($\dot{V}A$), alveolar hypoventilation may be defined as an increase in $\dot{V}CO_2/\dot{V}A$ (see Alveolar Air).

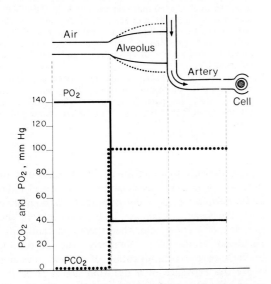

FIG. III-125. — *Alveolar hypoventilation.* Alveolar hypoventilation, shown as a decrease in the size of alveoli, is characterized by an increase in $PACO_2$ (100 mm Hg) and a decrease in PaO_2 (40 mm Hg). This magnitude of hypoventilation is directly related to the increase of $PaCO_2$ (see also Fig. III-123).

Decrease in $\dot{V}A$ may be measured by elevation of $PACO_2$ (Fig. III-123), which, in clinical situations, is estimated from measurement of $PaCO_2$. Reduction

of normal $\dot{V}A$ by half, doubles the $PACO_2$. Reciprocally, alveolar hypoventilation results in a decrease in PAO_2 and, secondarily in PaO_2.

Although an increase in $PaCO_2$ is proportional to a decrease in alveolar ventilation ($\dot{V}A$) a decrease in PaO_2 cannot be taken as a direct measure of the degree of hypoventilation because the latter value can be equally influenced by shunts or by disturbances of diffusion. Additionally PaO_2 is affected by uneven distribution of alveolar ventilation ($\dot{V}A$) in relation to pulmonary perfusion ($\dot{Q}$). It is possible to calculate the fractional part of the decrease in PAO_2 attributable to alveolar hypoventilation by utilizing the alveolar gas equation.

$$PAO_2 = PIO_2 - \frac{PACO_2}{R} \qquad \text{(eq. 2)}$$

Example: A five-day-old premature baby has been ventilated for hyaline membrane disease. After extubation, the infant's blood gases reflect chronic alveolar hypoventilation with an elevation of $PaCO_2$ to 90 mm Hg. The baby is breathing 30 % oxygen (barometric pressure of 747 mm Hg) but the PaO_2 is only 40 mm Hg. Is the decrease in PaO_2 explained solely by hypoventilation, or are other mechanisms of hypoxemia at work? In other words, what would the PaO_2 have been, if we were dealing exclusively with alveolar hypoventilation?

To clarify the situation we insert the respective values for PIO_2 and $PaCO_2$ in Equation 2.

PIO_2 can be calculated from the equation

$$PIO_2 = FIO_2 \times (PB - 47)$$
$$PIO_2 = 30 \times (747 - 47)$$
$$PIO_2 = 210 \text{ mm Hg}$$

as

$PaCO_2$ is known (90 mm Hg)

and

R is supposed to be 0.8

Equation 2 becomes:

$$PAO_2 = 210 - \frac{90}{0.8}$$
$$= 97.5 \text{ mm Hg}$$

Thus alveolar hypoventilation, in this instance, cannot explain the decrease in PaO_2 to 40 mm Hg, because with an FIO_2 of 30 %, the PaO_2 should equal 97.5 mm Hg. Other mechanisms of hypoxemia must be operating to explain the 57.5 mm Hg difference (97.5 — 40 mm Hg) that cannot be attributed to hypoventilation.

A question which is analogous to the previous one often comes up at the bedside: in the presence of an increased $PaCO_2$ (hypoventilation), what FIO_2

will be needed to correct the parallel decrease in PaO_2 to a "normal" value, for instance, of 80 mm Hg?

Example: A 1,500 gram premature is suffering from chronic hypoventilation characterized by an elevation in $PaCO_2$ to 70 mm Hg. Respiratory acidosis, in this example, is compensated because the pH is equal to 7.30 (barometric pressure equals 747 mm Hg).

Here we proceed to solve the alveolar gas equation (Equation 2) for FIO_2, since we know $PaCO_2$ (70 mm Hg) and we wish to obtain a PaO_2 of 80 mm Hg.

$$80 = FIO_2 \cdot (747 - 47) - \frac{70}{0.8}$$

$$FIO_2 = 23.9 \%$$

Thus an increase of 3 % in the oxygen in inspired air (23.9 — 20.9) should be sufficient to correct the hypoxemic consequences of a decrease in alveolar ventilation to almost half its initial value ($PACO_2$ = 70 mm Hg, instead of 40 mm Hg) (see Fig. III-123).

The more frequent types of acute alveolar hypoventilation in neonates are neonatal asphyxia and apnea. Chronic hypoventilation may occur after administration of medications which depress the centers of respiration, during respiratory airway obstruction, pneumothorax, and in association with respiratory distress syndrome.

As depicted in Figure III-123, oxygen therapy is corrective when the decrease in PaO_2 is secondary to alveolar hypoventilation, because the increase in PIO_2 compensates for the effect of hypoventilation on PAO_2. It should also be evident that oxygen therapy has no effect on CO_2 retention.

Disturbances
of alveolar capillary diffusion
(Fig. III-126)

One should consider a diffusion defect when there is an appreciable gradient between PAO_2 and PaO_2 (pressure of oxygen in the terminal pulmonary capillaries); for instance, when "thickness" of the alveolar capillary membranes is increased. The secondary decrease of PaO_2 (e. g. from 100-50 mm Hg) is not associated with an elevation of $PaCO_2$ because CO_2 diffuses 3 to 6 times more actively than oxygen [34, 56].

Since the transfer of oxygen from alveoli to pulmonary capillaries depends on the gradient of the partial pressures between the two regions (PAO_2-PcO_2), the difference between the PAO_2 and PcO_2

is far greater in hypoxemia than it is in normoxemia. Conversely, this gradient decreases with oxygen enrichment of inspired air.

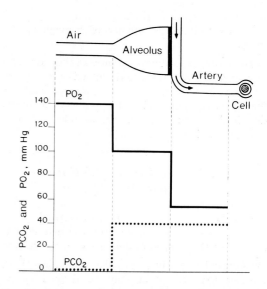

FIG. III-126. — *Abnormalities of diffusion.* Abnormalities of alveolocapillary diffusion are characterized by a decrease in PaO_2 (50 mm Hg) even though the $PaCO_2$ remains normal (40 mm Hg). The "barrier" to the diffusion of the alveolar O_2 in the pulmonary capillaries is such that equilibrium between the PO_2 in the terminal pulmonary capillaries (PcO_2) and the PaO_2 is not possible.

The gradient PaO_2-PcO_2, which is very small under physiological conditions, increases. PcO_2, and secondarily PaO_2, decrease. Since CO_2 diffusion is 3 to 6 times greater than O_2 [34, 56], $PaCO_2$ remains normal.

It is difficult to establish a clinical diagnosis of diffusion defect. The association of decreased PaO_2 and a normal $PaCO_2$ is not necessarily pathognomic since the same discrepancy also may occur in the presence of a shunt and when there is a ventilation perfusion abnormality. Similarly, the correction of PaO_2 by the administration of oxygen does not prove the existence of a diffusion defect since the same phenomenon is also observed in ventilation perfusion abnormalities and in variable shunts (see p. 513). The importance of the diffusion defect in human pathology has been emphasized in the past, both in adult and in neonatal patients [55, 175]. This mechanism of hypoxemia is not encountered as an isolated phenomenon in the newborn. In particular, it does not play a significant role in the hypoxemia associated with the respiratory distress syndrome [98].

The shunt of venous admixture
(Fig. III-127)

The term "shunt" is used to describe the passage of venous blood directly into the arterial blood without passing through ventilated regions of the lung. This diversion can occur in the lung itself (intrapulmonary shunt) or in the heart (intracardiac shunt). A shunt is said to be *fixed* when the part of the venous blood that is diverted to the arterial blood is constant and not influenced by any therapeutic maneuvers (e. g. the administration of oxygen or assisted ventilation). In all other states, a shunt is said to be *variable*.

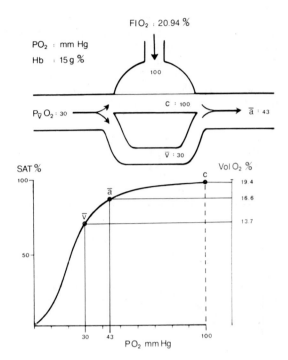

FIG. III-128. — *Illustration of the effect of a right-to-left shunt on PaO_2 in a 3 kg infant with cyanotic heart disease in room air.* A cardiac output of 500 ml/min is distributed equally in ventilated areas of the lung and the shunt. The mixture of 250 ml of blood coming from ventilated alveoli (c: PO_2: 100 mm Hg, O_2 content: 19.4 ml/100) with 250 ml of blood going through the shunt ($\bar{v}$: PO_2: 30 mm Hg, O_2 content: 13.7/100 ml) leads to a decrease in PaO_2 to 43 mm Hg.

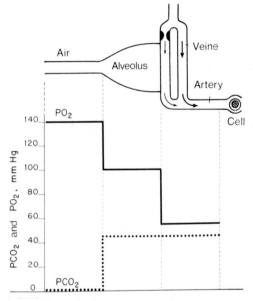

FIG. III-127. — *Shunt.* Shunt, or venous mixture, is characterized by a decrease of PaO_2 without a major change in $PaCO_2$. The mechanisms of these phenomena are illustrated in Figures III-128 and III-129.

The effect of a shunt on PaO_2 and $PaCO_2$ is illustrated in Figure III-127; the PaO_2 is decreased when $PaCO_2$ is normal. This discrepancy is illustrated in Figures III-128 and III-130. The schemes also serve as models for the calculation of the quantitative effect of a shunt on blood gases.

Effect of shunt on PaO_2 in air ($FIO_2 = 20.9$ %).

Example (Fig. III-128): A newborn at term weighing 3 kilograms has cyanotic congenital heart disease with a 50 % shunt. In the example the infant breathes air. Cardiac output is 500 ml/min the hemoglobin is 15 grams, and the mixed venous PO_2 ($P\overline{V}O_2$) is 30 mm Hg.

The blood leaving the lungs with a PaO_2 of 100 mm Hg (c) has an oxygen content of 19.4 ml/100 ml of blood (19.1 ml of oxygen bound to hemoglobin plus 0.3 ml of oxygen dissolved). The blood passing through the shunt at a PO_2 of 30 mm Hg ($\bar{v}$) has a total oxygen content of 13.7 ml/100 ml of blood (13.6 ml of oxygen bound to hemoglobin plus 0.1 ml of dissolved oxygen). Since there is a 50 % shunt, the pulmonary blood flow is equal to the flow through the shunt (250 ml/min), and the mean oxygen content of arterial blood is

$$\frac{19.4 + 13.7}{2} = 16.6 \text{ ml } (\bar{a}).$$

This oxygen content corresponds to a PO_2 of 43 mm Hg ($\bar{a}$), (read from the O_2 dissociation curve). Thus, the shunt of 50 % is responsible for a lowering of PaO_2 from 100 mm Hg to 43 mm Hg.

In this situation, the administration of oxygen in high concentration has no significant effect on PaO_2, unless the shunt is not fixed, and if the diversion is less than 50 % of the cardiac output. Except for the last caveat, oxygen therapy, even in concentrations over 80 % has little if any effect on PaO_2, as will be demonstrated in the following example.

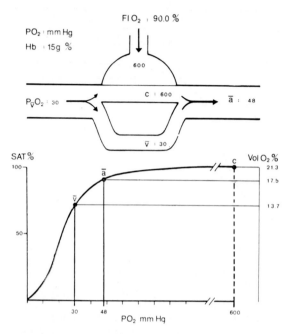

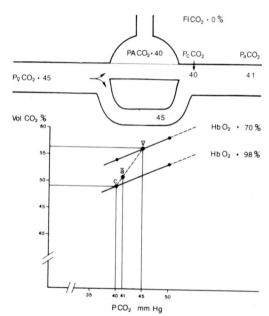

FIG. III-129. — *Effect of right-to-left shunt on PaO_2 in a 3 kg infant with cyanotic heart disease in 90 % O_2.* A cardiac output of 500 ml/min is distributed equally in ventilated areas of the lung and the shunt. The mixture of 250 ml of blood coming from ventilated alveoli (c: PO_2: 600 mm Hg, O_2 content: 21.3 ml/100) with 250 ml of blood going through the shunt ($\bar{v}$: PO_2: 30 mm Hg, O_2 content: 13.7 ml) leads to a PaO_2 of 48 mm Hg. As a result, the increase of PaO_2 from 100 mm Hg to 600 mm Hg (FIO_2 = 90 %) has produced only a minimal increase in PaO_2, from 43 mm Hg to 48 mm Hg (Fig. III-128).

Minimal effect of oxygen therapy (FIO_2 = 80 to 100 %) on PaO_2 in the presence of a shunt larger than 50 % of the cardiac output.

Example (Fig. III-129): The same newborn as in the previous example is given 90 % oxygen. What is the effect of this therapeutic move on the infant's PaO_2? The calculation is illustrated by Figure III-129. The increase in FIO_2 from 20.9 to 90 % raises PAO_2 and, secondarily, PcO_2 to 600 mm Hg (see calculation of PAO_2, Equation 2).

The oxygen content in the pulmonary capillary

blood (*c*) corresponds to a PcO_2 of 600 mm Hg (*i. e.* 21.3 ml of oxygen per 100 ml of blood + 19.5 ml oxygen bound to hemoglobin plus 1.8 ml of oxygen dissolved). The blood passing through the shunt has an oxygen content of 13.7 ml, as indicated by the previous example. Since pulmonary flow is equal to shunt flow, the mean oxygen content of the arterial blood is

$$\frac{21.3 + 13.7}{2} = 17.5 \text{ ml } (\bar{a}).$$

This oxygen content corresponds to a PO_2 of 48 mm Hg ($\bar{a}$). As a result, the increase of FIO_2 from 20.9 % to 90 % has only a minimal effect on PaO_2 (the increase being from 43 to 48 mm Hg).

FIG. III-130. — *Effect of right-to-left shunt on $PaCO_2$.* In a 3 kg infant with cyanotic heart disease, the cardiac output of 500 ml/min is equally distributed between the ventilated area of the lung and the shunt. The mixture of 250 ml of blood coming from ventilated alveoli (c: PCO_2: 40 mm Hg, O_2 content: 49 ml/100) with 250 ml of blood passing through the shunt ($\bar{v}$: PCO_2: 45 mm Hg, CO_2 content: 57 ml/100) leads to a modest increase in $PaCO_2$ to 41 mm Hg.

The lack of effect of shunt on $PaCO_2$. — The following example illustrates this phenomenon (Fig. III-130).

Example: The same newborn, as in the previous two examples, presents with the following values in alveolar air $PACO_2 = 40$ mm Hg, $P\bar{v}CO_2 = 45$ mm Hg.

What is the effect of the shunt on $PaCO_2$?

The blood that leaves the lung has a $PaCO_2$ of 40 mm Hg which corresponds to a CO_2 content of 49 ml (c) see the dissociation curve for CO_2 at saturation of oxygen of 98 %. The blood that crosses through the shunt at a $P\bar{v}CO_2$ of 45 mm Hg ($\bar{v}$) has a CO_2 content of 57 ml (see the dissociation curve for CO_2, for saturation of oxygen of 70 %). In the current example, pulmonary flow is equal to the flow through the shunt (250 ml/min), the mean content of CO_2 in arterial blood is equal to $\dfrac{57 + 49}{2}$ = 53 ml CO_2 per 100 ml blood.

The corresponding PCO_2 at this CO_2 content of 53 ml may be read from a mean curve obtained by joining the venous points ($\bar{v}$: PCO_2 45 mm Hg) to the end pulmonary capillary point (c: PCO_2 = 40 mm Hg). As one can estimate that the oxygen saturation in the resulting mixed arterial blood ($\bar{a}$) is approximately 90 % (see Fig. III-128), where the PaO_2 of 43 mm Hg corresponds to a saturation of about 90 %), the resulting PCO_2 is 41 mm Hg ($\bar{a}$).

Thus, a right-to-left shunt representing 50 % of the cardiac output, increases the $PaCO_2$ by 1 mm Hg (40 to 41 mm Hg). Usually, however, shunts lead to hypoxemia, the resulting hyperventilation (induced by the decreased PaO_2) may cause a secondary decrease of $PaCO_2$.

The association of a PaO_2 decrease with normal $PaCO_2$ is not pathognomonic of a shunt since the same discrepancy occurs in abnormalities of diffusion, and of ventilation perfusion ($\dot{V}A/\dot{Q}$). The persistence of hypoxemia unrelieved by the administration of oxygen in concentrations higher than 80 %, is typical of a venoarterial shunt. A shunt may occur in any of the cardio-respiratory disorders of the newborn. This circulatory abnormality is particularly common in hyaline membrane disease and in congenital heart disease. In fixed shunts, oxygen therapy has virtually no effect on PaO_2, unless the shunt is less than 50 % of cardiac output (see Fig. III-139).

High O_2 concentrations can thus be employed not only as a therapeutic agent, but also as a diagnostic tool to detect the presence of a shunt.

Disturbance of ventilation perfusion ($\dot{V}A/\dot{Q}$)

The efficiency of pulmonary gas exchange depends a great deal on optimal distribution of inspired air to perfused alveoli. Numerous intrinsic lung mechanisms tend to preserve the ventilation/perfusion relationship at a ratio of approximately 0.8. However, even in the normal subject, the distribution of ventilation and perfusion in the lung is uneven.

In pathologic states, the most frequent causes of hypoxemia are related to problems of distribution of $\dot{V}A/\dot{Q}$. The mechanism that leads to blood gas aberation following maldistribution is often misunderstood by the clinician with little experience in respiratory physiology. We will attempt to illustrate some effects with a simplified model taken from West's textbook [175].

Figure III-131 considers different types of alveoli perfused by the same venous blood ($P\bar{v}O_2$: 40 mm Hg, $P\bar{v}CO_2$: 45 mm Hg). Let us consider first case A, where $\dot{V}A/\dot{Q}$ is 0.8, PAO_2 and PaO_2 are 100 mm Hg and $PACO_2$ and $PaCO_2$ are 40 mm Hg, thus assuming perfect diffusion equilibrium. What happens when the relationship between $\dot{V}A$ and $\dot{Q}$ changes; for example, following bronchial obstruction (case B). In this situation $\dot{V}A$ decreases while $\dot{Q}$ remains normal. Consequently PAO_2 and PaO_2 diminish (48 mm Hg) because the ratio of alveolar ventilation ($\dot{V}A$) to oxygen consumption ($\dot{V}O_2$) is lowered, and $PACO_2$ and $PaCO_2$ increase reciprocally (43 mm Hg).

If the relationship $\dot{V}A/\dot{Q}$ falls to zero (case C) for example, when ventilation is impossible because of total bronchial obstruction, the pulmonary area is perfused by venous blood; both PaO_2 and $PaCO_2$ approximate their respective values in venous blood. We again have the situation of a shunt as discussed previously. Thus, the intra-pulmonary shunt represents the extreme form of $\dot{V}A/\dot{Q}$ disturbance where the ratio is equal to zero. Such an underperfused alveolus is not ventilated, and soon collapses (atelectasis).

Let us now consider the inverse situation: $\dot{V}A/\dot{Q}$ increases (case D), for example, because of diminished pulmonary perfusion ("vascular spasm") while ventilation remains even. In this case, both PAO_2 and PaO_2 increase because the relationship between alveolar ventilation ($\dot{V}A$) and oxygen consumption $\dot{V}O_2$ is increased. $PACO_2$ and $PaCO_2$ decrease because the relationship between $\dot{V}A$ and $\dot{V}CO_2$ is increased.

If the $\dot{V}A/\dot{Q}$ ratio rises to infinity (case E) for example when pulmonary perfusion ceases (e. g. emboli) while ventilation remains normal, PAO_2

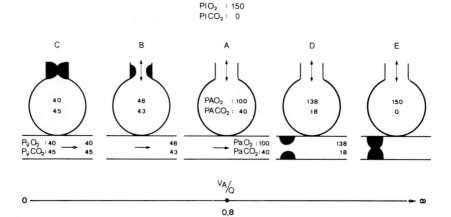

FIG. III-131. — *Effect of variations of the ration* $\dot{V}A$ *on alveolar and arterial gas* [176].

A : Normal situation $\dfrac{\dot{V}A}{\dot{Q}}$ $=0.8$, PAO_2, and $PaO_2 = 100$ mm Hg. $PACO_2$ and $PaCO_2 = 40$ mm Hg.

B : $\dfrac{\dot{V}A}{\dot{Q}} < 0.8$ after a decrease of $\dot{V}A$ because of a partial bronchial obstruction, $\dot{Q}$ remains unchanged. It is clear

that this situation, analogous to alveolar hypoventilation, is expected to cause a decrease in PAO_2 (48 mm Hg) and an increase in $PACO_2$ (43 mm Hg).

C : $\dfrac{\dot{V}A}{\dot{Q}} = 0$ after a total bronchial obstruction, $\dot{Q}$ again unchanged. Gaseous pressures are equal to venous pressures

(the situation that obtains in a shunt).

D : $\dfrac{\dot{V}A}{\dot{Q}} > 0.8$ after a decrease of $\dot{Q}$ because of vascular spasm, VA is unchanged here. The situation is analogous

to that in hyperventilation: PAO_2 increase (138 mm Hg) and $PACO_2$ decreases (18 mm Hg).

E : $\dfrac{\dot{V}A}{\dot{Q}} = \infty$, for example, if $\dot{Q}$ is very close to zero, because of pulmonary embolism, $\dot{V}A$ remains unchanged.

The values of the alveolar gas are those in inspired air. In conclusion [176], when the $\dot{V}A/\dot{Q}$ of a pulmonary unit is altered, the composition of the alveolar and arterial gas approaches that in venous blood ($\dot{V}A/\dot{Q} < 0.8$) or is close to that in inspired air (VA/Q > 0.8).

and $PACO_2$ are equal to their respective values in the inspired gas.

In summary when the $\dot{V}A/\dot{Q}$ ratio falls (relative hypoventilation), PaO_2 and $PaCO_2$ approach their corresponding venous blood values. When the ratio increases (relative hyperventilation) PaO_2 and $PaCO_2$ increase to their respective values in inspired gas.

Thus far, we have considered the total effect of the relationship between $\dot{V}A/\dot{Q}$. What happens, however, when the lung considered as a whole has a normal ratio of total ventilation to total perfusion but the ratio does not have the same value in all pulmonary units.

Two alveoli in Figure III-132 depict such a situation. The total alveolar ventilation (400 ml/min) and total perfusion (500 ml/min) are the values expected

in a newborn baby at term. The $\dot{V}A/\dot{Q}$ is 0.8. There is however a distribution abnormality since the $\dot{V}A/\dot{Q}$ is 1.4 $\left(\dfrac{350}{250}\right)$ in compartment I, and 0.2 $\left(\dfrac{50}{250}\right)$ in compartment II. This confusing disturbance is due to the irregularity of distribution of alveolar ventilation in the two compartments (e. g. adjacent to bronchial obstruction in compartment II). Let us suppose that $\dot{V}A$ in compartment I is seven times higher than in compartment II. What is the effect of this disturbance in the distribution of $\dot{V}A/\dot{Q}$ on the PaO_2 in admixed blood issuing from compartment I ($\dot{Q}$ I) and compartment II ($\dot{Q}$ II)? If there is no diffusion limitation, the PaO_2 of arterial blood coming from compartment I and II are equal to their respective PAO_2 in the respective

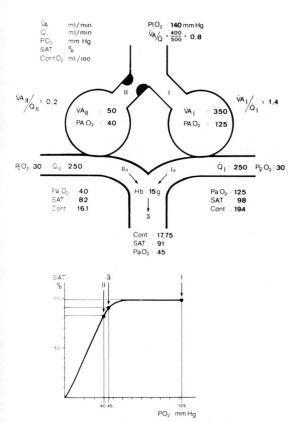

FIG. III-132. — Illustration of mechanisms by which an abnormality of $\dot{V}A/\dot{Q}$ distribution induces hypoxemia, at times when total alveolar ventilation and total pulmonary perfusion are normal. The lung is represented by 2 alveoli. Total alveolar ventilation (400 ml/min) and total perfusion (500 ml/min) are indicated as values seen in full-term neonates, $\dot{V}A/\dot{Q} = 0.8$. A decrease of $\dot{V}A$ in II leads to an abnormality of distribution as follows: $\dot{V}A/\dot{Q}$ I = 1.4, $\dot{V}A/\dot{Q}$ II = 0.2. This brings about arterial hypoxemia (PaO$_2$ of 45 mm Hg, see explanations in the text).

compartments. The oxygen saturation corresponding to this PaO$_2$ is determined by refering to the oxy-hemoglobin dissociation curve; the two oxygen contents are calculated assuming a hemoglobin of 15 g % (capacity for oxygen is 1.3 ml, per g of hemoglobin).

COMPARTMENT I. — The relative hyperventilation ($\dot{V}A$: 350 ml/min) leads to an elevated PaO$_2$ (from 100 to 125 mm Hg) and the latter value corresponds to 98 % saturation. Total oxygen content is 19.4 ml/100 ml of blood (19.1 ml of oxygen is bound to hemoglobin and 0.3 is dissolved).

COMPARTMENT II. — The relative hypoventilation ($\dot{V}A$: 50 ml/min) leads to a decrease of PaO$_2$ from 100 to 40 mm Hg. Here the total oxygen content is 16.1 ml/100 (16.0 ml is bound to hemoglobin and 0.1 ml is dissolved).

ARTERIAL BLOOD ($\bar{a}$). — On the assumption that perfusion ($\dot{Q}$) in compartments I and II is the same (250 ml/min), mean oxygen content in the arterial mixed blood ($\bar{a}$) is $\dfrac{19.4 + 16.1}{2} = 17.75$ ml O$_2$. This oxygen content corresponds to a saturation of 91 % and a PaO$_2$ of 45 mm Hg.

Conclusion. — When total alveolar ventilation/perfusion ratio in a lung is normal ($\dot{V}A/\dot{Q} = 0.8$), a disturbance in ventilation/perfusion ratio in two compartments (e. g. $\dot{V}A/\dot{Q} = 0.2$ and $\dot{V}A/\dot{Q} = 1.4$) leads to hypoxemia (e. g. PaO$_2$ of 45 mm Hg).

The construction of a model similar to the one in Figure III-132 would also allow us to demonstrate that this disturbance of distribution of $\dot{V}A/\dot{Q}$ causes an increase PaCO$_2$. It follows from implications of the slope of the CO$_2$ dissociation curve (Fig. III-130), that the increase in PCO$_2$ in the mixed arterial blood coming from compartments with unequal $\dot{V}A/\dot{Q}$ is less important than the decrease in PaO$_2$.

Diagnosis of $\dot{V}A/\dot{Q}$ abnormalities is difficult in practice. Simultaneous analyses of alveolar arterial gradients for O$_2$, CO$_2$ and N$_2$ and the washout studies of inert gases or radioactive gases used in pulmonary physiology studies are not practical in the course of everyday care [94].

Clinicians are well advised to suspect a distribution problem of $\dot{V}A/\dot{Q}$ when they encounter a significant decrease in PaO$_2$ associated with an elevation of PaCO$_2$. Administration of oxygen concentration of 80 to 100 % corrects the hypoxemia unless lung compartments with low $\dot{V}A/\dot{Q}$ are predominant. In the latter case, the situation is similar to the one in a shunt. The $\dot{V}A/\dot{Q}$ abnormalities are the most frequent cause of hypoxemia. They are usually seen in hyaline membrane disease and aspiration syndromes. In hyaline membrane disease, the decrease in functional residual capacity [96] goes along with $\dot{V}A/\dot{Q}$ abnormalities [38, 94] and shunts [172]. The increase in $\dot{V}A/\dot{Q}$ ratio secondary to pulmonary hypoperfusion is the predominant disorder [31, 38, 94].

In the meconium aspiration syndrome, the partial obstruction of the bronchioles by the meconium allows the inspired gas to enter the alveoli where it is trapped by the mechanical obstruction to normal expiration. The thorax is hyperexpanded and at the same time, the lung is hypoventilated. Hypoxemia associated with meconium aspiration is mainly caubed by a decrease in $\dot{V}A/\dot{Q}$ ratio [97]. Similar problems have been observed in transient tachypnea of the newborn [97], as well as in the Mikity-Wilson syndrome [94].

Tissue perfusion abnormalities
(Fig. III-133)

In the presence of perfusion abnormalities, blood gas values are normal. Under these circumstances the amount of oxygen delivered by the circulation does not meet cellular needs. Increased oxygen pressure in the arterial blood has virtually no effect on the hypoxia since the capacity of the oxygen transported by the hemoglobin is limited at PaO_2 over 80 mm Hg and the fact that the quantity of dissolvable oxygen is quite small.

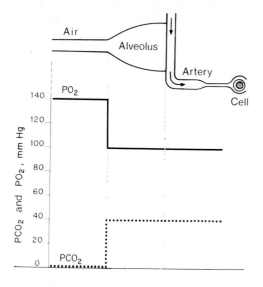

FIG. III-133. — *Illustration of a decrease in tissue prefusion or carrying capacity of Hb for O_2 (anemia). PaO_2 and $PaCO_2$ are normal.*

The effect of variations
in hemoglobin-oxygen affinity
or oxygen delivery
to the tissue is discussed
in chapter 25

OXYGEN ADMINISTRATION

Routes of administration

The routes of administration of oxygen vary according to the clinical situations that present themselves. Is the infant breathing spontaneously or must he or she be ventilated artificially? During spontaneous respiration, oxygen can be administered either in an incubator, by a hood that encloses the baby's head, by a mask applied to the face, or by nasal prongs under positive end-expiratory pressure. During assisted ventilation oxygen can be administered either by a tight fitting face mask, by orotracheal, or by nasotracheal tube. The choice of the method of oxygen administration depends on the indication for treatment.

Oxygen humidification
and warming

Regardless of the route of administration, the gaseous mixture containing oxygen should be humidified and warmed before it reaches the respiratory tract. *Humidification* prevents the drying of mucous membranes and reduces the chances of obstruction of endotracheal tubes by dried secretions; additionally, this measure reduces excessive loss of respiratory tract water during expiration. Adequate humidification can prevent up to 30 % of total water loss in the small premature [72].

Warming of the inspired air blocks the cold triggered increase in oxygen consumption [114]. It is recommended that the temperature of the gaseous mixture be maintained at or slightly lower than the level in the incubator. All tubes and containers used for warming and humidification should be sterilized regularly and the water used for humidification should be changed once a day.

Gas mixture

The optimal gas mixture for therapeutic use is achieved by using a source of pure oxygen and a source of compressed air. Mixing of the gases may take place in a humidification bottle or by the use of a blender. The gas mixtures achieved by the various devices even the most precise, vary by more than 10 %. The variation is also influenced by fluctuations in the system.

The oxygen concentration in the gas mixture should be measured regularly to ensure delivery of a stable mixture.

Oxygen concentration is usually measured at the bedside by either a paramagnetic or a polarographic method. The paramagnetic method requires intermittent sampling of a gas mixture. The polarographic method makes continuous monitoring possible, and alarm circuitry quickly detects inaccurate concentrations. Automatic servocontrol systems allowing instantaneous correction of the FIO_2 based on continuous PaO_2 measurement such as with a $tcPO_2$ monitor are currently under study.

When oxygen is administered by a hood around the baby's head, it is important to maintain a flow of at least 2 liters per minute [74] in order to prevent CO_2 accumulation [58].

THE DANGERS
OF OXYGEN THERAPY

The toxic effects of oxygen therapy were recognized from the first use of the gas. Priestly [139] already suspected in 1766 the "formation of a toxic substance to the organism" and such a complication was demonstrated by Bert (1878) [16]. The untoward effects are not the same at different barometric pressures (*i. e.* they are greater when pressures are high). As hyperbaric oxygen chambers are no longer used for newborn care, we will not discuss these environments or the toxic effects of oxygen at higher barometric pressures.

Mechanisms of toxicity

As previously indicated, oxygen occupies a crucial position in the mechanism of energy production since it is the final electron acceptor from the chain of cytochromes. Under usual conditions, most oxygen moieties combine with four electrons to form two molecules of water. However, occasionally molecules may accept only one, two or three electrons thus forming free radicals [39, 109]. In hyperoxia, the formation of these free radicals increases and signs of toxicity may then appear. The toxicity of oxygen has been attributed to four types of free radicals: the superoxide anion ($O_2^{\cdot}$), hydrogen peroxide (H_2O_2), hydroxide ion (OH), and lipidic radicals (L.). The superoxide anion ($O_2^{\cdot}$) is the product of the combination of one molecule of oxygen with an electron. Hydrogen peroxide is the product of the transformation of the superoxide

anion by superoxide dismutase as indicated in the following reaction:

$$O_2^{\cdot} + O_2^{\cdot} + 2H \rightarrow O_2 + H_2O_2$$
$$\uparrow$$
$$\text{superoxide dismutase}$$

The hydrogen peroxide (H_2O_2) formed by this reaction is degraded to water in the presence of catalase according to the reaction:

$$H_2O_2 \rightarrow H_2O + 1/2O_2$$
$$\uparrow$$
$$\text{catalase}$$

The free radicals of the hydroxide ion (OH) are produced as the result of the reaction of the superoxide anion ($O_2^{\cdot}$) and the hydrogen peroxide (H_2O_2) in the presence of trivalent iron (Fe^{3+}).

$$O_2^{\cdot} + H_2O_2 \rightarrow O_2 + OH + OH$$
$$\uparrow$$
$$Fe^{3+}$$

It is postulated that analogous reactions with desaturated lipids produce free lipidic radicals (L.) and the lipid peroxides ($LO_2^{\cdot}$) [164].

The natural mechanism of defense against oxygen toxicity consists of different systems of "detoxification": the superoxide dismutases, the catalases, glutathione reductase, NADPH and vitamin E [107]. An organism's tolerance for oxygen depends on the activity of these enzymatic systems of defense. Protective activity can be stimulated by short exposures to high concentrations of oxygen or by prolonged exposures to lower concentrations. A rat that breathes pure oxygen dies from pulmonary edema in five days, but survives in the same atmosphere if it is first conditioned for several days (by exposure to an FIO_2 of 80 % [120].

The toxic effects of oxygen are evident at molecular and tissue levels. On the molecular level, oxidation principally alters the function of enzymes that contain sulfhydril groups (e. g. those responsible for the metabolism of pyruvate in the tricarboxylic cycle and for the transport of electrons by the mitochondria) [59]. The inhibition of these enzymes leads to a decrease in energy-generating reactions [99, 113, 180]. Moreover, the peroxidation of lipids leads to an alteration of cellular membrane stability [164].

The most important tissue effects are those observed in lung and in brain.

The lung

By its exposed position in the cardiorespiratory complex the lung is subjected to the highest oxygen

pressures. The sequence of pulmonary cell alterations caused by pure oxygen has been particularly
well studied in the rat and the monkey [32, 83, 84].
The changes consist primarily of thinning and vacuolization of the capillary endothelium. These changes
can be observed after only a few hours of exposure
to 100 % oxygen. After two days there is interstitial
and alveolar edema, followed by alveolar cellular
desquamation and replacement of type I cells
by type II cells. After a few days of oxygen exposure
the alveolar epithelium is completely destroyed.
Intra-alveolar hemorrhages associated with the
formation of hyaline membranes are visible after
five days. If oxygen exposure continues, interstitial
fibrosis, atelectasis, and emphysema appear. The
general appearance of the lung is reminiscent of
that seen in bronchopulmonary dysplasia in the
newborn infant [161]. After 12 days of exposure,
air entry deteriorates and there is severe respiratory
distress. If oxygen concentrations are progressively
lowered these symptoms decrease and survival is
possible. After complete clinical recovery, histological preparations of the lungs reveal proliferative
changes in the alveolar capillary bed.

The effect of oxygen on the developing lung has
not been studied extensively. In the newly born rat,
administration of 45 % O_2 for 15 days changes the
time-table of development of the lung [12]. The
mechanism of the toxicity is related to a disturbance
of aerobic glycolysis, since O_2 exposure is associated
with a decrease in O_2 consumption and ATP production [43, 57, 108] as well as with an increased
glucose utilisation and lactate production [120, 169].

Furthermore oxygen interferes with the synthesis
of DNA in newborn mice [124] and decreases the
production of prostaglandins, serotonin and adrenalin in rat alveolar cells [18]. In the human, oxygen
causes a decrease in the production of mucous in
epithelial cells from the respiratory tract of neonates [19], but does not alter the production of surfactant [120, 121]. Regarding the effect of oxygen on
the lung in the human it is difficult to separate the
effect of an increase in oxygen tension in the inspired
air and the changes related to increase in oxygen
tension of arterial blood [135, 179].

The role of oxygen in human neonatal pulmonary
pathology has been questioned in regard to the
etiology of pulmonary hemorrhage [154] and in
bronchopulmonary dysplasia (BPD) [123]. Most
researchers on this topic agree that barotrauma
associated with mechanical ventilation is far more
important than oxygen exposure, particularly in
respect to BPD [141, 181]. However, it is difficult
to ignore experimental evidence in animals demonstrating that oxygen alone causes anatomical lesions

similar to those of bronchopulmonary dysplasia [121]
and that these lesions can be prevented in the rat
by the use of an anti-oxidant such as vitamin E [165].

Finally, Autor et al. [8] have demonstrated an
erythrocyte superoxide dismutase deficiency in
infants who have bronchopulmonary dysplasia.
This finding raises the suspicion that the protective
mechanisms which guard against the toxic effects of
oxygen may be inadequate in these infants. Note,
however that the protective action of vitamin E
in the newborn has not yet been well established.
Tocopherol therapy cannot be recommended [53, 54]
particularly since the side effects of vitamin E
administration are not yet known [137].

The eyes

The first collaborative study on retrolental fibroplasia, conducted in the years 1953 to 1954 [89],
demonstrated that oxygen administered at concentrations higher than 50 % for 28 days increased
the incidence of the disease in neonates weighing
less than 2,500 grams at birth who had survived
for at least 48 hours. Careful use of oxygen associated with the monitoring of arterial PO_2 has not
eliminated the condition. Aranda [5] reported that
33,8 % of premature infants weighing between
500 and 1,500 grams presented alterations of the
fundi in the eyes compatible to RLF, and 10 % of the
babies had cicatricial lesions. The incidence of the
disease has increased during the last decade [46, 64,
137 a, 162]. Experimental studies in animals [6, 7, 130]
and clinical studies in prematures [89, 90, 129, 130]
have suggested some risk factors. The toxic effect
of oxygen is thought to depend on the degree of
maturation of the retina since more than 20 % of
prematures of less than 1,500 grams show some
signs of RLF [90]. Exposure to FIO_2's higher than
50 % for 28 days increases the risk (23 % compared
to 7 % in the collaborative study [89]). But there is no
experimental proof that the risk if proportional to the
increased concentration of oxygen and the association with duration of oxygen exposure has never
been subjected to a critical test. The risk appeared
to be higher in twins enrolled in the 1953-1954
study [89]. Critical values of FIO_2, PaO_2 and O_2
content are simply not known [89, 90], however a
PaO_2 over 190 mm Hg is needed to produce retinal
vasoconstriction in the kitten [55 a]. The influence of
the decrease of affinity of hemoglobin for O_2 [2, 102]
following transfusion has been discussed. The
protective role of vitamin E on vascular changes
has been demonstrated in the animal model [136]
but it must be emphasized that neither the vita-

min E treated animals nor the controls developed cicatricial RLF with oxygen exposure. The role of vitamin E effectiveness and treatment in human RLF has been suspected for years [125] and is currently under investigation [81]. In the newborn kitten exposed to 80 % oxygen for 72 hours, vitamin E partially prevents the decrease of superoxide dismutase in the retina that is usually induced by hyperoxia [23] (the enzyme is essential in the detoxification of the free radical superoxide). Apnea, sepsis, intraventricular hemorrhages in premature infants are associated with a relatively high risk of RLF [65].

It may be that in addition to the oxidative effects of hyperoxia and the insufficiency of antioxidants, other factors are involved in the genesis of retrolental fibroplasia, since the disease has been observed in term infants (15 cases [14, 52] and in those who have cyanotic congenital heart disease [82]). Unfortunately (as noted above), experimental studies in animals have allowed us to reproduce only the vascular stages of RLF, cicatricial lesions have until recently not been produced in animals with oxygen exposure alone. The retinal alteration seen earliest during ophthalmoscopic examination is vasoconstriction of the terminal arterioles. If the administration of oxygen is discontinued, vasoconstriction does not go on to vaso-obliteration of the developing retinovascular network. The vaso-obliteration that occurs after continuous O_2 exposure is followed by wild vaso-proliferation in the retina, and new vessels breach the internal limiting membrane. Hemorrhages occur commonly during this proliferative phase. The vascular changes usually subside; common sequelae are dilatation and tortuosities of the retinal vessels [13]. In about 10-15 % of cases and for reasons that are not at all understood the vascular changes are followed by fibrotic organization: cicatricial retractions, and retinal detachment with secondary healing (cicatricial stage) [55 b].

We should emphasize the gaps in our knowledge: the cicatricial changes—blindness as the most serious complication in the disorder—are not necessary secondary to vasoconstriction, and the precise relationship between oxygen exposure and the cicatricial state has not been clearly established.

The brain

Those who are concerned with embryologic origins of vascular morphology have noted resemblances between the retinal and the cerebral circulation. The similarities of their physiological reactions make it highly plausible that hyperoxemia might cause aberations in the cerebrovascular system analogous to those observed in the immature retina. However, neither in the newborn animal exposed to oxygen, nor in the infants with RLF who come to necropsy, have proliferative vascular lesions of the cerebrovascular system analogous to those observed in the retina been found [7, 131]. Only in the baby mouse exposed to several days of oxygen has a decrease been seen in the capillary cortical density [68] analogous to that observed in the retina by Ashton [7]. Inhalation of 80 to 100 % O_2, with a corresponding elevation of the PaO_2 produces a decrease in cerebral blood flow of 10-15 % in the animal [86, 87] as well as in the human [73, 79, 80, 88, 101]. It should be noted that this effect is partly due to the decrease in $PaCO_2$ secondary to hyperventilation caused by the hyperoxia. In kittens elevation of PaO_2 to 350 mm Hg produces a decrease in the cerebral blood flow of 20 to 30 %, even in the presence of a normal PCO_2 [86, 87]. Recent observations in premature infants [4] suggest that elevation of PaO_2 above 150 mm Hg can be associated with anatomical alterations in the pontosubicular region.

Oxygen effect on regulation of respiration

Inhalation of 100 % O_2 in a full-term newborn is followed almost immediately by a decrease in tidal volume. After five minutes of oxygen exposure ventilation rises above normal and remains elevated during the exposure to oxygen. The immediate decrease in ventilation is due to the effects of O_2 on peripheral chemoreceptors [24, 40, 145, 146].

The mechanism responsible for the secondary increase in ventilation is unknown. A primary toxic effect of the oxygen on the lung is unlikely because the response is so rapid. It is not known whether or not there is a central effect of hyperoxemia. Recent work suggests [45] that cerebral vasoconstriction after an increase in PO_2 causes an increase in tissue PCO_2 triggering hyperventilation.

CONTROL OF OXYGEN THERAPY

As it is difficult to judge oxygenation solely from skin color or from cyanosis of the mucosa [61], all oxygen therapy should be controlled by monitoring PaO_2. When it is necessary to use supplemental oxygen for more than just a few hours, blood samples should be drawn via an umbilical catheter. In other situations, the method for checking PaO$_2$ should be chosen depending on the clinical state.

Umbilical arterial catheterization

The placement of an umbilical arterial line makes it possible to draw arterial blood or to continuously measure PaO$_2$ by means of an electrode [35]. The advantages of an umbilical arterial line are those of patient comfort, simultaneous measurement of acid-base equilibrium in blood samples, administration of fluid and medications, and continuous measurement of the arterial pressure. The disadvantages are the complications: vasospasm, thrombosis and infection [33, 91, 163, 171].

Vasospasm. — Pallor or cyanosis of the extremities, especially of the toes, indicates vasospasm. This problem usually appears soon after insertion of the catheter, often in association with bolus injections. The catheter should be withdrawn if cyanosis or pallor persists for more than a short period or after failure to induce reflex vasodilation by warming the other extremities.

The incidence of thrombosis found at autopsy, varies from 3,5 % [66] to 60 % [100]. In some it seems to be the cause of death [177]. Aortography in vivo has shown a frequency of 24 % in one study [60] and 95 % in another [122]. The radiologic abnormalities were associated with clinical signs of ischemia in only 10 % of instances. Thromboses seem to occur soon after catheter insertion [60]. Duration of catheter indwelling has been considered but does not seem to play a major role [60]. Thrombus formation can be prevented if one uses a catheter of silicone elastomere [22] (difficult to place) instead of a polyvinyl catheter, and also if one avoids antibiotic injections [116]. Infusion of heparinized solutions are without effect on the frequency of thrombosis [122]. The importance of the level of catheter position with respect to thrombotic complications has not been clearly determined [116].

Infection. — The incidence of bacterial colonization of the catheters approximates 60 % [95]. In 5 % of catheterized babies, bacteremia is disclosed by blood culture [138]. None of the following measures have any appreciable effect on bacterial colonization: catheter introduction before the age of 6 hours, withdrawal within 24 hours [95, 138], local or general antibiotic therapy [11, 17, 95, 138].

Even though umbilical catheterization has numerous advantages, the technique is associated with a relatively high frequency of major complications which are difficult to prevent. Therefore, the indications for this procedure must be carefully reviewed whenever it is considered. In our unit, it is reserved for the control of PO$_2$ when FIO$_2$ must be increased substantially. It appears that progress made with the use of tcPO$_2$ electrodes will decrease the indications for umbilical catheterization.

Sampling from peripheral arteries

Arterial blood can be obtained by puncture or catheterization of radial [25] or temporal arteries [152, 168]. Punctures of brachial and femoral arteries are more difficult and appear to be more dangerous [127]. The pain caused in the course of percutaneous arterial sampling can drastically change the PaO$_2$ and is therefore a disadvantage of these techniques. It should be noted that median nerve lesions and finger necrosis have been reported after radial artery puncture [28, 93]. These approaches are simply not practical or safe for oxygen therapy control over an extended period of time.

Transcutaneous method of PO$_2$ measurement (tcPO$_2$)

The measurement of tcPO$_2$ has been one of the more promising technological advances made in the control of oxygen therapy in newborns. Experiences with this approach in the last few years have been reported in detail [77]. The major advantages of this technique are those of continuous recording with an alarm system and the absence of major complications. When the peripheral circulation is in a normal state the correlation between tcPO$_2$ and PO$_2$ is satisfactory. Neverthless, arterial catheters are still needed in the acute phase of respiratory distress syndrome [50]. Use of capillary measurement of PO$_2$ to check PaO$_2$ is not recommended because of its potential inaccuracy [49].

The optimal limits of PaO$_2$

The American Academy of Pediatrics [1] recommends maintenance of PaO$_2$ within the range of limits observed in the asymptomatic fullterm neonate. Although these limits seem reasonable, it is possible that they are not optimal for sick neonates and particularly for prematurely-born infants.

High limits of PaO₂. — There is a limit above which the PaO₂ cannot be raised without producing retinal circulatory changes, a precursor to vascular RLF. In addition, hyperoxemia causes a decrease in cerebral perfusion as discussed above [101]. Finally, the oxidation of some enzymatic systems causes disorders of cellular metabolism (see above). The critically high PaO₂ in human subjects is not known. The first large scale experimental study of RLF in 1954 [89] compared the effects of two regimens of oxygen management on the retina: FIO₂ greater than versus less than 50 % (the technique of PaO₂ measurement had not been developed). A second study in 1977 [90] used an observational approach (rather than experimental methodology) in an effort to establish a correlation between the PaO₂, the length of exposure to the oxygen, and the incidence of RLF by retrospectively comparing the PaO₂ of babies less than 2,500 grams (who required oxygen treatment for various clinical conditions) with or without signs of RLF. That study revealed no apparent critical limit of the PaO₂ above which the risk of RLF increased significantly. The PaO₂ measurements were done on blood drawn intermittently. Only two circumstantial risk factors were noted: the infant's weight and the length of exposure to the oxygen. (Remember that the length of oxygen treatment was based on physician judgment and not according to an experimental protocol.) The weakness of this study design and conceivable explanations of failure to find an association have been discussed [103, 170]. Thus a critical limit of hyperoxemia has not been defined with respect to a defined clinical end point. Nevertheless, it seems reasonable to take into account that in neonatal blood, the capacity of hemoglobin to combine with oxygen is virtually at its maximum (95 % saturation) for PaO₂ at 70-80 mm Hg. Hence there is no physiological rationale to increase the PaO₂ to higher levels.

Lower limits for PaO₂. — The major risks associated with too low PaO₂ are those of increased mortality and increased neurological morbidity in survivors. In the first 1953-1954 RLF study [89] no differences in mortality (in the age interval 2-40 days) of babies receiving less than or more than 50 % oxygen were observed. It was concluded that the chances of survival did not decrease with the administration of oxygen at concentrations lower than 50%. In retrospect, it is clear that this optimistic conclusion was not justified [62], since the babies were admitted to the study at age 48 hours after the time of highest risk of death from hypoxia. Later observations suggested that mortality of

HMD-affected infants increased during the years when oxygen administration was curtailed: relatively low FIO₂ for relatively brief periods [10]. Systematic studies of neonatal mortality done in the United States, England and Wales during the years 1935-1970 [20] suggested that during the era of restricted oxygen use for every instance of blindness prevented there were 16 early neonatal deaths [41].

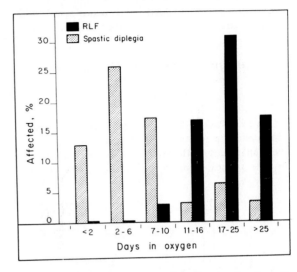

FIG. III-134. — *Relationship between the duration of oxygen therapy and the incidence of retrolental fibroplasia and spastic diplegia.* In 194 children, born at 31 or less weeks of gestation, RLF occured more often when the duration oxygen therapy (given for clinical indications in the neonatal period) was longer, but spastic diplegia occured less frequently [112a]. In infants born after 31 weeks gestation, the length of the oxygen therapy was unrelated to the incidence of spastic diplegia.

The association between hypoxemia and neurological problems in survivors was suspected by McDonald [110, 111, 112]. In 194 children aged 6-8 years and born before 37 weeks gestation, the incidence of spastic diplegia was inversely proportional to the duration of oxygen therapy (Fig. III-134). (Note the opposite relationship with respect to RLF when oxygen was given as needed [112 a].) The visually evoked EEG potential was found to be decreased in one study of full-term neonates when the PaO₂ was lower than 55 mm Hg [75]. After exposure to cold in another set of observations, the metabolic response decreased when the PaO₂ was between 55-45 mm Hg, and was abolished when PaO₂ was lower than 30 mm Hg [153].

At the latter limit lactic acid was found to be increased in young adults studied in conditions of simulated altitude [173]. Extrapolating from these various observations, it seems reasonable to propose that in newborns treated with oxygen, PaO_2 should be maintained in the neighbourhood of 50 to 80 mm Hg. Hopefully, the rather weak basis for this recommendation concerning a central facet of newborn care will be strengthened in the future (e. g. by a controlled study using continuous measurement of PaO_2 to determine—experimentally—the limits within which the risks of death and neurological and occular sequelae in survivors are the lowest).

Interpretation of PaO_2 changes during oxygen therapy
(Fig. III-135)

A rise in PaO_2 following oxygen therapy is usually interpreted as an objective indication that there has been an increase in the amount of oxygen transported to the tissues. This conclusion is, however, not

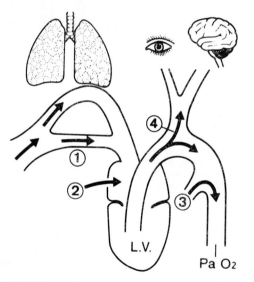

FIG. III-135. — *Illustrated here are the sites of various right-to-left shunts* (1, 2, 3) *in HMD and their influences on the arterial O_2 tension (PaO_2) in the aorta below the ductus.*

1. Intrapulmonary shunt.
2. Shunt through the foramen ovale.
3. Shunt through the ductus.
4. Circulatory flow above the ductus.

With a shunt through the ductus, the PaO_2 variations cannot be reliably interpreted. For example, an increase in PaO_2 means either *a*) better oxygenation of the brain (with or without a decrease in the total shunt) or *b*) worsening of cerebral oxygenation (following a decrease in perfusion of the cephalad part of the body). Also, with a right-to-left ductal shunt retinal hypoxemia may go undetected [59].

always justified, since elevations of PaO_2 are associated with decreased perfusion of some organs such as the retina and brain. Another interpretative difficulty is related to the fact that PaO_2 is usually measured in the aorta below the ductus; as a result, it is difficult to judge the state of oxygenation of the eye or brain when, for example, there is right-to-left shunting through the ductus arteriosus, a common occurence in HMD [118, 147, 157]. Under the latter conditions the measured aortic PaO_2 indicates oxygen status in the lower part of the body and underestimates the PaO_2 in the cephalic vasculature. Retinal hyperoxemia may go undetected. Additionally, in the presence of a right-to-left shunt through the ductus arteriosus, changes in aortic PaO_2 following therapeutic interventions are difficult to interpret. For example when treatment is given to a newborn with respiratory distress syndrome (breathing 80 % O_2), the PaO_2 may rise from 55 to 100 mm Hg: It is commonly concluded that such an incremental change is the result of a decrease in total right-to-left shunt and that the rise in PaO_2 signifies an improvement in the oxygenation of the tissues, especially the brain. But an identical change of aortic PaO_2 may come about as the result of either a change in the location of the right-to-left shunt or a decrease in cerebral blood flow.

For example, a decrease in ductal shunt associated with a parallel increase in the intrapulmonary shunt, could have the same effect on aortic PaO_2 (increase from 55 to 100 mm Hg); under these circumstances it is not necessary to postulate a change in total right-to-left shunt. The complexities have been discussed in detail by Gersony [59]. In such cases, total body oxygenation has improved even if the total quantity of blood passing through the shunts is still the same.

A decrease in cerebral blood flow following a therapeutic procedure may also cause a rise in aortic PaO_2 (again let us say from 55 to 100 mm Hg) and, once again, it is not necessary to postulate a change in right-to-left shunt. The reasoning is as follows: if some blood perfusing the cephalad sections of the body is diverted to the caudal areas, aortic PaO_2 will increase because pre-ductal PaO_2 is higher as consequence of a ductal right-to-left shunt. Under these latter circumstances the incremental rise in aortic PaO_2 does not signify a decrease in shunt, but is secondary to a decrease in cerebral oxygenation. In summary (Fig. III-135), an increase of PaO_2 in the abdominal aorta in the presence of a right-to-left shunt through the ductus, may indicate either an increase in cerebral oxygenation with a decrease in shunting, or a shift in the site of the shunting (ductal to intrapulmonary) or a decrease in cerebral blood flow, with a possible decrease in oxygenation. We should emphasize again that the last possibility must be given some consideration when judging the results of various therapeutic manœuvres, e.g. administration of oxygen [101], bicarbonate [105], vasoactive substances, tolazoline, prostaglandins, or assisted ventilation (particularly hyperventilation) [88, 106, 134]. The increase of aortic PaO_2 noted after these procedures is often interpreted as a sign of improved cerebral oxygenation, but, there is no assurance that such improvement has, in fact, taken place. It is equally possible that there has been a decrease in blood flow to the upper part of the body and attendant worsening of cerebral oxygenation. This gloomy interpretation is supported by observations concerning oxygen therapy, bicarbonate injections, or hyperventilation. All these well intended treatments may result in a decrease in cerebral blood flow [104, 105]. Detection of right-to-left shunt through the ductus is possible by simultaneous measurement of PaO_2 above and below the ductus; for example from information supplied by two transcutaneous monitors. Paired measurements of this kind do not, however, allow one to judge cerebral blood flow variations. Only direct measurement of flow can provide an answer to these vital questions. With the development of newer techniques for the measurement of cerebral blood flow by non-invasive methods (NMR and PET scanning) it may be possible to shed some light on such clinically important problems that arise in the routine care of sick neonates.

OXYGEN USE
IN SOME COMMON CLINICAL SITUATIONS

Acute neonatal asphyxia

Acute asphyxia in the immediate neonatal period is an example of alveolar hypoventilation associated with the presence of a variable shunt because of the transient persistence of the fetal circulation. Oxygen therapy plays a very important role in treatment here for a number of reasons. First it should be recalled, that the fetal lung receives only 7 % of the cardiac output and the placenta receives 40 % (Fig. III-136) [148]. At birth, the perfusion of the new oxygenator, the lung, becomes possible because of an acute drop in pulmonary vascular resistance (Fig. III-137).

This resistance depends on the following factors: 1) alveolar distention, 2) alveolar pressure of O_2

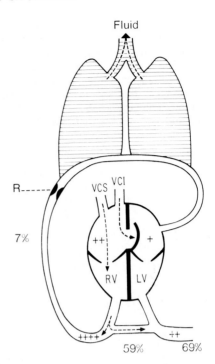

Fig. III-136. — *Fetal circulation.*

The fetal circulation is characterized by an increase in vascular resistance (R) in the lesser circulation producing shunts through the foramen ovale and the ductus arteriosus. Only 7 % of the cardiac output in the fetus goes through the lung [148].

and CO_2 (PAO_2, $PACO_2$), 3) arterial pressure of O_2 and CO_2 (PaO_2, $PaCO_2$) and arterial pH [29, 150]. Each of these factors is responsible for about one quarter of the total effect on the pulmonary vascular resistance. The effect of the change of the blood gas on the decrease in pulmonary vascular resistance is immediate; distention of the alveoli takes a few minutes to be effective [37]. By administering O_2 during acute neonatal asphyxia, the hypoxemic effects of alveolar hypoventilation and the shunt are corrected. The increase of oxygen concentration in inspired air compensates for a decrease of the PAO_2 due to the alveolar hypoventilation. The increase of PAO_2 and secondarily PaO_2, decreases pulmonary vascular resistance (Fig. III-137) which in turn causes a reduction in shunt at the foramen ovale and ductus arteriosus.

Oxygen must be administered by means of assisted ventilation using a mask or an endotracheal tube. The beneficial effects of O_2 on the adaptation of the pulmonary circulation are augmented by alveolar distention and by a decrease in $PACO_2$ and $PaCO_2$ which result from assisted ventilation. The optimal

O_2 concentration for these initial maneuvers are difficult to evaluate; these are clinical emergencies and PaO_2 is difficult to measure under such hectic conditions. The high risk of hypoxic damage associated with asphyxia leads to the reasonable proposal that assisted ventilation should begin with high O_2 concentrations until cyanosis disappears. The side-effects of relative brief periods of hyperoxemia

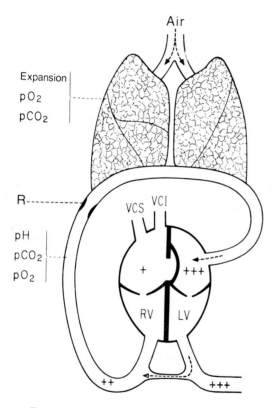

FIG. III-137. — *Mechanisms for the adaptation of the pulmonary circulation to extrauterine life.*

The adaptation of the pulmonary circulation to extrauterine life depends on a decrease in pulmonary vascular resistance (R). Factors implicated here are: A alveolar expansion by a gaseous mixture: Alveolar gas tensions (PAO_2 and $PACO_2$), arterial gas tensions (PaO_2 and $PaCO_2$) and arterial pH.

Closure of the foramen ovale. The increase in pulmonary blood flow after a fall in vascular resistance (R) causes a rise in pressure in the left atrium. When this pressure exceeds that in the right atrium, the foramen ovale closes.

Closure of the ductus. A decrease in pulmonary vascular resistance causes a fall in lesser circulation pressure to a value below that in the aorta. The right-to-left ductal shunt in utero changes direction (left-to-right) postnatally.

The increase in PO_2 and O_2 content in the ductus itself provokes closure by active contraction of musculature in the ductal wall.

induced under these circumstances are difficult to evaluate. But there is no evidence to suggest that short term elevation of PaO_2 in the lung and arterial blood can cause serious pulmonary lesions. Similarly there is no convincing evidence that such transitional hyperoxemia endangers the retina of premature infants. However, the frequency of retinal vascular alterations in premature infants not exposed to severe and prolonged hyperoxemia during their stay in the neonatal unit is relatively high [5] and it is conceivable that transitional hyperoxemia in the immediate postnatal period is a possible factor in the genesis of these disturbances. It should be emphasized that this, however, is entirely speculative. There are no critical studies of the matter. Acute hyperoxemia also causes a significant decrease in cerebral blood flow [101], thus it is recommended that prolonged O_2 inhalation without controlling PaO_2 should be avoided. Experiences using transcutaneous PO_2 monitoring (tcPO_2) during oxygen treatment in delivery rooms are in progress.

Hyaline membrane disease (HMD)

The hypoxia associated with HMD comes about as the result of the following mechanisms: alveolar hypoventilation, shunting, $\dot{V}A/\dot{Q}$ abnormalities, disorders of tissue-perfusion and increased hemoglobin affinity for O_2. Disturbances of alveolocapillary diffusion are not important [98]. The contribution of the tissue hypoperfusion and disturbances of hemoglobin affinity for O_2 are discussed in chapter 25.

It has been established that shunts are the most important causes of hypoxemia associated with this disease [31, 118, 119, 147, 149, 157, 160]. Anatomically, the shunts are either in the lung or through physiologic communications of the fetal circulation, *i. e.* foramen ovale and ductus arteriosus. The intrapulmonary shunts are secondary to atelectasis produced by the lack of surfactant. Shunts through the ductus and the foramen are the consequences of persistence of the fetal circulation, due to relative pulmonary hypertension associated with HMD [31, 157, 158, 160]. The proportional contribution of each of these shunts has not been clearly established. The situation varies, of course, not only from one infant to the other, but also in each infant during the course of the disease [140]. Published data concerning this issue are confusing; much depends on methods used to perform the relevant measurements.

Cardiac catheterization studies indicate that

HMD is associated with ductal shunting [117, 143]. Methods using dilution indicators seem to reveal the presence of a shunt through the foramen ovale, with or without shunt at the ductal site [157]. In certain cases 30 % of the pulmonary blood flow can go to nonventilated alveoli [174].

The hyperoxia test (see p. 528), has been used to estimate total shunting as well as the relative contribution of diversion through the ductus, by comparing PaO_2 in the aorta proximal and distal to the ductus [118, 147]. A total shunt of about 80 % of the cardiac output has been seen when the shunt through the ductus varied between 5 % and 20 %. A method of catheterizing pulmonary veins has permitted an estimate of the contribution of intrapulmonary shunts to the total shunt; values varying from 17 % to 75 % have been obtained [119]. It should be noted that the size of the shunts estimated by using the classical equation [15] may be in error (sometimes quite sizeable) [59] when a shunt at the ductus is present. There is evidence that the shunt through the ductus is systematically underestimated by a significant amount (6 % instead of 44 %) in an example noted by Gersony [59], and that the total shunt is somewhat overestimated (see p. 530).

The problems of the distribution of $\dot{V}A/\dot{Q}$ follow a time-course that is similar to that taken by shunts during the acute phase of HMD [38, 172]. However shunts disappear during the convalescent phase, while VA/Q problems remain operative for several weeks and constitute the principal cause of late hypoxemia [3, 128].

Alveolar hypoventilation is secondary to the decrease in pulmonary compliance (14 % to 20 % of normal [36, 172]) and to the increase in the ratio of physiological dead space (DV) to tidal volume (TV), For example, the proportion DV/TV (normal 0.3) may increase to 0.6 [85] and climb to values close to 0.8 [31]. Airway resistance during inspiration in HMD does not play a role in alveolar hypoventilation [36]. A decrease in alveolar ventilation in this disorder is sometimes seen in the early stages. Particularly in babies of less than 32 weeks gestation and in those with neonatal asphyxia. Alveolar hypoventilation is seen more frequently after the second to the third day of HMD. The functional deficit at this stage of the disease results from an increase in respiratory work (4 times the normal [36]). The degree of alveolar hypoventilation [159] and the decrease in pulmonary volume [172] are closely related to the increase in right-to-left shunts.

Oxygen therapy is the basic treatment for the hypoxemia associated with HMD. An increase in FIO_2 corrects for the decrease in the PAO_2 secondary to alveolar hypoventilation and to $\dot{V}A/\dot{Q}$ abnormalities. The increase in PAO_2 and pari passu, PaO_2 reduces pulmonary vascular resistance (Fig. III-137) [150]. The effect of the O_2 is enhanced by assisted ventilation since the correction of respiratory acidosis and alveolar expansion assist in the adaptative changes which must take place in the pulmonary circulation (Fig. III-136, III-137).

Pneumothorax

Hypoxemia caused by pneumothorax is secondary to alveolar hypoventilation, $\dot{V}A/\dot{Q}$ abnormalities and to shunting secondary to compression of pulmonary tissue by extrapulmonary air under tension.

In this condition oxygen therapy corrects hypoxemia due to alveolar hypoventilation and inequalities of $\dot{V}A/\dot{Q}$. Gas in the pleural space is reabsorbed relatively rapidly with O_2 therapy because of the reduced partial pressures of nitrogen that result from raising the FIO_2 [30]. When the partial pressure of nitrogen in alveolar air decreases, tension of this inert gas in arterial blood falls. A gradient difference in the partial pressure of nitrogen is thus established between blood perfusing the pleura surrounding the collection of air in the pneumothorax; as a consequence, nitrogen, which constitutes 80 % of the encapsulated air, is rapidly reabsorbed. The resulting decrease of volume causes an increase of the partial pressures of O_2 and CO_2, which then augments their reabsorption. Oxygen therapy for facilitation of reabsorption of a pneumothorax is probably contraindicated in the premature infant because of fears concerning the effects of hyperoxemia. The manœuver may be attempted in a full term baby, when a tension pneumothorax does not provoke serious respiratory acidosis and when oxygen administration does, in fact, correct the observed hypoxemia. When these preconditions are not met or when the infant is being mechanically ventilated, the pneumothorax must be evacuated by trans-thoracic aspiration. The ideal monitoring of every infant treated with O_2 for pneumothorax is with continuous measurements of PO_2, for example, with transcutaneous monitors [51, 77].

Idiopathic apnea of prematurity

Respiration in prematures is usually irregular, periodic and may be associated with repetitive apnea. Apnea, interruption of respiration for more than

20 seconds, is seen in more than 50 % of premature infants during the first weeks of life [44]. This manifestation rarely occurs after the 36th week of gestation. The temptation to use O_2 in the treatment of apnea is based on the following observations:

1. Apnea occurs only in babies with periodic breathing [115]. Since periodic breathing can be converted to regular rhythm by O_2 in high concentration [178], it seems reasonable to administer O_2 to prevent apnea.

2. Periodic breathing associated with apnea can be induced with mild hypoxia during the first, three weeks of life in the premature [143]. Moreover, hypoxia causes a decrease of the ventilatory response to CO_2 although in older infants, the same degree of hypoxia provokes hyperventilation as seen in the adult [144]. These observations suggest that chronic, subclinical hypoxic states are the cause of apnea and that O_2 administration can prevent respiratory arrest.

The dangers of such reasoning are now known: this was used as the rationale for the *routine and prolonged exposure* to high FIO_2 during the RLF-epidemic years 1942-1954 [156]. Recent surveys of the incidence of RLF suggest that the disorder is more frequent among premature infants with apnea [65]. The latter association is of particular interest because of Peabody's observation [133] that episodes of hyperoxemia are induced with particular frequency in premature infants with repetitive apnea. Finally, it has been suggested, that the administration of O_2 does reduce the frequency of apnea, but that the episodes that "break through" may be prolonged [115]. If this phenomenon is indeed common it raises further doubts about the advantages of oxygen treatment for the apnea-prone infant. For all of these reasons, it seems

justified to recommend against the use of O_2 to prevent apnea in normoxemic prematures. If the supplemental gas is used for other indications, PaO_2 should be continuously controlled by means of a transcutaneous monitor. In cases of serious apnea resistant to the usual measures of respiratory stimulation, mask ventilation is indicated using the same FIO_2 administered before mechanical assistance. Here again a continuous measurement of PO_2 with a transcutaneous monitor is the optimal method of surveillance for the premature infant with apnea.

UTILIZATION OF OXYGEN FOR DIAGNOSTIC STUDIES

Hyperoxia test. — Administration of O_2 for 15 to 20 minutes, at concentrations higher than 80 %, can correct hypoxemia due to alveolar hypoventilation, diffusion abnormalities and $\dot{V}A/\dot{Q}$ disturbances. Since O_2 administration has few if any effects on hypoxemia caused by shunts (Fig. III-129), the gas exposure can be used for the diagnosis of shunt as well as a test for assessing shunt size relative to cardiac flow. The rationale of the oxygen method is based on the Fick principle and calculations are made separately for the pulmonary and the systemic circulations [15]. The approach permits an estimate to be made of the volume of venous blood which has been mixed with arterial blood, without identifying the site of the admixture. The shunt equation was proposed in 1942 by Berggren [15] on the basis of studies done at the end of the last century [151].

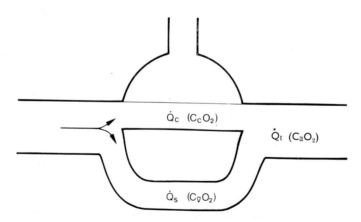

FIG. III-138. — *Illustrates the shunt equation* (see text p. 529).

$$\frac{\dot{Q}s}{\dot{Q}t} = \frac{CcO_2 - \bar{C}aO_2}{CcO_2 - \bar{C}vO_2}$$

$\dot{Q}s$ = blood flow via the shunt in ml/min.

$\dot{Q}t$ = total blood flow (cardiac flow) in ml/min.

CcO_2, $\bar{C}aO_2$, $\bar{C}vO_2$: content of O_2 in ml/100 ml of blood, in the capillary blood leaving the lung (CcO_2), the arterial blood ($\bar{C}aO_2$), and the mixed venous blood ($\bar{C}vO_2$). Berggren's equation follows from the following assumptions concerning function (Fig. III-138): the shunt ($\dot{Q}s$) is defined as the mixture of a certain quantity of non-arterialized blood in the lung with blood that was in contact with ventilated alveoli ($\dot{Q}c$) (alveoli-exposed capillary blood). The sum of capillary pulmonary blood flow ($\dot{Q}c$) and flow through the shunt ($\dot{Q}s$) is equal to the cardiac output ($\dot{Q}t$).

$$\dot{Q}c + \dot{Q}s = \dot{Q}t \qquad \text{(eq. 4)}$$

The "O_2 flow" in each of the defined compartments is equal to the blood flow times the O_2 concentration in the respective spaces. Thus,

$$\dot{Q}c \times CcO_2 + \dot{Q}s \times \bar{C}vO_2 = \dot{Q}t \times \bar{C}aO_2 \quad \text{(eq. 5)}$$

where CcO_2, $\bar{C}vO_2$ and $\bar{C}aO_2$ are, the O_2 contents in pulmonary capillaries, in mixed venous blood going through the shunt and in mixed arterial blood, respectively.

Because of Equation 4: $\dot{Q}c = \dot{Q}t + \dot{Q}s$, Equation 5 becomes

$$(\dot{Q}t - \dot{Q}s) \times CcO_2 + \dot{Q}s \times \bar{C}vO_2 = \dot{Q}t \times \bar{C}aO_2$$

or

$$\dot{Q}t \times (CcO_2 - \bar{C}aO_2) = \dot{Q}s \times (CcO_2 - \bar{C}vO_2).$$

From this last equation we can derive the shunt equation:

$$\frac{\dot{Q}s}{\dot{Q}t} = \frac{CcO_2 - \bar{C}aO_2}{CcO_2 - \bar{C}vO_2} \qquad \text{(eq. 3)}$$

If we know the O_2 content in capillary pulmonary blood (CcO_2) in arterial blood ($\bar{C}aO_2$), and in mixed venous blood (CvO_2), we can calculate the fractional part of the shunt ($\dot{Q}s$) as it relates to cardiac output ($\dot{Q}t$). Usually, CcO_2, $\bar{C}vO_2$ and $\bar{C}aO_2$ are not measured directly, but calculated as follows:

Calculation of CcO_2. — The terminal pulmonary capillary O_2 content (CcO_2) can be calculated if one knows the Hb concentration, O_2 saturation, and partial pressure of O_2 in the pulmonary capillaries (PcO_2). Hb concentration is measured routinely in peripheral blood, O_2 saturation is presumed to be 100 % during induced hyperoxemia. PcO_2 is equal to PAO_2, since, during hyperoxemia diffusion problems and $\dot{V}A/Q$ abnormalities are abolished. PAO_2 can be calculated by the alveolar gas equation (see Equation 2, above).

Calculation of $\bar{C}aO_2$. — O_2 content in the mixed arterial blood (CaO_2) can be calculated if Hb concentration, O_2 saturation, and PaO_2 are known. These parameters are routinely measured or derived.

Calculation of $\bar{C}vO_2$. — O_2 content in mixed venous blood ($\bar{C}vO_2$) is usually estimated on the basis of data obtained by right heart catheterization. Strang and MacLeish [159] estimated the arteriovenous difference in HMD to be 2 to 6 vol %. Usually, 3 vol % is used [119]. Thus knowing $\bar{C}aO_2$, one can calculate $\bar{C}vO_2$:

$$\bar{C}vO_2 \text{ (ml/100)} = \bar{C}aO_2 \text{ (ml/100)} - 3 \text{ ml } O_2/100.$$

Example of calculation of shunt. — A full-term newborn with respiratory distress after meconium aspiration, breathes 100 % O_2 at a barometric pressure of 747 mm Hg. Hb: 20 g %, PaO_2: 50 mm Hg, saturation: 90 %, PCO_2: 40 mm Hg.

As the baby is breathing 100 % oxygen, one can assume that the decrease in PaO_2 is entirely caused by shunt effect.

What is the size of the shunt? In Equation 3 insert the appropriate values for CcO_2, $\bar{C}aO_2$ and $\bar{C}vO_2$.

Calculation of CcO_2. — As discussed earlier, the calculation of CcO_2 requires that the value of the PcO_2 be known. At 100 % O_2, $PcO_2 = PAO_2$. PAO_2 can be calculated by using the alveolar gas equation (Equation 2, see p. 511).

$$PAO_2 = PIO_2 - \frac{PCO_2}{R}$$

R: respiratory quotient varies between 0.8 to 1.0.

$$PAO_2 = 100(747 - 47) - \frac{40}{0.8}$$

$$PAO_2 = 650 \text{ mm Hg}$$

or $\qquad PcO_2 = 650 \text{ mm Hg}$

What is the O_2 content (CcO_2) that corresponds to a PcO_2 of 650 mm Hg? $CcO_2 = O_2$ combined with Hb + dissolved O_2 (equation 6).

a) O_2 combined with Hb = Hb (gm %) × sat. (%) × O_2 capacity of Hb (ml O_2/gm Hb).

Now Hb: = 20 gm %, saturation: 100 %, capacity: 1.30 ml/g Hb. Therefore, O_2 combined with Hb (ml/100) = 20 × 100 × 1.30 = 26 ml O_2/100 ml blood.

b) Dissolved

O_2 (ml/100) = PcO_2 (mm Hg) × 0.003 ml/100 ml
                = 650 × 0.003
                = 1.95 ml O_2/100 ml blood.

Then, Equation 6 becomes:

CaO_2 = 26.0 + 1.95
        = 27.95 ml O_2/100 ml blood.

Calculation of CaO_2. — CaO_2 = O_2 combined with Hb + dissolved O_2 (Equation 7).

a) O_2 combined with Hb = Hb (g %) × sat. (%) × O_2 capacity of Hb (ml O_2/g Hb).

Now Hb: 20 g %, saturation: 90 % (PaO_2 = 50 mm Hg), capacity: 1.30 ml O_2/g Hb. Therefore, O_2 combined with Hb (ml/100) = 20 × 90 × 1.30 = 23.4 ml O_2/100 ml blood.

b) Dissolved

O_2 (ml/100) = PaO_2 × 0.003 ml/100 ml
               = 50 × 0.003
               = 0.15 ml O_2/100 ml blood.

Then, Equation 7 becomes:

CaO_2 = 23.40 + 0.15
        = 23.55 ml O_2/100 ml blood.

Calculation of $C\bar{v}O_2$. — If we assume an arterio-venous difference of 3 ml O_2/100

$C\bar{v}O_2$ = CaO_2 − 3
             = 23.55 − 3
             = 20.55 ml O_2/100 ml blood.

The respective values for CcO_2, $C\bar{a}O_2$, $C\bar{v}O_2$ can be inserted into the shunt equation (Equation 3):

$$\frac{\dot{Q}s}{\dot{Q}t} = \frac{CcO_2 - C\bar{a}O_2}{CcO_2 - C\bar{v}O_2}$$
$$= \frac{27.95 - 23.55}{27.95 - 20.55}$$
$$= \frac{4.4}{7.4}$$
$$60 \%$$

Thus, the affected newborn breathing 100 % O_2 who presents with a PaO_2 of 50 mm Hg, suffers from

a right-to-left shunt representing 60 % of the cardiac output.

In place of the laborious calculation for each case encountered, there is a graphic solution (Fig. III-139) which demonstrates the % shunt when knowing the FIO_2 and PaO_2.

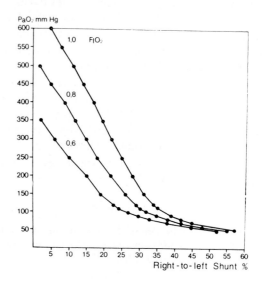

FIG. III-139. — *Estimation of right-to-left shunt by the O_2 method* [15].

Partial pressure of O_2 in arterial blood PaO_2 (mm Hg) in the presence of a right-to-left shunt (baby breathing 60 %, 80 %, or 100 % O_2). The lines of iso-shunt have been drawn by using Berggren's equation [15], if we assume: Hb 16 g %, arterio-venous difference: 4 volumes/100, pH: 7.40, PCO_2 40 mm Hg, t° 38° C, respiratory quotient: 0.8 [9].

Validity of the shunt equation. — It is important to note that the shunt equation, and therefore the graph of Figure III-139, cannot be used unless the arterial O_2 content perfusing the cephalad part of the body is the same as the O_2 content perfusing the caudal areas. A disparity comes about when there is a right-to-left shunt through the ductus and the shunt equation is thus invalid in this situation. We should emphasize here, that simultaneous measurement of PaO_2 above or below the ductus (tcPO_2) provides the clue needed to raise the possibility of a ductal shunt. Without this hint total shunt can be overestimated or underestimated by significant amounts. The magnitude of error that can occur using the shunt equation approach is especially large in certain conditions. An example was cited by Gersony [59] in which a 6 % shunt measured through the ductus using the usual shunt equation turned out to be about 40 % when the appropriate corrections were applied. Normograms that permit estimation of the size of the shunt in the presence of ductal shunting are illustrated in Gersony's studies [59].

APPENDIX

To facilitate the understanding of this chapter and the one on O_2 transport in the blood (Chapter 25), a glossary of important definition are listed below.

Affinity of Hb for O_2. — The strength with which Hb combines with O_2. A high affinity signifies that more molecules of O_2 are bound to Hb at any given PO_2. A relative decrease of Hb affinity for O_2 facilitates O_2 transport from arterial blood to the tissues.

Alveolar ventilation ($\dot{V}A$). — The proportion of inspired air which is distributed to perfused alveoli; expressed in ml of air per minute. Alveolar ventilation is not measured routinely. Its efficiency can be estimated by measuring PCO_2 in capillary or arterial blood.

Asphyxia. — Hypoxia caused by an acute insufficiency of alveolar ventilation. In asphyxia, hypoxemia is combined with hypercapnia.

Hypercapnia. — Respiratory acidosis; increase in PCO_2.

Hypocapnia. — Respiratory alkalosis; decrease in PCO_2.

Hypoxemia. — A quantity of O_2 in arterial blood that is insufficient for normal aerobic metabolism. This can be caused by a decrease in the arterial PO_2 or by a decrease in O_2 capacity of Hb.

Hypoxia. — Insufficiency of O_2 carried to cells for maintenance of normal aerobic metabolism.

O_2 blood content. — Also called O_2 blood concentration: content denotes ml O_2 carried by 100 ml blood. This term represents the sum of O_2 dissolved in plasma and O_2 carried by Hb. The latter quantity can be calculated if saturation (%), Hb concentration (Hb %), and the O_2 transport capacity (*i. e.* 1.30 per gram of the Hb at 100 % saturation) are known.

O_2 capacity. — Maximal quantity of O_2 (ml) that can be combined with Hb. This limit is reached when PO_2 is at or above 250 mm Hg. 1 g Hb combines with a maximum of 1.30 ml O_2 [47].

O_2 dissolved in the plasma. — Quantity, in ml, of O_2 molecules dissolved in the plasma. At 37° C,

0.3 ml O_2 are dissolved in 100 ml of plasma at a PO_2 of 100 mm Hg (normal alveolar pressure while breathing air).

Oxyhemoglobin-dissociation curve. — A graphic representation of the relation between PO_2 and quantity of O_2 combined with Hb, expressed in ml per 100 ml of blood or in Hb saturation.

P_{50}. — PO_2 when 50 % of Hb is combined with O_2.

PCO_2. — Partial pressure of CO_2 is the "strength" of the escaping tendency of molecules to leave their gaseous or liquid environment.

PO_2. — Partial pressure of O_2 is the "strength" of the escaping tendency of O_2 molecules to leave their gaseous or liquid environment. PO_2 measured with a platinum electrode in arterial blood, is one of the most frequently used parameters for assessing the body's oxygenation status. Arterial PO_2 (PaO_2) depends on alveolar ventilation, the pulmonary diffusion capacity, ventilation-perfusion. Ratio ($\dot{V}A/\dot{Q}$), and venous admixture in arterial blood (shunt).

PaO_2. — PO_2 in arterial blood, measured directly with an electrode, such as the Clark electrode.

PAO_2. — PO_2 in alveolar air, calculated when PIO_2 is known and PCO_2 is measured in capillary or arterial blood.

$$PAO_2 = PIO_2 - \frac{PCO_2}{R},$$

where

R = respiratory quotient = 0.8 to 1.0

PIO_2. — PO_2 in the inspired air, calculated by knowing barometric pressure (BP), O_2 fraction (%) in inspired air (FIO_2). $PIO_2 = $ (BP mm Hg − 47 mm Hg) $\times$ FIO_2, where 47 = pressure of saturated water vapor at 37° C.

Saturation (S %). — Fractional part of Hb combined with O_2, expressed in percent of O_2 transport capacity.

$$S \% = \frac{ml \text{ of } O_2 \text{ combined with Hb}}{capacity \times 100}$$

The saturation can be measured directly with a photometer.

Shunt. — Communication between the arterial and the venous limbs of the circulatory system (flow may take place in either direction). In the present chapter, the term shunt refers to net venous blood flow into arterial blood.

tcPO₂. — PO₂ measured by means of a warmed electrode placed on the skin. When peripheral perfusion is optimal, the tcPO₂ corresponds the PaO₂.

$\dot{V}A/\dot{Q}$. — Ratio of alveolar ventilation ($\dot{V}A$) to pulmonary perfusion ($\dot{Q}$). Normally, this value is 0.8.

*
* *

Note. — Data in the literature concerning the hemoglobin carrying capacity for O₂ vary between 1.24 and 1.39 ml O₂/g of hemoglobin. The number most frequently used has been the one proposed by Hüfner: 1.34 [78]. The differences between these estimates are probably explained by the presence of various substances in blood (e. g. derivates of hemoglobin that do not combine with O₂: hemoglobin, carboxyhemoglobin, methemoglobin) [47]. The recent studies of fetal blood by Gregory [63] estimate that Hb capacity is 1.31 and for adult blood 1.30 (though the number should be 1.39 based on the molecular weight of hemoglobin). We have chosen 1.30 for newborn blood.

REFERENCES

[1] AAP recommendations on oxygen use. Appendix 1 (Suppl.), *Pediatrics*, *57*, 635-637, 1976.
[2] ADAMKIN (D. H.), SHOTT (R. J.), COOK (L. N.), ANDREWS (B. F.). — Nonhyperoxic retrolental fibroplasia. *Pediatrics*, *60*, 828-830, 1977.
[3] ADAMSON (T. M.), HAWKER (J. M.), REYNOLDS, (E. O. R.), SHAW (J. L.). — Hypoxemia during recovery from severe hyaline membrane disease. *Pediatrics*, *44*, 168-178, 1969.
[4] ARANDA (J. V.), SAHEB (N.), STERN (L.), AVERY (M. E.). — Arterial oxygen tension and retinal vasoconstriction in newborn infants. *Am. J. Dis. Child.*, *122*, 189-194, 1971.
[5] ARANDA (J. V.). — In *Year Book of Pediatrics*, ed., F. A. Oski, Chicago, 1980, 26.
[6] ASHTON (N.), WARD (B.), SERPELL (C.). — Role of oxygen in the genesis of retrolental fibroplasia. A preliminary report. *Br. J. Ophthalmol.*, *37*, 513-520, 1953.
[7] ASHTON (N.), WARD (B.), SERPELL (C.). — Effect of oxygen on developing retinal vessels with particular reference to the problem of retrolental fibroplasia. *Br. J. Ophthalmol.*, *38*, 397-432, 1954.
[8] AUTOR (A. P.), FRANK (L.), ROBERTS (J. R.). — Developmental Characteristics of Pulmonary Superoxide Dismutase. Relationship to Idiopathic Respiratory Distress Syndrome. *Pediat. Res.*, *10*, 154-158, 1976.
[9] AVERY (M. E.), FLETCHER (B. D.). — The lung disorders in the newborn infant. Vol. I *in* the Series *Major Problems in Clinical Pediatrics*. W. B. Saunders Co., Toronto, Philadelphia, London, 67, 1974.
[10] AVERY (M. E.), OPPENHEIMER (E. H.). — Recent increase in mortality in hyaline membrane disease. *J. Pediatr.*, *57*, 553-559, 1960.
[11] BARD (H.), ALBERT (G.), TEASDALE (F.), DORAY (B.), MARTINEAU (B.). — Prophylactic antibiotics in chronic umbilical artery catheterization in respiratory distress syndrome. *Arch. Dis. Child.*, *48*, 630-635, 1973.
[12] BARTLETT (D. jr.). — Postnatal growth of the mammalian lung. Influence of low and high oxygen tensions. *Resp. Physiol.*, *9*, 58-64, 1970.
[13] BAUM (J. D.). — Retinal artery tortuosity in ex-premature infants. 18 year follow-up on eyes of premature infants. *Arch. Dis. Child.*, *46*, 247-252, 1971.
[14] BAUM (J. D.). — Retrolental fibroplasia. *Dev. Med. Child. Neurol.*, *21*, 385-387, 1979.
[15] BERGGREN (S. M.). — The oxygen deficit of arterial blood caused by non-ventilating parts of the lung. *Acta Physiol. Scand.*, vol. 4, suppl. 11, 1942.
[16] BERT (P.). — *La pression barométrique : Recherches de physiologie expérimentale*. G. Masson, Paris, 1137, 1878.
[17] BHATT (D. R.), HODGMAN (J. E.), TATTER (D.). — Evaluation of prophylatic antibiotic during umbilical catheterization in newborns. *Clin. Res.*, *18*, 217, 1970 (Abstr.).
[18] BLOCK (E. R.), FISHER (A. B.). — Depression of serotonin clearance by rat lungs after oxygen exposure. *J. Appl. Physiol.*, *42*, 33-38, 1977.
[19] BOAT (T. F.), KLEINERMAN (J. I.), FANAROFF (A. A.), MATTHEWS (L. W.). — Toxic effects of oxygen on cultured of human neonatal respiratory epithelium. *Pediat. Res.*, *7*, 607-615, 1973.
[20] BOLTON (D. P. G.), CROSS (K. W.). — Further observations on cost of preventing retrolental fibroplasia. *Lancet*, *1*, 445-448, 1974.
[21] BOOTHBY (C. B.), DESA (D. J.). — Massive pulmonary hemorrhage in the newborn. A changing pattern. *Arch. Dis. Child.*, *48*, 21-30, 1973.
[22] BORROS (S. J.), THOMPSON (T. R.), REYNOLDS (J. W.), JARVIS (C. W.), WILLIAMS (H. J.). — Reduced thrombus formation with silicone elastomere (silastic) umbilical artery catheters. *Pediatrics*, *56*, 981-986, 1975.
[23] BOUGLE (D.), VERT (P.), REICHART (E.), HARTEMANN (D.), HENG (E. L.). — Retinal superoxide dismutase activity in newborn kittens exposed to normobaric hyperoxia. Effect of vitamin E. *Pediat. Res.*, *16*, 400-402, 1982.
[24] BRADY (J. P.), COTTON (E. C.), TOOLEY (W. H.). — Chemoreflexes in the newborn infant: effects of 100 % oxygen on heart rate and ventilation. *J. Physiol. (London)*, *172*, 332-341, 1964.
[25] BUCCI (G.), SCALAMANDRÈ (A.), SAVIGNONI (P. G.), ORZALESI (M.), MENDICINI (M.). — Crib-side sampling of blood from the radial artery. *Pediatrics*, *37*, 497-498, 1966.
[26] BUDIN (P.). — *Le nourrisson*. Doin, Paris, 34, 1900.
[27] CAMPBELL (K.). — Intensive oxygen therapy as a possible cause of retrolental fibroplasia: A clinical approach. *Med. J. Australia*, *2*, 48-51, 1951.
[28] CARTWRIGHT (G. W.), SCHREINER (R. L.). — Major complication secondary to percutaneous Radial artery Catheterization in the Neonate. *Pediatrics*, *65*, 139-141, 1980.
[29] CASSIN (S.), DAWES (G. S.), MOTT (J. C.), ROSS (B. B.), STRANG (L. B.). — The vascular resistance of the fœtal and newly ventilated lung of the lamb. *J. Physiol.*, *171*, 61-79, 1964.

[30] CHERNICK (V.), AVERY (M. E.). — Spontaneous alveolar rupture at birth. *Pediatrics, 32*, 816-824, 1963.

[31] CHU (J.), CLEMENTS (J. A.), COTTON (E.), KLAUS (M. H.), SWEET (A. Y.), THOMAS (M. D.), TOOLEY (W. H.). — Preliminary report: The pulmonary hypoperfusion syndrome. *Pediatrics, 35*, 733-742, 1965.

[32] CLARK (J. M.), LAMBERTSEN (C. J.). — Pulmonary oxygen toxicity: A review. *Pharmacol. Rev., 23*, 37-133, 1971.

[33] COCHRAN (W. D.), DAVIS (H. T.), SMITH (C. A.). — Advantages and complications of umbilical artery catheterization in the newborn. *Pediatrics, 42*, 769-777, 1968.

[34] CONSTANTINE (H. P.), CRAW (M. R.), FORSTER (R. E.). — Rate of the reaction of carbon dioxide with human red blood cells. *Am. J. Physiol., 208*, 801-811, 1965.

[35] CONWAY (M.), DURBIN (G. M.), INGRAM (D.), McINTOCH (N.), PARKER (D.), REYNOLDS (E. O. R.), SOUTTER (L. P.). — Continuous monitoring of arterial oxygen tension using a catheter-tip polarographic electrode in infants. *Pediatrics, 57*, 244-250, 1976.

[36] COOK (C. D.), SUTHERLAND (J. M.), SEGAL (S.), CHERRY (R. B.), MEAD (J.), McILROY (M. B.), SMITH (C. A.). — Studies of respiratory physiology in the newborn infant. III. Measurements of the mechanics of respiration. *J. Clin. Invest., 36*, 440-448, 1957.

[37] COOK (C. D.), DRINKER (P. A.), JACOBSON (H. N.), LEVISON (H.), STRANG (L. B.). — Control of pulmonary blood flow in the fœtal and newly born lamb. *J. Physiol., 169*, 10-29, 1963.

[38] CORBET (A. J.), ROSS (J. A.), BEAUDRY (P. H.). — Ventilation-perfusion relationships as assessed by aADN$_2$ in hyaline membrane disease. *J. Appl. Physiol., 36*, 74-81, 1974.

[39] CRAPO (J. D.), TIERNEY (D. F.). — Superoxide dismutase and pulmonary oxygen toxicity. *Am. J. Physiol., 226*, 1401-1407, 1974.

[40] CROSS (K. W.), OPPÉ (T. E.). — The effect of inhalation of high and low concentrations of oxygen on the respiration of the premature infant. *J. Physiol., 117*, 38-55, 1952.

[41] CROSS (K. W.). — Cost of preventing retrolental fibroplasia. *Lancet, 2*, 954-956, 1973.

[42] CROSSE (V. M.), EVANS (Ph. J.). — Prevention of retrolental fibroplasia. *Arch. Ophthalmol., 48*, 83-87, 1952.

[43] CURRIE (W. D.), PRATT (P. C.), SANDERS (A. P.). — Hyperoxia and lung metabolism. *Chest, 66*, suppl., 19S-21S, 1974.

[44] DAILY (W. J. R.), KLAUS (M.), MEYER (H. B. P.). — Apnea in premature infants: Monitoring, incidence, heart rate changes and an effect of environmental temperature. *Pediatrics, 43*, 510-518, 1969.

[45] DAVI (M.), SANKARAN (K.), RIGATTO (H.). — Effect of inhaling 100 % O$_2$ on ventilation and acid-base balance in cerebrospinal fluid on neonates. *Biol. Neonate, 38*, 85-89, 1980.

[46] DE LEON (A. S.), ELLIOTT (J. H.), JONES (D. B.). — The resurgence of retrolental fibroplasia. *Pediat. Clin. North. Am., 17*, n° 2, 309-322, 1970.

[47] DIJKHUIZEN (P.), BUURSMA (A.), FONGERS (T. M. E.), GERDING (A. M.), OESEBURG (B.), ZIJLSTRA (W. G.). — The oxygen binding capacity of human haemoglobin. *Pfluegers Arch., 369*, 223-231, 1977.

[48] DUC (G.). — Assessment of hypoxia in the newborn. *Pediatrics, 48*, 469-481, 1971.

[49] DUC (G.), CUMARASAMY (N.). — Digital arteriolar oxygen tension as a guide to oxygen therapy of the newborn. *Biol. Neonate, 24*, 134-137, 1974.

[50] DUC (G.), FREI (H.), KLAR (H.), TUCHSCHMID (P.). — Reliability of continuous transcutaneous PO$_2$ (Hellige) in respiratory distress syndrome of the newborn. *Birth Defects: Original Article Series*, vol. XV, n° 4, 305-313, 1979.

[51] EBERHARD (P.), HAMMACKER (K.), MINDT (W.). — Methode zur kutanen Messung des Sauerstoffpartialdruckes. *Biomed Tech., 18*, 216-221, 1973.

[52] Editorial: Retrolental fibroplasia (RLF) unrelated to oxygen therapy. *Br. J. Ophthalmol., 58*, 487-489, 1974.

[53] EHRENKRANZ (R. A.), BONTA (B. W.), ABLOW (R. C.), WARSHAW (J. B.). — Amelioration of bronchopulmonary dysplasia after vitamin E administration: a preliminary report. *N. Engl. J. Med., 229*, 564-569, 1978.

[54] EHRENKRANZ (R. A.), ABLOW (R. C.), WARSHAW (J. B.). — Prevention of bronchopulmonary dysplasia with vitamin E administration during the acute stages of respiratory distress syndrome. *J. Pediatr., 95*, 873-878, 1979.

[55] FINLEY (T. N.), SWENSON (E. W.), COMROE J. H. Jr.). — The cause of arterial hypoxemia at rest in patients with « alveolar-capillary block syndrome ». *J. Clin. Invest., 41*, 618-622, 1962.

[55 a] FLOWER (R. W.), PATZ (A.). — Oxygen studies in retrolental fibroplasia: IX. The effects of elevated oxygen tension on retinal vascular dynamics in the kitten. *Arch. Ophthal., 85*, 197-203, 1971.

[55 b] FLYNN (J. T.), ESSNER (D.), ZESKIND (J.), MERRITT (J.), FLYNN (R.), WILLIAMS (M. S.). — Fluorescein angiography in retrolental fibroplasia: experience from 1969-1977. *Ophthalmology, 86*, 1700-1722, 1979.

[56] FORSTER (R. E.), CRANDALL (E. D.). — Pulmonary gas exchange. *Ann. Rev. Physiol., 38*, 69-93, 1976.

[57] GAIL (D. B.), MASSARO (D.). — Oxygen consumption by rat lung after *in vivo* hyperoxia. *Am. Rev. Respir. Dis., 113*, 8889-8891, 1976.

[58] GALE (R.), REDNER-CARMI (R.), GALE (J.). — Accumulation of carbon dioxide in oxygen hoods, infant cots and incubators. *Pediatrics, 60*, 453-456, 1977.

[59] GERSONY (W. M.), DUC (G. V.), DELL (R. B.), SINCLAIR (J. C.). — Oxygen method for calculation of the right to left shunt: new application in presence of right to left shunting through the ductus arteriosus. *Cardiovasc. Res., 6*, 423-438, 1972.

[60] GOETZMAN (B. W.), STADALNIK (R. C.), BOGREN (H. G.), BLANKENSHIP (W. J.), IKEDA (R. M.), THAYER (J.). — Thrombotic complications of umbilical artery catheters. A clinical and radiographic study. *Pediatrics, 56*, 374-379, 1975.

[61] GOLDMAN (H. I.), MARALIT (A.), SUN (S.), LANZKOWSY (P.). — Neonatal cyanosis and arterial oxygen saturation. *J. Pediatr., 82*, 319-324, 1973.

[62] GORDON (H. H.). — Oxygen therapy and survival rate in prematures (Letter). *Pediatrics, 19*, 967, 1957.

[63] GREGORY (I. C.). — The oxygen and carbon monoxide capacities of fœtal and adult blood. *J. Physiol., 236*, 625-634, 1974.

[64] GUNN (T. R.), ARANDA (J. V.), LITTLE (J.). — Incidence of retrolental fibroplasia. *Lancet, 1*, 216-217, 1978.

[65] GUNN (T. R.), EASDOWN (J.), OUTERBRIDGE (E. W.), ARANDA (J. V.). — Risk factors in retrolental fibroplasia. *Pediatrics*, 65, 1096-1100, 1980.

[66] GUPTA (J. M.), ROBERTON (N. R.), WIGGLESWORTH (J. S.). — Umbilical artery catheterization in the newborn. *Arch. Dis. Child.*, 43, 382-387, 1968.

[67] GUY (L. P.), LANMAN (J. T.), DANCIS (J.). — The possibility of total elimination of retrolental fibroplasia by oxygen restriction. *Pediatrics*, 17, 247-249, 1956.

[68] GYLLENSTEN (L. J.). — Influence of oxygen exposure on the postnatal vascularization of the cerebral cortex in mice. *Acta Morphol Neerl-Scand.*, 2, 289-298, 1959.

[69] HAUGGAARD (N.). — Cellular mechanisms of oxygen toxicity. *Physiol. Rev.*, 48, 311-373, 1968.

[70] HESS (J. H.). — *Premature and congenitally diseased infants*. Lea and Febiger, Philadelphia, 1922.

[71] HESS (J. H.). — Oxygen unit for premature and very young infants. *Am. J. Dis. Child.*, 47, 916-917, 1934 b.

[72] HEY (E. N.), KATZ (G.). — Evaporative water loss in the newborn baby. *J. Physiol. (London)*, 200, 605-619, 1969.

[73] HEYMAN (A.), PATTERSON (J. L. Jr.), DUKE (T. W.). — Cerebral circulation and metabolism in sickle cell and other chronic anemias, with observations on the effects of oxygen inhalation. *J. Clin. Invest.*, 31, 824-828, 1952.

[74] HODSON (W. A.), BELENKY (D. A.). — Management of respiratory problems. In: *Neonatology*. Ed. by G. B. Avery. J. B. Lippincott Company Philadelphia, 265-294, 1975.

[75] HREBEK (A.), KARLBERG (P.), KJELLMAR (I.), OLSSON (T.), RIHA (M.). — Clinical application of evoked EEG-responses in newborn infants: II. Idiopathic respiratory distress syndrome. *Dev. Med. Child. Neurol.*, 20, 619-626, 1978.

[76] HUCH (R.), HUCH (A.), LÜBBERS (D. W.). — Transcutaneous measurements of blood PO₂ (tcPO₂). Method and application in Perinatal Medicine. *J. Perinat. Med.*, 1, 183-191, 1973.

[77] HUCH (A.), HUCH (R.), LUCEY (J. F.). — Continuous transcutaneous blood gas monitoring. National Foundation, March of Dimes. *Birth Defects*, vol. XV, n° 4, 1979.

[78] HÜFNER (G.). — Noch ein Mal die Frage nach der « Sauerstoff-Kapazität des Blutfarbstoffes ». *Arch. Anat. Physiol.*, 217-224, 1903.

[79] JACOBSON (I.), HARPER (A. M.), McDOWALL (D. W.). — The effects of oxygen under pressure on cerebral blood-flow and cerebral venous oxygen tension. *Lancet*, 2, 249, 1963.

[80] JACOBSON (I.), HARPER (A. M.), McDOWALL (D. G.). — The effects of oxygen at 1 and 2 atmospheres on the blood flow and oxygen uptake of the cerebral cortex. *Surg. Gynec. Obstet.*, 119, 737-742, 1964.

[81] JOHNSON (L.), SCHAFFER (D.), BOGGS (T. R. Jr.). — The premature infant, vitamin E deficiency and retrolental fibroplasia. *Am. J. Clin. Nutr.*, 27, 1158-1173, 1974.

[82] KALINA (R. E.), HODSON (W. A.), MORGAN (B. C.). — Retrolental fibroplasia in a cyanotic infant. *Pediatrics*, 50, 765-768, 1972.

[83] KAPANCI (Y.), WEIBEL (E. R.), KAPLAN (H. P.), ROBINSON (F. R.). — Pathogenesis and reversibility of the pulmonary lesions of oxygen toxicity in

monkeys. II. Ultrastructural and morphometric studies. *Lab. Invest.*, 20, 101-118, 1969.

[84] KAPLAN (H. P.), ROBINSON (F. R.), KAPANCI (Y.), WEIBEL (E. R.). — Pathogenesis and reversibility of the pulmonary lesions of oxygen toxicity in monkeys. I. Clinical and light microscopic studies. *Lab. Invest.*, 20, 94-100, 1969.

[85] KARLBERG (P.), COOK (C. D.), O'BRIAN (D.), CHERRY (R. B.), SMITHS (C. A.). — Studies of respiratory physiology in the newborn infant. Observations during and after respiratory distress. *Acta Pediatr. Scand.*, 43, suppl. 100, 397-411, 1954.

[86] KENNEDY (C.), GRAVE (G. D.), JEHLE (J. W.). — Effect of hyperoxia on the cerebral circulation of the newborn puppy. *Pediat. Res.*, 5, 659-667, 1971.

[87] KENNEDY (C.), GRAVE (G. D.), SOKOLOFF (I.). — Alteration of local cerebral blood flow due to exposure of the newborn puppies to 80-90 % oxygen. *Eur. Neurol.*, 6, 137-140, 1971-1972.

[88] KETY (S. S.), SCHMIDT (C. F.). — The effects of altered arterial tensions of carbon dioxide and oxygen on cerebral blood flow and cerebral oxygen consumption of normal young men. *J. Clin. Invest.*, 27, 484-492, 1948.

[89] KINSEY (V. E.). — Etiology of retrolental fibroplasia and preliminary report of cooperative study of retrolental fibroplasia. *Tr. Am. Acad. Ophth. Otol.*, 59, 15-24, 1955.

[90] KINSEY (V. E.), ARNOLD (H. J.), KALINA (R. E.), STERN (L.), STHALMAN (M.), ODELL (G.), DRISCOLL (J. M.), ELLIOTT (J. H.), PAYNE (J.), PATZ (A.). — PaO₂ levels and retrolental fibroplasia. A report of the cooperative study. *Pediatrics*, 60, 655-668, 1977.

[91] KITTERMAN (J. A.), PHIBBS (R. H.), TOOLEY (W. H.). — Catheterization of umbilical vessels in newborn infants. *Pediatr. Clin. North Am.*, 17, 895-912, 1970.

[92] KLAUS (M.). — Respiratory function and pulmonary disease in the newborn. In *Pediatrics*, ed. H. L. Barnett, Appleton-Century-Crofts, 15th edition, New York, 1255-1261, 1972.

[93] KOENIGSBERGER (M. R.), MOESSINGER (A. C.). — Iatrogenic carpal tunnel syndrome in the newborn infant. *J. Pediatr.*, 91, 443-445, 1977.

[94] KRAUSS (A. N.), AULD (P. A.). — Ventilation-perfusion abnormalities in the premature infant: triple gradient. *Pediatr. Res.*, 3, 255-264, 1969.

[95] KRAUSS (A. N.), ALBERT (R. F.), KANNAN (M. M.). — Contamination of umbilical catheters in the newborn infant. *J. Pediatr.*, 77, 965-969, 1970.

[96] KRAUSS (A. N.), AULD (P. A.). — Measurement of functional residual capacity in distressed neonates by helium rebreathing. *J. Pediatr.*, 77, 228-232, 1970.

[97] KRAUSS (A. N.), SOODALTER (J. A.), AULD (P. A.). — Adjustment of ventilation and perfusion in the full-term normal and distressed neonate as determined by urinary alveolar nitrogen gradients. *Pediatrics*, 47, 865-869. 1971.

[98] KRAUSS (A. N.), KLAIN (D. B.), AULD (P. A. M.). — Carbon monoxide diffusing capacity in newborn infants. *Pediatr. Res.*, 10, 771-776, 1976.

[99] LAMBERTSEN (C. J.). — Effects of oxygen at high partial pressure in: *Handbook of Physiology*, Section 3, Respiration. Vol. II, 1027-1046, Washington, American Physiological Society, 1963.

[100] LARROCHE (J. Cl.). — Umbilical catheterization: its complications. *Biol. Neonate*, 16, 101-116, 1970.

[101] LEAHY (F.), SANKARAN (K.), CATES (D.), MAC CALLUM (M.), RIGATTO (H.). — Changes in cerebral blood flow in preterm infants during inhalation of CO₂ and 100 % O₂. *Clin. Res.*, 26, 879 A, 1978.

[102] LECHNER (D.), KALINA (R. E.), HODSON (W. A.). — Retrolental fibroplasia and factors influencing oxygen transport. *Pediatrics*, 59, 916-918, 1977.

[103] Les Chermignonards désenchantés. — Oxygen and retrolental fibroplasia: The questions persist. *Pediatrics*, 60, 753-754, 1977.

[104] LOU (H. C.), LASSEN (N. A.), FRIIS-HANSEN (B.). — Low cerebral blood flow in the hypotensive perinatal distress. *Acta Neurol. Scand.*, 56, 343-352, 1977.

[105] LOU (H. C.), LASSEN (N. A.), FRIIS-HANSEN (B.). — Decreased cerebral blood flow after administration of sodium bicarbonate in the distressed newborn infant. *Acta Neurol. Scand.*, 57, 239-247, 1978.

[106] LOU (H. C.), SKOV (H.), PEDERSEN (H.). — Low cerebral blood flow: A risk factor in the neonate. *J. Pediatr.*, 95, 606-609, 1979.

[107] LUCEY (J. A.). — Functional and structural aspects of membranes. A suggested structural role for Vitamin E in the control of membrane permeability and stability. *Ann. N. Y. Acad. Sci.*, 203, 4-11, 1972.

[108] MASSARO (G. D.), GAIL (D. B.), MASSARO (D.). — Lung oxygen consumption and mitochondria of alveolar epithelial and endothelial cells. *J. Appl. Physiol.*, 38, 588-592, 1975.

[109] McCORD (J.). — Superoxide, superoxide dismutase and oxygen toxicity. *Reviews in Biochemical Toxicology*, vol. I., ed. Hodgson (E.) et coll., 1979.

[110] McDONALD (A. D.). — Neurological and ophthalmic disorders in children of very low birthweight. *Br. Med. J.*, 1, 895-900, 1962.

[111] McDONALD (A. D.). — Cerebral palsy in children of very low birth weight. *Arch. Dis. Child.*, 38, 579-588, 1963.

[112] McDONALD (A. D.). — Oxygen treatment of premature babies and cerebral palsy. *Dev. Med. Child. Neurol.*, 6, 313-314, 1964.

[112 a] McDONALD (A. D.). — *Children of very low birth weight*. Heinemann Medical, London, 39, 1967.

[113] MENZEL (D. B.). — Toxicity of ozone, oxygen and radiation. *Ann. Rev. Pharmacol.*, 10, 379-394, 1970.

[114] MESTYAN (J.), JARAI (I.), BATA (G.), FEKETE (M.). — The significance of facial skin temperature in the chemical heat regulation of premature infants. *Biol. Neonate*, 7, 243-254, 1964.

[115] MILLER (H. C.), BEHRLE (F. C.), SMULL (N. W.). — Severe apnea and irregular respiratory rhythms among premature infants. *Pediatrics*, 23, 676-685, 1959.

[116] MOKROHISKY (S. T.), LEVINE (R. L.), BLUMHAGEN (J. D.), WESENBERG (R. L.), SIMMONS (M. A.). — Low positioning of umbilical-artery catheters increases associated complications in newborn infants. *N. Engl. J. Med.*, 299, 561-564, 1978.

[117] MOSS (A. J.), EMMANOUILIDES (G. C.), RETTORI (O.), HIGASHINO (S. M.), ADAMS (F. H.). — Postnatal circulatory and metabolic adjustments in normal and distressed premature infants. *Biol. Neonate*, 8, 177-197, 1965.

[118] MURDOCK (A. I.), SWYER (P. R.). — The contribution to venous admixture by shunting through the ductus arteriosus in infants with the respiratory distress syndrome of the newborn. *Biol. Neonate*, 13, 194-210, 1968.

[119] MURDOCK (A. J.), KIDD (B. S. L.), LLEWELLYN (M. A.), REID (M. McC.), SWYER (P. R.). — Intrapulmonary venous admixture in the respiratory distress syndrome. *Biol. Neonate*, 15, 1-7, 1970.

[120] MUSTAFA (M. G.), TIERNEY (D. F.). — Biochemical and metabolic changes in the lung with oxygen, ozone and nitrogen dioxide toxicity. *Am. Rev. Respir. Dis.*, 118, 1061-1090, 1978.

[121] NASH (G.), BLENNERHASSETT (J. B.), PONTOPPIDAN (H.). — Pulmonary lesions associated with oxygen therapy and artificial ventilation. *N. Engl. J. Med.*, 276, 368-374, 1967.

[122] NEAL (W. A.), REYNOLDS (J. W.), JARVIS (C. W.), WILLIAMS (H. J.). — Umbilical artery catheterization: demonstration of arterial thrombosis by aortography. *Pediatrics*, 50, 6-13, 1972.

[123] NORTHWAY (W. H. Jr.), ROSAN (R. C.), PORTER (D. Y.). — Pulmonary disease following respirator therapy of hyaline-membrane disease: bronchopulmonary dysplasia. *N. Engl. J. Med.*, 276, 357-368, 1967.

[124] NORTHWAY (W. H.), PETRICEKS (R.), SHAHINIAN (L.). — Quantitative aspect of oxygen toxicity in the newborn: Inhibition of lung DNA-synthesis in the mouse. *Pediatrics*, 50, 67-72, 1972.

[125] OWENS (W. C.), OWENS (E. U.). — Retrolental fibroplasia in premature infants: II. Studies on the prophylaxis of the disease: The use of alpha tocopheryl acetate. *Am. J. Ophth.*, 32, 1631-1637, 1949 b.

[126] OWENS (W. C.). — Spontaneous regression in retrolental fibroplasia. *Tr. Am. Ophth. Soc.*, 51, 555-579, 1953.

[127] PAPE (K. E.), ARMSTRONG (D. L.), FITZHARDINGE (P. M.). — Peripheral median nerve damage secondary to brachial arterial blood gas sampling. *J. Pediatr.*, 93, 852-856, 1978.

[128] PATHAK (A.), MORRISON (L.), PRUDENT (L. M.), CHERRY (R. B.), NELSON (N. M.). — Ventilatory disturbance and arterial-alveolar N₂ differences during recovery from hyaline membrane disease. *Pediatr. Res.*, 4, 479, 1970 (Abstr. 170).

[129] PATZ (A.), HOECK (L. E.), DE LA CRUZ (E.). — Studies on the effect of high oxygen administration in retrolental fibroplasia. I. Nursery Observations. *Am. J. Ophthalmol.*, 35, 1248-1253, 1952.

[130] PATZ (A.), EASTHAM (A.), HIGGINBOTHAM (D. H.), KLEH (T.). — Oxygen studies in retrolental fibroplasia. II. The production on the microscopic changes of retrolental fibroplasia in experimental animals. *Am. J. Ophthalmol.*, 36, 1511-1522, 1953.

[131] PATZ (A.). — The role of oxygen in retrolental fibroplasia. *Pediatrics*, 19, 504-524, 1957 a.

[132] PATZ (A.). — The effect of oxygen on immature retinal vessels. *Invest. Ophthal.*, 4, 988-999, 1965.

[133] PEABODY (J. L.), NEESE (A. L.), PHILIP (A. G. S.), LUCEY (J. F.), SOYKA (L. F.). — Transcutaneous oxygen monitoring in aminophylline-treated apneic infants. *Pediatrics*, 62, 698-701, 1978.

[134] PECKHAM (G. J.), FOX (W. W.). — Physiologic factors affecting pulmonary artery pressure in infants with persistent pulmonary hypertension. *J. Pediatr.*, 93, 1005-1010, 1978.

[135] PENROD (K.). — Lung damage by oxygen using differential catheterization. *Fed. Proc.*, 17, 123, 1958.

[136] PHELPS (D. L.), ROSENBAUM (A. L.). — The role of tocopherol in oxygen-induced retinopathy: kitten model. *Pediatrics*, 59 (suppl.), 998-1005, 1977.

[137] PHELPS (D. L.). — Toxicity of pharmacological parenteral doses of vitamin E in the neonatal kitten. *Pediatr. Res.*, *13*, 372, 1979.

[137 a] PHELPS (D. L.). — Retinopathy of prematurity: An estimate of vision loss in the United States, 1979. *Pediatrics*, *67*, 924-926, 1981.

[138] POWERS (W. F.), TOOLEY (W. H.). — Contamination of umbilical vessel catheters: encouraging information. *Pediatrics*, *49*, 470-471, 1972.

[139] PRIESTLY (J.). — *The discovery of oxygen* (1775). Alembic Club Reprints, No. 7. Chicago University of Chicago Press, 1906.

[140] PROD'HOM (L. S.), LEVISON (H.), CHERRY (R. B.), SMITH (C. A.). — Adjustment of ventilation, intra-pulmonary gas exchange and acid-base balance during the first day of life. Infants with early respiratory distress. *Pediatrics*, *35*, 662-676, 1965.

[141] REYNOLDS (E. O. R.), TAGHIZADEH (A.). — Improved prognosis of infants mechanically ventilated for hyaline membrane disease. *Arch. Dis. Child.*, *49*, 505-515, 1974.

[142] RIGATTO (H.), BRADY (J. P.). — Periodic breathing and apnea in preterm infants. I. Evidence for hypoventilation, possibly due to central respiratory depression. *Pediatrics*, *50*, 202-218, 1972.

[143] RIGATTO (H.), BRADY (J. P.). — Periodic breathing and apnea in preterm infants. II. Hypoxia as a primary event. *Pediatrics*, *50*, 219-228, 1972.

[144] RIGATTO (H.), DE LA TORRE VERDUZCO (R.), CATES (D. B.). — Effects of O_2 on the ventilatory response to CO_2 in preterm infants. *J. Appl. Physiol.*, *39*, 896-899, 1975.

[145] RIGATTO (H.), BRADY (J. P.), DE LA TORRE VERDUZCO (R.). — Chemoreceptor reflexes in preterm infants. I. The effect of gestational and postnatal age on the ventilatory response to inhalation of 100 % and 15 % oxygen. *Pediatrics*, *55*, 604-613, 1975.

[146] RIGATTO (H.), BRADY (J. P.), DE LA TORRE VERDUZCO (R.). — Chemoreceptor reflexes in preterm infants. II. The effect of gestational and postnatal age on the ventilatory response to inhaled carbon dioxide. *Pediatrics*, *55*, 614-620, 1975.

[147] ROBERTON (N. R.), DAHLENBURG (G. W.). — Ductus arteriosus shunts in the respiratory distress syndrome. *Pediatr. Res.*, *3*, 149-159, 1969.

[148] RUDOLPH (A. M.), AULD (P. A. M.), GOLINKO (R. J.), PAUL (M. H.). — Pulmonary vascular adjustments in the neonatal period. *Pediatrics*, *28*, 28-34, 1961.

[149] RUDOLPH (A. M.), DRORBAUGH (J. E.), AULD (P. A. M.), RUDOLPH (A. J.), NADAS (A. S.), SMITH (C. A.), HUBBELL (J. P.). — Studies on the circulation in the neonatal period. The circulation in the respiratory distress syndrome. *Pediatrics*, *27*, 551-566, 1961.

[150] RUDOLPH (A. M.), YUAN (S.). — Response of the pulmonary vasculature to hypoxia and H^+ Ion concentration changes. *J. Clin. Invest.*, *45*, 399-411, 1966.

[151] SACKUR. — Weiteres zur Lehre vom Pneumothorax. Virchow' Archiv für pathol. *Anatomie u. Physiologie*, *150*, 151-160, 1897.

[152] SCHLUETER (M. A.), JOHNSON (B. B.), SUDMAN (D. A.), WANG (L. Y.), NAMKUNG (P.), HEASLEY (S. V.), HADDOCK (S. A.), TOOLEY (W. H.). — Blood sampling from scalp arteries in infants. *Pediatrics*, *51*, 120-122, 1973.

[153] SCOPES (J. W.), AHMED (I.). — Indirect assessment of oxygen requirements in newborn babies by monitoring deep body temperature. *Arch. Dis. Child.*, *41*, 25-33, 1966.

[154] SHANKLIN (D. R.), WOLFSONS (S. L.). — Therapeutic oxygen as a possible cause of pulmonary hemorrhage in premature infants. *N. Engl. J. Med.*, *277*, 833-837, 1967.

[155] SILVERMAN (W. A.). — What is the present status of retrolental fibroplasia. In *Problems of neonatal intensive care units*. Rep. 59th Ross Conf. in Pediatric Research. Library of Congress, No. 53-22189, 57-63, 1969.

[156] SILVERMAN (W. J.). — *The lesson of retrolental fibroplasia*. Scientific American 236, No. 6, 100-107, 1977.

[157] STAHLMAN (M.), SHEPHARD (F. M.), YOUNG (W. C.), GRAY (J.), BLANKENSHIP (W.). — Assessment of the cardiovascular status of infants with hyaline membrane disease. In *The Heart and Circulation in the Newborn Infant*. Edited by D. E. Cassels, Grune and Stratton, New York, 121-140, 1966.

[158] STAHLMAN (M.), BLANKENSHIP (W. J.), SHEPHARD (F. M.), GRAY (J.), YOUNG (W. C.), MALAN (A. F.). — Circulatory studies in clinical hyaline membrane disease. *Biol. Neonate*, *20*, 300-320, 1972.

[159] STRANG (L. B.), MAC LEISH (M. H.). — Ventilatory failure and right-to-left shunt in newborn infants with respiratory distress. *Pediatrics*, *28*, 17-27, 1961.

[160] STRANG (L. B.). — The pulmonary circulation in the respiratory distress syndrome. *Pediatr. Clin. North. Am.*, *13*, 693-701, 1966.

[161] STRANG (L. B.). — *Neonatal respiration. Physiological and clinical studies*. Blackwell Scient. Publications, Oxford, London, Edinburgh, Melbourne, 236, 1977.

[162] SVEDBERGH (B.), LINDSTEDT (E.). — Retrolental fibroplasia in Sweden. *Acta Paediat. Scand.*, *62*, 458-464, 1973.

[163] SYMANSKY (M. R.), FOX (H. A.). — Umbilical vessel catheterization: indications, management, and evaluation of the technique. *J. Pediatr.*, *80*, 820-826, 1972.

[164] TAPPEL (A. L.). — Lipid peroxidation damage to cell components. *Fed. Proc.*, *32*, 1870-1874, 1973.

[165] TAYLOR (D. W.). — The effects of vitamin E and of methylene blue on the manifestations of oxygen poisoning in the rat. *J. Physiol.*, *131*, 200-206, 1956.

[166] TERRY (T. L.). — Extreme prematurity and fibroplastic overgrowth of persistent vascular sheath behind each crystalline lens. I. Preliminary report. *Am. J. Ophthalmol.*, *25*, 203-204, 1942.

[167] THIBEAULT (D. W.), POBLETE (E.), AULD (P. A. M.). — Alveolar-arterial oxygen difference in premature infants breathing 100 % oxygen. *J. Pediatr.*, *71*, 814-824, 1967.

[168] THOMSEN (A.). — Arterial blood sampling in small infants. *Acta Paediatr. Scand.*, *53*, 237-240, 1964.

[169] TIERNEY (D. F.). — Lactate metabolism in rat lung tissue. *Arch. Intern. Med.*, *127*, 858-860, 1971.

[170] TOOLEY (W. H.), HOFFMAN (J. I. E.). — Caution about statistics of retrolental fibroplasia study. *Pediatrics*, *60*, 754-756, 1977.

[171] TOOLEY (W. H.). — What is the risk of an umbilical artery catheter. *Pediatrics*, *50*, 1-2, 1972.

[172] TORI (C. A.), KRAUSS (A. N.), AULD (P. A. M.). — Serial studies of lung volume and $VA/\dot{Q}$ in hyaline membrane disease. *Pediatr. Res.*, *7*, 82-88, 1973.

[173] TUCHSCHMID (P.), BOUTELLIER (W.), KOLLER (E.A.), DUC (G. V.). — Comparison of hypoxantin lactate and ECG signs as indicators of hypoxia. *Pediatr. Res.*, *15*, 28-33, 1981.

[174] WALLGREN (G.), HANSON (J. S.), TABAKIN (B. S.), RÄIHÄ (N.), VAPAAVOURI (E.). — Quantitative studies of the human neonatal circulation. V. Hemodynamic findings in premature infants with and without respiratory distress. *Acta Paediat. Scand.*, suppl. *179*, 69-80, 1967.

[175] WEST (J. B.). — *Ventilation, blood flow and gas exchange*. Blackwell Scient. Publications, Oxford, Edinburgh, 12, 1967.

[176] WEST (J. B.). — *Respiratory Physiology*. Blackwell Scient. Publications, Oxford, Edinburgh, 58-59, 1974.

[177] WIGGER (H. J.), BRANSILVER (B. R.), BLANC (W. A.). — Thromboses due to catheterization in in-fants and children. *J. Pediatr.*, *76*, 1-11, 1970.

[178] WILSON (J. L.), LONG (S. B.), HOWARD (P. J.). — Respiration of premature infants. Response to variations of oxygen and to increased carbon dioxide in inspired air. *Am. J. Dis. Child.*, *63*, 1080-1085, 1942.

[179] WINTER (P. M.), GUPTA (R. K.), MICHALSKI (A. H.), LANPHIER (E. H.). — Modification of hyperbaric oxygen toxicity by experimental venous admixture. *J. Appl. Physiol.*, *23*, 954-963, 1967.

[180] WOLFE (W. G.), DEVRIES (W. C.). — Oxygen toxicity. *Ann. Rev. Med.*, *26*, 203-217, 1975.

[181] Workshop on bronchopulmonary dysplasia. *J. Pediatr.*, *95*, 815-919, 1979.

[182] YANKAUER (A.). — *Information memorandum*. New York State Health Dept. Febr. 17, 1955.

[183] YLPPO (A.). — Ueber Magenatmung beim Menschen. *Biochem. Zeitschr.*, *78*, 273-276, 1917.

27

Assisted ventilation in the newborn

P. MONIN, P. VERT

ABBREVIATIONS USED

AV	: Assisted ventilation.
BPD	: Bronchopulmonary dysplasia.
CNP	: Continuous negative airway pressure.
CPAP	: Continuous positive airway pressure.
FRC	: Functional residual capacity.
HMD	: Hyaline membrane disease.
HFO	: High frequency oscillations.
I/E	: Inspiratory/expiratory ratio.
IMV	: Intermittent mandatory ventilation.
IPPV	: Intermittent positive pressure ventilation.
INPV	: Intermittent negative pressure ventilation.
$PaCO_2$	: Arterial carbon dioxide tension.
PaO_2	: Arterial oxygen tension.
$PACO_2$	: Alveolar carbon dioxide tension.
PEEP	: Positive end expiratory pressure.
P_{50}	: Partial pressure of arterial oxygen necessary for a saturation of 50 %.

The reduction of mortality from respiratory distress in the newborn is to a considerable extent due to the development of artificial ventilation technics [16, 24, 67, 68]. Despite the beneficial results, these technics are also responsible for complications, which are sometimes severe [24, 58]. The aim of assisted ventilation (AV) is to re-establish alveolo-arterial gas exchange while awaiting resolution of the pulmonary disease. The pressure required for AV is different from that induced by the normal respiratory cycle. This pressure induces changes in the mechanics of breathing [6, 87] and intrathoracic haemodynamics [1, 25, 56, 66, 71]. In the newborn the more recent developments in AV include continuous positive airway pressure (CPAP) [46], intermittent mandatory ventilation (IMV) [63], high frequency ventilation [12] and more recently, high frequency oscillation (HFO) [21] and jet ventilation [102].

PHYSIOLOGICAL BASIS OF ASSISTED VENTILATION

Whatever its aetiology, respiratory insufficiency is characterized by a progressive increase in carbon dioxide partial pressure in arterial blood ($PaCO_2$), a reduction in arterial oxygen partial pressure (PaO_2) and a combined metabolic and respiratory acidosis. The alveolar hypoventilation responsible for these changes provides the rationale for AV.

AV and the mechanics of breathing

The pulmonary pressure. — In any technique of positive pressure ventilation, the airways pressure increases rapidly during inflation according to the flow and the mechanical properties of the lung-chest system. The airway pressure decreases as soon as the inflation stops and expiration begins. The latter is a passive process depending on lung-chest system elasticity which allows the lung to return towards its relaxation volume or functional residual capacity (FRC). The airway pressure reaches the barometric pressure or remains above it when a positive end expiratory pressure (PEEP) is added [89].

With negative pressure techniques, the airway pressure changes are much closer to those observed during spontaneous breathing [69, 72, 88]. Negative intra-tracheal pressure is not used in newborns because of the risk of atelectasis.

The airway pressure is not totally transmitted to the alveolar spaces [100]. The transmission is inversely related to airway resistance to air flow which causes a considerable loss [31]. The resistance is also related to the size of the intra-tracheal tube. At zero flow, the alveolar and airway pressures are identical. In some cases, especially with PEEP, the alveolar pressure can be greater than the pulmonary capillary pressure and arrest the perfusion (Fig. III-140).

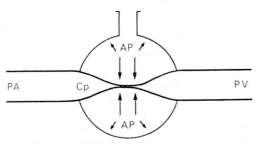

FIG. III-140. — *Effect of alveolar pressure on the pulmonary capillaries.* (A. P.: alveolar pressure, P. A.: pulmonary artery, Cp: pulmonary vessel, P. V.: pulmonary vein).

During spontaneous breathing, the intra-pleural pressure normally lower than barometric pressure decreases during inspiration [28, 44]. It increases above the barometric pressure during inflation with positive pressure ventilation and jeopardizes the venous return [1, 65]. This hemodynamic effect is related to the pressures applied on the lungs, the transmission of which is reduced in the intra-pleural space when lung compliance is low as in

hyaline membrane disease (HMD). During AV, the intra-pleural pressure also depends on the physical properties of the chest: the more rigid the chest, the higher is the rise in intra-pleural pressure during inflation [43]. This pressure is also considerably increased when the patient's respiratory rate is not synchronous with the respirator frequency [63, 86].

Lung volumes. — During AV, the tidal volume (V_T) depends on the ventilatory settings (peak inspiratory pressure, inspiration/expiration ratio, end expiratory pressure), the patient's airways and respiratory circuit resistances and leaks related to the use of uncuffed tracheal tubes.

To avoid thoracic distension which may induce hemodynamic disorders, the lungs should return to their initial volume during expiration. Because the expiratory flow is related only to the lung elasticity and dynamic resistance of the airway, expiration should be long enough to maintain the end expiration lung volume. The risk of overdistension is greater in the premature because of the small caliber of the airway [4, 44].

Lung compliance. — This depends on the lung's mechanical properties. It is considerably decreased in hyaline membrane disease [4]. The lung compliance changes are related to the specific volume pressure curve of the patient. The lung compliance is optimal for a lung volume identical to FRC. During AV, the alteration of the tensio-active properties of the alveolar layer of surfactant decrease lung compliance [99].

AV and hemodynamics

The lung capillaries are directly exposed to alveolar pressure. During positive pressure ventilation, the increase in alveolar pressure raises the resistance to blood flow into the capillaries: the elevation of pulmonary resistances and intra-pleural pressure increase the right atrial pressure which is in turn responsible for a drop in systemic venous return and cardiac output [1, 28, 47, 65, 70]. The fall in cardiac output is particularly evident when the adaptation mechanism (vasoconstriction) is jeopardized as during sepsis or following the administration of sedative drugs. The reduction in cardiac output is greater in hypovolemic and hypotensive patients [47, 58]. These hemodynamic disturbances differ according to the AV technic used. Also the addition of PEEP significantly increases the risk of hemodynamic adverse effects related to positive pressure ventilation (PPV) [25]. Continuous positive airway pressure or CPAP is less dangerous, because spontaneous breaths enhance the systemic venous return. Only the perithoracic negative pressure techniques are beneficial to cardiac output [26]. To avoid the hemodynamic adverse effects of AV the mean airway pressure should be decreased. Depending on blood gas changes, the pressure and/or the inspiratory duration should be reduced first [15, 17, 18]. IMV which allows spontaneous breaths minimizes the hemodynamic effects of AV [63].

ASSISTED VENTILATION TECHNIQUES

Continuous distending airway pressure

Introduced by Gregory in 1970 this technique decreases alveolar collapse by the application of a stable positive pressure into the airways [46]. This technique appears to be very efficient in HMD where the lack of surfactant is responsible for the alveolar collapse [4, 20]. Since its introduction, the technique, has been applied by different means to ellicit continuous lung distension [37, 42, 77, 91]. The elevation of the transpulmonary pressure provides the restoration of FRC [59].

Two methods are proposed: the delivery of a positive pressure into the airways or CPAP [46] or of a negative pressure around the body with the exception of the airway or CNP [88]. Properly applied, 50 to 60 % of CPAP is transmitted to the pleural space and œsophagus. Therefore it is possible experimentally to determine the optimal CPAP by œsophageal pressure measurement [14]. CPAP performed with a head box induces venous compression and is contraindicated because of the risk of intraventricular hemorrhage and hydrocephalus [97]. The face chamber or mask, responsible for cerebellar haemorrhages has also been abandoned [2, 78]. At present CPAP is performed either with an endotracheal tube or a nasal prong [61]. The latter device is less efficient in low birth weight babies ($<$ 1,000 g) than in larger ones. Despite an increase in airflow resistance and work of breathing the nasal prongs avoid the trauma of tracheal intubation [45]. However pressure drops secondary to the mouth opening are frequent. CPAP can also be applied directly into the pharynx. The use of an endotracheal tube however makes it possible to switch immediately from CPAP to IPPV. Conti-

nuous negative pressure, particularly efficient in babies with birth weight above 1,200 g is much less used; access to the baby is more difficult requiring CNP discontinuation and the risk of hypothermia [42, 69, 77].

HMD is the main indication for CPAP. The earlier CPAP is applied the better is the prognosis [24, 42, 91]. The reduction of the alveolar collapse saves surfactant during respiratory movements [99]. CPAP does not always increase alveolar ventilation, the latter may even be moderately reduced through a drop in V_T because of the distension of uncollapsed alveoli [90]. Also the effect of CPAP on $PaCO_2$ is generally moderate. In HMD with early use of CPAP, FIO_2 can be reduced more quickly which decreases the risk of retinopathy and bronchopulmonary dysplasia associated with hyperoxia [36]. However CPAP enhances the risk of intra-thoracic air block syndromes [9]. CPAP is also indicated for recurrent apnea of prematurity. By keeping an appropriate intra-thoracic volume CPAP stabilizes PaO_2 and improves the oxygenation of the respiratory centers highly sensitive to hypoxia in the premature [62]. CPAP also avoids progressive atelectasis of some alveolar areas secondary to the closure of distal airways. This phenomenon is common in the premature because the so called closing volume is very close to FRC. CPAP also stabilizes the ribcage and the subsequent disappearance of respiratory asynchronism between thoracic and abdominal movements reduces the risk of apnea [48, 62].

Intermittent positive pressure ventilation

Endotracheal intubation. — The insertion of an endotracheal tube is required for IPPV. This procedure needs a laryngoscope with a proper light source, Magill forceps, an O_2 source and an appropriate device for mask ventilation. The uncuffed tracheal tubes avoid the development of tracheal injuries which are induced by local compression of the mucosa. Prior to intubation, the size of the tube is selected according to the infant's weight and the length to be inserted is determined according to gestational age and weight (Fig. III-141). Mask ventilation for 2 to 3 minutes before the procedure reduces the hypoxic risk.

Following the aspiration of oropharyngeal nasal secretions and gastric content, the tracheal tube is introduced usually through the nasal route into the pharynx and then into the trachea under visual control [92]. The tube is then carefully fixed after the presence of symetrical ventilation has been

Distance (cm)

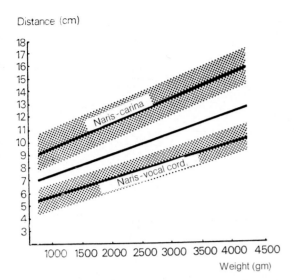

FIG. III-141. — *Changes in the narine-carina and narine-vocal cords distance according to weight.* Evaluation of the length of tracheal tube (COLDIRON et al., *Pediatrics, 41*, 823, 1968).

verified. The nasal route provides safer fixation which reduces the risk of unexpected extubation. The position of the tube's tip is then controlled by X-ray; it should be located at the level of the mid trachea approximating D_3. In it's maximal position, it should remain above the carina while being fixed [23, 60]. The extranasal portion of the tube is then regularly measured.

Despite the fixation of the tube, its tip position will be altered with flexion or extension movements of the neck. These movements carry the risk of selective intubation of the right main stem bronchus [30, 91, 93].

To avoid this complication, the infant's head should be placed in an intermediate position. The tube can be obstructed either by flexion or the accumulation of thick secretions or even blood. For these reasons, proper humidification of the gases and repeated endotracheal aspiration according to the amount of secretions are indicated. This amount is low early in the course of HMD and increases after the first 48 hours. Too frequent and unjustified aspirations lead to main stem bronchus injuries which may sometimes be responsible for haemorrhage or pneumothorax. The normal heating and humidification of gas which occurs in the nasal cavities and oropharynx is absent following intubation. In the trachea the inspired gas temperature is about 33° C and the relative humidity near 100 % [31, 51]. During AV, even with the use of a heating device for humidification, it is difficult to reach these

values. Depending on the length of the circuit and the low specific heat value of the gas, cooling and water condensation decrease humidity below 80 % at a temperature of 37° C (less than 40 mg of vapor water per liter of gas). The subsequent increase in the viscosity of the secretions reduces the ciliary activity. This justifies repeated instillations of saline water in the trachea every 2 or 3 hours. Physiotherapy is particularly helpful because the endotracheal tube makes cough inefficient [39, 40]. The procedures (manual or mechanical vibrations, thoracic pressures and provoked cough) should be preceeded by an instillation of 0.5 ml saline water which liquifies the secretions. Aspiration should be done under sterile conditions. The catheter is gently introduced as far as possible. To avoid any vacuum effect on the bronchial mucosa, the aspiration is begun only during the slow and progressive removal of the catheter out from the tube. A negative pressure of — 150 to 300 mm Hg for aspiration is usually appropriate. The higher the FIO_2, the higher is the risk of hypoxia during aspiration as shown by continuous recordings of transcutaneous PO_2 (Fig. III-142) [40]. The drop in $tcPO_2$ can be compensated for after aspiration by several gentle lung inflations which can be appropriate to ventilate atelectatic areas [31]. A moderate and transient increase in FIO_2 under control of transcutaneous PO_2 may also be indicated.

Indications for IPPV. — IPPV is indicated when spontaneous breathing is not sufficient or is absent as in the case of respiratory control disorders [35]. IPPV re-establishes alveolar ventilation, removes the CO_2 and brings O_2 into the alveolar spaces. Except for respiratory control disorders observed in patients with neurological disorders in whom the indication for IPPV is obvious, IPPV is always necessary when $PaCO_2$ is above 70 mm Hg. When $PaCO_2$ is between 40 and 70 mm Hg, the indication for IPPV depends on other biological parameters (pH, PaO_2) and on the clinical course.

A PaO_2 below 50 mm Hg at an FIO_2 of 1 also justifies IPPV. The final aim of IPPV is to keep $PaCO_2$ between 35 and 45 mm Hg and the PaO_2 between 50 and 70 mm Hg. These PaO_2 values are high enough in the newborn to obtain a normal oxygen saturation of arterial blood because the P_{50} (17 mm Hg) is lower than in adults (23 mm Hg).

The respirators used. — The respirators used in the newborn are generally separated into 2 groups, the volume delivered to the patient depending either on the pressure or on the volume delivered by the respirator. This distinction between volume and

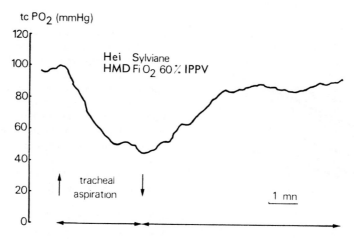

FIG. III-142. — *Effect of tracheal aspiration on transcutaneous oxygen partial pressure.*

pressure generators is complemented by considering the other characteristics of the respirators for flow and cycling methods which regulate the duration of insufflation.

The pressure generators such as the Bourns BP 200 provide a continuous flow. The inspiratory duration is limited. These respirators are considered mainly as flow generators. The insufflation is induced by closure of the expiratory circuit. The closure device is then removed at the end of the inspiratory duration. For this respirator, the tidal volume depends on the duration of insufflation during which positive pressure is applied and on the mechanical properties of the entire system (patient and circuit) where the pressure is delivered. When the respirator rate is high, the flow should be high enough to reach the required peak pressure rapidly to provide efficient ventilation. This is also the case when insufflation is very short. Cycling may also be pressure dependant. Insufflation is stopped as soon as the pressure reaches the present level. The closure of the inspiratory circuit of the respirator is obtained by a valve device depending on the pressure values.

The volume generators, whatever their peculiarities deliver a preset volume during every cycle. However the tidal volume actually insufflated into the patient's lungs is lower. These respirators which theoretically provide an unlimited pressure when they are acting strictly as volume generators are usually equiped with a special valve device limiting the insufflation pressure. The use of an uncuffed tube is also responsible for air leaks which are inversely related to lung compliance. The tidal volume is also related to the compressed gas volume which depends on the length and diameter of the circuit and on the internal compliance of the respirator. The

latter, for most of the respirators used is between 0.28 and 0.5 ml/cm H_2O.

Practically, whatever the respirator used, it should be possible to accurately adapt the FIO_2 between 0.21 and 1, to have various I/E ratios, a square pressure wave and be equiped with a security device limiting inspiratory pressure. A low inertia manometer is highly recommanded to measure the pressure changes in the circuit near the entrance of the tracheal tube. Control of the mean airway pressure is also recommended during AV. Alarms for pressures and temperatures are required as is a humidification device which is working properly. All the respirators used for the newborn should be able to provide PEEP. Aid to expiration is less useful except with high frequencies where it may reduce the PEEP to the required level.

Methods. — Artificial ventilation may be assisted or controlled. When assisted, the patient determines the rate of inflations. This method rapidly appeared inappropriate for the newborn. Not sensitive enough, the trigger system may induce hypoventilation. Too sensitive, the system is responsible for hyperventilation because of the high respiratory rate of patients with respiratory distress. In contrast, when ventilation is controlled, the respiratory rate is imposed by the respirator without any relationship to the spontaneous breaths of the patient. This is the method used for the newborn in various ways.

Intermittent mandatory ventilation (IMV), introduced by Kirby and De Lemos in 1972 [32, 63] is efficient in the newborn. IPPV and CPAP are associated and the patient, thanks to the low rate (5.15 cpm), is able to breathe spontaneously in the circuit while being submitted to CPAP. This method

TABLE I. — EFFECT OF WAVE FORMS USED DURING ASSISTED VENTILATION

Square wave		Sine wave	
Advantages	*Side effects*	*Advantages*	*Side effects*
— Higher mean airway pressure	— Increases risk for air-blocks	— More progressive use of airways pressure	— Lower mean airway pressure
— Improvement of distribution of ventilation	— Adverse effect on venous return	— Reduction of barotrauma	
— Reduces atelectasis			

enhances both oxygenation and CO_2 elimination. The hemodynamic effect of IPPV is also reduced because during spontaneous breaths the intra-pleural pressure provides for a favorable effect on venous return. IMV is indicated as soon as the evolution of RD is not controlled with CPAP or in the case of recurrent apnea in the premature. The method has significantly reduced mortality in the respiratory distress syndrome of the low birth weight newborn. Initially a rate of 5 to 15 c/min, an inspiratory duration of 1 sec, a peak inspiratory pressure of 20 to 25 cm H_2O and a PEEP of 4 cm H_2O are employed. The rate is then progressively increased if $PaCO_2$ remains high or rises further.

The efficacy of IPPV also depends on the pressure wave (table I) when AV was introduced, because of the high respiratory rate of the sick neonate, rapid insufflations at high frequencies associated with low I/E ratios were first proposed.

In the early seventies, Reynolds et al. proposed using lower peak pressures, lower rates and a prolonged inspiratory time [50, 80, 81]. These changes, decreased the barotrauma without any drop in oxygenation. The creation of a prolonged plateau of pressure during insufflation enhances the penetration of gas in the pulmonary areas with high resistance which provides lung aeration. With higher flow delivered by the respirator, the pressure plateau is reached earlier. The elevation of I/E ratio also increases PaO_2 and acts synergistically with PEEP on oxygenation (Fig. III-143). The square wave has significantly modified the prognosis of respiratory distress and has specifically reduced the risk of bronchopulmonary dysplasia [81].

High frequency ventilation initially proposed by Reynolds has recently been re-introduced by Bland and co-workers [12]. Mimicking the rapid respiratory pattern of the sick newborn this method associates low tidal volume, low peak pressures and

frequencies between 70 and 80 cycle/min. It has several advantages but also has disadvantages (table II). Several studies have demonstrated an evident improvement in the result [12, 18], particularly in the incidence of air block syndromes. Bland in a group of 23 cases of HMD observed a survival rate of 91 %. This method considered as being less responsible for barotrauma appears particularly indicated in cases of interstitial emphysema with a high risk for pneumothorax.

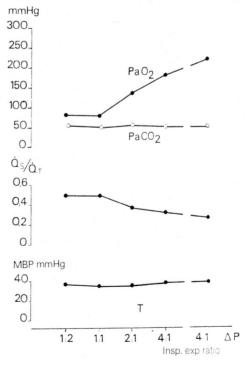

FIG. III-143. — *Effect of an increase in I/E ratio on blood gases, right to left shunt and mean systemic pressure* (from REYNOLDS E. O. R. [78]).

TABLE II. — EFFECTS OF THE FREQUENCY USED DURING ASSISTED VENTILATION
(BPD: bronchopulmonary dysplasia)

| Low frequency (< 40 cpm) | | High frequency (> 60 cpm) | |
Advantages	Side effects	Advantages	Side effects
— Useful for weaning — Used with square wave — May ↑ oxygenation	— May required a higher inspiratory pressure — The rise in inspiratory pressure increases the risk for barotrauma and BPD	— Allows the reduction of inspiratory pressure — Prevents atelectasis — ↓ barotrauma — Useful in case of persistant fetal circulation	— CO_2 retention — May produce iatrogenic respiratory alkalosis

Settings and surveillance of AV. — The initial setting of the respirator depends on the type of respiratory distress and on the infant concerned, *i. e.* premature or term baby. In the preterm, the most frequent cause of respiratory distress is HMD. In this case, except when AV is immediately indicated with IMV, the initial settings generally proposed are as follows. For most authors, the frequency is adjusted between 20 and 40 cpm, the inflation pressure between 20 and 25 cm H_2O, the PEEP between 2 and 4 cm H_2O and the I/E ratio at 1. The measurement of blood gases should be done within 15 or 20 minutes after the onset of AV and the settings modified according to the results. Eventually, PaO_2 and $PaCO_2$ may be continuously controlled with transcutaneous electrodes which provide for faster adaptation of FIO_2 and AV. Settings are mainly based on $PaCO_2$ which should be kept between 35 and 45 mm Hg. The changes in $PaCO_2$ are induced mainly by changes in respiratory rate. The peak pressure also modifies the minute ventilation and thus the I/E ratio which also modulates the airway pressure. The pH is usually corrected spontaneously if acidosis is related only to hypercapnia. When respiratory acidosis persists over 24 hours, it may be balanced by bicarbonate retention through the kidneys. A too rapid correction at the onset of AV runs the risk of metabolic alkalosis. Often, the acidosis observed during the course of respiratory distress is mixed because of an associated hypoxemia. When it is still possible the PaO_2 may be increased by elevation of FIO_2 or if FIO_2 is 1 and $PaCO_2$ normalized, increase in mean airway pressure induced by an elevation of inspiratory time, peak pressure or PEEP (Fig. III-144). The latter should never be above 6 cm H_2O. At any time, the mean airway pressure can be calculated according to the following formula:

$$MAP = \frac{f(ti)\,(\text{peak pressure}) + PEEP\,(60 - f(ti))}{60}$$

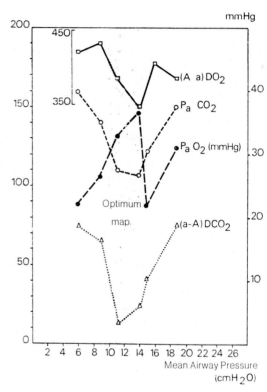

FIG. III-144. — *Relationship between mean airway pressure and oxygen and carbon-dioxide arterial partial pressure (PaO_2-$PaCO_2$) and the alveolo-arterial gradient for CO_2 (a-$ADCO_2$) (from* BOROS *et al. [13]).*

where f is the respiratory rate, ti the inspiratory duration and *PEEP* the end expiratory pressure.

The initial settings are different when AV is a consequence of a respiratory command disorder: *i. e.* in the case of apnea in prematures or in term babies with neurological problems. In this situation, the lungs are normal and the mechanical, properties of the ventilatory system are not modified the lung compliance is normal. Because of a high risk of respiratory alkalosis, the initial rate and peak pressure are lower (15 to 20 cpm, 15-20 cm H_2O). In term infants with respiratory distress related to meconium aspiration with a high risk of pneumothorax, lower pressures are recommended, and high frequency ventilation (70-80 cpm) seems appropriate [18]. In practice, during AV, several situations may occur in which the following approaches may be proposed.

— *Abrupt drop in PaO_2 with rise in $PaCO_2$:* This is related to the respirator itself or to the clinical course. By auscultation a misplacement or an obstruction of the tracheal tube should be excluded. The FIO_2 should be checked as should the integrity of the entire circuit. In this situation, blood gas values are normalized as soon as the ventilation is appropriate. If not, a pneumothorax or massive atelectasis should be considered.

— *Progressive drop in PaO_2 with clinical deterioration:* The fall in PaO_2 is related to an aggravation of the intrapulmonary shunt. Usually a worsening of the haemodynamic state is associated with a fall in systemic arterial pressure, the respirator settings are inappropriate. In these situations, when possible, FIO_2 or MAP should be increased. Blood gas measurements should be frequent enough to check the efficacy of the changes in ventilatory settings.

— *Rise in PaO_2:* This is related to a reduction in the intra-pulmonary shunt. The rise may be very rapid as shown by continuous recordings of $tcPO_2$. The drop in PaO_2 is obtained by decreasing FIO_2 then by a reduction of MAP. A careful attitude during this period of improvement will contribute to a reduction in the length of the intubation period.

— *Isolated changes in $PaCO_2$:* In case of hypercapnea, the alveolar ventilation can be increased through an increase in respiratory rate and/or in peak pressure which increases the tidal volume. The drop in $PaCO_2$ comes from hyperventilation and alkalosis is a potential danger through a reduction in cerebral blood flow and enhancement of hemoglobin affinity for oxygen. The persistance of hypocapnea despite the drop in ventilation sometimes justifies the addition of a dead space between the circuit and the tracheal tube. It is sometimes difficult to adapt the respirator rate completely to the patient's rate. Despite IMV, an asynchronism between the patient and the respirator may jeopardize gas exchange. In this situation, trials to stop spontaneous breathing are not realistic as long as hypercapnea or hypoxemia persist. Correct synchronisation between the patient and the respirator can be achieved by changes in respiratory settings. The increase in rate and peak pressure often provides a positive effect. The induction of moderate hypocapnea decreases the activity of the patient's respiratory centers and contributes to the disappearance of the asynchronism. The latter may also be eliminated with neuromuscular sedative drugs [86]. This treatment should therefore not be routinely recommended. Through their cardiovascular effects, these drugs are however sometimes responsible for haemodynamic disorders with a risk of intraventricular haemorrage [6]. The curare derivatives (e. g. pancuronium bromide) —have nevertheless been proposed to obtain—, when necessary, hyperventilation such as in the case of persistant fetal circulation [33]. When asynchronism is present, these drugs should be used only when the other reasons for blood gas disturbances (pneumothorax, tracheal tube displacement, or occlusion) are ruled out. They should be avoided if the ventilatory asynchronism is not responsible for any significant biological deterioration.

Weaning. — This should be tried as early as possible because of the risks directly related to the duration of AV. It is a progressive procedure largely simplified with IMV. Weaning should be considered as soon as the biological and clinical status are stabilized and regular spontaneous breathing movements return.

It is difficult to strictly apply any weaning rules. Often, during the recovery period in respiratory distress, hyperoxemia imposes a rapid reduction of FIO_2 [22, 36]. The PaO_2 is also reduced through a reduction of the mean airway pressure; this drop also decreases the risk of air block syndrome. The latter frequently occurs as the lung compliance improves. Following the reduction of the respiratory rate the onset of IMV requires a limitation in inspiratory duration. Definitive weaning can be carried out as soon as the rate is low enough (3 to 5 cpm). In some cases, it may be useful to keep a very low frequency AV for a prolonged period. This may avoid the occurence of a progressive atelectasis [99] which justifies an occasional deep insufflation to restore lung volume which cannot be done by the infant himself.

During the period with very low frequency ventilation or CPAP prior to extubation the quality of spontaneous breathing should be noted. The CPAP applied prior to the extubation should never be lower than 2 cm H_2O because of the tracheal tube resistances [10, 41, 49]. The functional evaluation of ventilation prior to weaning could theoretically, as shown by some studies [5], be a method to anticipate the outcome of weaning. When the ventilatory command is appropriate, it is reasonable to consider the weaning from AV before complete discontinuation of oxygen. Prior to the extubation, the stomach should be aspirated, and the bronchi and the upper airways cleaned. The tracheal tube is then progressively pulled out. The secretions accumulated at its tip are also removed by aspiration through a catheter inserted into the tracheal tube. The tip of the tube is then cut and cultured. The secretions accumulated in the nasal cavities are then cleaned with a soft catheter, which decrease the risk of obstructive apnea induced by high nasal resistance in the newborn unable to breath by mouth.

The risk of apnea and hypoventilation following extubation can be reduced by giving a single dose of 4 mg/kg of theophylline prior to extubation [5, 27]. Apnea may also be prevented by oscillating beds [37, 94] or nasal CPAP. When fatigue signs [75] such as polypnea, tachycardia or hypercapnia are present, the infant should be re-intubated after blood gas determination. After extubation, the work of breathing increases secondary to the elevation of airway resistances related to secretions; oxygen supplementation may be indicated. Atelectasis of the right upper lobe is particularly frequent and justifies physiotherapy after any extubation [38].

Intermittent negative pressure ventilation (INPV)

During intermittent negative pressure ventilation, the pressure changes during the respiratory cycle are close to those observed during spontaneous breathing [1, 72]. Introduced when neonatal resuscitation started it has been used with success by a number of teams [69, 77, 88]. This technique does not need any tracheal tube and subsequently is less liable to pneumothorax or other intrathoracic air block syndrome and to BPD [73]. The hypothesis of a better haemodynamic tolerance is not established because it is a pericorporeal negative pressure and not a strictly perithoracic one. The technique significantly reduces the saggital sinus venous pressure which could be beneficial in infants at neurological risk [98]. In a comparative study between IPPV and INPV the frequency of intraventricular haemorrage at autopsy was not however significantly different between the 2 groups [73].

Despite obvious success INPV is now little used as is CNP. This process has been accelerated by the improvement of IPPV techniques.

HIGH FREQUENCY OSCILLATIONS (HFO)

This is not really an AV technique. The pulmonary gases are submitted to high frequency oscillations (8-20 Hz or 480-1,200 cpm) which equilibrates the partial pressure in the entire system: respirator, circuit and patient's airways. This method introduced by Bryan [21] has provided encouraging results in small groups of patients [70].

This technique provides a more rapid reduction of FiO_2 and may reduce barotrauma. It seems to be particularly useful for the treatment or prevention of pulmonary interstitial emphysema ([101].

The technique of high frequency jet ventilation (HFJV) has been more recently proposed. It was previously used in adults with bronchopleural fistulas and other intractable pulmonary air leaks. Very small tidal volumes are delivered directly into the trachea using a special device or jet injector system, connected in parallel to a conventional infant ventilator and patient circuit providing end expiratory pressure and fresh air for spontaneous breaths. This technique has theorical advantages compared with current methods of conventional ventilation. HFJV systems have tiny compression volumes and minimal internal compliance. It is said to provide adequate ventilation using minimal proximal airway pressure [102], and seems useful in the case of pulmonary air leaks. But it may induce inflammatory injuries in the proximal trachea [103]. Since the number of patients treated is very low and only for short periods of time more investigations are needed to define the relative risks and benefits of these new techniques of treatment.

COMPLICATIONS OF ASSISTED VENTILATION

The intrathoracic air block syndromes [74] and bronchopulmonary dysplasia are considered elsewhere.

Sepsis

The tracheal tube is mobilized with head movements [27, 30] which enhance mucosal irritation with the occurrence of inflammatory injury. The tracheal suctioning adds to the trauma by a direct effect at the level of the main stem bronchus [95, 96]. These procedures induce the development of colonization in the airways, always present after 2 or 3 days following the intubation procedure [31]. Because of the risk of resistant bacterial selection, antibiotics should be given only if infection is present and obvious.

Ventilatory disorders

Localized hypoventilation may be induced either by poor positioning of the tracheal tube which can be located within the right main stem bronchus and be responsible for an overdistension of the inferior lobe with atelectasis of the upper right lobe and left lung. The tracheal tube or a lobar or main stem bronchus can also be occluded by a mucuous plug secondary to an accumulation of secretions. Atelectasis does not disappear immediately after the removal of the plug but only after several hours. Atelectasis, after extubation occurs frequently at the level of the right upper lobe [33] the secretions not being eliminated (drained) properly. Appropriate physiotherapy will reduce the frequency of these events.

Injuries to airways

The incidence of ulcerations, nasal, laryngeal or tracheal stenosis or tracheal dyskinesia is well known. It depends on the duration of tracheal intubation, the number and quality of tracheal tubes insertions and the route used [95].

Ulcerations occur when tracheal intubation is prolonged for at least 8 to 10 days. They are secondary to the ischemia of the mucosa induced by the direct pressure of the tube on the larynx, trachea or nasal wall. The tube movements facilitate the development of these ulcerations. They are located mainly on the endolaryngeal surface of the epiglottis, glottis, laryngeal surface of the arytenoid cartilages, postero-lateral wedges of the cricoid cartilage and trachea in contact with the cartilage rings. Posteriorly, these ulcerations occur at the level of the tip of the tube. There are aggravated by over-extension of the neck which raises the anterior pressure of the tube in the subglottic area. Tracheal ulceration is on rare occasion responsible for an œsophago-tracheal fistula [3]. The lesser lesions usually heal following extubation and a period of hypersecretion of the mucosa.

In the nasal cavities, a more or less important ulceration of the wall may sometimes be the origin of a stenosis [54]. In some cases, a deviation of the septum persists as a sequalae. Prolonged pressure of the tube on the nares may induce some degree of necrosis.

Less frequently, subglottic tracheal stenosis occurs during the healing process. This lesion is relatively stable. It appears clinically when laryngeal dyspnea occurs induced by inflammatory œdema or thickening of secretions. In case of stenosis a tracheal recalibration may need to be done.

The use of an orotracheal tube may be responsible for palate deformities [11, 34, 83].

Rare acute traumatic injuries

Pseudodiverticula of the pharynx and œsophagus located in the pre-vertebral space may be produced by the perforation of the posterior wall of the pharynx by the tracheal tube which produces the neo-cavity in the retropharyngeal area of the posterior part of the mediastinum. Tracheal or pharyngeal perforations are very rare. When present, they are usually produced by a traumatic intubation. These lesions are responsible for severe cardiorespiratory distress with cervical sub-cutaneous emphysema, pneumothorax and pneumomediastinum [52, 53, 84, 85]. The prognosis is relatively poor.

Fluid and electrolyte disorders

AV can induce a drop in urine output and œdema particularly when prolonged. The shift of fluid from the intravascular compartment is induced by the rise in intravascular pressures and the changes in the pressure gradient which according to Starlings law regulates the plasma fluid transfer in the capillary bed. The reduction of the circulating blood volume is a consequence of the adaptative mechanism: arterial vasoconstriction, increase in heart rate and reduction in urine output because of a secretion of antidiuretic hormone [8, 79]. The use of nebulizers can also sometimes induce fluid overload [31].

Long term sequelae

Other than in the case of broncho-pulmonary dysplasia, the infants treated with AV for respiratory distress may only show persistant minor disturbances [29, 55, 64]. They are more sensitive to infections. It is possible to show functional abnormalities in lung compliance and PaO_2 [13, 19].

CONCLUSION

AV is a complex therapeutic technique whose recent development in the newborn has led to a significant improvement in mortality and morbidity rate. These techniques can be dangerous if not properly used. Well trained teams with adequate logistic support are required. Only a major "investment" in material and personel can guarantee maximum benefit. This choice is a question of hospital policies and limits AV to larger neonatal care centers only. We must also remember that with the same devices a baby can be saved by a well trained team and lost by an ill trained one.

REFERENCES

[1] ANDERSEN (M. N.), KUCHIBA (K.). — Depression of the cardiac output with mechanical ventilation. Comparative studies of intermittent positive, positive-negative and assisted ventilation. *J. Thorac.-cardiovasc. Surg.*, 54, 182-190, 1967.

[2] AHLSTROM (H.), JONSON (B.), SVENNINGSEN (N. W.). — Continuous positive airways pressure treatment by a face mask chamber in idiopathic respiratory distress syndrome. *Arch. Dis. Child.*, 51, 13-21, 1976.

[3] APLIN (C. E.), SMITH (M.), HARRISON (R.). — Acquired tracheoœsophagial fistula in a premature infant. *J. Pediatr.*, 91, 993-994, 1977.

[4] AVERY (M. E.), FLETCHER (B. D.). — *The lungs and its disorders in the newborn infant.* Philadelphia, W. B. Saunders Co., 1974.

[5] BEN MILED (S.), MONIN (P.), SCHWEITZER (F.), VERT (P.). — Evaluation of Theophylline (T) as an adjunct agent in weaning preterm infants from ventilation. *Pediat. Res.*, 17, 4, abstract 1441, 327 A, 1983.

[6] BANCALARI (E.), GERHARDT (T.), FELLER (R.), GANNON (J.), MELNICK (G.), ABDENOUR (G.). — Muscle relaxation during IPPV in prematures with RDS. *Pediat. Res.*, 14, 590 (abst.), 1980.

[7] BARR (P. A.). — Weaning very low birth weight infants from mechanical ventilation using intermittent mandatory ventilation and theophylline. *Arch. Dis. Child.*, 53, 598-600, 1978.

[8] BARRATZ (R. A. D.), PHYLBIN (M.), PATTERSON (R. W.). — Plasma antidiuretic hormone and urinary output during continuous positive pressure breathing in dogs. *Anesthesiology*, 34, 510, 1971.

[9] BERG (T. J.), PAGTAKHAN (R. D.), REED (M. H.). — Bronchopulmonary dysplasia and lung rupture in hyaline membrane disease: Influence of continuous distending pressure. *Pediatrics*, 55, 51-54, 1976.

[10] BERMAN (L. S.), FOX (W. W.), RAPHAELY (R. C. R.), DOWNES (J. J.). — Optimum levels of CPAP for tracheal extubation in newborn infants. *J. Pediatr.*, 89, 109-112, 1976.

[11] BISKINIS (E.), HERZ (M.). — Acquired palatal groove after prolonged orotracheal intubation. *J. Pediat.*, 92, 512-513, 1978.

[12] BLAND (R.), KIM (M.), WOODSON (J. L.). — High frequency mechanical ventilation of low birth weight infants with respiratory failure from hyaline membrane disease. *Pediat. Res.*, 11, 531, 1977.

[13] BRYAN (M. H.), HARDIE (M. J.), REILLY (B. J.). — Pulmonary function studies during the first year of life in infant recovering from the respiratory distress syndrome. *Pediatrics*, 52, 169-178, 1973.

[14] BONTA (B. W.), UAUY (R.), WARSHAW (J. B.). — Determination of optimal continuous positive airway pressure for the treatment of idiopathic respiratory distress syndrome by measurement of œsophageal pressure. *J. Pediatr.*, 91, 449-454, 1977.

[15] BOROS (S. J.), MATALON (S. V.), EWALD (R.). — The effects of independent variations in inspiratory-expiratory ratio and end expiratory pressure during mechanical ventilation in hyaline membrane disease. The significance of mean airway pressure. *J. Pediatr.*, 91, 794-798, 1977.

[16] BOROS (S. J.), ORGILL (A. A.). — Mortality and morbidity associated with pressure and volume limited infant ventilators. *Am. J. Dis. Child.*, 132, 865-869, 1978.

[17] BOROS (S. J.). — Variations in inspiratory-expiratory ratio and airway pressure wave during mechanical ventilation. The significance of mean airway pressure. *J. Pediatr.*, 94, 114-117, 1979.

[18] BOROS (S. J.), CAMPBELL (K. A.). — A comparaison of the effects of high frequency-low tidal volume and low-frequency-high tidal volume mechanical ventilation. *J. Pediatr.*, 97, 108-112, 1980.

[19] BORKENSTEIN (J.), BORKENSTEIN (M.), ROSEGGER (H.). — Pulmonary function in long term survivors with artifical ventilation in the neonatal period. *Acta Paediatr. Scand.*, 69, 159-163, 1980.

[20] BOYLE (R. J.), OH (W.). — Respiratory distress syndrome. *Clinics in perinatology*, 5, 283-297, 1978.

[21] BOHN (D. J.), MIYASAKA (K.), MARCHAK (B. E.), THOMPSON (W. K.), FROESE (A. B.), BRYAN (A. C.). — Ventilation by high frequency oscillation. *J. Appl. Physiol.*, 48, 710-715, 1980.

[22] CLARK (J. M.), LAMBERTSEN (C. J.). — Pulmonary oxygen toxicity. *Pharmacol. Rev.*, 23, 37, 1971.

[23] COLDIRON (J.). — Estimation of nasotracheal tube length in neonates. *Pediatrics*, 41, 823-828, 1968.

[24] CORBET (A.), ANDAMS (J.). — Current therapy in hyaline membrane disease. *Clinics in perinatology*, 5, 299-316, 1978.

[25] COHEN (M. L.). — Clinical evidence for hemodynamic toxicity of PEEP. *Pediatr. Res.*, 7, 426 (abst.), 1973.

[26] COOK (T. I.). — A comparative study of pulmonary and circulatory effects of extra-thoracic assisted breathing and intermittent positive pressure breathing. *Int. Surg.*, 56, 63-67, 1971.

[27] COSTALOS (C.), HOULSKY (W. T.), MANCHETT (P.), LLOYD (D. I.). — Weaning very low birth weight infants from mechanical ventilation using intermittent mandatory ventilation and theophylline. *Arch. Dis. Child.*, 54, 404-405, 1979.

[28] COURNAND (A.), MOTHLEY (H. L.), BERTRAND (M.), KETELERS (J. Y.), DELOMEZ (M.). — Physiological studies of the effects of intermittent positive pression breathing. *Amer. J. Physiol.*, 152, 162-174, 1948.

[29] CRANCE (J. P.), KUHNAST (M.). — Étude des séquelles pulmonaires chez des enfants ayant sur-

vécu à une détresse respiratoire néonatale. In *Problème de Réanimation*, 6e série. T₂ LARCAN (A.), VERT (P.), éd., Spei, Paris, 441-450, 1970.

[30] DONN (S. M.), KUHNS (L. R.). — Mechanisms of endotracheal tube movement with change of head position in the neonate. *Pediatr. Radiol.*, 9, 37-40, 1980.

[31] DOWNES (J. J.), GOLDBERG (A. I.). — Airway management, mechanical ventilation and cardiopulmonary resuscitation. In *Pulmonary disease of the fetus, newborn and child.* SCARPELLI (E. M.), AULD (P. A. M.), GOLDMAN (H. S.), eds, Lea and Febiger, Philadelphia, 1978.

[32] DOWNS (J. B.), PERKINS (A. M.), MODELL (J. H.). — Intermittent mandatory ventilation. *Arch. Surg.*, 109, 519, 1974.

[33] DRUMMOND (W.), GREGORY (G.), HEYMANN (M.), PHIBBS (R.). — The effects of alkalosis on pulmonary artery pressure (PAP), systemic artery pressure (SAP) and PaO₂ in infants with persistant pulmonary hypertension (PPH). *Pediat. Res.*, 13, 493, 1979 (abst.).

[34] DUKE (P. M.), COULSON (J. D.), SANTOS (J. I.). — Cleft Palate associated with prolonged orotracheal intubation in infancy. *J. Pediatr.*, 89, 990-991, 1976.

[35] ENGSTRÖM (C. G.). — Treatment of severes cases of respiratory paralysis by the Engström Universal Respirator. *Br. J. Med.*, 2, 666, 1954.

[36] EHRENKRANZ (R. A.), ALBOW (R. C.), WARSHAW (J. B.). — Oxygen toxicity: The complication of oxygen use in the newborn infant. *Clinics in Perinatology*, 5, 437-450, 1978.

[37] FANAROFF (A. A.), CHA (C.), SOSA (R.) *et al.* — Controlled trial continuous negative external pressure in the treatment of severe respiratory distress syndrome. *J. Pediatr.*, 82, 921-928, 1973.

[38] FINER (N. N.), MORIARTEY (R. R.), BOYD (J.), PHILIPPS (H. J.), STEWART (A. R.), VILAN (O.). — Post extubation atelectasia: A retrospective review and a prospective controlled study. *J. Pediatr.*, 94, 110-113, 1979.

[39] FINER (N. M.), BOYD (J.). — Chest physiotherapy in neonates. *J. Pediatr.*, 92, 977-981, 1978.

[40] FOX (W. W.), SCHARTZ (J. G.), SHAFFER (T. H.). — Pulmonary physiotherapy in neonates. Physiologic changes and respiratory management. *J. Pediatr.*, 92, 977-981, 1978.

[41] FOX (W. W.), BERMAN (L. S.), DINWIDDIE (R.) *et al.* — Tracheal extubation of the neonate at 2-3 centimeters H₂O continuous positive airway pressure. *Pediatrics*, 59, 257-261, 1977.

[42] GERARD (P.), FOX (W. W.), OUTERBRIDGE (E. W.), BEAUDRY (P. H.), STERN (L.). — Early vs late introduction of continuous negative pressure in the management of the idiopathic respiratory distress syndrome. *J. Pediatr.*, 87, 591-595, 1975.

[43] GERHARDT (T.), BANCALARI (E.). — Chest wall compliance in full term and premature infants. *Acta Paediatr. Scand.*, 69, 359-364, 1980.

[44] GEUBELLE (F.), LAGNEAUX (D.). — *Aspects récents et méthodes d'investigation de la fonction respiratoire du nouveau-né.* éd., F. GEUBELLE, B. NELISSEN, Liège, 89, 1977.

[45] GOLDMAN (S. L.), BRADY (J. P.), DUMPIT (F. M.). — Increased work of breathing with nasal prongs. *Pediatrics*, 64, 160-164, 1979.

[46] GREGORY (G. A.), KITTERMAN (J. A.), PHIBBS (R. H.), TOOLEY (W. H.), HAMILTON (W. K.). —

Treatment of the idiopathic respiratory distress syndrome with continuous positive airway pressure. *New Engl. J. Med.*, 284, 1333-1340, 1971.

[47] GUYTON (A. C.), JONES (C. E.), COLEMAN (T. G.). — *Circulatory physiology. Cardiac output and its regulation.* 2nd Ed W. B. Saunders Co., 556 p, 1973.

[48] HAGAN (R.), BRYAN (A. C.), BRYAN (M. H.). — Neonatal chest wall afferents and regulation of respiration. *J. Appl. Physiol.*, 42, 362-366, 1977.

[49] HEGYI (T.), HYATT (M.). — Discontinuation of continuous positive airways pressure in infants with respiratory distress syndrome. *Arch. Dis. Child.*, 55, 722-724, 1980.

[50] HERMAN (S.), REYNOLDS (E. O. R.). — Methods for improving oxygenation in infants ventilated for severe hyaline membrane disease. *Arch. Dis. Child.*, 48, 612-617, 1973.

[51] HIRSH (J. A.), TOKAYER (J. L.), ROBINSON (M. J.), SACKNER (M. A.). — Effect of and subsequent humidification on tracheal mucous velocity in dogs. *J. Appl. Physiol.*, 39 (2), 242, 1975.

[52] JERLIN (S. P.), DAILLY (W. J. R.). — Tracheal perforation in the neonate. A complication of endotracheal intubation. *J. Pediatr.*, 86, 596-597, 1975.

[53] JOSHI (V. V.), MANDAVIA (S. G.), STERN (L.), WIGGLESWORTH (F. W.). — Acute lesions induced by endotracheal intubation. *Amer. J. Dis. Child.*, 124, 646-649, 1972.

[54] JUNG (A. L.), THOMAS (J. K.). — Stricture of the nasal vestibule. A complication of nasotracheal intubation in newborn infants. *J. Pediatr.*, 85, 412-414, 1974.

[55] KAMPER (J.). — Long-term prognosis of infants with severe idiopathic respiratory distress syndrome II. Cardiopulmonary outcome. *Acta Paediatr. Scand.*, 67, 71-76, 1978.

[56] KIRA (S.), HUKUSHIMA (Y.). — Effect of negative pressure inflation on pulmonary vascular flow. *J. Appl. Physiol.*, 25, 42-47, 1968.

[57] KORNER (A. F.), KRAEMER (H. C.), HAFFNER (M. E.), COSPER (L. M.). — Effects of waterbed flotation on premature infants. A pilot study. *Pediatrics*, 56, 361-367, 1975.

[58] KRAUSS (A. N.). — Assisted ventilation: a critical review clinics in perinatology. *Clinics in Perinatology*, 7, 61-74, 1980.

[59] KRAUSS (A. N.), AULD (P. A. M.). — Measurements of functional residual capacity in distress neonates by helium rebreathing. *J. Pediatr.*, 77, 228-232, 1970.

[60] KUHNS (L. R.), POZNANSKI (A. K.). — Endotracheal tube position in the infant. *J. Pediatr.*, 78, 99, 1971.

[61] KATTWINKEL (J.), FLEMING (D.), CHA (C.), FANAROFF (A. A.), KLAUS (M. H.). — A device for administering continuous positive airway pressure by the nasal route. *Pediatrics*, 52, 131-134, 1973.

[62] KATTWINKEL (J.). — Neonatal apnea. Pathogenesis and therapy. *J. Pediatr.*, 90, 342-347, 1977.

[63] KIRBY (R.), ROBINSON (E.), SCHULZ (J.), DE LEMOS (R. A. Jr.). — Continuous ventilation as an alternative to assisted or controlled ventilation in infants. *Anesthesia and analgesia*, 51, 871-875, 1972.

[64] LE LOC'H (H.), LALANDE (J.), DOYON (F.). — Enquête sur le devenir des nouveau-nés traités en unité de soins intensifs pour enfants. II. Séquelles respiratoires. *Arch. Franç. Ped.*, 35, 7-22, 1978.

[65] LENFANT (C.), HOWELL (B. T.). — Cardio-vascular adjustement in dogs during continuous pressure breathing. *J. Appl. Physiol.*, 15, 425-428, 1960.

[66] LINDE (L.), SIMMONS (D. H.), ELLMAN (E. L.). — Pulmonary hemodynamic during positive pressure breathing. *J. Appl. Physiol.*, 16, 644-646, 1961.

[67] LINDROTH (M.), SVINNINGSEN (N. W.), AHLSTROM (H.), JONSON (B.). — Evolution of mechanical ventilation in newborn infants. I. Techniques and Survival rates. *Acta Paediatr. Scand.*, 69, 143-149, 1980.

[68] LINDROTH (M.), SVINNINGSEN (N. W.), AHLSTROM (H.), JONSON (B.). — Evolution of mechanical ventilation in newborn infants. II. Pulmonary and neuro-development sequalae in relation to original diagnosis. *Acta Paediatr. Scand.*, 69, 151-158, 1980.

[69] MARCHAL (C.), VERT (P.), LEVEAU (P.), CRANCE (J. P.). — Traitement des détresses respiratoires néonatales. Utilisation d'un respirateur à dépression périthoracique. *Arch. Fr. Pédiatr.*, 30, 297-317, 1973.

[70] MARCHAK (B. E.), THOMPSON (W. K.), DUFFTY (P.), MIYAKI (T.), BRYAN (M. H.), BRYAN (A. C.), FROESE (A. B.). — Treatment of RDS by high frequency oscillations ventilation: a preliminary report. *J. Pediatr.*, 99, 287-292, 1981.

[71] MALONEY (J. V.), HANDFORD. — Circulatory responses to intermittent positive and alternating positive negative pressure respirators. *J. Appl. Physiol.*, 6, 453-459, 1954.

[72] MONIN (P.). — Étude expérimentale de la respiration en surpression chez le lapin. Comparaison de 2 techniques : pression positive intra-trachéale et dépression extra-corporelle. *Thèse Médecine Nancy*, 98, 1975.

[73] MONIN (P.), CASHORE (W. J.), HAKANSON (D. O.), COWETTE (R. M.), OH (W.). — Assisted ventilation in the neonate. Comparaison between positive and negative respirators. *Pediatr. Res.*, 10, 464, 1976 (abst.).

[74] MONIN (P.), VERT (P.). — Pneumothorax in the newborn, clinics and pathophysiology. *Clinics in Perinatology*, 5, 335-350, 1978.

[75] MULLER (N.), VOLGYSI (G.), BRYAN (M. H.), BRYAN (A. C.). — The consequence of diaphramatic muscle fatigue in the newborn infant. *J. Pediatr.*, 95, 793-797, 1979.

[76] NORTHWAY (W. H.), ROSAN (R. C.), POTER (D. Y.). — Pulmonary disease following respiratory therapy of hyaline membrane disease. Bronchopulmonary dysplasia. *New Engl. J. Med.*, 276, 357-368, 1967.

[77] OUTERBRIDGE (E. W.), ROLOF (D. W.), STERN (L.). — Continuous negative pressure in the management of severe respiratory distress syndrome. *J. Pediatr.*, 81, 384-391, 1972.

[78] PAPE (K. E.), AMSTRONG (D. L.), FITZHARDINGE (P. M.). — Central nervous system pathology associated with mask ventilation in the very low birth weight infant: a new etiology for intracerebellar haemorrhages. *Pediatrics*, 58, 473-483, 1976.

[79] POMAREDE (R.), MORIETTE (G.), CZERNICHOW (P.), RELIER (J. P.). — Étude de la vasopressine plasmatique chez les enfants prématurés soumis à la ventilation artificielle. *Arch. Franç. Péd.*, 35, 75-83, 1978.

[80] REYNOLDS (E. O. R.). — Effects of alterations in mechanical ventilator settings on pulmonary gas exchange in hyaline membrane disease. *Arch. Dis. Child.*, 46, 152-159, 1971.

[81] REYNOLDS (E. O. R.). — Pressure wave form and ventilator settings for mechanical ventilation in severe hyaline membrane disease. *International anesthesiology clinics*, 12, 259-280, 1974.

[82] ROY (R.), POWER (S. R. J.), FREUSTEL (P. J.), DUTTON (R. E.). — Pulmonary wedge catheterization during end expiratory pressure ventilation in the dog. *Anesthesiology*, 46, 385-393, 1977.

[83] SAUNDERS (B. S.), EASA (D.), SLAUGHTER (R. J.). — Acquired palatal groove in neonates. A report of two cases. *J. Pediatr.*, 89, 988-989, 1976.

[84] SCHILD (J. P.), WUILLOUD (A.), KOLLBERG (H.) et al. — Tracheal perforation as a complication of nasotracheal intubation in a neonate. *J. Pediatr.*, 88, 631-632, 1976.

[85] SERLIN (S. P.), DAILY (W. J. R.). — Tracheal perforation in the neonate. A complication of endotracheal intubation. *J. Pediatr.*, 86, 596-597, 1975.

[86] STARK (A. R.), BASCOM (R.), FRANTZ (I.). — Muscle relaxation in mechanically ventilated infants. *J. Pediatr.*, 94, 439-443, 1979.

[87] STAVIS (R. L.), KRAUSS (A. N.). — Complication of neonatal care. *Clinics in Perinatology*, 7, 107-124, 1980.

[88] STERN (L.). — Description and utilisation of the negative pressure apparatus. *Biol. Neonat.*, 16, 24-29, 1970.

[89] SUTER (P. M.), FAIRLEY (H. B.), ISEMBERG (M. D.). — Optimum end expiratory pressure in patient with acute pulmonary failure. *New Engl. J. Med.*, 292, 284-289, 1975.

[90] SPEIDEL (B. D.), DUNN (P. M.). — Effect of continuous positive airway pressure on breathing pattern of infants with respiratory distress syndrome. *Lancet*, 1, 302, 1975.

[91] TANSWELL (A. K.), CLUBB (R. A.), SMITH (B. T.), BOSTON (R. W.). — Individualized continuous distending pressure applied within 6 hours of delivery in infants with respiratory distress syndrome. *Arch. Dis. Child.*, 55, 33-39, 1980.

[92] TOCHEN (M. L.). — Orotracheal intubation in the newborn infant: a method for determining depth of tube insertion. *J. Pediatr.*, 95, 1050-1051, 1979.

[93] TODRES (I. D.), DE BROS (F.), KRAMER (S. S.), MOYLAN (F. M. B.), SCHANNON (D. C.). — Endotracheal tube displacement in the newborn infant. *J. Pediatr.*, 89, 126-127, 1976.

[94] TUCK (S.), MONIN (P.), DUVIVIER (G.), MAY (T.), VERT (P.). — The effect of a rocking bed on apnea of prematurity. *Arch. Dis. Child.*, 57, 475-477, 1982.

[95] TRAN VAN DUC, LE TSAN VINH, HUAULT (G.), THIEFFRY (S.). — Lésions laryngo-trachéales provoquées par l'intubation endotrachéale chez l'enfant. Étude anatomique. *Nouv. Pr. Méd.*, 3, 365-371, 1974.

[96] VAUGHAN (R. S.), MENKE (J. A.), GIACOIA (G. P.). — Pneumothorax. A complication of endotracheal tube suctionning. *J. Pediatr.*, 92, 633-634, 1978.

[97] VERT (P.), ANDRÉ (M.), SIBOUT (M.). — Continuous positive airway pressure and hydrocephalus. *Lancet*, 2, 319, 1973 (lettre).

[98] VERT (P.), MONIN (P.), SIBOUT (M.). — Intracranial venous pressure in newborn: variations in physiologic states and in neurological and respiratory disorders. In *Intensive Care in the newborn*,

STERN (L.) ed., Masson, New York, 185-196, 1976.

[99] WYSZOGRODSKI (I.), KYEI-ABOADGYE (K.), TAEUSCH (H. W.). — Surfactant inactivation by hyperventilation, conservation by end-expiratory pressure. *J. Appl. Physiol.*, *38*, 461, 1975.

[100] YU (V. Y. H.), FOLFE (P.). — Effect of continuous positive airway pressure breathing on cardio-respiratory function in infants with respiratory distress syndrome. *Acta Paediatr. Scand.*, *65*, 59, 1977.

[101] FRANTZ (I. D.), WERTHAMMER (J.), STARK (A. R.). — High frequency ventilation in premature infants with lung disease: adequate gas exchange at low tracheal pressure. *Pediatrics*, 1983, *71* (4), 483-488.

[102] POKORA (R.), BING (D.), MAMMEL (M.), BOROS (S.). — Neonatal high frequency jet ventilation. *Pediatrics*, 1983, *72* (1), 27-32.

[103] BOROS (S.), MAMMEL (M.), COLEMAN (J. M.), LEWALLEN (P. K.), GORDON (M. J.), BING (D. R.), OPHOVEN (J. P.). — Neonatal high frequency jet ventilation. Four years experience. *Pediatrics*, *75* (4), 657-663, 1985.

4

Neonatal infections

28

Neonatal immunity

M. XANTHOU

It is astonishing to think that as little as twenty years ago no precise function could be attributed to the lymphocyte. The lymphocyte remained a mystery, a cell whose morphology gave no clue as to its activities and which to the morbid anatomist appeared only as a "phlegmatic spectator passively watching the turbulent activity of the phagocytes" [12]. During the last 20 years, however, there has been an explosive development in immunology. It is a pity that its peculiar language has made it difficult for non-immunologists to follow the excitement.

During this period much original work has been done on the immunity of the neonate. It is the purpose of this chapter to try and bring to light the maturational deficiencies of the newborn that make him or her so susceptible to infections, hoping that the increased understanding will lead to the development of improved therapy of neonatal septicaemia through enhancement of the newborn's host-defense mechanisms.

General concepts of immunity

As defined by Bellanti [4]: "Immunity includes all those physiologic mechanisms that endow the animal with the capacity to recognize materials as foreign to itself and to neutralize eliminate or metabolize them with or without injury to its own tissues".

The material may interact with the host in a number of ways: (a) it may become localized or completely removed by phagocytes without any further response, (b) it may lead to a specific immune response in which case the material is referred to as an immunogen or antigen and (c) it may induce a state of unresponsiveness, after interaction with the host, in which case it is called a tolerogen. The resulting condition is referred to as immunologic tolerance.

Nonspecific immune responses follow exposure to foreign materials and while able to differentiate "self" from "nonself" they are not dependent upon specific recognition. Nonspecific immune mechanisms are enhanced by the development of specific immune responses which depend upon the exposure to a foreign substance and the subsequent recognition of memory and reaction to it. The specific responses are characterized by the induction and interaction of a variety of cell types specific for the inducing antigen. In general terms immunologic responses serve two major functions: (a) defence against pathogenic microorganisms, (b) preservation of homeostasis, aberrations of which leads to autoimmune or malignant diseases.

NONSPECIFIC IMMUNITY

Foreign substances may enter the body either naturally—i. e. through the respiratory or gastrointestinal tract—or artificially—i. e. through infection.

The best way to avoid infection is to prevent the pathogenic microorganisms from gaining access to the body. The skin, when intact, is impermeable to most infectious agents. Mucous, secreted by the membranes lining the inner surfaces of the body acts as a protective barrier as well. Finally other mechanical factors which help protect the epithelial surfaces and which contain bactericidal components are body fluids like tears, saliva and urine.

When microorganisms do penetrate the body two main defensive mechanisms exist: (a) the engulfment and digestion of microorganisms by cells called "phagocytes", (b) the destructive effect of soluble chemical factors such as bactericidal enzymes called "humoral mediators".

PHAGOCYTES AND THEIR FUNCTION

Phagocytic cells

It was approximately 100 years ago that Elia Metchnikoff published his observation on the bacteria killing capacity of mobile "microphages" and "macrophages". Today we believe that in the human, phagocytosis is carried out primarily by mononuclear phagocytes, neutrophils, and to a lesser extent, eosinophils.

Mononuclear phagocytes. — The mononuclear phagocytes are produced from a stem cell in the bone marrow. Bone-marrow promonocytes undergo proliferation and differentiate into blood monocytes which following a brief time in the blood (1-2 days)

migrate to the main site of their action in the tissues where they further differentiate into macrophages and constitute the so-called "mononuclear phagocyte system" (MPS) [9]. The term MPS has been suggested to replace the less precise term reticuloendothelial system (RES). The macrophages are present throughout the connective tissue and around the basement membrane of small blood vessels and are particularly concentrated in the lung (alveolar macrophages), liver (Kupffer cells), and lining of spleen sinusoids and lymph node medullary sinuses where they filter off foreign material.

Macrophages are long-lived cells and highly specialized to carry out their function in the ingestion and destruction of all foreign substances by the process of endocytosis. Thus, these cells remove and destroy certain bacteria, damaged cells, neoplastic cells and macromolecules. However, whereas the polymorphs provide the major defence against pyogenic bacteria, as a rough generalization it may be said that macrophages are at their best in combating those bacteria, viruses and protozoa which are capable of living within the cells of the host. Furthermore, the macrophages appear to have a more highly developed mechanism for dealing with lipid or waxy foreign materials.

Three volumetrically distinct subsets of human monocytes have been described; these subsets are termed M_1, M_2 and M_3 in order of increasing size. Functional diversity among these subsets is strongly suggested by the finding that the smaller M_1 and M_2 cells are less capable of ingesting carbonyl iron particles than the larger M_3 cells.

The circulating monocytes are attracted to an area of injury by a number of factors. It would appear that the marrow and spleen are the predominant sources of large mononuclear phagocytic cells which are mobilized to extravascular inflammatory sites. Once they get there they become activated, transform to tissue macrophages and assume heightened metabolic activity (activated macrophages) in order to ingest and kill the pathogenic organisms [5].

Polymorphonuclear leukocytes-neutrophils. — Of the three varieties of these cells—neutrophils, eosinophils and basophils—only the neutrophil and to a lesser extent, the eosinophil are primarily phagocytic. Unlike the macrophage the smaller polymorphonuclear neutrophil is a non-dividing short-lived cell with granules containing a wide range of bactericidal factors.

The neutrophils arise in the bone marrow from a common ancestral stem cell and after a series of divisions undergo maturation through a myeloblast $\rightarrow$ promyelocyte $\rightarrow$ metamyelocyte $\rightarrow$ band cell → mature polymorphonuclear phase. Using leukokinetic studies [14] it was found that the mean time required for myelocytes to divide, mature and appear in the blood is 11.4 days. There appears to be a large storage compartment in the bone marrow and increased demand for these cells is met acutely by accelerated release from the intramedullary reserves followed by increased myelopoiesis.

The neutrophils are approximately equally distributed between a circulating and a marginal blood pool. Cells exchange between these two pools with such rapidity that their sum, the total blood pool, can be considered as a kinetic unit. The marginal pool is probably diffusely distributed through the vascular system but the lungs may be a major site. The mean size of the total blood granulocyte pool in normal adults was found to be 70×10^7 cells/kg while the mean granulocyte turnover rate is 163×10^7 granulocytes/kg/day. From these findings it seems that the blood pool turns over 2.5 times per day and the average time which a neutrophil spends in the blood is 10.4 hours. Polymorphonuclear neutrophils are the dominant white cells in the blood stream normally accounting for 60 to 70 % of the total leucocyte count in human adults. Leaving the blood the polymorphonuclears enter the tissues where they complete their life span of a few days. The entire movement of granulocytes from marrow to tissues is uni-directional.

The normal mature granulocyte is therefore a cell which moves from the bone marrow via the blood to extravascular sites where it performes its phagocytic and bactericidal functions.

Eosinophils. — Polymorphonuclear eosinophils have a half life of approximately 30 minutes in the blood and of 12 days in tissues where they fulfill their major function. Major roles attributed to these cells are the ingestion of antigen-antibody complexes and their involvement in limiting inflammatory reactions [5].

Phagocytic-cell function

The phagocytes in order to perform their function must first reach the site of the foreign substance (chemotaxis), they must ingest it (phagocytosis) and finally they must destroy it (microbial killing).

Chemotaxis. — The directed attraction of cells towards chemical substances is known as chemotaxis. A second type of neutrophil movement is "random motility" which is characterized by non-direct movement.

Syndromes of defective chemotaxis include: (1) intrinsic cellular defects, (2) defects due to external inhibitors of locomotion and (3) defects resulting from a lack of chemotactic factors.

The polymorphonuclears respond to three different chemotactic stimuli derived from the complement system as well as from bacterial and lymphocyte derived factors. Chemotactic substances for monocytes and macrophages have also been found. These include products of the complement system as well as lymphocyte-derived factors—*i. e.* macrophage activity factor (MAF).

Phagocytosis and killing. — Before phagocytosis can occur, the microbe must first adhere to the surface of the polymorph or macrophage. The attachment between the microorganism and phagocyte can occur directly through unenhanced processes in which case it is largely dependent upon its surface properties to be phagocytosed. When certain serum proteins, e. g. complement or antibodies (opsonins) are present coating the bacterium, the attachment of the coated bacterium is facilitated by the surface receptors of the phagocytes. Phagocytes possess two types of receptors on their plasma membrane: (1) a receptor for the Fc fragment of an immunoglobulin molecule and (2) a receptor for the C_{3b} component of complement [42].

Ingestion is the next step in phagocytosis. A bacterium attached to the membrane initiates the ingestion phase in which it becomes engulfed by cytoplasmic processes and comes to be within the cell in a vacuole called a "phagosome". The lysosomal granules within the leucocytes then fuse with the vacuole to form a "phagolysosome" in which the ingested microbe is killed by many factors (Fig. IV-1). Both oxygen dependent and oxygen-independent antimicrobial mechanisms exist within phagocytic cells. Along with phagocytosis neutrophils show a burst of metabolic activity leading to increases in oxygen consumption, superoxide and hydrogen peroxide formation, and glucose metabolism through the hexose monophosphate shunt. The combination of peroxide, myeloperoxidase and halide ions constitute a potent halogenating system capable of killing both bacteria and viruses [42]. The oxygen-independent mechanisms consist of a low pH due to lactic acid production, a variety of proteolytic and other hydrolytic enzymes, lysozyme, bacteriostatic substances such as lactoferrin and cationic polypeptides, and myeloperoxidase.

During phagocytosis there is also an extracellular release of lysosomal constituents which may play an amplifying role. Thus the release of an endogenous pyrogen from the polymorphonuclears may

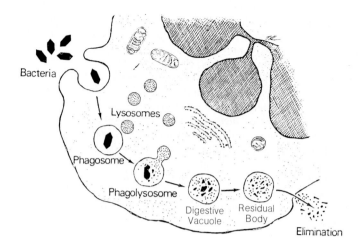

FIG. IV-1. — *Schematic representation of phagocytosis showing ingestion process and intracellular digestion.* (From BELLANTI, J. A.: *Immunology II*, 2nd ed., W. B. Saunders Company, Philadelphia, 1978).

explain the fever which often accompanies an infection.

The mononuclear phagocytes lack significant myeloperoxidase activity. Although little is known of the microbial mechanisms of mononuclear phagocytes at present, they do exhibit the metabolic burst displayed by neutrophils but to a lesser extent.

From all this it is clear that the phagocytic cells possess an impressive anti-microbial potential.

HUMORAL FACTORS

The complement system

Serum complement was discovered in the late 19th century because of its capacity to effect cytolysis, *i. e.* induce membrane damage in bacteria. The complement system consists of eleven serum proteins called "components". When one component is activated it acquires the ability to activate several molecules of the next component in the sequence; each of these is then able to act upon the next component and so on producing a cascade effect with amplification. The most abundant component C_3 is split either by the classical pathway ($C_{1,4,2}$) which is initiated by antibody or by the alternative pathway which is initiated by several non-immune mechanisms such as bacterial polysaccharides.

During complement activation several biologically active products are generated. One split product C_{3a} is chemotactic for polymorphonuclears and increases vascular permeability through histamine release from mast cells and basophils. The other product C_{3b} binds non-specifically to the antigen surface and

increases the attachment to the phagocytes because of C_{3b} receptors on the surface of these cells. Purified C_{3b} has been also shown to trigger extracellular release of lysosomal enzymes from macrophages and it is possible, but not yet established, that this could damage adhering microorganisms. Finally, C_{3b} generates C_{5b} which fires the remainder of the components to C_8 and C_9 thereby leading to cell death through membrane damage. Through these effects complement plays an important role in the defence against infection [24, 42].

Lysozyme

Of the soluble bactericidal factors the most abundant and widespread is the enzyme lysozyme (muramidase), a protein which hydrolyses the mucopeptide wall of susceptible bacteria; mostly gram-negative ones. Apart from its presence in the peripheral blood, lysozyme is present in high concentrations in several body secretions like saliva, tears and human milk.

Interferon

Interferon is an antiviral substance which being synthesized by cells in response to viral infection inhibits intracellular viral replication.

INFLAMMATORY RESPONSE

Following tissue injury, a variety of cellular and systemic events occur in which the host attempts to restore and maintain homeostasis. Mediators of the acute inflammatory response can be separated into vasopermeability factors (*i. e.* vasoactive amines) and leukotactic factors (*i. e.* complement). Thus the acute inflammatory response is characterized by dilatation of blood vessels and the outpouring of leukocytes and fluids. Within 30-60 minutes of injury neutrophilic granulocytes appear. The main function of these cells is to phagocytose and kill potentially dangerous agents, such as bacteria. Within 4-5 hours monocytes and lymphocytes will appear at the inflammatory site. Monocytes augment the defence by offering their own phagocytic function while lymphocytes respond to foreign agents by specific humoral and cell-mediated events [53].

SPECIFIC IMMUNITY

THE LYMPHOID SYSTEM

When a foreign substance enters the body as an antigen, two types of immunological reaction may occur: (1) The synthesis and release of free antibody into the blood and other body fluids, called "humoral antibody". This antibody acts in many different ways, for example by direct combination with and neutralization of bacterial toxins or, as we have seen, by coating bacteria to enhance their phagocytosis. (2) The production of sensitized lymphocytes which have antibody-like molecules on their surface called "cell-bound antibody". These are the effectors of cell-mediated immunity expressed in such reactions as controlling infections, rejecting foreign cells, limiting growth of malignant and altered cells and inhibiting the development of auto-immune phenomena.

The injection of a single dose of an antigen or immunogen into an immunocompetent animal will cause specific antibody to appear in the serum after a definite time. First exposure to an antigen has as a result the "primary response". The early primary response to most antigens is characterized by the predominance of IgM antibody. The IgG class of antibody appears somewhat later. Upon a second exposure to the same antigen weeks, months or even years later, there is a significantly enhanced response which is characterized by the accelerated appearance of immunocompetent cells and antibody. This is called "secondary response" and the type of antibody produced is predominantly of the IgG class. Thus the small lymphocytes carry the "memory" of the first contact with antigen. Immunologic memory may persist for many years and so provide long lasting immunity against infection. This particular lymphocyte function provides the principle for the use of immunizations and vaccinations. We can recognize at least three cell-types representing different phases in the differentiation of the immunocompetent cell: (*x*) virgin lymphocytes which have not yet experienced contact with antigen, (*y*) memory cells and (*z*) antibody-forming cells derived from *x* and *y* cells as a result of antigenic stimulation [22].

The lymphoid system consists of two components: (1) a central one involved in the differentiation of the lymphoid stem cells into lymphocytes and (2) a peripheral component in which these cells can subsequently react with antigen [5].

The central lymphoid system consists of three compartments: (*a*) the bone marrow, (*b*) the thymus and (*c*) a compartment whose identity is known with certainty only in birds (the bursa of Fabricius) and that in mammals is designated as the bursal equivalent tissue. In higher mammals, however, several sites have been postulated to contain this tissue including the gut-associated lymphoid tissues (GALT), the fetal liver, and the bone marrow.

The peripheral, or secondary, lymphoid tissue includes the lymph nodes, the spleen and unencapsulated tissue lining the respiratory, alimentary and genito-urinary tracts. In peripheral lymphoid tissues two types of lymphocytes may be found that are dependent upon their sites of differentiation in the central lymphoid component. One type which develops in the thymus and differentiates into small lymphocytes called T-lymphocytes. These cells are involved in antigen recognition and in cell mediated immune reactions (cellular immunity). The other population of lymphocytes is derived from stem cells, which differentiate in the bursa of Fabricius in birds and in the mammalian equivalent and consists of small lymphocytes called B-lymphocytes which in response to antigens are transformed into plasma cells and produce the humoral antibodies (humoral immunity) (Fig. IV-2).

Thus T-lymphocytes are particularly associated with immune responses which are conventionally described as cell-mediated, while B-lymphocytes are essential for humoral responses. This distinction, however, between "cell-mediated" and "humoral" responses is something of an over-simplification, if not a misconception. As we shall see, all types of immune response are the consequences of an interaction between antigens and cells. Furthermore, the effector mechanisms through which foreign antigens, whether soluble or cellular are eliminated, very often involve a combination of humoral and cell-mediated elements.

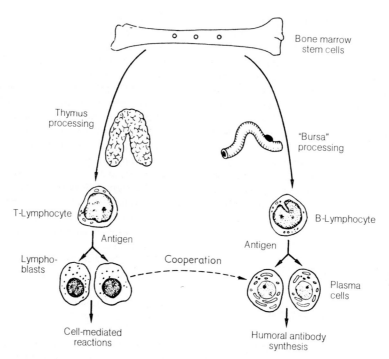

Fɪɢ. IV-2. — *Processing of bone marrow cells by thymus and gut-associated central lymphoid tissue to become immuno-competent T- and B-lymphocytes respectively.* Proliferation and transformation to cells of the lymphoblasts and plasma cell series occurs on antigenic stimulation. (From Roɪᴛᴛ I. M.: *Essential Immunology.* 3rd ed., Blackwell Scientific Publications, Oxford, 1978).

T-lymphocytes and B-lymphocytes

Antigens and receptors. — From the morphological point of view there is no difference between B and T-small lymphocytes examined by conventional light or electron microscopy but a variety of surface markers have been found to differentiate the two populations [42]. All B-cells have membrane-bound immunoglobulin synthesized by the cells themselves while T-cells do not. On the other hand human T-cells can form so called "spontaneous" rosettes with uncoated sheep erythrocytes, a useful identifying reaction of unexplained biological significance. At present, the method most often used for enumerating lymphocyte populations in human peripheral blood is fluorescent anti-immunoglobulin for B-cells and spontaneous rosette formation for T-cells. T-cells are the predominant type, comprising about 70 % of blood lymphocytes in adults. Values for T-cells and B-cells usually add up to a few per cent short of 100 %; the remaining lymphocyte like cells, negative on both counts, are termed "null-cells".

The histocompatibility antigens of the species are expressed on the surface of both B- and T-lymphocytes.

Maturation of T cells is associated with the presence of membrane antigens. Thus the TL antigen is present on the lymphocytes that enter the thymus but is lost on maturation in the gland. Ly antigens develop and are expressed on mature T-lymphocytes.

Various functional characteristics have been found to be associated with different Ly antigens and T-lymphocytes carrying such antigens can thus be divided into subpopulations. The functional activities of T-cells that can be defined on the basis of Ly markers are "helper cell activity" "cytotoxic activity" and "supressor cell activity" [53 *b*].

The main antigen-binding receptors on B-lymphocytes are immunoglobulins. Most of the B-cells also carry Fc receptors for the Fc portion of immunoglobulins and C_{3b} receptors for the third component of complement.

The nature of the receptor for antigen on T-lymphocytes is still uncertain. Recent work on the genetic control of the immune response has provided evidence that the antigen binding site on T cells is closely linked to a product of the gene complex controlling the histocompatibility antigens of the cell membrane.

Thus T-cells express receptors which recognize

products of the major histocompatibility complex on other lymphoid cells, such recognition being essential for cell-cooperation in the immune response.

An important advance is due to the development by Milstein and Kohler in Cambridge of cell lines capable of producing antibody of any required specificity, in cell culture conditions. These antibodies are called "monoclonal antibodies". The potential value of the technique is vast and will enable the identification of different antigens on cells, tumour antigens, microorganisms and their products. Regulation of the immune response by such antibodies is possible and the passive use of monoclonal antibodies for treatment of infections or tumours is a hopeful prospect [18 b, 53 b].

Blast transformation. — The recognition of an antigen (immunogen) by specific receptors on B- and T-lymphocytes leads to the initiation of a series of events in which the cells increase in size, the rate of DNA synthesis increases and mitosis occurs.

The addition of other agents, including certain plant proteins (i. e. phytohemagglutinin (PHA), concavalin-A (con A), Pokeweed mitogen (PWM) and endotoxin (lipopolysaccharide (LPS)) called mitogens, to cultures of nonsensitized lymphocytes may also initiate blast transformation in T- or B-cells. In addition to stimulating DNA synthesis in both T and B lymphocytes, certain mitogens such as insoluble Con A, will initiate synthesis and secretion of immunoglobulins in cultures of B-cells and others, such as PHA, will induce lymphokine production in cultures of T-cells [22].

Immunoglobulins. — The association of antibody activity with the classical γ-globulin fraction of serum was shown by Tiselius and Kabat in the early 1940's. In each species the immunoglobulin molecules can be divided into different classes according to their structure. Thus in the human, five major classes can be distinguished: immunoglobulin G (abbreviated to IgG), IgM, IgA, IgD and IgE [42].

The IgG antibodies can be split by papain into three fragments. Two of these are identical; they are able to combine with antigen and are called Fab (fragment antigen binding). The third fragment is called Fc (fragment crystallizable) and is able to bind to cells bearing Fc receptors such as phagocytes and B-lymphocytes.

There are perhaps 10^6 or more different immunoglobulin molecules in normal serum. IgG is the most abundant immunoglobulin particularly in the extravascular fluids where it combats pathogenic microorganisms and toxins. It is the only immunoglobulin that crosses the placenta. IgA exists mainly in the seromucus secretions where it represents the major immunoglobulin concerned in the defense of the external body surfaces. IgM is essentially intravascular. It is a very effective bacterial agglutinator and mediator of complement dependent cytolysis and is therefore a powerful weapon against septicaemia. IgD is largely present on lymphocytes and probably functions as an antigen receptor. Finally, IgE is important in certain parasitic infections and is responsible for the symptoms of atopic allergy.

The theories proposed for antibody formation fall into two categories that are based on the action of the antigen which can be either "selective" or "instructive" in the process of antibody formation. At present we favour the clonal selection model according to which the antigen selects a specific precursor cell that then proliferates into a clone of cells producing specific antibody.

Lymphokines. — As previously noted T-lymphocytes in response to antigens are incapable of differentiation into plasma cells but give rise to a cell capable of producing a variety of factors called lymphokines. Lymphokines trigger inflammatory or cell-mediated events. One lymphokine is transfer factor, a substance that has the capacity to transfer delayed hypersensitivity or homograft immunity to another non-reactive individual.

Other factors are the migration inhibitory factor (MIF) which inhibits the migration of normal macrophages and the macrophage activating factor (MAF) which induces the macrophages to become metabolically active and more effective in killing bacteria.

Lymphotoxin is a lymphokine associated with target cell injury and with inhibiting the capacity of cells to divide. Finally, several other chemotactic or mitogenic factors are released [6].

MACROPHAGES

It has been said that one of the most important properties of macrophages is their ability to engulf and remove foreign material. However, the large mononuclear cells of the monocyte-macrophage series play a central role in specific immunologic responses as well [22, 42].

Macrophages possess receptors for the third component of complement and Fc receptors. Antibodies of a variety of specificities can be attached to the macrophage surface through its Fc receptor and thus the macrophage becomes able to recognize, engulf and destroy antigenic substances.

Another most important function of macrophages is to "process" and subsequently "present" antigen to lymphocytes. Antigen taken up by free macrophages is partially degraded and partially fixed at or near the cell surface where it is thought to be in a strongly immunogenic state.

Finally, an additional function attributed to macrophages is the production of factors that influence the activity of lymphocytes (*i. e.* factors stimulating the proliferation of lymphocytes, factors suppressing their function, or stimulating the differentiation of memory B-lymphocytes into plasma cells).

CELL-MEDIATED CYTOTOXICITY

It is now well established that the in vitro destruction of target cells by specifically immune lymphoid cells may involve at least three main effector mechanisms [6, 12, 42].

(1) Direct lysis by immune cytotoxic lymphocytes sensitized to surface bound antigens such as those found on allograft or tumor cells.

(2) Antibody (normally IgG)-dependent lysis by nonimmune killer cells with receptors for the Fc portion of target-cell bound immunoglobulin, and

(3) Mitogen-induced lysis, such as the one which is elicited by the addition of PHA in lymphocyte cultures.

With respect to the first mechanism it seems that antigen-specific cytotoxic T-cells are the major mechanism in the immunological rejection of allografts or tumours. Thus a further activity of T-cells which has been well documented, is their ability to act as killer cells. Target cells are destroyed directly and/or through elaboration of specific cell products e. g. lymphokines.

Antibody-dependent cell-mediated cytotoxicity (ADCC) is a distinct cytotoxic mechanism in which target cells coated with low concentrations of IgG antibody can be killed "non-specifically" by a variety of cells possessing Fc receptors (Fig. IV-3). The nature of effector cells depends very much on the target cells used [29]. Studies using Chang human liver cells as targets have found a cell, morphologically indistinguishable from small lymphocytes, active in this sort of cytotoxicity, but which does not have the characteristics of either T- or B-lymphocytes. It was called K-cell (Killer-cell); however, its precise lineage is still uncertain. Chicken red blood cells which have been extensively used for ADCC are susceptible to lysis by K-cells but are also killed by adherent cells and possibly some B-lymphocytes. Rhesus positive human red blood cells in the presence of anti-A antibody are killed by monocytes but not by K-cells.

As to the third mechanism, lymphocytes can be rendered cytotoxic after stimulation with mitogen like PHA and then cause non specific lysis of target cells. The exact cells involved and the mechanisms of killing are not fully understood. It seems that when using human liver Chang-cells as targets about 2/3 of the effector cells bear Fc receptors and T-lymphocytes may be responsible for part of the activity.

Finally, another lymphocyte population has been recently discovered that cannot be identified as either T or B cells, K cells or macrophages by their surface markers. These are called "natural killer cells" or NK cells. These can destroy cells infected with a number of viruses without the help of complement or antibody. The cytotoxic ability of NK cells seems to be potentiated by interferon [3 b].

CELLCOOPERATION

Information regarding the mechanisms of cell cooperation involving macrophages, B-lymphocytes and T-lymphocytes has been obtained from both in vivo and in vitro experiments. In the 1960's it

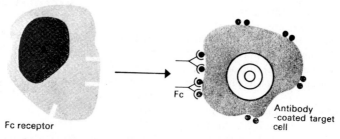

FIG. IV-3. — *Destruction of antibody coated target cell by immunodependant cell mediated cytotoxicity.* The membrane receptors for the Fc region of the immunoglobulin fix the effector cell to the antibody which is then killed by an extra-cellular mechanism. (After ROITT J. M.: *Essential Immunology.* 3rd ed., Blackwell, Oxford, 1978.

was found that thymus and bone marrow cells are necessary for the restoration of the immune response in immunodeficient animals. Following this it has been shown that depletion of spleen cell populations of macrophages resulted in suppression of their immune response. It is now quite clear that there are subpopulations of T-lymphocytes that influence the activity of other T-lymphocytes as well as B-lymphocytes [22]. Specific antigen receptors exist on the surface of both T- and B-lymphocytes. Certain antigens can directly stimulate the B-lymphocytes so that they will subsequently produce plasma cells and antibody (T-independent antigens). Other antigens require the interaction of T-lymphocytes which provide specific and non-specific helper substances that will induce B-lymphocytes to produce antibody (T-dependent antigens). At the moment of presentation of antigen three kinds of cells may be involved. Macrophages, which in some cases are essential for the processing of antigen, T-lymphocytes and B-lymphocytes.

During cell-cooperation there are two main mechanisms of action:

The first aims to increase the immune res-ponse. Stimulated macrophages release a factor (lymphocyte-activating factor or interleukin 1) which activates lymphocytes which in their turn release another factor (interleukin 2) which causes lymphocyte proliferation.

The second mechanism aims to decrease the immune response. Stimulated macrophages release postaglandin E_2 (PGE_2) which activates "suppressor" T-lymphocytes with end result suppression of the immune response [18 b].

Interferon appears to be a major stimulant of macrophages.

The interaction of T-cells in both their helper and suppressor function is under strict genetic control, which is mediated by genes that are located within the major histocompatibility complex. Approximately 10 genes control the overall antibody response to complex antigens; some affect macrophage antigen handling and some the rate of proliferation of differentiating B-cells [5].

However, it is important to note that cells cooperate with each other not only in specific immune responses. The interactions between specific and non-specific immune mechanisms is shown in Figure IV-4.

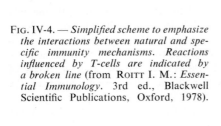

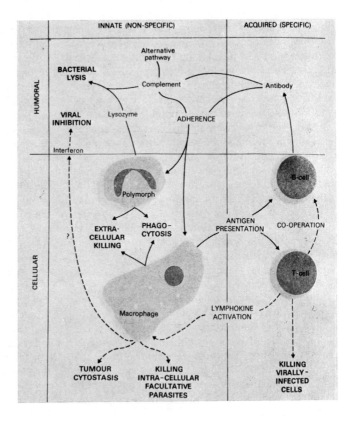

FIG. IV-4. — *Simplified scheme to emphasize the interactions between natural and specific immunity mechanisms. Reactions influenced by T-cells are indicated by a broken line* (from ROITT I. M.: *Essential Immunology*. 3rd ed., Blackwell Scientific Publications, Oxford, 1978).

Development of host defences and immunity of the neonate

THE LYMPHOID SYSTEM

Phylogeny of specific immunity

The development of the immune system depends on the pressures exerted by the environment and the survival of those life forms that are equiped for that particular environment [5].

Until recently it was thought that specific immune responses were confined to vertebrates. There is now evidence, however, that some invertebrates (i. e. tunicates) can reject foreign tissue. The earthworm has also been found able to develop transplantation immunity to tissues of the same or other species while permanently accepting autografts. These reactions are mediated by macrophage-like cells (coelomocytes) and possibly by humoral mediators. As there is no evidence that invertebrates have lymphocytes or immunoglobulins, it seems likely that specific immune responses evolved before the appearance of these two important immunological factors.

Among the vertebrates, all of them are capable of generating a specific immunologic response on antigenic challenge. Both B- and T-lymphocyte responses can be elicited even in the lowest vertebrate studied, the California hagfish. The thymus is the earliest lymphoid organ to appear in phylogeny and is present in the most primitive of vertebrates. Birds are the first vertebrates in which a clear dichotomy of the lymphoid system has been established and are unique in having two discrete central lymphoid organs, thymus and bursa, producing T- and B-lymphocytes respectively.

Mammals having abundant and highly organized lymphoid tissues can elaborate a variety of antibodies. It is of interest that the evolutionary order of appearance of immunoglobulin classes parallels that of the first antigenic exposure during the immune response. Thus, IgM appears in the most primitive vertebrates followed by IgG. IgA is only seen in mammals. IgD and IgE have only been found in man.

Ontogeny of T- and B-lymphocytes

The maturation of immunity in the human begins around the second to third months of gestation. The various cell types arise from a population of progenitor cells which are called "stem cells" or "hemocytoblasts" and which are located within the hematopoietic tissues of the developing embryo. Haemopoiesis originates in the early yolk sac but as embryogenesis proceeds, this function is taken over by the fetal liver and finally by the bone marrow where it continues throughout life [42].

Most if not all of the lymphocytes appearing in the thymus are derived from blood-borne stem cells. Stem cells from hematopoietic organs were found to enter the thymus around the eighth week of gestation. In the thymic cortical area which is an active site of lymphoid proliferation, distinctive surface antigens are acquired by these cells as is functional immunocompetence specific for T-lymphocytes. A thymic hormone, thymosin, has now been isolated and shown to promote the appearance of T-cell differentiation markers (Θ in the mouse, sheep cell receptors in the human, and so on). During cellular maturation, many of the lymphocytes die in the cortical areas; others migrate to the medulla of the thymic lobule. Mature T-lymphocytes leave the thymus through the blood stream and are distributed throughout the body but with particularly large concentrations in the paracortical areas of lymph nodes and the periarteriolar areas of the spleen. These areas are called "thymus-dependent areas". Some T-lymphocytes enter the lymphatics and return to the circulation via the thoracic duct. It is interesting to note that some of these circulating T-lymphocytes have relatively long lives, perhaps up to 10 years. This may explain the observation that removal of the thymus in humans produces no immediate immunologic deficit.

T-lymphocytes detected by the erythrocyte rosette forming technique (E-RFCs) appear initially in the thymus by 8-15 weeks of gestation and increase to their maximal percentage (65 to 100 % of thymocytes) by 18 weeks of gestation. After that E-RFCs appear in increasing quantities in the spleen and peripheral blood and decrease in the thymus gland. Thus the spleen by 18 weeks of gestation has only 5 % of T-lymphocytes but these increase to 10 %-30 % by 20 to 22 weeks. By 30-32 weeks the blood of prematurely born infants has near normal percentages of E-RFCs [49, 50].

B-lymphocytes are also derived from haemopoietic stem cells. Direct evidence for a separate lymphoid B stem cell is lacking. B-cell development occurs in various stages which can be distinguished on the basis of morphology and functional criteria. The first developmental stage is the rapidly dividing pre-B-cell which synthesizes cytoplasmic IgM but in contrast to B-lymphocytes does not have membrane associated immunoglobulins. Pre-B-lymphocytes first appear in the fetal liver at about the eighth week of gestation and are later maintained in the bone marrow. Following this, there is a stage of immature B-lymphocytes which express surface IgM but are immature in the sense of being very susceptible to inactivation by antigen binding. Finally, there is the stage of mature B-lymphocytes which express different classes of cell surface immunoglobulins and are able to differentiate into plasma cells synthesizing IgM, IgD, IgG, IgA or IgE immunoglobulins respectively.

B-lymphocytes identified by the presence of cell-surface immunoglobulins have been found in livers of 10 week fetuses and in spleens of 12 to 13 week fetuses. By 15 to 25 weeks of gestation 30 % to 45 % of spleen cells have surface immunoglobulin. B-lymphocytes are first detected in peripheral blood at 12 weeks of gestation and are essentially up to levels of normal newborns by 15 weeks. Thus, by the beginning of the second trimester of pregnancy the human fetus has an adult proportion of B-lymphocytes expressing different immunoglobulin classes and by the time of birth the neonate has a great variety of B-lymphocytes capable of recognizing virtually any antigenic determinant [27, 30].

As to the order of expression of various immunoglobulin classes data suggest that they develop in the order of IgM, IgG and IgA with cytoplasmic immunoglobulin preceding surface immunoglobulin. IgD-bearing B-lymphocytes follow IgM and do not clearly precede IgG or IgA. This differentiation is apparently antigen-independent and follows a specific chronology. The mechanism which regulates expression of immunoglobulin genes during B-lymphocyte differentiation is not yet clear.

B-lymphocytes after being processed in the "bursa equivalent" (probably represented by fetal liver and adult bone marrow) settle and proliferate in lymphoid organs other than the thymus. Like the T-lymphocytes they are localised to certain areas within these organs called "thymus independent areas". They are the predominant cell type in the primary follicles and with their progeny the plasma cells, in germinal centers and medullary cords. B-lymphocytes are also present in the thoracic duct lymph though in smaller numbers than T-lymphocytes. Some of them appear to participate in lymphocyte recirculation, but the majority are a more sessile population remaining fixed in lymph nodes, spleen and Peyer's patches. This is perhaps not surprising in relation to their principal function to respond to antigenic stimulation by secreting specific humoral antibody, a factor which is readily distributed via blood and lymph to sites from its production [12].

Lymphocyte numbers and subpopulations in peripheral blood

The first appearance of lymphocytes in fetal tissues is noted at approximately 40 days of gestation. There is subsequently a rapid rise of lymphoid cell levels in the blood until the 25th week of gestation. At birth the mean absolute lymphocyte values in prematures and full-terms are $3,700/mm^3$ and $5,700/mm^3$ respectively. After a drop during the first 3 days of life lymphocyte blood levels of $6,000/mm^3$ are reached around the 10th day. Premature babies have lower absolute values. Values of up to $10,000/mm^3$ have been found in healthy full-term neonates [55] (Fig. IV-5).

Several authors have studied T-lymphocyte numbers in cord blood or peripheral venous blood of newborns and have found conflicting results. The percentage of T-cell numbers has been found to be decreased or normal and particularly decreased in neonates small for gestational age. However, it should be noted that the absolute values of T-lymphocytes are generally increased when compared to those found in adults, due to the absolute lymphocytosis during the neonatal period. B-lymphocyte proportions as well as absolute values in neonatal cord or peripheral blood are greater than in adult blood. It is interesting that a rather high number of "null" cells has been found in neonatal blood. This might represent immature precursor cells [10, 30].

Subpopulations of T-lymphocytes have also been found in neonatal blood in the form of T-suppressor cells, T-helper cells and cytotoxic-T-lymphocytes.

During the last trimester of pregnancy and the neonatal period an activation of the T-suppressor

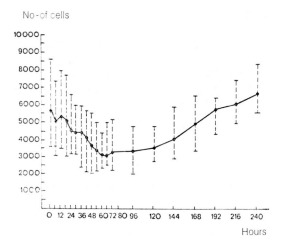

No- of cells

FIG. IV-5. — *Means and ranges of lymphocytes of 15 healthy full-term babies during the first 10 days of life* (from XANTHOU M.: Leucocyte blood picture in healthy full-term and premature babies during the neonatal period. *Archives of disease in Childhood*, 45, 242-249, 1970).

cells has been found probably related to the acceptance of the fetus by the mother [53 *b*].

Finally, the porportion of Fc-receptors and of complement receptors is significantly lower in neonatal than in adult lymphocytes [19]. This is attributed to the fact that either these cell-populations have not yet fully developed or that they do not have the appropriate stimulus to express membrane receptors.

Antigen recognition and response to specific and non-specific stimulation

During ontogeny, the specific recognition of allogenic cells appears almost as soon as the thymus becomes lymphoid. Among the methods used to measure antigen recognition is the mixed leukocyte culture (MLC). The MLC represents the recognition phase in the response of T-lymphocytes to foreign histocompatibility antigens in vitro. Histocompatibility antigens have been detected in the 6 weeks old foetus. Mixed lymphocyte culture reactions have been obtained with suspensions of fetal liver cells as early as 7.5-10 weeks gestation. Thymic lymphocytes have reacted in MLC at 12 and 16 weeks followed by blood and splenic lymphocytes becoming active in MLC reactions at 16 weeks.

The lymphocytes active in MLC reactions are capable of mounting a graft-versus-host (GVH) reaction. Splenic lymphocytes from 13-week-old human fetuses cause a local GVH reaction when implanted under a rat kidney capsule. Lymphocytes from 18 to 23 weeks old human fetuses are as reactive in GVH as adult human lymphocytes. Fetal thymus cells are less active than fetal spleen cells. Thus, there is much evidence that transplantation immunity in man develops at an early stage of gestation.

Antigen binding has been demonstrated in cells from fetal thymuses ranging from 10 to 30 weeks gestation. The number of antigen binding cells is higher in fetal thymuses as compared with cells from thymuses of children or adults.

Regarding the response of the lymphocytes to specific antigen stimulation we know that if the fetus is challenged in utero by an infection it will respond with antibody production largely of the IgM variety. Studies in fetal lambs and rats have shown a stepwise maturation of antibody responses during fetal life. This could represent differential maturation of T- and B-lymphocytes involved in the immune response or that the maturational component involves cells that prepare or process antigen, like the fetal macrophages, and has little to do with differential maturation of actual antibody-producing cells.

Although by mid gestation the human lymphoid tissue has matured sufficiently to respond to certain antigens, the actual synthesis of specific antibodies and the appearance of germinal centers in lymphoid tissues mainly occurs postnatally.

Normally, the immunological maturation appears to follow exposure of the gastrointestinal and respiratory tracts to such environmental antigens as food, bacteria, etc. Premature infants appear to elicit similar responses to those of mature ones suggesting that the interval from birth is more important than size or maturation. Studies in the neonatal period have shown that neonatal lymphocytes respond specifically to Salmonella antigen, following immunization of the host with typhoid vaccine, with blastogenesis comparable to that of adults. On the other hand, lymphocytes from non-immunized newborns fail to transform when cultured with tetanus or diphtheria toxoids. The acquisition of *Candida albicans* extract induced positive stimulation in approximately half of 37 healthy infants by a few weeks of age. More studies are needed to further clarify lymphocyte responses to specific antigenic stimulation in preterm and term neonates [10, 30, 49, 50].

In contrast to specific antigen-induced responses

mitogen induced responses have been extensively studied in neonates [11, 13, 58].

Lymphocyte proliferation following culture with soluble phytohaemaglutinin (PHA) is primarily a T-cell response while some B-cells may also be stimulated. Fetal thymocytes acquire the ability to respond to PHA at about 10-12 weeks of gestation. Two to four weeks later splenic and peripheral blood lymphocytes acquire PHA-responsiveness. A tendency for increased responsiveness of T-lymphocytes with increasing age of the fetus has been noted [36].

PHA responsiveness of cord or peripheral blood lymphocytes during the first days of life was found to be greater, equal to or less than that of adult lymphocytes. In most of these studies however the PHA-response had been measured in the presence of a single and often different dose of mitogen. The response of lymphocytes to PHA has the form of a curve. The necessity for dose-response measurements if meaningful data are to be obtained has recently been pointed out. The mean peak response of cord blood lymphocytes occurs at a lower PHA dose than that of adult lymphocytes [45].

In general, neonatal lymphocytes appear to have a good proliferating response to most PHA doses with the exception of diminished responses when high PHA doses are used during the first four days of life, and more so in premature neonates.

An interesting finding is the observation by many investigators of greater "spontaneous" transformation of neonatal blood lymphocytes when compared to those of adult blood. This higher spontaneous metabolic activity (increased DNA and RNA synthesis) could be attributed to the presence of immature stem cells and/or metabolically more active medium and large lymphocytes, in neonatal blood [49].

While PHA is mitogenic mainly for T-lymphocytes pokeweed mitogen (PWM) induces proliferation of both T- and B-lymphocytes in humans [21]. In 15-week old human fetuses, splenic and blood B-lymphocytes were triggered to differentiate into IgM or IgA producing plasma cells by stimulation with pokeweed mitogen. However, IgG and IgA responses were less than IgM. Exposure of neonatal B-lymphocytes either to specific antigens or to pokeweed mitogen elicited a quantitatively deficient response with respect to adult cells, in the number of B-lymphocytes that differentiated, and those cells that differentiated, were qualitatively different in being primarily of the IgM class. Furthermore, it was found that while adults show IgG activity within 5-15 days following immunization, only IgM is found in neonates for as long as 20 to 30 days following immunization. The period of prolonged IgM production lasts until 6 months of age. The qualitative and quantitative deficiencies in antibody responses of neonates, as compared to adults, appear to reflect regulatory interactions with T-lymphocytes and macrophages rather than the absence of B-lymphocytes capable of eliciting a response.

Fetal and neonatal immunoglobulin production

It is well known that fetal synthesis of IgG is minimal. However, passively transferred IgG from the maternal circulation occurs as early as the 38th day of gestation. The transfer of immunoglobulin IgG is accomplished by means of an active transport mechanism of this immunoglobulin through a receptor located on the Fc fragment of the molecule. IgG levels remain quite constant until the 17th week of gestation at which time a proportionate increase occurs with gestational age. At term, cord IgG levels are 5 to 10 % greater than corresponding maternal levels. Four subclasses of IgG have been recognized; IgG_1, IgG_2, IgG_3 and IgG_4. Placental transfer of all four IgG subclasses appears to be complete by term although some question remains about the transfer of IgG_2. During the neonatal period, levels of all IgG subclasses decrease sharply but IgG_3 falls off most rapidly, decreasing to approximately 50 % of term levels by 30 days postnatally.

IgG levels in premature infants may be proportionately decreased with the degree of prematurity. Babies small for gestational age have even lower levels which may reflect placental dysfunction. IgG synthesis by the neonate is governed by antigen stimulation so that in germ-free animals, for example, IgG levels are extremely low, but rise rapidly on transfer to a normal environment.

None of the other immunoglobulins has the ability to cross the placenta, and the low but significant levels of IgM in cord blood are synthesized by the baby. IgM immunoglobulin is found in fetal tissue at 10.5 weeks of gestation and continues at low levels through gestation. The normal fetus has sufficiently well established IgM synthesis so that nearly all fetuses have detectable levels of IgM in their serum by 30 weeks. Levels of IgM increase gradually during late gestation; at term birth, the mean level of IgM is 10 ± 5 mg/100 ml. An elevated cord IgM level suggests the possibility of a congenital infection. An elevated cord IgM level is not however, diagnostic, of a specific infection as specific antibodies are required for such a diagnosis. The levels of IgM immunoglobulin rise rapidly during the 4th and 7th post-natal days, possibly as a result of antigenic stimulation.

Synthesis of IgA is first detected at 30 weeks of gestation and then proceeds at such a limited rate that serum IgA is not usually detected until several days after birth, when levels are usually 1 to 5 mg/100 ml. Higher levels of IgA in cord blood are often indicative of a maternal-fetal transfusion. Secretory IgA (composed of two serum IgA molecules and a secretory component) is not detected in the fetus. It has been found in tears and saliva of neonates between the 2nd and 5th postnatal weeks.

The immunoglobulins IgD and IgE are found only in trace quantities in the fetus and in cord blood.

It is interesting to note that IgM globulins attain adult levels by one year of age, the IgG globulins by five to six years of age and the IgA globulins by 10 years of age. This pattern of appearance of immunoglobulins recapitulates that seen in phylogeny [30, 42, 48].

Production of lymphokines

Neonatal lymphocytes may synthesize some of but not all lymphokines as do adult lymphocytes [49]. Lymphotoxin production in the neonate is only about 40 % of the value for adult controls. Migration inhibition factor (MIF) production in PHA-stimulated neonatal and cord blood lymphocytes is about 10 % of that of adult lymphocytes. Classic interferon production appears to be normal by cord or neonatal leukocytes but immune interferon production following PHA stimulation seems to be markedly deficient in neonates. Little data exist on the relative production of other lymphokines by neonatal lymphocytes.

MONOCYTES-MACROPHAGES

Monocytes in the human first appear in the 4th month of gestation in the spleen and lymph nodes. Macrophage function has been little studied in human fetuses or neonates. There are however some interesting animal studies regarding these cells.

In neonatal rats macrophage function was found to be immature as evidenced by increased susceptibility to Listeria monocytogenes infections and diminished antibody production. These defects could be reversed by infusion of adult rat macrophages. Another example of deficient immune macrophage mechanisms in neonatal rats is the high degree of susceptibility of these animals to the induction of specific immunologic tolerance. Activation of macrophages (i. e. through injecting endotoxin) made the rats resistant to tolerance induction.

In rabbits it was found that there is an increase in functional pulmonary alveolar macrophages during the last trimester of gestation and the 1st post-natal week. The alveolar macrophages from neonatal rabbits were found to be relatively immature cells containing large quantities of phagocytosed surfactant, high activities of certain glycolytic and hydrolytic enzymes, normal phagocytic function and diminished chemotactic and bactericidal activities. Postnatally the cells undergo maturation and full development by 28 days. The ingested surfactant may be responsible for the diminished functional activities of these cells during the perinatal period and the changes in oxygen tension may be responsible for the induction of certain enzymes. Also interesting is the postulation that reduced alveolar macrophage numbers or their immature function could play a role in the pathogenesis of pulmonary neonatal illnesses such as idiopathic respiratory distress syndrome (I. R. D. S.), oxygen toxicity—in the form of bronchopulmonary dysplasia—and infections such as bronchopneumonia [7].

The results obtained in studies of human neonatal monocyte chemotaxis have so far been conflicting.

Cord blood monocytes have been found to be able to respond normally to lymphokines generated by adult lymphocytes. However, supernatants elicited from cord lymphocytes generated a very poor chemotactic response by neonatal monocytes in comparison to that generated by adult monocytes. Other investigators found that neonatal monocytes show normal movement.

The ingestion and intracellular multiplication of Toxoplasma gondii were found to be identical in human placental and adult monocytes; however, the rate of phagocytosing polystyrene spheres, in another study, was found to be considerably slower in neonatal monocytes than in those from adults [44]. The observation that monocytes are less efficient in the early stages of phagocytosis raises the question of what role phagocytic kinetics could play in neonatal sepsis. However, the ability of neonatal monocytes to kill Staph. aureus and E. coli has been reported to be satisfactory. Fc receptors and receptors for the third component of complement have been found on neonatal monocytes.

Finally, we have seen that macrophages play a central role not only in processing antigens but also in modulating antibody responses. In spite of the limited data in this respect there is a strong suspicion that human neonatal macrophages are deficient in this very important function. In neonates, the state of maturation of these cells may control the expression of immunocompetence to such an extent that primary defects in other cells of the newborn may be incorrectly suspected [7, 9, 10, 30, 49].

CELL-MEDIATED CYTOTOXICITY

Immunologically specific effector cells for cell-mediated cytotoxicity develop during the intrauterine life of the human fetus [18, 30]. PHA-induced cytotoxicity against chicken erythrocytes has been demonstrated by lymphocytes from bone marrow, spleen and blood of 14 to 18 weeks old human fetuses. Thymocytes from the same fetuses, however, failed to destroy target cells even though they showed a blastogenic response to PHA. On the contrary antibody-dependent cell-mediated cytotoxicity against lymphoblastoid targets could not be elicited by liver, spleen, thymus or bone marrow cells from human fetuses of 9-14 weeks gestation. Cytotoxic T-lymphocytes with specificity for allogenic target cells have been demonstrated in neonatal blood but no studies of their presence in fetal organs are reported. A number of studies however, indirectly support the development of this significant T-cell function during intrauterine life. Maternal lymphocytes frequently enter the fetal circulation. If such cells remained viable and proliferated they would be expected to mount a graft-versus host reaction. This does not happen, however, which suggests competent T-cell immunity by the fetus with the consequent ability to reject or inactivate the maternal lymphocytes. Further evidence of a good cell-mediated immune response during fetal life is the extreme rarity of GVH reactions in fetuses receiving intrauterine transfusions for severe Rhesus incompatibility.

The cytotoxic capacity of neonatal lymphocytes has been tested against a limited spectrum of target cells [11, 28, 47, 49, 58].

Cell-mediated lympholysis, a T-cell dependent process is qualitatively deficient in neonates when compared to adult lymphocytes. This was found after prior sensitization in mixed lymphocyte cultures with allogenic lymphocyte targets followed by lysis assayed against these targets to determine acquisition of specific sensitization. Deficient cell-mediated lympholysis has also been observed in neonatal mice for the first week.

PHA-induced cytotoxicity against Chang human liver cells was found to be very low in cord-blood of both full-term and preterm neonates. Through the neonatal period it rose but without reaching adult levels. PHA-induced cytotoxicity against chicken erythrocytes was found to be normal in cord-blood of full-term neonates; however, PHA-induced lysis of chicken erythrocytes can be mediated by a variety of cell types including, in addition to lymphocytes, polymorphonuclear cells, etc.

In the antibody-dependent system K-cells, cytotoxicity against Chang human liver cells, is readily detected among cord blood effector cells. However, during the first 4 days of life it was found to be low in fullterm and more so in premature neonates. Normal values were again obtained after the 4th day of life. In another study where the targets (Chang cells) were infected with *Herpes simplex* viruses the cytotoxicity of cord blood is found to be deficient [47]. Using human lymphocytes as targets sensitized with HLA- antibodies, antibody dependent cytotoxicity (ADCC) in cord blood and during the first two days of life was found to be very low.

Finally, the ADCC of neonatal cord and peripheral blood monocytes against human red blood cells used as targets was found to be satisfactory.

Most of these studies of cell-mediated cytotoxicity in neonates using various target cells indicate some degree of abnormality. These findings suggest either absence or functional immaturity of the sub-populations of cells involved. Alternatively inhibitory cells or factors may be present in the neonate's peripheral blood which affect the function of the involved cells.

HUMORAL FACTORS

The complement system

Complement analogs with physicochemical characteristics and functional properties have been found in invertebrates.

The synthesis of most complement components starts early in fetal life. Synthesis of C_3 in fetal tissues has been demonstrated by immunochemical techniques as early as $5\frac{1}{2}$ weeks of gestation, thus preceding that of immunoglobulins. The early synthesis of complement is evidently not related to the presence of antigen. Little or no placental transfer of maternal complement to the fetal circulation occurs. C_4 and C_2 are apparently produced by macrophages while C_3, C_5, C_6, C_9 and possibly C_2 are synthesized in the liver. Despite the early onset of complement synthesis, substantial quantities of complement do not appear in the serum until 12 to 14 weeks and then remain rather low until approximately 26-28 weeks of gestation at which point they increase markedly. At term total haemolytic complement titers and levels of individual components are 50 % to 60 % of the corresponding levels in normal adult serum or paired maternal serum. Post-natally there is a rapid increase in complement levels possibly due, in part, to complement proteins in colostrum or to the effect of extrauterine exposure to environmental antigens. Preterm neonates were found to have less whole complement activity and lower component concentrations than term infants.

About three-fourths of the normal neonates tested have had defective activity in the alternative pathway and significant correlation between activity and birth weight was found. Activity of the alternative pathway appears to be more frequently subnormal than that of the classical pathway. Factor B and properdin concentrations vary from about 35 % to 60 % and 35 % to 70 % of adult values respectively. Gestational age correlates with alternative pathway hemolytic activity and properdin concentration but not with concentration of factor B.

Whereas much quantitative data exists on complement components in the newborn [10, 24, 30], information on biologic activities is limited.

Lysozyme

Serum lysozyme levels at birth in full-term neonates are found to be similar or higher to those found in adults [57].

No correlation between the concentration of lysozyme in maternal and neonatal sera at delivery was demonstrated suggesting that the enzyme found is produced by the fetus.

The levels of the enzyme are subsequently found to fall during the neonatal period; in preterm neonates lysozyme levels on the first day of life are significantly lower than in term babies. They tend to rise during the first 5 days, by which time they have reached levels found in term babies.

With respect to secretory lysozyme, neonatal tears are found to contain less lysozyme than those of adults.

Interferon

The capacity to produce interferon seems to be present during early stages of fetal development. Animal experiments have shown that levels of interferon in mid and late gestation lambs were significantly higher than those found in adult sheep.

PHAGOCYTES

Phylogeny and ontogeny of non-specific immunity

Phagocytic cells constitute one of the most primitive host defence components. In protozoa foreign substances are ingested and digested by the entire cell. This event in unicellular organisms serves a nutritive function while in higher forms, the process has evolved to a defence function. It has long been known that phagocytosis occurs in invertebrates. In higher invertebrates there is a vascular system that allows phagocytosis to take place by both fixed and circulating cells. The presence of mobile phagocytic cells provides assistance to the slowly moving tissue histiocytes.

It is interesting that in phylogeny, the two most important non-specific factors, phagocytosis and the inflammatory response, are found in primitive life forms.

Neutrophils are found early in human ontogeny. Even in the early yolk sac stages of hematopoiesis, a few myelocytes are found in the blood islands. Granulocytic cells are first noted in the liver at about two months of gestation. By five months, the bone marrow becomes the chief synthetic organ. Myelopoiesis is 10 times more active in fetal than in adult blood. During the first half of gestation few granulocytes, not exceeding 1,000/mm³, circulate in the peripheral blood of the fetus. However, there is a rapid rise in their numbers during the last trimester of pregnancy so that at birth their absolute numbers exceed those found in the peripheral blood of adults [5, 10, 55].

The functional capabilities of fetal granulocytes to phagocytize and kill pathogenic microorganisms are not well studied; however, it is remarkable that as early as the 16th week of gestation a fetus is able to produce a polymorphonuclear leucocytosis of 5,000/mm³ or more, at an age when granulopoiesis is still confined to a small volume of bone marrow and spleen [48].

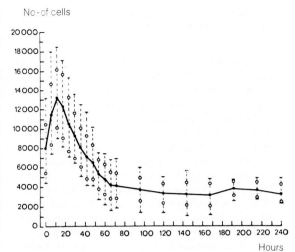

No-of cells

Hours

FIG. IV-6. — *Means, ranges and means ± 1 SD of neutrophils on 15 full-term healthy babies during the first 10 days of life.* (From XANTHOU M.: Leucocyte blood picture in healthy full-term and premature babies during neonatal period. *Archives of Disease in Childhood,* 45, 242-249, 1970).

Quantitation of phagocytes

At birth the polymorphonuclear neutrophils are the predominant cells found in the peripheral blood of neonates [55]. In full-terms the mean value is 8,000/mm³ and in prematures 5,000/mm³. Following birth, there is a marked increase in the absolute values reaching a peak at 12 hours of age in both full-terms and prematures (mean values 13,000/mm³ and 8,000/mm³ respectively). Subsequently there is a drop and by 72 hours of age the mean value in both full-terms and preterms is 4,000/mm³. Thereafter the counts remain quite steady, not exceeding 7,000/mm³ up to the end of the neonatal period (Fig. IV-6). The most plausible explanation for this enormous rise in neutrophils a few hours following birth seems to be their displacement from the marginal layer of vessels. This is known to happen after violent exercise in adults, and in the newborn may well reflect labors and childbirth which is by no means a passive process. Immature neutrophils as band forms, metamyelocytes, myelocytes and even blast cells can be found in healthy neonates during the first 3 days of life. This reflects the high hematopoietic activity of the bone marrow at term.

Eosinophils can be found in high absolute numbers throughout the neonatal period sometimes reaching 3,000/mm³.

As for the monocytes, their absolute values also show a small rise at 12 hours of life, with a sub-

sequent gradual fall until the third day of life both in preterm and full-term babies. High monocyte values can also be found in healthy neonates reaching 2,000/mm³.

At this point it is interesting to note briefly the most significant changes that take place in the bone marrow during this period. During the first month of life there is a significant decrease in the percentage of erythroblasts and granulocytes and an increase in small lymphocytes. While at the time of birth myeloid cells exceed both erythroblasts and lymphocytes several fold, after the first month the bone marrow becomes predominantly lymphocytic and remains so up to 18 months of age [43].

Phagocytic-cell function

Phagocytosis. — Several studies regarding the function of neonatal phagocytes have been reported [10, 31, 41].

Polymorphonuclear neutrophils of healthy neonates have been found to phagocytose pathogenic microorganisms normally or with decreased ability. Apart from the differences in the challenge particles and the conditions of the various experimental designs used, phagocytosis was found to be very dependent on the concentration of serum used in the assays. In the presence of normal serum concentrations the phagocytic activity of isolated neonatal polymorphonuclears against *E. coli, S. aureus, Serratia marcescens, S. pyogenes, Diplococcus pneumonia* and *Pseudomonas aeruginosa* was normal. In concentrations of serum less than 10 %, however, neonatal polymorphonuclears were less effective phagocytes than adult cells. Thus, the neonatal polymorph may be deficient in phagocytic activity providing the method used to measure phagocytosis is sensitive enough.

In premature neonates phagocytic activity of polymorphonuclear neutrophils was reported as normal by several investigators, and as relatively deficient by others. All these studies were performed with serum concentrations in excess of 10 %, however, there is no available basis for comparisons between deficient phagocytosis by polymorphs from term neonates and from prematures. Neonates small for gestational age have lower phagocytosis ability than normal for gestational age.

In order to understand phagocytic abnormalities better it is necessary to examine the chemotactic abilities of neonatal phagocytes as well as the opsonizing capacity of neonatal serum.

Chemotaxis. — In neonates, random mobility of neutrophils as measured by the capillary tube migration method, is reduced. In addition, neutrophil chemotaxis in the presence of chemotactic factors generated from standard pooled sera is lower in neonatal than adult neutrophils. Neonatal polymorphonuclears were found to be extremely "rigid" cells and this increased rigidity may contribute significantly to their impaired chemotaxis. Although there is general agreement that neonatal polymorphonuclears are relatively deficient in their ability to move toward defined chemotactic stimuli, the nature of this defect is not yet clear [30].

Apart from the intrinsic abnormalities of neonatal polymorphs there are chemotactic factor deficiencies in neonatal sera. Although these deficiencies have not been clearly defined it seems most likely that complement is involved.

As already noted the results obtained in studies of neonatal monocyte chemotaxis have so far been conflicting [30, 31].

Opsonization. — There is not much information available on the receptors of neonatal phagocytes. The percentage of neutrophils bearing Fc and complement receptors is similar in both cord and adult blood [40]. The Fc and C_3 receptors of phagocytic cells allow them to utilize specific immune recognition. Furthermore, evidence suggests that both in macrophages and neutrophils the complement receptors may be involved in the attachment phase of phagocytosis, whereas binding to the Fc receptor may be necessary for ingestion. Neonatal neutrophils appear to have a normal recognition system. They ingest both non-specifically coated particles, such as latex, and immune coated particles.

Opsonization (the coating of particles by serum factors) promotes immune-dependent phagocytosis. Opsonic serum factors consist of the heat stable specific antibodies IgM, IgG_1 and IgG_3 and of heat labile opsonic fragment of C_3 which can attach to particles by activation of complement by either the classical or alternative pathways. Several studies have shown significant deficiencies of opsonization by neonatal plasma or serum, and that these contribute to the impaired phagocytic function. The opsonic defects include deficiencies in both specific antibodies and complement components. Thus, the well known susceptibility of neonates to infection with gram-negative bacteria has been related to the lack of IgM antibodies which are known to be more efficient against gram-negative bacteria than IgG antibodies in their activation of complement, opsonic function and bactericidal capabilities. In other instances neonatal host resistance depends upon the placental transfer of specific IgG opsonins which may be lacking. Finally, repeated data suggest

deficiencies of complement-dependent opsonization in neonates [10, 31].

Intracellular killing. — Variable results regarding neonatal neutrophil bactericidal capacity have been reported [10, 30, 31, 41]. Normal activity has been reported for *S. aureus* and *E. coli*. For *P. aeruginosa* and *Candida albicans* the results have been conflicting. The decreased bactericidal activity exhibited by polymorphonuclears from normal neonates is not fully corrected when the microorganisms are opsonized by pooled adult sera. In a recent study, the rates of killing of ingested viable *P. aeruginosa* by polymorphs from premature infants and normal adults at 90 minutes were identical, by three hours. However, polymorphs from premature infants showed a decreased bactericidal rate. In another study of neutrophil bacteria ratios of 1 : 1 there was comparable killing in newborns and adults. However, at bacteria-neutrophil ratios of 100 : 1 markedly depressed bactericidal capacity was found in neonatal neutrophils.

The situation thus seems the same as with phagocytosis. When neonatal polymorphonuclears are subjected to increased demands then deficiencies in bactericidal activities become much more obvious and these may play a significant role in explaining compromise of neonatal host defence mechanisms. In favour of this postulate is the finding of markedly decreased bactericidal capacity unrelated to gestational age and birth weight in "stressed" neonates [30].

Metabolic activities. — Since metabolic processes underlie phagocytic and bactericidal function of neonatal phagocytes it is to be expected that the metabolic status of neonatal phagocytes will in several respects be different to that found in adult phagocytes [30, 34, 41]. Indeed, oxygen consumption, hexose monophosphate pathway activity and nitro-blue tetrazolium (NBT) reduction by neonatal leucocytes are significantly increased in the resting state when compared to those of adults. Neonatal granulocytes have also been found to have increased acid phosphatase and alkaline phosphatase activities as well as peroxidase activity. Furthermore, neonatal monocytes demonstrate higher peroxidase activity. However, decreased activity of the hexose monophosphate shunt pathway is found in phagocytosing polymorphonuclears of neonates compared with adult polymorphonuclears, although they utilize glucose and oxygen in similar amounts to those seen in adult leucocytes following phagocytosis. NTB reduction by cord blood monocytes has been found to equal to that of adult monocytes, and on in vitro stimulation cord blood granulocytes have been seen to display the same high NBT activity as those of the mothers and of healthy non-pregnant women. Finally, other work reports a significant defect in OH production of neonatal polymorpho-nuclears. This defect could underlie defective bactericidal activity of the relevant cells [2].

More work on metabolic activities of neonatal phagocytes needs to be done before we will be able to fully understand their functional defects.

INFLAMMATORY RESPONSE

The skin of the neonate is deficient in manifesting the inflammatory component of the immune response [30].

Experiments have been performed to assess the response to dermal infection with pneumonococci in weanling and adult rats. It was found that the weanling rats had: (a) delayed migration of leuko-cytes, (b) poor localization and increased spreading of bacteria and (c) an increased incidence of bac-teremia and death.

Several investigators have found that the response of human neonatal skin to irritants and their ability to localize inflammation is also deficient in comparison to adults. When inflammation is induced on neonatal skin by the skin window technique the shift from a predominantly granulocytic to a predo-minantly mononuclear cell response is slower and less intense in neonates than in adults. The difference in the mononuclear cell response of newborns and adults does not appear to be merely a reflection

of the number of those cells in the circulation, because, as we have seen, blood monocytes during the neonatal period exceed those found in the peri-pheral blood of adults. Furthermore, the deficiencies of neonatal polymorphonuclear in movement, phagocytosis and killing and those of the monocytes in antigen processing and perhaps in movement are likely to play a significant role in the diminished inflammatory response of the newborn and the decreased skin reactivity.

The skin response has been studied in premature and term neonates exposed to 2.4-dinitrochloro-benzene. It was found that delayed hypersensitivity can be induced in neonates (fullterm and preterm) but that they are inconsistent in this capacity, partly due to a diminished inflammatory response. Other investigators, as well, have come to the conclu-sion that the failure of the neonate to express cuta-neous hypersensitivity is attributable to skin-inflammatory factors as well as to immunologic factors. Neonates were given leucocytes or leucocyte transfer factor from PPD-positive mothers. Lympho-cytes subsequently obtained from the infants showed increased in vitro response to PPD by blast transformation. In contrast, the same infants showed no in vivo reactivity to PPD. When BCG was administered to a group of normal infants in vitro leucocyte responses to PPD preceded the development of positive skin tests by 1-3 weeks. These data thus demonstrated that antigen-respon-sive lymphocytes may be present in the newborn despite a negative skin test reaction.

Finally the deficient complement components as well as the deficiency of some of the coagulation factors—i. e. vitamin K-dependent factors—in neo-nates contribute to their diminished inflammatory response.

Fetomaternal relationships

It would be unsatisfactory to consider the develop-ment of immunity in the fetus and newborn in iso-lation from maternal influences [23, 42].

The most extensively studied but still unanswered problem in these relationships is how a fetus who inherits one half of its antigens from paternally controlled genes foreign to the mother can be tolerated successfully during pregnancy and is not rejected as an "allograft". We have seen that fetal cells possess histocompatibility antigens and can

recognize transplantation antigens and respond to mixed lymphocyte culture reactions from very early fetal life.

The acceptance of the fetus by the mother has in the past been attributed largely to the barrier function of the placenta. However, in the human haemochorial placenta, maternal blood with immu-nocompetent lymphocytes does circulate in contact with the fetal trophoblast and we now know that fetal and maternal cells are exchanged through the placenta and that both humoral and cellular immunity to fetal antigens develop in the mother. This process is referred to as "isoimmunization" and, as is well known, may lead to serious disease in the newborn such as haemolytic disease of the newborn, thrombocytopenia and leukopenia. On the other hand, it has been postulated that transfer of fetal lymphocytes to the mother may play a part in the acceptance of the fetus as a homograft, as the chronic intravenous administration of low dosages of transplantation antigens is conducive to a "specific" weakening of the ability to respond to tissue homografts.

Many speculations have been put forward to explain the acceptance of the fetus by its mother. These fall into two main categories: according to the first the trophoblast is immunologically privileged as:

(a) protection against attack by cytotoxic lymphocytes may be afforded by the barrier of sialic acid-rich mucopolysaccharide surrounding trophoblast cells,

(b) the trophoblast membranes produce a unique glycoprotein which inhibits the rejection reaction of lymphocytes while having no measurable effects on other lymphocyte reactions,

(c) trophoblast cells might be relatively resistant to T- or K-cell attack through a low density of the major histocompatibility complex (MHC) antigens,

(d) shedding of antigen could block aggressive T-lymphocytes on antibody and

(e) the placenta might produce a hormone which is locally immunosuppressive.

According to the second category, there are suppressor cells and other immunosuppressive factors in maternal and neonatal serum that do not allow the GVH reaction to take place [33]. A reduced lymphocyte mitotic response to PHA and reduced spontaneous rosette formation are found during the pregnancy which are attributed to plasma inhibitory factors. These factors can depress the response of lymphocytes from non-pregnant adults. Furthermore, suppressor cells are found in the mother which specifically prevent killing of paternal cells. These cells may prevent the mother's lymphocytes from reacting with antigens in the fetus that are inherited from the father.

On the other hand, active T-suppressor cells have been found in cord blood. These T-suppressor cells have been reported to inhibit both mitosis of and immunoglobulin production by lymphocytes from the mother. This inhibition could occur via a soluble suppressor factor. Neonatal lymphocytes

were found not only to suppress the blast transformation of their mother's lymphocytes but to inhibit the transformation of lymphocytes from other adult persons. A possible involvement of monocytes-macrophages as suppressor cells in this reaction has also been suggested.

Finally, substances like a fetoglycoprotein or prolactin found in maternal or neonatal sera have been reported to suppress lymphocyte proliferation.

TRANSPLACENTAL PASSAGE
OF ANTIGENS
AND ANTIBODIES

Another very interesting aspect of fetomaternal relationships is the effect of maternal antigens and antibodies that manage to cross the placenta, on the immunologic status of the fetus [5, 21, 30, 42]. There are different methods of transmission of maternal antibodies to the fetus in different species. In species with a large number of membranes between the maternal and fetal circulations, the colostrum is the main route of transfer. Conversely, as the number of layers of membranes decreases (i. e. in man) the transplacental route acquires greater importance. Thus, in man, as we have seen, the predominant transfer of antibody occurs via the passage of IgG immunoglobulin from the maternal circulation to that of the fetus, thus providing the fetus with a variety of antibodies which reflect most of the mother's experience with infectious agents. Maternal antibodies however have long been recognized to exert a suppressive effect on neonatal antibody formation. Thus, in the case of antibodies that are effectively transferred across the placenta, i. e. diphtheria, the immunosuppressive effects of maternal antibody may be substantial.

Apart from IgG no other classes of antibody are able to cross the placenta. The exclusion of other classes of antibody may be beneficial to the fetus in many cases. For example, the exclusion of the IgM isohaemagglutinins, leukoagglutinins or the IgE antibodies of allergy prevents disease that may be produced by these antibodies. However, it also prevents the passage of other beneficial maternal antibodies such as the IgM ones which are important in the bacterial defence against gram-negative bacteria.

With respect to the antigens, their transfer to the fetus from the maternal circulation provides a potential route by which the fetal immune system may be stimulated. Study of these relationships presents many complex immunologic and genetic problems, however, and few data are as yet available to define the extent of such interactions. In animal studies, immunization of mothers has led to offspring with enhanced or depressed responses. Direct evidence of placental passage of antigens in rat fetuses has been obtained. However, equivalent findings in man have not been reported although the apparent sharing of lymphocyte responses between mother and child might under some circumstances be due to antigen transfer.

Positive skin test reactions to common allergens are found in some newborns whose mothers had been immunized and are thought to be the result of passage of antigens via the placenta. In other human studies, fetal lymphocytes from cord blood responded on occasion to antigens that failed to elicit an immune response by corresponding maternal lymphocytes. These studies suggest that the fetal lymphocytes were stimulated by transplacental passage of antigen. Another interesting finding is that immunization of the fetus has been reported to occur via the amniotic fluid.

TRANSPLACENTAL PASSAGE OF VIRUSES

It is well known that some viruses are able to cross the placenta and directly infect the fœtus, the most common being rubella, cytomegalovirus and the infectious hepatitis virus. The fetal response depends upon the stage of gestation. Thus rubella in early gestation has a primarily teratogenic effect, in contrast, rubella in later pregnancy has primarily inflammatory effects (*i. e.* hepatitis, iridocyclitis, meningitis). These differences most probably result from a better cellular immune response in older fetuses.

Finally, in some instances the virus may alter normal immunologic development resulting in a permanent immunodeficiency state. The most common immunodeficiency associated with congenital rubella is the persistence of elevated levels of IgM through infancy with marked depression of IgE levels probably arising as a result of interference by the virus at a critical time when clonal differentiation from IgM-lymphocyte bearing cells to IgG lymphocyte and IgA lymphocyte bearing cells is occuring [10].

Neonatal immunity during bacterial infections

MAIN IMMUNOLOGIC MECHANISMS AGAINST BACTERIAL INFECTIONS

Microorganisms are kept out of the body by the skin, the secretion of mucous, bactericidal fluids, etc. If, however, penetration occurs, bacteria are destroyed by soluble factors such as complement and by phagocytosis with intracellular killing.

By activating the alternative complement pathway, phagocytic cells are attracted to the bacteria which adhere to the C_{3b} receptors and are engulfed. The antibody molecule is designed to attach to microorganisms which fail to activate the alternative pathway or the surface of phagocytic cells. In such circumstances the antibodies fix complement by the classical pathway and stimulate the phagocyte through its Fc receptor.

Humoral immunity to bacteria depends mainly upon the opsonizing mechanism of antibody to enhance phagocytosis, its ability to neutralize bacterial toxins and the lysis of cells through the terminal complement components plus lysozyme.

Thus, the participation of both non-specific and specific immune mechanisms occurs in all bacterial infections in man [42].

NEONATAL IMMUNOLOGIC DEFICIENCIES CAUSED BY BACTERIAL INFECTIONS

As discussed, healthy neonates present various immaturities in their immunologic mechanisms against bacterial infections. Thus, they have deficiencies in the alternative complement pathway, certain complement components, and low lysozyme levels. Furthermore, the function of their phagocytes and lymphocytes is deficient and the levels of most immunoglobulin classses are very low.

Bacterial infections further depress host defence mechanisms of the neonate resulting in their particularly high morbidity and mortality. The changes found in infection concern both cellular and humoral factors.

Cellular factors

There may be a remarkable increase in total neutrophil count. While in healthy babies the upper limit of normality is 7,000/mm³ after 72 hours of age, in newborns suffering from infection counts as high as 25,000/mm³ have been found. However, in neonates with very severe infections very low neutrophil counts, sometimes below 500/mm³ are often seen. Presumably as neutrophils are attracted to the site of infection, they leave the circulating neutrophil pool to reside initially in the marginal pool along the walls of the vessels, and then pass into the tissues. Release of marrow storage pools which contain mostly young or band-form neutrophils follows, sometimes with the appearance of even earlier myeloid precursors—such as pro-myelocytes or even myeloblasts—in the neonatal peripheral blood. Apart from changes in their numbers, neutrophils acquire morphologic changes during bacterial infections such as toxic granulation, vacuolization or the appearance of Döhle bodies [60].

Along with the drop in neutrophils during overwhelming infection there is often a considerable fall in the numbers of eosinophils and lymphocytes.

In adults with acute bacterial infections polymorphonuclear chemotaxis is usually enhanced and may become defective only in overwhelming infection, possibly because of marked endotoxemia. In contrast, in neonates the enhancement of PMN chemotaxis is observed only in those with superficial infections and without demonstrable bacteremia, whereas in those with proven sepsis a striking fall in chemotactic activity was constantly demonstrated. This could not be attributed to the presence of humoral factors [26].

Apart from deficient chemotactic ability decreased phagocytosis and bactericidal activity have been found in septicaemic as compared to healthy neonates. This must be partly due to the fact that PMN's from infected infants have less than normal enhancement of metabolic activity. In contrast to elevated NBT dye test results obtained during bacterial infection in older children and adults, in infected neonates the NBT-test is depressed as are the hexose monophosphate shunt values. These defects in metabolic activity reach values normal for neonates during recovery from infection [30].

The numbers of lymphocytes are also reduced in overwhelming infections. There is a drop in the number of lymphocytes forming sheep erythrocyte rosettes and particularly in those binding C_{3b} coated ox erythrocytes in neonates with acute septicaemia.

During acute bacterial infections the lymphocyte transformation to PHA was found to be much depressed in full-term and premature babies [59]. Deficient response to mitogen and antigens has also been found in adult patients suffering from meningitis [3]. The mechanisms causing this non-specific depression are not known; negative mediators may be produced or suppressor T-cells activated. A possible parallel in vivo is the temporary suppression of delayed type reactions which is best known in acute viral illness but has also been described in acute bacterial infections.

The antibody dependent and PHA-induced cytotoxicities of neonatal lymphocytes were also found to be very depressed in septicaemic neonates compared to those found in healthy ones [59]. The inhibition of immune responses by bacterial products and extracts has previously been reported. Lipopolysaccharide endotoxin has been shown to be capable of blocking in vitro and in vivo immune responses. Finally some strains of Pseudomonas aeruginosa contain a cytoplasmic material which suppresses skin graft rejection in rats and humans.

Humoral factors

During the course of neonatal septicaemia with group B streptococcus factor B was found to be depressed by 30-35 %, C_3 by 40-60 % and CH_{50} by 100 % when compared to their cord blood levels [16].

Thrombocytopenia and deficiencies of the blood coagulation system have also been reported to accompany neonatal septicaemia. An increased binding by the platelets of IgG either monomeric or in the form of immune complexes, may contribute to platelet destruction in septic thrombocytopenia. Abnormalities in blood coagulation frequently found are low factors V, XI and XII, low partial thromboplastin time and low kallikreinogen and kallikrein inhibitor levels. Abnormalities in the coagulation system in septicaemic neonates can lead to massive disseminated intravascular coagulation particularly in neonates who have had cardiovascular collapse [20, 60].

THE ROLE OF TRANSFUSIONS AND EXCHANGE TRANSFUSIONS IN THE ENHANCEMENT OF NEONATAL HOST-DEFENCES

The clinical improvement and reduction in mortality of patients who have been exchange-transfused for sepsis has been reported in both adults and neonates [39]. Furthermore, small blood transfusions have been widely used for the treatment of severe neonatal infection. However, the immunologic mechanisms through which the enhancement of neonatal host-defences is achieved by these procedures are not yet fully elucidated and it is a subject which attracts the attention of both immunologists and neonatologists at the moment.

Exchange transfusions

The changes in the various leucocyte types in the peripheral blood during and following exchange transfusion have not been studied in septicaemic neonates but they have been studied in neonates being exchange transfused for hyperbilirubinaemia [56]. The main findings were: (a) marked reduction in all cell types during the procedure with a significant difference in absolute values before and immediately after, (b) significantly lower values of the polymorphonuclear neutrophils and eosinophils in the baby's blood at the end of the exchange transfusion compared with those of the donor's blood, with the monocytes and lymphocytes showing no change, and (c) a remarkable rise in each cell type starting soon after the procedure and reaching a peak within the week following the exchange transfusion. Thus, apart from this brief period of mild leucopenia immediately after the exchange transfusion there is a significant rise in the absolute values of all cell types following it.

The rise in polymorphonuclear neutrophils at a postnatal age when their absolute numbers are normally found to be dropping could be due to the displacement of neutrophils from the marginal layer of vessels and other extravascular pools which have been estimated in adults to contain 20 times the total number of circulating leucocytes. Increased marrow production was excluded as no significant changes regarding any cell type were found in neonatal bone marrows before and 3-4 days following exchange transfusion for jaundice.

With respect to the significant rise in lymphocytes following exchange-transfusion it has been questioned whether these are the baby's own or the donor's lymphocytes which had proliferated through various immunologic stimuli. The use of chromosome markers in female jaundiced neonates who had been exchange transfused with male donor blood solved the problem as it was shown that less than 2 % of the lymphocytes found in the babies peripheral blood 12 hours following the procedure belonged to the donor. However, when the same chromosome studies were applied in neonates who were exchange transfused for septicaemia it was found that in neonates with overwhelming infections the percentage of donor's lymphocytes in the neonatal peripheral blood 12 hours following the exchange transfusion was much higher reaching up to 70 %. This shows the inability of the host defense mechanisms of the neonate depressed by severe infection to dispose of the donor lymphocytes.

Lysozyme blood serum levels were also studied in neonates exchange transfused for hyperbilirubinemia. The activity of the enzyme immediately following the procedure was higher than that in the donor's blood. The rise in enzyme activity coincided with the significant fall in the absolute neutrophil numbers in the baby's blood, indicating destruction of the donor's neutrophils with extracellular release of the enzyme. Three to five days following the exchange transfusion, while the neutrophil count rose significantly, the enzyme's activity fell returning to levels normal for age.

Furthermore, the effect of exchange transfusion for hyperbilirubinemia was studied on phagocytosis and intracellular killing of neonatal polymorphonuclears using *Candida albicans*. Although no change was found in the ability of PMN's to kill there was a significantly increased ability to phagocytose 72 hours following exchange transfusion. Since the addition of adult serum, whether in vivo or in vitro, does not increase intracellular killing of *Candida albicans* by neonatal leucocytes, the deficiency of that function during the neonatal period should rather be attributed to an intracellular defect than to a deficiency of serum factors.

In neonates exchange-transfused for septicaemia increases in components of complement and immunoglobulins have been reported by various investigators. One such study showed that provided the exchange transfusion was performed with fresh blood-stored for less than 24 hours—with adequate opsonization for yeast and/or donor granulocytes with normal maximum NBT reductive capacity—there was an improvement in the corresponding function in the neonate's circulation [35].

Lymphocyte function using the in vitro tests of their mitogenic response to PHA and their ability to elicit antibody-dependent and PHA-induced cytotoxicities has been studied both in jaundiced and septicaemic neonates. Exchange transfusion was found to significantly improve these cell functions in both groups of neonates as early as 12 hours following the procedure [59].

Apart from the probable activation of neonatal lymphocytes by adult lymphocytes, the improvement in the various cellular and humoral immunologic factors following exchange transfusion helps to restore lymphocyte function which is depressed because of the infection. As we have seen, lymphocyte function depends on: (a) other cell functions, like those of macrophages and (b) humoral immunologic components. For example, C_{3b} on the target cell enhances cytolysis by K-cells.

Finally, we have seen that severe neonatal infection is often accompanied by disseminated intravascular coagulation (DIC). Exchange transfusion with fresh blood in these babies provides clotting factors and platelets in addition to removing fibrin degradation products and some of the toxic factors causing DIC. Heparin in the donor blood is also useful as a means of arresting the consumptive process and isolated reports suggest that the response to heparin may be dramatic.

It is well known that resistent gram-negative bacteria may cause fatal septicaemia which cannot be controlled by antibiotics. Furthermore, bacteria and their toxins cause significant depression of the already immature host-defence mechanism of the neonate. Repeated exchange transfusion for the treatment of neonatal septicaemia not only removes bacteria and bacterial toxins from the neonatal circulation but greatly enhances its immune mechanisms, by provoking an increase in the numbers of the various circulating white cell types, by improving their function and by providing many other valuable humoral immunologic factors. As graft-versus-host disease is rarely seen in these babies, exchange transfusion will prove to be an important therapy for severe neonatal infection.

Transfusions

Leucocyte transfusions. — Leucocyte replacement therapy for neutropenic patients with infections was first attempted in 1934 and has been tried sporadically thereafter.

Large doses of PMN's (2×10^{10}/mm) can transiently clear established gram-negative bacteremia in leukopenic animals, even without adding antibiotics. Leucocyte transfusions in leukemic, infected, infants have shown remarkable results: within 36 hours there is normalization of temperature and disappearance of the symptoms of infection, healing of ulcerations and necrosis and a rise in leucocyte count in the peripheral blood. Leucocytes survived in recipients up to 8 days despite the fact that 1 hour after transfusion only 5 % of the infused leucocytes were found in the recipients blood. However, to noticeably increase, the leucocyte count in blood more than 1×10^{10} cells are needed.

Polymorphonuclear transfusions have been tried in severly infected neonates, with the speculation that the presence of normal or even increased numbers of functionally inactive polymorphonuclears equates a septic newborn to a neutropenic patient. Concentrated PMN's (2×10^{10}) were given to neonates not responsive to antibiotics. Clinical improvement was noticed within a few hours. Both chemotactic and killing values surpassed normal ranges [26]. However, it is very difficult to obtain such a large numbers of neutrophils from healthy donors.

Transfusions of fresh whole blood. — Transfusions of fresh whole blood were evaluated as a means of supplying opsonins and lessening the high mortality due to group-B streptococcal sepsis in neonates. Opsonic activity rose only when donor blood containing heat-stable antibody was given in high volume (> 40 % of blood volume) [46]. There are a few case reports of single children in whom C_3 function or T-lymphocyte function was restored after blood transfusion.

Interestingly, in adult medical and surgical patients blood transfusion has been shown to cause a significant rise in the PHA-response 6-8 days following the transfusion. An increase in atypical lymphocytes has also been noted. It appears that administration of even small amounts of blood causes definite immunologic stimulation in the recipient. Small blood transfusions of the order of 20 ml/kg do not appear to significantly affect lymphocyte function in anemic neonates as judged by their ability to respond to PHA or elicit cytotoxicity. However, depressed lymphocyte function in septicaemic neonates improves significantly with small blood transfusions [59].

Although work on the effect of blood transfusions on the immunologic mechanisms of the neonate is limited, it appears that it enhances them.

THE ROLE OF HUMAN MILK
IN THE ENHANCEMENT
OF NEONATAL HOST DEFENCES

The human neonate has poorly developed functional and differentiated mechanisms of secretory immunity of its own during the first few weeks of life [32]. There seems little doubt that the immunoglobulin synthesizing plasma cells arise only after antigenic stimulation. This is evidenced by the observation that the newborn of most species, including man and the mouse completely lack immunoglobulin-containing cells in mucosal sites such as the gastrointestinal tract.

During the first days of life the newborn is first exposed to colonization with microbial organisms and, shortly thereafter, to the ingested milk and other dietary proteins. The availability of immunologic factors in the mammary gland exosecretions may thus represent an evolutionary event to compensate through breast feeding for the transient deficiency of mucosal immunity in the neonate.

The contribution of colostrum to neonatal immunity involves both humoral and cellular factors. Initially the soluble host-resistance factors were studied [54].

Humoral factors

Human milk was found to be rich in human proteins which bind nutrients needed for the growth of certain bacteria and fungi [8].

The most important of these is the well known lactoferrin. Lysozyme was found in exceptionally large quantities in human milk and in the stools of breast-fed infants. The 3rd and 4th components of complement were also found in modest quantities. Finally, anti-viral agents, such as interferon and fatty acids exhibiting non-specific anti-viral properties, were found.

However, the most important of the soluble host-resistance factors in human milk are its antibodies with the principle immunoglobulin being the secretory IgA. An important characteristic of secretory IgA is that it is most resistant to digestion which explains how it is found in the stools of breast-fed infants.

The protective roles of secretory IgA include viral neutralization, bactericidal activity, aggregation of antigens and prevention of adherence of bacteria to epithelial cells. Another aspect of the protective role of IgA antibodies is the ability to promote phagocytosis, particularly by monocytes.

IgM and IgG antibodies are also found in human milk, but in small quantities.

It is interesting that in piglets and calves all the antibodies necessary for their protection are acquired from colostrum and milk by absorption through the intestinal wall during the first few hours of life. Deprivation of milk causes them to die from septicaemia. Until very recently it was believed that in human neonates immunoglobulins of breast-milk cannot cross the intestinal wall. However, colostral IgA has been found in the circulation of human neonates fed with colostrum between 18-24 hours after birth.

Cellular factors

The cells of human colostrum and milk have been little studied although they were discovered more than a century ago [37, 54]. The cells of human colostrum were first observed by the pioneer biologist-microscopist-photographer Alexandre Donné who is credited with obtaining their first photographic portrait in 1839. He called them "corpuscles" and was unable to distinguish their cellular nature. The "corpuscles" of Donné were found to be cells 20 years later, in 1868, when Beigel examined stained preparations of colostrum microscopically. The functions of the cells were not examined in those early studies and remained virtually unknown to immunologists. In 1966, Smith, in Goldman's laboratory, examining the "debris" that was obtained after centrifuging colostrum, was surprised to find what Donné had observed 122 years before. Phase microscopy revealed that colostrum was packed with living motile cells.

Because of the high fat content of colostrum, the usual cell-counting procedures are difficult and inaccurate. Consequently, alternate methods and staining procedures to those used for blood leucocytes have been devised, during which there is usually a loss of cells.

In general terms the total white cell count in colostrum has been found to vary from 1×10^5 to 1×10^7/ml and to decrease 5 to 10 times by the fifth post-partum day. The mean total WCC later on in milk ranges from 1×10^4 to 2×10^5/ml, but because of the increase in the quantity of milk offered, the total number of cells available to the neonate remains large.

The types of leucocytes seen in colostrum are usually monocytic macrophages 40-50 %, polymorphonuclear neutrophils 40-50 % and lymphocytes 5-10 %. Numerous epithelial cells and epithelial cell-fragments are also seen in human colostrum. Later on, human milk consists of 85 % monocytes or macrophages and 10-11 % small lymphocytes. Morphologically, the neutrophils are typical of those seen in the blood except that they contain numerous fat globules and fewer granules. Monocytes or macrophages also contain many fat globules and other granular material. The typical colostral corpuscle of Donné is a very large lipid laden monocyte. Lymphocytes appear similar to those found in the peripheral blood.

With respect to the function of milk leucocytes, the first cells studied were the lymphocytes [15]. Milk lymphocytes were found to consist of 50 %

T- and 50 % B-cells, half of which bear IgA immuno-globulin. Furthermore, human milk lymphocytes have been found to produce secretory IgA immuno-globulin, to release soluble mediators (MIF) and to produce interferon. They were shown to respond weakly to non-specific mitogens like PHA and to histocompatibility antigens on allogenic cells. However, they were found to have the ability to respond in vitro to various viral and microbial anti-gens like those of *E. coli*, candida, tetanus, strepto-kinase, mumps, measles, etc. Milk lymphocytes responded in vitro to different antigens than blood lymphocytes from the same individual.

It is interesting that T- or B-lymphocytes specific for the enteric antigens appear in the mammary secretions following gastrointestinal exposure to the antigen. Non pathogenic strains of *E. coli* adminis-tered to human pregnant volunteers led to the rapid appearance of colostral cells producing antibodies against the O antigen of the organism. This was probably due to a selective transfer of sensitized lymphocytes from the G. I. tract to the mammary gland. Thus, oral immunization or the presentation of antigen to the intestinal mucosa may be an important factor in the induction of colostral humo-ral immunity. Nature has appeared to endow the breast-milk with the special function of selecting only certain immunologic gifts for the neonate. Yet, it is through the same mechanism that the maternal milk may obtain antibodies against dietary antigens, including cow's milk proteins.

Finally, it was found that leucocytes in rats may be transmitted naturally from the mother's blood stream to the suckling's blood stream through the milk and in this way may be beneficial causing adap-tive immunity or harmful causing graft-versus host disease. We have no evidence so far that the human milk leucocytes cross the intestinal wall and enter the neonatal circulation. However, two neonates have been reported who after 5 weeks of nursing by tuberculin positive mothers developed a specific proliferative response to tuberculin.

The monocytic macrophages in breast milk are motile cells which adhere to glass. They have been shown to synthesize components of complement, lysozyme and lactoferrin and to serve as a transport vehicle capable of delayed immunoglobulin release.

In rats it has been demonstrated that a Klebsiella-induced necrotizing enterocolitis could be pre-vented by feeding rat colostral macrophages but not by feeding the soluble colostral factors [38]. These findings are in agreement with the observa-tion that necrotizing enterocolitis is infrequent in infants fed untreated breast milk. Human milk macrophages and neutrophils have been reported

to phagocytose and kill *Staph. aureus* and *E. coli* —in vitro—as effectively as blood leucocytes. However, other investigators have reported good phagocytosis, but poor intracellular killing of *E. coli* by colostral phagocytes. The antibody-dependent cytotoxicity of milk monocytes where human erythrocytes were used as targets was found to be lower than that elicited by peripheral blood monocytes. The ingestion of lipid by milk phagocytes may be the cause of their reduced killing power. It has been suggested that ingestion of lipids results in disruption of lysosomes and depletion of lysosomal enzymes.

Thus, human milk has the potential of enhancing, in a number of ways, the host defence mechanisms of the neonate. In support of this, epidemiologic studies have periodically suggested that breast fed infants have a lower mortality and morbidity from gastrointestinal infections, necrotizing entero-colitis and respiratory infections.

IMMUNE DEFICIENCY DISEASES OF THE NEONATE

Failure of the immunologic response to maintain homeostasis between the internal body environment and the external environment leads to an immuno-logic imbalance which are expressed as the immuno-logically mediated diseases. There may be failure to produce sufficient effector cells or cell products, or they may be defective in type. Depending on the level of the block of cellular development more or less complex and serious immune deficiency diseases have been described. The various immunodeficiency states are summarized in Figure IV-7.

Repeated infections and a predisposition to mali-gnant tumors and autoimmune diseases have been found in patients with immunodeficiency.

The diagnosis of immune deficiency diseases during the neonatal period is difficult for several reasons. Many immunologic mechanisms are imma-ture during this period of life and in some instances it is impossible to differentiate immaturity from abnormality. Secondly, placentally transferred ma-ternal cells and humoral factors influence the various diagnostic tests. Thirdly most newborns with immu-nodeficiency diseases appear normal clinically during the neonatal period.

Early diagnosis however is very important as it will result in caution regarding harmful blood or exchange transfusions and routine immunizations. Furthermore the known spectrum of pathogenic

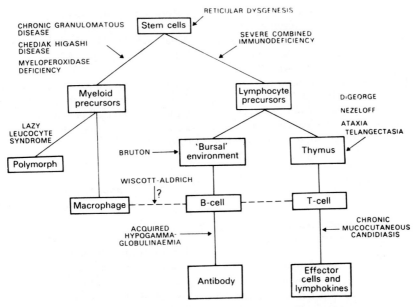

FIG. IV-7. — *The cellular basis of immunodeficiency states. The arrow indicates the type of cell or the differentiation process which is deficient.* (From ROITT H. M.: *Essential Immunology.* 3rd ed., Blackwell Scientific Publications, Oxford, 1978.

organisms specific to each of the various disease groups will help in the selection of the appropriate antibiotic treatment. Thus B-cell abnormalities are well known to be associated with encapsulated bacteria, T-cell disorders with fungi or viruses and neutrophil dysfunction with commensal bacteria. Finally, family counseling will be improved and the cases for prenatal diagnosis will be identified.

SEVERE COMBINED
IMMUNODEFICIENCY DISEASE (SCID)

Without proper differentiation of the common lymphoid stem cells, both T- and B-lymphocytes fail to develop and there is a severe combined immunodeficiency of both cellular and humoral responses [51, 52].

The rapidly fatal variant of severe combined immunodeficiency associated with lack of myeloid cell precursors is termed "reticular dysgenesis".

The frequent existence of a few T-lymphocytes and B-lymphocytes at birth argues against a complete absence of lymphoid stem cells in SCID. Different diseases with different causes are, at present, included in this syndrome but in all cases T-lymphocyte differentiation is prevented at an early stage. The spectrum of abnormalities found in the differentiation of the B-cell system probably results

either from an associated alteration of B-cell precursors or from the lack of normal T-lymphocytes.

Combined immunodeficiency occurs as an X-linked recessive, autosomal recessive and as sporadic forms. Some patients lack the enzyme adenosine deaminase (ADA) and some the enzyme purine nucleoside phosphorylase (PNP). Neonates with combined immunodeficiency disease and associated ADA or PNP deficiencies may be diagnosed at birth by red blood cell enzyme determinations. As PNP and ADA levels may also be determined in fibroblast cultures intrauterine diagnosis is possible when the family history is suggestive. ADA deficiency has been associated with both T- and B-cell deficiency while PNP deficiency has been mainly associated with T-cell deficiency.

Onset of symptoms frequently occurs during the first month of life. The most common findings are resistant diarrhoea with failure to thrive, rashes, perianal or perioral candidiasis and deficient lymphoid tissue. Without treatment, death is inevitable by 1 to 2 years of age.

Graft-versus host reactions are frequently encountered in patients with SCID. In neonates GVH reactions are induced by transplacental passage of maternal lymphocytes and their reaction against paternally inherited alloantigens of the fetus. Transfusion of blood or blood products may also induce GVH reactions in neonates with SCID.

The goal of treatment is to replace the missing components of the immune system. Transplantation of bone marrow or fetal liver from genotypically matched donors offers hope for patients with these disorders. Thymus transplantation, especially the use of cultured thymic epithelium, injection of thymocin and replacement of deficient enzymes is currently being evaluated.

PRIMARY DEFICIENCIES MAINLY AFFECTING T-CELLS

Di George syndrome. — The counterpart to neonatal thymectomy experiments is represented in man by a variety of syndromes in which there is congenital failure of thymic development. The most clearly characterized of these is Di George syndrome which is also the most clinically characteristic form of immunodeficiency occuring during the neonatal period [30].

In 1965, Di George [52] described the association between infection, absent thymus and congenital hypoparathyroidism in three infants. A variable severe dysembryogenesis of branchial pouches I to VI was postulated to explain the abnormalities.

Infants with Di George syndrome commonly present during the first week of life with congenital heart disease, neonatal tetany secondary to primary hypoparathyroidism and abnormal facies. Features of the abnormal facies may include hypertelorism, notched ear pinnae, micrognathia, antimongoloid slant of the eyes, fish shaped mouth and low set ears. Cardiac abnormalities, which are present in nearly all patients, have included right-sided aortic arch, aberrant left subclavian artery, right ventricular infundibular stenosis, ventricular septal defect, pulmonary artery atresia and hypoplastic pulmonary artery. The clinical expression of immune deficiency is similar to that of other syndromes with subnormal T-cell function. The patients usually develop oral candidiasis, chronic diarrhoea and failure to thrive during the first year of life. The overall health of the patient is also affected by the severity of the cardiovascular malformations and by the control of the hypocalcemia.

With the extensive evaluation of cellular immunity several descriptions of "partial" Di George syndrome have been reported.

Treatment by grafting neonatal thymus leads to restoration of immunocompetence but unless graft and donor are well matched, the thymus is ultimately rejected "by the ungrateful host cells it has helped to maturity" [42].

Other syndromes. — Other syndromes including T-cell disorders which present extremely rarely during the neonatal period are Nezelof's syndrome; ataxia telangiectasia and chronic mucocutaneous candidiasis.

PRIMARY DEFICIENCIES MAINLY AFFECTING B-CELLS

Congenital hypogammaglobulinaemias. — As with T-cell disorders a group of abnormalities of B-cell function have been described.

In Bruton's infantile sex-linked a-γ-globulinaemia the production of immunoglobulins is grossly depressed and no antibody production can be induced in response to antigenic stimulation. As T-cell mediated immune responses are normal this disease represents an experiment of nature which closely mimics the effect of bursectomy in birds.

It is now recognized that congenital hypogammaglobulinaemias are of several genetic types, including an X-linked recessive type (the Bruton's type) an autosomal recessive type, and a sporadic type.

Infants with this disorder do well during the first months of life. The maternally acquired IgG provides adequate protection during this time. After the maternal immunoglobulin is catabolized, severe suppurative recurrent infections with encapsulated pyogenic bacteria occur.

Treatment involves repeated administration of immune serum globulins to maintain adequate circulating levels.

Transient hypogammaglobulinaemias of infancy. — Immunoglobulin deficiency occurs naturally in human infants as the transplacentally acquired maternal IgG level wanes. Transient hypogammaglobulinaemia of infancy is a self-limited disorder, characterized by an abnormally prolonged delay in the onset of gamma globulin synthesis by the infant. Premature infants are particularly prone to this disorder as a result of diminished placental transport of IgG during gestation.

The disease occurs equally in both sexes. Following recovery by 9 to 15 months of age there is no evidence of permanent abnormality of the immune system. The etiology remains unknown; occasionally it is familial.

PRIMARY PHAGOCYTIC CELL DEFICIENCIES

Clinical diseases affecting phagocytes fall into two classes: (*a*) quantitative, *i. e.* those in which the total number of phagocytes are decreased and (*b*) qualitative, those in which the total number of phagocytes is normal but the cells are functionally defective.

Inherited neutropenias. — Inherited neutropenias occur either associated with stigmata of congenital syndromes or as isolated defects. There are X-linked recessive and autosomal dominant types. The pathogenesis may involve both diminished production and increased immune destruction.

Regardless of etiology most patients with neutropenia do not present with infection during the neonatal period. Infantile genetic agranulocytosis, a disease with an autosomal recessive mode of transmission found with a high frequency in Sweden, is an exception and frequently presents during the first month of life [25].

Neutropenias occuring in episodic fashion are referred to as cyclic. Some of the noncyclic ones follow a benign course with possible spontaneous cure in later childhood.

The diagnosis depends: (*a*) on family history, including parental consanguinity and (*b*) on haematologic studies, including bone marrow analysis. It is sometimes difficult to distinguish hereditary neutropenias from the transient neonatal neutropenias associated with maternal isoimmunization. In the latter the neutrophil count begins to rise after the first month of life along with the reduction of the maternally acquired IgG antileucocyte antibodies whose half life is 20 to 30 days.

Neutrophil transfusions have been used in the treatment of severe infections in patients with neutropenia.

Effective prevention of the hereditary neutropenias depends on genetic counseling.

Chronic granulomatous disease. — Chronic granulomatous disease is the prototype of defective bactericidal activity [30]. In this disease the monocytes and polymorphonuclears fail to produce hydrogen peroxide (H_2O_2) due to a defect in the respiratory enzymes normally activated by phagocytosis. Many bacteria produce H_2O_2 through their own metabolic processes and if they are catalase negative (as *H. influenzae*, *streptococci* and *pneumococci*) the bactericidal process continues normally. However if the bacteria are catalase positive (as

staphylococci and enteric organisms) the peroxide is destroyed and the bacteria will survive. Thus, polymorphonuclears from these patients phagocytose normally catalase positive organisms in the presence of antibody and complement but fail to kill them intracellularly.

Two genetic patterns of inheritance of CGD exist: X-linked and autosomal recessive.

The onset of symptoms is usually at about the age of one year, when the first recurrent and severe episodes of sepsis and disseminated abscesses occur. The characteristic suppurative granulomas are found throughout the body. They consist of inflammatory cells surrounding a necrotic central core. These granulomata are similar to those found in infectious granulomatosis. In infectious granulomatosis the microorganisms possess properties enabling them to resist phagocytic digestion by normal cells. In CGD, the metabolic abnormality of host cells allows persistence of organisms.

The diagnosis should be considered in a neonate when such a diagnosis has been previously made in a male member of the family. The diagnostic value of NBT dye reduction test in the neonate is questionable as neonatal leucocytes normally reduce NBT dye less effectively following phagocytic stimulation. However it is possible to diagnose CGD in newborns by testing the bactericidal capacity of their phagocytes.

For treatment of this disease high doses of bactericidal antibiotics are indicated.

The lazy-leucocyte syndrome. — The lazy-leucocyte syndrome represents an intrinsic defect of neutrophil chemotaxis. These patients suffer from low grade infections, are neutropenic and fail to generate inflammatory cells normally by the skin-window technique. The immaturity of the chemotactic function in normal neonates makes the diagnosis extremely difficult and it may not be confirmed until the patient is well beyond the neonatal period.

Wiscott-Aldrich syndrome. — The sex-linked recessive Wiscott-Aldrich syndrome is another immunodeficiency disorder which can be diagnosed during the neonatal period [52]. It is characterized by thrombocytopenia with a hemorrhagic tendency, eczema and immunodeficiency with recurrent infection.

This syndrome is associated with low IgM levels and poor antibody responses to many polysaccharides. Evidence that a vital defect in macrophage presentation of antigen underlies the disorder has been presented. It has also been related to defective monocyte chemotaxis [1].

Persistant thrombocytopenia of unknown etiology in a male infant suggests the diagnosis of Wiscott-Aldrich syndrome. Although cellular immunity may be relatively normal in these newborns small platelet size is characteristic. Therefore, in newborn male infants with persistent thrombocytopenia the diagnosis of Wiscott-Aldrich syndrome can be made by platelet sizing, in addition, intrauterine diagnosis may be feasible.

Treatment with transfer factor has been used in a number of patients with this syndrome and over 50 % have shown improvement in the susceptibility to infections and the chronic eczema, with reduction of their splenomegaly.

COMPLEMENT DISORDERS

Leiner's disease. — Congenital deficiencies have been described for all but the ninth component of complement. While any of these deficiencies can theoretically occur during the neonatal period only C_5 dysfunction (Leiner's disease) generally presents under the age of one month. The syndrome is characterized by severe seborrheic dermatitis, diarrhea, recurrent infections and marked dystrophy.

Seborrheic dermatitis is not enough to establish a diagnosis of Leiner's disease, the demonstration of deficient opsonic activity of the patient's serum is necessary. The dysfunction of C_5 is detected only by an assay which measures its biologic activity; quantitative levels of C_5 as measured by standard immunochemical techniques are often found to be within normal limits.

For treatment, whole blood or plasma transfusions are used. Fresh plasma or blood is satisfactory, whereas refrigirated plasma or blood over 24 hours old is not.

SECONDARY IMMUNODEFICIENCIES *

Some of the immunodeficiency syndromes which cannot be traced to a genetic defect may be acquired due to intrauterine infection. The timing of the injury during development is of particular importance. If it occurs before or during the maximum growth and development phase of a given organ, permanent damage and deficiency is to be expected.

Cell-mediated immunity may be impaired in a state of malnutrition as seen in small for dates neonates [17].

* See also section on AIDS by the author p. 659-661.

Finally other agents such as viral and other infections, cytotoxic drugs and corticosteroids can depress the immunologic responses of the neonates. Such secondary immunologic deficiencies are more common than the primary ones which are only rarely found.

REFERENCES

[1] ALTMAN (L. C.), SNYDERMAN (R.), BLAESE (R. M.). — Abnormalities of chemotactic lymphokine synthesis and mononuclear leukocyte chemotaxis in Wiscott-Aldrich syndrome. *Clin. Invest.*, 54, 486-493, 1974.

[2] AMBRUSO (D. R.), ALTENBURGER (K. M.), JOHNSTON (R. B.). — Defective oxidative metabolism in newborn neutrophils: Descrepancy between superoxide anion and hydroxyl radical generation. *Pediatrics* (suppl.), 722-725, 1979.

[3] ANDERSEN (V.), HANSEN (N. E.), KARLE (H.), LIND (I.), HOIBY (N.), WEEKE (B.). — Sequential studies of lymphocytes responsiveness and antibody formation in acute bacterial meningitis. *J. Exp. Immunol.*, 26, 469-477, 1976.

[3 bis] BACH (J. F.), LESAVRE (P.). — *Immunologie*. Flammarion, ed., Paris, 1982.

[4] BELLANTI (J. A.). — Introduction to immunology. In *Immunology II*, 2nd ed. BELLANTI (J. A.), ed. Saunders Co., Philadelphia, 1978.

[5] BELLANTI (J. A.). — General Immunobiology. In *Immunology II*, 2nd ed., BELLANTI (J. A.), ed. Saunders Co., Philadelphia, 1978.

[6] BELLANTI (J. A.), RAKLIN (R. E.). — Cell-mediated reactions. In *Immunology II*, 2nd ed., BELLANTI (J. A.), ed. Saunders Co., Philadelphia, 1978.

[7] BELLANTI (J. A.), NERURKAR (L. S.), ZELIGS (B. J.). — Host defences in the fetus and neonate: Studies of the alveolar macrophage during maturation. *Pediatrics*, 64 (suppl.), 726-739, 1979.

[8] BEZKOROVAINY (A.). — Human milk and colostrum proteins: A review. *J. Dairy Sci.*, 60, 1023-1037, 1977.

[9] BLAISE (R. M.), POPLAK (D. G.), MUCLIMADE (A. V.). — The mononuclear phagocyte system: Role in expression of immunocompetence on neonatal and adult life. *Pediatrics* (suppl.), 829-833, 1979.

[10] BOXER (L. A.). — Immunological function and leucocyte disorders in newborn infants. *Clin. Haematol.*, 7, 123-146, 1978.

[11] CAMPBELL (A. C.), WALLER (C.), WOOD (J.), AYNSLEY-GREEN (A.), YU (V.). — Lymphocyte subpopulations in the blood of newborn infants. *Clin. Exp. Immunol.*, 18, 469-482, 1974.

[12] CAMPBELL (A. C.). — Lymphocyte subpopulations and their measurement. P. H. D. *Thesis Oxford*, 1976.

[13] CARR (M. C.), STITES (D. P.), FUDENBERG (H. H.). — Cellular immune aspects of the human fetal-maternal relationship. I. *In vitro* response of cord blood lymphocytes to phytohemagglutinin. *Cell. Immunol.*, 5, 21-29, 1972.

[14] CARTWRIGHT (G. E.), ATHENS (J. W.), WINTROBE (M. M.). — The kinetics of granulopoiesis in normal man. *Blood*, 24, 780, 1964.

[15] DIAZ-JOUANEN (E.), WILLIAMS (R. C.). — T and B lymphocytes in human colostrum. *Clin. Immunol. Immunopathol.*, 3, 248-255, 1974.

[16] FENTON (L. J.), STRUNK (R. C.). — Complement activation and group B streptococcal infection in the newborn: Similarities to endotoxin shock. *Pediatrics, 60*, 901-907, 1977.

[17] FERGUSON (A. C.). — Prolonged impairment of cellular immunity in children with intrauterine growth retardation. *J. Pediatr., 93*, 52-56, 1978.

[18] GRANBERG (C.), MANNINEN (K.), TOIVANEN (P.). — Cell-mediated lympholysis by human neonatal lymphocytes. *Clin. Immunol. Immunopathol., 6*, 256-263, 1976.

[18 bis] GRISCELLI (C.). — Récepteurs membranaires lymphocytes. Leurs implications dans le développement immunologique. *Résumé 1er Congrès de la Société Française de Recherche en Pédiatrie*, Montpellier, 1983.

[19] HALLBERG (A.). — Receptors for immunoglobulin and complement on sheep RBC-binding lymphocytes in newborn infants. *Clin. Exp. Immunol., 34*, 69-77, 1978.

[20] HATHAWAY (W. E.), BONNAR (J.). — *Perinatal coagulation in monographs in neonatology*, HATHAWAY (W. E.), BONNAR (J.) eds. Grune and Stratton, New York, 1978.

[21] HAYWARD (A. R.), LYDYARD (P. B.). — B-cell function in the newborn. *Pediatrics, 64* (suppl.), 758-764, 1979.

[22] HERSCOWITZ (H. B.). — Immunophysiology: Cell function and cellular interactions. In *Immunology II*, 2nd ed., BELLANTI (J. A.) ed. Saunders Co., Philadelphia, 1978.

[23] HOWE (C. W. S.). — *Lymphocyte physiology during pregnancy: in vivo and in vitro studies in immunobiology of trophoblast.* EDWARDS (R. G.), HOWE (C. W. S.), JOHNSON (M. H.) eds. Cambridge University Press, Cambridge, 1975.

[24] JOHNSTON (R. V. Jr.), ALTENBURGER (K. M.), ATKINSON (A. W. Jr.), CURRY (R. H.). — Complement in the newborn infant. *Pediatrics, 64* (suppl.), 781-786, 1979.

[25] KOSTMANN (R.). — Infantile Genetic Agranulocytosis. *Acta Paediatr. Scand., 64*, 362-368, 1975.

[26] LAURENTI (F.), LAGRECA (G.), FERRO (R.), BUCCI (G.). — Transfusion of polymorphonuclear neutrophils in a premature infant with klebsiella sepsis. *Lancet, 2*, 111-112, 1978.

[27] LAWTON (A. R.), COOPER (M. D.). — Immunoglobulin genes and their expression. *Pediatrics, 64* (suppl.), 750-757, 1979.

[28] McCONNACHIE (P. R.), RACHELEFSKY (G.), STIEHM (E. R.), TERASAKI (P. I.). — Antibody-dependent lymphocyte killer function and age. *Pediatrics, 52*, 795-799, 1973.

[29] MacDONALD (H. R.), BONNARD (G. D.), SORDAT (B.), ZAWODNIK (S. A.). — Antibody-dependent cell-mediated cytotoxicity: Hererogeneity of effector cells in human peripheral blood. *Scand. J. Immunol., 4*, 488-497, 1975.

[30] MILLER (M. E.). — Host defences in the human neonate. In *Monographs in neonatology*, MILLER (M. E.) ed. Grune and Stratton, New York, 1978.

[31] MILLER (M. E.). — Phagocyte function in the neonate: Selected aspects. *Pediatrics, 64* (suppl.), 709-712, 1979.

[32] OGRA (P. L.). — Ontogeny of the local immune system. *Pediatrics, 64* (suppl.), 765-774, 1979.

[33] OLDING (L. B.), MURGITA (R. A.), WIGZELL (H.). — Mitogen-stimulated lymphoid cells from human newborns suppress the proliferation of maternal lymphocytes across the cell-impermeable membrane. *Immunology, 119*, 1109-1114, 1977.

[34] PARK (B. H.), HOLMES (B.), GOOD (R. A.). — Metabolic activities in leucocytes of newborn infants. *J. Pediatr.*, 237-241, 1970.

[35] PELET (B.). — Exchange transfusion in newborn infants: Effects on granulocyte function. *Arch. Dis. Child., 54*, 687-690, 1979.

[36] PRINDULL (G.). — Maturation of cellular and humoral immunity during human embryonic development. *Acta Paediatr. Scand., 63*, 607-675, 1974.

[37] PITTARD (W. B.). — Breast Milk Immunology. *Am. J. Dis. Child., 133*, 83-87, 1979.

[38] PITT (J.), BARLOW (B.), HEIRD (W. C.). — Protection against experimental necrotizing enterocolitis by maternal milk. I. Role of milk leukocytes. *Pediat. Res., 11*, 906-909, 1977.

[39] PROD'HOM (L. S.), LEMOS (L.), MAZOUNI (M.), TORRADO (A.). — Exchange tranfusions of fresh whole blood as treatment of severe neonatal septicaemia associated with sclerema neonatorum. *Current Topics in Pediatrics*, XVth International Congress of Pediatrics, New Delhi, India, 236, October 1977.

[40] PROSS (S. H.), HALLOCK (J. A.), ARMSTRONG (R.), FISHEL (C. W.). — Complement and Fc Receptors on Cord Blood and Adult Neutrophils. *Pediat. Res., 11*, 135-137, 1977.

[41] QUIE (P. G.), MILLS (E. L.). — Bactericidal and metabolic function of polymorphonuclear leukocytes. *Pediatrics, 64* (suppl.), 719-721, 1979.

[42] ROITT (I. M.). — *Essential Immunology*, 3rd ed. Blackwell Scientific Publications, Oxford, 1978.

[43] ROSSE (C.), KRAEMER (M. J.), DILLON (T. L.), McFARLAND (R.), SMITH (N. J.). — Bone marrow cell populations of normal infants: the predominance of lymphocyte. *J. Lab. Clin. Med., 89*, 1225-1240, 1977.

[44] SCHUIT (K. E.), POWELL (D. A.). — Phagocytic dysfunction in monocytes of normal newborn infants. *Pediatrics, 65*, 501-504, 1980.

[45] SEMENZATO (G.), PIOVESAN (A.), AMADORI (G.), COLOMBATTI (M.), GASPAROTTO (G.), RUBARTELLI (F. F.). — T cell immune function in newborn infants. *Biol. Neonate, 37*, 8-14, 1980.

[46] SHIGEOKA (A. D.), HALL (R. T.), HILL (H. R.). — Blood transfusion in group B streptococcal sepsis. *Lancet, 1*, 636-638, 1978.

[47] SHORE (S. L.), MILGROM (H.), WOOD (P. A.), NAHMIAS (A. J.). — Antibody-dependent cellular cytotoxicity to target cells infected with herpes simplex viruses: Functional adequacy of the neonate. *Pediatrics, 59*, 22-28, 1977.

[48] STIEHM (E. R.). — Fetal defence mechanisms. *Am. J. Dis. Child., 129*, 438-443, 1975.

[49] STIEHM (E. R.), WINTER (H. S.), BRYSON (Y. J.). — Cellular (T cell) immunity in the human newborn. *Pediatrics, 64* (suppl.), 814-821, 1979.

[50] STITES (D. P.), PAVIA (C. S.). — Ontogeny of human T cells. *Pediatrics, 64* (suppl.), 795-802, 1979.

[51] TOURAINE (J. L.). — Human T-lymphocyte differentiation in immunodeficiency diseases and after reconstitution by bone marrow or fetal thymus transplantation. *Clin. Immunol. Immunopathol., 12*, 228-237, 1979.

[52] WARA (D. W.), BARRETT (D. J.). — Cell-mediated immunity in the newborn: Clinical aspects. *Pediatrics, 64* (suppl.), 822-828, 1979.

[53] WARD (P. A.). — Mechanisms of tissue injury. In *Immunology II*, 2nd ed., BELLANTI (J. A.) ed. Saunders Co., Philadelphia, 1978.

[53 *bis*] WEIR (D. M.). — Immunology. An outline for students of Medicine and Biology. Churchill Livingstone, Edinburgh, London, Melbourne and New York, 1983.

[54] WELSH (J. K.), MAY (J. T.). — Anti-infective properties of breast milk. *J. Pediatr.*, *94*, 1-9, 1979.

[55] XANTHOU (M.). — Leukocyte blood picture in healthy full-term and premature babies during neonatal period. *Arch. Dis. Child.*, *45*, 242-249, 1970.

[56] XANTHOU (M.), NICOLOPOULOS (D.), GIZAS (A.), MATSANIOTIS (N.). — The response of leucocytes in the peripheral blood during and following exchange transfusion in the newborn. *Pediatrics*, *51*, 571-574, 1973.

[57] XANTHOU (M.), AGATHOPOULOS (A.), SAKELLA-RIOU (A.), ECONOMOU-MAVROU (C.), TSINGO-GLOU (S.), MATSANIOTIS (N.). — Serum levels of lysozyme in term and preterm newborns. *Arch. Dis. Child.*, *50*, 304-307, 1975

[58] XANTHOU (M.), MANDYLA-SFAGOU (H.), CAMPBELL (A. C.), WALLER (C. A.), ECONOMOU-MAVROU (C.), MATSANIOTIS (N.). — Lymphocyte subpopulations and their function in the blood of neonates. In *Intensive Care in Newborn*, STERN (L.), FRIIS-HANSEN (B.), KILDEBERG, eds. Masson, New York, 1976.

[59] XANTHOU (M.), MANDYLA-SFAGOU (H.), ECONO-MOU-MAVROU (C.), MATSANIOTIS (N.). — Lymphocyte function in anemic jaundiced and severely infected neonates: effect of transfusions and exchange transfusions. In *Intensive Care in the Newborn II*, STERN (L.), OH (W.), FRIIS-HANSEN (B.) eds. Masson, New York, 1978.

[60] ZIPURSKY (A.), JABER (H. M.). — The Haematology of bacterial infection in newborn infants. *Clin. Haematol.*, *7*, 175-193, 1978.

29

Bacterial infections in the newborn

A. CALAME, B. VAUDAUX

INTRODUCTION

Bacterial infections in the fetus and the neonate are frequent occurences. They are difficult to diagnose, have an apparently unpredictable course and the mortality is still high in spite of modern management.

These features have prompted many neonatologists to initiate early antibiotic therapy in any newborn likely to develop a bacterial infection.

Though seemingly prudent, this attitude is anything but innocuous, as exemplified by historical instances of sulfonamides (kernicterus) and chloramphenicol (gray syndrome).

We believe that the diversity of symptoms as well as the variability in the course and prognosis of bacterial infections can be understood and to some extent predicted on the basis of the routes of infection and the timing of the infectious process. The approach of early broad-spectrum, blind, antibiotic therapy ignores both the routes and the timing of the infection.

The purpose of this chapter is to depict a physiopathological and pathogenic approach to the problem of bacterial infections, with logical and practical consequences for diagnosis and management.

DEFINITION, INCIDENCE, MORTALITY

By definition, septicemias (positive blood cultures within the first 28 days of life with or without organ localisation) as well as bacteriologically proven organ infections without positive blood culture are included as bacterial infections.

The incidence of neonatal septicemia is generally estimated at about one case per thousand births [71]. Figures may differ according to local socio-economic conditions, hospital hygiene practices as well as the sample considered (healthy newborns, sick newborns, premature newborns). In a population of premature infants the incidence of bacterial infection is about 4 $\%_{oo}$ livebirths [72]. It may be as high as 164 $\%_{oo}$ in populations of very low birthweight infants [18].

The mortality rate from neonatal septicemia will depend on the route of infection, the timing of the infection in relation to birth, the infectious load and the newborn population under study. It is between 10 and 20 % for late postnatal infections and rises to 50 % for severe infections that are acquired in utero or intra partum by premature infants [99].

ENVIRONMENT OF THE FETUS AND NEWBORN. HOST RESPONSES TO INFECTION

Understanding the pathogenesis of fetal and neo-natal infections requires awareness of the following points:

— Anatomical and functional relationships between the fetus and its environment.

— Host responses of the fetus and term neonate to bacterial infections.

— Indigenous vaginal and cervical flora throughout pregnancy.

— Natural process of bacterial colonization of the newborn infant.

Anatomical and functional relationships between the fetus and its environment.

— The fetus is naturally protected from infections. Responsible for that protection are ana-tomical and functional barriers:

(*a*) The anatomical barriers consist of the fetal membranes and the placenta. Fetal membranes (amnion and chorion) keep the fetus separated from the maternal genital tract (Fig. IV-8). The placenta separates maternal from fetal blood. Throughout the second half of pregnancy, the placental barrier consists of three histologically distinct layers within villi: syncythiotrophoblast, connective tissue and capillary vascular endothelium.

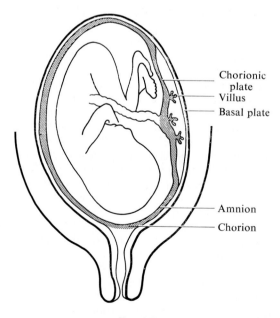

	Chorionic plate
	Villus
	Basal plate
	Amnion
	Chorion

FIG. IV-8.

(*b*) The functional barrier consists of the amniotic fluid that possesses bacteriostatic activity owing to the presence of lysozyme and transferrin as well as immune globulins [61]. This antibacterial activity increases progressively during pregnancy right up to term [23].

Host responses of the fetus and term newborn to bacterial infections.

— The three compartments of the immune system (*i. e.*: non specific immunity, humoral immunity, cell-mediated immunity) are not fully functional at birth. The fetus or neonate is in a position of lesser resistance against bacterial infections.

Lymphocytes can be identified in fetuses from the ninth gestational week. They are divided into two groups: T-cells that are responsible for cell-mediated immunity, and B-cells responsible for humoral immunity.

Cell-mediated immunity. — T-lymphocytes are effector cells for delayed hypersensitivity reactions. They participate in foreign tissue rejection reactions and, upon stimulation by mitogenic substances, produce chemical mediators termed lymphokines. They are also of utmost importance for protection against a large number of infectious agents.

Cell-mediated immunity is already well developed and functional at birth. This is evidenced by positive delayed hypersensitivity reactions, by the ability of cord blood lymphocytes to respond to phytohemag-glutinin or other mitogens' stimulation [66], and by a potential for rejection reactions [90].

Humoral immunity. — The fetus is capable of serum immune globulin production from the thirteenth week of gestation [121]. However, under normal conditions this production is very low as a result of the fetus being protected from antigenic agression.

The newborn infant's immune endowment nor-mally consists of IgG's of maternal origin that are acquired transplacentally. This transplacental trans-fer is an active process that involves a carrier attaching to the Fc fragment of the IgG's heavy chains. The intensity of this process is directly correlated to the degree of placental maturity [119]. Other classes of immune globulins (IgM, IgA...) cannot cross the placenta. Consequently, near term, IgG antibodies are at higher levels in fetal than in maternal blood, as opposed to IgM or IgA anti-bodies that are in very low concentrations in fetal blood.

Under normal conditions the newborn infant is protected by IgG's of maternal origin against a number of bacterial infections which the mother has previously experienced. However, the neonate can be remarkably susceptible to some agents, such as gram-negative rods, whose specific bactericidal antibodies belong mostly to the IgM class and thus are unable to cross the placenta.

The neonate will respond to a postnatal antigenic stimulus with an increase in IgM production. The IgM serum level normally builds up rapidly through the first few weeks of life and reaches a concentration of half the adult value between 3 and 6 months of age [54].

Secretory IgA antibodies can be detected in tears shortly after birth but the IgA serum level increases very slowly and attains adult values as late as at 12 to 16 years of age [114].

IgG antibodies of maternal origin are catabolized in the infant's reticuloendothelial system and have a half-life of approximately thirty days [45]. The newborn infant's own IgG production will replace a fraction of the amount of IgG's that are cleared. As a result, there is a continuous drop in IgG serum concentration until the third postnatal month. From that age on IgG levels rise gradually and eventually reach adult values around twelve to eighteen months of age.

Non specific immunity. — Leucocytes of neonates are deficient in their response to chemotactic stimuli and therefore cannot transit to and efficiently gather at inflammatory sites [82]. Their phagocytic and bactericidal activities appear to be normal in healthy and non stressed newborn infants [74].

The serum opsonization activity (*i. e.*: processing of bacteria for phagocytosis and intracellular killing) is deficient, owing to physiologically low IgM and complement levels and functional deficiencies of enzymatic systems responsible for complement activation (CH_{50}, C_5, C_3, Factor B) [81].

Special situations.

Premature infants. — The prematurely born infant is in a position of greater risk than is his term counterpart since some of the antiinfectious defense mechanisms develop during the last trimester of pregnancy. The following features characterize the premature newborn:

a) C_3 and opsonin levels are even lower, particularly in infants weighing less than 1,500 g [74].

b) The transplacental transfer of maternal IgG antibodies increases throughout pregnancy. Consequently, the lower the gestational age, the lower the cord blood IgG concentration [47].

c) The physiological postnatal drop in serum IgG

level is greater and IgM production in response to an antigenic stimulus is delayed and reduced as compared to that in term infants [126].

Small for gestational age infants. — Intrauterine growth retardation may be due to placental insufficiency or to a chronic fetal infection. In the former situation the active transfer of IgG from mother to fetus is diminished [27] whereas in the latter situation defense mechanisms are depressed.

Infected or stressed infants. — Polymorphonuclear leucocytes from infected or stressed neonates exhibit a functional defect with reduced intracellular bactericidal activity [107].

Vaginal and cervical flora in the pregnant woman. — Vaginal and cervical mucosal surfaces are physiologically inhabited by a great number of microbial species constituting the normal indigenous flora. Different individuals have different indigenous floras, as evidenced by the great variations, found in the literature, pertaining to the incidence of a given bacterial species [40]. The indigenous flora will be altered throughout a woman's life, showing a definite correlation with sexual hormone production: œstrogens appear to enhance genital bacterial colonization, that is they facilitate implantation and adherence of microorganisms on the epithelium. On the other hand, progesterone seems to decrease genital bacterial colonization [40].

The vaginal and cervical indigenous flora encompasses those microbial species that are indicated in Table I.

How much pregnancy will alter genital bacterial colonization is not fully understood yet. However one can stress the following points:

— The actual number of bacterial species in the genital flora diminishes from the end of the first trimester of pregnancy [40], this decrease is proportionally greater for anaerobes than aerobes.

— The incidence of anaerobes gradually increases from the onset of labor and throughout the puerperal period, particularly so for peptostreptococcus and bacteroides species [25].

Most bacterial species of the genital indigenous flora are potentially pathogenic for the neonate.

Bacterial colonization of the newborn infant. — Bacterial colonization is a natural phenomenon of bacterial implantation on the following surfaces in the neonate: skin, anterior nares, naso-pharynx, pharynx, intestinal lumen and digestive epithelium, vagina [128]. This process normally begins at birth, at the time of passage

TABLE I. — BACTERIAL INDIGENOUS FLORA IN THE FEMALE GENITAL TRACT

Aerobes		Anaerobes
Gram-positive cocci		

Staphylococcus epididermis
Staphylococcus aureus
Alpha-hemolytic streptococci
  (*Streptococcus pneumoniae* included)
Gamma-hemolytic streptococci
Beta-hemolytic streptococci
  (group A, B, C, E, F, G)
Group D streptococci
  (enterococcal and non-enterococcal)
		Peptococcus species
		Peptostreptococcus species

Gram-negative cocci		
Neisseria species Neisseria meningitidis		Veilonella species
Gram-positive rods		
Lactobacillus species Corynebacterium species Listeria monocytogenes		Clostridium species Clostridium perfringens Bifidobacterium species Eubacterium species
Gram-negative rods		
Escherichia coli Klebsiella species Enterobacter species Proteus species Pseudomonas species Haemophilus influenzae Haemophilus parainfluenzae		Bacteroides species Bacteroides fragilis Fusobacterium species
Mycoplasmas		
Mycoplasma hominis		

through the birth canal, and usually goes on for four days. Most of the definitive bacterial flora is already established on the fifth day of life.

This normal phenomenon may be altered or deviated and turned into an abnormal process. We consider the following colonization processes to be abnormal:

— Those starting before birth (premature colonization).

— Those involving a surface that physiologically should remain sterile (aberrant colonization).

— Those resulting in a marked predominance of one given bacterial species (unbalanced colonization).

The above three situations can be isolated or combined. Whatever might be the combination, as a rule only one bacterial species is involved in a process of abnormal colonization.

Pathogenesis of fetal and neonatal infections

Infections may be acquired by infants at different times in fetal or neonatal life:

— in utero (*i. e.*: until the end of the first stage of labor),

— intra partum (*i. e.*: during the second stage of labor),

— during the period of colonization (*i. e.*: from the end of the second stage of labor throughout the first four postnatal days),

— beyond the colonization period (*i. e.*: beyond the fourth day of life).

For each one of these four periods, three points

must be kept in mind in order to analyse the pathogenesis of fetal and neonatal infections and understand their clinical manifestations:

a) the source of the infection,

b) the portal of entry of the infection into the
fetus (or the neonate),

c) the route of spread of the infection within the
fetus (or the neonate).

INFECTIONS ACQUIRED IN UTERO

Sources. — Only two infectious sources can possibly present to a fetus:

— the maternal blood (in the course of a maternal
bacteremia),

— the maternal genital tract (physiologically
colonized with bacterial flora).

Portals of entry.

Transplacental route. — Transplacental penetration may occur in the course of a maternal bacteremia. It can occur in three different ways:

(1) Direct transvillous transfer of bacteria, that
is from the intervillous blood (*i. e.*: maternal)
to the intravillous blood (*i. e.*: fetal), with no
infectious focus established in the placenta
(Fig. IV-9).

(2) Deposition of bacteria in the basal plate of
the placenta and establishment of an infectious
focus which will progress through the intervillous

space (*i. e.*: maternal) and eventually reach the
intravillous blood (*i. e.*: fetal) (Fig. IV-9).

(3) Deposition of bacteria in the chorionic plate
and establishment of an infectious focus in the fetal
portion of the placenta, with eventual progression
through the chorion and amnion into the amniotic
fluid (Fig. IV-9).

It should be noted that, even though all three ave-
nues of penetration are anatomically transplacental,
they have different pathogenic consequences on the
fetus. The first will result in an umbilical bacteremia
that is simultaneous with and of the same duration
as the maternal bacteremia. The second will result
in an umbilical bacteremia that is delayed and of
longer duration than the maternal bacteremia.
The third will result in an infection of the amniotic
fluid.

Amniotic route. — The intrauterine infection
originating from the vagina or cervix must pass
across the chorion and amnion. The transfer of
bacteria through fetal membranes may occur not
only when membranes are ruptured but also when
they are intact. It is a known fact that, by term,
membranes may be impermeable to amniotic fluid
but permeable to the active penetration of bacteria.
This route of infection will always result in an
infection of the amniotic fluid (Fig. IV-10).

Routes of spread. — As noted above, bacterial infections present to the fetus either as a

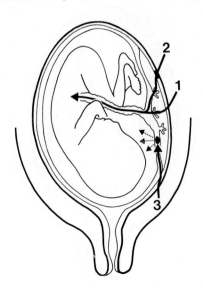

FIG. IV-9. — *Portals of entry for infections originating
from a maternal bacteremia: transplacental routes.*

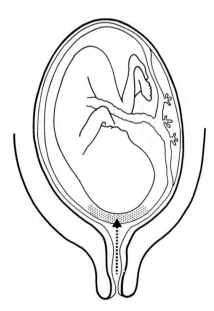

FIG. IV-10. — *Portals of entry for infections originating
from the maternal genital tract: amniotic route.*

bacteremia in the umbilical vein or as an infection of the amniotic fluid. Each of these two presentations will have different pathogenic effects on the fetus.

From an umbilical bacteremia. — A bacteremia in the umbilical vein will first reach the liver, then the inferior vena cava, the right side of the heart, the left side of the heart through the foramen ovale and, eventually, the systemic arterial circulation, resulting in a fetal bacteremia (Fig. IV-11). From that point, any fetal organ may be infected. The lung is at lesser risk owing to the small volume of pulmonary blood flow in intrauterine life.

A prolonged fetal bacteremia may result in a bacterial focus implanting within the renal parenchyma, bringing about a bacteriuria that in turn will cause an infection of the amniotic fluid. This sequence of events leads to an amplification of the infectious process (Fig. IV-12).

From an amniotic fluid infection. — Bacteria that are present in the amniotic fluid may be aspirated or swallowed by the fetus. Each of these processes results in a colonization and eventually an infection in the respiratory tract (pharynx, nasopharynx, middle ear, tracheo-bronchial tree, alveoli) and/or the digestive tract (lumen, epithelial surface) (Fig. IV-13).

Fetal pneumonia or enteritis may cause a secondary fetal bacteremia that will also bring about an amplification of the infectious process (Fig. IV-14).

The direct consequence of an amniotic fluid infection is the implantation of bacterial pathogens onto an epithelial surface in the fetus. In this situation, the bacterial colonization is always premature, and usually aberrant (*i. e.*: involving mucosal surfaces that should remain sterile, such as the tracheobronchial tree and alveoli), as well as unbalanced.

An infection of the amniotic fluid results in an anomalous colonization.

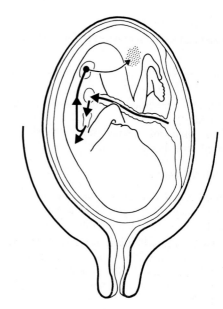

FIG. IV-12. — *Routes of spread: umbilical bacteremia and amplified fetal bacteremia.*

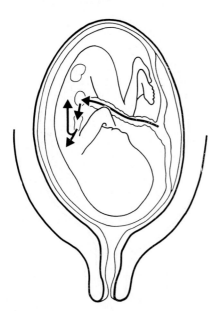

FIG. IV-11. — *Routes of spread: umbilical bacteremia and simple fetal bacteremia.*

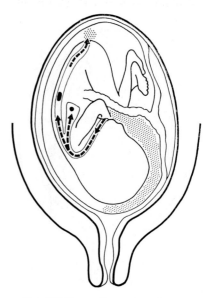

FIG. IV-13. — *Routes of spread: simple amniotic fluid infection.*

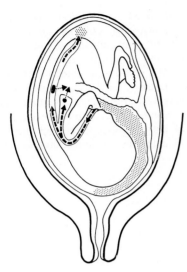

FIG. IV-14. — *Routes of spread: amplified amniotic fluid infection.*

INFECTIONS ACQUIRED INTRA PARTUM

Neonatal infections may be acquired at birth, during passage through the birth canal. These infections are in many ways similar to those acquired by the amniotic route.

Sources. — The infectious source is always the mother's cervical or vaginal flora.

Portals of entry. — The penetration of microorganisms into the fetus occurs as a result of contaminated genital secretions being aspirated all the way down to the bronchi or alveoli, at the time of the first inspiratory effort.

Routes of spread. — In this situation, neonatal infection is a direct consequence of an aberrant colonization of the infant's lower respiratory tract.

Intra partum aspiration of contaminated genital secretions results in an anomalous colonization.

INFECTIONS ACQUIRED DURING THE PERIOD OF COLONIZATION

We will consider separately infections that are acquired in the first four post-natal days, that is during the time necessary for a natural process of colonization to take place. The equilibrium of the bacterial flora is not yet achieved during that period, so that the slightest anomaly of colonization may bring about an infection, regardless of the bacterial pathogenicity.

The natural process of colonization may be altered by a number of different factors:

— A medical act or intervention in the neonate that would carry bacteria from physiologically colonized areas into areas that should remain sterile (iatrogenic aberrant colonization).

— The overexposure of the neonate to a given bacterial species, with eventual predominance of that particular species over the others (unbalanced colonization).

— The administration of antimicrobial drugs to the neonate that will cause a selection among bacterial species resulting in the predominance of resistant species (iatrogenic unbalanced colonization).

Sources. — The infectious source may be the maternal genital tract flora or any other flora that would be transmitted by the staff taking care of the infant or the equipment.

Portals of entry. — Penetration of microorganisms into the infant may occur through natural portals of entry (*i. e.*: aspiration, swallowing) or by way of iatrogenic interventions bypassing the infant's anatomical defenses (endotracheal intubation, umbilical arterial catheterization, continuous i. v. infusion, bladder catheterization).

Routes of spread. — Neonatal infection follows aberrant and/or unbalanced colonization in the infant.

Any iatrogenic action modifying the physiological process of colonization may result in anomalous colonization.

INFECTIONS ACQUIRED BEYOND THE PERIOD OF COLONIZATION

Infections that are acquired beyond the fourth day of life are caused either by bacteria with a high pathogenic potential or by microorganisms of low pathogenicity to which a given newborn is particularly susceptible (absence of passive transplacental immunity, breach in the infant's anatomical defenses, deficiency of the infant's active defense mechanisms).

Sources. — There are a number of possible infectious sources: the mother, the nursing or medical staff taking care of the infant, the nursery equipment, the infant's food...

Portals of entry. — Microorganisms will gain access to the infant by any of the following means:

— The respiratory route (broncho-pulmonary aspiration, endotracheal intubation, bronchial toileting).

— The enteric route (swallowing).

— The percutaneous route (i. m. or i. v. injection, venipuncture).

— The transurethral route (bladder catheterization).

Routes of spread. — Infections that are acquired beyond the period of colonization will exhibit a number of different clinical presentations: meningitis (the most frequent feature), osteomyelitis, arthritis... The pathogenic potential of microorganisms, the intensity of the infectious load and the state of passive transplacental immunity are essential in determining routes of spread and target organs. Portals of entry have a lesser importance in this scheme than in the first three situations.

Risk factors

Risk factors can be determined on the basis of environmental characteristics of the fetus and neonate, host responses to bacterial infections as well as pathogenic features. We define a risk factor as a condition increasing the probability for a fetus or a neonate to become infected.

A given risk factor does not necessarily apply to all periods of fetal and neonatal life alike, and different periods correspond to different risk factors.

We have considered in Table II only conditions that can easily be detected on clinical grounds alone.

TABLE II. — RISK FACTORS

In utero	Intra partum	During the period of colonization	Beyond the period of colonization
Maternal bacteremia. Vaginal and cervical infections. Prolonged rupture of membranes (>24 hours).	Vaginal and cervical infections. Prolonged labor.		
		Prematurity. Resuscitation of the newborn infant. Intensive care *. Prophylactic administration of antibiotics. Extensive mucous membrane or skin wounds and abrasions. Known contact with a source of infection **.	Prematurity. Prolonged intensive care *. Prophylactic administration of antibiotics. Extensive mucous membrane or skin wounds and abrasions. Known contact with a source of infection **.

* Endotracheal intubation, venous or arterial catheters, bladder catheters, chest tubes...
** Depending on local epidemiological conditions in the neonatal nursery.

Clinical approach

The clinical presentation of neonatal bacterial infections is usually described as being highly polymorphous, diverse and heterogenous, involving any organ or any combination of organs (Table III).

TABLE III. — NON-SPECIFIC CLINICAL MANIFESTATIONS OF BACTERIAL NEONATAL INFECTIONS

Circulatory signs	*Neurological signs*
— Cyanosis	— Lethargy/irritability
— Prolonged blanching following pressure on the skin	— Jitteriness/tremors/seizures
— Hypotension	— Decreased muscle tone/increased muscle tone
— Tachycardia/arrhythmia	— Abnormal eye movements
	— Full or bulging fontanelle
Respiratory signs	
— Tachypnea	
— Grunting	*Cutaneous signs*
— Nasal flaring	— Rashes
— Retractions	— Purpura
— Apnea spells	— Early jaundice / direct hyperbilirubinemia
	— Pustules
Abdominal signs	— Omphalitis
— Splenomegaly	— Sclerema
— Hepatomegaly	
	Constitutional signs
Gastrointestinal signs	— Poor temperature regulation (hypothermia/hyperthermia)
— Poor feeding	
— Prolonged, retarded or absent gastric emptying	
— Abdominal distension	
— Vomiting	
— Diarrhea	

However, we deem it justified to group neonatal infections into five distinct clinical pictures on the basis of pathogenic concepts and clinical manifestations:

1. Immediate systemic disease (*i. e.*: manifest immediately from birth).
2. Respiratory distress appearing within the first seven postnatal hours.
3. Respiratory distress and/or meningitis appearing between eight and thirty-six hours of age.
4. Systemic disease, with or without meningitis, appearing between thirty-six hours and five days of age.
5. Meningitis appearing after the fifth postnatal day.

This section will focus on several clinical examples of neonatal infections. The following cases have been drawn from the literature or from our own observations. For each case, we shall discuss the initial manifestations and the clinical course in view of the pathogenic concepts considered in the previous sections.

IMMEDIATE SYSTEMIC DISEASE

Case N⁰ 1 [12].

Presentation. — 20 year-old G 1 mother. At 34 weeks of gestation: fever of 39° C, shivering, vomiting, uterine cramps. A few hours after onset of symptoms: admission at a hospital where the amniotic fluid was found to be clear and fetal heart tones to be normal. 2 hours after admission: cessation of fetal heart tones. 12 hours after admission: spontaneous delivery of a 1,560 g stillborn infant. Cultures obtained: maternal blood, placental blood, fetal blood, amniotic fluid, fetal lungs and liver all growing *Listeria monocytogenes*.
Autopsy reveals miliary lesions containing gram-positive rods in the lungs, liver, spleen, pancreas, lymph nodes, adrenals and kidneys.
Examination of the placenta: chorioamnionitis, villositis and inflammation of the intervillous space.

Discussion. — This case is one extreme of the clinical picture which we have designated *immediate systemic disease*: generalised *Listeria monocytogenes* infection and death in utero.
The systemic involvement can be explained by an *umbilical bacteremia*. In the course of the ensueing fetal bacteremia, microorganisms implant in the kidneys, giving rise to a bacteriuria that will, in turn, lead to amniotic fluid infection and chorioamnionitis (the latter is usually asymptomatic in the mother). The infection in the amniotic fluid will induce a respiratory and digestive tract infection in the fetus, causing in turn a new fetal bacteremia. We have termed this process of self-maintenance of a fetal infection *amplified fetal bacteremia*.
The source of the initial umbilical bacteremia is a *primary maternal bacteremia* that was clinically not detected. The timing of this maternal bacteremia is difficult to assess since it was asymptomatic. However, one would suspect that the maternal bacteremia took place some 10 to 15 days prior to

delivery, as suggested by the finding of granulomatous lesions in the fetus.

The maternal febrile episode that occurred shortly before delivery signals a reinfection of the mother from the massively infected fetus and placenta. *The maternal bacteremia that is detected at the time of delivery is secondary.*

This 3-stage sequence of events (primary maternal bacteremia, amplified fetal bacteremia, secondary maternal bacteremia) is peculiar to maternal *Listeria monocytogenes* blood infections and readily explains the fatal outcome in this case.

It should be noted that this 3-stage process may be interrupted at any stage in its natural course by delivery. Thus the state of advance of the infectious process, and hence the completeness of the clinical picture, will then be directly correlated to the time interval elapsed between the time when the infection is acquired by the fetus and the time he is delivered. This is illustrated by the next case:

Case No 2 [122].

Presentation. — 34 year-old G 2 mother. Pregnancy was unremarkable until a few hours before delivery, at which time a 40° C fever was noted. Amoxicillin was given from the onset of fever. Onset of labor was spontaneous. There was a persistant fetal tachycardia. Rupture of membranes occurred spontaneously shortly before delivery. Amniotic fluid was meconium stained.

The infant was estimated at about 33 weeks of gestation; birth weight was 2,000 g; Apgar scores were 2, 3 and 6 at 1, 5 and 10 minutes respectively. The infant presented immediately with major respiratory distress, apneic spells and severe acidosis; endotracheal intubation and assisted ventilation were required from the 15th minute of life; a blood culture was then drawn, that grew *Listeria monocytogenes*; ampicillin and gentamicin were given as soon as blood cultures were obtained.

At 4 hours of life: transfer to another hospital where the following observations were made: hypothermia, tachycardia, marked cyanosis, no spontaneous breathing, diminished muscle tone, no primitive reflexes. Chest X-ray: bilateral infiltrate. CSF examination: 56 cells/mm³ (all mononuclear cells), low glucose. Direct smear of gastric fluid and meconium: numerous gram-positive rods. Cultures obtained (on antibiotics): blood and CSF remained sterile, meconium grew *Listeria monocytogenes*. Antibiotic regimen was continued (ampicillin and gentamicin). Exchange transfusion was performed at 10 hours of life. Course was progressively downhill with acidosis and hypoxemia out of control and intractable convulsions. Death occurred at 12 hours of age. Autopsy revealed listerial granulomas in the lungs, liver, spleen, kidneys and adrenals. Post mortem culture of brain grew *Listeria monocytogenes*.

Discussion. — This infant presented with an *immediate systemic disease*.

The existence of listerial granulomas indicates that the infection was acquired at least 10 days prior

to delivery and the generalized involvement implies a fetal bacteremia. Both features strongly suggest that there has been a *primary maternal bacteremia*, that was clinically undetected (such is often the case with *Listeria monocytogenes*). This primary maternal bacteremia is followed by an umbilical and then fetal bacteremia. Clinical and autopsy findings consistent with a pneumonia and an enteritis imply an amplification of the infectious process *(amplified fetal bacteremia)*.

It may happen that the primary *Listeria monocytogenes* bacteremia is particularly symptomatic in the mother, or that it brings about a detectable organ infection, so that appropriate therapy is started in the mother and, incidentally, influences the advance of the infectious process in the fetus. This situation is depicted in the next case:

Case No 3 [52].

Presentation. — 17 year-old mother. During the course of the 19th week of gestation: fever of 40° C, malaise, shivering, vomiting. Admission to a hospital 3 days after onset of symptoms; blood and urine cultures were then obtained and i. v. ampicillin immediately started for suspected pyelonephritis. Blood cultures grew *Listeria monocytogenes*. Ampicillin therapy was continued for 13 days. Pregnancy was brought to term with normal delivery of a healthy neonate.

Discussion. — This mother had a *Listeria monocytogenes* bacteremia, that was treated efficiently and on time. There is no way to be certain that an umbilical and fetal bacteremia actually occured in the fetus simultaneously with the primary maternal bacteremia. It is however very likely that it did happen in view of the very long interval between onset of maternal symptoms and the initiation of therapy (72 hours). Considering all we know about fetal *Listeria monocytogenes* infections acquired by way of umbilical bacteremia, it seems reasonable to assume that the maternal antibiotic treatment contributed to preventing the development of an infection in the fetus.

In our experience, the clinical picture of immediate systemic disease is oftentimes but not exclusively caused by *Listeria monocytogenes*. It may be due to another pathogen, such as in the following case:

Case No 4 [37].

Presentation. — Mother presenting with a febrile episode at the very end of pregnancy. A blood culture drawn at that time grew type 1 *Streptococcus pneumoniae*. Spontaneous delivery occurred within hours following onset of the fever.

Infant exhibited neurological abnormalities and apneic spells from birth on. Blood and CSF cultures obtained just after birth, grew type 1 *Streptococcus pneumoniae*.

Appropriate antibiotic therapy was started as soon as cultures were obtained. Outcome was favorable.

Discussion. — This mother suffered from a *Streptococcus pneumoniae* bacteremia shortly prior to delivery. The infant showed immediate signs of a *systemic disease.* Furthermore, the blood and CSF cultures were positive for a *Streptococcus pneumoniae* of the very same capsular type as the one obtained from the mother's blood. One must then suspect that the infection was acquired via a *simple umbilical bacteremia.*

The favorable outcome in this case may be accounted for by either of the following:

— the maternal febrile episode had attracted attention to a possible infection in the newborn,

— the maternal bacteremia that preceded the delivery was of short duration and allowed insufficient time for metastatic infectious foci to implant in the fetus,

— a simple umbilical bacteremia spares fetal lungs so that pulmonary disease does not intervene as a major aggravating factor.

RESPIRATORY DISTRESS MANIFESTING WITHIN THE FIRST SEVEN POST-NATAL HOURS

This clinical picture can be divided on the basis of clinical course into three distinct syndromes.

— Simple pneumonia.

— Pneumonia with secondary systemic manifestations.

— Diffuse pneumopathy radiologically consistent with hyaline membrane disease.

SIMPLE PNEUMONIA

Case N⁰ 5 [88].

Presentation. — Uneventful pregnancy. No febrile episode during labor. Cesarean section for prolonged labor and prolonged rupture of membranes (48 hours).

Vaginal delivery of a term infant. Apgar scores were 8 and 9 at 1 and 5 minutes respectively. Respiratory distress noticed shortly after birth. Assisted ventilation required from 4 hours of age. Chest X-ray: right-sided infiltrate. CSF examination: within normal limits. Cultures obtained: blood growing *Streptococcus pneumoniae*, CSF remained sterile. Penicillin and kanamycin were administered as soon as cultures had been obtained. Outcome was favorable.

Case N⁰ 6 [91].

Presentation. — 31 year-old G 3 mother. Uneventful pregnancy. Vaginal discharge for 2 days prior to delivery. Temperature spike at 39.6° C during labor. Forceps extraction. Cultures obtained during labor: blood remained sterile, vaginal secretions grew non typable *Haemophilus influenzae.* Penicillin and kanamycin administered to the mother after delivery.

Vaginal delivery of a term infant. Birth weight 3,400 g. Adjustment to extrauterine life difficult and required endotracheal intubation for a brief period. Increasing tachypnea noticed at 10 minutes of age. Chest X-ray: right middle and upper lobe infiltrate. Cultures obtained: blood, CSF and urine remained sterile; tip of the endotracheal tube, nose, throat, external auditory canal and umbilicus grew non typable *Haemophilus influenzae.* Penicillin and kanamycin given as soon as cultures obtained. Outcome was favorable. Culture of the fetal side of the placenta: non typable *Haemophilus influenzae.*

Discussion. — Both of these infants had a *pneumonia.* There is no evidence that a maternal bacteremia actually occured shortly before delivery; the mother of infant N° 5 was absolutely asymptomatic whereas the mother of infant N° 6 had a negative blood culture despite a fever spike during labor. The absence of a maternal bacteremia essentially rules out an umbilical bacteremia in the infant.

The marked predominance of respiratory manifestations suggests that there has been an *anomalous colonization in the lower airways* (aberrant colonization). This is substantiated, in infant N° 6, by the finding of the infecting agent in tracheal secretions obtained a few minutes after birth.

The occurrence of symptoms shortly after birth indicates that the colonization process took place *in utero* (premature colonization). This timing is confirmed by the cesarean section delivery of infant N° 5, which rules out intra partum colonization, and by the finding, in infant N° 6, of the infecting agent on several epithelial surfaces (nose, throat, external ear canal, umbilicus, fetal side of placenta), which is indicative of a vector role for the amniotic fluid.

The source of the infection can be precisely located for infant N° 6 in the maternal genital tract since the same organism was recovered from the mother and her neonate.

PNEUMONIA WITH SECONDARY SYSTEMIC MANIFESTATIONS

Case N⁰ 7 [3].

Presentation. — 22 year-old G 2 mother. Low grade fever and spontaneous onset of labor occurring shortly prior to e. d. c. Artificial rupture of membranes reveals thick meconium-stained fluid.

Vaginal delivery of a 3,580 g infant. Apgar scores were 8 and 7 at 1 and 5 minutes respectively. Immediate endotracheal intubation was performed for bronchial toilet and no meconium was visualised below the glottis. Frequent apneic spells and severe hypoxemia became manifest shortly after birth. Chest X-ray: bilateral confluent infiltrates. Ampicillin given from 6 hours of age. Assisted ventilation required by the second half of the first day. There was worsening of the hypoxemia (despite mechanical ventilation) attributed to persistant fetal circulation. Improvement followed tolazoline infusion. Ultimate outcome was favorable.

Cultures obtained: mother's cervix, infant's blood, skin and tracheal secretions (obtained by endotracheal tube just after birth) all grew *Listeria monocytogenes*; CSF remained sterile.

Case N⁰ 8 [4].

Presentation. — Uneventful pregnancy terminated by an elective cesarean section; rupture of membranes at the cesarean section. Delivery of a term infant presenting with respiratory distress immediately after birth. Apneic spells and hypotension became manifest during the first few hours of life. Chest X-ray: bilateral infiltrates. Cultures obtained: blood and nasopharynx grew non enterococcal group D streptococcus; CSF remained sterile. Ampicillin and gentamicin administered as soon as cultures obtained. Outcome was favorable.

Case N⁰ 9 [6].

Presentation. — 21 year-old G 1 mother. Uneventful pregnancy. Prolonged rupture of membranes (35 hours). Uneventful vaginal delivery. Cultures of lochiae: group G beta-hemolytic streptococcus.

Infant's gestational age was estimated at about 37 weeks; birth weight 2,600 g; Apgar scores 7 and 9 at 1 and 5 minutes respectively. Respiratory distress appeared shortly after birth and rapidly worsened with development of numerous apneic spells. Respiratory arrest occurred by 8 hours of age and required endotracheal intubation. Chest X-ray obtained just after intubation showed a bilateral infiltrate. Ampicillin and kanamycin started soon after X-rays had been taken. By 15 hours of age temperature noted to be around 37.8° C. Cultures obtained then (on antibiotics): tracheal secretions (by endotracheal tube), conjunctiva, external auditory canal, skin and rectum all grew group G beta-hemolytic streptococcus; blood, CSF and urine remained sterile. CSF examination within normal limits. Antibiotic regimen (ampicillin and gentamicin) continued for 14 days. Outcome was favorable.

Discussion. — All three infants presented with *pneumonia with secondary systemic manifestations* (arterial hypotension, apneic spells) occuring as complications. Bacteremias such as those observed in cases N⁰ˢ 7 and 8 are secondary to the pneumonia.

The initially predominating respiratory manifestations suggest that there has been an *anomalous colonization involving the lower airways* (aberrant colonization). This aberrant colonization process

in the lower respiratory tract is verified by the finding of the infecting agent in tracheal aspirate cultures.

The onset of the primary symptoms (*i. e.*: respiratory distress) soon after birth implies that this anomalous colonization took place *in utero* (premature colonization). The cesarean section delivery for infant N⁰ 8 and the finding in infant N⁰ 9 of the infecting agent on several epithelial surfaces (conjunctiva, external ear canal, skin and rectum) confirm the in utero timing of the anomalous colonization. Furthermore, the latter indicates a vector role for the amniotic fluid.

The mother of infant N⁰ 7 was the only one to be symptomatic; we ascribe the temperature rise in her case to a clinical chorio-amnionitis. For infants N⁰ˢ 7 and 9, the source of the infection is evidently situated in the maternal genital tract as evidenced by identical cultures from the mothers and their respective neonates.

DIFFUSE HYALINE-MEMBRANE-DISEASE-LIKE (HMD-LIKE) PNEUMOPATHY

Case N⁰ 10 [111].

Presentation. — 22 year-old G 3 mother. Onset of labor spontaneous at the 34th week of gestation. Labor inhibition started and remained effective for 3 days only. Membranes artificially ruptured 15 minutes prior to spontaneous vaginal delivery. Vaginal and cervical cultures obtained just after delivery grew non typable *Haemophilus influenzae*.

Infant's gestational age evaluated at around 34 weeks. Birth weight 2,000 g. Apgar scores 9 and 9 at 1 and 5 minutes respectively. Respiratory distress developed just after birth and progressively worsened with onset of apneic spells. Endotracheal intubation and assisted ventilation required from 5 hours of age. In addition to respiratory problems there was evidence of vascular collapse. Chest X-ray consistent with early hyaline membrane disease. Direct examination of gastric fluid showed numerous polymorphonuclear cells and small gram-negative rods. Cultures obtained: blood and gastric fluid grew non typable *Haemophilus influenzae*; urine and CSF remained sterile. Ampicillin and kanamycin were started as soon as cultures had been obtained. Clinical course was progressively downhill with severe acidosis and shock in spite of aggressive management. Death pronounced at 11 hours of age.

Autopsy revealed irregular fibrinous membranes covering the distal airways as well as foci of polymorphonuclear cells and macrophages in the lung parenchyma.

Case N⁰ 11 [4].

Presentation. — Uneventful pregnancy and delivery (no prolonged rupture of membranes).

Term infant presenting with respiratory distress soon after birth and developing, within hours, severe respiratory failure, apneic spells, vascular collapse and seizures.

Chest X-ray consistent with hyaline membrane disease. Cultures obtained: blood and CSF grew non enterococcal group D streptococcus. CSF examination: 2 cells/mm³, glucose 110 mg/dl (simultaneous blood glucose 112 mg/dl), protein 66 mg/dl. Penicillin given as soon as cultures obtained. Clinical course complicated and terminated with death on the 20th day.

Autopsy shows widespread bronchopneumonia and subarachnoid hemorrhage (but no leptomeningitis).

Discussion. — Both of these infants presented with *diffuse pneumonia that is radiologically compatible with hyaline membrane disease.*

In both cases the clinical course was rapidly and dramatically progressive and complicated by severe systemic manifestations (shock, apnea, uncontrolable acidosis). Neither infant seemed to have true hyaline membrane disease associated with a systemic infection; autopsy of infant N° 10 revealed no true hyaline membranes and the clinical course of infant N° 11 is different from that of hyaline membrane disease in term infants.

In both cases, we consider the bacteremia to be secondary to the infectious pneumopathy. There is no clinical evidence of a bacteremia occuring shortly before delivery in either of the mothers, which makes an umbilical bacteremia unlikely in their infants. The predominance of respiratory symptoms in the initial stage of the disease suggests that there has been an *anomalous colonization in the lower airways* (aberrant colonization). Culturing the infecting agent from the gastric fluid of infant N° 10 implies digestive colonization as well.

The occurence of primary symptoms (i. e.: respiratory distress) just after birth indicates that the colonization process took place *in utero* (premature colonization).

The source of infection must be located in the maternal genital tract; this is evidenced by case N° 10 in which the same organism was isolated from the mother's cervix and her newborn.

This syndrome of diffuse pneumopathy similiar to hyaline membrane disease is well recognized in group B beta-hemolytic streptococcus infections, and has been called "early septicemia". Clinical, radiological and histological similarities, as well as dissimilarities, between group B streptococcal infection and genuine HMD have been well studied [1, 56]. Distinctive features of the infection are the following:

(1) early onset of respiratory distress,
(2) very early onset of apneic spells,
(3) development of vascular collapse,
(4) early and dramatic aggravation of the infant's general condition.

We wish to emphasize that this diffuse HMD-like pneumopathy is by no means unique to group B streptococcal infection, as is clearly demonstrated by cases N⁰ˢ 10 and 11.

RESPIRATORY DISTRESS AND/OR MENINGITIS MANIFESTING BETWEEN 8 AND 36 HOURS OF AGE

Case N° 12 [98].

Presentation. — Spontaneous delivery of a term infant weighing 3,115 g. After delivery, mother spikes temperature to around 38.2° C and remains febrile for 7 hours.

Infant shows an easy adaptation to extrauterine conditions. Beginning at 32 hours of age, he develops a temperature around 38.2° C, a progressive respiratory distress, pulmonary rales and vomiting. Chest X-ray shows a bilateral confluent infiltrate. Cultures obtained: mother's vaginal secretions, infant's blood and throat grow *Listeria monocytogenes*; CSF remains sterile. Penicillin and streptomycin are then started and continued for 12 days. By 52 hours of age, the infant presents signs of vascular collapse and a low body temperature (35.5° C) for several hours; correction of the circulatory failure is first obtained by 60 hours of age and gradual improvement of the respiratory distress is observed even later. Ultimate outcome was favorable.

Case N° 13 [50].

Presentation. — Uneventful pregnancy and delivery. Routine culture of vaginal secretions grew group B beta-hemolytic streptococcus.

Term infant with a birth weight of 3,630 g and an easy adjustment to extrauterine life. Temperature instability, respiratory distress and seizures developed from 13 hours of age. Cultures obtained: CSF and umbilicus grew group B beta-hemolytic streptococcus. Penicillin given as soon as cultures obtained. Clinical course was downhill and death pronounced at 27 hours.

Autopsy reveals widespread bronchopneumonia, leptomeningitis, hypoxic encephalopathy and signs of disseminated intra-vascular coagulation.

Case N° 14 [71].

Presentation. — 18 year-old G 3 mother with uneventful pregnancy, labor and delivery. Isolated fever of around 38.5° C starting 9 hours after delivery. Cultures obtained: blood and urine remained sterile; lochiae grew type 3 *Streptococcus pneumoniae*.

Infant's gestational age estimated at 36 weeks. Birth weight 2,400 g. Apgar scores 8 and 9 at 1 and 5 minutes respectively. Apneic spells, cyanosis, lethargy and signs of vascular collapse developed from 30 hours of age. Chest X-ray obtained at that time shows a right-sided infiltrate. Cultures obtained: blood grew type 3

Streptococcus pneumoniae; CSF and urine remained sterile. Penicillin and gentamicin given as soon as cultures obtained. Outcome favorable.

Discussion. — All three infants presented with *pneumonia with secondary systemic manifestations* (apnea, temperature instability, shock, lethargy).

All three also had a secondary bacteremia originating from the pulmonary infection. *In infant N° 13 this bacteremia resulted in meningitis and in fatal disseminated intravascular coagulation ***.

There is no evidence of a maternal bacteremia occuring shortly before delivery, which makes an umbilical bacteremia in the fetus unlikely. The initially predominant pulmonary involvement suggests that there has been an *anomalous colonization in the lower airways* (aberrant colonization). Finding the infecting agent on the pharyngeal mucosa of infant N° 12 indicates colonization of the upper airways and strongly suggests distal respiratory colonization.

The rather long duration of the free interval between birth and onset of symptoms (from 13 to 32 hours in the above cases) makes it unlikely for the colonization process to have occured in utero which implies that it took place intra partum.

For all infants, the source of infection is clearly situated in the birth canal since the same agents were cultured from the mothers and their respective newborns.

Infections manifesting after 8 hours of age do not necessarily include a pneumopathy, as is shown in the next case:

Case N° 15 [46].

Presentation. — 30 year-old G 1 mother. Pregnancy, labor and delivery uneventful. 30 hours post-partum she became agitated and suddenly suffered a grand-mal seizure. CSF examination showed turbid fluid, 450 cells/mm³ (99 % polymorphonuclear cells) and gram-positive cocci on smear. Cultures obtained blood, urine and vaginal secretions grew group B beta-hemolytic streptococcus. Penicillin given as soon as cultures obtained. Outcome was favorable. Baby was a term infant with a birth weight of 3,475 g. Easy adjustment to extrauterine conditions. Routine physical examination performed at 8 hours of age entirely normal. Vomiting began by 18 hours of age. Irritability first noticed by the end of the first day. Convulsions observed at 28 hours. CSF examination at that time showed turbid fluid, 2,300 cells/mm³ (98 % polymorphonuclear cells) and gram-positive cocci in chains on smear. Cultures obtained: blood and CSF grew group B beta-hemolytic streptococcus. Ampicillin

---

* A consumption coagulopathy may complicate the clinical course of any neonatal systemic infection. It is usually associated with gram-negative bacterial infections [27] but has also been observed with gram-positive organisms [50, 89].

and gentamicin given as soon as cultures obtained. Ultimate outcome favorable but a slight developmental delay is noticed in subsequent examinations.

Discussion. — This infant presented with *bacteremia* and *meningitis*. So did his mother. The 30-hour delay between delivery and onset of symptoms in the mother implies that the maternal bacteremia took place *after* delivery. This rules out an umbilical bacteremia in the infant. The infection derives then from an *anomalous colonization*. This abnormal colonization process is unlikely to have occurred in the lower respiratory tract since there is no evidence of a pneumopathy. Considering that vomiting was the very first manifestation of the disease one might hypothesize that colonization took place in the digestive tract. The original description gives no clue supporting or refuting this assertion. The 18-hour delay between birth and onset of symptoms suggests that the colonization process occured intra partum and not in utero. The maternal genital origin of the infection is evidenced by culturing the same organism from the mother's vaginal secretions and the infant.

SYSTEMIC DISEASE,
WITH OR WITHOUT MENINGITIS,
MANIFESTING BETWEEN 36 HOURS
AND 5 DAYS OF AGE

Case N° 16 [62].

Presentation. — Uneventful pregnancy. Elective cesarean section delivery (for uterine malformation) of a 3,150 g infant. Apgar score 10 at 1 minute. Infant transfered to another hospital at 6 hours of age for moderate respiratory distress (in the same ambulance, but in a separate incubator, an infant with systemic *Listeria monocytogenes* infection, is transported both infants will be neighbors in the neonatal unit). Respiratory distress diagnosed as a transient tachypnea of the newborn due to slow resorbtion of lung fluid. All cultures that are routinely performed on admission in the neonatal unit proved negative.

On day 4 the infant spiked a temperature but no infectious focus could be detected. The CSF examination was normal and the CSF culture remained sterile. A blood culture was obtained, in which a positive result for *Listeria monocytogenes* was known 2 days later.

On day 6, before the blood culture result was known, the infant showed a sudden and dramatic aggravation of his general condition. The CSF examination revealed 1,600 cells per mm³ as well as gram-positive rods that were morphologically compatible with *Listeria monocytogenes*. In spite of appropriate antibiotic therapy started at that time, the infant showed a progressive downhill course and died on the 11th day.

Case N⁰ *17* [57].

Presentation. — 24 year-old G 1 mother with uneventful pregnancy and forceps extraction for prolonged rupture of membranes (28 hours).

Infant's gestational age estimated at 36 weeks. Birth weight 2,430 g. Apgar scores 8 and 10 at 1 and 5 minutes respectively. Cultures obtained soon after birth because of the history of prolonged rupture of membranes: blood, gastric fluid, external auditory canal, nasopharynx, umbilicus and placenta, all remained sterile.

By 48 hours of age the infant developed a pustule on the forceps mark as well as a bilateral purulent conjunctivitis. Later he became progressively lethargic. Cultures obtained: blood, nasopharynx, conjunctiva and pustule grew type *b Haemophilus influenzae*; CSF remained sterile. Methicillin and kanamycin given as soon as cultures obtained. Methicillin changed to ampicillin when cultures results are known. Outcome is favorable.

Case N⁰ *18* [100].

Presentation. — Term infant with an easy adaptation to extrauterine conditions.

Symptoms began during the 3rd day: respiratory distress, abdominal distention, 38.6° C temperature. Chest X-ray shows an infiltrate (of undetermined location). Cultures obtained: blood, CSF and nasopharynx grew *Streptococcus pneumoniae*. CSF examination: 4 cells/mm³ (all mononucleated cells), glucose 19 mg/dl (blood glucose 40 mg/dl), protein 35 mg/dl. Undetermined antibiotics were administered. Clinical course was very complicated with shock and temperature instability. Death occurred on day 4. Autopsy revealed a widespread pneumonia.

Discussion. — Each of these three infants presented a different disease picture (— bacteremia and meningitis for infant N° 16, — conjunctivitis, skin infection and secondary bacteremia for infant N° 17, — pneumonia, bacteremia and meningitis for infant N° 18) with a different clinical course (death 7 days after onset of symptoms for infant N° 16, survival with no residual damage for infant N° 17, death within hours of onset of symptoms for infant N° 18).

However, the following features are more important than these apparent dissimilarities:

— Onset of symptoms is between 36 hours and 5 days of age.

— Initial systemic manifestations include poor feeding, fever, lethargy...

— Late systemic manifestations are shock, apneic spells, temperature instability...

There are no grounds for suspecting maternal bacteremia occuring before delivery, which for practical purposes rules out an umbilical bacteremia in the infants. This infection must then originate from areas of *anomalous colonization*.

The prolonged free interval between birth and onset of symptoms (from 2 to 4 days) indicates that this abnormal colonization process did not occur in utero, nor intra partum. This point is supported by the cultures obtained just after birth being negative in infants N⁰ˢ 16 and 17 (no immediate postnatal cultures were obtained in infant N° 18). Therefore, the anomalous colonization process took place *during the period of colonization*.

In infant N° 17 the colonization by type *b Haemophilus influenzae* involved at least the skin, the conjunctiva and the nasopharynx. The addition of these three foci gave rise to an *unbalanced colonization* which, ultimately, caused a bacteremic infection.

In infant N° 18 the colonization by *Streptococcus pneumoniae* involved the upper respiratory tract, as shown by the positive culture of the nasopharynx. Two routes of spread may be postulated:

— A direct dissemination down the airways to the lungs *(aberrant colonization)* causing a pneumonia which, in turn, would give rise to a secondary bacteremia and then a meningitis.

— An excessive growth of *Streptococcus pneumoniae* on the nasopharyngeal mucosa *(unbalanced colonization)* initiating a bacteremia which, in turn, would cause pneumonia and meningitis.

MENINGITIS APPEARING
AFTER THE 5TH POSTNATAL DAY

Case N⁰ *19* [92].

Presentation. — 19 day-old infant admitted for fever, irritability and vomiting of 24 hours duration. Product of a normal term pregnancy and delivery. Birth weight 4,050 g. Physical examination on admission revealed a 39.4° C fever and a bulging fontanelle. CSF examination showed 2,200 cells/mm³ (all polymorphonuclear cells) and a low sugar. CSF culture grew *Listeria monocytogenes*. Appropriate antibiotics were administered and the outcome was favorable. (A vaginal culture was obtained from the mother 3 weeks post-partum and was negative for *Listeria monocytogenes*.)

Case N⁰ *20* [69].

Presentation. — 31 year-old G 4 mother with an uneventful twin pregnancy and delivery. (Routine cervical cultures obtained just after delivery showed no growth of *Neisseria meningitidis*). Twin A's birth weight was 2,550 g for a gestational age of 38 weeks. Apgar scores 7 and 9 at 1 and 5 minutes respectively.

A routine physical examination performed on day 7 was considered to be entirely normal. On day 15, he developed nasal congestion.

On day 17, he spiked a 40.8° C temperature and showed a bilateral conjunctivitis and a right otitis media. A few hours later, he presented with purpura and a bulging anterior fontanelle. CSF examination: 100 cells/mm³ (all polymorphonuclear cells), glucose 39 mg/dl (blood glucose 61 mg/dl), protein 85 mg/dl, gram-negative cocci on smear. Cultures obtained: blood, CSF, throat and conjunctiva grew group B *Neisseria meningitidis*. Penicillin and aminoglycosides administered as soon as cultures obtained. Soon after, cloramphenicol added to this antibiotic regimen. Fresh blood transfusions given. On day 19 he developed several generalized seizures. Progressive improvement occured from the 21st day of life and the ultimate outcome was favorable.

Case Nº 21 [100].

Presentation. — Uneventful pregnancy, labor and delivery of a healthy term newborn.

Onset of symptoms at 14 days of age: 38.9° C temperature, irritability, poor feeding. CSF examination: 645 cells/mm³ (predominantly mononucleated cells), glucose 32 mg/dl (blood glucose 58 mg/dl), protein 29 mg/dl, gram-positive cocci on smear. Cultures obtained: blood grew anaerobic *Streptococcus pneumoniae*; CSF sterile (it is not stated though whether CSF cultures were also processed under anaerobic conditions). Undetermined antibiotics administered. Favorable outcome.

Case Nº 22 [113].

Presentation. — Pregnancy, labor and delivery uneventful. (Routine vaginal cultures obtained soon after delivery showed no growth of group C beta-hemolytic streptococcus.)

Infant at term, weighed 3,180 g at birth and had an easy adjustment to extrauterine life.

He developed the first symptoms on day 13: poor feeding and lethargy alternating with irritability. On day 14, he spiked a 38.6° C temperature and showed tachypnea, marked lethargy and depressed reflexes. Chest X-ray normal. CSF examination revealed numerous polymorphonuclear cells and gram-positive cocci on smear. Cultures obtained: blood and CSF grew group C beta-hemolytic streptococcus. Penicillin given as soon as cultures obtained. Clinical course complicated with seizure activity for 7 days. Ultimate outcome favorable.

Case Nº 23 [42].

Presentation. — Mother with uneventful pregnancy, labor and delivery. Fever and vaginal discharge began 9 days post-partum. Infant at term, weighed 4,200 g and showed an easy adjustment to extrauterine conditions.

A 38° C temperature, poor feeding and irritibility were noticed from the 15th day of life, and vomiting started on the 18th day.

The infant was admitted to a hospital on the 21st postnatal day: physical examination revealed a fever, marked irritability and diminished muscle tone; CSF examination showed 400 cells/mm³ (all polymorphonuclear cells), protein 360 mg/dl (glucose not stated). Cultures obtained: blood, urine and CSF were sterile with conventional culture procedures. Gentamicin and cloxacillin were given as soon as cultures had been obtained.

The clinical condition remained stable and satisfactory between day 21 and day 31. CSF cultures obtained on 3 additional occasions showed no growth but there was a persistant cellular reaction in the spinal fluid. A sudden aggravation of the infant's general condition (fever, vomiting and convulsions) developed on day 31 and motivated transfer to another hospital. CSF examination in the other institution revealed 1,050 cells/mm³ (55 % polymorphonuclear, 45 % mononucleated cells), protein 130 mg/dl and glucose 50 mg/dl). A CSF culture was again obtained, which showed growth of *Mycoplasma hominis* 3 days later. Gentamicin and chloramphenicol were started as soon as cultures had been obtained. Chloramphenicol was changed to oxytetracycline when culture results were known. This appropriate antibiotic therapy for *Mycoplasma hominis* was administered for 21 days. On adequate therapy, a progressive improvement was noticed in the clinical condition and in the CSF parameters.

A follow-up examination at 10 months of age shows normal development with a slight residual right-sided hemiparesis.

Discussion. — Infants Nºs 19, 21 and 22 all present a similar clinical picture that is typical of *meningitis*. Clinical manifestations in infant Nº 20 are somewhat different though characteristic of *meningococcemia with an accompanying meningitis*. Clinical signs in infant Nº 23 are also suggestive of *meningitis*; in this last case, however, the clinical course was particularly insidious and protracted owing to partial treatment from the very beginning.

In all five infants, the timing of onset of symptoms (on days 13, 14, 17 and 18) indicates that the infections have been acquired beyond the period of colonization.

Not only are the above five cases similar to each other, they also share several common features with a disease called "late onset group B beta-hemolytic *Streptococcus meningitis*", as defined by Baker and co workers [11]:

— Uneventful perinatal period.

— Onset of symptoms beyond the tenth day of life.

— Mandatory symptoms: fever, poor feeding, vomiting, irritability or lethargy (alone or alternating).

— Optional though frequent symptoms: bulging of the anterior fontanelle, convulsions.

The pathogenic and clinical approach which has been depicted so far shows that infections that can be grouped in any of the defined five clinical pictures all derive from the same pathogenesis.

Accordingly, each clinical picture will correspond to one particular pathogenic mode and vice versa (see Table IV).

This approach enables one to estimate the extension of an infection, or its potential for extension:

— Infections that have been acquired by way of an umbilical bacteremia are immediately systemic.

TABLE IV. — Correspondance between clinical picture, pathogenic modes and timing of fetal and neonatal bacterial infections.

Clinical picture	Pathogenic mode and timing
Immediate systemic disease.	Umbilical → fetal bacteremia, simple or amplified.
Respiratory distress manifesting within the first 7 postnatal hours.	Anomalous colonization, in utero.
Respiratory distress and/or meningitis manifesting between 8 and 36 h of age.	Anomalous colonization, intra partum.
Systemic disease, with or without meningitis, manifesting between 36 h and 5 days of age.	Anomalous colonization, during the period of colonization.
Meningitis manifesting after the 5th day of life.	Infection acquired beyond the period of colonization.

They correspond to these diseases generally termed "early onset scepticemia".

— Infections that derive from anomalous colonization tend to be limited, in the initial stage, to the abnormally colonized organ. They possess though a potential for secondary extension.

— Infections that have been acquired beyond the period of colonization generally affect a target organ which oftentimes bears no relation to the portal of entry of the infection. These infections correspond to those diseases usually refered to as "late onset meningitis".

This approach furthermore shows that, in determining a given clinical picture, the infecting organism is not as important as the time at which it infects the fetus (or neonate) and the route by which it occurs. In other words, a given infecting agent is capable of causing different clinical pictures (such as exemplified by *Listeria monocytogenes*). On the other hand, different microorganisms can induce an identical clinical picture provided they occur at a similar period and through a similar route.

Two additional neonatal infections deserve comment: anaerobic infection and *Candida albicans* infection.

INFECTIONS DUE TO ANAEROBIC BACTERIA

Any neonatal infection may be caused by an anaerobic bacteria (see Table I).

The pathogenesis of anaerobic infections is in many respects identical to that of aerobic infections.

However, unlike what happens in aerobic infections, anaerobic bacteremias are frequently isolated and transitory, manifesting non-specific and non-dramatic clinical signs.

Anaerobic organ infections produce clinical manifestations that are very similar to those of aerobic infections. This is illustrated by the previously studied case N° 21 [100] (see p. 602) in which the infant showed a typical picture of meningitis starting after the fifth postnatal day.

The anaerobic etiology of a neonatal infection can be proved either by a positive bacterial culture or by the detection of microbial products by gas-liquid chromatography.

From a practical standpoint we are particularly suspicious of an anaerobic etiology in any of the following clinical situations:

(*a*) Neonate presenting a clinical picture of respiratory distress beginning at birth or during the first seven postnatal hours, and born to a mother with an anaerobic amnionitis.

The anaerobic etiology of an amniotic fluid infection is rather easy to suspect on clinical grounds alone owing to its foul odour. A good example of this situation is described in reference [102].

(*b*) Suspected or proven infection (on clinical and/or hematological grounds) in an infant already suffering from an ischemic enteropathy such as necrotizing enterocolitis.

(*c*) Subacute pneumopathy (on clinical or radiological grounds), oftentimes with a history of gastric fluid or milk aspiration, that is unresponsive to standard treatment (*i. e.*: physical therapy, bronchial toilet, broad spectrum antibiotics).

INFECTIONS DUE TO *CANDIDA ALBICANS*

The following features distinguish *C. albicans* infections from bacterial infections:

— Transplacental transfer of the infection

by way of an umbilical bacteremia does not occur.

— *C. albicans* exhibits a marked predilection for implanting on epithelial surfaces. Accordingly, the infection will usually affect integuments (including the amnion and the epithelial covering of the umbilical cord) and mucous membranes. Non mucosal epithelial surfaces (such as the synovia and ependyma) can be affected as a result of a prolonged fungemia. (A fungemia can occur as a consequence of an excessive growth of candida on a mucous membrane).

— The life cycle of *C. albicans* is much slower than that of bacteria, and is different from strain to strain. As a result, the latency period between the time of acquisition of the infection and the time of onset of symptoms is always prolonged and unpredictable.

With the exception of the umbilical bacteremia all pathogenic modes and timings that were defined for bacterial infections (see Table IV) also apply to candida infections.

However, because of the peculiarities mentioned above, the clinical pictures of *C. albicans* infections are somewhat different from those we have defined for bacterial infections. We distinguish the following three clinical pictures:

— Skin infection manifest at birth. (This skin infection is always associated with a digestive tract infection, and occasionally with a respiratory tract infection, both usually being asymptomatic).

— Simple digestive tract infection (thrush) manifesting after birth.

— Deep-seated organ infections manifesting after birth.

Skin infection manifest at birth

A candida infection that is evident at birth is actually present prior to birth. This is illustrated in the following case:

Case N° 24 [110].

Presentation. — 28 year-old G 2 mother. She had no clinical vulvovaginitis but vaginal cultures obtained soon after delivery were positive for *C. albicans*. Membranes artificially ruptured 29 minutes prior to delivery.

Vaginal delivery of an infant weighing 1,700 g estimated to be 31 weeks of gestation and easily adjusting to extrauterine conditions.

A macular, papular and vesicular rash was noticed at birth. It involved the entire body surface but was more pronounced in the intertriginous areas. There were a few pustules and areas of exfoliation. A perionychia and conjunctivitis were also present. Direct smears or cultures of skin, nails, meconium, vernix (sampled at the infant's

vulva) and conjunctiva showed and/or grew *C. albicans*. Spores of *C. albicans* were visualized in the epithelial layer of the umbilical cord. Treatment with nystatin p. o. and topically for 3 weeks. This infant never exhibited constitutional signs or fever. The course was characterized by a progressive improvement and healing of the skin lesions.

Discussion. — This neonate presented with a *Candida albicans infection of the skin, the conjunctiva and the digestive tract.*

Finding skin lesions at birth and detecting candida organisms in the first meconium discharged as well as in the umbilical cord suggests that this anomalous colonization process took place *in utero* (premature colonization) and implies a vector role for the amniotic fluid. The positive vaginal culture in the mother confirms the fact that the source of infection is located in the maternal genital tract.

Simple digestive tract infection manifesting after birth

This type of Candida infection may become apparent at any time after the beginning of the second postnatal week.

Case N° 25.

Presentation. — Term infant, product of an uneventful pregnancy, labor and delivery.

In the course of the third postnatal week, he developed numerous whitish plaques on the cheeks and tongue. These plaques were adherent to the underlying mucosa but could be removed, leaving an inflamed base. Though initially tiny and separate from each other, the plaques had a tendency to coalesce into larger spots. No associated fever or constitutional signs. Treatment was nystatin p. o. and topically over the affected mucous membranes.

Discussion. — This infant presents with *C. albicans stomatitis or thrush*. This infection is always the result of an *anomalous colonization of the buccal mucosa* (unbalanced colonization). The digestive mucosa and the intestinal lumen located distally are frequently colonized as well. The source of the infection might be the mother, the nursing (or medical) staff or the infant's clothing.

C. albicans stomatitis is a frequently observed but benign and self-limiting infection. However, extensive pharyngeal lesions can cause dysphagia.

Deep-seated organ infections manifesting after birth

In the presence of favorable conditions there may be an excessive growth of *C. albicans* on the buccal or intestinal mucous membranes. This overgrowth can, in turn, induce a fungemia. This is particularly the case when prolonged antibiotic therapy inhibits the normal intestinal flora, thus facilitating over-proliferation of candida organisms.

If the *Candida fungemia* lasts for an extended period of time, the infection may affect non-mucosal epithelial surfaces or any deep organ.

Case N° 26 [58].

Presentation. — Uneventful pregnancy and difficult vaginal delivery of a 3,345 g term infant.

Infant suffered perinatal distress due to thick meconium-stained amniotic fluid aspiration. Endotracheal intubation and assisted ventilation required right from birth. Culture of gastric fluid obtained 3 hours after birth grew *C. albicans.* Early neonatal period characterized by major respiratory distress secondary to meconium aspiration. Artificial ventilation required for 8 days. Ampicillin and kanamycin administered for 19 days, starting on day 1, and hydrocortisone for 14 days. On day 17, thrush noticed in the mouth.

On day 23, the infant spiked a temperature. Blood, urine and CSF cultures were obtained, and were sterile. Ampicillin and kanamycin again given and continued for 5 days (from day 23 to 27).

On day 30, the infant developed very loose stools. Stool cultures grew enteropathogenic *E. coli.* Neomycin, then polymyxin given orally.

On day 32, the umbilical arterial catheter and the endotracheal tube were removed and their tips sent for culture. Both of them grew *C. albicans.*

On day 37, an effusion was noticed in both knees. The following cultures were obtained: blood and urine were sterile; knee fluid and CSF grew *C. albicans.* CSF examination normal. X rays of knees revealed a symmetrical metaphysitis of the distal femur and proximal tibia and fibula. Intravenous amphotericin B was administered for a total of 10 weeks and the ultimate outcome was favorable.

Discussion. — This infant presented an *arthritis, an osteitis and a CSF candida infection.* (The latter is without obvious cytological or chemical or clinical manifestations). This case illustrates well the evident predilection of *C. albicans* for epithelial surfaces, whether they be mucosal (buccal cavity) or non-mucosal (synovia and ependyma).

All the conditions have been met for this type of pathology to occur:

— Anomalous digestive tract colonization. The absence of skin lesions evident at birth (or soon after) and the positive gastric fluid culture obtained at 3 hours of age suggest that this abnormal colonization process took place intra partum.

— Oral thrush noticed from day 17.

— Complicated perinatal and neonatal period requiring a number of agressive medical acts.

— Prolonged course of parenteral broad spectrum antibiotics, in addition to a course of oral non resorbable antibiotics.

— Administration of corticosteroid hormones.

One can also establish for *C. albicans* infections a correspondance between time of acquisition and pathogenic modes on the one hand and clinical pictures on the other hand (see Table V).

TABLE V. — CORRESPONDANCE BETWEEN CLINICAL PICTURES, PATHOGENIC MODES AND TIMING OF FETAL AND NEONATAL CANDIDA INFECTIONS.

Clinical picture	Pathogenic mode and timing
Skin infection (possibly associated with respiratory or digestive tract infection) manifest at birth.	Anomalous colonization, in utero.
Simple digestive tract infection manifesting after birth.	Anomalous colonization, intra partum or during the period of colonization or Infection acquired beyond the period of colonization.
Deep-seated organ infection manifesting after birth.	Anomalous colonization, intra partum or during the period of colonization or Infection acquired beyond the period of colonization + Prolonged fungemia.

Laboratory investigation

BACTERIAL CULTURES

When a neonatal bacterial infection is suspected aerobic and anaerobic cultures should be obtained immediately (*i. e.*: before antibiotics are administered to the infant). The following body fluids should be cultured:

— Blood, which should be drawn under strict antiseptic conditions and, whenever possible, from a peripheral venipuncture.
— Cerebrospinal fluid (CSF) obtained by lumbar puncture.
— Urine, which should be obtained by suprapubic bladder aspiration or under strict antiseptic conditions in a bag *.

Additional cultures from the infant (nasopharynx, throat, tracheal secretions, external auditory canal, umbilicus, stools...) or the mother (amniotic fluid, vaginal secretions) are helpful in estimating whether the colonization process is normal or abnormal. Accordingly, they help to understand the pathogenesis of the infectious process.

The direct examination of body fluids or secretions (CSF, urine, stool or any skin lesion) with smears and gram staining is very useful because it provides rapid information on the presence and the nature of an infecting bacterial pathogen.

Culturing a bacteria or detecting a bacterial antigen is essential in diagnosing neonatal bacterial infection. Microorganisms that are capable of causing neonatal infection originate either from the maternal genital tract (see Table I), or from the nursing (or medical) staff (e. g.: *Staphylococcus aureus*), or from the nursery equipment (e. g.: *Pseudomonas aeruginosa, Flavobacterium meningosepticum, Klebsiella pneumoniae...*) [109].

* The urine culture calls for three comments:
— it is oftentimes difficult to obtain,
— it causes excessive handling of the newborn with significant risk of hypothermia and hypooxygenation [123],
— a suprapubic bladder tap is not devoid of complications.

From a practical standpoint the initiation of antibiotic therapy should never be delayed because of technical problems in obtaining a proper urine sample.

We have previously arrived at the conclusion (see "clinical approach" section) that a given organism may cause different clinical pictures, and that identical clinical pictures may be caused by different pathogens. Consequently, for all practical purposes, identifying an infecting agent is essential in permitting us to selectively modify the initial antibiotic therapy from broad to narrow spectrum.

TABLE VI. — Prenatal and neonatal non-infectious conditions altering the white blood count.

	Observed alteration in the W.B.C.
Prenatal conditions	
— Maternal high blood pressure.	Neutropenia.
— Difficult or prolonged labor or delivery.	Increased ratio of NSN/SN.
— Administration of corticosteroid hormones to the mother.	Increased ratio of NSN/SN.
Neonatal conditions	
— Asphyxia (Apgar score $\leqslant$ 6 at 5 minutes).	Increased ratio of NSN/SN.
— Hemolytic disease (ABO or Rh fetal-maternal incompatibility).	Neutrophilia.
— Ventricular hemorrhage.	Increased ratio of NSN/SN.

NSN: non-segmented neutrophils.
SN: segmented neutrophils.

WHITE BLOOD COUNT

The usefulness of the white blood count in diagnosing neonatal bacterial infections has been much debated [124]. Responsible for this controversy are major discrepancies in absolute numbers of leucocytes and neutrophils throughout the first few postnatal days. Furthermore, it is well recognized that a number of prenatal and neonatal non-infectious conditions can induce a transient

TABLE VII. — Useful criteria for diagnosing neonatal septicemia

	First day of life	Second day of life	From the third day	From the tenth day
Non-segmented neutrophils (% of total number of leucocytes)	> 20	> 15	> 8 ——————→	
Ratio of non-segmented to segmented neutrophils (NSN/SN)	> 1/3	> 1/5		
Leucocytes (absolute number/mm³)	⩽ 4,000	——————————————————————→		
Platelets (absolute number/mm³)	< 100,000	——————————————————→ < 150,000		

Modified from Kuchler et al., 1976 [60].

alteration in the white blood count [70], and therefore complicate its interpretation (see Table VI).

Several investigators have the reexamined parameters of the neonatal white blood count and reviewed its usefulness in diagnosing bacterial infections [60, 67, 70]. The essential points are the following:

— The absolute numbers of leucocytes and neutrophils stabilize by the end of the first postnatal week [60, 67, 70, 129]. That makes interpretation of these numbers difficult during this period. A leucopenia (*i. e.*: < 4,000/mm³) or a neutropenia (*i. e.*: < 1,500/mm³) occuring beyond 72 hours of age is strongly suggestive of an infection (see Table VII). A non-infectious etiology for leucopenia or neutropenia can be thought of only when the ratio of non-segmented neutrophils to segmented neutrophils remains normal [67].

— The number of non-segmented neutrophils, expressed as a percentage of the total number of leucocytes, is elevated in 75 to 95 % of proven neonatal septicemias [60, 67]. Evidently, a valid enumeration of non-segmented neutrophils must be based on a strict definition of what is segmentation and what is not *. The following criteria are used to define an increase in the number of non-segmented neutrophils (expressed as a percentage of the total number of leucocytes): > 20 % on the first postnatal day, > 15 % on the second day, and > 8 % on the third day and thereafter [60, 67] (see Table VII).

* The following cells are defined as non-segmented: those whose nucleus is undivided, and those whose nuclear segments are connected by filaments that are at least on third as thick as the smallest segment.

— The ratio of non-segmented neutrophils to segmented neutrophils is also a valuable index of neonatal infection. It is elevated in 76 to 95 % of confirmed neonatal septicemias [60, 67]. The following criteria are used to define an increase in this ratio: > 1 : 3 on the first postnatal day, > 1 : 5 on the second day. Beyond the second day of life this parameter provides no reliable information (see Table VII).

— A thrombocytopenia is observed in 40 to 50 % of neonatal septicemias. The following criteria are used to define thrombocytopenia: < 100,000/mm³ from the first to the ninth postnatal day, < 150,000/mm³ on the tenth day and thereafter. Thrombocytopenia seems to occur somewhat more frequently in gram-negative bacterial infections [60] (see Table VII).

A bacterial infection is unlikely when there is no alteration in the white blood count [67, 70].

The timing of hematologic alterations during a proven bacterial infection is as follows:

— Increase in the absolute number of non-segmented neutrophils is usually observed within 24 hours after the onset of clinical symptoms [123]. Some investigators have stressed the possibility for this increase to precede the onset of symptoms [67]. This elevation in the absolute number of non-segmented neutrophils determines an early increase in the ratio of non-segmented to segmented neutrophils.

— Elevation in the absolute number of segmented neutrophils is inconstant and delayed [132].

— Leucopenia is also inconstant but appears early [67].

— Thrombocytopenia develops late in the course of an infection, and lasts for several days [60].

CEREBROSPINAL FLUID EXAMINATION

Essentially all neonates suspected of having a systemic infection should be subjected to a lumbar puncture and have the CSF examined. In addition to the aforementioned bacterial cultures and smears for gram stain one should obtain an enumeration of leucocytes (with differentiation into polymorphonuclear and mononucleated cells) and a determination of the sugar and protein levels. Knowing the simultaneous blood glucose level is essential in calculating the ratio of glycorrhachia over glycemia. Normal values for these parameters are given in Table VIII.

TABLE VIII. — NORMAL LABORATORY VALUES: CEREBROSPINAL FLUID

Parameter	Values in term newborns	Values in premature newborns
White blood cells (absolute number/mm³)		
mean	8.2	9.0
range	0-32	0-29
Polymorphonuclear cells (% of total leucocytes)	61.3	57.2
Protein (mg/dl)		
mean	90	115
range	20-170	65-150
Glucose (mg/dl)		
mean	52	50
range	34-119	24- 63
CSF glucose/blood glucose (%)		
mean	81	74
range	44-248	55-105

Modified from SARFF et al., 1976 [104].

Virtually all infants with bacteriologically proven meningitis show abnormal results in one or several of the above parameters [104]. On the other hand, an alteration in these parameters does not necessarily denote an acute bacterial meningitis; e. g.: a high CSF protein content may be observed in *Toxoplasma gondii* encephalitis [5] whereas a low CSF glucose level can result from an intracranial hemorrhage [31].

OTHER LABORATORY TESTS

Detection of bacterial antigens.

Capsular antigens. — Detecting a bacterial antigen in a body fluid (serum, CSF, urine) contributes to elucidating the bacterial etiology of an infection. Advantages of the antigen detection methods over conventional culture procedures are the following:

— Rapid results [38].

— Positive results even after bacteria have been killed and disintegrated (e. g.: by ongoing antibiotic treatment) [33].

— Possibility of serial quantitative measurements permitting establishment of a prognosis [34] or to assess the bacterial response to antiinfectious treatment [39, 75].

Several methods can be used for the detection of capsular antigens: counter-immunoelectrophoresis [9], latex agglutination [126] and staphylococcal coagglutination [115]. These methods have different sensitivities in detecting different antigens [117].

The following antigens have been found in infected newborns: *Escherichia coli* [75], group B beta-hemolytic streptococcus [35, 101, 108], *Listeria monocytogenes* [87], *Streptococcus pneumoniae* [96].

A number of other bacterial antigens have been identified in children and adults: type *b Haemophilus influenzae*, *Neisseria meningitidis*, *Pseudomonas aeruginosa*, *Klebsiella pneumoniae*, *Serratia marcescens...*, all these bacteria are capable of causing a neonatal infection.

Bacterial antigen detection should not substitute for but complement bacteriological cultures. We regard it as a useful and promising approach.

Bacterial endotoxins. — Endotoxins are constituents of gram-negative bacterial cell walls. They may be released in the blood stream in the course of a bacteremia or in the CSF in the course of a meningitis.

Endotoxins can be detected by the limulus lysate assay in serum or CSF [14]. With this method, endotoxins have been found in the CSF of 70 % of neonates with gram-negative bacterial meningitis [77].

The limulus lysate test is purely biological and, as such, of delicate interpretation.

Buffy coat examination. — Direct examination of the buffy coat after smears and appropriate staining (methylene blue, gram, wright) may reveal bacteria located within circulating neutrophilic leucocytes.

This technique has been proposed for early diagnosis of neonatal bacteremia [38].

In our experience it is useful and reliable only in massive and prolonged bacteremias.

Measurement of complement split products. — The complement system is physiologically activated in the course of a bacterial infection. Antigen-antibody complexes and endotoxins activate the "classical" pathway whereas some endotoxins activate the "alternative" pathway.

A recent report suggests that the presence of C3 split products in a newborn's serum, reflecting complement activation, is indicative of a bacteremia [32 a].

Detection and measurement of acute phase reactants.

Acute phase proteins. — In the presence of an acute inflammation, particularly of infectious origin, a number of different serum proteins become detectable or show increased levels: C-reactive-protein, orosomucoid, haptoglobin and fibrinogen.

Some studies suggest that, in newborn infants, high serum concentrations of these acute phase proteins should be considered as early evidence of a bacterial infection. Normal values and detailed information on sensitivity and specifity of different measurement techniques are proposed for C-reactive-protein [103 a, 103 b], fibrinogen [98 a], orosomucoid [45 a, 103 d] as well as haptoglobin [103 c].

Some reports emphasize the correlation between persistently elevated serum levels of C-R-P [103 a] or fibrinogen [29 a] and ongoing active infectious processes and suggest daily monitoring of acute phase proteins serum concentrations for evaluating antibacterial therapy efficacy [29 a] or identifying infectious relapses [103 a].

Erythrocyte sedimentation rate. — Although widely recognized as a valid non-specific indicator of inflammatory processes, the erythrocyte sedimentation rate in neonatal infections has received little attention. Determination of the sedimentation rate in the neonate requires micro-methods [2 a, 37 a].

Normal values are proposed for non-infected newborns, premature as well as term infants, showing that the sedimentation rate steadily increases with postnatal age [2 a, 37 a]. The highest normal value of the sedimentation rate in a non-infected neonate is 1 mm within 1 hour at one day of age and 17 mm within 1 hour at 14 days of age [2 a].

We consider the determination of the erythrocyte sedimentation rate to be less useful as a diagnostic aid than the measurement of acute phase proteins for the following two reasons: 1) The elevation of the sedimentation rate is a rather slow phenomenon occuring within 48 hours after onset of symptoms [2 a], and 2) The persistence of an elevated sedimentation rate does not necessarily correlate with an ongoing active infectious process [2 a]. Thus, in contradistinction to measurement of C-reactive-protein or fibrinogen, determination of the sedimentation rate cannot be considered useful as an early diagnostic procedure nor as a test of antibacterial therapy efficacy.

Measurement of metabolic activity in neutrophil leucocytes.

Nitroblue tetrazolium (NBT) reduction test. — The rate of NBT reduction by polymorphonuclear leucocytes is an index of their metabolic activity [94]. It is physiologically low (*i. e.*: 5 %) in healthy non-infected children but goes up during the course of a bacterial infection [10].

The baseline rate in healthy newborns has been much debated: most investigators now agree that it is physiologically high: 23.9 % in term infants and 27.8 % in premature neonates [7, 8]; even higher values have been reported [19].

Reduction rates in infected newborns are still disputed: some authors have reported lower rates (mean values around 13 %) [7, 8], while others have found higher rates (mean values around 60 %) [20].

Because of these uncertainties we do not consider this test useful for diagnosing neonatal infections [89].

Leucocyte alkaline phosphatase activity test. — Leucocyte alkaline phosphatase activity is physiologically low in healthy adults and children, and goes up during the course of a bacterial infection.

The baseline activity appears to be high in healthy non-infected newborns [32] and has been reported to be diminished in leucocytes from infected neonates [32].

TABLE IX

Antibiotic generic name	Daily dose depending on postnatal age (a) mg or unit/kg/day		Dosage interval depending on postnatal age (a)		Prefered route of administration (facultative routes)	Toxicity
	⩽ 7 days	> 7 days	⩽ 7 days	> 7 days		
Penicillin G	50,000 u (b)	75,000 u (b)	q 12 h	q 6 h	i. v. over 15-30 min (i. m.)	CNS irritation, seizures with doses greater than 250,000 u/kg
Ampicillin	50 mg (b)	75 mg (b)	q 12 h	q 6 h	i. v. over 15-30 min (i. m.)	
Amoxicillin	50 mg (b)	75 mg (b)	q 12 h	q 6 h	i. v. over 15-30 min (i. m.)	
Carbenicillin		400 mg		q 6 h	i. v. over 30 min (i. m.)	
Ticarcillin		250 mg		q 6 h	i. v. over 30 min (i. m.)	
Oxacillin	50 mg (b)	100 mg (b)	q 12 h	q 6 h	i. v. over 15-30 min (i. m.)	
Flucloxacillin	50 mg (b)	100 mg (b)	q 12 h	q 6 h	i. v. over 15-30 min (i. m.)	
Gentamicin	5 mg	7.5 mg	q 12 h	q 8 h	i. v. over 30-60 min (c) (i. m.) (intrathecal) (d) (intraventricular) (e)	Vestibular, cochlear, renal; serum levels: see Table X
Tobramycin	4 mg	6 mg	q 12 h	q 8 h	i. v. over 30-60 min (i. m.)	Vestibular, cochlear, renal; serum levels: see Table X
Amikacin	15 mg	20 mg	q 12 h	q 8 h	i. v. over 30-60 min (i. m.)	
Chloramphenicol birth weight ⩽ 2,000 g birth weight > 2,000 g	⩽ 14 days 25 mg 25 mg	> 14 days 25 mg 50 mg	⩽ 14 days q d q d	> 14 days q d q 12 h	i. v. over 15-30 min i. v. over 15-30 min	Gray syndrome (f); bone marrow depression; serum levels: see Table X

(a) Differential dosages and dosage intervals are derived from pharmacological studies showing that, in a newborn infant, the half-life in serum of an antibiotic is inversely correlated with birth weight and postnatal age.

(b) When meningeal infection is suspected (or proved): use daily dosages 2 to 3 times as large.

(c) Slow intravenous administration of aminoglycosides gives similar pharmacological results as observed after intramuscular injection [79]. We consider that constant intravenous infusion over a 15 to 30-minute period is more convenient than the i. m. route, particularly so for prolonged antibiotic therapy.

(d) Intrathecal injection of aminoglycosides does not improve the outcome of gram-negative meningitis [76].

(e) Intraventricular injection of aminoglycosides can be indicated when a gram-negative rod meningitis is unresponsive to systemic antibiotic therapy. Whichever technique of administration is prefered (repeated ventricular needle taps or implantation of a Rickham reservoir), the injection is a neurosurgical procedure and is not devoid of potential hazards [80].

(f) Early (reversible) symptoms: poor sucking, vomiting, diarrhea, abdominal distension, respiratory distress. Late symptoms: hypothermia, lethargy, cardiovascular collapse.

Therapy

CHOICE OF ANTIBIOTICS

Systemic infections.

Initial treatment. — The initial antibiotic regimen for treating a systemic neonatal infection must fulfill the following criteria:

— Possess a broad antibacterial spectrum; because the infecting agent is usually not yet identified when the decision is made to begin treatment, and because clinical features seldom give a clue as to the causative pathogen.

— Exert a bactericidal activity; because deficient chemotactic and opsonization activities make the neonate ill-prepared to kill bacteria, even those that are put into bacteriostasis.

— Be able to cross the blood-brain barrier and achieve therapeutic drug levels in the CSF; because central nervous system infection is often present, and, when not, always ominous.

— Be free of serious toxic effects.

The current antibiotic regimen meeting all the above conditions consists of a combination of an aminopenicillin and an aminoglycoside:

— The spectrum of antibacterial activity is wide enough to cover all gram-positive bacteria and many gram-negative organisms.

— Antibiotics from either class possess bactericidal properties and their combination has been shown to have a synergistic effect on some bacteria.

— Penetration of aminopenicillins into the CSF is satisfactory (*i. e.*: drug levels that are achieved in the CSF by parenteral administration of recommended doses are equal to or greater than the minimal inhibitory concentration of organisms causing most neonatal meningidities [55]. Conversely, penetration of aminoglycosides into the CSF is poor [73], and intrathecal [76] or intraventricular [65, 80] administration has been tried in an attempt to obviate this defect.

— Toxicity of aminopenicillins is essentially nil, as opposed to that of aminoglycosides that are

TABLE X. — Serum concentrations of antibiotics

	Gentamicin, Tobramycin	Chloramphenicol
Peak level	Should be measured 30 minutes following an i. v. injection or infusion; or 60 minutes following an i. m. injection.	Should be measured 30 minutes following an i. v. injection. (The combined use of enzyme-inducing drugs, such as phenobarbital, and chloramphenicol will result in decreased serum concentration of the antibiotic) [16].
Trough level	Should be measured just before a dose of the antibiotic is administered.	Should be measured just before a dose of the antibiotic is administered.
Therapeutic range	Peak level should be maintained between 4 and 6 μg/ml [93].	Peak level should be maintained between 10 and 25 μg/ml [78].
Toxicity	*Ototoxicity* When peak level is equal to or greater than 12 μg/ml [28]. *Nephrotoxicity* When trough level is equal to or greater than 2 μg/ml [28].	*Gray syndrome* When peak level is equal to or greater than 50 μg/ml [78].

well known for their undesirable side effects on renal and vestibular and cochlear functions [53, 28]. When recommended doses are used, this aminoglycoside toxicity is very low, and well out of proportion to the consequences arising from inappropriate treatment of a gram negative-infection in an infant. Furthermore it can be prevented by serial measurements in blood of drug levels, allowing adjustments of administered doses so that blood concentrations are kept within a therapeutic and subtoxic range (see Table X).

It is our practice to use a regimen combining ampicillin and gentamicin (see Table IX).

Amoxicillin appears to be a promising drug because of its bacterial spectrum somewhat wider than that of ampicillin and its faster in vitro bactericidal activity against *E. coli* and *Streptococcus pneumoniae* (see Table IX).

Aminoglycosides other than gentamicin (e. g.: tobramycin, amikacin) (see Table IX) have been recently made available and have not yet been used extensively in neonates. Their long term toxicity has not yet been fully investigated, though tobramycin is claimed to be the least nephrotoxic. We restrict their use to situations where gentamicin resistance is well known or strongly suspected. These situations are exceedingly rare during the initial phases of treatment.

Definitive treatment (selective). — The initial broad spectrum regimen should be changed to selective treatment when the causative pathogen is identified and the sensitivities to the antimicrobial drugs are determined. This selective antibiotic therapy should have a narrow spectrum, confined as much as possible to the infecting organism (see Table IX). The other three criteria mentioned earlier (i. e.: bactericidal activity, reasonable penetration into the CSF and low toxicity) should still be fulfilled.

It should be emphasized that this desire for reducing the spectrum of antimicrobial activity must be balanced against other considerations, such as:

— the single most active drug should not be relied on alone when its penetration into infected body fluids or tissues is known to be poor (e. g.: gentamicin in gram-negative bacterial meningitis);

— the combined use of an aminopenicillin and an aminoglycoside can be maintained if this association is known to have a synergistic effect on the infecting agent. Synergy has been reported in vitro and in vivo against *Listeria monocytogenes* [45, 85] and enterococci [84, 112].

Special situations

Anaerobic infections. — Antibiotics commonly used during the neonatal period (i. e.: aminopenicillins and aminoglycosides) are ineffective against most anaerobic bacteria.

When an anaerobic etiology is bacteriologically confirmed or clinically strongly suspected (see p. 603) chloramphenicol is the antibiotic of choice (see Table IX).

The toxicity of chloramphenicol is well recognized and potentially serious (bone marrow depression, gray syndrome) [116]. Furthermore, some of its pharmacological properties are undesirable for use in neonates (i. e.: high binding to plasma proteins, bacteriostatic activity).

Because of this chloramphenicol should not be administered when another antibiotic of equal efficiency is available and its use should be monitored by serial blood level assays [15] (see Table X).

Clindamycin and metronidazole are also active against most anaerobic bacteria. Both are claimed to have been used successfully in newborn infants [13, 48, 102]. However, because of the limited clinical experience and the lack of pharmacologic and toxicologic studies in neonates, the use of these drugs cannot yet be recommended.

Chronic lung infections. — *Pseudomonas aeruginosa*, *Klebsiella pneumoniae* and/or anaerobic bacteria are common causes of chronic pulmonary infections. These microorganisms show resistance to the aminopenicillins and variable susceptibility to gentamicin.

In these circumstances, it is our practice to use as a first line regimen a combination of tobramycin with ticarcillin (see Table X). Tobramycin is an aminoglycosidic antibiotic displaying the greatest in vitro activity against *Pseudomonas aeruginosa*. The combined use of tobramycin and ticarcillin appears to have an in vitro and in vivo synergestic effect against *Pseudomonas aeruginosa* [26]. Ticarcillin is active against a number of anaerobic bacteria (including *Bacteroides fragilis*) [103].

If a chronic lung infection appears to be clinically unresponsive to the combined tobramycin-ticarcillin regimen, we regard it as an anaerobic pulmonary infection and treat it accordingly.

"Candida albicans" infections. — Cutaneous or digestive *Candida albicans* infections are easily manageable though sometimes difficult to eradicate.

The treatment of choice is nystatin, topically or orally.

Conversely, systemic *Candida albicans* infections are difficult to control. Two drugs can be used in the neonate: amphotericin B and flucytosine (formerly called 5-fluorocytosine).

Amphotericin B is an active broad spectrum antifungal drug. However, it is toxic to the bone marrow and kidneys [22] and penetrates very poorly into the CSF: the CSF drug level is about 1/40 of the simultaneous serum concentration [120].

Amphotericin B therapy requires progressively increasing dosages with daily increments over the first week of therapy. Furthermore, the drug must be administered as a slow intravenous infusion (over 4 to 6 hours) and must be protected from light during the infusion. The practical use of amphotericin B is difficult owing to these technical requirements (see Table XI).

Flucytosine is a good antifungal drug. Its toxicity is low [120], and its penetration into the CSF and the brain tissue is excellent: the CSF drug level is equal to the simultaneous blood concentration [105].

It should not be considered an ideal drug however: not all *Candida albicans* strains are susceptible to flucytosine and a number of sensitive strains develop resistance during treatment. Consequently, flucytosine should not be used without prior in vitro testing of the infecting candida strain's sensitivity (see Table XI).

Amphotericin B and flucytosine show in vitro synergism against Candida species [86]. This charac-teristic has prompted some investigators to use them in combination for the treatment of *Candida meningitis* [24, 51].

EXCHANGE TRANSFUSION

Exchange transfusion can be beneficial in managing severe neonatal septicemia associated with sclerema or neutropenia [97, 118, 130, 67].

The following mechanisms have been credited for this beneficial effect:

— Shift of the oxygen dissociation curve to the right (because donor blood contains adult hemoglobin with lower oxygen affinity), and improvement of oxygen release into tissues [30].
— Removal of bacteria or bacterial toxins from the blood [68].
— Substitution of immune globulins, particularly IgM's [41].
— Substitution of opsonins and increase in the opsonizing capacity of the infant's serum [29].
— Enhancement of granulocyte functions (phagocytosis, intracellular killing) resulting from the substitution of humoral factors [12].
— Displacement of neutrophils from the marginating pool and of all leucocytes from the tissue pool [131].
— Substitution of clotting factors and removal

TABLE XI

Antifungal drug generic name	Daily dose (a) mg/kg/d	Dosage interval	Route of administration	Toxicity/caution
Amphotericin B	— On first day: 0.15 mg.	q d	IV over 6 h	— Renal, hematologic.
	— From second day: progressive daily increments up to:	q d		— When signs of toxicity are evident: doses should be reduced.
	— On 7th day: 1 mg.	q d		
	— From 8th day on: 1 mg.	q d		— Should always be diluted in 5 % dextrose.
	— After satisfactory clinical response: 1 mg/kg/2 days.	q 2 d		— Should be protected from light.
				— Highest total dosage: 35 mg/kg.
Flucytosine	100-150 mg.	q 6 h	p. o.	

(a) There are no pharmacological studies of antifungal drugs in newborn infants. Proposed doses and frequency of administration are extrapolated from adult standard dosages [22, 51].

of fibrin degradation products, resulting in a reduction in intravascular coagulation phenomena [2].

It has recently been shown that it is essential for the donor's white blood cells to be fully functional if the exchange transfusion is to be beneficial [95]. For practical purposes, we recommend that fresh whole blood stored for no more than 12 hours at 4° C be used, or that the donor's blood be tested for granulocyte functions.

It should be stressed that exchange transfusion is not a procedure without risk [12]. Potential risks are the following:

— Hemodynamic disturbances.
— Complications of venous or arterial umbilical catheters.
— Transmission of pathogens (Cytomegalovirus, Epstein-Barr virus, hepatitis B virus, HLTV III virus (AIDS), *Treponema pallidum*).
— Anaphylactic reactions.
— Undesirable immunologic side effects such as graft-versus-host-reactions and transfusion of anti-leucocyte agglutinins [12].
— Removal of specific antibodies produced by the neonate in response to the infection.

Exchange transfusion will lower serum and tissue levels of antibiotics, which is a drawback for a procedure meant to be antiinfectious.

Mean values of serum gentamicin concentration reductions reported in the literature range from 21 to 62 % [36, 59]. It has been noted that the total amount of gentamicin that is removed during an exchange transfusion is greater than that computed from the observed decline in plasma gentamicin levels. This finding suggests that the non-plasma compartment is partially depleted during exchange transfusion [59]. It may be necessary to perform two to three exchange transfusions within 24 hours to achieve clinical improvement. This obviously leads to a considerable loss of aminoglycosidic antibiotics.

Pending further data on aminoglycoside pharmacokinetics during exchange transfusion, we recommend that serum levels be monitored during the post-transfusion period and that dosages be adapted in order to achieve therapeutic blood concentrations (see Table X).

We are not aware of studies pertaining to pharmacokinetics of aminopenicillins during and following an exchange transfusion. Considering their extremely low toxicity, it is our practice to add into the donor blood an amount of aminopenicillin such that the antibiotic concentration be equal to the desired serum level.

Exchange transfusion is only an adjuvant therapy and its use should be restricted to severe neonatal septicemias associated with sclerema or neutropenia. In these situations it has been credited with a 50 % reduction in mortality rate [67].

TRANSFUSIONS

Granulocyte transfusions

Impaired metabolic activation and depressed intracellular bactericidal activity have been detected in neutrophils from stressed or infected neonates [107].

On the basis of these functional defects, some investigators have equated a sick and infected newborn to a neutropenic patient. This consideration has prompted these investigators to transfuse concentrated neutrophil granulocytes in infants with severe systemic infections. Clinical improvement has been reported to occur following these transfusions. This favorable clinical response seems to be related to the enhancement of bactericidal capacity in the neonate [63, 64].

Transfusion of neutrophil granulocytes is a technically complex procedure that is not available in every hospital.

Fresh whole blood transfusions

It has been observed that group B beta-hemolytic streptococcal systemic infections develop preferentially in newborn infants lacking specific opsonin antibodies to the infecting strain [49].

On the basis of this protective effect of opsonins, it has been suggested to transfuse fresh whole blood containing anti-group B streptococcal opsonins in severely ill infants infected with group B streptococcus [106].

The volume of transfusion should be 40 % or more of the newborn's blood volume to significantly enhance neonatal opsonic activity. Infants receiving blood which contains opsonic antibody to group B streptococci show a better survival rate.

It should be stressed that this procedure requires relatively large volumes of fresh whole blood and has potential hemodynamic side effects. Furthermore, the donor's blood must be screened for opsonin antibodies to group B streptococci.

PRACTICAL APPROACH

It is the purpose of this section to propose a practical approach to early diagnosis and correct management of neonatal infections. This approach rests upon pathogenic concepts, clinical features, laboratory parameters and therapeutic methods such as those described in the previous sections.

INITIAL ASSESSMENT
OF THE LEVEL OF PROBABILITY OF INFECTION
(See Table XII)

In order to establish the likelihood of a bacterial infection in a sick neonate, one should answer the following questions:

— Does the newborn present clinical signs (see Table III) or one of the clinical pictures (see p. 595) suggesting an infectious process?

— Are there risk factors (see Table II) or hematological findings (see Table VII) supporting this suspicion?

This two-step approach is necessary because none of the clinical signs or pictures described

earlier is by itself specific for an infectious process. By answering these questions, one can determine three levels of probability of a neonatal infection.

High probability (see Table XII). — The level of probability is defined as high in any of the following situations:

— The infant shows one of the five clinical pictures described earlier (see p. 595), with or without risk factors (see Table II), and the cell count is consistent with an infectious process (see Table VII). In our experience, clinical signs and hematologic evidence of an infection do correspond nicely, except in isolated pulmonary infections.

— The infant shows non-specific clinical signs (see Table III), with or without risk factors, and a cell blood count is consistent with an infectious process.

Moderate probability (see Table XII). — The level of probability is defined as moderate in any of the following situations:

— The infant shows one of the five clinical pictures described earlier or non-specific clinical signs, associated with risk factors, and the white cell count is normal.

— The infant shows no clinical manifestations,

TABLE XII. — INITIAL ASSESSMENT OF THE LEVEL OF PROBABILITY OF INFECTION

Level of probability		Initial criteria of infection			
		Clinical picture	Non-specific clinical manifestations	Risk factors	First W.B.C. count
High	1.1	+	+	+	+
	1.1	+	+	−	+
	1.2	−	+	+	+
	1.2	−	+	−	+
Moderate	2.1	+	+	+	−
	2.1	−	+	+	−
	2.2	+	+	−	−
	2.3	−	−	+	+
Low	3.1	−	+	−	−
	3.2	−	−	+	−
	3.3	−	−	−	+

+ : present or abnormal.
− : absent or normal.

but risk factors are present and the cell count is consistent with an infectious process.

— The infant shows no clinical manifestations, but risk factors are present and the cell count is consistent with an infectious process.

Low probability (see Table XII). — The level of probability is defined as low in any of the following situations:

— The infant shows non-specific clinical signs, without risk factors, and the white cell count is normal.

— Isolated risk factors are present.

— Hematologic evidence for an infectious process is discovered fortuitously in a healthy infant with no risk factors.

Determining the rate of probability of infection helps us modulate our attitude in terms of diagnosis and initial therapy. If the initial probability is high by our standards, we take it for granted that the neonate is infected. If the initial probability is moderate, we regard any aggravation, whether it be clinical or hematological, as evidence of an infection until proven otherwise. If the initial probability is low and a clinical or hematologic aggravation is then observed, we first look for non-infectious causes to explain this.

Obviously, there are situations where a cell count cannot be rapidly obtained or information on risk factors is not available, which makes it impossible to accurately determine the level of probability of infection. In such cases, laboratory work-up and antibiotic treatment must not be delayed if the clinical manifestations and course are at all compatible with a bacterial infection.

ATTITUDE WHEN THE PROBABILITY OF INFECTION IS HIGH
(See Table XIII)

In this situation, it is our practice to perform the following investigations without delay:

(1) Lumbar puncture, for cell count, chemical determinations and bacteriological work-up (gram stain and cultures) of the CSF.
(2) Blood cultures, both aerobic and anaerobic.
(3) Urine culture, provided the onset of treatment is not unduly delayed by technical difficulties.

Once this work-up has been done, we immediately initiate treatment with a broad spectrum antibiotic regimen (*i. e.*: aminopenicillin and an aminoglycoside, see p. 611 and Table IX).

TABLE XIII. — PROGRESSION TO DIAGNOSIS AND MANAGEMENT WHEN THE PROBABILITY OF INFECTION IS HIGH.

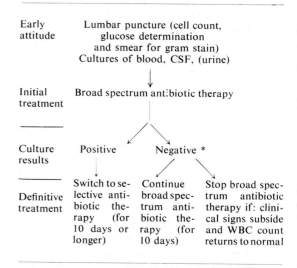

Early attitude	Lumbar puncture (cell count, glucose determination and smear for gram stain) Cultures of blood, CSF, (urine)		
Initial treatment	Broad spectrum antibiotic therapy		
Culture results	Positive	Negative *	
Definitive treatment	Switch to selective antibiotic therapy (for 10 days or longer)	Continue broad spectrum antibiotic therapy (for 10 days)	Stop broad spectrum antibiotic therapy if: clinical signs subside and WBC count returns to normal

* *Caution:* Cultures that are obtained from an infant who already was given an antibiotic or, shortly after birth, from an infant whose mother was on antibiotics are not reliable when negative.

We do not routinely perform an exchange transfusion because of the risks attached to this procedure: We restrict its use to severe infections associated with leucopenia and/or sclerema.

Proper monitoring and management require admission of these infants to a neonatal intensive care unit.

If culture results turn out positive we switch from the broad spectrum antibiotic regimen to a narrow spectrum drug aimed at the pathogen. We continue this selective antibiotic therapy for at least ten days.

If culture results turn out negative, we continue the broad spectrum regimen when any of the following conditions is met:

(1) Persistence of clinical signs and symptoms.
(2) Persistence of abnomalities in the peripheral white count and/or the CSF.
(3) Negative culture results are questioned when antibiotics have been administered before cultures were obtained (either to the infant or, shortly prior to delivery, to the mother).

If culture results turn out negative and the infant

has become asymptomatic and laboratory results are normal, we stop the (broad spectrum) antibiotic therapy.

ATTITUDE WHEN THE PROBABILITY OF INFECTION IS MODERATE
(See Table XIV)

In these circumstances we also routinely perform a lumbar puncture (for cell count, chemical determinations and bacteriological work-up of the CSF), blood cultures (both aerobic and anaerobic) and a urine culture.

However, we do not automatically begin antibiotic therapy. We consider that the use of a broad spectrum antibiotic regimen should be based on the clinical course or results of CSF examination or repeated white blood counts:

If the infant's clinical condition becomes worse, *or* any one of the laboratory results turns out to be abnormal, we regard these changes as evidence of an infectious process until proven otherwise. In other words, we consider that the probability of infection has shifted from moderate to high and start treating the infant accordingly (see p. 615).

If clinical manifestations remain stable, or regress, *and* all laboratory results are normal, we do not initiate antibiotic therapy, but rather keep the infant under close watch, monitoring clinical and laboratory parameters until culture results are available.

When cultures are reported as sterile we obviously do not begin treatment. When they show growth of an organism, we first strongly consider a contamination (type of pathogen, conditions of sampling, transporting and processing the specimen) before concluding in favor of treatment.

ATTITUDE WHEN THE PROBABILITY IS LOW

We perform no lumbar puncture, no blood culture and no urine culture in this situation, but simply repeat the white blood count. No antibiotics are given to the infant.

If there is any change in the infant's clinical condition (aggravation of findings already present or onset of new signs) we first look for non-infectious causes to explain the clinical course (*i. e.*: intracranial hemorrhage, cardiac failure, dehydration, pneumothorax...).

When none of these conditions can reasonably be held responsible for the observed clinical mani-

festations, we propose that the level of probability of infection be periodically reevaluated. These reevaluations should rest upon the clinical course, the possible occurence of new risk factors and the laboratory results, and can lead to either one of the following three conclusions:

— The probability of infection remains low and the infant is kept under close watch with no antibiotic treatment.
— The probability of infection becomes moderate and the infant is managed accordingly (see p. 615 and Table XIV).
— The probability of infection becomes high and the infant is immediately managed and treated accordingly (Table XIII).

TABLE XIV. — Progression to diagnosis and management when the probability of infection is moderate.

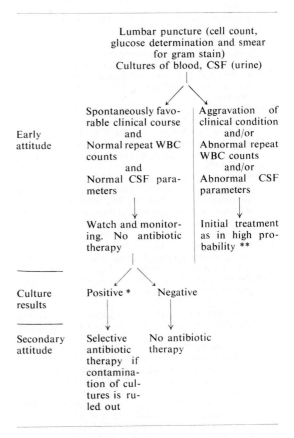

* *Caution:* the likelihood of contamination should always be evaluated in these circumstances.
** *See Table XIII.*

REFERENCES

[1] ABLOW (R. C.) et coll. — A comparison of early-onset group B streptococcal neonatal infection and the respiratory distress syndrom of the newborn. *N. Engl. J. Med.*, *294*, 65-70, 1976.

[2] ADAMKIN (D. H.). — New uses for exchange transfusion. *Pediatr. Clin. N. Am.*, *24*, 599-604, 1977.

[2 a] ADLER (S. M.) et coll. — The erythrocyte sedimentation rate in the newborn period. *J. Pediatr.*, *86*, 942-948, 1975.

[3] AHLFORS (Ch. E.) et coll. — Neonatal listeriosis. *Am. J. Dis. Child.*, *131*, 405-408, 1977.

[4] ALEXANDER (J. B.) et coll. — Early onset nonenterococcal group D streptococcal infection in the newborn infant. *J. Pediatr.*, *93*, 489-490, 1978.

[5] ALFORD (C. A.) et coll. — Congenital toxoplasmosis: clinical, laboratory and therapeutic considerations. *Bull. N. Y. Acad. Med.*, *50*, 160-181, 1974.

[6] ANCONA (R. J.) et coll. — Group G streptococcal pneumonia and sepsis in a newborn infant. *J. Clin. Microbiol.*, *10*, 758-759, 1979.

[7] ANDERSON (D. C.) et coll. — Leukocyte function in normal and infected neonate. *J. Pediatr.*, *85*, 420-425, 1974.

[8] ANDERSON (D. C.). — Use of NBT test in neonates. *J. Pediatr.*, *94*, 164, 1979.

[9] ANHALT (J. P.) et coll. — Detection of microbial antigen by counter immunoelectrophoresis. CUMITEH 8, 1-11, ASM, Washington, D. C., 1978.

[10] BAEHNER (R. L.). — Use of the nitroblue tetrazolium test in clinical pediatrics. *Am. J. Dis. Child.*, *128*, 449-451, 1974.

[11] BAKER (C. J.) et coll. — Suppurative meningitis due to streptococci of Lancefield group B: a study of 33 infants. *J. Pediatr.*, *82*, 724-729, 1973.

[12] BELOHRADSKY (B. H.) et coll. — Exchange transfusion in neonatal septicemia. *Infection*, *6*, 139s-144s, 1978.

[13] BERMAN (B. W.) et coll. — *Bacteroides fragilis* meningitis in a neonate successfully treated with metronidazole. *J. Pediatr.*, *93*, 793-795, 1978.

[14] BERMAN (N. S.) et coll. — Cerebrospinal fluid endotoxin concentration in Gram-negative bacterial meningitis. *J. Pediatr.*, *88*, 553-556, 1976.

[15] BLACK (S. B.) et coll. — The necessity for monitoring chloramphenicol levels when treating neonatal meningitis. *J. Pediatr.*, *92*, 235-236, 1978.

[16] BLOXHAM (R. A.) et coll. — Chloramphenicol and phenobarbitone, a drug interaction. *Arch. Dis. Child.*, *54*, 76-77, 1979.

[16 a] BRIGHAM (K. L.) et coll. — Increased sheep lung vascular permeability caused by *Escherichia coli* endotoxin. *Circ. Res.*, *45*, 292-297, 1979.

[17] BROMBERGER (P. A.) et coll. — Rapid detection of neonatal group B streptococcal infection by latex agglutination. *J. Pediatr.*, *96*, 104-106, 1980.

[18] BUETOW (K. C.) et coll. — Septicemia in premature infants. *Am. J. Dis. Child.*, *110*, 29-41, 1965.

[19] CHANDLER (B. D.) et coll. — Nitroblue tetrazolium test in neonates. *J. Pediatr.*, *92*, 638-640, 1978.

[20] CHANDLER (B. D.) et coll. — Use of NBT test in neonates: reply to a letter. *J. Pediatr.*, *94*, 164-165, 1979.

[21] CHANDRA (R. K.). — Levels of IgG subclasses, IgA, IgM, and tetanus antitoxin in paired maternal and fœtal sera: findings in healthy pregnancy and placental insufficiency. In *Maternofœtal Transmission of Immunoglobulins*. HEMMINGS (W. A.), ed., Cambridge University Press, Cambridge, 1976.

[22] CHERRY (J. D.) et coll. — Amphotericin B therapy in children. *J. Pediatr.*, *75*, 1063-1069, 1969.

[23] CHERRY (S. H.) et coll. — Lysozyme content of amniotic fluid. *Am. J. Obstet. Gynecol.*, *11*, 639, 1973.

[24] CHESNEY (P. J.) et coll. — Successful treatment of *Candida meningitis* with amphotericin B and 5-fluorocytosine in combination. *J. Pediatr.*, *89*, 1017-1019, 1976.

[25] CHOW (A. W.). — Anaerobic infections of the female genital tract: prospects and perspectives. *Obstet. Gynecol. Surv.*, *30*, 477-494, 1975.

[26] COMBER (K. R.) et coll. — Synergy between ticarcillin and tobramycin against *Pseudomonas aeruginosa* and *enterobacteriaceae in vitro* and *in vivo*. *Antimicrob. Agents Chemother.*, *11*, 956-964, 1977.

[27] CORRIGAN (J. J.) et coll. — Changes in the blood coagulation system associated with septicemia. *N. Engl. J. Med.*, *279*, 851-856, 1968.

[28] DAHLGREN (J. C.) et coll. — Gentamicin blood levels: a guide to nephrotoxicity. *Antimicrob. Agents Chemother.*, *8*, 58-62, 1975.

[29] DAVIS (A. T.) et coll. — Studies of opsonic activity for *E. coli* in premature infants after blood transfusion. In *Proceedings of the Meeting of the Society for Pediatric Research*, New Jersey, 223, 1971 (abstr.).

[29 a] DE GAMARRA (E.) et coll. — Surveillance du taux de fibrinogène chez le nouveau-né : intérêt au cours de l'évolution des infections bactériennes par contamination d'origine maternelle. *Arch. Fr. Pédiatr.*, *37*, 163-166, 1980.

[30] DELIVORIA-PAPADOPOULOS (M.) et coll. — Postnatal changes in oxygen transport of term, premature and sick infants: the role of red cell 2,3-diphospho-glycerate and adult hemoglobin. *Pediat. Res.*, *5*, 235-245, 1971.

[31] DEONNA (Th.) et coll. — Hypoglycorrachia in neonatal intracranial hemorrhage. *Helv. Paediat. Acta*, *32*, 351-361, 1971.

[32] DONATO (H.) et coll. — Leukocyte alkaline phosphatase activity in the diagnosis of neonatal bacterial infections. *J. Pediatr.*, *94*, 242-244, 1979.

[32 a] DREW (J. H.) et coll. — Complement activation: use in the diagnosis of infection in newborn infants. *Acta Paediat. Scand.*, *70*, 255-256, 1981.

[33] EDITORIAL. — Microbial antigen detection. *Lancet*, *2*, 138-139, 1974.

[34] EDITORIAL. — Diagnosis and prognosis in pyogenic meningitis. *Lancet*, *2*, 1277-1278, 1976.

[35] EDWARDS (M. S.) et coll. — Prospective diagnosis of early onset group B streptococcal infection by counter-current immunoelectrophoresis. *J. Pediatr.*, *94*, 286-288, 1979.

[36] EPSTEIN (M.) et coll. — Effect of exchange transfusion on serum aminoglycoside concentrations. *Pediatr. Res.*, *13*, 368, 1979 (abstr.).

[37] ESPAZE (E. P.) et coll. — Pneumococcies néonatales. *Nouv. Presse Méd.*, *6*, 2892, 1977.

[37 a] EVANS (H. E.) et coll. — The micro-erythrocyte sedimentation rate in newborn infants. *J. Pediatr.*, *76*, 448-451, 1970.

[38] FADEN (H. S.) et coll. — Early diagnosis of neonatal bacteremia by buffy coat examination. *Pediatr. Res.*, *9*, 340, 1975 (abstr.).

[39] FELDMANN (W. E.) et coll. — Relation of concentration of bacteria and bacterial antigen in cerebrospinal fluid to prognosis in patients with bacterial meningitis. *N. Engl. J. Med.*, 296, 433-435, 1977.

[39 a] FENTON (L. R.) et coll. — Complement activation and group B streptococcal infection in the newborn: similarities to endotoxin shock. *Pediatrics*, 60, 901-907, 1977.

[40] GALASK (R. P.) et coll. — Vaginal flora and its role in disease entities. *Clin. Obstet. Gynecol.*, 19, 61-68, 1976.

[41] GAUTIER (E.) et coll. — Unpublished results.

[42] GEWITZ (M.) et coll. — *Mycoplasma hominis.* A cause of neonatal meningitis. *Arch. Dis. Child.*, 54, 231-239, 1979.

[43] GITLIN (D.). — Development and metabolism of the immune globulins. In *Immunologic Incompetence.* Year Book Medical Publishers, Chicago, 1971.

[44] GORBACH (S. L.) et coll. — Rapid diagnosis of anaerobic infection by direct gas-liquid chromatography of clinical specimens. *J. Clin. Invest.*, 57, 478-484, 1976.

[45] GORDON (R. C.) et coll. — Influence of several antibiotics, singly and in combination, on the growth of *Listeria monocytogenes. J. Pediatr.*, 80, 667-670, 1972.

[45 a] GOTOH (H.) et coll. — Diagnostic significance of serum orosomucoid level in bacterial infections during neonatal period. *Acta Paediatr. Scand.*, 62, 629-632, 1973.

[46] GROSSMAN (J.) et coll. — Group B beta hemolytic streptococcal meningitis in mother and infant. *N. Engl. J. Med.*, 290, 387-388, 1974.

[47] GUDSON (J. P.). — Fetal and maternal immunoglobulin levels during pregnancy. *Am. J. Obstet. Gynecol.*, 103, 895-900, 1969.

[48] HARROD (J. R.) et coll. — Anaerobic infections in the newborn infant. *J. Pediatr.*, 85, 399-402, 1974.

[48 a] HELLERQVIST (C. G.) et coll. — Studies on group B beta-hemolytic streptococcus. I. Isolation and partial characterization of an extracellular toxin. *Pediatr. Res.*, 15, 892-898, 1981.

[49] HEMMING (V. G.) et coll. — Assessment of group B streptococcal opsonins in human and rabbit serum by neutrophil chemiluminescence. *J. Clin. Invest.*, 58, 1379-1387, 1976.

[50] HEY (D. H.) et coll. — Neonatal infections caused by group B streptococci. *Am. J. Obstet. Gynecol.*, 116, 43-47, 1973.

[51] HILL (H. R.) et coll. — Recovery from disseminated candidiasis in a premature neonate. *Pediatrics*, 53, 748-752, 1974.

[52] HUME (O. S.) et coll. — Maternal *Listeria monocytogenes* septicemia with sparing of the fetus. *Obstet. Gynecol.*, 48, 33s-34s, 1976.

[53] JACKSON (G. G.) et coll. — Ototoxicity of gentamicin in man. *J. Infect. Dis.*, 124, 130s-137s, 1971.

[54] JOHANSSON (S. G. O.) et coll. — Immunoglobulin levels in healthy children. *Acta Paediatr. Scand.*, 56, 572-579, 1967.

[55] KAPLAN (J. M.) et coll. — Pharmacologic studies in neonates given large dosages of ampicillin. *J. Pediatr.*, 84, 571-577, 1974.

[56] KATZENSTEIN (A. L.) et coll. — Pulmonary changes in neonatal sepsis due to group B beta-hemolytic streptococcus: relation to hyaline membrane disease. *J. Infect. Dis.*, 133, 430-435, 1976.

[57] KHURI-BULOS (N.) et coll. — Neonatal *Haemophilus influenzae* infection. *Am. J. Dis. Child.*, 129, 57-62, 1975.

[58] KLEIN (J. D.) et coll. — Neonatal candidiasis, meningitis, and arthritis. *J. Pediatr.*, 81, 31-34, 1972.

[59] KLIEGMAN (R. M.) et coll. — Pharmacokinetics of gentamicin during exchange transfusion in neonates. *J. Pediatr.*, 96, 927-930, 1980.

[59 a] KOH (K. S.) et coll. — The changing perinatal and maternal outcome in chorioamnionitis. *Obstet. Gynecol.*, 53, 730-734, 1979.

[60] KUCHLER (H.) et coll. — La formule sanguine dans le diagnostic précoce de la septicémie du nouveau-né. *Helv. Paediatr. Acta*, 31, 33-46, 1976.

[61] LARSEN (B.) et coll. — Host resistance to intra-amniotic infection. *Obstet. Gynecol. Surv.*, 30, 675-691, 1975.

[62] LAUGIER (J.) et coll. — Méningite du nouveau-né à *Listeria monocytogenes* et contamination en maternité. *Arch. Fr. Pédiatr.*, 35, 168-171, 1977.

[63] LAURENTI (F.) et coll. — Transfusion of polymorphonuclear neutrophils in a premature infant with *Klebsiella sepsis. Lancet*, 2, 111-112, 1978.

[64] LAURENTI (F.) et coll. — Functional activity of packed polymorphonuclear leukocytes obtained by leukafiltration. *Proceedings of the Annual Meeting of the European Society for Paediatric Research* (Abstract 85), Leuven, Belgium, September, 1979.

[65] LEE (E. L.) et coll. — Intraventricular chemotherapy in neonatal meningitis. *J. Pediatr.*, 91, 991-995, 1977.

[66] LEIKEN (S.) et coll. — Blast transformation of lymphocytes from newborn human infants. *J. Pediatr.*, 72, 510-517, 1968.

[67] LEMOS (L. A.). — Aspects hématologiques et cliniques des septicémies néonatales. *Thèse, Université de Lausanne*, 1977.

[68] LEVINSON (S. A.) et coll. — Effect of exchange transfusion with fresh blood on refractory septic shock. *Am. Surg.*, 38, 49-55, 1972.

[69] MANGINELLO (F. P.) et coll. — Neonatal meningococcal meningitis and meningococcemia. *Am. J. Dis. Child.*, 133, 651-652, 1979.

[70] MANROE (N. L.) et coll. — The neonatal blood count in health and disease. Reference values for neutrophilic cells. *J. Pediatr.*, 95, 89-98, 1979.

[71] McCARTHY (V. P.) et coll. — Endometritis and neonatal sepsis due to streptococcus pneumoniae. *Obstet. Gynecol.*, 53, 47s-49s, 1979.

[72] McCRACKEN (G. H.) et coll. — Changes in the pattern of neonatal septicemia and meningitis. *Am. J. Dis. Child.*, 112, 33-39, 1966.

[73] McCRACKEN (G. H.) et coll. — Gentamicin in the neonatal period. *Am. J. Dis. Child.*, 120, 524-533, 1970.

[74] McCRACKEN (G. H.) et coll. — Leukocyte function and the development of opsonic and complement activity in the neonate. *Am. J. Dis. Child.*, 121, 120-126, 1971.

[75] McCRACKEN (G. H.) et coll. — Relation between *Escherichia coli* K1 capsular polysaccharide antigen and clinical outcome in neonatal meningitis. *Lancet*, 2, 246-250, 1974.

[76] McCRACKEN (G. H.) et coll. — A controlled study of intrathecal antibiotic therapy in Gram-negative enteric meningitis of infancy. *J. Pediatr.*, 89, 66-72, 1976.

[77] McCRACKEN (G. H.) et coll. — Endotoxin in cerebrospinal fluid. Detection in neonates with

bacterial meningitis. *J. A. M. A.*, *235*, 617-620, 1976.

[78] McCRACKEN (G. H.) et coll. — *Antimicrobial Therapy for Newborns*, Grune and Stratton, N. Y., 1977.

[79] McCRACKEN (G. H.) et coll. — Intravenous administration of kanamycin and gentamicin in newborn infants. *Pediatrics*, *60*, 463-466, 1977.

[80] McCRACKEN (G. H.). — Intraventricular treatment of neonatal meningitis due to Gram-negative bacilli. *J. Pediatr.*, *91*, 1037-1038, 1977.

[81] MILLER (M. E.). — Demonstration and replacement of a functional defect of the fifth component of complement in newborn serum. A major tool in the therapy of neonatal septicemia. *Pediatr. Res.*, *5*, 379-380, 1971 (abstr.).

[82] MILLER (M. E.). — Chemotactic function in the human neonate: humoral and cellular aspects. *Pediatr. Res.*, *5*, 487-492, 1971.

[83] MILLER (R.) et coll. — Disseminated intraventricular coagulation in a newborn with *Listeria sepsis*. *J. Pediatr.*, *83*, 640-642, 1973.

[84] MOELLERING (R. C.) et coll. — Studies on antibiotic synergism against enterococci. I. Bacteriologic studies. *J. Lab. Clin. Med.*, *77*, 821-828, 1971.

[85] MOHAN (K.) et coll. — Synergism of penicillin and gentamicin against *Listeria monocytogenes* in *ex vivo* hemodialysis cultures. *J. Infect. Dis.*, *135*, 51-54, 1977.

[86] MONTGOMERIE (J. Z.) et coll. — Synergism of amphotericin B and 5-fluorocytosine for candida species. *J. Infect. Dis.*, *132*, 82-86, 1975.

[87] MOREL (A.) et coll. — Antigène soluble de *Listeria monocytogenes* dans un liquide céphalorachidien. *Nouv. Presse Méd.*, *7*, 2568-2569, 1978.

[88] MORIARTEY (R. R.) et coll. — Pneumococcal sepsis and pneumonia in the neonate. *Am. J. Dis. Child.*, *133*, 601-602, 1979.

[89] MORO SERRANO (M.) — La réduction du nitrobleu de tétrazoline par les granulocytes dans la période néonatale. *Thèse, Université de Lausanne*, 1976.

[90] NAIMAN (J. L.) et coll. — Possible graft-versus-host reaction after intrauterine transfusion for Rh erythroblastosis fetalis. *N. Engl. J. Med.*, *281*, 697-701, 1969.

[91] NICHOLLS (S. H.) et coll. — Perinatal infection caused by *Haemophilus influenzae*. *Arch. Dis. Child.*, *50*, 739-741, 1975.

[92] NICHOLS (W.) et coll. — *Listeria monocytogenes* meningitis. *J. Pediatr.*, *61*, 337-350, 1962.

[93] NOONE (P.) et coll. — Experience in monitoring gentamicin therapy during treatment of serious Gram negative sepsis. *Br. Med. J.*, *1*, 477-481, 1974.

[94] PARK (B. H.) et coll. — Metabolic activities in leukocytes of newborn infants. *J. Pediatr.*, *76*, 237-241, 1970.

[95] PELET (B.). — Exchange transfusion in newborn infants: effects on granulocyte function. *Arch. Dis. Child.*, *54*, 687-690, 1979.

[96] PELET (B.). — C3, factor B, α-1-antitrypsin in neonatal septicemia with sclerema; effects of exchange-transfusions and kinetic study of C3 using phenotypes as markers. *Arch. Dis. Child.*, *55*, 782-788, 1980.

[97] PROD'HOM (L. S.) et coll. — Care of the seriously ill neonate with hyline membrane disease and with sepsis (sclerema neonatorum). *Pediatrics*, *53*, 170-181, 1974.

[98] RAY (C. G.) et coll. — Neonatal listeriosis. *Pediatrics*, *34*, 378-392, 1964.

[98 *a*] RELIER (J. P.) et coll. — Intérêt de la mesure du taux de fibrinogène dans les infections néonatales par contamination maternelle. *Arch. Fr. Pediatr.*, *33*, 109-120, 1976.

[99] REMINGTON (J. S.) et coll. — *Infectious diseases of the fetus and newborn infant*. W. B. Saunders Company, Philadelphia, 1976.

[100] RHODES (P. G.) et coll. — Pneumococcal septicemia and meningitis in the neonate. *J. Pediatr.*, *86*, 593-595, 1975.

[101] RHODES (P. G.) et coll. — Countercurrent immuno-electropheresis of urine: a rapid diagnostic tool for group B streptococcal sepsis in the neonate. *J. Pediatr.*, *91*, 833, 1977.

[101 *a*] ROJAS (J.) et coll. — Studies on group B beta-hemolytic streptococcus. II. Effects on pulmonary hemodynamics and vascular permeability in unanesthetized sheep. *Pediatr. Res.*, *15*, 899-904, 1981.

[102] ROM (S.) et coll. — Anaerobic infection in a neonate. *Arch. Dis. Child.*, *52*, 740-741, 1977.

[103] ROY (I.) et coll. — *In vitro* activity of ticarcillin against anaerobic bacteria compared with that of carbenicillin and penicillin. *Antimicrob. Agents Chemother.*, *11*, 258-261, 1977.

[103 *a*] SABEL (K. G.) et coll. — The clinical usefulness of C-reactive protein determinations in bacterial meningitis and septicemia in infancy. *Acta Paediatr. Scand.*, *63*, 381-388, 1974.

[103 *b*] SABEL (K. G.) et coll. — C-reactive protein in early diagnosis of neonatal septicemia. *Acta Paediatr. Scand.*, *68*, 825-831, 1979.

[103 *c*] SALMI (T. T.). — Haptoglobin levels in the plasma of newborn infants, with special reference to infections. *Acta Paediatr. Scand.*, suppl. *241*, 1973.

[103 *d*] SANN (L.) et coll. — Étude de l'orosomucoïde chez le nouveau-né : intérêt dans le diagnostic des infections bactériennes. *Arch. Fr. Pédiatr.*, *33*, 961-971, 1976.

[104] SARFF (L. D.) et coll. — Cerebrospinal fluid evaluation in neonates: Comparison of high risk infants with and without meningitis. *J. Pediatr.*, *88*, 473-477, 1976.

[105] SHADOMY (S.). — *In vitro* studies with 5-fluorocytosine. *Appl. Microbiol.*, *17*, 871-877, 1969.

[106] SHIGEOKA (A. O.) et coll. — Blood transfusion in group B streptococcal sepsis. *Lancet*, *1*, 636-638, 1978.

[107] SHIGEOKA (A. O.) et coll. — Functional analysis of neutrophil granulocytes from healthy, infected, and stressed neonates. *J. Pediatr.*, *95*, 454-460, 1979.

[108] SIEGEL (J. D.) et coll. — Detection of group B streptococcal antigens in body fluids of neonates. *J. Pediatr.*, *93*, 491-492, 1978.

[109] SMITH (D. H.) et coll. — Epidemics of infectious diseases in newborn nurseries. *Clin. Obstet. Gynecol.*, *22*, 409-423, 1979.

[110] SONNENSCHEIN (H.) et coll. — Congenital cutaneous candidiasis. *Am. J. Dis. Child.*, *107*, 260-266, 1964.

[111] SPEER (M.) et coll. — *Haemophilus influenzae* infection in the neonate mimicking respiratory distress syndrome. *J. Pediatr.*, *93*, 295-296, 1978.

[111 *a*] STAHLMAN (M. T.) et coll. — Effects of group B streptococci on lung fluid balance in unanesthetized sheep. *Pediatr. Res.*, *11*, 506, 1977 (abstr.).

[112] STANFORD (H. C.) et coll. — Antibiotic synergism

of enterococci. *Arch. Intern. Med.*, *126*, 255-259, 1970.

[113] STEWARSSON-KRIEGER (P.) et coll. — Neonatal meningitis due to group C beta-hemolytic streptococcus. *J. Pediatr.*, *90*, 103-104, 1977.

[114] STIEHM (E. R.) et coll. — Serum levels of immune globulins in health and diseases. A survey. *Pediatrics*, *37*, 715-727, 1966.

[115] SUKSANONG (M.) et coll. — Detection of *Haemophilus influenzae* type *b* antigen in body fluids using specific antibody coated staphylococci. *J. Clin. Microbiol.*, *5*, 81-85, 1977.

[116] SUTHERLAND (J. M.). — Fatal cardiovascular collapse in infants receiving large amounts of chloramphenicol. *Am. J. Dis. Child.*, *97*, 761-767, 1959.

[117] THIRUMOORTHI (M. C.) et coll. — Comparison of staphylococcal coagglutination, latex agglutination and counter immunoelectrophoresis for bacterial antigen detection. *J. Clin. Microbiol.*, *9*, 28-32, 1979.

[118] TORRADO (A.) et coll. — L'exsanguinotransfusion comme moyen thérapeutique dans les sepsis néonatales compliquées de sclérème. *Helv. Paediatr. Acta*, suppl. *32*, 29-30, 1974 (abstr.).

[119] VAHLQUIST (B.). — The transfer of antibodies from mother to offspring. *Adv. Pediatr.*, *10*, 305-338, 1958.

[120] VAN DE VELDE (A. G.) et coll. — 5-fluorocytosine in the treatment of mycotic infection. *Ann. Intern. Med.*, *77*, 43-51, 1972.

[121] VAN FURTH (R.) et coll. — The immunological development of the human fetus. *J. Exp. Med.*, *122*, 1173-1188, 1965.

[122] VAUDAUX (B.). — Unpublished observation.

[123] VISSER (V. E.) et coll. — Urine culture in the evaluation of suspected neonatal sepsis. *J. Pediatr.*, *94*, 635-638, 1979.

[124] WEITZMAN (M.). — Diagnostic utility of white blood cell and differential cell counts. *Am. J. Dis. Child.*, *129*, 1183-1189, 1975.

[125] WERDER-KIND (H.). — Das serumeiweissbild beim Frühgeborenen. *Helv. Paediatr. Acta*, *18*, 450-460, 1963.

[126] WHITTLE (H. C.) et coll. — Rapid bacteriological diagnosis of pyogenic meningitis by latex agglutination. *Lancet*, *2*, 619-621, 1974.

[127] WILLIAMS (R. F.). — Colonization of the developing body by bacteria. In *Scientific Foundation of Peadiatrics*. DAVIS (J. A.), DOBBING (J.), eds. W. Heinemann Medical Books Ltd., London, 1974.

[128] YAMAZAKI (K.) et coll. — A placental view of diagnosis and pathogenesis of congenital listeriosis. *Am. J. Obstet. Gynecol.*, *129*, 703-705, 1977.

[129] XANTHOU (M.). — Leucocyte blood picture in healthy full term and premature babies during neonatal period. *Arch. Dis. Child.*, *45*, 242-249, 1970.

[130] XANTHOU (M.) et coll. — Exchange transfusion in severe neonatal infection with sclerema. *Arch. Dis. Child.*, *50*, 901-902, 1975.

[131] XANTHOU (M.) et coll. — The response of leucocytes in the peripheral blood during and following exchange transfusion in the newborn. *Pediatrics*, *51*, 570-574, 1973.

[132] ZIPURSKY (A.) et coll. — The hematology of bacterial infections in premature infants. *Pediatrics*, *57*, 839-853, 1976.

30

Special infections in the newborn (Syphilis, Tetanus, Tuberculosis)

Atties F. MALAN

Congenital syphilis

INTRODUCTION

Syphilis is one of the oldest diseases known to man, but its origins are obscure. It spread rapidly through the countries of Europe following the voyages of Columbus to the New World and was then referred to as the "new disease" and also called the Pox. The condition has had many synonyms over the centuries, and today still goes by different local names in many parts of the world. The name syphilis is derived from a poem written in 1530 [6] featuring a shepherd named Syphilus which set forth what was known about the disease at that time.

The earliest reference to congenital syphilis is probably that of Antonio Benivieni (1443-1502) who described a "fetus afflicted with the French disease" [4]. For centuries there was confusion over the transmission of the disease from mother to infant, and whether it was hereditary or congenital.

It was not until 1905 that the *Treponema pallidum* was discovered by Schaudinn and Hoffmann. In the following year von Wassermann, Neisser and Bruck demonstrated their serological test for syphilis. It was then apparent that for the infant to have congenital syphilis, the mother must first be infected.

Of all the ravages of syphilis, none is more disastrous than its effects on the fetus and the newborn infant. It is not surprising therefore, that premarital and antenatal serological testing is a legal requirement in certain countries. Unfortunately, syphilis is endemic in many parts of the world and there has been a resurgence of the condition in recent years. It is thus important that clinicians should be fully aware of the clinical features, diagnosis and management of congenital syphilis. The disease may appear in many and varied disguises, and those not familiar with the condition may not include syphilis in their initial differential diagnosis.

EPIDEMIOLOGY

Many factors, which vary from one community to another, influence the incidence of congenital syphilis in a particular area or country. The two major determinants are the prevalence of syphilis in child-bearing women and the effectiveness of antenatal care. Congenital syphilis can thus be seen as an index of public health care as well as the mores of a particular population.

Syphilis is endemic in certain areas and in these communities fetal death and congenital infection will be high. Such communities often lack adequate prenatal care and so compound the problem. If a woman has longstanding untreated syphilis she will develop a greater degree of immunity and subsequent pregnancies will, at least theoretically, be less likely to end in fetal death, or the birth of an affected infant.

In countries where statistics are available the incidence of syphilis, and thus congenital syphilis, has risen during the past two decades. This was in direct contrast to the hope that with the wide-spread availability and use of antibiotics, syphilis would be eradicated. There was indeed a decreased incidence in the 1940's and 1950's, but there has since been a resurgence in syphilis. Whether this is due to world-wide travel, the sexual revolution or a lack of sustained public health measures, is an open question.

The exact risk for the conceptus in untreated maternal syphilis is not well documented. Fiumara et al. [1] produced figures on the outcome of pregnancy in untreated maternal syphilis (Table I). If the mother has primary or secondary syphilis during the pregnancy, the incidence of death and congenital syphilis is considerably higher than if the mother has late syphilis. The notion that the fetus was protected by the layer of Langhans in the placenta if the mother has spirochetemia in the first 18 weeks of pregnancy, has now finally been disproved. It needs to be stated, however, that not every mother with untreated syphilis will have an affected infant, and that because of the sensitivity of the *T. pallidum* to penicillin even a single injection to the mother may alter the outcome. But if treatment is very late in pregnancy, or inadequate, congenital syphilis may still be seen.

The epidemiological factors involved are set out in Table II.

Failure to seek antenatal care or inadequate care due to the mother not being seen again are

TABLE I. — OUTCOME OF PREGNANCY IN UNTREATED SYPHILIS *

Status of mother	Conge-nital syphilis	Peri-natal death	Pre-mature infant	Normal infant
Untreated syphilis				
Primary or secondary	50 %	50 %		
Early latent	40 %	20 %	20 %	20 %
Late	10 %	11 %	9 %	70 %
Normal mother	0 %	1 %	8 %	91 %

* Modified from FIUMARA et al. [1].

TABLE II. — EPIDEMIOLOGY OF CONGENITAL SYPHILIS

	Fiumara [2]	Malan *
Failure to seek antenatal care.	30 %	24 %
Inadequate antenatal care . .	25 %	50 %
Failure to complete treatment.	17 %	13 %
Became infected subsequent to initial negative blood test. .	12 %	10 %
Failure of apparently adequate treatment.	3 %	3 %
Relapse or re-infection . . .	5 %	—
Diagnosis in infant doubtful. .	7 %	—

* Based on a series of 30 patients seen by the author.

responsible for the majority of infants with congenital syphilis. It can be seen in Table II that the practice of doing only one serological test does carry a risk but it is very small in relation to the large numbers so screened.

PATHOGENESIS AND PATHOLOGY

Syphilis is caused by the organism *Treponema pallidum* which is a thin, delicate, spiral organism about as long as the diameter of a normal red blood cell. For all practical purposes, fetal infection occurs only by transplacental passage of *T. pallidum* from an infected mother. Very rarely acquired syphilis may occur from direct contact with an infectious lesion during delivery through the birth canal.

The precise pathogenesis of congenital syphilis is still poorly understood. The morphological features are the result of inflammatory reaction to *T. pallidum* by an immunocompetent host, mainly that of plasma cells and lymphocyte infiltration. It is clear that the very early fetus does not react to spirochetemia and this had led to the belief that the layer of Langhans cells prevent the passage of the organism. The presence of *T. pallidum* has been demonstrated by means of silver and immuno-fluorescent stains in aborted fetuses as early as 9 week's gestation.

The inflammatory reaction in the placenta is villitis together with proliferation of stromal and endo- and perivascular tissues. The latter leads to vascular occlusion. Not only are the villous capillaries distended with inflammatory cells but they appear immature. These changes result in a disproportionately large placenta which is often pale and thicker than normal. Enlarged villi with relatively less blood in the capillaries are the cause of the pallor. An abnormally large placenta, especially in association with a growth retarded infant, should alert the attendant to the possibility of syphilis.

In the fetus the spirochetes disseminate widely. The pathogenic features seen are determined by the degree of host reaction and the organs most affected are the pancreas, liver, spleen, bone and kidney. The end result of the proliferative endarteritis is necrosis, atrophy and fibrosis. The mechanisms whereby the treponema causes tissue damage are not clearly understood but probably include humoral and cell-mediated immunologic responses. Total macroglobulin (IgM) is usually raised at birth or soon thereafter, and IgG production against reagin and treponemal antigens invariably occur.

The mortality in the infected fetus and newborn infant is high being around 30 % for each. The infant may be born with signs of early congenital syphilis, or may develop the signs only after several months. It is this wide variation in the clinical presentation that bedevils the recognition of congenital syphilis in the early weeks of life. If unrecognised and untreated the child may go on to develop late congenital syphilis with scarring of the initial lesions and phenomena attributed to hypersensitivity. The latter includes neurosyphilis, eighth nerve deafness, Clutton's joints and interstitial keratitis. The stigmata of late congenital syphilis present after 2 years of age, often around puberty.

CLINICAL FINDINGS

The clinical manifestations of congenital syphilis are extremely varied and the disease has been described as having "many faces". The spectrum seen ranges from macerated stillbirth or rapid neonatal death with gross signs, to the apparently normal infant in whom infection is proved only because investigation is indicated by positive maternal serological tests. In addition to the maternal antibody levels and host response, the timing of the placental transmission of organisms is presumably important in the clinical presentation at the time of delivery.

Although it is true that the clinical diagnosis becomes clearer with time, early suspicion of syphilis should be entertained in many infants. This will depend on the experience of the physician and a level of suspicion appropriate for the particular community.

The incidence of the manifestations of early congenital syphilis is given in Table III. The data are based on a series of 30 infants seen by the author and compared to that of Reynolds, Stagno

TABLE III. — MANIFESTATIONS
OF EARLY CONGENITAL SYPHILIS IN INFANTS

	Malan	Reynolds et al. [5] (modified)
Bone lesions (radiology) .	83 %	+ + + +
Preterm delivery . . .	82 %	+ +
Hepato-splenomegaly . .	76 %	+ + + +
Increased placental - fetal ratio	48 %	Not recorded
Skin lesions.	47 %	+ + +
Intrauterine growth retardation.	41 %	Not recorded
Pneumonitis (radiology).	39 %	+
Hepatitis.	37 %	+ +
Conjugated hyperbilirubinemia	30 %	+ +
Anemia	27 %	+ + +
Purpura	24 %	+
Edema	23 %	Not recorded
Bleeding diathesis . . .	20 %	Not recorded
Pseudoparesis	16 %	Not recorded
Mucocutaneous lesions .	10 %	+ +

Frequency classification: + 0-20 %, + + 21-50 %, + + + 51-75 %, + + + + 76-100 %.

and Alford [5]. If preterm delivery and bony lesions are included, then only one of the 30 infants had no abnormal findings except for serological tests. It goes without saying that the data are highly selective and asymptomatic cases could have been missed. In general, the findings in Table III are very consistent and in agreement with other publications [3].

Bone lesions. — Radiological lesions are the most frequent manifestation of congenital syphilis. The long bones are characteristically those most involved, and the femur more so than the tibia or humerus. The lesions are symmetrical and multiple, and are considered to be the result of a physio-pathological disturbance of endochondral and periostal bone formation. It is important to note that the changes are not specific for syphilis and similar lesions may be seen in other conditions, e. g. congenital rubella, cytomegalovirus, etc.

Many different lesions have been described and these may just be dependent on the duration of the disease rather than on its severity. Since the timing of fetal infection is hardly ever known, the post-conceptual age may be used as a guide to duration.

In preterm infants the predominant lesion is distal metaphyseal porosis or rarefaction (Fig. IV-15). Sometimes this porotic zone is associated with a band(s) of enhanced provisional calcifications. These may also be seen in the scapulae or pelvic bones.

In term infants, more florid changes are noted (Fig. IV-16). The zone of porosis is irregular with variable destruction (saw-tooth appearance). Wimberger's sign refers to destruction of the proximal medial metaphysis. Some of the latter changes could be explained by trauma to the weakened metaphyses.

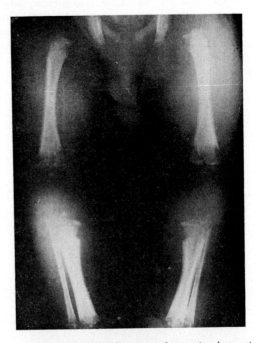

FIG. IV-16. — *Demineralization and extensive destruction of the metaphyses of the femurs and tibiae in a 2-day old term infant with syphilis. Early periosteal layering is present.*

Periostal layering (new bone formation) due to involvement of the diaphysis, is not very often seen early on but is the commonest bony abnormality noted after several months. This produces a double contour along the cortex of the bone shaft but does not extend to the terminal part of the metaphysis. The combination of both metaphyseal and diaphyseal lesions in multiple bones spells congenital syphilis until proved otherwise.

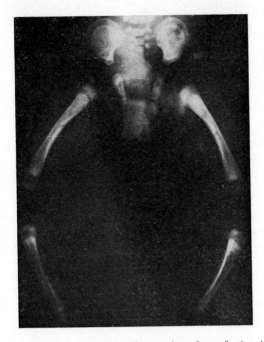

FIG. IV-15. — *Symmetrical metaphyseal rarefaction in an infant with congenital syphilis born at 30 weeks' gestation. The demineralization is most marked in the long bones but the pelvic bones are also involved.*

Preterm delivery. — This is a common finding and syphilis should be included in the causes of unexplained preterm delivery. It should be pointed out that the rate of preterm delivery is higher in underdeveloped countries than elsewhere and this may contribute to the very high percentage of preterm deliveries in Table III.

Hepato-splenomegaly. — Enlargement of both liver and spleen is the most consistent finding on physical examination. In a small number of cases ($\pm$ 15 %), only the spleen appears to be involved. Enlargement may be of any degree but is usually considerable (Fig. IV-17). Inflammatory changes as well as extra-medullary hematopoiesis are responsible for the organ enlargement, while silver stains demonstrate heavy infiltration with *T. pallidum* provided no antibiotics have been used. Organ consistency is firm but not hard. Congenital syphilis should certainly be thought of in any infant with unexplained hepato-splenomegaly.

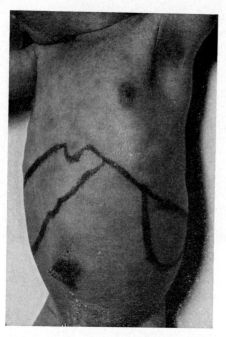

FIG. IV-17. — *Marked hepato-splenomegaly in a preterm infant with hemorrhagic skin lesions on the trunk. A diagnosis of syphilis was confirmed on serological tests.*

Placental size. — There is an increased placental-fetal ratio in about half of the infected infants. This is a most useful finding. The placenta appears pale and thicker than normal, and on handling, the tissues are very friable. The importance of inspection of the placenta after every delivery, and certainly in those babies with unexplained preterm delivery or physical signs, cannot be over-emphasized.

Skin lesions. — These are commonly seen and may be of different kinds.

Excessive cracking and peeling of the skin, especially of the hands and feet, is frequent. Almost total denudation is illustrated in Figures IV-18 and IV-19. This is more than the dryness and peeling found in growth retarded infants.

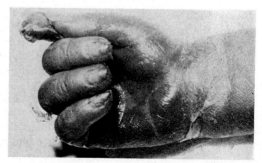

FIG. IV-18. — *Sloughing of the skin of the hand and fingers in congenital syphilis.*

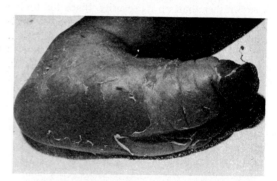

FIG. IV-19. — *Extensive peeling of the sole and toes in congenital syphilis.*

Pustular lesions teeming with spirochetes are sometimes present. When ruptured, they leave a denuded weeping area. Older books referred to this as pemphigus syphiliticus.

Maculopapular lesions are also seen. These are not as frequent in the author's experience, but this may be because they are less easily identified in patients with darker skin pigmentation. It has been suggested that this rash which is pink or red and oval in shape, precedes desquamation.

Very uncommonly annular or circinate cutaneous lesions are seen. "Blueberry muffin" lesions due to cutaneous hematopoiesis have also been observed.

Intrauterine growth retardation. — More than half of the growth retarded infants in our experience, were those in whom the placental-fetal ratio was also increased. This finding has not been a regular feature of congenital syphilis in the literature. It may be that factors affecting fetal growth are differently expressed in different populations.

Pneumonitis. — Mild to moderate pulmonary infiltrates are found in congenital syphilis. This is in keeping with the finding of syphilitic pneumonia at autopsy. The radiological changes, however, are not specific for syphilis.

Hepatitis and conjugated hyperbilirubinemia. — Abnormal liver function tests are frequently found. The hepatitis of congenital syphilis resembles other types of neonatal hepatitis with elevated enzyme levels, jaundice, low albumin levels and occasionally hypoglycemia. The picture of obstructive hyperbilirubinemia often persists for 1-2 months. In several of our patients abnormal liver function tests persisted for the first year of life before returning to normal. None of our children has developed cirrhosis.

Anemia. — It would appear that the spirochetes have a direct effect on the red blood cell with resultant hemolysis. Anemia has occasionally been described as the only sign of syphilitic infection in the newborn. There is an associated reticulocytosis.

Purpura and bleeding. — Thrombocytopenic purpura is not uncommon. The purpuric lesions may be small or large ecchymoses occurring mainly on the trunk, especially the abdomen. It is the author's belief that extensive purpura has a serious prognostic significance.

There may be an obvious bleeding diathesis with hemorrhage from the nose, mouth, or respiratory tract in some babies. It is not known to what extent this is due to a defect of clotting factors secondary to liver involvement or to disseminated intravascular coagulation. These infants do poorly and may die within hours of delivery.

Edema. — Generalised edema was seen in almost a quarter of our infants. It was associated with hypoalbuminemia of the order of 16 g/l and was strikingly extensive, sometimes including ascites. When severe enough the term hydrops fetalis is warranted. Congenital nephrosis or nephritis have been well documented but could not be substantiated as causes in the author's series. In none of the infants was there any proteinuria or hematuria. Serial estimations showed a rising serum albumin with gradual clearance of the edema.

Pseudoparesis. — The immobility of a limb, presumably due to painful bony lesions, is not frequently seen. It is usually unilateral and more often affects the upper limb. It may be confused with an Erb's palsy, but is painful on passive movement.

Mucocutaneous lesions. — Congenital syphilis may present as rhinitis ("snuffles") with a highly infectious nasal discharge which may be mucous, purulent or bloody. This appears not to be as common as previously reported.

Other findings. — Cerebro-spinal fluid abnormalities, indicative of asymptomatic involvement of the brain or spinal cord, are said to occur in 60 % of infants with congenital syphilis. An increase in protein and cells is usually found.

Ocular manifestations such as chorioretinitis and glaucoma have been reported but are infrequent although this may be due to lack of detailed examination.

DIAGNOSIS

In most instances the clinical findings and serologic tests are sufficient evidence for a confident diagnosis of congenital syphilis, and the correlation with autopsy findings very good. Actual demonstration of the *T. pallidum* itself is, of course, the only definitive test. In a small number of infants the diagnosis may be highly suggestive but the investigations not conclusive. One is then left with a possible or presumptive diagnosis of syphilis.

Much has been written about the difficulties of diagnosis of congenital syphilis in the neonate. The following is suggested as a logical approach:

Maternal history and serology. — It is clear that failure to seek antenatal care and an inadequate antenatal care program are the two most important epidemiological factors associated with congenital syphilis (Table II). If the mother has not been serologically tested antenatally, this should be done on blood taken at delivery. In instances of untreated or partially treated maternal syphilis the possibility of congenital infection should be suspected until disproved. There may be a history of rashes or mucocutaneous lesions during pregnancy or previous unexplained stillbirths, but the maternal serology remains the best screening procedure.

Clinical examination of infant and placenta.
— In practice the clinical appearance of the infant and the placenta are the most important pointers to congenital syphilis. Once the physician is familiar with the very varied presentation of the disease, he or she will develop an appropriate level of suspicion. Unexplained hepatosplenomegaly and skin lesions are the most frequent clinical signs (Table III). Others are indicated in the same Table. The various manifestations may appear singly or in any combination.

A large, pale and heavy placenta is highly suggestive of an intrauterine infection and the value of routine placental inspection should be stressed.

A few infants will appear completely normal but infection is suspected because of positive maternal serology. Failure to thrive if no other cause can be found, may occasionally indicate investigation for syphilis in an infant where the disease has not been suspected.

Radiology.
— There is no doubt that radiology of the long bones is a most useful confirmatory investigation in congenital syphilis. Although not completely diagnostic, the presence of bone lesions adds great weight to the clinical diagnosis. They are more extensive and more characteristic with advancing age. Radiological examination should therefore be part of the diagnostic work-up in infants where there is a possibility of congenital syphilis.

Laboratory investigations.

Skin lesions. — If pustules or bullae are present, direct darkfield illumination microscopy for spirochetes may be done. This requires experience and proper care since the fluid contains numerous very infective organisms. Immediate microscopic examination of the fluid is essential and if negative, the examination should be repeated. The scaly or denuded areas of skin do not appear to harbour organisms.

Placental histology. — It is most important that the placenta should be examined by an experienced pathologist. While the typical histologic features are not specific for syphilis, they are certainly compatible with the suspected diagnosis. Demonstration of T. pallidum by silver staining is possible in experienced hands and provides incontrovertible evidence.

IgM levels. — Immune serum macroglobulins are normally very low in the fetus and early neonatal life. This is due to the fact that maternal IgM does not cross the placenta and the fetus is not normally challenged to produce immunoglobulins. The finding of a raised IgM would strongly indicate the presence of a chronic intrauterine infection.

Most infants with congenital syphilis will have markedly raised IgM levels, usually above 60 IU/dl and reaching several hundreds. This was so in 17 out of 18 of our infants on whom the evaluation was made.

Low IgM levels are found in cases of overwhelming syphilitic infection with rapid death within hours of delivery. Other infants show a rise in IgM after several days or weeks which presumably is due to late infection or a delayed response.

It would seem that the serum IgM level is a good screening test in congenital syphilis. None of the other chronic intrauterine infections produce such high levels. The upper limit of normal for cord blood is around 27 IU/dl. A mild elevation ($\pm$ 40 IU/dl) for which no cause was apparent, has been found by the author in a small number of normal infants. It is possible that cord blood specimens may have become contaminated with maternal blood, and in a few cases that there was ABO blood group incompatibility.

Serology. — Serological tests are the principal laboratory aid in the diagnosis of syphilis. While they are extremely valuable in infants they may need to be interpreted in conjunction with the maternal serology and clinical findings.

There are several screening tests available such as the Venereal Disease Research Laboratory slide test (VDRL). These tests detect non-specific antibodies known as reagins. The quantitative VDRL is a good general test for the diagnosis of syphilis, keeping in mind that false positives do occur.

Specific treponemal antibodies are identified by a T. pallidum immobilization (TPI) test or the more commonly used fluorescent treponemal antibody absorption (FTA-ABS) test. The latter is sensitive and specific, and confirms the diagnosis of syphilis when there is doubt.

The VDRL and FTA-ABS detect both IgG and IgM classes of antibodies and since IgG is transferred across the placenta, the newborn infant's blood will passively show positive tests. A positive VDRL or FTA-ABS reaction in the infant is therefore not diagnostic of fetal infection. If the VDRL titre is considerably higher than that of the mother at the time of delivery, it is reasonably good evidence of *fetal* IgG production and hence of congenital syphilis. Transferred maternal antibodies should have disappeared by 3-4 months of age and a raised VDRL level after this time would indicate syphilis in the infant.

To overcome this difficulty in serological diagnosis, a test for *T. pallidum* IgM antibody is employed. This is called FTA-ABS (IgM) or FTA-IgM and assumes that macroglobulins are of fetal origin, and therefore diagnostic of congenital syphilis. On the face of it, the FTA-IgM test should be the final answer but false positives (reportedly 10 %) and negatives are found.

A false positive FTA-IgM is explicable in that the fetus or infant may make IgM antibody against the transferred IgG. The IgG antibody binds with the treponemal antigen and IgM in turn attaches itself to the IgG antibody. When fluorescent anti-human anti-M globulin is added it complexes with the above and gives a false positive test. The total serum IgM estimation will also be misleading in this situation. It is possible to identify this IgM anti-G antibody which is the rheumatoid factor, but no data are available on this point. It can be stated that the false positives are invariably found in situations where the mother either had a positive VDRL or was treated for syphilis, and are not seen in infants of healthy seronegative mothers. It may reflect subclinical or arrested infection.

It is more difficult to explain a negative FTA-IgM test (reportedly as high as 30 %) in the presence of other evidence of congenital syphilis. A negative FTA-IgM test may indicate overwhelming infection (akin to the low serum IgM) or represent a situation where the FTA-IgM becomes positive later on. A negative test in the face of strong evidence of congenital syphilis including raised serum IgM levels was seen in 5 out of 30 infants (16 %) in the author's series. Two infants died shortly after birth (autopsies confirmed the diagnosis), one had been treated in utero, and in two there was no explanation. It has been suggested that high levels of IgG antibody may competitively prevent the IgM from binding to the treponemal antibody. If this is so, then separation of the IgG and IgM classes of antibody in the infant's serum would be the answer. Techniques such as longer incubation and elution may also play a role in the actual test.

Cerebrospinal fluid. — A lumbar puncture is indicated in all infants with suspected syphilis. Not only will the finding of a raised protein and increased white cell count strengthen the case for congenital syphilis, but a VDRL should be done on the cerebrospinal fluid. It is generally agreed that if this is positive it is diagnostic of neurosyphilis, whether the patient is symptomatic or not. Many believe that false positive results do not occur in the spinal fluid.

Differential diagnosis. — The spectrum of differential diagnosis of early congenital syphilis is as wide as that of each of the clinical signs. In clinical practice, however, the main conditions to consider are those in the TORCH group *i. e.* toxoplasmosis, rubella, cytomegalovirus and herpes virus infection. Useful pointers to the diagnosis of congenital syphilis are the skin lesions, the placenta and the extensive bone lesions. Two other serious and multisystem diseases to keep in mind are bacterial septicemia and erythroblastosis fetalis.

PREVENTION AND TREATMENT

Congenital syphilis is preventable. Until infectious syphilis among adults has been eliminated, routine serological screening of every pregnant woman is mandatory. This should be done early in pregnancy and repeated in the third trimester or at delivery. If there is doubt about the VDRL test result, then the FTA-ABS should also be done. Where the mother is judged to have a recently acquired infection or a seropositive test, and has not been treated, she should be given a therapeutic course of penicillin.

Penicillin G, given parenterally, is the drug of choice in pregnancy. Benzathine penicillin G in a dose of 2.4-4.8 million units by deep intramuscular injection is advised. Some clinics give the penicillin at weekly intervals but if there is any doubt about patient compliance, 1.2 million units should be given into each buttock at the same visit. In the vast majority of instances this will cure fetal infection, especially if given early in pregnancy. Should the mother be allergic to penicillin, an alternative drug, preferably one not toxic to the fetus, must be used. Cephaloridine (0.5 g/day for 10 days intramuscularly) would appear to be satisfactory.

For congenital syphilis penicillin is still the drug of choice. Procaine penicillin G, 50,000 units/kg intramuscularly every day, for 10-14 days, is recommended. The same dosage of penicillin is obligatory if neurosyphilis is present or suspected in order to ensure adequate antibiotic levels in the spinal fluid.

Even if the serological tests are not conclusive, infants with clinical findings of congenital syphilis should be treated. This would in any event only happen in a small number of patients. If there is a history of maternal infection but the baby is clinically normal with negative blood tests, a wait and see policy may be adopted. The infant should then be followed up and the VDRL repeated.

It is recommended that all infants with congenital syphilis should be followed for 12 months to ensure that the VDRL titre falls progressively and the test ultimately becomes negative. Repeat lumbar puncture at 6 months is recommended if the earlier spinal fluid was abnormal. Although desirable, these recommendations are seldom carried out in practice. There is a paucity of data relating to the eventual outcome of infants treated for congenital syphilis. It is possible that treponemes may persist in some tissues such as the eye. Generally, if treatment is given while the baby is in utero or during the neonatal period, the prognosis in survivors is good. If the damage is severe, the baby may die despite adequate therapy.

Tetanus neonatorum

INTRODUCTION

There have been descriptions of tetanus in the literature since medical history first began. The relationship between a traumatic wound and subsequent locked teeth and jaws, opisthononos and death was recorded by Hippocrates. But it was not till 1884 that Nicolaier discovered the association between bacilli in the soil and tetanus in experimental animals. Rosenbach (1887) noted the drumstick appearance of the bacillus and ascribed this to spores. In 1890 Faber demonstrated tetanus toxin. In the same year Behring and Kitasato similarly discovered tetanus antitoxin in immune serum.

Prophylaxis against tetanus was first achieved by passive immunization with antitoxin produced by horses and cows. A major advance occurred in the 1920's when Descomby produced tetanus toxoid. He heated toxin and formaldehyde together and found that the resulting toxoid stimulated antibody formation in experimental animals. Although subsequently improved upon, toxoid remains the basis for active immunization. Despite being a totally preventable disease, tetanus remains a serious health problem worldwide. Fifty precent of reported deaths from the disease are in newborn infants, emphasizing the importance of neonatal tetanus in undeveloped countries.

EPIDEMIOLOGY

In many countries tetanus neonatorum has virtually been eliminated by active immunization programs. As immunization is primarily directed at children, and if antibody levels are not kept up in adults, women and their infants may be at increased risk due to declining immunity.

Where it does occur, tetanus neonatorum is an index of the general health care and socio-economic status of the community. In very poor countries it is estimated that up to 10 % of newborn infants die from tetanus; second only to preterm delivery as a cause of neonatal death.

In the neonate the portal of entry for the tetanus bacillus is the umbilicus. The incidence of tetanus neonatorum will thus be higher where there is inadequate cord care as in home deliveries without medical or nursing attendants. In many primitive societies various concoctions are placed on the umbilical stump and these have been known to include dung. In such communities it is improbable that the mothers will have been immunized. The incidence of tetanus is greater in countries with warm climates and in rural areas, probably because of enhanced spore formation by the bacillus and greater contact with the soil.

PATHOGENESIS

Tetanus is caused by a gram-positive bacillus, *Clostridium tetani*. It is an ubiquitous organism found in soil, dust and both animal and human feces. Under aerobic conditions the organism develops spores located at one end giving the characteristic drumstick appearance. These spores are highly resistant and can survive in the soil for many years. Being an obligate anaerobe, the organism thrives in deep wounds and necrotic tissues. The vegetative form of *C. tetani* produces two exotoxins, tetanolysin and tetanospasmin. The former is a hemolysin and is not involved in tetanus. Tetanospasmin is a soluble toxin, and next to botulinus toxin, is the most powerful poison known. It has a selective action on certain areas of the nervous system. These are the motor end plates in skeletal muscles, the spinal cord, the brain and the sympathetic nervous system. It is believed that when the toxin is released in the blood stream, it enters muscles and then reaches the central nervous system by spread along the neural pathway. The rate of spread is dependent on the quantity of toxin, the particular features of the neural pathway and muscle activity.

Tetanospasmin acts by interfering with inhibitory action at the synapses. Efferent output of motor neurones is increased and polysynaptic reflexes are enhanced resulting in unopposed muscular contraction. In the brain, toxin is bound to gangliosides. The mechanism whereby tetanospasmin produces sympathetic overactivity is not known. Once toxin is fixed to the central nervous system it cannot be neutralized by antitoxin.

CLINICAL FINDINGS

The generalised type of tetanus is the most common and the most severe form, and this form is invariably seen in the newborn. Exposure to the organism is usually taken to be at or shortly after birth, with a short incubation period. Signs may appear as early as the third day and peak around 6 to 7 days.

Diminished ability to suck and poor feeding are the earliest signs. Trismus is common and often precedes generalised rigidity because of the short neural pathway. Persistent trismus gives rise to the facial expression known as "risus sardonicus". The condition progresses to generalised rigidity with spasms which are exacerbated by any stimulus. Persistent flexion of the toes is also described. Spasms of the larynx result in inability to swallow while cyanotic episodes or apnoea are the result of involvement of the respiratory muscles. Complications may be vomiting with aspiration pneumonia, and dehydration due to poor intake and increased insensible water loss. Pyrexia is often present in severe cases.

The mortality in untreated tetanus neonatorum is very high, being over 90 %. The majority of deaths occur during the second week of life. Because of the very short incubation period, it is not clear whether the inverse relationship of incubation time to mortality observed in adults holds for the newborn infant. If the infant survives, there is gradual diminution of the spasms and rigidity from the end of the second week but the above signs may persist for up to four weeks or longer.

DIAGNOSIS

The diagnosis of tetanus neonatorum is a clinical one and is based on the presentation. A history of home delivery and inadequacy of maternal immunization are important factors about which to ask. Pathonomonic signs are persistent trismus and rigidity of the abdominal muscles between spasms. These are not found in generalised seizure spasms due to other causes. Attempts to culture *C. tetani* from the umbilicus are generally unsuccessful. Very little is known about electromyography or encephalography in tetanus neonatorum.

The differential diagnosis includes other causes of seizures in the newborn infant. Cerebral hypoxia, intracranial hemorrhage, meningitis, hypoglycemia, hypocalcemia, hypomagnesemia, septicemia and inborn errors of metabolism all should to be considered and excluded. Although the diagnosis may initially be missed in situations where the incidence is low, it should be high on the list in populations at risk for tetanus.

PREVENTION

Tetanus has rightly been described as an inexcusable disease, and this also holds true for tetanus neonatorum. Proper immunization of the pregnant woman worldwide would eliminate the disease. This requires much improved public health and obstetric care, and is an ideal very difficult to achieve.

Aseptic care of the umbilical stump is a sine qua non of good management. The use of a clean ligature and scissors or knife to cut the cord with subsequent application of spirits or alcohol would go a long way towards preventing tetanus neonatorum.

Tetanus antibody crosses the placenta and mothers adequately immunized confer a passive immunity to their infants. The possible interference of maternal antibody with subsequent infant immunization is purely academic in high risk situations. A maternal antitoxin level of 0.01 unit/ml at delivery is protective. This can be achieved by giving a single booster during delivery to a woman who has previously been immunized. In the non-immunized woman two injections of toxoid not less than one month apart will achieve the same result. This should preferably be done early in pregnancy, but even as late as six weeks before delivery enough antibody can be formed to protect the fetus. The need for two injections makes mass immunization difficult, especially in communities lacking a basic health care system. Research is now being directed towards finding a safe vaccine capable of producing primary immunization with a single injection. Active immunization during pregnancy has been shown to be effective in reducing the incidence and also the mortality from tetanus neonatorum.

MANAGEMENT

Tetanus is perhaps best regarded as a multisystem disease, and the affected infant should ideally be treated in an intensive care unit. It will immediately be apparent that where the incidence of tetanus neonatorum is highest, the facilities for treatment are lowest or non-existent. The management outlined here will, therefore, not be possible in many situations.

Antitoxin. — The newborn infant should be given 500 units of antitoxin to neutralise circulating toxin. Human tetanus immune globulin (TIG) is clearly preferable to animal antitoxin but is expensive and not always available. The antitoxin should be given intramuscularly in divided doses.

Antibiotics. — Procaine penicillin G 50-100,000 units/kg/day for 10-14 days intramuscularly is recommended to eliminate the vegetative forms of *C. tetani* and to control secondary infection. Alternatively aqueous penicillin G at the same dosage may be given if an intravenous infusion is being used.

Assisted ventilation. — If the facilities are available, total muscle paralysis with mechanical ventilation is the only treatment likely to be effective in severe cases. The introduction of this form of therapy in the late 1950's led to a dramatic fall in mortality. Indications for paralysis and ventilation are failure to control the frequency of spasms or the duration of spasms, leading to cyanosis and a drop in arterial oxygen levels below 50 mm Hg.

Neuromuscular blocking agents such as *d*-tubocurarine (0.2 mg/kg), alcuronium (0.1 mg/kg) or pancuronium (0.05 mg/kg) are used intravenously to curarise the infant. Mechanical ventilation is commenced after passing an endotracheal (or nasotracheal) tube. Subsequent tracheostomy has been preferred in most large series in the newborn. Tracheal stenosis, usually of the subglottis, is the most common complication of the procedure. The incidence of tracheal lesions or dysfunction is related to the frequency and duration of intubation and is more frequent in smaller infants. The initial intravenous therapy should be continued intramuscularly every 2 to 3 hours to control muscle rigidity sufficiently to allow for smooth ventilatory control. To ensure adequate ventilation continuous monitoring of blood gases is required. Efficient physiotherapy with bronchial toilet and frequent turning of the infant are most important. Pneumonia, pneumothorax or collapse of the right upper lobe are not infrequent complications and portable radiography is essential. There is a preference for volume ventilators, with intermittent sighing to lessen atelectasis and constant flow to allow spontaneous breathing, are both highly desirable. Assisted ventilation is usually required for 3-4 weeks.

Sedation. — Attempts to lessen the frequency and severity of spasms have not been very successful in the newborn. Diazepam, phenobarbitone, chlorpromazine and other drugs have been used. At effective levels they all produce undesirable side-effects, especially respiratory depression. However, an initial attempt to control spasms by sedatives and by reducing tactile and auditory stimuli is worthwhile in all instances.

An aggressive regimen of continuous intravenous infusion of diazepam (20-40 mg/kg/day) together with intragastric phenobarbitone (10-15 mg/kg/day), in 4 divided doses, has been reported to lower mortality and decrease the need for assisted ventilation. In a series of 19 infants so treated, the spasms were controlled in 12 while 7 required ventilation [1]. The side effects of severe drowsiness, coma and apnoeic episodes were reversible with reduction in the diazepam dosage, but presumably with a return of spasms.

General care. — Meticulous attention must be paid to all aspects of the infant's condition. This includes adequate fluid intake by intravenous infusion or nasogastric gavage and supplying the infant's nutritional requirements. The prevention of aspiration pneumonia by dealing with oral secretions, judicious feeding schedules and posturing require expert nursing care. Since tetanus does not confer permanent immunity, immunization with toxoid should always be commenced prior to discharge. Information on the long term neurological outcome of infants who have recovered from tetanus neonatorum is conspicuously absent.

Tuberculosis

INTRODUCTION

Tuberculosis is one of the most ancient diseases. It has been described by a host of writers from Hippocrates onwards, and was called "phthisis" by the Greeks. The name is derived from the Latin "tuberculum" meaning nodule. The Romans referred to the nodular disease in the lung as tuberculin. Because of its impact on societies, it was known in medieval times as the white plague and consumption. Although its communicable nature had been recognised in ancient times, the responsible organism was only isolated and described by Robert Koch, in 1882.

Congenital tuberculosis has very rarely been reported and most publications were before the era of chemotherapy. Unless there is a high index of suspicion, a timely diagnosis of congenital tuberculosis will seldom be made. Tuberculosis acquired in the neonatal period is more common but still a rare condition. Successful outcome depends on early and adequate treatment. The problem most often encountered in clinical practice is that of maternal tuberculosis during pregnancy and the physician needs to be clear about the approach to infants born of such mothers.

EPIDEMIOLOGY

Tuberculosis as a complication of pregnancy or as a disorder in the neonatal period, is clearly related to the incidence of tuberculosis in the general population. From being the leading cause of death at the end of the 19th century, tuberculosis is now an uncommon disease in developed countries. The decline has been attributed to many factors, the most important of which is probably an improved standard of living. In developing countries and in certain susceptible populations however, tuberculosis remains a major disease. It is in such communities that screening for tuberculosis in pregnancy is unfortunately not possible due to lack of health services.

No figures are available for congenital tuberculosis. For such a diagnosis to be made, the tuberculous nature of the lesions and evidence of in utero infection needs to be established. The routes of infection in the fetus and newborn infant are shown in Figure IV-20 [1]. Prenatal infection is very rare, even among infants born to mothers with active, untreated pulmonary tuberculosis, while genital tuberculosis often results in sterility, tubal implantations or miscarriages. Congenital infection is acquired either by hematogenous spread, primarily to the liver, or by inhalation of infected amniotic fluid. Infection acquired at or soon after delivery is more common and usually presents after the fourth week of life. The potential sources of infection are the cervix or vagina and infective adults, particularly the mother (Fig. IV-20). As already mentioned, the clinical diagnosis of congenital tuberculosis is seldom made and most reports are based on autopsy findings.

PATHOGENESIS AND PATHOLOGY

Although there are several *Mycobacterium bacilli*, human tuberculosis is predominantly caused by *Mycobacterium tuberculosis*. As the name implies, *M. tuberculosis* is a bacterial rod 2 to 4 microns long resembling a fungus. It is characterised by its acid fast staining properties (no discoloration by acid alcohol after fuchsin staining).

Tuberculosis is primarily a disease of the lungs and spread is by droplet inhalation into the alveoli. In the non-immune host the bacilli multiply and may then spread to neighbouring lymph nodes by the lymphatics or to distant sites via the blood stream.

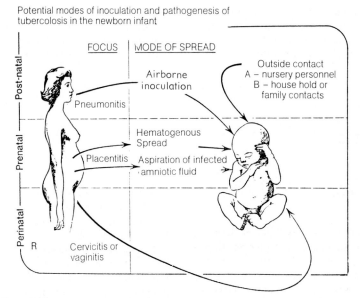

Potential modes of inoculation and pathogenesis of
tubercolosis in the newborn infant

Fig. IV-20. — *Sources of tuberculous infection in the fetus and newborn.*
Reprinted from infectious diseases of the fetus and newborn infant,
with permission of the publishers, W. B. Saunders Company.

The lung lesion and associated enlarged hilar lymph nodes are called the primary complex. The host response is that of a delayed hypersensitivity reaction. Macrophages organise to contain the bacilli and this results in an epithelioid nodule surrounded by lymphocytes. Some macrophages fuse to form the classical multinucleated giant cells. The nodule or tubercle undergoes central caseous necrosis and is finally sealed off by fibroblastic scar tissue.

Reactivation of old lesions is generally the cause of progressive tuberculosis. There is evidence that host resistance may be reduced in the puerperium due to the added burdens of infant care, nursing and sleep deprivation. Whether pregnancy itself influences pulmonary tuberculosis is doubtful. In a pregnant patient with tuberculosis, there may be hematogenous spread to the placenta and a tubercle may form. The fetal vessels supplied by this part of the placenta often undergo thrombosis, thereby preventing the spread of infection to the fetus. If not, the fetus is infected via the umbilical vein with involvement of the liver and lymph nodes. The lymph node at the junction of the cystic duct of the gall bladder and the common bile duct is the draining lymph node for the placental circulation. Hypersensitivity to *M. tuberculosis* cannot be transferred from mother to fetus, and the disease is therefore devastating in its effect. The usual picture is that of miliary tuberculosis including meningitis as a

result of hematogenous spread from the primary hepatic site. It is theoretically possible for the organisms to by-pass the liver and reach the lungs directly via the ductus venosus. In either event, the placenta often demonstrates the presence of acid-fast bacilli.

Amniotic fluid becomes infected when a tubercle ruptures into the amniotic cavity. This causes large numbers of bacilli to be aspirated by the fetus and results in extensive direct involvement of the lungs. There is no single primary complex in the fetus since the tuberculous foci are all at the same stage of development. Infected amniotic fluid may also be swallowed and result in lesions in the gastrointestinal tract. The tubercle bacillus is an obligate aerobe and this probably explains the rapid and usually fatal extension of congenital tuberculosis after birth. It may also explain the greater emphasis on pulmonary rather than hepatic lesions.

Infection from the cervix and vagina is extremely uncommon. Postnatal airborne infection is probably the most common cause of tuberculosis in young infants. Fortunately these latter categories are less severe and carry a better prognosis.

CLINICAL FINDINGS

The clinical signs of tuberculosis in the newborn period are rather non-specific. Congenital infection may present soon after birth but the infants often seem to be apparently well for about 2 weeks. The initial emphasis is on hepatosplenomegaly, jaundice and lymphadenopathy. Unexplained low birth weight has been suggested as an even earlier clue. A later presentation is with poor feeding, failure to thrive, loss of weight and apathy. If the infant lives long enough, respiratory signs predominate with dyspnoea causing difficulty with feeding, rib recession, cyanosis and sudden death related to cyanotic episodes. Auscultation of the chest is usually non-contributory. Unlike older children, the young infant seldom has pyrexia. Infection acquired at or after birth presents after the first month of life and extensive pulmonary involvement is the major finding. Unless the mother has known or overtly active disease, the possibility of tuberculosis will ordinarily not be considered in the very young infant.

DIAGNOSIS

Awareness of tuberculosis in the general population and a good medical history from the pregnant mother are important factors in the anticipation of congenital tuberculosis. Where the mother is known to have active tuberculosis it will be of value to examine the placenta and amniotic fluid for acid-fast bacilli. In most instances the placenta has been disposed of by the time the possibility of tuberculosis is even considered.

A definitive diagnosis of tuberculosis depends on demonstration of acid-fast bacilli. A liver biopsy is clearly not a desirable procedure and emphasis is therefore placed on microscopy and culture of gastric fluid. Unfortunately the positive yield from gastric aspirates in the newborn is rather low. Early chest radiography is also not very helpful. After several weeks, the diffuse, fine nodularity of miliary tuberculosis may be seen. Leucocyte counts do not help in this age period.

The tuberculin skin test is a major diagnostic aid in older children and adults, but is invariably negative in the newborn period. It may become positive after 3 to 5 weeks or may remain negative in the face of extensive disease. A lumbar puncture will show abnormalities in the CSF if the baby has meningitis and should therefore always be done. The likelihood of finding choroidal tubercles in the newborn ocular fundi is not known. A thorough investigation of the mother may provide sufficient evidence to begin therapy in the infant.

PREVENTION AND TREATMENT

During pregnancy. — It is undoubtedly better to identify and treat maternal tuberculosis during pregnancy than to attempt to deal with its serious consequences to the fetus and the newborn infant. Some form of screening is therefore required. The symptoms of sweating, fatigue and anorexia may be ascribed to pregnancy itself, but persistent cough and low grade fever should be investigated for tuberculosis. In a community with a low incidence of the disease, the tuberculin skin test is probably the best means of screening for infection. In populations where tuberculosis is common, most young adults are tuberculin positive. In these circumstances radiologic microfilm screening has been employed. Care must be taken to shield the developing fetus from irradiation. All positive skin reactors in the low incidence category and all those with suspicious microfilms should have a full-sized chest film taken. Appropriate culture for mycobacteria should also be done. Genital tuberculosis may go unnoticed if only microfilm screening is done.

Where there is evidence of tuberculous disease or sufficient suspicion of potential disease, the mother should be started on a chemotherapeutic regimen of isoniazid (300 mg/day) and para-aminosalicylic acid (12 g/day). Many would also add 50 mg pyridoxine per day. If the woman has advanced pulmonary tuberculosis, she should be hospitalised and the addition of streptomycin (2 g/day) to the above regimen be considered. Isoniazid and para-aminosalicylic acid readily cross the placental barrier but may be used in pregnancy, especially in the third trimester. There is no convincing evidence of an increase in congenital malformations with the use of these agents unlike ethionamide which is a potent teratogenic agent and should not be used. Streptomycin does cross to the fetus and may cause hearing loss, and should only be used in advanced disease preferably in the second half of pregnancy. Rifampicin has not been fully evaluated in pregnancy, but ethambutol has been used with no apparent effects on the fetus.

The newborn infant. — As a general rule, vaccination with the Calmette and Guerin attenuated bovine bacillus (BCG) should be a routine procedure for all infants born in communities with significant tuberculous infection. Given within a month of birth it will protect the infant against postnatal infection with *M. tuberculosis* and lessen the severity of such infection. Complications to BCG are now very uncommon and the only disadvantage is that of rendering the skin tuberculin test less easily interpreted. The tuberculin skin reaction after successful BCG vaccination is generally smaller than with active disease.

If the mother is found to have active tuberculosis and especially if she is sputum positive, the newborn infant should be separated from her at birth. If there is no evidence of congenital tuberculosis, BCG vaccination should be given immediately. The infant should remain separated from the mother until she has become sputum negative or received adequate initial therapy. The infant should be followed to ensure that signs of tuberculosis do not appear and that there is a positive tuberculin test indicating conversion following the BCG vaccination. The family should always be investigated for the source of the infectious contact.

Where the mother has active disease but has received treatment during pregnancy and is sputum negative, the infant need not be separated from her. He should receive chemoprophylaxis with isoniazid (5 mg/kg/day) fortwith and this should be continued for several months. The socioeconomic setting of tuberculous disease is usually such that breast feeding is highly desirable if at all possible. Breast feeding needs to be assessed in each situation, keeping in mind the drugs the mother is receiving. The infant should be seen regularly and BCG vaccination performed on cessation of isoniazid prophylaxis. The ideal would of course be to have an isoniazid-resistant strain of BCG to stimulate hypersensitivity and still allow isoniazid prophylaxis simultaneously.

In the situation where the mother has healed and inactive disease, BCG vaccination should be done and routine newborn care given. The mother and infant should be seen from time to time to ascertain that there has been no re-activation of the maternal lesions. The tuberculin skin test should be done after 6 to 8 weeks to document conversion. If negative, re-vaccination is indicated.

Congenital tuberculosis requires aggressive treatment. Because of its rarity and generally poor prognosis, the most effective treatment protocol has not been established. The following drugs have all been used in varying combinations: isoniazid (10-20 mg/kg/day), streptomycin sulphate (15 mg/kg/day), ethambutol (15 mg/kg/day) and rifampicin (15 mg/kg/day). If tuberculous meningitis is present, additional measures such as corticosteroids are indicated. The mortality in congenital tuberculosis is very high and the developmental outcome in survivors is unfortunately not very good.

Combinations of the above drugs are also used in acquired tuberculosis. Although still a very serious disease in the young infant, especially if meningitis is present, the prognosis is generally better than for congenital tuberculosis.

REFERENCES

Congenital syphilis

[1] FIUMARA (N. J.), FLEMIG (W. C.), DOWNING (J. G.), GOOD (F. L.). — The incidence of prenatal syphilis at the Boston City Hospital. *N. Engl. J. Med.*, *247*, 48-52, 1952.

[2] FIUMARA (N. J.). — Congenital syphilis in Massachusetts. *N. Engl. J. Med.*, *245*, 634-640, 1951.

[3] INGALL (D.), NORINS (L.). — *Infectious Diseases of the Fetus and Newborn Infant*, REMINGTON J. S. and KLEIN J. O. (eds), W. B. Saunders C., Philadelphia, 429, 1976.

[4] MAJOR (R. H.). — *A History of Medicine*, Vol. 1. Charles C. Thomas, Springfield, Illinois, 371, 1954.

[5] REYNOLDS (D. W.), STAGNO (S.), ALFORD (C. A.). — *Neonatology, Pathophysiology and Management of the Newborn*, AVERY G. B. (ed.), J. B. Lippincott C., Philadelphia, 609, 1975.

[6] TRUFFI (M.). — *Hieronymous Fracastor's Syphilis : A translation in prose*, 2nd ed., Urologic and Cutaneous Press, St Louis, 1931.

Tetanus neonatorum

[1] KHOO (B. H.), LEE (E. L.), LAM (K. L.). — Neonatal tetanus treated with high dosage diazepam. *Arch. Dis. Child.*, *53*, 737-739, 1978.

Tuberculosis

[1] HUBER (G. L.). — *Infectious Diseases of the Fetus and Newborn Infant*, REMINGTON J. S. and KLEIN J. O. (eds), W. B. Saunders C., Philadelphia, 472, 1976.

31

Fetal and neonatal viral infections

A. BOUE, C. MALBRUNOT

In 1941, Gregg, an Australian ophthalmologist, described 78 neonates who presented with a syndrome consisting of congenital cataract, cardiac malformations and low birth-weight for gestation. He related these abnormalities to maternal german measles (rubella) during the first trimester of pregnancy. In so doing, he opened a new chapter in fetal and neonatal pathology.

In the forty years following these observations, the risk which follows transmission by the mother of a viral infection has been documented by clinical, virological, immunological and epidemiological studies. Despite these, several gaps in our knowledge remain, in large measure due to the methodological problems inherent in this field of study. In the mother, clinically recognizable viral infection is rare (chickenpox, measles, mumps); several of these infections only present with non-specific symptoms (respiratory and intestinal syndromes, skin rashes). In fact, the largest number are asymptomatic (e. g. cytomegalovirus (CMV) infection). The problem is just as difficult if it is studied from the malformed neonate viewpoint. Apart from a few characteristic syndromes (congenital rubella, cytomegalic inclusion disease), many neurological, hepatic and other defects are common to different infections, whether by in utero or perinatal transmission. Also, the interpretation of retrospective studies of late appearing sequelae such as mental retardation and auditory damage remains difficult, even if based on biological criteria.

An analysis of the pathological processes involved in a viral infection in a child or adult normally presents a simple situation: in a subject susceptible to viral contamination without any previous specific, general or local defences, but with a normal capacity for an immune response, there is a general consistency in the evolution of the infection and the clinical signs.

On the other hand, for viral infections of the embryo, fetus and neonate, there exist complex systems for the transmission of the infection, as well as for the passive and acquired protection against it.

The great variety of different manifestations possible for the same viral infection results from the interaction of several factors:

The timing of the maternal viral infection with respect to the pregnancy, as well as the chronology of the path followed by the virus towards the fetus and neonate; the kind of immune reaction in the mother and its timing, these factors determining the time of passage of the maternal antibodies towards the fetus; and finally, the timing of the maturation of the fetal and infant immune responses.

The mother's infection may be primary, or a

reinfection, or a recurrence of a chronic viral infection (herpes, CMV), or a chronic carrier state (hepatitis B). The virus may be transmitted to the child directly by the hematogenous route, after a period of placental multiplication, by ascension through the membranes at the time of rupture, or quite simply at the time of delivery, from the infected genital tract.

Viral infection of embryonic and fetal tissues may occur prior to the passage of maternal specific immunoglobulins, but may also occur afterwards. In the latter case, fetal and neonatal protection is likely, but pathological changes may develop following the viral antigen-maternal antibody reaction in the child.

It is also known that pregnancy creates a some-what special immune state in the mother; the immune response to a viral infection may be different from that occurring with the same virus outside of pregnancy.

The last still poorly known factor is the maturation of the immune response during fetal life and the first few weeks of extra-uterine life. The effect of a viral infection on its progress is not clear, since it mobilises an immature immune system. Disease may thus develop in the newborn which will not be seen when the same virus infects a child only a few weeks older; the newborn will present specific pathological conditions such as with neonatal herpes, or as with the particular sensitivity of the newborn to the respiratory syncytial virus (RSV).

Rubella (German Measles)

Rubella causes a benign eruptive disease in children; however, during the first trimester of pregnancy, it carries a high risk for teratogenesis.

The rubella virus (rubivirus) is classed in the Togavirus family, which consists essentially of the viruses transmitted by arthropods (arbovirus).

EPIDEMIOLOGY

Because rubella gives such a mild clinical picture, and because of its common confusion with other viral eruptions, epidemiological data must be based on biological findings (isolation of the virus, serologic tests).

Normally, small yearly localised epidemic peaks occur, with an occasional great epidemic, such as in the United States in 1963-1964.

The seasonal factor is very important, rubella being prevalent in the spring. The first cases occur sporadically in December and January. Epidemic proportions arer eached from April to June. It is rare from July to November, even if many susceptible subjects remain after the spring epidemic. This seasonal outbreak most probably depends on climatic factors which favor transmission of the virus. This is confirmed by observations carried out in the southern hemisphere, where the epidemics occur during the southern spring (September to December).

Man is the only host; peak incidence occurs in 5 to 10 year old children, and is still common in children up to 15 years old. It thus occurs later than the other common childhood viral diseases. Serologic studies show the presence of specific antibodies in 25 % of 5 year old children, 50 % of 10 year olds and 75 % of 15 year olds.

Seroepidemiologic surveys in young women have shown that, on the whole, 8 to 9 pregnant women out of every 10 are immunised.

Transmission is airborne: the virus is present in the throat of children suffering from rubella for a period of 2 weeks, one week before and one after the skin rash. Congenitally infected neonates must not be forgotten as a possible source of infection.

CLINICAL PICTURE

The clinical picture of congenital rubella has been considerably enlarged since Gregg's description. Different syndromes are described:

A malformative syndrome initially described by Gregg, in which are associated:

— small birth weight, usually with a normal gestational age;

— cardiac malformations, mostly non-cyanotic,

the most common being a patent ductus arteriosus, followed by atrial and ventricular septal defects, and Fallot's tetralogy;

— eye malformations, essentially a cataract (bilateral in 70 % of cases), retinitis, which may be difficult to see if there is a cataract, but which can be the only eye defect; occasionally glaucoma may be present;

— auditory damage, with abnormalities of development of the cochlea and the organ of Corti.

The neonatal rubella syndrome, which may or may not be seen together with the malformative syndrome, consists of thrombocytopenic purpura which appears within the first 48 hours, usually disappearing spontaneously in one or two weeks. The number of platelets is usually between 60,000 and 100,000; the bone marrow shows a drop in megakaryocyte numbers. Hepatosplenomegaly may be associated with hepatitis also seen within the first 48 hours. Bone defects are a radiological finding, with alteration in the trabecular pattern in the metaphyses (Fig. IV-21). Other less common findings have been described, including lung and cerebro-

spinal fluid abnormalities. Central nervous system involvement is seen as early as the neonatal period, with signs of irritability, a tense anterior fontanelle and a rise in the protein content of the CSF from which the virus can be isolated.

Late appearing defects. — There are some relatively rare abnormalities that have been attached to congenital rubella because they are seen with other malformations (chronic rubella-like rash, interstitial pneumonia, hypogammaglobulinemia, diabetes mellitus). But two major complications predominate: — psychomotor problems: a third of the children followed up for congenital rubella show various degrees of psychomotor retardation and — auditory damage: apart from those cases where it is associated with other lesions and an early diagnosis is made, it has been shown that children at risk of contracting congenital rubella, but without recognizable defects at birth, can develop deafness during their first years of life. It seems likely that congenital rubella is responsible for approximately one quarter of the cases of congenital deafness of unknown etiology.

The frequencies and combinations of these clinical signs vary with the timing of examination of the child. Table I gives the frequencies of the main defects seen in 306 children born in the wake of the American epidemic of 1964 and followed up for 4 years by L. Z. Cooper in New York.

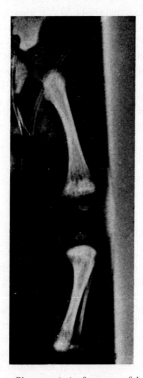

FIG. IV-21. — *Characteristic features of bone lesions in congenital rubella showing dense bands juxtaposed against zones of demineralization in the region of the metaphyses. These lesions may disappear within a few weeks.*

TABLE I. — FREQUENCIES OF THE MAIN CONSEQUENCES OF CONGENITAL RUBELLA IN 306 MALFORMED CHILDREN FOLLOWED UP FOR FOUR YEARS (According to L. Z. COOPER).

Deafness		252	82.3 %
Cardiopathy		182	59.4 %
Cataract { Bilateral		58	
{ Unilateral		50	267 87.2 %
Glaucoma		12	
Retinopathy alone		147	
Psychomotor retardation:			
— weak		84	
— mild		40	170 55.5 %
— severe		46	
Purpura		85	27.7 %
Death		61	19.9 %

Deafness is the only malformation in 68 children.
Cardiopathy is the only malformation in 7 children.

The severity of the malformations and their prevalence depend on the point in the pregnancy at which the infection occurred. The most serious

TABLE II. — CLINICAL CONSEQUENCES OF CONGENITAL RUBELLA
ACCORDING TO THE TIMING OF MATERNAL RUBELLA (according to L. Z. COOPER)

	Time in the pregnancy when rubella first appeared (weeks) *				
	2-4	5-8	9-12	13-16	>16
Neonatal purpura	14 (23 %)	43 (40 %)	7 (8 %)	2	0
Cardiopathy	34 (56 %)	62 (58 %)	17 (20 %)	2	1
Cataract and glaucoma	30 (50 %)	31 (29 %)	6 (7 %)	0	0
Deafness	50 (83 %)	76 (71 %)	55 (67 %)	21 (49 %)	0
Psychomotor retardation	34 (56 %)	63 (59 %)	20 (24 %)	11 (25 %)	0
Total number of children. .	60	106	82	43	16

* This division in weeks has been used to adapt the usual nomenclature of the months of pregnancy which are calculated from the date of the last period.

defects (cardiopathy, cataract) are essentially seen after rubella infection occurring during the first weeks of gestation (Table II).

Is it possible to estimate the teratogenic risk? Although the only available studies are retrospective, they furnish some valuable information: the risk is the same during epidemics as for sporadic cases. The first three months of pregnancy are the most risky, but it is impossible to precisely determine the end of this dangerous period. The risk seems to be particularly high during the first two months (up to the twelfth week of gestation); this is the time when the most serious malformations occur. Clinical studies have placed the teratogenic risk in this period at 30 to 80 % of births. However, more recent studies of aborted embryonic tissues have shown

TABLE III. — MALFORMATIONS SEEN IN CHILDREN EXPOSED TO THE RUBELLA VIRUS AT VARIOUS TIMES IN THE PREGNANCY. Prospective study by E. MILLER et al. (1982).

	≤ 12 weeks	13-16 weeks	17-22 weeks
Rate of congenital infection.	90 %	53 %	36 %
Number of seropositive children at birth	9	26	
Cardiopathies and other malformations	5	0	0
Deafness alone	4	9	0
Overall risk of malformation in all the children exposed to the virus	90 %	18 %	0 %

that the virus can be isolated in 90 % of cases.

The risk reduces during the third month of development and is quite small from the fourth month on (after the sixteenth week of pregnancy). This is due to two factors: a fall-off in the rate of fetal viral infection (about 50 %); also malformations do not always occur at this time in the infected fetus, and they are less severe, eye and cardiac lesions being absent, with hearing defects predominating (Table III). Despite a very good prospective study in England by Miller et al. (1982), more data is required to be able to assess the possible effects of the viral infection on the child's intellectual development.

PHYSIOPATHOLOGY
AND PATHOGENESIS

Maternal infection

The virus gains access to the lymphatic system via the nasopharyngeal mucosa where it fixes itself. This explains the adenopathy seen early during the period of invasion. There follows a period of viremia from the seventh or the ninth day, which continues until the rash appears. It is also on about the eighth day that the virus appears in the throat, where it remains for about a fortnight; virus titer is low at first, then becomes significant in the days immediately before and after the eruption. This represents the contagious period.

Antibodies appear at the same time as the rash.

The increase in antibody levels is usually very rapid, reaching high titres in a few days. This immune response is essentially made up of IgM antibodies which will remain for about one month; they are followed by specific IgG antibodies which will remain throughout the patient's life.

These antibody titres will fall during the months following the infection, but great variations are often seen. The mean antibody titres in subjects immune for several years lie between 1/80 and 1/640; lower or higher titres may be found.

Whereas other symptoms or complications of the disease can be attributed to viral proliferation in the tissues concerned (adenopathy, arthritis), the skin rash reflects the antigen-antibody interaction, variations in the equilibrium between antigen and antibodies being the determinants of the rash. This explains the high proportion of atypical cases, with no rash, as well as the prevention of the rash, but not of the viral infection, by gammaglobulins.

Reinfection is possible. Normally, in an immune subject, the virus is neutralized by the IgA antibodies present in mucosal secretions. In some cases, however, the virus may enter the mucosal cells and multiply therein. This viral infection can only be detected by routine serologic investigations which show a rise in antibody titres. Occasionally, the virus has been isolated from the throat where it is present in low titers and for a short time. These subjects are not contagious, and are asymptomatic.

The presence of specific antibodies and the immune memory which induces a rapid rise in antibody titres prevents the dissemination of the virus outside of the tissues where it was seeded at the time of contagion, as well as its hematogenous spread to the fetus.

Congenital infection

In the pregnant woman, the virus reaches the placenta and embryonic tissues during the viremic phase. When rubella occurs during the first ten weeks of pregnancy, the virus may be isolated from both the placenta and embryonic tissues; after the tenth week, it can be isolated more often from the former than the latter. This may explain the severity of rubella in the first two months, and the part the placenta may play in the following months.

Once the embryonic tissues have been infected, a chronic viral infection develops, which will remain throughout gestation. At birth, the virus is present in the throat, where it will be found for several weeks. Neonates with congenital rubella are contagious, and great care must be taken to protect the family members. After the sixth month, the virus can only rarely be isolated from the throat.

The presence of virus in the embryonic tissues during development explains the clinical signs of congenital rubella. It has been shown that the rubella virus acts on cellular division: In some tissues, the virus infecting as yet undifferentiated cells inhibits mitoses at the onset of differentiation; in others, damage in chromosome structure (breaks) leads to a slower rate of growth in that cell population, thus slowing down fetal growth and being responsible, among other things, for the low birth-weight.

The specific antibody titres evolve in a particular way. High titres of IgM antibodies as well as specific IgM antibodies are found from the time of birth on. These specific antibodies are made by the neonate: they will remain throughout the first years of life, being IgM initially and then IgG. The presence of specific antibodies after the sixth month confirms a case as congenital rubella.

DIAGNOSIS

Diagnosis of rubella infection in the pregnant mother

The clinical diagnosis is based on the differential diagnosis of a maculo-papular rash. However, it is almost impossible to make a positive diagnosis of rubella from clinical signs alone, except during a well defined epidemic, as normally seen at the end of winter and during springtime. Numerous other viruses, such as enterovirus, adenovirus, myxovirus, can give rubella-like skin rashes associated with the same clinical signs (adenopathy, arthralgia). They are responsible for a large proportion of false diagnoses. In addition, a large number of rubella cases are asymptomatic. For these reasons, the diagnosis should never be made on the strength of the clinical signs alone; laboratory investigations carried out under good conditions will give a reliable answer.

Biological diagnosis:

Isolating the virus is helpful in the differential diagnosis: but it is difficult, and requires particular cell systems. It is in fact almost never carried out. A virological search of throat samples can lead to the discovery of other viruses (enterovirus, adenovirus) which may be responsible for rubella-like rashes.

Serology is of great value, but only if some

essential rules have been followed: the samples must be taken at specific times, and the different serum titrations for one patient must always be carried out with the same test, even though the hemagglutination-inhibition test is well standardized.

The interpretation of serologic results depends on the early timing of the first blood sample. When it is taken less than ten days after exposure, serological tests will give the state of immunity of the woman at the time of exposure; if antibodies are present, in whatever titre, the mother is immune, the fetus is not at risk, and a second sample is not required. However, if antibodies are absent, the mother is susceptible to developing the infection and a second test a fortnight later is essential; it will show either a continued lack of antibodies which means that there has been no infection, or, more likely, that the suspected contact has had a rubella-like rash due to another virus; or, the appearance of specific antibodies which confirm a rubella infection.

More difficult is the interpretation of serological tests carried out later, either because the mother is seen too late (more than 10 to 15 days after the rash in the contagious child), or because the time of contamination cannot be determined exactly (child communities). It is then absolutely essential to carry out two tests a fortnight apart.

What will be found?

No antibodies; the patient is susceptible, but there has been no infection. Steady or increasing antibody titres are suspicious. However a high antibody titre, or a rapidly increasing titre cannot by itself define a rubella infection: there are great individual differences in the antibody titres of previously immune patients; also, the booster effect of a second infection simulates the rise in antibody titre of a primary infection. The presence of specific IgM antibodies can give an answer, as these are found only during the first infection, and for 4 to 6 weeks after the rash. Recent progress in fetal blood sampling techniques after the twentieth gestational week, and developments in specific IgM antibody titration (especially the "capture assay" with anti-μ antibodies) should allow for the diagnosis of viral infection to be carried out in the fetus. This should prove valuable for cases of maternal rubella during the third month of pregnancy in determining whether the fetus has been infected or not.

Diagnosis of congenital rubella

Clinical diagnosis. — The association of a cardiac and ocular malformative syndrome and fœtopathies (especially purpura) is highly suggestive. However, a biological diagnosis is necessary in the case of incomplete and uncharacteristic types (small birthweight, hepatic signs) which only suggest fetal disease of infectious origin.

Biological diagnosis. — The diagnosis is confirmed by serology alone, and more specifically, by the presence of specific IgM antibodies. The neonate has in fact received from its mother specific IgG antibodies usually in a high titre because of the recent infection; the neonate's immune response to the virus can only be shown by the presence of specific IgM antibodies.

PREVENTION
OF CONGENITAL RUBELLA

Vaccination. — The best way of avoiding congenital rubella is to assure that all women of procreative age have acquired specific immunity against the rubella virus. In an attempt to protect women, several different vaccination policies have been proposed:

(*a*) The vaccination program adopted by the American Health Authorities and applied since 1969, is the routine vaccination of all 1 to 12 year old children, boys and girls, so as to create an immune barrier against the spread of the virus which might contaminate susceptible pregnant women. The success of this programm depends on the efficiency of its organization, as such a vaccination campaign must reach at least 85 to 90 % of children to succeed.

(*b*) In some countries, adolescent girls are vaccinated when they are 12 to 14 year old, most of them by that time having been immunised by natural infection. For example, in France, 50 % of 10 year old children have antirubella antibodies, as do 75 % of those 15 years old. Routine vaccination without serological controls beforehand would immunise almost all the female population from the age of 15 years on.

(*c*) The vaccination of adult women is the most difficult problem encountered in using the live rubella vaccine. Its use must be on an individual case basis. Whereas serological tests are of no use in the routine vaccination of children or adolescents, they must be carried out in adult women; vaccination will then be reserved for the 10-20 % of susceptible women. The live rubella vaccine must be avoided in women who are at the beginning of their pregnancy or who could become pregnant in the weeks following its use, even if only for the fact that out of 100 "normal" pregnancies, 2 or 3 malformed children will be born in any case.

Despite this advice, women have been vaccinated with the live rubella vaccine only to discover afterwards they were pregnant at the time. During the early years of rubella vaccination, an abortion was recommended. However several hundred pregnancies where the seronegative mother was accidentally vaccinated at the start of pregnancy have now been taken to term with no malformations linked to an in utero rubella infection being reported.

There seems therefore to be little cause for concern for mothers vaccinated during pregnancy.

Passive immunisation. — It has been suggested that gamma globulins can only effectively protect the fetus if they are given in the first few days immediately after exposure (2 to 3 days at the most, according to trials in volunteers). Only gamma globulins with high antibody titres must be used. In any case, the antibody titre should be measured immediately before, as well as 2 and 4 weeks after the injection: gamma globulins can prevent the rash, and delay the formation of antibodies. In this case, a rubella infection which might reach the fetus can only be confirmed by serology.

Cytomegalovirus (CMV) infections

Cytomegaloviruses are so-called because they induce the formation of enlarged cells in infected tissues with a large intranuclear inclusion body. They belong to the herpes virus family. Although they are found in several animal species, they have great host specificity; the human CMV has no other reservoir than man, nor can it be transmitted to another species. Just as for the other herpes viruses, CMV infections are characterized by the lengthy presence of the virus and by periodic recurrences.

PATHOGENESIS

CMV is extremely fragile outside the host cell. This virtually excludes all airborne or water transmission. Contamination by CMV requires close intimate contact allowing the passage of the virus. Knowing the main excretory pathways for the virus leads to the identification of the various routes of contamination. The virus is usually isolated from urine. It has also been isolated from the throat, the uterine cervix, spermatic fluids and milk. Throughout pregnancy, the number of women with cervical CMV increases (Table IV). The virus has been isolated from 25 % of maternal milk samples taken 48 hours after delivery, and later.

There are no symptoms or signs which cause one to suspect a recurrence; indeed, the primary infection is most often asymptomatic. Only serology

TABLE IV. — FREQUENCY OF FINDING CMV AT THE UTERINE CERVIX ACCORDING TO THE TIME OF PREGNANCY.

| Study | Pregnant women | | | Non pregnant women |
	First trimester	Second trimester	Third trimester	
Stagno	1.6 %	6.1 %	11.3 %	9.4 %
Numazaki	0 %	9.6 %	27.8 %	—
Montgomery	2 %	7 %	12 %	—

can determine whether a subject has been infected or not. All patients with positive serology must be considered as potentially contagious. The period of viral excretion is usually very long. During the primary infection, in the congenital or neonatal types, the virus can be isolated throughout the first months and even the first years of life (up to 3 or 4 years). Viral excretion during recurrences is probably shorter, but still lasts weeks or months.

Outside of these periods of excretion of infectious viral particles, it is thought that the viral genome may be present in lymphocytes. Stimulating these lymphocytes leads to their division, and the synthesis of infectious viral particles from the viral genome contained within them. This is probably the mechanism responsible for post-transfusion CMV infections, the donor lymphocytes being stimulated by the foreign antigens of the recipient.

It is not known whether the immune system changes seen during pregnancy and the immune relationships between mother and fetus, play any part in the number of recurrences of CMV infection during pregnancy, and in the routes of transmission from the mother to the fetus.

EPIDEMIOLOGY

The first year of life. — Contamination is most often seen during the first months of life. Two factors in particular are involved:

The essential role of the mother as a source of virus. All studies show that only children with seropositive mothers are contaminated. Most of these infections occur in the first few weeks of life, the children developing their specific IgM antibodies between 3 and 6 months of age. The early infection time and the exclusive role of the mother makes one suspect the presence of CMV in the latter's genital tract. Weller went so far as to say that "the child is born within a sea of CMV". The virus is also found in the saliva and milk, but no study has yet been able to show conclusively their importance as a means of contamination.

Socio-economic factors also play an important part, on two levels:

(a) *The proportion of seropositive and therefore potentially contagious, mothers* is higher in lower income communities; this is often seen in African and Asian populations, where more than 90 % of the mothers are seropositive. Similar figures are found in the lower socioeconomic groups in industrialized societies. In high socioeconomic groups, less than 50 % of the mothers are seropositive.

(b) *The high rate of contamination during the first year of life.* In analyzing the risks of infection in children born of seropositive mothers, it appears that more than 70 % of the children are contaminated within the first year of life in African and Asian populations, compared with 25 to 40 % in lower socioeconomic groups, and only 10 % in higher class in industrialized societies (Table V).

Childhood, adolescence and adulthood. — Care must be taken in examining seroepidemiologic studies, because the increasing number of seropositive subjects with age depends on two factors, the relative importance of each being difficult to determine: on the one hand, primary infections occurring at all ages, and on the other hand, older people who will have had, during their

TABLE V. — SEROEPIDEMIOLOGY OF CMV INFECTIONS IN FRANCE

	French population		Migrant population	
	Number of cases tested	% of seropositive cases	Number of cases tested	% of seropositive cases
Paris and its suburbs				
Low socio-economic rank				
Mothers of 1 year old children (1974-1975) . . .	182	66	47	91
1 year old children (1974-1975)	182	13 (20 %)	47	38 (42 %)
Pregnant women (1978-1979)	194	59.8	225	94.2
Low and middle socio-economic ranks				
Pregnant women (1978-1979)	698	51.1	309	84.8
Middle socio-economic rank				
Mothers of 1 year old children (1974-1975) . . .	310	47	89	89
1 year old children (1974-1975)	310	5 (11 %)	89	22 (26 %)
Pregnant women (1978-1979)	445	41.1	128	85.9
Alsace, rural area				
Mothers of 1 year old children (1974-1975) . . .	339	46	26	96.2
1 year old children (1974-1975)	339	4 (9 %)	26	23 (24 %)
Pregnant women (1982)	303	39.6 %		

( ) Percentage of seropositive cases among children with a seropositive mother.

childhood, a greater risk of contamination than now occurs, thus giving a greater proportion of seropositive subjects in the older age groups.

Longitudinal studies carried out on groups of subjects followed up for several years will give a better idea of the risk of contamination in each age group. It has already been shown that sero-conversion is infrequent between the ages of 1 and 4; the mother is still the principal source of contamination, as during the first year of life. However, day nurseries and infant schools do not seem to facilitate contamination, quite the opposite of what is seen with most of the other childhood diseases.

During adolescence and adulthood, kissing and sexual intercourse may be sources of contamination, as they are for infectious mononucleosis, but no epidemiologic studies have been carried out to determine the rate of contamination in these age groups.

Risk factors of in utero transmission. — Because of its grave consequences, in utero infection is the main problem, the extent of which has been measured by routinely isolating virus from the urine of neonates. In utero CMV infection can lead to a very wide range of different effects in the neonate. Most often, it is asymptomatic, the diagnosis being made on virological and serological results. But the full clinical picture of cytomegalic inclusion disease can be seen with the diagnosis being made at birth. Its main clinical features are: low birth weight, hepatosplenomegaly, hyperbilirubinaemia, petechiae which appear a few hours after birth, associated with thrombocytopenia; chorioretinitis, microcephaly and paraventricular cerebral calcifications are often associated.

The relative importance of these signs varies from case to case; they may be seen with other signs: lethargy, feeding difficulties, convulsions, respiratory distress.

The immediate prognosis is poor. The longer term prognosis will depend essentially on the neurological sequellæ, such as mental retardation, paralyses, and spasticity.

Besides this generalised type of syndrome, other more localized forms exist where one organ system is more particularly involved (neurological and hepatic types with different prognoses).

Different routine virological studies in large numbers of neonates have shown that the virus can be isolated from the urine of 0.3-2 % of children studied.

In all of these studies, only a few rare cases of cytomegalic inclusion disease (CID) were reported, usually in less than 10 % of the children with virus present in their urine. Most of the children had no clinical signs of an in utero infection despite undeniable biological evidence of in utero infection. Prospective studies of these asymptomatic infected children have shown auditory defects, and even complete deafness, in 10 to 15 % of them.

Two questions need to be answered:

(1) Does the in utero infection follow a primary infection in the mother, or can it occur in a chronic carrier, or during a re-infection in an immune subject? After the birth of one child with CID, in utero infections with CMV have been detected during subsequent pregnancies, either by virological or serological studies. But in all of the carefully studied cases, the children had no clinical signs at birth.

(2) Are the effects on the fetus the same in both situations? If fetal infection can be seen during both primary infections and recurrences, the pathological effects of an in utero infection are only seen when the mother has biological signs of a primary infection (Stagno et al., 1982; Grant et al., 1981), in which case the fetal signs are seen in about 50 % of cases.

Its is not known as yet whether the auditory defects seen after congenital CMV infection result from viral contamination during a primary infection in the mother or during a recurrence.

Mental retardation has also been reported in these children. These studies must be interpreted very carefully, because transmission of the virus during a recurrence seems to be more frequent in lower socio-economic groups (single mothers, immigrant workers); the poor social background in which these children are brought up can have great influence on their mental development.

DIAGNOSIS

Laboratory investigations

Histopathology. — These methods are of interest in the absence of virology or serology. Cells from the urinary deposit stained with Giemsa, Papanicolaou or haematoxylin-eosin will show a very large intranuclear inclusion body taking up virtually all the nucleus. They are found in about half of the cases of CID. These inclusions can be ascribed to a CMV infection, because the other viral infections which give rise to intranuclear inclusion bodies only rarely cause this neonatal pathology. However, a negative urinary result cannot rule out the diagnosis which can be confirmed retrospectively by finding intranuclear inclusion bodies in various tissues.

Virology. — CMV can be grown on human fibroblast cell cultures, these being the only ones susceptible to the virus. Depending on the quantity of virus present in the inoculum, cytopathogenesis will occur within a few days, or weeks. Staining the cells shows up the characteristic lesions: small foci of cells, presenting a large intranuclear inclusion body surrounded by a clear halo. There are also intracytoplasmic condensations, giving a picture similar to inclusion bodies. All these characteristics together confirm the presence of CMV without carrying out identification by seroneutralization. Recently rapid detection of CMV in urine through DNA hybridization with a labelled probe has been proposed (Chan and Merigan, 1983).

To interpret these virology results, several factors must be kept in mind:

(*a*) The sampling quality: As CMV is extremely fragile outside the cell, urine is the best substance to use for its isolation; provided it arrives rapidly in the laboratory, and is sent in melting ice. It is always best to contact the virology laboratory beforehand to ensure the best sampling and transport conditions.

(*b*) The time of sampling: During both primary infections and recurrences, the virus may be excreted in the urine for months if not years. This is why isolating the virus to confirm a primary infection is in fact of little use, except in the first few weeks of life, when it confirms an in utero contamination. The number of viruses in the urine can be very important (10^5-10^6/ml). In the neonatal period, contamination leads to urinary viral excretion only from the second month; the viral numbers often being less important (10^3-10^4/ml).

Serology. — There are several serologic techniques available. Some can titrate specific IgM antibodies, and are therefore very useful in establishing a diagnosis (indirect haemaglutination, immunoenzymology).

Seroconversion confirming a primary infection is only rarely seen in successive tests. Seroconversion shown up by complement fixation must be viewed very critically. This method not being very sensitive, a rise in antibody titre found by other techniques, such as during a recurrence, may lead to a seroconversion demonstrated by complement fixation only. In the interpretation of positive serology, the antibody titre alone is not sufficient. In the neonate, a difference must be made between transmitted maternal antibodies and acquired antibodies, and later on, between a recurrent or a primary infection.

TREATMENT AND PREVENTION

Treatment. — The possibilities for treatment of CID by either antiviral substances or interferon have not been reliably assessed as yet.

Vaccination. — Vaccination against CMV has been suggested, on the same principles as for rubella. Vaccination trials have been carried out in volunteers with a living viral strain which had been passaged several times in human fibroblast cultures. Antibodies did appear after the subcutaneous injection of virus. It seems, however, premature to discuss vaccination trials, since several important factors have not yet been studied fully: e. g. the criteria and degree of attenuation of the virus used for vaccination; the characteristics of the latent infection caused by the "wild virus", and that of the infection that could follow from vaccination; the oncogenic properties of the herpes virus group.

Neonatal herpes

INTRODUCTION

The first cases of neonatal herpes were reported by Batignani (1934) and Haas (1935). Further clinical details have since, completed the picture and progress has been made in establishing the diagnosis by virology. Two problems remain however; its prevention i. e. detecting genital herpes in the pregnant woman and the steps that must be taken as a result, and its treatment.

THE VIRUS

The herpes-viruses, among which are included the cytomegalovirus, varicella-zoster virus, Epstein-Barr virus and herpes simplex virus are DNA viruses, which have an outer envelope. They multiply in the cell nucleus giving rise to inclusion bodies. Because of their envelope, they are very fragile. Their transmission in man often requires intimate contact. They tend to cause latent chronic infections, since they are able to survive throughout the life of the infected organism. Herpes simplex virus remains in latent form in the sensory ganglia of the cranial or vertebral nerve roots; under various circumstances, such as exposure to the sun, episodes in genital life, psychological stress, the virus reappears giving rise to recurrent herpes infection.

There are two different antigenic types of herpes simplex:

Type 1: Responsible for buccal infections (gingivostomatitis, recurrent oral herpes); ocular infections (follicular conjunctivitis, keratitis) and occasionally neonatal herpes;

Type 2: Responsible for genital infection, visible in men, often unseen in women. It is also the most common cause of neonatal herpes.

EPIDEMIOLOGY

Neonatal herpes is seen throughout the world, suggesting that the virus is ubiquitous. The rate of neonatal herpes infection has been established in the United States as 1 case of clinically diagnosed neonatal herpes for every 7,500 deliveries. In lower income groups, there are fewer cases even though there are a greater number of cases of genital herpes; but 80 % of these women have antiherpes antibodies, compared with 50 % in the higher income groups.

The rate is higher in the newborn of young primipara, who are more likely to develop a primary herpes infection. Herpes infections are seen more often in premature children than in children born at term. Neonatal herpes occurring in several children born successively of the same mother has not been reported.

Infections between the ages of 6 months and 14 years are mostly due to herpes 1: Herpes 2 infections appear later, after the commencement of sexual activity.

TRANSMISSION

Viral transmission can occur during the pregnancy, at the time of delivery and after birth.

During pregnancy. — At the beginning of pregnancy, primary maternal herpes can be transmitted to the embryo by the hematogenous route, and so lead to spontaneous abortion; the number of such miscarriages in women with genital herpes is three times greater than in controls. The virus has been grown from the products of conception. It is also possible that miscarriage may be due to the severity of the maternal infection. In some rare cases, the virus has been found in the fetal membranes and the amniotic fluid, but not in the fetal tissues.

— Primary maternal herpes during the first trimester of pregnancy may lead to congenital malformations. This has been shown in a few cases, where the neonate presented with microcephaly, cerebral calcifications, microphthalmia, a cutaneous vesicular rash; from which herpes virus type 1 or 2 could be grown.

— Herpes infection later on in the pregnancy can lead to stillbirth.

— Finally, if the mother develops a herpes infection right at the end of the pregnancy, the virus may be transmitted either by the transplacental route as for the cases described above, or by the ascending route in case of premature rupture of the membranes. In this case, the clinical signs will be present at birth.

At the time of delivery. — This is the most frequent kind of contamination. For this to occur, the virus must be present in the genital tract of the mother. It may be there as a result of a primary infection, or of a recurrence. In the former, the virus will be present in greater numbers and for longer (up to three months in case of a primary infection, and three weeks for a recurrence). The child is therefore at greater risk of contracting serious neonatal herpes if the mother has primary herpes at the time of delivery; this is particularly so as no maternal antiherpes antibodies will be present in the child's blood.

After birth. — The virus may be transmitted by direct contact with either the mother, or a member of the family, or a member of the health team. In actual fact, it seems the mother is virtually the only one to contaminate her child: 200 children and their mothers were followed up by serology up to the child's age of 4 years; for 131 seropositive mothers (*i. e.* potentially contagious), 80 children (61 %) had asymptomatic primary herpes infections; only 4 children (6 %) of the 67 seronegative mothers had such an infection. All the infections occurred in the first months of life.

CLINICAL PICTURE

Neonatal herpes can present with different clinical pictures, ranging from an asymptomatic infection to a localised condition, or even a general disease that can prove fatal or leave serious after-effects. On the whole, disseminated infection or central nervous system involvement most often leads to a fatal outcome, or else results in serious neurological and psychomotor consequences. Infections affecting only the skin, mouth or eyes have a better prognosis. However important psychomotor or ocular problems may be seen; they must be looked for carefully and for a long time after birth.

Generalised infections. — The first symptoms of herpes infection normally appear during the first week of life. But some may show signs from birth, and others may not show anything before the third week. Most often, the first signs are non specific, with anorexia, vomiting, lethargy, and pyrexia. Some children also have more specific signs, such as skin vesicles, buccal involvement, or keratitis. When the infection is fully established, all the organs are involved.

The disease progresses quickly in most cases, usually within the week, but some children die within a few hours after the onset of the initial symptoms. Mortality is about 80 %. Those children that do survive have, for the most part, significant mental retardation and/or ocular after effects such as chorioretinitis.

Localised infections. — They may be isolated or seen as several together. However, one can never be certain that a local infection will remain so; the risk of it becoming generalised is always present.

Central nervous system: symptoms usually occur later than with the generalized disease. In half the cases, the patient is at first irritable, lethargic; there are whole body tremors, and there may be focal or generalized convulsions. During the course of the illness, skin vesicles and rarely buccal and ocular manifestations, may be observed. In other cases, skin lesions appear first. In the cerebrospinal fluid, there is an increase in the leukocyte count due to a lymphocytosis as well as a rise in the protein content. The virus is only rarely isolated from the cerebrospinal fluid; this is quite the opposite to what is described in cases of neurological involvement in generalized infections. Non specific electroencephalographic changes are found in virtually all the children. The disease evolves towards a rapidly fatal outcome in 40 % of cases; of those who survive, many will show serious neurological sequelae (microcephaly, hydrocephaly, psychomotor retardation), or, more rarely, ocular problems (chorioretinitis, corneal scars, cataracts, blindness).

Eyes: Eye involvement may be the only sign, but it may be associated with central nervous involvement, or may be seen as part of a generalized infection: conjunctivitis, keratoconjunctivitis, chorioretinitis, keratitis. The usual after-effects are: chorioretinitis, cataracts, recurring herpes keratitis, and residual corneal scars.

Skin: a vesicular skin rash may be seen alone, but it may occur with other localised lesions. It may also be part of a generalized infection. The rash may vary from a few discrete and separate vesicles with an erythematous base measuring 1-2 mm in diameter, to bullous lesions more than 10 mm in diameter. They may be spread out, or grouped together by fours or fives. Rarely, a zoster-like rash can be seen; a generalized erythematous macular rash, which may give rise to vesicles a few days later. These may also be petechiae and purpura without the vesicular rash. The rash may recurr in the same, or different places at any time for at least five years after the initial infection. The prognosis is quite good, but subclinical ocular or central nervous lesions may exist. Long term follow-up is required to screen for psychomotor retardation and ocular lesions.

Buccal cavity: the mouth, tongue and larynx may be involved. Recurrences may occur. The buccal cavity may be involved alone or may be part of a generalized or localized infection.

DIAGNOSIS

This must be made as quickly as possible, so that therapy may be attempted.

Clinical diagnosis. — It is difficult to establish a firm clinical diagnosis because most cases present a non-specific syndrome, especially so in generalized infections. Even when specific lesions do exist (skin vesicles, eye involvement), they may be missed or thought to be due to some other cause. It is therefore important to question the mother concerning possible herpes infection, and in particular genital herpes, which might have occurred at one time or other in the mother's life, but more so towards the end of pregnancy. Genital herpes in the mother's sexual partner must also be asked about and looked for.

Biological diagnosis. — Despite the lengthy delay inherent in the different biological tests it is no longer of purely intellectual interest to prove the herpes infection. Various preventive and therapeutic measures are beginning to emerge.

Cytologic methods: Allow a quick presumptive diagnosis of infection by the Herpes simplex virus. The samples are obtained by scraping the base of vesicles, buccal ulcers, corneal or conjunctival lesions. To look for genital herpes, samples can be obtained from the lesions or from the cervico-vaginal secretions if no lesion can be seen. After fixing the smears with alcohol and staining with the Papanicolaou stain, giant multinucleated cells with intranuclear inclusion bodies may be seen. This is similar to the changes seen with the varicella zoster virus; the two infections can usually be differentiated on the basis of clinical and epidemiological data.

Virologic methods: The surest way of establishing that the neonatal illness is due to the herpes virus is to isolate and type the virus from samples from the neonate, the mother, and possibly her sexual partner. The samples must be obtained from several different places, thus increasing the chances of isolating the virus. This also gives an idea of the extent of the disease. If they cannot be studied in the hours that follow, the samples must be frozen at $-70°$ C ($-94°$ F). Samples taken with a swab can be kept at room temperature in Leibowitz-Emory transport medium. The samples are then used to inoculate tissue cultures. Cytopathogenesis is usually seen within 1-3 days. The nature of the virus is confirmed by immunofluorescence using specific monoclonal antibodies. The viral type is then obtained. If electron microscopy is available, herpes viral particles may be seen in various samples.

Serologic methods: These are of different value in the mother and the child.

— In the mother of a neonate with clinically evident infection, finding specific antiherpes IgM antibodies is a good argument for a presumptive diagnosis of neonatal herpes.

— In the neonate, serologic tests cannot give a diagnosis because of the presence of transmitted maternal antibodies. In the case of contamination at birth, studies have shown that IgM antibodies appear 2-3 weeks after birth and last for 6-12 months.

These tests are therefore really only useful in establishing a retrospective diagnosis e. g.:

— finding antiherpes type 2 antibodies during the first year of life is indirect evidence of perinatal herpes infection, knowing the route of transmission of this virus;

— finding specific antiherpes IgM antibodies in the serum of children less than six months old is also indirect evidence of perinatal infection.

The methods used most often are complement fixation, passive haemaglutination and immuno-enzymology.

TREATMENT

Here the problems are far from resolved. There is firstly the problem of effectiveness of the treatment:

— For the treatment to be effective, it must be given as early as possible so that the virus has not spread to the entire body;

— however, all the details of the immune mechanisms involved in herpes infection are not known; it is possible that treatment may depress that host immune response, thereby allowing the spread of the virus;

— despite treatment, a large number of children survive with serious after-effects. There is additionally the problem of drug toxicity.

Specific treatment. — Three drugs have been successively studied: iododesoxyuridine (IDU), cytosine-arabinoside (Ara-C), and adenine-arabinoside (Ara-A). All inhibit herpes virus multiplication in vitro, and act on viral DNA synthesis.

IDU given parenterally is the most toxic of the three. It acts on the rapidly growing cells such as the bone marrow, liver, intestine, hair. It is now used only for the local treatment of ocular herpes in the neonate. Ara-C is also toxic, and seems to depress the immune response, especially antibody synthesis.

The more recent Ara-A has a number of advantages compared with the other two: its metabolite, hypoxanthine has some antiviral activity; it is less toxic and immunodepressant than the other two. A dose of 15 mg/kg/day is given intravenously every 12 hours for 5 to 10 days. Some neurological complications have been reported e. g. ataxia, paraesthesiae, encephalopathy. Although results seem promising, more study is required to be able to come to a final conclusion concerning this drug.

In addition to the above three drugs, there is a guanine derivative, acycloguanosine (Acyclovir), which inhibits viral DNA polymerase. This is due to its transformation into a triphosphate derivative by a viral thymidine kinase. A dose of 5-15 mg/kg/day has been given to neonates with herpes for 5-10 days. It is not as toxic and acts on both types of herpes virus, whereas Ara-A acts only on type 1. The only disadvantage seems to be the presence of thymidine kinase deficient viral mutants, against which the drug is inactive. Although this drug too seems promising because of its low toxicity and greater efficacy, more trials with greater numbers of children must be carried out to decide on its value in the treatment of neonatal herpes. The efficacy of gammaglobulins in the treatment of neonatal herpes has not yet been established.

Other treatment. — This depends on strict clinical and biological monitoring of the neonate and the evolution of the disease. Biological disorders can thus be identified and treated rapidly. Appropriate antibiotics may be given early if a bacterial opportunistic infection occurs. Anticonvulsants may be useful. The child's clinical state will determine the other treatment required: oxygen, controlled ventilation, etc.

PREVENTION

Because of the problems encountered in the treatment of this infection, the difficulty of carrying out vaccination because of the possible oncogenic properties of the vaccine, and the impossibility of fully eradicating the virus in the mother, attention must be focused on its prevention.

At the beginning of pregnancy. — A careful gynaecological examination must be carried out to look for genital herpes; cervicovaginal smears and serologic tests must be perfomed if there exists the least doubt. It is essential to know at this time whether the infection is primary or a recurrence. A therapeutic abortion is not justified if genital herpes is discovered within the first months; if the pregnancy should end in a miscarriage or a stillbirth, samples should be obtained for cytologic and virologic studies.

At the end of pregnancy. — The presence or absence of the virus in the genital tract of the mother in the eighth and ninth month must be determined. Should the virus be present, the indications for caesarian section need to be considered, as this may prevent the child being contamined in the passage through the genital tract. Not all authors are agreed on this, but should a *c*-section be decided on, it must be carried out early enough to prevent contamination after any possible premature rupture of the membranes. The presence of virus in the amniotic fluid may be determined by amniocentesis. If this proves to be positive, caesarian section is of no use.

After birth. — It is known that some children have been infected by their mother or the staff. Before deciding whether the children of mothers with herpes must be isolated, large scale epidemiologic studies are needed.

Varicella-zoster

Chickenpox (varicella), is one of the most contagious and most frequent of the childhood infectious diseases. Few adults remain susceptible and chickenpox is only rarely seen in pregnant women; its incidence as studied by Sever was 0.7 per 1,000 pregnancies.

INTRAUTERINE INFECTION

About ten cases of fetal involvement in maternal chickenpox occurring between the eighth and fifteenth week of pregnancy have been reported from various parts of the world. The clinical picture described was virtually the same everywhere: small birthweight, large cutaneous scars, resulting from the rash, with muscular atrophy, hypoplasia and even atrophy and paralysis of a limb, rudimentary digits, convulsions and psychomotor retardation, chorioretinitis and cataracts. The condition is fatal in about half the cases. The virologic proof of neonatal varicella was obtained in a few of these cases. It seems certain therefore that a serious fetal syndrome can occur after exposure and infection at the start of pregnancy. The actual size of the problem has yet to be assessed. None of the prospective studies available at the moment show a significant increase in the number of congenital malformations or of fetal pathology after varicella occurring at the start of the pregnancy. The risk appears to be rather small, and a therapeutic abortion is not justified. It is possible to follow fetal growth by ultrasound and in particular, limb development. The malformations seen in the rare cases described can thus be diagnosed early; as a result, the mother will be reassured if the limbs are developing normally.

As for zoster occurring at the start of pregnancy, there is probably no fetal risk. Shingles is a recurrence of a varicella infection occurring in an immune subject with circulating antibodies. The virus being present only in one neural territory cannot reach the fetus.

PERINATAL INFECTION

Varicella can occur in the days before delivery, and the infection can then be transmitted to the neonate. The risk is significant; neonatal chickenpox is seen in 17 % of cases, with varying clinical features, from standard chickenpox with complete cure, to serious infection with disseminated cutaneous lesions and visceral involvement; the latter has a mortality rate of 15-30 %.

An important factor in the prognosis is shown in Table VI: the time of the rash in the mother determines the time of the infection in the neonate and its severity. If the maternal infection occurred more than five days before birth, the neonate may have received some protection from the transmitted maternal antibodies; this probably explains why these cases are not so serious. Because the skin rash is so characteristic in chickenpox, laboratory investigations are of little use (viral isolation or serology), especially as they are not easily available to all practitioners.

TABLE VI. — MATERNAL CHICKENPOX NEAR THE END OF PREGNANCY AND THE OUTCOME FOR THE NEONATE. According to GERSHON (50 cases).

Time of the rash	Outcome for the neonate		
	Number of cases	Mortality	
		Number	%
Maternal chickenpox more than 5 days before birth and neonatal chickenpox within the first four days of life. . .	27	0	0
Maternal chickenpox less than 5 days before birth and neonatal chickenpox 5 to 10 days after birth	23	7	28

PREVENTION

Because of the possible consequences of maternal varicella, prevention is a must; it may be carried out on two levels: protecting the pregnant mother from possible contagion, and protecting the neonate from maternal infection occurring at the end of pregnancy. A pregnant woman with no history of chickenpox in childhood who has been in contact with a possible source of virus at the start of pregnancy or near the end of term may be offered passive

immunization with specific gammaglobulins if seen within three days after the contact. When varicella has occurred in the days preceeding delivery, the child must be isolated, and should also receive specific gammaglobulins. This will either prevent all clinical signs, or at least, attenuate them.

Neonatal hepatitis B (HB)

INTRODUCTION

Our knowledge of the hepatitis A and B viruses has increased considerably in the last few years; as a result, some neonatal hepatitis, up to now of unknown origin, has at last been labelled.

Transmission from mother to child has also been studied. This mostly concerns mothers who are chronic carriers of the HBs antigen (HBsAg); these women make up a large proportion of the population of some countries. It is within these populations that the problems of prevention are encountered, both for the child and for the community where attempts are made to reduce the carrier rate below the present mean of 10 % in Africa and Asia.

THE VIRUS

Three antigen antibody systems have been identified in connection with HB:

The surface HBsAg and its antibody: the HBsAg is located on the surface of the virus. It is linked to particles which are antigenically identical, but morphologically different (particles and tubules, 22 nm in diameter, Dane's particles, 42 nm across); these appear briefly in the serum of people with acute hepatitis, and for rather longer in patients who are chronically infected.

A specific antigenic determinant "*a*" is found in all HBs positive sera; two other mutually exclusive determinants exist, "*d*" or "*y*", "*w*" or "*r*". The possible phenotypes are therefore *adw, adr, ayw* and *ayr*. These are only of epidemiologic interest, as markers. The anti-HBs antibody is found after the HBsAg has disappeared, it affords protection against further infection by the HB virus.

The HBc antigen (HBcAg): is thought to make up the core of Dane's particles. This core, 28 nm in diameter, is seen in the nuclei of hepatocytes during an acute infection with hepatitis B. The anti-HBc antibody may be seen during the acute episode; it is always present in chronic carriers.

Unlike the other two antigens, **the "e" antigen** is a soluble component found in the serum of some patients with chronic HB. It has been suggested that the formation of anti-*e* antibody signals the end of the chronic carrier state.

EPIDEMIOLOGY, TRANSMISSION

Vertical transmission of the HB virus, *i. e.* mother to child, can be seen in 2 circumstances: (1) The mother has acute hepatitis during her pregnancy; this is the greatest risk;

(2) The mother is an asymptomatic chronic carrier of the HBsAg.

The mother has acute hepatitis during her pregnancy. — During the first six months of pregnancy, the risk of infection for the child is similar to that for children of chronic carrier mothers. The risk is much greater for the child (40 %) if the mother has hepatitis during the last three months of her pregnancy, or during the two months that follow delivery.

The mother is an asymptomatic chronic carrier. — In this case, geographic factors play an important part. In western countries, HBsAg transmission by the mother to her child is relatively rare (5 %); however, in Asian countries, where the carrier rate is very high, the transmission rate is also high. Half the children of carrier mothers become HBs carriers during their first year of life. It has been noticed that when the neonate is a carrier, the older sibs are too; and when the neonate is free of HBs, so are the older sibs. This leads to the suggestion that some mothers are "HBs transmitters" and others "HBs non-transmitters". Research has shown that mothers with the "*e*" Ag transmit the HBsAg more often than women who have anti-*e* antibodies. The serum level of HBsAg seems to play a part in determining HBsAg transmission to the neonate: the higher the level, the greater the number of cases of transmission.

Infection may occur:

In utero by the transplacental route: not all authors are agreed on this route. An argument in its favour is the fact that a mother who develops acute hepatitis at the start of pregnancy and becomes HBs negative after delivery, gives birth to a child who is HBsAg positive. Against it is the fact that transmission during the first six months of pregnancy is rare.

At the time of delivery: this is the time when contamination is the most frequent, as shown by the incubation periods of neonatal hepatitis. Two routes may be involved: orally, by swallowing secretions containing the virus, or parenterally, such as when there is a scalp wound.

Postnatally: transfusions play a lessening part here, because of the care taken in screening for the HBsAg in the blood used.

Breast feeding does not seem to play an important part in HBsAg transmission.

CLINICAL FEATURES

The clinical picture that follows infection with the HB virus varies: there may be no clinical or biological signs, or hepatitis with antigen briefly present in the serum, followed by the development of anti-HBsAg antibody, or acute or overwhelming hepatitis, or chronic persistant hepatitis in children who become chronic HBsAg carriers.

The incubation period is usually 2-3 months. Most neonates who become HBs positive after vertical transmission remain anicteric, with no clinical signs of acute hepatitis. They remain HBsAg positive for long periods, even up to several years. There may be a transient rise in the transaminases. Severe or fatal hepatitis is exceedingly rare. Some studies have shown that children with low birth weight or a gestational age of less than 37 weeks are more prone to becoming HBsAg positive. In fact, these early deliveries are probably more due to the mother's acute illness than to the fetal infection.

We now have some information on possible long term effects of these chronic carrier states: chronic hepatitis, cirrhosis and hepatic carcinoma.

DIAGNOSIS

In the children of mothers who have had acute hepatitis during their pregnancy, or who are healthy carriers, the diagnosis will be made on finding the HBsAg in the serum of the child at birth and then during the first months of life. The antigen will be revealed by the following techniques, in order of increasing sensitivity: double immunodiffusion in a gel medium, electrosyneresis, complement fixation, reverse haemagglutination, and finally radioimmunoassay. The presence of HBsAg in the cord blood is no proof of transplacental transmission; to confirm the latter, the HBsAg must be present in the child's serum at a later date. A rise in the hepatic transaminases must also be looked for.

TREATMENT. PREVENTION

There is no specific therapy at the moment, except for symptomatic treatment. Prevention, largely concerns children born of mothers who had acute hepatitis during the pregnancy. Prevention for children born of chronic carrier mothers will probably have to be limited to some groups defined from recent clinical experiences. Prevention is recommended: (1) when a mother is HBsAg positive and Hbe positive, (2) when a mother is HBsAg positive and has anti-*e* antibodies and belongs to a high risk population, such as the Asian group.

Untill recently prevention was based on the use of specific rather than standard immunoglobulins given within the first 48 hours after birth (0.5 ml/kg) and then 0.15 ml/kg every month for six months. It has now been recommended to associate vaccination with HB vaccine.

CONCLUSION

It seems possible to hope that, in the years to come, with the results of present research, it will be possible to predict which mother is a transmitter or a non-transmitter. Also, better neonatal HB prevention protocols with specific anti-HB immunoglobulins associated with hepatitis B vaccine will be developed along with our increasing clinical experience.

Mumps

Manson's and Siegel's epidemiologic studies have shown that there is a sharp increase in spontaneous abortions after maternal mumps in the first three months of pregnancy about 2 weeks after the acute illness. According to Siegel, these may be due to the action of the virus on ovarian function leading to hormonal changes which do not allow the continuance of the pregnancy. They however failed to show any malformative action of mumps on the embryo.

Different studies, in particular, St Geme's, have shown, by using skin tests with the viral antigen, that endocardial fibroelastosis in infants and mumps are linked. These authors believe that it follows from a fetal viral myocarditis associated with a secondary immune deficiency. But no virologic proof has been obtained (viral culture, acquired antiviral antibodies) and other studies have not confirmed these results.

Hamster embryos experimentally inoculated with mumps virus develop hydrocephalus, and the hen embryo shows myocarditis and immune disorders. Although this experimental work is important, it is difficult to extrapolate it to human pathology. Moreover, epidemiological data is not in favour of a viral action on the human embryo. Studies carried out with live attenuated mumps virus given to women prior to abortion has shown the presence of the virus in the placenta, but not in the embryonic tissues. Hydrocephalus has been seen to occur in the hamster embryo after intra amniotic inoculation with the vaccine virus.

Influenza

Influenza can be serious for the mother because of the importance of its general symptoms and its toxic syndrome. This was seen during the pandemics of 1918 and 1958 when there was a high maternal mortality. Influenza can also affect fetal development. Because of the impressive statistics of the influenza pandemics, a number of studies have been carried out on the possible effects of the infection on the pregnancy and the fetus: retrospective studies on entire populations or on individuals as well as prospective studies in the latter, with the diagnosis being based on clinical data (case history) and on serological data (serum tests in the post partum period). The conclusion in half the studies is that there is a link between influenza during pregnancy and fetal morbidity. Malformations have been particularly carefully looked for; it seems that central nervous system malformations appear to be prominent. In actual fact, this relationship has only been found in Northern and English-speaking countries, where the incidence of these malformations is already high; but they are the only countries where such studies have as yet been carried out. Of four prospective studies based on serological diagnosis, three concluded that there is a link between influenza and fetal morbidity, in two between influenza and a low birth weight, and only in one between influenza and fetal malformations. There are two possible explanations for this link between influenza during pregnancy and fetal morbidity:

(1) The influenza virus may act directly on the fetus. The experimental intracerebral inoculation

of influenza virus in Rhesus monkey fetuses has led to the development of bilateral hydrocephalus. However the experimental methodology used is questionable. Moreover it is too far removed from the natural infection to be of value in considering the situation in man. It therefore seems there are few arguments in favour of this theory.

(2) Influenza may modify the maternal environment as a result of pyrexia, drug taking and circulating toxins. These factors may well lead to fetal morbidity. Saxen's work seems to support this idea; he blames the drugs taken by mothers with influenza during the first three months of pregnancy.

Fedrick and Alberman (1972) opened another chapter in the influenza during pregnancy story when they noted a strong link between influenza during pregnancy and childhood leukemias. In the British perinatal study, the incidence of acute lymphoid leukemia in children of mothers who claimed to have had influenza during their pregnancy (1957 pandemic) was significantly increased, whereas that of other cancers was not increased.

Precise epidemiologic studies are needed to confirm or contradict these findings. In all influenza studies, the antigenic variations of the virus must be taken into account; some of the viral strains may have different effects on the fetus or on the mother.

Conclusion. — No teratogenic action of the influenza virus has been conclusively shown. However, the illness seen in the second half of the pregnancy can, via the toxic syndrome it produces, affect the placenta and fetus, leading to fetal hypotrophy. It seems therefore logical to vaccinate susceptible pregnant women against influenza, especially as the vaccine is a killed one and thus can be given with a relative degree of safety.

Enteroviruses

INTRAUTERINE INFECTION

The enteroviruses belong to the picornaviruses, which also include the rhinoviruses, and perhaps the hepatitis A virus. There are about sixty enteroviruses pathogenic for man, among which are the poliomyelitis virus, the Coxsackie viruses and the ECHO viruses. Enterovirus infections are common and ubiquitous. In the adult, their most serious effects are neurological. However, enterovirus infections are mostly asymptomatic or only mildly so, giving rise to influenza-like syndromes. It is likely that the virus can reach the fetus because there is a viraemia at the start of the illness.

Before poliomyelitis vaccination was available, cases of poliomyelitis with paralysis were seen in pregnant women, with spontaneous abortions and deaths in utero being reported, probably due to an indirect effect of the disease. No congenital malformations have however been reported. Similarly, no embryonic or fetal morbidity has ever been reported after vaccinating the mother with live attenuated poliovirus in the course of pregnancy.

As for the Coxsackie and ECHO viruses, an epidemiologic study carried out over several years and based on routine serology throughout pregnancy suggests that some Coxsackie viruses (B3 and B4) may be responsible for some congenital cardiac malformations (0.9 % after a Coxsackie B3 infection against 0.5 % in the control group). But this has not been confirmed by others.

In fact, there is as yet no clinical or epidemiological evidence to show that enteroviruses may be responsible for fetal morbidity if the infection occurs at the start of or during pregnancy.

NEONATAL INFECTION

Because infections with Coxsackie viruses groups A and B and Echoviruses are so common and so contagious, especially in the summer and fall in the temperate zones of the northern hemisphere, the neonate is at risk of contracting such an infection from his immediate environment, his mother or the health team. Many virologic studies have shown that these neonatal infections often occur at the same time as there is wide dissemination of the virus in the maternity unit. As with older children and adults, these infections are for the most part asymptomatic, cr only mildly so (pyrexia, diarrhea, macular rash) with a favourable outcome.

A few isolated cases of more serious illness (meningitis, interstitial pneumonia, hepatitis) have been linked to infections by various ECHO viruses. No one characteristic clinical syndrome or particular frequency can be given to a particular serologic type of virus; similarly for Coxsackie A viruses.

On the other hand, Coxsackie B viruses have been held responsible for small epidemics of neonatal myocarditis. The disease appears between the third and eighth day of life, with signs of infection, such as pyrexia, diarrhea, failure to gain weight. Menin-

geal involvement may be found biologically although clinically it is often not apparent. In most cases, the illness will evolve favorably without any neurological sequelæ. In a few cases, after 2-7 days, a more serious second period begins, with cardiac signs predominating: tachycardia, respiratory distress, dulling of heart sounds, dysrythmias... together with neurologic and sometimes hepatic signs. The prognosis is not at all certain: sudden collapse, progressive heart failure, or cure. It is the Coxsackie B3 and B4 viruses which are mainly responsible for this serious illness. The B2 and B5 viruses have also been implicated.

Rotaviruses and viruses responsible for diarrhea

Until recently, the problem of the aetiology of neonatal diarrheas was unresolved. In the absence of bacteria, viruses were often held to be responsible; but it was not until 1973 that this was confirmed by electron microscopy. The viruses involved are: the rotaviruses, astroviruses and adenoviruses.

ROTAVIRUSES

The virus. — It was at first found that this virus was responsible for diarrhea in the young of many animal species: mice, green monkeys, calves. Flewett and Bishop were the first to find rotaviruses in the fæces of children with acute gastroenteritis. It is a double stranded RNA virus. It is called rotavirus because of its morphology (rota = wheel); it has a central core 38 nm diameter, icosahedral, surrounded by a double layer of capsomeres. The inner capsomeres resemble wheel spokes, and the outer layer a wheel rim. The total diameter of the viral particle is 60-65 nm. The inner capsid carries the group specific antigens and the outer capsid the species or type specific antigens. Two serological types are now recognised and at least a third may exist. The outer capsid seems essential for the particle's infectivity.

Physiopathology. — Rotaviruses multiply in the intestinal epithelial cells, especially in the duodenum and upper jejunum. They accumulate in cyto-

plasmic vesicles which are in fact outgrowths of the endoplasmic reticulum. The cells involved are the epithelial cells with a brush border; the microvilli regress as the infection progresses. The brush border then disappears totally, and the viral particles pass into the intestinal lumen through the destroyed cytoplasmic membrane. These cells produce disaccharidases. There thus follows a deficient absorption of disaccharides, giving rise to an osmotic diarrhea.

Clinical features. — In children 6 months to 2 years old, rotavirus diarrhea can be quite serious, producing dehydration and requiring intensive care. In the neonate, it is exceedingly serious. The incubation period is 1-2 days. The diarrhea lasts about 12-48 hours (5-8 days in children 6 months to 2 years of age). During the acute phase, neonates excrete 10^9-10^{10} viral particles per gram of fæces; very quickly, these numbers fall off below the limit of detection by electron microscopy. There is no relationship between the number of viral particles excreted and the severity of the clinical features. Occasionally, one sees pyrexia, vomiting or irritability. The infants may quickly recover their original birth weight.

Epidemiology. — Rotaviruses are ubiquitous: epidemic gastroenteritis due to this virus has been reported from all parts of the world. For children over the age of 6 months, there is an increase in the number of cases in winter time. This seasonal variation is less marked for neonates. In fact, the virus enters maternity units via the personnel, the parents, and especially the siblings. It then remains, creating an endemic over several months, occasionally giving small epidemics. Many neonates excrete the virus (50 %) but few have symptoms. Once the virus is within the confines of the maternity unit, it is difficult to get rid of. Only a complete disinfection will do so. If the virus is not present in the maternity unit, the neonates do not excrete it.

The diarrhea is no more frequent or more severe in children of low birth weight or in premature babies.

It seems that infants breast fed excrete the virus less often, and have less viral diarrhea than children who are bottle fed. The secretory IgA present in the colostrum probably plays an important part in the protection against the diarrhea by acting at the intestinal level. Specific antibodies do not protect if there are no local antibodies present. In milk, the level of IgA antibodies falls off rapidly within the first week. This probably means that another specific antiviral agent as yet unknown exists.

In fact, according to a recent study, the kind of feeding is not the only factor involved in neonatal rotavirus diarrhea. More diarrheas are seen in children requiring special care from the time of birth and in children who are in contact with other neonates, who are cared for by the health team. Breast feeding does not protect all children from diarrhea.

Of the two serotypes identified, type 2 is responsible for 75 % of rotavirus diarrheas and type 1 for 25 %. By the age of 18 months, 85 % of children have antibodies against both types. It would seem therefore that the clinical expression of type 2 is greater than that of type 1. The antibodies appear within the fortnight following the infection, remain at a high titre for a few weeks, and then fall off over a year to reach very low titres. Reinfections with the same serological type are rare, but there is no crossed immunity and infections with the other type are possible.

Diagnosis. — This must be made quickly, especially during epidemics in nurseries or maternity units, so as to avoid the large scale use of antibiotics which might lead to the appearance of multi-resistant germs. There are for the moment no routine cell culture systems which allow in vitro viral multiplication. In any case, this would take several days.

Electron microscopy usually shows the typical virions in the fæces. The minimum level of detection is 10^5 particles per gram of fæces. This technique can be made more specific by using immune electron microscopy. The fæcal extract is first treated with specific immune serum. The viral particles are then aggregated by the antibodies. Not only are these aggregates easier to see, but the technique gives immunologic proof of the nature of the virus. This is, however, expensive. Other techniques have been suggested:

— Immunoelectrophoresis has become the most frequently used.

— Solid phase radio-immunoassay is very precise, very sensitive, but requires an expensive scintillation counter.

— The ELISA technique: an antigen antibody reaction is made to occur; antibody fixation on the antigen is shown by an enzymatic method.

Serology is of only limited interest because of the speed with which the answer must be obtained. It is based on a complement fixation method, where the antigen is either of human origin from fæcal extract containing the rotavirus, or of bovine origin, which is very close antigenically to the former. However, the sensitivity of this method is poor. Other techniques, such as indirect immunofluorescence and the ELISA technique, appear to be more promising.

Treatment. — There is no specific treatment. Neonates with rotavirus diarrhoea must be watched very carefully. If need be, rehydration may thus be started as soon as required. The giving of milk and other disaccharides is usually halted. Oral rehydration is carried out with water containing 5 % glucose and electrolytes. Excessive amounts of glucose must be avoided as it is absorbed by the same route as lactose. If necessary, the unit must be disinfected.

Prevention. — No definite protocol has yet been defined. Some authors have however reported a lesser incidence of rotavirus diarrhea in maternity units where visits are restricted; especially those of young children.

OTHER VIRUSES

Parvoviruses. — These viruses, including Norwalk's agent, have been found by electron microscopy in the fæces of children and adults with gastroenteritis. But it seems they are found just as often in control groups at the same time. The part they play in neonatal diarrheas has not yet been established.

Astroviruses. — The name comes from their shape which resembles a star. They have been found in some maternity units during epidemics of gastroenteritis. However it seems their presence alone is not enough to cause diarrhea. Other, as yet unknown, factors are probably required. They may be associated with rotaviruses. They are found in both the control and disease groups.

Enteroviruses and adenoviruses. — These most probably cause some diarrheas: they are found in great numbers in the faeces of a few cases. There is also seroconversion after such diarrhea, but its incidence is not known; it probably is not very high.

Coronavirus. — These were recently found during an epidemic of ulcerative necrotising enterocolitis in a maternity unit. But they are probably not the only agent involved, clostridial bacteria being likely candidates. The diagnosis is made on electron microscopy of fæces. They have a typical shape 60-120 nm diameter, with 6 nm projections all round.

CONCLUSION

Despite progress that has been made, the triggering and risk factors for diarrheal epidemics in nurseries still need to be understood before an effective prevention protocol can be established.

REFERENCES

BATIGNANI (A.). — Conjunctivite da virus erpetico in neonato. *Boll. Ocul.*, 13, 1217-1220, 1934.

BEASLEY (R. P.), LEE (G.), ROAN (H.), HWANG (L.), LAN (C.), HUANG (F.), CHEN (C.). — Prevention of perinatally transmitted Hepatitis B virus infections with Hepatitis B Immune Globulin and Hepatitis B Vaccine. *Lancet*, 2, 1983.

BISHOP (R. F.), DAVIDSON (G. P.), HOLMES (J. H.), TOWNLEY (R. R. W.), RUCK (B. J.). — Importance of a new virus in acute sporadic enteritis in children. *Lancet*, 1, 242-245, 1975.

BISHOP (R. F.), CAMERON (D. J. S.), VEENSTRA (A. A.), BARNES (G. L.). — Diarrhea and Rotavirus Infection associated with differing regimens for post-natal care of new-born babies. *J. Cl. Microb.*, 9, 525-529, 1979.

BOXALL (E. H.). — Vertical transmission of Hepatitis-B Surface Antigen. *Biomedicine*, 26, 12-15, 1977.

BRICOUT (F.), DUSSAIX (E.), NICOLAS (J. C.), HURAUX (J. M.), BEFEKADU (E.). — Diarrhées infantiles et rotavirus, étude sérologique rétrospective (1971-1975). *Path. Biol.*, 25, 43-45, 1976.

BROWN (G.), KARUNAS (R. S.). — Relationship of congenital anomalies and maternal infection with selected enteroviruses. *Am. J. Epidemiol.*, 95, 207-217, 1972.

CAMERON (D. J. S.), BISHOP (R. F.), VEENSTRA (A. A.), BARNES (G. L.). — Non-cultivable viruses and neonatal diarrhea: fifteen-month survey in a new-born special care nursery. *J. Cl. Microbiol.*, 8, 93-98, 1978.

CHANG (Te-Wen), O'KEEFE (P.). — Cesarean section and genital herpes. *N. Engl. J. Med.*, 296, 573, 1977.

CHIN (J.). — Prevention of chronic Hepatitis B virus infection from mothers to infants in the United States. *Pediatrics*, 71, 289-292, 1980.

CHOU (S.), MERIGNAN (T. C.). — Rapid detection and quantitation of human cytomegalovirus in urine through DNA hybridization. *N. Engl. J. Med.*, 308, 921-923, 1983.

CHRYSTIE (J. L.), TOTTERDELL (B.), BANATVALA (J. E.). — Rotavirus infections in a maternity unit. *Arch. Dis. Child.*, 51, 924-928, 1976.

COOPER (L. Z.). — Congenital rubella in the United States. KRUGMAN S. and GERSHON A. A., eds., *Infections of the fetus and newborn*, Alan R. Liss, New York, 1-21, 1975.

DERSO (A.), BOXALL (E. H.), TARLOW (M. J.), FLEWETT (T. H.). — Transmission of HbSAg from mother to infant in four ethnic groups. *Brit. Med.*, 1, 949-952, 1978.

DU PASQUIER (R.). — La varicelle et l'herpès chez la femme enceinte. *Médecine périnatale*, 7es Journées Nationales, Arnette, Édit., Paris, 1978.

DUPUY (J. M.). — Contamination par le virus de l'hépatite B en période néonatale. *Médecine périnatale*, 7es Journées Nationales, Arnette, Édit., Paris, 1978.

FEDRICK (J.), ALBERMAN (E. D.). — Reported influenza and subsequent cancer in the child. *Brit. Med. J.*, 2, 485-488, 1972.

FLEWETT (T. H.), WOODE (G. N.). — The Rotaviruses, Brief Review. *Arch. Vir.*, 57, 1-23, 1978.

FREYMUTH (F.), LALOUM (D.), KOBILINSKY (G.), DELAVENNE (J.), DENIS (A.), BOUTARD (P.), GANDON (S.). — Infections à virus Coxsackie et virus Echo de la femme enceinte et du nouveau-né. *Médecine Périnatale*, 7es Journées, O. DUBOIS et J. M. THOULON, éd., Arnette, Paris, 153-165, 1978.

GERETY (R. J.), SCHWEITZER (J. L.). — Viral Hepatitis type B during pregnancy, the neonatal period and infancy. *J. Pediat.*, 90, 368-374, 1977.

GERSHON (A. A.). — Varicella in mother and infant: problems old and new. KRUGMAN S. and GERSHON A. A., eds., *Infections of the fetus and newborn*, Alan R. Liss, New York, 79-95, 1975.

GERSONY (W. M.), KATZ (S. L.), NADAS (A. S.). — Endocardial fibroelastosis and mumps virus. *Pediatrics*, 37, 430-434, 1966.

GOUDEAU (A.). — Transmission mère-enfant du virus de l'hépatite B. Perspectives de prévention de l'infection néonatale. *Presse Méd.*, 11, 3051-3054, 1982.

GRANT (S.), EDMOND (E.), SYNUE (J.). — A prospective study of cytomegalovirus infection in pregnancy: laboratory evidence of congenital infection following maternal primary and reactivated infection. *J. Infection*, 3, 24-31, 1981.

GREGG (N. M.). — Congenital rubella following german measles in the mother. *Trans. Ophthalmol. Soc. Aust*, 3, 35-46, 1941.

HAAS (G. M.). — Hepato-adrenal necrosis with intranuclear inclusion bodies. Report of a case. *Amer. J. Path.*, 11, 127-142, 1975.

HARDY (J.), AZAROWICZ (E. N.), MANNINI (A.). — The effect of asian influenza on the outcome of pregnancies. *Amer. J. Publ. Health, 51,* 1182-1188, 1961.

KARKINEN-JAASKELAINEN (M.), SAXEN (L.). — Maternal influenza drug consumption and congenital defects of the central nervous system. *Amer. J. Obstet. Gynec., 118,* 815-818, 1974.

KILHAM (L.), MARGOLIS (G.). — Induction of congenital hydrocephalus in hamsters with attenuated and natural strains of mumps virus. *J. Infect. Dis., 132,* 462-466, 1975.

MAC CALLUM (F. O.), PARTRIDGE (J. W.). — Fetal-maternal relationships in *Herpes simplex. Arch. Dis. Child., 43,* 265-267, 1968.

MANSON (M. M.), LOGAN (W. P. D.), LOY (R. M.). — Rubella and other virus infections during pregnancy. *Rep. Publ. Hlth. Med. Subj.,* n° 101, 1960.

MILLER (E.), CRADOCK-WATSON (J. E.), POLLOCK (T. M.). — Consequences of confirmed maternal rubella at successive stages of pregnancy. *Lancet,* 2, 781-784, 1982.

MONTGOMERY (J.), GEAR (J.), PRINSLOO (F.), KAHN (M.), KIRSCH (Z.). — Myocarditis of the newborn. *S. Afr. Med. J., 29,* 608-612, 1955.

MURPHY (A. M.), ALBREY (M. B.), CREWE (E. B.). — Rotavirus infections of neonates. *Lancet,* 2, 1149-1150, 1977.

MYERS (J. D.). — Congenital varicella in term infants: risk reconsidered. *J. Infect. Dis., 129,* 215-217, 1974.

NAIB (Z. M.), NAHMIAS (A. J.), JOSEY (W. E.), WHEELER (J. H.). — Association of maternal genital herpetic infection with spontaneous abortion. *Obstet. Gynecol., 35,* 260-263, 1970.

NUMAZAKI (Y.), YANS (N.), MORIZUKA (T.), TAKAR (S.), ISHIDA (N.). — Primary infection with human cytomegalovirus: virus isolation from healthy infants and pregnant women. *Am. J. Epidemiol., 91,* 410-417, 1970.

OKADA (K.), KAMIYAMA (I.), INOMATA (M.), IMAI MITSUNOBU, MIYAKAWA (Y.), MAYUMI (M.). — e Antigen and anti-e in the serum of asymptomatic carrier mothers as indicators of positive and negative transmission of Hepatitis-B virus to their infants. *N. Engl. J. Med., 294,* 746-749, 1976.

ROSENDAHL (C.), KERTSCHMER (R.), KOCHEN (M. M.), WEGSCHEIDER (K.), KAISER (D.). — Avoidance of perinatal transmission of Hepatitis B virus: Is passive immunization always necessary? *Lancet, 1,* 1127-1129, 1983.

SAIGAL (S.), LUNYK (O.), LARKE (R. P. B.), CHERNESKY (M. A.). — The outcome of children with congenital cytomegalovirus infection. *Amer. J. Dis. Child., 136,* 896-901, 1982.

SAXEN (L.), HJELT (L.), SJOSTEDT (J. E.). — Asian influenza during pregnancy and congenital malformations. *Acta Pathol. Microb. Scand., 49,* 114-126, 1960.

SEVER (J.), WHITE (L. R.). — Intrauterine viral infections. *Am. Rev. Med., 19,* 471-486, 1968.

SIEGEL (M.). — Congenital malformations following chickenpox, measles, mumps and hepatitis. *JAMA, 226,* 1521-1524, 1973.

SIEGEL (M.), FIERST (H. T.), PEREN (N. G.). — Comparative fetal mortality in maternal virus diseases. *N. Engl. J. Med., 274,* 768-771, 1966.

SPIRA (A.), BOUE (A.), DUROS (C.), COULON (M.), GUEGUEN (S.), DREYFUS (J.), SCHNEEGANS (P.). — Grippe et grossesse, relation avec le poids de naissance et le poids du placenta. *J. Gyn. Obst. Biol. Repr., 6,* 289-300, 1977.

STAGNO (S.), PASS (R. F.), DWORSKY (M. E.), HENDERSON (R. E.), MOORE (E. G.), WALTON (P. D.), ALFORD (C. A.). — Congenital cytomegalovirus infection, the relative importance of primary and recurrent maternal infection. *N. Engl. J. Med., 16,* 945-949, 1982.

ST GEME (J. W.), NOREN (G. R.), ADAMS (P.). — Proposed embryopathic relation between mumps virus and primary endocardial fibroelastosis. *N. Engl. J. Med., 275,* 339-347, 1966.

TADA (H.), YANAGIDA (M.), MISHINA (J.), FUJII (T.), BABA (K.), ISHIKAWA (S.), AIHARA (S.), TSUDA (F.), MIYAKAWA (Y.), MAYUMI (M.). — Combined passive and active immunization for preventing perinatal transmission of Hepatitis B virus carrier State. *Pediatrics, 70,* 613-619, 1982.

WALKER-SMITH (J.). — Rotavirus gastro-enteritis. *Arch. Dis. Child., 53,* 355-362, 1978.

WELLER (T. H.). — The cytomegalovirus: ubiquitous agents with protean clinical manifestations. *N. Engl. J. Med., 285,* 203-214, 267-274, 1971.

WILSON (M. G.), STEIN (A. M.). — Teratogenic effects of asian influenza. *JAMA, 210,* 336-337, 1969.

YAMAUCHI (T.), ST GEME (J. W.), OH (W.), DAVIS (C. M. C.). — The biological and biochemical pathogenesis of mumps virus induced embryonic growth retardation. *Pediat. Dis., 9,* 30-34, 1975.

YAMAUCHI (T.), WILSON (C.), ST GEME (J. W.). — Transmission of live, attenuated mumps virus to human placenta. *N. Engl. J. Med.,* 710-712, 1974.

YEAJER (A. S.). — Use of acyclovir in premature and term neonates. *Amer. J. Med., 96,* 205-209, 1982.

Acquired immune deficiency syndrome (AIDS)

M. XANTHOU

AIDS was first recognised as an entity in the latter half of 1979. The clinical presentation includes an acquired immunodeficiency and recurrent opportunistic infections often associated with unusual malignant neoplasms or autoimmune phenomena.

Luc Montagnier and his group in Paris and R. C. Gallo et al. in the States identified the causative agent, a virus of the retrovirus family, in 1983 and 1984 respectively [2, 5]. As retroviruses infect a cell their genetic code carried on RNA is transcribed "backward" into DNA. In some cases the DNA is integrated into the host cell's chromosomes in the form of a sequence known as a provirus. Later the host cell transcribes the viral genes and synthesizes the proteins they encode, which are assembled into new viruses [7].

In the case of the AIDS retrovirus immunosuppression results from viral infection of T_4 lymphocytes (Helper T-cells). A region of the cell membrane associated with the T_4 marker acts as a receptor for the virus. The reduction of the T_4-cell population has consequences that reflect its important place in the immune system. Lacking T_4-cell help, B cells are unable to produce adequate quantities of specific antibody to the AIDS virus or other infections. The cytotoxic and suppressor T-cell responses are similarly hampered. The B cells of AIDS patients continuously secrete large amounts of nonspecific immunoglobulin because they do not receive the suppressor T-cell signal to stop. With the loss of T_4 cells the level of interleukin-2 falls slowing the clonal expansion of mature T cells and depressing the activity of natural killer cells and macrophages which this protein normally stimulates. Apart from T_4 cells it is likely that macrophages, platelets and B cells serve as reservoir of the virus [4, 7].

The virus is ordinarily transmitted in adults only though the blood or through sexual intercourse. The screening of donated blood for evidence of AIDS infection has drastically reduced the risk in blood recipients. The groups at highest risk for infection include homosexual and bisexual men, abusers of injected drugs, the sexual partners of people in AIDS risk groups and children born to mothers at risk. It seems that a vertical transplacental transmission of virus is possible [6] as is transmission of virus via cervical secretions during delivery [3].

Since the disease was first recognized the number of cases has risen; in the U. S. alone the number of patients reached 14,000 by late 1985. The prevalence of antibody among individuals at risk for the disease has led to estimates that between one and two million people in U. S. alone are infected with the AIDS virus. Some of them may never show symptoms even though retroviral infections persist for life. For others the incubation period may vary from several months to decades. The mortality rate of the illness has been reported as 49 % for adults and 69 % for children [8].

Pediatric AIDS represents only 1 % of the cases. In United States 72 % of the pediatric patients came from families in which one or both parents had AIDS or were at increased risk for developing AIDS, 13 % had received transfusions of blood or blood compo-

nents before their onset of illness and 5 % had hemophilia [8].

Because neonates and in particular premature infants are relatively immunodeficient they are probably especially susceptible to AIDS. The long latent period observed in adults between infection and development of clinical AIDS is absent and the disease presents during the first few months of life.

Affected infants have all been observed within the first few months of life to have recurrent or chronic opportunistic infections, failure to thrive, hepatosplenomegaly, generalized lymphadenopathy, pneumonia and or encephalitis. Apart from the usual agents responsible for opportunistic infections like pneumocystis carini, herpes viruses, cytomegalovirus and C. albicans, bacterial infections and gram-negative sepsis have been found in these infants [9].

Immunologic studies showed most of the infants to have polyclonal hypergammaglobulinemia, decreased helper/suppressor T-cell ratios and decreased responses of peripheral blood mononuclear cells to mitogens and antigens. The first detectable immunologic abnormality was an early elevation of serum IgG and IgM which occured at 2 months of age. Abnormalities of T-cells were not present until 5 months of age. Lymphopenia was not as common as it is in adult patients [1].

The difficulty that one faces in making a diagnosis of AIDS in an infant is related to the fact that a number of congenital immune deficiencies and congenital viral infections that result in immune deficiencies can be seen in infants. During early infancy detection of antibodies to the AIDS retrovirus doesn't establishe the diagnosis as passive transfer of maternal IgG may occur. Isolation of the virus is essential. Early diagnosis of pediatric AIDS is important in identifying immunodeficient patients who have unique medical and social problems.

Regarding treatment, physicians usually concentrate on the clinical manifestations of the disease, such as infection and malignancies, that develop because of the immune deficiency. Other treatment strategies have attempted to restore immune function. Bone-marrow transplants and injections of white cells have been tried. Patients have also been given interleukin-2 and interferons to stimulate their immune system. These efforts have not proved to be successful so far. Other investigators are searching for a weapon against the virus itself. Ribavirin, HPA-23, 3'-azido-3'-deoxythymidine have been used; however most drugs that inhibit viral replication also hinder the growth of the host's own immune cells.

The creation of an AIDS vaccine is not easy as the AIDS virus has great genetic variability. However efforts are being made in that direction at present [7].

REFERENCES

[1] AMMANN (A. J.). — The Acquired Immunodeficiency Syndrome in Infants and Children. *Annals of Internal Medicine, 103,* 734-737, 1985.

[2] BARIE-SINOUSSI (F.), CHERMANN (J. C.), REY (F.), NUGEYRE (M. T.), CHAMARET (S.), GRYEST (J.), DANGUET (C.), AXLER-BLIN (L.), VEZINET-BRUN (F.), ROUZIOUX (C.), ROSENBAUM (W.), MONTAGNIER (L.). — Isolation of a T-lymphotropic retrovirus from a patient at risk for acquired immune deficiency syndrome (AIDS). *Science, 220,* 868-870, 1983.

[3] COWAN (M. J.), HELLMAN (D.), CHUDWIN (D.), WASA (D. W.), CHANG (R. S.), AMMANN (A. J.). — Maternal transmission of acquired immune deficiency syndrome. *Pediatrics, 73,* 382-386, 1984.

[4] FAUCI (A. S.). — Immunologic abnormalities in the acquired immunodeficiency syndrome (AIDS). *Clinical Research, 32,* 491-492, 1984.

[5] GALLO (R. C.), SAJAHUDDIN (S. Z.), POPOVIC (M.), SHEARER (G. M.), KAPLAN (M.), HAYNER (B. F.), PALKER (T. J.), REDFIELD (K.), OLESKE (J.), SAFAI (B.), WHITE (G.), FOSTER (P.), MARKHAM (P. D.). — Frequent detection and isolation of cytopathic retroviruses (HTLV-III) from patients with AIDS and at risk for AIDS. *Science, 224,* 500-503, 1984.

[6] LAPOINTE (N.), MICHAUD (J.), PEKOVIC (D.), CHAUSSEAU (J. P.), DUPUY (J. M.). — Transplacental transmission of HTLV-III virus. *New Engl. J. Med., 312,* 1325-1326, 1985.

[7] LAURENCE (J.). — The Immune System in AIDS. *Scientific American, 253,* 70-79, 1985.

[8] *Morbidity and Mortality Weekly Report, 34,* 245-248, 1985.

[9] SCOTT (G. B.), BUCK (B. E.), LETERMAN (J. G.), BLOOM (F. I.), PARKS (W. P.). — Acquired immunodeficiency syndrome in infants. *N. Engl. J. Medicine, 310,* 76-81, 1984.

32

Congenital toxoplasmosis

G. DESMONTS, J. S. REMINGTON, J. COUVREUR

THE ORGANISM, ITS TRANSMISSION AND THE PREVENTION OF INFECTION

Toxoplasma is a coccidian, the life cycle of which involves the cat and its prey animals. Schizogeny and gametogeny take place in the small intestine of the cat and end in the formation of oocysts which are shed in the feces and which survive and remain potentially infectious for months or even years in soil. This is a source of infection for rodents, birds, and domestic animals. In their tissues, Toxoplasma are able to multiply intracellularly; this form of the organism is termed trophozoite or tachyzoite. The organisms then encyst in tissue cells. Cysts persist as viable parasites throughout the life of their host, mainly in brain, heart, and skeletal muscle. Cats which hunt or which are fed raw meat become infected, and the cycle is renewed.

Humans are a dead end in the life cycle, and are frequently infected due to the numerous sources of the parasite and the susceptibility of humans to different forms of Toxoplasma gondii (Table I). As can be seen in Table I, the primary forms of the organism responsible for the frequency of infection in the general population are the cyst and oocyst, but the cyst form, present in meat, is likely the main source of infection in populations which consume undercooked meat. An example is France where the prevalence of Toxoplasma infection among adults is over 75 %. The probable main source of infection in populations which for economic reasons or cultural habits, either seldom consume meat, or, if they do, consume meat which is well cooked is the oocyst. Examples are certain low income populations such as in Central America where the prevalence of infection is very high due to poor conditions of hygiene and close contact with feral cats and certain developed countries such as Great Britain, where the prevalence of infection is low (approximately 20 %) and where contact with feral cats is possibly less frequent and eating of grossly undercooked meat relatively uncommon.

The following advice should be given to pregnant women in order to prevent infection:

— Cook meat thoroughly (over 70° C) or eat meat which has been previously frozen (below — 30° C).

— Wear gloves, or thoroughly wash hands after handling raw meat, or when working in the garden.

— It would seem prudent not to have a pet cat at home. If one is present, it should be fed canned or cooked food and not allowed to hunt.

— A pregnant woman at risk (seronegative) should not handle nor clean the cat litterbox.

CONGENITAL TRANSMISSION OF TOXOPLASMA

The prevalence of Toxoplasma antibodies among most human populations reflects the fact that infec-

TABLE I. — THE DIFFERENT FORMS OF TOXOPLASMA GONDII AND THEIR ROLE IN TRANSMISSION TO HUMANS

Forms of organism	Congenital infection	Accidental or professional	Alimentary (ingestion)	Respiratory (inhalation)
Tachyzoite Present in the blood stream and tissues in the early days of infection; frail	+	Blood transfusion (leukocytes) Laboratory workers Veterinarians	No	No
Cyst Persist in brain and muscle; relatively resistant to digestion but not to heat and not to freezing	No	Veterinarians Butchers Trappers Organ transplant recipients	+ (Undercooked meat)	No
Oocyst Resistant to antiseptics, but not to heat, freezing, and prolonged drying Persist for years in moist soil	No	Laboratory workers Garden and field workers	+ (Contamination of food e. g. by cockroaches) (Geophagia: severe cases when associated with other parasites)	(Dust? in special circumstances of cohabitation with cats)

tion with Toxoplasma is widespread. A significant proportion, and even the majority of women of child bearing age in France, have been infected by the parasite. These women probably harbor cysts in their tissues including their uterine muscle. Despite this, congenital toxoplasmosis is infrequent. Thus, it seems evident that transmission of parasites from mother to fetus occurs only under certain specific conditions of maternal infection. The explanation for this comes from the results of studies of acquired Toxoplasma infection in pregnant women.

INFECTION OF THE PLACENTA

There is an excellent correlation between the isolation of Toxoplasma from placental tissue and infection in the neonate. As a rule, if Toxoplasma is isolated, infection of the infant has occured; if Toxoplasma is not isolated, infection of the infant has not occured. Since few infants, if any, escape the infection when the parasite is present in the placenta, infection of this tissue appears to be an event which must occur between the time of infection of the mother and subsequent infection of the fetus. An appreciation of this fact is important to our understanding of the pathogenesis of the congenital infection.

The frequency of placental infection, and thus of fetal infection varies greatly and depends upon the time that the pregnant woman becomes infected. There are few reports of isolation of parasites from placentas of women with chronic infection. In our own experience, we have not isolated Toxoplasma when the infection was acquired before pregnancy. In contrast, positive results are frequently obtained when the infection was acquired during pregnancy. The frequency of successful isolation of Toxoplasma depends upon the time during pregnancy when primary infection of the mother occurs. The later the infection is acquired, the more frequently are parasites isolated from the placenta (Table II). The proportion of infected neonates follows the same pattern and increases as the duration of pregnancy increases before primary maternal infection occurs (Table III).

If we consider only the higher incidence of neonatal Toxoplasma infection which results when maternal infection occurs late in gestation, an explanation might be that Toxoplasma more readily crosses placental tissue as the duration of pregnancy continues. However, it is not only that crossing the placenta becomes more frequent but also that placental infection occurs more frequently. A possible explanation may be that the volume of blood which flows through the placenta increases during

TABLE II. — ATTEMPTS TO ISOLATE TOXOPLASMA * FROM THE PLACENTA AT TIME OF DELIVERY OF WOMEN WHO ACQUIRED TOXOPLASMA INFECTION DURING PREGNANCY **

Maternal treatment during pregnancy	Trimester during which maternal infection was acquired							
	I No.		II No.		III No.		Total	
	Exam.	Posit.	Exam.	Posit.	Exam.	Posit.	Exam.	Posit.
None	16	4 (25 %)	13	7 (54 %)	23	15 (65 %)	52	25 (50 %)
Spiramycin	89	7 (8 %)	144	28 (19 %)	36	16 (44 %)	269	51 (19 %)
Total	105	11 (10 %)	157	35 (22 %)	59	31 (53 %)	321	77 (24 %)

* By mouse inoculation.
** Adapted from DESMONTS, G. and COUVREUR, J.: Congenital toxoplasmosis: a prospective study of the offspring of 542 women who acquired toxoplasmosis during pregnancy. Pathophysiology of congenital disease. In THALHAMMER, O., BAUMGARTEN, K. and POLLAK, A., (eds.): Perinatal Medicine, Sixth European Congress, Stuttgart, Georg Thieme Publishers, 1979, pp. 51-60.

TABLE III. — FREQUENCY OF CONGENITAL TRANSMISSION AND OF STILLBIRTH, CLINICAL CONGENITAL TOXOPLASMOSIS, AND SUBCLINICAL INFECTION AMONG OFFSPRING OF WOMEN WHO ACQUIRED TOXOPLASMA INFECTION DURING PREGNANCY *.

Outcome in offspring	Trimester during which maternal infection was acquired			
	I No. (%)	II No. (%)	III No. (%)	Total No. (%)
No congenital Toxoplasma infection	109 (86)	173 (71)	52 (41)	334 (67)
Congenital toxoplasmosis				
— subclinical	3 (2)	49 (20)	68 (53)	120 (24)
— mild	1 (1)	13 (5)	8 (6)	22 (4)
— severe	7 (6)	6 (2)	0 (0)	13 (3)
Stillbirth or perinatal death	6 (5)	5 (2)	0 (0)	11 (2)
Total	126 (100)	246 (100)	128 (100)	500 (100)

(*) Adapted from DESMONTS, G. and COUVREUR, J.: Congenital toxoplasmosis: a prospective study of the offspring of 542 women who acquired toxoplasmosis during pregnancy. In THALHAMMER, O., BAUMGARTEN, K. and POLLAK, A. (eds.): Perinatal Medicine, Sixth European Congress, Stuttgart, Georg Thieme Publishers, 1979, pp. 51-60.

gestation and thereby increases the likelihood of localization of the parasites in placental tissue during maternal parasitemia.

MATERNAL PARASITEMIA

A construct may be conceived in which transmission of Toxoplasma from mother to fetus depends upon two factors: (1) the placenta and its volume and (2) the duration and magnitude of maternal parasitemia.

There are no systematic studies of attempts to define the duration of parasitemia following primary infection with Toxoplasma in humans. In isolated cases, parasitemia has been found for at least ten days. We have systematically attempted to isolate Toxoplasma from the first sample of blood drawn from women who seroconverted; all of these attempts were negative (in contrast, when using the same technique, Toxoplasma were easily and frequently isolated from the blood clot of samples drawn from neonates with congenital infection).

We consider that the data which exist at present support the concept that parasitemia in naturally acquired human Toxoplasma infection is of short duration and that, as a rule, is not present once antibodies are demonstrable in the serum.

Recurrent parasitemia has been observed during chronic infection in small laboratory animals and in humans. The latter probably occurs rarely and mainly in immunosuppressed individuals. Such recurrent parasitemia might explain the exceptional cases in which Toxoplasma infection acquired before pregnancy was reported to have been transmitted to the fetus.

In summary, congenital Toxoplasma infection results from localization and multiplication of Toxoplasma in the placenta. This placentitis is a result of the parasitemia which occurs in the pregnant woman. As a clinical guideline, parasitemia in otherwise normal humans should be considered to occur only during the first few days of infection. Thus, the risk of placentitis and, as a consequence, the transmission of the parasite to the fetus is high only for those women who become infected for the first time during gestation; the later the infection is acquired, the higher the risk of transmission to the fetus.

CONGENITAL TOXOPLASMOSIS: PATHOGENESIS OF CONGENITAL INFECTION AND DISEASE DUE TO TOXOPLASMA

The pathogenesis of toxoplasmosis is related both to the virulence of the parasite and to the competence of the defence mechanisms of the host (*i. e.* the inflammatory response to invasion by the parasite, as well as the ability of the host to recognize certain antigens of the organism, both early and late during the infection).

Parasites multiply intracellularly and cause host cell disruption. Some strains are more virulent than others but the vast majority isolated in nature are of low virulence at least for small laboratory animals. Intracellular multiplication of tachyzoites ceases with development of host immunity and encystment of the parasites occurs. As a consequence, Toxoplasma infection reaches a stage in which parasites are tolerated by the host tissues as long as the organisms remain intracellularly or within cysts. Latent Toxoplasma infection is an almost perfect example of equilibrium between a parasite and its hosts, an "equilibrium" which appears to be a tolerance due to the inability to the recognize foreign antigen on the surface of cysts.

If the immune response is delayed or is abnormal, tachyzoites continue to multiply and result in continued cell destruction during the initial infection and in larger number of cysts in the latent infection (which will result in there being more foreign

antigen in the tissues of the chronically infected host and in a higher risk that eye or C. N. S. lesions will occur during the chronic stage of the infection).

Various factors may help to explain why the fetus is a more susceptible host than the mother. Parasites are transmitted directly through the bloodstream via the umbilical vein, to an immunologically immature and small host. (Young animals as a rule are more susceptible to Toxoplasma than are adults—example e. g. chickens versus hens; baby rats versus mature rats.)

Passively transmitted maternal IgG possibly has an immunosuppressive effect. While IgG probably affords some protection, such antibodies will also inhibit recognition of Toxoplasma antigen as being foreign and thereby delay an active immune response and modify the pattern of disease.

Systematic surveys among infants born of mothers who acquired Toxoplasma infection during pregnancy have shown that congenital Toxoplasma infection is usually mild or even clinically inapparent: the child may be completely free of signs of the infection. In contrast, clinically severe disease has been observed only in a minority of cases (Table III).

The clinical pattern of congenital toxoplasmosis differs markedly from one case to another and depends on the time during gestation the infection is transmitted to the fetus. This is shown in Table IV. If maternal infection acquired during the first half of pregnancy is transmitted to the fetus, disease in the fetus will be severe and will often result in fetal death or stillbirth. If born alive, signs of severe fetopathy will be present in the newborn with obvious ocular and cerebral lesions. If maternal infection is acquired later in pregnancy (third trimester), the neonate will most often be without signs of infection. Severe clinical disease is seldom observed in this circumstance. If severe, the clinical pattern is more suggestive of neonatal septicemia than of toxoplasmosis.

From these data it can be deduced that while the risk of transmission of Toxoplasma is greatest when maternal infection is acquired during the last months of pregnancy, the frequency of severe fetal disease is markedly less among the infected offspring than among infected infants born of mothers who acquire their infection early in pregnancy. Thus, there is a high risk period for pregnant women, during which, if the infection is acquired, the result will often be delivery of a child with overt, severe, clinical disease. This high risk period includes weeks 10 to 24 of gestation; if the infection is acquired by the mother before 10 weeks, fetal infection may be severe but is infrequent. If acquired after 24 weeks, infection of the fetus is frequent but seldom severe.

TABLE IV. — Effect of trimester during which maternal infection was acquired on relative frequency of stillbirth and on different clinical aspects of congenital toxoplasmosis among the 166 children who either died or were proved to be infected (*).

Outcome in offspring	Trimester during which maternal infection was acquired			
	I	II	III	Total
	No. (%)	No. (%)	No. (%)	No. (%)
Congenital toxoplasmosis				
— subclinical	3 (18)	49 (67)	68 (89)	120 (72)
— mild	1 (6)	13 (18)	8 (11)	22 (13)
— severe	7 (41)	6 (8)	0 (0)	13 (8)
Stillbirth or perinatal death	6 (35)	5 (7)	0 (0)	11 (7)
Total	17 (100)	73 (100)	76 (100)	166 (100)

* Adapted from Desmonts, G. and Couvreur, J.: Congenital toxoplasmosis: a prospective study of the offspring of 542 women who acquired toxoplasmosis during pregnancy. Pathophysiology of congenital disease. In Thalhammer, O., Baumgarten, K. and Pollak, A. (eds.): *Perinatal Medicine*, Sixth European Congress, Stuttgart, Georg Thieme Publishers, 1979, pp. 51-60.
The 334 children born alive and not infected who are listed in Table III are excluded from this table.

DATA OBTAINED FROM STUDY OF INDUCED ABORTIONS

The risk of giving birth to a child with congenital toxoplasmosis has often been considered as an indication for induced abortion. Placental and/or fetal tissues obtained from 139 such abortions were inoculated into mice in an attempt to isolate Toxoplasma. In 47 cases, maternal infection was probably acquired shortly before pregnancy as judged by serological and/or clinical data. Toxoplasma was not isolated in this group. In 92 cases, maternal infection was definitely acquired after the beginning of pregnancy. Nine (9 %) of the inoculations from this group were positive. In six of these nine, it was possible to inoculate the placental and fetal tissues separately. In two cases the placentas were positive and the fetal tissues negative. (The fetuses were macroscopically normal). This clearly demonstrates that there is a delay between placental and fetal

infection. In four cases, isolation of the organism from fetal tissues proved that the infection was transmitted before the abortion had been induced. In these four cases, the fetus had overt signs of the infection which consisted mainly of a considerably enlarged liver and, in two cases, of large necrotic foci in the brain. These results support the clinical observation that when Toxoplasma is transmitted early during fetal life, the infection will be clinically apparent in the newborn.

SUBCLINICAL CONGENITAL TOXOPLASMA INFECTION

Prospective studies of acquired Toxoplasma infection in pregnant women have revealed that subclinical infection is the most frequent pattern of congenital infection in the newborn, and that congenital infection sometimes remains subclinical even if treatment is not given to the mother during pregnancy or to the child after birth. This fact was established in studies in which samples of sera drawn during pregnancy were stored and studied some months following delivery. Children were examined a few months and at times over a period of a year after birth. It was surprising in some cases to observe definite evidence that maternal infection acquired during pregnancy had been transmitted to the fetus without observing any signs or symptoms of the congenital infection in their infant (Table XI untreated group).

Congenital Toxoplasma infection may be subclinical for different reasons. For instance, transmission of Toxoplasma may occur early and thereby induce fetal disease which is mild and the lesions of which are cured without sequelae before delivery. This probably happens in a few cases where the mother is treated early following acquisition of the infection.

Another circumstance is when transmission has been delayed. The parasites remain localized to the placenta without reaching the fetal bloodstream until the last days of pregnancy or during labour. We consider the accumulated data to suggest that this is probably what occurs most frequently. As a result, the child is born without clinically apparent lesions. Infection occurs during a period when passive humoral immunity due to transfer of maternal IgG is already present. This antibody prob bly results in some degree of protection (but also m ay suppress active immunization).

The consequences of infection in the neonate will also differ in relationship to the degree of maturity

TABLE V

Mother	Placenta No localization in the placenta	Fetus No congenital infection		Infant
Acquisition of toxoplasma infection	Localization in the placenta	Early transmission:	Fetal disease	Fetal death Overt toxoplasmosis in the newborn
Parasitemia	Placentitis	Delayed transmission	No fetal disease	Premature: late onset of overt disease
			Subclinical infection associated with passive immunity in the newborn	Full term infant: subclinical infection. Possible discovery of sequelae in chilhood or adulthood. Possible occurence of relapses of ocular disease.

of the infant's immune system at birth. Premature infants born of mothers with infection acquired late in pregnancy will be prone to develop delayed and more severe disease during the first weeks or months of life. Full term infants will be more likely to remain asymptomatic during infancy, but as a consequence of subclinical infection many will be discovered to have retinal scars in later life. Even when subclinical in the newborn, congenital Toxoplasma infection is a cause of lesions during its chronic stage; untoward sequelae are detected in about 60 % of untreated cases.

A summary of these points on transmission and pathogenesis of congenital toxoplasmosis is given in Table V.

PATHOLOGY
AND CLINICAL MANIFESTATIONS

The genesis of the natural infection is comparable to that observed in experimental toxoplasmosis in susceptible laboratory animals. The organisms reach all organs, including the brain, via the bloodstream, but the distribution of parasites and lesions varies considerably and depends on a variety of factors: the virulence of the infecting strain, the number of parasites actually transmitted from the mother to the fetus, the time during pregnancy when maternal infection occured, the duration of placental delay before transmission of parasites to the fetus, the developmental maturity of the infant's immune

system, the amount of passively transmitted IgG antibodies at the time of transmission and the duration of fetal infection before birth. These different factors result in a disease with protean manifestations. Extraneural lesions may be severe in some cases and may even predominate. More frequently however, the disease in infants reflects damage to the Central Nervous System and is manifested clinically mainly as an encephalomyelitis.

SUMMARY
OF THE MAIN PATHOLOGICAL FINDINGS
AND
OF THE RELATED CLINICAL MANIFESTATIONS

Central nervous system: necrotic encephalomyelitis.

— Miliary granuloma scattered in the brain and spinal cord.

— Extensive necrosis of brain parenchyma due to vascular involvment by lesions.

— Periventricular vasculitis and ulcers on the walls of the ventricles.

— Cellular reactions in the meninges with lymphocytes, plasma cells, and eosinophils.

— *Calcifications* within zones of necrosis.

— Periaqueductal vasculitis and inflammatory *obstruction* of the *aqueduct of Sylvius*.

Signs related to central nervous system lesions include:

— Convulsive seizures, lethargy, hypertonia or

hypotonia, paralysis, respiratory distress, dysregulation of body temperature.

— *Abnormal cerebrospinal fluid* (CSF): xanthochromia, mononuclear pleocytosis, a very high protein content (sometimes grams per ml in severe cases). A moderately elevated protein content is a common feature even in infants with subclinical infection.

— Microcephaly is a possible consequence of brain atrophy due to extensive necrotic lesions.

— *Hydrocephalus* is related mainly to the obstruction of the aqueduct of Sylvius. It may become manifest late in children with otherwise discrete central nervous system lesions, and little or no clinical manifestations.

Eye: Focal necrotizing retinochoroiditis.

— The primary and principal lesions are in the retina and choroid. Intraocular inflammation may result in cataract formation and in an arrest in development of the eye (microphthalmia).

Foci of retinitis are situated either near the posterior pole, or peripherally; œdematous foci with indistinct borders are seen in acute lesions whereas older ones are sharply outlined and characterized by accumulation of choroidal pigment. Inflammatory exudate sometimes makes visualization of the fundus impossible. Healed lesions are seen as pigmented scars surrounded by normal retina. In older infants and children, signs due to involvment of the retina often occur as strabismus and nystagmus.

Other viscera.

Skin. — Maculopapular rash, jaundice, purpura, ecchymoses.

Abdomen.

Ascites: a peritoneal exudate is present in cases with severe systemic disease and has been detected by echography during pregnancy. This procedure permits an early consideration of the possibility of fetal infection.

Liver may be considerably enlarged. Hepatomegaly accompanied by erythropoiesis, hepatocellular degenerative changes with or without interstitial cellular infiltrations; areas of necrosis and calcified foci have also been observed. Hepatic cirrhosis has also been observed as a sequel to congenital toxoplasmosis.

Spleen is often enlarged, with engorgement of splenic pulp and erythropoiesis.

Kidneys: foci of hematopoiesis and focal glomerulitis have been observed. In a few cases a nephrotic syndrome has occured.

Thorax.

Lungs: interstitial pneumonia: alveolar septa are widened, œdematous and infiltrated with mononuclear cells and some eosinophils. The pneumonic process is usually not a prominent part of the generalized disease.

Heart: parasites are always present in the form of cysts in myocardial fibres. There are focal areas of infiltration with lymphocytes, plasma cells, mononuclear cells and eosinophiles. Myocarditis is probably produced by disruption of parasitized cells which results in liberation of the organisms. This release of parasites causes inflammation in the surrounding tissues.

Other tissues.

Skeletal muscles: lesions analogous to those which are seen in the myocardium.

Bones: radiographic signs may be present and may reveal bands of metaphyseal lucency and irregularity of the epiphyseal line of provisional calcification.

Blood: thrombocytopenia is frequently noted, even in subclinical cases. Leukocytosis or leukopenia. eosinophilia and hemolytic anemia may also be associated with congenital toxoplasmosis. An intravascular coagulation syndrome has been observed in severe systemic neonatal toxoplasmosis. Clinically this resembles bacterial sepsis from which it must be differentiated.

Immunoglobulin abnormalities: an increase in IgG and IgM levels, macroglobulinemia, hypergammaglobulinemia related to the presence of monoclonal immunoglobulin and delayed development of IgA all may occur.

CLINICAL PATTERNS

One can schematically describe different patterns of congenital disease:

Neurological disease in the infant.

— In this form the infant may have hydrocephalus or microcephaly, microphthalmia and/or retinochoroiditis. These signs may be present either at birth, or hydrocephalus may be discovered only after a period of a few months during which the child was considered to have developed normally (delayed congenital toxoplasmosis).

Severe systemic disease. — These infants may have purpura, jaundice and hepatosplenomegaly. Uveitis and/or enlargement of the cerebral ventricles may or may not be present in these infants.

Mild disease, with isolated signs. — Jaundice and/or thrombocytopenic purpura are signs which are sometimes noted during the first weeks of life in children who are discovered later to have the retinal scars of toxoplasmic chorioretinitis.

TABLE VI. — PROSPECTIVE STUDY OF INFANTS BORN TO WOMEN WHO ACQUIRED TOXOPLASMA INFECTION DURING PREGNANCY: SIGNS AND SYMPTOMS IN 108 INFANTS WITH PROVEN CONGENITAL INFECTION *.

Finding	No. examined	No. positive (%)
Prematurity { birth weight below 2,500 g	108	4 (3.7)
birth weight of 2,500 g to 3,000 g		7 (6.5)
Dysmaturity (intrauterine growth retardation)	108	3 (2.7)
Postmaturity	108	9 (8.3)
Icterus	107	12 (11.2)
Hepatosplenomegaly	108	5 (4.6)
Thrombocytopenic purpura	108	2 (1.8)
Abnormal blood count (anemia, eosinophilia)	105	5 (4.8)
Microcephaly	108	9 (8.3)
Hydrocephaly	108	4 (3.7)
Hypotonia	108	7 (6.5)
Convulsions	108	5 (4.6)
Psychomotor retardation	108	5 (4.6)
Intracranial calcifications on X-ray	103	16 (15.5)
Abnormal EEG	95	8 (8.4)
Abnormal CSF { pleocytosis	94	32 (34.0)
increased protein level		32 (34.0)
Microphthalmia	108	4 (3.7)
Strabismus	108	9 (8.3)
Chorioretinitis { unilateral	108	21 (19.4)
bilateral		6 (5.5)

* Adapted from SZUSTERKAC, *A propos de 124 cas de toxoplasmose congénitale*. Thèse Faculté de Médecine Saint-Antoine, Paris, 1980. Étudiant service Éditeur.

The relative frequency of this attenuated form of congenital toxoplasmosis and of subclinical congenital toxoplasma infection is shown in Table VI.

DIAGNOSIS

DIAGNOSTIC METHODS

Parasitological methods

Microscopic examination. — Smears or histological sections of tissues may be examined for the presence of the parasite. These methods are most commonly used for postmortem examination. Using these methods the pathogenicity of Toxoplasma for humans and the pathological picture of congenital toxoplasmosis were first described.

Tachyzoites are found on smears of tissue obtained at the periphery of necrotic foci present in brain. Histologic demonstration of cysts is possible in normal tissues some distance from necrotic areas. Tachyzoites are not easily identified. Oval shaped cysts situated inside fibers in sections of skeletal and heart muscle are also easily demonstrated. Experience is necessary for recognition of these forms of the organism. In the literature, microphotographs of "Toxoplasma" not infrequently suggest that the authors misdiagnosed the infection and described artifacts.

The fluorescent antibody technique or the peroxidase anti-peroxidase method has been suggested as increasing the sensitivity and specificity of detecting the organism in tissue smears or histologic sections.

Isolation procedures. — Isolation of the parasites provides definite proof of the identity of the organism seen in smears or histological sections, but the main purpose of this procedure is to prove the presence of Toxoplasma in tissues in which they are difficult to find microscopically (e. g. in lymph nodes of patients with acquired toxoplasmosis).

Inoculation of placental tissue into mice should be performed whenever possible when acute Toxoplasma infection is diagnosed in the mother during pregnancy. Approximately 100 g of placenta should be kept without fixative and stored at 4° C until it can be digested with trypsin and inoculated into mice. Unfortunately, availability of results of this procedure are slow. Mice must be observed for as long as six weeks before assessing a negative result. By that time, the child is one and a half months old. The result is, however, important, even at that age.

If positive, the risk of congenital infection is so high that treatment must be continued even if the child still has no clinical signs of the infection. If negative, a clinically normal child is probably not infected; this is not definitely proven since isolation procedures may fail either due to technical problems or to the fact that the mother was treated during pregnancy.

Cerebrospinal fluid, cord blood or blood drawn from the newborn should also be inoculated into mice. The clot may be triturated and inoculated after the serum has been withdrawn. When blood has been obtained during the first days of life, positive results are obtained in nearly half the cases.

Demonstration of antibodies in serum-methods

A wide variety of serological methods are used to demonstrate the presence of antibodies to Toxoplasma. In the three methods most widely used, the dye test, the immunofluorescent antibody test (IFA) and the agglutination test, the whole parasite, either alive or formalin fixed is employed as the antigen. In the other methods, the indirect hemagglutination test, complement fixation test and enzyme linked immunoabsorbent assay (ELISA), antigenic extracts obtained from lysed parasites are used.

Dye test (Sabin and Feldman, 1948). — This test is based on the observation that Toxoplasma, once altered by antibodies, do not stain with alkaline methylene blue. This is due to the lysis of the organisms; the membrane is disrupted due to activation of the complement system after the formation of antigen-antibody complexes on the surface of the parasite. The antibodies which act in this test are mainly IgG (but probably not subclass IV, which do not activate the complement system). The dye test is a very sensitive and quantitatively accurate method, since it is possible to exactly determine the end point of the reaction (lysis of 50 % of parasites). Due to its accuracy and its specificity, the dye test is often considered as the reference method. The drawback is that live, and therefore infectious, parasites have to be used.

Immunofluorescent antibody test. — The specific reaction between the antigenic sites of the cell membrane of Toxoplasma and the patient's antibodies can be detected by a fluorescein tagged antiserum prepared against human Ig. The antiserum may be directed against all classes of Ig (conventional IFA test) or against a single class of Ig (e. g.

IgM IFA test, or IgG IFA test). Slide preparations of killed Toxoplasma and tagged antihuman Ig sera are commercially available and this method is now widely used despite its drawbacks: it is not very precise and the end point of a titer in two-fold dilutions is difficult to read. This is the reason why threefold or even fourfold dilutions are most commonly used. At times, it is also difficult to objectively distinguish between a weakly positive result and a negative one.

Agglutination test. — This test employs whole parasites which have been preserved in formalin. In the absence of antibodies, a smooth button is observed at the bottom of the wells in a microtiter plate. In the presence of antibodies, a carpet of agglutinated parasites is observed. The method is very sensitive to IgM antibodies. Unfortunately, non-specific agglutination has been observed in individuals devoid of antibodies in the dye test or IFA test. This is due to "naturally occuring" IgM Toxoplasma agglutinins which probably bind to antigens present at the anterior pole of the parasite (this binding is also responsible for the "polar staining" observed in the IFA test). False positive results due to these "natural antibodies" may be avoided if the agglutination test is performed in a buffer containing 2 mercapto-ethanol. When this is done, the agglutination method has proven to be very sensitive for detection of IgG antibodies to Toxoplasma. The method is simple to perform and readily adaptable for wide scale screening of pregnant women. It is also accurate and valuable for the quantitative study of IgG antibodies directed towards the antigen of the membrane of Toxoplasma.

Complement fixation test and hemagglutination test. — Antigenic extracts from the lysed parasite are used for both methods. Depending on how they are prepared, the remnants of membranes and their antigens are either retained or excluded. As a consequence, the results may be different from one technique to the other. If remnants of parasite membrane are present they closely parallel the dye test results both quantitatively and qualitatively. In contrast, the results are very different from those of the dye test if the antigen preparation consists mainly of cytoplasmic components.

Enzyme linked immunoabsorbent assay (ELISA). — The ELISA has recently been adapted to serodiagnosis of toxoplasmosis. Results with this method will vary depending on the antigen preparation used. It should prove to be a very useful test as our knowledge of the different antigens of the parasite increases.

Quantitative study of IgG: the "antibody load". — Most of the IgG present in newborn serum has been transferred from the mother through the placenta. Some synthesis may also have occured during fetal life and progressively increases during the first months of life. The amount of IgG present in the serum depends on the age of the infant and may differ considerably from one patient to another. The level of IgG is higher in the newborn child than in the mother due to concentration of IgG by the placenta; it is much lower after a few months of age. These differences are so important that they must be taken into account when evaluating serologic test results.

If a comparison is to be made between the antibody titer of the mother and child or between two samples drawn from the same infant at different ages, it is necessary to determine the level of total IgG in the different samples. This must be performed in order to appreciate whether the differences between levels of IgG are sufficient to explain differences in specific antibody titers. This is accomplished by computing the ratio of specific antibody to total IgG, which may be expressed by the number of units of specific antibody per milligram of IgG. This ratio has been termed "the specific antibody load of IgG". Total IgG may be measured by immunodiffusion. A quantitatively accurate method must be used for measurement of specific antibodies to allow one to obtain a clear cut end point in sera run in twofold dilutions. Both the dye test and the agglutination test have given reliable results for this purpose.

Tests for IgM antibodies. — These tests are important in the diagnosis of congenital Toxoplasma infection since IgM does not normally pass the placental barrier (except if there is a placental leak). As a consequence, the presence of IgM antibodies is definite proof of antibody synthesis by the fetus, and thus of congenital infection.

Exclusion chromatography, with specific serologic testing of the fractions, can demonstrate the presence of toxoplasma antibodies in the IgM fractions. It is necessary to prove that this antibody activity is not related to the contamination of these fractions by IgG. Such methods are too cumbersome for routine examination of numerous samples of sera.

IgM fluorescent antibody test: this method is simple and specific but it sometimes fails to demonstrate IgM antibodies in the presence of a high titer of IgG antibodies in patient serum. High titer (or high avidity) IgG antibodies result in competition for the antigenic sites on the parasite membrane which inhibits binding of IgM antibodies.

False positive reactions may be observed in newborn sera when IgM antibodies (rheumatoid factor) to maternal IgG are present. This is mainly observed in patients with fœtopathy. IgG Toxoplasma antibodies of maternal origin combine with antigens of the parasite and the newborn's rheumatoid factor in turn reacts with the IgG. The fluorescein tagged anti-IgM antiserum then detects the infant's rheumatoid factor which causes a false positive reaction.

Immunoabsorbent assays (ISA): The initial step in these assays is to coat the wells of microtiter plates with specific antibodies to human IgM. The patient's serum is then added and its IgM binds to the antibodies coating the plate. The wells are then washed; in this way, IgG is eliminated and the wells remain coated with the patient's pure IgM. Different procedures may be used to test the presence of specific antibodies in this IgM:

In the double sandwich ELISA, soluble Toxoplasma antigen is first added, and then an enzyme labelled antibody preparation to Toxoplasma. In the reverse enzyme immuno assay (reverse EIA) the soluble antigen itself is labelled with the enzyme.

In the immunabosorbent agglutination assay (ISAgA), formalin treated Toxoplasma (agglutination antigen) are added: they become attached to the wells of antibody to Toxoplasma present in the IgM.

These methods are significantly more sensitive and specific than the IgM IFA test, due to the separation of IgM from IgG, and thus to the absence of inhibition by competition. Separation from IgG also eliminates false positive reactions due to the presence of rheumatoid factor.

Tests of cell mediated immunity

Toxoplasmin skin test. — Infection with Toxoplasma results in the development of cell-mediated immunity, which may be demonstrated by a skin test. In a small series of cases, we have not observed a single positive test in infants with congenital Toxoplasma infection before the end of the first year of life: the skin test is probably not useful for diagnosis of the infection in the neonate.

Antigen specific lymphocyte transformation. — This method may be used for the diagnosis and is a sensitive indicator of congenital Toxoplasma infection as it proved positive in 84 % of cases studied. The method is specific and should be performed when technically possible. Initial results suggest that this method may be negative in very young infants.

Demonstration of antigen in body fluids and of antigenemia

The presence of antigen resulting from parasite lysis was demonstrated in the cerebrospinal fluid of infants with congenital toxoplasmosis by Frenkel. This was done by inoculating the fluid into allergic guinea pigs. Recently, an enzyme linked immuno-absorbent assay has been used to demonstrate Toxoplasma antigen in CSF, in amniotic fluid and in serum. The usefulness of this method for diagnosis of congenital toxoplasmosis remains to be defined.

ANTIBODY RESPONSE IN CONGENITALLY INFECTED INFANTS

The antibody response of an adult to the acquired infection may be described as follows: IgM and IgG antibodies directed towards antigens of the parasite membrane are detectable first. Later, antibodies to intracellular "soluble" antigens are demonstrable. The level of IgM antibodies rises rapidly. The rise in IgG antibodies is slow but protracted. Due to the suppressive effect of IgG on IgM synthesis, titers in the tests for IgM antibodies decrease and finally become negative. The titer of IgG antibodies rises during the first weeks of infection (8 or more), remains steady for several months or even years and then decreases slowly. They remain weakly positive for years, probably, as a rule, for the life of the host.

The antibody response of a congenitally infected child may differ for a number of reasons: the immunologic immaturity of the fetus and infant; the suppressive effect of maternal IgG which is probably most important when maternal antibodies have been transferred to the fetus before transmission of the parasite; in some cases, the severity of a heavy infection; specific treatment which the mother, and the fetus as a consequence, received during pregnancy and the child received after birth.

One may schematically describe *three stages* in the antibody response to congenital Toxoplasma infection:

The *first stage* comprises the first weeks and months of life. It may last up to the tenth month. During this stage, the antibody response may be strikingly different from one patient to another. In some patients, the response may be completely suppressed with no evidence of synthesis of IgM or IgG antibody; the antibodies present in the child's serum seem to be solely of maternal origin. In other newborns a definite and strong antibody response may be observed, parallel to that which is observed following an acquired infection in the adult, and including both IgM and IgG antibodies. In most cases however the observed antibody response is weak, delayed, or incomplete; some infants do synthesize IgM antibodies, others do not. In addition, synthesis of IgG antibodies may sometimes be present without any evidence of synthesis of IgM antibody. The antibody response is also labile and easily suppressed when the child remains on treatment.

It should be noted that a strong production of antibody or, on the contrary the absence of any specific antibody synthesis, may be observed in infants with subclinical infection and in those with severe clinical congenital disease as well. In severe congenital cases, this lack of specific antibody response may often be associated with hypergammaglobulinemia with a monoclonal IgG component which does not apparently contain specific antitoxoplasma antibodies.

Specific IgG antibody synthesis, when weak, is difficult to assess as long as passive antibodies of maternal origin are present. As a consequence, in the absence of IgM antibodies, a definitive serological diagnosis of congenital Toxoplasma infection may be delayed for several months (sometimes for as long as 6 to 10 months). This is especially true in treated children.

The special feature of the *second stage* is the occurrence of very active synthesis of IgG antibodies. This occurs between 10 months and two years of age in both treated and untreated children. The titer of antibodies which may have decreased during the first months of life or may have remained stable at the same level, rises strikingly to a very high level. This late response is most often due to IgG antibodies. IgM antibodies are seldom present. The reasons for this phenomenon are unclear. It may be related to the persistence of parasites in the tissues of the infected child, and possibly to their limited multiplication. The latter is known to occur after cessation of treatment. It may also be related to the accomplishment of some immunologic ability which improves the recognition, killing and lysis of parasites, thus increasing the antigenic stimulus. The infection itself is known to cause immunosuppression probably due to suppressor cells. Thus, this may also be due to a release of the immunosuppression of infection.

During the *third stage*, the antibody titer decreases slowly to low levels. This does not differ from what is observed following the acquired infection, except for the fact that serologic relapses—that is, late increases in titers—appears to be much more frequent following congenital than acquired infection. These serologic relapses may or may not be associated with recurrent relapses of chronic Toxoplasma infection while the relapses of clinical disease, when present, are accompanied as a rule by evidence of a local increase in antibody synthesis in the aqueous humour and, to a lesser degree, in cerebrospinal fluid.

DISCUSSION OF DIAGNOSIS

When one considers the diagnosis of neonatal Toxoplasma infection, two different situations must be taken into account: (1) when a newborn baby has signs which suggest a fœtopathy which might be due to Toxoplasma infection. (2) When an apparently normal baby is born of a woman who is known to have acquired primary Toxoplasma infection during pregnancy.

In a similar manner, two sets of data should be considered: (1) data obtained from the clinical examination of the child and (2) serologic results obtained in the mother. However, even with these considerations the diagnosis will only be established if parasites are isolated from the child, and/or, if synthesis of specific antibodies is demonstrable.

Clinical data

Overt fœtopathy. — Congenital toxoplasmosis has protean manifestations; the clinical signs may vary considerably, ranging from subclinical infection to severe systemic disease, or to neurologic syndromes due to widespread destruction of the central nervous system. Among infectious agents which may be associated with similar patterns of neonatal disease, cytomegalovirus is the most frequent, and many signs are shared by infants with congenital cytomegalovirus infection and congenital Toxoplasma infection. Herpes simplex virus infection, rubella, syphilis and bacterial sepsis must at times also be considered.

Without discussing the details of the signs or symptoms which are more or less frequently associated with one or another of these infections, it should be noted that a systemic disease with rash, spleen and liver enlargement, is more often related to cytomegalovirus infection than to toxoplasmosis. In contrast, a disease with hydrocephaly, intracranial calcifications, microphthalmia, and chorioretinitis, is much more often due to Toxoplasma than to cytomegalovirus; each of these syndromes may, however, be caused by either of these agents.

Subclinical infection. — At the present time, the most frequent problem in France is to recognize the presence of subclinical infection in a newborn or in an infant born to a woman known to have acquired Toxoplasma infection during pregnancy. The infant may appear to be normal but may be infected as established by serologic data (presence of IgM antibodies), or by results of attempts at isolation of the parasite. A careful examination must be performed to evaluate the consequences of possible lesions, if any are present. Table VI shows the results of examination of 108 infants who were examined because a diagnosis of acute Toxoplasma infection was made in their mothers during gestation, and in whom the diagnosis of congenital infection was established during the first weeks of life.

The number of cases with chorioretinitis (25 %) and particularly with abnormal spinal fluids (34 %) is important. This last abnormality suggests that subclinical encephalitis is a frequent manifestation of the infection. This silent encephalitis may sometimes result in an obstruction of the aqueduct of Sylvius. For this reason, computed tomography examination should be performed in every case of proven congenital Toxoplasma infection even if subclinical, to evaluate the ventricles for early evidence of obstruction and possible indication for surgical intervention. This procedure may reveal calcifications which are not demonstrable or are easily missed with standard radiography.

Data obtained from examination of the mother

Interpretation of serologic results obtained in the mother obviously differ depending on the circumstances. If the problem is to establish the diagnosis is an infant with a clinical picture which suggests congenital toxoplasmosis and who was born from a mother who had never been examined before, a high titer of antibodies in maternal serum strongly suggests that the infant has congenital toxoplasmosis. However this occurs relatively infrequently today in France where systematic examinations are performed during pregnancy. The birth of a child with congenital toxoplasmosis is seldom not predictable. The severe, obvious cases of toxoplasmic fœtopathy which are sometimes observed, are most often born to mothers who have failed to be systematically examined during their pregnancy and treated when infection occurs. Serologic test results in these cases are described and evaluated in Table VII.

TABLE VII. — DIAGNOSIS OF CONGENITAL TOXOPLAS-
MOSIS IN AN INFANT WITH OVERT CLINICAL DISEASE.
GUIDELINES FOR INTERPRETATION OF SEROLOGICAL
RESULTS OBTAINED IN THE MOTHER FOR THE FIRST TIME
AT THE TIME OF DELIVERY (UNTREATED MOTHER).

Serological results Antibodies		
IgG	IgM	Conclusion
> 300 iu	+	Recent infection in mother
> 1,000 iu	0	Congenital disease in the child is probably toxoplasmosis
0	0	Recent infection in mother is
< 300 iu	0	excluded. Congenital toxoplasmosis is unlikely
< 300 iu	+	Mother may have been infect-
0	+	ed very recently. The diagnosis should be established by demonstration of a rise in IgG titer in a second serum sample obtained after 2 or 3 weeks. Congenital toxoplasmosis is a likely diagnosis if the neonate has signs of severe or mild systemic disease

The most frequent problem in countries where women are systematically examined during pregnancy is to decide if an apparently normal child is infected. To make this decision, the titer of maternal antibodies is unfortunately not helpful since the infants are known to have been born of mothers who acquired Toxoplasma infection during gestation and therefore to have a high titer. Nevertheless, valuable information may be obtained from serological test titers which had been performed during pregnancy (cf. Table VIII).

Biological diagnosis of infection in the child

Definitive establishment of the diagnosis of Toxoplasma infection, whether overt or subclinical,

depends on the demonstration of Toxoplasma and/or of a specific immune response (antibody production) in the child. Diagnosis is sometimes established at the time of delivery if antibody synthesis during fetal life has been sufficiently active. This is discussed in Table IX. If inoculation of blood or placental tissue has been performed, the result is obtained after six weeks at the latest, and is discussed in Table X. If the diagnosis is not established when the child is 6 weeks old, a close follow up of the serological test titer evolution is necessary. Examinations should be performed monthly, or at least every two months in order to follow the evolution of the "immune load". Figures IV-22, IV-23 and IV-24 are schematic curves depicting what is observed when antibodies are solely of maternal origin (Fig. IV-22), when production of IgG specific antibodies in the infant has occured early (Fig. IV-23); and when this production is delayed (Fig. IV-24).

TABLE VIII. — DIAGNOSIS OF TOXOPLASMA INFECTION IN
A CHILD WHOSE CLINICAL EXAMINATION IS NORMAL OR
IN WHOM SIGNS WHICH ARE UNCOMMON IN CONGENITAL
TOXOPLASMOSIS ARE PRESENT. GUIDELINES FOR INTER-
PRETATION OF MATERNAL SEROLOGICAL TEST RESULTS
OBTAINED DURING PREGNANCY.

Maternal serological test titer	Duration of pregnancy when observed	Subclinical infection in the child
Strongly positive but not rising	Before 14th week	±
	After 14th week	+
Definite serologic conversion from negative to positive	Before 14th week	+
	Between 14th and 26th week	+ +
	After 26th week	+ + +

± = highly improbable
+ + + = probable

In treated children, development of a specific antibody response may sometimes be very slow, weak and delayed. The serologic tests may even become completely negative. These negative results may be transient. If they persist, this suggests that the infection has been eradicated in the infant; this can only be assessed if definitive parasitologic evidence for infection was previously established.

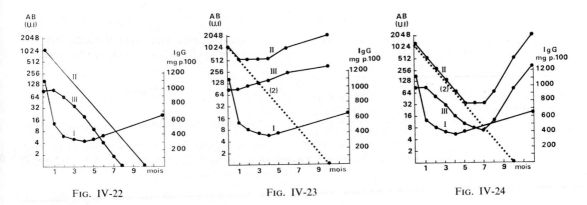

FIG. IV-22   FIG. IV-23   FIG. IV-24

Fɪɢ. IV-22. — *IgG and toxoplasma antibodies: uninfected child.* Curve I: mg of IgG/100.
Curve II: I. U. of toxoplasma antibody per ml. Curve III: I. U. of toxoplasma antibody per mg of IgG.

Fɪɢ. IV-23. — *Antibodies in congenital toxoplasmosis (cases with early synthesis of antibodies).* Curve I: mg of IgG/100.
Curve II: I. U. of toxoplasma antibody per ml, (2) expected titer if antibodies were maternal in origin. Curve III: I. U. of toxoplasma antibody per mg of IgG.

Fɪɢ. IV-24. — *Antibodies in congenital toxoplasmosis (cases with delayed synthesis * of antibodies).* Curve I: mg of IgG/ 100. Curve II: I. U. of toxoplasma antibody per ml, (2) expected titer if antibodies were maternal in origin. Curve III: I. U. of toxoplasma antibody per mg of IgG.

* Synthesis is usually not delayed more than 3 or 4 months, if the child receives no treatment. It may be delayed up to the 6th or 9th month, if treated.

TABLE IX. — Cᴏᴍᴘᴀʀɪsᴏɴ ʙᴇᴛᴡᴇᴇɴ ᴍᴀᴛᴇʀɴᴀʟ ᴀɴᴅ ᴄᴏʀᴅ (ᴏʀ ɴᴇᴏɴᴀᴛᴀʟ) sᴇʀᴜᴍ
ꜰᴏʀ ᴅᴇᴍᴏɴsᴛʀᴀᴛɪᴏɴ ᴏꜰ ᴀɴᴛɪʙᴏᴅʏ ᴘʀᴏᴅᴜᴄᴛɪᴏɴ ᴅᴜʀɪɴɢ ꜰᴇᴛᴀʟ ʟɪꜰᴇ.

IgM:	*IgG:*
IgM antibodies do not cross the placental barrier. If present, they have been synthesized by the fetus.	The immune load of the child, if greater than that of the mother, demonstrates IgG antibody synthesis by the fetus.

Methods:	*Limits:*	*Limits:*
IgM immunofluorescent antibody test	— Positive in only 25 % of neonates with congenital Toxoplasma infection. A negative test does not exclude infection. — Possible false positive result, related to antibodies against maternal IgG.	— This is only observed in treated cases when the maternal titer has remained low (below 400 iu/ml), due to treatment. — Reliable only if titration of antibodies is accurate. — Differences are sometimes observed even if the infant is not infected possibly due to the heterogeneousness of Toxoplasma antibodies, and to the different rate of transfer of the different subclasses of antibodies.
Immunoabsorbent assay (ELISA or ISAGA)	— Positive in 70 % of cases. — Very sensitive, even to a minimal placental leak: it should be repeated after 1 or 2 weeks.	

The antibody load of the child is significant when it is at least four times that of the mother.

TABLE X. — Attempts at isolation of parasites. Discussion of results

Cord (or neonatal) blood *or cerebrospinal fluid*	If positive, child is infected. Results are negative in about 50 % of cases when blood is used and in the majority of cases when CSF is used.
Placenta	Negative: Does not definitely exclude infection in the child: false negative results may be obtained in about 15 % of cases due to technical difficulties — volume of tissue sample was too small, — poor conditions of preservation, or due to treatment during pregnancy.
	Positive: Does not definitely prove infection in the child, as parasites might not have been transmitted. Yet infection is present in over 95 % of such children.

THERAPY

Specific therapy is recommended in every case of congenital toxoplasmosis or congenital Toxoplasma infection, even when it is subclinical or inapparent.

Pyrimethamine plus sulfonamides (sulfadiazine, sulfadimerazine) act synergistically. This drug combination results not only in survival, but also in radical cure of animals with the experimental infection.

Trimethoprim plus sulfamethoxazole are also synergistic in vitro, but their effectiveness in congenital toxoplasmosis has not been demonstrated.

Spiramycin has proved active against Toxoplasma in animal experiments but is less active than pyrimethamine plus sulfonamides.

GUIDELINES FOR THE TREATMENT OF CONGENITAL TOXOPLASMOSIS

Drugs

Pyrimethamine + Sulfadiazine: 21-day course

(*a*) Pyrimethamine: 1 mg/kg/day, oral route. (Since the half-life of the drug is 4 to 5 days, the dose can be given every 2 to 3 or even 4 days).

(*b*) Sulfadiazine: 50 to 100 mg/kg/day, oral route in two daily divided doses.

Spiramycin: 30- to 45-day course. 100 mg/kg/day, oral route in two daily divided doses.

Corticosteroids (prednisone or methylprednisolone): 1 to 2 mg/kg/day, oral route in two divided doses. Continued until the inflammatory process (e. g., high cerebrospinal fluid protein, chorioretinitis) has subsided; dosage then to be tapered progressively to zero.

Folinic acid: 5 mg twice weekly during pyrimethamine treatment.

Indications

Overt congenital toxoplasmosis: Pyrimethamine + sulfadiazine: 21 days. Folinic acid to be given as soon as possible. During the first year of life, the child is given 3 to 4 courses of pyrimethamine + sulfadiazine, separated by spiramycin courses of 30 to 45 days. No treatment is usually given after 12 months of age.

Overt congenital toxoplasmosis with evidence of inflammatory process: (chorioretinitis, high cerebrospinal fluid protein content, generalized infection, jaundice): As above + corticosteroid treatment.

Subclinical but definite congenital toxoplasmosis: As above for overt congenital cases.

Healthy newborn in whom serologic testing has not provided definitive results but definite maternal infection was acquired during pregnancy: one course of pyrimethamine + sulfadiazine for 21 days, followed by spiramycin. Then wait for laboratory evidence for the diagnosis.

Healthy newborn born to a mother with high dye-test titer-date of maternal infection undetermined: Spiramycin alone, until laboratory evidence for the diagnosis is definitive. It must be borne in mind that in certain cases, the indication for treatment is difficult to define due to the lack of information about the pregnancy and lack of isolation attempts from the corresponding placenta.

PROGNOSIS OF CONGENITAL TOXOPLASMA INFECTION WITH SPECIAL REFERENCE TO TREATMENT

Three different problems which relate to this subject will be addressed:

— prognosis for a neonate who was infected during fetal life;

— prognosis of congenital toxoplasmosis;

— prognosis of subclinical congenital infection.

Prognosis for the neonate infected during fetal life

It can be seen in Table II that the frequency of placentitis (and thus of transmission) is definitely reduced when the mother receives spiramycin treatment during pregnancy. In order to appreciate the possible role of maternal treatment with spiramycin on the pattern of congenital infection, cases in which transmission had occured have been classified into two groups which correspond to untreated and treated mothers (Table XI). There was no difference in the proportion of mild and subclinical cases between these 2 groups. However, the number of still-births decreased and the proportion of children born alive with severe disease was slightly increased in the treated group. This suggests that in some instances treatment might have prevented fetal death, but that it was insufficient or undertaken too late to prevent severe damage. If a method becomes available for prenatal diagnosis of fetal infection, it might allow for more effective drugs (e. g., pyrimethamine plus sulfonamides) to be used.

Prognosis of congenital toxoplasmosis

The studies by Eichenwald, in 1947, of 156 children with proven congenital toxoplasmosis, most of whom were followed from birth to 5 (or more) years of age, revealed that the spontaneous evolution of congenital toxoplasmosis is severe: the mortality rate was 12 %; 85 % of survivors were mentally retarded; 75 % developed convulsions, spasticity and paralyses; and 50 % had severely impaired vision.

This severe outcome is not surprising in view of the extensive necrotic lesions probably present in the central nervous system of these infants. As far as it is possible to ascertain their presence in newborn infants with congenital toxoplasmosis (CT scan), it may be evident that the damage is irreversible in many cases.

In other infants that present with neurologic disturbances which suggest severe encephalitis, a good response to medical treatment (with surgery, if necessary, for obstructive hydrocephalus) has

TABLE XI. — Effect of treatment with spiramycin on the relative frequency of still-birth and different aspects of congenital toxoplasma infection

		Mother treated during pregnancy					
		No		Yes		Total	
		No.	(%)	No.	(%)	No.	(%)
Congenital subclinical infection		64	(68)	65	(72)	129	(70)
Congenital toxoplasmosis { mild		14	(15)	13	(14)	27	(15)
{ severe		7	(7)	10	(11)	17	(9)
Stillbirth or perinatal death		9	(10)	3	(3)	12	(6)
Total		94	(100)	91	(100)	185	(100)

been observed. In a few cases, even medical treatment alone has been sufficient to allow for an improvement of an obstructed aqueduct of Sylvius. In these circumstances, neurologic signs were probably due mainly to inflammatory encephalitis with limited necrotic lesions, and to the increased intracranial pressure. The evolution of these cases is often surprisingly good, with normal mental development on follow up. The prognosis for vision depends on the location of the retinal scars.

Prognosis of subclinical and inapparent congenital infection

It is now well established that sequelae of congenital toxoplasmosis (mainly ocular but sometimes neurologic) may occur years after birth in children with subclinical congenital Toxoplasma infection. The exact incidence of these sequelae is unknown since such data would necessarily come from prospective studies of untreated cases. Such a study is no longer ethically feasible since it is known that these children so often end up mentally retarded or blind. Some data are however available: the diagnosis was prospectively established in 13 among 23 children studied by Wilson and co-authors. These children were either untreated or had received treatment of short duration. On follow up, chorioretinitis was discovered in 11 (85 %) and neurologic sequelae in 5 (38 %) of the 13 children.

De Roever-Bonnet and co-authors have performed repeated ocular examinations in 12 children with inapparent congenital infection, who were born during a prospective study of toxoplasma infection in pregnancy. These children were not treated. 8 (67 %) were later discovered to have chorioretinitis and in 5 of them relapses occured.

These findings are strikingly different from what is observed among children with subclinical congenital Toxoplasma infection who received treatment from birth to the end of the first year of life. Follow up of these children is still in progress, but the observed incidence of chorioretinitis is probably well below 5 % in this group.

REFERENCES

[1] REMINGTON (J. S.), DESMONTS (G.). — Toxoplasmosis. In *Infectious diseases of the fetus and newborn infant.* Second edition. J. S. REMINGTON and J. O. KLEIN, eds. Philadelphia, W. B. Saunders Co., 193-263, 1983.

[2] KRAUBIG (H.). — Praventive behandlung der konnatalen toxoplasmose. In *Toxoplasmose; Praktische Fragen und Ergebnisse.* KIRCHOFF, H. and KRAUBIG, H., eds. Stuttgart, Georg Thieme Verlag, 104-122, 1966.

[3] DESMONTS (G.), COUVREUR (J.). — Congenital toxoplasmosis: A prospective study of 378 pregnancies. *N. Engl. J. Med.,* 290, 1110, 1974.

[4] KOPPE (J. G.), KLOOSTERMAN (G. J.), de ROEVER-BONNET (H.), ECKERT-STROINK (J. A.), LOEWER-SIEGER (D. H.), de BRUIJNE (J. I.). — Toxoplasmosis and pregnancy, with a long-term follow-up of the children. *Europ. J. Obstet. Gynecol. Reprod. Biol.,* 4, 101, 1974.

[5] De ROEVER-BONNET (H.), KOPPE (J. G.), LOEWER-SIEGER (D. H.). — Follow-up of children with congenital Toxoplasma infections and children who became serologically negative after one year of age, all born in 1964-1965. In *Perinatal Medicine,* Sixth European Congress. THALHAMMER, O., BAUMGARTEN, K. and POLLAK, A., eds. Stuttgart, Georg Thieme Publishers, 61-75, 1979.

[6] FRENKEL (J. K.). — Toxoplasma in and around us. *Bioscience,* 23, 343, 1973.

[7] WILSON (C. B.), REMINGTON (J. S.). — What can be done to prevent congenital toxoplasmosis? *Am. J. Obstet. Gynecol.,* 138, 357-363, 1980.

[8] WILSON (C. B.), REMINGTON (J. S.), STAGNO (S.), REYNOLDS (D. W.). — Development of adverse sequelae in children born with subclinical congenital Toxoplasma infection. *Pediatrics,* 66, 767-774, 1980.

[9] EICHENWALD (H.). — A study of congenital toxoplasmosis. In *Human toxoplasmosis.* SIIM, J. C., ed. Copenhagen, Munksgaard, 41-49, 1960.

5

Hematology – Oncology

Hematology of the newborn

Alvin ZIPURSKY

General principles for the assessment of anemia in newborn infants

THE HEMOGLOBIN CONCENTRATION OF BLOOD DURING THE EARLY DAYS OF LIFE

Anemia may be defined as a hemoglobin concentration or a red blood cell count below the normal range for a given individual. In the newborn infant normal values differ from those of adults and they change rapidly after birth. Therefore, assessment of anemia in the neonatal period requires knowledge of the normal concentration of hemoglobin at birth and of changes that occur thereafter.

The normal blood hemoglobin concentration in newborn infants

The hemoglobin concentration of infants during the first days of life is dependent not only on the concentration of hemoglobin in cord blood at the moment of birth but also on the amount of blood received from the placenta immediately after birth, in other words, the placental transfusion.

The normal cord blood hemoglobin concentration. — The values for cord blood hemoglobin shown in Figure V-1 are similar to those reported in the literature [1]. The concentration of hemoglobin in the cord blood is, of course, unrelated to the placental transfusion but rather reflects the hemoglobin concentration of the fetus. Cord blood hemoglobin values above or below normal represent *fetal polycythemia or fetal anemia* respectively.

The cord blood hemoglobin may rise slightly with gestational age although there is no significant change after the 34th week [2]. It has been suggested that prior to the 34th week the hemoglobin concentration may be slightly lower, particularly in female newborns [2]. Infants who are small for gestational age seem to have slightly higher cord hemoglobin levels than normal [2].

The placental transfusion. — This factor must be considered in assessing hemoglobin concentrations after birth. In the normal full term infant 50-125 ml of placental blood are transferred following vaginal delivery. Approximately 75 % of this transfusion occurs in the first minute and the remainder within

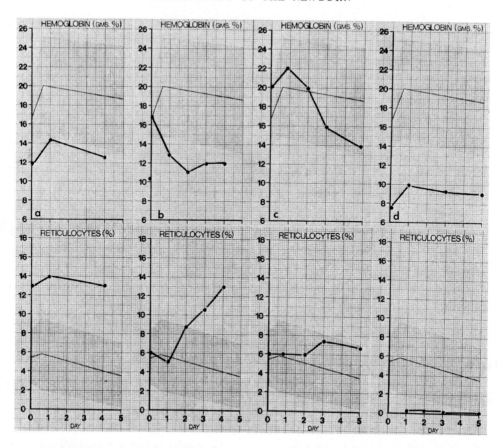

FIG. V-1. — *Hemoglobin and reticulocyte counts in newborn infants during the first five days of life.* In the background the solid lines represent means and the shaded areas include 95 % of the values found on 163 normal term infants. The first point "Day 0" are cord blood values. The other values are capillary blood values. •—• in each figure represents the data in each child described below.

(*a*) An infant born after a transplacental hemorrhage of 200 ml of fetal blood into the maternal circulation. It is presumed that the hemorrhage occurred for several days prior to delivery inasmuch as anemia ("fetal anemia") and reticulocytosis was evident in the cord blood.

(*b*) An infant born following massive blood loss as a result of a tear and hemorrhage from a placental vessel at or around the time of delivery. The baby was in shock at birth but was not anemic at that time (cord blood hemoglobin was normal). As the plasma volume increased to compensate for the hypovolemia, anemia appeared. Reticulocytosis was evident several days later.

(*c*) An infant who developed a gastro-intestinal hemorrhage on the second day of life. The fall of hemoglobin concentration was substantial (8.0 gms/dl) but all results were in the "normal range".

(*d*) An infant born with a low cord hemoglobin ("fetal anemia") and subsequent neonatal anemia. No reticulocyte response was evident, suggestive of bone marrow failure. A case of Blackfan-Diamond syndrome (Congenital Hypoplastic Anemia).

five minutes. This "transfusion" presumably results from the early constriction of the umbilical artery (preventing return of blood from the fetus) together with compression of the placenta by the contracting uterus. It follows therefore that anything that interferes with this placental transfusion will result in a lower hemoglobin level in the newborn. This can occur either as a result of early cord clamping or after cesarean section when the infant has been held above the uterus.

Conversely, the hemoglobin concentration may be very high in newborn infants as a result of late cord clamping and cord stripping, cesarean section with maintenance of the infant below the level of the uterus after delivery, or perinatal asphyxia which results in a greater placental transfusion.

The significance of changes in hemoglobin concentration

In the first five days of life hemoglobin concentrations may differ greatly among infants and also may show considerable day-to-day changes. In babies under study we have found it valuable to graph the hemoglobin concentration against normal values for the first five days of life (Fig. V-1). The changes after birth include a rise in hemoglobin concentration during the first day of life due in part to the shift in sampling from venous (cord) to capillary blood (Fig. V-2) and also to the normal placental transfusion at birth. In the case shown in Figure V-1a, the hemoglobin concentration of cord blood is abnormally low, representing "fetal anemia". Fetal anemia is followed by neonatal anemia despite the normal rise in hemoglobin concentration secondary to the placental transfusion. Figure V-1b displays the changes in hemoglobin concentration which occur in a child who had bled from a torn umbilical cord immediately before delivery. The child was hypotensive at birth because of an acute depletion in blood volume, but the hemoglobin concentration was normal in the cord blood. In the early hours of life as the plasma volume increased to compensate for the vascular depletion, the hemoglobin concentration fell and anemia appeared.

The assessment of hemoglobin concentrations in newborns demands not only knowledge of normal absolute values, but also the pattern of change that occurs. The case described in Figure V-1c is that of an infant whose hemoglobin value was in the normal range during the first five days of life; however, the hemoglobin concentration fell more rapidly than normal.

ERRORS IN THE ASSESSMENT OF ANEMIA IN NEWBORN INFANTS

Despite knowledge of normal values the assessment of hemoglobin concentrations is often difficult or confusing in the newborn period because of technical errors, blood loss due to sampling, and changes in the vascular space and blood volume.

Technical errors.

Capillary versus venous sampling. — In newborn infants the hemoglobin concentrations of blood taken from capillary punctures are significantly higher than those of venous samples [3]. These differences are shown in some of our own studies in Figure V-2. The reason for this difference appears to be a relatively sluggish circulation in the capillaries of the heel of the newborn infant which results in slow mixing of plasma within the relatively stagnant capillary bed. Hemoglobin values taken from pre-warmed heels will approximate those of venous blood.

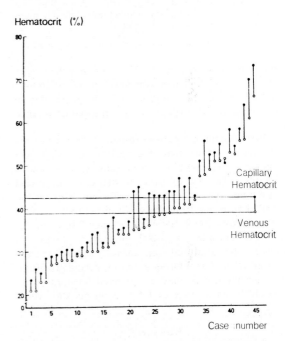

FIG. V-2. — *Simultaneous capillary and venous hemoglobin concentrations in 45 newborn infants during the first six weeks of life.* The black circles represent capillary values and the open circles simultaneous venous values. The vertical bars display the extent of the differences. The differences between the parallel horizontal lines represent the average capillary-venous differential [102].

Compounding the problem of sampling site is *the error of the technique* itself. The extent of this error is shown in Table I. It can be seen that there is an error in duplicate hemoglobin testing using either automatic or manual testing. That error is relatively small as shown in Table I. However, the error associated with multiple sampling (that is from duplicate punctures) is considerable. The significance of the errors inherent in sampling can be appreciated if we consider an example. If in a baby the true hemoglobin value is 18 g/dl, the errors associated with sampling could produce results

TABLE I

The error of five determinations of hemoglobin concentrations in each of 20 samples of blood.

95 % confidence limits = ± .13 g/dl

The error of duplicate capillary hemoglobin samples in 25 normal newborn infants.

95 % confidence limits = ± 1.7 g/dl

Example: In a baby whose true hemoglobin was 16 g/dl, 95 % of capillary hemoglobin determinations would vary from 14.3 to 17.7 g/dl.

that ranged (inclusive of 95 % of samples) from 16.28 to 19.72. Those are very great differences indeed and must be considered in the interpretation of changes in hemoglobin values in newborn infants.

Blood sampling and transfusion. — We turn now to factors other than technical errors that will influence hemoglobin concentrations in newborn infants. The first of these is the effect of blood sampling and of blood transfusion. Unlike the well child or adult, in the small ill premature infant these factors are of major importance. For example, let us consider a 1,000 premature infant in whom the total red cell mass is approximately 35 ml (Fig. V-3). During a 10 day period, 15-20 ml of red blood cells may be removed for study (that would be an average of 1.5 to 2 ml per day which

would not be an unusual amount). Anemia surely would result from the less of that quantity of blood. That this is not an uncommon problem is shown in Figure V-3 where the volumes of red blood cells sampled from a population of premature infants in a neonatal intensive care unit are recorded. In a large proportion of infants the volume of red cells removed was greater than their total red cell mass. It follows therefore that *anemia in newborn infants cannot be assessed without an accurate determination of the volumes of blood sampled or transfused.*

Growth and total body red cell mass. — The assessment of anemia in the early weeks of life also must include an analysis of growth. As we shall discuss later (see "Physiologic Anemia of Infancy"), red cell production diminishes during the early weeks of life and in the face of rapid growth hemoglobin levels can fall quickly. This is shown graphically in Figure V-4 where the growth pattern of a small premature infant is shown. We observe that in the third week as the growth rate accelerates the decline in hemoglobin concentration becomes more rapid. Thus, by the fifth week hemoglobin concentration continues to decline despite an increase in red cell production. On first consideration, the presence of a high reticulocyte count and a falling or stable hemoglobin concentration is suggestive of a shortened red cell life span (hemorrhage or hemolysis). In this instance, however, the combination of a falling hemoglobin despite a high reticulocyte count results from the rapidly expanding blood volume as

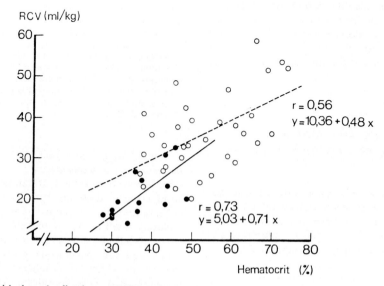

FIG. V-3. — *Total body red cell volume (RCV) and venous hematocrit values in a series of newborn infants.* The open circles represent infants at days 1-5 and the closed circles represent infants at six weeks of age. The poor correlation between venous hematocrit and RCV is evident at both ages.

evidenced by the continuous increase in red cell mass during that time. It can be concluded therefore that the assessment of anemia in the neonatal period demands appreciation of body growth.

Rapid changes in blood volume are seen in the newborn infant during acute illness. In association with severe infections or central nervous system disease inappropriate secretion of antidiuretic

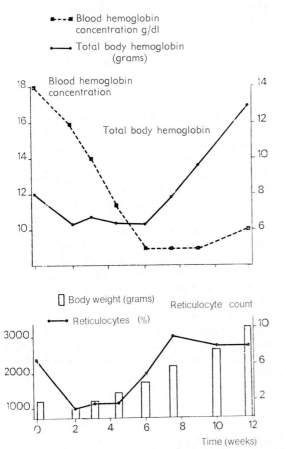

Fig. V-4. — *Changes in total body hemoglobin, blood hemoglobin concentration, reticulocyte count and body weight in a hypothetical premature infant.* The vertical bars represent the infant's body weight. Note that during the first six weeks of life the blood hemoglobin concentration and total body hemoglobin fall as a result of decreased red blood cell production (as evidenced by the low reticulocyte count). The more rapid decline in blood hemoglobin concentration in the third to sixth week is the result of the increasing body size and therefore "dilution" of the hemoglobin mass. After six weeks hemoglobin production increases as evidenced by the increased reticulocyte count and the rapid increase in total body hemoglobin. The blood hemoglobin' concentrations during that period rises only slightly or not at all because the total body size increases at approximately the same rate as the total body hemoglobin mass.

hormone can occur [4] with substantial fluid retention, expansion of the plasma volume, and a dilutional anemia.

All the above observations suggest that hemoglobin concentration can fall to "anemic" levels despite stable or rising total body red cell mass. Hence, assessment of anemia demands appreciation of changes in body weight and plasma volume of the baby.

THE RELATIONSHIP OF RED CELL MASS AND HEMOGLOBIN CONCENTRATION

There is one additional difficulty in the assessment of anemia in newborn infants. In adults a low hemoglobin concentration is interpreted as a reflection of a diminished red cell mass since the correlation between red cell mass and hemoglobin concentration in adults is quite good [5]. There is a lower correlation in newborn infants either at birth or at six weeks of age, as shown in Figure V-3. This low correlation which has been found in other studies [6] means that two infants with similar blood hemoglobin concentrations may have very different total red cell masses. It also means that the vascular space of the newborn must be considerably more accommodating than that of adults. In this way a given red cell mass may be sufficiently diluted by a large plasma volume in one infant so that "anemia" exists, whereas in another the same red cell mass is associated with a "normal" hemoglobin concentration. It is difficult to apply the latter data to the assessment of anemia in individual patients. Nevertheless, appreciation of the wide range in red cell mass which may be represented by an individual hemoglobin concentration is important for an understanding of the significance of a specific hemoglobin concentration, or a change in the hemoglobin concentration of a given patient.

PRINCIPLES IN THE ASSESSMENT OF ANEMIA IN NEWBORN INFANTS

The above considerations may be simplified into a series of principles which should be applied when anemia is studied in newborn infants. These principles are as follows:

(*i*) Fetal anemia must be distinguished from anemia which develops after delivery.

(ii) The blood hemoglobin concentration of a given patient must be assessed in the light of the normal pattern of changes which occur during the early days of life.

(iii) Technical errors in the determination of hemoglobin concentrations in newborn infants are very large.

(iv) Anemia cannot be assessed without accurate knowledge of the volumes of blood sampled and transfused.

(v) Changes in the hemoglobin concentration cannot be assessed without accurate knowledge of changes in body weight.

TABLE II. — NUCLEATED RED BLOOD CELL COUNTS IN 163 NORMAL FULL TERM NEWBORN INFANTS

	Mean	± S. D.
Day 0 *	830/mm³	850/mm³
Day 1	150/mm³	480/mm³
Day 5	10/mm³	45/mm³

* Day 0 sample = cord blood. Days 1 and 5 = capillary samples.

THE RESPONSE TO ANEMIA IN NEWBORN INFANTS

In the newborn and fetus, red blood cell production can be increased in response to anemia. In the fetus erythropoietin is produced, and consequently erythropoiesis can increase as necessary [7]. This increase will manifest in the peripheral blood as an elevation in the number of reticulocytes and nucleated red blood cells. The appearance of nucleated red blood cells (erythroblastosis) as a response to anemia is characteristic of the fetus and newborn infant since it occurs only rarely in older children and adults, usually only in association with abnormal erythropoiesis. Normal values for nucleated red blood cells in the blood of newborn infants are shown in Table II. We have found the use of the graph shown in Figure V-1 valuable in practice for appreciating the reticulocyte response to anemia in the fetus and newborn. This is illustrated in the series of cases shown in Figure V-1 in which the response to fetal and neonatal anemia is depicted. In Figure V-1a, anemia developed in utero and there was sufficient time for a reticulocyte response to occur. In contrast, infants who have suffered blood loss at or around the time of delivery (Fig. V-1b) will have a normal reticulocyte count at birth with reticulocytosis appearing only several days after delivery. The presence of fetal and neonatal anemia together with low reticulocyte counts is suggestive of bone marrow failure as shown in Figure V-1d, where this has occured as a result of a congenital hypoplastic anemia. Thus, careful attention to the pattern of hemoglobin and reticulocyte values during the early days of life along with reference to normal values offers a rational approach to the interpretation of anemia in newborn infants.

Hemolytic disease in newborn infants

A significant shortening of red cell life span in the absence of hemorrhage is referred to as hemolytic disease. Such diseases are common in the newborn and are major causes of anemia and hyperbilirubinemia during that period.

The study of a hemolytic process involves two main principles: the first is the detection of evidence of increased red blood cell destruction; the second involves a study of the red blood cells themselves to determine whether they are intrinsically abnormal or whether some external factor is acting upon them. These are general principles that apply to patients of any age; however certain features of the neonatal period affect the expression and interpretation of hemolytic disease and therefore require specific consideration.

Evidence of an increased rate of erythrocyte destruction in newborn infants

A low or stable body hemoglobin concentration together with an elevated reticulocyte count indicates an increased rate of erythrocyte turnover. In the absence of blood loss this suggests a hemolytic process. Therefore, bearing in mind the factors outlined in the previous section, careful consideration of hemoglobin concentrations and reticulocyte numbers may provide the first evidence of a hemolytic process. Evidence of increased red cell destruction in a given patient will vary depending on whether erythrocyte destruction occurs in the bloodstream (intravascular hemolysis) or in the reticuloendothelial system (extravascular hemolysis).

Extravascular erythrocyte destruction. — Erythrocytes destroyed outside the bloodstream are digested by the macrophages of the spleen, liver and bone marrow (*i. e.* the reticuloendothelial system). As a result bilirubin is produced, passes into the blood in its unconjugated form, is taken up by the liver and excreted into the bowel. Accordingly, a high level of unconjugated bilirubin is a characteristic feature of an extravascular hemolytic process. In adults serum bilirubin levels seldom exceed 5 mg/dl as a result of a hemolytic process. However, in newborn infants much higher levels may develop rapidly because of the limited ability of the liver of the newborn to take up, conjugate and excrete bilirubin. It follows therefore that the appearance of hyperbilirubinemia in a newborn infant is not a specific sign of a hemolytic process since it may arise for many other reasons. There are, however, certain characteristics to hemolytic hyperbilirubinemia. These include an elevated cord blood bilirubin (more than 3 mg/dl) and the appearance of jaundice during the first 24 hours of life.

In the adult excessive bilirubin production and excretion causes an elevation of the bilirubin breakdown product urobilinogen in both stool and urine. During the early days of life, however, the assessment of urobilinogen excretion is of no value in the diagnosis of hemolytic disease since the bacterial flora upon which urobilinogen production is dependent are incompletely developed in newborns.

Intravascular erythrocyte destruction. — When red blood cells are lysed within the blood stream hemoglobin is released. Characteristically, this hemoglobin binds to haptoglobin and the complex is metabolized by the liver. As a result plasma haptoglobin levels fall, and if hemolysis continues free (unbound) hemoglobin levels increase. This in turn will result in hemoglobinuria, the formation of methemalbumin and consumption of hemopexin (the heme-binding protein) in plasma. Thus, in adults intravascular hemolysis is evidenced by high levels of plasma hemoglobin and methemalbumin,

low levels of plasma haptoglobin and hemopexin and hemoglobinuria.

In the newborn infant these signs are of relatively little value. In many normal newborn infants haptoglobin is absent from the plasma. In our studies of full term and premature infants we found that a high proportion of normal infants had all the above signs of intravascular hemolysis without other evidence of hemolytic disease.

Abnormalities of erythrocytes as evidence of a hemolytic process

Because the indices of erythrocyte destruction in newborn infants are not specific, they are of limited value in the diagnosis of hemolytic disease. Therefore, additional evidence is required. This includes a critical assessment of hemoglobin and reticulocyte values, as well as direct evidence of abnormalities of the red blood cells.

The assessment of erythrocyte morphology is important in the diagnosis of hemolytic disease. Traditionally this is done by examination of the two-dimensional shape of erythrocytes on a stained blood smear. In the newborn infant erythrocyte shape is different than in adults (Table III) and interpretation requires adequate assessment and quantitations of the three dimensional shape of the erythrocyte population (Fig. V-5). Accordingly in

TABLE III. — ERYTHROCYTE DIFFERENTIAL COUNTS IN ADULTS, FULL TERM AND PREMATURE INFANTS

	Adult (53) % *	Full term (31) %	Premature (52) %
Discocyte	78 (42-94)	43 (18-62)	39.5 (18-57)
Bowl	18 (4-50)	40 (14-58)	29 (13-53)
Disc-Bowl	2 (0-4)	2 (0-5)	3 (0-10)
Spherocyte	0 (0-0)	0 (0-1)	0 (0-3)
Echinocyte	0 (0-3)	1 (0-4)	5.5 (1-23)
Acanthocyte	0 (0-1)	1 (0-2)	0 (0-2)
Dacrocyte	0 (0-1)	1 (0-3)	1 (0-5)
Keratocyte	0 (0-1)	2 (0-5)	3 (0-7)
Schizocyte	0 (0-1)	0 (0-2)	2 (0-5)
Knizocyte	1 (0-5)	3 (0-8)	1 (0-6)
Immature erythrocyte	0 (0-0)	0 (0-2)	4 (1-11)

* Median values (%); the figures in brackets represent the 5 %-95 % range.

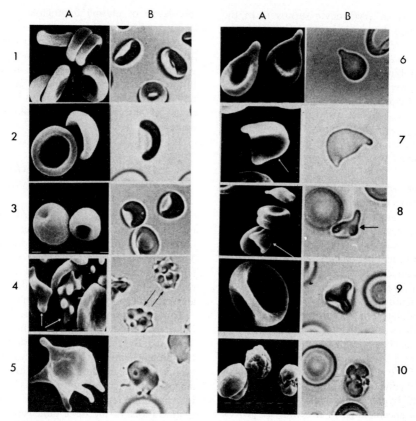

Fig. V-5. — *The three-dimensional appearance of erythrocytes as seen by scanning electron microscopy* (A) *and by light microscopy of glutaraldehyde-fixed cells* (B). The terminology used to describe the cells is that of Bessis [104], with the exception of 2 and 10.

1 A & B. Discocytes
2 A & B. Bowl
3 A & B. Spherocytes
4 A & B. Echinocytes
5 A & B. Acanthocyte

6 A & B. Dacrocyte
7 A & B. Keratocyte
8 A & B. Schizocyte
9 A & B. Knizocyte
10 A & B. Immature Erythrocyte.

the following sections erythrocyte shape in disease is described in both two and three dimensions.

The normal three-dimensional appearance of red blood cells is shown in Figure V-5 and normal values for erythrocyte differential counts are shown in Table III.

Principles in the assessment of hemolytic disease in newborn infants

(*a*) A hemolytic process may manifest as either a low or normal hemoglobin concentration in the presence of an increased reticulocyte count.

(*b*) Increased numbers of nucleated red blood cells ("erythroblastosis") appear as evidence of increased red cell production in hemolytic disease.

Erythroblastosis however also occurs in response to hemorrhage and as an acute stress response in asphyxia and therefore cannot be considered as specific for hemolytic disease.

(*c*) Hyperbilirubinemia may be a sign of hemolytic anemia, however a hemolytic anemia can develop without hyperbilirubinemia and conversely hyperbilirubinemia may result from causes other than hemolytic disease.

(*d*) An abnormal rise of bilirubin levels in the first 24 hours of life and an elevated cord blood bilirubin concentration strongly suggests hemolytic disease.

(*e*) Evidence of intravascular hemolysis (hemoglobinemia, methemalbuminemia and a decrease of plasma haptoglobin and hemopexin) are seen in normal infants and are of little value in the diagnosis of hemolytic disease in newborns.

(*f*) The study of erythrocyte morphology is important in the diagnosis of hemolytic disease. The standard stained blood smear is usually of little value for this purpose. Where possible, three dimensional assessment of erythrocyte shapes should be employed.

CAUSES OF HEMOLYTIC DISEASE IN NEWBORN INFANTS

Hemolytic disease may result from an abnormality of the red blood cell itself, or because of factors acting upon the red blood cell.

HEMOLYTIC DISEASES DUE TO INTRINSIC ABNORMALITIES OF THE RED BLOOD CELL

In this group of diseases the abnormalities of the red blood cell are intrinsic and inherited. If the erythrocyte is considered as a membrane containing a solution of hemoglobin and enzyme systems, these inherited intracorpuscular disorders may be classified as abnormalities of: (1) membrane structure, (2) enzymes, and (3) hemoglobin.

Congenital hemolytic anemia due to abnormalities of membrane structure

Hereditary spherocytosis. — In this disease, inherited as an autosomal dominant trait, the erythrocytes have an abnormal shape (Fig. V-6), an increased osmotic fragility and a shortened life span caused by entrapment and destruction by the spleen. The disease may manifest in the newborn by severe hyperbilirubinemia, and less frequently by anemia [8]. ABO incompatibility hemolytic disease must be excluded since the hematologic picture (spherocytosis, early jaundice, increased erythrocyte osmotic fragility) is similar in the two diseases. Diagnosis is aided by the finding of the disease in one of the parents, although in approximately 25 % of the cases, there is no evidence of the disease in other members of the family [9].

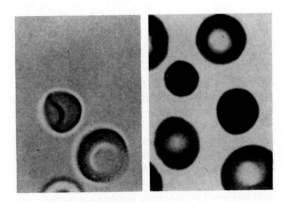

Fig. V-6. — *The erythrocytes of a patient with hereditary spherocytosis as seen on a stained blood smear and by three dimensional viewing of glutaraldehyde-fixed cells.*

Hereditary elliptocytosis. — In adults, this autosomal dominant disorder of membrane structure is usually harmless although a hemolytic process, similar to that of hereditary spherocytosis, can occur in patients whose cells are predominantly elliptical or oval (ovalocytosis). A hemolytic process in newborn infants with hereditary elliptocytosis in which the clinical picture is similar to those described above for hereditary spherocytosis [10] has been reported. In the blood of these newborns there are not only elliptocytes but also grossly distorted cells.

Hemolytic disease of the newborn due to abnormalities in metabolism or enzyme function

The red blood cell is dependent on intracellular metabolism both for its viability and for specific functions such as ion transport, shape and maintenance of hemoglobin in its functional state. The commonest disorder of erythrocyte enzyme function is glucose 6-phosphate dehydrogenase deficiency (see below). Other abnormalities in erythrocyte enzyme function have been described and in adults and older children they are rare causes of hemolytic disease. In each of these disorders hemolytic disease of the newborn has occurred. However, these are very rare causes of disease in the newborn. Accordingly, they will not be reviewed in detail here. They are transmitted as autosomal recessive disorders and should be considered in a well-documented hemolytic anemia when an intracorpuscular defect of the red blood cell is detected which is neither an abnormality of membrane structure nor shape nor hemoglobin synthesis. Of the many such disorders that have been reported, the commonest is pyruvate kinase deficiency which itself has an incidence of less than 1 in 20,000 of the population.

Glucose 6-phosphate dehydrogenase deficiency. — The major function of the red blood cell is the delivery of oxygen to the tissues. The cell, therefore, is constantly exposed to oxygen and its membrane and cytoplasm are subjected to oxidative damage. Oxidation causes the formation of precipitates of denatured hemoglobin (Heinz bodies) (Fig. V-7) which appear to be associated with a shortened life span in vivo. The red blood cell has a metabolic system which can prevent oxidative damage (Fig. V-8). Glucose 6-phosphate dehydrogenase is an enzyme in this system and when absent, there is a risk of oxidative damage to the red cell, particularly if exposed to chemicals or drugs (see Table IV) capable of causing oxidative injury.

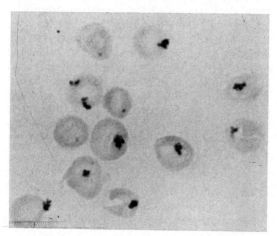

FIG. V-7. — *Heinz bodies in a newborn who developed a hemolytic anaemia following exposure to mothballs (naphthalene).*

TABLE IV. — DRUGS CAPABLE OF PRODUCING HEMO-LYTIC ANAEMIA IN PATIENTS WHOSE RED BLOOD CELLS ARE DEFICIENT IN GLUCOSE-6-PHOSPHATE DEHYDRO-GENASE.

Antimalarials:
  Primaquine
  Pamaquine
  Pentaquine
  Plasmoquine
  Quinocide
  Quinacrine (Atabrine)
  Quinine (C)

Sulfonamides:
  Sulfanilamide
  N^2 Acetylsulfanilamide
  Sulfacetamide (Sulamyd)
  Sulfamethoxypyridazine
    (Kynex, Midicel)
  Salicylazosulfapyridine
    (Azulfidine)
  Sulfisoxazole (Gantri-sin)
  Sulfapyridine

Nitrofurans:
  Nitrofurantoin (Fura-dantin)
  Furazolidone (Furoxone)
  Furaltadone (Altafur)
  Nitrofurazone (Furacin)

Antipyretics and analgesics:
  Acetylsalicylic acid (in large doses)
  Acetanilide
  Acetophenetidin (Phena-cetin)
  Antipyrine (C)
  Aminopyrine (C)
  p-Aminosalicylic acid

Sulfones

Others:
  Dimercaprol (BAL)
  Methylene blue
  Naphthalene
  Phenylhydrazine
  Acetylphenhydrazine
  Probenecid
  Vitamin K (large doses of water soluble ana-logues)
  Chloramphenicol (C)
  Quinidine (C)
  Fava beans (C)
  Chloroquine
  Nalidixic acid (Negram)
  Orinase

Infections:
  Respiratory viruses
  Infectious hepatitis
  Infectious mononucleo-sis
  Bacterial pneumonias

Diabetic acidosis

(C), to date, only Caucasians from: OSKI, F. A. and NAIMAN, J. L. (103).

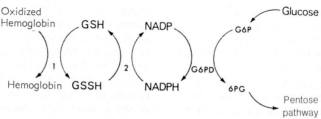

FIG. V-8. — *Protection against oxidative stress in red blood cells.* The red blood cell is constantly exposed to oxygen. As a result, there is formation of hydrogen peroxide (H_2O_2), lipid peroxides in the membrane and oxidized products of hemoglobin such as methemoglobin and Heinz bodies. To prevent the formation of and to reduce such oxidized products, the red blood cell has a system in which a series of enzyme steps link the metabolism of glucose through the pentose pathway to the reduction of oxidized products in the red blood cell. (1) = Glutathione Peroxidase; (2) = Glutathione Reductase; G6PD = glucose-6-phosphate dehydrogenase; GSH = reduced glutathione; GSSG = oxidized glutathione; NADP = nicotinamide-adenine-dinucleotide phosphate; NADPH = nicotinamide-adenine-dinucleotide phosphate, reduced; G6P = glucose-6-phosphate; 6PG = 6-phospho-gluconic acid.

Glucose 6-phosphate dehydrogenase (G6PD) deficiency is a common genetic disorder affecting millions of people in the world. There are three major types of deficiency, all of which are inherited as a sex linked recessive disorder. The most severe deficiency occurs rarely and is associated with a chronic hemolytic anemia. In that group the subject has a mild to moderate anemia throughout life and may have severe hemolytic disease as a newborn. A second group is that affecting Orientals (5.5 % of Chinese) as well as many populations in the Middle East and Mediterranean region (0.7-3 % of Greeks; the highest incidence being 53 % in Kurds). These subjects are healthy but are at risk of developing a hemolytic anemia when exposed to oxidative drugs or chemicals (e. g. sulpha drugs, fava beans, etc.). The anemia may be of sudden onset and may be very severe. In the absence of drug exposure, hemoglobin levels are normal, although there is evidence that red cell life span is slightly shorter than normal.

The third group affects Blacks (e. g. 10-14 % of American Blacks) in whom the severity of the defect is not as great as in the other two groups. Anemia appears only with drug exposure, is less severe than that of the Asian-Mediterranean type and tends to be self-limited.

Glucose 6-phosphate dehydrogenase deficiency and neonatal jaundice. — Because their erythrocytes have a diminished capacity to deal with oxidative stress (Fig. V-8) as a result of lower levels of gluta-thione peroxidase, catalase as well as a relative deficiency of Vitamin E, newborn infants with G6PD deficiency are at greater risk of developing hemolytic anemia than are adults. Indeed it would appear that G6PD deficiency is associated with an increased incidence of neonatal hyperbilirubinemia. This is particularly the case in the more severe type affecting the Asian and Mediterranean groups. Hyperbilirubinemia in G6PD-deficient males has been reported in newborns in Greece, Italy, Singapore and Taiwan [11, 12]. Although the hyper-bilirubinemia is largely the result of G6PD deficiency, there is a tendency for the jaundice to occur more frequently in particular families and communities [13], indicating that genetic and environmental factors must influence the incidence of the disease. In this group of patients, jaundice may be very severe and may lead to kernicterus [14]. In most of these instances, the hemoglobin and reticulocyte counts are normal, although in some reported cases the cord blood contains increased bilirubin and decreased hemoglobin levels, suggesting the presence of a mild hemolytic process in utero. There is,

however, no evidence of intravascular hemolysis in most of these cases. Black full term infants in North America with G6PD deficiency do not develop hyperbilirubinemia more frequently than normal infants, although the incidence may be slightly higher in prematures [15]. It has been reported from Africa, however, that black males with G6PD deficiency have a significantly higher incidence of hyperbilirubinemia than controls [16].

Clinical manifestations. — The jaundice that occurs in these babies appears to be an accentuation of the physiologic jaundice of newborns, although jaundice may appear in some during the first 24 hours. As noted above, there is seldom evidence of a hemolytic process. Abnormal erythrocyte mor-phology has been documented during hemolytic episodes in adults, but this is seldom described in newborns. However, in some instances a more severe hemolytic anemia may appear with evidence of abnormal erythrocyte morphology (Fig. V-6) and of Heinz bodies (Fig. V-7) in the peripheral blood and intravascular hemolysis. In these babies this may be a result of exposure to drugs or chemicals (e. g. Naphthalene in mothballs) which may have occurred [17].

Diagnosis. — The presence of unexplained hyper-bilirubinemia in an infant of a high-risk population group may suggest glucose 6-phosphate dehydroge-nase deficiency. The enzyme defect can be detected by one of the many screening tests now available such as that of Motulsky et al. [18] or Brewer et al. [19]. It should be added, however, that the finding of glucose 6-phosphate dehydrogenase deficiency in a jaundiced infant does not in itself prove that the jaundice was due to the enzyme defect. Rather, all other causes of jaundice must first be excluded. Since it is a sex linked recessive disorder, it is most severe and frequent in males. However females may be affected as well, since such females will have two populations of erythrocytes. one with normal and one with low levels of G6PD in keeping with the Lyon hypothesis concerning the occurence of sex linked recessive disorders in females.

Treatment. — The treatment is that of hyper-bilirubinemia which is described elsewhere in this book. In addition, drugs and chemicals likely to produce hemolytic anemia (Table IV) should be avoided in these patients.

Principals concerning G6PD deficiency:

(*i*) G6PD deficiency is a sex linked recessive disor-der affecting millions of people throughout the world.

(*ii*) In the type affecting populations in Asia and

the Mediterranean region, neonatal hyperbilirubinemia occurs frequently and may be severe.

(*iii*) In the type of defect commonly affecting Blacks, neonatal hyperbilirubinemia is uncommon but may occur in certain populations in full term babies and is probably more frequent in premature babies.

(*iv*) In all glucose 6-phosphate dehydrogenase deficient newborn infants, there is a risk of severe hemolytic anemia if exposure to oxygen and chemicals occurs. Under these circumstances the hemolytic anemia may manifest with Heinz bodies and evidence of intravascular hemolysis.

Neonatal hemolytic disease due to disorders of hemoglobin synthesis

The hemoglobin disorders, particularly thalassemia and sickle cell disease, are major problems in adults and children; however in newborn infants they cause relatively little disease. What are the reasons for this?

Hemoglobin is composed of four polypeptide chains and four heme molecules. Hemoglobin A is composed of two alpha and two beta chains (α_2 and β_2); hemoglobin F has two alpha and two gamma chains (α_2 and γ_2) and hemoglobin A_2 has two alpha and two delta chains (α_2 and δ_2).

In adults approximately 97 % of the hemoglobin of the red blood cell is hemoglobin A (α_2, β_2), 2.5 % is hemoglobin A_2 (α_2, δ_2) and 0.5 % hemoglobin F (α_2 and γ_2). In the newborn infant, approximately 70 % is hemoglobin F, 29 % is hemoglobin A and 0.5 % is hemoglobin A_2. Hemoglobin structure and the factors controlling the rates of synthesis of adult and fetal hemoglobins are reviewed elsewhere [20] and will not be discussed here. The change from predominantly hemoglobin F synthesis begins in utero at about the 34th week of gestation (therefore premature infants have a higher concentration of hemoglobin F than infants born at term) and the adult pattern is reached between the third and sixth month of postnatal life. The hemoglobin of the newborn infant has, in comparison to the hemoglobin of adults, a lower percentage of beta chains, a higher percentage of gamma chains and an equal percentage of alpha chains. Accordingly, the following principals should characterize the manifestations of the hemoglobin disorders at birth:

— Disorders of beta chain structure (e. g. sickle cell anemia) or beta chain synthesis (e. g. beta thalassemia) do not manifest as disease in the newborn period.

— Abnormalities of gamma chain synthesis may manifest in the newborn but clear up in the first few months of life as the normal switch from hemoglobin F to hemoglobin A is completed.

— Disorders of alpha chain structure or synthesis (e. g. alpha thalassemia) do manifest in the newborn.

Beta chain disorders. — Structural defects (such as sickle cell disease) as well as disorders of synthesis rate (beta thalassemia) rarely manifest in the newborn. Thalassemia has been diagnosed as early as the second month of life [21]. Patients with sickle cell disease are usually well during the first month although cases of jaundice and systemic signs during the neonatal period have been reported [22].

Gamma chain disorders. — A case has been described of hypochromic microcytic anemia in a newborn infant with reduced gamma (and beta) chain synthesis. This disorder improved in the first month of life and was considered to have been a case of gamma-beta thalassemia [23]. Though many structural defects of gamma chain synthesis in newborns occur [24] and are transient they rarely cause disease, although a case of Heinz body hemolytic anemia with an unstable hemoglobin (gamma chain abnormality) has been reported [25].

Alpha chain disorders. — There are many structural defects of alpha chains that occur and have been found in the newborn [24, 26]. They rarely, if ever, cause significant disease; however, an abnormality of hemoglobin synthesis, namely alpha thalassemia does manifest itself and can have serious effects on the newborn. Alpha thalassemia includes a group of diseases in which there is defective synthesis of the alpha polypeptide chains of hemoglobin. Synthesis of these chains is determined by two pairs of alpha genes, one on each of the number sixteen chromosomes. The alpha thalassemia diseases are caused by a deletion of one or more of these four alpha genes; the severity of the disease in the newborn and in the adult is dependent on the number of genes deleted, as shown in Table V. If one gene is absent the patient is hematologically normal, but as a newborn will have a slight elevation of Bart's hemoglobin (γ_4). If two genes are absent (either two missing from one chromosome or one from each of the two chromosomes) the patient has alpha thalassemia trait which manifests as microcytosis in the newborn (MCV < 95 μ^3) [27]. We have observed some of these patients to develop mild hyperbilirubinemia and anemia in the newborn. If three genes are deleted the patient has hemo-

TABLE V. — The manifestations of alpha thalassemia at birth [28, 29]

Genotype *	Anaemia	Jaundice	MCV	Barts **	Adult phenotype
αα, αα	−	−	106 ± 4.4	0	Normal
αα, α-	−	−	106 ± 4.4	0-2 %	Normal hematology
αα, - - *** or α-, α-	±	±	< 95	2-9 %	Mild microcytic Anemia
α-, - -	+	+	< 95	2 %	Hemolytic anaemia (Hemoglobin H disease)
- -. - -	+ +	+ +	< 95	> 80 %	Death at birth (Hydrops fetalis)

* α refers to a gene for the alpha chain of globin; normally there are two alpha genes on each ≠ 16 chromosome, hence αα/αα; - refers to the absence of an alpha gene.

** Haemoglobin Barts consists of four beta polypeptide and presumably occurs in these diseases because of the reduced production of alpha chains.

*** The group consisting of two gene deletions may be of two types. In the cis form αα, - - the deletions are on the same chromosome; this is the type found in orientals. In the trans form α-, α- one deletion is on each of the number 16 chromosomes; this is the type found in Blacks.

globin H (β_4) disease, a lifelong hemolytic anemia which manifests in the newborn as jaundice and microcytic anemia. If all four genes are abnormal the patient can form neither hemoglobin A nor F (since both contain alpha genes), is either born dead or severely hydropic, dying shortly after birth. The hemoglobin of such infants is predominantly hemoglobin Barts (γ_4).

The genetics of these diseases are consistent with the above theory. Thus, a patient with hemoglobin H disease (-/-, -/α) has parents one of whom is a "silent carrier" (-α, αα) and one who has alpha thalassemia trait (- -, αα); the patient with the homozygous form of alpha thalassemia (- -, - -) must have parents both of whom have alpha thalassemia trait (- -, αα). It is now believed that the alpha thalassemia trait which is found in 2 % of Blacks [28] is in the form (trans) in which one abnormal gene is present in each of the two chromosomes (-α, -α) and that the cis form (- -, αα) does not occur in Blacks. Hence homozygous alpha thalassemia and hemoglobin H disease are not found in Blacks.

The incidence of alpha thalassemia trait has been estimated from a percentage of infants having hemoglobin Barts in their blood at birth (Table V). Using this, it is estimated that 2-10 % of Blacks have alpha thalassemia trait (trans form -α, -α). The cis form (- -, αα) of alpha thalassemia occurs in various percentages in populations in South-East Asia and the Mediterranean region.

ISOIMMUNE HEMOLYTIC DISEASE OF THE NEWBORN

Isoimmune or alloimmune hemolytic disease of the newborn refers to those diseases in which maternal antibodies cross the placenta to enter the fetal circulation and thereby destroy fetal erythrocytes. The group includes Rh disease, ABO incompatibility hemolytic disease and diseases due to minor group antibodies.

Rh hemolytic disease

This disease is often referred to as "erythroblastosis fetalis" or simply "hemolytic disease of the newborn". It was first discovered and defined in 1940 and soon recognized as a major cause of perinatal mortality and morbidity. In the ensuing 30 years methods of effective diagnosis, treatment and prevention were developed. The remarkable progress in the control and eradication of this disease is shown in Figure V-9.

Despite the progress made cases still occur and it is necessary therefore to understand fully the nature of the disease and the methods of diagnosis and treatment. A detailed account of Rh disease is presented elsewhere [30].

The Genetics of Rh Disease. — "Rh positive" erythrocytes refer to those which contain the Rh_O

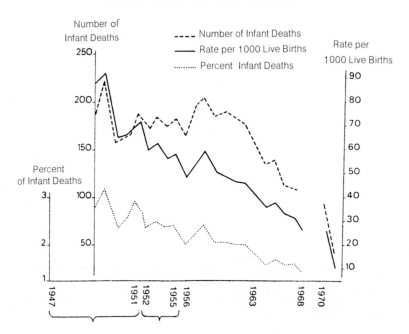

Fig. V-9. — *The decline in infant deaths due to Rh disease in California.* The decline appears to be due to improved techniques of care of the newborn and of the fetus and finally as a result of prevention of Rh immunization (from Hawes, W. E. and Mordaunt, V. L., *Calif. Med., 118, 28, 1973*).

(or D) antigen. The erythrocytes of the Rh subject lack that antigen. Since the D antigen is genetically determined and dominant the Rh positive subject may be homozygous (D/D) or heterozygous (D/d); the Rh negative subject is (d/d).

The Rh system is very complex and includes many related antigens, such as CcEe; however in this section we shall restrict discussion to the D antigen and refer to it as D or Rh positive and to the antibody as anti-D or anti-Rh. The Rh negative phenotype (d/d) is found in approximately 15 % of Caucasians and 5 % of Blacks; it is very rare in the Japanese and Chinese populations.

The pathogenesis of Rh disease. — Rh disease is due to the passage of anti-D antibodies from an Rh negative mother to her Rh positive fetus, resulting in red cell destruction and a hemolytic anemia. Normally there is no anti-D (Rh) antibody in the plasma of Rh negative subjects.

Anti-D antibodies appear only after immunization by Rh positive erythrocytes. In pregnant women such immunization results from the transplacental passage of fetal erythrocytes into the maternal circulation. Months after such an event anti-D antibodies will appear. Most of the significant transplacental hemorrhages occur late in pregnancy, so that in most of the immunized women the antibodies

first will appear post-partum. Some women, although previously immunized, will not have antibodies demonstrable in their plasma until a subsequent Rh positive pregnancy during which antibodies will appear as a result of a booster effect of a transplacental hemorrhage. In these ways approximately 15 % of Rh negative women carrying an Rh positive fetus will become immunized. Since antibodies usually appear post-partum, the first Rh positive baby is rarely affected. There are exceptions however; occasionally antibodies appear during a first pregnancy so that it is possible for Rh disease to develop in a first child. In addition, Rh immunization occurs following abortion in about 5 % of cases.

Rh immunization manifests itself by the appearance first of an immunoglobulin M (IgM) type of anti-D and later by an immunoglobulin G (IgG) anti-D. The reason for distinguishing these two types of antibody is that IgM does not cross the placenta, whereas IgG does. The two antibodies can be distinguished by laboratory techniques. Classically, IgM antibodies agglutinate erythrocytes suspended in saline and for this reason they were described initially as "saline" or "complete" antibodies. Since IgG anti-D does not agglutinate cells in saline, detection requires more sensitive techniques such as the Coombs test. In this technique serum containing IgG anti-D is incubated with Rh (D) positive erythrocytes whereby the anti-D binds to the cells. The cells then are washed and incubated with an anti-IgG antibody which causes agglutination of the sensitized cells.

The level of IgG anti-D in the plasma of the mother is important because that will determine the amount of antibody that crosses the placenta which will in turn affect the amount of antibody that binds to the erythrocyte. *Anti-D sensitized cells have shortened red cell life-spans and the shortening is directly related to the amount of antibody on the cell. Thus the level of maternal anti-D is directly related to the severity of Rh disease in the fetus.* Although this relationship is not absolute it is valuable in understanding the nature of the disease, as well as in selecting those pregnancies that are at risk and require more specific diagnostic study.

Rh disease in the fetus and newborn therefore is simply a result of anti-D sensitization of the red blood cells with consequent shortening of their lifespan and development of a hemolytic anemia. The consequences of this hemolytic anemia may be (*a*) intrauterine death, (*b*) a live born infant with severe anemia, (*c*) a live born infant who develops severe hyperbilirubinemia.

In the fetus a hemolytic process causes some elevation of plasma bilirubin, but, since bilirubin is cleared by the placenta hyperbilirubinemia is not a problem in utero. However anemia may be very severe and may culminate in a state of generalized edema referred to as hydrops fetalis. Death may ensue, or the severely afflicted infant may be delivered and die shortly thereafter.

Less severe forms of Rh disease occur. In these there may be mild or moderate anemia in utero, hepatosplenomegaly and moderate elevation of serum bilirubin. In such cases the infants' problems begin after birth since they cannot adequately clear bilirubin. In utero the placenta clears bilirubin, but after birth the baby's limited bilirubin clearance mechanisms must deal with the high bilirubin production secondary to hemolytic disease. Hyperbilirubinemia results and if untreated will rapidly reach high levels which can produce kernicterus and death.

Thus the spectrum of Rh disease extends from those born with little or no evidence of hemolytic disease to those who die in utero with hydrops fetalis. It is estimated that 40 % of immunized pregnancies will result in live births who require no therapy; 14 % will result in stillbirths. The remainder have disease of intermediate severity.

Diagnosis of Rh disease

Rh disease in the fetus should be suspected in any Rh negative pregnant woman who has anti-D anti-bodies in her plasma. If the father is homozygous Rh positive (D/D) it is certain that the infant will be Rh positive (D/d) and will be affected. If the father is heterozygous Rh positive (D/d) there is a 50 % chance that the fetus will be Rh positive and therefore affected.

If Rh antibodies are detected in the mother she must be followed carefully at two week intervals from the 20th week of gestation. If the level of antibody by the Coombs test in the serum is greater than 1/8 the fetus is at risk of disease which may be fatal in utero. This means that the severity of disease in the fetus must be determined by performing an amniocentesis at the 22nd week, and thereafter as necessary. Analysis of the amnionitic fluid for bilirubin provides an accurate estimate of the severity of disease in the fetus and therefore of its prognosis (Fig. V-10).

If it is determined that disease is not severe the pregnancy can be allowed to continue to term. If disease is severe and the baby is sufficiently mature (greater than 34 weeks and with a mature lecithin/sphyngomyelin (L/S) ratio in the amniotic fluid) delivery can be induced to prevent intrauterine death. If, however, the baby is less mature and there is impending death, intrauterine transfusion can be performed. Thus by judicious use of amniocentesis, premature delivery and intrauterine transfusion, most, but not all, fetal deaths can be prevented.

In the infant born with Rh disease the erythrocytes will be Rh positive and anti-D antibody can be demonstrated on their surface by reacting the cells with anti-IgG antibody (*i. e.* a positive direct Coombs test). The cord blood may have an elevated level of serum bilirubin and a lowered level of hemoglobin. Increased red cell production, including increased numbers of normoblasts ("erythroblastosis") and reticulocytes is seen. Hepatosplenomegaly is found.

Treatment of Rh disease. — The degree of the above changes reflects the severity of the disease and will determine the need for therapy. In infants who do not have profound anemia the major risk is hyperbilirubinemia. As it develops, light therapy can be given; however, if the serum bilirubin level reaches 20 mg/dl, exchange transfusion should be carried out. The considerations regarding such treatment are the same as for other causes of hyperbilirubinemia with one additional consideration. If an exchange transfusion is required, it is best to do this as soon as possible to avoid severe hyperbilirubinemia since it is better to remove "potential" bilirubin (*i. e.* sensitized red cells) early than to permit the accumulation of bilirubin in plasma and

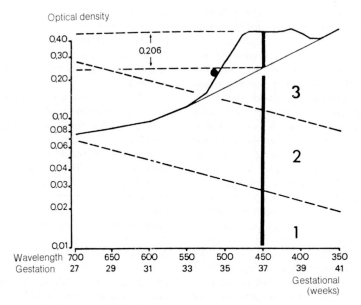

Fig. V-10. — *The spectrophotometric method of estimating amniotic fluid bilirubin levels*. The optical density is measured from wavelength 350 mμ to 700 mμ. The optical density rise at 450 mμ (due to bilirubin) is measured by the rise in optical density at that point above the projected base line. The graph shown is of the amniotic fluid of a woman at 34.5 weeks gestation. The optical density at 450 mμ in this case was 0.206. The value 0.206 is then plotted on the graph superimposed in this figure and shown in slanted broken lines that delineate three zones, 1, 2 and 3. In this case, 0.206 lies in zone 3. Zone 3 represents severe disease with impending fetal death. Zone 2 represents less severe disease, and zone 1 indicates an Rh-negative infant or one with very mild disease. The calculated optical density must be plotted in this way because the density decreases with gestational age (from Bow-MAN, J. M. and POLLACK, J. M., *Pediatrics, 35*, 815, 1965).

tissue from which it is less efficiently removed.

If the hemoglobin of cord blood is less than 10.5 g/dl, or if the cord bilirubin is greater than 4.5 mg/dl, exchange transfusion should be carried out as soon as possible. For other babies the bilirubin level must be followed every six to eight hours to determine its rate of rise. Graphs are available on which the serum bilirubin levels can be plotted to determine the need for an exchange transfusion.

The physiology of *exchange transfusion* and details of its performance are described elsewhere [30]. The procedure itself is simple in concept: small volumes of blood (20 ml in full-term infants) are removed and replaced by an equal volume of donor blood. An exchange transfusion equal to two times the blood volume (*i. e.* 180 ml per kg) affects exchange of approximately 90 % of the circulating red blood cells by donor cells. The removal of bilirubin, however, is not as complete, averaging approximately 50 % because bilirubin is distributed in at least 3 pools in the body, bound to albumin either within the intravascular space or in extravascular sites; the third portion is presumably in the tissues in a slowly equilibrating pool.

As a result, exchange transfusion removes only

50 % of the bilirubin of the body and is often followed by a rapid rebound in bilirubin levels which occurs within the first hour following exchange transfusion. Accordingly, as noted above, when exchange transfusion is required, it is advisable to do this as soon as possible. In this way, "potential bilirubin", that is red blood cells, can be removed more effectively than tissue bilirubin. Exchange transfusion removes only 50 % of anti-D from the body. As a result residual antibody can contribute to subsequent hemolysis of Rh positive cells and may thereby contribute to the rebound hyperbilirubinemia noted above.

Other blood cells are removed during an exchange transfusion, and as a result, a transient neutropenia frequently occurs. This seldom causes significant problems. Thrombocytopenia also may occur after exchange transfusion and may last for several days. This is less likely to occur if fresh blood is used for exchange transfusion.

At times, exchange transfusion is also used for the treatment of severe anemia such as that associated with hydrops fetalis. In these infants, anemia may be profound and the infants may be near death. Treatment consists of management of the severe acidosis, and initial correction of the anemia with packed red blood cells followed by exchange transfusion [30].

Complications of Rh disease

Hemorrhagic diathesis. — A bleeding disorder can complicate severe cases of Rh hemolytic disease. The picture usually includes severe thrombocytopenia with or without laboratory evidence of intravascular coagulation. It is possible that intravascular coagulation results directly from intravascular hemolysis, however, it is likely also that intravascular coagulation results from the state of cardiovascular collapse found in some of these severely ill infants. If thrombocytopenia is a major problem, exchange transfusion should be followed by a platelet infusion if necessary. Consumptive coagulopathy due to intravascular coagulation should be treated by exchange transfusion and heparin therapy is not necessary.

Obstructive jaundice. — This disorder occurs not infrequently in severe cases of Rh hemolytic disease in newborns. The obstructive jaundice is apparent at birth since the levels of direct bilirubin in cord blood are elevated. There is no structural explanation for the phenomenon since liver function tests are otherwise normal. Functionally, this finding may reflect an imbalance between hepatic conjugation and excretion of bilirubin. No specific therapy appears necessary for this self-limited complication.

Hypoglycemia. — This may appear during the first 24 hours of life of patients with Rh hemolytic disease, and may be intensified following the hyperglycemia which is associated with an exchange transfusion. Severe Rh disease has been shown to be associated with hyperinsulinemia in the fetus and newborn, possibly as a result of glutathione derived from broken down red blood cells acting as a stimulator for insulin release and islet cell hyperplasia. In the postexchange hyperglycemia occurring as a result of the excess glucose concentration in the dextrose containing preservative mixtures, a delayed reactive hyperinsulinemia may result in a postexchange hypoglycemic reaction. Accordingly, the blood glucose of these infants should be monitored closely.

Late anemia. — Anemia may develop within the first weeks of life in affected babies. This may occur either following exchange transfusion or in those babies who have not been transfused. The latter group may be seen more frequently now because of the use of phototherapy which may control hyperbilirubinemia even though hemolysis

continues. The reason for the late anemia, therefore, is the continued destruction of Rh positive erythrocytes and reticulocytes by residual anti-D antibody.

Prevention of Rh immunization. — The pathogenesis of Rh disease has been described earlier in this section. Anti-D antibodies develop in the Rh negative mother as a result of the entry of Rh positive erythrocytes into the maternal circulation. This process of immunization occurs mainly towards the end of pregnancy, so that antibodies usually develop after the first sensitizing pregnancy. Research done in New York and Liverpool proved that the administration of anti-D antibodies to the Rh negative mother after delivery prevented immunization [30]. This dramatic development has profoundly reduced the incidence of Rh immunization so that Rh disease has virtually disappeared. Initially, 300 micrograms of anti-D were given as a gamma-globulin preparation to women immediately post-partum. It is now recommended that 100 micrograms is satisfactory [31]. In some pregnancies (approximately 1 out of every 250 in our experience) large transplacental hemorrhages occur (greater than 30 ml) and for such women, 300 micrograms may not be sufficient to prevent immunization. For those women larger doses must be given. These women can be detected by screening for large transplacental hemorrhages after delivery, using the acid elution technique [31a].

Rh immunization will also develop in 5 % of Rh negative women following therapeutic or spontaneous abortion. Accordingly, such women should be protected as well [31].

All of the above techniques have reduced Rh immunization from 15 % of Rh negative women delivering Rh positive babies to 1.5 %. It now appears that this residual group is immunized prior to delivery rendering post-partum prevention too late. A programme of treatment with 300 micrograms of anti-D at the 28th week of gestation has resulted in the prevention of most of these cases [31].

Principles in the prevention of Rh immunization

— The Rh group of all pregnant women should be determined.

— Those women delivering Rh positive babies should receive gamma-globulin containing anti-D antibodies within the first 72 hours post-partum. In most series, 250-300 micrograms have been used but 100 micrograms appears to be satisfactory.

— Large transplacental hemorrhages should be detected by the Kleihauer technique. If found, the woman should receive anti-D gamma-globulin in a dose of 10 micrograms per ml of fetal hemorrhage.

— All Rh negative women should receive 100 micrograms of anti-D following an abortion.

— All Rh negative women should receive 100 micrograms of anti-D following amniocentesis.

— To prevent ante-partum immunization anti-D gamma-globulin should be given at the 28th week of pregnancy in a dose of 300 micrograms.

ABO hemolytic disease

ABO hemolytic disease occurs in group A or B newborn infants of group O mothers. This combination exists in 15 % of pregnancies, yet ABO hemolytic disease is diagnosed in only 3 % of pregnancies and exchange transfusion for this disease is required in only 1 in 1,000 pregnancies. The disease occurs more frequently and is more severe in Black populations [30, 32].

The plasma of group O mothers contains anti-A and anti-B as naturally occurring antibodies. This differs therefore from Rh antibodies which develop only after immunization by Rh positive erythrocytes. The anti-A and anti-B antibodies occur as IgG, IgA and IgM molecules. However, only the IgG molecules cross the placenta and cause disease in the fœtus. For this reason, it has been difficult to relate the severity of the disease in newborns to the level of anti-A or anti-B in the maternal plasma. The relationship between disease and the level of IgG anti-A or B is closer, but such testing is difficult, and the relationship is not absolute; hence the testing for IgG anti-A or B in maternal plasma has been of little practical value.

The disease itself is caused by the entry of IgG anti-A or B into the fœtal circulation, which sensitizes the fœtal erythrocytes, resulting in their destruction. The disease process therefore is similar to Rh disease. The difference is that ABO disease is rarely very severe; profound anemia is uncommon and death due to anemia does not occur. Since most group O women have IgG anti-A in their circulation, it is not surprising that evidence of sensitization (direct Coombs Test or the elution of anti-A or B from the cells) is found in most of their A or B newborns [32].

Clinical features. — ABO hemolytic disease classically manifests as jaundice during the first 24 hours of life ("icterus praecox"). Cord bilirubin levels are also elevated [30, 32]. The peripheral blood shows slight or no anemia and a variable elevation of the reticulocyte count. The Coombs test is positive and anti-A or B can be eluted from the cells. As noted above, these tests are positive

in a high proportion of incompatible infants, most of whom do *not* have disease. It is clear, therefore, that the finding of erythrocyte sensitization is not specific for the diagnosis of *disease*.

We believe that microspherocytosis is an important feature of ABO hemolytic disease. Such cells are evident on stained blood smears (Fig. V-6). It is our contention [33], however, that microspherocytes can be detected and quantitated better by the assessment of the three-dimensional shape of the red blood cells as shown in Figure V-6. Using this technique, the number of spherocytes is significantly increased in severe ABO hemolytic disease [33]. Since most A or B infants of Group O mothers have sensitized erythrocytes, it is not surprising that most may have some degree of ABO hemolytic disease. To prove that jaundice in a newborn infant is due exclusively to ABO hemolytic disease is difficult and therefore demands *exclusion of other causes of hyperbilirubinemia* before the diagnosis can be accepted.

Hemolytic disease due to blood group antibodies other than anti-D, anti-A or anti-B

Hemolytic disease due to minor group antibodies is uncommon. Queenan et al. [34] studied 15,378 pregnancies and found 31 babies who were Coombs positive because of minor group antibodies. Five of these children required exchange transfusions. The types of antibodies found in 30 cases has been described by Giblett [35]: 14 were due to Anti-c, 9 to Anti-E, 2 to Anti-Ce, 2 to Anti-Kell and 1 each to Anti-Fy$_a$, Anti-Jk$_a$ and Anti-U.

The diagnosis and treatment of these diseases is similar to that for Rh hemolytic disease. Although the diseases are infrequent, it is recommended that all women (both Rh negative and Rh positive) be screened at the 34th week of pregnancy for minor group antibodies.

MISCELLANEOUS CAUSES OF HEMOLYTIC ANEMIA

Microangiopathic hemolytic anemia. — There are two major causes of this relatively rare disorder in newborn infants. The first is that associated with giant hemangioma (the Kasabach-Merritt syndrome) [36]. In these cases, the child is born with a massive hemangioma and the major problem is thrombocytopenia. However, hemolytic anemia associated with abnormal red cell shape (fragments) has been reported [37].

A second condition in which this occurs is that associated with a placental chorioangioma [38]. Here the hematologic picture is similar to that noted in the presence of giant hemangiomas.

Infantile pyknocytosis. — In this syndrome, initially described by Tuffy et al. [39], abnormally shaped red blood cells (see Fig. V-11) are associated with hyperbilirubinemia. On careful review of the literature there is little clear delineation of the nature of this disorder. It has been reported in association with Vitamin E deficiency [40] no evident disease [41], bacterial infection [41] and G6PD deficiency [42]. The inability to clearly define the shape of the cells found normally in premature infants makes it difficult to define this syndrome further. Complete definition of this problem will require careful description of morphologic abnormalities in premature infants using quantitative techniques for the evaluation of red cell shape (see section on Vitamin E deficiency anemia).

Bacterial infections. — Although frequently considered, it is our experience that in newborn infants hemolytic anemia is rarely due to bacterial sepsis. The one notable exception is the profound hemolytic anemia with spherocytosis and intravascular hemolysis due to Clostridium Welchi septicemia.

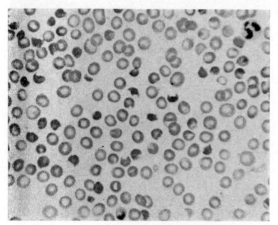

Fig. V-11. — *Erythrocytes of a patient with "infantile pyknocytosis".*

ANEMIA DUE TO BLOOD LOSS

The response of the fetus and newborn infant to blood loss is similar to that of adults. Sudden loss of large volumes of blood produces an acute reduction in circulating blood volume (but not in blood hemoglobin concentration) which can cause shock or death. In the ensuing hours, as the plasma volume expands to correct this hypovolemia the hemoglobin concentration falls and *anemia* becomes evident. Anemia in the fetus and newborn stimulates the production of erythropoietin within 24 hours and this is turn results in increased red cell production for the correction of the anemia. The situation is somewhat more complicated in the newborn for two reasons. The first is that many of the bleeding episodes that occur do so in utero where one cannot observe the above changes. Secondly, substantial hemorrhage in the fetus and newborn can occur and yet not be evident. This includes bleeding into the mother, into the placenta, into a twin or into a body cavity. Accordingly, in this section we shall first discuss the response of the fetus and newborn to hemorrhage and then discuss the various forms of hemorrhage that may occur.

The response of the fetus and newborn to hemorrhage

The response of the fetus to hemorrhage is like that of the adult in that it is dependent on the size and rapidity of the hemorrhage. For example, transplacental hemorrhage can occur during the third trimester of pregnancy; if massive, death results [43]. If less severe, anemia ensues and the infant responds by increasing red cell production which is evidenced by a reticulocytosis; if production is adequate the hemoglobin and reticulocytosis levels return to normal [44] (Fig. V-1).

If the bleeding occurs at delivery the newborn may show evidence of hypovolemia (but not anemia). In the first few hours of life anemia appears as the plasma volume expands and reticulocytosis develops thereafter (Fig. V-1).

Causes of hemorrhagic anemia

Bleeding into the maternal circulation. — In our experience, large transplacental hemorrhages (greater than 30 ml of fetal blood) occur in one in 250 pregnancies and thereby constitutes the commonest cause of fetal and neonatal hemorrhagic anemia. The clinical expression of this disorder has been described in the section above and is outlined in Figure V-1. Diagnosis is made by demonstrating fetal cells in the maternal circulation by means of the acid elution test of Kleihauer (Fig. V-12),

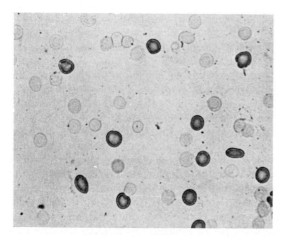

FIG. V-12. — *The acid elution technique of distinguishing fetal from adult erythrocytes.* The densely stained cells are cells containing fetal haemoglobin which was not eluted by the acid phosphate buffer wash. The ghost-like cells are cells which had contained adult haemoglobin which was eluted by the buffer wash.

When the baby is ABO-incompatible with the mother (e. g. baby A and mother O), fetal erythrocytes may not be demonstrable.

Bleeding into the placenta. — Although not common, large bleeds into the placental substance in association with anemia have been reported.

Bleeding into a twin. — Twin to twin transfusions are not uncommon in identical twins. In the majority of identical twin pregnancies there is evidence of vascular anastomosis within the placenta. Rausen et al. found evidence of a twin to twin transfusion (as evidenced by a hemoglobin difference between twins of greater than 5 g %) in 15 % of monochorional twins [45]. Over 50 % of those babies died. In the survivors, anemia can be profound with the other twin showing polycythemia.

It is likely that there are two types of such transfusions [46]. In one the fetal-fetal transfusion has occurred at the time of delivery, and, depending on the time of each clamping, one of the infants may retain much of the blood from the placenta and from the other twin. One infant thereby becomes polycythemic and plethoric and the other may develop shock and anemia. In these babies there is little difference in body weight between donor and recipient. In the other form, twin-twin transfusion occurs during intra-uterine life. Here the donor infant tends to be very much smaller than the recipient and shows signs of increased red cell production.

Bleeding from the placenta. — Bleeding may occur from a placental vessel, particularly in association with a velamentous insertion of the cord (Fig. V-13). The importance of this form of bleeding is that it may be massive and, if draining out through the maternal vagina, can be detected antepartum. Accordingly, all abnormal antepartum hemorrhage should be screened for fetal erythrocytes by the Kleihauer technique. The finding of substantial amounts of fetal blood in the vaginal bleeding is an indication for emergency intervention. Velamentous insertion of the cord may also be associated with vasa praevia, where the placental vessels cross the cervical os and may be torn during labour or delivery.

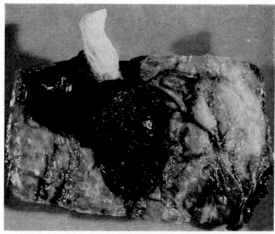

FIG. V-13. — *The placenta of a patient who was born anaemic and in shock.* There is evidence of haemorrhage from a surface placental vessel (photograph courtesy of Dr. DEREK DE SA).

Bleeding from the umbilical vessel. — The umbilical cord may be torn during delivery either because of undue trauma, a short cord or an abnormality of the vessels. Hypovolemia followed by anemia may result.

Bleeding into the fetus or newborn. — As mentioned above, hemorrhage can occur internally and may not be readily evident.

Bleeding into the head: Anemia may develop after birth following blood loss under the galeal aponeurosis (sub-galeal) or under the periostium (cephalohematoma). Intracranial hemorrhage may appear after traumatic delivery. Because of the relatively large size of the cranium in newborns, a sufficiently large volume of blood may accumulate with relatively few signs other than anemia. Intra-cerebral (or intraventricular) hemorrhage can occur, particularly in premature infants. Clinical signs are usually gross and of greater significance than the anemia.

Hemorrhage into the chest: Intrapulmonary hemorrhage may occur; however, this is usually in ill premature infants. The hemorrhage is now thought to be a hemorrhagic pulmonary edema [47], and therefore the anemia is of relatively little significance.

Hemorrhage into the abdomen: Massive hemor-rhage may occur, particularly after traumatic delivery, into the adrenals, spleen or liver, without overt signs other than anemia. Subcapsular hema-tomas of the liver manifesting only as anemia may subsequently rupture with ensuing shock. Gastro-intestinal hemorrhages do occur rarely in newborns, and are usually from a stress ulcer in the stomach. Blood in the vomitus or stool of newborn infants must be analyzed to determine whether it is of fetal or maternal (swallowed at delivery or during feeding from a bleeding nipple) origin. The Apt test [48] rapidly distinguishes fetal from adult blood on the basis of the resistance of fetal blood to denaturation by alkali. This test should be applied im-mediately whenever bloody stools or vomitus appear.

ANEMIA DUE TO FAILURE OF PRODUCTION AT BIRTH

This is a very uncommon cause of anemia. In Figure V-1, three cases from our nursery are shown. Anemia, with evidence of poor red cell production, was noted in these patients in our nursery. All three represent cases of Blackfan-Diamond syn-drome who developed sustained failure of red cell production and required repeated transfusions. Failure of red cell production at birth occurs rarely as a result of iron deficiency secondary to trans-placental hemorrhage. Anemia due to production failure occurs also as a result of bone marrow repla-cement by those conditions described in the section dealing with amegakaryocytic thrombocytopenia.

PHYSIOLOGIC ANEMIA OF INFANCY

The newborn infant is born with a hemoglobin concentration that is significantly greater than that of

the adult. Red cell production is active in utero as evidenced by the expanding hemoglobin mass, and by the high reticulocyte (Fig. V-1) and normoblast counts (Table II) at birth. Shortly after birth, possibly because the child now enters an oxygen rich environment, there is a dramatic change. Normoblast counts drop rapidly (Table II), as do reticulocytes (Fig. V-1). As a result of both this drop in red cell production and rapid growth, the concentration of hemoglobin (or number of red blood cells) in the peripheral blood begins to fall, as shown in Figure V-4. In full-term infants this fall causes hemoglobin levels to reach average values of approximately 12 g by 6 weeks of age (Fig. V-14).

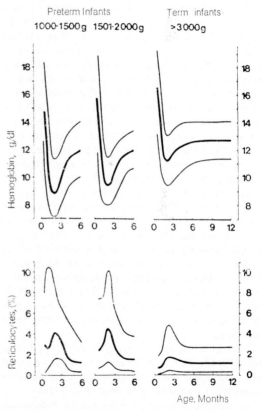

FIG. V-14. — *Hemoglobin concentration and reticulocyte counts in preterm and term infants.* Median values and 95 % confidence limits are indicated for each of the three birth weight categories (from DALLMAN, P. R., *Ann. Rev. Med., 32,* 143, 1981).

This stage is referred to as the physiologic anemia of infancy. In premature infants, the physiologic anemia is more severe (Fig. V-14). The major cause of the more rapid fall in premature infants is the relatively greater rate of growth as compared ot full-term infants. Consider the full-term infant who in 6 weeks may grow from 3,000 g to 4,500 g, a 50 % increase. During the same period the 1,000 g infant may grow to 2,000 g, or a 100 % increase, together with a corresponding increase in blood volume, and consequently a greater fall in hemoglobin concentration. The physiologic anemia in premature infants may also be more severe because the life span of their erythrocytes is significantly shorter than that of full-term infants.

Erythrocyte production in utero and after birth

It would appear that red cell production in utero is associated with erythropoietin production by the fœtus [7]. If, for any reason, red cell production must be increased in utero (e. g. secondary to hemolytic disease), erythropoietin levels are increased. After birth, presumably as a result of the higher oxygen content in the blood of the newborn compared to that of the fœtus, erythropoietin production and red cell production decline. For the next 4-6 weeks, erythropoietin production remains low, but as the hemoglobin falls, production increases, as shown in Figures V-14, V-15. It would appear, therefore, that the hemoglobin level at which erythropoietin production occurs is lower during the first 4-6 weeks of life than the level in adults (14-16 g per dl), or in infancy and childhood of 11-13 g per dl. That erythropoietin can be produced, however, during the first 6 weeks of life is evidenced by the fact that hypoxia (as in cyanotic heart disease) can stimulate erythropoietin production. Thus infants with cyanotic heart disease have hemoglobin levels which remain elevated during the first 6 weeks of life and "physiologic anemia" does not appear.

After birth, in association with the low erythropoietin levels there is a fall in the reticulocyte count and a decline in the levels of blood and total body hemoglobin concentrations (Fig. V-4, V-14).

As anemia develops, erythropoietin production begins to increase, as evidenced by the increasing levels of erythropoietin in the plasma as the haemoglobin concentration falls (Fig. V-15). It is of interest also that the stimulus to erythropoiesis is not only the low hemoglobin level, but also the ability of the blood to deliver (unload) oxygen to the tissues. This is also shown in Figure V-15 where erythropoietin levels are lower in infants whose blood contains predominantly hemoglobin A because they had received an exchange transfusion shortly after birth.

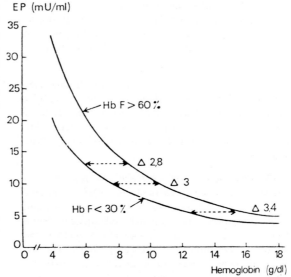

FIG. V-15. — The relationship between plasma erythropoietin (E. P.) concentrations and blood hemoglobin in two groups of infants; in one the hemoglobin F concentration was greater than 70 % and in the other (because of exchange transfusion) the hemoglobin F concentration was less than 30 %. It can be seen that erythropoietin levels increase as the hemoglobin level falls. The same erythropoietin levels were found at higher hemoglobin concentrations in those infants whose blood contained more than 70 % hemoglobin F. The difference (Δ) in hemoglobin levels associated with given erythropoietin concentrations are shown by the horizontal dotted lines (from STOCKMAN, J. A. III, GARCIA, J. F. and OSKI, F. A., New Engl. J. Med., 296, 647, 1977).

In Figure V-4, it can be seen that erythropoiesis increases after the fourth week of life as evidenced by the reticulocyte response. In the case displayed in Figure V-4, during the sixth and seventh week of life, there is a high reticulocyte count with no change in hemoglobin concentration. At any other time of life, that combination (increased red cell production with no increase in hemoglobin concentration) means the red cell life span has been shortened as a result of either hemorrhage or hemolysis. In this case, the reason is that the infant is growing rapidly and although the total body hemoglobin is increasing, the concentration of hemoglobin in the blood is falling. This is a common phenomenon during the first weeks of life and teaches us that anemia in premature infants cannot be assessed properly without accurate consideration of changes in body weight and thereby of total hemoglobin mass.

The physiologic anemia of infancy and particularly that of prematurity, therefore, is a normal phenomena due to diminished erythropoiesis and rapid growth during the first six weeks of life. It is clear that in sick and small premature infants, this anemia is intensified by blood sampling. It is not clear at this time whether these anemic babies should be transfused and, if so, at what level. This topic has been debated recently with some evidence suggesting benefit from transfusion [50]; the issue however is not settled particularly in view of the potential dangers of transfusion. At present it is the usual practice to consider transfusion when the patient's hemoglobin concentration falls below 7 g per dl. The indications for transfusion should be the same as for any other age.

There is no other therapy indicated for the physiologic anemia of infancy. Iron, copper, cobalt, pyridoxine and folic acid have all been tried without effect. The role of Vitamin E therapy will be discussed in the following section.

LATE ANEMIA
OF THE NEWBORN INFANT

During the first six weeks of life anemia may develop which is more severe than that of the physiologic anemia described in the previous section. Clearly, any of the causes of anemia described in the section on neonatal anemia may also cause anemia in the subsequent weeks of life. There are, however, two significant forms of anemia which develop during the first six weeks of life and deserve separate consideration. The first occurs in children with hemolytic disease and the second is related to nutritional deficiency.

Hemolytic disease

Hemolytic disease, particularly when due to Rh immunization, may be a cause of late anemia. Initially, this was observed following exchange transfusion, and presumably represents the continued presence of the anti-D antibody destroying any new Rh positive red cells produced. It has now become more frequent in milder forms of Rh disease (and other types of hemolytic disease) which are treated with light therapy [51]. The disease in such infants manifests during the first days of life as hyperbilirubinaemia, which is treated and controlled by light therapy. However, anemia may gradually appear. Accordingly, all patients with hemolytic disease should be followed carefully during the first weeks of life to be certain that a late anemia does not appear.

Nutritional deficiency

The rapidly growing newborn infant, particularly the premature infant, is susceptible to the development of a nutritional deficiency.

Folic acid deficiency. — Folic acid deficiency, defined by adult standards, occurs in premature infants. Although serum and red cell folate levels are normal at birth, it has been reported that the majority of premature infants have serum folic acid levels below normal adult levels by 1-3 months of age [52]. Cases of folic acid deficiency are not common, but have been reported in premature infants in the first 2 months of life, particularly those suffering from diarrhoea, infections or receiving antibiotic therapy [53]. It is recommended therefore that such infants should receive a prophylactic dose of 1 mg of folic acid to prevent the appearance of a deficiency state.

Copper deficiency. — Infants of low birthweight fed by parenteral nutrition have been reported to develop a state of copper deficiency [54]. This is characterized by the presence of anemia, neutropenia and rachitic-like changes in the bone.

Vitamin E deficiency. — Vitamin E levels in the plasma and tissue of newborn and premature infants in particular are significantly lower than adult values. This state of Vitamin E deficiency persists during the first few weeks of life; it has been suggested that it is associated with a hemolytic anemia which manifests at 4-6 weeks of age [55]. Furthermore, it has been reported that this anemia is associated with abnormal erythrocyte morphology as well as with thrombocytosis [55]. The anemia is most evident in infants whose birthweights are less than 1,500 g. There are recent reports that the anemia is intensified by oral iron therapy [56] and feedings high in linoleic acid [57], and that Vitamin E therapy given to such infants results in a hemoglobin level which is 1-1.5 g higher at 6 weeks of age than in control groups. Studies in our own laboratory (in a large randomized controlled trial) suggest that Vitamin E therapy in newborn infants of birth weight less than 1,500 g does not affect the development of anemia during the first six weeks of life [58]. At the present time, therefore, there is no reason to employ Vitamin E therapy for the prevention of anemia in newborn infants.

POLYCYTHEMIA

Polycythemia in newborn infants is defined as a capillary hemoglobin above the normal range shown in Figure V-1. Because of the error associated with capillary sampling, the increased hemoglobin should be confirmed by venous sampling; a venous hemoglobin of 22 g/dl or higher is considered to be abnormal.

The causes of polycythemia are:

— Excessive production in utero, and
— Excessive transfusion.

Excessive production

This occurs in response to hypoxemia in utero and presumably occurs for similar reasons in small-for-gestational age infants [59]. It has been noted also in newborns with down syndrome [60] and in infants of diabetic mothers [61], although the polycythemia in this situation may be due to reduced plasma volume.

Excessive transfusion

This may result from twin to twin transfusion in utero or at delivery (see above) or where there is a mother-to-fœtus transfusion [62]. Excessive placental transfusion also may produce polycythemia; this occurs following caesarian section when the infant is held below the mother, or more particularly following deliveries associated with intrauterine hypoxia [63]. In the latter instance, the amount of blood left in the placenta following ligation of the cord is significantly less than normal [63].

Clinically, patients with polycythemia may appear cyanosed, plethoric, tachypneic, excessively irritable and in congestive failure. Most of these patients, however, do not have abnormal signs and do not require therapy. Thus, Weinberger and Olieinick [64] studied 44,683 infants and detected 418 (0.09 %) with hematocrits greater than 77 % (hemoglobin concentration 26 g/dl or greater), a value above the normal range shown in Figure V-1. They did not find any difference in the morbidity or mortality of this group when compared to those with lower hemoglobin. On the other hand, Gross et al. [65] reported a series of polycythemic infants with abnormal signs and symptoms who had permanent neurologic sequelae. Others have reported

an increased frequency of thromboses in polycythemic newborns [66]. In association with polycythemia, the incidence of thrombocytopenia, hyperbilirubinemia and hypoglycemia is higher than in normal newborns. When treatment is considered necessary, partial exchange transfusion has been suggested [65], whereby blood is removed and replaced by plasma. This is based on the assumption that the symptoms are due to the high hematocrit hence hyperviscosity. We have observed extraordinarily high blood volumes in these patients and believe that consideration should be given to the possibility that the plethoric state (high blood *volume*) may be the cause of the tachypnea and congestive failure. If this is true simple venesection would seem more appropriate. Clearly, there is no definitive answer and each infant should be treated cautiously on the basis of clinical findings. Where feasible, circulating blood volumes should be determined as well.

NEUTROPHILS
IN NEWBORN INFANTS

The normal number of segmented and band (non-segmented, young) neutrophils is shown in Figure V-16. The values therein are for full-term infants, however similar values were found in premature infants.

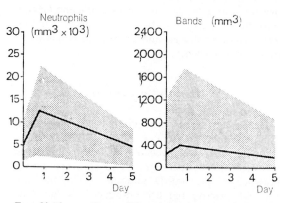

Fig. V-16. — *Neutrophil and band counts during the first five days of life in 163 normal full term infants.* The first point "Day 0" are cord blood values. The second point represents a capillary blood sample taken 4-24 hours after birth. The mean time of sampling was 14 hours; however, there was no difference in the values from 4-24 hours. The third point is a capillary blood sample taken on day 5. The dark solid lines represent means and the shaded areas include 95 % of the values.

Bacterial infection

In severe infections, the first hematologic change is a fall in neutrophils [67], in part due to their utilization and in part as a result of bacterial induced complement activation [68]. Then young (band) neutrophils are released into the circulation so that the ratio of band/segmented neutrophils becomes abnormally high (greater than 0.3). Thereafter, as the absolute numbers of bands increase, they exceed the normal limits (Fig. V-16). Finally, the total neutrophil count may or may not exceed the values shown in Figure V-16. It is this latter feature that distinguishes the neutrophil response to infection of newborns from that of adults. Because the reserve of neutrophils in the bone marrow is low in newborns [67], infection is often not associated with an abnormally high neutrophil count, in contrast to the characteristic neutrophilia of infection in adults. It should be added also that the neutrophil response in newborns is frequently associated with the appearance of very immature cells, myelocytes, promyelocytes and myeloblasts.

Neutropenia

As mentioned above, profound neutropenia is seen as an early response to bacterial infection. The low neutrophil count is often accompanied by or followed within hours by the remainder of the neutrophil response, namely a shift in the band/segmented neutrophil ratio and an elevation in total band cells.

In contrast, *isoimmune neutropenia* may appear in association with severe infection and there is need therefore to distinguish this situation from the neutropenia of sepsis. The presence of young neutrophils in the circulation is unlikely in isoimmune neutropenia and the transient nature of the neutropenia of sepsis is usually evident.

Isoimmune neutropenia occurs as a result of

maternal antibodies to the neutrophils of the infant [69], hence its pathogenesis is similar to isoimmune (alloimmune) hemolytic disease or thrombocytopenia in newborns. As with these disorders, although the newborn may be ill with infection in the early days of life, neutrophil numbers gradually improve, presumably as the maternal neutrophil antibodies disappear from the infant's circulation.

Congenital leukemia

This is an extremely rare disorder where the predominant form of leukemia, unlike childhood leukemia of other ages, is acute myeloblastic leukemia. In both acute myeloblastic and acute lymphoblastic congenital leukemia, the prognosis is poor. The manifestations of the disease are identical to those of leukemia at other times of life.

There are, however, a number of disorders which can appear very similar to acute leukemia in the newborn period. Thus, congenital infections, such as cytomegalovirus disease, toxoplasmosis and syphilis may manifest as hepatosplenomegaly with a pronounced leukemoid response in the peripheral blood. Severe bacterial infections may also manifest in this way.

Special mention should be made of the "transient leukemia" picture that is seen in patients with Down's syndrome. Although the incidence of acute and congenital leukemia is higher in Down's syndrome [70], there is, in addition, an unusual syndrome in which a classic picture of acute myeloblastic leukemia appears, and then, over the subsequent weeks, regresses and disappears [71]. It is not clear whether this form of "transient leukemia" represents true leukemia. It does, however, cause a diagnostic and therapeutic problem in assessing the significance of a leukemia-like picture in patients with Down syndrome. While treatment of acute leukemia in the newborn is the same as for that of the older child, the prognosis is worse.

Hemorrhagic disorders in newborn infants

Ill and premature newborn infants frequently suffer from hemorrhage. Bleeding occurs in some as a result of trauma or hypoxia; in others, bleeding is the result of a hemorrhagic diathesis. In both

instances, the incompletely developed hemostatic system of the newborn may contribute to the clinical and laboratory manifestations of these diseases.

In this section the hemostatic system of the newborn will be examined to determine how it differs from that of adults. This is of considerable importance in the diagnosis of neonatal hemorrhagic problems and in the genesis of certain disorders. Parenthetically, it should be noted that although the hemostatic system is incompletely developed at birth, uncontrolled bleeding is rare in normal infants. Furthermore, it is a general experience that complex surgery can be performed during the neonatal period without undue bleeding. It may be concluded therefore that the normal newborn infant is not a "bleeder".

Hemostasis involves both platelets and the blood coagulation system. Accordingly, the following sections will deal separately with diseases due to abnormalities of each of these systems.

STUDY
OF THE BLOOD COAGULATION SYSTEM
IN THE NEWBORN INFANT

Many of the hemorrhagic disorders of the newborn are complex and require both detailed clinical and laboratory investigation. Laboratory testing requires microtechnology together with knowledge of normal values for the particular infant under study. In our own laboratory, we have developed microtechnology by a simple adaptation of tests

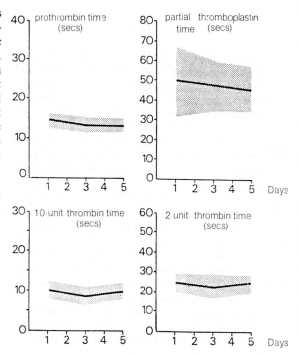

FIG. V-17. — *Coagulation screening tests in newborn infants.* These graphs show the results of studies on venous blood samples of 46 full term (> 37 weeks) normal infants on days 1, 3 and 5. Day 1 samples were obtained between 4 and 24 hours of age. The solid line represents the mean and the shaded areas include 95 % of the values. These graphs are used in our clinical units for the display of test results on individual patients.

TABLE VI. — VOLUMES OF PLASMA
REQUIRED FOR VARIOUS COAGULATION TESTS

Coagulation test	Amount of plasma needed (μl)
Prothrombin time.	20
Kaolin-cephalin time (APPT) . .	20
Thrombin time	40
Fibrinogen.	20
Factors: VIII	15
IX	15
X.	15
II, V, VII and X . . .	15
XI	15
XII	15
Antithrombin III, α_2 macroglobulin,	
α_1 antitrypsin	5
Fibrin degradation products (FDP).	25
Total (μl)	220

used for adults [72]. Using these methods, a wide battery of tests can be performed on 0.2 ml of plasma as outlined in Table VI. Normal values for full-term and premature infants using these techniques are shown in Figures V-17 and V-18 and Table VII. There are several important features to these data. It should be noted that the prothrombin time in both full-term and premature infants is only slightly different than the adult range of 10-12 seconds. The partial thromboplastin time which is commonly used as a screening test in adults and older children is much longer in newborn infants, particularly those of low birth weight. It is our impression that those children with a long partial thromboplastin time often are not particularly prone to hemorrhagic phenomena. We believe that this anomaly is due to low levels of contact factors (factors XI, XII, pre-kallikrein and low molecular weight kininogen [73]). As a result, we consider that the partial thromboplastin time is of little value in the newborn. The two unit thrombin time is a valuable screening test since it

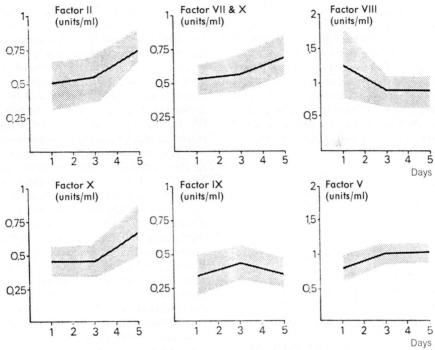

FIG. V-18. — *Specific assays for Factors II, VII, X, X, VIII, IX and V for the same normals referred to in Figure V-17.*

TABLE VII. — Normal values for adults, full-term, and premature infants

Coagulation tests	Control adults			Full-term babies			"Disease-free" prematures			Significance *, **
	No. studied	Mean	+ SD	No. studied	Mean	+ SD	No. studied	Mean	+ SD	
Prothrombin time (sec)	34	12	1	50	14	1.3	22	14	1.3	NS
APTT (sec) ***	113	42	4	48	51	10.0	20	57	10.5	NS
Thrombin clotting time										
10 U (sec)	25	10	1	47	10	1.6	10	11	2.6	NS
2 U (sec)	25	25	2	46	23	2.9	22	23	2.4	NS
Factors:										
II (%)	38	81	17	49	50	14.5	22	31	8.6	$p < 0.001$
V (%)	38	90	19	44	79	17.0	22	70	22.0	NS
VII + X (%)	36	93	20	49	54	12.2	22	37	11.0	$p < 0.001$
X (%)	54	89	23	49	45	12	22	31	9.0	$p < 0.001$
VIII (%)	76	87	27	49	126	56	21	116	73.0	NS
IX (%)	38	99	23	49	35	12.6	22	28	11.0	$p < 0.5$
Antithrombin III (%)	66	99	10	18	58	9.6	17	33	9	$p < 0.001$
α_1 Antitrypsin (%)	66	94	20	18	88	20.5	19	92	34	NS
α_2 Macroglobulin (%)	66	98	20	—	—	—	16	77	32	—
Fibrinogen (mg/dl)	31	319	180	—	—	—	19	282	131	—
FDP (µg/ml)	52	6	3	—	—	—	18	14	11	—

* Full-term and premature infants were compared using the unpaired student *t*-test.
** NS = Not significant.
*** Kaolin-activated partial thromboplastin time.

can also detect heparin contamination and fibrinogen deficiency [72].

The specific coagulation factors shown in Figure V-18 and in Table VII are, in many instances, different from those of adults. The variation and significance of these have been reported by others [73]. However, in this chapter, they are considered in regard to the evaluation of specific coagulation problems in the newborn. Table VIII shows the use of screening tests in the diagnosis of hemorrhagic disorders in newborn infants.

TABLE VIII. — Laboratory screening tests
for bleeding newborn infants

	T. C. P.	D. I. C.	K-Def.	Hep.	Haemophilia
Platelet count	AB	AB/N	N	N	N
Plasma fibrinogen	N	AB	N	N	N
Prothrombin time	N	AB	AB	AB/N	N
Partial thromboplastin time *	N	AB/N	AB/N	AB/N	AB/N
Thrombin time	N	AB	N	AB	N

Abbreviations

T. C. P.: thrombocytopenia
D. I. C.: disseminated intravascular coagulation
K-Def. : Vitamin K deficiency ("hemorrhagic disease of the newborn")
Hep.   : heparin in the blood sample
AB   : abnormal
N   : normal
AB/N   : the test may or may not be abnormal in the particular condition

* The partial thromboplastin test in the newborn is of little value because of its wide range in normals (Table II, Fig. V-1).

HEMORRHAGE
DUE TO ABNORMALITIES
IN THE BLOOD COAGULATION SYSTEM

VITAMIN K DEFICIENCY

Hemorrhagic disease of the newborn.
— The low levels of blood coagulation factors found in newborn infants and shown in Figure V-18 and Table VII are due largely to "immaturity" of the

newborn, presumably in the necessary enzyme systems. Vitamin K deficiency has been invoked as an additional cause of the low levels of Vitamin K dependent clotting factors (factors II, VII, IX and X) which occur at birth. Early studies of the blood coagulation system in the newborn demonstrated a relatively long prothrombin time at birth which was prolonged even further during the first few days of life. During that period it was noted also that many newborns had a tendency to spontaneous hemorrhages. This was referred to as hemorrhagic disease of the newborn. Studies completed over 30 years ago showed that the administration of Vitamin K at birth prevented both the prolongation of the prothrombin time and the appearance of hemorrhagic disease of the newborn [74]. It was shown in those studies and in more recent ones [75] that the fall in prothrombin activity in newborn infants was more severe in those babies who were fed breast milk than those placed immediately on cow's milk. Cow's milk contains more Vitamin K and supports the development of bacterial flora which itself can manufacture Vitamin K within the bowel.

Because of the above studies and considerations it has been a generally accepted procedure to administer 1 mg of the naturally occurring fat-soluble analogue Vitamin K_1 oxide at birth. As a result, hemorrhagic disease of the newborn has virtually disappeared. Recent studies have questioned whether normal newborn infants are, in fact, Vitamin K deficient. In Vitamin K deficiency the activity of Vitamin K dependent coagulation factors is reduced and these factors can be detected in normal levels in the plasma by immunologic means. In the newborn, however, the immunologic as well as the biologic activity of the Vitamin K dependent factors are reduced, suggesting that the newborn is not Vitamin K deficient [76-79]. These reports also suggest that the Vitamin K dependent coagulation factors do not change as a result of Vitamin K therapy at birth. As a result of these findings the rationale of administering Vitamin K prophylactically to newborn infants has been questioned. But these observations are of a preliminary nature; the substantial number of clinical trials which demonstrate the effectiveness of Vitamin K [80], plus the virtual disappearance of hemorrhagic disease of the newborn would seem to indicate the wisdom of continuing with prophylactic Vitamin K for all newborn infants.

There is another possible explanation for the conflicting views concerning the significance of Vitamin K deficiency in newborn infants: Vitamin K deficiency hemorrhagic disease has been observed in babies whose mothers have been on the anticonvulsants phenobarbital and/or Dilantin [81]. This relationship is sufficiently significant to suggest that mothers on anticonvulsants should receive supplemental Vitamin K in the last weeks of pregnancy. This raises the possibility that hemorrhagic disease of the newborn may occur only in certain infants, possibly because of drugs or other factors in the mother's circulation, which may explain why Vitamin K prophylaxis is effective in preventing hemorrhagic disease of the newborn, even though most newborn infants may not be truly Vitamin K deficient.

Late hemorrhagic disease of the newborn infants. — In addition to the Vitamin K deficiency which manifests in the first days of life, there are now numerous reports of Vitamin K deficiency hemorrhagic disease manifesting later, namely at 4-6 weeks of age [82, 83]. The majority of these babies had not received Vitamin K at birth and had been breast fed or had received milk which was low in Vitamin K. Many of these infants also had suffered from diarrhoea and had been on antibiotic therapy, which would have interfered with the production and absorption of Vitamin K in the bowel. These observations should alert one not only to the possibility of Vitamin K deficiency in a bleeding baby at 4-6 weeks of age, but also to the need for prophylactic Vitamin K for infants who have suffered from severe diarrhoea and infection during the first two months of life.

DISSEMINATED INTRAVASCULAR COAGULATION (D. I. C.)

Cardiovascular collapse syndrome of newborn infants. — Much has been written about D. I. C. in newborn infants. Its occurrence has been described in babies suffering from severe asphyxia, viral disease, bacterial infections, hemorrhagic shock, cardiovascular disease, erythroblastosis and infants born after abruptio placentae, toxaemic pregnancy and the presence of a dead twin sibling [84]. Indeed there are many causes, and it has been difficult to determine a common denominator that renders the newborn so prone to D. I. C. as a result of such a diverse group of disorders.

Our own studies [84] indicate that the only major cause of significant D. I. C. in infants is cardiovascular collapse. We reached the following conclusions:

(1) A profound form of D. I. C. occurs in newborn infants which is characterized by consumption of coagulation factors (particularly fibrinogen), ischemic necrosis of organs and a hemorrhagic diathesis. Platelet counts may be normal or only slightly reduced.

(2) This disorder must be distinguished from the predominantly thrombocytopenic syndrome seen in bacterial sepsis (see Section on thrombocytopenia due to bacterial infections).

(3) The cardiovascular collapse group includes only those patients with the following clinical conditions:

— an Apgar of 0 or 1; or
— an episode of cardiac arrest; or
— a state of profound hypotension with imperceptible pulses, and a grossly compromised peripheral circulation.

The many causes of the collapse include bacterial shock, severe hemorrhage, hypoplastic left heart syndrome, asphyxia neonatorum and intracranial hemorrhage.

(4) In our experience the cardiovascular collapse syndrome underlies virtually all cases of D. I. C. seen in newborn infants. We believe it is the causative mechanism in the wide variety of diseases associated with D. I. C. described at the beginning of this section.

In Table IX the clinical and coagulation observations of a typical case are shown.

This case demonstrates the central feature of this syndrome:

— The onset is sudden and results from an episode of cardiovascular collapse.
— The laboratory findings include consumption of fibrinogen and other coagulation factors (fibrin split products usually appear in the plasma; platelet counts may be normal or only slightly reduced).
— A bleeding diathesis appears which may be profound.
— The laboratory abnormalities and bleeding diathesis can be corrected by exchange transfusion and usually do not recur.

This patient also had signs of organ damage (hematuria, oliguria) which, together with the underlying primary disease, may result in death [84].

MISCELLANEOUS CAUSES OF A HEMORRHAGIC DIATHESIS

Heparin. — Bleeding may occur in babies who are inadvertently given excessive doses of heparin;

TABLE IX. — BLOOD COAGULATION TESTS IN A 3,560 G NEWBORN INFANT, RESUSCITATED AFTER A TRAUMATIC DELIVERY AND A STATE OF COLLAPSE SHORTLY AFTER BIRTH.

Time after collapse (hours)	P. T. * (secs)	T. T. (secs)	Fibrinogen mg/dl	Factor V (%)
2	38	62		10
7	28	36	69	17
Exchange transfusion				
9	15	20	144	33
16	18	30	162	30
112	14	25	178	68

* P. T. = prothrombin time; T. T. = 2 unit thrombin time (for normal values see Table VII).

Note: In this patient the first coagulation study was done two hours after collapse, and it is evident that the syndrome appeared quickly. From the time that the first sample was studied until preparation for exchange transfusion (an interval of 5 hours), there appears to be improvement in the prothrombin and thrombin times. Exchange transfusion corrected the coagulation defect and the haemorrhagic diathesis and there was no recurrence.

this can occur, for example, when heparin is used to flush out catheters. A bleeding diathesis due to heparin intoxication is unusual in our experience, however, what is common is heparin contamination of samples used for coagulation testing. Since heparin is used so frequently in the newborn (to flush out catheters, for blood gas sampling, etc.), heparin contamination must be ruled out in any blood sample from a newborn infant. This can be done most conveniently and quickly using the 2-unit thrombin time [72].

Liver disease. — Bleeding due to liver disease can result from Vitamin K deficiency or from decreased production of coagulation factors. Therapy should include the administration of Vitamin K plus replacement with plasma if necessary. Because liver disease may be associated with low antithrombin 3 levels, factor IX concentrates should not be used because of their thrombogenic potential [85].

INHERITED BLEEDING DISORDERS

Newborn infants with hemophilia A (AHG or factor VIII deficiency) or hemophilia B (Christmas

disease or factor IX deficiency) are theoretically at risk of bleeding, since neither factor VIII or factor IX cross the placenta. It is surprising, therefore, that hemorrhage is relatively uncommon in hemophiliacs during the newborn period. The incidence of neonatal hemorrhage in congenital bleeding disorders is shown in Table X [86]. It is evident that most babies with congenital bleeding disorders do not bleed in the newborn period. Nevertheless, bleeding can occur and does so in 10 % of patients with hemophilia. Patients with fibrinogen deficiency frequently bleed during the newborn period, and it is of interest that in factor XIII deficiency virtually all of the patients have bleeding in the newborn, particularly from the umbilical cord. Bleeding manifestations in these disorders include bleeding into the subcutaneous tissues, umbilical hemorrhage, intracranial bleeds, as well as a variety of internal bleeds. Abnormalities of platelet function do not usually manifest in the newborn period. In one

TABLE X. — BLEEDING IN NEWBORN INFANTS WITH HEREDITARY HEMORRHAGIC DISORDERS

Deficiency	No. studied	No. with bleeding	%
Fibrinogen	55	37	67
Prothrombin	10	1	10
Factor V	39	2	5
Factor VII	49	9	18
Factors VIII and IX (hemophilia)	630	63	10
Factor X	38	15	39
Factor XI	160	4	2
Factor XIII	9	9	100

study no bleeding was noted in 8 infants with thrombasthenia or in 11 patients with Von Willebrand's disease [87].

Management of these patients depends on the nature of the disorder in order that specific replacement therapy may be given. Since these congenital bleeding disorders can manifest in the newborn, an unexplained hemorrhagic diathesis in any newborn requires a complete study of his or her coagulation system [72].

A not uncommon problem is the birth of a child into a family who is already known to have a hemorrhagic disorder. Under these circumstances, it is appropriate to attempt to determine the type of defect. To permit extensive studies without the need for what might be a traumatic venipuncture, cord blood may be obtained at the time of delivery. Most hemorrhagic disorders can be diagnosed at birth, although there may be difficulties in diagnosing factor IX deficiency, since factor IX levels in normal newborn infants may be low (Fig. V-18). It may not be possible to obtain a definitive diagnosis of factor IX deficiency until these infants are several months old.

PLATELET DISORDERS IN NEWBORN INFANTS

Platelets are formed by megakaryocytes in the bone marrow. After release from the marrow, platelets live in the circulation for 7-10 days. Any disease which interferes with megakaryocyte function can cause thrombocytopenia because of *production failure*. Any process which *destroys or consumes* platelets and thereby shortens their average lifespan can produce thrombocytopenia.

Platelet production can be increased to compensate for a shortened lifespan. This is evidenced by increased numbers of megakaryocytes in the marrow and by the release of larger platelets into the circulation (megathrombocytes).

Thrombocytopenia represents a reduction in platelet numbers below that which is normal. The normal values for platelets in full-term and premature infants have been the subject of many studies [73]. Normally, platelet counts are greater than 150,000/mm^3; we consider significant thrombocytopenia to be present if the platelet count is less than 100,000/mm^3. It should be noted that bleeding from thrombocytopenia itself in both newborns and adults rarely occurs unless the platelet count is less than 40,000/mm^3.

THROMBOCYTOPENIA DUE TO DECREASED PRODUCTION OF PLATELETS

This group of diseases is an uncommon cause of thrombocytopenia in newborn infants. The onset of the disease may occur at birth or it may gradually appear in the early days of life. This group is characterized by having a normal lifespan of platelets and decreased numbers of megakaryocytes in the marrow. The reduction of megakaryocytes in the marrow may be due to primary hypoplasia or may be secondary to replacement of the marrow by leukemic cells or by histiocytes.

Congenital amegakaryocytic hypoplasia. — This group of diseases of unknown etiology are characterized by thrombocytopenia and a bone marrow with reduced numbers of megakaryocytes but no abnormal cells. There may or may not be associated congenital anomalies.

With congenital anomalies:

Thrombocytopenia, absent radii syndrome. — These infants are born with thrombocytopenia and bilateral absence of the radii and other skeletal anomalies. Inheritance is thought to be recessive. Bleeding may be severe and fatal. A minority of cases may improve after the first year of life.

Fanconi's syndrome. — This syndrome of pancytopenia with multiple congenital anomalies rarely begins in the newborn.

Without congenital anomalies. — Isolated thrombocytopenia without congenital anomalies has been reported. In some instances this has progressed to become pancytopenia, whereas in others it has cleared spontaneously.

Congenital leukemia. — As in any leukemia, thrombocytopenia occurs in association with marrow replacement by leukemic cells. It is of interest that there may be more apparent purpura than would be expected from the thrombocytopenia. This is due to leukemic infiltrates into the skin which are similar to those seen in congenital viral disease with purpura (see below).

Congenital histiocytosis. — In this acute disease, extensive infiltration of the liver and spleen is associated with reduced numbers of megakaryocytes in the marrow. Cutaneous hemorrhages are often severe and the extensive petechial rash is often more severe than the degree of thrombocytopenia would suggest. Again, this is due to tissue infiltration by abnormal cells.

Osteopetrosis. — Because of bone marrow replacement this disease has been associated with thrombocytopenia which is usually mild if present at all at birth.

THROMBOCYTOPENIA DUE TO INCREASED DESTRUCTION OR CONSUMPTION OF PLATELETS

As mentioned earlier, platelets survive 7-10 days in the circulation. A minor reduction of platelet life

span can be compensated for by increased produc_
tion, as evidenced by increased numbers of megakaryocytes in the marrow and young large platelets
(megathrombocytes) in the peripheral blood. Platelet
life span can be shortened because of the action of
antibodies (immune thrombocytopenia), consumption by intravascular coagulation or by a combination of these and possibly other mechanisms, as in
severe infections. These are the commonest forms
of thrombocytopenia and deserve careful attention.

Thrombocytopenia
due to anti-platelet antibodies

In these cases, the mother's blood contains anti-
platelet antibodies of the immunoglobulin G type
which can cross the placenta and affect the baby.
There are two major types of this disorder, namely
those in which the mother has an antibody against
her own platelets as well as the baby's platelets
(autoimmune thrombocytopenia), and those in
which the antibody is directed only against the
baby's platelets (alloimmune or isoimmune thrombocytopenia).

Autoimmune thrombocytopenia. — This not uncommon disorder affects women in the childbearing
age, causing thrombocytopenia. Since the antibodies
in this disease are of the immunoglobulin G type,
which can cross the placenta, the foetus is at risk of
developing thrombocytopenia. Indeed, if the
mother's platelet count is less than 100,000, over
40 % of the patients will have thrombocytopenia [88].
This is usually evident at birth, although in some
instances the lowest level may not be reached
until the third or fourth day of life. The thrombocytopenia may be severe in these cases, with values
below 20,000/mm³. Death may occur as a result of
intracranial hemorrhage which may occur shortly
after birth, as a result of trauma during delivery, or
may not be evident until after the third day of life.
Intracranial hemorrhage has occurred after Caesarian section and has been reported to occur in utero.
The overall risk of neonatal thrombocytopenia
secondary to autoimmune disease has been studied [88]. In 51 pregnancies in 29 women, all of whom
were delivered vaginally, 50 % of the infants were
found to be thrombocytopenic. One infant developed
intracranial hemorrhage at 60 hours of age. There
were no deaths and no problems with the mothers.
In these cases, thrombocytopenia may occur in the
newborn even though the maternal platelet counts
are normal. If the mother's platelet production
can compensate for antibody-induced thrombo-

cytopenia, then she may have a normal platelet
count despite immunoglobulin G anti-platelet antibodies in the circulation. Under these circumstances
the baby may be thrombocytopenic. This is seen
most commonly in women whose autoimmune
thrombocytopenia has gone into remission following
a splenectomy.
There is no clearcut treatment of this disease. It
has been suggested that thrombocytopenic infants
should be delivered by Caesarian section. For this
purpose, it has been suggested that a scalp puncture
platelet count should be done in early labour [88].
If the platelet count is less than 50,000, Caesarian
section is recommended. The argument against
this is:

— The lack of evidence that Caesarian section is
safer than vaginal delivery.

— The occurrence of intracranial hemorrhage
in utero [89] or after Caesarian section [88].

In addition, there is a real surgical risk in the
thrombocytopenic mother. It would seem preferable
to attempt as gentle a delivery as possible and then
observe the infant. Platelet transfusions are of little
value because survival of platelets is very short.
Steroid therapy (Prednisone, 2 mg per kilo per day
in 3 divided doses each day) can be tried, and is
thought to help reduce the likelihood of severe
hemorrhage. If there is an indication of severe
hemorrhage then therapy by exchange transfusion
and platelet infusions is recommended.

Alloimmune thrombocytopenia. — In our experience the commonest cause of immune thrombocytopenia in newborn infants is the transplacental
passage of allo-antibodies directed against an antigen on the platelets of the baby which is not present
on the platelets of the mother. It is believed that in
this disorder the mother is immunized by the
transplacental passage of platelets bearing a paternal
antigen which she lacks. Antibodies thus formed
can affect the foetus and cause thrombocytopenia
even in a first pregnancy.
The antigen is usually PL^A1, a platelet antigen
present in 98 % of the population. Other antigens
are rarely involved. Alloimmune thrombocytopenia
may be severe and can be fatal. In one major review
of this topic, intracranial hemorrhage occurred in 8
out of 55 cases; the mortality rate in that series
was 12.7 % [90].
Characteristically, the infant at birth has many
petechiae, although they may not appear until 24
or 48 hours later. Large platelets (megathrombocytes)
may be present in the peripheral blood smear and
megakaryocytes should be found in bone marrow

aspirates. Bone marrow aspirates are often reported to have decreased numbers of megakaryocytes; however, it is likely that such observations reflect the difficulty of obtaining technically satisfactory marrow aspirates in newborn infants.

Alloimmune thrombocytopenia in newborn infants differs from that associated with autoimmune thrombocytopenia in the mother. In the latter group in most instances, the mother's platelet count will be reduced where there is a history of thrombocytopenic purpura. The two conditions can be distinguished by searching for platelet antibodies. In alloimmune disease, antibodies will be found on the platelets of the baby and in the serum of the mother, but not on her platelets. Where the cause is autoimmune thrombocytopenia in the mother, antibodies are found in the serum of the mother and on the platelets of both the mother and baby [91].

This disease is treated by transfusing the infant with maternal platelets. The mother can donate a unit (200-250 ml) of platelet rich plasma by plasmapheresis. The plasma should be centrifuged and all plasma removed, leaving the platelet concentrate. The platelets should be Rh compatible and fresh frozen, group AB plasma should be added to a total volume of approximately 30 ml. The infant should receive 10 ml per kilo of this platelet suspension.

Drug induced thrombocytopenia. — Thrombocytopenia in adults can occur as a result of the ingestion of certain drugs (e. g. Sedormid, Quinidine). In these patients platelets are destroyed when the drug unites with the antibody to form a complex which is destructive to the platelet. If mothers possess such an antibody and receive the drug, both of which can cross the placenta, thrombocytopenia may develop in the baby. This has been reported with quinine [24]. Treatment is similar to that described for autoimmune thrombocytopenia.

Thrombocytopenia due to infections

Bacterial infections. — This is now the commonest cause of thrombocytopenia in newborn infants. During severe bacterial infections in newborns or in adults, thrombocytopenia can develop and is often severe. In our own experience [67], thrombocytopenia occurs in approximately 50 % of infants with severe bacterial infections (septicemia, meningitis or peritonitis). In most instances, the platelet count is below 50,000/mm^3 and develops rapidly, suggesting shortened platelet survival and therefore

destruction. Platelet transfusions produce only transient elevations of platelet counts, again suggesting platelet destruction.

While the mechanism of thrombocytopenia is unknown, it has been suggested that endotoxin or other bacterial products may cause platelet aggregation either directly or indirectly by endothelial damage or by causing disseminated intravascular coagulation (D. I. C.). In our opinion, the role of D. I. C. in this process is not a significant one [84]. The process is to be distinguished from that described in association with cardiovascular collapse. In sepsis, thrombocytopenia may be very severe, but, the evidence of disseminated intravascular coagulation is minimal [67]. It has been suggested also that bacteria may cause thrombocytopenia as a result of the production of neuraminidase which causes removal of sialic acid from the surface of platelets, which, in turn, causes a shortening of platelet life span [93]. Whatever the cause, thrombocytopenia is frequent and may last 7-10 days. It can be very severe with platelet counts below 10,000/mm^3. Surprisingly, however, petechial eruptions and hemorrhagic diathesis are rare under these circumstances, hence treatment of the thrombocytopenia is not mandatory. In our own experience with the very ill and premature infant at risk of intracerebral or intrapulmonary hemorrhage we have employed platelet infusions with variable success. In necrotizing enterocolitis, thrombocytopenia occurs in a manner similar to that found in association with bacterial infections. Indeed, the hematologic picture of necrotizing enterocolitis is in every way similar to that of bacterial infections.

Thrombocytopenia due to congenital and acquired viral disease. — Congenital rubella and cytomegalic inclusion virus diseases frequently are associated with thrombocytopenia. The cause of thrombocytopenia in these conditions is not always clear. Hepatosplenomegaly is a frequent feature of this disorder, and may be responsible for the thrombocytopenia. Indeed, the thrombocytopenia in these diseases may not be as severe as the cutaneous hemorrhagic lesions would suggest. These lesions are often severe and striking ("blueberry muffin" lesions) and are actually more than just hemorrhagic lesions. It would appear that they represent cutaneous infiltrates, often with nucleated red blood cells, suggesting dermal erythropoiesis [94]. A generalized bleeding tendency is unusual in these disorders. The thrombocytopenia may last up to six months and does not usually require therapy.

Thrombocytopenia also occurs in newborn infants as a result of viral disease acquired after birth, either from human contact, or as a result of blood transfusions. In this group, we have seen instances of cytomegalovirus, Echo 11 virus, Coxsackie B and Epstein-Barr virus diseases. The thrombocytopenia is transient, disappearing after several weeks, and is associated with the appearance of atypical lymphocytes in the peripheral blood.

Thrombocytopenia due to toxoplasmosis or syphilis is similar to that found in congenital viral disease.

Thrombocytopenia in association with giant hemangioma

Large cavernous hemangiomas may be associated with moderate or severe thrombocytopenia. The cause appears to be platelet aggregation and deposition in the tortuous vasculature of these tumours. As a result, there may also be evidence of intravascular coagulation and a microangiopathic hemolytic anemia (with fragmented red blood cells). The tumours are usually cutaneous, and therefore obvious, but the syndrome has been reported with hemangiomas of the liver or spleen. Therapy, if necessary (usually it is not) is directed primarily at the tumour.

Thrombocytopenia due to disseminated intravascular coagulation

The major problem in this disorder is the consumption of coagulation factors, although thrombocytopenia may be prolonged and require replacement therapy.

Miscellaneous causes of thrombocytopenia in newborn infants

There are numerous additional causes of thrombocytopenia which usually are not severe and are included here for completeness.

Splenomegaly causes mild thrombocytopenia in any subject, including newborns, as a result of expansion of the platelet pool. Bleeding is uncommon.

Polycythemia occurs primarily in infants who suffer from intrauterine hypoxia or are small for gestational age. The thrombocytopenia appears to parallel the increased hematocrit and is not usually associated with bleeding [66].

Light therapy for jaundice has been associated with the development of a mild thrombocytopenia, once again, unassociated with hemorrhagic disorders [95].

Chromosome disorders have been associated with the appearance of thrombocytopenia [96].

The Wiscott-Aldrich syndrome may manifest at birth. In this multisystem disorder, diminished resistance to infection is the major problem, however, a hemorrhagic diathesis occurs due to thrombocytopenia and minute platelets in the circulation.

Bleeding due to abnormalities in platelet function

Inherited. — As noted above it is unusual for congenital disorders of platelet function (e. g. thrombasthenia) to manifest in the newborn.

Acquired. — There are now several reports that aspirin therapy given to the mother interferes with platelet function in newborns [97] and may cause a mild hemorrhagic diathesis [98]. The significance of this problem is not clear at this time. Indomethacin has been used in the treatment of patent ductus arteriosus in newborns and has been associated with a bleeding diathesis [99]. Penicillin and related drugs interfere with platelet function [100]. We have observed a prolonged bleeding time in newborn infants receiving high doses of penicillin as well as the development of a mild bleeding tendency in association with such therapy [101].

REFERENCES

[1] O'BRIEN (R. T.), PEARSON (H. A.). — Physiologic anemia of the newborn infant. *J. Pediatr.*, 79, 132, 1971.
[2] BURMAN (D.), MORRIS (A. F.). — Cord hemoglobin in low birth weight infants. *Arch. Dis. Child.*, 49, 382, 1974.
[3] MOLLISON (P. L.). — *Blood Transfusion in Clinical Medicine.* Oxford, Blackwell Scientific Publications Ltd., 2nd Ed., 432, 1956.
[4] MOYLAN (F. M. B.), HERRIN (J. T.), KRISHNA-MOORTHY (K.), SHANNON (D. C.). — Inappropriate antidiuretic hormone secretion in premature infants with cerebral injury. *Am. J. Dis. Child.*, 132, 399, 1978.
[5] MOLLISON (P. L.). — *Blood Transfusion in Clinical Medicine.* Oxford, Blackwell Scientific Publications Ltd., 5th Ed., 1972.

[6] Faxelius (G.), Raye (J.), Gutberlet (R.), Swanstrom (S.), Tsiantos (A.), Dolanski (E.), Dehan (M.), Dyer (N.), Lindstrom (D.), Brill (A. B.), Stahlman (M.). — Red cell volume measurements and acute blood loss in high risk newborn infants. J. Pediatr., 90, 273, 1977.

[7] Stockman (J. A. III), Garcia (J. F.), Oski (F. A.). — Anemia of prematurity. Factors governing the erythropoietin response. N. Engl. J. Med., 296, 647, 1977.

[8] Stamey (C. C.), Diamond (L. K.). — Congenital hemolytic anemia in the newborn. Am. J. Dis. Child., 94, 616, 1957.

[9] Morton (N. E.), MacKinney (A. A.) et coll. — Genetics of spherocytosis. Am. J. Hum. Genet., 14, 170, 1962.

[10] Austin (R. F.), Desfarges (J. F.). — Hereditary elliptocytosis: an unusual presentation of hemolysis in the newborn associated with transient morphologic abnormalities. Pediatrics, 44, 196, 1969.

[11] Doxiadis (S. A.), Valaes (T.), Karaklis (A.), Starrakakis (D.). — Risk of severe jaundice in glucose-6-phosphate dehydrogenase deficiency of the newborn. Lancet, 2, 1210, 1964.

[12] Lu Tsung-Cho, Wei Huoyao, Blackwell (R. Q.). — Increased incidence of severe hyperbilirubinemia among newborn Chinese infants with G6PD deficiency. Pediatrics, 37, 994, 1966.

[13] Fessas (P.), Doxiadis (S.), Valaes (T.). — Neonatal jaundice in glucose-6-phosphate dehydrogenase-deficient infants. Br. Med. J., 2, 1359. 1962.

[14] Necheles (T.), Rai (U. S.), Valaes (T.). — The role of hemolysis in neonatal hyperbilirubinemia as reflected in carboxyhaemoglobin levels. Acta Paediatr. Scand., 65, 361, 1976.

[15] Eshgapour (E.), Oski (F. A.), Williams (M.). — The relationship of glucose-6-phosphate dehydrogenase deficiency to hyperbilirubinemia in Negro premature infants. J. Pediatr., 70, 595, 1967.

[16] Bienzle (U.), Effiong (C.), Luzzatto (L.). — Erythrocyte glucose-6-phosphate dehydrogenase deficiency (G6PD type A) and neonatal jaundice. Acta Paediatr. Scand., 65, 701, 1976.

[17] Valaes (T.), Doxiadis (S. A.), Fessas (P.). — Acute hemolysis due to naphthalene inhalation. J. Pediatr., 63, 904, 1963.

[18] Beutler (E.), Mitchell (M.). — Special modifications of the fluorescent screening method for glucose-6-phosphate dehydrogenase deficiency. Blood, 32, 816, 1968.

[19] Motulsky (A. G.), Campbell-Kraut (J. M.). — Population genetics of glucose-6-phosphate dehydrogenase deficiency of the red cell. In: Proceedings of Conference on Genetic Polymorphisms and Geographic Variations in Disease. Blumberg (B. S.) (ed.), New York, Grune and Stratton, 159, 1961.

[20] Bunn (H. F.). — Hemoglobin structure and function. In Hematology of Infancy and Childhood. Nathan (D. G.) and Oski (F. A.) (eds), Philadelphia, W. B. Saunders Co., 643, 1981.

[21] Erlandson (M. E.), Hilgartner (M.). — Hemolytic disease in the neonatal period. J. Pediat., 54, 566, 1959.

[22] Hegyi (T.), Delphin (E. S.), Bank (A.), Polin (R. A.), Bland (W. A.). — Sickle cell anemia in the newborn. Pediatrics, 60, 213, 1977.

[23] Kan (Y. W.), Forget (B. G.), Nathan (D. G.). — Gamma-beta Thalassemia: A cause of hemolytic disease of the newborn. N. Engl. J. Med., 286, 129, 1972.

[24] Stockman (J. A. III), Oski (F. A.). — Erythrocytes of the human neonate. In: Current Topics in Hematology. Piomelli (S.) and Yachnin (S.). Alan R. Liss Inc., New York, 1, 193, 1978.

[25] Lee-Potter (J. P.), Deacon-Smith (R. A.), Simpkiss (M. J.), Kamuzova (H.), Lehmann (H.). — J. Clin. Pathol., 28, 317, 1975.

[26] Minnich (V.), Cordonnier (J. K.), Williams (W. J.), Moore (C. V.). — Alpha, beta and gamma hemoglobin polypeptide chains during the neonatal period with a description of a fetal form of hemoglobin D. St. Louis. Blood, 19, 137, 1962.

[27] Schmaier (A. H.), Maurer (H. M.), Johnston (C. L.), Scott (P. B.). — Alpha thalassemia screening in neonates by mean corpuscular volume and mean corpuscular hemoglobin concentration. J. Pediatr., 83, 794, 1973.

[28] Friedman (S.), Atwater (J.), Gill (F. M.), Schwarz (E.). — Alpha thalassemia in Negro infants. Ped. Res., 8, 955, 1974.

[29] Higgs (D. R.), Pressley (L.), Clegg (J. B.), Weatherall (D. J.), Higgs (S.), Carey (P.), Sergeant (G. R.). — Detection of alpha thalassemia in Negro infants. Br. J. Haematol., 46, 39, 1980.

[30] Zipursky (A.). — Isoimmune hemolytic diseases. In: Hematology of Infancy and Childhood, Nathan, (D. G.) and Oski (F. A.). W. B. Saunders Co., Philadelphia, 50, 1981.

[31] RH Conference. — McMaster University, 1977. Vox Sang., 36, 50, 1979.

[31 a] Zipursky (A.). — The universal prevention of Rh immunization. Clin. Obstet. and Gynec., 14, 869, 1971.

[32] Desjardins (L.), Blajchman (M.). — The spectrum of ABO hemolytic disease. J. Pediatr., 95, 447, 1979.

[33] Zipursky (A.), Chintu (C.). — The quantitation of spherocytes in ABO hemolytic disease. J. Pediatr., 94, 965, 1979.

[34] Queenan (J. T.), Smith (B. D.). — Irregular antibodies in the obstetric patient. Obstet. Gynecol., 34, 767, 1969.

[35] Giblett (E. R.). — Blood group antibodies causing hemolytic disease of the newborn. Clin. Obstet. Gynecol., 7, 1044, 1964.

[36] Kasabach (H. H.), Merritt (K. K.). — Hemangioma with extensive purpura. Am. J. Dis. Child., 59, 1063, 1964.

[37] Propp (R. P.), Scharfman (W. B.). — Hemangioma-thrombocytopenia syndrome associated with microangiopathic hemolytic anemia. Blood, 28, 623, 1966.

[38] Bauer (C. R.), Fojaco (R. M.), Bancalari (L.), Fernandez-Roche (L.). — Microangiopathic hemolytic anemia and thrombocytopenia in a neonate associated with a large placental chorioangioma. Pediatrics, 62, 574, 1978.

[39] Tuffy (P.), Brown (A. K.), Zuelzer (W. W.). — Infantile pyknocytosis. A common erythrocyte abnormality of the first trimester. Am. J. Dis. Child., 98, 227, 1959.

[40] Oski (F. A.), Barness (L. A.). — Vitamin E deficiency: A previously unrecognized cause of hemolytic anemia in the premature infant. J. Pediatr., 70, 211, 1967.

[41] KEIMOWITZ (R.), DESFORGES (J. F.). — Infantile pyknocytosis. *N. Engl. J. Med.*, *273*, 1152, 1965.

[42] ZANNOS-MARIOLEA (L.), KATAMIS (C.), PADOUCIS (M.). — Infantile pyknocytosis and glucose-6-phosphate dehydrogenase deficiency. *Br. J. Haemat.*, *8*, 258, 1962.

[43] VAN DE PUTTE (I.), RENAER (M.), VERMYLEN (C.). — Counting fetal erythrocytes as a diagnostic aid in perinatal death and morbidity. *Am. J. Obstet. Gynecol.*, *114*, 850, 1972.

[44] PAI (M. K. R.), BEDRITIS (I.), ZIPURSKY (A.). — Massive transplacental hemorrhage: Clinical manifestations in the newborn. *Can. Med. Assoc. J.*, *112*, 585, 1975.

[45] RAUSEN (A. R.), SKI (M.), STRAUSS (L.). — Twin transfusion syndrome. *J. Pediatr.*, *66*, 613, 1965.

[46] TAN (K. L.), TAN (R.), TAN (S. H.), TAN (A. M.). — The twin transfusion syndrome. Clinical observations on 35 affected pairs. *Clin. Pediatr.*, *18*, 111, 1979.

[47] BOOTHBY (C. B.), SA (D. J. DE). — Massive pulmonary haemorrhage in the newborn. A changing pattern. *Arch. Dis. Child.*, *48*, 21, 1973.

[48] ABT (L.), DOWNEY (W. S. Jr.). — Melena neonatorum, the swallowed blood syndrome. *J. Pediatr.*, *47*, 6, 1955.

[49] ZIPURSKY (A.). — The erythrocytes of the newborn infant. *Semin. Hematol.*, *2*, 167, 1965.

[50] WARDROP (C. A.), HOLLAND (B. M.). — Nonphysiological anemia of prematurity. *Arch. Dis. Child.*, *53*, 855, 1978.

[51] LANZKOWSKY (P.), SALEMI (M.) et al. — Phototherapy, a note of caution. *Pediatrics*, *48*, 914, 1970.

[52] SHOJANIA (A. M.), GROSS (S.). — Folic acid deficiency and prematurity. *J. Pediatr.*, *64*, 323, 1964.

[53] HOFFBRAND (A. V.). — Folate deficiency in premature infants. *Arch. Dis. Child.*, *45*, 441, 1970.

[54] CORDANO (A.), BAERTL (J. M.) et coll. — Copper deficiency in infancy. *Pediatrics*, *34*, 324, 1964.

[55] OSKI (F. A.), BARNESS (L. A.). — Vitamin E Deficiency: a previously unrecognized cause of hemolytic anemia in the premature infant. *J. Pediatr.*, *70*, 211, 1967.

[56] MELHORN (D. K.), GROSS (S.). — Vitamin E-dependency in the premature infant. Effects of large doses of medicinal iron. *J. Pediatr.*, *79*, 569, 1971.

[57] WILLIAMS (M. L.), SHOTT (R. J.), O'NEAL (P. L.), OSKI (F. A.). — Role of dietary iron and fat on Vitamin E deficiency of infancy. *N. Engl. J. Med.*, *292*, 887, 1975.

[58] BLANCHETTE (V.), BELL (E.), NAHMIAS (C.), GARNETT (S.), MILNER (R.), ZIPURSKY (A.). — A randomized control trial of Vitamin E therapy in the prevention of anemia in low birth weight infants. *Pediatr. Res.*, *14*, 591, 1980.

[59] HUMBERT (J. R.), ABELSON (H.), HATHAWAY (W. E.), BATTAGLIA (F. C.). — Polycythemia in small for gestational age infants. *J. Pediatr.*, *75*, 812, 1969.

[60] WEINBERGER (M. M.), OLEINICK (A.). — Congenital marrow dysfunction in Down's Syndrome. *J. Pediatr.*, *77*, 273, 1970.

[61] KLEBE (J. G.), INGOMAR (C. J.), NORGAARD-PEDERSEN (B.). — Blood volumes in premature infants of diabetic and non-diabetic mothers, correlated with the time clamping of the umbilical cord. *Acta Paediatr. Scand.*, *61*, 549, 1972.

[62] MICHAEL (A. F. Jr.), MAUER (A. M.). — Maternal-fetal transfusion as a cause of plethora in the neonatal period. *Pediatrics*, *28*, 458, 1961.

[63] PHILIPS, ALISTAIR (G. S.), YEE (A. B.) et al. — Placental transfusion as an intrauterine phenomenon in deliveries complicated by fœtal distress. *Brit. Med. J.*, *2*, 11, 1969.

[64] WEINBERGER (M. M.), OLEINICK (A.). — Neonatal polycythemia. *Clin. Res.*, *29*, 209, 1971.

[65] GROSS (G. P.), HATHAWAY (W. F.), McGAUGHEY (H. R.). — Hyperviscosity in the neonate. *J. Pediatr.*, *82*, 1004, 1973.

[66] HENRIKSSON (P.). — Hyperviscosity of the blood and haemostasis in the newborn infant. *Acta Paediatr. Scand.*, *68*, 701, 1979.

[67] ZIPURSKY (A.), JABER (H. M.). — The haematology of bacterial infections in newborn infants. *Clin. Hematol.*, *7*, 175, 1978.

[68] GOLDBLUM (S. E.), REED (W. P.), SOPHER (R. L.), PALMER (D. L.). — Pneumococcus-induced granulocytopenia and pulmonary leukostasis in rabbits. *J. Lab. Clin. Med.*, *97*, 278, 1981.

[69] LALEZARI (P.), RADEL (E.). — Neutrophil specific antigens: Immunology and clinical significance. *Semin. Hematol.*, *11*, 281, 1971.

[70] HOLLAND (W.), DOLL (R.), CARTER (C. O.). — The mortality from leukemia and other cancers among patients with Down's syndrome and among their parents. *Br. J. Cancer*, *16*, 178, 1962.

[71] WEINSTEIN (H. J.). — Congenital leukaemia and the neonatal myeloproliferative disorders associated wtih Down's syndrome. *Clin. Haematol.*, *7*, 147, 1978.

[72] JOHNSTON (M.), ZIPURSKY (A.). — Microtechnology for the study of the blood coagulation system in newborn infants. *Can. J. Med. Technol.*, *42*, Issue 6, 133, 1980.

[73] HATHAWAY (W. E.), BONNAR (J.). — *Perinatal Coagulation*. Grune and Stratton Inc., New York, 1978.

[74] DAM (H.), DUGGVE (H.), LARSEN (H.), PLUM (P.). — The relation of Vitamin K deficiency to Hemorrhagic Disease of the Newborn. *Adv. Paedr.*, *5*, 129, 1952.

[75] SUTHERLAND (J. M.), GLUECK (H. I.), GLESER (G.). — Hemorrhagic disease of the newborn. Breast feeding as a necessary factor in the pathogenesis. *Am. J. Dis. Child.*, *113*, 524, 1967.

[76] MALIA (R. G.), PRESTON (F. E.), MITCHELL (V. E.). — Evidence against Vitamin K deficiency in normal neonates. *Thromb. Haemost.*, *44*, 159, 1980.

[77] VAN DOORM (J. M.), MULLER (A. D.), HEMKER (H. C.). — Vitamin-K deficiency in the newborn. *Lancet*, *1*, 852, 1977.

[78] GOBEL (U.), SONNENSCHEIN-KOSENOW (S.), PETRICH (C.), VON VOSS (H.). — Vitamin-K deficiency in the newborn. *Lancet*, *2*, 187, 1977.

[79] MORI (P. G.), BISOGNI (C.), ODINO (S.), TONINE (G. P.), BOERI (E.), SERRA (G.), ROMANO (C.). — Vitamin-K deficiency in the newborn. *Lancet*, *2*, 188, 1977.

[80] VEST (M.). — Vitamin K in medical practice: pediatrics. *Vitam. Horm.*, *24*, 649, 1963.

[81] BLEYER (W. A.), SKINNER (A. L.). — Fetal neonatal hemorrhage after maternal anticonvulsant therapy. *J. Am. Med. Assoc.*, *235*, 626, 1976.

[82] GOLDMAN (H. I.), DEPOSITO (F.). — Hypoprothrombinemic bleeding in young infants. *Am. J. Dis. Child.*, *111*, 430, 1966.

[83] MINFORD (A. M. B.), EDEN (O. B.). — Haemorrhage responsive to Vitamin K in a 6 week old infant. *Arch. Dis. Child.*, *54*, 310, 1979.

[84] ZIPURSKY (A.), DE SA (D.), HSU (E.), JOHNSTON (M.), MILNER (R.). — Clinical and laboratory diagnosis of hemostatic disorder in newborn infants. *Am. J. Ped. Hem. Onc.*, *1*, 217, 1979.

[85] GILL (F. M.). — Transfusion therapy for coagulation disorders in the newborn infant. In SHERWOOD (W. C.) and COHEN (A.).: *Transfusion Therapy*, Masson Publishing, USA, Inc., New York, 75, 1980.

[86] KUNZER (W.). — Die Blutgerrinung bei Neuegeborenen und Ihre Störungen. *Wien. Klin. Wchnschr.*, *80*, 159, 1968.

[87] CROIZAT (P.), REVOL (L.), FAVRE-GILLY (J.), THOUVEREZ (J. P.), BELLEVILLE (J.). — Les hémorragies néonatales dans les diethèses hémorragiques congénitales. *Nouv. Rev. Franc. Hemat.*, *4*, 181, 1964.

[88] JONES (R. W.), ASHER (M. I.), RUTHERFORD (C. J.), MUNRO (H. M.). — Autoimmune (idiopathic) thrombocytopenic purpura in pregnancy and the newborn. *Br. J. Obstet. Gynaecol.*, *84*, 679, 1977.

[89] SCOTT (J. R.), CRUICKSHANK (D. R.), KOCHENOUR (N. K.), PITKIN (R. M.), WARENSKI (J. C.). — Fetal platelet counts in the mana ement of immunologic thrombocytopenic purpura. *Am. J. Obstet. Gynecol.*, *136*, 495, 1980.

[90] PEARSON (H. A.), SHULMAN (N. R.), MARDER (V. S.). — Isoimmune neonatal thrombocytopenic purpura. Clinical and therapeutic considerations. *Blood*, *23*, 154, 1964.

[91] KELTON (J. G.), BLANCHETTE (V. S.), WILSON (W. E.), POWERS (P.), PAI (K. R. M.), EFFER (S. B.), BARR (R. D.). — Neonatal thrombocytopenia due to passive immunization. *N. Engl. J. Med.*, *302*, 1401, 1980.

[92] MAUER (A. M.), DE VAUX (W.), LAKEY (M. E.). — Neonatal and maternal thrombocytopenia due to quinine. *Pediatrics*, *19*, 84, 1957.

[93] SCOTT (S.), REIMERS (H. J.), CHERNESKY (M. A.), GREENBERG (J. P.), KINLOUGH-RATHBONE (R. L.) PACKHAM (M. A.), MUSTARD (J. F.). — Effect of viruses on platelet aggregation and platelet survival in rabbits. *Blood*, *52*, 47, 1978.

[94] BROUGH (A. J.), JONES (D.), PAGE (R. H.), MIZUKAMI (I.). — Dermal erythropoiesis in neonatal infants. *Pediatrics*, *40*, 627, 1967.

[95] MAURER (H. M.), FRATKIN (M.), MCWILLIAMS (N. B.), KIRKPATRICK (B.), DRAP (D.), HAGERGINS (J.), HUNTER (C. R.). — Effects of phototherapy on platelet counts in low birthweight infants and on platelet production and life span in rabbits. *Pediatrics*, *57*, 506, 1976.

[96] THÜRING (W.), TÖNZ (O.). — Neonatale Thrombozytenwerte bei Kindern mit Down-Syndrom und anderen autosomalen Trisomien. *Helv. Paediatr. Acta*, *34*, 545, 1979.

[97] CORBY (D. G.), SCHULMAN (I.). — The effects of antenatal drug administration on aggregations of platelets of newborn infants. *J. Pediatr.*, *79*, 307, 1971.

[98] BLEYER (W. A.), BRECKENRIDGE (R. T.). — Studies on the detection of adverse drug reactions in the newborn. II. The effects of prenatal aspirin on newborn hemostasis. *J. Am. Med. Assoc.*, *213*, 2049, 1970.

[99] FRIEDMAN (Z.), WHITMAN (V.). — Indomethacin disposition in premature infants: bleeding due to platelet dysfunction after single doses of indomethacin. *Pediatr. Res.*, *12*, 405, 1978.

[100] BROWN (C. H. III), BRADSHAW (M. W.). — Defective platelet function following the administration of penicillin compounds. *Blood*, *47*, 949, 1976.

[101] VENTURELLI (J.), ZIPURSKY (A.). — Unpublished observations.

[102] BLANCHETTE (V.), ZIPURSKY (A.). — Unpublished observations.

[103] OSKI (F. A.), NAIMAN (J. L.). — *Hematologic Problems in the Newborn*. W. B. Saunders, Co., 2nd Ed., 1972.

[104] BESSIS (M.). — *Red cell shapes*. An illustrated classification and its rationale. Red cell shape. Physiology, Pathology, Ultrastructure. M. BESSIS, R. I. WEED and P. F. LEBLOND (eds). Springer Verlag, New York, 1-25, 1973.

34

Neonatal oncology

Danièle OLIVE
Pierre BORDIGONI and Elisabeth LEMOINE

Introduction, incidence, epidemiology

INTRODUCTION

Malignant diseases are relatively uncommon in newborn infants, and generally show the same distribution and histological features as in older children. Nevertheless we consider this separate chapter to be important, for the following reasons:

Epidemiologic: the congenital, or very early post-natal, occurrence of cancer, sometimes in association with malformations, make it an excellent model for the study of (*a*) *genetic factors* responsible for a cancer or a predisposing state, and, (*b*) *oncogenic and/or teratogenic agents*, whether physical, chemical, or infectious, which may have damaged the parental germinal cells, or the developing fœtus.

Pathologic: in the neonatal period, malignant proliferations must be distinguished from certain dysplastic states (abnormalities of differentiation or proliferation) which may themselves be pre-malignant.

Clinical and therapeutic: the spontaneous regression or maturation of certain tumors is a pheno-menon peculiar to infancy. Current research is concerned with identifying the mechanisms involved, so as to adapt treatment to the anomalies of cellular behaviour and minimise short and long-term harm to the patient.

Despite a generally favourable prognosis, based on Bolande's concept [16] of the relative "*benignity*" of neonatal tumours, tumour behaviour is some-times identical with that observed in older children. The prognostic factors are not yet clearly defined.

It is impossible to over-emphasise *the risks* incurred by the too rigid application in neonates, *of therapeutic protocols* used for infants and older children. *Chemotherapy* may cause serious (and sometimes rapidly fatal) complications, because of the neonate's poor haematological, gastrointestinal, and neurological tolerance. It is recommended that the usual dosages of drugs be reduced by 25 to 75 %. *Radiotherapy* is only rarely used, because of its immediate and late complications. The choice of energies, volume irradiated, fields, and dose delivered depends primarily on the age of the infant.

Finally, *surgical treatment* of a neonatal tumour must be undertaken by a paediatric surgeon who is experienced not only in neonatal surgery, but also in paediatric oncology. At this age, surgery has a major, and often unique, place in the diagnosis and treatment of malignant tumours. This may involve emergency surgery (for example in large cephalic or sacrococygeal teratomata), but in other cases the surgeon must know when to defer his operation, or plan it in stages. All biopsies and excisions must be done in close collaboration with the pathologist; who should receive all the excised tissue, well orientated, kept at a suitable temperature, and placed in appropriate fixatives for light and electron microscopy; and if necessary for immunological and biochemical studies.

Although the diagnosis of neonatal malignancy may easily be made in a neonatal unit, it is desirable that the immediate and long term management be undertaken by a multidisciplinary paediatric oncology team, preferably based in a children's hospital with facilities for medical and surgical intensive care of the newborn [49].

INCIDENCE

According to the Childhood Tumor Register established in Manchester in 1954, based on a stable, homogenous population of 1 million subjects *under the age of 15 years*, the mean annual incidence of cancer in childhood is 1 new case in 10,000 children [72].

In Europe and the USA [72, 138], leukaemias account for 30 to 35 % of all malignancies, followed by cerebral tumours (20 %), lymphomas (15 %), neuroblastomas (10 %), nephroblastomas (8 to 10 %) and embryonic sarcomas (10 %).

Published studies have yielded various estimates of the frequency of malignant tumours in *the first month of life* [6, 7, 12, 43, 132]. The study of Fraumeni and Miller [43] published in 1969, was based on the examination of 21,659 death certificates of children under 15 years of age dying of cancer between 1960 and 1964. 130 (0,6 %) of these were less than 28 days old, the total deaths from cancer at this age being 6.24 per million live births. The commonest cause of death from cancer was leukaemia (33.9 %), followed by neuroblastomas (20.8 %), sarcomas (9.2 %), hepatic tumours (7 %), teratomas (6.9 %), Wilms tumours (6.9 %), cerebral tumours (5.4 %), and other tumours (9.2 %).

According to the report of the British Paediatric Pathology Society published in 1978 [7] the incidence of benign and malignant tumours diagnosed during the first month of life is between 1 in 12,500 and 1 in 17,300 births. In this study, based on clinical and histological records, benign and malignant teratomas are the most frequent (24 %) followed closely by neuroblastomas (23 %), then soft tissue sarcomas (8 %), Wilms tumours and mesoblastic nephromas (7 %), cerebral tumours (6 %), leukaemias (6 %), and finally miscellaneous tumours (5 %) (histiocytosis X, haemangiomatosis, hepatoblastoma, retinoblastoma).

The Third National Cancer Survey compared the true incidence and the mortality from cancers in the first month and the first year of life. This study, undertaken between 1969 and 1971, was based on the collection of clinical, biochemical and histological data [6]. The annual incidence of neonatal cancers was estimated at 36.5 per million live-births, or 1 case in 27,400 births. This figure is clearly lower than that of the British study, which included both benign and malignant tumours.

In children under 12 months (including neonates) the incidence of cancer is 6 times greater than in the neonatal period (183.4 cases per year per million live-births), but the relative incidence of different types is the same; in the newborn it is as follows: neuroblastoma (21 cases out of 39), leukaemias (5 in 39), renal tumours (5 in 39), sarcomas (4 in 39), other tumours (4 in 39). There is a slightly higher incidence in males (35 % more than in females) and in white races (28 % more than in Blacks).

EPIDEMIOLOGY

Half of neonatal cancers are discovered on the first day of life and 2/3 during the first week [6]. This suggests that genetic factors, and physical, chemical and infectious agents may be responsible for lesions of the parental germinal cells or for damage to the fetus, either direct or transplacental [10, 77, 99, 108]. In this context, the role of the obstetrician and neonatologist is three fold:

— for genetic counselling they must know the mode of transmission of the hereditary cancers and of conditions predisposing to cancer;
— they can contribute to the detection and prevention of cancers induced by the physical and chemical agents used in pregnant women and newborn babies;
— finally, they must participate in the immediate and long term surveillance of children born after cure of a parental cancer.

We will discuss in turn, genetically determined cancers, the oncogenic role of environmental factors liable to damage the fetus in utero; and finally the question of pregnancy, and of the off-spring of patients being treated for, or considered cured of cancer.

Hereditary cancers
(10, 39, 58, 108)

They are transmitted as an autosomal dominant.

The cancer may be the essential manifestation of the mutant gene. — Apart from certain cancers of the alimentary tract often associated with polyposis, the best example is *retinoblastoma*. 40 % of retinoblastomas are hereditary. They may be familial or sporadic, unilateral or more commonly bilateral and sometimes multifocal. They present early. Penetrance is high (80-90 %). 60 % of retinoblastomas are not hereditary and these are always unilateral [17, 39, 46].

The mutant gene can be situated on the long arm of chromosome 13 in relation to a deletion whose importance determines the severity of the malformations sometimes associated; microcephaly, mental retardation, hypertelorism, abnormalities of the maxilla, aplasia of the thumb [28, 68, 113]. This mutant gene also predisposes to the occurrence of other tumours, in 5 % of cases (osteosarcoma in irradiated areas, leukaemia). Knudson's *theory of carcinogenesis* [67, 69] was based on data obtained from the study of retinoblastomas. According to this theory, the appearance of a tumour requires at least 2 mutational events. The first mutation predisposes the cell to cancer, and the second mutation triggers off the proliferation. *In hereditary forms*, the first mutation is prezygotic and is transmitted to all the fetal germinal and somatic cells; the second mutation is somatic, affecting only the retinal cells. This appears to be confirmed by the early presentation and multifocal nature of these tumours. *In the non-hereditary forms*, both mutations are somatic. Other theories involve the concepts of delayed mutation [54] and of genetically transmitted resistance to tumour formation [84].

The importance of genetic counselling in retinoblastoma must be emphasized. This should take account of the age at diagnosis, whether the tumour is unilateral or bilateral, the number of tumour sites and, above all, the family tree after ophtalmological examination of the family [17]. In bilateral forms, sporadic or familial, 40 to 50 % of the descendants are likely to be affected. Even in unilateral and apparently sporadic forms, some cases are hereditary, which accounts for the 8 to 10 % transmission in

these cases. Genetic counselling is sometimes difficult when cases are recorded in distant relatives.

Knudson and Strong's theory probably applies to other embryonic tumours of childhood. 30-35 % of nephroblastomas should be inherited, with a 60 % penetrance. The descendants of patients successfully treated for bilateral nephroblastomas will perhaps confirm this [69]. Similarly 20-30 % of neuroblastomas may be hereditary, with a penetrance of 50-60 % [70].

There may be a systemic disorder characterised by abnormalities of development and by cancers which are often multiple. — This applies to: (I) *Basal-cell naevomatosis*, in which-cell epitheliomas and medulloblastomas may be associated with numerous abnormalities; bony, neurological, cutaneous, ovarian. (II) *Poly-endocrine adenomatosis* or *apudomas*, of which the 3 types (Werner's, Sipple's, and Gorlin's syndromes) differ occording to the nature of the benign and malignant endocrine tumours, and the associated malformations [8]. (III) *Neurocutaneous melanosis*.

Hereditary preneoplastic syndromes

These constitute a state predisposing to cancer.

Phakomatoses (transmitted as an autosomal dominant):

Von Recklinghausen's disease is a systemic neurocristopathy, transmitted as an autosomal dominant with strong penetrance and variable expression, affecting 1 in 3,000 people. The tumours are usually benign, but their functional prognosis may be poor (e. g. gliomas of the optic pathways or spinal tumours). Apart from neurofibrosarcomas and malignant schwannomas, neuroblastomas and rhabdomyosarcomas have been described [82]. About 30 cases of leukaemia have also been reported, mainly chronic myeloid and myelomonocytic, as well as three transient leukaemoid states [5].

Cerebral tumours (gliomas, ependymomas) and cardiac rhabdomyosarcomas are found in 1 to 3 % of patients with Bourneville's *tuberous sclerosis*, whereas cutaneous tumours (lipomas, haemangiomas, fibromas, adenoma sebaceum) do not degenerate.

Apart from haemangioblastomas of the retina and the central nervous system, *Von Hippel Lindau's disease* may be complicated by pheochromocytomas and ependymomas.

There is a small risk of malignancy in *multiple exostoses* (5 to 10 % chrondrosarcomas), and in the *Peutz-Jegher syndrome* 5 to 10 % develop ovarian cancers.

Genodermatoses. — We will concentrate mainly on xeroderma pigmentosum, an autosomal recessive condition, which may be complicated after exposure of the skin to ultraviolet light, by prickle cell and basal cell epitheliomas, melanomas, and occasionally sarcomas. Genotypic and phenotypic heterogeneity is attested to by the variability of the enzymatic defects, which hinder the repair of DNA altered by ultraviolet rays. Prenatal diagnosis is possible. These patients have increased susceptibility to neoplastic transformation induced by the SV 40 virus, and also to chromosomal breakages and exchanges between sister chromatids on exposure to physical (radiation) or chemical (Cyclophosphamide) agents.

Chromosome-breakage-syndromes [44]. — These are essentially represented by Fanconi's syndrome, Bloom's syndrome and ataxia-telangiectasia, which are transmitted as autosomal recessives. This instability is also described in basal-cell naevomatosis, Incontinentia pigmenti, scleroderma, progeria and congenital dyskeratosis.

In Fanconi's disease various malformations are associated with a progressive marrow aplasia, and, in 10-15 % cases, with leukaemias or hepatic tumours. The risk of cancer is also increased in heterozygotes.

Bloom's syndrome is characterized by dwarfism, telangiectatic erythema of the face with photosensitivity, and a risk of cancer in 20 % of cases (half being leukaemia).

In ataxia-telangiectasia, the risk of malignancy (8-10 % have leukaemias and lymphomas) is related to disorders of cellular differentiation, the immune deficiency (thymic dysplasia), and chromosomal instability.

In these 3 conditions, apart from spontaneous chromosomal instability, in vitro studies have shown an increased susceptibility to acquired chromosomal or chromatid breakages and rearrangements, exchange of material between chromatid sisters and partial endo-reduplications, provoked by radiation and alkylating agents [28, 126, 133].

Certain congenital immune defects are complicated by lymphomas and leukaemias, and more rarely by epitheliomas, cerebral tumours and mesenchymatous tumours. Spector et al. have recorded 257 cases in a World Register between 1947 and 1977 [128].

Among the congenital immune deficiencies, the greatest risk of cancer occurs in the Wiskott-Aldrich syndrome (15 %), then in ataxia-telangiectasia (10 %), Chediak-Higashi syndrome, and IgA deficiency; to these must be added the X linked lympho-proliferative syndrome, with abnormal sensitivity to Epstein-Barr virus [48].

Certain metabolic diseases causing liver damage may lead to the development of hepatocarcinomas and hepatoblastomas. This applies to tyrosinosis [134], the glycogenoses, galactosemia, Wilson's disease, alpha-1-antitrypsin deficiency [8], hypermethioninaemia, and Fabry's disease.

Twin studies

The same condition affecting two monozygotic twins is clearly in favour of the role of genetic factors [85, 92]. Thus, in leukaemia, when one twin is affected in the first year of life, the risk for the other twin is very high, approaching 100 %, the risk diminishes progressively with age, to disappear at the age of seven.

Familial susceptibility
[10, 19, 33, 41, 51, 58, 76, 77, 80, 86, 89, 105, 108, 111]

"Cancer families" are well described; sometimes the same type of cancer has developed in several members of the family (for example: cancer of the breast, the digestive tract, leukaemia), sometimes the cancers are different and occasionally multiple, for example: cerebral tumours associated with skeletal tumours, soft tissue sarcomas, and Hodgkin's disease. The existence of biological markers, such as carcino-embryonic antigen, or of a chromosomal abnormality, or the recognition of a defect in DNA repair, could permit identification of subjects at risk [19, 34].

The risks of a second cancer developing in the same sibship is 1 in 100 according to Schweisguth [121]; 38 cases in 5,000 were reported by Li [86]. Draper considers that the risk is twice that for a control population [26]. However, the risk is so small that parents should not be dissuaded from having further children.

Cancers and malformations

Chromosomal aberrations. — In Down syndrome, whether a free trisomy 21, a translocation or a mosaic, the risk of acute leukaemia is multiplied 15-20 times; this is myeloblastic in type in 60 % of cases. Transitory neonatal leucoblastoses are also described, resulting from a disorder of regulation of hematopoiesis. Mongolism also predisposes to other tumours: — renal, ocular and cerebral [91, 137].

We have already mentioned the association between *chromosome 13 deletion and retinoblastoma*; the extent of psychomotor retardation and of malformations, depends on the size of the deletion. It is one of the rare tumours where the study of the karyotype may be used for genetic counselling in sporadic forms, identifying subjects at risk [38, 68, 139].

There appears to be a parallel in the recent description [19 b] of an autosomal translocation between chromosomes 3 and 8, associated with *familial renal disorders* (carcinomas and cysts).

Finally, a few cases of *Wilms' tumours* have been found to be associated with unequivocal chromosomal anomalies: (47, 18+), (47, 8+), (46, 11 p⁻); in the latter, the tumour is associated with aniridia [113].

Klinefelter's syndrome predisposes to breast cancer and to leukaemias.

In patients with *mixed gonadal dysgenesis* (phenotype female, gonadal atresia; genotype 46, XY or 45, X/46, XY) there is an increased risk of gonadoblastomas (arising from germinal cells, interstitial cells and/or Sertoli granulosa cells) and of endometrial carcinoma. The risk is principally related to the presence of the Y chromosome, and increases with age, to reach more than 50 % after 30 years. This makes early removal of the gonads necessary in these patients [24, 65, 99].

Congenital aniridia. — The incidence of aniridia is 1.8 per 100,000 births, and 1.1 to 1.4 % in patients with nephroblastoma. Classically it occurs sporadically, and is associated with various malformations: cataract, anomalies of the ears, microcephaly, neurological and growth retardation, urogenital disorders, and, in some cases, 11 p⁻ deletion [27, 42, 139].

In a pair of monozygous twins with aniridia, the occurrence of nephroblastoma in only one of them supports Knudson and Strong's theory: — a parental germinal mutation is responsible for the aniridia and predisposes to nephroblastoma; a second somatic mutation is responsible for the development of the tumour [85].

Growth disorders. — *Hemihypertrophy* is associated with nephroblastoma, tumours of the adrenal cortex, hepatoblastoma and pheochromocytoma [87, 90, 120]. Hamartomas, abnormalities of pigmentation and multilocular renal cysts are frequently found, either in the patient or his family.

The same tumours are found in *Wiedeman-Beckwith syndrome* (gigantism with visceromegaly). The risk increases from 10 to 25 % when there is associated hemihypertrophy [127].

In ectopic testes the incidence of tumours is increased 30 to 40 times.

Some cancers have been reported in **various malformation syndromes**: — leukaemias in Schwachman's syndrome [6], leukaemias in Rubinstein-Taybi's syndrome [61], tumours of the liver with cerebral gigantism, renal tumours and teratomas in urogenital and/or vertebral malformations, leukaemia in Poland's syndrome, and tumours associated with cerebral malformations.

The association between malformations and tumours, in the same patient or in his family is interesting as it may make earlier diagnosis of the tumours possible. It also demonstrates the links which exist between teratogenesis and oncogenesis and the interaction of genetic with environmental factors. This can be demonstrated in certain experimental models, such as the opossum. As the young opossum lives for 2 months in his mother's marsupial pouch, it is accessible to the effect of chemical agents such as nitroso-ureas, which can induce urogenital malformations, hamartomas and malignant embryonic tumours [60].

The role of environmental factors

Ionizing radiation (diagnostic radiation, radioactive fall-out). — According to the retrospective study published in 1956 by Stewart et al. the risk of developing cancer before the age of 10 is multiplied by 2 after antenatal irradiation [130]. This agrees with the conclusion of MacMahon [83] and of a recent prospective study [124]. However, the analysis of a subsequent prospective study (Oxford Childhood Cancer Survey) showed only a slight increase in the number of cancers found in children after irradiation in utero, the risk being calculated as 0.5 % for a radiation dose of 2 rads [14, 66, 129]. It must also be pointed out that the children irradiated in utero in Hiroshima and Nagasaki have not been found to have an increased risk of cancer [101].

Chemical agents. — Medication, accidental or occupational exposure to certain chemical agents [40, 58, 94, 100, 116].

Numerous animal experiments have demonstrated the possibility of induction of cancers by carcinogenic substances transmitted transplacentally or in the mother's milk [62]. These tumours may even be transmitted to succeeding generations. In man, diethylstilbestrol is the prime example of transplacental carcinogenesis. Other drugs, notably diphenylhydantoin, are under suspicion.

The carcinogenic effect of diethylstilbestrol (DES) has been known in the mouse since 1963 and was suggested in man in 1971 by Herbst [2, 53]. He found an increased incidence of vaginal adenocarcinoma in girls aged 13 to 25, whose mothers had been treated with DES before the 18th week of pregnancy. The register of these tumours showed that the risk remained small (1 °/$_{oo}$) compared with the incidence of vaginal adenoses induced by DES; 50 % of adenocarcinomas developed from this pre-existing dysplasia which is recognised as a precursor. It is interesting to note that cancers and malformations (vaginal adenosis, uterine hypoplasia, and also epididymal cysts, micropenis, testicular hypoplasia) arise from the exposure to the drug in the same period [13, 55].

In adults and older children, *Diphenylhydantoin (DPH)* is responsible for immunologic disorders and benign or malignant lympho-proliferative syndromes. There have been 6 recent reports of malignant tumours occuring in patients whose mothers received DPH during pregnancy. Apart from one malignant mesenchymoma diagnosed at 18 years of age [15] and one extra-renal Wilms' tumor [130 b], the other 4 tumours were all neuroblastomas, diagnosed at 36 months [106], 7 days [123], 35 months [122], and 1 day of age [3]. Only the first case died. The malformations due to DPH were present and in one case there was also fetal alcohol syndrome [122]. The carcinogenic, mutagenic and teratogenic action of DPH may be related to intermediate metabolites, the epoxides, or to an alteration of folic acid metabolism. Nevertheless, these facts must be interpreted with caution; they may be due to coincidence or the interaction of various factors e. g. the epilepsy itself or other drugs [45, 50, 116 135].

Immunosuppressive drugs given to a pregnant woman after the second trimester can induce immunologic defects in the foetus [21]; a carcinogenic effect has not yet been reported.

Hepatoblastoma has been reported following the taking of *oral contraceptives* during the first trimester of pregnancy [104]. This is similar to the benign and malignant hepatic tumours which have been described after treatment with œstrogens and androgens in children and adults [88].

It is possible that *maternal alcoholism and cigarette smoking* may have a predisposing role adding to other factors [30, 59, 63]. Finally, we should consider the possible carcinogenic role of substances such as *vinyl chloride* in the working environment of pregnant women.

Viruses. — A number of inconclusive studies have attempted to establish a relationship between maternal viral infections and cancer in the child; influenza and leukaemias, chicken pox and cerebral tumours [2, 32, 47, 73, 112].

CANCER AND PREGNANCY

We will discuss the two problems which interest the paediatrician and the obstetrician: the risk to the foetus in the case of active cancer in the mother; and advice about embarking on pregnancy to a patient who has been "cured" of cancer.

Fœtal risk in maternal cancer

Early data emphasized the high incidence of spontaneous abortion, and of fœtal distress. With modern means of surveillance, some of these high-risk pregnancies can result in the birth of normal infants, but the mother's chances of survival should not be prejudiced by therapeutic abstinence.

Materno-fœtal transmission of cancer. — The placenta is an effective barrier, so that there is only a very small risk of tumour being transmitted to the foetus by placental metastasis and invasion of the chorionic villi, unless there is an abnormality of placental permeability, or an immune deficit [109, 110].

With respect to *solid tumours*, Potter and Schoeneman [107], in a review of the literature in 1970, found 24 untreated maternal cancers (all metastatic) transmitted to the placenta (examined in 18 cases) and/or the fœtus.

There were 11 cases of melanoma. 8 infants were born with disseminated cancer (7 melanomas and 1 lymphoma); 2 of whom survived after regression of the tumour. 11 infants were unaffected. 6 died of fœtal distress.

Placental choriocarcinoma, despite its trophoblastic origin, only rarely spreads to the fœtus: in

9 cases collected by Kalifa et al., death was always noted [64]. Diagnosis in the fœtus may sometimes lead to the discovery of the mother's tumour (by measurement of beta HCG).

"Transmission" of *acute lymphoblastic leukaemia* has been reported in 2 cases, detected in the infant some months after birth [11, 22].

Fœto-maternal transmission of cancer. — This situation has not been observed, despite extension to the fœtal villi of neonatal neuroblastomas and metastatic malignant melanomas. However, Kremp et al. have reported a case of neonatal malignant histiocytosis which led to detection of a partial myeloblastosis in the mother, preceding by 4 months the development of an acute myeloblastic leukaemia [71].

Therapeutic risk. — This problem arises, either when a cancer is discovered during pregnancy, or when a woman becomes pregnant on maintenance chemotherapy. Sterility is not invariable. We have encountered this situation several times in adolescents being treated for leukaemia.

(1) *Risks of irradiation.* — Apart from the carcinogenic risk (cf. p. 722), irradiation may cause death of the products of conception, disorders of growth and development, sterility, and genetic mutations. The effects of irradiation on the fœtus are well known from animal experimentation and from the study of survivors of atomic explosions. The risk of death is greatest at the pre-implantation stage. During organogenesis the risks are of cerebral malformations (microcephaly), and ocular and skeletal malformations. Later irradiation affects fœtal development [98, 131, 197]. Consequently, radiotherapy must be avoided during the first trimester. Mediastinal, and, a fortiori, cervical irradiation become possible later.

The minimum dose liable to result in malformations is difficult to define, but it is reasonable to offer abortion if the gravid uterus has received a single dose of 10 rads. In relation to this, we point out that the dose received during a radiological examination (which sometimes occurs at the beginning of an unrecognised pregnancy) is usually less than 5-10 rads.

The administration of ^{131}I is contra-indicated during pregnancy and breast feeding; destruction of the thyroid occurs from the third month of gestation [117].

(2) *Risks of antimitotic chemotherapy.* — All antimitotics must be avoided during the first tri-

mester. They may be administered during the 3rd trimester, but during the second, disorders may develop [20, 25, 31, 102, 103, 115, 116, 118, 125]. They inhibit cellular multiplication and alter the integrity of the cellular genome by mutagenic effects.

The risk depends on placental permeability, the physico-chemical properties of the drugs (substances diffuse more easily if of molecular weight less than 600, if fat-soluble, and if they have a high dissociation constant) and fœtal pharmacokinetics.

Although the results of animal experiments cannot always be extrapolated to humans, it is safe to say that the greatest risk is associated with *folate antagonists* (administration of methotrexate between the 3rd and 8th weeks of pregnancy causes abortion or cerebral malformations in 50 % of cases). The risk is less with *alkylating agents* (nitrogen mustards, cyclophosphamide), and the pervinca alkaloids, and is unknown for antibiotics. The danger appears to be very slight with 6-mercaptopurine, chlorambucil and busulphan; however, the latter drug can sterilise the fœtal gonads [136].

It is wise to avoid administering *corticosteroids* during the first trimester unless absolutely necessary, but the risk of abortion and malformation (cleft palate) observed in animals, has not been established in man.

Offspring of patients "cured" of cancer
[9, 35]

If the treatment of cancer has permitted normal puberty, without impairing fertility [56, 74, 114], it is difficult to assess the risks to any offspring (insufficient length of follow-up, modification of therapeutic protocols).

We have already considered the *risk of transmission of a hereditary cancer, or of a predisposing state,* and have stressed the importance of genetic counselling in cases of retinoblastoma (cf. p. 720).

The risk of abortions, of malformations and of cancer in the offspring can be related to numerical or structural chromosomal abnormalities, to genetic mutations, and to defects in DNA repair, secondary to the effects of radiotherapy or chemotherapy on the parental gametes [23, 29, 36, 37, 75, 93, 94, 95, 125].

Chromosomal aberrations in somatic cells are found in 65-70 % of subjects treated with chemo and/or radiotherapy and persist for 5-10 years after cessation of treatment [28, 95, 126]; these anomalies are considered to be secondary to treatment; they may reflect individual sensitivity of the subject to the lesions induced by mutagenic agents. It is likely that similar abnormalities affect the gametes, increasing the risk of malformations or of cancers in the descendants. Nevertheless, an analysis of published data encourages cautious optimism, and overall, the percentage of malformations and abortions is comparable with that of a control population, both after irradiation [57], and after chemotherapy for placental choriocarcinoma [4, 64, 115], acute leukaemia [96], or solid tumours [35, 78].

It is possible that combined radiotherapy and chemotherapy carry a higher risk to the offspring, as is suggested, for example, after the treatment of Hodgkin's disease [57].

In conclusion, there is no formal contra-indication to pregnancy following the treatment of cancer considered "cured", except when the history or the results of investigations (spontaneous or provoked chromosomal anomalies, defects of DNA repair, transformation by SV 40 virus, biological markers) establish the likelihood of transmission either of a hereditary cancer, or of a specific sensitivity to mutagenic and oncogenic agents [28, 44, 51, 95, 126, 133, 137].

Amniocentesis may be indicated mainly in cases where somatic chromosomal abnormalities persist in either the mother or father, after cessation of treatment.

REFERENCES

[1] Advisory Committee on the biological effects of ionizing radiations: the effects on populations of exposure to low levels of ionizing radiation. *Natl. Acad. Sci. Nal. Res. Council., Washington*, D. C., 1972.

[2] ADELSTEIN (A. M.), DONOVAN (J. W.). — Malignant disease in children whose mothers had chickenpox mumps or rubella in pregnancy. *Br. Med. J.*, 4, 629, 1972.

[3] ALLEN (R. W.), BUEHLER (B.), OGDEN (B.), BENTLEY (F. G.), JUNG (A. L.). — Fetal hydantoin syndrome, neuroblastoma and hemorrhagic disease. *Pediatr. Res.*, 14, 530, 1980.

[4] AMIEL (J. L.), TURSZ (Th.), DROZ (J. P.). — Tumeurs placentaires et maternités. *Bull. Cancer*, 66, 186-188, 1979.

[5] BADER (J. L.), MILLER (R. W.). — Neurofibromatosis in childhood leukemia. *J. Pediatr.*, 92, 925-929, 1978.

[6] BADER (J. L.), MILLER (R. W.). — US cancer incidence and mortality in the first year of life. *Am. J. Dis. Child.*, 133, 157-159, 1979.

[7] BARSON (A. J.). — Congenital neoplasia: the Society's experience (Abstract). *Arch. Dis. Child.*, 53, 436, 1978.

[8] BAYLIN (S. B.). — The multiple endocrine neoplasia syndrome. Implications for the study of inherited tumors. *Semin. Oncol.*, 5, 35-45, 1978.

[9] BENDER (R. A.), YOUNG (R. C.). — Effects on cancer treatment in individual and generational genetics. *Semin. Oncol.*, 5, 47-56, 1978.

[10] BERGSMA (D.). — *Cancer and Genetics.* New York, Alan R. Liss, 12, 1976.

[11] BERNARD (J.), JACQUILLAT (Cl.), CHAVELET (F.), BOIRON (M.), STOICHKOV (Y.), TANZER (J.). — Leucémie aiguë d'une enfant de 5 mois née d'une mère atteinte de leucémie aiguë au moment de l'accouchement. *Nouv. Rev. Fr. Hématol.*, 4, 140-146, 1964.

[12] BERTOLONE (S.). — Neonatal oncology. *Pediatr. Clin. North. Amer.*, 24, 585-598, 1977.

[13] BIBBO (M.), HAENSZEL (W. M.), WIED (J. L.), HUBBY (M.), HERBST (A. L.). — A twenty-five-year follow-up study of women exposed to diethylstilbestrol during pregnancy. *N. Engl. J. Med.*, 298, 763-767, 1978.

[14] BITHELL (J. F.), STEWART (A. M.). — Prenatal irradiation and childhood malignancy: a review of Bristish data from the Oxford survey. *Br. J. Cancer*, 31, 271-287, 1975.

[15] BLATTNER (W. A.), HENSON (D. E.), YOUNG (R. C.), FRAUMENI (J. F.). — Malignant mesenchymoma and birth defect. *J. A. M. A.*, 238, 334-335, 1977.

[16] BOLANDE (R. P.). — Benignity of neonatal tumors and concept of cancer repression in early life. *Am. J. Dis. Child.*, 122, 12-14, 1971.

[17] BRIARD-GUILLEMOT (M. L.), VOINAITI-PELLIE (C.), FEINGOLD (J.), HAYE (C.), FREZAL (J.). — Le conseil génétique dans le rétinoblastome. *Ann. Ocul.*, 209, 717-723, 1976.

[18] CAPIZZI (R. L.). — Hematologic neoplasms during pregnancy. In: *Cancer Chemotherapy*, BRODSKY (I.), KAHN (B. S.) and MOYER (J. H.) Eds. New York, Grune et Stratton, 131-146, 1972.

[19] CHENG (W. S.), MULVIHILL (J. J.), GREENE (M. H.), PICKLE (L. W.), TSAI (S.), WHANG PENG (J.). — Sister chromatid exchanges and chromosomes in chronic myelogenous leukemia and cancer families. *Int. J. Cancer*, 23, 8-13, 1979.

[19 bis] COHEN (A. J.), LI (F. P.), BERG (S.). — Hereditary renal-cell carcinoma associated with a chromosomal translocation. *N. Engl. J. Med.*, 301, 592-595, 1979.

[20] COLBERT (N.), NAJMAN (A.), GORIN (N. N.), BLUM (F.), TREISSER (A.), LASFARGUES (G.), CLOUP (M.), BARRAT (H.), DUHAMEL (G.). — Leucémie aiguë au cours de la grossesse: évolution favorable de la gestation chez 2 malades traitées par chimiothérapie. *Nouv. Presse Méd.*, 9, 175-178, 1980.

[21] COTE (C. J.), MEUWISSEN (H. J.), PICKERING (R. J.). — Effects on the neonate of prednisone and azathioprine administered to the mother during pregnancy. *J. Pediatr.*, 85, 324-328, 1974.

[22] CRAMBLETT (H. G.), FRIEDMAN (J. L.), NAJJAR (C.). — Leukemia in an infant born of a mother with leukemia. *N. Engl. J. Med.*, 259, 727-729, 1958.

[23] DIATLOFF (C.), MACIEIRA-COELHO (A.). — Effect of low-dose-rate irradiation on the division potential of cells *in vitro*. V. Human skin fibroblasts from donors with a high risk of cancer. *J. Nal. Cancer Inst.*, 63, 55-59, 1979.

[24] DONAHOE (P. K.), CRAWFORD (J. D.), HENDREN (W. H.). — Mixed gonadal dysgenesis, pathogenesis, and management. *J. Pediatr. Surg.*, 14, 287-300, 1979.

[25] DONEY (K. C.), KRAEMER (K. G.), SHEPARD (T. H.). — Combination chemotherapy for acute myelocytic leukemia during pregnancy: three case reports. *Cancer Treat. Rep.*, 63, 369-371, 1979.

[26] DRAPER (G. J.), HEAF (M. M.), KINNIER-WILSON (L. M.). — Occurrence of childhood cancers among sibs and estimation of familial risks. *J. Med. Genet.*, 14, 81-90, 1977.

[27] DUTAU (G.), ZAYSSE (Ph.), RIBOT (C.), CARTON (M.), JUSKIEWENSKI (S.), ROCHICCIOLI (P.). — Le syndrome aniridie-néphroblastome. *J. Genet. Hum.*, 43, 43-54, 1976.

[28] DUTRILLAUX (B.), DUBOS (C.), VIEGAS-PEGUIGNOT (E.), BURIOT (D.). — Partial endoreduplication: a new cytogenetic anomaly possibly related to a DNA repair defect. *Ann. Genet.*, 22, 25-29, 1979.

[29] EVANS (H. J.). — Effects on ionizing radiation on mammalian chromosomes. In: *Chromosome and cancer*, GERMAN (J.) Ed. John Wiley and Sons. New York, 191, 1974.

[30] EVERSON (R. B.). — Individuals transplacentally exposed to maternal smoking may be at increased cancer risk in adult life. *Lancet*, II, 123-127, 1980.

[31] FALKSON (H. C.), SIMSONS (I. W.), FALKSON (G.). — Non Hodgkin's lymphoma in pregnancy. *Cancer*, 45, 1679-1682, 1980.

[32] FEDRICK (J.), ALBERMAN (E. D.). — Reported influenza in pregnancy and subsequent cancer in the child. *Br. Med. J.*, 2, 485-488, 1972.

[33] FEINGOLD (J.). — Génétique et cancers humains : méthodologie d'étude. *Bull. Cancer*, 65, 73-77, 1978.

[34] FELBERT (N. T.), MICHELSON (J. B.), SHIELDS (J. A.). — CEA family syndrome: Abnormal carcino-embryonic antigen (CEA) levels in asymptomatic retinoblastoma family members. *Cancer*, 37, 1397-1402, 1976.

[35] FLAMANT (F.), SCHWEISGUTH (O.). — Descendance et grossesse future chez les enfants traités pour cancer. *Bull. Cancer*, 1966, 171-176. 1979.

[36] FOREST (H. A.), NORMAN (A.), BASS (D.), OKU (C.). — Chromosome damage in infants and children after cardiac catheterization and angiocardiography. *Pediatrics*, 62, 312-316, 1978.

[37] FOX (B. W.). — DNA Repair after drugs and radiation. *Int. J. Radiat. Oncol. Biol. Phys.*, 4, 65-69, 1978.

[38] FRANCKE (U.), KUNG (F.). — Sporadic bilateral retinoblastoma and 13 *q*-chromosomal deletion. *Med. Pediat. Oncol.*, 2, 379-385, 1976.

[39] FRANÇOIS (J.), BIES (S. DE), MATTON (M.). — Genetic aspects of childhood tumours. *Acta Genet. Med. Gemellol.*, 24, 145-149, 1975.

[40] FRAUMENI (J. F.). — Chemical in human teratogenesis and transplacental carcinogenesis. *Pediatrics*, 53, 807-812, 1974.

[41] FRAUMENI (J. F.). — Multiple primary neoplasms: relationship to familial cancer. In: *Multiple Primary Malignant Tumors*, SEVERI (L.) Ed. Perugia, Perugia University. 177-184, 1975.

[42] FRAUMENI (J. F.), GLASS (A. G.). — Wilms' tumor and congenital aniridia. *J. A. M. A.*, 206, 825-828, 1968.

[43] FRAUMENI (J. F.), MILLER (R. W.). — Cancer deaths in the newborn. *Am. J. Dis. Child.*, 117, 186-189, 1969.

[44] GERMAN (J.). — Genes which increase chromosomal instability in somatic cells and predispose to cancer. In: *Progress in Medical Genetics*, STEIN-BERG (A. G.) and BEARN (A. G.) Ed. Vol. VIII, Grune et Stratton, New York, 61-101, 1972.

[45] GOLD (E.), GORDI (F. L.), TONASIA (J.), SZKLO (M.). — Increased risks of brain tumors in children exposed to barbiturates. *J. Nal. Cancer Inst.*, 61, 1031-1034, 1978.

[46] GORDON (H.). — Family studies in retinoblastoma. Birth defects: original article. *Series X*, 10, 185-190, 1974.

[47] HAKULINEN (T.), HOVI (L.), KARKININ (M.), JAASKELAINEN (M.), PENTTINEN (R.). — Association between influenza during pregnancy and childhood leukaemia. *Br. Med. J.*, 4, 265-267, 1973.

[48] HAMILTON (J. K.), PAQUIN (L. A.), SULLIVAN (J. L.), MAURER (A. H. S.), CRUSY (F. G.). — X-linked lymphoproliferative syndrome registry report. *J. Pediatr.*, 96, 669-673, 1980.

[49] HAMMOND (G. D.), BLEYER (W. A.), HARTMANN (J. R.), HAYS (D. M.), JENKIN (R. D. T.). — The team approach to the management of pediatric cancer. *Cancer*, 41, 29-35, 1978.

[50] HANSON (J. W.), MYRIANTHOPOULOS (N. C.), HARVEY (M. A.), SMITH (D. W.). — Risks to the offspring of women treated with hydantoin anticonvulsants, with emphasis on the fetal hydantoin syndrom. *J. Pediatr.*, 89, 662-668, 1976.

[51] HARRIS (C. C.), MULVIHILL (J. J.), THORGEIRSSON (S. S.), MINNA (J. D.). — Individual differences in cancer susceptibility. *Ann. Intern. Med.*, 92, 809-825, 1980.

[52] HERBST (A. L.), SCULLY (R. E.), ROBBOY (S. J.). — Prenatal diethylstilbesteal exposure and human genital tract anomalies. *J. Natl. Cancer Inst. Monogr.*, 51, 25-35, 1979.

[53] HERBST (A. L.), ULFELDER (H.), POSKANZER (D. C.). — Adenocarcinoma of the vagina. *N. Engl. J. Med.*, 284, 878-881, 1971.

[54] HERRMANN (I.). — Delayed mutation as a cause of retinoblastoma: application to genetic counseling. In: *Cancer and Genetics*, BERGSMA (D.) Ed. New York, Alan R. Liss. Inc., 79-90, 1976.

[55] HILGERS (R. D.). — Prenatal oncogenesis and the development of malignant tumors in the infant and adolescent vagina. A review and hypothesis. *Gynec. Oncol.*, 5, 262-272, 1977.

[56] HIMELSTEIN-BRAW (R.), PETERS (H.), FABER (M.). — Morphological study of the ovaries of leukaemia children. *Br. J. Cancer*, 38, 82-87, 1978.

[57] HOLMES (G. E.), HOLMES (F. F.). — Pregnancy outcome of patients treated for Hodgkin's disease. *Cancer*, 41, 1317-1322, 1978.

[58] HOOVER (R.), FRAUMENI (J. F.). — Drugs. In: *Persons at high risk of cancer. An approach to cancer etiology and control*, FRAUMENI (J. F.) Ed. New York, Academic Press, 185-198, 1975.

[59] HORNSTEIN (L.), CROW (E. C.), GRUPPO (R.). — Adrenal carcinoma in a child with history of fetal alcohol syndrome. *Lancet*, 2, 1292-1293, 1977.

[60] JERGELSKI (W.), HUDSON (P. M.), FALK (H. L.). — Embryonal neoplasms in the opossum: a new model for solid tumors of infancy and childhood. *Science*, 193, 328-331, 1976.

[61] JONAS (D. M.), HEILBRON (D. C.), ABTIN (A. R.). — Rubinstein-Taybi syndrome and acute leukemia. *J. Pediatr.*, 92, 851-852, 1978.

[62] JONES (A. H.), FANTEL (A. G.), KOCAN (R. A.), JUCHAU (H. R.). — Bioactivation of procarcinogens in mutagens in human fetal and placental tissues. *Life Sci.*, 21, 1831-1836, 1977.

[63] KAHN (A.), BADER (J. L.), HOY (G. R.), SINKS (J. F.). — Hepatoblastoma in child with fetal alcohol syndrome. *Lancet*, *1*, 1403-1404, 1979.

[64] KALIFA (C.), BRULE (F.), BAILLIF (P.), CAILLAUD (J. M.), SCHWEISGUTH (O.). — Métastases chez un nourrisson d'un choriocarcinome placentaire. *Arch. Fr. Pédiat.*, *38*, 351-352, 1981.

[65] KHODR (J. S.), CADENA (G. D.), ONG (T. C.), SILER-KHODR (T. M.). — Y-autosome translocation gonadal dysgenesis and gonadoblastoma. *Am. J. Dis. Child.*, *133*, 277-282, 1979.

[66] KNEALE (G. W.), STEWART (A. M.). — Age variation in the cancer risks from fœtal irradiation. *Br. J. Cancer*, *35*, 501-510, 1977.

[67] KNUDSON (A. G.). — Mutation and human cancer. *Adv. Cancer Res.*, *17*, 317-352, 1973.

[68] KNUDSON (A. G.), MEADOWS (A. T.), NICHOLS (W. W.), HILL (R.). — Chromosomal deletion and retinoblastoma. *N. Engl. J. Med.*, *295*, 1120-1123, 1976.

[69] KNUDSON (A. G.), STRONG (L. C.). — Mutation and cancer: a model for Wilms' tumor of the kidney. *J. Nal. Cancer Inst.*, *48*, 313-324, 1972.

[70] KNUDSON (A. G.), STRONG (L. C.). — Mutation and cancer: neuroblastoma and pheochromocytoma. *J. Hum. Genet.*, *24*, 514-532, 1972.

[71] KREMP (L.), MACART (M.), HOPFNER (C.), FLANDRIN (G.), BERNARD (J.). — Découverte simultanée d'une hémopathie maligne chez un nouveau-né et d'un syndrome préleucémique chez la mère. *Nouv. Rev. Fr. Hémat.*, *20*, 349-357, 1978.

[72] LECK (I.), BIRCH (J. M.), MARSDEN (H. B.), STEWARD (J. K.). — Methods of classifying and ascertaining children's tumors. *Br. J. Cancer*, *34*, 69-82, 1976.

[73] LECK (I.), STEWARD (J. K.). — Incidence of neoplasms in children born after influenza epidemics. *Br. Med. J.*, *4*, 631-634, 1972.

[74] LENDON (M.), HANN (I. M.), PALMER (M. K.), SHALET (S. M.), JONES (P. H. M.). — Testicular histology after combination chemotherapy in childhood for acute lymphoblastic leukaemia. *Lancet*, *2*, 439-441, 1978.

[75] LEWIS (E. B.). — Possible genetic consequences of irradiation of tumors in childhood. *Radiology*, *114*, 147-153, 1975.

[76] LI (F. P.). — Investigative approach to familial cancer: Clinical studies. In: *Genetics of Human Cancer*, MULVIHILL (J. J.), MILLER (R. W.), FRAUMENI (J. F.) Eds. Raven Press, New York, 262-280, 1977.

[77] LI (F. P.). — Host factors in the development of childhood cancer. *Semin. Oncol.*, *5*, 17-23, 1978.

[78] LI (F. P.), FINE (W.), JAFFE (N.), HOLMES (G. E.), HOLPES (F. F.). — Offspring of patients treated for cancer in childhood. *J. Nal. Cancer Inst.*, *62*, 1193-1197, 1979.

[79] LI (F. P.), FRAUMENI (J. F.). — Familial breast cancer, soft tissue sarcomas and other neoplasms. *Ann. Intern. Med.*, *83*, 833-834, 1975.

[80] LI (F. P.), TUCKER (M. A.), FRAUMENI (J. F.). — Childhood cancer in sibs. *J. Pediatr.*, *88*, 419-423, 1976.

[81] LIEBERMAN (J.), SILTON (R. M.), AGLIOZZO (C. M.), McMATHON (J.). — Hepatocellular carcinoma and intermediate alpha 1 antitrypsin deficiency (MZ phenotype). *Am. J. Clin. Pathol.*, *64*, 304-310 1975.

[82] McKEEN (E. A.), BODURTHA (J.), MEADOWS (A. T.), DOUGLASS (E. C.), MULVIHILL (J. J.). — Rhabdomyosarcoma complicating multiple neurofibromatosis. *J. Pediatr.*, *93*, 992-993, 1978.

[83] McMAHON (B.). — Prenatal X-ray exposure and childhood cancer. *J. Nal. Cancer Inst.*, *28*, 1173-1191, 1962.

[84] MATSUNAGA (E. I.). — Hereditary retinoblastoma: host resistance and age at onset. *J. Nal. Cancer Inst.*, *63*, 933-939, 1979.

[85] MAURER (H. S.), PENDERGRASS (T. W.), BORGES (W.), HONIG (G. R.). — The role of genetic factors in the etiology of Wilms' tumor. Two pairs of monozygous twins with congenital abnormalities (aniridia-hemihypertrophy) and discordance for Wilms' tumor. *Cancer*, *43*, 205-208, 1979.

[86] MEADOWS (A. T.), LI (F. P.), STRONG (L. C.), SCHWEISGUTH (O.), BAUME (S.). — Childhood cancer in siblings (abstr.). *Pediatr. Res.*, *10*, 455, 1976.

[87] MEADOWS (A. T.), LICHTENFELD (J. L.), KOOP (C. E.). — Wilms' tumor in three children of a woman with congenital hemihypertrophy. *N. Engl. J. Med.*, *291*, 23-24, 1974.

[88] MEADOWS (A. T.), NEIMANN (J. L.), VALDES-DAPENA (M.). — Hepatoma associated with androgen therapy for aplastic anemia. *J. Pediatr.*, 109-110, *84*, 1974.

[89] MEISNER (L. F.), GILBERT (E.), RIS (H. W.), HAVERTY (G.). — Genetic mechanisms in cancer predisposition. Report of a cancer family. *Cancer*, *43*, 679-689, 1979.

[90] MILLER (R. W.). — Relation between cancer and congenital defects. An epidemiologic evaluation. *J. Natl. Cancer Inst.*, *40*, 1079-1085, 1968.

[91] MILLER (R. W.). — Neoplasia and Down's syndrome. *Ann. N. Y. Acad. Sci.*, *171*, 637-644, 1970.

[92] MILLER (R. W.). — Deaths from childhood leukemia and solid tumors among twins and other sibs in the US, 1960-1967. *J. Natl. Cancer Inst.*, *46*, 203-209, 1971.

[93] MILLER (R. W.). — Radiation induced cancer. *J. Natl. Cancer Inst.*, *49*, 1221-1227, 1972.

[94] MILLER (R. W.). — The discovery of human Teratogens, Carcinogens, and Mutagens: Lessons for the Future. In: *Chemical-Mutagens*, HOLLAENDER (A.) and SERRES (F. J. DE), Eds. Plenum Publishing Corporation, 101-126, 1978.

[95] MILLER (R. W.), HILL (R. B.), NICHOLS (W. W.), MEADOWS (A. T.). — Acute and long-term cytogenetic effects of childhood cancer chemotherapy and radiotherapy. *Cancer Res.*, *38*, 3241-3246, 1978.

[96] MOE (P. J.), LETHINEN (M.), WEJELIUS (R.), FRIMAN (S.), KRUGER (A.), BERG (A.). — Progeny of survivors of acute lymphocytic leukemia. *Acta Pediat. Scand.*, *68*, 300-303, 1979.

[97] MOLE (R. H.). — Antenatal irradiation and childhood cancer: causation or coincidence? *Br. J. Cancer*, *30*, 199-208, 1974.

[98] MOLE (R. H.). — Radiation effects on pre-natal development and their radiological significance. *Br. J. Radiol.*, *52*, 89-101, 1979.

[99] MULVIHILL (J. J.), MILLER (R. W.), FRAUMENI (J. F.). — *Genetics of human cancer*. New York, Raven Press, 1977.

[100] NAPALKOV (N. P.). — Some general considerations on the problem of transplacental carcinogenesis. In: *Transplacental Carcinogenesis*, TOMATIS (L.), and

MOHR (U.) Eds. Scientific Publication, n° 4, Intern. Agency for Research in Cancer, Lyon, 1-13, 1973.

[101] NEEL (J. V.), KATO (H.), SCHULL (W. J.). — Mortality in the children of atomic bomb survivors and controls. *Genetics*, 76, 311-326, 1974.

[102] NICHOLSON (H. O.). — Cytotoxic drugs in pregnancy. Review of reported cases. *J. Obstet. Gynaecol. Brit. Commonw.*, 75, 307-312, 1968.

[103] NISHIMURA (H.), TANIMURA (T.). — *Clinical aspects of the teratogenicity of drugs*. Amsterdam, Excerpta Medica, 453, 1968.

[104] OTTEN (J.), SMEIS (R.), DE JAGER (R.). — Hepatoblastoma in an infant after contraception intake during pregnancy. *N. Engl. J. Med.*, 297, 22, 1977.

[105] PARRY (D. M.), MULVIHILL (J. J.), MILLER (R. W.), SPIEGEL (R. J.). — Sarcomas in a child and his father. An etiologic consultation. *Am. J. Dis. Child.*, 133, 130-133, 1979.

[106] PENDERGRASS (T. W.), HANSON (J. W.). — Fetal hydantoin syndrome and neuroblastoma. *Lancet*, 2, 150, 1976.

[107] POTTER (J. F.), SCHOENEMAN (M.). — Metastases of maternal cancer to the placenta and fœtus. *Cancer*, 25, 380-388, 1970.

[108] PURTILO (D. T.), PAQUIN (L.), GINDHART (T.). — Genetics of neoplasia. Impact of ecogenetics on oncogenesis. A review. *Am. J. Pathol.*, 91, 109-187, 1978.

[109] QUERLEU (D.), CAPPELAERE (P.), CREPIN (G.), DEMAILLE (A.). — *Cancers et grossesse*. Masson éd., Paris, 372, 1978.

[110] QUERLEU (D.), VASSEUR (J. J.), TRIPLET (I.), DEMAILLE (M.), CREPIN (G.), DEMAILLE (A.). — Les métastases placentaires. *Rev. Fr. Gynécol. Obstét.*, 72, 565-577, 1977.

[111] RAGHAVAN (D.), JELIHOVSKY (T.), FOX (R. M.). — Father-son testicular malignancy. Does genetic anticipation occur? *Cancer*, 45, 1005-1009, 1980.

[112] RANDOLPH (V. L.), HEALTH (C. W.). — Influenza during pregnancy in relation to subsequent childhood leukemia and childhood. *Am. J. Epidemiol.*, 100, 399-409, 1974.

[113] RICCARDI (V. M.), SUJANSKY (E.), SMITH (A. C.), FRANCK (E. U.). — Chromosomal imbalance in the aniridia-Wilms' tumor association: 11 p. interstitial deletion. *Pediatrics*, 61, 604-610, 1978.

[114] SCHILSKY (R. L.), LEWIS (B. J.), SHERINS (R. J.), YOUNG (R. C.). — Gonadal dysfunction in patients, receiving chemotherapy for cancer. *Ann. Intern. Med.*, 93 (Part 1), 109-114, 1980.

[115] ROSS (G. T.). — Congenital anomalies among children born of mothers receiving chemotherapy for gestational trophoblastic neoplasms. *Cancer*, 37, 1043-1047, 1976.

[116] SANDERS (R. W.), DRAPER (G. J.). — Childhood cancer and drugs in pregnancy. *Br. Med. J.*, 1, 717-718, 1979.

[117] SARKAR (S. D.), BEIERWALTES (W. H.), GILL (S. P.). — Subsequent fertility and birth histories of children and adolescents treated with I 131 for thyroid cancer. *J. Nucl. Med.*, 17, 460-464, 1976.

[118] SCHAISON (G.), JACQUILLAT (C.), AUCLERC (G.), WEIL (M.). — Les risques fœto-embryonnaires des chimiothérapies. *Bull. Cancer*, 66, 165-170, 1979.

[119] SHERWOOD (T.). — Diagnostic radiation risks (Annotation). *Arch. Dis. Child.*, 55, 249-251, 1980.

[120] SCHNAKENBURG (K. VON), MUELLER (M.), DOERNER (K.). — Congenital hemihypertrophy and malignant giant pheochromocytoma: a previously undescribed coincidence. *Europ. J. Pediatr.*, 122, 263, 1976.

[121] SCHWEISGUTH (O.). — Épidémiologie. In: *Tumeurs solides de l'enfant*. Flammarion Médecine Science éd., 13-18, 1979.

[122] SEELER (R. A.), ISRAEL (J. N.), ROYAL (J. E.), KAYE (C. I.), RAO (S.), ABULABAN (M.). — Ganglioneuroblastoma and fetal hydantoin-alcohol syndrome. *Pediatrics*, 63, 524-527, 1979.

[123] SHERMAN (S.), ROISEN (N.). — Fetal hydantoin syndrome and neuroblastoma. *Lancet*, 2, 517, 1976.

[124] SHIONO (P. H.), CHUNG (C. S.), MYRIANT-HOPOULOS (N. C.). — Preconception radiation, intrauterine diagnostic radiation and childhood neoplasic. *J. Natl. Cancer Inst.*, 65, 681-686, 1980.

[125] SIEBER (S. M.), ADAMSON (R. H.). — Toxicity of anti-neoplastic agents in man. Chromosomal aberrations, antifertility effects congenital malformations and carcinogenetic potential. *Adv. Cancer Res.*, 22, 57-155, 1975.

[126] SOLOMON (E.), BOBROW (M.). — Sister chromatid exchanges. A sensitive assay of agents damaging human chromosomes. *Mutat. Res.*, 30, 273-278, 1975.

[127] SOTELO-AVILA (C.), GONZALEZ-CRUSSI (F.), FOWLER (J. W.). — Complete and incomplete forms of Beckwith-Wiedemann syndrome: their oncogenic potential. *J. Pediatr.*, 96, 47-50, 1980.

[128] SPECTOR (B. D.), PERRY (G. S.), KERSEY (J. H.). — Genetically determined immunodeficiency disease (GDID) and malignancy: Report from the immunodeficiency-cancer registry. *Clin. Immunol. Immunopathol.*, 11, 12-29, 1978.

[129] STEWART (A.), KNEALE (G. W.). — Radiation dose effects in relation to obstetric X-rays and childhood cancers. *Lancet*, 1, 1185-1188, 1970.

[130] STEWART (A.), WEBB (J.), GILES (D.), HEWITT (D.). — Malignant disease in childhood and diagnostic irradiation *in utero. Lancet*, II, 447, 1956.

[130 bis] TAYLOR (W. F.). — Fetal hydantoin syndrome and extrarenal Wilms' tumor. *Lancet*, II, 481-482, 1980.

[131] TUBIANA (M.). — Problèmes posés par l'irradiation des femmes enceintes. Effets des radiations ionisantes sur l'embryon et le fœtus. *Bull. Cancer*, 66, 155-164, 1979.

[132] WELLS (H. G.). — Occurrence and significance of congenital malignant neoplasms. *Arch. Pathol.*, 30, 535-601, 1940.

[133] WEICHSELBAUM (R. R.), LITTLE (J. B.). — Familial retinoblastoma and ataxia telangiectasia. Human models for the study of DNA damage and repair. *Cancer*, 45, 775-779, 1980.

[134] WEINBERG (A. G.), MIZE (C. E.), WORTHEN (H. G.). — The occurrence of hepatoma in the chronic form of hereditary tyrosinemia. *J. Pediatr.*, 88, 434-438, 1976.

[135] WHITE (S. J.), McLEAN (A. E. M.), HOWLAND (C.). — Anticonvulsant drugs and cancer. A cohort study in patients with severe epilepsy. *Lancet*, 2, 458-461, 1979.

[136] WILLIAMS (D. W.). — Busulfan in early pregnancy. *Obstet. Gynecol.*, 27, 738-740, 1966.

[137] YOTTI (L. P.), GLOVERT (W.), TROSKI (S. E.),

SEGAL (D. J.). — Comparative study of X-Ray and UV induced cytotoxicity, DNA repair, and mutagenesis in Down's syndrome and normal fibroblasts. *Pediat. Res.*, *14*, 88-92, 1980.

[138] YOUNG (J. L.), MILLER (R. W.). — Incidence of malignant tumors in US children. *J. Pediatr.*, *86*, 254-258, 1975.

[139] YUNIS (J. J.), RAMSAY (N.). — Retinoblastoma and subband deletion of chromosome 13. *Am. J. Dis. Child.*, *132*, 161-163, 1978.

Neuroblastomas

DEFINITION, OCCURRENCE, EPIDEMIOLOGY

Neuroblastomas are malignant embryonic tumours of cells originating from the neural crest, forming the sympathetic ganglia and the adrenal medulla. They account for 7-10 % of all cancers in children, and 50 % in the newborn [5, 19, 36, 85, 101]. They must be distinguished from "neuroblastoma in situ", described by Beckwith and Perrin, at autopsy, in 1 in 250 newborns and infants dying before the age of 3 months from various causes; and whose incidence is 40 times greater than that of true neuroblastomas [6, 83, 94]. These nodules are thought to be either (*a*) remnants of nodules normally present in the fœtal adrenals up to 20 weeks gestation, or (*b*) dysplastic features, or (*c*) true malignant tumours evolving spontaneously towards regression or maturation [11, 34, 74, 91].

Neuroblastomas occur a little more frequently in boys (sex ratio 1.3 M/1 F), but this does not apply to the neonatal period.

If Knudson's theory is applicable to neuroblastomas [49, 50, 51], it would follow that certain cases are *genetically determined* (dominant germinal mutation) as evidenced by occasional reports of familial forms, affecting several siblings or vertically transmitted [3, 17, 27, 38, 42, 99, 100], bilateral and/or multifocal cases, and the association with other clinical manifestations of a neural crest disorder—Von Reckinghausen's disease, haemangiomas, Hirschsprung's disease, polyadenomatosis—and disorders of the autonomic nervous system [11, 92, 99].

The aetiological factors responsible for acquired forms are not known; however, there has been observed an association between 4 neuroblastomas (2 neonatal), and a syndrome of malformations ascribable to the transplacental passage of diphenylhydantoin.

Finally, there has been one autopsy report of a neonate with toxoplasmosis, a ganglioneuroma and an adenoma of the contralateral adrenal cortex [29].

HISTOGENESIS AND PATHOLOGY
[97]

Neuroblastomas result from a disorder of differentiation and maturation of the sympathogonias derived from the neural crest. These cells normally give rise to two cell lines; the chromaffin cells of the adrenal medulla and of chromaffin bodies (e. g. the organ of Zuckerkandl), and the sympathoblasts which form the sympathetic nervous system. The neuroblastomas essentially belong to the latter line, but may also contain chromaffin material (Table I).

TABLE I. — HISTOGENESIS OF SYMPATHETIC TUMOURS

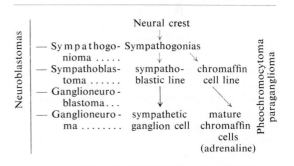

Macroscopic appearances: The size of neuroblastomas is very variable, and unrelated to the risk of metastatic spread; they are irregular shaped, soft or heterogeneous, yellowish-grey, with haemorrhagic, cystic or calcified areas. The tumour capsule or the limits of the affected organ are often breached, with local and regional extension (lymph nodes, spinal canal, kidneys, blood vessels).

Light microscopy: Neuroblastomas are rich in "lymphocyte-like" round cells, with clear cytoplasm and a dark nucleus, sometimes grouped into lobules. They may form rosettes; silver stains confirm the neural origin of the fibrillary matrix. Maturation is manifested by an increase in cell size, and in the quantity of fibrillar substance. Thus, ganglioneuroblastomas contain nests of undifferentiated cells as well as ganglion cells of differing maturity. The prognostic significance of lymphoid infiltration has not been proven [60].

Electron microscopy. — This confirms the correlation between histogenesis, biochemistry and morphology (APUD cell concept), demonstrating neurosecretory granules, in which dopamine is converted to noradrenaline and the latter is stored. The number of granules and the development of the neurofilaments and neurotubules are related to tumour differentiation [79].

REGRESSION AND MATURATION

Whether spontaneous, or a result of treatment, these phenomena are manifested by a haemorrhagic necrosis with fibrosis and calcification, or transformation into a benign ganglioneuroma (Bolande). Rare in other malignant tumours, they occur mainly in neonates and young infants [23, 24]. This may be related to the regression of "in situ" tumours. Prognosis and treatment would be greatly improved by an understanding of the immunologic, metabolic and genetic mechanisms involved [75].

Immunologic factors [8, 41]. — Although the nature and specificity of tumour antigens has not been clearly elucidated, there is in vitro evidence that the patient's lymphocytes and antibodies have cytotoxic and cytostatic effects on the tumour cells, and that these are associated with a favourable prognosis. In contrast, during active growth, blocking factors may mask the antigenic sites (antigen-antibody complexes) or inhibit the action of lymphocytes and macrophages. Helson has suggested that blocking agents crossing the placenta may explain neuroblastomas in situ, and their possible regression after birth [41]. However, there is no clear immunological evidence to account for the favourable prognosis of neuroblastomas in the young infant.

Biological factors. — *Nerve growth factor* induces maturation of immature neuroblasts in vitro [33]. No evidence has been found in humans, either in vitro or in vivo of deficiency of this factor,

nor of any abnormality of receptors, inhibitory activity, or protective effect [63].

It is possible to study the *biochemical properties* of differentiating tumour cells in vitro using cultures of human neuroblastoma cell lines.

Prasad et al. [72] consider that *cyclic AMP (CAMP)* has a determining role in the organisation of the microtubules and microfilaments necessary for the expression of differentiated phenotypes. Drugs which modify the activity of CAMP phosphodiesterase and increase levels of CAMP, might potentially have therapeutic value.

The degree of differentiation of neuroblastic cells may also be distinguished according to modification of their *membrane structure* relating to surface glycoproteins [32] and their electric charge, or to the secretory granules which reflect metabolic activity.

In summary, the abnormal behaviour of neuroblastic cells, probably due to alterations of the membrane, and of their environment, are secondary to genetic mutations inhibiting cellular differentiation and provoking malignant changes with their morphological, biochemical and immunological consequences. Cytogenetic studies have not yet resulted in localisation of the mutant gene, because of the variability and inconstancy of the abnormalities observed in tumour cells. Cellular hybridisation techniques may prove to be helpful.

Genetic factors. — Knudson and Meadows [50] theory of malignancy in two stages of mutation provides an attractive explanation for the maturation observed in certain early disseminated neuroblastomas (stage IV_s). These would not be regarded as metastases but merely as multiple malignant or non malignant tumours. A first mutation would be responsible for a block in differentiation, with abnormal proliferation of neural crest cells. These would evolve spontaneously towards maturation, unless a second mutation occurs, which is responsible for malignancy. The study of G6PD isoenzymes in the tumour cells of a female patient should allow the first mutation to be situated before the X inactivation (multicellular tumour), or after it (monoclonal tumour). In the first case there is a germinal mutation which carries a risk for subsequent generations. In the second case, both mutations are somatic.

Apart from its genetic implications, this hypothesis poses the problem of the possible mutagenic role of therapeutic agents; these could induce the second mutation in cells already predisposed, and explain the occurrence of a second cancer or of late relapse.

Thus, neuroblastoma constitutes a model of fundamental interest in the fields of early detection, and of the understanding of cellular abnormalities, which arise from hereditary or acquired errors of differentiation (malformations, benign tumours) and give rise to cancer [45].

BIOLOGICAL DIAGNOSIS

The excretion of catecholamines and their metabolites. — Neuroblastic cells have the necessary enzymes for the synthesis and the degradation of catecholamines (Table II). Despite increased synthesis, neuroblastomas differ from pheochromocytomas in that adrenaline and noradrenaline are not stored but rapidly degraded in tumour tissue into VMA and MHPG, which are non-hypertensive. Dopamine itself is converted mainly into HVA and also into MHPE.

90-95 % of neuroblastomas are characterised by increased excretion of catecholamines and their derivatives. Those usually measured are dopamine, noradrenaline, HVA, VMA and MHPG, and, in some cases, rarer metabolites. Measurements are made, either on a 24 hour urine collection (collected in the dark at 4° C and at pH 4) or an a random sample, in which case it is related to urinary creatinine. Two dimensional chromatography is the most commonly used method of measurement.

This may be preceded by a La Brosse test, or spot-test—these are colorometric reactions using diazo-paranitroaniline [56]. Interpretation of the results must take account of age [31].

Apart from its diagnostic value, the measurement of catecholamine metabolite levels is also important for following the evolution of the tumour, assessing the effect of treatment, and detecting relapse. The unfavourable significance of a VMA/HVA ratio < 1 at diagnosis is disputed [57]. In stage IV_s (abdominal), very high levels are classically found, but have little relation to evolution. Cervical and thoracic tumours are less often secretory, perhaps because they originate from spinal ganglia, whose cells are depleted of tyrosine-hydroxylase.

Serum levels of catecholamines, apart from dopamine, are of little diagnostic value. This also applies to dopamine-β-hydroxylase [15].

Abnormal excretion of *cystathionine* in the urine, related to increased catechol-O-methyl-transferase activity, is not specific, but may be useful for surveillance of tumours which do not secrete much.

Systematic screening for neuroblastoma has been suggested using either a spot-test, or measurement of HVA and VMA, 3 times a year in the first year of life, and then twice yearly until the age of 5 years. However, in spite of better prognosis due to earlier detection, it is debatable whether this meets the other generally accepted criteria for a mass screening programme (reliability, easiness, acceptable cost) [37].

TABLE II. — METABOLISM OF CATECHOLAMINES

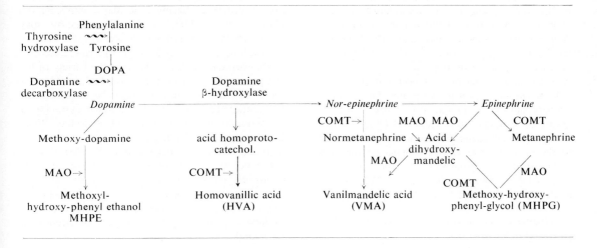

MAO : monoaminoxidase.   COMT : catechol-O-methyltransferase.

Haematologic manifestations [73]. — *Anaemia* is common and may sometimes dominate the clinical picture. Anaemia is not always due to bone marrow invasion, but often to dyserythropoeisis, and can be misdiagnosed as erythroblastosis fœtalis [2, 25, 65, 96]. Sometimes it is of a haemolytic type; the erythrocytes are spiky and fragmented, and the overall clinical picture is of a micro-angiopathy. The effect on the *white cells* also depends on the state of the marrow. It is not certain that a raised lymphocyte count implies a better prognosis. With regard to lymphoblastic infiltration of the bone-marrow, which is perhaps evidence of an immunological reaction, this must be interpreted in relation to the age of the child (physiological lymphoblastosis in the very young infant) and distinguished from partial tumour invasion. *Thrombocytopenia* can be of central or peripheral origin. There may be *thrombocytosis*.

Other investigations. — In the acute phase of the condition, increased levels of orosomucoid, alpha-1-antitrypsin, ferritin and the presence of circulating immune complexes, have been reported [30].

A connection has been found between immunologic status and prognosis; but this has not been adequately studied in the neonatal period.

CLINICAL FEATURES

In utero, the development of a neuroblastoma in the fœtus can give rise to neuro-vegetative disorders in the mother, due to the liberation of catecholamines which can be estimated in the urine [98]. A disseminated tumour may cause fœtal death [9, 66, 71] or simulate erythroblastosis fœtalis. Despite metastatic invasion of the chorionic villi, tumour spread to the mother has not been reported [93].

In the neonate, clinical symptoms depend on the primary site of the tumour, on its size, and on the nature of its metastases. Table III (from Pochedly [70]) gives the incidence of neuroblastomas according to the primary site. The percentage of abdomino-pelvic forms is a little higher in the newborn. In cases of bilateral adrenal tumours (5 %) the diagnosis is usually made before 6 months [54].

Abdominal neuroblastomas and Pepper's syndrome [13, 20, 62, 95].

Clinical features. — As in the older child, the commonest site of neuroblastoma is the retro-

TABLE III. — OCCURRENCE ACCORDING TO PRIMARY SITE (from POCHEDLY [70])

Site	% in neonates	% in children of all ages
Head	3.0	0.2
Neck	3.0	3.2
Thorax	10.3	14.6
Abdomen	72.3	65.5
Pelvis	8.6	4.5
Unknown	3.0	12.0
Total no. of cases . . .	68	1,303

peritoneal region. It usually arises from the adrenal gland or retroperitoneal sympathetic ganglia. Presenting signs are abdominal distension, sometimes causing dystocia or respiratory disorders; detection on routine clinical or radiological (calcification) examination; and occasionally a picture of adrenal haemorrhage and/or haemoperitoneum [67]. Pepper's syndrome may sometimes be associated with an extra-abdominal neuroblastoma; the primary tumour may also be undetectable.

In more than 60 % of cases, this primary tumour is associated with, and even masked by, rapidly increasing hepatomegaly. This can cause considerable abdominal distension with collateral circulation, sometimes ascites, alimentary difficulties, respiratory distress, and renal failure. Jaundice is not usually present, nor are there any serious effects on hepatic function. Anaemia, which can be severe, and disorders of haemostasis may complicate the clinical picture [26]. Further investigation may show subcutaneous tumour nodules or bone-marrow infiltration; bony metastases are, as a rule, absent.

Diagnostic difficulties arise from the variety of the symptomatology; the retroperitoneal and para-renal site of the tumour must be defined. The differential diagnosis includes adrenal cysts [4] or haematomas, lymphangiomas and teratomas. When hepatomegaly is the presenting sign, a metabolic disorder is often suspected, but this does not fit with the rapid progression. Sometimes an erroneous diagnosis is made of septicaemia, or of a haematological malignancy, because of the haematological abnormalities. Finally, it is important to exclude a primary hepatic tumour, particularly a haemangio-endothelioma.

Further investigations are straight forward (cf. Table IV).

Once neuroblastoma is suspected, the spot-test, followed by a *quantitative estimation of catecholamine metabolites* confirms the diagnosis, as there is usually massive excretion.

Plain X-ray of the abdomen may demonstrate homogeneous posterior tumour opacity, obscuring the shadow of the psoas. All or part of this may contain granular or cloudy calcifications, which are often better seen on soft-tissue X-rays. Hepatomegaly may obscure the tumour. Intra-hepatic calcification is rare.

Intravenous urography may show ureteric and renal displacement, without pelvicalyceal disorganization or amputation, confirming the retroperitoneal and extra-renal origin of the primary tumour, or compression of one or both kidneys, with backward displacement due to hepatomegaly, and pelvicalyceal stretching. Interpretation may be difficult in cases of pelvi-ureteric dilatation (malformations, compression by tumour or lymph nodes), of bilateral renal displacement and/or deformation, or in the absence of definite abnormalities (very small tumours, coeliac origin).

Abdominal echotomography and C. T. scanning confirm and complete the urographic data by defining the size and extent of the tumour.

Venous or umbilical arterial angiography are not indicated after catecholamine estimation.

Liver scan shows heterogenous uptake and/or liver displacement by a posterior tumour. It is not helpful in diagnosis, but may be used to follow tumour evolution and the effects of treatment (radiotherapy).

Pelvic neuroblastomas [7]. — Pelvic neuroblastomas arise from sacral sympathetic ganglia or the organ of Zukerkandl. They present with signs of compression, which may be

— venous and lymphatic, causing peripheral œdema which may extend to the external genitalia and the upper thighs,

— bladder compression causing dysuria, retention and infection,

— rectal or spinal compression. Rectal examination confirms the presacral site of the tumour.

Intravenous urography, retrograde cystography, and barium enema, as well as echotomography, enable the extent of the tumour to be defined.

Differential diagnosis is mainly with teratomas. Alpha-1-fœtoprotein and catecholamine estimations are helpful diagnostic aids, but the decision to proceed with surgery must be made rapidly.

Cervical neuroblastomas [12, 46]. — According to their site, these tumours may present in the following ways: (1) as hard and irregular cervical or subclavicular swellings, (2) with heterochromia of the iris, (3) with respiratory difficulties due to tracheal compression, (4) with œdema of the arm, (5) with swallowing difficulty due to XII nerve paralysis, or œsophageal displacement, (6) with Horner's syndrome (ptosis, enophtalmos, myosis).

Even in the absence of a palpable tumour, neuroblastoma must be suspected in Horner's syndrome, and the child investigated.

Investigations to determine the site of the tumour include radiographs of the neck (A. P. and lateral), barium swallow, and thyroid scan.

In neonates, teratoma, vascular tumours, sternomastoid haematoma and branchial cysts must all be excluded.

Thoracic neuroblastomas [88]. — Presenting symptoms are more dramatic in the neonate and young infant than in children over 5 years old. Respiratory difficulties, sometimes severe, stridor, or signs of vascular and nerve compression, lead to the discovery of a round mass in the posterior mediastinum. The trachea and œsophagus are displaced and the bony thorax is sometimes deformed. The ribs may be separated and eroded in contact with the tumour. A pleural effusion may be present. Differential diagnosis is with a teratoma, œsophageal duplication, vascular tumour, and bronchogenic cyst.

Miscellaneous and dumb-bell tumours:

— Some neuroblastomas are cervico-mediastinal, or thoraco-abdominal, single or multiple [58, 78].

— Retro-orbital [61], pneumogastric [80], scrotal [70] and peri-umbilical tumours have been reported in neonates. One case was associated with homocystinuria [64], and another with hyperplasia of the islets of Langerhans [70].

— Signs of *cord compression* may point to an intra-spinal extradural neuroblastoma, either isolated, or secondary to extension of a prevertebral thoracic or abdominal tumour, through the intervertebral foramina. In neonates clinical signs may be unrecognised; limb hypotonia, sphincter disturbances or sensory abnormalities. Spinal X-rays show enlargement of the intervertebral foramina, erosion of the pedicles and widening of the interpedicular space. A negative sign, which is important in differential diagnosis, is the absence of vertebral malformations, which would suggest a benign tumour (epidermoid cyst). Cerebrospinal fluid albumin concentration may be raised, but must be interpreted in relation to the age of the child. Myelography confirms the level and the extra-dural nature of the compression.

Catecholamine levels are normal when the tumour arises from a spinal ganglion.

Metastases. — Metastases occur in 50 % of neonatal cases. In this age group, they are classically hepatic (Pepper's syndrome) and subcutaneous, whereas in children over the age of 2, the metastases are usually bony (Hutchinson's syndrome).

Concerning *massive hepatic infiltration*, several theories have attempted to explain its occurence in relation to the fœtal circulation. Liver involvement in Pepper's syndrome can actually be considered as a primary rather than metastatic tumor.

Subcutaneous nodules occur in one third of congenital neuroblastomas and may be the presenting feature [39, 89]. They are firm, mobile, non tender, sometimes bluish in colour; they average 0.5 to 1 cm in diameter and may be situated anywhere. On palpation, the overlying skin may redden and then blanch for 30 to 60', because of vasoconstriction due to the local release of catecholamines. Biopsy distinguishes them from angiomas and from haematological malignancies. They may disappear spontaneously, or mature. In one case, we have noted the appearance of multiple subcutaneous ganglioneuromas, 16 years after the diagnosis of a neonatal multifocal subcutaneous neuroblastoma, which resolved without treatment...

Bone-marrow infiltration can occur in the absence of bony lesions. When this is partial, trephine marrow biopsy may be necessary. The prognosis seems less favourable when there is massive infiltration.

Bony metastases are rare in neonates, but have the same characteristics and bad prognosis as in children over two years old. They are diffuse, often symmetrical, osteolytic lesions, with cortical destruction and periosteal reaction, found in the skull, the pelvis and the long bones. Technetium 99 scan may confirm the radiologic findings. These lesions may be confused with the following conditions:
— osteomyelitis, Caffey's cortical hyperostosis, toxic or viral embryopathy, and haematological malignancy.

Prognostic factors

Overall prognosis of neuroblastomas

[14, 20, 47, 102]. — Survival for 2 years is generally considered equivalent to cure because of the rapid deterioration of unfavourable cases. Nevertheless, very late recurrences may occur [53, 77].

Retrospective analysis of several large series, shows that the following parameters have prognostic value: — the stage of extension of the tumour (cf. Table V), the age of the child, the site of the primary tumour, and the site of the metastases.

TABLE V. — Classification of neuroblastomas according to anatomical features [22]

Stage I	: tumour limited to organ of origin
Stage II	: tumour spreading beyond organ of origin but not crossing the midline
Stage III	: tumour with local extension crossing the midline
Stage IV	: presence of metastases distant from the primary tumour: — lymph nodes, bone-marrow, liver...
Stage IV$_s$	: stage I or II tumours, associated with metastases limited to the liver, skin and bone-marrow, but without skeletal metastases

Effect of age: the 2 year survival rate is 72 % for presentation between 0 and 11 months, 38 % from 12 to 23 months, and 12 % after 2 years old.

Effect of site: thoracic and pelvic forms have a better prognosis than abdominal forms; cervical forms nearly always have an excellent prognosis.

Effect of the stage of extension: survival rates are 80-90 % for stages I and II, 30 % for stage III, 60-70 % for stage IV$_s$, and 5 % for stage IV. The stage is linked to the site and also to the age. The role played by other factors has not been established: — the sex of the child [47], the degree of histological maturation [60, 79], the immunological stage [30, 69], the HVA/VMA ratio [57].

The prognosis of neuroblastomas in the first year of life. — The favourable prognosis associated with this group is related to the high incidence of stage IV_s tumours which represent 60 % of cases; they do not perhaps always have the significance of a malignant tumour. Bony involvement is rare at this age and its prognosis is not as bad as in a child greater than 1 year of age [76, 91]. The definition of stage IV_s should perhaps be modified to reflect the poorer prognosis associated with bone-marrow infiltration when it is massive.

In the neonatal period (and also the first 3 months of life), the mortality rate is clearly higher (50-60 %) than between 3 and 12 months; this is due to the respiratory, alimentary and renal complications arising from compression by the tumour, and to haemorraghic and infectious complications of therapy.

TREATMENT

In the infant and child the general principles of treatment of neuroblastomas are as follows: — in stages I, II and III, excision of the primary tumour together with radiotherapy and/or chemotherapy to residual microscopic and macroscopic tumour sites. In stage IV predominantly chemotherapy is used [21, 27, 103].

In the newborn, the choice of treatment is influenced by the following factors; the severe functional effects of bulky tumours, the site of metastases, the poor tolerance of chemotherapy and radiotherapy, and finally, the possibility of spontaneous regression. At present it is still not possible to distinguish between tumours which are truly malignant, and those which are more related to a dysplastic state.

Stage IV_s [17, 18, 21, 34, 62, 74, 86]. — Certain cases undergo spontaneous regression, but this is neither constant nor predictable.

Pepper's syndrome: the rapid increase in abdominal size due to hepatomegaly can compromise respiratory, digestive, and renal function, and may necessitate respiratory assistance and continuous enteral feeding. Incision of the abdominal wall, with or without the temporary insertion of an inert material, has been carried out in some cases, despite the risk of infection [35, 84]. *Early surgical intervention*, aimed at diagnosis or excision, is contraindicated. If necessary, radiotherapy may accelerate regression of the hepatomegaly. Small doses are recommended (5-10 Gy) over 8-10 days (1-1.5 Gy per session) given via lateral fields to the anterior 2/3 of the liver, sparing the kidneys, ovaries and colon.

Chemotherapy may be used, especially when there is bone-marrow involvement. Drugs used are; Vincristine (VCR), Cyclophosphamide (CPM), epipodophyllotoxine (VM 26), Diethylcarboxamide (DTIC), and Doxorubicine (DXR) taking account of their toxicity to the nervous system (VCR, VM 26), the alimentary tract (DTIC), the heart (DXR), and the liver, bladder and bone-marrow (CPM). The dosage must be reduced by 50 % for the first treatment and modified according to haematological tolerance and hepatic and renal function, which govern drug elimination. The duration of chemotherapy (whose indications are at present not precisely defined), depends on the tumour regression and catecholamine excretion (several weeks to several months).

Ablation of the primary tumour is usually performed after regression of hepatomegaly, especially if abdominal catecholamine excretion persists, even if there are radiological signs of regression and calcification. Liver biopsy may show fibrotic areas but there is no hepatocellular damage, and, curiously, the tumour cells disappear without tending to mature.

In the very rare stage IV_s *cases without clinical evidence of liver involvement*, it is usual to proceed to excision of the primary tumour as soon as the diagnosis is made. Hepatic infiltration is sometimes only revealed by biopsy. The use of chemotherapy depends on post operative catecholamine concentrations, and/or the presence of bone-marrow infiltration.

Stages I-II (localised forms). — Surgical excision is the only treatment. Radiotherapy is useless and dangerous. Cautious chemotherapy may be considered in cases where there are microscopic tumour residues, according to catecholamine levels.

Stage III (local-regional spread). — Complete excision is not possible without major risks (vascular, nervous). Excision can if necessary be done in 2 stages, following reduction of the tumour volume using chemotherapy, but avoiding irradiation.

Dumb-bell tumours. — Decompressive laminectomy with excision of the tumour must be rapidly performed. The pre-vertebral tumour is subsequently treated according to its stage. These tumours may be completely calcified, and their excision unjustified.

Stage IV [28, 40, 43, 103]. — Chemotherapy is the only initial treatment. If remission is achieved, surgical excision may be considered.

New therapeutic perspectives. — Their objectives are: — to promote maturation of neuroblastomas [55, 63]. Nerve growth factor and drugs which increase cyclic AMP levels (e. g. papaverine) have not however given in vivo the effects anticipated from in vitro experiments; — the selective destruction of neuroblastic cells [40]; — the stimulation of host defence mechanisms [8, 68].

RESULTS

Publications concerning the newborn are few, and heterogeneous. Some predate the considerable recent advances in neonatal intensive care, the importance of which we have seen in the treatment of large tumours. This explains the poor survival rate (30-40 %) in neonatal stage IV$_s$, with or without treatment, in the series of Evans [21], Murthy et al. [67], Grosfeld et al. [35], Schneider et al. [85].

Improvement of results depends on close medical and surgical collaboration for intensive care, selection of the optimum timing and extent of surgical excision, and the choice or rejection of additional treatment.

MEANS OF SURVEILLANCE

In the short and medium term, this is done by monitoring urinary catecholamine excretione very 8 to 15 days during the first three months, then monthly for one year, and bi-monthly in the second year. Ultrasound scanning is better than radiological examination for assessing the size of the liver and of tumour tissue left in situ (at first weekly, then monthly, then every 2 to 3 months for 18 months to 2 years).

In the long term, it is important to assess the possible effects of treatment on growth, and renal, hepatic, and gonadal function. Finally, study of descendants of cured subjects should permit confirmation of the hereditary nature of certain neuroblastomas.

REFERENCES

[1] NEUROBLASTOMA, 5th Symposium of the International Society of Paediatric Oncology. *Oncol. Maandschr. Kindergeneesk, 42,* 365, 1974.

[2] ANDERS (D.), KINDERMANN (G.), PFEIFER (U.). — Metastasasizing fetal neuroblastoma with involvement of the placenta simulating fetal erythroblastosis. *J. Pediatr., 82,* 50-53, 1973.

[3] ARENSON (E. B.), HUTTER (J. J.), RESTUCCIA (R. D.), HOLTON (C. P.). — Neuroblastoma in father and son. *J. Amer. Med. Ass., 235,* 727-729, 1976.

[4] BABIN (J. P.), ALLAIN (D.), DEMARQUEZ (J. L.), BONDONNY (J. M.), LEGER (H.), MARTIN (C.). — Les kystes de la surrénale chez le nouveau-né. A propos de 2 cas. *Arch. Fr. Pediatr., 34,* 130-142, 1977.

[5] BADER (J. L.), MILLER (R. W.). — US cancer incidence and mortality in the first year of life. *Am. J. Dis. Child., 133,* 157-159, 1979.

[6] BECKWITH (J. B.), PERRIN (E. V.). — *In situ* neuroblastomas: a contribution to the natural history of neural crest tumors. *Am. J. Pathol., 43,* 1089-1104, 1963.

[7] BENSAHEL (H.), BOUREAU (M.). — Perspectives diagnostiques et pronostiques des neuroblastomes pelviens purs du nouveau-né. *Ann. Chir. Infant., 13,* 37-44, 1972.

[8] BERNSTEIN (I.), HELLSTROM (I.), HELLSTROM (K. E.), WRITE (T. W.). — Immunity to tumors antigens: potential implications in human neuroblastoma. *J. Natl. Cancer Inst., 57,* 711-715, 1976.

[9] BIRNER (W.). — Neuroblastoma as a cause of antenatal death. *Am. J. Obst. Gynec., 82,* 1388-1391, 1961.

[10] BOLANDE (R. P.). — Benignity of neonatal tumors and concept of cancer repression in early life. *Am. J. Dis. Child., 122,* 12-14, 1971.

[11] BOLANDE (R. P.). — The neurocristopathies. A unifying concept of disease arising in neural crest maldevelopment. *Hum. Pathol., 5,* 409-429, 1974.

[12] BONAMICO (M.), COZZI (F.). — Ganglioneuroblastoma of the neck in a newborn. *Minerva Pediat., 24,* 266-270, 1972.

[13] BOND (J. V.). — Neuroblastoma metastatic to the liver in infants. *Arch. Dis. Child., 51,* 879-882, 1976.

[14] BRESLON (N.), MCCANN (B.). — Statistical instigation of prognosis for children with neuroblastoma. *Cancer Res., 31,* 2098-2103, 1971.

[15] BREWSTER (M. A.), BERRY (D. H.). — Serial studies of serum Dopamine-B-hydroxylase and urinary vanillylmandelic and homovanillic acids in neuroblastoma. *Med. Ped. Oncol., 6,* 93-99, 1979.

[16] CATALANO (P. W.), NEWTON (W. A. Jr), WILLIAMS (T. E.), CLATWORTHY (H. W.), KILMAN (J. W.). — Reasonable surgery for thoracic neuroblastoma in infants and children. *J. Thorac. Cardiovasc. Surg., 76,* 459-464, 1978.

[17] CHATTEN (J.), VOORHESS (M. L.). — Familial neuroblastoma. Report of a kindred with multiple disorders, including neuroblastomas in four siblings. *N. Engl. J. Med., 277,* 1230-1236, 1967.

[18] D'ANGIO (G. K.), EVANS (A. E.), KOOP (C. E.). — Special pattern of a widespread neuroblastoma with a favourable prognosis. *Lancet, 1,* 1046-1049, 1971.

[19] EVANS (A. R.). — Congenital neuroblastoma. *J. Clin. Path., 18,* 54-62, 1965.

[20] EVANS (A. E.). — Staging and treatment of neuroblastoma. *Cancer, 45,* 1799-1802, 1980.

[21] EVANS (A. E.), CHATTEN (J.), D'ANGIO (J. G.), GERSON (J. M.), ROBINSON (J.), SCHNAUFER (L.). — A review of stage IVs neuroblastoma patients at the Children's Hospital of Philadelphia. *Cancer, 45,* 833-839, 1980.

[22] EVANS (A. E.), D'ANGIO (G. J.), RANDOLPH (P. H.). — A proposed staging for children with neuroblastoma. *Cancer*, 27, 374-378, 1971.

[23] EVANS (A. E.), GERSON (J.), SCHNAUFER (L.). — Spontaneous regression of neuroblastoma. *Natl. Cancer Int. Monogr.*, 44, 49-54, 1976.

[24] EVERSON (T. C.), COLE (W. H.). — *Spontaneous regression of cancer*. Saunders W. B. Co. ed., Philadelphia, 1966.

[25] FALKENBURG (L. W.), KAY (M. N.). — A case of congenital sympathogonioma (neuroblastoma) of the right adrenal simulating erythroblastosis fetalis. *J. Pediatr.*, 42, 462-465, 1953.

[26] FAXELIUS (G.), TAGER-NILSSON (A. C.), WILHELMSSON (S.), ASTRÖM (L.). — Disseminated intravascular coagulation and congenital neuroblastoma. *Acta Paediatr. Scand.*, 64, 667-670, 1975.

[27] FEINGOLD (M.), GHERODI (G.), SIMONS (C.). — Familial neuroblastoma and trisomy 13 (letter to the editor). *Am. J. Dis. Child.*, 121, 451, 1971.

[28] FINKLESTEIN (J. Z.), KLEMPERER (M. R.), EVANS (A.), BERNSTEIN (I.), LEIKIN (S.), McCREDIE (S.), GROSFELD (J.), HITTLE (R.), WEINER (J.), SATHER (H.), HAMMOND (D.). — Multiagent chemotherapy for children with metastatic neuroblastoma: a report from *Childrens Cancer Study Group Med. Ped. Oncol.*, 6, 179-187, 1979.

[29] GERSHANIK (J. J.), ELMORE (M.), LEVKOFF (A. B.). — Congenital concurrence of adrenal cortical tumor, ganglioneuroma, and toxoplasmosis. *Pediatrics*, 51, 705-709, 1973.

[30] GERSON (J.), EVANS (A. E.), ROSEN (F.). — The prognostic value of acute phase reactants in patients with neuroblastoma. *Cancer*, 40, 1655-1656, 1977.

[31] GITLOW (F. E.), DZIEDZIC (L. B.), DZIEDZIC (S. W.). — Catecholamine metabolism in neuroblastoma, 115-154. In *Neuroblastoma*, POCHEDLY (C.), ed. Arnold Publ., London, 1977.

[32] GLICK (M. C.), GLYCO (S.). — Proteins on the surface on neuroblastoma cells. *J. Natl. Cancer Inst.*, 57, 653-658, 1976.

[33] GOLDSTEIN (M.). — Neuroblastoma cells in tissue culture. *J. Pediatr. Surg.*, 3, 166-169, 1968.

[34] GRIFFIN (M.), BOLANDE (R.). — Familial neuroblastoma with regression and maturation to ganglioneurofibroma. *Pediatrics*, 43, 377-382, 1969.

[35] GROSFELD (J. L.), SCHATZLEIN (M.), BALLANTINE (T. V. N.), WEETMAN (R. M.), BAEHNER (R. L.). — Metastatic neuroblastoma: factors influencing survival. *J. Pediatr. Surg.*, 13, 59-65, 1978.

[36] GUIN (D. H.), GILBERT (E. S.), JONES (B.). — Incidental neuroblastoma in infants. *Am. J. Clin. Pathol.*, 51, 126-136, 1969.

[37] HALLETT (G. W.). — Urine VMA screening for neuroblastoma; is it worth the cost? *Pediatrics*, 51, 757, 1973.

[38] HARDY (P.), NESBIT (M.). — Familial neuroblastoma; report of a kindred with a high incidence of infantile tumors. *J. Pediatr.*, 80, 74-77, 1972.

[39] HAWTHORNE (H.), NELSON (K.), WITZLEBEN (C.), GIANGIACOMA (J.). — Blanching subcutaneous nodules in neonatal neuroblastoma. *J. Pediatr.*, 77, 297-300, 1970.

[40] HAYES (F. A.), GREEN (A. A.), MAUER (A. M.). — Correlation of cell kinetic and clinical response to chemotherapy in disseminated neuroblastoma. *Cancer Res.*, 37, 3766-3770, 1977.

[41] HELSON (L.). — Regression of neuroblastomas. *Lancet*, 1, 1075-1076, 1971.

[42] HELSON (L.), BLASCO (P.), MORPHY (M. L.). — Familial neuroblastoma (abstr.). *Clin. Res.*, 17 614, 1969.

[43] HELSON (L.), HELSON (C.), PETERSON (R. S.), DAS (S. K.). — A rationale for the treatment of metastatic neuroblastoma. *J. Nal. Cancer Inst.*, 57, 727-729, 1976.

[44] HRABOVSKY (E.), JONES (B.). — Congenital intraspinal neuroblastoma. *Amer. J. Dis. Child.*, 133, 73-75, 1979.

[45] JAFFE (N.). — Neuroblastoma: review of the literature and an examination of factors contributing to its enigmatic character. *Cancer Treat. Rev.*, 3, 61-82, 1976.

[46] JAFFE (N.), CASSADY (R.), FILLER (R. M.), PETERSEN (R.), TRAGGIS (D.). — Heterochromia and Horner syndrome associated with cervical and mediastinal neuroblastoma. *J. Pediatr.*, 87, 75-77. 1975.

[47] KINNIER (R.), WILSON (L. M.), DRAPER (G. J.). — Neuroblastoma, its natural history and prognosis: a study of 487 cases. *Br. Med. J.*, 3, 301-307, 1974.

[48] KING (D.), GOODMAN (J.), HAWK (T.), BOLES (E. T.), SAYERS (M. P.). — Dumbell neuroblastomas in children. *Arch. Surg.*, 110, 888-891, 1975.

[49] KNUDSON (A. G.), MEADOWS (A. T.). — Developmental genetics of neuroblastoma. *J. Nal. Cancer Inst.*, 57, 675-682, 1976.

[50] KNUDSON (A. G.), MEADOWS (A. T.). — Regression of neuroblastoma IV-S. A genetic hypothesis. *N. Engl. J. Med.*, 302, 1254-1256, 1980.

[51] KNUDSON (A. G.), STRONG (L. C.). — Mutation and cancer: neuroblastoma and pheochromocytoma. *Am. J. Hum. Genet.*, 24, 514-532, 1972.

[52] KLEIN (H.), PLOECHL (E.). — Familiaeres neuroblastom der Nebennieren beim neugeborenen Muench. *Med. Wschr.*, 116, 1163-1168, 1974.

[53] KONRAD (T. N.), SINGHER (L. J.), NEERHOUT (R. C.). — Late death from neuroblastoma. *J. Pediatr.*, 82. 80-81, 1973.

[54] KRAMER (S. A.), BRADFORD (W. D.). ANDERSON (E. E.). — Bilateral adrenal neuroblastoma. *Cancer*, 45, 2208-2212, 1980.

[55] KUMAR (S.), STEWARD (J. K.), WAGHE (M. A.), PEARSON (D.), EDWARDS (D. C.), FENTON (E. L.), GRIFFIN (A. H.). — The administration of nerve growth factor to children with widespread neuroblastoma. *J. Pediatr. Surg.*, 5, 18-22, 1970.

[56] LA BROSSE (E. H.), COMOY (E.), BOHUON (C.), ZUCKER (J. M.), SCHWEISGUTH (O.). — Catecholamine metabolism in neuroblastoma. *J. Nal. Cancer Inst.*, 57, 633-638, 1976.

[57] LAUG (W. E.), SLEGEL (S. E.). — Initial urinary catecholamine metabolite concentrations and prognosis in neuroblastoma. *Pediatrics*, 62, 77-83 1978.

[58] LEAPE (L. L.), LOWMAN (J. T.), LOVELAND (G. C.). — Multifocal non disseminated neuroblastoma; report of 2 cases in siblings. *J. Pediatr.*, 92, 75-77, 1978.

[59] LEPINTRE (J.), SCHWEISGUTH (O.), LABRUNE (M.), LEMERLE (J.). — Les neuroblastomes en sablier. Étude de 22 cas. *Arch. Franç. Pédiat.*, 26, 829-847, 1969.

[60] MÄKINEN (J.). — Microscopic patterns as a guide to prognosis of neuroblastoma in childhood. *Cancer*, 29, 1637-1646, 1972.

[61] MEHTA (M.), BUBARIWALLA (R.). — Neuroblastoma in the newborn. *Indian. Pediatr.*, 8, 74-75, 1971.

[62] MESSICA (Cl.). — Étude de 18 cas de syndrome de Pepper (sympathoblastome avec métastases hépatiques du nourrisson). *Thèse Méd.*, *Paris*, 1970.

[63] MOBLEY (W. C.), SERVER (A. C.), ISHII (D. N.), RIOPELLE (R. J.), SHOOTER (E. M.). — Nerve growth factor. *N. Engl. J. Med.*, *297*, 1096-1104, 1977 (1ʳᵉ partie); *297*, 1149-1158, 1977 (2ᵉ partie); *297*, 1211-1218, 1977 (3ᵉ partie).

[64] MONCH (E.), STEFAN (H.), KASER (H.). — Neuroblastoma of the Pepper type with homocysteinuria. *Helv. Pediat. Acta*, *25*, 530-541, 1970.

[65] MOSS (T. J.), KAPLAN (L.). — Association of hydrops fetalis with congenital neuroblastoma. *Amer. J. Obstet. Gynec.*, *132*, 905-906, 1978.

[66] MULLER (M.). — Metastatic neuroblastoma with intra-uterine stillbirth. *Zbl. Allg. Path.*, *108*, 356-358, 1966.

[67] MURTHY (T. V. W.), IRVING (I. M.), LISTER (J.). — Massive adrenal hemorrhage in neonatal neuroblastoma. *J. Pediatr. Surg.*, *13*, 31-34, 1978.

[68] NECHELES (T. S.), RAUSEN (A. R.), KUNG (F. H.), POCHEDLY (C.). — Immunochemotherapy in advanced neuroblastoma. *Cancer*, *41*, 1282-1288, 1978.

[69] ORGEL (H. A.), HAMBURGER (R. N.), MENDELSON (L. M.), MILLER (J. R.), KUNG (F. H.). — Antibody responses in normal infants and in infants receiving chemotherapy for congenital neuroblastoma. *Cancer*, *40*, 994-997, 1977.

[70] POCHEDLY (C.). — *Neuroblastoma*. Arnold Publ., London, 1977.

[71] POTTER (E.), PARISH (J. M.). — Neuroblastoma, ganglioneuroma, and fibroneuroma in a stillborn fetus. *Amer. J. Path.*, *18*, 141-151, 1942.

[72] PRASAD (K. N.), SAHU (S. K.), SINHA (P. K.). — Cyclic nucleotids in the regulation of expression of differentiated functions in neuroblastoma cells. *J. Nal. Cancer Inst.*, *57*, 619-629, 1976.

[73] QUINN (J. J.), ALTMAN (A. J.). — The multiple hematologic manifestations of neuroblastoma. *Am. J. Pediatr. Hematol. Oncol.*, *1*, 210-215, 1979.

[74] RANGECROFT (L.), LAUDER (I.), WAGGET (J.). — Spontaneous maturation of stage IV-S neuroblastoma. *Arch. Dis. Child.*, *53*, 815-817, 1978.

[75] RAYBAUD (Cl.), BERNARD (J. L.). — Le neuroblastome. *Arch. Franç. Pédiat.*, *36*, 837-852, 1979.

[76] REILLY (D.), NESBIT (M. E.), KRIVIT (W.). — Cure of 3 patients who had squelettal metastasis in disseminated neuroblastoma. *Pediatrics*, *41*, 47-51, 1968.

[77] RICHARDS (M. J. S.), JOO (P.), GILBERT (E. F.). — The rare problem of late recurrence in neuroblastoma. *Cancer*, *38*, 1847-1852, 1976.

[78] ROBERTS (F. F.), LEE (K. R.). — Familial neuroblastome presenting as multiple tumors. *Radiology*, *116*, 133, 1975.

[79] ROMANSKY (S. J.), CROCKER (D. W.), SHAW (K. N. F.). — Ultrastructural studies on neuroblastoma. Evaluation of cyto-differenciation and correlation of morphology and biochemical and survival data. *Cancer*, *42*, 2392-2398, 1978.

[80] ROSEDALE (R.). — Neuroblastoma of nodose ganglion of infant vagus nerve. *Arch. Otolaryng.*, *80*, 454-459, 1964.

[81] ROTHNER (A. D.). — Congenital « dumbbell » neuroblastoma with paraplegia. *Clin. Pediatr.*, *10*, 235-237, 1971.

[82] SIMPSON (T.), LYNN (H.), MILLS (S.). — Congenital neuroblastoma in the scrotum. *Clin. Pediatr.*, *8*, 174-175, 1969.

[83] SHANKLIN (D. R.), SOTELO-AVILA (C.). — *In situ*

tumors in fetuses, newborns and young infants. *Biol. Neonate*, *14*, 286-316, 1969.

[84] SCHNAUFER (L.), KOOP (C.). — Silastic abdominal patch for temporary hepotomegaly in stage IV-S neuroblastoma. *J. Pediatr. Surg.*, *10*, 73-75, 1975.

[85] SCHNEIDER (K. M.), BECKER (J. M.), KRASNA (I. H.). — Neonatal neuroblastoma. *Pediatrics*, *36*, 359-366, 1965.

[86] SCHWARTZ (A. D.), DADA-ZADEH (L.), LEE (H.), SWANEY (J. J.). — Spontaneous regression of disseminated neuroblastoma. *J. Pediatr.*, *85*, 760-763, 1974.

[87] SCHWEISGUTH (O.). — Tumeurs de la crête neurale. In *Tumeurs solides de l'enfant*. Flammarion Médecine-Sciences, 165-189, 1979.

[88] SCHWEISGUTH (O.), MATHÉ (Y.), GIRENAULT (P.), BINET (J.). — Intra-thoracic neurogenic tumors in infants and children. A study of 40 cases. *Ann. Surg.*, *150*, 29-41, 1959.

[89] SHOWN (T.), DURFEE (M.). — Blueberry muffin baby; neonatal neuroblastoma with subcutaneous metastases. *J. Urol.*, *104*, 193-195, 1970.

[90] SHUANGSHOTTI (S.), EKARAPBANICH (S.). — Congenital neuroblastoma and hyperplasia of islets of Langerhans in an infant. *Clin. Pediatr.*, *11*, 241-243, 1972.

[91] SITARZ (A. L.), SANTULLI (T. V.), WIGGER (H. J.), BERDON (W. E.). — Complete maturation of neuroblastoma with bone metastases in documented stages. *J. Pediatr. Surg.*, *10*, 533-536, 1975.

[92] STEWARD (V. M.), JEVTIC (M. M.). — Derangement of neuronal migration in a child with multiple congenital anomalies, two congenital neoplasms, without apparent chromosomal abnormalities. *J. Neuropathol. Exp. Neurol.*, *38*, 259-285, 1979.

[93] STRAUSS (L.), DRISCOLL (S.). — Congenital neuroblastoma involving the placenta; report of 2 cases. *Pediatrics*, *34*, 23-31, 1964.

[94] TURKEL (S. D.), ITABASHI (H. H.). — The natural history of neuroblastic cells in the fetal adrenal gland. *Am. J. Pathol.*, *76*, 225-243, 1974.

[95] UCHINO (J.), HATA (Y.), KASAI (I.). — Stage IVs neuroblastoma. *J. Pediatr. Surg.*, *13*, 167, 1978.

[96] VAN DER SLIKKE (J. W.), BALK (A. G.). — Hydramnios with hydrops fetalis and disseminated fetal neuroblastoma. *Obstet. Gynecol.*, *55*, 250-253, 1980.

[97] VILDE (F.), NEZELOF (C.). — Les neuroblastomes de l'enfant. Étude anatomo-clinique de 46 observations. *Ann. Anat. Pathol.*, *20*, 305-326, 1975.

[98] VOUTE (P.), WADMAN (S.), VON PATTERN (W.). — Congenital neuroblastoma; symptoms in the mother during pregnancy. *Clin. Pediatr.*, *9*, 206-207, 1970.

[99] WITZLEBEN (C. L.), LANDY (R. A.). — Disseminated neuroblastoma in a child with von Recklinghausen's disease. *Cancer*, *34*, 786, 1974.

[100] WONG (K. Y.), HANENSON (I. B.), LAMPKIN (B. C.). — Familial neuroblastoma. *Am. J. Dis. Child.*, *121*, 254-258, 1974.

[101] YOUNG (J. L.), MILLER (R. W.). — Incidence of malignant tumors in US children. *J. Pediatr.*, *86*, 254-258, 1974.

[102] ZUCKER (J. M.). — Retrospective study of 462 neuroblastomas treated between 1950-1970. In 5th Symposium of the International Society of Paediatric Oncology, Maandschr. *Kindergeneesk*, *42*, 369-385, 1974.

[103] ZUCKER (J. M.), MERCIER (J. C.). — Chimiothérapie lourde dans le neuroblastome. *Arch. Franç. Pédiatr.*, *33*, 355, 1976.

Nephroblastomas and related renal tumours

DEFINITION, INCIDENCE, EPIDEMIOLOGY
[1, 33, 46, 47, 78, 85, 91]

Nephroblastomas are embryonic malignant tumours, arising from the metanephrogenic blastoma which, between the 8th and 34th week of gestation, forms the epithelial components of the kidneys and supporting tissue. Its incidence appears to be constant, which excludes a major role for exogenous aetiological factors. In the Manchester Register, it is 5 per 1,000,000 children under 15 years old, constituting 5.4 % of all childhood cancers and 8.9 % of solid tumours [91]. Both sexes are equally affected. 80 % of children are less than 5 years old at the time of diagnosis, 15-20 % are less than 1 year old. In the newborn, Fraumeni and Miller [36] analyzing 21,659 death-certificates of newborn infants between 1960 and 1964, found only 9 Wilms' tumours out of 130 cases of congenital cancer. Bader and Miller reported 5 cases out of 39 cases of cancer diagnosed in the first month of life [1].

Although congenital Wilms' tumours are very rare, it is much commoner at this age to find renal tumours which are considered benign (mesoblastic nephromas), and abnormalities of maturation and differentiation of the renal blastema, which are thought to be possible precursors of Wilms' tumours (nodular blastema and nephroblastomatosis).

Early recognition of these lesions should permit identification of patients at risk. This is sometimes possible by the identification of familial factors, malformations, and growth anomalies, which are now known to be associated with Wilms' tumours and their precursor states [60 bis].

Hereditary forms. — By analogy with retinoblastoma, Knudson and Strong [56] postulate that nephroblastoma is secondary to 2 mutations. They suggest that the first is germinal in about 38 % of cases: 63 % of carriers of the mutant gene should have a risk of tumour; 15 % of them have bilateral tumours, and the age at diagnosis is earlier than in sporadic forms. In 62 % of cases the 2 mutations should be somatic, and the tumour is single and not transmissible. According to these theoretical data, all subjects cured of bilateral tumours and about 30 % of those cured of a unilateral tumour

would transmit the mutant gene to half of their descendants giving them a 63 % tumour risk.

This deserves confirmation; nevertheless familial forms affecting several siblings (less than 1 % of cases) or transmitted through 2 or 3 generations are known [16, 20, 53, 55, 64, 83]. Further, concordance in some monozygotic twins (inconstant) is evidence of prezygotic factors in some cases [22]; whereas the difference in their occurrence may signify that only the ill-twin has been the target of the 2nd mutation [66 bis].

Associated malformations. — These have been reported in 16.2 % of cases by Pendergrass et al. [73] and in 13 % by Lemerle et al. [61].

Congenital aniridia (hypoplasia or absence of the iris): this is linked to an autosomal dominant mutation, although some autosomal recessive cases have been reported [30]. The incidence in the general population is 1 per 50,000 newborn infants. It is 1,000 times more frequent in patients with nephroblastoma [61, 69, 73]. Only the sporadic form, which accounts for 1/3 of cases, appears to be associated with this tumour, for which the risk of occurrence was evaluated at 33 % by Fraumeni and Glass [35]. Other malformations are often associated [32, 44, 69, 75]. These are, in order of frequency:—ocular abnormalities—cataract or glaucoma (78 %), psychomotor retardation with microcephaly and facial dysmorphia (71 %), abnormalities of the external ear (35 %), growth retardation (28 %), genital (28 %) and urinary malformations, with hypospadias and horse-shoe kidney (21 %).

In monozygotic twins with aniridia, with or without other associated malformations, there is discordance for the risk of nephroblastoma. Knudson and Strong [56] postulate that, in these cases, aniridia is due to the first germinal mutation and that a Wilms' tumour only occurs following a second somatic mutation in predisposed cells.

These concepts may lead us to revise the idea that only sporadic cases of aniridia are linked with nephroblastoma, and to predict the risk of tumour in descendants.

The overall incidence of *hemihypertrophy* is 1 in 1,430 children followed to the age of 6 years;

the incidence is 2.9-3.1 % in children with nephro-blastoma [61, 72]. It is also associated with an increased incidence of adrenal cortical adenomas, hepatoblastomas and multiple tumours [69]. Hemi-hypertrophy is usually noted at ages between 1 and 3 years, but sometimes much later [50]. It is rarely diagnosed at birth. It can be limited to one limb or even a limb segment.

Certain forms are familial; Meadows et al. [67] reported a woman with hemihypertrophy, 3 of whose 5 children had Wilms' tumours, despite the absence of hemihypertrophy. However, Knudson and Strong [56], on the basis of the age of occurence of the tumours and the discordance in the mono-zygotic twins, consider that in the majority of cases, this association is due to two somatic post-zygotic mutations, and is therefore not transmissible.

Wiedeman-Beckwith's syndrome [9, 74] pre-disposes to the same tumours as hemihypertrophy (with which it may be associated). The incidence of nephroblastoma is 10-25 %.

Various genito-urinary anomalies (cryptorchidism, sexual ambiguity, horse-shoe kidney, ectopic kidney, pelvic-ureteric duplication, nephrotic syndrome, etc.) are found in 5-8 % of cases [3, 29].

Finally the association of nephroblastomas with *neurofibromatosis* [80 *bis*], *haemangiomas* [65], *naevi* [68], *fibromas and lipomas* is evidence of various embryonal tumors with abnormalities of differen-tiation.

Various chromosomal abnormalities have been described in association with Wilms' tumour: Turner's syndrome, XX/XY mosaic [28, 77], trisomy 18 [38, 63], translocation B-C [40]. *Interstitial 11 p⁻ deletion* is more specifically associated with the syndrome aniridia/Wilms' tumour [92].

WILMS' TUMOUR
[42, 44, 47, 52, 59, 60, 61, 62, 70, 76, 77, 78, 87, 89, 90]

Apart from its rarity, its fairly frequent association with malformations, and its generally favourable prognosis, Wilms' tumour in the newborn does not have any specific clinical characteristics and presents essentially the same therapeutic problems as in children less than 6 months old.

Clinical picture. — With the exception of a few cases of hydramnios and dystocia [11], the usual clinical presentation is by palpation of a lum-bar tumour. Its volume is very variable, but may cause respiratory embarassment. The consistency is firm and the surface is smooth or lumpy. Haematuria and hypertension may occur.

Biochemical investigations are essentially nega-tive; renal function is unsually normal and cate-cholamine concentrations are not elevated.

Diagnosis is made by intravenous urography. The affected kidney is of increased volume and abnormally lumpy. According to the size and site of the tumour there may be pelvi-calyceal distortion, calyceal amputation, ureteric distortion or delayed excretion. Calcification is rare. Where there is a non-functioning kidney, pelvi-calyceal dilatation, or doubt about the integrity of the contralateral kidney, angiography should be performed. This demonstrates a pathological tumour circulation in the renal cortex or medulla [23]. However, some tumours may appear poorly vascularised or even cystic. Ultra-sound and/or computerised tomographic scans are reliable and less invasive means of distinguishing Wilms' tumour from cystic dysplasia. This is the major differential diagnosis apart from mesoblastic nephroma, whose clinical, radiological and angio-graphic features may be identical (see below).

Search for hepatic and pulmonary metastases is likely to be negative. Two cases have been reported of congenital nephroblastoma, associated with hydrocephalus and a second primary tumour in the posterior fossa [54, 87].

Surgical excision and pathological fea-tures. — Once the diagnosis of an intra-renal solid tumour has been established (and/or if it is in doubt) the initial treatment is surgical, without any preoperative radiotherapy or chemotherapy, because of the frequency of mesoblastic nephroma at this age.

Nephrectomy is performed via a transperitoneal laparotomy, taking care to avoid tumour rupture. Biopsies are taken from the tumour bed and from suspect lymph nodes. Markers are inserted. The other kidney is examined and biopsied if any abnormality of its surface is found. As far as we are aware, no case of true bilateral nephroblastoma has been reported in a neonate, although blastematous nodules may be found in the contralateral kidney.

The tumour, of variable size, compresses and distorts the remaining parenchyma, from which it is separated by a fibrous pseudo-capsule which may be invaded by tumour cells. These may also extend into the perirenal fat, blood vessels and local lymph glands. On section the tumour has a grey/pink irregular surface with haemorrhagic and cystic zones. *Histological examination* classically reveals undifferentiated blastema cells, structures providing evidence of epithelial differentiation (immature glomerular tubules, cystic structures) and mesenchymatous fibroblastic tissue which may include cartilagenous and bony elements, and striated muscle.

Prognosis is partly related to the degree of epithelial differentiation [21]. Recent studies emphasize the adverse prognosis associated with aortic lumbar lymph node involvement and with two particular histological types of tumour; the anaplastic and sarcomatous forms [7].

Indications for further treatment according to prognostic factors. — At present, the treatment of nephroblastoma depends on the age of the child, staging of tumour spread, and the histological data [19, 25, 26, 52, 59, 60, 62, 70].

Age: for children under 1 year the 2 year survival rate is 90 %. There are no specific data for neonatal forms.

Staging: this depends on the operative and macroscopic findings.

The classification used is that of the National Wilms' Tumour Study Group (N.W.T.S.G.).

Stage I : tumour limited to the kidney and completely excised.

Stage II : tumour extending beyond the kidney, but excision macroscopically complete.

Stage III : tumour with local/regional extension precluding complete excision.

Stage IV : presence of blood-borne metastases.

Stage V : bilateral nephroblastoma (does not take account of the extent of each tumour).

Other prognostic factors have recently been defined. Taken in conjunction with the stage of the tumour, they identify patients with an increased risk of metastases. Local or regional lymph node involvement carries an adverse prognosis, as do two specific histological forms, the anaplastic form and the sarcomatous form. The latter commonly occurs in children under 2 years, and may sometimes be confused with mesoblastic nephroma (see below).

Current methods of treatment are based on the results of phase III trials organised by American (N. W. T. S. G.) and European (S. I. O. P.) cooperative studies.

In general terms, these have shown:

— that irradiation is unnecessary for stage I tumours;

— the value of chemotherapy, *pre-operatively*, to avoid rupture of the tumour (except in cases of diagnostic uncertainty, and in children under 1 year) and *post-operatively*, to prevent and/or destroy metastases;

— that Vincristine and Actinomycin D have an additive effect when used in combination;

— that chemotherapy may reduce the indications for, and the dosage of irradiation, except in cases of lymph node involvement, unfavourable histology, local and regional extension.

Because of the exceptional features of congenital Wilms' tumours it is only possible to give some general principles of treatment. Obviously it is desirable not to overtreat patients who are going to recover, because of the stage and histology of their tumour, but the risks of relapse and metastases, even at this age, must be recognised.

In stage I no post operative treatment appears necessary.

In stage II treatment with Vincristine and Actinomycin D is probably sufficient, without irradiation. The standard dosage is reduced by a least 50 % because of poor haematologic, digestive, and neurologic tolerance in infants.

In stage III it is undoubtedly preferable to combine chemotherapy with radiotherapy, delivering a dose of 20 grays, via two anterior and posterior fields, according to initial tumour-size, without exceeding 1 gray per session or 5 sessions per week.

Complications, both early (haematologic, digestive, hepatic), and late (digestive, orthopedic, gonadal) may occur [76, 91]. The duration of chemotherapy is 6-12 months.

It is unnecessary to consider the treatment of stages IV and V, which are thought not to occur in the first month of life.

Follow up of the child relies on abdominal echotomography, and/or computerised tomography, and intravenous urography, to assess the compensatory hypertrophy of the remaining kidney, and for detection of bilateral tumours (5-10 % of cases). Chest X-ray is required every 6 weeks for 12 to 15 months. Renal function, blood pressure, ^{197}Hg Cl_2 uptake by the remaining kidney, and the effect of treatment on growth, the digestive tract, the liver and the ovaries, must also be monitored.

Results. — The 2 year survival rate for infants with Wilms' tumour under 12 months of age is 90 %. This is identical with that for stage I tumours. 2 year survival is equivalent to cure.

MESOBLASTIC NEPHROMA
[5, 6, 7, 8, 11, 12, 13, 14, 15, 31, 37, 41, 66,
71, 72, 80, 81, 85, 88, 89]

Definition. Incidence. — This tumour, which is always unilateral and essentially mesenchymatous in nature, is the commonest congenital renal tumour. In the series of 622 renal tumours registered by the S. I. O. P., there are 9 mesoblastic nephromas out of 48 tumours diagnosed before the age of 6 months. It accounts for 20-50 % of all renal tumours at this age, and, overall, half of published cases are neonatal [61].

It has often been confused with Wilms' tumour, from which it must be distinguished by its pathological features, and its favourable prognosis. It has also been called fibrosarcoma, fibroma, congenital leiomyoma or rhabdomyoma, leiomyomatous hamartoma and fœtal mesenchymatous hamartoma. The term mesoblastic nephroma has been used since Bolande et al. published their work in 1967 [15]. The relations between this tumour and nephroblastoma are controversial. Bolande regards it as a tumour of the metanephric blastema [13, 14]. Wigger [89], and Bogdan [12] believe that this tumour is a hamartoma consisting of cells arising from the first stage of connective tissue differentiation, which having originated from secondary mesenchyme is incapable of forming epithelial tissue, as is confirmed by electron microscopy.

Clinical features. — 50 % of cases are diagnosed during the first month of life, most commonly at birth. The presenting clinical sign is an abdominal mass, slight more often on the left, which may, because of its size, cause respiratory embarassment or hypertension [5]. Haematuria is rare. Intravenous urographic findings are similar to those in nephroblastoma, with pelvicalyceal distortion, amputation, and delayed excretion. Echotomography and/or computerised tomography exclude cystic malformations, and make angiography unnecessary.

Pathological features [6, 13, 14, 41, 80].

Macroscopically, the kidney is deformed by a tumour which is often large. On section it occupies 60-80 % of the renal parenchyma, from which it is not separated by a capsule. It is yellow/grey or red/grey in colour, firm. fasciculated and remi-

niscent of a uterine fibroid. There are no haemorrhagic or necrotic areas, and it may contain small cysts.

Histologically, the tumour is composed of elongated fusiform cells, which are fibroplastic or smooth muscular in type, and generally show few mitoses. These enclose occasional scattered islets of epithelial cells which are immature, cystic or dysplastic and of tubular or glomerular appearance. The tumour interdigitates with the cortex without forming a capsule. Some mesoblastic nephromas infiltrate and cross the renal capsule and extend around the renal pedicle or into the perirenal fat.

In principle, a mesoblastic nephroma is easily distinguished from a Wilms' tumour by the absence of malignant epithelial cells and of a capsule. However, problems may arise in forms which contain foci of cells with intense mitotic activity. These must not be confused with the sarcomatous type of nephroblastoma described by Beckwith and Palmer, occuring mostly before 2 years, and carrying a poor prognosis [7].

It should be remembered that inappropriate pre-operative treatment (chemotherapy, radiotherapy) can give the false impression of a mesenchymatous tumour, because the blastematous islets have disappeared.

It is therefore important to perform both a wide initial excision without tumour residue, and skilled histological examination, before assuming that the tumour is benign and that excision alone is sufficient treatment.

Treatment. Results. — Pre-operative chemotherapy or radiotherapy is contraindicated, because they may compromise both histological interpretation, and the quality of survival. *Nephrectomy is the first, and in principle, the only treatment.* Partial resection is not usually possible, because the tumour is usually large and its demarcation from the remaining parenchyma poor.

After nephrectomy, *no further treatment* is necessary if the histological results are clear cut. In the study of Suzuki et al., all 11 cases of mesoblastic nephroma (9 neonatal) were cured by nephrectomy [81]. Follow up was for 4 to 17 years in nine cases. Only 2 patients received Actinomycin D; but chemotherapy is certainly more dangerous than useful [15, 27, 76, 91].

The benign nature of this tumour has sometimes been questioned, and 4 cases of *local or regional recurrence* have been reported [15, 37, 86]. These have been attributed, either to incomplete initial excision, or to doubtful histological interpretation or to the existence of intermediate forms between benign mesoblastic nephroma and the sarcomatous forms of Wilms' tumour.

BLASTEMATOUS NODULES AND NEPHROBLASTOMATOSIS
[14, 17, 64 *bis*, 77, 79, 89]

Persistent metanephric blastema refers to the finding of accumulations of metanephric blastema in infants and children beyond 36 weeks gestation. Two main patterns of distribution are observed: *superficial multifocal nephroblastomatosis and the diffuse form.*

Superficial multifocal nephroblastomatosis [4, 57, 60 *bis*, 63, 64, 64 *bis*, 65, 74, 88] is
characterized by persistent nodular renal blastema located in a subcapsular position, and along the columns of Bertin. Its rate based on pediatric necropsies is 0.49 %; it reaches 0.9 % in children less than 3 months [64 *bis*]. Its relationship to Wilms tumor is clearly defined: nodular blastema could accompany 30 to 50 % of Wilms tumor and all bilateral cases [27, 64 *bis*]; moreover, beyond 3 to 4 months of age nephroblastomatosis is always associated with Wilms' tumor. According to the model defined by Knudson and Strong, nephroblastomatosis is considered as the consequence of the first mutation: a genetic defect of differentiation frequently associated with a familial incidence and congenital anomalies: hemihypertrophy [18, 27], Wiedeman-Beckwith syndrome [4, 43, 64, 64 *bis*, 74], genital ambiguity [18, 27], Klippel-Trenaunay syndrome [65], 18-trisomy syndrome [63]. One can see the interest in defining environmental factors to explain the second mutation leading to cancer: the role of progestative drugs, excess of coffee and tea during pregnancy is under study [60 *bis*].

Superficial multifocal nephroblastomatosis has three major *histological features.*

Nodularblastema is defined as circumscribed collections of immature (sometimes epithelial) cells, of 100 to 300 μ in diameter; mitotic activity is very low; there is no conjunctive tissue.

Wilms' tumorlets measure more than 0.3 to 0.5 cm in diameter; they are composed of blastemal or epithelial tissue; they are regarded as truly neoplastic, but without metastatic potential.

Metanephric hamartomas contain sclerosed stomal and epithelial cellular components of an adenomatous, papillar or tubular type. They may replace nodular blastema and Wilms' tumorlets after spontaneous regression or successful chemotherapy.

Therapeutically, some Wilms' tumorlets may be excised when they are discovered during surgical treatment of Wilms' tumor; furthermore it is admitted that chemotherapy is able to provoke the regression of multifocal nephroblastomatosis. However careful follow up by echotomography, computerized tomography and intravenous pyelography is necessary.

Diffuse nephroblastomatosis [18, 27, 43, 48, 64 *bis*, 84, 88, 89] is characterized by the confluence of persistent metanephric nodular blastema: The term nephroblastomatosis was used initially by Hou and Holman [48] to refer only to this type of lesion; however, it differs from multifocal nephroblastomatosis only by the quantity and the arrangement of the persistent blastema. A diffuse form may follow the multifocal type, or be associated simultaneously in the same patient. Both may have a familial incidence, as has been reported by Perlman et al. [74] and by Liban et al. [64]. Thus it seems justified to use the term nephroblastomatosis refering to both multifocal and diffuse forms.

The first observation published by Hou and Holman [48] in 1961 concerns an infant dead at 13 hours of life of respiratory distress; the entire kidney was replaced by blastema, which characterised an exceptionally diffuse pannephric nephroblastomatosis incompatible with life.

In other cases, blastemal tissue constitutes a layer (20 % of kidney), external to normal parenchyma; only some ten cases have been reported but others may have been misdiagnosed as bilateral Wilms' tumours.

From a clinical point of view, diffuse nephroblastomatosis gives bilateral nephromegaly often asymetric, sometimes associated with hypertension and malformations. Intravenous pyelography is often suggestive of polycystic kidneys, but this diagnosis may be excluded by echotomography and/or computerised tomography. Renal angiography demonstrates peripheral vascular abnormalities (fine, stretched vessels), and in the nephrogram phase, a clear band, 0.5 to 1 cm wide, corresponding to the hypoperfused cortex contrasting with the normal medulla [18].

Definitive diagnosis depends on histology. Laparotomy, permitting exploration and biopsy of both kidneys, is indicated when bilateral nephroblastoma is a diagnostic possibility. In fact, in published cases, this problem has not arisen in the neonatal period, but only after the age of 3 months.

Pathological data: the kidneys are enlarged and abnormally lobulated. The tumour diffusely invades the subcortical zone, within which it is confined. It is homogeneous, pink in colour, and distinct from the underlying normal parenchyma. The embryonic epithelial cells are organised into tubules and immature glomeruli, without atypical cells, or abundant mitoses. The primary mesenchyme is not represented, and there are no haemorrhages or necrotic areas.

The principles of treatment are based upon the diffuse nature of the lesions and the possibility of spontaneous regression, but also on the risk of the development of a Wilms' tumour. Nearly all patients received treatment at various stages, so that the natural history of nephroblastomatosis is not well known. A few cases, well documented with angiographic and histological data (open biopsy and repeated needle biopsies) have enabled the evolution of the nodular blastema to be followed either towards massive nephroblastomatosis and Wilms' tumour, or regression under the influence of treatment [18, 27, 43, 84]. When evolution is favourable, the kidney(s) become(s) progressively smaller, and there is progressive subscapular fibrosis, enclosing small islets of atrophic and sclerotic tubules and glomeruli, or occasional immature epithelial cells. Calcification is not unusual.

Treatment relies mainly on chemotherapy, using Vincristine combined with Actinomycin D for 6 to 12 months [43, 57]. Radiotherapy has been used but its hazards seem to outweigh its benefits. Overall the prognosis is good. Follow-up relies mainly on intravenous urography, echotomography and/or computerised tomography. Repeated percutaneous renal biopsies have been suggested, but their interpretation may be difficult due to persisting islets of embryonic cells, whose immediate and long term significance is not clearly established. It may be preferable to perform a second laparotomy after 6 to 12 months.

WELL DIFFERENTIATED EPITHELIAL NEPHROBLASTOMAS

There is controversy over whether well differentiated epithelial nephroblastomas should be classified as tumours or dysplasias. The monomorphic or nephroblastic variety, and the so-called "rosette"

form described by Chatten [21] which account for 10 % of the total, occur before the age of 1 year, and have an excellent prognosis with a cure rate of 90-100 %.

Polycystic nephroblastoma, or partially differentiated cystic nephroblastoma, or cystic nephroma [2, 14, 24, 34, 39, 42, 52, 58] is an encapsulated cystic tumour occuring before the age of 2 years. The cysts are bounded by an epithelium, and are separated by septa containing partially differentiated or immature elements originating from the metanephric blastema. In principle, this distinguishes this tumour from a solitary multilocular cyst of the kidney, but the boundaries between neoplastic and cystic lesions are not always very clear.

Cystic nephromas and multilocular cysts present clinically and radiologically like classical Wilms' tumours. Echotomographic findings are sometimes ambiguous, because of the large number of small cystic structures. The avascularity of this tumour, not always demonstrated by angiography, theoretically distinguishes it from a nephroblastoma, but computerised tomography is the only reliable method of preoperative diagnosis. Total or partial nephrectomy is always curative.

REFERENCES

[1] BADER (J. L.), MILLER (R. W.). — US Cancer incidence and mortality in the first year of life. *Am. J. Dis. Child.*, *133*, 155-159, 1979.

[2] BALDAUF (M. C.), SCHULZ (D. M.). — Multilocular cyst of the kidney. Report of 3 cases with review of the literature. *Am. J. Clin. Pathol.*, *65*, 93-102, 1976.

[3] BARAKAT (K. Y.), PAPADOPOULOU (Z. L.), CHANDRA (R. S.), HOLLERMAN (C. E.), CALGANO (P. L.). — Pseudohermaphroditism, nephron disorder and Wilms' tumor: a unifying concept. *Pediatrics*, *54*, 366-369, 1974.

[4] BAR-ZIV (J.), HIRSCH (M.), PERLMAN (M.). — Bilateral nephroblastomatosis. *Pediatr. Radiol.*, *3*, 85-88, 1975.

[5] BAUER (J. H.), DURHAM (J.), MILES (J.), HAKAMI (N.), GROSHONG (T.). — Congenital mesoblastic nephroma presenting with primary reninism. *J. Pediatr.*, *95*, 268-272, 1979.

[6] BECKWITH (J. B.). — Mesenchymal renal neoplasms of infancy revisited (editorial). *J. Pediatr. Surg.*, *9*, 803-805, 1974.

[7] BECKWITH (J. B.), PALMER (N. F.). — Histopathology and prognosis of Wilms' tumor. Results from the first National Wilms' tumor study. *Cancer*, *41*, 1937-1948, 1978.

[8] BERDON (W. E.), WIGGER (H. J.), BAKER (D. H.). — Fetal renal hamartoma; a benign tumor to be distinguished from Wilms' tumor. *Am. J. Roentgenol. Radium Ther. Nucl. Med.*, *118*, 18-27, 1973.

[9] BETEND (B.), BRUNAT (M.), DAVID (L.), LESBROS (F.), HERMIER (M.). — Association d'un néphroblastome

bifocal à un syndrome de Wiedemann-Beckwith. *Arch. Fr. Pédiatr.*, *33*, 683-691, 1976.

[10] BISHOP (H. C.), TEFFT (M.), EVANS (A. E.). — Survival in bilateral Wilms' tumor. Review of 30 National Wilms' tumor study cases. *J. Pediatr., Surg.*, *12*, 631-637, 1979.

[11] BLANK (E.), NEERHOUT (R. C.), BERRY (K. A.). — Congenital mesoblastic nephroma and polyhydramnios. *J. A. M. A.*, *240*, 1504-1505, 1978.

[12] BOGDAN (R.), TAYLOR (D. E. M.), MOSTOFI (F. K.). — Leiomyomatous hamartoma of the kidney. *Cancer*, *31*, 462-467, 1973.

[13] BOLANDE (R. P.). — Congenital mesoblastic nephroma of infancy. *Perspect. Pediatr. Pathol.*, *1*, 227-250, 1973.

[14] BOLANDE (R. P.). — Neoplasia in early life and its relationship to teratogenesis. *Perspect. Pediatr. Pathol.*, *3*, 145-183, 1976.

[15] BOLANDE (R. P.), BROUGH (A. J.), IZANT (R.). — Congenital mesoblastic nephroma of infancy; a report of 8 cases and relationship to Wilms' tumor. *Pediatrics*, *40*, 272-278, 1967.

[16] BOND (J. V.). — Wilms' tumor, hypospadias and cryptorchidism in twins. *Arch. Dis. Child.*, *52*, 243, 1977.

[17] BOVE (K. E.), MCADAMS (A. J.). — The nephroblastomatosis complex and its relationship to Wilms' tumor. A clinicopathological treatise. *Perspect. Pediatr. Pathol.*, *3*, 185-223, 1976.

[18] BRANTLEY (R. E.), SIMSON (L. P.). — Angiography and histopathology of nephroblastomatosis. *Radiology*, *120*, 151-154, 1976.

[19] BRESLOW (N. E.), PALMER (M. F.), HILL (L. R.), BURING (J.), D'ANGIO (J. G.). — Wilms' tumor: prognostic factors for patients without metastases at diagnosis. Results of the national Wilms' tumor study. *Cancer*, *42*, 1577-1589, 1978.

[20] BROWN (W. T.), PURANIK (S. R.), ALTMAN (D. H.), HARTIN (H. C.). — Wilms' tumor in three successive generations. *Surgery*, *72*, 756-761, 1972.

[21] CHATTEN (J.). — Epithelial differentiation in Wilms' tumor: a clinico-pathologic appraisal. *Perspect., Pediatr. Pathol.*, *3*, 225-254, 1976.

[22] COTLIER (E.), ROSE (M.), MOEL (S. A). — Aniridia, cataracts, and Wilms' tumor in monozygous twins. *Am. J. Ophtal.*, *86*, 129-132, 1978.

[23] CREMIN (B. J.), KASCHULA (R. O.). — Arteriography in Wilms' tumor; the results of 13 cases and comparaison with renal dysplasia. *Br. J. Radiol.*, *45*, 425-432, 1972.

[24] CROUZET (A.), PASQUIER (D.), DYON (J. F.), BOST (M.), BAUDAIN (Ph.). — Kyste multiloculaire ou néphroblastome plurikystique? *Pédiatrie*, *35*, 359-364, 1980.

[25] D'ANGIO (G. J.), EVANS (A. E.), BRESLOW (N.), BECKWITH (B.), BISHOP (H.), FEIGL (P.), GOODWIN (W.), LEAPE (L. L.), SINKS (L. F.), SUTOW (W.), TEFT (M.), WOLFF (J.). — The treatment of Wilms' tumor results of the national Wilms' tumor study. *Cancer, 38*, 633-646, 1976.

[26] D'ANGIO (G. J.), BECKWITH (J. B.), BRESLOW (N. E.), BISHOP (H. C.), EVANS (A. E.), SAREWELL (V.), FERNBACH (D.), GOODWIN (W. E.), JONES (B.), LEAPE (L. L.), PALMER (N. F.), TEFFT (M.), WOLFF (J. A.). — Wilms' tumor: an update. *Cancer*, *45*, 1791-1798, 1980.

[27] DE CHADAREVIAN (J. P.), FLETCHER (B. D.), CHATTEN (J.), RABINOVITCH (H. H.). — Massive infantile nephroblastomatosis. A clinical, radiological, and pathological analysis of four cases. *Cancer*, *39*, 2294-2305, 1977.

[28] DENYS (P.), MALVAUX (P.), VAN DEN BERGHE (H.), TANGHE (W.), PROESMANS (W.) — Association d'un syndrome anatomo-pathologique de pseudohermaphrodisme masculin, d'une tumeur de Wilms, d'une néphropathie parenchymateuse, et d'un mosaïcisme XX/XY. *Arch. Fr. Pediatr.*, *24*, 729-739, 1967.

[29] DRASH (A.), SHERMAN (F.), HARTMANN (W. H.), BLIZZARD (R. M.). — A syndrome of pseudohermaphroditism, Wilms' tumor, hypertension, and degenerative renal disease. *J. Pediatr.*, *76*, 585-593, 1970.

[30] DUTAU (G.), ZAYSSE (Ph.), RIBOT (C.), CARTON (M.), JUSKIEWENSKI (S.), ROCHICCIOLO (T.). — Le syndrome aniridie-néphroblastome. *J. Genet. Hum.*, *42*, 43-54, 1976.

[31] EIDELMAN (A.), SIBI (J.), VURE (E.), KOHN (R.), TIEDER (M.). — The management of benign renal tumors of infancy. Case report of congenital mesoblastic nephroma (leiomyomatous hamartoma). *Helv. Paediatr. Acta*, *30*, 169-174, 1975.

[32] EVANS (D. I. K.), HOLZEL (A.). — Wilms' aniridia syndrome with transient hypo-globulinaemia of infancy. *Arch. Dis. Child.*, *48*, 645-646, 1973.

[33] FAVARA (B. E.), JOHNSON (W.), ITO (J.). — Renal tumors in the neonatal period. *Cancer*, *22*, 845-855, 1968.

[34] FOBI (M.), MAHOUR (G. H.), ISAACS (H.). — Multilocular cyst of the kidney. *J. Pediatr. Surg.*, *14*, 282-286, 1979.

[35] FRAUMENI (J. F.), GLASS (A. G.). — Wilms' tumor and congenital aniridia. *J. A. M. A.*, *206*, 825-828, 1968.

[36] FRAUMENI (J. F.), MILLER (R. W.). — Cancer deaths in the newborn. *Am. J. Dis. Child.*, *117*, 186-189, 1969.

[37] FU (Y. S.), KAY (S.). — Congenital mesoblastic nephroma and its recurrence. *Arch. Pathol.*, *96*, 66-70, 1973.

[38] GEISER (C. F.), SCHINDLER (A. M.). — Long survival in a male with 18-trisomy syndrome and Wilms' tumor. *Pediatrics*, *44*, 111-115, 1969.

[39] GALLO (G. E.), PENCHANSKY (L.). — Cystic nephroma. *Cancer*, *39*, 1322-1327, 1977.

[40] GIANGIACOMO (J.), PENCHANSKY (L.), MONTELEONE (P. L.), THOMPSON (J.). — Bilateral neonatal Wilms' tumor with B-C chromosomal translocation. *J. Pediatr.*, *86*, 98-102, 1975.

[41] GILLY (J.), BOUVIER (R.), BERARD (J.). — Néphromes mésoblastiques. A propos de 6 cas. *Ann. Chir. Pédiatr.*, *21*, 275-279, 1980.

[42] GOLDSCHMIDT (H.), BACHMAN (K. D.). — Der Wilms' tumor beim neugeborenen. *Schweiz. Med. Wochenschr.*, *104*, 658-662, 1974.

[43] HADDY (T. B.), BAILIE (M. D.), BERNSTEIN (J.), KAUFMAN (D. B.), ROUS (S. N.). — Bilateral, diffuse nephroblastomatosis: report of a case managed with chemotherapy. *J. Pediatr.*, *90*, 784-786, 1977.

[44] HAICKEN (B. N.), MILLER (D. R.). — Simultaneous occurrence of congenital aniridia, hamartoma and Wilms' tumor. *J. Pediatr.*, *78*, 497-502, 1971.

[45] HAVERS (W.), STAMBOLIS (C.). — Benign cystic nephroblastoma. *Europ. J. Pediatr.*, *231*, 119-123, 1979.

[46] HILTON (C.), KEELING (J. W.). — Neonatal renal tumors. *Br. J. Urol.*, *46*, 157-161, 1973.

[47] HOLLAND (T.). — *Clinical and biochemical manifestations of Wilms' tumor*. In POCHEDLY (C.),

MILLER (D.), ed. Wilms' tumor, John Wiley and Sons, New York, 11-30, 1976.

[48] HOU (L. T.), HOLMAN (R. L.). — Bilateral nephroblastomatosis in a premature infant. J. Pathol. Bacteriol., 82, 249-255, 1961.

[49] JAGASIA (K. H.), THERMAN (W. G.), PICKETT (E.), GRABSTALDT (H.). — Bilateral Wilms' tumor in children. J. Pediatr., 65, 371-376, 1964.

[50] JANIK (J. S.), SEELER (R. A.). — Delayed onset of hemihypertrophy in Wilms' tumor. J. Pediatr. Surg., 11, 581-582, 1976.

[51] JAVADPOUR (M.), BUSH (I. M.). — Induction and treatment of Wilms' tumor by transplantation or renal blastema in a new experimental model. J. Urol., 107, 931-937, 1972.

[52] JOHNSON (D. G.). — Treatment of Wilms' tumor in children. World. J. Surg., 4, 5-13, 1980.

[53] JUBERG (R. C.), MARTIN (E. C. S.), HUNDLEY (J. R.). — Familial occurrence of Wilms' tumor: nephroblastoma in one of monozygous twins and in another sibling. Am. J. Hum. Genet., 27, 155-164, 1975.

[54] KALOUSEK (D. K.), CHADAREVIAN (J. P. DE), MACKIE (G. G.), BOLANDE (R. P.). — Metastatic infantile Wilms' tumor and hydrocephalus. A case report with review of the literature. Cancer, 39, 1312-1316, 1977.

[55] KAUFMAN (R. L.), VIETTI (D. J.), WABNER (C. I.). — Wilms' tumor in father and son. Lancet, 1, 43, 1973.

[56] KNUDSON (A. G.), STRONG (L. C.). — Mutation and cancer: a model for Wilms' tumor of the kidney. J. Natl. Cancer Inst., 48, 313-324, 1972.

[56 bis] KULKARNI (R.), BAILIE (M. D.), BERNSTEIN (J.). — Progression of nephroblastomatosis to Wilms' tumor. J. Pediatr., 96, 178, 1980.

[57] KUMAR (A. P. M.), PRATT (C. B.), COBURN (T. P.), JOHNSON (W.). — Treatment strategy for nodular renal blastoma and nephroblastomatosis associated with Wilms' tumor. J. Pediatr. Surg., 13, 281-285, 1978.

[58] KYAW (M. M.). — The radiological diagnosis of congenital multicystic kidney; « radiological trial ». Clin. Radiol., 25, 45-62, 1974.

[59] LEAPE (L. L.), BRESLOW (M. E.), BISHOP (H. C.). — The surgical treatment of Wilms' tumor: results of the National Wilms' Tumor Study. Am. J. Surg., 187, 351-356, 1978.

[60] LEDLIE (E. M.), MYNORS (L. S.), DRAPER (G. J.). GORBACH (P. D.). — Natural history and treatment of Wilms' tumor: an analysis of 335 cases occurring in England and Wales 1962-1966. Br. Med. J., 4, 195-200, 1970.

[60 bis] LE MASTERS (G. K.), BOVE (K. E.). — Genetic/environmental significance of multifocal nodular renal blastema. Am. J. Pediatr. Hematol. Oncol., 2, 81-87, 1980.

[61] LEMERLE (J.), TOURNADE (M. F.), GÉRARD-MARCHANT (R.), FLAMANT (R.), SARRAZIN (D.), FLAMANT (F.), LEMERLE (M.), JUNDT (R.), ZUCKER (J. M.), SCHWEISGUTH (O.). — Wilms' tumor: natural history and pronostic factors. A retrospective study of 248 cases treated at the Institut Gustave-Roussy, 1952-1967. Cancer, 37, 2557-2566, 1976.

[62] LEMERLE (J.), VOUTE (P. A.), TOURNADE (M. F.), DELEMARRE (J. F. M.), JEREB (B.), AHSTROM (L.), FLAMANT (R.), GÉRARD-MARCHANT (R.). — Radiotherapy, single versus multiple courses of actinomycin D, in the treatment of Wilms' tumor. Preliminary results of a controlled clinical trial conducte-

bly the international society of paediatric oncology (SIOP). Cancer, 38, 647-654, 1976.

[63] LEWIS (A. J.). — The pathology of 18-trisomy. J. Pediatr., 65, 92-101, 1964.

[64] LIBAN (E.), KOZENITZKY (I. L.). — Metanephric hamartomas and nephroblastomatosis in siblings. Cancer, 25, 885-888, 1970.

[64 bis] MACHIN (G. A.). — Persistent renal blastema (nephroblastomatosis) as a frequent precursor of Wilms' tumor; a pathological and clinical review. Part 1. Nephroblastomatosis in context of embryology and genetics. Am. J. Pediatr. Hematol. Oncol., 2, 165-172, 1980. Part 2. Significance of nephroblastomatosis in the genesis of Wilms' tumor. Am. J. Pediatr. Hematol. Oncol., 2, 253-261, 1980. Part 3. Clinical aspects of nephroblastomatosis. Am. J. Pediatr. Hematol. Oncol., 2, 353-362, 1980.

[65] MANKAD (V. N.), GRAY (G. F.), MILLER (D. R.). — Bilateral nephroblastomatosis and Klippel-Trenaunay syndrome. Cancer, 33, 1462-1467, 1974.

[66] MCCUNE (W. R.), GALLEHER (E. P.), WOOD (C.). — Leiomyoma of kidney in a newborn infant. J. Urol., 91, 646-648, 1964.

[66 bis] MAURER (H. S.), PENDERGRASS (T. W.), BOYES (W.). — The role of genetic factors in the etiology of Wilms' tumor. Cancer, 43, 205-208, 1979.

[67] MEADOWS (A. R.), LICHTENFELD (J. L.), EVERETT DOOP (C.). — Wilms' tumor in three children of a woman with congenital hemihypertrophy. N. Engl. J. Med., 291, 23-24, 1974.

[68] MEADOWS (A. R.), JARRETT (P.). — Pigmented nevi, Wilms' tumor, and second malignant neoplasms. J. Pediatr., 93, 889-890, 1978.

[69] MILLER (R. W.), FRAUMENI (J. F.), MANNING (M. D.). — Association of Wilms' tumor with aniridia hemihypertrophy and other congenital malformations. N. Engl. J. Med., 270, 922-927, 1964.

[70] MORRIS-JONES (P. H.). — Med. Res. Council's Working Party in Embryonal tumors in childhood: management of Nephroblastoma in childhood. Arch. Dis. Child., 53, 112-119, 1978.

[71] OSHI (W. W.), KAY (S.), MILSTEN (R.), KOONTZ (W. W.), MCWILLIAMS (N. B.). — Congenital mesoblastic nephroma of infancy: report of a case with unusual clinical behaviour. Am. J. Clin. Pathol., 60, 811-816, 1973.

[72] PENCHANSKY (L.), GALLO (G.). — Leiomyomatous tumors of infant kidney. J. Pediatr., 89, 320-326, 1976.

[73] PENDERGRASS (T. W.). — Congenital anomalies in children with Wilms' tumor: a new survey. Cancer, 37, 403-409, 1976.

[74] PERLMAN (M.), LEVIN (M.), WITTELS (B.). — Syndrome of fetal gigantism, renal hamartomas and nephroblastomatosis with Wilms' tumor. Cancer, 35, 1212-1217, 1975.

[75] PILLING (G. P.). — Wilms' tumor in seven children with congenital aniridia. J. Pediatr. Surg., 10, 31-36, 1975.

[76] POCHEDLY (C.), COLLUTTI (J. A.), KENIGSBERG (K.), LOESEVITZ (A.). — Hazard of chemotherapy in congenital Wilms' tumor. J. Pediatr., 79, 708-709, 1971.

[77] POCHEDLY (C.), MILLER (D.). — Wilms' tumor. New York, John Wiley and Sons Inc., 239 p., 1976.

[78] RICHMOND (H.), DOUGALL (A. J.). — Neonatal renal tumors. J. Pediatr. Surg., 513-518, 1970.

[79] SHANKLIN (D. R.), SOTELO-AVILA (C.). — In situ

tumors in fetuses, newborns and young infants. *Biol. Neonate*, *14*, 286-316, 1969.

[80] SHEN (S. C.), YUNIS (E. J.). — A study of the cellularity and ultrastructure of congenital mesoblastic nephroma. *Cancer*, *45*, 306-314, 1980.

[80 bis] STAY (E. J.), VAWTER (G.). — The relationship between nephroblastoma and neurofibromatosis (von Recklinghausen's disease). *Cancer*, *39*, 2550-2555, 1977.

[81] SUZUKI (H.), YAMASHITA (O.), SAKAKURA (K.), AMANO (S.), HONZUMI (M.). — Congenital mesoblastic nephroma: report of a case and clinical analysis of 11 cases in Japan. *Z. Kinderchir.*, *27*, 64-68, 1979.

[82] TAXY (J. B.), FILMER (R. B.). — Glomerulocystic kidney, report of a case. *Arch. Pathol. Lab. Med.*, *100*, 186-188, 1976.

[83] TEBBI (K.), GROSS (S.). — Wilms' tumor in a mother and child. *J. Pediatr.*, *92*, 1026-1027, 1978.

[84] TELANDER (R. I.), GILCHRIST (G. S.), BURGERT (E. O.), KELALIS (P. P.), GOELLNER (J. R.). — Bilateral massive nephroblastomatosis in infancy. *J. Pediatr. Surg.*, *13*, 163-166, 1978.

[85] WAISMAN (J.), COOPER (P. H.). — Renal neoplasms of the newborn. *J. Pediatr. Surg.*, *5*, 407-412, 1970.

[86] WALKER (D.), RICHARD (G. A.). — Fetal hamartoma of the kidney; recurrence and death of patient. *J. Urol.*, *110*, 352-353, 1974.

[87] WEXLER (H. A.), POOLE (C. A.), FOJACO (R. M.). — Metastatic neonatal Wilms' tumor: a case report with review of the literature. *Pediatr. Radiol.*, *3*, 179-181, 1975.

[88] WIGGER (H. J.). — Fetal mesenchymal hamartoma of kidney. A tumor of secondary mesenchyma. *Cancer*, *36*, 1002-1008, 1975.

[89] WIGGER (H. J.). — *Histopathology of Wilms' tumor and related lesions*, 105-131. *In* POCHEDLY (C.), MILLER (D.), ed. New York, John Wiley and Sons Inc., 1976.

[90] WRIGHT (E. S.). — Congenital Wilm's tumors: case report. *Br. J. Urol.*, *42*, 270-272, 1970.

[91] YOUNG (D.), WILLIAMS (D.). — Malignant renal tumors in infancy and childhood. *Br. J. Hosp. Med.*, *2*, 741, 1969.

[92] YUNIS (J. J.), RAMSAY (N. K. C.). — Familial occurrence of the aniridia-Wilms' tumor syndrome with deletion 11. 13-14. 1. *J. Pediatr.*, *96*, 1027-1030 1980.

Teratomas

DEFINITION. INCIDENCE PATHOLOGICAL FEATURES

Teratomas (from the Greek teratos: monster) are tumours derived from multipotential cells, composed in variable proportions, of tissues originating from endodermal, mesodermal and ectodermal layers, some of which are foreign to the site in which they are found [6]. They are thereby distinguished from heterotopias and choristomas, which are malformations and proliferations of a tissue or organ in an abnormal anatomical position, and from hamartomas, which are proliferative malformations of a tissue normally present in the organ of origin. They also differ from blastematous tumours which originate from embryonic tissue already orientated towards a specific type of histogenesis. Although Willis regards all teratomas as congenital [68], only some of them are discovered in the neonatal period: these are primarily sacrococcygeal, cervical, and nasopharyngeal teratomas. Testicular teratomas are usually discovered before two years of age, while the ovarian and mediastinal teratomas are usually found after 5 years of age [71].

In the British Paediatric Pathological Society study, teratomas accounted for 24 % of all benign and malignant tumours diagnosed in the first month of life [10]. Fraumeni and Miller attributed, 6.9 % of neonatal tumour deaths to teratomas. In this study, 8.1 % of children under 5 years of age with teratomas died in the first month of life [26, 27].

Females are more often affected than males, particularly by sacro-coccygeal forms (70 %), whereas gastric and cerebral teratomas are more common in boys. More than 90 % of neonatal teratomas are benign.

Teratomas are classified into three histological types, of prognostic importance [9, 16, 23, 24]; their potential depends on the presence of embryonic or poorly differentiated tissues, which are liable to degenerate.

Mature teratomas (or dermoid cysts). — These are always benign, and are formed of mature multi-tissular elements, with alternating solid and cystic zones, together with organoid structures which are often well differentiated. Some areas may seem immature, but their stage of differentiation corresponds to the age of the child. An unusual, highly differentiated form of mature teratoma has been described (the "fœtus in fetu") of which about thirty cases have been published [8, 43, 44, 48]. It consists of a differentiated vertebrate parasitic structure usually situated in the abdominal cavity, and more rarely in the skull, on the face or in the scrotum. This teratoma represents a mono-zygous twin (of the same chromosomal sex), whose development has arrested after accidental impri-sonment within the carrier.

Mixed teratomas contain mature tissue, toge-ther with components that are truly immature, not frankly malignant.

Malignant teratomas are not always pluri-tissular. Malignancy is confirmed by the following histological tissues: embryonal carcinoma, chorio-carcinoma and particularly yolk sac tumor.

Pathological examination of a teratoma must be meticulous, because of the frequent co-existence of mature, immature and frankly malignant zones.

SACRO-COCCYGEAL TERATOMAS
[1, 2, 4, 13, 17, 18, 24, 30 32,
34, 35, 40, 46, 53, 60, 67, 69]

Incidence. Epidemiology. — Sacro-coccy-geal teratomas, whose incidence is estimated by Berry to be 1 per 35,000 births, account for 40-65 % of teratomas in children [12]. Two thirds are disco-vered in the neonatal period. In 10-50 % of cases there is an increased incidence of twin pregnancies in the family [52].

Associated malformations occur in 5-25 % of cases [26], in the patients and their family. These are, in order of frequency: skeletal abnormalities, uro-genital, intestinal and cardiac malformations; angiomas and naevi are often found in relation to the teratoma. Ganick et al. found a translocation 46 G/G in a neonate with a teratoma and ano-rectal abnormalities [28]. Ashcraft and Holder have described a syndrome, transmitted as an autosomal dominant over 3 generations, in which a sacro-coccygeal teratoma was associated with local bony anomalies, vesico-ureteric reflux and ano-rectal stenosis [5].

No exogenous factors have been demonstrated to have an aetiologic role, except possibly for acetazolamide in one case [72].

Clinical picture. — The symptomatology differs according to the origin and mode of extension of the tumour. Various types are recognised. Extra-pelvic tumours which develop more or less in the midline, correspond to Altman's type I [1]. This external tumour may have an intra-pelvic extension, which must not be overlooked (and is then of Altman type II). Other teratomas develop mainly within the pelvis, growing out laterally towards the buttock (Altman type III); and finally, some are purely intra-pelvic (Altman type IV).

The exteriorised forms (types I and II) represent 82 % of these neonatal teratomas. The tumour is implanted between the anus and the coccyx. It may be of considerable size, and causes dystocia in 10-15 % of cases [38]. The diagnosis can be made in utero by echography, which is often done because of hydramnios. Its consistency is heterogeneous and the surface may be lumpy or smooth. The skin has a tendency to ulcerate, to bleed, and to become secondarily infected. The anus is pushed forward to lie in the same plane as the umbilicus and the external genitalia, which excludes myelo-menin-gocoele. On rectal examination, which is sometimes difficult, an extension of the tumour between the sacrum and rectum may be palpable; this intra-pelvic tumour is usually well delimited and does not extend beyond the sacral promontory.

Predominantly intra-pelvic teratomas are much rarer in the neonatal period. Attention is drawn by a small, lateral, swelling usually situated in the infero-medial quadrant of the buttock. Rectal examination reveals a pre-sacral tumour, sometimes poorly defined, which may extend into the retro-peritoneal space.

Purely intra-pelvic teratomas are rarer still. Diagnosis is made later, as a result of signs of bladder, rectal or spinal cord compression.

The importance of careful routine clinical exa-mination of the buttocks and perineal area in the neonate should be remembered; in looking for mal-formations, asymetry, cutaneous angiomas, coccy-geal dimple, abnormal buttock fold, pilonidal sinus pigmented naevus, displacement of the anus, reten-tion of urine, and lower limb paralysis.

Investigations. — Investigations should include the following:

Biochemical investigations. — Apart from the estimation of urinary catecholamine metabolite concentrations to exclude a pelvic neuroblastoma, and evaluation of renal function, measurement of the alpha-1-fœto-protein and Beta-2-Human Chorio-nic Gonadotropin (β_2HCG) is helpful.

Radiology, echotomography, and/or computerised tomography, are necessary to define the extent of the tumour. Pelvic X-rays, in cases of exteriorised tumour, show a mass of soft-tissue density over the postero-inferior part of the coccyx, which is displaced backwards. Calcification and osteoid areas are seen in 30 to 60 % of tumours and would indicate a more favourable prognosis. Views of the lumbo-sacral spine, show a backward tilt of the coccyx, and, when there is pelvic extension, loss of the sacral concavity. Bony erosion and/or lytic lesions may be seen where the tumour is in contact with the vertebral bodies, the sacrum, the coccyx and the ischium. Malformations of the lower lumbar vertebrae and the sacro-coccygeal region may be seen.

Abdomino-pelvic ultrasound (and/or computerised tomographic scans) define the extent of the tumour in the pelvis and/or in the retro-peritoneal region. They also establish the nature of the tumour (solid, cystic or calcified), and may show lymph node or hepatic metastases.

Intravenous urography is not essential in purely extra-pelvic tumours. However it is necessary in order to assess compression or invasion of the bladder, displacement of the ureters, and possible ureteric dilatation and hydronephrosis, in the case of intra-pelvic tumours.

Barium enema may demonstrate anterior and/or lateral displacement of the rectum, whose wall may be infiltrated.

Myelography is indicated where there is neurological deficit, bony invasion, hydrocephalus, or diagnostic uncertainty with regard to an anterior meningocoele [21, 47].

Differential diagnosis. — Sacro-coccygeal teratomas in neonates pose few problems in differential diagnosis.

With *a tumour of the buttock*, soft tissue sarcoma, haemangioma, and abscess must be excluded.

With *intra-pelvic tumours*, apart from the above-mentioned conditions, an erroneous diagnosis of anterior or posterior meningocoele can be made. Pelvic neuroblastomas are difficult to distinguish from teratomas, if catecholamine levels are not raised; but, in either case, surgical excision is necessary. Finally, occasional chordomas have been reported [57, 66].

Treatment. — Surgical excision must be decided upon as quickly as possible, as soon as investigations are complete and the infant has been adequately resuscitated. Analysis of 11 published series shows that less than 10 % of sacro-coccygeal teratomas coming to operation in the neonatal period are malignant. After 3 months, the risk of malignancy is between 25 and 75 %. Operative techniques, described by Gross [35] and modified by Hendren [37], depend on the anatomical type of the teratoma. In the predominantly extra-pelvic forms (types I and II) the tumour and the coccyx, to which it is adherent, must be removed en bloc, and a careful search made for a possible intraspinal extension.

For the abdomino-pelvic tumours (types III and IV) excision of the pelvic portion necessitates an abdomino-perineal approach, in one or two stages.

Post-operative complications observed in 5 to 8 % of patients include: delayed wound haeling; urinary complications, bladder paralysis, which may be transient or permanent, due to lesions of the hypogastric or sacral nerve plexuses and finally, intestinal complications [41, 69]. Recurrences of the tumour may occur—the risk increases to 30-40 % when excision is incomplete, leaving the coccyx, or because of failure to recognize an anterior or intraspinal extension; or in the event of tumour spillage at operation. However, even after satisfactory excision there is a 5-10 % recurrence rate, sometimes local and benign, and sometimes malignant—either local or distant (lungs, liver, bones, lymph nodes).

Additional post-operative treatment is only considered in the unusual malignant neonatal teratomas, which are never completely excised, and when alpha-1-fœto-protein secretion remains raised.

It is best to avoid radiotherapy at this age, as its benefits have not been demonstrated. In combination with chemotherapy, it may cause death as surely as the tumour itself. Adjuvant chemotherapy which has given some encouraging results in older children, may be tried [19]. Active drugs are: Methotrexate, Actinomycin D, Cyclophosphamide, Bleomycin and Vincristine. The toxicity of Doxorubicine and Cis Platinum makes their use dangerous in the newborn. Primary chemotherapy after biopsy could theoretically be indicated to allow secondary excision of a pelvic tumour. Obviously, chemotherapy must be used for the exceptional case of metastatic disease.

Prognostic factors. — These are: the age (less than 1 month) at diagnosis and at operation, the absence of intra-pelvic extension, the quality of the resection and mature tissue components. Although teratomas containing elements of the vitelline sac are frankly malignant, the significance of immature (notably neuroid) elements in a mixed teratoma is sometimes doubtful.

Results and follow-up. — 85-90 % of mature teratomas are completely curable. Benign or malignant recurrences occur in 5-10 % of cases, always within 2-3 years.

Follow-up is based on monthly clinical examination (including rectal examination), echotomography and estimations of alpha-1-fœto-protein and βHCG concentrations.

CERVICO-FACIAL TERATOMAS

This is the second most common site in the newborn and in this site both sexes are equally affected. These tumours may be solid but are more often cystic and always benign. They are either dermoid tumours arising from ecto- and mesodermic layers, or teratomas, arising from all three layers; sometimes having an immature component with neuroid immature elements.

They may arise in the **lateral cervical region** [25, 31, 33, 36, 49, 58, 59]. Because of their large size they may cause hydramnios, and be detected by echotomography [58]. The cervical mass, which can extend to the mandible, the clavicle and retrosternally, carries a risk of dystocia, and of neonatal respiratory distress from tracheal compression which is often fatal (50 % of cases in Partlow's series) [54]. Apart from these acute events, isolated disorders of swallowing or of cry may be noted. Cervical and thoracic radiographs, and barium swallow, define the extent of the tumour and the degree of compression. Calcification is present in 40-45 % of cases. The differential diagnosis includes lymphangiomas, cystic hygromas, congenital goitres, thyroglossal cysts, branchial cysts, and the unusual neonatal adenocarcinoma of the parotid. Surgical excision must not be delayed and leads to cure in 90 % of cases.

Naso-pharyngeal teratomas may arise from the tongue, nasopharynx, palate or tonsils [15, 36, 63]. They may have an intra-cranial component which follows the cranio-pharyngeal canal [70]. A particular form of these are the epignaths, which are teratomas, attached by a pedicle to the basilar portion of the occipital bone and coming out via the buccal orifice. Epignaths are highly differentiated tumours which may have a crude fœtal axial organization. The clinical signs are respiratory distress, swallowing disorders, and nasal obstruction with rhinorrhœa. In a case of ours, a 2 months old girl spontaneously expelled a mature teratoma, which had caused nasal obstruction with purulent nasal discharge from the first day of life. Careful radiological investigation is required. Examination of the posterior-nasal space under general anaesthesia

is needed to find the tumour, and detection may be difficult, especially if it is small, non-calcified and pedunculated. Surgical excision should preclude recurrence or degeneration, although these may occur when excision has been incomplete. Computerised tomography is of value in ensuring that an intra-cranial or contralateral extension is not missed.

Benign teratomas of the orbit present with exophtalmos. About 50 cases have been reported. Plain radiography, computerised tomography. and if necessary angiography, are used to detect intra-cranial or contralateral extensions [11, 39].

INTRA-CRANIAL TERATOMAS
(cf. p. 758)
MEDIASTINAL TERATOMAS [62]

Seibert et al. [62] reported 30 cases in children under 2 years of age, of whom four were neonates. These tumours cause respiratory distress by tracheal compression and diminution of pulmonary vital capacity. The position in the mid-anterior mediastinum, the presence of calcification, and tracheal displacement and/or compression enable simple thymic hypertrophy, neuroblastoma, or lymphangioma to be excluded. Surgical excision of these tumours, which are always benign, is often difficult.

PERICARDIAL TERATOMAS [3, 56]

50 % of reported intra-pericardial teratomas were discovered in the neonatal period, both sexes being equally affected. These benign tumours are pedunculated, usually attached to the ascending aorta, and often associated with a massive pericardial effusion. They present with severe respiratory distress. Echocardiography and cine-angiocardiography enable the diagnosis to be made and exclude myocardial tumours (mainly rhabdomyomas). Surgical excision must not be delayed; it is curative and also removes intra-pericardial bronchogenic cysts.

GASTRIC TERATOMAS [50, 51]

60 % of gastric teratomas are found in neonates, in whom about 20 cases have been reported. They

were all boys. The presenting features include an abdominal mass, sometimes very large and causing dystocia, vomiting, respiratory difficulty, and sometimes gastro-intestinal haemorrhage. These teratomas are usually situated on the posterior aspect of the lesser curve of the stomach. The diagnosis is suggested by the presence of calcification, osteoid zones, and teeth, which reflect the benign nature of the tumour. Excision of the tumour or partial gastrectomy is curative.

RETRO-PERITONEAL TERATOMAS

About ten cases have been published [4, 24, 55]. In two cases the teratomas were malignant. These tumours present as an abdominal mass, often very large, resulting in signs of compression of the alimentary, and the urinary tracts. Surgical excision is curative in most cases, but dissection of the tumour is often difficult.

HEPATIC TERATOMAS [20, 22, 65]

Four cases have been reported by Dische [22]; in one case, the tumour was associated with a cervical teratoma and was part of a trisomy 18; in another case it was associated with a teratoma of the cord. These 4 tumours were benign; in contrast with the commonly malignant character (40 % of cases) of hepatic teratomas in older children [70].

TERATOMAS OF THE SPINAL CORD

Zwartverwer et al. collected 10 cases out of 16 neonatal intraspinal tumours, the others being sarcomas, neuroblastomas and gliomas [73]. These teratomas are associated with motor disorders and overlying cutaneous abnormalities. One case was associated with a lumbar myelo-meningocoele. Diagnosis depends on myelography, and necessitates laminectomy and rapid excision of the tumour to improve the neurological state.

Finally, **renal** [7, 45] and **abdominal wall teratomas** have been reported [14]. To our knowledge, gonadal teratoma has not been diagnosed in the neonatal period; this contrasts with the relative frequency of benign ovarian cysts [29, 43].

REFERENCES

[1] ALTMAN (R. P.), RANDOLPH (J. G.), LILLY (J. R.). — Sacrococcygeal teratomas: American Academy of Pediatrics Surgical Section Survey, 1973. *J. Pediatr. Surg.*, 9, 389-398, 1974.

[2] APPLEBAUM (H.), EXELBY (P. R.), WOLLNER (N.). — Malignant presacral teratoma in children. *J. Pediatr. Surg.*, 14, 352-355, 1979.

[3] ARCINIEGAS (E.), HATIMI (M.), FARVOTI (Z. Q.), GREEN (E. W.). — Intrapericardial teratomas in infancy. *J. Thorac. Cardiovasc. Surg.*, 79, 306-311, 1980.

[4] ARNHEIM (E. E.). — Retroperitoneal teratomas in infancy and childhood. *Pediatrics*, 8, 309-312, 1951.

[5] ASHCRAFT (K. W.), HOLDER (T. M.). — Hereditary presacral teratoma. *J. Pediatr. Surg.*, 9, 691-697, 1974.

[6] ASHLEY (D. J. B.). — Origin of teratomas. *Cancer*, 32, 390-394, 1973.

[7] AUBERT (J.), CASAMAYOU (J.), DENIS (P.), HOPPLER (A.), PAYER (J.). — Intrarenal teratoma in a newborn child. *Eur. Urol.*, 4, 306-308, 1978.

[8] BACHELIER (C.). — Fœtus *in fetu*. Étude clinique, radiologique, anatomo-pathologique et revue de la littérature à propos d'un cas. *Thèse Méd., Tours.* n° 224, 1977.

[9] BALE (P. M.), PAINTER (D. M.), COHEN (D.). — Teratomas in childhood. *Pathology*, 7, 209-218, 1975.

[10] BARSON (A. J.). — Congenital neoplasia: the Society's experience (abstract). *Arch. Dis. Child.*, 53, 436, 1978.

[11] BARTHOLDSON (L.), JOHANSON (B.), MORTENSON (K.). — Congenital teratoma of the orbit-case report: mainly clinical and therapeutic aspect. *Scand. J. Plast. Reconstr. Surg.*, 1, 90-96, 1967.

[12] BERRY (C. L.), KEELING (J.), HILTON (C.). — Teratomata in infancy and childhood: A review of 91 cases. *J. Pathol.*, 98, 241-252, 1969.

[13] BLANCHARD (H.), COLLIN (P. P.), GUERIN (A.), PERREAULT (G.), CLERMONT (J.), GARANCE (P.). — Tératome sacro-coccygien chez l'enfant. Étude clinique et artériographique. *Union Méd. Can.*, 100, 1311-1320, 1971.

[14] BOISRAMÉ (M.), SOUTOUL (J. H.). — Omphalocèle géante congénitale et tératome pariétal. *Bull. Féd. Soc. Gynécol. Obstét. Lang. Fr.*, 18, 425, 1966.

[15] CALCATERRA (T.). — Teratomas of the nasopharynx. *Ann. Otol. Rhinol. Laryngol.*, 78, 165-171, 1969.

[16] CARNEY (J. A.), THOMPSON (D. P.), JOHNSON (C. L.), LYNN (H. B.). — Teratomas in children: clinical and pathological aspects. *J. Pediatr. Surg.*, 7, 271-282, 1972.

[17] CHRÉTIEN (P. B.), MILAM (J. D.), FOOTE (F. W.), MILLER (T. R.). — Embryonal adenocarcinomas (a type of malignant teratoma) of the sacrococcygeal region: Clinical and pathological aspects of 21 cases. *Cancer*, 26, 522-535, 1970.

[18] CLAY (A.), DUPONT (A.), HOUCKE (M.), DEBEUGNY (P.). — Les tératomes sacro-coccygiens de l'enfant. Étude de 15 cas. *Lille Méd.*, 12, 33-38, 1967.

[19] D'ANGIO (G. J.), RANCY (R. B. Jr.), SCHRAUFER (L.), BISHOP (H. C.), LITTMAN (P.). — Management of children with sacro-coccygeal teratomas. *Proc. Am. Assoc. Cancer Res.*, 21, 386, 1980.

[20] DEROIN (F.). — Les tératomes abdominaux du nouveau-né. A propos d'une observation de tératome hépatique avec perforation digestive. *Thèse Méd., Tours,* n° 5, 1976.

[21] DILLARD (B. M.), MAYER (J. H.), MACALISTER (W. H.), MACGAVRIN (M.), STROMINGER (D. B.). — Sacrococcygeal teratomas in children. *J. Pediatr. Surg.,* 5, 53-59, 1970.

[22] DISCHE (M. R.), GARDNER (H. A.). — Mixed teratoid tumors of the liver and neck in trisomy 13. *Am. J. Clin. Pathol.,* 69, 631-637, 1978.

[23] DONNELLAN (W. A.), SWENSON (O.). — Benign and malignant sacrococcygeal teratomas. *Surgery,* 64, 834-846, 1968.

[24] ENGELS (R. M.), ELKINS (R. C.), FLETCHER (B. D.). — Retroperitoneal teratomas: a review of literature and presentation of an unusual case. *Cancer,* 22, 1068-1073, 1968.

[25] FELDER (H.). — Benign congenital neoplasms: dermoids and teratomas. *Arch. Otolaryngol.,* 101, 333-334, 1975.

[26] FRAUMENI (J. F.), LI (F. P.), DALAGER (N.). — Teratomas in children: epidemiologic features. *J. Natl. Cancer Inst.,* 51, 1425-1430, 1973.

[27] FRAUMENI (J. F.), MILLER (R. W.). — Cancer deaths in the newborn. *Am. J. Dis. Child.,* 117, 186-189, 1969.

[28] GANICK (D. J.), GILBERT (E. F.), OPITZ (J. M.). — Teratomas in children and young adults. *Med. Ped. Oncol.,* 6, 235-242, 1979.

[29] GAUTHIER (F.), VALAYER (J.), BIENAYMÉ (J.). — Tumeurs et kystes de l'ovaire du nouveau-né, du nourrisson et de l'enfant. *Chir. Pédiatr.,* 20, 75-83, 1979.

[30] GHAZALI (S.). — Prescacral teratomas in children. *J. Pediatr. Surg.,* 8, 915-918, 1973.

[31] GIFFORD (G. H.), MACCOLLUM (R. V.), BAEHNER (R. L.). — Facial teratoma in the newborn. Report of 5 cases. *Plast. Reconstr. Surg.,* 49, 616-621, 1972.

[32] GONZALEZ-CRUSSIF (F.), WINKLER (R. F.), MIRKIN (D. L.). — Sacrococcygeal teratomas in infants and children. Relationship of histology and prognosis in 40 cases. *Arch. Pathol. Lab. Med.,* 102, 420-425, 1978.

[33] GOODWIN (B. D.), GAY (B. B.). — The roentgen diagnosis of teratoma of the thyroid region. *Am. J. Roentgenol.,* 95, 25-31, 1965.

[34] GROSFELD (J. L.), BALLANTINE (R. V. N.), LOWE (D.), BAEHNER (R. L.). — Benign and malignant teratomas in children. Analysis of 85 patients. *Surgery,* 80, 297-305, 1976.

[35] GROSS (R. E.), CLATWORTHY (H. W. Jr.), MEEKER (I. A.). — Sacrococcygeal teratomas in infants and children: a report of 40 cases. *Surg. Gynecol. Obstet.,* 92, 341-354, 1951.

[36] HAWKINS (D. B.), PARK (R.). — Teratoma of the pharynx and neck. *Ann. Otorhinolaryngol.,* 81, 848-853, 1972.

[37] HENDREN (W. H.), HENDERSON (B. M.). — The surgical management of sacrococcygeal teratomas with intra-pelvic extension. *Ann. Surg.,* 171, 77-84, 1970.

[38] HORGER (E. O.). — Prenatal diagnosis of sacrococcygeal teratomas. *Am. J. Obstet. Gynecol.,* 134, 228-229, 1979.

[39] HOWARD (G. M.). — Congenital teratoma of the orbit. *Arch. Ophtalmol.,* 73, 350-352, 1965.

[40] IZANT (R. J.), FILSTON (H. C.). — Sacrococcygeal teratomas: Analysis of 43 cases. *Am. J. Surg.,* 130, 617-621, 1975.

[41] KIRK (D.), LISTER (J.). — Urinary complications of sacrococcygeal teratomas. *Z. Kinderchir.,* 18, 294-304, 1976.

[42] KNOX (A. S. S.), WEBB (A. S.). — The clinical features and treatment of fœtus *in fetu:* 2 cases reports and a review of the literature. *J. Pediatr. Surg.,* 10, 483-489, 1975.

[43] KOROBKIN (M.), DE LORIMIER (A. A.), GOODING (C. A.). — Ovarian cyst presenting within neonatal period. *Br. J. Radiol.,* 43, 820-823, 1970.

[44] LORD (J. M.). — Intra-abdominal fœtus *in fetu.* *J. Pathol. Bacteriol.,* 72, 627-641, 1956.

[45] MACCURDY (J.). — Renal neoplasm in childhood. *J. Pathol.,* 59, 623-626, 1934.

[46] MAHOUR (G. H.), LANDING (B. H.), WOOLLEY (M. M.). — Teratomas in children: clinico-pathologic studies in 133 patients. *Z. Kinderchir.,* 23, 365-379, 1978.

[47] MITGANG (R. N.). — Teratoma occurring within a myelomeningocele. *J. Neurosurg.,* 37, 448-451, 1972.

[48] MORAGAS (A.), VIDAL (M. T.). — Giant congenital intra-cranial teratoma. *Helv. Paediatr. Acta,* 24, 106-110, 1969.

[49] MORGON (A.), MULLER (J. P.). — A propos d'un cas de tératome cervical antérieur chez un nourrisson. *J. Fr. Otorhinolaryngol.,* 27, 568-570, 1978.

[50] MORRISON (L.), SNODGRAFF (P.), WISEMAN (H.). — Gastric teratoma. Report of a case and a review of the literature. *Clin. Pediatr.,* 14, 712-718, 1975.

[51] NANDY (A. K.). — Teratoma of the stomach. *J. Pediatr. Surg.,* 9, 563-564, 1974.

[52] NIX (W. L.), STENBER (C. P.), HAWKINS (E. P.), STENBACH (W. A.), POKORNY (W. J.), FERNBACH (D. J.). — Sacrococcygeal chordoma in a neonate with multiple anomalies. *J. Pediatr.,* 93, 995-997, 1978.

[53] PANTOJA (E.). — Sacrococcygeal teratomas in infancy and childhood. *N. Y. State J. Med.,* 78, 813-816, 1978.

[54] PARTLOW (W. F.), TAYBI (H.). — Teratomas in infants and children. *Am. J. Roentgenol.,* 112, 155-166, 1971.

[55] PELLERIN (D.), BERTIN (P.), GROSS (P.). — Les tératomes abdominaux (extra-gonadiques) rétro-péritonéaux de l'enfant. *Ann. Chir. Inf.,* 14, 157-168, 1973.

[56] PERNOT (Cl.), TREHEUX (A.), BRETAGNE (M. C.), WORMS (A. M.). — Tumeurs primitives cardiaques et intra-péricardiques de l'enfant. A propos de 6 observations du CHU de Nancy. *J. Radiol. Électr.,* 53, 115-123, 1972.

[57] RICHARDS (A. T.), STRICKE (L.), SPITZ (L.). — Sacrococcygeal chordomas in children. *J. Pediatr. Surg.,* 8, 911-913, 1973.

[58] ROSENFELD (C. R.), COLN (C. D.), DUENHOELTER (J. H.). — Fetal cervical teratoma as a cause of polyhydramnios. *Pediatrics,* 64, 176-179, 1979.

[59] SHAH (B. L.), VASAN (U.), RAYE (J. R.). — Teratoma of the tonsil in a premature infant. Case report and review of the literature. *Am. J. Dis. Child.,* 133, 79-80, 1979.

[60] SCHEY (W. L.), SHKOLNIK (A.), WHITE (H.). — Clinical and radiographic considerations of sacrococcygeal teratomas: An analysis of 26 new cases and review of the literature. *Radiology,* 125, 189-195, 1977.

[61] SCHMID (W.), MÜHLERTHALER (J. P.). — High amniotic fluid alpha 1 fetoprotein in a case of fetal sacrococcygeal teratoma. *Hum. Genet.*, 26, 353-354, 1975.

[62] SEIBERT (J. J.), MARVIN (W. J.), ROSE (E. F.), SCHIEKEN (R. M.). — Mediastinal teratoma: a rare cause of severe respiratory distress in the newborn. *J. Pediatr. Surg.*, 11, 253-255, 1976.

[63] STEICHEN (F. M.), EINHORN (A. H.), FELLINI (A.), FEIND (C. R.). — Congenital retropharyngeal neurofibroma causing laryngeal obstruction in a newborn. *J. Pediatr. Surg.*, 6, 480-483, 1971.

[64] TEFFT (M.), WAWTER (G.), NEUHAUSER (E. B. D.). — Unusual facial tumors in the newborn. *Am. J. Roentgenol.*, 95, 32-40, 1965.

[65] TODANI (T.), TABUCHI (K.), WATANABE (Y.). — True hepatic teratoma with high alpha-feto-protein in serum. *J. Pediatr. Surg.*, 12, 591-592, 1977.

[66] TUSHIDA (Y.), URANO (Y.), ENDO (Y.). — A study on alpha-fetoprotein and endodermal sinus-tumors. *J. Pediatr. Surg.*, 10, 501-506, 1975.

[67] WALDHAUSEN (J. A.), KOLMAN (J. W.), VELLIOS (F.),

BATTERSBY (J. S.). — Sacrococcygeal teratoma. *Surgery*, 54, 933-941, 1963.

[68] WILLIS (R. A.). — Teratomas. In *Atlas of tumor. Pathology*, sect. III, fasc. 9, Washington (D. D.), Armed Forces Institute of Pathology, 1951.

[69] WILLITAL (G. H.), MEIER (H.), SCHNEIDER (H.). — Sakrokoksygeale Teratome. Diagnostik und Therapie. *Z. Kinderchir.*, 25, 113-125, 1978.

[70] WILSON (J. W.), GEHWEILER (J.). — Teratoma of the face associated with a patent canal extending into the cranial cavity in a 3 weeks old child. *J. Pediatr. Surg.*, 5, 349-359, 1970.

[71] WOOLLEY (M. M.). — Malignant teratomas in infancy and childhood. *World J. Surg.*, 4, 39-47, 1980.

[72] WORSHAM (G. Jr.), BECKMAN (E. N.), MITCHELL (E. H.). — Sacrococcygeal teratoma in a neonate. Association with maternal use of acetazolamide. *J. A. M. A.*, 240, 251-252, 1978.

[73] ZWARTVERWER (F. L.), KAPLAN (A. M.), MONTGOMERY (C. H), HERTEL (G. A.), SPATARO (J.). — Meningeal sarcoma of the spinal cord in a newborn. *Arch. Neurol.*, 85, 844-846, 1978.

Soft tissue tumours

Soft tissue tumours are derived from the primitive mesenchyme, and may arise wherever there is connective tissue. They are very rare in the newborn and consist mainly of fibroblastic tumours and rhabdomyosarcomas or embryonic sarcomas.

FIBROBLASTIC TUMOURS

Fibroblastic tumours are characterised by a combination of fibroblastic cells (arranged more or less tightly in bundles), an interstitial substance giving rise to collagen fibers and reticulin, and elastic fibers.

In the newborn, they are usually benign tumours, whose number and site make it possible to distinguish several types of congenital fibromatoses.

Congenital fibroblastic sarcomas have also been described. It is not always easy to distinguish them from certain aggressive fibromatoses.

Congenital fibromatoses [1, 2, 4, 6, 10, 12, 13, 14, 18, 22, 24, 26, 28, 29, 30, 32, 33, 36, 38, 39, 41, 47, 49]. — In a major study by Dehner and Askin of 66 fibroblastic tumours observed in a 20 year period in children under 15 years, 10 % involved the newborn, and both sexes were equally affected [13].

Familial cases affecting several siblings have been reported [3, 10, 24, 29] and autosomal dominant transmission is suggested. The aetiology is unknown, and so are the mechanisms of regression of lesions which are usually disseminated [5, 41, 49]. In the light of ultrastructural and immunofluorescent studies, details have been given of the *cellular constitution* of the lesions which are regarded as mesenchymal hamartomas [5]. Part of the predominant fibroblastic component seems to have the characteristics of myo-fibroblasts (fibrocontractile cells of mesenchymal origin), which appear to play a part in the regression and disappearance of these hamartomas [3, 4, 5, 28, 36]. Some evidence [37] suggests a relationship between these tumours and fœtal exposure to œstrogens; this needs to be confirmed by study of the hormone receptors in the myofibroblasts [41].

The lesions are present from birth, or in the first week of life; always before 6 weeks.

Subcutaneous or intra-muscular tumours form firm nodules of variable size, covered by normal skin. They are mainly found in the head and neck, but also on the abdominal wall, the back and the limbs. Their limits are variably well-defined, and their number varies from one (solitary fibromatosis) to more than 10. They may initially increase rapidly in size.

Apart from defining the extent of the soft tissue

tumours (for which soft tissue radiographs are of value) radiological investigation [10, 24] may lead to the discovery of *bony lesions* in the metaphyses of long bones, and also in the flat bones and vertebrae. These take the form of more or less regular round lacunae, bordered by a dense zone, from which clefts may originate. Fractures may occur [29]. Bony lesions may be in continuity with soft tissue lesions or quite separate. Periosteal reactions and cortical hyperostosis are sometimes present [18, 36].

Visceral involvement seems commonly to affect the *lungs*, causing respiratory distress which is usually rapidly fatal [41]. The radiological picture may be one of interstitial pneumonia, but the fibrous nodules may not be visible and only be discovered at autopsy. Pulmonary involvement may be associated with *myocardial infiltration*. It should be remembered that 70 % of cardiac tumours are rhabdomyomas and 25 % are fibromas [38]. Infiltration of the *alimentary tract* is equally common, but is usually asymptomatic. It is found on radiological examination (filling defects) or endoscopy.

Miscellaneous other sites have been reported; the orbit, gums, larynx, thyroid, thymus, pancreas, peritoneum, and adrenal glands. Involvement of the liver, spleen, kidneys and lymph nodes is very rare; and involvement of the central nervous system has not been described. Familusi et al. reported a case with involvement of the tendons and joint capsules, of the gums and of the lamina propria, which caused cystic dilatation of the intestinal lymphatics [18].

It is conventional to distinguish two clinical forms, according to these different sites.

Diffuse or multiple fibromatosis only affects the soft tissues and/or the skeleton. The lesions are usually multiple, but a *single lesion* may be the only manifestation [28]. The outlook is usually good, with progressive spontaneous regression of the lesions in a few months [33, 41, 44, 49].

In generalised fibromatosis, the lesions described above are associated with visceral involvement, which is responsible for the gravity of the prognosis [47]. Death, which is usual within a few days or weeks, is not related to any more aggressive histological features than in the preceding form. Furthermore, spontaneous regression is possible.

These two forms are not really different, and the prognosis of congenital fibromatosis depends, above all, on the site and size of the lesions, and on their functional effects [28, 29, 41].

Differential diagnosis is with histiocytosis X and neuroblastoma, because of the subcutaneous and bony lesions. If the lesion arises in soft tissues,

possibilities include other fibrous tumours (at this age essentially fibrous hamartoma and fibrosarcoma) and other benign or malignant soft-tissue tumours (haemangiopericytoma, rhabdomyosarcoma). Sterno-mastoid haematoma gives rise to a fibrous swelling which regresses, and should be distinguished from a solitary congenital fibromatosis.

The indication for a wide, formal, surgical excision in the older child hardly applies in the newborn when the lesions are multiple. Surgery may be considered later for residual lesions. Radiotherapy must not be used and corticosteroids are of no value [4, 18].

Congenital fibrosarcoma [2, 9, 11, 13, 26, 32, 40, 42, 46]. — Although the overall *incidence* of fibrosarcomas in children is very low, the majority occur in the first 2 years of life [9, 46] and even at birth.

In a study of 53 cases of childhood fibrosarcomas collected over 27 years, Chung and Enzinger found 20 congenital fibrosarcomas [9]. This proportion is similar to that observed by Soule and Pritchard who reported 40 congenital fibrosarcomas out of 110 cases in children under 15 years [40, 46].

In the two series there was a *slight male predominance* (60 %). *Familial* associations of fibrosarcoma with bone and cerebral tumours are known [3].

This tumour principally affects the distal extremities of the lower limbs, presenting as an ill-defined, rapidly growing, irregular swelling, which invades the neighbouring tissues and may ulcerate.

Whether the tumour is congenital or not, the overall incidence of lymph node or blood borne metastases is low in children under 5 years old. It was 7.3 % in Soule and Pritchard's series [46], and 8.3 % in that of Chung and Enzinger [9]. It is difficult to evaluate the prognosis at the time of making a therapeutic decision [13]. The risk of recurrence is not affected by the initial site or size of the tumour, nor by whether it is congenital or not.

The histological diagnosis is based on the very cellular nature of the proliferation, increased mitotic activity, and the presence of atypical cells. The richness of the collagen fibres in reticulin, and ultrastructural studies, enable the tumours to be distinguished according to their degree of differentiation, and is helpful in the differential diagnosis with malignant mesenchymoma, haemangiosarcoma and haemangiopericytoma, rhabdomyosarcoma, neurogenic tumours, and fibromatosis [9, 20, 32].

The choice of treatment must take account of the small risk of metastases and should preferably, if possible, be conservative [2, 9, 16, 46]. The high local recurrence rate (54 % in Soule and Pritchard's series [46]), which is not related to the risk of metastases, may ultimately lead to more radical surgery. Radiotherapy is not indicated when the excision is adequate, and chemotherapy is not justified in the neonatal period. Follow-up must be regular and continued for at least 3 to 5 years because of the risk of metastases, of late recurrences [42], and perhaps of a second tumour [9]. The 5 year survival rate was 84 % in the 48 children under 5 followed up by Chung and Enzinger [9]. They found no difference according to whether the diagnosis was made neonatally or later.

EMBRYONAL RHABDOMYOSARCOMAS (RMS)

Embryonal rhabdomyosarcomas are malignant mesenchymal tumours containing a more or less immature component of striated muscular tissue looking like fœtal rhabdomyoblasts. In embryonal sarcomas (usually included in this group of tumours), muscular striation is difficult to detect without ultramicroscopic or immunological (using anti-myosin serum) examinations [21]. *Incidence of* RMS in USA and Europe is 10 to 15 % of solid tumours in children less than 15 years, but they are rare in neonates; at that age a dozen cases have been published [7, 25, 27]. The role of *genetic factors* is advocated because of the agregation of RMS and other tumors (brain tumors, breast cancers, adreno-cortical tumors) in sibships and families. Moreover some cases are associated with neurofibromatosis [31], naevomatosis [45], brain and lung malformations [50].

Pathological data are the following:

— *Macroscopically*, RMS is either a massive, firm, infiltrative tumor or it has a polypoid aspect (botryoid sarcoma) within a cavity.

— *Microscopically*, several types are observed according to cellular density, degree of myoblastic maturation and correlation with macroscopic type. Thus RMS are classified according to the following types *: loose, botryoid or not (25 %), dense (60 %) and alveolar of Riopelle and Theriault (15 %). Ultrastructural examinations aim at demonstrating the presence of myofilaments and primitive Z bands in tumoral cells, thereby comparing types of RMS to

---

* Classification of International Society of Pediatric Oncology.

---

successive steps of fœtal rhabdomyoblast differentiation.

Metastases by the hematogenous and lymphatic route affect lungs, liver, bones, soft tissues and heart. Alveolar RMS particularly involve bone-marrow and lymph nodes.

The general distribution of RMS according to the primary site shows that 40 to 50 % affect head and neck (35 % ear, nose, throat; 10-15 % orbit); 15-20 % originate in the urogenital sinus, 15 % in limbs, 20 % in miscellaneous sites: thorax, retroperitoneal region, biliary ducts, trunk walls, testicular and funicular envelopes.

Clinical features are variable, depending on the primary site; it is redundant to describe them, as their incidence is rare in newborns. At that age [7, 25], orbital invasion (orbit and lids) is the common site. As in older children, the major sign is an external large tumour, located either inside the eye-lid or more often behind the eye responsible for a quickly evolutive exophtalmos. Orbital X-rays, computerized tomography, cytology or cerebro-spinal fluid allow one to detect loco-regional extension. Biopsy confirms the diagnosis; the approach depending on the tumor site and attempts not to touch the globe [19].

The aim of treatment is to obtain local control, to prevent metastases and to avoid major sequelæ [23, 34]. Surgical excision, usually partial, must be followed by chemotherapy. Its effects on survival rate are clearly demonstrated in older children; nevertheless we need to indicate once more its poor tolerance in newborns. Radiotherapy currently used in the treatment of orbital RMS of children, needs to be avoided in infants.

Prognosis is poor, differing from results obtained in older children (75 % cure-rate in orbital RMS). Out of 11 reported orbital RMS, only one patient is a long term survivor [25].

REFERENCES

[1] BAER (J. W.), RADKOWSKI (M. A.). — Congenital multiple fibromatosis: a case report with review of the world literature. *Am. J. Roentgenol.*, *118*, 200-205, 1973.

[2] BALSAVER (A. M.), BUTLER (J. J.), MARTIN (R. G.). — Congenital fibrosarcoma. *Cancer*, *20*, 1607-1616, 1967.

[3] BARTLETT (R. C.), OTIS (R. D.), LAAKSO (A. O.). — Multiple congenital neoplasms of soft tissues.

Report of 4 cases in a family. *Cancer*, *14*, 913-920, 1961.

[4] BEATTY (E. C.). — Congenital generalized fibromatosis in infancy. *Am. J. Dis. Child.*, *103*, 620-624, 1962.

[5] BENJAMIN (S. P.), MERCER (R. D.), HAWK (W. A.). — Myofibroblastic contraction in spontaneous regression of multiple congenital mesenchymal hamartomas. *Cancer*, *40*, 2343-2352, 1977.

[6] BERLAND (H.), SACREZ (R.), WEITZENBLUM (S.), BUCK (P.), PHILIPPE (E.), BERGER (J.). — A propos de deux cas de fibromatose de l'enfant à localisation profonde. *Ann. Pédiatr.*, *19*, 197-205, 1972.

[7] BOIE (W.), KUHNER (U.), FOET (K.). — Rhabdomyosarkom bei Neugeborenen. *Pädiatr. Prax.*, 421-425, 1979.

[8] CHRISTENSEN (E.), HJGAARD (K.), SMITH (W. C. C.). — Congenital malignant mesenchymal tumors in a two month old child. *Acta Pathol. Microbiol. Scand.*, *53*, 237, 1961.

[9] CHUNG (E. B.), ENZINGER (F. M.). — Infantile fibrosarcoma. *Cancer*, *38*, 729-739, 1976.

[10] CONDON (V. R.), ALLEN (R. P.). — Congenital generalized fibromatosis: case report with roentgen manifestations. *Radiology*, *76*, 444-448, 1961.

[11] DAHL (I.), SAVE-SODERBERGH (J.), ANGERVALL (I.). — Fibrosarcoma in early infancy. *Pathol. Eur.*, *8*, 193-209, 1973.

[12] DAUDET (M.), CHAPPUIS (B. S.), ROSENBERG (D.), MAMELLE (J. C.). — Fibromatose congénitale multiple. *Ann. Chir. Infant*, *10*, 273-282, 1969.

[13] DEHNER (L. P.), ASKIN (F. B.). — Tumors of fibrous tissue origin in childhood. A clinicopathologic study of cutaneous and soft tissue neoplasms in 66 children. *Cancer*, *38*, 888-900, 1976.

[14] DRESCHER (E.), WOYKE (S.), MARKIEVICZ (C.), TEGI (S.). — Juvenile fibromatosis in siblings (fibromatosis hyalinica multiplex juvenilis). *J. Pediatr. Surg.*, *2*, 427-430, 1967.

[15] DREYFUS (M. L.). — Congenital sarcoma. *J. Pediatr.*, *34*, 583-587, 1949.

[16] EXELBY (P. R.), KNAPPER (W. H.), HUVOS (A. G.), BEATTIE (E. J.). — Soft tissue fibrosarcoma in children. *J. Pediatr. Surg.*, *8*, 415-420, 1973.

[17] FAHEY (J. J.), BOLLINGER (J. A.). — Congenital sarcoma of foot. Case report and review of literature. *Am. J. Dis. Child.*, *86*, 23-27, 1953.

[18] FAMILUSI (J. B.), NOTTIDGE (V. A.), ANTIA (A. U.), ATTAH (E. B.). — Congenital generalized fibromatosis. An african case with gingival hypertrophy and other unusual features. *Am. J. Dis. Child.*, *130*, 1215-1217, 1976.

[19] FLAMANT (F.), BLOCH-MICHEL (E.), LEMAISTRE (D.) et coll. — Actual treatment of rhabdomyosarcoma of the orbit in children. *J. Fr. Ophtalmol.*, *1*, 451, 1978.

[20] GONZALEZ-CRUSSI (F.). — Ultrastructure of congenital fibrosarcoma. *Cancer*, *26*, 1289-1299, 1970.

[21] GONZALEZ-CRUSSI (F.), BLACK-SCHAFFER (S.). — Rhabdomyosarcoma of infancy and childhood. Problems of morphologic classification. *Am. J. Surg. Pathol.*, *3*, 157-171, 1979.

[22] GOSLEE (L.), CLERMONT (V.), BERNSTEIN (J.), WOOLLEY (P. V.). — Superficial connective tissue tumors in early infancy. A study of fibromatosis and lipoblastomatosis. *J. Pediatr.*, *65*, 377-387, 1964.

[23] GREEN (D. M.), JAFFE (N.). — Progress and controversy in the treatment of childhood rhabdomyosarcoma. *Cancer Treat. Rev.*, *5*, 7, 1978.

[24] HEIPLE (K. G.), PERRIN (E.), AIKAWA (M.). — Congenital generalized fibromatosis. A case limited to osseous lesions. *J. Bone Joint Surg.*, *54*, 663-669, 1972.

[25] HARLOW (P. J.), KAUFMAN (F. R.), SIEGEL (S. E.), QUEVEDO (E.). — Orbital rhabdomyosarcoma in a neonate. *Med. Pediatr. Oncol.*, *7*, 123-126, 1979.

[26] KAUFFMANN (S. L.), STAOUT (A. P.). — Congenital mesenchymal tumors. *Cancer*, *18*, 460-476, 1965.

[27] KHAN (A.), HOY (G.), SINKS (L. F.). — Unexpected favorable outcome of congenital stage III Rhabdomyosarcoma. *CA-A*, *30*, 189-190, 1980.

[28] KINDBLOM (L. G.), TERMEN (G.), SAVE SOVERBERGH (J.), ANGERVALL (L.). — Congenital solitary fibromatosis of soft tissue, a variant of congenital generalized fibromatosis. 2 case reports. *Acta Pathol. Microbiol. Scand.*, *85*, 640-648, 1977.

[29] LAURAS (B.), FREYCON (F.), NIVELON (J. L.), BATTIN (J.), GILLY (J.), IZAC (M.). — Fibromatose congénitale généralisée. A propos de 3 observations. *Pédiatrie*, *31/4*, 327-335, 1976.

[30] LEGALL (Y.), SCHNEEGANS (E.), BUCK (P.). — Les tumeurs fibromateuses de la première enfance. *Ann. Chir. Inf.*, *3*, 105-114, 1962.

[31] McKENN (E. A.), BODURTHA (J.), MEADOWS (A. T.). — Rhabdomyosarcoma complicating multiple neurofibromatosis. *J. Pediatr.*, *93*, 992, 1978.

[32] MAMELLE (J. C.), SALLE (B.), DAUDET (M.), ROSENBERG (D.), BRUNAT (M.), MONNET (P.). — Fibrosarcome et fibromatose congénitaux. *Ann. Pédiatr.*, *16/4*, 1031-1037, 1969.

[33] MANDE (R.), HENNEQUET (A.), LOUBRY (E.), CLOUP (M.), MARIE (J.). — Fibromatose congénitale diffuse du nouveau-né à évolution régressive. *Ann. Pédiatr.*, *45*, 690-700, 1965.

[34] MAURER (H. M.), MOON (T.), DONALDSON (M.) et coll. — The Intergroup Rhabdomyosarcoma Study. *Cancer*, *40*, 2015, 1977.

[35] MILLER (R. W.), DALAGER (M. A.). — Fatal rhabdomyosarcoma among children in the United States, 1960-1969. *Cancer*, *34*, 1897, 1974.

[36] MORETTIN (L. B.), MUELLER (E.), SCHREIBER (M.). — Generalized hamartomatosis (congenital generalized fibromatosis). *Am. J. Roentgenol.*, *114*, 722-734, 1972.

[37] NADEL (E. M.). — Histopathology of œstrogen induced tumours in guinea pigs. *J. Nal. Cancer Inst.*, *10*, 1043-1051, 1950.

[38] OLIVA (P. B.), BRECKINRIDGE (J. C.), JOHNSON (M. L.), BRANTIGAN (C. I.), O'MEARA (O. P.). — Left ventricular outflow obstruction produced by a pedunculated fibroma in a newborn. *Chest*, *74*, 590-592, 1978.

[39] PLASCHKES (J.). — Congenital fibromatosis: localized and generalized forms. *J. Pediatr. Surg.*, *9*, 95-101, 1974.

[40] PRITCHARD (D. S.), SOULE (E. H.), TAYLOR (W. F.). — Fibrosarcoma. A clinicopathologic and statistical study of 199 tumors of the soft tissues of the extremities and trunk. *Cancer*, *33*, 888-897, 1974.

[41] ROGGLI (V. L.), KIM (H. S.), HAWKINS (E.). — Congenital generalized fibromatosis with visceral involvement. A case report. *Cancer*, *45*, 954-960, 1980.

[42] ROOTMAN (J.), CARVOUNIS (E. P.), DOLMAN (C. L.), DIMMICK (J. E.). — Congenital fibrosarcoma metastatic to the choroid. *Am. J. Ophtalmol.*, *87*, 632-638, 1979.

[43] ROSENBERG (H. S.), STENBACK (W. A.), SPJUT (H. J.). — The fibromatoses of infancy and childhood. *In*

Rosenberg (H. S.), Bolande (R. P.), ed. *Perspectives in pediatric pathology*, Vol. 4, ed. Chicago: Yearbook Medical Publishers, 1978.

[44] Schaffzin (E. A.), Chung (S. M. K.), Kaye (R.). — Congenital generalized fibromatosis with complete spontaneous regression. A case report. *J. Bone Jt. Surg.*, 54, 657-662, 1972.

[45] Schweisguth (O.), Gérard-Marchant (R.), Lemerle (J.). — Nævomatose baso-cellulaire. Association à un rhabdomyosarcome congénital. *Arch. Franç. Pédiatr.*, 25, 1083, 1968.

[46] Soule (E. H.), Pritchard (D. J.). — Fibrosarcoma in infants and children. A review of 110 cases. *Cancer*, 40, 1711-1721, 1977.

[47] Stout (A. P.). — Juvenile fibromatosis. *Cancer*, 7, 953-978, 1954.

[48] Stout (A. P.), Lattes (R.). — Tumors of the soft tissues. *Atlas of Tumor Pathology*, Series 2. Fascicle 1, Washington (D. C.), Armed Forces Institute of Pathology, 1967.

[49] Teng (P.), Warden (M. J.), Cohen (W. L.). — Congenital generalized fibromatosis (renal and skeletal) with complete spontaneous regression. *J. Pediatr.*, 62, 748-753, 1963.

[50] Veda (K.), Gruppo (R.), Unger (F.), Martin (L.), Bove (K.). — Rhabdomyosarcoma of lung arising in congenital cystic adenomatoid malformation. *Cancer*, 40, 383-388, 1977.

Cerebral tumours

GENERAL FEATURES
INCIDENCE. SITE

Since the first case of teratoma described by Maier in 1861 [37], it appears that 1.9-5.8 % of cerebral tumours in children are diagnosed before the age of one year [11, 18, 20, 37]; among these, 5-10 % are found in the neonatal period [8, 21]. They account for 5.4 % of neonatal deaths from cancer, and 0.34 deaths per million live births per year.

In 25 % of cases the diagnosis is only made at autopsy. In 30 % it is made in the first month of life, and in 45 %, despite signs and symptoms which began in the neonatal period, the diagnosis is made later [15].

Of the 166 published cases we have analysed [3, 8, 14, 15, 33, 35, 36, 37], 60 % of tumours were supratentorial. This distribution differs from that seen in infants and children (cf. Table VI), and is due to the predominance of teratomas, which are almost exclusively supratentorial. These constitute 38 % of neonatal cerebral tumours; gliomas account for 38 % and medulloblastomas for 14 %. The percentage of teratomas is particularly high in Japan (61.9 % according to Takaku [36]).

CLINICAL SIGNS AND DIAGNOSIS

Presentation is usually the same, with increased cranial volume, and hydrocephalus which is sometimes the cause of hydramnios and dystocia. Intra-

TABLE VI. — Distribution according to histological diagnosis of 166 neonatal cerebral tumours collected from the literature.

Teratomas		64 cases
Gliomas		47 cases
Ependymomas	13	
(ependymoblastomas)	22	
Astrocytomas:	34	
— malignant	3	
— oligodendroglioma	1	
— brain-stem gliomas	9	
— gliosarcomas	2	
— benign astrocytomas	19	
Medulloblastomas		23 cases
Craniopharyngiomas		7 cases
Papilloma of the choroid plexus		6 cases
Meningiomas		6 cases
Vascular tumours		4 cases
Haemangio pericytomas	2	
Cavernous haemangiomas	2	
Miscellaneous		9 cases
Neuroepithelioma	1	
Pinealoblastoma	1	
Osteoma	1	
Adamantimoma	1	
Metastases:	5	
— Wilms	2	
— Cutaneous angiosarcoma	1	
— Placental choriocarcinoma	2	

cranial hypertension (I.C.H.) is commonly found, and is characterised by the rarity of papilloedema and the frequency of vomiting. The I.C.H. is often rapidly progressive, requiring early insertion of a cerebrospinal fluid shunt.

Hemiplegia, convulsions, cerebellar syndrome (essentially suspected because of hypotonia), opisthotonic crises, disorders of consciousness (sometimes due to neurogenic hypernatraemia [34] and cranial nerve palsies [32, 33] are less common and often difficult to diagnose at this age.

Finally, the newborn infant may have a more or less severe, non-specific, "neurological syndrome" often aggravated by a difficult delivery, with or without focal neurological signs. This is often responsible for respiratory distress, which may necessitate artificial ventilation [23].

Skull X-rays, as well as confirming widening of the sutures, may show tumour calcification, which favours a teratoma, or a rare craniopharyngioma. Raised cerebrospinal fluid protein levels, often impairing the function of internal shunts, is particularly common in medulloblastomas [6], and teratomas [14]. It is sometimes accompanied by hypercytosis or even a meningeal blastosis. Meningeal haemorrhage may both reveal the tumour, and be a source of diagnostic error [30].

Because cerebral tumours are unusual in the neonatal period, the symptoms more often suggest hydrocephalus, due to malformation or infection, bacterial meningitis, viral infection, toxoplasmosis, and, above all, acute or chronic cerebral hypoxia with or without haemorrhage.

Although transillumination is a simple and useful test, echotomography and computerised tomography remains the key examination, especially as it may, at this age, be performed without general anaesthesia.

CLINICAL COURSE
AND PRINCIPLES OF TREATMENT

The outlook is extremely poor. 25 % of affected infants are still-born, and 90 % die within a year, whatever the type of tumour. A few operations have been attempted, and these were reviewed by Takaku [37]. He recorded only 6 total excisions, amongst which were the only four cases to survive beyond the first year (2 teratomas and 2 choroid plexus papillomas).

As a rule, total excision is impractical because of the precarious state of the infant, due to the delay in diagnosis.

Some patients have been treated by irradiation, for indications, and by techniques, which varied considerably.

PATHOLOGICAL TYPES
OF CONGENITAL CEREBRAL TUMOURS

Teratomas [3, 9, 12, 14, 15, 26, 27, 31, 36, 38, 39]. — These account for more than one third of neonatal cerebral tumours (cf. Table VI). They sometimes have an extracranial component (orbit, nasal cavity). They arise from the region of the pineal gland and the third ventricle, although they occasionally occur in atypical sites such as the brain stem [36]. Most are histologically benign, although their volume is sometimes such (sometimes with the "fœtus in fetu" type) that the fœtus dies in utero. They may sometimes replace the entire cerebral mass. At times they present with a rapidly fatal neonatal hydrocephalus; or with a progressive hydrocephalus, which is diagnosed later.

Surgery has only been possible on rare occasions (7/64) [14, 31, 58], most tumours being too large to be resectable. Of seven excisions, 4 were partial and 3 total. The latter resulted in the only two cases of prolonged survival (18 and 24 months) [37].

Gliomas [3, 8, 15, 21, 25, 30, 31, 33, 37]. — These represent 28 % of neonatal cerebral tumours (cf. Table VI) and include:

— *Ependymomas*, of which we have found 13 published cases [1, 3, 7, 8, 13, 15, 22, 26, 37]. 11 of the 13 were supra-tentorial [7], and benign. They were rapidly fatal despite some attempts at surgical excision [1] and radiotherapy [13].

— *Astrocytomas* [3, 8, 15, 21, 26, 30, 31, 33, 37] of which we have discovered 34 cases. 12 were situated in the posterior fossa, 9 in the brain stem [10, 20, 24, 32, 37], and 3 in the cerebellar hemispheres. Most were histologically benign; 5 were malignant, of which one was in the brain stem [23].

All attempts at surgery have ended in failure.

Medulloblastomas [3, 6, 8, 15, 16, 26, 28, 35, 37]. 23 cases were collected. One case was associated with a glioblastoma multiforme [37]. They account for 14 % of congenital cerebral tumours. Familial neonatal medulloblastoma [6, 36], and associated multiple malformations, have been described.

Taboada [35] emphasised the diagnostic value of the combination of opisthotonic crises with downward deviation of the gaze, resulting from mesencephalic compression by a tumour of the vermis. These are rare clinical signs in older children.

Despite some attempts at neurosurgery [35, 36] and/or cerebral irradiation [28] they are invariably fatal.

Craniopharyngiomas [4, 5, 15, 35, 37, 40]. These are exceptional, as only 7 cases (4 girls, 3 boys) have been reported. The modes of presentation are varied: dystocia and hydrocephalus (in 3 cases out of 7), respiratory distress, generalised hypotonia, exophtalmia and convulsions. Cerebral calcification is usually present. Death within 3 months, despite attempts at surgery, remains the rule.

Meningiomas [2, 15, 29, 33]. Meningioma is an unusual tumour in children; of 16 cases collected by Amano, 6 were neonatal. These were benign cystic tumours, of a fibroblastic type [2]. A meningeal sarcoma has been described [29].

Miscellaneous tumours. — Other rare tumours have been reported such as vascular neoplasms, (4 cases); haemangiopericytoma, cavernous haemangioma [3, 15, 37], choroid plexus papillomas (6 cases) [25, 26, 37], and tumours considered to be metastases (5 cases), from Wilms' tumours * [17, 41], placental choriocarcinomas [16, 19] and a cutaneous angiosarcoma [8].

REFERENCES

[1] ABBOTT (M.), NAMITRI (H.). — Congenital ependymoma: case report. *J. Neurosurg.*, 28, 162-165, 1968.

[2] AMANO (K.), MIURA (N.), TAJIKA (Y.), MATSUMORI (K.), KUBO (O.), KOBAYASHI (N.), KITAMURA (K.). — Cystic meningioma in a 10 month old infant: case report. *J. Neurosurg.*, 52, 829-833, 1980.

[3] ARNSTEIN (L. H.), BOLDREY (E.), NAFFZIGER (H. C.). — A case report and survey of brain tumors during the neonatal period. *J. Neurosurg.*, 8, 315-319, 1951.

[4] AZAR-KIA (B.), KRISHMAN (U. R.), SCHECHTER (M. M.). — Neonatal craniopharyngioma: case report. *J. Neurosurg.*, 42, 91-93, 1975.

[5] BAUDON (J. J.), PIGOT (J. Y.), LE BESNERAIS (Y.), LEGER (A.). — Hydrocéphalie néonatale par craniopharyngiome. *Arch. Fr. Pédiatr.*, 30, 563, 1973.

[6] BELAMARIC (J.), CHAU (A. S.). — Medulloblastoma in newborn sisters: report of two cases. *J. Neurosurg.*, 30, 76-79, 1969.

[7] CHUSID (J. G.), DE GUITTEREZ-MAHOMEY (C. G.), CARVERY (T. Q.). — Ependymoma of the cerebellopontine angle in an infant. *Neurology*, 6, 152-156, 1956.

[8] FESSARD (C.). — Les tumeurs cérébrales des deux premières années de la vie : 66 observations anatomocliniques. *Ann. Pédiatr.*, 16, 290-302, 1966.

[9] FINCK (F. M.), ANTIN (R.). — Intracranial teratomas of the newborn. *Am. J. Dis. Child.*, 109, 439-442, 1965.

[10] FUSTE (F. G.), SNYDER (D. E.), PRICE (A.). — Congenital spongioblastoma of the pons. *Am. J. Clin. Pathol.*, 47, 790-796, 1967.

[11] GOLD (E. B.). — Patterns of incidence of brain tumors in children. *Ann. Neurol.*, 5, 565-568, 1979.

[12] GREENHOUSE (A. H.), NEUBUERGER (K. T.). — Intracranial teratomata of the newborn. *Arch. Neurol. (Chicago)*, 3, 718-724, 1960.

[13] GRUSZKIEWICZ (J.), DORON (Y.), PEYSER (E.). — Congenital ependymoma in a child. *Neur. Chir.*, 12, 227-231, 1969.

[14] HIRSH (L. F.), RORKE (L. B.), SCHMIDEK (H. H.). — Unusual cause of relapsing hydrocephalus: congenital intracranial teratoma. *Arch. Neurol. (Chicago)*, 34, 505-507, 1977.

[15] JELLINGER (K.), SUNDER-PLASSMANN (M.). — Connatal intracranial tumors. *Neuropaediatr e*, 4, 46-63, 1973.

[16] KADIN (M. E.), RUBINSTEIN (L. J.), NELSON (J. S.). — Neonatal cerebellar medulloblastoma originating from the fetal external granular layer. *J. Neuropathol. Exp. Neurol.*, 29, 583-600, 1970.

[17] KALOUSEK (D. K.), DECHADAREVIAN (J. P.), BOLANDE (R. P.). — Letters to the editors. *Pediatr. Radiol.*, 4, 124, 1976.

[18] KEITH (H. M.), CRAIG (W., McK.), KERNOHAN (J. W.). — Brain tumors in children. *Pediatrics*, 3, 839-844, 1949.

[19] KELLY (D. L.), KUSHNER (J.), McLEAN (W. T.). — Neonatal intracranial choriocarcinoma: case report. *J. Neurosurg.*, 35, 461-471, 1971.

[20] KOOS (W. Th.), MILLER (M. H.). — *Intracrania Tumors of Infants and Children*. St Louis, C. V. Mosby Company, 1971.

[21] LIN (S. R.), LEE (K. F.), O'HARA (A. E.). — Congenital astrocytomas: the roentgenographic manifestations. *Am. J. Roentgenol.*, 115, 78-85, 1972.

[22] LORENTZEN (M.). — Congenital ependymoblastoma. *Acta Neuropathol.*, 49, 71-84, 1980.

[23] LUSE (S. A.), TEITELBAUM (S.). — Congenital glioma of brain-stem. *Arch. Neurol. (Chicago)*, 18, 196-201, 1968.

[24] MASSON (A.), HELDT (N.), CRONMULLER (G.), SCHNEEGANS (E.). — Astrocytome congénital du tronc cérébral. *Ann. Pédiatr.*, 18, 789-795, 1971.

[25] MATSON (D. D.). — Intracranial tumors of the first two years of life. *West. J., Surg. Gyn.*, 72, 117-122, 1964.

[26] MOLZ (G.), BISWAS (R. K.), KONNATALER. — Ependymom der Grosshirnmaflager bei einem Frühgeborenen. *Z. Allg. Pathol.*, 115, 439-444, 1972.

[27] MORAGAS (A.), VIDAL (M. T.). — Giant congenital intra-cranial teratoma. *Helv. Paediatr. Acta*, 24, 106-110, 1969.

[28] PAPADAKIS (N.), MILLAN (J.), GRADY (D. F.), SEGERBERG (L. H.). — Medulloblastoma of the neonatal period and early infancy: report of 2 cases. *J. Neurosurg.*, 34, 88-91, 1971.

[29] REIGH (E. E.), DECKER (J. T.). — Meningeal sarcoma in a two weeks old infant simulating hydrocephalus. *J. Neurosurg.*, 19, 427, 1962.

[30] ROTHMAN (S. M.), NELSON (J. S.), DE VIVO (D. C.),

* At the present time, they are considered as multiple primary tumours.

COXE (W. S.). — Congenital astrocytoma presenting with intracerebral hematoma. *J. Neurosurg.*, *51*, 237-239, 1979.

[31] SATO (O.), TAMURA (A.), SANO (K.). — Brain tumors of early infants. *Child's Brain*, *1*, 121-125, 1975.

[32] SIEBEN (R. L.). ISHII (N.). — Brain stem glioma causing failure to thrive. *Pediatrics*, *47*, 451-455, 1971.

[33] SOLITARE (G. B.), KRIGMAN (M. R.). — Congenital intracranial neoplasm. *J. Neuropath. Exp. Neurol.*, *23*, 280-292, 1964.

[34] TABADDOR (K.), SHULMAN (K.), DAL CANTO (M. C.). — Neonatal craniopharyngioma. *Am. J. Dis. Child.*, *128*, 381-383, 1974.

[35] TABOADA (D.), FROUFE (A.), ALONSO (A.), ALVAREZ (J.), MURO (D.), VILA (M.). — Congenital medulloblastoma: report of two cases. *Pediatr. Radiol.*, *9*, 5-10, 1980.

[36] TAKAKU (A.), MITA (R.), SUSUKI (J.). — Intracranial teratoma in early infancy. *J. Neurosurg.*, *38*, 265-268, 1973.

[37] TAKAKU (A.), KODAMA (N.), OHARA (H.), HORI (S.). — Brain tumor in newborn babies. *Child's Brain*, *4*, 365-375, 1978.

[38] TAMURA (H.). — Intracranial teratoma in fetal life and infancy. *Obstet. Gynecol.*, *27*, 134-141, 1966.

[39] VRAA-JENSEN (J.). — Massive congenital intracranial teratoma. *Acta Neuropathol.*, *30*, 271-276, 1974.

[40] WEBER (F.), MORI (Y.). — Craniopharyngiome congénital géant. *Helv. Paediatr. Acta*, *31*, 261-270, 1976.

[41] WEXLER (H. A.), POOLE (C. A.), FOJACO (R. M.). — Metastatic neonatal Wilms' tumor: a case report with review of the literature. *Pediatr. Radiol.*, *3*, 179-181, 1975.

Congenital leukaemias

INCIDENCE AND EPIDEMIOLOGY

The incidence of congenital leukaemia seems to be low; Pierce [40] noted 1 case per 37,000 births between 1948 and 1958, but the condition may have gone unrecognised, because of confusion with other neonatal conditions. Two thirds of the 200 known cases were published between 1960 and 1980. A large number of these are collected in the general reviews of Bernhard [6], Pierce [40], Gaillard [24], Fournier [23], Buhler [13], Bernard [5]. Boys seem to be slightly more often affected than girls.

The role of genetic and environmental factors has been raised.

Genetic factors. — In 15 % of cases, congenital leukaemia is associated with *trisomy 21* [3, 5, 17, 22, 31, 34, 36, 43]. The karyotype of the leukaemic cells may show additional anomalies, such as an extra Group C chromosome [31], or diploidisation of the supernumerary chromosome, giving karyotypes with 49-54 chromosomes [36]. Immunological disorders may favour leukaemic transformation in some subjects [51].

Other malformations are reported: trisomy D [48], trisomy E [20], organomegaly [16], Bonnevie-Ulrich syndrome [41], bilateral absence of the radii [6], Klippel-Feil syndrome [6], Ellis Van Creveld syndrome [39], and renal dysembryoplasia [45].

Familial forms and parental consanguinity are rare [10]. The 4 affected siblings described by

Campbell et al. had familial lymphohistiocytosis rather than leukaemia [14].

When monozygous *twins* are both affected, genetic factors may be considered, without however excluding the possibility of extrinsic factors acting in utero. If one of a pair of twins has congenital leukaemia, there appears to be a very high risk that the other will be affected during the first year of life. Simultaneous and early presentation in both twins is in favour of a prenatal aetiology [15, 29, 33, 37, 46, 56]. It is interesting to note the presence of identical cytogenetic anomalies in the leukaemic cells of both twins, which is evidence in favour of the monoclonal origin of the condition affecting one cell, whose proliferation is followed by migration to the other twin as a result of vascular exchanges [15].

Although the *transplacental passage of maternal leukaemic cells* can be demonstrated by quinacrine marking techniques, there are no known cases of congenital leukaemia in infants born to leukaemic mothers [1, 7, 8, 35]. However two cases of acute lymphoblastic leukaemia diagnosed in the mother at the time of delivery have been followed 9 months later by a leukaemia of the same type in the child [4, 18].

Environmental factors. — The role of physical factors and viruses in the induction of congenital leukaemias is not absolutely established. Cases of congenital leukaemia following intrauterine *irradiation* have been described [21, 32, 37, 38, 49]. The role played by *maternal infections* is unknown.

CLINICAL SIGNS
[13, 16, 24, 28, 54, 58]

The infants are generally born at term and are of normal birth-weight. Some are still-born [30]. Hydramnios is sometimes noted towards the end of pregnancy [13, 32].

The initial signs are variable, and include purpura, ecchymoses, alimentary disorders, abdominal distension, and respiratory disorders. *The clinical picture* develops and deteriorates rapidly, dominated by cutaneous, abdominal, and haemorrhagic manifestations. Abdominal distension with collateral circulation is characteristic. It seems to be due to a combination of several factors: hepatosplenomegaly, present in 85 % of cases, compression from abdominal lymphadenopathy, intestinal distension and ascites. Petechial or ecchymotic purpura is often associated with other haemorrhagic phenomena: epistaxis, bleeding from the gums; haematemesis, melaena, and meningeal haemorrhages.

Cutaneous nodules consisting of non-haemorrhagic tumours, are specific leukaemic lesions, present in 80 % of cases. They may lie in the epidermis which they indurate and may ulcerate, or in the dermis and hypodermis into which they are often inset, with an ill defined boundary. Their size is variable. Their colour differs according to their depth: if hypodermic, they are only palpable; in the dermis they are covered with copper or buff-coloured skin; the superficial nodules are reddish purple, with a red centre (sometimes yellowish if they are secondarily infected). These two types of purpuric and nodular lesions usually co-exist; they may occur over the whole body, not sparing the face and scalp. The mucous membranes are only rarely affected by nodular lesions.

Other parts of the clinical picture are not constant; moderate *peripheral lymphadenopathy* is present in one third of cases. Mediastinal lymph node enlargement is rare. *Pulmonary involvement*, demonstrated in many cases at autopsy, has no specific radiological features. Dyspnoea results from several causes: diffuse parenchymal infiltration, superinfection, cardiac malformation, severe anaemia, and respiratory distress due to hyperleucocytosis.

Meningeal involvement is probably more common than is reported in the literature; in contrast, ocular involvement with exophtalmos is extremely rare. *Renal infiltration* may be manifested by two masses

filling the lumbar fossae; the testes may also be affected. *Bony involvement* gives a radiological picture of linear rarefaction at the metaphyses. The general condition is altered by the haematologic state, secondary infection and alimentary disorders.

HAEMATOLOGICAL SIGNS

Anaemia is absent or mild in the first few hours after birth, but is then rapidly revealed. The platelet count is usually diminished. There is no exact correlation between thrombocytopenia and the severity of the haemorrhagic phenomena. *Hyperleucocytosis* is the rule; the white cell count may reach between 50,000 and 1 million/mm^3; leucopenia is unusual. Atypical cells are nearly always present and their percentage is very high.

The diagnosis is established by examination of the *marrow*. The extreme difficulty of a purely morphologic cytological classification makes the relative incidence of various types uncertain. In 1972 Rosner collected the data of the "Acute leukemia Group B", and noted that 58 % were granulocytic and 42 % lymphoblastic [43]. Cytochemical and immunological studies afford a more precise means of classification [16, 27, 58].

Granulocytic leukaemias of the newborn may be purely myeloblastic with monomorphic proliferation of myeloblasts, or resemble chronic myeloid leukaemia with proliferation of myeloblasts, promyelocytes and myelocytes without a hiatus and with a marrow picture identical to the blood film. Nevertheless, it is an acute leukaemia whose course, although less fulminating than that of the pure myeloblastic form, is rapidly fatal. In newborns with Down syndrome leukaemia is nearly always of the myeloblastic type.

The blood and marrow findings are usually sufficient for the diagnosis. Skin biopsies show a disordered blast cell infiltration in all layers, without peri-adnexial organisation, and lymph node biopsy (or puncture) shows a diffuse blast cell infiltration with destruction of the architecture. At autopsy, histologic studies of the liver, spleen, lungs, kidneys and testes show the same type of picture.

Cytogenetic study of the marrow (directly) and the blood (directly or in the presence of phytohaemaglutinin) is useful to demonstrate, apart from any constitutional chromosomal aberration, the presence of abnormalities confined to the leukaemic cells [9, 27, 42, 47, 53, 59]. It is recommended to analyse the parents chromosomes: if abnormal chromosomal breakages are observed, fœtal transformation by an environmental factor may be involved [27].

We have seen the value of the karyotype in determining the monoclonal origin of the leukaemic proliferation in twins [15, 46]. Finally, the appearance of new cytogenetic abnormalities in the course of a neonatal leucoblastosis, may throw doubt on its apparently transitory nature, and suggest a true haematological malignancy.

COURSE AND TREATMENT
[5, 10, 23, 24, 27, 28, 38, 58]

The time course of neonatal leukaemias is generally very short; 20 % of deaths occur in the first week, and only 4 % after 3 months. The average survival time is 3 weeks. The causes of death are multiple: haemorrhages, secondary infection, and respiratory, hepatic and renal failure.

Transfusions only correct anaemia; exchange transfusions are useful in case of respiratory distress due to hyperleucocytosis. De Carvalho reported a remission of six years in a Down syndrome Infant treated with injections of his mother's serum, because of its cytotoxic action on the child's lymphoid cells [19].

Various chemotherapeutic regimes have been attempted: either with a single drug: corticosteroids or Cytosine-Arabinoside; or using 2 drugs: corticosteroids with 6-Mercaptopurine, or with Vincristine; or finally using multiple chemotherapy, combining Daunorubicin, Cytosine-Arabinoside and corticosteroids.

Results are disappointing; when remissions are obtained, they do not usually exceed one month. Although the various drugs used have an undoubted effect upon the leukaemic process, we must stress their life-threatening toxicity.

DIFFERENTIAL DIAGNOSIS

Several neonatal conditions may simulate leukaemia. The marrow response of a newborn infant to infection, hypoxia or severe haemolysis frequently combines a leukaemoid reaction with the passage of red cell and granulocytic precursors into the peripheral blood. This leuco-erythroblastic reaction may wrongly suggest malignant blood disease; it is therefore wise to exclude viral or bacterial septicaemia, toxoplasmosis and syphilis by specific virological, bacteriological and serological tests.

Severe fœto-maternal incompatibility is excluded by appropriate immunological tests.

Neuroblastoma may cause diagnostic problems because of the similarity of the clinical signs: hepatomegaly, cutaneous nodules, and sometimes massive marrow infiltration by atypical cells. The discovery of a primary tumor, and above all the increased urinary excretion of catecholamines, confirm the diagnosis.

Malignant histiocytosis of which the clinical signs are little different, is confirmed by histological and/or cytological examination of the skin which demonstrates, in the deep dermis, a perivascular histiocytic infiltrate.

In Down syndrome, it is difficult to distinguish genuine congenital leukaemia from a *spontaneously regressing leucoblastosis*, which is a haematologic state of doubtful significance, reported for the first time in 1954 by Shunk and Lehman [50], then analysed in 1963 by Ross et al., who suggested the term "labile granulopoiesis" [44]. Since then, numerous attempts have been made to define the nature of this haematological disorder, which has a favourable prognosis, although sometimes a true leukaemia develops later [2, 12, 21, 26, 45, 50, 55, 57].

The clinical and haematological signs are usually present at birth or in the first week of life: pallor, possibly a haemorrhagic syndrome, and above all hepatosplenomegaly are the essential features. Lymphadenomegaly and cutaneous signs are possible but unusual and the clinical impression is generally of a less severe illness than with leukaemia [21].

Haematologically, apart from the anaemia and thrombocytopenia, which as a rule are moderate and inconstant; there is a variable leucocytosis which may exceed $10^5/mm^3$, and a leucoblastosis whose level may exceed that in the marrow [17]. The absolute number of polymorphonuclear neutrophils may be normal. The leucoblastic proliferation is made up of myeloblasts and/or undifferentiated cells. Cytogenetic examination is useful to demonstrate, the 21-trisomy, even in spite of a normal phenotype (mosaicism) and then to hope for a spontaneous cure [12].

Diagnostically, it is appropriate to exclude a leukaemoid reaction secondary to an infectious or immunological process. These may stimulate haemopoiesis, the regulation of which is poor in Down syndrome. In the event of death, the only findings at autopsy are myeloid metaplasia of the liver and spleen, myelofibrosis, and the absence of blast cell infiltration of the viscera.

Only symptomatic treatment is therefore justified, although some patients have been treated with corticosteroids and/or antimitotics.

Autopsies performed on children who have died from malformations or infections, some time after a neonatal leucoblastosis, have confirmed the total disappearance of the blastic process [17, 44, 50].

A true myeloblastic (or, much more rarely, lymphoblastic) leukaemia may nevertheless develop after several months or years of remission. Sequential cytogenetic studies are of value in demonstrating a clonal change in this type of clinical course [17, 31, 36]. In contrast, when complete remission of the leucoblastosis occurs, there is disappearance of the abnormalities which were additional to the trisomy 21.

The significance of this neonatal haematological disorder in Down Syndrome is not clear. The ultimate development of leukaemia in certain cases, and the cytogenetic data, are in favour of a genuine neonatal leukaemic process; but it is more likely to be an abnormality of haemopoiesis, occuring in trisomy 21; characterized by a transitory excess of development of trisomic cells. These cells can be related to other abnormalities such as the low level of polymorphonuclear lobulation, leucocyte and erythrocyte enzymatic abnormalities, and functional lymphocyte deficiency of these patients.

REFERENCES

[1] ALLAN (J.). — Leukemia and pregnancy. *Br. Med. J.*, *2*, 1080-1082, 1954.

[2] BEHRMAN (R.), SIGLER (A. T.), PATCHEFSKY (A. S.). — Abnormal hematopoiesis in 2 of 3 siblings with mongolism. *J. Pediatr.*, *68*, 569-577, 1966.

[3] BERGER (R.), WEISGERBER (G.), BERNARD (J.). — Évolution clonale au cours d'une leucémie aiguë chez l'enfant mongolien. *Nouv. Rev. Fr. Hématol.*, *2*, 229-236, 1973.

[4] BERNARD (J.), JACQUILLAT (C.), CHAVELET (F.), BOIRON (M.), STOITCHKOV (Y.), TANZER (J.). — Leucémie aiguë d'une enfant de 5 mois née d'une mère atteinte de leucémie aiguë au moment de l'accouchement. *Nouv. Rev. Fr. Hématol.*, *4*, 140-146, 1964.

[5] BERNARD (J.). — Leucémies aiguës du nouveau-né et du très jeune enfant. *Méd. Inf.*, *72*, 457-471, 1965.

[6] BERNHARD (W. G.), GORE (L.), KILBY (R. A.). — Congenital leukemia. *Blood*, *6*, 990-1001, 1951.

[7] BIERMAN (H. R.), AGGELER (P. M.), THELANDER (H.), KELLY (K. H.), CORDES (F. L.). — Leukemia and pregnancy. A problem in transmission in man. *J. Am. Med. Ass.*, *161*, 220-223, 1956.

[8] BILSKI-PASQUIER (G.), CHARON (P.), BOUSSER (J.). — Leucose et grossesse. *Nouv. Rev. Fr. Hématol.*, *2*, 289-311, 1962.

[9] BJÖNNESS (H.). — Congenital leukemia with chromosome aberrations (trisomy G) in a non-mongoloid child. *Helv. Paediatr. Acta*, *29*, 457-470, 1974.

[10] BOUTON (M. J.), PHILIPPS (H. J.), SMITHELLS (R. W.), WALKER (S.). — Congenital leukaemia with parental consanguinity. Case report with chromosomes studies. *Br. Med. J.*, *3*, 866, 1967.

[11] BRESCIA (M. A.), SANTORA (E.), SARNATARO (V. F.), HEIGHTS (J.), FLUSHING (N. Y.). — Congenital leukemia. *J. Pediatr.*, *55*, 35-41, 1959.

[12] BRODEUR (G. M.), DAHL (G. V.), WILLIAMS (D. L.) TIPTON (R. E.), KALWINSKY (D. K.). — Transient leukemoid reaction and trisomy 21 mosaicism in a phenotypically normal newborn. *Blood*, *55*, 691-693, 1980.

[13] BUHLER (M.), LANDOLT (R.). — Kongenitale Leukämie. *Helv. Paediat. Acta*, *25*, 173-193, 1970.

[14] CAMPBELL (W. A. B.), MACAFEE (A. L.), WADE (W. G.). — Familial neonatal leukemia. *Arch. Dis. Child.*, *37*, 93-98, 1962.

[15] CHAGANTI (R. S. K.), MILLER (D. R.), MEYERS (P. A.) GERMAN (J.). — Cytogenetic evidence of the intrauterine origin of acute leukemia in monozygotic twins. *N. Engl. J. Med.*, *300*, 1032-1034, 1979.

[16] CHU (J. Y.), O'CONNOR (D. M.), BLAIR (J.). — Congenital leukemia. *Proc. Amer. Ass. Cancer Res.*, *18*, 299, 1977.

[17] CONEN (P. E.), ERKMAN (B.). — Combined mongolism and leukemia. *Am. J. Dis. Child.*, *112*, 429-443, 1966.

[18] CRAMBLETT (H. G.). — Leukemia in an infant born of a mother with leukemia. *N. Engl. J. Med.*, *259*, 729, 1958.

[19] DE CARVALHO (S.). — Natural history of congenital leukemia. *Oncology*, *27*, 52-63, 1973.

[20] DJERNES (B. W.), SOUKUP (S. W.), BOVE (W. E.), WONG (K. Y.). — Congenital leukemia associated with mosaic trisomy 9. *J. Pediatr.*, *8*, 596-597, 1976.

[21] ENGEL (R. R.), HAMMOND (D.), EITZMAN (C. V.), PEARSON (H.), KRIVIT (W.). — Transient congenital leukemia in 7 infants with mongolism *J. Pediatr.*, 303-305, 1964.

[22] FABIA (J.), DROLETTE (M.). — Malformations and leukemia in children with Down's syndrome. *Pediatrics*, *45*, 60-70, 1970.

[23] FOURNIER (A.), ROLLET (M.), PAULI (A.), COUSIN (J.). — Les hémopathies malignes de la période néonatale. A propos d'une observation chez un garçon de 25 jours. *J. Sci. Méd. Lille*, *86*, 205-321, 1968.

[24] GAILLARD (L.), MOURIQUAND (C.), DELPHIN (D.), BRUGIÈRE (J.). — Leucoses et réticuloses histiomonocytaires aiguës congénitales. A propos de 3 observations. *Sem. Hôp.*, *4*, 255-267, 1961.

[25] GARDAIS (J.), LARGET-PIET (L.), LEROUX (J. P.), VIDAL (J. L.). — Leucoblastose néonatale transitoire, puis leucose aiguë chez un trisomique 21. *Ann. Pediatr.*, *16*, 780-785, 1969.

[26] GERMAIN (D.), MONNET (P.), ROUX (J. F.), SALLE (B.), ROSENBERG (D.), BERGER (C. L.), DAVID (M.). — Les leucoblastoses transitoires de la trisomie 21. *Ann. Pediatr.*, *26/27*, 504-510, 1967.

[27] GILGENKRANTZ (S.), BENZ (E.), CHICLET (A. M.), BUISINE (J.), GRÉGOIRE (M. J.), OLIVE (D.), STREIFF (F.). — Leucémie aiguë lymphoblastique congénitale avec remaniements chromosomiques comportant une translocation 4-22. *Comm. Soc. Fr. Hématol.*, *Poitiers*, 1980.

[27 *bis*] GOH (K.), LEE (H.), KLEMPERER (M.). — Evidence of clastogens in acute leukemia. Chromosomal abnormalities in healthy parents of congenital leukemic patients. *Cancer*, 46, 109-117, 1980.

[28] HAAR (J.). — Congenital leukemia. *Acta Paediatr. Scand.*, 60, 720-723, 1971.

[29] HILTON (H. B.), LEWIS (I. C.), TROWELL (H. R.). — C group trisomy in identical twins with acute leukemia. *Blood*, 35, 222-226, 1970.

[30] HOGG (G. R.), SCHMIDT (D. A.). — Myelogenous leukaemia in a stillborn infant. *Can. Med. Assoc. J.*, 78, 421-423, 1958.

[31] HONDA (F.), PUNNET (H. H.), CHARNEY (E.), MILLER (G.), THIEDE (H. A.). — Serial cytogenetic and hematologic studies on a mongol with trisomy 21 and acute congenital leukemia. *J. Pediatr.*, 65, 880-887, 1964.

[32] IRWIN (L.), CAMPBELL (J. W.). — Congenital leukemia. *Afr. Med. J.*, 71, 1445-1446, 1978.

[33] KEITH (L.), BROWN (E. R.), AMES (B.), STOTSKY (M.), KEITH (D. M.). — Leukemia in twins: antenatal and postnatal factors. *Acta Genet. Med. Gemellol.*, 20, 9-22, 1971.

[34] KRIVIT (W.), GOOD (R. A.). — Simultaneous occurrence of mongolism and leukemia. *Am. J. Dis. Child.*, 94, 289-293, 1957.

[35] LEE (R. A.), JOHNSON (C. E.), HANLON (D. G.). — Leukemia during pregnancy. *Am. J. Obstet. Gynec.*, 84, 455-458, 1962.

[36] LEJEUNE (J.), BERGER (R.), HAINES (M.), LAFOURCADE (Y.), VIALATTE (Y.), SATGE (P.), TURPIN (R.). — Constitution d'un clone à 54 chromosomes au cours d'une leucoblastose congénitale chez une enfant mongolienne. *C. R. Acad. Sc.*, 256, 1195-1197, 1963.

[37] MACMAHON (B.), LEVY (M. A.). — Prenatal origin of childhood leukemia: evidence from twins. *N. Engl. J. Med.*, 270, 1082-1085, 1964.

[38] MATTELAER (P. M.). — Leukemia in the perinatal period. *Ann. Paediatr.*, 203, 124-136, 1964.

[39] MILLER (D. R.), NEWSTEAD (G. J.), YOUNG (L. W.). — Perinatal leukemia with a possible variant of the Ellis-Van Creveld syndrome. *J. Pediatr.*, 74, 300-303, 1969.

[40] PIERCE (M. I.). — Leukemia in the newborn infant. *J. Pediatr.*, 54, 691-706, 1959.

[41] PRIDIE (G.), DUMITRESCUPIRVU (D.). — Leucemia acuta, sindrom Bonnevie-Ullrich la un nou nascut. *Pediatria*, 10. 345. 1961.

[42] PONZONE (A.), DE SANCTIS (C.), FABRIS (C.), CIRIOTTI (G.), FRANCESCHINI (P.). — Blast cell proliferation in perinatal leukemia with chromosomal translocation (Bq +; Dq −). *Helv. Paediatr. Acta*, 27, 3-13, 1972.

[43] ROSNER (F.), LEE (S. L.). — Down's syndrome and acute leukemia: myeloblastic or lymphoblastic? *Am. J. Med.*, 53, 203-218, 1972.

[44] ROSS (J. D.), MOLONEY (W. C.), DESFORGES (J. R.).

— Ineffective regulation of granulopoiesis masquerading as congenital leukemia in a mongoloid child. *J. Pediatr.*, 63, 1-10, 1963.

[45] SALEUN (J. P.), ALIX (D.), LEROY (J. P.), BARET (M.), BALQUET (G.), CASTEL (Y.). — Leucoblastose transitoire et dysembryoplasie rénale chez un trisomique 21. *Ann. Pediatr.*, 22, 543-550, 1975.

[46] SANDBERG (A. A.), CORTNER (J.), TAKAGI (N.), MOGHADAM (M. A.), CROSSWHITE (L. H.). — Differences in chromosome constitution of twins with acute leukemia. *N. Engl. J. Med.*, 275, 809-812, 1966.

[47] SANDBERG (A. A.). — In *The chromosomes in human cancer and leukemia*. Elsevier, ed. New York, 322-323, 1980.

[48] SCHADE (H.), SCHOELLER (L.), SCHULTZE (K. W. D.). — Trisomie (Patau) mit kongenitaler myeloischer Leukemia. *Med. Welt*, 5, 2690, 1962.

[49] SCHULERI (E.), MAGHERU (H.). — Un cas de leucémie aiguë granulocytaire chez un nourrisson, probablement congénitale, et produite par l'exposition répétée de la mère aux rayons X pendant la grossesse. *Arch. Anat. Path.*, 19, 25-29, 1971.

[50] SHUNK (G. J.), LEHMAN (W. L.). — Mongolism and congenital leukemia. *J. A. M. A.*, 155, 596, 1954.

[51] SUTNICK (A. I.), LONGON (W. T.), BLUMBERG (B. S.), GERSTLEY (B. J. S.). — Susceptibility to leukaemia: immunologic factors in Down's syndrome. *J. Natl. Cancer Inst.*, 47, 923-933, 1971.

[52] SVARCH (E.), TORRE (E. DE LA). — Myelomonocytic leukaemia with a preleukaemic syndrome and Phi chromosome in monozygotic twins. *Arch. Dis. Child.*, 52, 72-74, 1977.

[53] VAN DEN BERGHE (H.), FRYNS (J.), VERRESEN (H.). — Congenital leukemia with 46, XX, t (Bq − Cq) cells. *J. Med. Gen.*, 9, 468-484, 1972.

[54] WAGNER (H. P.), TONZ (D.), GREYERZ-GLOOR (R.). — Congenital lymphoid leukemia. *Helv. Paediatr. Acta*, 6, 591-611, 1968.

[55] WEINSTEIN (H. J.). — Congenital leukaemia and the neonatal myeloproliferative disorders associated with Down's syndrome. *Clin. Haematol.*, 7, 147-154, 1978.

[56] WEGELIUS (R.). — Discordant leukaemia in twins. A report of 2 cases including one of congenital leukaemia. *Ann. Paediatr. Fenn.*, 6, 227, 1960.

[57] WEISGERBER (C.), SCHAISON (G.), TANZER (J.). — Leucémies aiguës des mongoliens. *Actualités Hématologiques*, Paris, Masson éd., 5e série, 143, 1971.

[58] WOLK (J. A.). — Congenital and neonatal leukemia. Lymphocytic or myelocytic? *Am. J. Dis. Child.*, 128, 864-866, 1974.

[59] ZUSSMAN (W. V.), KHAN (A.), SHAYESTEH. — Congenital leukemia. Report of a case with chromosome abnormalities. *Cancer*, 8, 1227-1233, 1967.

Congenital histiocytoses

This term is used for conditions, which are apparently primary and of unknown aetiology, characterised by local or disseminated proliferation of non malignant histiocytes. Cytological, immunological, and functional study of these histiocytes makes it possible to distinguish two different

conditions: — histiocytosis X and malignant histiocytosis [6, 13].

It is difficult to know their relative incidence in
the newborn; in fact, the similarities of their clinical
features and evolution has led to their being confused, both with each other, and with certain reactive
histiocytoses.

HISTIOCYTOSIS X

Definition. Incidence. Epidemiology.
— Lichtenstein [30], in 1953, suggested the term
histiocytosis X to group together Abt-Letterer-
Siwe disease, Hand-Schuller-Christian disease and
eosinophilic granuloma, all conditions characterised
by local or diffuse proliferation of (usually differentiated) histiocytes, with a subacute or chronic
course, sometimes ending in death despite the non
malignant nature of the proliferation. The unique-
ness of the clinical manifestations depends on the
presence in the cytoplasm of these histiocytes of
tubular inclusions, the X bodies identical to the
granules of Langerhans' cells which are histiocytes
normally present in the skin, and in small numbers
in lung and lymph nodes [4, 35, 52].

Nezelof regards as disseminated histiocytoses X
all forms which affect at least 2 different tissue types
or organs [35, 36]. These disseminated forms, which
are twice as common in males, are found especially
in young children. Of the 50 cases reported by
Nezelof et al., 35 were in children under 2 years,
19 between 0 and 6 months, and 8 of the 50 cases
(16 %) were neonatal [36]. The incidence of congenital histiocytosis X, which is always disseminated,
is therefore not negligable; in all, 40 cases have been
reported, but it is probable that not all have been
published, and that some have gone unrecognised [20].

The appearance of the first clinical signs at birth
suggests an intra-uterine onset; however, aetiological
enquires are mostly negative. Common viral infections (influenza, herpes, smallpox vaccination) are
reported [33, 53]. No malformation is associated
with this condition. Rare familial cases have occured
affecting two siblings or two monozygous twins [7,
19, 23, 41].

Clinical picture. — Affected infants are
usually born at term, and of appropriate birthweight.
Cases of intra-uterine death [16], prematurity [14],
and dysmaturity [15] appear to be rare; they are
associated from the outset with dramatic symptoms.

Cutaneous manifestations are the earliest and are
almost always present.

They are variable, ranging from papules, to
bullous lesions which crust rapidly, and squamous
lesions resembling seborrhoeic eczema. The lesions
are often purpuric. Often numerous, they are found
mainly on the trunk, on the buttocks and skin folds,
but may also be present on the scalp and limbs.
Less typical chamois-yellow or violaceous nodular
lesions are often associated [5, 8, 15, 16, 17, 28, 29,
32, 51]. On the mucous membranes, specific lesions
create ulcers [14, 33, 36, 46]. Fever, hepato-splenomegaly with or without jaundice, and local or
diffuse lymphadenopathy, present in 2/3 of cases,
may appear secondarily. Pulmonary manifestations,
apparent in about 50 % of cases, are rarely early.
They may be purely radiological, in the form of a
disseminated reticulonodular pattern. Cough, dyspnoea and cyanosis indicate severe involvement;
both lung fields are then riddled with bullous micro-
cavities giving a "bees nest" or honey-comb appearance [22]. A fatal outcome may be hastened by
rupture of an emphysematous bulla into the pleura
or mediastinum [8, 46]. Hypertrophy of the thymus
is uncommon [8, 22, 42, 45]. Bony involvement may
manifest clinically as swellings, particularly in the
skull vault [5, 42], or as loss of bone substance [34].
The radiological picture is of a punched out lesion
of variable size, with well defined edges, sometimes
polycyclical or encircled by a hatched border. The
bones which are most often involved are the skull
(vault, orbit, mastoid), and the flat bones (pelvis,
scapula, clavicle and ribs). Mastoiditis occurs in
1/4 of cases. The other manifestations, diabetes
insipidus, and ocular lesions [34, 36] are rare, and
only occur after several months or years.

*Haematological and histological fea-
tures.* — Moderate anaemia is present in one half
of cases, together with a variable leucocytosis and
sometimes a slight monocytosis. Severe anaemia
and thrombocytopenia are signs of hysticocytic
invasion of the bone-marrow. This poses the problem
of forms on the border line with or confused with
malignant histiocytosis.

Careful immunological investigations are useful,
since a recent study has brought out suppressive
T cell deficiency [37 *bis*].

*Histological examination under the light micro-
scope of a skin biopsy* shows infiltration of the
superficial dermis by differentiated histiocytes
without malignant characteristics. They have pale
or acidophyllic cytoplasm, an oval or kidney shaped
nucleus, with fine regular chromatin, and a nucleolus
which is not easily visible. Some multinucleated

cells are seen, but mitotic figures are rare. Phagocytosis is limited to the ingestion of a few erythrocytes or haemosiderin. The infiltrate is accompanied
by a small proportion of eosinophils and of multinucleated giant cells. More or less fibrosis and
necrosis has been noted... Similar proliferation is
found in lymph nodes, liver, spleen, lung and bones.

Ultrastructural study shows the cytoplasmic X
bodies (or Birbeck granules) which are trilamellar
structures, of variable length, but constant width
of 400-450 Å resembling a zipfastener [4]. Langerhans' cells may also be characterized by their
enzymatic activity and membrane complement
receptors.

Clinical course and treatment. — The
adverse prognostic criteria in histiocytosis X [27, 31,
36, 37, 50] include a young age, the number of
organs involved and their functional impairment.
This accounts for the high mortality rate, of over
65 %: 35 % before the second month [5, 8, 14, 22,
28, 41, 45, 46], and 30 % between the 2nd and
6th months [22, 33, 36, 45, 46, 53]. Death is usually
due to respiratory complications, to extension of
the skin lesions leading to progressive cachexia
and to infections promoted by immuno-suppressive
therapy [33].

More favourable cases have a chronic course
which may end in recovery [7, 17, 34, 36, 51].
Nevertheless there is a serious risk of disabling
sequelæ: diabetes insipidus, blindness, deafness,
orthopaedic complications, growth retardation,
and psychomotor retardation [36].

Treatment based on corticosteroids and antimitotic
drugs (Vinblastine and Vincristine sulphate) does
not seem to have improved survival, as half of
the treated cases have died. However, spectacular
improvements in the cutaneous and lymph node
lesions have been observed [15, 32, 33, 42]. Corticosteroids and/or chemotherapy should therefore
always be attempted, but not continued if ineffective
because of the risks of iatrogenic infections or haemorrhagic complications. Current interest lies in the
attempt to treat patients with thymic factor [37 *bis*].

CONGENITAL MALIGNANT
HISTIOCYTOSIS

Definition. Occurence. Epidemiology.
— Malignant histiocytosis, which is still called leukaemic reticulo-endotheliosis, or histiocyto-medul-
lary reticulosis of Scott and Robb-Smith [47] is a

proliferation of atypical histiocytes and their
precursors [40, 54, 55]. It occurs mainly between the
ages of 10 and 30 years, and seems to be unusual
in the newborn. Since the first case, reported by
Sacrez and Frühling in 1954 [43], about ten cases
have been published; furthermore there has often
been confusion with congenital Letterer-Siwe disease [1, 2, 16, 18, 24, 25, 26, 32, 44, 49]. Both sexes
are equally affected. In one case, Ahnquist and
Holyoke noted anti-poliomyelitis and anti-influenza
vaccination during pregnancy [1]. In the case reported
by Kremp et al. a pre-leukaemic state was discovered
in the mother of an infant with congenital malignant
histiocytosis, and acute myeloblastic leukaemia
was confirmed 4 months later [24].

Clinical picture. — Of the 10 cases we have
analysed, 6 were infants of normal birth weight, born
at term. One infant was still-born at term [1], and
the three others were either premature or dysmature [18, 24, 49]. In all ten cases the signs were
present from birth. The most constant sign is a
specific skin rash, consisting of disseminated haemorrhagic nodules, penetrating into the deep
dermis, which may ulcerate. They are dark brown,
blue-black, or wine-coloured, and vary in diameter
from a few millimetres to 5 cms. These lesions may
involve the mucous membranes. Hepatomegaly is
almost constant, associated with splenomegaly,
and sometimes with neoplastic lymph nodes.
Respiratory disorders, jaundice, irregular fever,
and neurological abnormalities complete a clinical
picture, whose gravity is obvious. Chest radiographs
may show thymic enlargement and a fine disseminated reticulo-nodular pattern. Bone involvement has
not been noted, except in the case of Amato, who
found tiny punched-out lesions dispersed through
all the long bones and flat bones [2]. Meningeal
involvement must be sought routinely by lumbar
puncture; in two cases there was ocular infiltration [26, 44], and in another there was diffuse
infiltration of cerebral tissue [26].

***Haematological and cytological fea-
tures*** are as follows:

Anaemia is at first mild and regenerative, sometimes with considerable reticulocytosis, but rapidly
deteriorates. *Thrombocytopenia* occurs early. Coagulation disorders, of a disseminated intravascular
coagulation type, are possible [2]. *Leucocytosis, or
leucopenia* may occur with variable and fluctuating
numbers of atypical cells. These are cells of the
histiomonocytic line, or undifferentiated cells. There
may also be an increased number of normal cir-

culating monocytes and numerous early and dystrophic cells of the granulocytic series, at various stages of maturation hence the term reticulo-myelosis. Serum and urinary lysozyme level is increased.

The bone-marrow is polymorphic, with the different haematological cell lines all represented. There may be some hyperactivity, in the form of erythroblastosis. Sometimes the marrow appears normal, and the minimal histiocytic infiltration has to be carefully sought. Occasionally this infiltration is massive with large basophilic cells, whose distorted nuclei have one or several nucleoli and irregular chromatin.

Histological study of a cutaneous nodule shows, in all cases, a proliferation of cells of histiocytic type in the deep dermis, mainly perivascular and periadnexial. These cells have an atypical nucleus and cytoplasm, with thickening of the nuclear membrane, irregular chromatin, and an easily visible, irregular nucleolus. There are numerous mitoses, and phagocytosis, mainly of red corpuscles, is frequent. *In the lymph nodes*, histiocytic infiltration is mainly in the medullary sinuses (hence the term histiocytic medullary reticulosis).

Cytochemical and immunological studies may help to identify the histiocyte, when the morphology alone is insufficient.

Cytochemistry: *positivity for esterases with the substrate α naphtyl acetate or α naphtyl butyrate and inhibition by sodium fluoride is pathognomonic; acid phosphatases are positive, with inhibition by L-tartric acid; PAS reaction is positive and peroxydase weakly positive.*

Immunology: *receptors are present for the F_c fraction of IgG (EA rosettes), and for the C1q fraction of complement.*

Course and treatment. — The condition appears uniformly fatal in the first 10 days, with respiratory and renal failure, infection or haemorrhage, in spite of corticosteroids: 6-mercaptopurine [49], and Vinblastine sulphate [24]. Protocols for intensive multiple chemotherapy, used in the treatment of lymphomas, give fairly encouraging results in adults and children [9, 55], but are difficult to apply to the newborn.

DIFFERENTIAL DIAGNOSIS OF NEONATAL HISTIOCYTOSES

The reticulo-histiocytoses of storage diseases can present differential diagnostic problems in the infant and the older child, but are practically never considered in the neonatal period, although a few very early cases of xantho-granuloma or juvenile lipid granuloma have been reported.

Reactive histiocytoses constitute the main diagnostic problems.

Congenital infections, either bacterial, or, more especially, viral and parasitic, cause, particularly if chronic, reticulo-histiocytic stimulation. This results in a clinical picture which can resemble Letterer-Siwe disease or even malignant histiocytosis. The distinction can generally be made by careful search for an infectious agent and characterisation of the histiocytic proliferation, by light and electron microscopy, and by modern immunological studies.

Certain congenital immune deficiencies, characterised by a proliferation if macrophages, have also initially been confused with Letterer-Siwe disease [11, 12, 48].

Familial lympho-histiocytosis (or Farquar and Claireaux's haemophagocytic reticulosis) is usually inherited as an autosomal recessive and presents in the first 6 months of life [3, 35, 38, 39]. There is fever, pallor, purpura, erythematous or maculo-papular skin rash, hepatosplenomegaly, meningo-encephalitis, anaemia with marrow erythroblastosis, thrombocytopenia and neutropenia, with relative lymphocytosis and monocytosis. Histologically, there is a mixed infiltration of many viscera by lymphocytes and histiocytes; the histiocytes show frequent haemophagocytosis, but are cytologically normal.

Congenital leukaemias obviously present differential diagnostic problems with malignant histiocytosis because of their clinical similarities. The diagnosis may usually be established from the marrow origin of the blast proliferation, the monomorphic nature of the marrow infiltrate, and the cytochemical and immunological findings. Certain myeloblastic leucoses with a polymorphic proliferation of the entire granular series, may be difficult to distinguish from those malignant histiocytoses which are accompanied by a strong myeloid reaction.

Finally, histiocytosis X and congenital malignant histiocytoses differ in the following ways: in malignant histiocytosis the cutaneous lesions are always nodular and situated in the deep dermis. In histiocytosis X they are maculopapular and always in the superficial dermis; haematological disorders are always marked in malignant histiocytosis X. The clinical course is devastating in malignant histiocytosis, more prolonged in histiocytosis X. The histiocytes have atypical nucleus and cytoplasm in malignant histiocytosis but are relatively well differentiated in Letterer-Siwe disease; X bodies are present in histiocytosis X, although this is not an infallible criterion.

REFERENCES

[1] AHNQUIST (G.), HOLYOKE (J. B.). — Congenital Letterer-Siwe disease reticuloendotheliosis in a term stillborn infant. J. Pediatr., 57, 897-903, 1960.
[2] AMATO (M.). — Diagnostic différentiel entre l'histiocytopathie maligne du nouveau-né et la leucémie congénitale. Arch. Fr. Pédiatr., 21, 212-218, 1964.
[3] BARTH (R. F.), BERGARA (G. G.), KHURANA (S. K.), LOWMA (J. T.), BECKWITH (J. B.). — Rapidly fatal familial histiocytosis associated with eosinophilia and primary immunological deficiency. Lancet, 2, 503-506, 1972.
[4] BASSET (F.), NEZELOF (C.). — L'histiocytose X. Microscopie électronique, culture in vitro et histoenzymologie. Discussion à propos de 21 cas. Rev. Fr. Étude Clin. Biol., 14, 31-45, 1969.
[5] BATSON (R.), SHAPIRO (J.), CHRISTIE (A.), RILEY (H. D.). — Acute non-lipid disseminated reticuloendotheliosis. Am. J. Dis. Child., 90, 323-343, 1955.
[6] BENZ (E.). — Les histiocytoses tumorales de l'enfant. Thèse Méd., Nancy, 242 p., 1980.
[7] BIERMAN (H. R.). — Apparent cure of Letterer-Siwe disease. Seventeen year survival of identic twins with non lipoid reticulo-endotheliosis. J. Am. Med. Assoc., 396, 368-370, 1966.
[8] BONSTEIN (H.). — Un cas de maladie de Letterer-Siwe chez un nouveau-né. Ann. Anat. Pathol., 3, 362-374, 1956.
[9] BYRNE (G. E.), RAPPAPORT (H.). — Malignant histiocytosis. In Malignant diseases of the hematopoietic system. Gann Monograph on Cancer Research 15 Tokyo, University of Tokyo Press, 15, 143-153, 1973.
[10] CALVANI (M.), LOTTI (A.), TADDEINI (R.). — Istiocitopatia congenita maligna del neonato. Contribute clinico ad anatomo-istologica. Paediatria, 70, 1136-1146, 1962.
[11] CEDERBAUM (S. D.), NIWAYAMA (G.), STIEHM (R.), NEERHOUT (R. C.), AMMANN (A. J.), BERMAN (W.). — Combined immunodeficiency presented as the Letterer-Siwe syndrome. J. Pediatr., 85, 4, 466-471, 1974.
[12] CLAMAN (H. N.), SUVATTE (V.), GITHENS (J. H.), HATHAWAY (W. E.). — Histiocytic reaction in dysgamma-globulinemia and congenital rubella. Pediatrics, 46, 89-96, 1970.
[13] CLINE (M. J.), GOLDE (D. W.). — A review and reevaluation of the histiocytic disorders. Am. J. Med., 55, 49-60, 1973.
[14] COHEN (D. M.), MITCHELL (C. B.), ALEXANDER (J. W.). — Letterer-Siwe disease in a newborn. Arch. Pathol., 81, 347-350, 1966.
[15] DALTROFF (G.), WILLARD (D.), MESSER (J.), OBERLING (F.). — An observation of neonatal reticulosis. Sacrez disease. Acta Paediatr. Belg., 29, 4, 223-230, 1976.

[16] DLUHOS (M.), SCHEJBAL (V.). — Morbus Abt-Letterer-Siwe congenitus. Kind. Arz. Prax., 30, 431-436, 1962.
[17] DOSMONS (S.), BURIOT (D.), BONIFACE (N.), BOMBART (M.), ALIX (D.), GRISCELLI (C.). — Histiocytoses X précoces avec nodules dermiques. Évolution favorable. Ann. Dermatol. Vénérol., 105, 87-89, 1978.
[18] FONTAN (A.), VERGER (P.), LEGER (H.), PERY (P.). — Réticulomyélose congénitale chez un enfant prématuré. Pédiatrie, 13, 527, 1968.
[19] FRISSEL (E.), BJORKSTEN (B.), HOLMGREN (G.), AMGSTROM (T.). — Familial occurrence of histiocytosis X. Clin. Genet., 11, 163-170, 1977.
[20] GLASS (A. G.), MILLER (R. W.). — US Mortality from Letterer-Siwe, 1960-1964. Pediatrics, 42, 364-368, 1968.
[21] GUBERT (J. P.), VIGNES (B.), OLIVIER (C.), HAYAT (B.), BABINET (J. M.). — La maladie de Letterer-Siwe néonatale. Ann. Pediatr., 21, 719-522, 1974.
[22] HAMILTON (W.). — Congenital Letterer-Siwe disease. Scot. Med. J., 6, 575-577, 1961.
[23] JUBERG (R. C.), KLOEPFER (H. W.), OBERMAN (H. A.). — Genetic determination of acute disseminated histiocytosis X (Letterer-Siwe syndrome). Pediatrics, 45, 5, 753-765, 1970.
[24] KREMP (L.), MACART (M.), HOPFNER (C.), FLANDRIN (G.), BERNARD (J.). — Découverte simultanée d'une hémopathie maligne chez un nouveau-né et d'un syndrome préleucémique chez la mère. Nouv. Rev. Fr. Hématol., 20, 3, 349-357, 1978.
[25] KUCHEMANN (K.). — Congenital Letterer-Siwe disease. Beitr. Pathol., 151, 405-411, 1974.
[26] LAHAV (M.), ALBERT (D. M.). — Unusual ocular involvement in acute disseminated histiocytosis X. Arch. Ophtalmol., 91, 455-458, 1974.
[27] LAHEY (M. E.). — Histiocytosis X: an analysis of prognostic factors. J. Pediatr., 87, 184-189, 1975.
[28] LANE (C. W.), SLITH (M. G.). — Cutaneous manifestations of chronic idiopathic lipoidosis. Arch. Derm. Syph., 39, 617-644, 1959.
[29] LAURET (Ph.), HENOCQ (A.), DE MENIBUS (C. H.), THEMINE (E.). — Histiocytose X congénitale, à propos d'un nouveau cas. Bull. Soc. Franç. Derm. Syph. 81, 247-251, 1974.
[30] LICHTENSTEIN (L.). — Histiocytosis X: integration of eosinophilic granuloma of bone Letterer-Siwe's disease and Hand-Shüller-Christian disease as related manifestations of a single nosologic entity. Arch. Pathol., 56, 84-102, 1953.
[31] LUCAYA (X.). — Histiocytosis X. Am. J. Dis. Child., 121, 289-295, 1971.
[32] LYONNET (R.), SAVOYE (J.), MOREL (P.), MICHEL (P. J.). — Réticulose histiomonocytaire maligne congénitale (Letterer-Siwe) avec formations nodulaires très nombreuses disséminées sur le tégument chez un nouveau-né. Évolution apyrétique et régressive sous l'influence de la corticothérapie à hautes doses soutenue depuis 4 mois et demi. Bull. Soc. Fr. Derm. Syph., 68, 736-737, 1961.
[33] MALLET (R.), BACH (Ch.), SARRUT (S.), DRESCH (C.). — Une observation de maladie de Letterer-Siwe congénitale. Traitement par Prednisone. Surinfection terminale par pneumocystis carinii. Ann. Pediatr., 41, 531-540, 1965.
[34] MOZZICONACCI (P.), OFFRET (G.), FOREST (A.), ATTAL (C.), GIRARD (F.), HAYEM (F.), PHAM HUU TRUNG. — Histiocytose X avec lésions oculaires. Étude anatomique. Ann. Pédiatr., 21, 348-355, 1966.
[35] NEZELOF (C.). — Les réticulo-histiocytoses de

l'enfant : nosologie et classification. *Arch. Fr. Pédiatr.*, *36*, 6, 629-639, 1979.

[36] NEZELOF (C.), FRILEUX-HERBET (F.), CRONIER-SACHOT (J.). — Disseminated histiocytosis X. Analysis of prognostic factc 's based on a retrospective study of 50 cases. *Cancer*, *44*, 1824-1838, 1979.

[37] OBERMAN (H. A.). — Idiopathic histiocytosis. A clinico-pathologic study of 40 cases and review of literature on eosinophilic granuloma of bone, Letterer-Siwe disease and Hand-Schüller-Christian disease. *Pediatrics*, *28*, 307-327, 1961.

[37 bis] OSBAND (M. E.), LIPTON (J. M.), LAVIN (P.), LEVEY (R.), VAWTER (G.), GREENBERGER (J. S.), McCAFFREY (R. P.), PARKMAN (R.). — Histiocytosis X: demonstration of abnormal immunity, T-cell histamine H2-receptor deficiency, and successful treatment with thymic extract. *N. Engl. J. Med.*, *304*, 146-153, 1981.

[38] PERRY (M.), HARRISON (E.), BURGET (O.), GILGHUST (G.). — Familial erythrophagocytic lymphohistiocytosis. Report of two cases and clinicopathologic review. *Cancer*, *38*, 209-218, 1976.

[39] PUISSAN (C. H.), PETIT (J.), MARESCHAL (B.), AUDEBERT (M.), REGUET (Cl.), RISBOURG (B.). — Lympho-histiocytose familiale. *Ann. Pédiatr.*, *25*, 119-125, 1978.

[40] RAPPAPORT (H.). — Tumors of the hematopoietic system, 3 fasc., 8. *Atlas of Tumor Pathology*. Ed. Armed forces institute of pathology. Washington, 1966.

[41] ROGERS (D. L.), BENSON (T. E.). — Familial Letterer-Siwe disease. Report of a case. *J. Pediatr.*, *60*, 550-554, 1962.

[42] ROSSIER (A.), CALDERA (R.), LE TAN VINH, NEZELOF (C.), BASSET (F.). — Histiocytose néonatale à localisations multiples avec présence de filaments d'apparence virale dans les lésions cytologiques. Effet de la vincaleucoblastine. *Bull. Hém. Soc. Méd. Hôp. Paris*, *117*, 393-397, 1966.

[43] SACREZ (R.), FRUHLING (L.), HEUMANN (G.), CAHN (R.). — Réticulohistiocytose maligne à forme cutanée et hématologique chez un nouveau-né. *Arch. Fr. Pédiatr.*, *11*, 141-144, 1954.

[44] SACREZ (R.), WILLARD (D.), LEVY (J. M.), SUAREZ (J.). — La réticulohistiocytose maligne du nouveau-né. *Pédiatrie*, *19*, 103-111, 1964.

[45] SAENGER (E. L.), JOHANSMANN (R. J.). — Letterer-Siwe's disease. Problems in diagnosis and treatment. *Am. J. Roentgenol.*, *71*, 472-483, 1954.

[46] SCHAFER (E. I.). — Non lipid reticulo-endotheliosis (Letterer-Siwe disease). Report of 3 cases. *Am. J. Pathol.*, *25*, 59-73, 1949.

[47] SCOTT (R. B.), ROBBSMITH (A. H. T.). — Histiocytic medullary reticulosis. *Lancet*, *2*, 194-198, 1939.

[48] SCOTT (H.), MOYNAHAN (E. J.), RISDON (R. A.), HARVEY (B. A.), SOOTHILL (J. F.). — Familial opsonisation defect associated with fatal infantile dermatitis infections and histiocytosis. *Arch. Dis. Child.*, *50*, 4, 311-317, 1975.

[49] SKODACEK (G.), BABALA (J.). — Angeborene leukämische Retikulose (Myelo Retikulose) bei einem frühgeborenen Saügling. *Neoplasma (Bratislava)*, *11*, 199-206, 1964.

[50] SIMS (D. G.). — Histiocytosis X: Follow-up of 43 cases. *Arch. Dis. Child.*, *52*, 433-440, 1977.

[51] STEWART (W.), SEASSARD (C.), LAURET (B. T.), BOULLIEM (C.), SOUBRANE (J. C.). — Histiocytose X congénitale purement cutanée à évolution bénigne. *Bull. Soc. Derm. Syph.*, *80*, 438-443, 1973.

[52] STINGL (G.), KATZ (S. I.), SHEVACH (E.), ROSENTHAL (A.), GREEN (I.). — Analogous functions of macrophages and Langerhans cells in the initiation of the immune response. *J. Invest. Dermatol.*, *71*, 59-64, 1978.

[53] VISSIAN (I.), ROVINSKI (J.), LANIER (M.). — A propos de deux observations de maladie de Letterer-Siwe. *Ann. Derm. Syph.*, *91*, 263-277, 1964.

[54] WARNKE (R.), KIM (H.), DORFMAN (R. F.). — Malignant histiocytosis (Histiocytic medullary reticulosis). Clinico-pathologic study of 29 cases. *Cancei*, *35*, 215-230, 1975.

[55] ZUCKER (J. M.), CAILLAUX (J. M.), VANEL (D.), GÉRARD-MARCHANT (R.). — Malignant histiocytosis in childhood: Clinical study and therapeutic results in 22 cases. *Cancer*, *45*, 2821-2829, 1980.

6

Metabolism and Endocrinology

35

Thermoregulation in the newborn

Paul R. SWYER

The thermal environment of the newborn

THE INTRAUTERINE ENVIRONMENT AND THE TRANSITION TO EXTRAUTERINE LIFE

The fetus lives in a thermally constant and protected environment. The body temperature of the fetus is approximately 0.5° C higher than that of the mother, ensuring dissipation of the heat resulting from fetal metabolic processes mainly through heat exchange in the placenta, mediated by placental blood flow [1]. However, maternal pyrexia can temporarily reverse the temperature gradient and cause fetal pyrexia which may be manifested by fetal tachycardia.

COLD STRESS AT BIRTH

At the time of delivery the newborn enters an environment some 12° C cooler (e. g., 25° C vs 37° C), and is moreover wet with amniotic fluid and so subject to evaporative as well as radiative and convective heat loss. Dahm and James [2] have demonstrated both the marked reductions in newborn body temperature (Fig. VI-1) and the mitigation of heat loss by different methods of heat conservation in the delivery room. Calculations from their data shows heat losses up to 100 cal/ kg.min (144 kcal/kg.d), a rate of heat loss almost three times as great as the usual resting metabolic heat production [3]. Each fall of 1° C in core temperature implies a loss of 900 cal/kg. For a term newborn at 28° C and 50 % relative humidity, heat losses are 50 cal/kg.min (84 % dry, 16 % wet loss) equivalent to 72 kcal/kg.d [4].

Such rates of heat loss exceed an infant's ability to increase heat production even when postnatal adaptation to extrauterine life has been completed and may result in failure of adequate compensatory heat production with cardiorespiratory failure, hypoglycaemia and acidosis.

These dangers are augmented for the premature or low birth weight infant whose higher surface area to body weight ratio, lower body fat insulation, higher peripheral blood flow and immature homeostatic reflexes promote heat loss under cool condi-

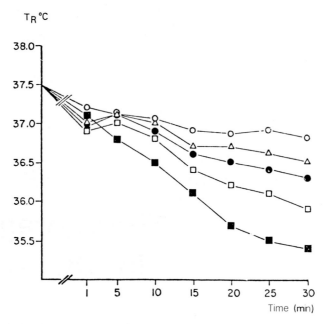

FIG. VI-1. — *Mean deep body temperatures (T$_R$) of each group during the first 30 minutes of life.* T$_R$ is on the ordinate and minutes post-delivery on the abscissa. ■ wet infants in room air; □ dry infants in room air; ● wet infants under the radiant heater; △ dry infants wrapped in a blanket, ○ dry infants under the radiant heater. Reproduced with permission from DAHM L. S. & JAMES L. S.: *Pediatrics,* 49, 504, April 1972.

tions. Despite the special mechanism of brown fat thermogenesis there is a reduced ability to increase metabolism to defend body temperature because of relatively restricted energy substrate reserves and cardiopulmonary function, poor musculature and inability to shiver. The more premature and the more underweight the infant, the more exaggerated are all these handicaps, and the greater their contribution to morbidity and mortality, especially when potentiated by asphyxia.

AVOIDANCE OF COLD STRESS AT BIRTH

Measures to conserve heat at delivery are therefore extremely important to the well being of the newborn, particularly if the infant happens to be asphyxiated, of low birth weight, or both.

The data quoted from Dahm and James [2] suggests that heat conservation is best served by immediately drying the neonate, by wrapping in a warm towel and transferring the infant immediately to the mother's arms for skin to skin contact with both warmly covered, or to a prewarmed incubator at the thermoneutral temperature.

Should resuscitation be necessary, it is advanta-

geous, particularly for premature or compromised infants, to have a resuscitation room immediately adjacent to the delivery room kept at a relatively warmer air temperature of approximately 28° C where the dried infant can be immediately placed under a radiant heater for the necessary resuscitative procedures.

POSTNATAL THERMOREGULATION

The temperature of the infant will depend on the balance between metabolic heat production and heat loss (or gain) from the environment. This balance will be determined by a complex of biological factors intrinsic to the infant and by extrinsic factors related to the physical laws governing energy exchange with the environment by radiation, convection, evaporation and conduction.

The general equation describing thermal equilibrium with the environment is [5, 6, 7]:

Equation 1.

$$\dot{Q} \text{ met} = \dot{Q} \text{ loss} + \dot{Q} \text{ storage}$$

where $\dot{Q}$ met = metabolic heat production per unit time,

$\dot{Q}$ loss   = heat loss per unit time,

$\dot{Q}$ storage = heat stored or lost per unit time (may have a +ve or −ve sign).

In thermal equilibrium, heat storage is zero and heat loss is equal to the total metabolic heat production. This is the usual physiologic equilibrium condition. Heat loss exceeding heat production by metabolic processes results in a fall of body temperature, while heat storage is manifested by a rise in body temperature.

Change in the total heat content of the body can be calculated according to the following formula:

Equation 2.

$$\Delta s = m_b \times c_b \times \frac{(0.6\Delta T_{int} + 0.4\Delta \overline{Tsk})}{\Delta t}$$

where Δs = change in heat content, either positive (storage) or negative (loss) (kcal/unit time),

m_b = body weight (kg),

c_b = specific heat of body mass (0.84 kcal/ kg/° C),

ΔT_{int} = change in core temperature,

$\Delta \overline{Tsk}$ = variation of mean skin temperature,

Δt = time interval.

Thus it is necessary to consider both the level of metabolic heat production and the amount of heat loss in delineating the energy balance equation of the newborn.

METABOLIC HEAT PRODUCTION

The homeothermic state is a fundamental physiological imperative for the newborn [8] and thermoregulatory adjustments in heat production have a high priority in the hierarchy of demands on metabolisable energy sources, ranking only behind the basal metabolic demands of continuing vital organ function. It is only after these two demands have been met that energy substrate can be used for growth. Glass and his colleagues [9] have clearly demonstrated the operation of this hierarchy in showing that premature infants reared in cooler incubators grew less well than controls reared at a warmer temperature, because extra energy substrate was used to defend the body temperature under the cooler conditions. It was also shown that a compensating increase in energy intake in the cool environment

restored the control rate of growth, by supplying extra energy substrate sufficient to satisfy the demands of both defence of body temperature and of new tissue deposition.

The level of heat production is also directly dependent on the level of energy intake. Serial studies in our laboratory [54] linking energy intake with metabolic heat production measured by indirect calorimetry at thermoneutrality clearly define the dependence of metabolic heat production on energy intake foreshadowed by Bhakoo and Scopes [10]. From Figure VI-2 it can clearly be seen that metabolic heat production parallels energy intake as well as rate of growth in relation to age.

There is a sharp increase in the first two weeks of life followed by a levelling off after three weeks. But for a steady energy intake of 140 kcal/kg.d received at 12, 35 or 52 days, the weight gain is constant at 17 g/kg.d and the metabolic rate is stable between 61 and 65 kcal/kg.d showing that age has no direct effect on metabolic state.

Thus, in the first days of life, when energy intake is low, metabolic heat production also tends to be low and the infant is more dependent on the neuroendocrine activation of brown fat thermogenesis in the event of cold stress. Similarly, the strict maintenance of thermoneutral conditions, especially for low birth weight infants, can be expected to conserve body heat and place least demands for body temperature maintenance on the low rate of metabolic heat production prevalent at this time.

HEAT LOSSES

On the negative side of the heat balance (Equation 1) are the body heat losses.

An overall controlled heat loss is a fundamental characteristic of all homeotherms and represents the essential provision for the dissipation of metabolic heat. At raised environmental temperature or lowered body temperature (for example, during rewarming from hypothermia), the usual direction of heat flow from the body core to the exterior is reversed and heat storage rather than heat loss takes place with a concomitant rise in core temperature. Such a reversal in the usual direction of heat flow must be temporary and reversible or death will ensue from overheating.

The physical and physiological factors governing neonatal heat loss have been well reviewed [8]. Thermal exchange with the environment is determined by the balance between metabolic heat production, and heat losses mediated by the following factors: tissue conductance; the internal temperature gradient (ITG, core temperature—mean skin temperature) environmental insulation; and the external

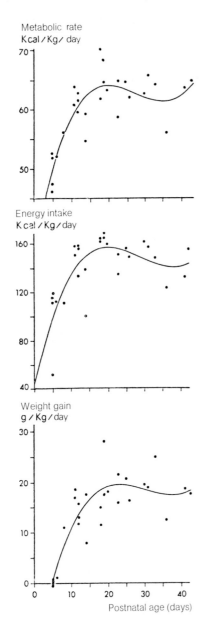

FIG. VI-2. — *Polynomial regression analysis showing in 28 studies the similar pattern of lines of best fit between metabolic rate (kcal/kg/day), energy intake (kcal/kg/day) and weight gain (g/kg/day) with increasing postnatal age (A).* MR = 0.00165, A³ − 0.138A² + 3.56A + 35.4; r = 0.85, p > 0.001; EI = 0.00591A³ − 0.516A² + 13.61A + 44.6; r = 0.74, p < 0.001; WtG = 0.00138A³ − 0.126A² + 3.65A − 14.5; r = 0.86, p < 0.001. Reproduced with permission form CHESSEX P. et al., *J. Peds.*, 99, 761, 1981.

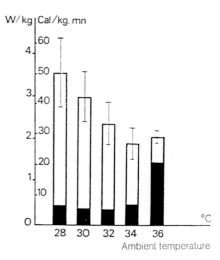

FIG. VI-3. — *Total heat loss (± SEM) expressed in W/kg and kcal/kg/min at various ambient temperatures (28°-36° C).* Evaporative heat loss is in black, dry heat loss in white. Derived from a study of 69 normal infants of 37-42 weeks gestation who were 8-24 hours old. Reproduced with permission from RYSER G. & JÉQUIER E., *Eur. J. Clin. Invest.*, 2, 176, 1972.

temperature gradient (ETG, mean skin temperature—operative environmental temperature). These heat losses have been quantified by direct calorimetry by Day [11], Ryser and Jéquier [4] and Hey and associates [12-14].

Evaporative, dry and total heat losses of normal newborns averaging 15 hours of age and 3.2 kg in weight at ambient T° C of 28°-36° are shown in Figure VI-3. Total heat loss varies from 30 to 50 cal/kg.min.

Term healthy infants attain thermal equilibrium at an environmental temperature of 32° C (Fig. VI-4). Heat transfer above and below this temperature is graphically shown as the interval between metabolic heat production (M) and heat loss ($\dot{Q}$) in Figure VI-4. Below an ambient temperature of 32° C there is overall heat debt, while above 32° C there tends to be a reversal to heat gain; however, over the hour depicted in the study [4], heat transfer comes into equilibrium, due to physiologic homeostatic adjustments increasing heat loss and diminishing metabolism.

The influence of environmentally imposed changes in the ETG on wet and dry heat loss can be seen in Figure VI-5. There is a direct linear increase in dry heat loss by approximately 10-fold as ETG increases from 0.8° C to 6.2° C, and as ambient temperature reduces from 36° C to 28° C [4].

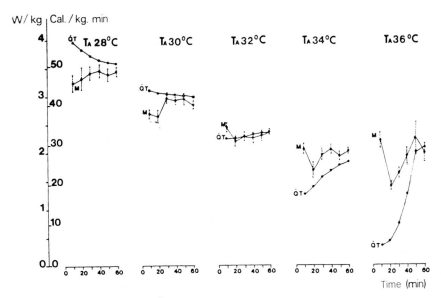

FIG. VI-4. — *Evolution of the total heat loss ($\dot{Q}T$), the metabolic rate (M), and the heat storage (interval between $\dot{Q}T$ and M) measured every 10 minutes during 1 hour at different T_A of 28° C-36° C. The metabolic rate is minimal at a T_A of 34° and 36° C, but the heat storage is positive. At a T_A of 32° C, the mean heat storage during the whole exposure is near zero. Subjects as in figure VI-3. Reproduced with permission from* RYSER G. & JÉQUIER E., *Eur. J. Clin. Invest., 2, 176, 1972.*

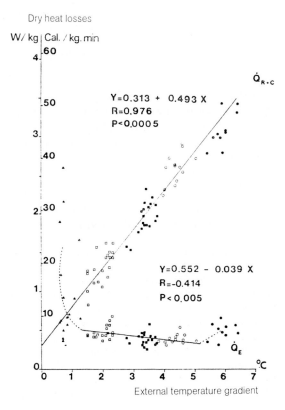

Over a range of ETG from 1.3° C in a warm environment to 5.2° C in a cool environment there is only a minimal reduction in a low level of evaporative loss. However, below an ETG of 1.3° C there is a sharp increase due to sweating and hyperventilatory loss, while above an ETG of 5.3° C the infant increases respiratory evaporative loss due to discomfort, with consequent restlessness and hyperventilation.

In order adequately to dissipate metabolic heat, a minimal external temperature gradient is necessary which depends on body size [12-15]. At from 1.0 kg to 2.5 kg body weights, ETG's ranging from 1.5° to 3° to 4° C are necessary (Fig. VI-5). Suitable

FIG. VI-5. — *Relationship between dry heat loss ($\dot{Q}_R + C$, upper regression line) and the external temperature gradient (ETG), and relationship between evaporative heat loss $\dot{Q}_E$, lower regression line) and ETG at various TA:* •, 28° C; ○, 30° C; ■, 32° C; □, 34° C; ▲, 36° C ($\dot{Q}_E + C$); △, 36° C ($\dot{Q}_E$). *The increase in $\dot{Q}_E$ by sweating at a TA of 36° C (△) is shown by the dotted line; note the increase in $\dot{Q}_E$ (due to higher respiratory heat loss and restlessness) at a TA of 28° C. Derived from a study of 69 normal infants of 37-42 weeks gestation who were 8-24 hours old. Reproduced with permission from* RYSER G. & JÉQUIER E., *Eur. J. Clin. Invest., 2, 176, 1972.*

TABLE I. — Operative environmental temperatures

The mean temperature needed to provide thermal neutrality for a healthy baby nursed naked in draught-free surroundings of uniform temperature and moderate humidity after birth.

To estimate operative temperature in a single-walled incubator subtract 1° C from incubator air temperature for every 7° C by which this temperature exceeds room temperature.

Body weight (kg)	35° C	34° C	33° C	32° C
1.0	For 10 days	After 10 days	After 3 weeks	After 5 weeks
1.5	—	For 10 days	After 10 days	After 4 weeks
2.0	—	For 2 days	After 2 days	After 3 weeks
> 2.5	—	—	For 2 days	After 2 days

operative environmental temperatures to ensure these ETG's are shown in Table I.

Modulation of heat losses with variation of operative environmental temperature and ETG is accomplished by changes in tissue insulation brought about by alterations in cutaneous blood flow and hence thermal conductance. These relationships can be seen in Table II which shows reductions in blood flow and cutaneous conductance at low ambient temperatures and marked increases in a warm environment, but constant values at a T_A of, or just below 32° C in normal term infants.

TABLE II. — Changes in cutaneous thermal conductance and in blood flow from skin at different ambient temperatures (T_A).

Exposure time was 30-60 minutes. Values are means ± SEM. Negative values indicate a decrease during this period; positive values indicate an increase. Subjects were 69 normal infants of 37-42 weeks gestation who were 8-24 hours old.

T_A (°C)	Cutaneous conductance (cal/sec/m²/°C)	Skin blood flow (ml/m²/min)
28	−0.29 ± 0.12	− 18.95 ± 7.84
30	−0.09 ± 0,07	− 5.88 ± 4.57
32	+0.25 ± 0.09	+ 16.34 ± 5.88
34	+0.48 ± 0.13	+ 31.37 ± 8.49
36	+3.12 ± 0.65	+203.95 ± 42.49

Reproduced with permission from Ryser G. and Jéquier E., *Eur. J. Clin. Invest.*, 2, 176, 1972.

Figure VI-6 shows the relationship between cutaneous thermal conductance, ITG, and T_A at or near a steady thermal state. At a T_A of 30° C cuta-

neous conductance reaches a minimum of 0.0041 kcal/sec/m²/°C. This represents the thermal conductivity of the subcutaneous tissue since the blood flow becomes negligible at 30° C. As the T_A rises and the ITG narrows to about 1.8° C there is a progressive increase in conductance (and cutaneous blood flow) to maximal values of 0.015-0.019 kcal/sec/m²/°C as the ITG reduces to about 0.6° C at a T_A of 36° C. This represents a fourfold increase in tissue conductance, corresponding to a skin blood flow of greater than 200 ml/m²/min, or about 4 % of the resting neonatal left ventricular output (see Table II). Judging from measurements of total limb (calf) blood flow under hyperthermic conditions (20 ml/100 g tissue/min at 40° C versus 9.6 ml/100 g tissue/min at 36° C) [16], this figure is not maximal at a T_A of 36° C.

Conductance (and skin blood flow) is at a low value of approximately 0.005 kcal/sec/m²/°C at a $T\overline{sk}$ of 33.5° C-36° C. Above a T_A 36.3° C, a $T\overline{sk}$ of 36.3° C or an ITG of 1° C, there is a progressive vasodilatation and an increase in blood flow and tissue conductance (Fig. VI-6).

Modulation of heat loss in response to cooling

Control of body temperature under conditions of cold stress is the result of a complex interaction of neural, endocrine, and metabolic factors. In the newborn, physiologic and anatomic maturational factors are also involved, manifested by the ability to regulate and redistribute blood flow and increase oxygen uptake and metabolic heat production. The efficiency of these adjustments is related to gestational age at birth, but more importantly to postnatal age. Figure VI-7 shows the ability of newborn kittens to defend body temperature and

Conductance = cal/sec/m²/°C

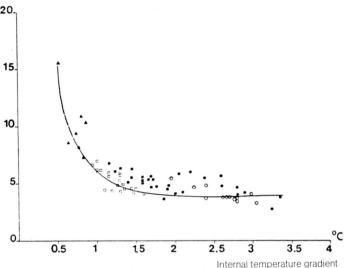

Internal temperature gradient

FIG. VI-6. — *Relationship between total cutaneous thermal conductance and the internal temperature gradient (ITG) at or near a thermal steady state.* Conductance increases sharply when ITG reaches 1.0° C. The minimal conductance of 4 cal/sec/m² corresponds to the thermal conductivity of the subcutaneous tissues. Newborns at various T_A: ●, 28° C; ○, 30° C; ■, 32° C; □, 34° C; △, 36° C. Reproduced with permission from RYSER G. & JÉQUIER E., *Eur. J. Clin. Invest.*, 2, 176, 1972.

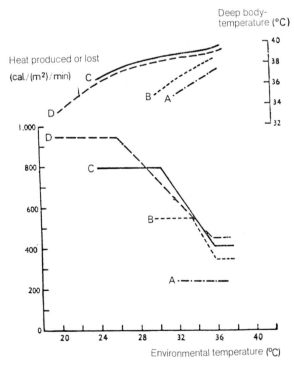

increase thermogenesis progressively from the first to the fifth day of postnatal life [17]. A similarly increased capacity to thermoregulate with age is evidenced by the progressive decrease in the required operative environmental temperature in human infants [12]. Previous exposure to a cold stress has a facilitative effect on thermogenesis as manifested by an increased resistance to the fall in body temperature when exposed to a later episode of cold stress [9].

The presence of normal thyroid function would appear to be a prerequisite for satisfactory defense against cold stress [18, 19].

There are a number of stages that can be identified in the progressive recruitment of heat-conserving mechanisms under cold stress. First an attempt is

FIG. VI-7. — *Heat production and body temperature related to environmental temperature in a single newborn kitten at various ages.*

A: 3 hours after birth.
B: 2 days of age.
C: 4 days of age.
D: 7 days of age.
Reproduced with permission from HILL J. R., *Br. Med. Bull.*, 17, 164, 1961.

made to diminish surface area for heat loss by huddling in the nest in the case of animals, or by adoption of a flexed posture. The newborn and particularly the premature infant is handicapped in this respect as he lacks the muscle mass and power to change posture effectively and habitually lies in an extended position.

The next stage is a reduction in cutaneous blood flow as a result of peripheral vasoconstriction, thereby decreasing thermal conductance. Cutaneous thermal conductance decreases to a minimum of about 4.11 ± 0.17 cal/sec/m²/°C at an ambient temperature of 30° C. The vasoconstriction responsible is mediated by a sympathetic neural reflex triggered by stimulation of skin thermoreceptors when skin temperature falls. By these means the tissue insulation is increased, reducing conductive and convective losses. Concomitantly, as a result of thermoreceptor stimulation, there is an increase in activity in the sympathetic nervous system and an outpouring of catecholamines, chiefly noradrenaline, by the adrenal glands. Noradrenaline stimulates adenylcyclase in the brown fat to increase CAMP, triggering lipolytic cycles that, providing both oxygen and glucose are available, are strongly thermogenic. There is vasodilatation and an increase in blood flow in brown fat up to 1/4 of the total cardiac output [55]. Simultaneously, ventilation is stimulated and oxygen uptake increases to cover the oxidative needs of glycolysis and lipolysis. Relatively moderate cold stress (for example, exposure to a 25° C-28° C environment) will provoke an increase in oxygen uptake and metabolism up to threefold, thereby tripling heat production. The simultaneous reduction in heat loss and the increased thermogenesis conserves deep body temperature in a heat-losing environment.

If the degree and duration of cold stress exceed the compensating ability of the infant, there is progressive decompensation, manifested by a fall in core temperature, respiratory failure, recurrent apnoea, heart failure, exhaustion of carbohydrate and lipid metabolic substrates, inefficient anaerobic metabolism with lactic acidosis, and finally death.

The onset of such decompensation has widespread adverse effects of a more subtle nature. These include an increased susceptibility to infection, particularly pneumonia, and to bleeding, particularly pulmonary and intracranial.

The mortality of sick and low birth weight infants is greatly increased by cold stress [20-25]. Perlstein et al. [26] have shown that a close control of the thermal environment by computer programming significantly reduces the mortality rate in infants suffering from the respiratory distress syndrome.

Enhancement of heat-losing mechanisms in a hot environment

The physiologic mechanisms responsible for increasing heat losses in a warm environment again are the result of a complex interaction of the central nervous system and hormonal factors. The infant's extended posture maximizes surface area for heat loss. As the ETG diminishes and the ITG approaches 1° C with a rise in core temperature toward 37.3° C, there is a marked increase in cutaneous blood flow up to about 200 ml/m²/min, thereby increasing cutaneous thermal conductance [4, 27]. Sweating begins first on the forehead about 35-40 minutes after exposure to an ambient temperature of 37° C, reaching maximal values of evaporative loss at about four times higher than basal 35 minutes after the onset of sweating [27]. Infants small for gestational age have a somewhat slower onset of sweating, 55-60 minutes after exposure to the hot environment; however, sweat rate increases more rapidly and the maximal value of five-fold is somewhat higher than that for full term infants [27]. Premature infants have a reaction similar to that of infants small for gestational age with regard to onset, but the maximal rate of sweating is significantly lower than in either of the other two groups.

There are two types of sweat response. More commonly there is a repeated stepwise increase in evaporative heat loss followed by a plateau; less common is a rapid and continuously increasing sweat production. The first area to sweat is the forehead, followed in order by the upper arms, hands, thighs, feet, and finally the abdomen. Using the hypothesis that the set point is the trigger for the onset of sweating, the threshold body temperature for sweating is lowest on the forehead and increases in the order given for each separate area of the body. The set point for sweating varies with postnatal age [27]. The threshold temperature for sweating is significantly lower on the third day than on the first day ($p < 0.05$) but both basal and maximal values of evaporation heat loss are unchanged with age [27]. Some infants have shown a statistically significant increase in the set point with age. In these infants there was a significantly greater weight loss from the first to the third day ($p < 0.05$). The increase in the set point for sweating therefore may be related to a greater weight loss, presumably due to dehydration [27]. The increase in set point has the effect of reducing losses due to sweating, thereby conserving body water stores.

The threshold body temperatures for sweating decrease and the maximal sweat production increases with increasing postnatal age. The functional development and maximal capacity for sweating are also dependent on gestational age [11]. The very small premature infant (less than 30 weeks' gestation) has no or very poorly developed sweat glands [28]. There is also evidence from local pharmacologic stimulation by epinephrine, acetylcholine, nicotine, and pilocarpine that there is a functional maturation of glandular activity with increasing gestational age [29]. Appearance and maturation of sweat glands proceeds from the center to the periphery in the same order as recruitment of sweating, *i. e.*, from the forehead, the upper arm, hand, thigh, foot and abdomen. While in the infant at term the number of sweat glands per square centimeter of skin surface on the thigh (414/cm²) is 6.5 times that of the adult, the mean peak sweat rate on pharmacologic stimulation is only 1/3 that of the adult at 2.4 nl/gland/min [28]. Despite the apparent lack of functional sweat glands in the premature, large water losses occur through the skin (presumably by transudative evaporation), particularly under conditions of increased radiant heat input (e. g., under bilirubin lights or radiant heaters) [30, 31]. As much as 120 ml/kg.d may be lost by prematures in this way (equivalent to 70 kcal/kg.d) [30]. In contrast, the maximal water loss of the term infant has been calculated as 70 nl/cm²/min by sweating [31]. If this rate could be sustained over 24 hours it would correspond to 57 ml/kg.d or 33 kcal/kg.d. This is a substantially lower rate of evaporative heat loss than maximally achieved by the premature and in any case represents a theoretical maximum that is probably not sustained in practice.

Failure of adequate heat loss in warm conditions

If heat gain exceeds heat loss in a warm environment the core temperature rises; there is a reduction in the ITG or even a reversal, so that the mean skin temperature is higher than the core temperature. The infant becomes restless, cardiac output increases, and the infant hyperventilates. If the heat stress continues the infant will develop hyperpyrexia, sweat, become dehydrated, and eventually die from cardiorespiratory failure in "heat stroke".

SUMMARY OF ADJUSTMENTS TO HEAT AND COLD STRESSES

The range of thermal conditions from cold to heat stress and their physiologic consequences are summarized in Figure VI-8 [32].

INFLUENCE OF PREMATURITY AND BODY SIZE ON THERMOREGULATORY ADJUSTMENTS: BODY SURFACE AREA, BODY WEIGHT AND BODY CONTOUR

The surface area/body weight ratio of a 2 kg infant at 0.078 m²/kg is three times the 0.025 m²/kg of a 75 kg adult man. It is proportionately higher for the very low birth weight infant (< 1,500 g) than for the term infant.

Heat is lost from the body surface (including the respiratory tract) by radiation (60-70 %), convection and evaporation (15-25 %) and conduction (< 3 %) at 50 % relative humidity in an incubator (single walled) at the thermoneutral temperature. The effective surface area is a major component controlling the extent of these losses (Fig. VI-8) [15]. The smaller the infant the larger is the surface area for heat exchange in relation to its size.

Convective heat exchange is also enhanced by the shorter radius of curvature of the smaller infant's body surfaces.

Adoption of a flexed position under conditions of cold stress is a familiar strategy to limit heat loss which can be observed in newborns. By this means exposed surface area is limited to conserve body heat.

BODY COMPOSITION

Energy stores:

Table III shows the relative body composition of infants of 1, 2 and 3.5 kg body weight respectively. The Table shows the changes in body content of protein, fat and carbohydrate in the approximately 7 weeks necessary for a 1 kg infant to grow to 2 kg.

It can be appreciated that the energy substrate reserves of fat and carbohydrate are extremely curtailed for the very low birth weight infant. The white fat organ of the 1 kg 28 week premature

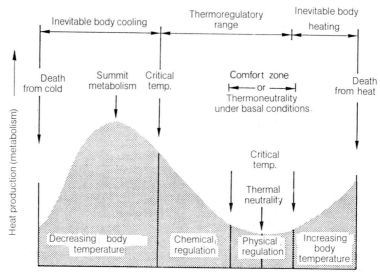

FIG. VI-8. — *Homeothermic model.*

Reproduced with permission from Sinclair J. C., in Goodwin et al. (eds): *Perinatal Medicine*, Williams & Wilkins, Baltimore, 1976. (After Brody S., 1945).

TABLE III. — Body composition
of infants weighing 1, 2 and 3.5 kg.

	Infant		
	1 kg	2 kg	3,5 kg
Water	860	1,620	2,400
Fat	10	100	560
Protein	85	230	390
CH$_2$O	4.5	9	34
Calories	460	1,900	6,950
Non protein calories . .	110	970	5,350

Reproduced with permission from Sinclair J. C. et al., *Ped. Clin. N. Amer.*, 17, 863-893, 1970. From data of Widdowson E. M. and Spray C. M., *Arch. Dis. Child.*, 26, 205-214, 1951.

is practically nonexistent, the 10 g of total body fat content being confined to the brown fat depots. Nevertheless, Heim and others [33] have clearly demonstrated an ability to activate thermogenesis in brown fat in response to cold stress in such infants, though lack of insulating subcutaneous white fat is clearly conducive to a more rapid fall in body temperature. Even when present, white adipose tissue yields energy substrate preferentially to a starvation stimulus rather than to cold stress.

Carbohydrate stores are similarly minimal in the 1 kg infant, only about 1/3 being immediately available as liver glycogen. Hence, infants in this weight category develop hypoglycaemia as an immediate response to cold stress rather than the increasing blood sugar levels characteristic of more mature and larger infants [33]. In both cases, however, one can expect rapid depletion leading to hypoglycaemia with continued cold stress.

Thus the very low birth weight infant is hampered in responding to cold by a deficiency of both carbohydrate and lipid energy substrate as well as by the frequently low calorie intake associated with feeding difficulty in this group. Malfunctional handicaps relating to poorly developed neuroendocrine control of thermoregulation compound the problem of developing an adequate thermogenic response to cold stress in the very low birth weight infant.

ORGAN PROPORTIONS AND CONTRIBUTION OF THE BRAIN TO HEAT PRODUCTION AND HEAT LOSS IN THE VERY LOW BIRTH WEIGHT INFANT

Gruenwald [35] has assessed the relative weights of viscera in low birth weight infants of appropriate weight for gestational age (AGA) compared with infants small for gestational age (SGA). He has

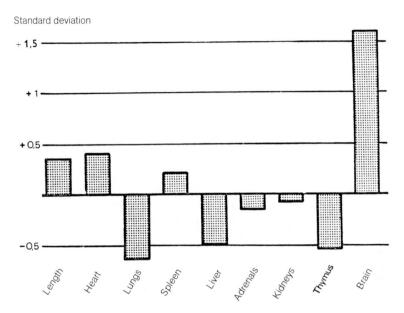

Fig. VI-9. — *Chronic fetal distress and placental insufficiency.* Deviation of organ weights and body length of infants with a score of − 2 from values for normal (score 0) infants of similar birthweight, expressed as fractions of the respective standard deviations. Each block is the mean of 6 values for 250 gram weight groups from 1,250 to 2,500 grams. Reproduced with permission from GRUENWALD P., *Biol. Neonat.*, 5, 215, 1963, S. Karger A. G, Basel.

demonstrated that the major difference resides in the larger brain and somewhat smaller liver of the SGA compared with the AGA infant of similar weight (Fig. VI-9). Cooke et al. [34] have demonstrated that the brain weighs approximately 20 g/kg more in the SGA compared with the AGA. Data obtained in our own laboratory as well as elsewhere [36, 38] suggests that brain heat production accounts for at least 55 % of total metabolic heat production in the newborn. Dissipation of heat from the uninsulated skull of the newborn will take place very readily under conditions of cool temperature and high surface air velocity which may obtain under modern conditions of oxygen administration in head hoods, where high air/oxygen mix flows are often used with inadequate heating and possibly with poor humidification, promoting evaporative and convective heat loss. The use of a simple head covering will go far to prevent this source of heat loss [37].

TISSUE INSULATION
AND BLOOD FLOW

Increase in tissue insulation due to enhanced thickness of subcutaneous fat with maturity and postnatal growth can be expected to contribute to thermal conservation, though precise data on tissue heat conductance as a function of skin fold thickness are not available. For term infants, skin conductance is 5 cal/sec/m²/°C in the thermoneutral temperature zone and mean skinfold thickness is approximately 4 mm [39]. This rate of loss would amount to approximately 60 cal/min (86.4 kcal/d) for such an infant. As ambient temperature rises, so does mean skin temperature, skin blood flow and skin heat conductance (Fig. VI-10) by more than threefold.

Under cooler ambient conditions than thermoneutral, e. g. (< 30° C) skin blood flow is at minimal levels and skin conductance falls minimally below the thermoneutral level, providing little additional protection against cold stress.

EXTRINSIC FACTORS
IN NEWBORN THERMOREGULATION

Heat exchange with the environment is mediated by radiation, convection, conduction and evaporation (The reader should consult alternative texts for the physical laws which govern the transfer

Conductance cal/sec/m²/°C

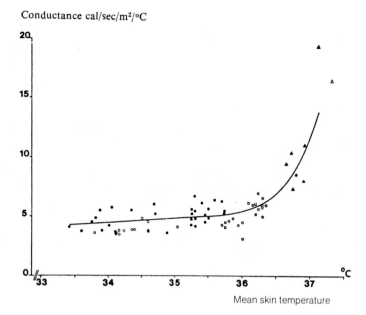

Mean skin temperature

FIG. VI-10. — *Relationship between total cutaneous thermal conductance and mean skin temperature at or near a thermal steady state.* Conductance increases sharply when the mean skin temperature reaches 36.3° C. Newborns at various T_A: ●, 28° C; ○, 30° C; ■, 32° C; □, 34° C; Δ, 36° C. Subjects as in Figure VI-3. Reproduced with permission from RYSER G. & JÉQUIER E., *Eur. J. Clin. Invest.*, 2, 176, 1972.

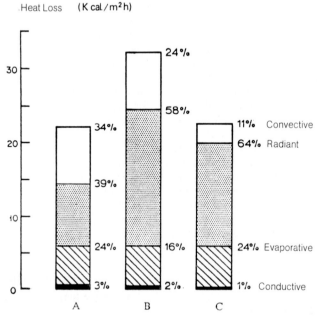

FIG. VI-11. — *Heat loss from a naked 4-day-old baby weighing 1.5 kg with a rectal temperature of 37° C in draught-free surroundings of moderate humidity (50 % relative humidity).* A. Heat loss by conduction, convection, radiation and evaporation in a thermoneutral environment of uniform temperature (34° C). B. Heat loss within a single-walled commercial incubator having the same air temperature (34° C) when room temperature is low. C. Heat loss in a similar incubator after increasing air temperature 2° C. Reproduced with permission from HEY E. N. in AUSTIN C. R. (ed.), *The Mammalian Fetus in vitro.* London, Chapman & Hall, 1976.

of energy by these processes) [8]. The general equation which describes heat transfer is:

Equation 3.

$$\dot{Q} = K(\Delta t)$$

where $\dot{Q}$ = energy transfer/unit time,

$\quad\quad$ K = a radiative, convective, conductive or evaporative constant,

$\quad\quad$ Δt = temperature gradient for energy transfer.

The nature of the constants differ according to the physical mode of heat transfer, but will have components relating to surface area, geometry, conductance and specific heat appropriate to the mode of energy transfer.

Hey [15] has quantitated losses by these means under standardised conditions (Fig. VI-11).

The neutral thermal environment is defined by the International Union of Physiological Societies as [6, 56]. "The range of ambient temperature within which metabolic rate is at a minimum and within which temperature regulation is achieved by non-evaporative physical processes alone, the individual being in thermal equilibrium with the environment."

The thermoneutral zone is bounded by an upper and a lower critical temperature. The upper critical temperature is the ambient temperature above which thermoregulatory evaporative heat loss is recruited. The lower critical temperature is the ambient temperature below which the rate of metabolic heat production of a resting thermoregulating individual increases to maintain thermal balance. Related to the neutral thermal environment, but somewhat wider, is the zone of thermal comfort. Some animals, given a choice, will seek preferentially an environmental temperature somewhat lower than neutral. A zone of minimal heat production is also defined as the range of environmental temperature over which heat production is kept at a minimum by a combination of vasodilatation, postural change and increased evaporative heat loss [13]. It is wider than the thermoneutral zone. Under clinical conditions it would be advantageous to have a single temperature term to describe the net effect of the environment on energy exchange that would take account of radiant, convective, and conductive losses imposed by environmental conditions, perhaps modified by the size, posture and radius of curvature of the infant. This definition is obviously impossible to meet clinically, but an operative temperature (T_0) for incubators [12] taking account of both convective and radiant losses (conductive losses are usually less than 3 %) is defined as follows:

Equation 4.

$$T_0 = \frac{K_{rad}T_w + K_{conv}T_A}{K_{rad} + K_{conv}}$$

where T_0 $\quad$ = operative temperature,

$\quad\quad$ K_{rad} $\;$ = radiant constant,

$\quad\quad$ K_{conv} = convective constant,

$\quad\quad$ T_w $\quad$ = internal wall temperature,

$\quad\quad$ T_A $\quad$ = ambient air temperature.

T_0 is thus a weighted mean of the air and wall temperatures in proportion (usually 6 : 4) to the relative magnitudes of radiant and convective heat losses [8]. The T_0 may be estimated for single-walled warm-air incubators by subtracting 1° C from the incubator air temperature (T_A) for every 7° C by which this temperature exceeds the room air temperature (T_{RA}):

Equation 5.

$$T_0 = T_A - \frac{(T_A - T_{RA})}{7}$$

The T_0 required for thermoneutrality is also an inverse function of both body weight and postnatal age and can be calculated by the use of the above relationship (Equation 5) and Table I which takes account of weight and age [13].

The newborn infant is extremely sensitive to fluctuations of body temperature and it has been found that when deep body temperature is below 36° C or above 37.8° C the mortality rate increases [11]. This zone (36°-37.8° C) is therefore described as the *optimal body temperature* for survival and will usually be attained under approximately thermoneutral conditions [13].

Heat flow from the core to the skin surface will depend on the difference between the core temperature and the mean skin temperature. The mean skin temperature in infants can be computed with the use of the following weighting factors [41]:

Forehead. .	23 %		Thigh. . .	23 %
Upper arm .	11 %		Hand . . .	5 %
Abdomen. .	33 %		Foot . . .	5 %

These factors are applied to the skin temperature at each site in order to compute a mean skin temperature.

Heat loss occurs by evaporation though the mucous membranes of the respiratory tract to the extent of 5-10 % of total heat loss at 50 % relative humidity between 28-36° C ambient temperature; evaporation into the moving air front through the skin accounts for 15-25 % of total heat losses according to environmental conditions of temperature, speed of air flow and relative humidity in normal term infants [45]. For each gram of water evaporated 0.58 kcal is lost. Increasing relative humidity to 100 % effectively prevents evaporative loss and the use of high relative humidity in incubators for very low birth weight infants is an effective heat conserving strategy.

Internal factors controlling evaporative loss relate to the control of sweating as well as to increased water permeability of newborn skin, particularly the premature's. Below a certain ambient temperature, designated the "set point" for sweating, evaporation through the skin is "insensible". However, insensible loss is particularly important in premature infants who have little or no development of the sweat glands but whose skin layers are extremely thin and permeable [40, 42]. Up to 120 ml of water/kg.d can be lost through the skin, which is equivalent to a loss of approximately 70 kcal/kg.d, a figure in excess of half the usually recommended intake of 120 kcal/kg.d for the premature infant [30].

In more mature infants with developed sweat glands, sweating occurs when the set point for sweating is exceeded. Evaporative heat loss is recruited at an ambient temperature of 34° C by the activation of a small number of sweat glands on the forehead. In term infants overt sweating begins at a T_A of 36° C and usually coincides with an esophageal or core temperature of 37.5° C; even more precisely, sweating commences when the ITG reaches 0.68° C. In prematures and certain term infants with cerebral dysfunction, sweating and cutaneous vasodilation does not appear even at core temperatures of 37.5° C, indicating defective control mechanisms due to a compromised central control, compounded in the case of prematures by defective effector units (deficient sweat glands) [28].

Maturational factors are influential in the control of evaporative heat loss: e. g., prematures have increased skin permeability to insensible loss, their sweat glands develop only with advancing postnatal age, the central regulatory mechanisms improve with maturation.

In a heat-gaining environment thermally induced hyperpnea (panting) takes place. Thermal hyperpnea constitutes an important means by which heat losses can be increased in certain animals (e. g., the dog), but it is much less important for humans; it is relatively more important for infants than adults, however, because of their disproportionately higher minute volumes of respiration. At a T_A of 36° C and a relative humidity of 50 % there is an enhanced respiratory water loss as a consequence of an increased minute ventilation [45]. The respiratory rate is slightly increased but the main augmentation is in the tidal volume.

At a constant relative humidity of 50 % the total respiratory heat loss varies from 10.4 % of the total metabolic heat production to 6.81 % at a T_A of 28° C to 36° C. Increases in minute volume up to threefold, observed under various pathologic conditions in the newborn, augment these losses proportionately. Increasing the relative humidity of the air breathed reduces the evaporative component of the respiratory heat loss to negligible proportions. On the other hand, hyperventilation in low relative humidity, particularly in the cold, substantially augments evaporative water loss from the respiratory tract to over 40 % of the total evaporative heat loss, probably corresponding to more than 0.22 W/kg (0.00315 kcal/kg/min) [45].

IMPLICATIONS
FOR THE THERMAL ENVIRONMENT
OF NEWBORNS
UNDER CLINICAL CONDITIONS

For the healthy term infant a satisfactory thermal environment approximating the thermoneutral and thus ensuring thermal equilibrium can be attained by light clothing and cotton blankets at an ambient temperature of 18° C-22° C with a relative humidity of 40-60 %.

More controversial are the requirements for the sick, the premature, or the infant small for gestational age. Many such infants, especially those over 1,800 g in weight, can be satisfactorily nursed clad and in bassinets, though it would be advisable to maintain the environmental temperature at somewhat higher levels of 20° C-25° C and the relative humidity at approximately 50 %.

Infant less than 1,800 g in birth weight, particularly if they are ill, require close observation of their activity, colour, posture, behaviour, and response to therapy. Under these circumstances it may be desirable to nurse them naked in transparent walled incubators within a controlled microclimate. Unfortunately, the engineering requirements to achieve the total environment that will minimise heat loss while providing for visual and electronic monitoring, satisfactory gas exchange, and accessibility for nursing and medical procedures (including radiographic) are difficult to fulfill. Most modern incubators use either a single-walled transparent enclosure heated by warmed recirculating air or consist of open bassinettes heated solely by radiation.

Warm air incubators cause a variable and to some extent unpredictable but certainly elevated radiant heat loss for the infant since the internal surface of the single wall takes up a relatively cool temperature intermediate between the air temperature within the incubator and that in the room. Such radiant heat loss can be compensated for by increasing the air temperature, thereby diminishing convective losses (Fig. VI-11). However, relative humidity within the incubator needs to be controlled at a relatively high level (50-80 %) to minimize evaporative heat loss. This requirement presents a problem in ensuring an environment free of bacterial pathogens, since evaporating water reservoirs used for this purpose may rapidly become colonised with potentially pathogenic hydrophilic organisms (e. g., Klebsiella, Pseudomonas) within hours. Consequently, it is preferable to supply warmed, humidified, filtered air or an air/oxygen mixture from an external sterile source while monitoring both incubator air temperature and relative humidity. There are often variable environmental conditions in the room containing the incubators—for example, sunlight or shade, or proximity to cold windows or hot radiators in winter. Internal transparent plastic heat shields obviate abnormally high radiant heat loss to incubator walls but present access problems.

An alternative has been the introduction of infant servocontrolled incubators whose air temperatures are controlled by comparing the infant's own temperature (usually anterior abdominal skin) with an arbitrary "set point" designated as consistent with thermoneutrality (usually 35° C-36° C) depending on size. An error signal then activates or cuts the heating cycle. Some practical objections to the servocontrol principle can be raised. There are technical difficulties in the continuous measurement of skin temperature. Care must be taken to ensure that the thermistor is protected from direct radiant heat by suitable shielding, and that it is attached to exposed skin and not protected by contact with the mattress. In the presence of fever, the servoloop will promote cooling which may be inappropriate. It can also be questioned whether it is appropriate to use a single skin temperature location to control the thermal cycle as the skin surface represents a mosaic of different temperatures. Nevertheless, the reports by Buetow et al. [24] and Day et al. [22] of controlled trials of servocontrolled incubator heating systems, and the study by Perlstein et al. [26] of a computer-controlled thermal environment for infants with respiratory distress syndrome suggest that automatic feedback (servocontrol) of environmental heating results in a significantly lower mortality.

Are there advantages of proportional control versus on/off control of incubator temperature? Evidence on this point is scanty. Observations [8] in our unit suggest that proportional servocontrol in convectively heated incubators is clearly superior to on/off servocontrol insofar as it induces narrower fluctuations in incubator temperature and consequently a steadier and lower metabolic rate, as judged by concomitant changes in oxygen uptake (Fig. IV-12) [8]. However, a formal controlled trial of proportional versus on/off servocontrol in relation to outcome has not yet been performed.

Are radiant heaters as effective as convectively warmed incubators or is a combination of the two desirable? Again, there has been no controlled trial to answer these questions in terms of the mortality and/or morbidity. Radiant heat alone has been used to minimize heat loss from a naked infant in an open bassinette. While minimal rates of oxygen uptake (and metabolism) can be achieved under certain ambient air temperature conditions, it is highly questionable whether radiant heating is physiologically desirable in the long term. It is undoubtedly useful for short-term exposure, for example during resuscitation or minor operative procedures, but it is likely that metabolism is inhibited by activation of superficial thermoceptors [48] (particularly on the face, in the distribution of the fifth cranial nerve [47]) even though core temperature may be low and there is active peripheral vasoconstriction in a relatively cool air environment [49]. Furthermore, unusually high evaporative water losses are a consequence of radiant heating [43, 44]. Despite the high radiant input, overall this thermal environment often promotes heat loss, particularly in infants weighing less than 1,500 g. A radiant heat input high enough to prevent heat loss presents a danger of skin burn. Overheating and hyperthermia can also result from malfunction, displacement of the skin thermistor, radiofrequency interference [50], or manual operation without monitoring skin and body temperature.

It is thus likely that for better control of the infant's microclimate a combination of warm air conditioning and infant servocontrolled radiant heat input is to be prefered. Such a unit has been designed and operated successfully [51], but has not been produced commercially. A randomized controlled trial evaluating such a unit against conventional radiant and convectively warmed incubators is desirable.

CONCLUSIONS

The term newborn has attributes of form and function that render the maintenance of homeo-

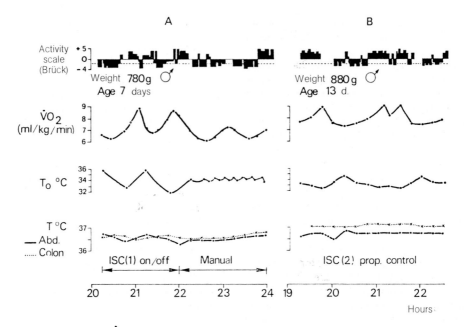

FIG. VI-12. — *Oxygen uptake ($\dot{V}O_2$) as a reflection of metabolic rate in thermal environments determined by on/off servocontrol with a set point of 36.5° C abdominal skin temperature and a manual set point of 34° C operative ambient temperature ($T_0°$ C), and, 6 days later, proportional servocontrol in a convectively heated incubator with an abdominal skin set point of 36.5° C.* Activity scale is that of Brück; the dotted line indicates the boundary between — 2 and — 3 on the scale. Note the wide fluctuations in T_0 and the slightly phase-shifted increase in $\dot{V}O_2$ in response to descending T_0 and abdominal skin temperature in the on/off servocontrolled mode (40 % of minimal level). On switching to a manual set point T_0 of 34° C the temperature remains more constant and $\dot{V}O_2$ fluctuation diminishes to 18 % of the minimal level, which is itself lower. One week later the same patient on proportional servocontrol, also with an abdominal skin set point of 36.5° C, shows similar but less marked fluctuations (25 % of the minimal level) than on/off servocontrol; note the higher colonic temperature and the steadier abdominal skin temperature.

thermy more fragile than in later life. The physical principles underlying energy exchange with the environment, particularly heat loss, are such that small body mass, relatively increased surface area, and effective radius of curvature promote the exchange of energy with the environment to a greater extent than is the case in later and larger life.

Physiologically the mature infant at birth possesses the necessary sensory, motor, and integrative mechanisms to modulate heat exchange, including heat loss, but only within more restricted limits than in adult life.

The premature infant, appropriately grown for gestational age, has not only the physical disadvantage of small body size and relatively large surface area, but also morphologic (e. g., undeveloped sweat glands), functional (e. g., relatively higher peripheral blood flow) [16], and regulatory (e. g., deficient summit metabolism) characteristics related to immaturity that render maintenance of homeothermy in a thermal environment other than neutral

even more precarious than for the term or undergrown but more mature infant.

The infant who is small for gestational age shares the premature's disadvantage of small body size but has a relatively more mature physiologic modulating system for energy exchange. Relatively lower body water enhances his or her susceptibility to the ill effects of increased thermoregulatory heat losses by sweating in a warm environment, though this is minimized by a higher set point temperature for sweating.

Illness in the newborn, particularly when associated with prematurity or intrauterine growth retardation, still further compounds the problems in maintenance of homeothermy. Thus, central regulatory mechanisms (e. g., upward shift of the set point with fever), energy substrate reserves (depletion from feeding difficulties), cardiorespiratory function, and oxygen uptake (e. g., in respiratory distress syndrome [52], or congenital heart disease [53]) may all be adversely affected, with potentially serious consequences for the defense of body temperature under thermally stressfull conditions. Failure, to avoid such thermal stress by appropriate management of the environment may strongly prejudice survival and predispose to subsequent morbidity.

An appreciation of the physical and physiologic principles underlying the maintenance of the homeothermic state as set out in this chapter should enable the caretaker to understand and manage the thermal environment of the newborn in such a way as to minimize harmful thermal stresses, particularly cold, and aid the infant to make a satisfactory transition from the thermally protected intrauterine environment to the more thermally variable conditions of extrauterine life.

REFERENCES

[1] ADAMSONS (K. Jr.). — The role of thermal factors in fetal and neonatal life. *Ped. Clin. N. Amer.*, 13, 599-619, 1966.

[2] DAHM (L. S.), JAMES (L. S.). — Newborn temperature and calculated heat loss in the delivery room. *Pediatrics*, 49, 504-513, 1972.

[3] REICHMAN (B. L.), CHESSEX (P.), PUTET (G.), VERELLEN (G. J. E.), SMITH (J. M.), HEIM (T.), SWYER (P. R.). — Partition of energy metabolism and energy cost of growth in the very low birthweight infant. *Pediatrics*, 69, 446-451, 1982.

[4] RYSER (G.), JÉQUIER (E.). — Study by direct calorimetry of thermal balance on the first day of life. *Eur. J. Clin. Invest.*, 2, 176-187, 1972.

[5] HARDY (J. D.), SODERSTROM (G. F.). — Heat loss from the nude body and peripheral blood flow at temperatures of 22° to 35° C. *J. Nutr.*, 16, 493-510, 1938.

[6] HARDY (J. C.), GAGGE (A. P.), RAPP (G. M.). — Proposed standard system of symbols for thermal physiology. *J. Appl. Physiol.*, 27, 439-440, 1969.

[7] STOLWIJK (J. A.), HARDY (J. D.). — Partitional calorimetric studies of responses of man to thermal transients. *J. Appl. Physiol.*, 21, 967-977, 1966.

[8] SWYER (P. R.). — Heat loss after birth. In SINCLAIR (J. C.), ed. *Temperature Regulation and Energy Metabolism in the Newborn*, 91-128, 1978.

[9] GLASS (L.), SILVERMAN (W. A.), SINCLAIR (J. C.). — Effect of the thermal environment on cold resistance and growth of small infants after the first week of life. *Pediatrics*, 41, 1033-1046, 1968.

[10] BHAKOO (N. N.), SCOPES (J. W.). — Minimal rates of oxygen consumption in small-for-dates babies during the first week of life. *Arch. Dis. Child.*, 49, 583, 1974.

[11] DAY (R.). — Respiratory metabolism in infancy and childhood. XXVII. Regulation of body temperature of premature infants. *Am. J. Dis. Child.*, 65, 376-398, 1943.

[12] HEY (E.N.), MOUNT (L. E.). — Heat loss from babies in incubators. *Arch. Dis. Child.*, 42, 75-84, 1967.

[13] HEY (E.). — Thermal neutrality. *Br. Med. Bull.*, 31, 69-74, 1975.

[14] HEY (E. N.), O'CONNELL (B.). — Oxygen consumption and heat balance in the cot-nursed baby. *Arch. Dis. Child.*, 45, 335-343, 1970.

[15] HEY (E.). — Physiological principles involved in the care of the preterm human infant. In AUSTIN (C. R.), ed. *The Mammalian Fetus* in vitro. London, Chapman and Hall, 251, 1976.

[16] KIDD (L.), LEVISON (H.), GEMMEL (P.) et coll. — Limb blood flow in the normal and sick newborn. *Am. J. Dis. Child.*, 112, 402-407, 1966.

[17] HILL (J. R.). — Reaction of the newborn animal to environmental temperature. *Br. Med. Bull.*, 17, 164-167, 1961.

[18] SACK (J.), BEAUDRY (M.), DE LAMATER (P. V.) et coll. — Umbilical cord cutting triggers hypertriiodothyronemia and nonshivering thermogenesis in the newborn lamb. *Ped. Res.*, 10, 169-175, 1976.

[19] FISHER (D. A.), ODDIE (T. H.), MAKOSKI (E.). — The influence of environmental temperature on thyroid, adrenal, and water metabolism in the newborn human infant. *Pediatrics*, 37, 583-591, 1966.

[20] BUDIN (P. C.). — The nursling. *The feeding and hygiene of premature and full term infants* (MALONEY (W. J.), trans.). London, Caxton, 1907.

[21] CHANCE (G. W.), O'BRIEN (M. J.), SWYER (P. R.). — Transportation of sick neonates: an unsatisfactory aspect of medical care. *Can. Med. Assoc. J.*, 109, 847-851, 1973.

[22] DAY (R. L.), CALIGUIRI (L.), KAMENSKI (C.) et coll. — Body temperature and survival of premature infants. *Pediatrics*, 34, 171-181, 1964.

[23] JOLLY (H.), MOLYNEUX (P.), NEWELL (D. J.). — A controlled study of the effect of temperature on premature babies. *J. Pediatr.*, 60, 889-894, 1962.

[24] BUETOW (K. C.), KLEIN (P. H.), KLEIN (S. W.). — Effect of maintenance of « normal » skin temperature on survival of infants of low birth weight. *Pediatrics*, 34, 163-170, 1964.

[25] SILVERMAN (W. A.), FERTIG (J. W.), BERGER (A. P.). — The influence of the thermal environment upon the survival of newly born premature infants. *Pediatrics*, 22, 876-886, 1958.

[26] PERLSTEIN (P. H.), EDWARDS (N. K.), ATHERTON (H. D.) et coll. — Computer-assisted newborn intensive care. *Pediatrics*, 57, 494-501, 1976.

[27] SULYOK (E.), JÉQUIER (E.), PROD'HOM (L. S.). — Thermal balance of the newborn infant in a heat-gaining environment. *Ped. Res.*, 7, 888-900, 1973.

[28] FOSTER (K. G.), HEY (E. N.), KATZ (G.). — The response of the sweat glands of the newborn baby to thermal stimuli and to intradermal acetylcholine. *J. Physiol.*, 203, 13-29, 1969.

[29] GREEN (M.), BEHRENDT (H.). — Drug induced localised sweating in neonates: responses to exogenous and endogenous acetylcholine. *Am. J. Dis. Child.*, 120, 434-438, 1970.

[30] FANAROFF (A. A.), WALD (E. H.), GRUBER (H. S.) et coll. — Insensible water loss in low birth weight infants. *Pediatrics*, 50, 236-246, 1972.

[31] HEY (E. N.), KATZ (G.). — Evaporative water loss in the newborn baby. *J. Physiol. (Lond.)*, 200, 605-619, 1969.

[32] BRODY (S.). — *Bioenergetics and Growth*, New York, Reinhold, 1945.

[33] HEIM (T.), CSER (A.), JASZAI (V.) et coll. — Energy metabolism and thermal homeostasis in the newborn. In STERN (L.). *Intensive Care in the Newborn II*, 275, 1978.

[34] COOKE (R. W. I.), LUCAS (A.), YUDKIN (P. L. N.) et coll. — Head circumference as an index of brain weight in the fetus and newborn. *Earl. Hum. Dev.*, *1/2*, 145, 1977.

[35] GRUENWALD (P.). — Chronic fetal distress and placental insufficiency. *Biol. Neonat.*, *5*, 215-265, 1963.

[36] STRATTON (D.). — Aural temperature of the newborn infant. *Arch. Dis. Child.*, *52*, 865-869, 1977.

[37] CHAPUT DE SAINTONGE (D. M.), CROSS (K. W.), HATHORN (M. K. M.) et coll. — Hats for the newborn infant. *Br. Med. J.*, *2*, 570, 1979.

[38] OLESEN (J.), PAULSON (O. B.), LASSEN (N. A.). — Regional cerebral blood flow in man determined by the initial slope of the clearance of intra-arterially injected Xe-133. *Stroke*, *2*, 519, 1971.

[39] REICHMAN (B. L.), CHESSEX (P.), PUTET (G.), VEREL-LEN (G.), SMITH (J. M.), HEIM (T.), SWYER (P. R.). — Diet, fat accretion and growth in premature infants. *N. Engl. J. Med.*, *305*, 1495, 1981.

[40] YASHIRO (K.), ADAMS (F. H.), EMMANOUILIDES (G. D.) et coll. — Preliminary studies on the thermal environment of low-birth-weight infants. *J. Ped.*, *82*, 991-994, 1973.

[41] SILVERMAN (W. A.), AGATE (F. J. Jr.). — Variation in cold resistance among small newborn infants. *Biol. Neonate.*, *6*, 113-127, 1964.

[42] NACHMAN (R. L.), ESTERLY (N. B.). — Increased skin permeability in preterm infants. *J. Ped.*, *79*, 628-632, 1971.

[43] KATZMAN (G. H.). — Insensible water loss by small infant in radiant heater. *J. Ped.*, *83*, 1094, 1973.

[44] WU (P. Y.), HODGMAN (J. E.). — Insensible water loss in preterm infants: changes with postnatal development and non-ionizing radiant energy. *Pediatrics*, *54*, 704-712, 1974.

[45] SULYOK (E.), JÉQUIER (E.), PROD'HOM (L. S.). — Respiratory contribution to the thermal balance of the newborn infant under various ambient conditions. *Pediatrics*, *51*, 641-650, 1973.

[46] PERLSTEIN (P. H.), EDWARDS (N. K.), SUTHER-LAND (J. M.). — Apnoea in premature infants and incubator-air-temperature changes. *N. Engl. J. Med.*, *282*, 461-466, 1970.

[47] BRUCK (K.). — Temperature regulation in the newborn infant. *Biol. Neonat.*, *3*, 65-119, 1951.

[48] MESTYAN (J.), JARAI (I.), BATA (B.) et coll. — Surface temperature and the metabolic response to cold of hypothermic premature infants. *Biol. Neonat.*, *7*, 230-242, 1964.

[49] LEVISON (H.), LINSAO (L.), SWYER (P. R.). — A comparison of infra-red and convective heating for newborn infants. *Lancet*, *2*, 1346-1348, 1966.

[50] SEGAL (S.), HALE (D. R.). — Inactivation of infant thermal control by hospital paging system. *Can. Paed. Soc. Prog. Abst.*, *73*, 1977.

[51] AGATE (R. J. Jr.), SILVERMAN (W. A.). — The control of body temperature in the small newborn infant by low-energy infra-red radiation. *Pediatrics*, *31*, 725, 1963.

[52] LEVISON (H.), DELIVORIA-PAPADOPOULOS (M.), SWYER (P. R.). — Oxygen consumption in newly born infants with the respiratory distress syndrome. *Biol. Neonat.*, *7*, 255-269, 1964.

[53] LEVISON (H.), DELIVORIA-PAPADOPOULOS (M.), SWYER (P. R.). — Variations in oxygen consumption in the infant with hypoxaemia due to cardiopulmonary disease. *Acta Paed. Scand.*, *54*, 369-374, 1965.

[54] CHESSEX (P.), REICHMAN (B. L.), VERELLEN (G. J. E.) et coll. — Influence of postnatal age, energy intake, and weight gain on energy metabolism in the very low-birth-weight infant. *J. Ped.*, *99*, 761, 1981.

[55] HULL (D.). — Storage and supply of fatty acids before and after birth. *Br. Med. Bull.*, *31*, 32-36, 1975.

[56] BLIGH (J.), JOHNSON (K. G.). — Glossary of terms for thermal physiology. *J. Appl. Physiol.*, *35*, 941-946, 1973.

36

Neonatal hyperbilirubinemia

William J. CASHORE and Leo STERN

INTRODUCTION

Neonatal jaundice is one of the most common conditions encountered in the newborn nursery. Most cases are benign and self limited and result from a physiologic delay in the maturation of the hepatic and gastrointestinal mechanisms for the conjugation and excretion of bilirubin; however, at very high plasma levels (*i. e.,* > 15-20 mg/dl) or in severly compromised newborns, bilirubin is potentially toxic to the central nervous system and perhaps to other organs. Since in many cases of "physiologic" jaundice the serum bilirubin level tends to rise until approximately the fourth postnatal day, and since the usual length of stay for maternity patients is now 3-4 days in many hospitals, a number of infants found to be jaundiced in the hospital may be discharged while their serum bilirubin levels are still increasing. Whether in or out of the hospital, such infants must be followed closely until it is certain that the origin and course of their jaundice is benign and the serum bilirubin concentration has either stabilized or decreased to a safe level. The infant's physician must maintain a proper balance between the recognition of the benign character of most cases of "physiologic" neonatal jaundice and concern for the potential toxicity of uncontrolled bilirubin levels or hyperbilirubinemia associated with a number of pathophysiologic condi-tions. In the following pages we shall discuss the origin and disposal of bilirubin in the newborn, some current hypotheses for the mechanism of bilirubin toxicity, and some contemporary approaches to the management of the jaundiced newborn.

FORMATION AND CHEMICAL PROPERTIES OF BILIRUBIN

Bilirubin, a degradation product of heme, is a weakly polar tetrapyrrole of molecular weight 585. Although unconjugated bilirubin has often been described as lipid soluble, Brodersen has shown that bilirubin is practically insoluble in animal fat and is more soluble in weakly polar than in non-polar solvents [1]. In fact, bilirubin-IXα, the usual confor-mation of unconjugated bilirubin, might best be described as a weakly polar weak acid of low solu-bility in water at neutral pH, rather than as a lipo-philic or lipid soluble molecule. Unconjugated bilirubin has an orange-yellow color and a charac-teristic spectrum with maximum absorbance at 455-460 nm when bound to serum albumin. The solubility and transport of bilirubin in the extra-cellular water is enhanced by its high affinity for albumin [2]. Bilirubin also has a high affinity for certain membrane phospholipids [3] and for a specific binding protein (Y-protein, or ligandin) within the hepatocyte [4]. The affinity of bilirubin for extracellular transport proteins (albumin and ligandin) explain the efficient transport of this relatively insoluble molecule in the body water, and its affinity for certain membrane components may be responsible for the development of visible jaundice in skin and fatty tissues. The relationship of bilirubin's physical and chemical properties to its toxicity will be explored in a later section of this chapter.

Bilirubin is a metabolic product of heme, the major source of which is the normal destruction of erythrocytes. Small amounts of heme and consequently of bilirubin also result from ineffective erythropoiesis or from the turnover of heme in oxygen dependent electron transport systems [5]. Hemolysis increases the rate of release of heme and production of bilirubin. Since the average time of survival of red cells is 88 days in the fetus and newborn versus 120 days in the adult, bilirubin production is more rapid in the fetus and newborn than in the adult [6, 7].

CONJUGATION
AND EXCRETION OF BILIRUBIN

The oxidation of heme to biliverdin and the reduction of biliverdin to bilirubin take place in the reticuloendothelial system. Bilirubin, bound to albumin, is transported in the plasma to the hepatocytes, where a specific binding protein (the Y-protein, or ligandin) acts as a receptor for bilirubin within the liver cell. In the microsomal system of the liver cell, the conjugation of bilirubin with UDP glucuronic acid is catalyzed by the enzyme glucuronyl transferase [8]. Bilirubin diglucuronide (conjugated or "direct acting" bilirubin) is more water soluble than unconjugated bilirubin and is excreted from the liver cells into the bile canaliculi, and then from the bile ducts into the small bowel. Within the small bowel, a series of reactions partly catalyzed by bacterial enzymes converts bilirubin to biliverdin, then to urobilinogen and stercobilinogen, the form in which it is usually eliminated from the bowel. If the intestinal bacteria are absent, bilirubin may remain unchanged in the small bowel and in the stool of the newborn infant. Since the bowel is sterile prior to birth, the meconium contains considerable amounts of bilirubin.

The fetus eliminates bilirubin via the placenta and the maternal circulation, since the intestinal route

for bilirubin elimination is not functioning during fetal life. Unconjugated bilirubin crosses the placental membranes more readily than conjugated bilirubin because of its solubility and polar characteristics, so that bilirubin in the fetus must remain unconjugated for placental excretion of bilirubin to take place. During some cases of antibody-induced hemolytic disease in the fetus, conjugated or direct acting bilirubin appears in the fetal circulation; this may be seen for example in response to intrauterine transfusions for severe Rh sensitization. In such cases, the conjugated bilirubin is not readily excreted by the placenta and tends to remain in the fetal circulation, so that the infant is born with a high direct acting fraction of bilirubin in the cord blood.

Unconjugated bilirubin appears in the amniotic fluid after the twelfth week of gestation; diffusion of bilirubin across the skin and across the membranes of the placenta and umbilical cord appears to be the most likely mechanism for the appearance of bilirubin in amniotic fluid at this time [9]. The bilirubin concentration of amniotic fluid falls in a predictable way with increasing gestational age, and abnormal accumulations of bilirubin in amniotic fluid, as described by Liley [10], have long been used to predict the severity of Rh hemolytic disease in the fetus. A high intestinal obstruction or other lesion producing major impairment of fetal swallowing may be associated with an increased concentration of unconjugated bilirubin in amniotic fluid [11]. The decrease in amniotic fluid bilirubin concentration usually found as gestational age increases is probably caused by a rapidly increasing volume of amniotic fluid as the fetus approaches term.

TOXICITY OF BILIRUBIN

The toxicity of bilirubin to the central nervous system was described in the early 1900's by Schmorl [12] but the deposition of bilirubin in the tissues of severely jaundiced newborns was first recognized some years earlier. The association of a specific syndrome of bilirubin neurotoxicity with hemolytic disease of the newborn was described in the 1920's and the 1930's by several authors, preceding by several years the recognition that Rh sensitization was the major cause of severe neonatal hemolytic disease [13]. Before the effective treatment of Rh hemolytic disease and its later prenatal prevention became clinical realities, severe hyperbilirubinemia due to hemolytic disease of the newborn was a major cause of neurological handicap in newborn infants and children.

Bilirubin encephalopathy is caused by the entry of bilirubin into the central nervous system. The characteristic signs in the newborn are lethargy and poor sucking, followed by opisthotonos, athetosis, spasticity, and seizures. Gastric and/or pulmonary hemorrhage sometimes accompany the abnormal neurological findings [14]. Acute bilirubin encephalopathy is rapidly fatal in more than 50 % of cases particularly in low birth weight infants; survivors may have varying combinations of athetosis, clumsiness, spasticity, disturbances of gait and balance, 8th nerve deafness, paralysis of upward gaze and mental retardation [15]. The term "kernicterus" used to describe the characteristic bilirubin staining of lower brain nuclei in bilirubin encephalopathy [12] is also often used to describe the clinical syndrome of acute bilirubin toxicity. At postmortem examination, Kernicterus is characterized by selective bilirubin staining of brain nuclei, including the basal ganglia, globus pallidus, putamen, the caudate nucleus, the cerebellum, and the auditory nucleus of the 8th nerve. Cortical staining is also occasionally seen. Clinically, the abnormal neurologic findings associated with bilirubin toxicity are consistent with damage to the areas which appear most likely to be stained with bilirubin at autopsy.

Before exchange transfusion was developed as an effective treatment of jaundice associated with Rh sensitized erythroblastosis, kernicterus occurred in approximately 15 % of cases of neonatal Rh disease [16]. As exchange transfusion and the subsequent prevention of Rh disease by maternal immunization dramatically reduced the incidence of kernicterus due to jaundice in Rh erythroblastosis, kernicterus began to be recognized in low birth weight infants with indirect bilirubin concentrations considerably lower than those considered hazardous for term erythroblastotic infants [17, 18]. Predisposing events, such as asphyxia and acidosis appeared to be responsible for an increased susceptibility of the brain to bilirubin and increased risk of kernicterus in low birth weight infants described during the 1960's and 1970's.

In vivo and in vitro experiments using animal models have identified the uptake of bilirubin into the brain under various conditions and have revealed some of the toxic mechanisms responsible for bilirubin encephalopathy. These experiments have demonstrated the toxicity of unconjugated bilirubin to intact brain cells and the enhancement of bilirubin toxicity in the presence of asphyxia or acidosis. However, the exact mechanism of bilirubin toxicity is not yet precisely known. Unbound conjugated bilirubin at high concentrations can uncouple mitochondrial oxidative phosphorylation [19], but this effect has not been seen in brain extracts from animals made toxic by infusing lower doses of bilirubin, and appears to be absent at "free" bilirubin levels likely to be seen within the central nervous system [20]. Bilirubin also increases the oxidation of glucose without increasing basal glucose transport, inhibits membrane adenylate cyclase and inhibits lipolysis mediated by triglyceride lipase in fat cells [21]. These findings suggest that bilirubin toxicity may occur partly because of bilirubin stimulated increases in the cell's consumption of oxygen, energy and substrates, under conditions in which oxygen and substrates are not readily restored. The finding that bilirubin interferes with the metabolism, both of glucose and of cyclic AMP, dictates that bilirubin is potentially toxic to a number of metabolic processes in the cells.

Within the cell, bilirubin aggregates and occasionally crystallizes at mitochondrial membranes, and most metabolic studies show it to be a mitochondrial poison. The straightening and swelling of complexly folded mitochondrial membranes suggest that bilirubin encephalopathy may be associated with abnormalities of water transport into and out of mitochondria, with possible abnormalities of electrolyte transport at mitochondrial membranes, and with probable uncoupling of a number of mitochondrial reactions.

There are several possible ways in which bilirubin might enter the brain. First, it is appropriate to review the protection normally afforded by the blood-brain barrier. The terminal capillary blood supply to the brain has "tight" endothelial junctions, and a high level of metabolic activity in the endothelium of the same capillaries [22]. The blood-brain barrier shows the combined properties of an anatomic diffusion barrier and a metabolic pump. Several events might permit entry of bilirubin into the brain: (1) breakdown of barrier permeability by temporary or permanent opening of tight junctions; (2) injury to the metabolic pump by *hypoxia* and acidosis; (3) a concentration of unbound bilirubin exceeding the solubility of bilirubin or the ability of the metabolic pump to exclude it from the brain, with aggregation of bilirubin at the junctions between capillaries and cells.

Diffusion of unconjugated, unbound bilirubin across the blood-brain barrier as "free" bilirubin is the most likely mechanism by which toxic levels of bilirubin enter the brain. This mechanism is suggested by the animal experiments of Diamond and Schmid [23], showing the toxicity of infused bilirubin not bound to albumin and the protective effect of albumin in an animal model, as well as by other experiments and by clinical observations which show that sulfa drugs displace bilirubin from albumin and simultaneously increase the uptake of bilirubin by the brain [24, 25]. More recently, however, the possibility that bilirubin may cross the blood-brain barrier in association with albumin during opening of the blood-brain barrier has been raised [26]. Reversible opening of the blood-brain barrier to large molecules such as albumin can be demonstrated with marked osmotic shifts, or with some changes in the circulation and perfusion pressures within the brain [27]. It has been suggested by some that reversible opening of the blood-brain barrier to the bilirubin-albumin complex may better explain some of the observed cases of kernicterus in small preterm infants with asphyxia, sepsis, acidosis, or shock than would the diffusion of large amounts of free bilirubin at low total bilirubin concentration. While it is correct that kernicterus now appears more frequent in very ill premature infants with total bilirubin levels well below 20 mg/dl than in healthy term infants with extremely high indirect bilirubin levels, both experimental evidence and clinical observations suggest that large amounts of bilirubin may be transferred from the plasma to the tissues at low bilirubin concentrations in the presence of reduced binding affinity of albumin (often for unknown reasons) [28], or the presence of known displacers of bilirubin such as salicylates [29] and sulfa drugs. At present, the controversy concerning the mechanism of kernicterus at low bilirubin levels is still unresolved, and both mechanisms (penetration of bound bilirubin or unbound bilirubin across the blood-brain barrier) may be considered possible.

Brodersen has suggested that the toxicity of bilirubin is related to its lack of solubility in water and its affinity for membrane components regardless of the mechanisms by which it enters the brain [30]. Because of its low solubility, bilirubin tends to exist in a supersaturated solution with a strong tendency to aggregate at membrane surfaces. Since the aqueous solubility of bilirubin is markedly pH dependent, even a small decrease in pH greatly increases the likelihood that bilirubin will precipitate. In Brodersen's model, the tendency of bilirubin to precipitate is considered constant, and depends on the pH, the total bilirubin concentration, and the number of reserve albumin sites available to bind additional bilirubin, irrespective of the actual free bilirubin concentration. These relationships are expressed in the equation:

$$I = \log \frac{B}{p} - 2\,pH + 15.5$$

in which I is an index indicating the relative likelihood of bilirubin precipitation under the defined conditions; B is the total concentration of unconjugated bilirubin; p is the reserve albumin concentration available for additional binding of unconjugated bilirubin; and the factor 15.5 is a constant related to the solubility of bilirubin in water and its affinity for serum albumin. According to this equation, an increase in total bilirubin, a decrease in reserve albumin, or a fall in pH would all increase the likelihood that bilirubin would precipitate in the tissues. Either hypothesis (*i. e.*, the entry of bound bilirubin or the entry of free bilirubin) for the mechanism by which bilirubin crosses the blood-brain barrier would be consistent with this theoretical model, since it is the supersaturation of bilirubin in the plasma, rather than its free concentration which governs its tendency to deposit in the tissues. However, if bilirubin did enter the central nervous system as bound bilirubin it would then have to dissociate from albumin in order to fix to the tissues and produce its metabolic toxicity.

In cases of kernicterus occuring at low unconjugated bilirubin levels in low birth weight infants, acidosis is a common associated finding and may be an important predisposing factor. Although a lowering of pH itself does not promote the dissociation of bilirubin from albumin, acidosis may increase the permeability of the blood-brain barrier and may also increase the tendency of the bilirubin to precipitate or aggregate in cells [31]. Furthermore, by interfering with the metabolism of cells or the integrity of the cell membrane, acidosis may make the cells in the brain more vulnerable to the toxic action of bilirubin.

THE BINDING OF BILIRUBIN TO ALBUMIN

Although relatively insoluble in water at physiologic pH, bilirubin is transported in the plasma tightly bound to albumin. The concentration of unbound bilirubin present in equilibrium with the bound in the plasma is usually 2.0 µg/100 ml or less so that all but a small fraction of the plasma bilirubin is bound to albumin. In the physiologic state, binding of bilirubin to protein appears to protect the CNS against kernicterus; bilirubin that is tightly bound to albumin is unable to diffuse into the CNS. In general, binding of bilirubin to protein also appears necessary for the transport of large amounts of relatively insoluble bilirubin in the plasma, so that binding is important in the excretion as well as in the toxicity of bilirubin.

Albumin has one binding site with a high affinity for bilirubin and additional bilirubin binding sites (definitely one and probably two) of considerably lower affinity [2]. Normally, the concentration of albumin is approximately 3.5 g/100 ml (500 μM/liter) in the serum. This means that under physiologic conditions, most of the bilirubin in the plasma is bound to the high affinity site on albumin. Theoretically, one mole of albumin should bind and transport one mole of bilirubin with high affinity; this would mean that a serum with an albumin concentration of 3.5 gm/100 ml should bind up to 29 mg/100 ml of bilirubin at its primary site. However, clinical and laboratory experience with neonatal serum have shown that the actual bilirubin binding capacity of infants' serum albumin is usually only 50-90 % of what is theoretically predicted [28, 32-34]. In sick infants, the binding ability of serum albumin is usually lower than in well infants [28, 32]. Under these circumstances, some of the bilirubin present in neonatal serum may be bound to secondary rather than primary albumin sites, and may be identifiable as "loosely bound" bilirubin. In clinical situations in which the risk of kernicterus is presumably high, such as acidosis or asphyxia, the identification of high concentrations of "loosely bound" or "unbound" (free) bilirubin has sometimes appeared to correlate better with the incidence of kernicterus at total bilirubin levels below 15-20 mg/100 ml, than has the total or the indirect bilirubin concentration itself [33-35].

The reason for reduced albumin binding of bilirubin in newborn and premature infants is not known. Although serum albumin concentration is lower in the infant than in the adult and still lower in the premature than in the term infant, as noted above the number of binding sites available for binding of bilirubin appears to be reduced relative to the albumin concentration present. Larger and older infants with severe asphyxia and respiratory distress often seem to have lower binding capacities than smaller and less mature infants who are well, even though the total albumin concentrations may be higher in the larger infants [28]. Although some workers have speculated that there may be maturational differences in the structure of albumin to account for its changing affinity for bilirubin and some drugs, the structural differences which might be responsible have not been identified so far. Increasing affinity of bilirubin for albumin with increasing postnatal age [36] and especially with recovery from serious neonatal illness [37] suggests that endogenous metabolic products may block the

albumin binding sites for bilirubin during periods of stress or abnormal metabolism.

Certain substances are known to compete with bilirubin for its binding sites on serum albumin. This competition may occur if a drug can occupy the bilirubin binding sites in direct competition, or if it can change the geometry of the albumin molecule so that bilirubin is less readily bound. Among the substances known to compete for the bilirubin binding sites on albumin are hematin, salicylates, sulfonamides, furosemide, and benzoate used to preserve certain drugs which are stored in multiple injection vials, such as diazepam and plasma expanders. The potential ability of a drug to displace bilirubin from albumin should be considered before that drug is given to a newborn infant or to mothers, either antepartum or during lactation. Unfortunately, many commonly used drugs, or their vehicles and preservatives, have not been studied adequately in this respect.

A variety of in vitro tests have been devised for the measurement of free bilirubin concentrations in the plasma or the availability of bilirubin binding sites on serum albumin of newborn infants. These tests are used to assess the risk of kernicterus in neonatal jaundice by estimating either the concentration of unbound bilirubin or the remaining albumin sites available, and can also be used to estimate the availability of competing substances, such as drugs, to displace bilirubin from albumin. The binding tests in use employ several different features: (1) an attempt to separate and measure loosely bound or free bilirubin (peroxidase oxidation or Sephadex gel filtration). (2) Estimation of the reserve, or the remaining sites available for bilirubin in a serum sample, by addition of a dye analogue of bilirubin or bilirubin itself (the HBABA dye test, albumin titration with Direct Yellow 7 dye, and several fluorometric methods for the titration of bilirubin and albumin). (3) Analysis of the bilirubin spectrum, using a spectral shift or difference spectroscopy to demonstrate the adequacy or inadequacy of albumin binding of bilirubin or displacement of bilirubin from albumin by a competing substance. (4) Use of a selective trace ligand—a trace amount of a small molecule bound to the albumin site for bilirubin in a predictable way and displaced in a measurable quantity from albumin by bilirubin or one of its competitors.

The various methods briefly described here, the terminology used in those methods, and list of references describing them are given in Table I. The variety of binding tests available and their lack of universal acceptance indicate that different investigators have entertained different hypotheses con-

TABLE I. — IN VITRO TESTS OF BILIRUBIN BINDING TO ALBUMIN

Method	Measures
A. Measurement of free or loosely bound bilirubin.	
1. Sephadex gel filtration [33, 34].	Free and loosely bound bilirubin.
2. Horseradish perioxidase oxidation [38].	Free bilirubin.
Both methods also estimate reserve and total bilirubin binding capacity by titration with excess bilirubin.	
B. Dye test for reserve binding capacity.	
1. Hydroxy-benzeneazo benzoic acid (HBABA) [39].	Reserve dye binding sites, some not identical to bilirubin sites.
2. Titration with direct yellow 7 [40].	Binding of dye to primary and secondary albumin sites.
C. Fluorescence techniques.	
1. Fluorescence quenching of albumin by bilirubin [41].	Affinity of bilirubin for albumin and effects of competitors.
2. Whole blood fluorometry [42, 43].	Bound bilirubin, reserve and total binding capacity of primary site.
D. Spectral analysis.	
1. Difference spectroscopy and circular dichroism [44, 45].	Affinity of bilirubin and effect of competitors at albumin sites.
2. Saturation index (BR displacement by salicylate at OD 460) [46].	Displacement of bilirubin from weaker sites—indirectly estimates reserve binding at weaker sites.
E. Selective trace ligand.	
1. Electron—labeled spin resonance [47].	Reserve albumin at high-affinity sites.
2. Dialysis of trace ligand ^{14}C-monoacetyl diamino diphenyl sulfone [48].	Reserve albumin at high-affinity sites.

cerning this problem, have approached the problem of bilirubin binding to albumin in different ways, and are not yet in agreement as to which of these tests might prove most suitable in a clinical setting for predicting the risk of kernicterus in the newborn [49, 50]. Among the problems cited are those of sample dilution, the addition of excess bilirubin to specimens, and the use of dyes or other substances which may not be exclusively bound at the bilirubin sites on albumin. Nevertheless, available clinical evidence does suggest that the risk for kernicterus in a newborn is greatly increased once the available high affinity binding sites on albumin are saturated with bilirubin [28, 34, 35]. Especially among premature and sick infants, there appear to be marked differences between subjects in the bilirubin binding capabilities of their albumin. Once the high affinity sites are saturated with bilirubin, secondary binding sites appear to offer much less protection, since the remaining bilirubin is more weakly bound and more readily diffusible. At physiologic pH, the free bilirubin concentration in equilibrium with weak binding sites on albumin rapidly approaches or exceeds the limits of bilirubin solubility [1]. In addition to differences between individual infants in the binding of bilirubin to albumin and in the reserve albumin available for further binding of

bilirubin, various types of injury to the CNS, pathophysiologic changes in the plasma or elsewhere, or disturbances of circulation (especially in cerebral circulation) may contribute to differences in the vulnerability of individuals to kernicterus. For example, when there are wide changes in mean blood pressure, the cerebral circulation of newborn animals (and probably newborn human infants) may become pressure-passive, and leaks may develop in the blood-brain barrier as the capillary integrity of the blood-brain barrier is temporarily lost [27]. In the asphyxiated infant, rapid changes in pH, PCO_2, or blood pressure may allow temporary opening of the blood-brain barrier to the bilirubin-albumin complex. In addition, under these conditions the lack of an essential substrate for oxidative metabolism, such as glucose or oxygen itself, or the malfunctioning of an important activating or transport mechanism, such as the membrane system for the production of cyclic AMP, may locally increase vulnerability of the tissues to injury by bilirubin or other toxins. Therefore, the binding of bilirubin by albumin in the plasma may not wholly protect the infant from bilirubin encephalopathy under adverse pathophysiologic conditions. Even if the bilirubin-albumin complex enters the brain under some conditions, the ability of bilirubin to dissociate from albumin under those conditions might still be important, since bilirubin would probably have to bind or precipitate elsewhere in order to be toxic. The precise relationships between binding of bilirubin in the plasma and events in the tissues predisposing to bilirubin toxicity are not yet completely understood.

BILIRUBIN METABOLISM
IN THE NEWBORN

At birth, serum bilirubin levels in cord blood are approximately 1.5-2.0 mg per 100 ml [51]. Higher cord bilirubin levels are usually associated with intrauterine hemolysis. Bilirubin is produced at an average rate of 8.5 mg/kg/day [6, 7]. Since in most infants the conjugating system for bilirubin is not yet fully matured, in most healthy term infants the bilirubin levels will rise slowly to mean levels of 6-7 mg per 100 ml at approximately 72 hours of age [52]. The serum bilirubin level then remains on a plateau for a day or two, then falls to normal levels by the end of the first week. Clinically, bilirubin levels in the range of 5-8 mg per 100 ml are barely visible in most newborns. In "physiologic" jaundice, the usual rate of increase of serum bilirubin does not exceed 5 mg per 100 ml per day (0.2 mg per 100 ml per hour), and nearly all the bilirubin accumulated in the serum is of the indirect acting or unconjugated variety. Serum indirect bilirubin levels in excess of 15 mg per 100 ml occur in only 3 % of otherwise normal term babies [53]. The reason for marked individual differences in the levels of neonatal jaundice appears to be the interaction between the rate of bilirubin formation and the rate of conjugation and excretion of bilirubin by the liver; both the rate of formation and the rate of its elimination may vary widely between individuals. Even from day to day in the same subject, there may be marked differences in hepatic glucuronyl transferase activity, as shown by Stern et al. [54], and the differences in enzyme activity between individuals may vary even more widely. The conjugation of bilirubin by the liver may further be influenced by the mother's intake of enzyme inducing drugs (such as phenobarbital or alcohol), which may cross the placenta or be present in the breast milk. In addition to enzyme inducing substances, enzyme inhibiting substances may appear in breast milk in some cases. Finally, in the intestine conjugated bilirubin may be deconjugated by beta-glucuronidase in the small bowel; this unconjugated bilirubin

may be reabsorbed and recycled. The rate of increase in serum bilirubin in a term infant may be considered greater than the expected physiologic rate if: (1) the cord bilirubin is 3 mg per 100 ml or greater. (2) Clinically obvious jaundice appears on the first day. (3) The indirect bilirubin concentration exceeds 15 mg per 100 ml at any time. (4) The direct bilirubin conjugation persistently exceeds 1 mg per 100 ml or (5) jaundice is clinically evident during the second week after birth.

Preterm infants initially show a rate of bilirubin accumulation similar to that of term infants, but the mature mechanisms of bilirubin conjugation and excretion may be delayed for a week or more; although they have similar cord blood bilirubin values and similar serum bilirubin levels during the first few days, the indirect bilirubin levels often continue to rise until the end of the first week, and clinically evident jaundice during the second week is not unusual in infants less than 36 weeks gestation. Before phototherapy was widely used to treat jaundice in premature infants, average bilirubin levels in preterm infants were approximately 11 mg per 100 ml, and approximately 18 % of white infants and 9 % of black preterm infants had peak bilirubin levels higher than 15 mg per 100 ml towards the end of the first week after birth [55, 56]. The principal reason for these higher bilirubin levels in preterm infants appears to be a delay in maturation of the conjugating system. Several other contributing factors include bruising at delivery, possibly a higher incidence of hemolysis due to nonspecific causes, and a delay in excretion of bilirubin caused by a delay in the onset of feeding, so that bilirubin present in the bowel may be absorbed and recirculated. It is also worth noting that generalized cutaneous jaundice seems to appear at lower bilirubin levels in preterm than in term infants; this may be due to the thinner skin and smaller amounts of depot fat in the preterm infant, so that jaundice becomes visible earlier. Infants of diabetic mothers and infants with polycythemia have higher bilirubin levels than other infants of comparable gestation and birth weight [57, 58]. Despite their somatic overgrowth, infants of diabetic mothers tend to have an immature conjugation and excretion system. Intrauterine growth retardation and prolonged placental transfusion are two conditions associated with neonatal polycythemia; in this condition, the increased red cell load appears to result in an increased rate of bilirubin production [58].

Prolonged unconjugated hyperbilirubinemia occurs in some breast feeding infants whose mothers appear to secrete high levels of an inhibitor substance in the breast milk. $3\alpha20\beta$ pregnanediol is one recognized inhibitor of hepatic glucuronyl transferase found in the breast milk of some mothers [59], but does not appear to account for all cases of protracted jaundice in breast feeding infants [60]. More recently, Gartner has demonstrated that variations in fatty acid composition of some breast milks may enhance intestinal reabsorbtion of bilirubin and persistence of jaundice in infants receiving those milks [61]. Early onset hyperbilirubinemia appears somewhat more common in some populations of breast fed mothers, although specific inhibitors of bilirubin conjugation and excretion cannot be identified in all cases. The suspect inhibitor of bilirubin conjugation (3α20β pregnanediol) is only demonstrable once lactation is well established. The overall incidence of neonatal jaundice due to breast feeding is estimated at about 2 % [53].

HEMOLYTIC DISEASES
OF THE NEWBORN

Isoimmune hemolytic diseases of the newborn are caused by transplacental passage of maternal antibodies against fetal cells of a major or a minor blood group incompatible with the mother. The two most common manifestations of hemolytic disease of the newborn are ABO Hemolytic Disease, which is far more common, and Rh Erythroblastosis, which is now fortunately rare. Most cases of ABO Hemolysis are found in Type A or B babies of Type O mothers and are caused by transfer to the infant of preexisting maternal anti-A or anti-B antibodies. It is possible that much of the antibody transfer takes place late in pregnancy (perhaps at or near parturition), because there is seldom prenatal evidence of a severely affected fetus. The infants are usually well at birth, and severe anemia is unusual. ABO incompatibility cannot be detected prenatally from maternal titers of anti-A or anti-B, since these are already high in the Type O mother. At first, the direct Coombs' test on the infant's cells is variably positive, often weakly positive because the neonatal cell contains fewer A or B antigen sites than the adult red cell [62]. The indirect Coombs' test, at least, should always be positive for the diagnosis to be made. There are many A or B infants born to Type O mothers without clinical or laboratory evidence of blood group incompatibility, so that the diagnosis must be made by means of a positive Coombs' test, symptoms in the infant and hemolysis on a peripheral blood smear.

Neonatal hemolytic disease associated with both

ABO and Rh antibody induced hemolysis is characterized by a rapid early rise in serum indirect bilirubin levels. This early rapid increase in jaundice may exceed 1 mg % per hour. Infants with hemolytic disease of the newborn may become visibly jaundiced within the first few hours of life and may be quite markedly jaundiced by the end of the first day. Without treatment, indirect bilirubin levels due to ABO or Rh hemolytic disease may exceed 20 mg % by the second day of postnatal life. It is important to follow these patients for hyperbilirubinemia from an early age; if the infant is born in a hospital where diagnostic and treatment facilities are not adequate for close observation and early treatment of the baby, it is important to transfer the baby to a referral center early in the course of the disease and before the hyperbilirubinemia has become severe and out of control.

Although ABO and Rh hemolytic disease can both be present with anemia, severe hyperbilirubinemia, and hepatosplenomegaly, their presentation and postnatal course are usually quite different. The differences will be noted in the following two paragraphs.

Infants with ABO disease are only slightly anemic at birth, or sometimes have no anemia at all [62, 63]. The indirect bilirubin level in the cord blood is usually normal or only slightly elevated. There may be slight to moderate hepatosplenomegaly, and sometimes there is splenomegaly without hepatic enlargement. The direct Coombs' test is usually weakly positive (for the reasons cited above) or in some mild cases, is even negative; the indirect Coombs' test is positive, showing an incompatibility between the infant's serum and the cells of the infant's major blood group (A or B). The peripheral blood smear may show many spherocytes and cell fragments but the number of immature red cells is not usually increased. The indirect bilirubin level tends to increase rapidly during the first 48 hours. After that, the rate of increase in bilirubin decreases markedly in most normal infants, and a plateau level is reached by the beginning of the third day. There are several likely reasons for this pattern of jaundice in ABO incompatibility. The sensitized cells undergo rather rapid intravascular hemolysis and the antigen antibody complexes are then removed by the spleen, so that the rate of further hemolysis tends to decrease after the initial hemolytic episode. In addition, A and B antigen substance is found in other tissues, so that some of the antibody may fix to tissue sites other than red cells. After the fourth to fifth postnatal day, the signs of rapid hemolysis tend to decrease and the circulating antibody may fall to undetectable levels. Because hemolysis in ABO hemolytic disease tends to be early, rapid, and short-lived, evidence of prolonged hemolysis and of late anemia occurs only in a minority of cases.

In Rh hemolytic disease, sensitization of the Rh negative mother usually occurs by accidental exposure to Rh positive blood [64]. The most common sensitizing event appears to be a fetal to maternal transfusion of Rh positive blood, most often occurring at parturition of an infant who is himself/herself unaffected.

A subsequent pregnancy with an Rh positive fetus then evokes an antibody response early in the gestation so that antibody mediated destruction of Rh positive fetal erythrocytes begins some weeks before birth. The elevation of the maternal antibody titer, the gestational age at which antibodies first cross the placenta to the fetus, and the resulting hemolytic anemia may be mild to moderate or may be so severe as to be fatal even before term. The accumulation of bilirubin in the fetal plasma and tissues likewise begins before birth in many cases. Many erythroblastotic infants have cord indirect bilirubin levels between 3-8 mg per 100 ml. The subsequent increase in bilirubin levels tends to be rapid, often exceeding 1 mg %/hour [65]. However, as in all cases of neonatal jaundice, the rapidity of onset, eventual severity, and duration of the hyperbilirubinemia associated with hemolysis depends not only on the rate of hemolysis, but on the rate of bilirubin conjugation and excretion by the fetus or newborn. As previously noted, this can be highly variable and in itself may account for some of the wide individual variation in bilirubin levels seen in Rh erythroblastotic infants at comparable levels of hemoglobin. In general, compared with ABO blood group incompatibility, the course of jaundice in infants with Rh blood incompatibility tends to be more severe and more prolonged. Because of the high titer of antibody present long before birth, hemolysis and jaundice may persist for many days, and several exchange transfusions may be needed for clinical management. Even after the hepatic system for conjugation and excretion of bilirubin matures, late anemia is common. The presence of many nucleated red cells (erythroblasts) on peripheral blood smear indicates a long standing hemolytic process.

MANAGEMENT OF RH ERYTHROBLASTOSIS

Prevention of Rh sensitization and of erythroblastosis fetalis is the goal of management of the Rh negative pregnant woman. The routine use of Rh immune antiglobin given in the immediate post-partum period to Rh negative mothers who have delivered Rh positive infants has reduced the incidence of Rh D erythroblastosis fetalis by approximately 95 %, compared to the incidence of Rh erythroblastosis seen in North America between the 1930's and 1950's [66, 67]. For an effective approach to prevention, it is imperative that the blood types of all mothers be known at the time of delivery to the medical personnel attending or supervising the delivery. The means to determine major and Rh blood group and Rh antibody titer should be routinely available in all settings where obstetrics is practiced, and the results of typing should be available to the birth attendant within 24 hours after delivery. In the United States, it is customary to give Rh immune antiglobulin within three days of delivery, but the immunization is still effective up to a week after delivery, so that failure to obtain the mother's blood group and Rh titer during the first three days is not a contraindication to giving the vaccine later. It is best to obtain the mother's blood type and her Rh antibody titer at the beginning of her prenatal care, and this information should be forwarded to the hospital where the birth will take place. It is now considered appropriate by many authorities to administer small doses of Rh immune globulin even before delivery, immediately after a variety of obstetrical accidents (such as first or early second trimester bleeding) or intervention such as amniocentesis [68]. It is also considered appropriate to give Rh immune antiglobulin to any Rh negative woman whose pregnancy terminates early, whether the termination of the pregnancy is spontaneous or induced. In doubtful cases, the dose of Rh immune globulin (that is, whether the dose needs to be smaller or larger than the standard dose) can sometimes be estimated by a differential count of the number of fetal cells per one-thousand maternal red cells in the maternal circulation. Several methods are now commercially available for estimating the volume of a potential fetal transfusion to the mother following abortion, amniocentesis, premature separation of the placenta, or even a normal delivery. The cost of these diagnostic and therapeutic measures is far less than the cost would be of caring for a potentially preventable case of neonatal erythroblastosis.

In spite of attempts at prevention of Rh erythroblastosis by the use of Rh immune globulin, a small residual percentage of Rh negative mothers (approximately 0.5-1 % of all Rh negative pregnant women) present with a positive anti-Rh titer in the absence of any suspicion of Rh sensitization. Many of these present with a positive Rh titer during the first pregnancy, while a few present unexpectedly with Rh antibody titers during a subsequent pregnancy after a negative titer and unaffected first infant during the first pregnancy. The first group (those presenting already sensitized in the first pregnancy) may have been sensitized by maternal to fetal transfusions of Rh positive maternal blood at the time when they were born or by early fetal to maternal hemorrhage during the first trimester of their first pregnancy. The second group represents failures of Rh immune globulin administration, either because the Rh immune globulin was never given or was given improperly or, in most cases, because the size of the fetal to maternal hemorrhage at parturition of an earlier infant was larger than estimated and the dose of Rh immune globulin given was therefore not large enough. This small residue of cases of Rh erythroblastosis continue to represent a problem for the obstetrician and for the pediatrician so that it is still pertinent to review the basic aspects of management of the Rh sensitized pregnancy and the Rh erythroblastotic newborn.

The prenatal management of the Rh sensitized patient requires that serial Rh antibody titers in the mother be followed by the obstetrician during the second and third trimesters of pregnancy. Rising titers generally signal that the condition of the fetus is worsening, and may be accompanied by polyhydramnios and evidence on X-ray or ultrasound examination of fetal organomegaly or edema. In addition to the maternal antibody titers, the bilirubin content of the amniotic fluid can be measured by serial amniocentesis, according to the method first described by Liley [10]. A marked increase in titer, a marked increase in amniotic fluid bilirubin (or its failure to decrease in a physiologic manner towards the end of pregnancy), polyhydramnios, or early signs of fetal hepatosplenomegaly or edema are all signs of progressive hemolysis and a worsening fetal condition. If biochemical maturation of the lung is shown by testing the amniotic fluid for surfactant [69], or if early maturation of the lung can be induced by corticosteroids [70], an early delivery is indicated. The goal of the prospective management of the Rh sensitized pregnancy is to select a time for the delivery of the infant before severe anemia or hydrops fetalis with stillbirth occur, but late enough to avoid the hazards of severe immunity. This requires close monitoring of the pregnancy, careful planning including consultation with persons experienced in the management of Rh disease, serial Rh titers, and scheduled amniocentesis for measurement of amniotic fluid bilirubin

and of fetal pulmonary maturation. High resolution ultrasonography may also prove helpful in detecting the early onset of polyhydramnios, fetal organ enlargement, or subcutaneous edema. In the most severe forms of Rh erythroblastosis erythropoiesis is profoundly affected, and even the immature forms of the red cells are rapidly destroyed by the antibodies. Severely affected infants may be remarkably anemic and jaundiced even at birth, with massive hepatosplenomegaly, decreased serum albumin and a strongly positive Coombs' test. The most severely affected fetuses become profoundly anemic even before the 32nd week of gestation. The mortality of infants severely affected early in the third trimester of pregnancy is extremely high. Although early maturation of the fetal lung by the use of corticosteroids or other drugs may increase the safety of a preterm delivery either by the induction of labor or by cesarean section; in the most severely affected infants one or more intrauterine intraperitoneal transfusions of Rh negative packed cells may become necessary [71]. This was formerly a common procedure but is now less often done since the techniques of early fetal lung maturation and neonatal intensive care have made preterm delivery a much safer alternative than in the past.

At delivery, the hemoglobin, hematocrit, bilirubin, blood type, and Rh antibody status (with both a direct and indirect Coombs' test) should be performed on cord blood as rapidly as possible. A careful record should be kept of the time at which each test was performed, so that subsequent changes in bilirubin values, hemoglobin, and hematocrit, can be closely followed. Early exchange transfusion is the treatment of choice for moderately or severely affected cases. The criteria for early exchange transfusions may vary somewhat among different institutions but in general an early exchange transfusion is recommended for one or more of the following [65]: (1) cord indirect reacting bilirubin greater than 5.0 mg per 100 ml; (2) cord hemoglobin concentration of 10 mg per 100 ml or less; (3) a rate of rise for indirect reacting bilirubin of 1 mg per 100 ml/hr or greater; (4) after 12 hours of age, an indirect reacting bilirubin concentration greater than one-half of the infant's postnatal age in hours; (5) evidence of cardiovascular or multi-system involvement (edema, ascites, cardiac failure); (6) in addition, an exchange transfusion is considered the treatment of choice for an indirect bilirubin concentration of 20 mg/100 ml or greater at any time during the first week. Formerly, the outcome in about one-third of Rh sensitized pregnancies was stillbirth or postnatal death of the infant with a very high mortality of live-born but severely affected infants. If the fetal lung can be matured, early delivery of an affected fetus before the development of fetal hydrops may obviate much of the need for intensive treatment. In this context, it is worth noting that the incidence of respiratory distress syndrome appears to be higher in erythroblastotic infants than in non affected infants of the same gestational age, so that particular attention must be paid to fetal lung maturation if an early delivery is considered [72]. The approaching onset of severe anema or fetal hydrops is often marked by a sharp increase in maternal titer during the third trimester, sometimes by hydramnios, and by a marked increase in the amniotic bilirubin levels which may move rapidly towards or into Liley Zone III [10]. In choosing the best time for delivery, the risk of pulmonary immaturity versus the risk of continued deterioration of the fetus should be considered; the route of delivery (cesarean section or induction of labor) is a secondary consideration.

Infants with Rh erythroblastosis should be delivered in a well equipped and fully staffed tertiary perinatal center, and a physician should attend the delivery. Even in the moderately to severely affected infant, stabilization of temperature and immediate treatment of cardiac and respiratory problems should precede attempts at early exchange transfusion. The most severely affected infant may require immediate resuscitation, ventilation, and respiratory support and also, rapid replacement of red cell volume within the first few hours after birth. This is often done by means of a partial exchange transfusion in which a volume of 30-50 ml/kg of the infant's whole blood are replaced by an equal volume of packed red cells. Cardiac failure in such infants results from severe anemia with defective oxygen transport, as well as hypoalbuminemia from massive hepatic congestion. While specific therapy for cardiac failure may be of some value, replacement of oxygen carrying capacity and respiratory support until the red cell and plasma volumes can be restored toward normal represent the optimal treatment of the underlying disorder, with the use of digoxin and other medications specifically directed towards the treatment of cardiac failure only as symptomatic rather than definitive treatment. Infants with an Apgar score of seven or greater and a cord hematocrit above 30 % will benefit more from a few hours of observation and stabilization before exchange transfusion than they will from a transfusion quickly done under suboptimal conditions and without the necessary supporting information to stabilize the infant.

Incompatibility of major blood groups between the mother and the fetus offers the fetus some protection against Rh sensitization because the incompatible fetal cells of an A or B positive fetus are rapidly removed from the circulation of an O negative mother. Because of this, the Rh positive fetus, type A or B, with an O Rh negative mother, is less likely to have Rh erythroblastosis than would a type O fetus of the same mother.

Erythroblastosis can also be caused by maternal fetal incompatibility for minor blood groups other than the Rh (D) blood group system or the ABO system. Such cases are relatively rare, but make up an increasingly important portion of cases of erythroblastosis, as anti-Rh (D) sensitization decreases as a result of successful immunization. Sensitization to the Rh subgroups C, D^u and E can occur in a similar way to sensitization to Rh group D, and once sensitization is established, the pattern of hemolytic disease in the newborn can repeat in successive pregnancies. Even rarer causes of maternal fetal blood group incompatibility are found in the Kell Duffy, and Lewis blood groups. In the course of prenatal care, screening for the major groups, the Rh (D) blood type, and the anti-D titer are mandatory procedures in rendering good care, but sensitization to the rarer minor group may be obscured unless there is a well-equipped serology laboratory with an experienced staff available, and unless the index of suspicion is high on the part of the personnel caring for the pregnant woman.

Severe intrauterine hemolysis may also result from congenital infections, particularly congenital syphilis, and from congenital defects of hemoglobin synthesis, of which the most frequent manifestation is homozygous alpha thalassemia (Hemoglobin Barts). Most congenital infections and alpha thalassemia are associated with a high incidence of stillbirth due to hydrops. Very few infants affected with alpha thalassemia are born alive, and those born alive may survive only a few hours at most. Some infants with congenital syphilis may also be severely affected by hemolytic anemia. It is therefore necessary to perform serologic testing during pregnancy as an indication of need for treatment. Unless the mother is also symptomatic (e. g., polyhydramnios) alpha thalassemia is not usually suspected before birth without a prior family history. The postnatal management of severe anemia due to congenital syphilis or to defects of red cell synthesis is the same as described above. Unfortunately, no surviving cases of neonatal homozygous alpha thalassemia have been reported.

TREATMENT
OF NEONATAL JAUNDICE

When serum indirect reacting bilirubin levels are rising rapidly or markedly elevated due to any cause, exchange transfusion remains the treatment of choice for the rapid reduction of serum bilirubin levels and the prevention of kernicterus [65]. This technique, which produced a dramatic decline in the incidence of bilirubin encephalopathy when first used in the 1950's [73], continues to serve as the standard for comparison with other treatments from the standpoint of rapidity, safety, and efficacy in lowering serum bilirubin levels. At present the other major therapeutic technique for reducing serum bilirubin levels is phototherapy [74], which is effective but does not act as quickly as exchange transfusion. Additional treatments, such as the use of phenobarbital or other medications to increase the rapidity of clearance of bilirubin either from the circulation or from the GI tract are at present still considered preventative or auxiliary measures rather than definitive treatments for hyperbilirubinemia. In the care of the jaundiced infant, investigation and detection of the cause of hyperbilirubinemia are of more aid in managing the underlying disorder than in managing the jaundice itself. Treatment of the jaundice as a separate problem must be directed towards keeping the bilirubin level acceptably low, or reducing it promptly if it has risen to dangerously high levels. For these purposes, the therapies mentioned above (exchange transfusion and phototherapy) are the treatments of choice regardless of the underlying causes of the jaundice once the bilirubin has risen rapidly or to very high levels. Irrespective of the cause of the jaundice, the threshold for bilirubin encephalopathy is probably the same for any given infant.

An extensive differential diagnosis of the causes of neonatal jaundice need not be reviewed in detail here. Most diagnostic procedures undertaken in the nursery are intended to reveal a rather limited number of causes. The causes underlying the majority of cases of neonatal hyperbilirubinemia are listed in Table II.

The single most effective screening test for hyperbilirubinemia is to inspect hospitalized infants daily in well-lighted surroundings. It is also easier to identify neonatal jaundice by inspection if the walls and ceilings of the nursery are of a non-reflecting neutral color, than if the walls are of bright or strong colors masking the faint yellow

TABLE II. — CAUSES
OF NEONATAL HYPERBILIRUBINEMIA

1. Hemolysis induced by maternal antibodies:
   (*a*) Rh (D) hemolytic disease.
   (*b*) ABO incompatibility.
   (*c*) Other (rare blood groups).
2. Hereditary defects of the red cell, including alpha-thalassemia, hereditary spherocytosis, glucose-6-phosphate dehydrogenase deficiency, pyruvate kinase deficiency, glutathione reductase deficiency.
3. Congenital or neonatal infection.
4. Enclosed hemorrhage.
5. Metabolic disorders (galactosemia, congenital hypothyroidism).
6. Extrahepatic or intrahepatic bile duct obstruction (elevated direct bilirubin).
7. Persistent jaundice due to a breast milk inhibitor of bilirubin conjugation and excretion.
8. Hepatic dysfunction associated with prolonged intravenous nutrition.

appearance of the jaundiced infant. At the usual physiologic levels of serum bilirubin an infant will have only slight facial jaundice and jaundice of the sclerae. If the trunk or thighs are jaundiced, especially if this jaundice is evident on the first or second day, bilirubin levels are usually higher and such findings may indicate hyperbilirubinemia. In small prematures generalized jaundice is usually seen at lower bilirubin levels than in term infants, probably because of their thinner skin and smaller amount of depot fat.

Measurements of serum bilirubin levels should be available at all times in the hospital laboratory on microsamples of serum (0.1 ml or less), and direct as well as total bilirubin levels should be reported. In planning management, it is useful to determine the rate of increase in serum bilirubin by plotting the change of bilirubin concentration against the time interval since the last bilirubin measurement, keeping in mind that the maximum physiologic rate of increase for bilirubin is about 0.2 mg/100 ml/hr. If the rate of rise in bilirubin is plotted, this allows a rough prediction of the course of the hyperbilirubinemia and may assist in choosing the best time to order the next test. Since the error of the test is between 5-10 %, measurements taken too frequently may be superflous and unproductive if the rate of change is slow. On the other hand, if the rate of change appears rapid or unpredictable, a long delay between measurements may endanger the patient. When possible, the tests should be ordered well in advance of planned discharge from the hospital to avoid unnecessary delays if the result is normal or to permit repetition of the tests or initiation of therapy if the bilirubin level is unexpectedly high.

Based on the current available information, it seems appropriate to keep indirect bilirubin values below 10 mg/100 ml in infants of 1,000 g, below 15 mg/100 ml in infants of 1,500 g, below 17-18 ml in infants of 1,500-2,500 g, and less than 20 mg/100 ml in term infants. It is important to note that these rough guidelines have not been developed as the result of a large controlled prospective study, but rather are based on clinical experience and case reports of kernicterus at low bilirubin levels [17, 18, 28]. However, the available information in the literature and in our own experience does indicate that low birth weight infants are less likely to tolerate high bilirubin levels than are healthy term infants. A more sensitive approach than these admittedly imprecise guidelines may be found by use of one or more of the bilirubin binding tests reported by many authors. These tests can give some indication of the extent of albumin saturation with bilirubin or of additional albumin binding sites available and allow some estimation of the margin of safety for the infant. At present, however, none of the available binding tests can be used as an absolute guide to therapy, because clinical deterioration of the infant, physiologic or chemical changes affecting the level and binding ability of serum albumin, or the unavoidable use of a potentially displacing drug may lower the threshold at which kernicterus is possible and at which exchange transfusion should be considered.

An exchange transfusion is the treatment of choice when clinical and/or laboratory findings indicate an indirect bilirubin level which is already hazardous. This procedure results in a prompt decrease in plasma bilirubin levels as the patient's bilirubin-loaded albumin is exchanged for fresh unsaturated albumin, cells susceptible to hemolysis are exchanged for cells not sensitized to the antibody causing the hemolysis, and bilirubin re-equilibrates from the tissues to the plasma compartment within several hours after the transfusion. For treating hyperbilirubinemia the usual practice is to exchange twice the infant's blood volume (2×80 or 160 ml/kg) via the umbilical artery or vein. Heparinized or citrate phosphate dextrose preserved blood may be used; it is best to avoid acid citrate dextrose blood since the pH of that blood is approximately 6.0. For the purpose of lowering bilirubin levels, freshly drawn blood is not considered necessary, but the freshest possible blood available (3 days old or less) is preferred. For infants of 3,000-3,500 g or larger, a complete double volume exchange transfusion will require more than

one unit (450 ml) of blood; however, the use of a second unit of blood with its attendant expenses and risks is not usually warranted in such cases, since most of the intravascular red cells and albumin are effectively replaced after one and one-half blood volumes have been exchanged. Occasionally, it becomes necessary to use a second unit of blood for an effective exchange transfusion of a very large baby (4,000-4,500 gms or larger). The umbilical vein is the route preferred by most experienced operators [65], although a freshly placed indwelling arterial catheter can be used with caution if the blood is filtered. Occasionally it becomes necessary to perform an exchange transfusion via a peripheral venous cutdown in a larger or older child whose umbilical vessels are no longer accessible. However, this is seldom necessary during the immediate newborn period or during the first week after birth. While standard practice in neonatal hyperbilirubinemia is to perform a double volume exchange transfusion, not all exchange transfusions performed for other purposes require exactly the same volumes. When an exchange transfusion is performed to replace red cells, white cells, platelets, or clotting factors, a single volume exchange transfusion is often sufficient. If the exchange transfusion is performed for the removal of other toxins, for example, to lower high magnesium levels resulting from the administration of large maternal doses of magnesium sulfate, the volume of the exchange transfusion may be judged according to the clinical response.

The effect on serum bilirubin of a double volume exchange is to lower the serum bilirubin levels to about 50-55 % of the pre-exchange level. Since approximately half of the albumin in the extracellular water is outside the vascular compartment, within an hour after completion of the exchange transfusion serum bilirubin levels rise again by about one-third the amount of the decrease produced by the exchange transfusion. For example, if the exchange transfusion lowers serum bilirubin levels from 20 mg/100 ml to 11 mg/100 ml a "rebound" to 14 mg/100 ml is to be expected. The subsequent rate of rise in bilirubin can then be calculated after the rebound has been taken into account, so that further steps in therapy may be planned.

The recognized complications of exchange transfusion (hypocalcemia, hyperkalemia, hypoglycemia, hypovolemia or hypervolemia) are rare in healthy infants and treatable if promptly identified. The cost and time required for an exchange transfusion and the fact that it is an invasive procedure are outweighed by its effectiveness. Other treatments for jaundice act a great deal more slowly and do not provide for the rapid re-equilibration of high tissue levels of bilirubin with the plasma or for the rapid binding of high levels of unbound bilirubin to fresh albumin.

Phototherapy acts by isomerizing bilirubin to a water soluble form which can be excreted by the hepatocyte into the biliary system and the small bowel without the need to conjugate indirect reacting bilirubin [76]. At the level of the cutaneous circulation, the major effect of phototherapy at wavelengths of 400-500 nm is to isomerize bilirubin with a smaller fraction of the bilirubin broken down into water soluble and presumably harmless dipyrroles. The action of phototherapy is much slower than that of exchange transfusion, so that the therapy must be planned in anticipation of high bilirubin levels; the action of phototherapy in the usual doses is to stabilize the bilirubin level or to slow further increases in serum bilirubin rather than to lower serum bilirubin levels dramatically. For this reason, phototherapy is not an acceptable substitute for exchange transfusion once the serum indirect bilirubin has already reached presumably dangerous levels. The effectiveness of phototherapy depends on the area of skin exposed, the number and intensity of fluorescent bulbs used, and their distance from the infant [77]. In our nursery, we use at least eight 200-watt fluorescent bulbs at a distance not greater than 50 cm from an infant who is totally undressed. In addition to shielding the lightbulbs themselves, phototherapy should be given in transparent closed incubators to avoid accidents with the equipment. Since the infants are kept in closed incubators, it is also necessary to pay close attention to temperature stability, particularly in the larger infants. The major complications seem to be related to increased insensible water loss by two routes: in small infants, transcutaneous insensible water loss is markedly increased [78]. In most infants, the increased flow of bile pigments also results in increased water loss in the stool, with a characteristic dark green "phototherapy" stool often being seen [79]. Other notable complications include a fine maculo-papular rash in a small percentage of patients and the "bronzed baby syndrome" in some patients who have direct as well as indirect bilirubinemia [80]. To date, no serious permanent harm has been reported from any of these complications. The possibility exists of retinal damage from prolonged exposure to bright light, and therefore, the eyes of the newborn are patched during phototherapy. Follow-up studies have not revealed any indications of permanent retinal damage in humans [81]. While in general the fall in bilirubin level is related to the duration of light exposure,

it has been shown that intermittent phototherapy is effective, so that the infant may be removed from under the phototherapy lamps for brief periods for purposes of feeding, bathing, dressing, and increased maternal attachment.

The most appropriate use of phototherapy is in the early treatment of infants who are clinically unstable and for whom the risk of exchange transfusion is considered unacceptably high. Early phototherapy is often ineffective in preventing the initial exchange transfusion for antibody induced hemolysis from Rh or ABO hemolytic disease and is not the primary therapy of choice for those conditions. In the treatment of antibody hemolysis, exchange transfusion not only lowers the serum bilirubin rapidly, but also carries the added benefit of removing some of the antibody and replacing many of the vulnerable circulating red cells. In hemolytic diseases of the newborn, the early use of phototherapy may mask the true rate of bilirubin accumulation without preventing an eventual exchange transfusion, and at times may allow the progression of the hemolytic anemia which could be more effectively treated by exchange transfusion. In the management of idiopathic hyperbilirubinemia in healthy term and preterm infants, phototherapy will stabilize the bilirubin level and reduce the peak level of indirect bilirubin but the infant may remain exposed to moderately high levels of jaundice for several days. When phototherapy does not appear able to stabilize the serum bilirubin at an acceptable level within a reasonable length of time (12-24 hours), then the performance of exchange transfusion according to established criteria may be a quicker, safer and more effective treatment.

Besides the rapid production of bilirubin by rapid hemolysis, there are several other reasons why phototherapy may appear ineffective or less than optimally effective under certain circumstances. The most obvious reason is an inadequate dose of light due to insufficient strength of the light bulbs, insufficient exposure of skin, or a distance too great between the lights and the skin surface [77]. Even fluctuations in hospital line voltage may change the light intensity sufficiently to decrease the effectiveness of phototherapy. In some infants, the cause of jaundice (for example, a breast milk factor prolonging the period of physiologic jaundice, a hepatic or high intestinal obstruction, rapid destruction of red cells in an enclosed hemorrhage, or a metabolic disease such galactosemia) persisting even while phototherapy is given may reduce its effectiveness. The bilirubin photoisomer excreted via the liver into the small bowel may be reabsorbed in the face of decreased bowel motility or the absence of bacteria able to oxidize it to harmless products; this may be especially the case in low birth weight infants who are not fed.

Although exact procedures vary between hospitals, moderately jaundiced infants may be sent home from the hospital if the bilirubin level is stable or falling and if the cause of the jaundice has been determined. We usually discharge healthy term infants on the third or fourth hospital day if bilirubin levels are stable at 12-13 mg/100 ml out of phototherapy for the preceding 24 hours. If the indirect bilirubin is 15 mg/100 ml or greater on the third hospital day, we prefer to keep the baby in the hospital for at least 24 hours of further observation. We do not usually keep healthy infants with moderately elevated but stable bilirubin levels of 12-15 mg/% under phototherapy beyond the third to fourth day, but prefer to observe such infants and even to send them home unless the bilirubin levels are continuing to rise. When distances are short and hospital facilities are available, many moderately jaundiced infants may be discharged if the parents are cooperative and well informed and are properly instructed to bring their infant back to the hospital for follow-up bilirubin determinations as an outpatient.

In our opinion then, the ideal candidates for phototherapy include: (1) low birth weight infants in whom the risks of exchange transfusion may be unacceptably high; these infants may be placed under phototherapy as a preventative measure as early as the first hospital day to keep their bilirubin level as low as possible; (2) term infants with jaundice of sudden onset, for example, from an enclosed hemorrhage, provided they are not shown to have hemolytic anemia characterized by rapid early hemolysis and an early onset of jaundice. An example would be the infant with a serum indirect bilirubin level between 10-12 mg/% on the second hospital day, with no other condition necessitating an exchange transfusion. In such cases, 24 hours of phototherapy may stabilize the bilirubin level below the point at which the infant would have to be kept in the hospital. We would probably not place this same infant under phototherapy with a stable bilirubin level of 12-14 mg/% on the third or fourth hospital day; (3) a third group eligible for phototherapy would be those infants requiring prospective treatment with an obvious underlying cause for jaundice, but whose parents have strong religious objections to the use of blood transfusions; (4) finally, certain infants with hereditary defects of bilirubin conjugation may be treated with phototherapy over a long period of time to prevent an uncontrollable rise in serum bilirubin levels leading to kernicterus.

When a factor in the breast milk is causing prolonged neonatal jaundice, temporary cessation of breast feeding for 24-48 hours is often followed promptly by a fall in serum bilirubin concentration. The mother should be encouraged to resume nursing within 48-72 hours. Resumption of nursing at this point is usually safe since hepatic maturation following cessation of breast feeding is usually sufficient to overcome the inhibitor effect. It is only rarely necessary to discontinue breast feeding entirely because of persistent neonatal jaundice. Many infants who develop early jaundice while breast feeding are actually preterm infants of 35-37 weeks gestation and of 2,400-2,800 gm birth weight. A careful analysis of the problem in these infants will often show that they do not suck well, that milk production in the mother is sometimes sub-optimal for the first few days, and that weight loss in the nursery has been excessive. While in most cases the mothers of these infants should be encouraged to continue nursing, at times it becomes necessary to intervene with alternative forms of feeding, especially using a softer nipple so that the infant's intake is increased. Jaundice in these cases may be due more to dehydration and to the immaturity of the infant's hepatic conjugating system than to a factor in the breast milk itself.

A number of other therapies have been suggested for neonatal jaundice. These include the use of activated charcoal [82], cholestyramine, or agar [83] to decrease the enterohepatic recirculation of bilirubin and to increase its excretion. Phenobarbital (in addition to a number of other compounds) given to the mother or to the baby early in the hospital course, induces the activity of hepatic glucuronyl transferase, and may lower peak bilirubin concentrations [84]. Given to an infant who already has hyperbilirubinemia, enzyme induction with phenobarbital is not usually rapid enough to be effective. While this therapy is not widely used in North America, in underdeveloped areas where geography and hospital facilities prevent a prolonged stay for mother or infant or hinder prompt recognition and treatment of severe jaundice, phenobarbital may have some advantages, especially if given to the mother shortly before delivery. This therapy has been found beneficial in several areas of the world where severe idiopathic unconjugated hyperbilirubinemia is more common than it is in North America, and where medical facilities are not always available for the performance of exchange transfusions or phototherapy [84]. A review of the treatments of neonatal jaundice without exchange transfusion suggests that, while the rate of bilirubin formation in the newborn cannot be controlled, its rate of excretion can be affected by a number of therapeutic modalities. Further understanding of the chemistry and physiology of the bilirubin molecule and of the nature of prolonged hyperbilirubinemia in certain infants may allow more precise matching of the therapy to the cause of the jaundice in some newborns.

REFERENCES

[1] BRODERSEN (R.). — Bilirubin solubility and interaction with albumin and phospholipid. *J. Biol. Chem.*, *254*, 2364, 1979.

[2] JACOBSEN (J.). — Binding of bilirubin to human serum albumin: determination of the dissociation constants. *FEBS Lett.*, *5*, 112, 1969.

[3] NAGAOKA (S.), COWGER (M.). — Interaction of bilirubin with lipids studied by fluorescence quenching method. *J. Biol. Chem.* *253*, 2009, 1979.

[4] LEVI (A. J.), GATMAITAN (Z.), ARIAS (I. M.). — Two hepatic cytoplasmic fractions, Y and Z, and their possible role in the hepatic uptake of bilirubin, sulfobromphthalein, and other anions. *J. Clin. Invest.*, *45*, 2156, 1969.

[5] SCHMID (R.). — Hyperbilirubinemia. In STANBURY (J. B.), WYNGAARDEN (J. B.), FREDERICKSON (D. S.), eds.: *The Metabolic Basis of Inherited Disease*, 3rd ed., New York, McGraw-Hill, 1141-1178, 1972.

[6] MAISELS (M. J.), PATHAK (A.), NELSON (N. M.) et coll. — Endogenous production of carbon monoxide in normal and erythroblastotic newborn infants. *J. Clin. Invest.*, *50*, 1, 1971.

[7] BARTOLETTI (A. L.), STEVENSON (D. K.), OSTRANDER (C. R.), JOHNSON (J. D.). — Pulmonary excretion of carbon monoxide in the human infant as an index of bilirubin production. I. Effects of gestational and postnatal age and some common neonatal abnormalities. *J. Pediatr.*, *94*, 952, 1979.

[8] BROWN (A. K.), ZUELZER, (W. W.). — Studies on the neonatal development of the glucuronide conjugating system. *J. Clin. Invest.*, *37*, 322, 1958.

[9] BROWN (A. K.), SCOGGIN (W. A.). — Studies of bilirubin and water transfer across umbilical cord and fetal skin. *Proc. Soc. Ped. Res.*, Atlantic City, New Jersey, 264, 1971.

[10] LILEY (A. W.). — Liquor amnii analysis in the management of the pregnancy complicated by Rhesus sensitization. *Am. J. Obstet. Gynecol.*, *82*, 1359, 1961.

[11] GOODLIN (R.), LLOYD (D.). — Fetal tracheal excretion of bilirubin. *Biol. Neonate*, *12*, 1, 1968.

[12] SCHMORL (G.). — Zur Kenntnis des Icterus neonatorum. *Verh. Deutsch. Ges. Path.*, *6*, 109, 1903.

[13] MOLLISON (P. L.), CUTBUSH (M.). — Hemolytic disease of the newborn: criteria of severity. *Brit. Med. J.*, *1*, 123, 1949.

[14] OSKI (F. A.), NAIMAN (J. L.). — *Hematologic problems in the newborn*, 2nd ed., Philadelphia, Saunders (W. B.), 191, 1972.

[15] GERVER (J. M.), DAY (R.). — Intelligence quotient of children who have recovered from erythroblastosis fetalis. *J. Pediatr.*, *36*, 342, 1950.

[16] DAY (R.), HARRIS (M. S.). — Intelligence quotients of children recovered from erythroblastosis fetalis since the introduction of exchange transfusion. *Pediatrics*, *13*, 333, 1954.

[17] STERN (L.), DENTON (R. L.). — Kernicterus in small premature infants. *Pediatrics*, *35*, 483, 1965.

[18] GARTNER (L. M.), SNYDER (R. N.), CHABON (R. S.), BERNSTEIN (J.). — Kernicterus: high incidence in premature infants with low serum bilirubin concentrations. *Pediatrics*, *45*, 906, 1970.

[19] COWGER (M. L.). — Mechanism of bilirubin toxicity in tissue culture cells: factors that affect toxicity, reversibility by albumin, and comparison with other respiratory poisons and surfactants. *Biochem. Med.*, *5*, 1, 1971.

[20] DIAMOND (I.), SCHMID (R.). — Oxidative phosphorylation in experimental bilirubin encephalopathy. *Science*, *155*, 1288, 1967.

[21] SHEPHERD (R. E.), MORENO (F. J.), CASHORE (W. J.), FAIN (J. N.). — Effects of bilirubin on fat cell metabolism and lipolysis. *Am. J. Physiol.*, *237*, E504-E508, 1979.

[22] GOLDSTEIN (G. W.), WOLINSKY (J. S.), CSEJTEY (J.), DIAMOND (I.). — Isolation of metabolically active capillaries from rat brain. *J. Neurochem.*, *25*, 715, 1975.

[23] DIAMOND (I.), SCHMID (R.). — Experimental bilirubin encephalopathy. The mode of entry of bilirubin-^{14}C into the central nervous system. *J. Clin. Invest.*, *45*, 678, 1966.

[24] ØIE (S.), LEVY (G.). — Effect of sulfisoxazole on pharmacokinetics of free and plasma protein-bound bilirubin in experimental unconjugated hyperbilirubinemia. *J. Pharmaceut. Sci.*, *68*, 6, 1979.

[25] SILVERMAN (W. A.), ANDERSEN (D. H.), BLANC (W. A.), CROZIER (D. N.). — A difference in mortality rates and incidence of kernicterus among premature infants allotted to two prophylactic antibacterial regimens. *Pediatrics*, *18*, 614, 1956.

[26] LEVINE (R. L.). — Bilirubin: worked out years ago? *Pediatrics*, *64*, 380, 1979.

[27] RAPOPORT (S. I.). — *The Blood-Brain Barrier in Physiology and Medicine*. Raven Press, New York, N. Y., 87-152, 1976.

[28] CASHORE (W. J.). — Free bilirubin concentrations and bilirubin binding affinity in term and pre-term infants. *J. Pediatr.*, *96*, 521, 1980.

[29] ØIE (S.), LEVY (G.). — Effect of salicylic acid on pharmacokinetics of free and plasma protein-bound bilirubin in experimental unconjugated hyperbilirubinemia. *J. Pharmaceut. Sci.*, *68*, 1, 1979.

[30] BRODERSEN (R.). — Bilirubin transport in the newborn infant, reviewed with relation to kernicterus. *J. Pediatr.*, *96*, 349, 1980.

[31] NELSON (T.), JACOBSEN (J.), WENNBERG (R. P.). — Effect of *p*H on the interaction of bilirubin with albumin and tissue culture cells. *Pediatr. Res.*, *8*, 963, 1974.

[32] CASHORE (W. J.), HORWICH (A.), KAROTKIN (E. H.), OH (W.). — The influence of gestational age and clinical status on bilirubin binding capacity in newborn infants determined by Sephadex G-25 gel filtration technique. *Am. J. Dis. Child.*, *131*, 898, 1977.

[33] SCHIFF (D.), CHAN (G.), STERN (L.). — Sephadex G-25 quantitative estimation of free bilirubin potential in jaundiced infants' sera: a guide to the prevention of kernicterus. *J. Lab. Clin. Med.*, *80*, 455, 1972.

[34] KAPITULNIK (J.), VALAES (T.), KAUFMANN (N. A.) et al. — Clinical evaluation of Sephadex gel filtration in the estimation of bilirubin binding in

serum in neonatal jaundice. *Arch. Dis. Child.*, *49*, 886, 1974.

[35] ODELL (G. B.), STOREY (G. N. B.), ROSENBERG (L. A.). — Studies in kernicterus. III. The saturation of serum proteins with bilirubin during neonatal life and its relation to brain damage at 5 years. *J. Pediatr.*, *76*, 12, 1970.

[36] KAPITULNIK (J.), HORNER-MIBASHAN (R.), BLOND-HEIM (S. H.) *et al.* — Increase in bilirubin-binding affinity of serum with age of infant. *J. Pediatr.*, *86*, 442, 1975.

[37] CASHORE (W. J.), HORWICH (A.), LATERRA (J.), OH (W.). — Effect of postnatal age and clinical status of newborn infants on bilirubin-binding capacity. *Biol. Neonate*, *32*, 304, 1977.

[38] JACOBSEN (J.), WENNBERG (R. P.). — Determination of unbound bilirubin in the serum of newborns. *Clin. Chem.*, *20*, 783, 1974.

[39] PORTER (E. G.), WATERS (W. J.). — A rapid micromethod for measuring the reserve binding capacity in serum from newborn infants with hyperbilirubinemia. *J. Lab. Clin. Med.*, *67*, 660, 1966.

[40] LEE (K. S.), GARTNER (L. M.), ZARAFU (I.). — Fluorescent dye method for the determination of the bilirubin binding capacity of serum albumin. *J. Pediatr.*, *86*, 280, 1975.

[41] LEVINE (R. L.). — Fluorescence-quenching studies of the binding of bilirubin to albumin. *Clin. Chem.*, *23*, 2292, 1977.

[42] LAMOLA (A. A.), EISINGER (J.), BLUMBERG (W. E.), PATEL (S. C.), FLORES (J.). — Fluorometric study of the partition of bilirubin among blood components: basis for rapid microassays of bilirubin and bilirubin binding capacity in whole blood. *Anal. Biochem.*, *101*, 25, 1979.

[43] CASHORE (W. J.), OH (W.), BLUMBERG (W. E.) *et al.* — Rapid fluorometric assay of bilirubin and bilirubin binding capacity in blood of jaundiced neonates: comparisons with other methods. *Pediatrics*, *66*, 411, 1980.

[44] BERDE (C. B.), HUDSON (B. S.), SIMONI (R. D.), SKLAR (L. A.). — Human serum albumin: spectroscopic studies of binding and proximity relationships for fatty acids and bilirubin. *J. Biol. Chem.*, *254*, 391, 1979.

[45] BEAVER (G. H.), D'ALBIS (A.), GRATZER (W. B.). — The interaction of bilirubin with human serum albumin. *Eur. J. Biochem.*, *32*, 500, 1973.

[46] ODELL (G. B.), COHEN (S. N.), KELLY (P. C.). — Studies in kernicterus. II. The determination of the saturation of serum albumin with bilirubin. *J. Pediatr.*, *74*, 214, 1969.

[47] HSIA (J. C.), KWAN (N. H.), ER (S. S.) *et al.* — Development of a spin assay for reserve bilirubin loading capacity of human serum. *Proc. Natl. Acad. Sci. USA*, *75*, 1542, 1978.

[48] BRODERSEN (R.). — Determination of the vacant amount of high-affinity bilirubin binding site on serum albumin. *Acta Pharmac. Tox.*, *42*, 153, 1978.

[49] CASHORE (W. J.), GARTNER (L. M.), OH (W.), STERN (L.). — Clinical application of neonatal bilirubin-binding determinations: current status. *J. Pediatr.*, *93*, 827, 1978.

[50] GITZELMANN-CUMARASWAMY (N.), KUENZLE (C. C.). — Bilirubin binding tests: living up to expectations? *Pediatrics*, *64*, 375, 1979.

[51] BROWN (A. K.), MCGAUGHEY (H. S.). — Observations on maternal fetal, and placental bilirubin concentrations at the time of delivery. *Am. J. Dis. Child.*, *100*, 574, 1960.

[52] DAHMS (B. B.), KRAUSS (A. N.), GARTNER (L. M.) *et al.* — Breast feeding and serum bilirubin values during the first 4 days of life. *J. Pediatr.*, *83*, 1049, 1973.

[53] MAISELS (M. J.). — Neonatal jaundice. *In* AVERY (G. B.), Ed.: *Neonatology*, 2nd ed., Philadelphia and Toronto, J. B. Lippincott Co., 473-544, 1981.

[54] STERN (L.), KHANNA (N. N.), LEVY (G.), YAFFE (S. J.). — Effect of phenobarbital on hyperbilirubinemia and glucuronide formation in newborns. *Am. J. Dis. Child.*, *120*, 26, 1970.

[55] BROWN (A. K.). — Perinatal aspects of bilirubin metabolism. *In* WYNN (R. M.), ed., *Obstet. Gynecol. Annual.*, *4*, 191, 1975.

[56] BROWN (A. K.). — Neonatal jaundice. *Pediatr. Clin. N. Am.*, *9*, 575, 1962.

[57] TAYLOR (P. M.), WOLFSON (J. H.), BRIGHT (N. H.) et coll. — Hyperbilirubinemia in infants of diabetic mothers. *Biol. Neonate*, *5*, 289, 1963.

[58] SAIGAL (S.), O'NEILL (A.), SURAINDER (Y. A.) *et al.* — Placental transfusion and hyperbilirubinemia in the premature. *Pediatrics*, *49*, 406, 1972.

[59] ARIAS (I. M.), GARTNER (L. M.), SEIFTER (S.) *et al.* — Prolonged neonatal inconjugated hyperbilirubinemia associated with breast feeding and a steroid pregnane-3α20β diol, in maternal milk that inhibits glucuronide formation *in vitro*. *J. Clin. Invest.*, *43*, 2037, 1964.

[60] RAMOS (A.), SILVERBERG (M.), STERN (L.). — Pregnanediols and neonatal hyperbilirubinemia. *Am. J. Dis. Child.*, *113*, 353, 1966.

[61] GARTNER (L. M.), LEE (K. S.). — Effect of starvation and milk feeding on intestinal bilirubin absorption. *Pediatr. Res.*, *14*, 498, 1980 (Abstract).

[62] ZIPURSKY (A.). — *In* NATHAN (D.) and OSKI (F. H.), Eds.: *Hematology of Infancy and Childhood*, 2nd ed., Philadelphia, W. B. Saunders Co., 78-80, 1981.

[63] OSKI (F. A.), NAIMAN (J. L.). — *Hematologic Problems in the Newborn*, 2nd ed., Philadelphia, W. B. Saunders Co., 226-232, 1972.

[64] COHEN (F.), ZUELZER (W. W.), GUSTAFSON (D. C.), EVANS (M. M.). — Mechanisms of isoimmunization I. The transplacental passage of fetal erythrocytes in heterospecific pregnancies. *Blood*, *23*, 621, 1964.

[65] ALLEN (F. H.), DIAMOND (L. K.). — *Erythroblastosis Fetalis, Including Exchange Transfusion Technique.* Boston, Little Brown, 1958.

[66] ZIPURSKY (A.), ISRAELS (L. G.). — The pathogenesis and prevention of Rh immunization. *Can. Med. Assoc. J.*, *97*, 1245, 1967.

[67] Combined Study. — Prevention of Rh-haemolytic disease: final results of the « high risk » clinical trial. A combined study from centres in England and Baltimore. *Br. Med. J.. 2*, 607, 1971.

[68] BUCHANAN (D. I.), BELL (R. E.), BECK (R. P.), TAYLOR (W. C.). — Use of different doses of anti-Rh IgG in the prevention of Rh isoimmunization. *Lancet*, *2*, 288, 1969.

[69] GLUCK (L.), KULOVICH (M. V.), BORER (R. C.) et coll. — Diagnosis of the respiratory distress syndrome by amniocentesis. *Am. J. Obstet. Gynecol.*, *109*, 440, 1971.

[70] LIGGINS (G. C.), HOWIE (R. N.). — A controlled trial of antepartum glucocorticoid treatment for prevention of the respiratory distress syndrome in premature infants. *Pediatrics*, *50*, 515, 1972.

[71] LUCEY (J. F.). — Diagnosis and treatment of the fetus with erythroblastosis. *Pediatr. Clin. N. Am.*, *13*, 117, 1966.

[72] PHIBBS (R. H.), JOHNSON (P.), KITTERMAN (J. A.), GREGORY (G. A.), TOOLEY (W. H.). — Cardiorespiratory status of erythroblastotic infants. I. Relationship of gestational age, severity of hemolytic disease, and birth asphyxia to idiopathic respiratory distress syndrome and survival. *Pediatrics*, *45*, 9, 1972.

[73] ALLEN (F. H. J.), DIAMOND (L. K.), VAUGHAN (V. C. III). — Erythroblastosis fetalis. VI. Prevention of kernicterus. *Am. J. Dis. Child.*, *80*, 779, 1950.

[74] CREMER (R. J.), PERRYMAN (P. W.), RICHARDS (D. H.). — Influence of light on the hyperbilirubinemia of infants. *Lancet*, *1*, 1094, 1958.

[75] SCHIFF (D.), ARANDA (J. V.), COLLE (E.), STERN (L.). — Metabolic effects of exchange transfusions. I. Effect of citrated and of heparinized blood on glucose, non-esterified fatty acids, 2-(4 hydroxybenzeneazo) benzoic acid binding, and insulin. *J. Pediatr.*, *78*, 603, 1971.

[76] MCDONAGH (A. F.), PALMA (L. A.), LIGHTNER (D. A.). — Blue light and bilirubin excretion. *Science*, *208*, 145, 1980.

[77] BONTA (B. W.), WARSHAW (J. B.). — Importance of radiant flux in the treatment of hyperbilirubinemia: failure of overhead phototherapy units in intensive care units. *Pediatrics*, *57*, 502, 1976.

[78] BELL (E. F.), NEIDRICH (G. A.), CASHORE (W. J.), OH (W.). — Combined effect of radiant warmer and phototherapy on insensible water loss in low birth weight infants. *J. Pediatr.*, *94*, 810, 1979.

[79] RUBALTELLI (F. F.), LARGAJOLLI (G.). — Effect of light exposure on gut transit time in jaundiced newborns. *Acta Paediatr. Scand.*, *62*, 146, 1973.

[80] KOPELMAN (A. E.), BROWN (R. S.), ODELL (G. B.). — The « bronze » baby syndrome: a complication of phototherapy. *J. Pediatr.*, *81*, 466, 1972.

[81] DOBSON (V.), COWETT (R. M.), RIGGS (L. A.). — Long-term effect of phototherapy on visual function. *J. Pediatr.*, *86*, 555. 1975.

[82] ULSTROM (R. A.), EISENKLAM (E.). — The enterohepatic shunting of bilirubin in the newborn infant. I. Use of oral activated charcoal to reduce normal serum bilirubin values. *J. Pediatr.*, *65*, 27, 1964.

[83] POLAND (R. D.), ODELL (G. B.). — Physiologic jaundice: the enterohepatic circulation of bilirubin. *N. Engl. J. Med.*, *284*, 1, 1971.

[84] VALAES (T.), KIPONROS (K.), PETMEZAKI (S.) *et al.* — Effectiveness and safety of prenatal phenobarbital for the prevention of neonatal jaundice. *Pediatr. Res.*, *14*, 947, 1980.

37

Glucose metabolism and homeostasis

Richard M. COWETT and Robert SCHWARTZ

INTRODUCTION

The neonate is born not only with the requirement of providing itself with substrate, especially carbohydrate for energy and growth, but also with the necessity of maintaining a balance between glucose deficiency and excess. The conceptus' dependence on the maternal organism for continuous substrate delivery in utero may be contrasted with the variable and intermittent exogenous oral intake by the neonate. Maturation of neonatal carbohydrate homeostasis results from a balance between substrate availability and coordination of developing hormonal, enzymatic, and neural systems. The number of conditions producing or associated with neonatal hypo- or hyperglycemia, especially in the sick term or low birth weight infant, emphasizes the vulnerability of the neonate to carbohydrate disequilibrium. These concepts have recently been presented elsewhere [31].

Glucose homeostasis in the fetus

The neonate depends upon substrate previously acquired and accumulated in utero to support carbohydrate needs in the period immediately following delivery. Until recently, exogenous glucose (from the mother) was thought to be the only substrate utilized in fetal oxidative reactions. This was based on the original work of Bohr and others who estimated the respiratory quotient (R/Q) to be one, and who found a rapid rate of glucose utilization, which was in excess of the utilization rate of other substrates [12]. Subsequent investigations have suggested that the R/Q is high, but less than one. Furthermore, carbon balance data support the conclusion that glucose uptake may represent only 23 % of fetal carbon uptake [60]. Other substrates such as lactate and amino acids have also been considered as important for fetal oxidative reactions in the fetal lamb, especially in the fasted state [55].

Maternal glucose delivery to the fetus is controlled by factors influencing blood flow and maternal glucose concentration. Analyses of factors affecting delivery of glucose are limited. In studies in late gestation using fetal lambs, glucose turnover rates with labelled substrate have been compared to umbilical glucose uptake rates. In some studies it has been suggested that fetal gluconeogenesis and not simply exogenous glucose delivery may provide important contributions to fetal glucose homeostasis [12]. These data indicate that the simple dependency relationship of the fetus on the mother for substrate delivery may, in fact, be much more complex [56].

However, recent studies have analyzed glucose kinetics by evaluation of double labelled tracers in the pregnant ewe and her conceptus. In the fed state all fetal glucose turnover was derived from the mother through placental transfer without any evidence of fetal glucose production. Simultaneously with maternal fetal glucose transfer, fetal maternal glucose transfer equalled approximately 50 % of the total glucose transferred to the fetus from the mother. These authors concluded that fetal glucose production did not occur [6]. This was subsequently reaffirmed by the same authors when pregnant animals were made hypoglycemic using exogenous insulin [5]. Further analyses will be required to evaluate the contradictions between the various investigations in this area.

A number of hormones are thought to play major roles in utero. Of particular importance, in addition to pancreatic hormones, are hormones secreted by the placenta, anterior pituitary and the adrenal cortex [28, 64]. In early to mid-pregnancy, increased tissue glycogen storage and a suppressed maternal fasting plasma glucose concentration are related to secretion of estrogen and progesterone [64]. The anabolic effects of these steroids plus induction of increased B cell insulin secretion result in reduced hepatic glucose production and peripheral glucose utilization [28, 80, 94, 140].

During the last trimester of pregnancy, other hormones achieve maximum concentration, and the emergence of insulin antagonism and resistance results in deterioration of glucose tolerance in the mother [64]. Human chorionic somatomammotropin (HCS) and prolactin have been implicated as significant. Beck and Daughaday initially noted that HCS is diabetogenic [15] and is produced in quantities exceeding any other polypeptide hormone in late pregnancy [66]. Increasing in amount in parallel with an increase in placental mass, HCS results in "contrainsulin" effects such as an impaired glucose uptake as well as stimulation of maternal free fatty acid (FFA) release [42]. The hormone may act to insure a steady source of glucose for the fetus while insulin may function as a fluctuating modifier of the effects of HCS on the maternal organism [65].

Another hormone whose concentration is altered in late pregnancy is cortisol. Kalkhoff et al. suggest that this steroid may counteract the sex steroids and insulin with respect to hepatic glucose production and peripheral uptake of glucose in late pregnancy [64].

The integration of these effects results in an adequate supply of glucose for the fetus since insulin increases glycogen, fat, and protein synthesis while human chorionic somatomammotropin decreases maternal glucose utilization [119].

The role of insulin in fetal glucose homeostasis has also received considerable attention, but the results are conflicting. While earlier work suggested that insulin may not control the rate of fetal glucose utilization, other investigations utilizing the chronically catheterized lamb fetus as a model suggest that infusion of insulin into the fetal circulation leads to an increase in glucose uptake and utilization. Although this possible mechanism of action of insulin requires further elaboration, these findings would correlate with the well-accepted growth promoting effect of insulin in utero [55].

The factors which influence fetal insulin secretion are equally important [91]. Insulin is present in the fetal pancreas as early as the tenth gestational week and in the fetal plasma from the twelfth week of gestation [100, 127]. The placenta is known to be impermeable to insulin transfer [103]. A number of reports have suggested that fetal insulin may be more responsive to amino acid stimulation than to glucose in utero [52, 112]. Further work is also required to substantiate their findings. A recent review has evaluated the current data of the various hormonal influences (insulin and glucagon) in utero and neonatally [123].

Glucose homeostasis at delivery

At the time of birth, the plasma glucose concentration is euglycemic in the range of 70-80 % of the maternal concentration. The last maternal meal, the length of labor, the mode of delivery, and the type of intravenous fluid administration to the mother all influence the actual concentration [44]. Heretofore, glucose has been considered to be the major substrate for brain oxidative metabolism, since this requires a constant supply of glucose, although ketones, glycerol and lactate can support these metabolic needs [111]. Glucose is extracted at a given rate/unit time irrespective of its concentration in the blood, as long as a minimum amount is available [82].

Evaluation of the adaptation from fetal to neonatal life has been studied in neonatal lambs by analyzing the significance of the plasma glucagon elevations known to occur in a number of species including the human after delivery. An adrenergic mechanism has been postulated as responsible for not only the observed surge in plasma glucagon, but also for the maintenance of the low plasma insulin levels noted. Lipolysis, glycogenolysis and ketogenesis are favored and may be part of the adaptation from fetal to the neonatal period [51].

In the immediate neonatal period, the concentration of glucose in the newborn declines to approximately 50 mg/dl by two hours of age but equilibrates at approximately 70 mg/dl by 72 hours after birth [27]. The actual concentration may be further influenced by environmental temperature and heat loss sustained by the infant (see below). Cornblath and Reisner evaluated the blood glucose concentration over time in an analysis of both term and low birth weight neonates and suggested that concentrations below 40 mg/dl or greater than 125 mg/dl are abnormal after three days of age [26] (see Fig. IV-13).

If oral nutrients cannot be provided as required, the neonatal liver and possibly the kidney may provide glucose by either of two major pathways: (1) lysis of glycogen stored by the fetal liver, or (2) hepatic conversion of amino acids and/or glycerol from lipolysis and/or lactate and pyruvate (via the Cori cycle) to glucose [1]. These reactions

are shown in Figure IV-14 [90]. However, glycogenolysis rapidly decreases glycogen stores and is unable to sustain glucose homeostasis for more than several hours. Previously, neonatal gluconeogenesis was thought to be deficient since neither amino acids, lactate, or pyruvate were actively converted to glucose immediately; however, direct measurement of gluconeogenesis has been reported by six hours after birth in the human newborn [47].

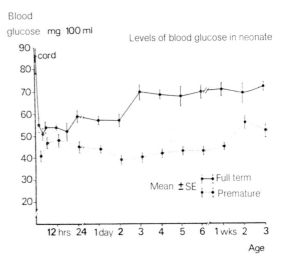

FIG. VI-13. — *Blood glucose concentrations in 179 full-term infants weighing > 2.5 kg (206 determinations) and in 104 low birthweight infants weighing < 2.5 kg (442 determinations) during the neonatal period* [26].

It has been suggested that the maternal hormonal substrate balance primarily regulates fetal glucose concentration and that vaginal delivery causes a readjustment to develop subsequent control [87]. The repetitive occurrence of wide variations in neonatal glucose concentration and the delayed disappearance of an acute exogenous glucose load in both term and preterm infants indicate that the regulation of carbohydrate metabolism is relatively poorly developed in the newborn at birth [118].

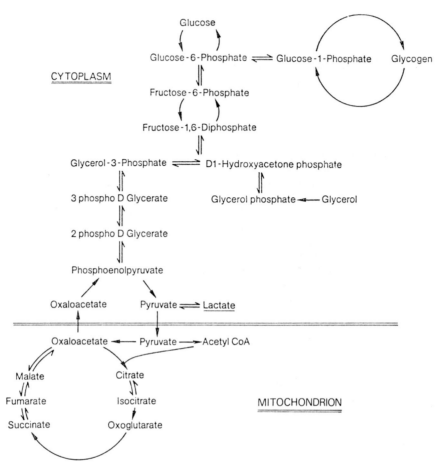

Pathways of glycolysis and gluconeogenesis

FIG. VI-14. — *Pathways of glycolysis and gluconeogenesis in liver and kidney cortex* [90].

Glucose homeostasis in the newborn

In the adult, control of homeostasis is precise and fine control of endogenous hepatic (splanchnic) glucose production is characteristic of the mature (adult) response to either glucose deprivation or exogenous administration. When glucose is infused at a rate equal to or greater than endogenous glucose production, hepatic production of glucose will be diminished [33, 78, 122, 126, 130].

Initially, indirect methodology incorporating stepwise incremental glucose infusions was employed to determine the rate of basal glucose output in the infant in contrast to the adult [2]. Studies in the neonatal puppy utilizing ^{14}C-glucose and the prime plus constant infusion technique have shown that basal glucose production is 2-3 times the adult value expressed/unit body weight [70]. These studies were dependent upon the assumption that the newborn was as sensitive as the adult to minute changes in glucose concentration. Subsequent studies in puppies and in the lamb have suggested that precise regulation of glucose homeostasis is not fully developed [33, 130, 135]. Hepatic suppression of endogenous glucose production does not occur promptly in the neonatal period.

In a more recent study, metabolic fuel and hormone responses to fasting were evaluated in 45 healthy infants at the end of an eight hour fast after birth. The infants were term and preterm AGA and SGA. Plasma glucose concentrations ($\leqslant 40$ mg/dl) were noted by eight hours in a number of infants in all groups, and the fuel and hormone patterns of the premature and SGA infants were similar to those seen in the term AGA infants. In these infants, the capacity for hepatic ketone synthesis appeared to be restricted as was the capacity for hepatic glucose synthesis from lactate and alanine, which would account for the presence of the hypoglycemia noted [125].

There are a number of other studies of glucose homeostasis in the human newborn using stable non-radioactive isotopes such as deuterium at the sixth carbon of glucose [19, 20], ^{13}C at carbon 1 [62, 63] and uniformly ^{13}C labelled glucose [32, 35]. The values obtained range from 2.5 to 6.1 mg/kg/min depending on the age of the newborn, the label used, and the general medical condition of the infant.

There is also data evaluating the autonomic and enzymatic control of neonatal glucose homeostasis, suggesting that glycogenolysis is insufficient to maintain glucose production [24]. Other studies of glucose kinetics have focused on the developmental maturation of the newborn liver and have provided quantitative data concerning steady state hepatic glucose output and peripheral utilization. There is evidence that hepatic unresponsiveness to insulin may be a major factor responsible for the inefficiency in glucose homeostasis noted in the neonatal lamb model [33, 130]. Evaluation of opposing or synergistic hormonal, neural, metabolic, and enzymatic systems is required to understand the maturation of neonatal glucose homeostasis.

HYPOGLYCEMIA IN THE NEWBORN

Hypoglycemia is usually defined as $\leqslant 25$ mg/dl in plasma in the low birth weight infant and $\leqslant 35$ mg/dl in plasma of the term infant at $\leqslant 72$ hours of age. After 72 hours, plasma glucose concentration should be $\geqslant 45$ mg/dl [26]. The main clinical difficulty with these definitions is the non-specific nature of symptomatology, which includes the signs and symptoms listed in Table I. These difficulties are compounded by the occurrence of symptoms at different levels of blood glucose in different infants

TABLE I. — SIGNS AND SYMPTOMS OF NEONATAL HYPOGLYCEMIA

Abnormal cry	Hypothermia
Apathy	Hypotonia
Apnea	Jitteryness
Cardiac arrest	Lethargy
Convulsions	Tremors
Cyanosis	Tachypnea

and the lack of a universal threshold below or above which symptomatology may occur.

Further difficulties may result from lack of attention to the details of laboratory measurement of glucose. One of the most troublesome problems is the failure to measure the glucose concentration rapidly enough so that subsequent blood cell oxidation of glucose results in falsely low plasma values. A number of centers use the Dextrostix * technique, which is reliable if directions are followed carefully. Abnormally low or high values need to be corroborated with laboratory determination of glucose concentration prior to correction of the suspected hypoglycemia unless the patient is symptomatic. It is important also to remember that blood glucose concentration is usually 10-15 % lower than the corresponding plasma glucose value.

A number of different classifications have been employed to categorize the various causes of hypoglycemia seen in the neonatal period. Cornblath and Schwartz [27] and others [45, 53] analyzed the various causes on the basis of clinical course, emphasizing time of presentation, duration, severity, and response to therapy. Another schema considers the biochemical and physiologic parameters and evaluates the relationship between hepatic production and/or uptake in contrast to peripheral utilization [86, 115]. Differentiation of the various causes on the basis of biochemical and physiological parameters would compare decreased hepatic glucose production due to enzymatic or substrate deficiencies to those secondary to increased insulin concentration. Inadequate glucose production includes those conditions involving decreased availability of substrate (*i. e.* glycogen, lactate, glycerol and amino acids), altered sensitivity to neural or hormonal factors, and/or immature or altered enzymatic pathways (*i. e.* gluconeogenesis and/or increased peripheral utilization rates).

* Ames Co.

IMPRECISE/DIMINISHED
HEPATIC GLUCOSE PRODUCTION

Neonatal hypoglycemia secondary to causes other than insulin excess relates primarily to that of diminished hepatic glucose production. The role of hepatic control of glucose homeostasis and its relationship to disequilibrium in the neonate has only recently been subjected to study [30]. Conditions in the newborn which produce hypoglycemia relating to either imprecise control of glucose production or diminished substrate availability include: prematurely born infants appropriate for gestational age (AGA), small for gestational age infants (SGA), perinatally stressed and asphyxiated infants, cold stressed infants and neonates with congenital heart disease and/or sepsis. Infants may also be hypoglycemic because of glucagon deficiency or deficits in intermediary metabolic pathways such as glycogen storage disease type I or fructose 1,6 diphosphatase deficiency reflecting a series of hereditary metabolic disorders in which hypoglycemia may be the initial or most obvious presenting feature.

Preterm appropriate
for gestational age infants
(AGA)

The appropriate for gestational age infant born before term may develop hypoglycemia. While the first report of this entity concerned small for gestational age infants [25] subsequent studies documented hypoglycemia in the low birth weight infant who was appropriate for gestational age. In 1968, Raivio and Hallman reported a frequency of 1.4 % in these infants [98]. Fluge also reported that as many as 14 % of AGA infants showed evidence of neonatal hypoglycemia [45].

The diminished oral and parenteral intake in the low birth weight infant in combination with the decreased concentration of substrates may explain the lower plasma glucose seen in these infants and their propensity to hypoglycemia. Functionally immature gluconeogenic and glycogenolytic enzyme systems present in the neonate potentiate these difficulties. The relatively increased size of the brain (13 % of the body mass in the newborn versus 2 % in the adult) may be responsible for the greater proportion of glucose consumption during periods of fasting, an effect magnified in the low birth weight infant.

Small for gestational age infants
(SGA)

Many centers have reported a relatively high frequency of hypoglycemia in SGA infants since Cornblath et al. in 1959 described its occurrence in eight infants born to mothers with toxemia [25]. Lubchenko and Bard [77], deLeeuw and deVries [37], and others have all substantiated the occurrence of hypoglycemia in these infants. Toxemia has been repeatedly reported to be associated with this occurrence and the incidence of hypoglycemia was highest (61 %) in those infants born to mothers with relatively low urinary estriols, compared to a frequency of 19 % in infants born to mothers with normal estriol levels [25, 37, 69]. Reduction in energy reserves manifested as decreased glycogen deposition combined with increased utilization of substrate may result in the appearance of the hypoglycemia.

There have also been a number of studies evaluating the intermediary metabolism of substrate available postnatally. A functional delay in the development of phosphoenolpyruvate carboxykinase (PEPCK), thought to be the rate limiting enzyme of gluconeogenesis, in SGA infants was suggested by Haymond et al. [57]. This was substantiated by Williams et al. who studied the effect of oral alanine feeding on glucose homeostasis in the SGA infant compared to AGA infants [144]. Oral alanine feeding enhanced plasma glucagon in both groups but only stimulated hepatic glucose output in the AGA infants.

The effect of intravenous glucagon on plasma amino acids has been evaluated in various types of infants including the SGA infant. SGA infants in the first hours of life had significantly less total amino acids compared to a comparable group of AGA infants; although the response to glucagon in the SGA infants mimiced the control (AGA) group. It is speculated that the inability of the SGA infant to extract specific gluconeogenic amino acids could account for the susceptibility to hypoglycemia in these stressed infants [101].

The role of glucagon was also evaluated by Mestyan et al. by measuring 17 amino acids before and during glucagon infusion in normoglycemic and hypoglycemic SGA infants [83]. In the normoglycemic group most amino acid concentrations declined significantly but this did not occur in the SGA infants who were hypoglycemic. Although the effect was transient in nature, these results reinforce the importance of glucagon in acute changes of hepatic glucose homeostasis. This importance was also demonstrated in neonatal lambs between one and three days of age with infusions of somato-statin alone or in combination with insulin and glucagon during an acute two hour interval. Plasma glucose concentration fell when both insulin and glucagon were suppressed acutely suggesting that the latter is of importance in maintaining glucose concentration during short-term fasting. It was suggested that the ratio between the two hormones acutely affected glucose homeostasis [124].

The secretion of glucagon and insulin has been evaluated in SGA infants. Both SGA and AGA infants, after being fed oral glucose and protein (1 g/kg each after a 4 hour fast) had similar secretions of both pancreatic hormones. The authors speculated that the instability of glucose metabolism in the SGA infant followed from the rapid disappearance rate of glucose and probably also because of a transient deficiency of hepatic gluconeogenic enzymes but not from altered secretory patterns of the hormones [104].

Infants Experiencing perinatal stress/hypoxia

Infants who develop an increased rate of utilization of glucose may be prone to hypoglycemia. Since the low birth weight infant is subject to hypoxia, the combination of decreased substrate availability and an increased rate of utilization may result in hypoglycemia. An increased rate of anaerobic glycolysis in combination with an increased rate of glycogenolysis is probably the underlying biochemical mechanism. Two moles of ATP are generated by the Embden Meyerhof anaerobic pathway. Thus, 18 times more glucose is required to generate the same amount of ATP in contrast to aerobic oxidation which results in 36 moles of ATP. In addition, increased lactate production may result in an associated acidosis. Beard has emphasized the association between hypoxia and hypoglycemia in the low birth weight infant and noted increased metabolic needs out of proportion to substrate availability [13, 14]. The difficulties are all accentuated in infants who are clinically compromised and are thus unable to replace substrate from the usual exogenous (oral) sources. What may complicate the situation even further is the inability of hypoxic infants to tolerate an oral glucose load. Metabolic acidosis and lactic acidemia were noted during the first 24 hours of life in four term and eleven preterm infants whose Apgars had been ≤ 5 at one minute after birth and who were fed oral glucose loads [132]. Thus, not only may endogenous stores be depleted, but also these infants may be unable to tolerate an exogenous load.

Cold stressed infants

Hypoglycemia has been identified in infants who experience cold injury. Mann and Elliott described fourteen infants who suffered neonatal cold injury following prolonged exposure to environmental temperatures below 90° F (32.2° C) [79]. Marked hypoglycemia was documented in three of six infants in whom it was measured. The hypoglycemia is presumed to be the result of free fatty acid elevation secondary to a cold induced norepinephrine response [109]. Recognition of the potential association of hypoglycemia following cold stress should result in parenteral treatment if necessary in conjunction with the warming of the infant. In addition, this relationship needs to be considered in the evaluation of blood glucose levels in infants with either temperature instability or who are in a suboptimal thermal environment.

Neonatal sepsis

Neonatal sepsis has been identified with increased frequency in association with hypoglycemia. Yeung noted the association in 20 of 56 infants with signs of sepsis [147]. He suggested that inadequate caloric intake in these infected infants may predispose to hypoglycemia. The possibility of an increased metabolic rate was suggested because of the infusion of ≥ 100 kcal/kg/day by the intravenous route to these infants. A decreased rate of gluconeogenesis has also been documented in laboratory animals following gram negative bacterial infection [71]. The possibility of increased peripheral utilization because of enhanced insulin sensitivity in sepsis has been considered [148]. It is likely that one or more of these factors will operate in specific circumstances to produce the resultant hypoglycemia (see also causes of Neonatal Hyperglycemia).

Infants with congenital heart disease/ congestive heart failure

An inverse relationship has been noted between the concentration of cardiac glycogen and the level of maturity, resulting in low levels in the offspring in mammalian species born with relative maturity, *i. e.* man, monkey, sheep, etc. These reserves are rapidly depleted during anoxia [117]. Benzing et al. reported on a series of 27 patients in whom the simultaneous occurrence of hypoglycemia and acute congestive heart failure was noted in association with congenital heart disease [17]. Reduced dietary intake in association with diminished hepatic glycogen resulted in hypoglycemia. This has been further substantiated by Amatayakul et al. who noted the association of congestive heart failure with hypoglycemia in infants without significant heart defects [4]. The pathophysiology of hypoglycemia in cyanotic congenital heart disease has been studied by Haymond et al. [58]. Six subjects were evaluated between 13 and 67 months of age. Glucose and alanine turnover studies utilizing stable isotope labelled glucose in these infants were compared to controls. A subtle defect in hepatic extraction of gluconeogenic substrates was suspected, possibly secondary to decreased hepatic perfusion. It is apparent that the presence of either hypoglycemia or congestive heart failure should be considered when one or the other appears. The interrelationship of hypoglycemia and pulmonary edema has recently been emphasized. Unfortunately, it was unclear whether the pulmonary edema was secondary to the hypoglycemia or due to treatment of the hypoglycemia since 20 % glucose in water was administered through an umbilical venous catheter into a branch of the left pulmonary vein [67].

Infants manifesting defective gluconeogenesis/glycogenolysis

Hypoglycemia has been noted in infants unable to sustain normal gluconeogenesis. Glucagon is influential in hepatic glucose production since it enhances glycogenolysis and gluconeogenesis. A recent report has documented an infant with isolated glucagon deficiency and neonatal hypoglycemia. The diagnosis was based on a low basal glucagon concentration as well as a diminished response to hypoglycemia and alanine infusion, both potent stimulators of glucagon secretion, in an infant in whom normal insulin secretion was present [137]. Vidnes has also reported on three infants with persistent neonatal hypoglycemia, one of whom evidenced an abnormal subcellular distribution of PEPCK in the extramitochondrial fraction [138, 139].

A specific enzymatic deficiency that may affect gluconeogenesis in the neonate is type I glycogen storage disease (glucose-6-phosphatase deficiency). The deficiency is an autosomal recessive genetic defect with may occasionally present in the neonatal period with severe hypoglycemia and hepatomegaly [27]. A second enzymatic defect, fructose-

1,6-diphosphatase deficiency, has also been associated with hypoglycemia [93, 99].

Galactosemia may present in infants early with septicemia and hepatocellular jaundice and later (1 month) with cataract formation. In some infants, hypoglycemic symptoms have been reported and a positive reducing test in the urine (to copper or iron) noted. The usual biochemical defect is that of galactose-1-phosphate uridyl transferase. The diagnosis involves the demonstration of a low true glucose level (glucose oxidase) in the presence of normal total hexoses together with the determination of the enzymatic defect, which can be analyzed in both red and white blood cells. Exclusion of milk and milk products (lactose) is the current treatment. Because early intervention is preventative, routine neonatal screening has been recommended [75].

Hereditary fructose intolerance has also been documented after the neonatal period, particularly in infants who ingest fruits or juices. The major intolerance is due to fructose-1-phosphate accumulation secondary to fructose-1-phosphate aldolase deficiency. The hypoglycemia is secondary to an inhibition of hepatic glucose release and absence of a hyperglycemic response to glucagon following ingestion or parenteral administration of fructose.

HYPERINSULINISM

Hypoglycemia following increased plasma insulin has now been associated with several discrete disorders of the islets including the infant of the diabetic mother, infants with hemolytic disease of the newborn, pancreatic nesidioblastosis, discrete or multiple islet cell adenomatosis, and infants undergoing exchange transfusions. The infant with Beckwith Wiedemann Syndrome should also be considered along with other causes of hyperinsulinemic hypoglycemia.

The infant of the diabetic mother

Because of the importance of this clinical problem, we shall discuss: the infant of the diabetic mother (IDM) at length. The IDM has been the subject of a detailed review elsewhere [113]. Although most IDM's have an uneventful perinatal course, there is an increased risk for untoward complications in both previously identified as well as undiagnosed diabetes during pregnancy.

Perinatal mortality and morbidity. — Infants of diabetic mothers have a greater morbidity than infants of non-diabetic women (Table II). More than 40 % of infants of insulin-dependent diabetic women may experience an uneventful clinical course and a much higher percentage (80 %) of infants of gestationally (chemically) diabetic women do well. The more closely metabolically controlled the diabetic pregnant patient, the greater the potential for a normal infant [95].

TABLE II. — POTENTIAL MORBIDITIES
IN THE IDM

Asphyxia neonatorum	Macrosomia
Birth injury	Neurological instability
Congenital anomalies	Polycythemia and hyperviscosity
Heart failure	
Hyperbilirubinemia	Respiratory distress/respiratory distress syndrome
Hypocalcemia	
Hypoglycemia	Small left colon syndrome
Increased blood volume	Transient hematuria

Studies of perinatal morbidity and mortality from multiple centers attest to the success of the above principle. Pedersen et al. published a review of their experience over a 26 year period with an analysis of 920 diabetic pregnancies [95]. Perinatal mortality varied directly with maternal severity of diabetes, as judged by two commonly used maternal classification schema: White's classification of diabetes in pregnancy, and the Prognostically Bad Signs in Pregnancy (PBSP) classification. The White classification is based on the duration of diabetes and the presence of late vascular complications while the PBSP classification includes abnormalities of the current pregnancy, including clinical pyelonephritis, precoma, severe acidosis, mild to severe preeclampsia, and "neglectors". The risk to the fetus was increased when the PBSP classification was "added" to the White classification. While these investigators noted an improvement in non-diabetic pregnancy outcome during this same period, they emphasized that the improved recognition of the various classes of diabetes combined with increased experience were the major reasons for the improved results in the diabetic pregnancies.

Of equal importance, the frequency of macrosomia decreased; however, the rate was still twice as high as that in infants born to non-diabetic women. In a recent survey of macrosomic infants (LGA > 95 percentile weight) for gestational age, we have confirmed that most such infants are from obese mothers, not all of whom have glucose intolerance as judged by postpartum glycohemoglobin studies. Nevertheless, the gestational diabetic remains often undiagnosed and may have an infant at greater risk for perinatal complications [95, 142].

Pathogenesis of the effects of maternal diabetes on the fetus. — As yet, no single pathogenesis has been clearly defined to explain the diverse problems observed in IDM's. Nevertheless, many of the effects can be attributed to maternal metabolic (glucose) control. Pedersen emphasized the relationship between maternal glucose concentration and neonatal hypoglycemia [95]. His simplified hypothesis recognized that maternal hyperglycemia was paralleled by fetal hyperglycemia, which stimulated the fetal pancreas, resulting in islet cell hypertrophy and beta cell hyperplasia with increased insulin content. Upon separation of the fetus from the mother, the former no longer is supported by placental glucose transfer resulting in neonatal hypoglycemia.

Hyperinsulinemia in utero affects diverse organ systems including the placenta. Insulin acts as the primary anabolic hormone of fetal growth and development resulting in visceromegaly (especially heart and liver) and macrosomia. In the presence of excess substrate (glucose), increased fat synthesis and deposition occur during the third trimester. Fetal macrosomia is reflected by increased body fat, muscle mass, and organomegaly, but not in increased size of the brain or kidneys [131]. After delivery, there is a rapid fall in plasma glucose with persistently low concentrations of plasma free fatty acids (FFA), glycerol and betahydroxybutyrate. In response to an intravenous glucose stimulus, plasma insulin-like activity is increased as are plasma immunoreactive insulin (determined in the absence of maternal insulin antibodies) and plasma C-peptide.

The response to an oral glucose load results in an earlier plasma insulin rise compared to normal infants, although the area under the insulin curve is similar. The response to an acute intravenous bolus of glucose in IDM's compared to normals is a rapid rate of glucose disappearance from the plasma. In contrast, the rise in plasma glucose concentration following stepwise hourly increases in the rate of continuously infused glucose results in elevations even at low rates, i. e. 4-6 mg/kg.min. The latter may be attributed to a persistence of hepatic glucose response which differs from the normal infant. In fact, kinetic studies in the initial six hours after delivery indicate a hepatic glucose production of approximately half that observed in normal infants [63]. Our own studies with $D[U^{-13}C]$-glucose, however, have revealed a heterogeneous

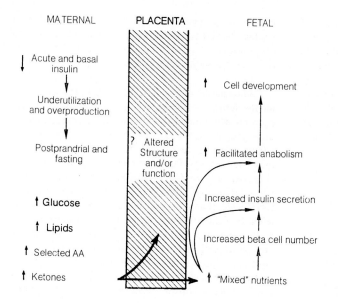

FIG. VI-15. — *Fetal development in insulino-penic diabetic pregnancy utilizing maternal mixed nutrients as controlling factors (after* MILNER *[85]).*

hepatic response so that suppression of hepatic glucose output is not a consistent occurrence, which may reflect the prior maternal metabolic condition [32].

On the basis of animal and in vitro studies of the isolated pancreas, the simplified hyperglycemia-hyperinsulinemia hypothesis has been expanded to include maternal "mixed nutrients" as controlling factors (Fig. VI-15). Of the major maternal nutrients (glucose, fatty acids, ketones, and amino acids), it is likely that, in addition to glucose, amino acids are important in maturation of the fetal beta cell and release of insulin. While ketones readily cross the placenta and may provide substrate, they do not affect insulin secretion. With the exception of essential fatty acids, long chain fatty acids do not cross the placenta in sufficient quantities to influence growth and development in utero [85].

Congenital anomalies in IDM's. — While most of the morbidity and mortality data for the IDM have shown definite improvement with time, congenital anomalies remain as the major unexplained problem. The three to four fold increase in the incidence of congenital anomalies in the offspring of diabetic women has continued to be noted in most centers and currently is the most frequent contributor to perinatal mortality. This comes at a time when these centers are reporting perinatal mortalities in offspring of insulin-dependent diabetic women that are no different from non-diabetics after correction for deaths due to congenital anomalies [48].

Although anomalies in offspring of diabetic mothers encompass a spectrum of organ systems rather than a specific, discrete syndrome, some individual patterns tend to occur more frequently. major, Thus congenital heart disease, musculoskeletal deformities, including the caudal regression syndrome and central nervous system deformities (anencephally, spina bifida, hydrocephalus), have been reported. Based on these findings, the critical period of teratogenesis for the pregnant diabetic has been inferred to take place before the seventh week following conception [84].

One rare congenital defect that is increased in IDM's is the small left colon syndrome. The etiology of this deformity is obscure. With conservative medical management, the condition usually resolves spontaneously within the neonatal period [36].

Although cardiac hypertrophy apart from congenital heart disease has been recognized in autopsies of IDM's for the past three decades, it has only been more recently that attention has been directed at a peculiar form of subaortic stenosis similar to the idiopathic hypertrophic subaortic stenosis found in adults. Propranolol appears to be the therapeutic drug of choice. Clinically, this disorder resolves spontaneously over a period of weeks to months with correction of the echocardiographic features as well.

Macrosomia, birth injury, asphyxia, and respiratory distress syndrome. — At birth, the infant of the poorly controlled diabetic patient will often appear macrosomic in contrast to infants born to the well-controlled diabetic and the non-diabetic, non-obese mother. At birth, one consequence of undetected fetal macrosomia may be a difficult vaginal delivery due to shoulder dystocia with resultant birth injury and/or asphyxia. These potential birth injuries include: cephalohematoma, subdural hemorrhage, facial palsy, ocular hemorrhage, clavicular fracture and brachial plexus injuries. Injury to the brachial plexus may appear with a variety of presentations because the nerves of the brachial plexus may be variably damaged. In addition to the obvious injury to the nerves of the arm, diaphragmatic paralysis occurs if the phrenic nerve is affected. Because of the associated organomegaly in IDM's, hemorrhage into the abdominal organs is possible, specifically liver and adrenals. Hemorrhage into the external genitalia of these large infants has also been reported.

Asphyxia, probably the result of relative macrosomia, may have diverse consequences for the infant. Acutely it may affect respiratory, renal, and central nervous system functions. Thus, decreased fluid intake is usually recommended until the degree of injury to the renal and central nervous systems can be ascertained. An important complication of asphyxia in the newborn may be later respiratory difficulties.

Respiratory distress, including Respiratory Distress Syndrome (RDS), is a frequent and potentially severe complication in the infant of the diabetic mother. While the clinical association has been long recognized, more recent investigations have increased our understanding of the pathophysiological interrelationships. Neonatal RDS, the pathological correlate of which is hyaline membrane disease, develops because of lung immaturity in the newborn and remains a major cause of mortality in the newborn. The problem of RDS is covered in more detail in Chapter 19.

While the increased susceptibility to RDS has been suspected in the infant of the diabetic mother (IDM), a retrospective analysis by Robert et al. [102] evaluated the relative risk of RDS in the IDM in a large series of diabetic pregnancies from the Joslin Clinic and the Boston Hospital for Women. The relative risk of RDS in IDM's was higher in comparison to infants of non-diabetic mothers. If one excluded specific confounding variables including gestational age, delivery by cesarean section, presence of labor, birth weight, sex, Apgar score at five minutes, antepartum hemorrhage, presence of hydramnios, maternal anemia and maternal age, the relative risk was 5.6 times higher in the infant of the diabetic mother. This effect was primarily confined to infants whose gestational age was ⩽ 38 weeks. Present obstetrical

management, however, has been noted to reduce the frequency of RDS.

The trend to deliver diabetic patients later in gestation rather than earlier is increasing. Previously, early delivery was advised to diminish the risk of intrauterine fetal death, but increasing assessment of fetal well being (estriols, ultrasound, stress and non-stress testing, etc.) affords the obstetrician the opportunity of delivering the patient at the optimal time.

Hypoglycemia. — A rapid fall in plasma glucose concentration following delivery is characteristic of the infant of the diabetic mother. Values less than 35 mg/dl in term infants and less than 25 mg/dl in preterm infants are abnormal and may occur within 30 minutes after clamping the umbilical vessels. Factors which are known to influence the degree of hypoglycemia include: prior maternal glucose homeostasis and maternal glycemia during delivery. An inadequately controlled pregnant diabetic will have stimulated the fetal pancreas to synthesize excessive insulin, which may be readily released. Administration of intravenous dextrose during the intrapartum period, which results in maternal hyperglycemia (> 125 mg/dl), will be reflected in the fetus and will exaggerate the infant's normal post-delivery fall in plasma glucose concentration. In addition, hypoglycemia may persist for 48 hours or may develop after 24 hours [113].

Most infants of diabetic mothers are asymptomatic with very low plasma glucose levels. This may be due to the initial brain stores of glycogen; however, the exact biochemistry is as yet undefined. Signs and symptoms which may be observed are non-specific and include tachypnea, apnea, tremulousness, sweating, irritability and seizures.

Hypocalcemia and hypomagnesemia. — In addition to hypoglycemia, hypocalcemia ranks as one of the major metabolic derangements observed in the IDM. Tsang has shown that there are a number of neonates who are prone to hypocalcemia—particularly the prematurely born, the infant who is asphyxiated and the infant of the diabetic mother [134].

Approximately 50 % of infants born to insulin-dependent diabetic women develop hypocalcemia (⩽ 7 mg/dl) during the first three days of life. This high incidence of hypocalcemia is not seen in infants of gestational diabetic women when compared to controls. Evaluation of the mechanism(s) has failed to establish prematurity or asphyxia per se (both of which may be present in IDM's) as the cause. However, the frequency and severity of serum hypocalcemia is directly related to the severity of the diabetes and potentiated if birth asphyxia is superimposed on the clinical state. It has been postulated that the mechanism at least partially responsible for hypocalcemia is the hyperphosphatemia, which is present through 48 hours of age.

In the infant of the insulin-dependent diabetic, a failure of the appropriate rise in PTH concentration in response to hypocalcemia has been reported in contrast to both infants of gestational diabetics and non-diabetics. The PTH response in the normal infant, which occurs on the second to third day does not occur in the infant of the insulin-dependent diabetic patient until 48 hours or later on the third to fourth day. As yet, the etiology of these differences is not known. This subject is considered in detail elsewhere [133].

Hypomagnesemia ($\leqslant$ 1.5 mg/dl) has been found in as many as 33 % of IDM's. As with hypocalcemia, the frequency and severity of clinical symptoms is correlated with the maternal status. Tsang has correlated the neonatal magnesium concentration with that in the mother, as well as with the maternal insulin requirements and concentration of intravenous glucose administered to the infant [134].

Hyperbilirubinemia and polycythemia. — Hyperbilirubinemia is observed more frequently in the IDM than in the normal infant. Although a number of hypotheses have been suggested, the pathogenesis remains uncertain [113].

The polycythemia frequently observed in IDM's may well be the most important factor associated with hyperbilirubinemia. Venous hematocrits $\geqslant 65\%$ have been observed in 20-40 % of IDM's during the first days of life and have sometimes been associated with signs and symptoms of neonatal hyperviscosity such as jitteriness, seizures, tachypnea, priapism and oliguria. Therapy with the use of a partial exchange transfusion (10-15 % of total blood volume) through the umbilical vein using plasmanate or 5 % albumin has been associated with a rapid resolution of symptoms. Careful studies examining the relationship of neonatal hyperviscosity to maternal blood glucose control and/or other perinatal factors associated with the diabetic pregnancy have not been done as yet.

Recent indirect evidence for fetal hypoxia in IDM's may explain the neonatal polycythemia and hyperbilirubinemia. Umbilical cord erythropoietin levels measured at birth using a highly sensitive and specific radioimmunoassay for this hormone, which is stimulated by hypoxia, have been found to be above the narrow range for controls in one-third of a group of 61 IDM's. Moreover, there was an association with relative hyperinsulinemia at birth. Fetal monkeys made hyperinsulinemic in the last third of gestation in the absence of maternal diabetes have been shown to have markedly elevated plasma erythropoietin levels as well as other evidence of increased fetal erythropoiesis such as elevated reticulocyte counts [141].

A final consideration is the concept of ineffective erythropoiesis in IDM's. Increased ineffective erythropoiesis, defined as erythroid precursors harbored in body organs such as the liver and spleen and not released into the peripheral circulation, has been postulated as an etiology for the observed increased bilirubin levels in the IDM's [129].

Renal vein thrombosis. — Renal vein thrombosis is a severe, life-threatening but rare occurrence in the perinatal period. Its occurrence is more frequently associated with maternal diabetes mellitus than in the normal population [9].

The pathogenesis of this lesion remains obscure although most speculation has centered around the possible etiologic role of polycythemia (vide supra). Sludging of blood combined with a further reduction in cardiac output as a result of diabetic cardiomyopathy may be contributing factors. Why this lesion shows selectivity for the kidneys and not other organs is obscure. Birth trauma is an unlikely initiating factor since this lesion has been observed in both stillborns and IDM's delivered by cesarean section.

In the liveborn infant, the diagnosis is usually made in the first hours or days of life with the findings of hematuria and flank mass(es) as the most salient features. Therapy is aimed at careful fluid and electrolyte management and correction of polycythemia with a plasma exchange. A pediatric surgical consultation is indicated for evaluation of possible renal excision. The role of heparinization in the therapy of this entity remains controversial.

Long-term prognosis and follow-up. — The previous discussion has concerned only problems encountered during the neonatal period. Of equal concern and perhaps of greater ultimate importance are the long-term effects on growth and development, on psychosocial intellectual capabilities and finally on the risk to the infant of subsequently developing diabetes. One of the important factors influencing long-term prognosis is the improvement in management of the pregnant diabetic and her infant. Assuming that many of the deleterious effects of the diabetic pregnancy are being modified by normalization of metabolic status in both the pregnant woman and her conceptus, the poor prognoses that have been reported in previous retrospective studies should be ameliorated in future prospective evaluations.

There are few prospective studies of growth and development of the IDM. Farquhar's analysis of 231 of a group of 329 infants is significant in that more children up to 15 years of age fell below the third percentile for height than exceeded the 97th percentile (21 vs. 5) [41]. Weight, in contrast, seemed to be equally divided both above and below the normal range. This was confirmed by evaluating the weight to height index of each child expressed as a percentage of the 50th percentile for age and sex. Evaluation by these parameters suggested that excessive weight is almost ten times more common than unusually low weight. Farquhar suggests that this may represent a potential "return to obesity" noted at birth in this group of infants. In another study, Bibergeil noted that height was elevated in 16.7 % but below normal in 9.3 %. Newborns greater than 4 kg evidenced significant elevations of height or weight at time of entrance to school [18].

In consideration of neuropsychological development, it is important to note that the high frequency of congenital malformations may be directly or indirectly associated with neuropsychological handicaps. In one series, Yssing found that 36 % (265 children) had evidence of cerebral dysfunction or related conditions [149]. Cerebral palsy and epilepsy were found to be three to five times higher in comparison to the normal population, but mental retardation was not noted to be different. When present, the difficulties seemed to be related to extremes of maternal age, severity of diabetes, low birth weight for gestational age, or complications during pregnancy.

The question of whether the IDM has an increased likelihood of becoming diabetic is important and has been the subject of a number of analyses [120]. Previously, 4-6 % of siblings of diabetic individuals have developed diabetes. While family aggregates do exist, transmitted both through and within generations, a simple mode of inheritance is inconsistent with the reported data. Some have suggested that a polygenic multifactorial model best explains the reported observations. From recent studies of IDM's, the prevalence of Type I, insulin-dependent, juvenile diabetes among offspring of diabetic mothers was approximately 1.0 %. Thus, it appears that the infant born to a mother with diabetes is at increased risk for developing the disease in comparison to the normal population.

Rh incompatibility

Hyperinsulinism has been implicated as the cause of the hypoglycemia seen in infants with severe Rh isoimmunization [11, 88, 92, 108]. These children are invariably severely affected by their disease, with profound anemia and hepatosplenomegaly at birth. The shock and collapse seen on occasion may be caused primarily by the profound hypoglycemia, and, under such circumstances, glucose administration in addition to measures taken to correct the anemia may be critical. The IDM and severely Rh-affected infant share several pathologic hallmarks. In addition to the hyperinsulinism and islet cell hyperplasia, both show almost identical edematous placental changes. The IDM, just as the Rh-affected counterpart, has excessive islands of extramedullary hematopoiesis in both liver and spleen. Although this latter finding may be the result of insulin stimulation, the precise cause of the hyperinsulinism itself in the Rh-affected infant is uncertain. It has been suggested that an increase in glutathione resulting from massive hemolysis of red blood cells may act as a stimulus to insulin release.

Metabolic effects of exchange transfusions

Hypoglycemia, although not often considered, may be a significant problem following exchange transfusion. In this connection, the exchange blood and its preservatives are more critically important in the newborn in whom a double volume washout is being undertaken than in an adult, who is receiving 450 ml of the blood/preservative mixture to be diluted in a total five litres or more.

Heparinized blood contains no added glucose. Moreover, the heparin, by raising the free fatty acid levels, contributes to the hypoglycemic potential of the transfusion blood, so that under some circumstances (e. g., severe Rh incompatibility with hyperinsulinism) its use would be contraindicated unless a concomitant IV glucose infusion is administered to both prevent and/or treat the hypoglycemia [105]. With citrated blood, acid citrate dextrose (ACD) or citrate phosphate dextrose (CPD), the added dextrose will yield a blood preservative mixture containing as much as 300 mg/dl glucose. In this situation, although immediate hypoglycemia is not a problem, the high glucose load results in a reactive insulin response. This response lags behind the glucose infusion so that when the glucose "bolus" is suddenly terminated at the end of the exchange procedure, a state of hyperinsulinism ensues. Studies documenting this occurrence have shown a precipitous two-hour post-exchange fall in blood glucose to levels below that present prior to undertaking the exchange procedure [106]. Once again, the severely Rh-affected infant is at greatest risk, but even mildly affected and non-erythroblastotic exchanged infants may respond in such a manner as well. Recognition of this possibility should lead to its detection and treatment.

Beckwith-Wiedemann syndrome

In 1964, Beckwith and associates described a syndrome characterized by omphalocele, muscular macroglossia and visceromegaly [16]. Wiedemann almost simultaneously described a similar clinical picture in three siblings [143]. It was subsequently shown that hypoglycemia may be an associated metabolic component of this syndrome, occurring in approximately 50 % of the cases reported, with hyperinsulinism responsible for both the hypoglycemia and the somatic and visceral growth abnormalities. Pathologically, islet cell hyperplasia of the pancreas has been demonstrated in these infants, although the etiology of the syndrome remains unclear. The hypoglycemia, which is ultimately self-limiting, may be relatively protracted and difficult to control. In a carefully studied patient, with resistant hypoglycemia and hyperinsulinism, Schiff and co-workers [107] were ultimately able to achieve adequate control of glucose levels with a combination of Sus-phrine * and diazoxide therapy, that suppressed both basal insulin release and that in the postprandial state. The infant presented at birth with an umbilical hernia, macroglossia and hepatosplenomegaly as well as hyperinsulinism and severe, persistent hypoglycemia. Normal glucose control was achieved by one month of age. At six months, somatic growth was normal, hepatosplenomegaly had receded, but the macroglossia was still present. At two years of age growth was normal, and the tongue, although still large, could be kept within the mouth without any evidence of malocclusion.

Nesidioblastosis, islet cell adenomas

Although rare at any age in childhood, infants with nesidioblastosis [59, 114, 145], discrete islet

* Sus-phrine: 1 : 200 Epinephrine, Aqueous Suspension, Cooper Laboratories, Inc.

cell adenoma [10, 23], or adenomatosis [54] have been reported and successfully treated. Hyperinsulinism without other apparent cause and resistant hypoglycemia should raise these rare but, nevertheless, real possibilities. Preoperative confirmation may be sought either by means of regular GI radiographic studies, peritoneal air insufflation, abdominal angiography, and/or ultrasound examination, but surgical exploration may be necessary as a definitive diagnostic as well as therapeutic measure.

Other causes of hyperinsulinism and hypoglycemia

Isolated instances have also been reported which mimic the problem of insulin excess and resultant hypoglycemia. Zucker et al. have reported symptomatic neonatal hypoglycemia in association with maternal administration of chloropropamide [151]. This resulted in stimulation of both the maternal as well as the fetal beta cells. Because the teratogenicity of the drug is a concern, its use is limited, especially since control of glucose is insufficient for the management of diabetes in pregnancy. Benzothiadiazide diuretics have also been implicated in stimulating insulin secretion [116]. It has been suggested that the drug produces elevated maternal blood glucose levels and results in stimulation of the fetal islets with subsequent neonatal hypoglycemia. There is also a report of an infant in whom hypoglycemia may have been due to an insulin releasing substance, possibly from the gut [128].

Hypoglycemia has been noted in individuals who are sensitive to leucine. This amino acid, among others, is known to be associated with increased insulin release and may be seen following ingestion of milk [22]. A fourth defect of leucine metabolism, 3-hydroxy-3-methylglutaryl CoA lyase deficiency has been reported. Hypoglycemia was noted along with a characteristic excretory pattern of organic acids, but the exact mechanism resulting in the hypoglycemia was not apparent [110]. Reports also note the potential of hypoglycemia after betasympathomimetic tocolytic therapy, which is being used increasingly to inhibit premature onset of labor. While the specific mechanism of action is not known, a possible explanation of the relationship involves increased pancreatic secretion of insulin in response to a specific glucose concentration [40].

Another cause of relative hyperinsulinism was reported secondary to malposition of an umbilical artery catheter. In an infant requiring supplemental oxygen because of increasing respiratory distress, hypoglycemia was relieved only when a "high" catheter was repositioned from T 11-12 to L 4. Following repositioning of the catheter, the child became euglycemic. The mechanism of the hypoglycemia was postulated to be excessive insulin secretion following infusion into the celiac axis [89].

Neonatal hypoglycemia has also been associated with administration of salicylates [96], with the suggested mechanism being an uncoupling of mitochondrial oxidative phosphorylation. The association of congenital adrenal hyperplasia and hypoglycemia has been recorded [49].

EVALUATION OF NEONATAL HYPOGLYCEMIA

As in other areas of neonatology, a detailed maternal history as well as a thorough physical examination are important in determining the probability of neonatal hypoglycemia and its etiology. Maternal history, which includes family or maternal history of diabetes or other glucose intolerance, drug ingestion (chloropropamide, benzothiadiazide diuretics and salicylates), and blood group incompatibility (Rh) or preeclampsia should alert the physician to the potential problems of hypoglycemia. Perinatal history, including birth asphyxia and/or trauma and the presence of cold injury is of further importance is establishing the possibility.

A thorough physical exam will indicate whether an infant is AGA, SGA or LGA and also what the gestational age of the infant is. The appearance of the infant of the diabetic mother from class A or B versus classes C-F is well recognized, as is the infant with Beckwith-Wiedemann syndrome. Prolonged jaundice and failure to thrive suggest galactosemia while the infant with unexplained hepatomegaly should be considered for the possibility of glycogen storage disease.

Most etiologies of hypoglycemia should be apparent following a detailed maternal history, review of labor and delivery, and physical examination of the infant. However, appropriate laboratory studies may include plasma glucose, insulin, glucagon, lactate, alanine, ketones, free fatty acids, and pH as well as cortisol, growth hormone, and thyroid function studies in some cases. Tolerance tests such as glucose, galactose, fructose, glucagon, insulin and tolbutamide are usually reserved to confirm suspected diagnoses. In a recent report Finegold et al. evaluated the use of glucagon infusions as a means of diagnosing hyperinsulinism [43]. Suggesting that hyperinsuli-

nism would inhibit glycogenolysis, they found elevated glycemic responses to glucagon during hypoglycemia in infants with hyperinsulinemic hyperinsulinism. In comparison, in normal fasting children, continued mobilization of liver glycogen stores lead to a marked reduction in the glycemic response to glucagon as the plasma glucose level approaches 40 mg/dl. Further details of specific diagnostic tests can be found elsewhere [27]. In some research laboratories, stable non-radioactive isotopes are being utilized to analyze glucose kinetics (turnover).

HYPERGLYCEMIA IN THE NEWBORN

Hyperglycemia may also be a problem for the newborn because of the potential for an osmotic diuresis and resultant dehydration [39, 46, 73]. Gentz and Cornblath [50] reviewed hyperglycemia in SGA newborns with transient neonatal diabetes in the first six weeks of life. Symptoms included failure to thrive and dehydration, in spite of adequate oral intake. Insulin was utilized to treat the extreme hyperglycemia noted without concomitant ketosis or acidosis. Subsequently, others have confirmed the presence of this entity and suggested that deficient insulin secretion or production of a biologically inactive from of insulin was responsible for its appearance [72, 121]. The association of hyperglycemia and a chromosome deletion (46, XXDq⁻) on number 13 has also been reported in an infant who was small for gestational age [74].

Of current interest, in veiw of the widespread use of parenteral alimentation to nourish low birth weight infants, are the increasing number of reports documenting the occurrence of hyperglycemia. Dweck and Cassady reported on 43 of 50 infants who weighed 1,000 g or less who showed plasma glucose concentrations of 125 mg/dl or greater during parenteral glucose administration. Thirty-six of these infants had plasma glucose levels > 300 mg/dl, usually within 24 hours of age [39]. Diminished tolerance to glucose was inferred in these very low birth weight infants who did not manifest the well known adult Staub Traugott effect (*i. e.* lower blood glucose concentration and increasingly rapid disappearance rates of glucose following its repeated administration) [38].

Hyperglycemia was evaluated by Zarif et al. by measuring glucose and insulin and growth hormone during the first five days of life prospectively in low birth weight infants receiving a parenteral or oral glucose load or a combination of both [150]. Hyperglycemia was noted in 32 of 75 infants and an association was noted between death and hyperglycemia. Insulin and growth hormone responses were not felt to be of etiologic significance, but the authors did note that most infants had been stressed suggesting the possibility of increased cortisol and/or catecholamine secretion.

Exogenous insulin as a treatment for hyperglycemia specifically to increase glucose disposal was evaluated in eight low birth weight infants < 1,500 g by Pollak et al. [97]. A saline placebo was given during infusion of 14 mg/kg/min of exogenous glucose on day one and was followed on day two by 10 mU/kg/min of insulin infused over 50 minutes under similar conditions of glucose administration. Normoglycemia resulted from the exogenous administration of the insulin. The authors speculated that hyperglycemia during exogenous infusion of glucose was either the result of persistent endogenous hepatic glucose production or decreased peripheral utilization, but the two entities could not be differentiated. It appeared, however, that an elevated plasma insulin concentration was required to achieve appropriate control of glucose homeostasis.

A second series of studies defined tolerance for glucose in 35 clinically healthy appropriate for gestational age infants weighing 750 to 1,500 g between 3 and 38 days of age [29]. Infants were given graded doses of glucose at either 8, 11 or 14 mg/kg/min

for three hours by continuous peripheral intravenous infusion. Plasma glucose and insulin concentrations and timed urine volume and glucose concentrations were measured. Nine infants received 8 mg/kg/min and, in these infants, plasma glucose and insulin concentrations were similar in the steady state period of analysis. None of these infants evidenced hyperglycemia. In contrast, 10 infants receiving 14 mg/kg/min of exogenous glucose developed significantly higher plasma glucose and insulin responses in contrast to the infants receiving 8 mg/kg/min of exogenous glucose. Sixteen infants received 11 mg/kg/min and the plasma glucose concentration significantly increased to 140-160 mg/dl in a comparable time period, but the plasma insulin concentrations were not significantly different from baseline. Half of these infants developed hyperglycemia (plasma glucose concentration > 150 mg/dl) with concomitant glucosuria. At the time of study, all of these infants had been clinically asymptomatic for at least 48 hours prior to the study but had been clinically ill prior to that time (see Table III). These findings parallel the work of others who have also suggested that clinical morbidity could unfavorably affect glucose homeostasis in the newborn [76].

There is also a case report of an infant who had culture proven *E. coli* sepsis in association with clinical evidence of hyperglycemia. Since the infant's plasma insulin levels were correspondingly low,

TABLE III. — FREQUENCY OF DIFFERENT CLINICAL MORBIDITIES * (N = 35)

Group	Glucose infusion rate (mg/kg/min)	No glyco-suria	Glyco-suria	Frequency ** Low	Frequency ** High	Statistical significance
1 (n = 9)	8	9	0	4	5	None
2A (n = 9)	11	9	0	9	0	$p < .05$
2B (n = 7)	11	0	7	2	5	None
3 (n = 10)	14	0	10	8	2	None

* Clinical morbidities include the following: Apgar score ≤ 6 at 1 min; Apgar score ≤ 6 at 5 min; sepsis or necrotizing enterocolitis; apnea ≥ 4/24 hrs; respiratory distress syndrome requiring use of respirator; hypocalcemia ≤ 7 mg/100 ml; serum bilirubin ≥ 10 mg/100 ml at 48 hrs; patent ductus arteriosus with congestive heart failure.
** Low frequency = 1 to 2 clinical morbidities; high frequency = 3 to 8 clinical morbidities.
(Reference [29]).

the authors postulated an inadequate insulin response as a mechanism of the observed hyperglycemia [61]. Stable isotope tracer analyses and other techniques will provide differentiation of the characteristics of glucose metabolism in these infants and should help explain the clinical appearance of hyperglycemia.

TREATMENT

The treatment of neonatal hypo- and hyperglycemia begins with identification of its potential in the infant at risk, documentation of its presence by appropriate laboratory measurement (Dextrostix and confirmatory blood or plasma glucose determinations) and corrective measures to either raise or lower blood or plasma glucose concentration.

Feedings generally are advocated as either 5 % D and W or formula but probably should only be utilized to maintain a glucose concentration in the euglycemic range. Using 6 mg/kg/min as the concentration of glucose required to maintain glucose homeostasis, it is unreasonable to expect that oral feedings alone will provide for adequate glucose intake in infants who are hypoglycemic. We advocate parenteral (intravenous) treatment of the hypoglycemic condition using a constant infusion pump to avoid fluctuations in the rate of infusion that would result in irregular rates of endogenous insulin release. Oral feedings should be initiated as tolerated. Repeated documentation of blood or plasma glucose concentration should be an integral part of the treatment of any infant. The glucose infusions should be gradually reduced rather than abruptly terminated to avoid sudden reactive hypoglycemia due to "uncovered" hyperinsulinism. Once oral feedings are initiated, evaluation of the glucose concentration just prior to a subsequent feeding provides an analysis of the infant's status.

Parenteral therapy should begin with 6 mg/kg/min followed by graded increases to achieve euglycemia with the minimum concentration of glucose required. A peripheral vein rather than an umbilical vessel is the preferred route of infusion, however, concentrations greater than 15-20 mg/kg/min are probably contraindicated by either route. Other than in an emergency, concentrations greater than that should probably only be given using a central venous approach. Acute administration of 25 % glucose by bolus infusions of 0.25-1.0 g/kg, if required for relief of acute symptoms (seizures, etc.), must be followed by parenteral infusion until the effect of the bolus infusion on pancreatic insulin release is no longer apparent.

Calculation of parenteral glucose therapy must include the actual concentration of glucose present in the administered fluids. A hydrated form of glucose, Dextrose (molecular weight 198), is used by most manufacturers to prepare the parenteral fluid so that the actual amount of sugar available is approximately 10 % less [34]. Thus, it is of particular concern when very low birth weight or severely hypoglycemic infants are being treated.

Treatment with a number of specific agents is indicated when parenteral therapy above 15 mg/kg/min is not effective in maintaining euglycemia. Corticosteroids have been shown to be effective in the therapy of hypoglycemia. Although several glucose-producing reactions are enhanced by the steroids, the major effect is probably that of gluconeogenesis from non-carbohydrate (protein) sources. The alleged "superiority" of ACTH over cortisone was in all likelihood the result of the use of crude hog pituitary extract, from which the patient received the added benefit of "pollutant" growth hormone. Current preparations afford no advantage between the two. Hydrocortisone is given at a dose of 5 mg/kg/day either by IV or orally every 12 hours or prednisone at a dose of 2 mg/kg/day orally. As with all forms of therapy, gradual diminution of the dosage administered in concert with decreasing parenteral concentration of glucose and increasing oral intake of nutrients will successfully allow weaning of the infant.

Glucagon provides a highly effective method of releasing glycogen from the liver and can be utilized as a therapeutic means of assessing whether or not the liver contains adequate stores. Thus, its failure in some IUGR infants is considered to be evidence for a lack of hepatic glycogen stores in these children. In normal infants, as well as in the infant of the diabetic mother, there is often a failure to respond to the usual small doses (30 µg/kg) despite the presence of more than adequate hepatic glycogen stores. Both groups of infants will frequently respond to higher doses (300 µg/kg) with a prolonged and sustained hyperglycemia (see above), so that the higher dose might well be used as initial therapy in the IDM [146].

Like glucagon, epinephrine is capable of promoting glycogen to glucose conversion, but in far smaller quantities. For this effect, therefore, glucagon is the drug of choice. The hyperglycemic potential of epinephrine in blocking glucose uptake by peripheral muscle presupposes an adequate blood level to start with and is, therefore, of little practical benefit in the hypoglycemic state.

Phenobarbital, commonly used in the treatment of seizures, may have value if these are of hypoglycemic origin and glucose is maintained, over and above its effect as a sedative agent alone. Experimentally (in hypoglycemic animals) phenobarbital appears to increase the amount of glucose in the brain, at a given blood level [81]. The effect is not caused by a decrease in metabolic demand by the brain under these conditions, suggesting that glucose transport into the brain may be enhanced by an enzyme system induced by the barbiturate. These observations would explain the frequently seen diminution in severity and intensity of hypoglycemic seizures following phenobarbital therapy in the absence of any effect of the drug on blood glucose levels.

Diazoxide, in a dose of 10-15 mg/kg/day, probably exerts its effect by suppressing pancreatic insulin secretion, although some have suggested a direct effect on hepatic glucose production [136]. The drug should be used only when other methods have failed [3].

Surgical intervention is indicated with nesidioblastosis or when an islet cell adenoma or adenomatosis has been confirmed. Several reports have documented the use of somatostatin in place of surgical removal of pancreatic tissue because of the precarious clinical condition of the patients involved. In one case, somatostatin alone was able to suppress insulin release resulting in only one episode of hypoglycemia during an interruption of the infusion. In another case, glucagon was required to be simultaneously infused to prevent hypoglycemia. In both cases, surgical removal of pancreatic tissue was subsequently possible [21, 68].

The treatment of hyperglycemia is usually successfully accomplished by lowering the concentration of parenteral glucose administered; however, at least 60 kcal/kg/day of carbohydrate or fat are required to spare protein for subsequent somatic growth [7]. Before lowering the concentration of parenteral glucose administered on the basis of hyperglycemia alone, measurement of urine concentration and volume is required to confirm the presence of an osmotic diuresis, which may be absent in the very low birth weight infant [29]. The absolute level of hyperglycemia at which untoward CNS effects are first manifest has not been documented in the human. However, the presence of intracranial bleeding has been reported in newborn puppies in whom acute hyperglycemia was produced by "standard regimens" of glucose therapy [8]. Caution and further evaluation are necessary to define the effect of acute and chronic hyperglycemia on the central nervous system of the infant at risk.

REFERENCES

[1] ADAM (P. A. J.). — Control of glucose metabolism in the human fetus and newborn infant. *Adv. Metab. Disord.*, 5, 184-275, 1971.

[2] ADAM (P. A. J.), KING (K. C.), SCHWARTZ (R.). — Model for the investigation of intractable hypoglycemia: Insulin-glucose interrelationship during steady state infusions. *Pediatrics*, 41, 91-105, 1968.

[3] ALTSZULER (N.), HAMPSHIRE (J.), MORARU (E.). — On the mechanism of diazoxide-induced hyperglycemia. *Diabetes*, 26, 931-935, 1977.

[4] AMATAYAKUL (O.), CUMMING (G. R.), HAWORTH (J. C.). — Association of hypoglycemia with cardiac enlargement and heart failure in newborn infants. *Arch. Dis. Child.*, 45, 717-720, 1970.

[5] ANAND (R. S.), GANGULI (S.), SPERLING (M. A.). — Effect of insulin-induced maternal hypoglycemia on glucose turnover in maternal and fetal sheep. *Am. J. Physiol.*, 238, E524-532, 1980.

[6] ANAND (R. S.), SPERLING (M. A.), GANGULI (S.), NATHANIELSZ (P. W.). — Bidirectional placental transfer of glucose and its turnover in fetal and maternal sheep. *Pediatr. Res.*, 13, 783-787, 1979.

[7] ANDERSEN (T. L.), MUTTART (C. R.), BEIBER (M. A.), NICHOLSON (J. D.), HEIRD (W. C.). — A controlled trial of glucose versus glucose and amino acids in premature infants. *J. Pediatr.*, 94, 947-951, 1979.

[8] ARANT (B. S. Jr.), GOOCH (W. M. III). — Effects of acute hyperglycemia on brains of neonatal puppies. *Pediatr. Res.*, 13, 488, 1979 (Abstract).

[9] AVERY (M. E.), OPPENHEIMER (E. H.), GORDON (H. H.). — Renal vein thrombous in newborn infants of diabetics mothers. *N. Engl. J. Med.*, 265, 1134-1138, 1957.

[10] BAERENTSEN (H.). — Case report: Neonatal hypoglycemia due to an islet cell adenoma. *Acta Paediatr. Scand.*, 62, 207-210, 1973.

[11] BARRETT (C. T.), OLIVER (T. K. Jr.). — Hypoglycemia and hyperinsulinism in infants with erythroblastosis fetalis. *N. Engl. J. Med.*, 278, 1260-1263, 1968.

[12] BATTAGLIA (F. C.), MESCHIA (G.). — Principle substrates of fetal metabolism. *Physiol. Rev.*, 58, 499-527, 1978.

[13] BEARD (A. G.). — Neonatal hypoglycemia. *J. Perinat. Med.*, 3, 219-225, 1975.

[14] BEARD (A. G.), PANOS (T. C.), MARASIGAN (B. V.) et coll. — Perinatal stress and the premature neonate. II. Effect of fluid and caloric deprivation on blood glucose. *J. Pediatr.*, 68, 329-343, 1966.

[15] BECK (P.), DAUGHADAY (W. H.). — Human placental lactogen: Studies of its acute metabolic effects and disposition in man. *J. Clin. Invest.*, 46, 103-111, 1967.

[16] BECKWITH (J. B.), WANG (C. I.), DONNEL (G. N.), GWIN (J. L.). — Hyperplastic fetal visceromegaly with macroglossia, omphalocele, cytomegaly of adrenal fetal cortex, postnatal somatic gigantism, and other abnormalities. Newly recognized syndrome. *Proc. Am. Pediatr. Soc., Seattle*, June 16-18, 1964 (abstract 41).

[17] BENZING (G.), SCHUBERT (W.), HUG (G.) et al. — Simultaneous hypoglycemia and acute congestive heart failure. *Circulation*, 40, 209-216, 1972.

[18] BIBERGEIL (H.), GÖDEL (E.), AMENDT (P.). — Diabetes and pregnancy; In: *Early and late Pro-*

gnoses of children of Diabetic Mothers, CAMERINI-DAVALOS (R. A.) and COLE (H. S.) (Eds.), Academic Press, Inc., New York, 427-434, 1975.

[19] BIER (D. M.), ARNOLD (K. J.), SHERMAN (W. R.) et al. — *In vivo* measurement of glucose and alanine metabolism with stable isotopic tracers. *Diabetes*, 26, 1005-1015, 1977.

[20] BIER (D. M.), LEAKE (R. D.), HAYMOND (M. W.) et al. — Measurement of « true » glucose production rates in infancy and childhood with 6,6-dideuteroglucose. *Diabetes*, 26, 1016-1023, 1977.

[21] BLOOMGARDEN (R. T.), SUNDELL (H.), ROGERS (L. W.), O'NEILL (J. A.), LILJENQUIST (J. E.). — Treatment of intractable neonatal hypoglycemia with somatostatin plus glucagon. *J. Pediatr.*, 96, 148-151, 1980.

[22] BROWN (R. E.), YOUNG (R. B.). — A possible role for the exocrine pancreas in the pathogenesis of neonatal leucine sensitive hypoglycemia. *Am. J. Digest. Dis.*, 15, 65-72, 1970.

[23] BURST (N. R. M.), CAMPBELL (J. R.), CASTRO (A.). — Congenital islet cell adenoma causing hypoglycemia in a newborn. *Pediatrics*, 47, 605-610, 1971.

[24] CHLEBOWSKI (R. T.), ADAM (P. A. J.). — Glucose production in the newborn dog. II. Evaluation of autonomic and enzymatic control in the isolated perfused canine liver. *Pediatr. Res.*, 9, 821-828, 1975.

[25] CORNBLATH (M.), ODELL (G. B.), LEVIN (E. Y.). — Symptomatic neonatal hypoglycemia associated with toxemia of pregnancy. *J. Pediatr.*, 55, 545-562, 1959.

[26] CORNBLATH (M.), REISNER (S. H.). — Blood glucose in the neonate and its clinical significance. *N. Engl. J. Med.*, 273, 378-381, 1965.

[27] CORNBLATH (M.), SCHWARTZ (R.). — *Disorders of Carbohydrate Metabolism in Infancy*, 2nd ed., W. B. Saunders Co., Philadelphia, 1976.

[28] COSTRINI (N. V.), KALKHOFF (R. K.). — Relative effects of pregnancy, estradiol and progesterone on plasma insulin and pancreatic islet insulin secretion. *J. Clin. Invest.*, 50, 992-999, 1971.

[29] COWETT (R. M.), OH (W.), POLLAK (A.), SCHWARTZ (R.), STONESTREET (B. S.). — Glucose disposal of low birth weight infants: Steady state hyperglycemia produced by constant intravenous glucose infusion. *Pediatrics*, 63, 389-396, 1979.

[30] COWETT (R. M.), SCHWARTZ (R.). — The role of hepatic control of glucose homeostasis in the etiology of neonatal hypo- and hyperglycemia. *Semin. Perinatol.*, 3, 327-340, 1979.

[31] COWETT (R. M.), STERN (L.). — Carbohydrate homeostasis in the fetus and newborn. In *Neonatology*, 2nd ed., AVERY (G.) (Ed.), Lippincott, Philadelphia, 1981.

[32] COWETT (R. M.), SUSA (J. B.), GILETTI (B.) et al. — Glucose kinetics in infants of diabetic mothers. *Amer J. Obstet. Gynecol.* 146, 781-786, 1983.

[33] COWETT (R. M.), SUSA (J. B.), OH (W.), SCHWARTZ (R.). — Endogenous glucose production during constant glucose infusion in the newborn lamb. *Pediatr. Res.*, 12, 853-857, 1978.

[34] COWETT (R. M.), SUSA (J. B.), SCHWARTZ (R.), OH (W.). — Concentration of parenteral glucose solution. *Pediatrics*, 59, 791, 1977.

[35] COWETT (R. M.), SUSA (J. B.), KAHN (C. B.) et al. — Glucose kinetic in non diabetic and diabetic women during the third trimester of pregnancy. *Amer J. Obstet. Gynecol.* 146, 773-780, 1983.

[36] DAVIS (W. S.), CAMPBELL (J. B.). — Neonatal small left colon syndrome. *Am. J. Dis. Child.*, 129, 1024-1027, 1975.

[37] DELEEUW (R.), DEVRIES (I. L.). — Hypoglycemia in small for dates newborn infants. *Pediatrics*, 58, 18-22, 1976.

[38] DWECK (H. S.), BRANS (Y. W.), SUMNERS (J. E.) et al. — Glucose intolerance in infants of very low birth weight. II. Intravenous glucose tolerance tests in infants of birth weights 500-1,380 grams. *Biol. Neonate*, 30, 261-267, 1976.

[39] DWECK (H. S.), CASSADY (G.). — Glucose intolerance in infants of very low birth weight. I. Incidence of hyperglycemia in infants of birth weights 1,100 grams or less. *Pediatrics*, 53, 189-195, 1974.

[40] EPSTEIN (M. F.), NICHOLLS (E.), STUBBLEFIELD (P. G.). — Neonatal hypoglycemia after beta-sympathomimetic tocolytic therapy. *J. Pediatr.*, 94, 449-453, 1979.

[41] FARQUHAR (J. W.). — Prognosis for babies born to diabetic mothers in Edinburgh. *Arch. Dis. Childh.*, 44, 36-47, 1969.

[42] FELIG (P.). — Energy balance and fuel homeostasis in pregnancy. In *The Endocrine Milieu of Pregnancy, Puerperium and Childhood*, JAFFE (R. B.) (Ed.),Third Ross Conference on Obstetric Research, 60-67, 1974.

[43] FINEGOLD (D. N.), STANLEY (C. A.), BAKER (L.). — Glycemic response to glucagon during fasting hypoglycemia: An aid in the diagnosis of hyperinsulinism. *J. Pediatr.*, 96, 257-259, 1980.

[44] FISHER (D. A.). — Perinatal insulin, glucagon and carbohydrate metabolism. In: *Perinatal Endocrinology*, BLOOM (R. S.), SINCLAIR (J. C.) and WARSHAW (J. B.) (Ed.), Mead Johnson Symposium in Perinatal and Developmental Medicine, No. 8, 30-37, 1975.

[45] FLUGE (G.). — Clinical aspects of neonatal hypoglycemia. *Acta Paediatr. Scand.*, 63, 826-832, 1974.

[46] FOX (H. A.), KRASNA (I. H.). — Total intravenous nutrition by peripheral vein in neonatal surgical patients. *Pediatrics*, 52, 14-20, 1973.

[47] FRAZER (T. E.), KARL (I. E.), HILLMAN (L. S.) et al. — Direct measurement of gluconeogenesis from (2,3-$^{13}C_2$) alanine in the human neonate. *Amer J. Physiol.* 240, E 615-621, 1981.

[48] GABBE (S. G.). — The diagnosis of glucose intolerance in pregnancy. Its impact on the fetus and the neonate. In: *Early Detection of Potential Diabetics: The Problems and the Promise*, GRAVE (G. D.) (Ed.), Raven Press, New York, 131-142, 1979.

[49] GEMELLI (M.), DELUCA (F.), BARBERIO (G.). — Hypoglycemia and congenital adrenal hyperplasia. *Acta Paediatr. Scand.*, 68, 285-286, 1979.

[50] GENTZ (J. C. H.), CORNBLATH (M.). — Transient diabetes of the newborn. *Adv. Pediatr.*, 16, 345-363, 1969.

[51] GRAJWER (L. A.), SPERLING (M. A.), SACK (J.), FISHER (D.). — Possible mechanisms and significance of the neonatal surge in glucagon secretion: Studies in newborn lambs. *Pediatr. Res.*, 11, 833-836, 1977.

[52] GRASSO (S.), PALUMBO (G.), RUGOLO (S.), CIANCI (A.), TUMENO (G.), REITANO (G.). — Human fetal insulin secretion in response to maternal glucose and leucine administration. *Pediatr. Res.*, 14, 782-783, 1980.

[53] GUTBERLET (R. L.), CORNBLATH (M.). — Neonatal hypoglycemia revisited, 1975. *Pediatrics*, 58, 1-17, 1976.

[54] HABBICK (B. J.), CRAM (R. W.), MILLER (K. R.). — Neonatal hypoglycemia resulting from islet cell adenomatosis. *Am. J. Dis. Child.*, 131, 210-212, 1977.

[55] HAY (W. W. Jr.). — Fetal glucose metabolism. *Semin. Perinatol.*, 3, 157-177, 1979.

[56] HAY (W. W. Jr.), SPARKS (J.), QUISELL (B.) et al. — Simultaneous measurements of umbilical uptake/fetal utilization rate. and fetal turnover rate of glucose. *Am. J. Physiol.*, 240 E, 662-668, 1981.

[57] HAYMOND (M. W.), KARL (I. E.), PAGLIARA (A. S.). — Increased gluconeogenic substrate in the small for gestational age infant. *N. Engl. J. Med.*, 291, 322-328, 1974.

[58] HAYMOND (M. W.), STRAUSS (A. W.), ARNOLD (K. J.), BIER (D. M.). — Glucose homeostasis in children with severe cyanotic congenital heart disease. *J. Pediatr.*, 95, 220-227, 1979.

[59] HERTZ (P. U.), KOPPEL (G.), HACKE (W. H.) et al. — Nesidioblastosis: The pathologic basis of persistent hyperinsulinemic hypoglycemia in infants. *Diabetes*, 20, 632-642, 1977.

[60] JAMES (E. J.), RAYE (J. R.), GRESHAM (E. L.) et al. — Fetal O_2 consumption, CO_2 production and glucose uptake in a chronic sheep preparation. *Pediatrics*, 50, 361-371, 1972.

[61] JAMES (T. III), BLESSA (M.), BOGGS (T. R. Jr.). — Recurrent hyperglycemia associated with sepsis in a neonate. *Am. J. Dis. Child.*, 133, 645-646, 1979.

[62] KALHAN (S. C.), SAVIN (S. M.), ADAM (P. A. J.). — Measurement of glucose turnover in the human newborn with glucose-1-^{13}C. *J. Clin. Endocrinol. Metab.*, 43, 704-707, 1976.

[63] KALHAN (S. C.), SAVIN (S. M.), ADAM (P. A. J.). — Attenuated glucose production rate in newborn infants of insulin dependent diabetic mothers. *N. Engl. J. Med.*, 296, 375-376, 1977.

[64] KALKHOFF (R. K.), KESSEBAK (A. H.), KIM (H. J.). — Carbohydrate and lipid metabolism during normal pregnancy. Relationship to gestational hormone action. In: *The Diabetic Pregnancy. A Perinatal Perspective*, MERKATZ (I. R.) and ADAM (P. A. J.) (Eds.), Grune and Stratton, New York, 3-22, 1979.

[65] KAPLAN (S. L.). — Human chorionic somatomamotropin: Secretion, biological effects and physiologic significance. In: *The Endocrine Milieu of Pregnancy, Puerperium and Childhood*, JAFFE (R. B.) (Ed.), Third Ross Conference on Obstetric Research, 75-80, 1974.

[66] KAPLAN (S. L.), GURPIDE (E.), SCIARRA (J. J.) et al. — Metabolic clearance rate and production of chorionic growth hormone prolactin in late pregnancy. *J. Clin. Endocrinol. Metab.*, 28, 1450-1460, 1968.

[67] KERKERING (K. W.), ROBERTSON (L. W.), KODROFF (M. B.), MUELLER (D. G.), KIRKPATRICK (B. V.). — Grand Round Series: Hypoglycemia and unilateral pulmonary edema in a newborn. *Pediatrics*, 65, 326-330, 1980.

[68] KITSON (H. F.), McCROSSIN (R. B.), JIMENEZ (M.), MIDDLETON (A.), SILINK (M.). — Somatostatin treatment of insulin excess due to β-cell adenoma in a neonate. *J. Pediatr.*, 96, 145-148, 1980.

[69] KOIVISTO (M.), JOUPPILA (P.). — Neonatal hypo-glycemia and maternal toxaemia. *Acta Paediatr. Scand.*, 63, 743-749. 1974.

[70] KORNHAUSER (D.), ADAM (P. A. J.), SCHWARTZ (R.). — Glucose production and utilization in the newborn puppy. *Pediatr. Res.*, 4, 120-128, 1974.

[71] LaNOUE (K. F.), MASON (A. D. Jr.), DANIELS (J. P.). — The impairment of glucogenesis by gram negative infection. *Metabolism*, 17, 606-611, 1968.

[72] LeDUNE (M. A.). — Insulin studies in temporary neonatal hyperglycemia. *Arch. Dis. Childh.*, 16, 393-394, 1971.

[73] LeDUNE (M. A.). — Intravenous glucose tolerance and plasma insulin studies in small for date infants. *Arch. Dis. Childh.*, 47, 111-114, 1972.

[74] LEISTO (J.), RAIVIO (K.), KROHN (K.). — Neonatal hyperglycemia and chromosome deletion (46, xx, Dq⁻). *J. Pediatr.*, 88, 989-990, 1976.

[75] LEVY (H. L.), HAMMERSEN (G.). — Newborn screening for galactosemia and other galactose metabolic defects. *J. Pediatr.*, 92, 871-877. 1978.

[76] LILIEN (L. D.), ROSENFIELD (R. L.), BACCARO (M. M.). — Hyperglycemia in stressed small premature neonates. *J. Pediatr.*, 94, 454-459, 1979.

[77] LUBCHENCO (L. O.), BARD (H.). — Incidence of hypoglycemia in newborn infants classified by birth weight and gestational age. *Pediatrics*, 47, 831-838, 1971.

[78] MADISON (L. L.). — Role of insulin in the hepatic handling of glucose. *Arch. Intern. Med.*, 123, 284-292, 1969.

[79] MANN (T. P.), ELLIOTT (R. I. K). — Neonatal cold injury due to accidental exposure to cold. *Lancet*, 1, 229, 1957.

[80] MATUTI (M. L.), KALKHOFF (R. K.). — Sex steroid influence on hepatic gluconeogenesis and glycogen formation. *Endocrinology*, 92, 762-768, 1973.

[81] MAYMAN (C. I.). — Carbohydrate metabolism in the brain of experimental animals. In: *Studies in Physiology*, HILDES (J. A.), NAIMARK (A.) and FERGUSON (M. H.) (Eds.), University of Manitoba Press, Winnipeg, 83-92, 1969.

[82] McILWAIN (H.). — *Biochemistry and the Central Nervous System*, Churchill-Livingstone, Edinburgh, 1971.

[83] MESTYAN (M. J.), SCHULTZ (K.), SOLTESZ (G.) et al. — The metabolic effects of glucagon infusion in normoglycaemic and hypoglycaemic small for gestational age infants. II. Changes in plasma amino acids. *Acta Paediatr. Acad. Sci. Hung*, 17, 245-253, 1976.

[84] MILLS (J. L.), BAKER (L.), GOLDMAN (A. S.). — Malformations in infants of diabetic mothers occur before the seventh gestational week. Implications for treatment. *Diabetes*, 28, 292-293, 1979.

[85] MILNER (R. D. G.). — Amino acids and beta cell growth in structure and function. In: *The Diabetic Pregnancy. A Perinatal Perspective*, MERKATZ (I. R.) and ADAM (P. A. J.) (Eds.), Grune and Stratton, New York, 145, 1979.

[86] MILNER (R. D. G.). — Annotation-Neonatal hypoglycemia. A critical appraisal. *Arch. Dis. Childh.*, 47, 679-682, 1972.

[87] MILNER (R. D. G.). — The growth and development of the endocrine pancreas. In: *Scientific Foundations in Pediatrics*, DAVIS (J. A.) and DOBBING (J.) (Eds.), W. B. Saunders, Philadelphia, 507-513, 1974.

[88] MØLSTED-PEDERSEN (L.), TRAUTNER (H.), JØRGENSEN (K. R.). — Plasma insulin and K values during

intravenous glucose tolerance test in newborn infants with erythroblastosis fœtalis. *Acta Paediatr. Scand.*, *62*, 11-16, 1973.

[89] NAGEL (J. W.), SIMS (J. S.), APLIN (C. E. II), WESTMARK (E. R.). — Refractory hypoglycemia associated with a malpositioned umbilical artery catheter. *Pediatrics*, *64*, 315-317, 1979.

[90] NEWSHOLME (E. D.), START (C.). — *Regulation in Metabolism*, John Wiley and Sons Co., London, 272, 1973.

[91] OBENSHAIN (S. S.), ADAM (P. A. J.), KING (K. C.), TERAMO (K.), RAIVIO (K. O.), RAIHA (N.), SCHWARTZ (R.). — Human fetal insulin response to sustained maternal hyperglycemia. *N. Engl. J. Med.*, *283*, 566-570, 1970.

[92] OH (W.), YAP (L. L.), D'AMODIO (M. D.). — Hypoglycemia in severely affected Rh erythroblastotic infants. *J. Pediatr.*, *74*, 813, 1969 (Abstract).

[93] PAGLIARA (A. S.), KARL (I. E.), KEATING (J. P.), BROWN (R. I.), KIPNIS (D. M.). — Hepatic fructose-1,6-diphosphatase deficiency: A cause of lactic acidosis and hypoglycemia in infancy. *J. Clin. Invest.*, *51*, 2115-2123, 1972.

[94] PAUL (P. K.). — Dynamics of hepatic glycogen, œtrogen and pregnancy. *Acta Endocrinol.*, *71*, 385-392, 1972.

[95] PEDERSEN (J.). — *The Pregnant Diabetic and Her Newborn. Problems and Management*, Williams and Wilkins, Baltimore, 1977.

[96] PICKERING (D.). — Neonatal hypoglycemia due to salicylate poisoning. *Proc. R. Soc. Med.*, *61*, 1256, 1968.

[97] POLLAK (A.), COWETT (R. M.), SCHWARTZ (R.), OH (W.). — Glucose disposal in low birth weight infants during steady state hyperglycemia: Effects of exogenous insulin administration. *Pediatrics*, *61*, 546-549, 1978.

[98] RAIVIO (K. O.), HALLMAN (N.). — Neonatal hypoglycemia. I. Occurrence of hypoglycemia in patients with various neonatal disorders. *Acta Paediatr. Scand.*, *57*, 517-521, 1968.

[99] RALLESON (M. L.), MUKLE (A. W.), ZIGRANG (W. D.). — Hypoglycemia and lactic acidosis associated with fructose-1,6-diphosphatase deficiency. *J. Pediatr.*, *94*, 933-936, 1979.

[100] RASTOGI (G. K.), LETARTE (J.), FRASER (T. R.). — Immunoreactive insulin content of 203 pancreases from fœtuses of healthy mothers. *Diabetologia*, *6*, 445-446, 1970.

[101] REISNER (S. H.), ARANDA (J. V.), COLLE (E.) *et al.* — The effect of intravenous glucagon on plasma amino acids in the newborn. *Pediatr. Res.*, *7*, 184-191, 1973.

[102] ROBERT (M. F.), NEFF (R. K.), HUBBELL (J. P.) *et al.* — Association between maternal diabetes and the respiratory distress syndrome in the newborn. *N. Engl. J. Med.*, *294*, 357-360, 1976.

[103] SABATA (V.), FRERICHS (H.), WOLF (H.), STUBBE (P.). — Insulin and glucose levels in umbilical cord blood after infusions of glucose with insulin to women in labor. *J. Obstet. Gynaecol. Br. Comm.*, *77*, 121-128, 1970.

[104] SALLE (B. L.), RUITON-UGLIENGO (A.). — Effects of oral glucose and protein load on plasma glucagon and insulin concentrations in small for gestational age infants. *Pediatr. Res.*, *11*, 108-112, 1977.

[105] SCHIFF (D.), ARANDA (J. V.), CHAN (G.), COLLE (E.), STERN (L.). — Metabolic effects of exchange

transfusions. I. Effect of citrated and of heparinized blood on glucose, non-esterified fatty acids, 2-(4 hydroxybenzeneazo) benzoic acid binding and insulin. *J. Pediatr.*, *78*, 603-609, 1971.

[106] SCHIFF (D.), ARANDA (J. V.), COLLE (E.), STERN (L.). — Metabolic effects of exchange transfusion. II. Delayed hypoglycemia following exchange transfusion with citrated blood. *J. Pediatr.*, *79*, 589-593, 1971.

[107] SCHIFF (D.), COLLE (E. C.), WELLS (D.), STERN (L.). — Metabolic aspects of the Beckwith-Wiedemann syndrome. *J. Pediatr.*, *82*, 258-267, 1973.

[108] SCHIFF (D.), LOWY (C.). — Hypoglycemia and excretion of insulin in urine in hemolytic disease of the newborn. *Pediatr. Res.*, *4*, 280-285, 1970.

[109] SCHIFF (D.), STERN (L.), LEDUC (J.). — Chemical thermogenesis in newborn infants: Catecholamine excretion and the plasma non-esterified fatty acid response to cold exposure. *Pediatrics*, *37*, 577-582, 1966.

[110] SCHUTGENS (R. B. H.), HEYMANS (H.), KETEL (A.), VEDER (H. A.), DURAN (M.), KETTING (D.), WADMAN (S. K.). — Lethal hypoglycemia in a child with a deficiency of 3-hydroxy-3-methyl glutaryl coenzyme A lyase. *J. Pediatr.*, *94*, 89-91, 1979.

[111] SCHWARTZ (A. L.). — The metabolism of carbohydrate. In: *Disorders of Carbohydrate Metabolism in Infancy*, CORNBLATH (M.) and SCHWARTZ (R.) (Eds.), W. B. Saunders, Philadelphia, 3-23, 1976.

[112] SCHWARTZ (R.). — Islet responsiveness of the human fetus in utero. In: *Early Diabetes in Early Life*, CAMERINI-DAVALOS (R.) and COLE (H. S.) (Eds.), Academic Press, Inc., New York, 127-134, 1975.

[113] SCHWARTZ (R.), COWETT (R. M.), WIDNESS (J. A.). — Infants of diabetic mothers. In: *Diabetes Mellitus and Obesity*, BRODOFF (B. N.) and BLEICHER (S. J.) (Eds.), Williams and Wilkins, Baltimore, 1982, 601-610.

[114] SCHWARTZ (S. S.), RICH (B. H.), LUCKY (A. W.) et coll. — Familial nesibioblastosis: Severe neonatal hypoglycemia in two families. *J. Pediatr.*, *95*, 44-53, 1979.

[115] SENIOR (B.). — Current concepts. Neonatal hypoglycemia. *N. Engl. J. Med.*, *289*, 790-793, 1973.

[116] SENIOR (B.), SLONE (D.), SHAPIRO (S.). et coll. — Benzothiadiazides and neonatal hypoglycemia. *Lancet*, *2*, 377, 1976.

[117] SHELLEY (H. J.). — Glycogen reserves and their changes at birth and in anoxia. *Br. Med. Bull.*, *17*, 137-143, 1961.

[118] SHELLEY (H. J.), BASSETT (J. M.). — Control of carbohydrate metabolism in the fetus and newborn. *Br. Med. Bull.*, *31*, 37-43, 1975.

[119] SIMMONS (M. A.), JONES (M. D. Jr.), BATTAGLIA (F. C.) *et al.* — Insulin effect on fetal glucose utilization. *Pediatr. Res.*, *12*, 90-92, 1978.

[120] SIMPSON (S. L.). — Genetics of diabetes mellitus and anomalies in offspring of diabetic mothers. In: *The Diabetic Pregnancy. A Perinatal Perspective*, MERKATZ (I. R.) and ADAM (P. A. J.) (Eds.). Grune and Stratton, New York, 235-248, 1979.

[121] SODOYEZ-GOFFAUX (F.), SODOYEZ (J. C.). — Transient diabetes mellitus in a neonate. *J. Pediatr.*, *91*, 395-399, 1977.

[122] SOSKIN (S.), ESSEX (H. E.), HERRICK (J. F.) *et al.* — The mechanism of regulation of the blood sugar by the liver. *Am. J. Physiol.*, *124*, 558-567, 1938.

[123] SPERLING (M. A.). — Carbohydrate metabolism, glucagon, insulin and somatostatin. In: *Maternal-Fetal Endocrinology*, TULCHINSKY (D.) and RYAN (K. J.) (Eds.), W. B. Saunders, 333-354, 1980.

[124] SPERLING (M. A.), GRAJWER (L.), LEAKE (R. D.) et coll. — Effects of somatostatin (SRIF) infusion on glucose homeostasis in newborn lambs: Evidence for a significant role of glucagon. *Pediatr. Res., 11*, 962-967, 1977.

[125] STANLEY (C. A.), ANDAY (E. K.), BAKER (L.), DELIVORIA-PAPADOPOLOUS (M.). — Metabolic fuel and hormone responses to fasting in newborn infants. *Pediatrics, 64*, 613-619, 1979.

[126] STEELE (R.). — Influences of glucose loading and of injected insulin on hepatic glucose output. *Ann. N. Y. Acad. Sci., 82*, 420-430, 1959.

[127] STEINKE (J.), DRISCOLL (S. G.). — The extractable insulin content of pancreas from fetuses and infants of diabetic and control mothers. *Diabetes, 14*, 573-578, 1965.

[128] STERN (C.). — Idiopathic hypoglycemia. *Proc. R. Soc. Med., 66*, 345-346, 1973.

[129] STEVENSON (D. K.), BARTOLETTI (A. L.), OSTRANDER (C. R.) et al. — Pulmonary excretion of carbon monoxide in the human infant as an index of bilirubin prediction. II. Infants of diabetic mothers. *J. Pediatr., 94*, 956-958, 1979.

[130] SUSA (J. B.), COWETT (R. M.), OH (W.), SCHWARTZ (R.). — Suppression of gluconeogenesis and endogenous glucose production by exogenous insulin administration in the newborn lamb. *Pediatr. Res., 13*, 594-599, 1979.

[131] SUSA (J. B.), MCCORMICK (K. L.), WIDNESS (J. A.), SINGER (D. B.), OH (W.), ADAMSONS (K.), SCHWARTZ (R.). — Chronic hyperinsulinemia in the fetal rhesus monkey. Effects on fetal growth and composition. *Diabetes, 28*, 1058-1063, 1979.

[132] TEJANI (N.), LIPSHITZ (F.), HARPER (R. G.). — The response to an oral glucose load during convalescence from hypoxia in newborn infants. *J. Pediatr., 94*, 792-796, 1979.

[133] TSANG (R. C.), BROWN (D. R.), STEICHEN (J. J.). — Diabetes and calcium. Calcium disturbances in infants of diabetic mothers. In: *The Diabetic Pregnancy. A Perinatal Perspective*, MERKATZ (I. R.) and ADAM. (P. A. J.) (Eds.), Grune and Stratton, New York, 207-226, 1979.

[134] TSANG (R. C.), STEICHEN (J. J.), BROWN (D. R.). — Perinatal calcium homeostasis. Neonatal hypocalcemia and bone demineralization. *Clin. Perinatol., 4*, 385-409, 1977.

[135] VARMA (S.), NICKERSON (H.), COWAN (J. S.) et coll. — Homeostatic response to glucose loading in newborn and young dogs. *Metabolism, 22*, 1367-1375, 1973.

[136] VICTORIN (L. H.), THORELL (J. I.). — Plasma insulin and blood glucose during long-term treatment with diazoxide for infant hypoglycemia. Case Report. *Acta Paediatr. Scand., 63*, 302-306, 1974.

[137] VIDNES (J.), ØYASÆTER (S.). — Glucagon deficiency causing severe neonatal hypoglycemia in a patient with normal insulin secretion. *Pediatr. Res., 11*, 943-949, 1977.

[138] VIDNES (J.), SØVIK (O.). — Gluconeogenesis in infancy and childhood. II. Studies on the glucose production from alanine in three cases of persistent neonatal hypoglycaemia. *Acta Paediatr. Scand., 65*, 297-305, 1976.

[139] VIDNES (J.), SØVIK (O.). — Gluconeogenesis in infancy and childhood. III. Deficiency of the extramitochondrial form of hepatic phosphoenolpyruvate carboxykinase in a case of persistent neonatal hypoglycaemia. *Acta Paediatr. Scand., 65*, 307-312, 1976.

[140] WALAAS (O.). — Effect of œstrogens on the glycogen content of rat liver. *Acta Endocrinol., 10*, 193-200, 1952.

[141] WIDNESS (J. A.), SUSA (J. B.), GARCIA (J. F.) et al. — Increased erythropoiesis and elevated erythropoietin in infants born to diabetics mothers and in hyperinsulinemic rhesus fetuses. *J. Clin. Invest. 67*, 637-642, 1981.

[142] WIDNESS (J. A.), SCHWARTZ (H. C.), ZELLER (W. P.), OH (W.), SCHWARTZ (R.). — Glycohemoglobin (Hb A$_{Ic}$) in postpartum women. *Obstet. Gynecol. 57*, 414-421, 1981.

[143] WIEDEMANN (H. R.). — Complexe malformatif familial avec hernie ombilicale et macroglossie, un syndrome nouveau? *J. Genet. Hum., 13*, 223-228, 1964.

[144] WILLIAMS (P. R.), FISER (R. H. Jr.), SPERLING (M. A.) et al. — Effects of oral alanine feeding on blood glucose, plasma glucagon, and insulin concentrations in small for gestational age infants. *N. Engl. J. Med., 292*, 612-614, 1975.

[145] WOO (D.), SCOPES (J. W.), POLAK (J. M.). — Idiopathic hypoglycemia in sibs with morphological evidence of nesidioblastosis of the pancreas. *Arch. Dis. Childh., 51*, 528-531, 1976.

[146] WU (P. Y.), MODANLOU (H.), KARELITZ (M.). — Effect of glucagon on blood glucose homeostasis in infants of diabetic mothers. *Acta Paediatr. Scand., 64*, 441-445, 1975.

[147] YEUNG (C. Y.). — Hypoglycemia in neonatal sepsis. *J. Pediatr., 77*, 812-817, 1970.

[148] YEUNG (C. Y.), LEE (V. M. Y.), YEUNG (C. M.). — Glucose disappearance rate in neonatal infection. *J. Pediatr., 83*, 486-489, 1973.

[149] YSSING (M.). — Long-term prognosis of children born to mothers diabetic when pregnant. In: *Early Diabetes in Early Life*, CAMERINI-DAVALOS (R. A.) and COLE (H. S.) (Eds.), Academic Press, Inc., New York, 575-586, 1975.

[150] ZARIF (M.), PILDES (R. S.), VIDYASAGAR (D.). — Insulin and growth hormone responses in neonatal hyperglycemia. *Diabetes, 25*, 428-433, 1976.

[151] ZUCKER (P.), SIMON (G.). — Prolonged symptomatic neonatal hypoglycemia associated with maternal chloropropamide therapy. *Pediatrics, 42*, 824-825, 1968.

38

Calcium, phosphorus, magnesium and vitamin D

Jacques SENTERRE and Bernard SALLE

Several reasons justify considering the metabolism of calcium, phosphorus and magnesium together. Contrary to most other electrolytes, these minerals occur in the body fluids in the form of divalent ions. Furthermore their homeostasis involves the same three hormones: parathormone, calcitonin, and vitamin D which act essentially on the three effector organs, bone, the intestine and the kidney.

Perinatal physiology

CALCIUM

About 99 % of body calcium is located in the skeleton. In *plasma*, the concentration of total calcium is approximately 2.5 mmol/l (10 mg/dl) (Table I). Calcium in plasma is found in three forms: ionized calcium (48 %) non-ionized calcium (42 %) which is bound essentially to albumin, and finally, chelated or complexed calcium (10 %) which is found in the form of minimaly dissociated calcium salts. Contrary to ionized or complexed calcium, the calcium bound to proteins is non diffusable and non ultrafiltrable (Table II). Ionized calcium constitutes the most important fraction physiologically.

TABLE I. — CONVERSION FACTORS FOR CALCIUM, PHOSPHORUS AND MAGNESIUM CONCENTRATION

Element	Atomic weight	mmol/l	= mEq/l	= mg/l
Ca	40	1	2	40
P	31	1	1.8 *	31
Mg	24	1	2	24

* At pH 7.4.

TABLE II. — PLASMA DISTRIBUTION OF CALCIUM,
PHOSPHORUS AND MAGNESIUM

TABLE II. — PLASMA DISTRIBUTION OF CALCIUM,
PHOSPHORUS AND MAGNESIUM

Fraction	Ca	P	Mg
Ionized *	48 %	85 %	60 %
Complexed *	10 %	5 %	15 %
Bound to protein **	42 %	10 %	25 %

* Diffusible.
** Non diffusible.

The amounts of ionized and non-ionized fractions in the plasma depend essentially on the concentration of albumin and on the pH. All increases in the concentration of hydrogen ions diminish the link between calcium and albumin, and increase the amount of ionized calcium; alkalosis has the opposite effect.

In the *cells*, the greater portion of the calcium is transported actively in the mitochondria and sarcoplasmic reticulum. The concentration of calcium in cystosol is in fact extremely weak, several thousand times less than that of extracellular liquid. At the cellular and subcellular level, ionized calcium plays an essential role, however, in the integrity and permeability of membranes, binding aggregation and intracellular communication, cellular division, muscular contraction, blood coagulation, hormonal responses, etc. All these phenomena are preceeded by a transitory rise in intracellular calcium level. In response to a neural stimulus, for example, the concentration of calcium in the muscular cells increases more than one thousand times, resulting in the activation of the enzymes concerned in the biological phenomena. Calcium acts, not by direct intervention, but by reversibly fixing proteins called "calciproteins", such as calmodulin, for example. In fact, the nervous system and the hormones transmit primary information which is received by the cells, which is then transmitted by the intermediary of a second messager in which cyclic AMP and calciproteins play an essential role.

During *pregnancy*, the maternal total calcium in plasma decreases parallel to the fall in albumin. In the fetus, calcemia increases progressively from 1.5 mmol/l (6 mg/dl) in mid gestation, to reach 2 to 2.25 mmol/l (8 to 9 mg/dl) in premature infants [1] and 2.75 to 3 mmol/l (11 to 12 mg/dl) in full term infants [2, 3]. The active transport of the mother's calcium to the fetus represents 50 mg per day at 20 weeks of gestation, and 350 mg per day at 36 weeks. At the end of pregnancy, the quantity of calcium fixed by the fetus diminishes parallel to the slowing down of fetal growth. The total accumulation of calcium in the fetus is of the order of 30 g of which 80 % is fixed during the last trimester of pregnancy [4].

This amount represents 2.5 % of the maternal total calcium. In full term newborns, calcemia diminishes during the two first days of life to about 2.25 mmol/l (9 mg/dl). This reduction brings into play all the factors of regulation, in particular the hormonal secretions, which progressively re-establish the concentration of ionized calcium to a normal value [5, 6].

PHOSPHORUS

About 85 % of body phosphorus is found in the skeleton. In *plasma*, phosphorus can be divided into one fraction which is insoluble in acid (about 2.6 mmol/l) constituted mainly by phospho-lipids, and a fraction which is soluble in acid (about 1.3 mmol/l) constituted by all the inorganic phosphates and a small quantity of organic ester phosphorus. Like calcemia, inorganic phosphates of the plasma are found in three forms (Table II). At pH 7.4 the phosphates are divided into 80 % divalent ions (HPO^-_4) and 20 % monovalent ions ($H_2PO^-_4$), the result of which is that the apparent valence is 1.8 (Table I).

In the *cells*, the greater part of the phosphorus is in the form of organic compounds. The total concentration of inorganic phosphorus is higher in the cell than in the extracellular fluid, and phosphates are usually considered as the principal intracellular anions. Moreover, the fraction free in cytosol is lower, by about half, than the concentration in the extracellular fluid. Most inorganic phosphates of the cells form complexes with calcium and magnesium or are included inside mitochondria or other organelles.

The mitochondria accumulate calcium ions and phosphate together to form tricalcic amorphous and insoluble phosphates; consequently, a deficiency of intracellular phosphate can reduce calcium incorporation by the mitochondria. They also participate directly in the phosphorylation of glycogen to glucose-1-phosphate.

During *pregnancy* the maternal phosphorus in the plasma is little changed. In the fetus, the concentration of inorganic phosphorus in the plasma is high in mid gestation (5 mmol/l or 15 mg/dl) then decreases progressively to between 1.8 and 2.3 mmol/l (5.5 to 7 mg/dl) at term. It has been suggested that this fetal hyperphosphatemia could prevent the loss of calcium in the urine due to the relative inactivity and weightlessness in the uterus. In the full term newborn, the plasma phosphorus is stable or rises in the first days of life according to the state of the kidneys and the phosphorus content of food [6].

MAGNESIUM

About 65 % of body magnesium is found in the skeleton. In *plasma*, magnesium is also found in three forms (Table II). The organism contains 40 times less magnesium than calcium. However, except for bone, tissues contain more magnesium than calcium; on a millimolar basis, muscle, for example, contains 5 times more and the brain 3 times as much.

In the *cells*, the concentration of free magnesium in cytosol is weak, close to or less than that of extracellular fluid. Like calcium and phosphorus, the greater part of magnesium is included in the mitochondria or forms complexes with proteins or other ions such as phosphates and ATP. From the metabolic point of view, magnesium acts as a chelating agent in numerous biological systems and is essential for the activity of several enzymes.

During *pregnancy*, the concentration of magnesium in the plasma decreases parallel to that of calcium, by about 10 %. Hypoalbuminemia and hemodilution are particularly responsible for this diminution. Like calcium and phosphorus, magnesium is actively transported from the mother to the fetus. At term, the body of the newborn contains about 500 mg of magnesium. At birth, the plasma level of magnesium is correlated with that of the mother, but tends to be slightly higher [1, 3]. Under normal conditions it hardly changes during the first days of life.

PARATHORMONE

Parathormone is a polypeptide consisting of 84 amino acids, synthetized in the parathyroid glands from high weight molecular precursors. PTH includes an amino-terminal extremity consisting of 34 amino acids which represents the biologically active fraction of the molecule. The secretion of PTH is controlled primarily by the concentration of ionized calcium in the blood, and to a lesser degree, by that of magnesium. However, in the case of severe magnesium deficiency the secretion of PTH would be disrupted.

PTH circulates in the plasma reversibly linked to alpha-globulins; it is rapidly metabolized by the kidney and the liver (half-life: 20 min). The main metabolite is a molecule of approximately 7,000 daltons molecular weight, which is characterized by a carboxy-terminal extremity. This fragment is biologically inactive but its half-life is at least 20 times longer than that of the native hormone.

From the metabolic point of view, the most obvious effect of PTH deficiency is a fall in calcemia and a rise in phosphates. The endogenous secretion of PTH prevents these disorders by continually acting on the bone and kidney, by a mechanism which activates the adenylcyclase of the membrane and increases membrane permeability to calcium [8]. In bone PTH favours resorption by increasing the activity and number of osteoclasts. This effect is rapid and requires the presence of 1.25 dihydroxycholecalciferol. This bone resorption may result in an increase in hydroxyprolinuria. In the kidney, PTH decreases tubular reabsorption not only of phosphates but also sodium, potassium, bicarbonates and amino acids, and increases the tubular reabsorption of calcium, magnesium and glucose. Moreover, in primary hyperparathyroidism, the induced hypercalcemia can exceed the renal capacity for reabsorption and lead to hypercalciuria. Furthermore, in the mitochondria of the proximal tubules, PTH activates the 1-alpha-hydroxylase and induces the synthesis of 1.25 dihydroxycholecalciferol from 25-hydroxycholecalciferol. In this way it induces the intestinal absorption of calcium, phosphorus and magnesium.

The plasma level of PTH can be assayed by radioimmunologic methods. Moreover, the concentrations differ according to the antiserum used. In fact, some measure the native hormone, others, the biologically active amino-terminal fragment, whose half life is short, and others only recognize the carboxyterminal fragment of the molecule, which persists for a long time, but which is no longer biologically active.

During *pregnancy*, it is classical to consider that the progressive fall in calcium and phosphorus in plasma, is accompanied by a rise of plasma circulating PTH, particularly during the latter part of gestation, but recent studies do not confirm this [1]. PTH does not rise despite the reduction in calcemia, probably because ionized calcium remains at a normal level. PTH does not cross the placenta, and no correlation exists between the parathormone level in cord blood and that of the mother. The human fetus can secrete parathormone as is evident in the case of maternal hypoparathyroidism not treated during pregnancy. In the *newborn* PTH is often undetectable in cord blood, but increases parallel to the fall in calcemia and the increase in calcitonin; this phenomenon is more rapid and more marked in prematures [9].

CALCITONIN

Calcitonin (CT) is a polypeptide consisting of 32 amino acids secreted in the form of a pro-hormone by the parafollicular cells (C cells) of the thyroid. In numerous animal species, CT results in a fall in the concentration of calcium and phosphorus in plasma, but in man, this only occurs with pharmacologic doses.

This action would result, on the one hand, in the inhibition of bone resorption induced by PTH, and on the other, in an increase of mineralization processes. In the kidney, CT, like PTH, increases the urinary excretion of sodium and phosphorus; contrariwise, it inhibits the reabsorption of calcium and magnesium. There are multiple immunoreactive forms of CT in the circulation, all with high molecular weights, which could be either the precursors or the polymers of CT. In contrast, to PTH, the entire molecule is required to obtain biological activity. The synthesis of CT is much less coupled to its secretion than in the case of PTH, and large quantities of CT can be accumulated in the thyroid gland. The concentration of CT in plasma can be determined by radioimmunologic means, but in adults it is often undetectable even with the most sensitive assays. This could be due to an extremely rapid catabolism (half life is 10 min) probably in the kidney. The immuno-reactive concentrations are however 50 to 100 times weaker than those determined by biological assays. It is not known if this discordance is due to technical artefacts, or to the existence of another, as yet unidentified, hypocalcemic hormone [10].

During *pregnancy* calcitoninemia is not high. In the fetus, the appearance of cells containing CT occurs around the 14th week, and the dosage in the cord blood demonstrates the secretion of immuno-reactive CT during fetal life from the 28th week of gestation [9]. In the full term *newborn* CT rises in the first 48 hours of life, and then falls to become once again undetectable at the end of the first week. This phenomenon is as well more marked in premature infants.

VITAMIN D

Vitamin D3 or cholecalciferol (CC) and vitamin D2 or ergocalciferol (EC) have similar properties in man.

CC can be synthesized in skin from 7-dihydrocholesterol which is transformed into precholecalciferol by the action of ultra-violet rays of 290-300 nm wave length. One international unit of vitamin D corresponds to 0.025 µg (Table III).

TABLE III. — CONVERSION FACTORS FOR VITAMIN D UNITS

mmol	=	µg	=	IU
1		0.384		15.4
2.6		1		40
0.065		0.025		1

Vitamin D is absorbed in the digestive tract by the biliary salts, mainly taurocholates, and is carried into the intestinal lymphatics by lipoproteins. Either, absorbed in the digestive tract or produced in the skin, it is linked in the plasma to an alpha-globulin called transcalciferin or "D-binding-protein". In order to act on the target organs, vitamin D must be metabolised into more polar derivates. This metabolism consists in a double hydroxylation: the first step takes place on the carbon-25 in the microsomes of the hepatic cells and leads to the synthesis of 25-hydroxycholecalciferol (HCC), the second step occurs in the mitochondria of the proximal renal tubular cells, and leads to the synthesis of 1.25-dihydroxycholecalciferol (1.25-DHCC) by the action of a-alpha-hydroxylase [11]. 1.25-DHCC is considered to be the principal metabolite responsible for the physiologic activities of vitamin D. The regulation of the metabolism of vitamin D is still not well defined. The half-life of vitamin D3 is from 6 to 8 hours.

Under normal conditions, only a small fraction of the vitamin D is 25-hydroxylated; the rest is partly stored in adipose tissue, and partly excreted in the bile, in the form of inactive glucuronoconjugates. The production of 25-HCC is probably regulated by a delayed action mechanism, but in reality, large doses of vitamin D raising the level of 25-HCC, can legitimately be considered as a worthwhile index of the nutritional state of vitamin D. The physiological level of 25-HCC doesn't seem to have any biological activity. In blood, 25-HCC is linked to the same protein as vitamin D. This is normally only saturated at about 2 %; the result being that the concentration of free 25-HCC is extremely weak. Only a small fraction is retained by the kidney, the rest being partly excreted in the feces after an entero-hepatic cycle, or stocked in muscle. The half-life of 25-HCC is about 21-25 days. In the case of euparathyroidism, normocalcemia and normophosphatemia, the activity of renal 24-hydroxylase becomes preponderant, and leads to the synthesis of 24.25-dihydroxycholecalciferol. In the case of depletion of vitamin D, hypocalcemia, hypophosphatemia or hyperparathyroidism, renal 1α-hydroxylase is activated and 25-HCC is transformed into 1.25-DHCC. This metabolite increases calcemia by increasing the intestinal absorption of calcium, by potentiating the action of PTH on bone resorption and perhaps by favouring tubular reabsorption of calcium. By the same mechanism, it increases the concentration of inorganic phosphorus in the plasma. Furthermore, 1.25-DHCC inhibits the secretion of PTH and probably its own synthesis. The half-life of this metabolite is from 10 to 12 hours [12].

The role of 24.25-DHCC is still disputed, but this metabolite could intervene in bone formation of conjugation cartilage. What becomes of 1.25-DHCC is unknown. Several metabolites are excreted in the feces and urine, and it has been shown that the lateral chain is oxidized with the formation of CO_2 from carbon 26 and 27. The kidney can also synthesize 1.24.25-DHCC from 24.25-DHCC. Elsewhere, all subjects synthesize 25.26-DHCC, but the role and the place of production of this metabolite remain unknown.

In *pregnancy*, the need for vitamin D is increased, and the production of 1.25-DHCC stimulated, resulting in greater intestinal absorption and bone mobilization of calcium and phosphorus, thus satisfying the mineral needs of the fetus. The maternal level of 25-HCC varies according to sunlight exposure and exogenous supplies of vitamin D [13, 14]. The level of 24.-25-DHCC is comparable to that of the adult or slightly less [15]. On the other hand, the serum level of 1.25-DHCC rises to values of more than 60 pg/ml at the end of gestation [16]; this increased production of 1.25-DHCC is linked to the reduction of extracellular calcium, due to the continual transfer of calcium for the mineralisation of the fetus. The increase in the sexual and growth hormone levels might also play a role in this increased production of 1.25-DHCC. Furthermore, recent studies suggest that the placenta could be a production site of 1.25-DHCC. This could play a direct role in the transport of calcium from the mother to the fetus. The role of vitamin D metabolites in the mineralization of the fetal skeleton is poorly understood. In renal agenesis (Potter's syndrome) plasma 1.25-DHCC is very low but detectable and calcium, bone mineralization and size

at birth are normal. Some authors have suggested that bone growth in the fetus could depend on 24.25-DHCC, but this remains a very controversial subject.

In *newborns* both fullterm and premature infants, the plasma concentration of 25-HCC in cord blood

TABLE IV. — MEANS ± 1 SEM OF BLOOD CALCIUM, PHOSPHORUS, MAGNESIUM AND VITAMIN D METABOLITE CONCENTRATIONS IN MATERNAL VENOUS BLOOD AND CORD BLOOD FOR 20 PREMATURE INFANTS OF 34 ± 2 WEEKS GESTATIONAL AGE.

	Mother	*Cord*
Calcium (mmol/l)	1.98 ± 0.07	2.38 ± 0.12
Phosphorus (mmol/l)	1.06 ± 0.04	1.62 ± 0.07
Magnesium (mmol/l)	0.68 ± 0.04	0.72 ± 0.02
25-(OH) D (µg/l)	18 ± 12	12 ± 2
24,25-(OH)$_2$ D (µg/l)	1.3 ± 0.3	0.8 ± 0.2
1,25-(OH)$_2$ D (ng/l)	59 ± 5	34 ± 4

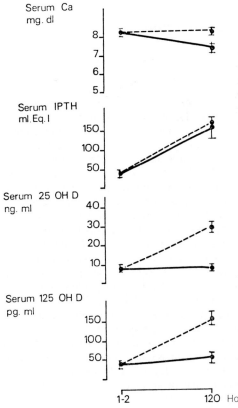

FIG. VI-16. — *Evolution of blood calcium, immunoreactive parathormone, 25 hydroxy and 1.25 Dihydroxy vitamin D levels in 2 groups of premature children fed human milk, one group receiving 2,000 IU of vitamin (- - - - -) and the other without supplemental Vitamin D (———).*

is correlated with that of the mother, but the cord level is lower because of a lesser concentration of the protein linking vitamin D [13, 14, 15]. Thus it is highly likely that there is transplacental passage of vitamin D and/or 25-hydroxy-vitamin D; 24.25- and 1.25-DHCC are also detectable in cord blood (Table IV). Some authors find a significant correlation between maternal and cord levels for these two vitamin D metabolites, but for others, this correlation does not exist. The metabolism of vitamin D in the neonatal period remains a controversial subject. Recent studies indicate that prematures, like full term newborns, are capable of synthesizing

25-HCC and 1.25-DHCC at birth [2, 17]. In fact, provided the supply of vitamin D is adequate, plasma concentrations of 25-HCC and 1.25-DHCC increase in the first days after birth. This increase is due to the diminution of calcemia, and a rise in the serum concentration of parathormone (Fig. VI-16). This physiological phenomenon plays a role in the maintenance of calcemia by stimulating bone resorption and favouring the intestinal absorption of calcium and phosphorus. Furthermore, the gut of prematures responds to oral administration of 1.25-DHCC with a significant increase in the absorption of calcium [18].

Problems in homeostasis of calcium, phosphorus and magnesium

EARLY NEONATAL HYPOCALCEMIA

Definition

Early neonatal hypocalcemia occurs spontaneously during the first 48 hours of life in nearly half of all prematures, infants born of diabetic mothers, and newborns showing signs of perinatal asphyxia. It is rare, however, in the normal full term newborn.

It is generally considered that only newborns with calcemia below 1.87 or even 1.75 mmol/l (7.5-7 mg/dl) have hypocalcemia. Although acceptable from a clinical point of view, this definition is disputable. Physiologically calcemia is in fact an important mineral in the physiological equilibrium; any drop in calcemia results in the disturbance of neuromotor functions, cellular growth, hormonal secretions, stability of cellular membranes, and enzyme activities. The presence of high cord calcemia at birth indicates that, during the last weeks of fetal life, the physiological level of calcemia is at a comparable level to that observed in children and adults. Furthermore, the premature newborn, like the fullterm newborn, is quick to normalize the situation, as after a few day it's calcemia reaches a level similar to that of an older infant.

Physiopathology

In the full term newborn, cord hypercalcemia is followed by a moderate reduction of calcemia,

which reaches its nadir during the course of the second day of life with a mean level of approximately 2.25 mmol/l (9 mg/dl). Calcemia is normalized in the great majority of infants before the end of the first week [5, 6].

This change from the intra-uterine situation, where calcemia depends essentially on the maternal calcium supply, to extra-uterine life, where it becomes suddenly dependent on food supply, and bone reserves, leads us to think that the hormonal regulation of calcemia is functional in the full term newborn.

Ideally, hypocalcemia should be defined in terms of physiologically active calcium, meaning the concentration of ionized calcium. In fact, the concentration of total calcium can be lowered, for example in the case of hypo-albuminemia, without the concentration of ionized calcium being affected. On the other hand, the concentration of ionized calcium can be raised or decreased according to blood pH without the concentration of total calcium being modified.

The reduction of ionized calcium is favoured by an increase of pH following an injection of bicarbonate, by forming calcium complexes in the case of exchange-transfusions with citrated blood, perfusions of albumin, or with the elevation of circulatory free fatty acids.

In the premature, hypocalcemia is often considered as physiological because of its high frequency. In fact, in the absence of a calcium supply, calcemia falls below 1.75 mmol/l (7 mg/dl) in about 50 %

of premature infants [19]. Longitudinal studies performed during the first 24 hours of life, have demonstrated that hypocalcemia in prematures takes place in the first 12 hours [20], during which time the mean amplitude and fall of calcemia is approximately 0.5 mmol/l; a further very moderate reduction follows up to the 24th hour of life.

After the 48th hour, a progressive increase begins in most infants, reaching normal values around the end of the first week.

The pathogenic mechanism of early neonatal hypocalcemia has been much discussed. Understanding has greatly progressed with the miniaturisation of hormonal measurements. Albuminemia, phosphatemia and magnesemia undergo no noticeable modification whilst it takes place. Hyperphosphatemia can however be an aggravating factor, favoured, for example, by neonatal anoxia.

The parathyroids seem to function and longitudinal studies made during the first hours of life demonstrate that the majority of prematures show a rapid increase in immunoreactive parathormone levels in serum, already significant after the 5th hour [9, 20, 22, 23] (Fig. VI-16). Following the decrease in calcemia, it can be concluded that the parathyroids of prematures act by increasing the secretion of PTH, which is contrary to the concept of parathyroid inertia, usually attributed to these infants. However, the lower the gestational age, the weaker this response seems. Furthermore, if the bone system of the newborn is capable of responding to PTH, the renal response, on the contrary, seems limited during the first 48 hours of life, as confirmed by low urinary excretion of phosphorus and cyclic AMP [24].

One of the most frequently advanced arguments for the explanation of this hypocalcemia, has been the immaturity of the activation system of vitamin D; first immaturity of hepatic 25-hydroxylation was considered, then immaturity of renal 1-alpha-hydroxylation. The arguments in favour of these immature enzymes were essentially indirect, and were based on the observation of a certain limitation in the reduction of calcemia when pharmacologic doses of 25-HCC or 1.25-DHCC were administered early. Given the doses used, none of the results acquired in these conditions were physiological. In fact, the assay of vitamin D metabolites indicates that vitamin D is correctly absorbed, and no impairment exists either in 25-hydroxylation or in 1.25-hydroxylation, at least in the premature infant having a gestational age of more than 30 weeks. These infants, in fact, when given a daily oral dose of vitamin D3 rapidly increase their plasma levels of 25-HCC and 1.25-DHCC (Fig. VI-16). The level

of 1.25-DHCC in plasma observed at the 72nd hour of life is higher than normal, indicating that the PTH secreted by these infants activates renal 1-alpha-hydroxylation [17].

The third hormonal factor which draws attention is calcitonin. Hypercalcitoninemia accompanies early neonatal hypocalcemia in prematures. Longitudinal studies have demonstrated that this hypercalcitoninemia takes place following a latent period of 2 to 3 hours after birth. The level of CT in plasma rises very rapidly, reaching maximal values between the 12th and the 24th hour (Fig. VI-17) [9, 20].

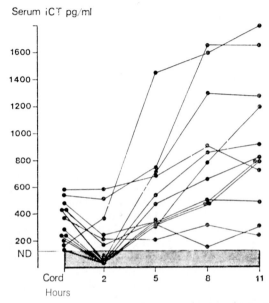

Serum iCT pg/ml

FIG. VI-17. — *Evolution of immunoreactive calcitonin during the first 11 hours of life.*

With the exception of the secretions of certain cancers, at no other time in extra-uterine life do we see CT plasma levels as high as during this period; values can exceed 1,000 pg/ml in some prematures whilst the normal level in adults is less than 100 pg, even 50 pg/ml. The amplitude of the CT peak is even higher for prematures with a lower gestational age. These high levels stay at a plateau until about the 36th hour, then diminish rapidly to low values after the 3rd or 4th day of life [21]. Knowing the antagonistic effect of CT on the bone activity of PTH, we can presume that this hypercalcitoninemia contributes in some degree to the causation and maintenance of hypocalcemia in the premature. The factor or factors which are at the origin of this hypercalcitoninemia, are at present unknown.

The main factor in early neonatal hypocalcemia in the premature is the sudden interruption of calcium at birth, in an infant with full skeletal growth and whose need of calcium is very great. The parathyroid secretion is rapidly exceeded by this sudden imbalance and its efficiency is possibly inhibited by the occurence of hypercalcitoninemia. The central role played by this interruption in the etiology of early neonatal hypocalcemia can explain a fact observed by several authors—that of the relation between the severity of hypocalcemia in the premature during the 2nd day of life, and the cord calcemia; the lower the cord calcemia, the more severe the hypocalcemia [20]. One may wonder why this reduction of calcemia is not present in full term newborns; this probably results from the fact that intra-uterine growth slows down a great deal at the end of gestation, and the calcium needs of the full term newborn are thus considerably reduced. This phenomenon shows us the physiological preparation for the first days of fasting, for which the premature is not, of course, prepared.

It is classic to isolate the hypocalcemia of *newborns of diabetic mothers*, by considering that it has a special pathogenesis. In fact, the great majority of these infants are like most prematures, with an early reduction of calcemia followed by a progressive correction after the 3rd day of life. An early rise of PTH levels in plasma indicates a good parathyroid response, the rise of CT levels in plasma is similar to that observed in "normal" prematures of the same gestational age, as is the rapid rise in plasma levels of 1.25-DHCC in the presence of a vitamin D3 supplement. It seems then, that the newborn of a diabetic mother has early hypocalcemia due, above all, to the interruption of calcium supply, this undoubtedly having special importance due to the occurence of macrosomia in these infants [25].

Symptomatology

Early hypocalcemia is usually asymptomatic. Contrary to late neonatal hypocalcemia, it is rarely responsible for convulsions. Moreover, if the infants are carefully observed, neuromuscular signs are not rare, but are not very specific. The most frequent symptoms are hyperexcitability with jitteriness, trembling of the extremities, tachypnea and eventually episodes of apnea, tachycardia and digestive disorders. These symptoms can only be viably related to hypocalcemia if they disappear when calcemia returns to normal.

The determination of calcemia must be included in systematic biological surveillance tests of prematures or infants at risk during the first two days of life. Calcemia between 12 and 24 hours constitutes a good prognostic sign; if it is below 2 mmol/l (8 mg/dl) prophylactic treatment must be envisaged. In case of convulsions, lumbar puncture is indicated essentially in search of another cause. The electro-encephalogram, if used at the moment of hypocalcemia, can show wave points which can only be connected to this disorder if they disappear with the correction of the calcemia. The electrocardiogram may show a prolongation of the QT interval, but this is not constant.

Treatment

The lack of calcium appears as the predominant etiological factor in early neonatal hypocalcemia, and the supply of calcium must be the main treatment. The (intra-muscular) administration of parathormone is illogical, costly and of very ephemeral value.

Parenteral administration of calcium. — Continuous intravenous administration of calcium at a dose of 30 mg calcium/kg/24 hr has proved efficient in the prevention of hypocalcemia [26]. In case of emergency, rapid administration of calcium at a dose of 5 mg/kg/min may be considered. It must be stressed that in cases of peripheral infusion, the extravasation of calcium into the sub-cutaneous tissue can cause severe tissue necrosis. Infusion via the umbilical vessels may result in hepatic necrosis if the catheter is placed in a branch of the portal vein, and vasomotor spasms in case of infusion via the umbilical artery.

Acute administration of calcium must always be carried out slowly with half diluted solutions of 10 % calcium glutonate or 1 % calcium chloride (1 ml/kg/min). The latter acts more rapidly on the concentration of ionized calcium, because, contrary to gluconate, the anion is not catabolized. Calcium gluconate or chloride are not compatible with solutions of sodium bicarbonate because they form a calcium carbonate precipitate. In the presence of metabolic acidosis, bicarbonate can be replaced by lactate. Acute injection of calcium can only be effected with cardiac monitoring, to screen the eventual occurence of bradycardia or arrhythmia. This risk is even greater in the presence of digitalis. The prophylactic injection of 1 ml of 10 % calcium gluconate or of 1 % calcium chloride in the course of exchange transfusions is currently recommended. Recent studies however show that this prophylaxis hardly modifies the level of ionized calcium and that the parathyroid response remains at maximum level in the course of the exchange.

Enteral administration of calcium. — Some authors recommend early oral supplementation of calcium at a dose of 70 to 100 mg/kg/day [27]. However, this induces a rise in gastric acidity and gastrin secretion. Furthermore, calcium salts considerably raise the osmolarity of the diet, and could favour the formation of a lactobezoar or the occurence of necrotizing enterocolitis. The calcium content of different calcium salts is detailed in Table V. Calcium chloride is effective but irritating to the stomach and vomiting often occurs. Solutions of only 2 % maximum can be used. Furthermore, if the treatment is continued for more than 3 or 4 days, there is a risk of hyperchloremic acidosis. Calcium lactate has fewer secondary effects, but the classic solution of 6 % is not very stable, and it is better to use the powdered form which can be administered incidentally with milk. Calcium glu-

conate, or calcium glubionate in ampoules of 10 % can also be used but this only supplies 9 mg of calcium element per ml.

Administration of vitamin D or its metabolites. — An early supply of vitamin D can be useful to favour the synthesis of 1.25-DHCC which increases digestive absorption of calcium and PTH action in bone. In fact, prematures like full term newborns are capable, after the 30th week of gestation, of absorbing and synthesizing 25-HCC and 1.25-DHCC from vitamin D [17]. The recommended dose varies from 25 to 50 μg (1,000 to 2,000 I. U.) per day according to the season. It is correct that with pharmacologic doses, 25-HCC (250 μg/day) and 1.25-DHCC (0.5 to 1 mg/day) can limit early neonatal hypocalcemia [28]. However, these metabolites run the risk of secondary hypercalcemia, more or less prolonged with hypercalciuria and nephrocalcinosis. Because of its good resorption and rapid action, 25-HCC may be given at a dose of 10 μg (400 I. U.) per day for the first 2 or 3 days of life, with the aim above all, of avoiding that the early neonatal hypocalcemia be prolonged into late neonatal hypocalcemia.

TABLE V. — CALCIUM CONTENT
OF VARIOUS CALCIUM SALTS

Anhydrous calcium salt	Calcium content	
	mmol/g	mg/g
Carbonate	10	400
Chloride	9	360
Citrate	5.2	210
Lactate	3.2	130
Gluconate	2.2	90

LATE NEONATAL HYPOCALCEMIA

Physiopathology

Late neonatal hypocalcemia most often occurs towards the end of the first week of life, but can be present, as early as the third day of life, or later, near the end of the first month (Table VI). It is observed particularly in full term infants born in

TABLE VI. — TYPES OF NEONATAL HYPOCALCAEMIA

	Early	Late
Age (days)	0-2	3-21
Patients	Premature infants	Full-term neonates
Contributing factors	Maternal diabetes mellitus, perinatal asphyxia	Artificial feeding, maternal hyperparathyroidism, primary hypoparathyroidism, hypomagnesaemia
Season	Independent	End of winter-early spring
Frequency	+++	+
Symptoms	+	+++
Phosphatemia	N or ↑	↑
iPTH	↑	↓
iCT	↑	N
Physiopathology	Low calcium intake (hypercalcitoninaemia)	Hypoparathyroidism (hypovitaminosis D, phosphorus overload)

winter or early spring and artificially fed. In prematures and newborns of diabetic mothers, it often follows early neonatal hypocalcemia.

The dominant pathogenic element is parathyroid insufficiency which is manifested by abnormally low PTH plasma levels along with the hypocalcemia [29, 30]. This hypoparathyroidism also reduces renal 1α-hydroxylase activity and the synthesis of 1.25-DHCC. In the situation of parathyroid insufficiency, several factors can aggravate or unmask hypocalcemia: the phosphorus content of artificial feeding and an early deficiency of vitamin D due to maternal deficiency, are the two principal favouring factors. Prolonged hypocalcemia with tetany has also been observed in newborns of mothers treated with anticonvulsivants for several years, which induces an increase in the hydroxylation of vitamin D into inactive metabolites. The mechanism of this transitory hypoparathyroidism is unknown. The pathogenesis can be considered in the light of hypoparathyroidism and hypocalcemia observed in newborns of hyperparathyroid mothers. In these infants, in fact, the parathyroid activity is at rest during fetal life, under the effect of the maternal hypercalcemia, which hinders parathormone reactivity for 2 or 3 months after birth.

The secretion and peripherical activity of PTH being dependant on magnesium ion, one must always remember the possibility of primary hypomagnesemia linked to congenital difficulty in the absorption of magnesium, as an explanation for late neonatal hypocalcemia, and any unresponsiveness to classical treatment should lead to measurement of the serum magnesium level which is very low in primary hypomagnesemia [31, 32].

Finally, neonatal hypocalcemia can be the result of true hypoparathyroidism. This can be sporadic or sex linked. Agenesis of the parathyroids may be associated with anomalies of the aortic arch and with an absence of the thymus resulting in a profound deficiency of cellular immunity. This congenital dysplasia constitutes the Di George syndrome.

Symptomatology

Contrary to early neonatal hypocalcemia, late neonatal hypocalcemia is often revealed by convulsions, of which it is a not infrequent cause at this age. The convulsions are often of short duration but repetitive; they can be focal, multifocal or generalized. During the interval phase, there is usually no generalized hypotonia; the infant remains alert and often presents an increase in extensor tone, rapid reflexes and clonus [29]. In some cases, hypo-

calcemia manifests as digestive and cardiorespiratory difficulties; a presentation as tachycardia with superficial respiration and even sometimes signs of cardiac failure with a picture of respiratory distress may be observed. In contrast, the classic signs of tetany: carpopedal spasm, Chvostek's sign and laryngospasm are usually absent. The neurological prognosis of hypocalcemic convulsions is considerably better than that of hypoglycemic convulsions. When hypocalcemia is prolonged hypoplasia of the milk teeth can be observed. Calcium determination can confirm or reveal late neonatal hypocalcemia in asymptomatic forms. It is necessary to measure plasma phosphorus and magnesium, because two thirds of hypocalcemia is accompanied by hyperphosphatemia, and one third by hypomagnesemia. In the absence of a measurement of ionized calcium, this can be estimated from the measurement of pH and protein. Ideally, the examination is completed by a measurement of alkaline phosphatase; PTH and the metabolites of vitamin D. The E. E. G. is abnormal in more than half the cases. The E. C. G. can show a prolongation of the QT interval as hypocalcemia prolongs venticular systole. In cases of convulsions one must perform a lumbar puncture. In the cerebro-spinal fluid, the variations in the concentration of calcium (about 50 % of the calcemia) and of magnesium (about 125 % of the magnesemia) are less marked than in the blood because the homeostasis is regulated by an active transport process. Furthermore, it is useful to X-ray the thorax to eliminate the Di George syndrome. Finally, late neonatal hypocalcemia is sometimes the only revealing sign of maternal hyperparathyroidism which can be confirmed by plasma measurements of calcium, phosphorus, phosphatase and parathormone in the mother.

Treatment

The treatment of late neonatal hypocalcemia is both preventive and curative. Prophylaxis consists of providing a sufficient supply of vitamin D at birth, or even better, at the end of pregnancy, particularly if sunlight exposure is reduced, or if the mother has received anticonvulsants. In the rare case where the mother has a parathyroid adenoma, neonatal hypoparathyroidism can be avoided by its removal during pregnancy. In full term newborns, as well as in prematures, human milk feeding, with its high calcium/phosphorus ratio, reduces the frequency of late neonatal hypocalcemia. Finally all parenteral feeding should contain a balanced phosphorus and calcium supply.

The treatment of late neonatal hypocalcemia combines that of transient hypoparathyroidism and rests essentially on the supply of calcium, vitamin D and eventually parathormone. In case of emergency, intravenous calcium is necessary to arrest clinical manifestations. It should be used in the same modality as that described for the treatment of early neonatal hypocalcemia.

In case of a severe deficiency associated with magnesium deficiency, calcemia can only be re-established by the correction of the hypomagnesemia. In the case of hyperphosphatemia, the phosphorus food supply must be reduced by using human milk or infant formulas with a high calcium: phosphorus ratio. An oral supplement of calcium at a dose of 70 to 100 mg/kg/day is often necessary.

The administration of vitamin D at a dose of 100 to 150 μg (4,000 to 6,000 I. U.) per day, or of 25-hydroxycholecalciferol in a dose of 25 to 50 μg/day followed by a progressive reduction once the calcemia is normalized, is often effective. However, it is certain that the best treatment for transient hypoparathyroidism is the concomitant administration of 1.25-dihydroxycholecalciferol or of 1-alpha-hydroxycholecalciferol in a dose of 0.5 to 2 μg per 24 hours for several days [30]. The very short half-life of these metabolites of vitamin D removes the risk of prolonged hypercalcemia. Before the availability of these active metabolites of vitamin D, dihydroxytachysterol, which is an analogue of the structure of 1.25-DHCC was successfully used in a dose of 50 to 100 μg/day.

The intra-muscular injection of parathormone in a dose of 5 I. U. per kg is effective but costly and its effects only last a few hours.

As a general rule, once corrected, hypocalcemia does not tend to reappear. However, the newborn of a mother with a parathyroid adenoma may present with hypoparathyroidism necessitating treatment for several weeks. Finally the rare cases of true hypoparathyroidism require uninterrupted treatment.

HYPERCALCEMIA

Physiopathology

In the neonatal period, hypercalcemia is rare and is often of iatrogenic origin (Table VII). It is generally explained by a relative deficiency in phosphorus supply during parenteral or oral feeding. It can also be due to an overdose of vitamin D or its metabolites, or to untimely injections of calcium salts or parathormone. However, when an injection of calcium gluconate is given during exchange transfusions with citrated blood, the level of total calcium will be high whilst the level of ionized calcium will remain low.

TABLE VII. — MAIN CAUSES OF HYPERCALCAEMIA

Low phosphorus intake
Vitamin D overdose
Parathormone injections
Primary hyperparathyroidism
Secondary hyperparathyroidism
Idiopathic childhood hypercalcaemia
Hypophosphatasia
Calcified fatty necrosis
Blue diaper syndrome

Rarely, neonatal hypercalcemia is due to a primary adenoma or a diffuse hyperplasia of the parathyroids, which can be either sporadic or herediraty. Secondary hypoparathyroidism, observed in infants born of hyperparathyroid mothers is generally manifested by serious bone demineralization with normo- or hypercalcemia.

Idiopathic infantile hypercalcemia usually appears after a few months. However, neonatal forms have been described. It can be caused by a transient disorder in the homeostasis mechanism of the secretion of parathormone and the metabolism of vitamin D. In rare cases, prolonged hypercalcemia can be found in newborns with large areas of calcified sub-cutaneous steatonecrosis.

Inexplicable hypercalcemia is found in most cases of hypophosphatasia with precocious manifestations (before 6 months). This rare illness is characterized by an absence of alkaline phosphatase of bone origin, an enchondral defect in ossification, and radiological signs similar to rickets.

Blue diaper syndrome which classically associates hypercalcemia and nephrocalcinosis is due to a deficiency in the absorption of tryptophan which is degraded by the bacteria of the intestinal tract into indol derivatives. These are responsible for the indicanuria with blue coloration of the diapers. In this disorder, hypercalcemia generally only appears after several months.

Symptomatology

Moderate hypercalcemia is usually asymptomatic. Beyond 3.5 mmol/l (14 mg/dl) it is revealed by digestive difficulties: anorexia, constipation and vomiting, and renal manifestations: polyuria and polydipsia. Cardiac findings are frequent: hypertension, arrythmia with shortening of the S. T. segment on the E. C. G. Neurologic manifestations are characterized by hypotonia, pseudo-paralysis, or in contrast, hyperirritability and convulsions. Hypercalcemia rapidly results in a halt in staturo-ponderal growth, nephrocalcinosis and calcium deposits in the tissues.

All hypercalcemia must be documented by a complete ionogram with measurements of calcium, phosphorus and magnesium in the blood and urine to which must be added the determination of plasma levels of alkaline phosphatase, parathormone and if possible the metabolites of vitamin D. A check on renal function and an X-ray of the skeleton must also be carried out.

Iatrogenic hypercalcemia is accompanied by hypercalciuria and hypophosphatemia. An adenoma or diffuse hyperplasia of the parathyroids is shown by an increase in alkaline phosphatase and a high level of parathormone. Severe idiopathic neonatal hypercalcemia is characterized by the Elfin-face syndrome, staturo-ponderal and mental retardation and a systolic murmur due to aortic supravalvular stenosis (Williams-Beuren syndrome).

Treatment

In iatrogenic cases, hypercalcemia is often moderate and can be corrected by rebalancing the supplies of calcium and phosphorus and by adaptation of the dose of vitamin D or its metabolites. Severe hypercalcemia, which accompanies dehydration with hyperthermia and collapse, constitutes a medical emergency. The treatment must, first and foremost, correct the hydration and electrolyte disturbances. In case of associated severe renal insufficiency, an exchange transfusion is indicated, or eventually peritoneal dialysis. A reduction in calcemia can be obtained by sequestering the intravascular calcium, by increasing the calciuria, by favouring the bone fixation of calcium or by diminishing the intestinal absorption. If the calcemia is very high (5 mmol/l) there is considerable risk of cardiac arrest. Under these conditions a continuous injection of an aqueous solution of EDTA in a dose of 5 g/l will immediately reduce the level of ionized calcium in the plasma, by forming soluble inert complexes, but this effect is transient. A massive increase in calciuria can be obtained by the administration of furosemide at a dose of 2 mg/kg every 4 hours, with control of hydration and electrolyte losses. The use of 2 u/kg of calcitonin every 8 hours can be effective, particularly if the hypercalcemia is secondary to an

increased osteolysis. In the case of hypervitaminosis D, a dose of 1 mg/kg/day of prednisolone can inhibit the intestinal absorption of calcium. In some cases of hypophosphatasia, corticoids improve the X-ray changes and rapidly bring calcemia back to normal values. In the case of primary hyperparathyroidism, surgical treatment is necessary.

HYPOPHOSPHATEMIA

Neonatal hypophosphatemia can be defined as a serum level of inorganic phosphorus less than 1.3 mmol/l (4 mg/dl).

In practice, it is essentially secondary to a deficient phosphorus supply. It is often observed during parenteral feeding with solutions short of phosphorus or unbalanced in calcium and phosphorus. It is not rare in prematures fed with human milk, particularly when this has been enriched with proteins and/or calcium. Hypophosphatemia due to lack of supply, occurs together with hypercalcemia, hypercalciuria and a urinary excretion absent or very low in phosphorus. Despite hypercalcemia and the inhibition of the secretion of parathormone, bone resorption is increased and alkaline phosphatase activity is high, perhaps because of an increased synthesis of 1.25-dihydroxyvitamin D. Hypophosphatemia associated with hypercalcemia can also be observed in primary hyperparathyroidism because of the diminished renal tubular reabsorption of phosphorus.

Hypophosphatemia is classic in rickets due to a lack of vitamin D, and can appear very early in prematures. It generally appears after the neonatal period in the case of vitamin D-resistant rickets secondary to the diminution of tubular reabsorption of phosphates. This is found in sex linked hypophosphatemia and in the Fanconi syndromes, idiopathic or secondary to inborn errors of metabolism (cystinosis, tyrosinosis, Lowe's syndrome, Wilson's disease, fructosemia) (Table VIII).

Hypophosphatemia is usually asymptomatic. However, when it is severe, it can result in a diminution of the concentration of ATP in all tissues and the amount of 2.3-DPG in erythrocytes; this is shown by muscular weakness, apathy, and a reduction of oxygen delivered to the tissues. Chronic hypophosphatemia also results in hypomineralization of bone and stops growth.

The treatment of neonatal hypophosphatemia rests particularly on the adaptation of the phosphorus supply during oral or parenteral feeding and the eventual correction of the lack of vitamin D.

Hypophosphatemia:

Low phosphorus intake
Hypovitaminosis D
Primary hyperparathyroidism
Secondary hyperparathyroidism
Sex linked hypophosphataemia
Fanconi syndromes

Hyperphosphatemia:

Phosphorus-rich diet
Anoxia and acidosis
Neonatal renal failure
Hypervitaminosis D
Primary hypoparathyroidism
Secondary hypoparathyroidism

HYPERPHOSPHATEMIA

The two principal causes of hyperphosphatemia, in the newborn, e. g. a level of inorganic phosphorus in plasma greater than 2.8 mmol/l (8.7 mg/dl), are a deficiency of secretion or a lack of peripheral activity of parathormone and renal insufficiency (Table VIII).

In the first days of life, hyperphosphatemia is most often secondary to neonatal asphyxia with loss of intra-cellular phosphorus to the extra-cellular compartment, together with a slight decrease in renal glomerular filtration. After the first days, hyperphosphatemia is essentially observed in infants fed formula milk rich in phosphorus. In the case of renal immaturity, transient hypoparathyroidism or lack of vitamin D (which affects the absorption of calcium more than that of phosphorus), this high supply of phosphorus can produce hyperphosphatemia and symptomatic secondary hypocalcemia.

Treatment consists of reducing the phosphorus supply by giving preference to breast milk or infant formulas with a high calcium/phosphorus ratio. In the case of lack of vitamin D, the administration of vitamin D3 can also reduce the overload of phosphorus in the organism by increasing intestinal absorption of calcium, thus favoring phosphorus and calcium retention in the skeleton.

HYPOMAGNESEMIA

In the newborn, hypomagnesemia (magnesium less than 0.6 mmol/l or 1.4 mg/dl) often accompanies hypocalcemia. This is in part explicable by the fact that magnesium ions are not substituted for calcium ions in the cells [33]. In some cases hypomagnesemia is secondary to a maternal lack of magnesium; it is not rare in infants of diabetic mothers and in newborns with intra-uterine growth retardation. A drop of magnesium in the plasma can also be observed in the course of repeated exchange transfusions with citrated blood, in the acute correction of acidosis by alkaline buffers, or in the course of parenteral feeding completely bereft of magnesium (Table IX). Hypomagnesemia can also be secondary to increased urinary excretion of magnesium from a defect of tubular reabsorption following the administration of nephrotoxic antibiotics, diuretics or diphenylhydantoin.

Hypomagnesaemia:

Low magnesium intake
Maternal magnesium deficiency
Repeated exchange transfusions with citrated blood
Diuretics, nephrotoxic antibiotics and diphenyl-hydantoin
Chronic congenital hypomagnesaemia due to intestinal malabsorption

Hypermagnesaemia:

Treatment of maternal eclampsia with magnesium sulphate
Antacids
Anoxia, acidosis, renal failure

Chronic congenital hypomagnesemia is rare. This hereditary sex linked disorder is due to a deficiency in the intestinal transport of magnesium rapidly manifested by the near disappearance of magnesemia (below 0.4 mmol/l or 1 mg/dl) and severe hypocalcemia [34].

The symptoms of hypomagnesemia are often confounded with those of the hypocalcemia which accompanies it. The Na^+, K^+, ATPase which maintain a high concentration of potassium and a low concentration of sodium in the cell, is activated by magnesium; consequently, in cases of magnesium deficiency, there is a reduction of potassium and intracellular magnesium and a risk of cardiac difficulties, greatly accentuated by the administration of digitalis. In the case of profound magnesium deficiency, calcemia can only be restored by the administration of magnesium. In the presence of symptoms of tetany, it is necessary to obtain a plasma measurement of both ions. The concentration of magnesium in the erythrocyte diminishes more slowly and to a lesser degree than in the plasma; because of this the level of intra-erythrocyte magnesium is not a sufficient measure of an acute deficiency of magnesium.

The emergency treatment of symptomatic hypomagnesemia with hypocalcemia and convulsions rests on the parenteral administration of magnesium sulfate which gives 20 mg of elemental Mg per 100 mg; the slow administration of 0.3 ml/kg of a 15 % solution intravenously, or 0.1 ml/kg of a 50 % solution intramuscularly every 8 to 12 hours, generally permits the correction of hypomagnesemia, but the intravenous route is preferable because of the risk of local necrosis at the point of injection.

The treatment must be followed by the oral administration of 100 mg of magnesium per kg per day, in the form of sulfate or lactate for a few days in transient hypomagnesemia and permanently in chronic congenital hypomagnesemia. Some authors have recommended the use of magnesium to treat symptomatic hypocalcemia in newborns, including cases where serum magnesium is normal, but this approach does not seem logical. An overdose of magnesium causes hypotonia, easily corrected by calcium salts.

HYPERMAGNESEMIA

Hypermagnesemia is occasionally observed in newborns of mothers who have received injections of magnesium sulfate for the treatment of eclampsia (Table IX). There are no symptoms and no treatment is required as long as the plasma concentration of magnesium remains below 2.5 mmol/l (6 mg/dl) beyond that concentration, the curariform effect of magnesium can bring about respiratory depression, lethargy and hypotonia.

Hypermagnesemia can also result in intraventricular conduction difficulties and ganglionic paralysis with delayed meconium elimination. Some cases of hypermagnesemia have recently been described following the use of antacid preparations containing magnesium for the treatment of gastric hemorrages in newborns treated with tolazoline.

The treatment of severe hypermagnesemia rests on the intravenous administration of calcium salts and eventually on exchange-transfusion with citrated blood, which has the ability both to remove the magnesium from the body in addition to inactivating excess amounts by binding to the citrate.

The requirements for calcium, phosphorus, magnesium and vitamin D

THE NEEDS
OF FULL TERM NEWBORNS

Breast milk constitutes the physiological food for a fullterm newborn. Mature milk contains per 100 ml, 25 to 30 mg of calcium, 12 to 15 mg of phosphorus and 2.5 to 3 mg of magnesium. Under normal conditions more than two thirds of the calcium and magnesium, and about 90 % of the phosphorus are absorbed by the intestine and practically all the minerals absorbed are retained in the organism for growth. Thanks to its high calcium phosphorus ratio, breast milk entails no overload of phosphorus, and prevents neonatal hypocalcemia.

Preparations based on cows milk are richer in minerals. In the absence of a lack of vitamin D, these are usually well absorbed and the amounts retained are higher than those observed during breast feeding. This is shown by a slighter drop in bone density, observed either by X-ray or by the measurement of bone mineral content during the first months of life (Fig. VI-18). However, the calcium phosphorus ratio is usually lower in these preparations than in maternal milk. The absorption of phosphorus always being higher than that of calcium, this carries the risk of a phosphorus overload, which can result in hyperphosphatemia, hyperphosphaturia and eventually, hypocalcemia. It is therefore undesirable to feed fullterm newborns preparations rich in minerals; if breast feeding is not possible, it is better to use formula milk with a calcium phosphorus ratio close to the 2/1 of maternal milk.

Although the real need is probably less, the daily prophylactic dose of vitamin D generally recommended is 10 μg (400 I. U.) per day in the form of

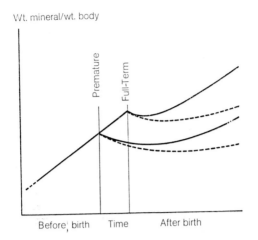

Wt. mineral/wt. body

Premature

Full-Term

Before birth   Time   After birth

FIG. VI-18. — *Evolution in body content of calcium per kg body weight in premature infants and full-term neonates fed maternal milk (- - - - -) or calcium-rich milks.*

vitamin D3 (cholecalciferol) or D2 (ergocalciferol). This daily dose must be administered systematically from birth to the end of the first year in the form of hydrosoluble preparations of vitamin D. Intermittent administration of large doses of vitamin D must be avoided, as their resorption is variable and can risk overdosage. Certain formula milks are enriched in vitamin D by 1 microgram or 40 I. U. per 100 ml. Although the risk of overdosage is minimal with these milks, the daily prophylactic dose of vitamin D can be reduced by half. Like cows milk, breast milk contains only 1 to 2 I. U. of vitamin D per 100 ml. Some studies have suggested that breast milk can contain nearly 40 I. U. of vitamin D sulphate and non negligible quantities of hydroxylated derivates of vitamin D in the aqueous phase. Recent studies using more specific measurement techniques have not confirmed these observations. Although rare, cases of rickets have been described in infants breastfed for a long time. In practice, there are grounds for administering a daily prophylactic dose of vitamin D to breastfed infants.

THE NEEDS OF THE PREMATURE

During pregnancy the fetus accumulates about 30 g of calcium, 17 g of phosphorus, and 0.8 g of magnesium [4, 36]. More than two thirds of these minerals are acquired during the last trimester of gestation; the retention is exponential between 26 and 36 weeks then it decreases progressively to the end of pregnancy (Table X). From this we can easily see that the mineral needs of prematures are

higher than those of fullterm newborns; it is not rare to observe early signs of osteopenia or rickets in prematures of low birth weight. The optimal mineral supply for these infants, however, is a controversial subject. In 1919, Yllpö [37] already doubted that breast milk could cover the phosphocalcic needs of prematures. Metabolic studies performed on breastfed prematures show that the intestinal absorption coefficient of calcium is high (50 to 80 %) but the calcium retention is limited (15 to 25 mg/kg/day) because the calcium supply is very low and calciuria is abnormaly high [38, 39].

TABLE X. — MINERAL RETENTION (mg kg^{-1} day^{-1}) IN THE FŒTUS AND BREASTFED FULLTERM NEONATE

Age	Ca	P	Mg
30 weeks.	122	65	3.5
35 weeks.	168	86	3.8
40 weeks.	89	48	1.9
1-4 months	30	20	1.6

This hypercalciuria is explained by a deficient phosphorus supply. In fact, the low quantity of phosphorus supplied by the mother's milk is well absorbed, but given the degree of nitrogenous anabolism, phosphorus is used preferentially for cellular growth. In these conditions, there is not sufficient phosphorus left to fix all the calcium absorbed; this shows in a drop in phosphatemia, almost absent phosphaturia, hypercalcemia and above all, hypercalciuria [40]. This deficient phosphorus supply also explains the high magnesium content of urine. The milk of mothers prematurely delivered again accentuates this relative deficiency of phosphorus, because the milk is rich in nitrogen and in electrolytes but not in minerals.

One must beware of the high calciuria and the risk of nephrocalcinosis in prematures fed from bank human milk enriched with protein and/or calcium. In practice, it is useful to add phosphorus to breast milk for prematures, in the form of, for example, a molar solution of dipotassium phosphate or disodium phosphate. This supplies 31 mg of elemental phosphorus and 2 mmol of cation per ml. As a general rule, the addition of 2 to 3 ml of this solution per litre of milk, is sufficient to normalize calciuria and phosphatemia [41, 42, 46].

Cow's milk preparations are richer in minerals than breast milk. However, the phosphorus and calcium retention is not necessary better with these preparations. The intestinal absorption of calcium is influenced by numerous factors, such as the calcium phosphorus ratio in the milk, the presence of lactose, the digestive secretion of endogenous calcium, the presence of steatorrhea, the vitamin D supply and the postconceptional age [42, 43, 44]. Metabolic balance studies have shown that, in prematures as in older infants, 1.25-dihydroxyvitamin D is the main factor in the intestinal absorption of calcium [18]. The plasma level of 1.25-DHCC is substrate dependant. The fullterm newborn's need of vitamin D is of the order of 400 I. U. per day, whilst it is at a minimum of 1,200 in prematures. In the case of lack of vitamin D, it is not rare to observe a negative calcium balance, the faecal loss of calcium being greater than the ingested quantity because of a deficiency in the reabsorption of endogenous calcium. Steatorrhea, which is not negligible in prematures also favours the faecal loss of calcium. Moreover, the frequent correlation observed between the faecal loss of calcium and fats is not solely explicable by the formation of insoluble calcium soaps.

In fact, calcium inhibits the activity of pancreatic and prepyloric lipase; because of this, milks rich in calcium favour steatorrhea, principally in the form of triglycerides.

The use of formulas containing well absorbed fats such as medium chain triglycerides improves not only the intestinal absorption coefficient of fats, but also that of calcium [41].

In contrast to calcium, phosphorus is always well absorbed, even in the case of vitamin D deficiency. In prematures, even more than in full term newborns, milks rich in phosphorus or with a low calcium/phosphorus ratio entail the risk of hyperphosphatemia, hypocalcemia, and metabolic acidosis secondary to a urinary excretion high in sodium phosphates because of an impaired production of amonium ions. Some infant formulas specially adapted for prematures, are very rich in minerals; control studies have demonstrated that the calcium retention is similar or even superior to that of the fetus in utero. However, the phosphorus retention and the bone density measurements do not differ from those observed with classical milks, which casts a doubt on the reality of the high calcium balance [41]. It must not be forgotten that the calcium salts added to milk are not very soluble. By falling quickly to the bottom of the container, they also favour a relative overload of phosphorus. Milks rich in protein and in minerals can also favour the appearance of lactobezoars and the occurrence of necrotizing enterocolitis. In fact, it is neither useful nor necessary to try to obtain the same bone mineralization as in utero, in the very premature. The deposition of calcium in the form of hydroxyapatites also involves a non-

negligible amount of hydrogen ions (2 mEq/100 mg of calcium). As long as the vitamin D supply is adequate, satisfactory bone mineralisation can be obtained in prematures receiving 100 to 150 mg of calcium and 50 to 80 mg of phosphorus per kg per day.

NEEDS IN PARENTERAL FEEDING

To maintain the homeostasis of minerals, and to assure a satisfactory mineralization of the skeleton, it is necessary to supply calcium, phosphorus, magnesium and vitamin D in prematures receiving total parenteral feeding. A supply of calcium of the order of 45 mg/kg/day, in the form of gluconate, and magnesium of the order of 5 mg/kg/day, in the form of sulphate, will avoid hypocalcemia and hypomagnesemia and insure satisfactory mineralization of the skeleton. In these conditions, it is imperative to supply phosphorus as well, in the form of potassium, sodium or sodium potassium phosphates. Keeping in mind the fact that tissues fix about 8 mg of phosphorus per 100 mg of nitrogen retained, and bone 45 mg of phosphorus per 100 mg of calcium, the phosphorus needs are also of the order of 45 mg/kg/day when the calcium supply is 45 mg/kg/day and the nitrogen supply 400 mg/kg/day.

Our experience shows that ready to use solutions containing calcium, phosphorus and magnesium can be prepared if the calcium is added at the beginning of the preparation, with the amino acids, and the phosphorus at the end of the preparation; under these conditions no precipitates of calcium phosphate are formed. Infusions of bicarbonate are not compatible with calcium salts and the bicarbonate must be otherwise administered, or replaced by lactate.

REFERENCES

[1] DELVIN (E. E.), GLORIEUX (F. H.), SALLE (B. L.), DAVID (L.), VARENNE (J. P.). — Control of vitamin D metabolism in preterm infants; fœtomaternal relationships. *Arch. Dis. Child.*, 57, 754-757, 1982.
[2] STEICHEN (J. J.), TSANG (R. C.), GRATTON (T. L.), HAMSTRA (A.), DELUCA (H. F.). — Vitamin D homeostasis in the perinatal period 1.25-dihydroxyvitamin D in maternal, cord and neonatal blood. *N. Engl. J. Med.*, 302, 315-319, 1980.
[3] PITKIN (R. M.), CRUIKSHANK (D. P.), SCHAUBERGER (C. W.), REYNOLDS (W.), WILLIAMS (G. A.), HARGIS (G. K.). — Fetal calcitropic hormones and neonatal calcium homeostasis. *Pediatrics*, 66, 77-82, 1980.
[4] WIDDOWSON (E. M.), DICKERSON (J. T.). — Chemical composition of the body. In: *Mineral metabolism*, COMAR (C. L.) and BRONNER (F.), eds. Academic Press, New York, vol. 2, part. A, chapter 17, 1961.

[5] BAGNOLI (F.). — Calcium homeostasis in the first days of life in relation to feedind. *Eur. J. Pediatr.*, *144*, 41, 1985.

[6] DAVID (L.), ANAST (C. S.). — Calcium metabolism in newborn infants: the interrelation ship of parathyroid function and calcium, magnesium and phosphorus metabolism in normal « sick », and hypocalcemic newborns. *J. Clin. Invest.*, *54*, 287-296, 1974.

[7] GLEN (D. W.), MacGREGOR (R. R.), CHU (L. L.), HUANG (D. W.), ANAST (C. S.), HAMILTON (J. W.). — Biosynthesis of proparathormone and parathormone chemistry, physiology and role in calcium regulation. *Am. J. Med.*, *56*, 767, 1974.

[8] HAMBURGER (R. J.), LAWSON (N. L.), SCHWARTZ (J. H.). — Response of parathormone in defined segments of proximal tubule. *Am. J. Physiol.*, *230*, 286, 1976.

[9] DAVID (L.), SALLE (B. L.), CHOPARD (P.), GRAF-MEYER (D.). — Studies on circulating immunoreactive calcitonin in low birth weight infants during the first 48 hours of life. *Helv. Paediatr. Acta*, *32*, 39, 1977.

[10] RIORDON (J. L.), AMBUCH (G. D.). — Mode of action of thyrocalcitonin. *Endocrinology*,*82*,377,1968.

[11] DELUCA (H. F.), SCHNOES (H. K.). — Metabolism and mechanism of action of vitamin D. *Ann. Rev. Biochem.*, *45*, 631, 1976.

[12] DELUCA (H. F.). — Vitamin D metabolism. *Clin. Endocrinol. (suppl.)*, *7*, 15, 1977.

[13] MILLNON (L. S.), HADDAD (J. G.). — Human perinatal vitamin D metabolism 1.25-hydroxyvitamin D in maternal cord blood. *J. Pediatr.*, *84*, 742, 1974.

[14] BOUILLON (R.), VAN ASSCHE (F. A.), VAN BAELEN (H.), HEYNS (W.), DE MOOR (P.). — Influence of the vitamin D binding protein on the serum concentration of 1.25-dihydroxyvitamin D_3 concentration. *J. Clin. Invest.*, *67*, 589, 1981.

[15] WEISMAN (Y.), OCCHIPINTI (M.), KNOX (G.), REITER (E.), ROOT (A.). — Concentrations of 24-25-dihydroxyvitamin D and 25-hydroxyvitamin D in paired maternal-cord sera. *Am. J. Obstet. Gynecol.*, *130*, 1073, 1978.

[16] KUMAR (R.), COHEN (W. R.), SILVA (P.), EPSTEIN (F. H.). — Elevated 1.25-dihydroxyvitamin D plasma levels in normal human pregnancy and lactation. *J. Clin. Invest.*, *63*, 342, 1979.

[17] GLORIEUX (F.), SALLE (B. L.), DELVIN (E.), DAVID (L.). — Vitamin D metabolism in preterm infants: serum calcitriol levels during the first five days of life. *J. Pediatr.*, *99*, 640-643, 1981.

[18] SENTERRE (J.), DAVID (L.), SALLE (B. L.). — Effects of 1.25-dihydroxychole-calciferol on calcium, phosphorus and magnesium balance, and on circulating parathyroid hormone and calcitonin in preterm infants. In: *Intensive Care in the newborn* III. STERN (L.) and SALLE (B.), eds., Masson, New York, 115-125, 1981.

[19] ROSLI (A.), FANCONI (A.). — Neonatal hypocalcemia. « Early type » in low birth weight newborns. *Helv. Paediatr. Acta*, *28*, 443-457, 1973.

[20] DAVID (L.), SALLE (B. L.), PUTET (G.), GRAFMEYER (D.). — Serum immunoreactive calcitonin in low birth weight infants. Description of early changes; effect of intravenous calcium infusion; relationships with early changes in serum calcium, phosphorus, magnesium, parathyroid hormone and gastrin levels. *Pediatr. Res.*, *15*, 803-808, 1981.

[21] SALLE (B. L.), DAVID (L.), GLORIEUX (F. H.), DELVIN (E.), SENTERRE (J.), RENAUD (H.). — Early oral administration of vitamin D and its metabolites in premature neonates. Effect on mineral homeostasis. *Pediatr. Res.*, *16*, 75-78, 1982.

[22] HILLMAN (L. S.), ROJANASATHIT (S.), SLATOPOLSKY (E.), HADDAD (J. G.). — Serial measurements of serum calcium, magnesium, parathyroid hormone, calcitonin and 25-hydroxyvitamin D in premature infants during the first week of life. *Pediatr. Res.*, *11*, 739-744, 1977.

[23] ANAST (C. S.), DIRKSEN (H.). — Studies related to the pathogenesis of neonatal hypocalcemia. In: *Endocrinology of calcium metabolism*, COPP (D. H.) and TALMAGE (R. V.), eds. Excerpta Medica Foundation, Amsterdam, *421*, 12-17, 1978.

[24] LINARELLI (L. G.), BOBIK (C.), BOBIK (J.). — Urinary *c*AMP and renal responsiveness to parathormone in premature hypocalcemic infants. *Pediatr. Res.*, *7*, 329-101, 1973.

[25] SALLE (B. L.), DAVID (L.), GLORIEUX (F. H.), DELVIN (E. E.), LOUIS (J. J.), TRONCY (G.). — Hypocalcemia in infants of diabetic mothers. Studies in circulating calciotropic hormone concentrations. *Acta Paediatr. Scand.*, *71*, 573-577, 1982.

[26] SALLE (B. L.), DAVID (B. L.), CHOPARD (J. P.), GRAFMEYER (D. C.), RENAUD (H.). — Prevention of early neonatal hypocalcemia in low birth weight infants with continuous calcium infusion: effect on serum calcium, phosphorus, magnesium and circulating immunoreactive parathyroid hormone and calcitonin. *Pediatr. Res.*, *11*, 1180-1185, 1977.

[27] SANN (L.), DAVID (L.), CHAYVIALLE (J. A.), LASNE (Y.), BETHENOD (M.). — Effect of early oral calcium supplementation on serum calcium and immunoreactive calcitonin concentration in preterm infants. *Arch. Dis. Child.*, *55*, 611-615, 1980.

[28] CHAN (G. M.), TSANG (R. C.), CHEN (I. W.), DELUCA (H. F.), STEICHEN (J. J.). — The effect of 1.25 (OH)$_2$ vitamin D_3 supplementation in premature infants. *J. Pediatr.*, *93*, 91-96, 1978.

[29] FANCONI (A.), PRADER (A.). — Transient congenital idiopathic hypoparathyrodism. *Helv. Paediatr. Acta*, *22*, 331-344, 1967.

[30] DAVID (L.), SALLE (B. L.), VARENNE (P.), GLORIEUX (F. H.), DELVIN (E. E.). — Treatment of late neonatal hypocalcemia with 1-alpha-hydroxycholecalciferol (10HCC). *Pediatr. Res.*, *15*, 1222, 1981 (abstract).

[31] DAVID (L.), CHAPUIS (M. D.), COLLOMBEL (C.), RACLE (B.), RACLE (P.), FRANÇOIS (R.). — Étude du mécanisme pathogénique de l'hypocalcémie dans l'hypomagnésémie primitive. *Arch. Franç. Péd.*, *32*, 803-814, 1975.

[32] ANAST (C. S.), WINNACKER (J. L.), FORTE (L. R.), BURNS (T. W.). — Impaired release of parathyroid hormone in magnesium deficiency. *J. Clin. Endocrinol. Metab.*, *42*, 707, 1976.

[33] SALET (J.), FOURNET (J. P.). — Les hypomagnésémies néonatales. *Ann. Pédiatr.*, *17*, 837 (11), 1970.

[34] PAUNIER (L.), RADDE (I. C.), KOOH (S. W.), CONEN (P. E.), FRASER (D.). — Primary hypomagnesemia with secondary hypocalcemia in an infant. *Pediatrics*, *41*, 385-402, 1968.

[35] SHAW (J. C. L.). — Evidence for defection skeletal mineralization in low birth weight infant: the absorption of calcium and fat. *Pediatrics*, *57*, 16-25, 1976.

[36] Widdowson (E. M.). — Absorption and excretion of fat, nitrogen and minerals from « filled » milks by babies one-week-old. *Lancet*, 2, 1099-1105, 1965.

[37] Yllpö (A.). — Das Wachstum der Frühgeboren von der Geburt bis zum Schulalter. *Z. Kinderheilk.*, 24, 111, 1919.

[38] Rowe (J. C.), Wood (D. H.), Rowe (D. W.), Reisz (L. G.). — Nutritional hypophosphatemic rickets in a premature infant fed breast milk. *N. Engl. J. Med.*, 300, 293-295, 1979.

[39] Sagy (M.), Birenbaum (E.), Balin (A.), Orda (S.), Barzilay (Z.), Brish (M.). — Phosphate depletion syndrome in a premature infant fed human milk. *J. Pediatr.*, 96, 683-685, 1980.

[40] Barltrop (D.), Oppe (T. E.). — Calcium and fat absorption by low birth weight infants from a calcium-supplemented milk formula. *Arch. Dis. Child.*, 48, 580-582, 1973.

[41] Senterre (J.), Salle (B.). — Calcium and phosphorus economy of the preterm infant and its interaction with vitamin D and its metabolites. *Acta Paediatr. Scand.*, suppl. 296, 85-92, 1982.

[42] Barltrop (D.), Oppe (T. E.). — Absorption of fat and calcium by low birth weight infants from milks containing butter fat and olive oil. *Arch. Dis. Child.*, 48, 496-501, 1973.

[43] Barness (L. P.), Morrow (G. III.), Solverio (J.), Finnegan (L. P.), Heitman (S. E.). — Calcium and fat absorption from infant formulas. *Pediatrics*, 54, 217-221, 1979.

[44] Day (G. M.), Chance (G. W.), Radde (I. C.), Reilly (B. J.), Park (E.), Sheepers (J.). — Growth and mineral metabolism in very low birth weight infants. II. Effects of calcium supplementation on growth and divalent cations. *Pediatr. Res.*, 9, 568-575, 1975.

[45] Greer (F. R.), Steichen (J. J.), Tsang (R. C.). — Calcium and phosphate supplements in breast milk-related rickets. *Am. J. Dis. Child.*, 136, 581-583, 1982.

[46] Senterre (J.), Putet (G.), Salle (B.), Rigo (J.). — Effects of vitamin D and phosphorus supplementation on calcium retention in preterm infants fed banked human milk. *J. Pediatr.*, 103, 305-307, 1983.

39

Water and electrolyte metabolism and therapy

William OH

The principles of fluid and electrolyte treatment in the neonatal period are similar to those established for older children, except for some variations and specific features of body composition, physiologic water and electrolyte losses such as insensible water loss, and the neuroendocrine control of fluid and electrolyte balance.

A major consideration in handling fluid and electrolyte problems in the neonate is the relative limitation in renal function, particularly in preterm, low-birth-weight infants, which leaves less room for errors in calculation. It is well known that the renal concentrating and diluting capacity in the presence of fluid restriction and overhydration respectively are not as well developed in the neonate when compared with adults or older children. Therefore, to appropriately manage parenteral fluid therapy in the neonate, the clinician should have a fundamental knowledge of these limitations. In addition, he or she should develop a system of approach so that the handling of the fluid and electrolyte problem is a combination of mathematical calculation of fluid and electrolyte for replacement of deficit, and provision of intake to balance output, along with clinical assessments to monitor the appropriate response to treatment. Furthermore, there are important differences in body composition, neuro-endocrine control of body fluid changes and insensible water losses in the newborn, particularly in low birth weight infants, which makes it more difficult and more challenging to manage fluid and electrolyte problems in the neonatal period.

BODY COMPOSITION IN THE FETAL AND NEONATAL PERIOD

Changes in body fluid during growth

In the early stages of fetal development, water constitutes a large portion of the body composition [1]. It has been estimated that total body water (TBW) is high: 94 % of the body weight during the third month of fetal life. As the gestational age increases, the TBW gradually declines, so that if a fetus is born prematurely at 32 weeks of gestation, the TBW is approximately 80 %, and at term the TBW decreases to about 78 % (Fig. VI-19). The changes during growth also assume certain characteristics. Extracellular water (ECW) decreases from 60 % body weight at the fifth month of fetal life

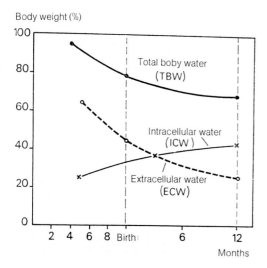

FIG. VI-19. — *Alteration in body fluid during fetal life and in the first year.*

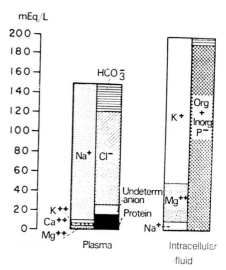

FIG. VI-20. — *Ionic distributions in the various body fluid compartments.*

to about 45 % at term, and intracellular water (ICW) increases from 25 % in the fifth month of fetal life to approximately 33 % at birth.

A contraction of ECW normally occurs during the first few days of life. In low birth weight infants, 32 to 34 weeks of gestation, the ECW declines from 45 % to 39 % at the end of the first week of life [2]. This reduction of ECW is accompanied by an improvement in renal function [3]. Fluid therapy in low birth weight infants should be such that the net fluid balance in the first week of life should allow for a contraction of ECW [4]; failure to do so may be associated with adverse cardiopulmonary complications, such as an in increase in the incidence of symptomatic patent ductus arteriosus and necrotizing enterocolitis [5, 6].

Characteristics of solute distribution in body fluid

As shown in Figure VI-20, the major cation in the plasma is sodium. Potassium, calcium and magnesium constitute the balance of the cation fraction. The anion is primarily chloride, with protein, bicarbonate and some undetermined anion constituting the smaller fraction of the total anions. The interstitial fluid has a similar solute composition to that of the plasma except that its protein content is lower. The ICW contains K^+ and Mg^+ as its primary cations, while organic phosphate and inorganic phosphate are the major anions, with bicarbonate contributing a smaller fraction.

The electrolyte composition in the body fluid of the newborn infant also largely depends on the gestational age. Per unit body weight, a preterm, low birth weight infant has a larger extracellular ion content than a term infant simply on the basis of larger ECW. Conversely, the ICW electrolyte content is lower in a preterm infant because of a smaller ICW. These concepts are important considerations when calculating electrolyte losses for replacement and during parenteral fluid therapy.

Because fetal fluid and electrolyte balance in utero also depends on maternal homeostasis and placental exchange, the neonatal fluid and electrolyte status at birth is influenced significantly by the maternal fluid and electrolyte state.

INSENSIBLE WATER LOSS IN THE NEONATAL PERIOD

Data on insensible water loss (IWL) in newborn infants has been well established by several authors. Because of differences in methodology, technique, and study designs, normal values proposed range from 0.7 to 1.6 g/kg/hour [7, 10, 13, 14]. There is also a considerable degree of controversy as to the appropriate units for expressing IWL. Theoretically, caloric expenditure is the ideal reference unit for IWL, because the latter depends almost entirely on the evaporative heat loss through the skin and respiratory tract. Because heat loss is also closely related to body weight and surface area, most studies in the past have used these two parameters as units of expressing IWL.However, it has recently been shown that within the range of 1 to 4 kg body weight, the variations in expressing the metabolic rate on the basis of body weight or surface area are significant and that the least degree of error is achieved when the calculation of metabolic rate is based on body weight minus extracellular fluid [8]. Unfortunately, the latter parameter (ECW) is not readily available in the daily care of infants, therefore, for practical reasons, body weight would still be the most desirable parameter for expressing IWL and heat expenditure.

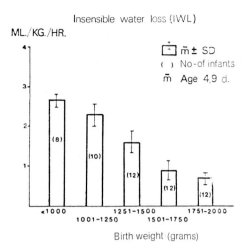

Insensible water loss (IWL)

ML./KG./HR.

$\bar{m}\pm$ SD
( ) No-of infants
$\bar{m}$ Age 4,9 d.

Birth weight (grams)

FIG. VI-21. — *Insensible water loss and birth weight.*

TABLE I. — FACTORS
AFFECTING INSENSIBLE WATER LOSS (IWL)

Changes in IWL

Increase	*Decrease*
Decreasing maturity	High relative humidity in environment
Ambient temperature in incubator exceeds neutral thermal zone	Use of double wall incubator
Fever	Use of plastic heat shield
Low relative humidity in environment	Respirator
Radiant warmer	
Phototherapy	

Several factors may increase the IWL in infants while others may reduce it. Table I shows the various factors that may influence IWL in the neonate. It is known that the IWL is inversely proportional to birth weight or gestational age (Fig. IV-21) [9, 10]. The reasons for the greater IWL in very low birth weight infants include increased permeability of the skin epidermis to water, larger body surface area per unit of weight, and greater skin blood flow relative to metabolic rate. Although not proven beyond doubt, it has been suggested that the higher respiratory rate in the low birth weight infant may partially account for the higher IWL. Fever increases the IWL by increasing metabolic rate; it has also been shown that elevation of ambient temperature above the range of the neutral thermal environment will result in a significant and proportional increase

in IWL. The study by Bell and coworkers [11] has shown that when the ambient thermal environment exceeds 1° C above the range of thermal neutrality in low birth weight infants, an incremental increase in IWL occurs. However, oxygen consumption (heat production) was unchanged. This series of observations clearly demonstrates the close relationship between ambient thermal environment and fluid balance in infants.

Use of a radiant warmer [12] and phototherapy [13] also increases IWL significantly. The mechanism is generally considered as an increase of heat expenditures (including evaporative heat loss) when radiant energy is absorbed by infants subjected to phototherapy or who are nursed under a radiant warmer. In addition, peripheral blood flow increases during phototherapy [15, 16]. The radiant warmer may also participate in this mechanism. Infants nursed in a radiant warmer and treated with phototherapy triple their IWL when compared with the values obtained when they are maintained in an incubator at a neutral thermal environment, and are not receiving phototherapy [18].

Factors that may reduce IWL include the use of a heat shield, high relative humidity in the ambient environment, and utilization during assisted ventilation of humidified gas. Heat shields reduce IWL by half in low birth weight infants but not in large sized infants [9, 17]. High ambient relative humidity reduces IWL by 30 % [7]. In a ventilator when the inspired air is properly warmed and humidified (which is mandatory for proper respiratory care), evaporative water loss through the respiratory tract can be completely eliminated, hence reducing the IWL.

It becomes obvious that in calculating maintenance fluid for infants with various clinical conditions and environmental factors, the amount of IWL will vary and should be modified accordingly. This consideration becomes more critical when the infant's fluid intake is solely derived from a parenteral route.

ENDOCRINE CONTROL
OF FLUID AND ELECTROLYTE BALANCE

The pituitary (antidiuretic hormone), adrenal cortex (mineralocorticoids) and parathyroid glands are the three major endocrine organs that regulate the water and electrolyte balance in the body fluid. In the human newborn, the pattern of antidiuretic hormone (ADH) secretion and metabolism is not well established. Indirect evidence, based on data obtained by water deprivation and loading, suggests that neonates can regulate water balance by means of ADH control in the same manner as adults do, although within a certain physiologic limitation. For example, the urinary concentrating mechanism of a newborn infant is limited to a maximum of 800 mOsm/l on water deprivation, while in the adult, a urine concentration of 1,200 mOsm/l can be achieved on the same challenge [19]. On water loading, the newborn infant can attain its maximal diluting mechanism only at 5 days of age or older [20]. It is not clear whether ADH deficiency or inadequate renal tubular function is the primary reason for the lack of appropriate concentrating and diluting response to water deprivation or loading, although it is conceivable that both hormonal and end-organ factors are responsible for such a phenomenon.

The role of mineralocorticoids such as aldosterone in the regulation of electrolyte balance, particularly sodium, has been reported by several workers. Beitins and coworkers demonstrated the high level of serum aldosterone in the neonate [21]; in preterm, low birth weight infants, the feedback mechanism between Na intake, Na excretion and serum aldosterone level is intact and appropriate [22].

Data on serum parathyroid hormone levels in the newborn infant are now available [23]. The evidence suggests that newborn infants may have relative and transient hypoparathyroidism [23], accounting for the frequent occurrence of hypocalcemia in infants associated with high risk factors such as diabetic pregnancy, toxemia, and in preterm, low birth weight infants with respiratory distress syndrome [24].

PRINCIPLES
OF FLUID AND ELECTROLYTE THERAPY

As in older children, three essential steps should be followed in the treatment of infants with fluid and electrolyte disorders.

(*a*) Estimate the quantity of fluid and electrolyte losses.

(*b*) Calculate fluid and electrolytes for replacement of losses, maintenance and replacement of current abnormal losses.

(*c*) Institute a system of monitoring the adequacy of therapy.

Estimate of fluid loss

Fluid loss is conveniently estimated on the basis of degree of dehydration. If sequential data on body weight are available, a reduction in body weight during a short period of time will generally provide an accurate assessment of the degree of dehydration. In this context, those who treat newborn infants for fluid and electrolyte problems will have a distinct advantage, in that they can readily obtain daily body weight measurements to assess the degree of aberration in fluid balance (dehydration or overhydration). However, it should be pointed out that during the first week to 10 days of life, a 5 % to 10 % reduction in body weight is considered normal because it represents the normal contraction of body fluid and tissue breakdown during a catabolic state. Hence, during the first week of life, dehydration is considered when weight loss exceeds 10 % to 15 % of the birth weight. A useful graph that can assist in interpreting hydration status is the "Dancis Growth Chart" (Fig. VI-22) [25]. The chart depicts the normal body weight changes in infants of various birth weight categories during the first month of life. The daily weight can be plotted on this graph; if the infants' body weight deviates above or below the normal growth pattern, one may suspect the possibility of fluid overload or dehydration respectively.

In the absence of body weight data, clinical evaluation of physical signs may provide an approximate estimation of the degree of dehydration, particularly in cases of isotonic dehydration. Dry skin, dry mucous membranes and a slightly sunken fontanelle are signs of 5 % dehydration; loose abdominal skin turgor, a markedly sunken fontanelle and eyeballs,

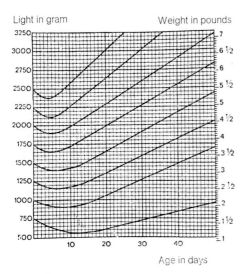

Light in gram   Weight in pounds

Age in days

FIG. VI-22. — *Weight changes during the first month of life.*

severe oliguria, and signs of circulatory insufficiency (*i. e.*, tachycardia, mottled skin, hypotension) are evidence of 10 % dehydration; clinical signs of shock and a generally moribund-looking infant usually indicate 15 % dehydration or greater.

Calculation of fluid deficit for replacement

Fluid deficit is calculated on the basis of estimated degree of dehydration. If an accurate weight change has been obtained during the dehydration period, the difference in weight can be considered as the amount of fluid deficit. If such an observation is unavailable, the use of clinical signs for the estimation of percentage of dehydration will suffice.

However, it is well recognized that the signs of dehydration are difficult to assess in infants particularly those who are of low birth weight or clinically ill. Thus, the weight changes are important data for the assessment of the degree of dehydration. Once again, it is important to recognize that the percentage dehydration in the first weeks of life should be calculated in the context of weight loss exceeding the normally observed 5 to 10 % reduction in body weight. If this concept is not maintained, overcorrection of a fluid deficit may result in serious overhydration. The rapidity of deficit replacement depends on the severity of the dehydration. As a rule, dehydration of acute onset and of short duration requires a more rapid correction and vice versa. The exception to this rule is found in the case of

hypertonic dehydration, in which an exceedingly rapid expansion of body fluid may result in convulsions.

Estimate of electrolyte loss

The nature and extent of electrolyte disturbances along with fluid disorders can often be determined by a carefully obtained clinical history and physical examination, and by measurement of serum electrolytes. Using serum Na values as the criteria, the type of electrolyte disturbance is divided into isotonic or isonatremic (serum sodium within normal range of 131-149 mOsm/l), hypotonic or hyponatremic (serum Na < 130 mOsm/l) and hypertonic or hypernatremic (serum Na > 150 mOsm/l). Electrolyte disorders depend on the nature of the underlying causes of fluid and solute abnormalities. For instance, severe diarrhea usually leads to isotonic dehydration; prolonged febrile illness with diarrhea, and inappropriate use of milk formulas are common causes of hypertonic dehydration; and inappropriate parenteral fluid administration, central nervous system disease, and fluid overload to the mother prior to the delivery of the infant are frequently associated with hypotonic dehydration [26].

In addition, physical signs may provide a lead to the type of dehydration present (e. g., doughy and thickened skin turgor in hypertonic dehydration) and the diagnosis can be confirmed by serum electrolyte determination. With the current availability of micromethods, electrolyte determinations are feasible even in infants of the smallest size. It should also be stressed that in neonates with severe underlying pathology such as sepsis, respiratory distress syndrome, and so on, the clinical signs, particularly those related to central nervous system manifestations, may not be readily discernible. Therefore, it is of the utmost importance that serum electrolytes be determined before initial fluid therapy can be serially monitored during the course of treatment.

Fluid and electrolyte maintenance

IWL, urinary water loss, stool water loss, and water for tissue growth are the four components to be considered in calculating the daily maintenance fluid requirement. Stool water loss averages approximately 5 to 10 ml/kg/day, while water for tissue growth is about 20 ml/kg/day; assuming 70 % of 30 g/kg/day new tissue (average weight gain in growth) is water. In the first 10 days of life, stool water loss is minimal and the infant is not in a growth phase. Therefore, the two main components that need to be accounted for are IWL and urinary water loss.

In a full term infant under basal conditions, IWL is approximately 20 ml/kg/day [7]. Urinary water loss will depend on the amount of the renal solute load. The latter is in turn dependent on the exogenous solute intake and the solute derived endogenously from the metabolic process. In most term infants receiving parenteral fluid administration, one should provide 10 % glucose and 2 to 3 mmol/kg/day of Na and K, which would provide a solute load of approximately 15 mOsm/kg/day. Because urinary concentration in the newborn infant generally ranges from 280 to 300 mOsm/l, an allowance of approximately 50-70 ml/kg/day of fluid for the formation of urine would be appropriate. Hence, in a term infant, the initial fluid prescription for maintenance would be 70 ml/kg/day during the first day and would increase to 80, 90 and 120 ml/kg/day on days 3, 5 and 7 respectively. The increment is to fulfill the requirement generated by an increasing solute load and the amount of water loss by an increasing volume of stool. In older, orally fed infants, the maintenance fluid requirement is between 120 and 150 ml/kg/day because of a larger solute intake and the water requirement for growth.

In low birth weight infants, the maintenance fluid requirements are larger because of a higher IWL. The inverse correlation between IWL and birth weight (and gestational age) has been well documented (Fig. VI-21) [10]. Therefore, the IWL component of the maintenance fluid should be increased proportionately with decreasing birth weight or gestation. It should be pointed out that the IWL data of Wu et al. [10] were obtained with the infants in an incubator under a certain set of environmental settings with reference to ambient temperature and relative humidity. Thus the IWL allowance for individual infants under various environmental settings may be different and should be modified accordingly. For instance, in infants cared for under a radiant warmer *or* receiving phototherapy, the allowance for IWL should be increased by 50 % of its basal values. The combination of both increases the IWL by 100 %. Elevation of ambient temperature above the range of thermal neutrality [27], also increases the IWL significantly [11, 28]. Therefore, one of the important aspects in maintaining IWL within a normal range is to constantly focus attention on appropriate temperature control, maintaining the incubator temperature within the neutral thermal zone.

As stated previously there are a number of factors that may reduce the IWL: high humidity and the use of a plastic heat shield can reduce the IWL by 50 % in the low birth weight infant [9] and, if the infants are being artificially ventilated, the warmed and fully humidified inspired air in the respirator will completely eliminate the respiratory component (30 %) of the IWL.

In infants with perinatal asphyxia, it is highly desirable to restrict the fluid intake during the first 24 to 48 hours of life in anticipation of the potential development of acute renal insufficiency as a result of renal injury or inappropriate ADH secretion, the latter as a consequence of central nervous system injury. Both conditions may result in oliguria and anuria, hence, the fluid restriction. The fluid prescription can be revised upward when normal urinary flow is established during the second and third day of life.

The electrolyte requirements for maintenance primarily involve Na^+, K^+ and Cl^-, which represent the amount of losses through the kidney and in the stool. Based on balance study data, this amount is constant and similar to those of older infants at 2 to 3 mmol/kg/24 hours for each of the elements. Since the infant's body composition is such that a large ECW is present at birth and needs to be mobilized and removed from the body within the first few days of life, it is generally not necessary to supplement with sodium during the first day or two days of life.

Concurrent abnormal losses

It is important that current abnormal losses be replaced during the course of parenteral fluid therapy. This usually involves accurate collection and estimation of abnormal fluid and electrolyte losses, such as vomiting, diarrhea, bile, or ileostomy drainage. The fluid replacement should correspond to the estimated amount of fluid loss. Solute replacement should correspond to the estimated solute content of the fluid loss. The approximate electrolyte content of each kind of drainage is listed in Table II.

Monitoring the effectiveness of parenteral fluid therapy

During the course of parenteral fluid therapy, detailed and organized data collection can clearly reflect the effectiveness of treatment. Data to be collected at a designated interval should include intake, output, body weight changes, urinary specific gravity (or osmolarity), serum electrolytes including blood urea nitrogen, and clinical assess-

TABLE II. — ELECTROLYTE CONTENT
OF VARIOUS FLUIDS

Fluid	Na	K (mmol/l)	Cl
Gastric	20- 80	5-20	100-150
Small intestine. . .	100-140	5-15	90-120
Bile	120-140	5-15	90-120
Ileostomy	45-135	3-15	20-120
Diarrheal stool . .	10- 90	10-80	10-110

ment for the presence of edema, dehydration, or evidence of acute water overload. The interrelationships among the various parameters are shown in Figure VI-23. Frequent causes of inadequate fluid administration are underestimation of fluid requirement for maintenance, and neglect in replacing the abnormal concurrent losses during the therapy period. These factors will result in the reduction of urine volume, an increase in urine specific gravity and, if these compensatory steps are inadequate, a significant weight loss with clinical signs of dehydration. If an excessive amount of fluid is administered, the urine volume will be high and the urine specific gravity low. If these compensations are tested to the maximum, fluid retention will take place resulting in edema and weight gain. If the rate of overhydration is rapid, pulmonary edema and congestive heart failure may occur, particularly in ill neonates with underlying cardiopulmonary

disorders. Once again, it is important to recognize the fact that the neonatal kidney has a limited capacity for compensation when inadequate or excess fluids are given; early and prompt identification of inappropriate amounts of fluid administration is critical to minimize complications.

Urinary specific gravity is a convenient and accurate approximation of urinary solute excretion. An exception to the rule would be in cases of significant glycosuria in which a high specific gravity may be observed, reflecting the presence of glucose rather than electrolytes. Specific gravity should be determined at 6 to 8 hour intervals with the use of a reflectometer. Normally, the range of urinary specific gravity in the newborn is between 1.008 and 1.012.

Stationary weight or appropriate weight gain (or weight loss in the first week of life), when fluid therapy is being instituted, without clinical evidence of fluid overload or dehydration and maintenance of urinary specific gravity at 1.008 to 1.012 would indicate success in maintaining fluid balance. Serial daily serum electrolyte determinations would provide evidence of electrolyte balance (or imbalance).

During the first week of life, a 5 % to 10 % weight loss is considered physiologic and is partly the allowance for the normal contraction of the extracellular fluid. Therefore, in using weight changes as an index for fluid balance, a weight loss of 1 % to 2 % per day should be considered normal. In fact, a rigid insistence on maintaining a zero weight (or fluid) balance during the first week of life may lead to fluid overload.

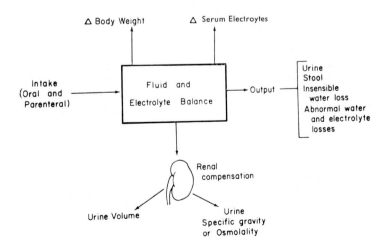

FIG. VI-23. — A system of monitoring fluid and electrolyte therapy.

ACID BASE BALANCE

The buffer system (primarily bicarbonate and its weak acid counterpart, carbonic acid), renal and respiratory compensations, are the three major mechanisms responsible for the maintenance of normal acid base equilibrium in the body fluids. H^+ changes in the body fluid follow the Henderson-Hasselbach equation:

$$pH = 6.1 + \log \frac{HCO^-_3}{H_2CO_3 \text{ or } (S.P_{CO_2})}$$

where 6.1 is the pK constant of carbonic acid, $S.P_{CO_2}$ the amount of CO_2 dissolved in the body fluid which is nearly equivalent to the amount of total weak acid (H_2CO_3). It can be seen from this formula that any increase or reduction of the $^-HCO_3$ fraction in the buffer compartment will result in alkalosis or acidosis respectively. Because H_2CO_3 is interchangeably related to P_{CO_2} under the constant influence of a catalyst, carbonic anhydrase, any alteration in P_{CO_2} in the body fluid would also alter the pH values. Hence, hyperventilation with reduction of P_{CO_2} will result in respiratory alkalosis, and hypoventilation with hypercarbia will result in respiratory acidosis.

A good example of respiratory alkalosis is that of an infant who is hyperventilated with a mechanical ventilator (respirator). In respiratory distress syndrome, the respiratory component of the acidosis is caused by retention of CO_2 in the body fluid as a result of pulmonary insufficiency. Metabolic acidosis is also seen in respiratory distress syndrome as a result of significant lactic acidemia, the latter as a result of anaerobic metabolism under hypoxemic conditions. An excellent example of metabolic alkalosis occurs in infants with congenital pyloric stenosis. In these cases, the abnormal loss of gastric contents by persistent vomiting results in a marked excess of bicarbonate content in the body fluids in amounts exceeding the bicarbonate excreting capacity of the kidney.

In all instances of acid base disturbance, a compensatory mechanism takes effect either via the lung or the kidney. If the compensatory mechanism is adequate, the pH value may be normalized at the expense of an altered bicarbonate or carbonic acid concentration. In this instance, the acid base disturbances are termed compensated. For instance, if a neonate with respiratory distress syndrome has the following acid base values: pH = 7.38, P_{CO_2} = 32 torr, bicarbonate content = 15 mmol/l, and

acid base deficit = − 10 mmol/l, the acid base status would be considered as compensated metabolic acidosis. Hyperventilation results in lower P_{CO_2} compensation for the reduced bicarbonate content (base deficit), hence normalizing the pH values.

SPECIFIC CLINICAL CONDITIONS WITH FLUID AND ELECTROLYTE PROBLEMS

Respiratory distress syndrome (hyaline membrane disease)

Earlier studies by Cort had shown that in respiratory distress syndrome (RDS), renal function is markedly reduced and that hyperkalemia and hyperphosphatemia are common occurrences [29]. More recent observations, however, seem to indicate that if the cardiorespiratory status is kept within the physiologic range, the renal function in RDS infants is comparable to non-RDS infants within the same range of gestational age [30]. Also, with appropriate fluid and electrolyte management by the parenteral route, there is less likelihood of hyperkalemia, hyperphosphatemia and azotemia as previously reported by Usher [31].

The parenteral solution should include fluid and electrolytes for maintenance, taking into consideration the variable requirement for IWL as a result of the infant's physiologic and pathologic status and environment.

Because limitation in renal concentration capability is characteristic of preterm infants with or without RDS, it is apparent that adequate fluid intake is essential to maintain an appropriate fluid balance. The precise volumes required will vary from one infant to another depending on the gestation, birth weight, presence or absence of perinatal asphyxia, environmental factors (e. g., radiant warmer versus incubator), and all the factors cited previously that may affect the fluid requirement of preterm infants. In general, an infant weighing 1,500 g with RDS, but without perinatal asphyxia, who is being cared for in an incubator should receive a fluid volume of 70 ml/kg during the first day as a 5 % to 10 % glucose solution. This will fulfill the requirement for IWL (35-40 ml/kg/day) and urinary water loss (40-45 ml/kg/day for a solute load of 5 to 10 mOsm/kg/day) and allow for an anticipated body weight loss of 1 % (10 gm), resulting from the removal of ECW from the body. The amount of fluid administration in the subsequent days should be guided by a careful monitoring of intake, output, body weight changes, urine specific gravity, and serum electrolyte determinations. To assure accurate parenteral fluid intake, a calibrated infusion pump should be used. For urine collection, a pediatric urine collector may be used in the larger preterm infant. To avoid skin irritation and excoriation from frequent changing of the urine collector, the urine can be aspirated from the collector from time to time for volume determination through a feeding tube placed within the urine bag. In very small male infants in whom urine collector application is impractical, an appropriate size test tube may be fitted onto the penis for urine collection (Fig. IV-24).

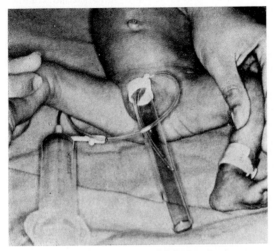

Fig. VI-24. — *Urine collection
in small male infants.*

Urine volumes, urine specific gravity, and changes in body weight are the three important guidelines for fluid calculation. During the first week of life, the infant should lose approximately 10 to 20 g/kg/day. If, at the same time, the urine volume and specific gravity are within the normal range (40-50 ml/kg/day and 1.008-1.012, respectively), the fluid intake of the previous 24 hours can be continued for the next 24 hours. Day to day adjustment of the fluid intake may be made according to these three parameters.

Moderate to severe forms of RDS are associated with a significant incidence of pulmonary edema from left to right shunting across the patent ductus arteriosus (PDA) [32, 33]. It has further been shown that fluid overload may enhance the occurrence of this complication [34]. Bell and associates, in a randomized study, showed that a high fluid intake increases the incidence of PDA and left to right shunt [5].

This study clearly emphasizes the importance of careful monitoring of fluid and electrolyte intake in high risk infants to avoid cardiopulmonary complications.

During the first 12 to 24 hours of life, it is usually not necessary to add Na to the parenteral fluid, particularly if it is anticipated that Na bicarbonate may be used for the treatment of metabolic acidosis. Potassium supplementation (2 mmol/kg/24 hr) should be added as soon as the infant voids unless serum K^+ is elevated. Sodium (in the form of NaCl) should be added starting on the second day of age at a dose of 2 to 3 mmol/kg/24 hours.

Serial serum electrolyte determinations should be done at 24 to 48 hour intervals. Hyperkalemia may occasionally occur; in such instances, supplemental K in the parenteral fluid should be discontinued until the serum K level returns to normal.

RDS is commonly associated with a combined respiratory and metabolic acidosis resulting from hypercarbia and lactic acidemia respectively. In severe RDS, when the acidosis is predominantly respiratory, some form of assisted ventilation should be instituted. On the other hand, if the acidosis is primarily metabolic, Na bicarbonate (0.9 M $NaHCO_3$) may be used as a buffer to correct the acidotic state. The dose of $NaHCO_3$ should be calculated on the basis of the following formula:

dose of $NaHCO_3$ (mmol)
$$= \text{base deficit (mmol/l)} \times \text{body weight} \times 0.4$$

The common clinical practice is to calculate the base deficit from the pH and Pa_{CO_2} by using an appropriate nomogram [35]. Base deficit may also be derived from a known pH and plasma CO_2 content or bicarbonate concentration. The 0.4 value in the formula represents the bicarbonate space which is confined mostly to the extracellular fluid compartment. It should be noted that there is some disagreement on the true bicarbonate space, the values ranging from 0.3 to 0.6 of body weight.

The calculated $NaHCO_3$ dose may be given intravenously at a rate of 1 mmol/min or by slow infusion over a 2 to 3 hour period. The use of $NaHCO_3$ is not without risk. Bolus infusion of large amounts of $NaHCO_3$ is known to produce significant changes in the osomolar concentration in the intravascular compartment [36] which may result in a sudden alteration in osmotic balance between the intra- and extracellular fluid compartments, leading to intracranial hemorrhage [37]. Thus $NaHCO_3$ should not be used indiscriminately. As a matter of fact, a more important task in the treatment of RDS is to provide optimal tissue oxygenation by continuously monitoring and ensuring adequate arterial blood pressure, oxygen tension, and hemoglobin mass. If tissue hypoxia is avoided, the occurrence of metabolic acidosis can be minimized, hence, reducing the need for $NaHCO_3$ administration.

Because of its buffering effect on the carbon dioxide, Tris (hydroxymethyl) aminomethane (THAM) has been suggested for the treatment of respiratory acidosis. However, the effect of THAM on reducing plasma CO_2 is at most transient and would require a large continuous dose of THAM to effectively neutralize the CO_2 accumulated as a result of respiratory insufficiency. The dose needed to accomplish this would far exceed the therapeutic safety of THAM. Furthermore, because of its corrosive quality, local tissue sloughing may occur if subcutaneous infiltration takes place. Hence, in treating the acidosis of RDS, THAM should not be used.

Congenital pyloric stenosis

The magnitude of fluid and electrolyte disturbance in congenital pyloric stenosis depends entirely on the duration and severity of its main symptom, vomiting. In severe and persistent vomiting, the electrolyte abnormality is usually that of hypochloremic alkalosis and hypokalemia. Studies have shown that in infants with severe vomiting caused by congenital pyloric stenosis, intracellular Na is increased and K is decreased [38]. The intracellular K deficiency is frequently reflected in the form of low serum K. An ECG may also show evidence of intracellular hypopotassemia with depressed and wide T waves and prolongation of the S-T segment. These infants usually appear chronically dehydrated and emaciated. The metabolic alkalosis leads to lethargy, stridor, shallow and slow respiration, and, in some cases, tetany. Serum electrolyte determination reveals in addition to low K, a high pH (> 7.50), low chloride (< 90 mmol/l), and elevated bicarbonate or CO_2 content; serum Na level may be within the normal range.

Parenteral therapy consists of fluid replacement of the calculated deficit and maintenance. The chloride deficit should be corrected with the use of NaCl. When the infant's urination is established, KCl should be added to the parenteral fluid. Specific treatment of the metabolic alkalosis with such agents as ammonium chloride is usually not necessary. In most instances, cessation of vomiting by withholding oral intake, correction of dehydration, and replacement of Cl and K deficits by providing NaCl and KCl respectively will restore the blood pH value to

within the normal range. Complete correction of intracellular electrolyte abnormalities, particularly the K deficit, may take 7 to 10 days. Surgical correction of the congenital pyloric stenosis is however advisable after 24 to 48 hours of parenteral fluid therapy.

Diarrhea dehydration

The principle of parenteral fluid therapy for diarrheal dehydration in the neonate is generally similar to that of older infants and children. Because of lower physiologic reserves, severe dehydration without prompt treatment in the neonate may quickly lead to contraction of intravascular volume, shock, and cardiorespiratory arrest. Therefore, the handling of moderate to severe dehydration from diarrhea requires exquisite skill both in initiating a parenteral fluid line and in the prompt expansion of the intravascular space.

Following stabilization, an estimate of fluid and electrolyte deficits should be made according to the methods described in this chapter, and appropriate fluid and electrolytes given parenterally to cover deficit, maintenance requirement and concurrent abnormal losses such as persistent diarrhea, during the repair period. Metabolic acidosis is a frequent finding in diarrheal dehydration. However, it frequently does not require specific correction with the use of a buffer, such as sodium bicarbonate or lactate, because correction of the dehydration and maintenance of positive fluid and electrolyte balance will normalize the acid base status with 24 to 48 hours.

Institution of oral fluid intake should be carried out with extreme care. The infant's gastrointestinal tract is frequently in a precarious state following a diarrheal episode. Introduction of oral intake sooner than indicated frequently leads to recurrence of diarrhea, which may proceed into a protracted diarrheal state. The latter is a serious and difficult problem to handle, particularly in a very young and small infant. A vicious cycle of diarrhea, starvation, malnutrition, and more diarrhea may necessitate a very long period of fasting and the use of intravenous alimentation.

The appropriate period of fasting depends on the severity of the diarrheal episode. As a rule, a more severe diarrheal state will require a longer period of fasting and vice versa. Also, the number of diarrheal stools following fasting will provide a good guideline for the duration of fasting. It should also be pointed out that in prolonged diarrheal states, a transient lactase deficiency can occur [39], which may require the use of a lactose-free milk formula during the resumption of milk intake [40].

Parenteral alimentation

The pioneer work by Dudrick and coworkers in experimental animals [41] and subsequently by his colleagues in infants [42] has shown that metabolic needs and a normal growth rate can be sustained by parenteral hyperalimentation alone. This is achieved by parenterally feeding infants with hypertonic glucose, protein hydrolysate, trace elements, and vitamins along with fresh plasma transfusions at regular intervals.

In low birth weight infants, total parenteral alimentation is not routinely used because of the perceived high rates of complication and the technical difficulty of placing central venous catheters in a small infant [43]. In these infants, parenteral nutrition through a peripheral vein is preferred. With this form of parenteral nutrition, the glucose concentration in the infusate is generally limited to 12 % because a higher glucose concentration carries the risk of tissue sloughing if infiltration of the intravenous site occurs. Because of the limitation in glucose concentration, the caloric intake of infants receiving nutritional support solely from this route is often inadequate. This problem is heightened by our axiom of not giving too much fluid, and the frequent occurrence of hyperglycemia in these infants when a large dose of glucose is given [44, 45]. Under the circumstances, it may be necessary to use intravenous fat emulsion as a supplemental source of calories. A 10 or 20 % solution of commercially available intravenous fat emulsion may be used. The dose ranges from 1 to 4 g/kg/day depending on the infant's caloric and fluid need. The usual precautions and monitoring for toxicity should be observed when intravenous fat emulsion is infused. Giving an intravenous fat emulsion also resolves the problem of essential fatty acid deficiency that occurs when infants receive a prolonged period of parenteral nutrition without fat [46]. It has been estimated that supplying 4 % of the caloric intake in the form of an intravenous fat emulsion is sufficient to prevent the development of biochemical or clinical essential fatty acid deficiency.

FLUID AND ELECTROLYTE MANAGEMENT OF NEONATAL SURGICAL PATIENTS

If the surgical condition results in an abnormal loss of fluid and electrolytes, leading to a significant degree of dehydration and electrolyte aberration, the repair of the deficit should be achieved before surgery. For example, in congenital pyloric stenosis with severe dehydration and electrolyte disturbance, the surgical repair of the pyloric stenosis should be postponed for a 48 to 72 hour period while fluid and electrolyte therapy is in progress. Failure to do so may result in a stormy postoperative course.

During surgery, the calculated fluid and electrolyte requirements and rate of administration should be continued. The anesthesiologist and the members of the surgical team should be apprised of the plan for the parenteral fluid therapy in order to avoid unnecessary errors in the administration of parenteral fluid resulting from lack of communication. Any abnormal fluid loss, blood loss, or both should be recorded and repaired either during surgery or immediately thereafter.

During the first 2 postoperative days, some infants, particularly those who have received general anesthesia, may have reduced urine flow as a result of increased secretion of ADH [47]. It has also been shown that for unknown reasons, IWL in the postoperative neonate is significantly reduced [48]. Therefore, during the immediate postoperative period (24 hr), the parenteral fluid intake should be reduced to avoid overhydration and water intoxication. Again, a system of careful monitoring of fluid and electrolyte balance is an important step in the day-to-day calculation of fluid and electrolyte needs.

TECHNICAL ASPECTS OF PARENTERAL FLUID THERAPY

Blood sampling

Because of their size and often precarious state, blood sampling for electrolyte analysis in newborn infants can impose a serious problem. The antecubital vein or superficial veins on the hands or feet are by far the safest site for blood sampling. Unfortunately, in small infants, it is often difficult to obtain an adequate blood specimen from this site. The femoral vein is a convenient site for blood sampling; however, proximity to the femoral artery and the risk of traumatizing the hip joint and its surrounding bony structures make this method of blood sampling undesirable, particularly in the small neonate. External jugular vein puncture is a good choice in large and older infants if free of cardiorespiratory symptoms. Internal jugular vein puncture should be avoided in newborn infants because of the risk of incurring injury to adjacent structures such as the trachea, carotid artery, or vagus nerve.

It is apparent from the above discussion that sampling capillary blood by heel puncture is by far the least traumatic method of blood letting in the newborn period. The correlations between capillary and venous blood samples in regard to electrolyte values are satisfactory. The validity of the capillary blood samples can be further enhanced by warming the heel with a warmed, wet towel (40° C) for 5 to 10 minutes. The latter procedure will improve local circulation which, in turn, will partially abolish the capillary-venous difference of various parameters including hematocrit. Because the amount of blood obtained by heel puncture is limited, the neonatal service should be supported by a laboratory capable of performing microanalysis. For infants who require frequent monitoring of arterial acid-base and blood-gas values, an indwelling catheter- (size 3.5 or 5.0 F) may be inserted into the umbilical artery and retrogradely passed into the aorta just above the diaphragm. For occasional sampling of arterial blood for blood-gas analysis, direct arterial puncture of the temporal, radial, or brachial arteries may be carried out using a butterfly needle inserted against the arterial inflow. Skill and experience are obviously necessary. Complications such as arteriospasm, bleeding, or infection are rare.

Intravenous fluid infusion

In infants, the branches of the superficial temporal vein and facial vein are the most commonly used sites for intravenous infusion. With practice and skill, a suitable size scalp vein needle can be inserted into these venous tributaries with ease. The needle can be immobilized by appropriate taping. Infusion of hypertonic parenteral solutions such as 0.9 M $NaHCO_3$ or 50 % glucose and calcium containing solution should be avoided. Infiltration of these solutions into the subcutaneous tissue may result in sloughing and necrosis to the adjacent tissue. Veins in the antecubital fossa or dorsal of the hands and feet are also appropriate sites for intravenous infusion. However, subcutaneous infiltration is more common in these sites because of the relative difficulty in the immobilization of the infusion needle.

The umbilical vein has long been a favorite site for intravenous infusion because of the relative ease in placing a catheter in this vessel. However, recent reports have documented the complications arising from umbilical venous catheterization and fluid infusion, including infection, hepatic necrosis, and

phlebitis. If the use of umbilical venous infusion is mandatory for lack of other alternative sites. the catheter tip should be placed in the inferior vena cava through the ductus venosus. If the latter cannot be entered, one should avoid placing the catheter in the hepatic portal sinuses, particularly if infusion of hypertonic solution such as $NaHCO_3$ is anticipated. In any case, the position of the catheter should always be determined or confirmed radiologically. In general, the umbilical vein as an infusion site should be used only as a last resort and only in case of emergency.

Cutdown by way of a peripheral vein (saphenous, basilic, cephalic, or external jugular) should be used only in infants who may require a prolonged period of intravenous infusion. Infection is the most common complication from this route of parenteral infusion. Meticulous aseptic care of the cutdown sites and frequent dressing changes will reduce the incidence of local and systemic infection.

In all cases of parenteral fluid infusion, a constant infusion pump should be employed, along with a volumetric chamber, to assure a constant rate of infusion. A fluctuating infusion rate may result in erratic blood glucose values and overhydration. The latter may significantly alter the cardiorespiratory status of a sick neonate with congestive heart failure and pulmonary edema.

References

[1] FRIIS-HANSEN (B.). — Body composition during growth. *Pediatrics* (Suppl.), *47*, 264, 1971.
[2] KAGAN (B. M.), STANINCOVA (V.), FELIX (N. S.), HODGMAN (J.), KALMAN (D.). — Body composition of premature infants: Relation to nutrition. *Am. J. Clin. Nutr.*, *25*, 1153, 1972.
[3] OH (W.), OH (M. A.), LIND (J.). — Renal function and blood volume in newborn infant related to placental transfusion. *Acta Paediatr. Scand.*, *56*, 197, 1966.
[4] STONESTREET (B. S.), BELL (E. F.), WARBURTON (D.), OH (W.). — Renal response in low birthweight neonates. Results of prolonged intake of two different amounts of fluid and sodium. *Am. J. Dis. Child.*, *137*, 215, 1983.
[5] BELL (E. F.), WARBURTON (D.), STONESTREET (B. S.), OH (W.). — Effect of fluid administration on the development of symptomatic patent ductus arteriosus and congestive heart failure in premature infants. *N. Engl. J. Med.*, *302*, 598-604, 1980.
[6] BELL (E. F.), WARBURTON (D.), STONESTREET (B. S.), OH (W.). — High volume fluid intake predisposes premature infants to necrotizing enterocolitis. *Lancet*, *2*, 90, 1979.
[7] HEY (E. N.), KATZ (G.). — Evaporative water loss in the newborn baby. *J. Physiol.*, *200*, 605, 1969.
[8] SINCLAIR (J. C.), SCOPES (J. W.), SILVERMAN (W. A.).

— Metabolic reference standards for the neonate. *Pediatrics*, 39, 724, 1967.

[9] FANAROFF (A. A.), WALD (M.), BRUBER (H. S.), KLAUS (M. H.). — Insensible water loss in low birth weight infants. *Pediatrics*, 50, 236, 1972.

[10] WU (P. Y. K.), HODGMAN (J. E.). — Insensible water loss in preterm infants: Changes with postnatal development and non-ionizing radiant energy. *Pediatrics*, 54, 704, 1974.

[11] BELL (E. F.), GRAY (J. C.), WEINSTEIN (M.), OH (W.). — The effects of thermal environment on heat balance and insensible water loss in low-birth-weight infants. *J. Pediatr.*, 96, 452-459, 1980.

[12] WILLIAMS (P. R.), OH (W.). — The effects of radiant warmer on insensible weight loss in newborn infant. *Am. J. Dis. Child.*, 128, 511, 1974.

[13] OH (W.), KARECKI (H.). — Phototherapy and insensible water loss in the newborn infant. *Am. J. Dis. Child.*, 124, 230, 1972.

[14] ZWEYMULLER (E.), PREINING (O.). — The insensible water loss in the newborn infant. *Acta Paediatr. Scand.* (Suppl.), 205, 1970.

[15] OH (W.), YAO (A. C.), HANSON (J. S.), LIND (J.). — Peripheral circulatory response to phototherapy in newborn infants. *Acta Paediatr. Scand.*, 62, 49, 1973.

[16] WU (P. Y. K.), WONG (W. H.), HODGMAN (J. E.), LEVAN (N. E.). — Changes in blood flow in the skin and muscle with phototherapy. *Pediatr. Res.*, 8, 257, 1974.

[17] BELL (E. F.), WEINSTEIN (M. R.), OH (W.). — Heat balance in premature infants: Comparative effects of convectively heated incubator and radiant warmer, with and without plastic heat shield. *J. Pediatr.*, 96, 46-465, 1980.

[18] BELL (E. F.), NEIDICH (G. A.), CASHORE (W. J.), OH (W.). — Combined effect of radiant warmer and phototherapy on insensible water loss in low birth weight infants. *J. Pediatr.*, 94, 810-813, 1979.

[19] CALCAGNO (P. L.), RUBIN (M. I.), WEINTRAUB (D. H.). — Studies on the renal concentrating and diluting mechanisms in the premature infant. *J. Clin. Invest.*, 33, 91, 1954.

[20] MCCANCE (R. A.), NAYLOR (N. J.), WIDDOWSON (E. M.). — Response to infants to a large dose of water. *Arch. Dis. Child.*, 29, 104, 1954.

[21] BEITINS (I. Z.), BAYARD (F.), LEVITSKY (L.), ANCES (I. G.), KOWARSKI (A.), MIGEON (C. J.). — Plasma aldosterone concentration at delivery and during the newborn period. *J. Clin. Invest.*, 51, 386, 1972.

[22] SIEGEL (S. R.), FISHER (D. A.), OH (W.). — Serum aldosterone levels related to sodium balance in the newborn infant. *Pediatrics*, 53, 410, 1974.

[23] TSANG (R. C.), LIGHT (I. J.), SUTHERLAND (J. M.), KLEINMAN (L. I.). — Possible pathogenic factors in neonatal hypocalcemia of prematurity. *J. Pediatr.*, 82, 423, 1973.

[24] TSANG (R.), OH (W.). — Neonatal hypocalcemia in low birth weight infants. *Pediatrics*, 45, 773, 1970.

[25] DANCIS (J.), O'CONNELL (J. R.), HALT (L. E. Jr). — A grid for recording the weight of premature infants. *J. Pediatr.*, 33, 570, 1948.

[26] ALSTATT (L. B.). — Transplacental hyponatremia in the newborn infant. *J. Pediatr.*, 66, 985, 1965.

[27] BRUCK (K.), PARMELEE (A. H.), BRUCK (M.). — Neutral temperature range and range of « thermal comfort » in premature infants. *Biol. Neonate*, 4, 32, 1962.

[28] HEY (E. N.), KATZ (G.). — Optimum thermal environment for naked babies. *Arch. Dis. Child.*, 45, 328, 1970.

[29] CORT (R. L.). — Renal function in the respiratory distress syndrome. *Acta Paediatr. Scand.*, 51, 343, 1961.

[30] SIEGEL (S. R.), FISHER (D. A.), OH (W.). — Renal function and serum aldosterone levels in infants with respiratory distress syndrome. *J. Pediatr.*, 83, 854, 1973.

[31] USHER (R.). — Reduction in mortality from respiratory distress syndrome and prematurity with early administration of intravenous glucose and sodium bicarbonate. *Pediatrics*, 32, 966, 1963.

[32] KITTERMAN (J. A.), EDMUNDS (L. H. Jr.), GREGORY (G. A.), HEYMAN (M. N.), TOOLEY (W. H.), RUDOLPH (A. M.). — Patent ductus arteriosus in premature infants. Incidence relation to pulmonary disease and management. *N. Engl. J. Med.*, 287, 473, 1972.

[33] THIBEAULT (D. W.), EMMANOUILIDES (G. C.), DODGE (M. E.), CACHMAN (R. S.). — Early functional closure of the ductus arteriosus associated with decreased severity of respiratory distress syndrome in preterm infants. *Am. J. Dis. Child.*, 131, 741, 1977.

[34] STEVENSON (J. G.). — Fluid administration in the association of patent ductus arteriosus complicating respiratory distress syndrome. *J. Pediatr.*, 90, 257, 1977.

[35] SIGGARD-ANDERSEN (O.). — The *p*H-log *p*CO₂ blood acid base nomogram revised. *Scand. J. Clin. Lab. Invest.*, 14, 598, 1962.

[36] SIEGEL (S. R.), PHELPS (D. L.), LEAKE (R. D.), OH (W.). — The effects of rapid infusion of hypertonic sodium bicarbonate in infants with respiratory distress. *Pediatrics*, 51, 651-654, 1973.

[37] SIMMONS (N. A.), ADCOCK (E. W. III), BARD (H.) et coll. — Hypernatremia and intracranial hemorrhage in neonates. *N. Engl. J. Med.*, 291, 1974.

[38] BENSON (C. D.), LLOYD (J. R.). — Infantile pyloric stenosis. *Am. J. Surg.*, 107, 429, 1964.

[39] SUNSHINE (P.), KRETCHMER (N.). — Studies of small intestine during development. III. Infantile diarrhea associated with intolerance to disaccharides. *Pediatrics*, 34, 38, 1964.

[40] LEAKE (R. D.), SCHROEDER (K. C.), BENTON (D. A.), OH (W.). — Soy-based formula in the treatment of infantile diarrhea. *Am. J. Dis. Child.*, 127, 373-376, 1974.

[41] DUDRICK (S. J.), WILMORE (D. W.), VARS (H. M.). — Long term total parenteral nutrition with growth in puppies and positive nitrogen balance in patients. *Surg. Forum*, 18, 356, 1967.

[42] WILMORE (D. W.), GROFF (D. B.), BISHOP (H. C.), DUDRICK (S. J.). — Total parenteral nutrition in infants with catastrophic gastro-intestinal anomalies. *J. Pediatr. Surg.*, 4, 181, 1969.

[43] DRISCOLL (J. M.), HEIRD (W. C.), SCHULLINGER (J. N.), GONGAWARE (R. D.), WINTER (R. W.). — Total intravenous alimentation in low birth weight infants: A preliminary report. *J. Pediatr.*, 81, 145, 1972.

[44] DWECK (H. S.), CASSADY (G.). — Glucose intolerance in infants of very low birth weights 1,100 grams or less. *Pediatrics*, 53, 189, 1974.

[45] COWETT (R. M.), OH (W.), POLLAK (A.), SCHWARTZ

(R.), STONESTREET (B. S.). — Glucose disposal of low birth weight infant: Steady state hyperglycemia produced by constant intravenous glucose infusion. *Pediatrics*, *63*, 389-396, 1979.

[46] FRIEDMAN (Z.), DANON (A.), STAHLMAN (M. T.), OATES (J. A.). — Rapid onset of essential fatty acid deficiency in the newborn. *Pediatrics*, *58*, 640, 1976.

[47] BENNETT (E. J.), DAUGHETY (M. J.), JENKINS (M. T.). — Fluid requirement for neonatal anesthesia and operation. *Anesthesiology*, *32*, 343, 1970.

[48] LESTER (J.). — Insensible water loss in infants. *J. Pediatr. Surg.*, *2*, 483, 1967.

40

Endocrine disorders
in the newborn

Problems related to thyroid
and adrenal disorders in the neonatal period

Maguelone G. FOREST

The many causes of hyper- or hypofunction of the thyroid or adrenal glands are each relatively rare but not uncommon endocrine disorders in the newborn infant. The rather non specific manner in which the newborn responds to almost any systemic insult greatly complicates the recognition of any endocrine dysfunction in this period of life. However, entirely missing the diagnosis or making it far too late, will often have tragic consequences: either rapid death or irreversible or lasting effects on the child's development, growth, mentation, sexual orientation and on the family psychologic balance. The importance of complete and careful physical examination of any baby, at birth and during the neonatal period should not be underestimated. When clinical findings call for attention the diagnosis is only established by hormonal measurements, dynamic testing or morphological studies which still may have considerable technical difficulties and are best performed in specialized centres. The accumulating knowledge of the feto-maternal relationship and of the perinatal changes in function are essential to understand the pathogenesis and plan rational diagnosis and proper therapy of any neonatal endocrine dysfunction.

Thyroid

The adaptation of thyroid function to the new endocrine and metabolic exigencies of birth, in particular, thermogenesis represents one of the most significant aspects in the general scheme of neonatal adaptation to extra-uterine life.

Developments in experimental and clinical research

have demonstrated findings of fundamental importance concerning materno-fetal relationships during pregnancy and fetal and neonatal thyroid function which refutes most concepts held in the past on this subject. As we believe that their precise knowledge is fundamental to understanding the approach to the management of thyroid problems in the neonatal period, we shall first present the newer concepts in thyroid physiology during fetal and neonatal periods.

NORMAL DEVELOPMENT

ANATOMICAL AND BIOCHEMICAL DEVELOPMENT OF THE HYPOTHALAMIC-PITUITARY-THYROID (HPT) AXIS

The thyroid gland. — The thyroid is one of the largest endocrine glands weighing approximately 1.5 g at birth [84] and 15-25 g in normal adults. It is constituted of two lateral lobes, lying along the lower half of the lateral margins of the thyroid cartilage, joined by a thin band of tissue, the isthmus, just below the cricoid cartilage.

The definitive thyroid is normally constituted by the association of 2 anlages, a principal median one and two lateral ones [48, 61]. The first anlage is visible in the 16-17 day embryo (2 mm) as a median outpouching of the endoderm of the primitive buccal cavity (tongue base) in contact with the endothelium of the developing heart. The primordium develops as a flasklike vesicle with a narrow connection with the buccal cavity. This median diverticulum undergoes relative caudal displacement and the primitive stalk elongates (thyroglossal duct). As the developing thyroid becomes hollow and bilobed it also migrates caudally and comes in contact with the lateral anlages originating from ultimobranchial portions of the fourth pharyngeal pouches. The latter contribute to the parathyroid glands (which normally remain situated on or beneath the posterior surface of the thyroid lobes) and to the parafollicular cells (thyrocalcitonin secreting component) which become incorporated within the developing lateral lobes. The fusion is complete by the 9th week (48 mm). About a week earlier, the thyroid gland has reached its final position in the anterior lower neck and weighs 1-2 mg. Meanwhile the stalk ruptures (around 40 days) and normally undergoes dissolution leaving 2 remnants, the foramen caecum at its point of origin,

the junction of the midline and the posterior third of the tongue; its lower portion will form the pyramidal lobe of the thyroid in a midline superior projection from the isthmus, It will gradually atrophy later in life.

Remnants of the thyroglossal duct are not uncommon (20 % of routine autopsies). Thyroid tissue may develop near the foramen caecum and constitute the sole functioning tissue (lingual thyroid). Rarely some thyroid tissue migrates along with the cardiovascular structures within the mediastinum. More frequently, remnants of the duct will later give rise to thyroglossal cysts.

In contrast, defective development of the thyroid gland will constitute the bulk of congenital hypothyroidism (cryptothyroid) whether the gland is in the lingual, hyoidal or subhyoidal position with a variety of structural and functional abnormalities.

Concomitantly with its anatomic development histologic maturation of the thyroid gland proceeds. Three phases are described: (a) precolloid (47-72 days) during which small intracellular canaliculi appear and accumulate colloid material, (b) beginning colloid (73-80 days) when the colloid material becomes organized into extracellular colloid spaces and (c) the follicular growth phase (beyond 80 days and continuing until the end of uterine life). At this stage, iodide concentration and thyroxine (T_4) synthesis are present [2, 140], showing full functional capacity of the gland as it will remain throughout life. Thyroid synthesis, as reflected by fetal blood levels of T_4, increases with fetal age.

The pituitary gland. — Classically, it also derives from a dorsal ectodermal outpocketing of the primitive oral cavity, called Rathke's pouch, and a neuroectodermal funnel-shaped thickening in the floor of the third cerebral ventricle, the infundibulum. Recent evidence suggests that Rathke's pouch may arise from neuroectodermal tissue, the most caudal extension of the ventral neural bridge [151]. Hence, both the hypothalamus and the adenohypophysis can be regarded as derivatives of a common neuroectodermal embryologic anlage [113].

Rathke's pouch is visible by the first month of pregnancy. During the second month, it separates from the stomadeum and establishes contact with the primitive infundibular process, the future neurohypophysis. Between the latter and the lumen of the pouch, the intermediate lobe will form, while the anterior lobe will derive from the anterior limb of the pouch. By the 7th week the sphenoid bone begins to develop, first as a cartilaginous plate at the base of the skull, then slowly the pituitary fossa is formed.

The ventral connection of the pituitary with the pharyngeal region is obliterated by the 12th week. A month later the gland has attained its adult form and is enclosed in the bony sella turcica [109]. From then until term, the pituitary increases about 30 fold in weight gradually filling the sella turcica.

Concomitantly with the proliferation of epithelial cells penetrating the surrounding mesenchyme from the bulk of the anterior lobe [4] the epithelial cells continue to proliferate and differentiate until term.

By the end of the 3rd month the anterior pituitary consists of a large number of epithelial cells arranged in follicles and cords, with vascular mesenchymal tissue dispersed between them [4]. Cell differentiation can be observed as early as the 7th week, basophilic (8 weeks) and eosinophilic cells (9-10 weeks) become visible but most of the cells remain chromophobic. This classification has now been abandonned since there is no relationship between particular staining and function. Classification of the pituitary cells is actually made on histochemical studies [5]. Thyrotropin stimulating hormone (TSH) is identifiable by 10-12 weeks, essentially in the anterior region of the adenohypophysis [51]. The other pituitary hormones are also all present [82].

The hypothalamus — This is the first of the prosencephalon region to differentiate [165]. It is identifiable at 22 days as an appenendage of the forebrain (the most caudal part of the neural tube), telencephalon and diencephalon being formed about a week later and the third ventricle by 5 weeks. The basal hypothalamus, or median eminence, develops from the floor of the diencephalon which overlies Rathke's pouch. At 34 days primitive fiber tracts and neuroblasts are already differentiated in the primordial hypothalamus [105]. Between 6 and 12 weeks of gestation the median eminence undergoes rapid differentiation: specific nuclei (supraoptic, paraventricular, dorsomedial, arcuate and mammilary) are fully developed by 100 days' gestation. The fibers of the supra-optic tract can be identified at about 12 weeks [51]. At this time, thyrotropin releasing hormone (TRH) or factor (TRF) as well as other hypothalamic hormones [82] and neurotransmitters (dopamine, serotonin and norepinephrine) all become detectable [5, 70, 105].

The hypothalamo-hypophyseal-portal system. — It would appear that both the anterior pituitary and the median eminence are well vascularized by the 3rd month of gestation. The hypothalamic-hypophyseal portal connections are established at mid-gestation, but the secondary plexus in the adenohypophysis develops from about 20 weeks to term [42]. It remains a good possibility that the median eminence and the pituitary may be in communication much earlier in development, by simple local diffusion of factors, as the two tissues develop in close proximity to one other. The recent demonstration of a retrograde blood flow from the pituitary to the brain [108] suggests a further potential mechanism of pituitary-hypothalamic interaction [8, 9].

MATURATION OF THE HPT AXIS

This is a complex series of interrelated events which have been classified by Fisher et al. (cf. review in [49] and [51]) in 3 overlapping stages:

— The first *(first trimester of gestation)* represents fetal organogenesis of the thyroid and pituitary glands.
— The second involves maturation of the hypothalamic function and development of the pituitary portal vascular system *(from 10 to 35 weeks of gestation)*.
— During the third *(from 30 week's gestation to 1 month of postnatal life)*, there is maturation of peripheral metabolism (liver maturation) and development of the thyroid-hormonal response in target tissues. Superimposed is a maturation of the neuroendocrine control of thyroid secretions.

Thyroid hormone secretion is normally regulated by a feedback system between the hypothalamus, the pituitary gland and the thyroid (Fig. VI-25). TSH is the main hormone controlling both the growth and secretion of the thyroid gland. During fetal life the 3 components of the HPT axis develop independently. Indeed, from experimental evidence [51] and consideration of "experiments of the nature" such as anencephaly [92], pituitary aplasia [15, 132] and hypothalamic hypopituitarism [82] it is concluded that pituitary TSH is not necessary for normal thyroid development as a thyroid gland develops relatively normally in size and histology in the absence of, or with low TSH secretion. But a minimal level of circulating fetal TSH is essential for maintaining normal development and function of the thyroid gland near term. TRH is detected in the hypothalamus very early in gestation (5 weeks), TRH receptors are present by 10-14 weeks gestation in the pituitary [60]; preterm babies are responsive to TRH stimulation [76]. A role for TRH in fetal thyroid development is not established.

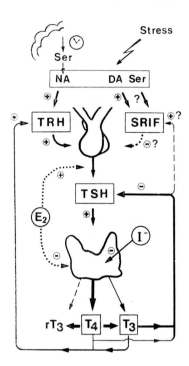

FIG. VI-25. — *The hypothalamic-pituitary-thyroid axis.*
Thyroid hormones, T_3 and T_4, have a negative feed-back action on the pituitary secretion of TSH but a positive feed-back control of the hypothalamus. Estrogens enhance the pituitary response to TRH by stimulating specific receptors. Iodide (I^-) blocks thyroid hormone biosynthesis (autoregulation). The catecholamines from the central nervous system, Noradrenaline (NA), dopamine (DA), Serotonin (Ser) modulate the release of hypothalamic TRH. Somatostatin (SRIF) inhibits the release of TSH in response to TRH. See text for other legends and abbreviations.

In contrast, the negative feedback control exerted by thyroid hormones on TSH secretion is progressively established during the second half of gestation and seems essentially mature by 1 month of age. Plasma levels of FSH are significantly higher in the fetus than in the mother and the ratio free T_4/TSH rises progressively from 0.17 at 30 week's gestation to 1.3 at 1 month of age ($\sim$ 1 in the adult) [51].

Maturation of thyroid biosynthesis and metabolism.

— It is beyond the scope of this chapter to review the normal biosynthesis and metabolism of thyroid hormones (see reviews [27, 38, 58, 136]). In brief, thyroid hormone synthesis and release requires the combination of 4 functions: thyroglobulin (Tg) synthesis; trapping of iodide and iodination of thyrosyl residues on Tg; simultaneous transfer of Tg in the colloid lumen and of colloid

material in the follicular cell; release of thyroid hormones.

Normal thyroid function depends on sufficient dietary iodine intake (reflected by urinary iodide excretion) which is irregular and often precarious; its intestinal absorption is complete. Iodine is *trapped* as an anion (iodide) in the thyroid. The thyroid follicular cells can concentrate up to 40 times the blood levels.

Organic *binding* of trapped iodide occurs rapidly. This requires the *oxidation* of iodide by a peroxidase enzyme system, allowing for the spontaneous iodination of tyrosyl groups on the Tg molecule. In the case of a deficit in peroxidase enzyme the trapped but unbound iodide can be discharged by the administration of perchlorate. *Coupling* of monoiodotyrosine (MIT) and diiodotyrosine (DIT) residues results in the formation of 3,5,3',5'-tetraiodothyronine (T_4) and 3,5,3'-triiodothyronine (T_3). The latter, still linked to Tg are stored in the thyroid colloid. Absorption into the follicular cell, and proteolysis of Tg, result in the liberation of T_4 and T_3 (in a molar ratio of 85 to 9) together with small amounts of Tg and iodotyrosines [27]. Most of the latter are deiodinated within the cell by a dehydrogenase, the iodide being reutilized for further biosynthesis. When this last step is impaired, DIT and MIT escape into the circulation with the end result of iodine deficiency.

TSH stimulates all steps in the biosynthesis of T_4 and T_3. Other thyroid stimulators are known, either of placental origin or of an immunologic nature (see below). Intraglandular iodide plays an important role in autoregulation of thyroid function exclusive of variations in serum TSH [71]. Acute exposure to a large dose of iodide inhibits thyroid hormone synthesis (Wolff-Chaikoff effect) and secretion. In contrast, iodide deficiency induces autoregulatory enhancement of iodide transport, increases the responsiveness of the iodide trap to the raised levels of TSH which follow the deficiency, and favors T_3 synthesis. Oestrogens are considered to directly inhibit thyroid hormone release but to increase the TSH response to TRH stimulation (Fig. VI-25).

Metabolism of T_4 and T_3 includes deiodination, side chain metabolism (direct deamination, transamination, decarboxylation), or renal sulfoconjugation and hepatic glycuronidation of the phenyl group.

Sequential monodeiodination is the most important pathway [27]. The initial steps probably involve two separate enzymes, the alpha ring monodeiodinase ($T_4 \rightarrow rT_3$) and the beta ring monodeiodinase ($T_4 \rightarrow T_3$). Further deiodination follows. The initial step is important providing both the "activation" of T_4 to T_3 (more potent) and its inactivation as 3,3′,5′-triiodothyronine or reverse T_3 (rT_3, of no biological activity), in equal proportions. As a result 60-80 % of the plasma levels of T_3 are provided by peripheral conversion and little from direct glandular secretion.

In the fetus: Thyroid secretion begins early in fetal life. Tg is synthetized at about 4 weeks. The thyroid gland traps iodine as early as 10 weeks. Around the 12th week, T_4 and specific binding proteins, thyroxin binding globulin (TBG) and thyroxin binding pre-albumin (TBPA) appear in fetal blood. These proteins together with T_4 increase progressively, therefore the free T_4 (FT_4) parallels T_4 production.

In contrast, *fetal metabolism is characterized by a stage of T_3 deficiency.* Virtually no T_3 is produced until after the 30th week. Due to relative inactivity of the β-monodeiodinase, T_4 metabolism is oriented in the production of rT_3, resulting in rT_3 concentrations that exceed T_3 by several fold. The change with gestational age in hormone concentrations is well documented [B] and is illustrated in Figure VI-26.

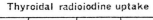

Thyroidal radioiodine uptake

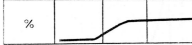

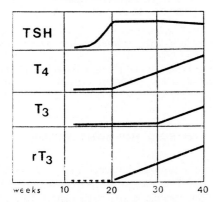

FIG. VI-26. — *Schematic illustration of the changes in fetal thyroidal radioiodine uptake, and in fetal serum levels of TSH, T_4, T_3 and rT_3 occuring during gestation.* Diagram drawn after the data of Fisher et al. [51].

During the last trimester the rate of T_3 production appears to increase and both the T_4/T_3 and rT_3/T_3 ratios decrease. The developing thyroid gland lacks the autoregulatory mechanism described earlier, and is susceptible to iodine induced inhibition of

thyroid biosynthesis. The fetus does not seem to acquire the capacity to defend itself against the suppressive effect of excessive iodide until after birth [21, 153].

FETAL THYROID FUNCTION

It is autonomous, independant of maternal thyroid function. The fetus has to depend mainly on its own thyroid function: the placenta acts as a barrier for TSH and TBG (Table I). Although T_4 and T_3 can pass the placental barrier the amounts are insufficient for fetal needs (see review in [63]), TRH can cross in both directions, but the amounts are not likely to be sufficient for fetal pituitary stimulation. The reality of the existence of a hormone chorionic thyrotropin hormone (hCT) now appears dubious (artefact of purification?). Indeed, it now appears that human chorionic gonadotropin (hCG) itself has some weak thyrotropic activity (1/4,000 that of pituitary TSH) [152].

TABLE I. — TRANSPLACENTAL TRANSFER FROM THE MOTHER TO THE FETUS

Hypothalamic-pituitary-thyroid axis	
TRH	Good
TSH	No *
Iodide	Rapid (active)
Iodotyrosines Tyrosine analogs	Good
T_4	Very poor
T_3	Poor and late
TBG	No *
Hypothalamic-pituitary-adrenal axis	
CRF	?
ACTH	No *
Cortisol	Excellent with active inactivation to cortisone
Cortisone	Yes
Dexamethasone Betamethasone	Good
CBG	No *

* No for negligible or not existent.

The fœtus is entirely dependent on the mother for its iodine supply. The placenta plays an active role in trapping maternal iodide and concentrating it in the fœtal compartment. It can also inactivate T_3.

In contrast, the placental barrier is permeable to immunoglobulins [14, 88, 96], iodide [47, 153] synthetic antithyroid agents [17, 25], anti-convulsant drugs, all molecules which may have various and adverse effects on fetal thyroid function.

ADAPTATION TO EXTRAUTERINE LIFE

This stage is characterized by two well-documented (cf. reviews in [51] and [B]) but still not fully understood phenomena: There is first an acute release of TSH with a subsequent response of T_4 and an early rise in serum T_3 concentration (Fig. VI-27). Peak serum TSH (combined with a prolactin surge) occurs 30′ after birth, reaching values 10-15 times higher than in the cord. TSH rapidly decreases during the first 24 hours, then more slowly over the first 5 days of life [22]. According to Fischer [49], the initial TSH surge would be a response of the newborn to cooling in the extra-uterine environment. Prevention of cooling does not prevent the TSH surge which appears related to umbilical cord cutting [130]. This neuroendocrine phenomenon does not exist in anencephalic babies (Czernichow in [A]). There is an early (1-4 h) T_3 surge, perhaps due to either a sudden increase in peripheral conversion of T_4 into T_3 or a discharge of thyroid stores, which is followed by a more gradual rise [49]. Peak T_3 levels observed at 24-36 hours, concomitantly with that of T_4, would represent an increase in both thyroidal secretion and peripheral conversion of T_4 to T_3. After the first week of life, T_3 serum levels increase 50-70 % with a maximum at the end of the 2nd month [51]. The high levels of rT_3 are unchanged until 4-5 days of life decreasing rapidly thereafter.

It is important to know that blood levels of T_4, T_3, rT_3, but not that of TBG, vary with gestational age, birth weight and postnatal morbidity [51, 75-78]. At birth, in premature and small-for-gestational age babies, serum levels of T_4 and T_3 are lower, that of rT_3 higher than in full-term infants. That of TSH are not measurably lower. Postnatal changes are not identical. TSH and T_4 postnatal changes are qualitatively similar but their rise is blunted. The early rise of T_3 does occur as in fullterm babies but T_3 levels fall off, increasing slowly from 3-4 days of life to normal postnatal values [49]. As a result of this identifiably different pattern in premature babies, normal postnatal values of T_3 and T_4 are only reached after approximately 6-8 weeks of life [31, 74], whereas TSH levels are normalized within 5 days [51]. In contrast, the higher than normal rT_3 levels drop in 2-4 days to values similar to that of full term babies and thereafter follows the same evolution [49] (Fig. VI-27).

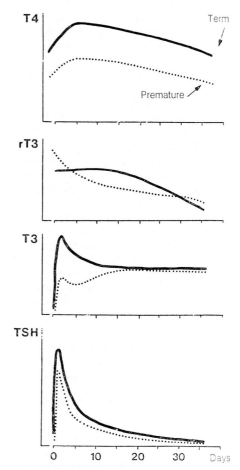

FIG. VI-27. — *Relative changes in serum levels of thyroid hormones and TSH occuring during the first month of postnatal life.*

Patterns of evolution and absolute values differ between full-term (—) and premature (· · ·) newborn infants. Diagram drawn after the data of FISHER et al. [49].

THYROID HORMONE ACTION

Thyroid hormones influence many processes of metabolism. They increase oxygen consumption, heat production, cardiac output (see review [10, 149]). They also have a developmental action on bone maturation, the central nervous system [68] and lung. In the latter they influence permeability to drugs [65] and the production of the sulfactant factor by type II pneumocytes [164]. Prenatal somatic growth is not dependent on fetal thyroid function. At birth, hypothyroid neonates usually have a relatively high normal weight and length for gestational age [95].

The most serious consequence of fetal hypothyroidism is the damage to the central nervous system which is the cause of mental retardation and other neurological manifestations. Neuronal multiplication occurs from 1 to 18 gestational weeks. Brain growth begins prenatally and continues until the 2nd postnatal year while myelinization continues longer. At birth, the brain has already reached one fourth of its adult weight and half of the postnatal brain growth is completed by 6 months of age. The cerebellum has a shorter and more rapid growth period [43]. Thyroid deficiency results in retardation of cerebellar nerve cell migration and growth, and a delay in dendritic arborization and synaptogenesis, providing explanations for the common occurence of ataxia and nystagmus. The effect of treatment on the development of dendrites seems to depend on the age of starting treatment. After a certain age it is no longer effective (Morreale de Escolar in [D], p. 25-50).

Iodine is also necessary for early fetal brain development in man: several iodine deficiency may lead to mental deficiency, deaf-mutism, spastic diplegia and squint, even in the absence of hypothyroidism. Correction of iodine deficiency in late pregnancy will not prevent the condition. Neither will the clinical features be reversible by thyroid hormone. The irreversible effect of severe iodine deficiency indicates that iodine is necessary for brain growth at the time of neuroblast multiplication.

ABNORMAL THYROID FUNCTION IN THE NEWBORN

Because of the various and rapid neonatal changes in thyroid function associated with gestational age and postnatal morbidity which complicate the appraisal of thyroid function in the neonatal period, both congenital hypo- and hyperthyroidism still present clinical and laboratory problems in diagnosis. Precise diagnosis is however mandatory since all thyroid diseases are serious problems in the newborn.

CONGENITAL AND NEONATAL HYPOTHYROIDISM

Aetiologies and pathogenesis

Neonatal thyroid hypofunction encompasses a collective group of disorders either genetic or prenatally acquired (congenital), or postnatally acquired and manifest in the neonatal period. They result

from various underlying causes. Congenital hypothyroidism is often classified as to the site of disturbance in the HPT axis: in the thyroid itself (primary), the pituitary (secondary) or the hypothalamus (tertiary). We have rather used a classification based on three different pathogenic conditions:

— fetal origin (life long disease),
— maternal origin (more or less serious transitory disease),
— post-natally acquired (usually less severe transitory disease).

The causes of hypothyroid states are given in detail in Table II. This impressive list must not withhold from us knowledge of what is the real problem in the newborn: *Primary hypothyroidism is by far the most frequent cause* [20]. It is a permanent disorder for which both early diagnosis and treatment are mandatory, Indeed, it is a serious health problem since hypofunction of the thyroid gland during fetal life or infancy results in mental retardation and other neurological sequelae.

Defective organogenesis of the thyroid. — Whatever its anatomical variety (Table II) this is the most frequent cause of sporadic hypothyroidism, particularly in countries where the dietary iodine intake is adequate. The underlying cause is unknown. The causal role of maternal autoimmunization [14] is no longer conceivable: transplacental transfer of maternal thyroid antibodies to the fetus does occur [14] but does not always result in fetal hypothyroidism [44]. Moreover, it would only represent about 1 % of congenital hypothyroidism [44] and is usually transitory [127]. The reason for a female to male ratio of about 2-4 : 1 [40, 50, 104, 118] is also unclear. Racial differences [16], seasonal [99], familial occurence [145, 161] and positive association with certain types (AW24) of human leucocyte antigen (HLA) [100] suggest that both genetic backgrounds and environmental factors contribute to the cause of the disease, but does not explain its pathogenic process.

Dyshormonogenesis. — This is the second most frequent cause of permanent congenital hypothyroidism. Defects are hereditary and often familial. The sex ratio is close to one [D]. Earlier classifications of inherited metabolic errors of thyroid hormone biosynthesis based essentially on the various biochemical steps of iodine metabolism are still considered as a framework for assessing the causative disorder but have been unable to classify about 50 % of the patients. In two recent authoritative

TABLE II. — CAUSES OF HYPOTHYROID STATES IN THE INFANT AND CHILD

A. *Congenital*

1. *Fetal origin:* fetal defective thyroid function due to:
   a) *Defect in morphogenesis*
      1. *of the thyroid gland* (sporadic, might also be familial, with autosomal recessive inheritance) [145].
         — total: athyreosis
         — partial: — hypoplastic thyroid gland in normal location
                     — hemiagenesis of the thyroid (exceptional) [98]
         — ectopic thyroid gland (cryptothyroid) [83]
      2. *of the pituitary* (sporadic or autosomic recessive) [27, 132]
         — total: — anencephaly [64] (lethal)
                   — pituitary agenesis or aplasia [101] not always lethal [132
                   — familial hypoplasia of the sella turcica [142]
                   — pituitary hypofunction in an enlarged sella [111]
         — ectopia of the pituitary gland [46]
      3. *of the hypothalamic region*
         — midline defects, septo-optic dysplasia, optic nerve hypoplasia associated or not with agenesis of the septum pellucidum [112]
         — hypothalamic deficiency associated with cleft lip and palate [120] or holoprosencephaly [81]
   b) *Genetic defect in thyroid hormone biosynthesis* [106, 133]
      — usually autosomal recessive inheritance
      — several defects have been recognized, see Table III for details
   c) *Tissue unresponsiveness*
      — TSH unresponsiveness [147]
      — peripheral resistance to thyroid hormones [122]

2. *Maternal origin:* adverse effect on fetal thyroid function due to:
   a) iatrogenic destruction of the fetal thyroid by ^{131}I treatment of the mother [53]
   b) deficient supply in iodide: endemic cretinism [154]
   c) excess of iodine supply: maternal ingestion of iodine containing drugs [79]
   d) maternal ingestion of antithyroid drugs [17] or dietary goitrogens
   e) maternal autoimmune thyroiditis: placental transfer of maternal thyroid antibodies [88] or immunoglobulins [96]

B. *Acquired*

1. Transient hypothyroidism: — due to prematurity
                             — associated with respiratory distress syndrome [137]
                             — idiopathic

2. Autoimmune thyroiditis (Hashimoto's disease)

3. Exogenous causes: — excess of iodine supply [23], accident of amniofetography [129]
                     — iodine deficiency (endemic goiter)

4. Iatrogenic: partial or total thyroidectomy, head or neck irradiation [32], various drugs (PAS, lithium...)

5. Associated: — with other endocrinopathies: Schmidt's syndrome, congenital adrenal hyperplasia [18], type II Albright osteodystrophy [37], Klinefelter's syndrome [19]
               — with collagen vascular disease [126]
               — with cystinosis [24]
               — with chronic renal failure [93]
               — with Farber's disease [155]

reviews [106, 133], it has been proposed that quantitative, as well as qualitative defects in Tg synthesis may cause the same clinical picture as intrathyroid iodine metabolism defects. Iodinated Tg being the normal precursor of thyroid hormones, may in fact be considered as a prothyroid hormone. Thus, diminished or absent Tg synthesis could theoretically originate from a defect at each step of protein synthesis. More detailed classification of actual and potential molecular mechanisms has been offered [106, 133] (Table III). Recognition of the etiologic defect in any patient with dyshormonogenesis awaits further progresses in molecular biology.

TABLE III. — CONGENITAL BIOSYNTHETIC DEFECTS
IN THYROID HORMONE SYNTHESIS AND ACTION [106, 133].

"Classical" denomination and site of defect	Biochemical defect	Occurence	Plasma hormone levels		^{131}I uptake	Other findings of diagnostic value	Treatment
			TSH	$T_3 + T_4$			
Intrathyroidal iodine metabolism 1. Trapping defect [33]	I-transport membrane defect?	Very rare	↗↗	↘	↘	— Uptake not stimulated by TSH — Also affects salivary gland, buccal mucosa... Low I salivary/plasma ratio	Massive doses of iodine (10 mg/day)
2. Iodine organification defect [97]	a) Real peroxidase defect b) Or defective oxidation with normal peroxidase activity *	Rare	N or ↗	N or ↘	↗	Positive ClO_4 discharge test: discharge of non organic iodine after potassium perchlorate administration No formation of iodotyrosines	T_4
3. Iodotyrosine dehalogenase defect [128]	Defect in dehalogenase	Quite rare	N or ↗	N or ↘	↗↗ But rapid turnover	High serum level of iodinated tyrosines Urinary excretion of labeled MIT + DIT injected I. V.	High doses of iodine
*Biosynthesis of thyroid proteins *** 4. Iodothyrosyl coupling defect [102]	Insufficient coupling of iodothyrosyl sites into T_3 and T_4 unknown mechanism	Rare	N or ↗	N or ↘	↗ Low turnover	Negative ClO_4 discharge test	T_4
5. Plasma iodoproteins defect [55]	Unknown mechanism	Quite rare	↗	N or ↘	↗	Elevated PBI due to abnormal iodinated peptides (butanol insoluble in plasma)	T_4
6. Thyroglobulin synthesis defect [135]	Tg-gene absent? mRNA deficient or abnormal?	Not really known***	↗	↘	↗	Increased urinary excretion of iodohistidine following I.V. injection of ^{131}I	T_4
TSH unresponsiveness [11, 147]	TSH binding defect?	Exceptional	N or ↗	↘	↘	Uptake not stimulated by TSH	T_4
Peripheral resistance to thyroid hormones [89, 122]	Decreased affinity of receptor for T_3	Very rare	↗	↗↗	↗	TSH not suppressed by T_3 Exaggerated TSH response to TRH	Not necessary

* This is the case in Pendred syndrome (association of nerve deafness) which appears to be inherited as an autosomal dominant trait [148]; all other defects are autosomal recessive disorders.

** Defects n° 4-6 might represent a group of diseases in which the thyroglobulin synthesis is defective or aberrant and which could be influenced by other 1 to 3 defects.

*** Might encompass the unclassified (as many as 50 %) forms of inherited goiters [133].

Endemic cretinism * (cf. review in 39). Is due to iodine deficiency. In addition to severe fetal and neonatal hypothyroid function, iodine deficiency appears to be itself an additional factor in brain damage (see above). Both sexes are equally affected.

For some reason, cretinism strikes only a part of the population living in a severely deficient iodine area, although the total population has some biochemical or clinical thyroid dysfunction. Endemic cretinism is also aggravated by or is the result of both borderline normal iodine intake and prevalent food habits, such as soybean, which enhances fecal loss of thyroid hormones, or rutabaga, white turnip containing antithyroid agents or cabbage which provides a high thiocyanate supply [41]. According to the 1960 WHO's report 200 millions people are still exposed to the risk of endemic cretinism. It is often claimed that severe cretinism no longer exists in Europe. However endemic goiter is still a serious health problem in some parts of many European countries [41]. Transient neonatal hypothyroidism is related to borderline iodine deficiency which is still prevalent in Europe, as opposed to North America.

Iodine intoxication. — Is one of the most frequent cause of iatrogenic hypothyroidism either congenital (maternal intake of iodine containing expectorants, iodine containing röntgen contrasts used in amniofetography), or neonatally acquired (most often iodine alcohol skin application).

The mechanism of the Wolff-Chaikoff [163] blockade of hormone synthesis is uncertain: blockade of oxidation of iodine or preventing its binding to tyrosyl residues? In long term intoxication, iodine uptake decreases and, as a consequence, the intrathyroid content of iodine is reduced. Chronic exposure to moderate doses stimulates, then decreases iodothyronine synthesis.

The rare occurence of such a pathologic condition relative to the frequency of inadvertant exposure to iodine excess either of maternal origin (various drugs) or neonatal (skin absorption) is totally unexplained. Individual susceptibility is demonstrated by hypothyroidism occuring in only one of a pair of twins after amniofetography, or the higher occurence in prematures. The thyroid dysfunction is usually transient.

Defect in thyroid hormone action. — The underlying causes are summarized in Table III. They are extremely rare. Only a few cases of thyroidgland unresponsiveness to TSH in association with congenital hypothyroidism have been reported. Peripheral thyroid hormone unresponsiveness may lead to either hypothyroidism or to TSH-dependent hyperthyroidism [57]. Neither one has been described in the newborn.

Secondary and tertiary hypothyroidism. — Impairment of thyroid function results from decreased effective stimulation of the thyroid. This is a very heterogenous group of clinical manifestations: sporadic or familial deficiency in TRH or isolated deficiency in TSH secretion are very rare. In other instances, deficient TSH secretion is associated with either multiple pituitary deficiencies or various morphological malformations (see References in Table II for more details). In all cases, either hypothyroidism is not the major clinical problem or is expressed later in life. The combined incidence of such abnormalities is close to one in 110,000 births [D].

Acquired hypothyroidism. — Except for the neonatally iatrogenic causes discussed above, in all other conditions hypothyroidism develops in childhood (2-6 yrs) or later in life and is therefore not a neonatal problem.

Thyroid hormone-binding alterations. — Absence or partial deficiency of the principal thyroid hormone carrier protein, TBG, is an inherited disorder. It was first recognized in adult patients and described in several families. The introduction of neonatal mass-screening programs for congenital hypothyroidism based on serum T_4 determination has revealed that the situation is rather frequent occuring in about 1 in 10,000 live births [D, 50].

The condition is characterized by low or absent TBG, low T_4-T_3, normal TSH, normal thyroid hormone binding prealbumin (TBPA), and normal albumin. This is not a thyroid function disease since the free fractions of both T_4 and T_3 are normal as are the TSH responses to TRH, and since the individuals are clinically euthyroid. Both sexes are equally affected but the deficiency is often quan-

---

* It is important to mention that the word *cretinism* is not used with the same meaning throughout the literature.

In Europe, *"cretinism"* means mental retardation whatever its causes; the expression *"endemic cretinism"* specifically designates the triad mental retardation, goiter and hypothyroidism due to iodine deficiency. The Anglo-saxon equivalent of the latter is usually *"goitrous cretinism"*.

In contrast, in the United States, the other expressions *"sporadic cretinism"*, or simply *"cretinism"*, unambiguously refer to congenital hypothyroidism, even in the absence of manifest mental retardation (B). These terms are unclear and nonspecific in Europe, and seldom used.

titatively more pronounced in males than in females [78]. Congenital hyper-TBG-emia has also been described [124]. Pedigree studies have shown that the genetic locus for TBG resides on the X chromosome [124]. Both abnormalities in TBG hepatic synthesis are X-linked dominant inherited conditions.

A familial disturbance in TBPA has recently been reported [66], the increase in both TBPA and TBG binding produces an increase in total T_4 but no signs of hyperthyroidism (normal free T_4).

Congenital absence of albumin (analbuminemia) has little effect on thyroid hormone levels since both TBG and TBPA levels are concomitantly increased.

Thyroid hormone protein binding is also affected in malnutrition, hypoproteinemia, active acromegaly, nephrotic syndrome, major illness and by drugs (androgens, anabolic steroids, prednisone, diphenylhydantoin).

In none of the above conditions is the thyroid function per se impaired. Nevertheless, it is important to be aware of the modifications in total to free thyroid hormone ratio that they govern, when interpreting laboratory data, particularly when clinical and hormonal findings seem discordant.

Clinical findings

Three basic notions are worth remembering: (*a*) Early clinical diagnosis of congenital hypothyroidism is *difficult* and very often missed before 3 months of age. (*b*) The clinical syndrome varies to a great extent according to the severity and the onset of hypothyroidism, age at first examination and the time elapsed during which the untreated disease will progress and lead to a more uniform and typical symptomatology. (*c*) It is useless and illusory to describe clinical etiological forms, since the clinical findings calling for attention are, in all cases, the end-result of the common problem that is thyroid hormone deficiency. On the other hand, because of the seriousness of the affection and the great benefit of early treatment, the first priority is to assess the state of hypothyroidism. An etiological diagnosis may be considered as a next step. However, the etiological significance of palpating a thyroid gland or finding a goiter should not be disregarded. In newborns, goiters may present as the prevalent sign. This clinical form will be discussed in a subsequent section.

Deficiency in thyroid hormone affects a number of functions among which are somatic growth, bone maturation, the cardiovascular system and neurological and mental development. In the early postnatal period clinical diagnosis is still always a difficult problem because the disease can be asymptomatic for a certain period of time, and only lead to a few abnormal signs or symptoms which, in addition, are rather nonspecific, Intrauterine somatic growth is usually normal. This is why, in the last 2 or 3 decades, efforts have been devoted to thoroughly evaluate the significance of the presence and/or association of subtle abnormalities in morphology, comportment and basic functions [94, 95, 119, 144]. Smith et al. [144], from a retrospective study, have insisted on the orienting value of the association of 1-7 symptoms (mean = 3) in the first week of life, which are by decreasing frequency (%): icterus > 3 days (73 %); oedema (53 %); prolonged gestation > 42 weeks, abdominal distension (47 %); poor feeding, vomiting (40 %); lag in stooling > 20 hrs, hypothermia (36 %), large (> 0.5 cm) posterior fontanel, respiratory distress, peripheral cyanosis (33 %); hypoactivity, lethargy and birth weight > 4 kg (27 %). Unfortunately, the significance of prevalent clinical findings varies considerably between studies [94, 95, 118, 119, 144]. More recently Letarte et al. have proposed the use of a clinical scoring index, similar to the performance of the Apgar scores, on admission to the nursery, in the hope that it can led one to suspect the diagnosis of hypothyroidism in the early neonatal period (Table IV).

TABLE IV. — Neonatal hypothyroid index

	Score
Umbilical hernia	0.8
Feeding problems	0.9
Hypotonia	0.9
Constipation *	1.0
Enlarged tongue *	1.1
Inactivity	1.1
Skin mottling	1.1
Dry skin *	1.4
Open posterior fontanel	1.4
Typical facies	2.8
Total	12.5

* Only symptom correlated with T_3 levels.
** Only two symptoms *not* correlated with T_4 levels (adapted from Letarte et al., in ref. [D], pp. 225-235).

To illustrate the difficulties of early detection of hypothyroidism based on clinical findings alone, we report the experience of Price et al. [118]. In a careful prospective study of 40 hypothyroid infants diagnosed at neonatal screening and examined at 6-118 days of age (mean 21.5), except for umbilical hernia and jaundice, they found a lower incidence of abnormal signs than did MacFaul and Grant [94] within the first month of life. Moreover only 22.5 % of their patients had 2 or more of the Smith et al. criteria [144] and only 15 % fulfill the criteria of the scoring index established by Letarte et al. (Table IV), despite the fact that both reference criteria were established for neonates less than one week of age and their patients were much older. Skeletal maturation was also normal in 24 % of the cases.

The early findings described above precede the development of signs which are more obvious for the disease: hypothermia, oedema, peripheral cyanosis, hoarse cry due to laryngeal oedema, constipation, abnormal body proportions (brachyskelia, increased head circumference), typical facies with a low nasal bridge and a large protruding tongue (Fig. VI-28), slowing rate of growth and relatively conserved weight gain contrasting with persistent feeding problems or anorexia. The pulse rate is slow and congenital heart block may occasionally supervene.

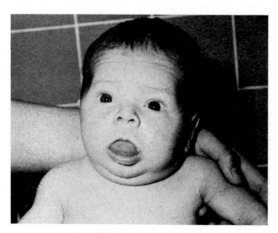

FIG. VI-28. — *Typical facies*
of severe congenital hypothyroidism.
Note in this 2 month old infant, low nasal bridge, œdema of the face, protruding tongue and macroglossia.

When treatment is delayed, growth retardation and poor mental development to severe mental retardation become more obvious, as do other neurologic handicaps: cerebellar ataxia, fine and gross motor disturbances, strabismus, nystagmus and behavior problems (Fig. VI-29). Even in less severe forms, delay in speech, primary enuresis, difficulties in thought, in concentration, in orienting time and space, slow movement and hyperkinesis are typically observed in young hypothyroid children. In children over one year of age a characteristic muscular hypertrophy of the limbs develops (Kocher-Debré-Semelaigne syndrome).

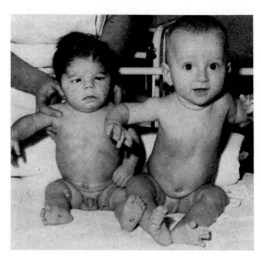

FIG. VI-29. — *Hypothyroid infant 6 month old (left) in comparison with a normal baby of the same age (right).*
Brachyskely, short stature, nystagmus, abdominal dilatation, hypotonia are manifest (Courtesy of Dr. M. BETHENOD, Hôpital Debrousse, Lyon).

The beneficial influence of breast feeding on the mitigation and/or prevention of hypothyroidism in the newborn is highly controversial. In any case the mother's milk content of T_4/T_3 is not high enough to insure more than 10 % of neonatal needs. Artificial milks do not contain thyroid hormones.

A search for predisposing factors such as: Maternal diet and diseases, drug ingestion, maternal or neonatal exposure to iodine containing röntgen contrast media, parental consanguinity and family history of thyroid disease, may orient the etiological diagnosis and or future decisions (see below, discussion on prenatal diagnosis).

In severely affected or untreated newborns serious complications may occur: suffocation due to milk inhalation, sudden vascular collapse, seizures, cutaneous and pulmonary infections, septicemia, intestinal occlusion with all its potential complications, intestinal perforation, peritonitis...; rapid or sudden death are not uncommon.

Other findings

Widespread skeletal abnormalities are observed: not only is *bone maturation usually retarded* but ossification of the epiphyseal centres is irregular which causes the fragmentation of the epiphysis; femoral and humeral *epiphysial dysgenesis* are characteristic. There is also an *increased bone density* especially at the base of the skull and around the orbits. As a result of the combination of these 3 abnormalities, marked deformation of the bones eventually occurs, especially in the femoral neck and lumbar vertebrae. An enlarged sella turcica is not uncommon (increased volume of the pituitary?).

The electrocardiogram (ECG) often shows signs of sinus bradycardia. Slowing of alpha wave activity and generalized reduction of amplitude are typical findings on electroencephalography (EEG). Examination of the achiles reflex is not recomended in newborns or young infants: Impractical to manage, it is an unnecessary stress.

Laboratory investigations

Assessing the state of hypothyroidism. — In contrast with a difficult clinical diagnosis, biochemical evidence of impaired thyroid function is *simple* to perform and *easy* to establish. It is essentially based on the measurement of both thyroid hormones and TSH concentrations in the blood, with the help of the newly introduced radioimmunological methods (RIA). From a practical standpoint all older methods are becoming obsolete.

The simultaneous findings of low T_4 and T_3 levels are sufficient proof of primary hypothyroidism. There is enough evidence to make the general statement that both abnormalities are correlated with the severity and the time of onset of the disease rather than with its cause. However, T_4-T_3 levels are often not drastically reduced and are always still detectable, even in patients later proven to be athyreotic. The reason for this is unclear. The decreases in T_3 and T_4 levels are not always parallel. From the knowledge of the physiological backgrounds (see above) reflection of thyroid hormone secretion is given by T_4 levels, that of peripheral metabolism by T_3 levels. Theoretically measurement of T_4 levels would be sufficient. However, measurement of both T_4 and T_3 is very helpful in clarifying the transient states of hypothyroidism which will be discussed in a further section.

Blood and urinary determinations. — Whatever the parameters chosen for study, they should not cause

delay in the initiation of treatment. However some are not widely available.

Total T_4-T_3 serum levels: Determination of T_4 rather than T_3, or both when possible by RIA, is mandatory. When interpreting the results, one should keep in mind the discrete variations which normally occur according to age and prematurity (Fig. VI-27), or intercurrent stress [1]. Rather than reporting here detailed reference values in the neonatal period, we advise the clinician to interpret the data with the help of the local laboratory which has previously established its own reference values. Indeed, with the same physiological profiles, absolute figures of reference values vary to a significant extent in the literature according to sampling time [107], to series number, methods and possibly geographic distribution in term [B, D, 3, 12, 22, 45, 52, 72, 74, 77] or preterm newborn infants [1, 12, 31, 77, 86, 156] or sick newborn infants [1, 77, 86]. Between 2 months and 2 years of age the range of normal values is usually 5-15 µg/dl (69-200 nmol/l) for T_4 and 80-230 ng/dl for T_3 (1.3-3.5 nmol/l).

Free T_4 and T_3: These are reduced in proportion to the total levels [45, 52], except in TBG deficient patients [78] (see above). This determination is not widely available and not necessary for the diagnosis when TSH is unambiguously elevated.

Measurement of rT_3 [22, 72]: This has no diagnostic value in hypothyroidism.

TSH levels: These are almost always of diagnostic value. Basal levels must also be interpreted with caution in relation to physiological variations during the first week of life [22, 31, 77, 86, 131, 156]. It is also worth noting that falsely high values, persisting for several months, have been observed in infants whose mother received microbial vaccines during pregnancy and likely developed antibodies interfering with the TSH assay [56].

Normal TSH and low T_4 levels, or subnormal T_4 levels and moderately elevated TSH does not always contradict the diagnosis of primary hypothyroidism. This may correspond to less severe or compensated hypothyroid states. In this situation the *TRH test* is helpful, showing an exagerated TSH rise [75]. Indeed, in primary hypothyroidism the TSH rise response to a TRH stimulation test is always exagerated both in amplitude and duration. When basal TSH levels are unambiguously high, the TRH stimulation test is unnecessary. In contrast, it is helpful to distinguish secondary and tertiary hypothyroidism. In both conditions, serum levels of T_4 and TSH are usually low but the TSH response to TRH stimulation differs: in the former, the TSH response is always blunted or absent while in the latter the response can be delayed, exaggerated and prolonged [54].

Normal TSH basal values are rather stable after the 5th day of life and according to the laboratory less than 5 to 15 μU/ml. After IV injection of 7 μg/kg of TRH the peak TSH response in our experience is 17 ± 5 μU/ml at 30', with a return to less than 10 μU/ml at 120' [35]. The response in full term [75, 77], preterm [77], small-for-date [77] infants is similar to that of older children or adults.

Prolactin (PRL) [22, 103, 131]: Basal levels are high in primary hypothyroidism and occasionally in hypothalamic disorders [150]; in both instances the PRL response follows the same pattern as TSH after TRH injection [103]. Basal PRL levels are extremely high (230-795 ng/ml) in the newborn, depending on gestational age and weight, while the PRL response to TRH is not [103]. It is only after 6 months of age that basal levels drop to adult levels (< 10 to < 20 ng/ml according to laboratory).

Growth hormone (GH): In primary hypothyroid patients the GH response to various stimulation tests is diminished and returns to normal after thyroid hormone treatment [36]. A paradoxical GH response to TRH is seen in about half of the cases [29]. This determination is not however of any diagnostic help, except in those patients suspected of secondary or tertiary hypothyroidism, for whom further search for deficiencies in other pituitary hormones, adrenocorticotrophic hormone (ACTH) in particular, is recommended.

Thyroglobulin (Tg): Tg levels in blood can now be measured and their physiological variations in the newborn have been described [85, 117]. The presence of Tg in blood reflects that of a functioning thyroid tissue and therefore its absence has been suggested as reflecting thyroid aplasia [110]. This measurement is so far not a routine procedure and its diagnostic value has not yet been evaluated.

TBG: This can be measured directly by RIA or indirectly by estimating its binding capacity (TBC). As mentioned above, its measurement is only indicated when a deficiency in TBG is suspected. Normal values are 12-30 mg/litre.

Iodine status: Can be evaluated by measurement of serum protein-bound iodine (PBI) (normal values after 1 week = 4.8 μg/dl) and 24 hr urinary iodine excretion. One should be aware of the interference of iodine medications and of iodine containing röentgen contrast agents used even several days

or weeks previously. When these potential "artefacts" have been eliminated, the measurement of these 2 parameters is only useful when a dyshormonogenesis is suspected (Table IV). An elevation in serum PBI, but not in serum T_4, is indicative of a defect in thyroglobulin synthesis.

Other findings. — These include normochromic anemia, elevated cholesterol levels (not in young infants however), excessively positive calcium balance but usually normal calcemia and phosphatemia. The cortisol production rate is decreased and cortisol metabolism is slowed. The latter is due to relative 11β-hydroxydehydrogenase deficiency. Hence, urinary excretion of 17-hydroxysteroids (17OHCS) and 17-ketosteroids (17KS) is reduced but plasma cortisol is maintained at about normal levels [13].

X-ray examination

The cardiac shadow is increased. Estimation of bone age [139] (left foot, hip and knee in newborns) and the presence or the absence of bone deformations (dysgenesis of the epiphysial hip center; coxa vara or coxa plana...) will give some information about the onset, hence of the severity of the disease. A search for craniofacial abnormalities should also be made.

When and how to perform thyroid scanning?

Scintiscaning of the neck region after injection or ingestion of radioactive iodine or sodium pertechnetate technetium 99 m (technetium for short) is an important test to determine the precise anatomical diagnosis. In cases of defective embryogenesis, the most frequent cause of congenital hypothyroidism, it will often provide a definitive diagnosis.

Radioactive ^{131}I-iodine thyroid uptake is no longer recomended because of its radiation hazard, the lack of specificity and the length of duration of the test. Its use should be abandoned in newborn infants.

According to recent experiences [6, 118], both technetium and ^{123}I-iodine, isotopes with much shorter half-lifes (6 and 13 hrs respectively), give a rapid diagnosis and reliable scans. In addition, ^{123}I uptake can be used the first 24 hours after administration for turnover studies [157].

When hypothyroidism is confirmed biologically in a newborn infant, the major concern is not to delay the onset of treatment. There is some debate in the literature as to whether it is opportune to perform a scintiscan or to begin treatment immediately. However, modern scintiscans do give rapid anatomical diagnosis, therefore enable treatment to be started immediately, the delay in treatment being reasonably short. It is only when a *normal size* thyroid gland is found in a normal position that it is necessary to await the results of further hormonal testing ro tule out transient hypothyroidism. In our opinion which agrees with that of many pediatric endocrinologists, a scintiscan should be performed in all but two conditions: (*a*) if the child is severely ill; (*b*) if there is no close facility to perform the test; an hypothyroid infant should not be travelling back and forth in somewhat stressing conditions. Under these conditions treatment is started. Diagnosis can be completed after 2-3 years, an age at which there is no harm in stopping the treatment for a few weeks.

Diagnostic approach to etiologic diagnosis

From the long, though not exhaustive, above list of laboratory procedures and findings it must not be concluded that this represents standard thyroid function testing. There is no routine procedure in assessing thyroid function in an infant or child. *Diagnosis must be conducted step by step and the number of tests kept to the essential minimum.* An outline of a rational approach to the etiological diagnosis is given in Table V.

Special mention is made of the case of probable thyroid hormone dysgenesis: it may often be suspected on family history and clinical grounds.

Indeed, a variably hypertrophied thyroid gland is found in patients with dyshormonogenesis. In newborns the gland is usually not so enlarged but it can always be palpated by careful examination: because of the shortness of the neck it may be unnoticeable but the infant should be patiently examined in full extension of the neck.

When by eliminating other causes, a diagnosis of dyshormonogenesis becomes more than likely (Table V), determination of thyroid antibodies is not necessary in the newborn for two reasons: (*a*) in the neonatal period circulating antibodies might be of maternal origin and these will disappear in a few weeks or months [44]; (*b*) autoimmune thyroiditis is not seen in early infancy.

The next step in the diagnosis, that of the site of the hormonogenesis defect, will require extensive investigations (Table III) which are often disappointing and should not interfere with an early start of therapy. Treatment should be started immediately. More precise diagnosis must await an older age.

Differential diagnosis

From a practical stand point there should be no differential diagnosis. Determination of cord or serum T_4 levels is so easy and unexpenssive that it should be done in any condition where an hypothyroid state is suspected, even on weak clinical grounds. If the clinician does not have close laboratory facilities, dried blood samples (after heelprick puncture, deposit a few drops of blood on filter paper, wait for drying and send) can be sent by regular mail, safely with no problems of conservation of T_4 [91].

TABLE V. — OUTLINE OF A PRACTICAL APPROACH TO THE ASSESSMENT OF THE HYPOFUNCTIONING NON GOITROUS THYROID GLAND

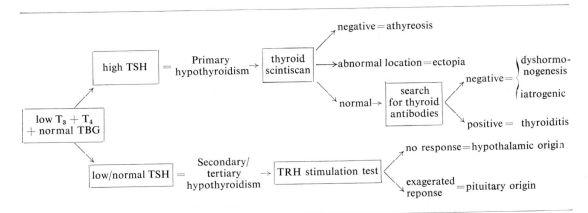

However, some features of overt hypothyroidism have, in the past, been mistaken for other diseases:

— For example, severe constipation might have been falsely attributed to megacolon (pseudomegacolon).

— Protruding tongue, depressed nasal bridge, and umbilical hernia are features in common with the Beckwith-Wiedemann syndrome of autosomal dominant inheritance [7, 162]. One sixth of the patients with this syndrome have been misdiagnosed as cases of congenital hyperthyroidism, in spite of overgrowth, hemi-hypertrophy, abnormalities of genitalia... but normal intellectual development; in the absence of hypoglycemic episodes.

Prenatal diagnosis of congenital hypothyroidism

There seems to be little demand for such diagnosis. Indeed, congenital hypothyroidism is mostly sporadic or due to iodine deficiency. The latter is known and can be prevented by normalizing iodine dietary content, while the former is unpredictable. However a rare, but familial occurence of thyroid dyshormonogenesis has been well documented in 10 families containing two or more children affected with either ectopic or athyreotic congenital hypothyroidism (see review in [161]). The incidence of consanguinous marriage in those families is suggestive of an autosomal recessive inheritance pattern. On the other hand, when hypothyroidism is associated with inborn errors in thyroid hormone biosynthesis (autosomal recessive inheritance) there is a 25 % risk for the child to be born with the disease. Other circumstances for which prenatal screening would be suitable are a family history of thyreopathology, treatment with iodides, radioactive iodine or antithyroid drugs during pregnancy.

Because of this, attempts have been made to provide for antenatal diagnosis. Until now the premises are meager and moreover, if done, it would only be late in pregnancy. Indeed, as mentioned earlier, fetal thyroid secretions are low until the 20-22th weeks of pregnancy and serum T_3 (active form) only begins to rise at about 30 weeks of gestation. In contradiction to earlier reports [B, 26], it would seem that amniotic fluid concentrations of T_4 and T_3 follow the same temporal pattern as that in fetal serum [87]. Technical difficulties are involved, since some laboratories have not been able to detect either T_4 fluctuations or T_3 concentrations in the amniotic fluid [26]. The need for a great number of observations to detect temporal variations in T_4, and of a sensitive technique to be able to detect T_3 in amniotic fluid, together with the variability in the absolute values obtained from one laboratory to the other (rT_3 in particular), emphasizes the potential difficulties of estimating amniotic fluid thyroid hormone levels. However, because rT_3 can easily be measured and because its temporal pattern in the amniotic fluid also ressembles that seen in fetal plasma, it has been proposed for prenatal screening. The recent report of a premature newborn infant with congenital hypothyroidism (and sepsis) presenting with very high levels of rT_3 in cord blood [59] has raised much discussion about the usefulness of rT_3 in the prenatal diagnosis of hypothyroidism. The doubts have been reinforced when a preliminary attempt at prenatal diagnosis based on amniotic fluid levels or rT_3 failed to detect an hypothyroid foetus [90].

On the other hand, if a reliable method is established in the future, management of the situation will still remain difficult. We do not yet know with certainty at what time of intrauterine life the development of the nervous system becomes thyroid-dependent, although it is believed that the last 4-8 weeks are the critical period. There will be little time between diagnostic and therapeutic decisions. Because of the specific materno-fetal relationships and placental barrier to thyroid hormones it would be illusory to hope to prevent hypothyroidism by treating the mother. Attempts at treating the foetus in utero directly have been disappointing [67] and repeated amniocenteses is not without risks.

Despite the limitation of our present knowledge and because scientific discoveries are constantly made, genetic counselling of the parents for future pregnancies is highly recommended when an hereditary defect is suspected.

Treatment

There is only one treatment for primary congenital hypothyroidism: i.e. medical thyroid replacement therapy for life. As soon as hypothyroidism is diagnosed in a newborn, hormonal treatment should be started without delay. Substitutive thyroid therapy is commonly considered as one of the least complicated of hormonal therapies. There are however some recent developments about what form of medication to use, its optimal dosage, on the risks of under-treatment or overtreatment, and the choice of the best parameter for controlling the adequacy of treatment, that need some consideration.

Common forms of thyroid hormone medications and their advantages and disadvantages. — A number of thyroid hormone preparations are commercially available. In pediatric practice only three are usually considered:

Dessiccated thyroid which has been extensively used for many years (as early as 1880), is a mixture of iodinated proteins, tyrosines and thyronines, extracted from ovine or porcine thyroid glands. Fabrication control of this medication is made according to either the United States or the International pharmacopeia standards which are both based essentially on the organic iodine content of the tablets (0.2 ± 0.03 %). In no country is there any specification of their precise hormonal content. A recent study has attracted attention to the fact that when T_4-T_3 are measured, there are notable variations (16-101 %) in hormonal content among generic thyroid preparations issued either by the same or by different manufacturers, despite a constant organic iodine content [121]. The wide variation in T_4/T_3 content of the drug, may well explain the unusually high requirements seen in some patients. The use of this form of medication is nowadays controversial [73]. It has however satisfied many pediatricians in the past and still does.

The only advantages of this form of treatment are in fact its low cost and the long-term experience of clinical control of the effects of treatment acquired by those pediatricians who have used it for many years. The dosages have been for long purely empirical. Since the recent wide spread of laboratory facilities, attempts at rationalizing the optimal dose have made in children by estimating the average dose of desiccated thyroid necessary to bring TSH back to normal values [160], to maintain T_4 levels above the lower limits of normal for age [80, 160] or both [80, 143]. Daily doses ranging from 8.5 ± 0.86 cg/m² to 10 cg/m² have been given as recommended dosages [80, 143, 160]. Similar studies have not been made in newborns. With this form of therapy, a constant finding is that normalized T_4 levels are accompanied by higher than normal T_3 levels [116]. On clinical grounds, that is euthyroidism, it is accepted that such an unphysiologic hormonal status is of no consequence for the child. This has not really been precisely studied.

Synthetic racemic thyroxine. — Solutions or tablets containing an equal mixture of levothyroxine (L-T_4) and dextrothyroxine (D-T_4). Textbooks classically refer to the former as being the only "active" physiological hormone and to the latter as being "inactive".

The recent use of biochemical criteria for assessing the biological activity of thyroid hormone preparations in vivo has begun to adjust our knowledge to more precise facts. A recent study has clearly shown that both T_4 isomers given separately are effective in lowering serum TSH, cholesterol, triglycerides and phospholipid levels and in stimulating metabolic rate, although in a ratio of 27 to one in favor of L-T_4 [62]. Differences in metabolism and disappearance rates in blood between the isomers render it difficult to assign their relative therapeutic efficiency when given in equal amounts. Moreover, one should be aware of the fact that D-T_4 interfers with the measurement of blood T_4 levels. Therefore, when this medication is used (commonly in France) and serum T_4 determined for controlling the adequacy of treatment, it is recommended to draw the blood 24 hours after the last oral dose to minimize and standardize the amount of D-T_4 so inwillingly measured, and only to correct the reference norms by a factor of about 1.4 [141]. This correction factor takes into account the differences in elimination half-lives between D-T_4 (one day) and L-T_4 (7 days). The technical problem mentioned above may also be overcome by the measurement of free T_4 which is not influenced by D-T_4; but this assay is more complicated and not widely available.

Synthetic levothyroxine sodium (L-T_4). — Used for several years in the United States, it has been recently introduced in Europe. The optimal daily dose has been a matter of debate. At first it was felt, and even advised, that treatment should achieve slightly above normal T_4 levels to compensate for the lack of T_3 and obtain an euthyroid status. This is now known to be incorrect inasmuch as it has been established that the main source of circulating T_3 arises from peripheral conversion of T_4 (see above). Recent studies in children, based on the minimal dose of L-T_4 effective in suppressing TSH to normal values in serum, have reassessed the optimality of previously calculated daily requirements (5-10 µg/kg between 2 to 15 yrs of age, [B]) to much lower dosages: 3.78 ± 0.6 µg/kg/day or 104.6 ± 5.2 µg/m² of body surface area [125]. Similar findings have been obtained by others ([30, 116] and Ref. in [125]). With the use of L-T_4, there is no problem in measuring T_4 serum levels, and as peripheral metabolism of T_4 is normal in treated hypothyroid children, normalized serum T_3 levels are normally obtained.

Synthetic triiodothyronine sodium (T_3). — On the theoretical background of T_3 being the active thyroid hormone one might be tempted to prefer the use of T_3. In fact, the drug has a short half-life which produces fluctuations in blood levels (maximal 1 to 5 hours after administration) and makes difficult the routine evaluation of such uneven hormonal levels. Other disadvantages are its cost and the fact that serum T_4 levels, the most reliable and generally available thyroid test, cannot be used to control the adequacy of treatment. T_3 might however be useful when, particularly in newborns, a rapid hormonal effect is desirable. Its short life also allows for a more rapid escape from hormone action, if complications are to occur during therapy [30].

Choice of replacement agent. — For the reasons discussed above, the American Academy of Pediatrics * Committee on Drugs recommends L-T_4 as the drug of choice for the treatment of hypothyroidism [30]. This recommendation is receiving increasing agreement [D, 116]. In Europe, France in particular, the use of desiccated thyroid is still common practice for treating hypothyroid children, and keeps its supporters [143, 160]. Nevertheless, treatment of newborn infants diagnosed on a neonatal screening basis is nowadays most usually begun with L-T_4. Finally, an early proposal of starting neonatal treatment of an hypothyroid infant with 25 µg of L-T_4 and 15 µg of T_3 daily for 2 weeks, then to discontinue T_3 and increase L-T_4 (Guyda in [D], p. 247-261) has not been pursued.

Optimal dosage in newborns. — This has not been studied as strictly as in children or adults. It is felt that daily requirements are slightly higher during the first few months of life than later on. One argument in favor of this view is that larger doses of thyroid hormones are apparently necessary to suppress TSH in infancy than later in life. Indeed, in spite of normalized T_3/T_4 levels, TSH only returns to normal for age by 6-12 months of age in apparently well controlled hypothyroid infants [D]. For others, this phenomenon is only the expression of a higher threshold of sensitivity of the HPT axis at this age [134], or is secondary to cellular hyperplasia of the TSH-secreting pituitary cells which may require some time to be suppressed by normal thyroid hormone levels. In support of this interpretation is the longer time required for TSH suppression in those newborns with the most severe clinical signs of hypothyroidism [D].

To summarize current concepts [D, 30] *the scheme for early treatment of congenital hypothyroidism is:*

— Full therapeutic doses can be started at once when the disease is recognized before the development of significant complications (myocardial

* American Academy of Pediatrics, Committee on Drugs.

involvement, anemia...) except in infants with secondary or tertiary hypothyroidism. In the latter cases, impairment of adrenal function may be latent, or marked. Because initiation of thyroid hormone therapy rapidly increases the hepatic metabolism of cortisol (see above) adrenal insufficiency must be considered as a potential additional risk. Therefore, in such instances, thyroid hormones are started only after 2-3 days of cortisol therapy (at physiological doses), to prevent an acute adrenal crisis (see below).

— The initial dosage in otherwise healthy fullterm babies averages 37.5 µg per day [20-50] in a single oral dose. The dose may be increased slightly thereafter if necessary but a L-T_4 dose of 50 µg/day is generally adequate during the entire first year of life. After this, the dose is increased to 3-5 µg/kg/day until the average adult dose is attained, that is to say that the daily dose would be 75-100 µg from 1 to 5 years and 100-150 µg from 6 to 12 years. Adult doses are around 150 µg per day. In prematures weighting less than 2 kg, or infants at risk for cardiac failure, the initial dose should not exceed 25 µg per day but can be increased to 50 µg in 4-6 weeks (5 additional µg per week). If the infant cannot take oral medication, the IV route can be used as well. Dosages are only reduced to 75 % of the oral doses and caution should be taken to use *a freshly* prepared solution.

Control of treatment. — Initiation of treatment can exceptionally be undertaken at home. When signs of severe hypothyroidism are present, it is mandatory to initiate therapy in an equiped hospital environment. The first follow up visit is made six weeks later, a time when full effect of the hormonotherapy will, or should, be seen.

By using the scheme proposed above not all infants would be ideally controlled. There are evident individual variations (differences in oral absorption or needs?). The ideal dose for each patient should be adjusted and closely checked by both biological and clinical criteria.

To summarize the long discussions in the literature and what has been learned from recent and extensive experiences of treating those infants diagnosed very early in life, through screening programs, it does appear that both TSH and T_4 levels are the only useful biological criteria to use in the newborn. *TSH must not however be used as the sole criterion of adequacy.* TSH is, indeed, a sensitive indicator of undertreatment, but, when found in the normal range for age, it is not able to detect overtreatment. Also, the slow response of TSH to a readjusted dose imposes a delay of at least 2 weeks before rechecking the hormonal status. Determinations of serum T_4 levels clearly indicate when physiological levels are attained. Unfortunately there are situations which do appear discordant: TSH levels might remain elevated or in the not-too-far-above normal range and T_4 levels be normal. By now, it is known that this situation is commonly observed in the newborn infant [138]. Then, one should rely completely on T_4 levels, particularly when the child is euthyroid, and not attempt to suppress TSH to the normal range for age. This will make the child at risk for overtreatment. In other occasional circumstances, normal T_4 can be seen in clinically hypo- or hyperthyroid patients. Adjustement to a proper dosage should then be guided by clinical criteria. There is a general consensus that, indeed the *definitive criteria of adequate replacement therapy are clinical:* signs and symptoms of hypo- or hyperthyroidism, physical development, growth and bone maturation. Among those, normal growth and bone maturation are still the best indicators of proper treatment. Follow-up should be done regularly (at least every 2-3 months in infants, and 2-3 times a year until age 2-3), including carefully history, measurement of height, weight, head circumference, systematic physical and neurological examinations, laboratory evaluation and less frequent bone age evaluation.

If some of the above cited discrepancies remain unexplained, and in any case in situations such as prematurity, dysmaturity, respiratory distress in which the management of treatment remains controversial (see below) specialized advice should be requested.

Risks of treatment. — A continuation of the state of hypothyroidism has obviously to be avoided by giving the child sufficient hormonotherapy. In the past, it has been recommended that the patient should be kept on the slight overdose side, particularly in early infancy, to insure the best mental development possible, the belief being that slight underdose was harmful but slight overdosage was not. These concepts must be reconsidered. Indeed, if excessive dosages have led to overt iatrogenic hyperthyroidism with advanced bone maturation and premature craniosynostosis [115], it now also appears that slight overdosage, even if not clinically evident, might be as harmful as undertreatment.

Recent studies indicate that, in fact, hazards of overtreating an hypothyroid infant might have been overlooked: hyperactivity and irreversible perceptual motor problems and mild mental retardation are long term sequellæ of neonatal thyrotoxicosis [69]. There is experimental evidence in the rat, that T_3

may decrease cell number in the cerebellum while also advancing cell differentiation.

In conclusion, in the modern concept of monitoring thyroid hormone replacement therapy, *overtreatment should be as carefully avoided as undertreatment* [159]. Finally one should keep in mind that some drugs may alter the metabolism of thyroid hormones and vice versa. For instance, phenobarbital accelerates T_4 metabolism while salicylate or phenytoin may alter thyroxin binding to TBG (thus necessitating measurement of free T_4 instead of total T_4 as a control parameter). Diarrhea, malabsorption or high soybean content in food all are causes of reduced intestinal absorption of thyroid hormones. In the case of intercurrent disease, T_4 should usually not be stopped. High fever should not affect thyroid hormone treatment given at physiological dosage. Any reason for it must be looked for and treated specifically. The requirements for vitamin D are the same as in any newborn. Treatment should not however be started immediately because of the risks of hypercalcemia. When the child has reached an equilibrium of euthyroidism (about $\leqslant 2$ months) then vitamin D is given at the usual dosages.

Treatment of other etiologies. — Treatment of secondary or tertiary hypothyroidism does not differ essentially from that of primary hypothyroidism. Associated pituitary deficiencies require specific treatments.

Insufficient dietary iodine intake has to be supplemented for. There is no general consensus however on how to administer iodine in neonatal goiter, this therapy being anyhow seldom actually used. In some cases of dyshormonogenesis, high dosage of iodine is the only recommended treatment (cf. Table III). In all the others, treatment is thyroid hormone supplementation.

Prognosis

Congenital hypothyroidism is a serious health problem, but is the most common preventable cause of mental retardation. However, prognosis is conditioned by the adequacy of treatment and the time elapsed between the onset (in utero or post-natally) of the thyroid deficiency and the beginning of hormonal therapy. Based on clinical observations it has been perceived for a long time that hypothyroidism originating at or before birth leads to severe neurophysiological disorders and to mental retardation, while hypothyroidism starting in late infancy had less long-term consequences. Retrospective clinical studies [119] have suggested that starting treatment before the 3rd month of life will improve the prognosis. Doubts as to the existence of a strict correlation between precocity and success of treatment have been expressed. Indeed, the anatomical or functional alterations of fetal hypothyroidism causing the most severe abnormalities in the mental development of the child are already present at birth, but clinical manifestations usually appear at a later time. Therefore despite considerable attention to the problem, the purely clinical diagnosis of congenital hypothyroidism is made, in the majority of cases, after the third month of life, an age at which the treatment is obviously already too late and the consequences for the psychoneurological development of the child are often severe and irreversible. On the other hand, the disease is frequent. Based on *clinical screening* the incidence of the disease is estimated at 1 patient per 6,500-9,500 newborns. In an effort to prevent the irreversible brain damage physicians have continuously striven for early diagnosis and treatment. As soon as sensitive and specific radioimmunoassays for measuring T_3 and T_4 in biological fluids became available, experimental screening programs for neonatal hypothyroidism were started [50] and successively developed. Neonatal screening has now extended to many countries and totally changed the conditions of diagnosis and treatment of congenital hypothyroidism which now is regarded as a *social problem*. Thus a discussion on the subject cannot be omitted.

Neonatal screening

The 10-year experience of neonatal screening programs has recently been summarized [D]. It is beyond the scope of this chapter to discuss its technical aspects. Suffice it to say that neonatal screening is based on the measurement of either T_4 or TSH on blood samples collected on filter paper at the time samples for phenylketonuria (PKU) screening are obtained. Both methods are efficient but present their own advantages and disadvantages. Screening based on T_4 determination (mostly used in North America) is cheaper but is hampered by a higher recall rate than does the method based on TSH determination (most widely developed in Europe). The latter test is an extremely sensitive method for detection of athyreotic patients but will not detect secondary or tertiary hypothyroidism. In contrast, the T_4 test will screen all patients with congenital TBG deficiency (1/10,000 to 14,000 births), the screening of which is not needed and requires further testing for establishing the correct diagnosis.

Neonatal screening of over 5 million newborns has provided some interesting epidemiological information: The screening *prevalence* (proportion of a defined group having a condition at one point in time) was found to be significantly higher (1/3,500-4,500) than the clinical *incidence* (proportion of a defined group developing a condition within a stated period) in the first two years of life (1/6,900). Among several possible explanations for this apparent difference, the fact has to be considered that neonatal screening will detect cases of biochemical hypothyroidism, which probably would never have led to clear clinical manifestations or are merely transient.

These transient abnormalities now recognized in the neonatal period have been classified into 4 groups according to the biochemical pattern observed and recently reviewed [49]. In fact, in only the first two is transient hypothyroid function observed:

Transient hypothyroidism. — The abnormality is characterized by low serum T_4 and high TSH concentrations. As, the infants are usually classified as having primary hypothyroidism, a definite diagnosis should be provided. The condition is referred as to "transient hypothyroidism" or "early neonatal acquired hypothyroidism" since hypothyroidism may develop during the first few days of life. This heterogenous group also includes iatrogenic transient hypothyroidism (exposure to iodine, antithyroid drugs), borderline iodine deficiency or mild thyroid hormone synthesis defects (Table VI). The prevalence varies from 1 in 40,000 to 150,000 births. Usually these infants have been treated on the same schedule as given to primary hypothyroid patients (detailed above). Treatment is stopped later on, and the return to normal thyroid function assessed by thyroid function testing.

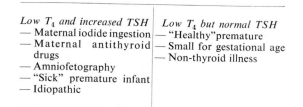

TABLE VI. — Causes
of transient hypothyroid states

Low T_4 and increased TSH	Low T_4 but normal TSH
— Maternal iodide ingestion	— "Healthy" premature
— Maternal antithyroid drugs	— Small for gestational age
— Amniofetography	— Non-thyroid illness
— "Sick" premature infant	
— Idiopathic	

Transient hypothyroxinemia. — This is characterized by low T_4 levels, low free T_4 values, normal TSH levels and normal response of both T_4 and TSH to TRH. The condition is mostly seen in premature babies and usually normalized within the first week of life (Table VI). The biological pattern ressembles hypothalamic (tertiary) hypothyroidism and is thus explained by hypothalamic immaturity. The prevalence approximates one in 6,000 births. No treatment is needed, except for a careful check of the recovering thyroid function.

Transient hyperthyrotropinemia. — A transient increase in TSH has in fact been found in many other infants in whom the TSH levels might be considerable, but T_4 is normal. Its prevalence, estimated only in Japan, would be one in 19,000 newborns. The mechanism of the disorder is not understood. In some cases it may be an artefactual problem (discussed above) in the measurement of TSH. The condition usually does not need treatment. However, the defect should be differentiated from thyroid ectopia which may also present with normal T_4 and elevated TSH levels. Thus scintiscan studies may be necessary and should be recommended.

Euthyroid sick syndrome. — This is characterized by low T_4 and low T_3 levels for gestational age but normal FT_4 and normal TSH. Found in euthyroid premature infants, the condition appears to result from a non-thyroid illness on various aspects of thyroid metabolism and is explained on the basis of a protective mechanism reducing the metabolic rate during illness. Thyroid treatment is highly controversial: advantageous for some authors, deleterious for others. It seems advisable not to recommend hormonal treatment unless hypothyroidism is really documented in these infants.

From the review of the abundant literature on this newly opened field, it would seem that many children have received hormonal treatment only on the findings of transient biochemical abnormalities. Whether in such cases treatment is unnecessary or even harmful is not really established. It is clear that clinicians now face a new situation: the biological diagnosis of hypothyroidism before any clinical manifestations. Clinical and laboratory investigations of hypothyroid infants detected by screening programs are currently attempting to correlate clinical and hormonal status. The main conclusion is that the severity of hypothyroidism and T_4/T_3 levels are correlated, athyreotic infants presenting with the lowest T_4 and the highest TSH. This reemphasizes the need for hastening the start of treatment. At present, the mean age at starting treatment is 25-30 days, a time when most infants

do not have any noticeable clinical signs of hypothyroidism.

Neonatal screening has also confirmed that primary hypothyroidism is the main cause (86-91 %) of congenital hypothyroidism: about 74 % of the affected children have primary thyroid dysgenesis, 13 % thyroid dyshormonogenesis, 3-4 % secondary-tertiary hypothyroidism and the remainder have transient hypothyroidism secondary to intrauterine goitrogen exposure in most cases [50].

It already seems that mental development is improved in the early treated infants. However, the follow up studies have not yet been carried for a period of time long enough to draw definitive conclusions.

INFANTS OF HYPOTHYROID MOTHERS

With adequate and early treatment there will be complete catch up of growth and physical development. The onset of puberty might be either advanced or delayed in few inadequately treated patients [34] but is usually normal. In *primary hypothyroidism* pubertal development usually proceeds normally even though somewhat slowly [34] and fertility is the normal outcome. Because of the autonomy of its thyroid function in utero (see above) the fœtus of an hypothyroid mother does not have thyroid problems unless an inherited disease is the cause of hypothyroidism in the mother (dyshormonogenesis).

An exception is in the children born to a hypothyroid mother with Hashimoto's disease *(acquired autoimmune thyroiditis)* who possesses TSH-binding-inhibitor immunoglobulins (TSIs). These antibodies can pass through the placenta and render the fetal thyroid unresponsive to TSH stimulation [96], thus causing fetal as well as neonatal hypothyroidism. At birth, the neonates have a clear clinical and biological pattern of hypothyroidism. However, the impairment of thyroid function appears reversible, as gradual disappearance of the antibodies over 6-15 months of age is accompanied by a gradual return to normal and persisting euthyroid function, with normal physical and mental development after discontinuing thyroid hormone therapy [96].

In iodine deficiency areas fertility is not a problem. The child is expected to suffer from iodine deficiency as well as his mother. However, for obvious individual susceptibility and environmental factors, most subjects with obvious thyromegaly do not suffer from overt hypothyroidism (only 10-20 %). There is also no close relation between maternal thyroid hypofunction and the risk for the child to develop hypothyroidism before or after birth. The major risk is neonatal goiter (see below). In the areas (Latin America and South Pacific) where endemic cretinism is expressed rather as a neurological defect (neurological form) than as thyroid deficiency, the newborns almost never show hypothyroidism at birth.

In the other secondary or tertiary forms there is most always an association of TSH deficiency and other pituitary hormone deficiency. Fertility in the mother depends on specific treatment.

In the older literature, and more recently in endemic cretinism areas, a high frequency of spontaneous abortions and a significantly higher rate of malformations of all kinds in the children born to hypothyroid mothers have been reported. To our knowledge this aspect has not been studied in the light of modern physiopathological concepts. It is possible that these deleterious outcomes might rather be associated with fertility problems, or result from specific teratogenic effects of iodide deprivation per se than be the consequence of maternal thyroid hypofunction (with or without hormonal treatment).

NEONATAL GOITERS

Neonatal goiters are rare but not exceptional, and are always *serious* or life-threatening disorders. This clinical situation is peculiar because its seriousness does not depend on the underlying cause, nor on its association with hypothyroidism or not, but depends on the specific anatomical extent of an hypertrophied thyroid gland in the newborn.

Pathogenesis. Etiology

Hypertrophy of the gland results from numerous causes which are listed in Table VII. They all have in common an hyperstimulation of the thyroid gland by either fetal TSH or by maternal TSH-like antibodies. In the first instance and whatever the cause, fetal or neonatal thyroid hormone biosynthesis is blocked and thus hypothyroidism is present. This is the most frequent situation. In contrast, the transplacental passage of maternal antibodies overstimulating a normally secreting fetal thyroid gland results in a state of hyperthyroidism. In exceptional cases, there is no thyroid dysfunction (idiopathic) and the cause of the goiter is unclear, Intratracheal thyroid goiter might be one of those. It likely results from a dysmorphogenetic process:

either the thyroid tissue is entrapped within the developing trachea or invades the trachea.

The most frequent cause is *iatrogenic*: maternal ingestion of iodine containing drugs. Often the medication appears so trivial (expectorants) that it is not reported on questioning. A more recently recognized cause of neonatal iodine intoxication is the cutaneous use of iodine alcohol or iodine containing disinfectants. As a result of the infant's skin well known permeability a massive cutaneous iodine absorption leads to overloading of the thyroid, and by the Wolff-Chaikoff effect stimulates TSH secretion (see above). There is however some unexplained pathogenic process, that is the relatively small number of infants who have suffered from serious iodine intoxication, compared with the large number of those who have been exposed to this routine, apparently harmless practice. Individual susceptibility is likely involved. It is also possible that in more babies than generally thought the use of iodine disinfectants has led to unrecognized, slight, transient thyroid disorders. It is thus recommended to avoid any post-natal use of iodine-containing disinfectants in neonates, particularly in prematures, and, when necessary, to use such antiseptics with great caution during the neonatal period.

TABLE VII. — ETIOLOGY OF GOITER IN NEONATES

A. *Associated with hypothyroidism*

1. *Accidental iodine overdose:* by far the most frequent cause; complete remission is usual
   — maternal ingestion of iodine containing drugs during pregnancy
   — neonatal intoxication, most frequently by cutaneous absorption of iodine (skin disinfectant)

2. *Iodine deficiency during fetal life of maternal origin*
   — deficient maternal dietary intake: in iodine deficient, goitrous endemic areas
   — maternal misuse of drugs (lithium, cobalt, PAS, sulfonamides, sulfones) or abuse of thiocyanate containing food (crucifera, soybean)

3. *Dyshormonogenesis* (hereditary)

4. *Graves' disease in the mother*
   — treated with iodine (same mechanism as in 1)
   — treated with antithyroid agents (transplacental or milk transfer)

B. *Associated with hyperthyroidism*

5. *Graves' disease in the mother:* untreated or counted as cured (transplacental transfer of TSH-stimulating immunoglobulins)

6. *True Graves' disease of neonatal onset*

Apart from iatrogenic causes, and unless the mother is hyperthyroid herself and has been treated with either iodine or antithyroid drugs (see below), the presence of a goiter in a newborn is diagnostic of fetal thyroid dysfunction (Table VII) which has been discussed above.

Clinical findings and diagnosis

The prevalent feature is an acute respiratory, or cardio-respiratory distress, occuring in the first few hours or days of life. Sometimes the baby is born apparently dead necessitating prolonged neonatal resuscitation. If the cause is not recognized promptly, the respiratory distress does not respond to the usual treatment and its rapid aggravation may appear unexplained. Severe attacks of apnea, cyanosis, swallowing difficulties, episodes of suffocation and cardiomegaly are observed.

The volume of the goiter is variable: it may be enormous, developed prenatally, extending into the neck and head posteriorily, a cause of dystocia by presentation of the face at delivery. It may be large, and/or develop rapidly within a week in cases of postnatal iodine exposure. It presents then, as a mass around the neck and calls for attention. Unfortunately it may also be unnoticed at first because of the shortness of the newborn's neck or because of the baby's dorsal position (Fig. VI-30).

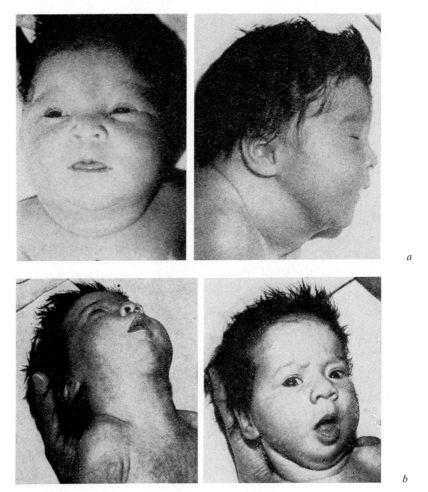

a

b

FIG. VI-30. — *Clinical aspects of neonatal goiters.*

(*a*) Neonatal goiter with overt signs of hypothyroidism before one week of age (from JOB et al., Ref. with permission).
(*b*) Persisting features after a month of thyroid hormone treatment: note the anxious look, the somewhat gross features but no signs of hypothyroidism, the goiter encircling the neck laterally and the difficulty to notice (but not to palpate) the goiter when the head is in hyperextension (Reproduced from GIORNO et al., *La Médecine infantile*, 1979, *86*, p. 1116, with permission).

In practice, the clinical difficulty is to promptly relate the respiratory problems to the presence of a goiter. In the newborn the hypertrophied thyroid gland does not project as anteriorily as in children or adults. Hypertrophy of the gland mainly proceeds in the posterior lobes, encircling and compressing the trachea. Myxœdematous infiltration of the tracheal walls may also contribute to further reducing the lumen of the trachea. Signs of hypothyroidism may be present (pallor, abdominal distension, œdema, hypoactivity, retarded bone maturation). They may be either evident, rather modest and recognized retrospectively, or totally absent.

When a neck mass in found, the second step is to recognize its thyroid nature. The first examination to perform is a lateral X-ray of the neck [79]. It is usually diagnostic, showing a pretracheal mass, surrounding the trachea and a narrowed lumen. Tracheomalacia may be associated. These findings usually make unnecessary the practice of other anatomical tests such as echotomography or scintiscan. The latter may however be useful when the goiter is modest and the clinical symptoms less severe.

Recognition of the thyroid nature of the neck mass is sufficient to eliminate other causes of respiratory distress or cervical tumors (lymphangioma, teratoma, lymph nodes, cervical duplication of the œsophagus...). Although rare, congenital neoplasms of the thyroid have however been described including Hürthle cell tumors as well as adenocarcinomas. A teratoma may be suspected when calcification in the cervical region is found. Diagnosis is confirmed at biopsy.

When hypothyroidism is associated with the goiter, it is necessary to evaluate the baby's thyroid function, as discussed above. In all instances, maternal history should be documented: thyroid disease, treatment. Adsorption of iodine containing drugs is often difficult to document because, as mentioned above, it is a long-life "minor habit". Iodine intoxication is best proven by determination of iodinemia or iodinuria in both mother and child which will be found to be well above the normal range, and progressively decrease in the newborn. The less frequent cases in which the mother has a history of Graves' disease will be discussed below.

Treatment and evolution

In the case of respiratory distress, treatment is an *emergency*. It consists of the administration of thyroid hormones *intra-muscularly*, for more rapid action and because of the secretion-swallowing difficulties. There is no standard treatment. Some

have used IM T_4 (DL) at a total dose of 0.5 mg/day or 1 mg/m^2/day, or T_3 (3 µg/kg), for a few days, then conventional oral therapy [23, 79]. Intubation and mechanical ventilation may be necessary. The response to hormonal treatment is usually rapid and the goiter's volume decreases. However dyspnea and tracheal congestion may persist for several weeks, while it takes the thyroid gland several months to return slowly to a normal size (Fig. VI-30). Fœtuses or neonates exposed to iodine intoxication will not all present with such a dramatic scene, but all have a goiter, and evidence of hypothyroid function (low T_4, high TSH). The severity of thyroid dysfunction is usually correlated to the degree of prematurity.

When there is no respiratory distress, treatment may not be necessary. In few weeks or months, thyroid function will resume. Thyroid hormonal treatment may be indicated (conventional regimen) when biological signs of hypothyroidism persist at repeated testing.

Duration of treatment depends on the cause: usually 6-12 months in those infants exposed to iodine intoxication or maternal transfer of antithyroid agents, but it is for life in primary hypothyroidism. Management of hyperthyroidism, when present, is discussed below.

Prognosis

Is firstly conditioned by the gravity and result of the respiratory distress's consequences. Dystocia, tragic deliveries, repetitive anoxic episodes are responsible for brain damage even in the absence of hypothyroidism.

In the most common cases, iodide intoxication or maternal antithyroid agents, hypothyroidism is transient and thyroid function usually recovers fully within some months. In the other cases, long-term prognosis is related to the cause; primary fetal hypothyroidism, discussed above, or neonatal hyperthyroidism discussed below.

NEONATAL HYPERTHYROIDISM

This is a serious and potential life-threatening condition. Congenital hyperthyroidism should be considered in the newborn of any mother with a history of treated or active Graves' disease. It is a rare disorder occuring in one of 70 infants born to thyrotoxic mothers, with increasing frequency when the mother is treated during pregnancy. Maternal thyroid autoimmune disease is however not always associated. The incidence is strikingly the same in males and females as opposed to that seen later in life when the sex ratio of females to males ranges from 3 : 1 to 4 : 1 in childhood and is 7 : 1 by the adult years. Familial incidence has been noted from the earliest description of the disease (see review in [69 *bis*]).

Etiology and pathogenesis

Congenital Graves' disease represent a heterogeneous population with different pathogenic mechanisms and probably a superimposed spectrum of disease with a similar cause. A transient self-limited variety of neonatal thyrotoxicosis may occur in infants of mothers who are receiving iodine or antithyroid drugs during pregnancy. Both goitrogenic compounds cross the placenta, thus inducing excessive secretion of TSH by the fetal pituitary gland which in turn leads to development of a fetal goiter (see above). At birth, with removal of the effects of the drugs the infant's hyperplastic thyroid gland is stimulated by a transient persistance of increased TSH secretion. The large quantities of T_4 thus released into the circulation and the postnatal "turn-on" of T_4 to T_3 peripheral conversion are responsible for a brief period of thyrotoxic symptoms seen in some newborns. The onset is usually delayed a few days but there is no explanation for the delayed appearance of goiter seen in some cases, nor of the occasional occurence of such complications in infants born to treated mothers with Graves' disease.

It is currently accepted that Graves' disease is a thyroid autoimmune disease, secondary to the production of thyroid stimulating immunoglobulins (TSI) of the IgG class which are antibodies to the TSH receptor and possess the capacity of stimulating the thyroid cells [158]. As a consequence of sustained thyroid stimulation thyroid hormones are produced in excessive amounts and pituitary secretion of TSH is suppressed. The same mechanism is believed to be at play in most infants with neonatal hypertoxicosis with the difference that the autoantibodies are not produced by the infant but transmitted transplacentally from the mother to the foetus, as suggested by the tendency for the disease to occur in infants born to women with high TSI levels, the equal male and female incidence, and the transient nature of the disease in many cases. Such an hypothesis does not however explain either the 4 to 6 months duration of the disease nor its recurrence or persistance for several years. Inherent thyroid hypersensitivity to TSI or inherent thyroid hyperactivity unrelated to TSI have been suggested to explain the first situation [D, E]. As an explanation for the second situation it has been proposed that TSI serves as an immunological marker or inciting agent in a genetically preselected population of infants who will ultimately develop true Graves' disease [69 *bis*].

Clinical findings

Typical signs may be classified into three groups each of them being potentially the prominent clinical feature:

— *Signs of thyrotoxicosis:* high incidence of congenital anomalies, premature birth, intrauterine growth retardation, failure to thrive, vomiting, diarrhea, exophtalmos, hyperactivity, hyperirritability, tremor, excessive perspiration and sometimes hyperthermia.

— *A goiter* of variable size is present in at least half of the cases [69] but thyroid size is seldom large enough to lead to respiratory distress and all the findings described above.

— *Signs of sympathetic hyperstimulation,* among which marked *tachycardia,* is the prominent one (sometimes over 200 beats/minute) with cardiovascular failure (polypnea, cardiomegaly, hepatosplenomegaly).

Bone age is often advanced, synostosis at birth and frontal bossing are less frequent but highly suspicious of the disease. Increased size of the thymus, spleen, and lymph nodes may be readily seen.

However, the diagnosis is often *difficult* in the first few days of life. No single sign nor symptom is diagnostic and neither exophtalmos or thyromegaly need be present. Moreover, the onset of clinical symptoms may be delayed for 7-10 days for reasons which are not yet understood.

As neonatal thyrotoxicosis should be suspected in any infant born to a mother with a history of treated or active Graves' disease, careful and repeated clinical examination will usually reveal the progression of the signs of thyrotoxicosis (Fig. VI-31) tachycardia, exophtalmos, irritability, ravenous appetite with excessive weight loss.

Laboratory findings

When neonatal thyrotoxicosis is suspected to occur in a newborn the first hormonal investigations should be made on the cord blood. Elevated serum

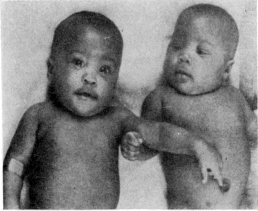

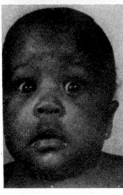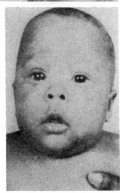

FIG. VI-31. — *Congenital Graves disease in one of a pair of monozygotic female twins pictured at birth (top pannel) and at 5 months of age (bottom)*. The mother affected with Graves disease received 150-300 mg of PTU daily throughout pregnancy. Both twins had elevated TSH levels but only one (on the left side) developed clinical and laboratory signs of hyperthyroidism, the other being euthyroid. Note in the affected baby the prominent and staring eyes (tachycardia and hyperactivity were also present). Clinical signs were more pronounced at 5 months of age (Reproduced from HOLLINGWORTH et al., Ref. [69], with permission).

levels of total and free T_4 and T_3 with low or unmeasurable TSH levels are sufficient proof and treatment should follow. Thyroid hormones and TSH may however be low normal or elevated depending upon the cause and the degree of in utero thyroid suppression (maternal treatment) or stimulation (maternal stimulating IgG) and be non informative during the first few days of life. Repeated hormone studies are required showing the progressive rise in serum T_3 to thyrotoxic levels, with or without a progressive rise in T_4, and no TSH response to TRH stimulation.

Scintiscan studies are not necessary. In early life, thyroid radioactive iodine uptake will not differentiate thyrotoxic from normal infants since thyroid uptake is normally very high ($\geqslant 90$ %) in this period.

A search for circulating antibodies in both mother and child will only be of retrospective help to establish an etiological diagnosis since the results take 1 to 2 weeks. Several types of antibodies may be found: *microsomal antithyroid antibodies* are found in all newborn populations, normal, hypothyroid and hyperthyroid, with about the same frequency ($\leqslant 15$ %). Transferred from the mother through the placenta, they do not give any valuable information in the neonatal period.

The various names given to the TSIs are related to the methods, used to show a biological or biochemical property similar to that of TSH (binding to thyroid cell membranes or functional response of thyroid cells) rather than to identify any one of the different molecules which constitute the heterogenous group of thyroid antibodies. There are at least 7 different assays for measuring thyroid stimulating immunoglobulins, but only four have been applied to understanding the problem of neonatal hyperthyroidism:

(*a*) LATS *(long acting thyroid stimulator)* is measured by a technique involving in vivo stimulation of the thyroid of the mouse; (*b*) LATS-P *(long acting stimulating protector)* primarily reflects binding to a component of a homogenate of human thyroid preventing ("protecting") the subsequent binding of LATS; (*c*) The assay of TSI is essentially a receptor-binding procedure; (*d*) The term TSAb *(thyroid-stimulating antibody)* is used when the capacity of stimulating human thyroid slices in vitro is measured as an increase in the concentration of cyclic AMP [94 *bis*].

All tests are not always positive in the same patient. Estimation of LATS (the most commonly used) in both mother and child is not always positive and LATS titers are not well correlated with thyrotoxic intensity or incidence. Some LATS-positive mothers have been observed to have euthyroid infants and inversely some normal euthyroid mothers may give birth to infants with neonatal Graves' disease. False positive results with LATS-P and TSI are possible, and not all high concentrations of TSAb will necessarily correlate with a positive LATS. It seems, however, that high concentrations of TSAb are required both to produce the neonatal syndrome and to give a positive LATS assay. Therefore the association of positive LATS with neonatal hyperthyroidism results in early recognition of the disease [94 *bis*].

Treatment

Delay in clinical symptoms during the first week of life and the rapid evolution of thyrotoxicosis thereafter complicate the treatment which must be rapid and vigourous. It includes the association of antithyroid agents and iodine, sedatives, and digitilization.

Among the antithyroid drugs of the thionamide class, propyl-thiouracil (PTU) is preferable to methimazole (1-2 mg/kg/day) because it inhibits the peripheral conversion of T_4 to T_3 in addition to inhibiting the synthesis of thyroid hormones [B]. It should be administered in doses of 5 to 10 mg/kg/day in three 8-hourly divided doses. In such countries as France, where PTU is no longer available, carbimazole (5-10 mg/day) or benzylthiouracil (5-10 mg/kg/day) are the most frequently used antithyroids.

Iodine, which until 1945 was the major chemotherapeutic agent for thyrotoxicosis, is still used in combination with the antithyroid drug because it potentiates its inhibition of the thyroid gland and in addition virtually immediately blocks the release of thyroid hormones. Concentrated iodine solution (126 mg/ml), Lugol's solution containing a mixture of 5 % iodine and 10 % potassium iodine, is given in doses of 8 mg iodine every eight hours (1 drop). If a therapeutic response is not observed within 24-48 hours the dose of both drugs can be increased by 50-100 %.

Glucocorticoids may be useful in severe cases, as these compounds acutely inhibit thyroid hormone secretion. The normal 2 mg/kg/day dose of Prednisone seems appropriate, although the minimal effective dose has not been established.

Propanolol hydrochloride is useful in controlling sympathetic overstimulation, and is used to bring the cardiac rate into a range appropriate for age and to combat high output failure. The recommended dose is 2 mg/kg/day in 3 divided doses.

In cases of cardiac failure *digitalization* may be used according to conventional regimens. Treatment should not include both digitalis and propanolol. If the latter is chosen, digitalis should be discontinued. One must also be aware of the possibility of coexistent congenital heart disease as the explanation for cardiac failure which is refractory to treatment. Voluminous goiter and tracheal obstruction may necessitate intubation and mechanical ventilation. Adequate nutrition is also important with supply of sufficient calories and free water to meet the demands of an increased metabolic rate.

There are no clear guidelines as to how long one needs to continue treatment of neonatal hyperthyroidism. Iodine administration as well as propanolol or digitalis, is usually discontinued as soon as toxic symptoms are under control. Sedation with reserpine may temporarily be advisable as adjunct therapy. It is extremely important for the antithyroid treatment to be adjusted so as to keep the T_4 levels within the normal range because iatrogenic hypothyroidism should be avoided. The need for frequent reevaluation of the hormonal status is thus apparent.

The half-life disappearance of the maternally transferred immunoglobulins is about two weeks and a 16 fold decrease in TSI levels would be expected by 8 weeks of age. Determination of TSI levels is however not a useful criteria for discontinuing the treatment since there is no correlation between the infant's levels of TSI and the evaluation of its thyroid problem. Therefore treatment is best stopped when both clinical euthyroidism is obtained and thyroid function returned to normal (T_3, T_4, TSH levels and TSH response to TRH).

Preventive treatment of neonatal hyperthyroidism is extremely difficult (see below). It is best achieved by advising against a new pregnancy in women with Graves' disease.

Evolution and prognosis

Neonatal hyperthyroidism is a serious disease with a high rate of mortality in utero or postnatally and significant morbidity. The first few days of life are a critical period during which death may result from tracheal compression and asphyxia, congestive cardiac failure, idiopathic thrombocytopenic purpura or infections (about 20 % of the cases). The course of the disease is variable and unpredictable. The disease may be a transient disorder or it may be a persistant disease as it is in later life. Indeed if in many instances (30 %) the symptoms are transient and subside within 1 to 3 months [B] in parallel with the levels and duration of TSI activity, the disease lasts more than six months in 15-25 % of the patients and in about 1/4 of the cases clinical manifestations may for persist several months or be recurrent over several years [69 *bis*]. In such instances the diagnosis of true Graves' disease with neonatal onset is likely.

The most serious complication is premature craniostenosis that may result in inadequate cerebral development; hyperactivity, growth retardation, irreversible perceptual motor problems and mild mental retardation even in the absence of premature craniostenosis are believed to be long term sequelae of neonatal thyrotoxicosis [69 *bis*].

INFANT OF THE HYPERTHYROID MOTHER

Maternal hyperthyroidism is present in about 1 in 2,000 pregnancies. Fertility rate is low in hyperthyroid mothers. The greatest threat to the foetus is maternal hyperthyroidism per se which results in increased frequencies of abortion and premature birth. Having a mother with Graves' disease is a difficult situation for a surviving foetus: she will be the source of problems and offer no help. Indeed, whatever the state of the mother's illness, the foetus is at risk of having either hypothyroidism or hyperthyroidism. In the case where the mother has active Graves' disease, all forms of treatment that she is receiving are potentially harmful for the foetus: iodine, radioactive iodine or antithyroid drugs cross the placenta (destroying or blocking the fetal thyroid gland) but maternal thyroid hormones do not. Antithyroid drugs are nowadays the only treatment used for treating the mother. Large doses of propylthiouracil (PTU) given to the mother, whether she remains hyperthyroid or is euthyroid, will result in overt fetal hypothyroidism, neonatal goiter with the tragic consequences discussed above. The underlying thyroid problem is however short-lived, the child's thyroid gland recovers its function within a few days to 2 weeks of life. The question whether a transient, usually mild, reduction of fetal serum T_4 levels, is of any long-term consequence to the infant is not completely answered. But there is no clinical evidence that "minimal brain dysfunction" is implicated. The blockage of foetal function is proportional to the dose of PTU that the mother is taking, although there are again marked individual susceptibilities [123]. At all events one should try to reduce to the minimum the dose of PTU that the mother is taking. Mild maternal hyperthyroidism would be of no consequence for the foetus.

Propanolol treatment of a mother with active Graves' disease is also a factor aggravating fetal and placental malnutrition through enhancement of uterine smooth muscle tone and by contributing to neurological depression, bradycardia and hypoglycemia at birth.

Regardless of the state or the course of the Graves' disease, even in an apparently cured situation, there may be a variety of antibodies still produced by the mother, which all cross the placental barrier. High maternal levels of serum long-acting thyroid stimulator (TSI) will invariably produce fetal hyperthyroidism [169]. Measurement of TSI or LATS is becoming a practice in late pregnancy of mothers

with Graves' disease in order to estimate the risk for the child and to insure close neonatal observation. It has been proposed that if high levels of TSI are present, the mother should be given a small dose of PTU in order to treat the foetus [123]. However the dose and/or effectiveness of PTU that the fetus will receive is unpredictable and the risk for the fetus to develop hyperthyroidism cannot be estimated. Twins exposed to the same intrauterine environment may respond differently to TSI (Fig. VI-31) or PTU [123], suggesting genetic predispositions to autoimmune disorders with clinical expression requiring an additional triggering event [69 *bis*]. It would thus appear that the risk of overtreating many normal fetuses is greater than that of preventing hyperthyroidism in a few others.

There is an additional risk for a child born to an euthyroid apparently cured mother with Graves' disease: a susceptibility to Graves' disease inherited in a autosomal dominant manner [69 *bis*]. Despite accumulating evidence (family studies, strong association with HLA-RD W 3) that Graves' disease is a genetic disorder, the mechanism of action of possible disease susceptibility genes is totally unknown. Nevertheless, the last, but not the least risk for the child is to develop true Graves' disease in the neonatal period or later in life.

REFERENCES

I. *General reading.*

[A] BERTRAND (J.), RAPPAPORT (R.), SIZONENKO (P. C.). — *Endocrinologie pédiatrique : physiologie, physiopathologie, clinique.* Payot, Lausanne, 1981.
[B] FISHER (D. A.), BURROW (G. N.). — *Perinatal thyroid physiology and disease.* Raven Press, New York, 1975.
[C] LEE (P. A.), PLOTNICK (L. P.), KOWARSKI (A. A.), MIGEON (C. J.). — *Congenital adrenal hyperplasia : a quarter of century later.* University Park Press, Baltimore, 1977.
[D] BURROW (G. N.), DUSSAULT (J. H.). — *Neonatal thyroid screening.* Raven Press, New York, 1980.
[E] NEW (M. I.), FISER (R. H. Jr.). — *Diabetes and other endocrine disorders during pregnancy and in the newborn.* ALAN (R.), Liss Inc., New York, 1976.

II. *Thyroid.*

[1] ABBASSI (V.), MERCHANT (K.), ABRAMSON (D.). — Postnatal triiodothyronine concentrations in healthy preterm infants and in infants with respiratory distress syndrome. *Ped. Res., 11,* 802-804, 1977.
[2] ABOUL-KHAIN (S. A.), BUCHANAN (T. J.), CROOKS (J.), TURNBULL (A. C.). — Structural and functional development of the human fetal thyroid. *Clin. Sci. Mol. Med., 31,* 915, 1966.

[3] ABUID (J.), STINSON (D. A.), LARSEN (P. R.). — Serum triiodothyronine and thyroxine in the neonate and acute increases in these hormones following delivery. *J. Clin. Invest.*, *52*, 1105-1119, 1973.

[4] ANDERSON (H.), VON BÜLLOW (F. A.), HØLLGARD (K.). — The histochemical and ultrastructural basis of the cellular function of the human fetal adenohypophysis. *Prog. Histochem. Cytochem.*, *1*, 153-184, 1970.

[5] BAKER (B. L.), JAFFE (R. B.). — The genesis of cell types in the adenohypophysis of the human fetus as observed by immunocytochemistry. *Am. J. Anat.*, *143*, 137-162, 1975.

[6] BAUMAN (R. A.), BODE (H. H.)., HAYEK (A.), CRAWFORD (J. D.). — Technetium 99 m pertechnetate scans in congenital hypothyroidism. *J. Pediatr.*, *89*, 269-271, 1976.

[7] BECKWITH (J. B.). — Macroglossia, omphalocele, adrenal cytomegaly, gigantism and hyperplastic micromegaly. *Birth Defects*, *5*, 188-196, 1969.

[8] BERGLAND (R. M.), PAGE (R. B.). — Pituitary-brain vascular relations: a new paradigm. *Science*, *204*, 18-24, 1979.

[9] BERGLAND (R. M.), PAGE (R. B.). — Can the pituitary secrete directly to the brain? (Affirmative anatomical evidence). *Endocrinology*, *102*, 1325-1338, 1978.

[10] BERNAL (J.), REFETOFF (S.). — The action of thyroid hormone. *Clin. Endocrinol.*, *6*, 227-249, 1977.

[11] BERNAL (J.), REFETOFF (S.), DEGROOT (L. J.). — Abnormalities of triiodothyronine binding to lymphocyte and fibroblast nuclei from a patient with peripheral tissue resistance to thyroid hormone action. *J. Clin. Endocrinol. Metab.*, *47*, 1266-1272, 1978.

[12] BERNARD (B.), ODDIE (T. H.), FISCHER (D. A.). — Correlation between gestational age, weight, or ponderosity and serum thyroxine concentration at birth. *J. Pediatr.*, *91*, 199-203, 1977.

[13] BERTRAND (J.). — Intérêt de l'étude de la dégradation de l'hydrocortisone dans le myxœdème de l'enfant. *Arch. Fr. Ped.*, *16*, 1-9, 1959.

[14] BLIZZARD (R. M.), CHANDLER (R. W.), LANDING (B. H.), PELTIT (M. O.), WEST (C. D.). — Maternal autoimmunization as a probable cause of athyreotic cretinism. *N. Engl. J. Med.*, *263*, 327-336, 1960.

[15] BREWER (D. B.). — Congenital absence of the pituitary gland and its consequences. *J. Pathol. Bacteriol.*, *73*, 59-67, 1956.

[16] BROWN (A. L.), FERNHOFF (P. M.), MILNER (J.), McEWEN (C.), ELSAS (L. S.). — Racial differences in the incidence of congenital hypothyroidism. *J. Pediatr.*, *99*, 934-936, 1981.

[17] BURROW (G. N.). — Neonatal goiter after maternal propylthiouracil therapy. *J. Clin. Endocrinol. Metab.*, *25*, 1103-1108, 1965.

[18] CABEN (L. A.), FERMAGLICH (D. R.), CRIGLER (J. F.). — Congenital hypothyroidism and congenital adreno-cortical hyperplasia in an infant: Diagnostic and metabolic implications. *J. Pediatr.*, *90*, 77-79, 1977.

[19] CAMPBELL (W. A.), PRICE (W. H.). — Congenital hypothyroidism in Klinefelter's syndrome. *J. Med. Genet.*, *16*, 439-442, 1979.

[20] CARR (E. A.), BEIERWALTES (W. H.), NEEL (J. V.), DAVIDSON (R.), LOWREY (G. H.), DODSON (V. N.), TAUTON (J. H.). — The various types of thyroid

malfunction in cretinism and their relative frequency. *Pediatrics*, *28*, 1-6, 1961.

[21] CASTAING (H.), FOURNET (J. P.), LÉGER (F. A.), KIESGEN (F.), PIELTE (C.), DUPART (M. C.), SAVOIE (J. C.). — Thyroid of the newborn and postnatal iodine overload. *Arch. Fr. Péd.*, *36*, 356-368, 1979.

[22] CAVALLO (L.), MARGIOTTA (W.), KERNKAMP (C.), PUGLIESE (G.). — Serum levels of thyrotropin, thyroxine 3,3′,5-triiodothyronine and 3,3′5′,-triiodothyronine (reverse T$_3$) in the first six days of life. *Acta Paediat. Scand.*, *69*, 43-47, 1980.

[23] CHABROLLE (J. P.), ROSSIER (A.). — Goiter and hypothyroidism in the newborn after cutaneous absorption of iodine. *Arch. Dis. Childh.*, *53*, 495-498, 1978.

[24] CHAN (A. M.), LYNCH (M. J. G.), BAILEY (J. D.), EZRIN (C.), FRASER (D.). — Hypothyroidism in cystinosis. *Am. J. Med.*, *48*, 678-692, 1970.

[25] CHERON (R. G.), KAPLAN (M. M.), LARSEN (P. R.), SELENKOW (H. A.), CRIGLER (J. F. Jr.). — Neonatal thyroid function after propylthiouracil therapy for maternal Graves' disease. *N. Engl. J. Med.*, *304*, 525-528, 1981.

[26] CHOPRA (I. S.), CRANDALL, (B. F.). — Thyroid hormones and thyrotropin in amniotic fluid. *N. Engl. J. Med.*, *293*, 740-743, 1975.

[27] CHOPRA (I. J.), SOLOMON (D. H.), CHOPRA (U.), WU (S. Y.), FISHER (D. A.), NAKAMURA (Y.). — Pathways of metabolism thyroid hormones. *Rec. Prog. Horm. Res.*, *34*, 521-567, 1978.

[28] CODACCIONI (J. L.), CARAYON (P.), MICHAEL-BECHET (M.), FOUCAULT (F.), LEFORT (G.), PIERRON (H.). — Congenital hypothyroidism associated with thyrotropin unresponsiveness and thyroid cell membrane alterations. *J. Clin. Endocrinol. Metab.*, *50*, 932-937, 1980.

[29] COLLU (R.), LEBŒUF (G.), LETARTE (J.), DUCHARME (J. R.). — Increase in plasma growth hormone levels following thyrotropin-releasing hormone injection in children with primary hypothyroidism. *J. Clin. Endocrinol. Metab.*, *44*, 743-747, 1977.

[30] Committee on Drugs, Treatment of congenital hypothyroidism. *Pediatrics*, *62*, 413-417, 1978.

[31] CUESTAS (R. A.). — Thyroid function in healthy premature infants. *J. Pediatr.*, *92*, 963-967, 1978.

[32] CZERNICHOW (P.), CACHIN (O.), RAPPAPORT (R.), FLAMANT (F.), SARRAZIN (D.), SCHWEISGUTH (O.). — Séquelles endocriniennes des irradiations de la tête et du cou pour tumeurs extra-crâniennes. *Arch. Fr. Péd.*, *34*, 104-114, 1977.

[33] DALLOT (C.), LABRUNE (B.), COURPOTIN (C.), LÉGER (A.), GRENET (P.). — Hypothyroïdie par trouble congénital de la captation des iodures. *Arch. Fr. Péd.*, *37*, 597-601, 1980.

[34] DAVID (M.), AUGAY (C.), SEMPÉ (M.), PAVIA (C.), BIRON (A.), JEUNE (M.). — Description de la puberté dans les hypothyroïdies congénitales; à propos de 95 observations. *Pédiatrie*, *34*, 403-417, 1979.

[35] DAVID (M.), FLORET (D.), GHALI (I.), CLAUSTRAT (B.), BIRON (A.), DAVID (L.). — Le test au TRF (thyrotropin releasing factor) dans les insuffisances antéhypophysaires chez l'enfant. *Pédiatrie*, *33*, 163-172, 1978.

[36] DAVID (M.), HAOUR (F.), SCHEDEWIE (H.). — Hormone de croissance et hypothyroïdie chez l'enfant. Influence du traitement sur la réponse à la stimulation. *Ann. Pédiat.*, *17*, 100-110, 1970.

[37] DAVID (M.), MADJAR (J. J.), FLORET (D.), SANN (L.), TERRIER (M.), JEUNE (M.). — Ostéodystrophie d'Albright type II et hypothyroïdie par déficit en TSH. *Arch. Fr. Péd.*, 34, 108-129, 1977.

[38] DEGROOT (L. J.), NIEPOMNISCZE (H.). — Biosynthesis of thyroid hormones: basic and clinical aspects. *Metabolism*, 26, 665-718, 1977.

[39] DELANGE (F.), ERMANS (A. M.). — Endemic goiterandcretinism. Naturally occurring goitrigens. *Pharmac. Ther.*, C 1, 57, 1976.

[40] DELANGE (F.), ILLIG (R.), ROCHICCIOLI (P.), BROCK-JACOBSEN (B.). — Progress-report 1980 in neonatal thyroid screening in Europe. *Acta Paediat. Scand.*, 70, 1-2, 1981.

[41] DELANGE (F.), VIGNERI (R.), TRIMARCHI (F.), FILETTI (S.), PEZZINO (V.), SQUATRITO (S.), BOURDOUX (P.), ERMANS (A. M.). — Etiological factors of endemic goiters in North-eastern Sicily. *J. Endocrinol. Invest.*, 2, 137-142, 1978.

[42] D'ESPINASSE (P. G.). — The development of the hypophysial portal system in man. *J. Anat.*, 68, 11-18, 1933.

[43] DOBBING (J.), SANDS (J.). — Quantitative growth and development of human brain. *Arch. Dis. Childh.*, 48, 757-767, 1973.

[44] DUSSAULT (J. H.), LETARTE (J.), GUYDA (H.), LABERGE (C.). — Lack of influence of thyroid antibodies on thyroid function in the newborn infant and on a mass screening program for congenital hypothyroidism. *J. Pediatr.*, 96, 385-389, 1980.

[45] ERENBERG (A.), PHELPS (D. L.), LAM (R.), FISHER (D. A.). — Total and free thyroid hormone concentrations in the neonatal period. *Pediatrics*, 53, 211-216, 1974.

[46] ERLICH (R. M.). — Ectopic and hypoplastic pituitary with adrenal hypoplasma; case report. *J. Pediatr.*, 57, 377-384, 1957.

[47] EXSS (R.), GRAEWE (B.). — Congenital athyroidism in the newborn infant from intrauterine radioiodine action. *Biol. Neonate*, 24, 289-291, 1974.

[48] FISHER (D. A.), DUSSAULT (J. M.). — Development of the mammalian thyroid gland. In: *Handbook of Physiology*, Section 7, GREER (M. A.) and SOLOMON (D. M.) (Eds.). American Physiological Society, Washington, DC, vol. 3, 21-38, 1974.

[49] FISHER (D. A.), KLEIN (A. H.). — Thyroid development and disorders of thyroid function in the newborn. *N. Engl. J. Med.*, 304, 702-712, 1981.

[50] FISHER (D. A.), DUSSAULT (J. H.), FOLEY (T. P.), KLEIN (A. H.), LAFRANCHI (S.), LARSEN (P. R.), MITCHELL (M. L.), MURPHEY (W. H.), WALFISH (P. G.). — Screening for congenital hypothyroidism. Results of screening 1,000,000 North American infants. *J. Pediatr.*, 94, 700-705, 1979.

[51] FISHER (D. A.), DUSSAULT (J. H.), SACK (J.), CHOPRA (I. J.). — Ontogenesis of hypothalamic-pituitary-thyroid function and metabolism in man, sheep and rat. *Rec. Prog. Horm. Res.*, 33, 59-116, 1977.

[52] FISHER (D. A.), SACK (J.), ODDIE (T. H.), PEKARY (A. E.), HERSHMAN (J. M.), LAM (R. W.), PARSLOW (M. E.). — Serum T_4, TBG, T_3 uptake T_3, reverse T_3 and TSH concentrations in children for one fo fifteen years of age. *J. Clin. Endocrinol. Metab.*, 45, 191-198, 1977.

[53] FISHER (W. C.), WOORHESS (M. L.), GARDNER (L. I.). — Congenital hypothyroidism in infant following maternal $I^{(131)}$ therapy. *J. Pediatr.*, 62, 132-146, 1963.

[54] FOLEY (T. P. Jr), OWINGS (J.), HAYFORD (J. T.), BLIZZARD (R. M.). — Serum thyrotropin responses to synthetic thyrotropin-releasing hormone in normal children and hypopituitary patients; a new test to distinguish primary releasing hormone deficiency from primary pituitary hormone deficiency. *J. Clin. Invest.*, 51, 431-437, 1972.

[55] GATTEREAU (A.), BENARD (B.), BELLABARA (D.), VERDY (M.), BRUN (D.). — Congenital goitre in four euthyroid siblings with glandular and circulating iodoproteins and defective iodothyronine synthesis. *J. Clin. Endocrinol. Metab.*, 37, 118-128, 1973.

[56] GENDREL (D.), FEINSTEIN (M. C.), GRENIER (J.), ROGER (M.), INGRAND (J.), CHAUSSAIN (J. L.), CANLORBE (P.), JOB (J. C.). — Falsely elevated serum thyrotropin (TSH) in newborns infants: transfer from mothers to infants of a factor interfering in the TSH radioimmunoassay. *J. Clin. Endocrinol. Metab.*, 52, 62-65, 1981.

[57] GERSHENGORN (M. C.), WEINTRAUB (B. D.). — Thyrotropin-induced hyperthyroidism caused by selective pituitary resistance to thyroid hormone: a new syndrome of « inappropriate secretion of TSH ». *J. Clin. Invest.*, 56, 633-642, 1975.

[58] GERSHENGORN (M. C.), GLINOER (D.), ROBBINS (J.). — Transport and metabolism of thyroid hormones. In: *The Thyroid Gland*, DE VISSCHER (M.) (Ed.). Raven Press, 81-121, 1980.

[59] GINSBERG (J.), WALFISH (P. G.), CHOPRA (I. J.). — Cord blood, reverse T_3 in normal, premature, euthyroid low T_4 and hypothyroid newborns. *J. Endocrinol. Invest.*, 1, 73-77, 1978.

[60] GOODYER (C. G.), HALL (C. S. G.), GUYDA (H.), ROBERT (F.), GIROUD (C. J. P.). — Human fetal pituitary in culture hormone secretion and response to somatostatin, luteinizing hormone releasing factor, thyrotropin releasing factor and dibutyryl cyclic AMP. *J. Clin. Endocrinol. Metab.*, 45, 73-85, 1977.

[61] GORBMAN (A.). — *Comparative anatomy and physiology of the thyroid*, WERNER (S. C.) and INGBAR (S. H.) (Eds.). Harper and Row, New York, 22, 1978.

[62] GORMAN (C. A.), JIANG (N.-S.), ELLEFSON (R. D.), ELVEBACK (L. R.). — Comparative effectiveness of dextrothyroxine and levothyroxine in correcting hypothyroidism and lowering blood lipid levels in hypothyroid patients. *J. Clin. Endocrinol. Metab.*, 49, 1-7, 1979.

[63] GOSLINGS (B. M.). — Placental transfer of thyroid hormones. In: *Brain Development and Thyroid Deficiency*, QUERIDO (A.) and SWAAB (D. F.) (Eds.). North Holland, Amsterdam, 15-18, 1975.

[64] GRASSO (S.), FILETTI (S.), MAZZONE (D.), PEZZINO (V.), VIGO (P.), VIGNERI (R.). — Thyroid pituitary function in eight anencephalic infants. *Acta Endocrinol.*, 93, 396-401, 1980.

[65] HEMBERGER (J. A.), SCHANKER (L. S.). — Effect of thyroxine on permeability of the neonatal rat lung to drugs. *Biol. Neonate*, 34, 299-303, 1978.

[66] HENNEMANN (G.), DOCTER (R.), KRENNING (E. P.), BOS (G.), OTTEN (M.), VISSER (T. J.). — Raised total thyroxine and free thyroxine index but normal free thyroxine: a serum abnormality due to inherited increased affinity of iodothyronines for serum-binding proteins. *Lancet*, 1, 639-642, 1979.

[67] HERLE (A. J. VAN), YOUNG (R. T.), FISHER (D. A.), ULLER (R. P.), BRINKMAN III (C. R.). — Intra-

uterine treatment of a hypothyroid fetus. *J. Clin. Endocrinol. Metab.*, 40, 474-477, 1975.

[68] HETZEL (B. S.), HAY (I. D.). — Thyroid function, iodine nutrition and fetal brain development. *Clin. Endocrinol.*, 11, 445-460, 1979.

[69] HOLLINGSWORTH (D. R.), MABRY (C. C.), REID (M. C.). — Congenital Graves' disease. In: *Problems in Paediatric Endocrinology*, LACAUZA (C.) and ROOT (A. W.) (Eds.). Academic Press, London, 169-191, 1980.

[69 bis] HOLLINGSWORTH (D. R.), MABRY (C. C.). — Congenital Graves' disease. Four familial cases with long-term follow-up and perspective. *Am. J. Dis. Child.*, 130, 148-155, 1976.

[70] HYYPPÄ (M.). — Hypothalamic monoamines in human fœtuses. *Neuroendocrinology*, 9, 257-266, 1972.

[71] INGBAR (S. H.). — Autoregulation of the thyroid: response to iodide excess and depletion. *Mayo Clin. Proc.*, 47, 814-823, 1972.

[72] ISAAC (R. M.), HAYEK (A.), STANDEFER (J. C.), EATON (R. P.). — Reverse triiodothyronine to triiodothyronine ratio and gestational age. *J. Pediatr.*, 94, 477-479, 1979.

[73] JACKSON (I. M. D.), COBB (W. E.). — Why does anyone still use desicated thyroid VSP? *Am. J. Med.*, 64, 284-288, 1978.

[74] JACOBSEN (B. B.), HUMMER (L.). — Changes in serum concentrations of thyroid hormones and thyroid hormone-binding proteins during early infancy. *Acta Paediat. Scand.*, 68, 411-418, 1979.

[75] JACOBSEN (B. B.), ANDERSON (H.), DIGE-PETERSEN (H.), HUMMER (L.). — Thyrotropin response to thyrotropin-releasing hormone in full-term, euthyroid and hypothyroid newborns. *Acta Paediat. Scand.*, 65, 433-438, 1976.

[76] JACOBSEN (B. B.), ANDERSEN (H.), DIGE-PETERSEN (H.), HUMMER (L.). — Pituitary-thyroid responsiveness to thyrotrophin-releasing hormone in preterm and small-for-gestational age newborns. *Acta Paediat. Scand.*, 66, 541-548, 1977.

[77] JACOBSEN (B. B.), ANDERSEN (H. J.), PEITERSEN (B.), DIGE-PETERSEN (H.), HUMMER (L.). — Serum levels of thyrotropin, thyroxine and triiodothyronine in full-term, small-for-gestational age and preterm newborn babies. *Acta Paediat. Scand.*, 66, 681-687, 1977.

[78] JACOBSEN (B. B.), HANDSTED (L. C.), BRANDT (N. J.), HAAHR (J.), HUMMER (L.), MUNKER (T.), SORENSEN (S. S.). — Thyroxine binding globulin deficiency in early childhood. Post-natal changes in serum concentrations of thyroid hormones and thyroid hormone-binding globulins. *Acta Paediat. Scand.*, 70, 155-159, 1981.

[79] JOB (J. C.), BOCQUENTUR (F.), CANLORBE (P.). — Les goîtres du nouveau-né. *Arch. Fr. Péd.*, 31, 127-136, 1974.

[80] JOB (J. C.), BINET (E.), CANLORBE (P.), ROSSIER (A.). — Traitement des hypothyroïdies de l'enfant. Valeur du taux sérique de la thyréostimuline. *Nouv. Presse Méd.*, 1, 305-308, 1972.

[81] KAPLAN (S. L.), GRUMBACH (M. M.), HOYT (W. F.). — A syndrome of hypopituitary dwarfism hypoplane of optic nerves, and malformation of prosencephalon: report of 6 patients. *Ped. Res.*, 4, 480, 1970.

[82] KAPLAN (S. L.), GRUMBACH (M. M.), AUBERT (M. L.). — The ontogenesis of pituitary hormones and hypothalamic factors in the human fetus: maturation of the central nervous system, regulation of the anterior pituitary function. *Rec. Prog. Horm. Res.*, 32, 161-243, 1976.

[83] KAPLAN (M.), KAULI (R.), LUBIN (E.), GRUNEBAUM (M.), LARON (Z.). — Ectopic thyroid gland: a clinical study of 30 children and review. *J. Pediatr.*, 92, 205-209, 1978.

[84] KAY (C.), ABRAHAM (S.), McCLAIN (P.). — The weight of normal thyroid glands in children. *Arch. Path. (Lab. Med.)*, 82, 349, 1966.

[85] KET (J. L.), DE VIJLDER (J. M.), BIKKER (H.), GONS (M. H.), TEGELAERS (W. H. H.). — Serum thyroglobulin levels: the physiological decrease in infancy and the absence in athyroidism. *J. Clin. Endocrinol. Metab.*, 53, 1301-1303, 1981.

[86] KLEIN (A. H.), FOLEY (B.), KENNY (F. M.), FISCHER (D. A.). — Thyroid hormone and TSH responses to parturition in premature infants with and without the respiratory distress syndrome. *Pediatrics*, 63, 380-385, 1979.

[87] KLEIN (A. H.), MURPHEY (B. E. P.), ODDIE (F. H.), FISHER (D. A.). — Amniotic fluid thyroid hormone concentrations during human gestation. *Am. J. Obstet. Gynecol.*, 136, 626-630, 1980.

[88] KÖNING (M. P.), GUZLER (E.), VASSELLA (F.). — Transitory hypothyroidism in a child born to a mother with circulating thyroid antibodies. *Ann. Endocrinol. Paris*, 38, 57A. 1977.

[89] LAMBERG (B. A.). — Congenital euthyroid goitre and partial peripheral resistance to thyroid hormones. *Lancet*, 1, 854-857, 1973.

[90] LANDAU (H.), SACK (J.), FRUCHT (H.), PALTI (Z.), HOCKNER-CELNIKIER (D.), ROSENMANN (A.). — Amniotic fluid 3,3',5'-triiodothyronine in the detection of congenital hypothyroidism. *J. Clin. Endocrinol. Metab.*, 50, 799-801, 1980.

[91] LARSSON (A.), LJUNGGREN (J. G.), LUNDBEY (K.). — TSH and thyroxine in stored neonatal filter-paper blood samples from patients with congenital hypothyroidism. *Acta Paediat. Scand.*, 71, 39-41, 1982.

[92] LEMIRE (R. J.), BECKWITH (J. B.), WARKANY (J.). — *Anencephaly*. Raven Press, New York, 1978.

[93] LIM (V. S.), FANG (V. S.), KATZ (A. I.), REFETOFF (S.). — Thyroid dysfunction in chronic renal failure. *J. Clin. Invest.*, 60, 522-534, 1977.

[94] MACFAUL (R.), GRANT (D. B.). — Early detection of congenital hypothyroidism *Arch. Dis. Child.*, 52, 87-88, 1977.

[94 bis] MACKENZIE (J. M.), ZAKARIJA (M.). — Pathogenesis of neonatal Graves' disease. *J. Endocrinol. Invest.*, 2, 183-189, 1978.

[95] MÄENPÄÄ (J.). — Congenital hypothyroidism: aetiological and clinical aspects. *Arch. Dis. Childh.*, 47, 914-923, 1972.

[96] MATSUURA (N.), YAMADA (Y.), NOHARA (Y.), KONISHI (J.), KASAGI (K.), ENDO (K.), KOJIMA (H.), WATAYA (K.). — Familal neonatal transient hypothyroidism due to maternal TSH-binding inhibitor immunoglobulins. *N. Engl. J. Med.*, 303, 738-741, 1980.

[97] MEDEIROS-NETO (G. A.), KNOBEL (M.), YAMAMOTO (K.), CAVALIERE (H.), KALLAS (W.). — Deficient thyroid peroxidase causing organification defect and goitrous hypothyroidism. *J. Endocrinol. Invest.*, 2, 353-357, 1979.

[98] MELNICK (J. C.), STEMKOWSKI (P. E.). — Thyroid hemiagenesis (Hockey stick sign): A review of the world literature and a report of four cases. *J. Clin. Endocrinol. Metab.*, 52, 247-251, 1981.

[99] MIYAI (K.), ICHIHARA (K.), AMINO (N.). — Seasonality of birth in sporadic cretinism. *Early Human Dev.*, 3, 85-88, 1978.

[100] MIYAI (F.), MIZUTA (H.), NOSE (O.), FUKUNISHI (T.), HIRAI (T.), MATSUDA (S.), TSURUHARA (T.). — Increased frequency of HLA-AW24 in congenital hypothyroidism in Japan. *N. Engl. J. Med.*, 303, 226, 1980.

[101] MONCRIEFF (M. W.), HILL (D. S.), ARCHER (J.), ARTHUR (J. H.). — Congenital absence of pituitary gland and adrenal hypoplasia. *Arch. Dis. Childh.*, 47, 136-137, 1972.

[102] MORRIS (J. H.). — Defective coupling of iodotyrosine in familial goiters. *Arch. Intern. Med.*, 114, 417-423, 1964.

[103] MUSSA (G. C.), BONA (G.), SILVESTRO (L.), FABRIS (C.). — Prolactin in perinatal age. In: *Problems in Pediatric Endocrinology*. LA CAUZA (C.) and ROOT (A. W.) (Eds.). Academic Press, London, 253-271, 1980.

[104] Newborn Committee of the European Thyroid Association, Neonatal screening for congenital hypothyroidism in Europe. *Acta Endocrinol. (Kbh)*, Suppl. 223, 1-29, 1979.

[105] NOBIN (A.), BJORKLUND (A.). — Topography of the monoamine neuron systems in the human brain as revealed in fetuses. *Acta Physiol. Scand. Suppl.*, 388, 1-40, 1973.

[106] NUNEZ (J.). — Iodination and thyroid hormone synthesis. In: *The Thyroid Gland*. DEVISSCHER (M.) (Ed.). Raven Press, New York, 39-59, 1980.

[107] ODDIE (T. H.), BERNARD (B.), PRESLEY (M.), KLEIN (A. M.), FISHER (D. A.). — Damped oscillations in serum thyroid hormone levels of normal newborn infants. *J. Clin. Endocrinol. Metab.*, 47, 61-65, 1978.

[108] OLIVER (D.), MICAL (R. S.), PORTER (J. C.). — Hypothalamic-pituitary vasculature. Evidence of retrograde blood blow in the pituitary stalk. *Endocrinology*, 95, 1499-1505, 1974.

[109] O'RHAHILLY (R.), GARDNER (E.). — The initial development of the human brain. *Acta Anat.*, 104, 123-133, 1979.

[110] OSOTIMEHIN (B.), BLACK (E. G.), HOFFENBERG (R.). — Thyroglobulin concentration in neonatal blood: a possible test for neonatal hypothyroidism. *Brit. Med. J.*, 2, 1467-1468, 1978.

[111] PARKS (J. S.), TENORE (A.), BONGIOVANNI (A. M.), KIRKLAND (R. T.). — Familial hypopituitarism with large sella turcica. *N. Engl. J. Med.*, 298, 698-702, 1978.

[112] PATEL (H.), TZE (W. J.), CRICHTON (J. U.), McCORMICK (A. Q.), ROBINSON (G. C.), DOLMAN (C. L.). — Optic nerve hypoplasia with hypopituitarism. Septo-optic dysplasia with hypopituitarism. *Am. J. Dis. Child.*, 129, 175-180, 1975.

[113] PEARSE (A. G. E.). — *The endocrine division o the nervous system*. A concept and its verification in molecular endocrinology. MACINTYRE (I.) and STELKE (M.) (Eds.). Elsevier/North Holland, Amsterdam, 3-18, 1979.

[114] PEARSE (A. G. E.), TAKOR TAKOR (T.). — The embryology of the diffuse neuroendocrine system and its relationship to the common peptides. *Fed. Proc.*, 38, 2288-2294, 1979.

[115] PENFOLD (J. L.), SIMPSON (D. A.). — Premature craniosynostosis. A complication of thyroid replacement therapy. *J. Pediatr.*, 86, 360-363, 1975.

[116] PENNY (R.), FRASIER (S. D.). — Elevated serum concentrations of triiodothyronine in hypothyroid patients. Values for patients receiving USP thyroid. *Am. J. Dis. Child.*, 134, 16-18, 1980.

[117] PEZZINO (V.), FILETTI (S.), BELFIORE (A.), PROTO (S.), DONZELLI (G.), VIGNERI (R.). — Serum thyroglobulin levels in the newborn. *J. Clin. Endocrinol. Metab.*, 52, 364-366, 1981.

[118] PRICE (D. A.), EHRLICH (R. M.), WALFISH (P. G.). — Congenital hypothyroidism. Clinical and laboratory characteristics in infants detected by neonatal screening. *Arch. Dis. Childh.*, 56, 845-851, 1981.

[119] RAITI (S.), NEWNS (G. H.). — Cretinism: early diagnosis and its relation to mental prognosis. *Arch. Dis. Childh.*, 46, 692-694, 1971.

[120] ROITMAN (A.), LARON (Z.). — Hypothalamopituitary hormone insufficiency associated with cleft lip and palate. *Arch. Dis. Childh.*, 53, 952-955, 1978.

[121] REES-JONES (R. W.), ROLLA (A. R.), LARSEN (P. R.). — Hormonal content of thyroid replacement preparations. *J. A. M. A.*, 243, 549-550, 1980.

[122] REFETOFF (S.), DEWIND (L. T.), DEGROOT (L. J.). — Familial syndrome combining deafmutism, stippled epiphyses, goiter and abnormally high PBI: possible target organ refractoriness to thyroid hormones. *J. Clin. Endocrinol. Metab.*, 27, 279-294, 1967.

[123] REFETOFF (S.), OCHI (Y.), SELENKOW (H. A.), ROSENFIELD (R. L.). — Neonatal hypothyroidism and goiter in one infant of each of two sets of twins due to maternal therapy with antithyroid drugs. *J. Pediatr.*, 85, 240-244, 1974.

[124] REFETOFF (S.), ROBIN (N. I.), ALPER (C. A.). — Study of four kindreds with inherited thyroxine binding globulin abnormalities. Possible mutation of a single gene locus. *J. Clin. Invest.*, 51, 848-867, 1972.

[125] REZVANI (I.), DIGEORGE (A. M.). — Reassessment of the daily dose of oral thyroxine for replacement therapy in hypothyroid children. *J. Pediatr.*, 90, 291-297, 1977.

[126] RICHARDS (G. E.), PACHMAN (L. M.), GREEN (O. C.). — Symptomatic hypothyroidism in children with collagen disease. *J. Pediatr.*, 87, 82-84, 1975.

[127] RITZÉN (E. M.), MAHLER (H.), ALVERYD (A.). — Transitory congenital hypothyroidism and maternal thyroiditis. *Acta Paediat. Scand.*, 70, 765-766, 1981.

[128] ROCHICCIOLI (P.), DUTAU (G.). — Trouble de l'hormonosynthèse thyroïdienne par déficit en iodotyrosine déshalogénase. *Arch. Fr. Péd.*, 31, 25-36, 1974.

[129] RODESCH (F.), CANNS (M.), ERMANS (A. M.), DODRON (J.), DELANGE (F.). — Adverse effect of amniofetography on fetal thyroid function. *Am. J. Obstet. Gynecol.*, 126, 723-727, 1976.

[130] SACK (J.), BEAUDRY (M.), DELAMATER (P. V.), OH (W.), FISCHER (D. A.). — Umbilical cord cutting triggers hypertriiodothyroninemia and nonshivering thermogenesis in the newborn lamb. *Ped. Res.*, 10, 169-175, 1976.

[131] SACK (J.), FISHER (D. A.), WANG (C. C.). — Serum thyrotropin, prolactin and growth hormone levels during the early neonatal period in the human infants. *J. Pediatr.*, 89, 298-300, 1976.

[132] SADEGHI-NEJAD (A.), SENIOR (B.). — A familial syndrome of isolated « aplasia » of the anterior pituitary. *J. Pediatr.*, *84*, 79-84, 1974.

[133] SALVATORE (G.), STANBURY (J. B.), RALL (J. E.). — Inherited defects of thyroid hormone biosynthesis. In: *The Thyroid Gland*. DEVISSCHER (M.) (Ed.). Raven Press, New York, 443-487, 1980.

[134] SATO (T.), SUZUKI (Y.), TAKETANI (T.), ISHIGURO (K.), NAKOJIMA (H.). — Age-related changes in pituitary threshold for TSH release during thyroxine replacement therapy for cretinism. *J. Clin. Endocrinol. Metab.*, *44*, 553-559, 1977.

[135] SAVOIE (J. C.), MASSIN (J. P.), SAVOIE (F.). — Studies on mono and diiodohistidine. II. Congenital goitrous hypothyroidism with thyroglobulin defect and iodohistidine-rich iodoalbumin production. *J. Clin. Invest.*, *52*, 116-125, 1972.

[136] SCHIMMEL (M.), UTIGER (R. D.). — Thyroidal and peripheral production of thyroid hormones. Review of recent findings and their clinical implications. *Ann. Intern. Med.*, *87*, 760-768, 1977.

[137] SCHÖNBERGER (W.), GRIMM (W.), GEMPP (W.), DINKEL (E.). — Transient hypothyroidism associated with prematurity, sepsis and respiratory distress. *Eur. J. Ped.*, *132*, 85-92, 1979.

[138] SCHULTZ (R. M.), GLASSMAN (M. S.), MACGILLIVRAY (M. H.). — Elevated threshold for thyrotropin suppression in congenital hypothyroidism. *Am. J. Dis. Child.*, *134*, 19-20, 1980.

[139] SÉNÉCAL (J.), GROSSE (M. C.), VINCENT (A.), SIMON (J.), LEFRECHE (J. N.). — Maturation osseuse du fœtus et du nouveau-né. *Arch. Fr. Péd.*, *34*, 424-438, 1977.

[140] SHEPARD (T. H.). — Onset of function in the human fetal thyroid: biochemical and radio-autographic studies from organ culture. *J. Clin. Endocrinol. Metab.*, *27*, 945-958, 1967.

[141] SIMONIN (R.), HEIM (M.). — Variations nycthémérales du taux de thyroxine totale sérique lors du traitement des hypothyroïdies pour la dl-thyroxine en gouttes. *Rev. Fr. Endocrinol. Clin.*, *21*, 159-160, 1980.

[142] SIPPONEN (P.), SIMILÄ (S.), COLLAN (Y.), AUTERE (T.), HERVA (R.). — Familial syndrome with panhypopituitarism, hypoplasia of the hypophysis and poorly developed sella turcica. *Arch. Dis. Childh.*, *53*, 664-667, 1978.

[143] SIZONENKO (P. C.), GRETILLAT (A.), PAUNIER (L.). — Value of serum thyroxine measurement for the management of congenital hypothyroidism in children. *Helv. Paediat. Acta*, *33*, 341-350, 1978.

[144] SMITH (D. W.), KLEIN (A. M.), HENDERSON (J. R.), MYRIANTHPOULOS (N. C.). — Congenital hypothyroidism: signs and symptoms in the newborn period. *J. Pediatr.*, *87*, 958-962, 1975.

[145] STÄGER (J.), FROESCH (E. R.). — Congenital familial thyroid aplasia. *Acta Endocrinol.*, *96*, 188-191, 1981.

[146] STANBURY (J. H.), AIGINGER (P.), HARBISON (M. D.). — Familial goiter and related disorders. In: *Endocrinology*. DEGROOT (L. J.), CAHILL (C. F. Jr.) and ODELL (W. D.) (Eds.). Grune and Stratton, New York, 523-529, 1979.

[147] STANBURY (J. B.), ROCMANS (P.), BUHLER (U. K.), OCHI (Y.). — Congenital hypothyroidism with impaired thyroid response to thyrotropin. *N. Engl. J. Med.*, *279*, 1132-1136, 1968.

[148] STEELE (M. W.). — Genetics of congenital deafness. *Ped. Clin. North Am.*, *28*, 973-980, 1981.

[149] STERLING (K.). — Thyroid hormone action at the cellular level. *N. Engl. J. Med.*, *300*, 117-123 and 173-177, 1978.

[150] SUTER (S. N.), KAPLAN (S. L.), AUBERT (M. L.), GRUMBACH (M. M.). — Plasma prolactin and thyrotropin and the response to thyrotropin-releasing factor in children with primary and hypothalamic hypothyroidism. *J. Clin. Endocrinol. Metab.*, *47*, 1015-1020, 1978.

[151] TAKOR TAKOR (T.), PEARSE (A. G. E.). — Neuroectodermal origin of avian hypothalamohypophyseal complex: the role of the ventral neural ridge. *J. Embryol. Exp. Morphol.*, *34*, 311-325, 1975.

[152] TALIADOUROS (G. S.), CANFIELD (R. S.), NISULA (B. C.). — Thyroid stimulating activity of chorionic gonadotropin and luteinizing hormone. *J. Clin. Endocrinol. Metab.*, *47*, 855-860, 1978.

[153] THEODOROPOULOS (T.), BRAVERMAN (L. E.), VOGENAKIS (A. G.). — Iodide-induced hypothyroidism: a potential hazard during perinatal life. *Science*, *205*, 502-503, 1979.

[154] THILLY (C. H.), DELANGE (F.), LAGASSE (R.), BOURDOUX (P.), RAMIOUL (L.), BERQUIST (H.), ERMANS (A. M.). — Fetal hypothyroidism and maternal thyroid status in severe endemic goiter. *J. Clin. Endocrinol. Metab.*, *47*, 354-360, 1978.

[155] TORPET (L. S.). — Farber's disease with athyreosis. *Acta Faediat. Scand.*, *67*, 113-116, 1978.

[156] UHRMANN (S.), MARKS (K. H.), MAISELS (M. J.), FRIEDMAN (Z.), MURRAY (F.), KUHN (H.), KAPLAN (M.), UTIGER (R.). — Thyroid function in the preterm infant. A longitudinal assessment. *J. Pediatr.*, *92*, 968-973, 1978.

[157] VALLÉE (G.). — Exploration du corps thyroïde chez l'enfant. *Arch. Fr. Péd.*, *33*, 997-1002, 1976.

[158] VOLPÉ (R.). — The pathogenesis of Graves' disease: an overview. *Clin. Endocrinol. Metab.*, *7*, 3-29, 1978.

[159] WEICHSEL (M. E.). — Thyroid hormone replacement therapy in the perinatal period: neurologic considerations. *J. Ped.*, *92*, 1035-1038, 1978.

[160] WEILL (J.), DEBRUXELLES (P.), FULLA (Y.), DUBOIS (G.), PONTE (C.). — Surveillance biologique des hypothyroïdies primitives de l'enfant sous traitement par extraits thyroïdiens. *Arch. Fr. Péd.*, *37*, 29-34, 1980.

[161] WHITE (C. W.), WIEDERMANN (B. L.), KIRKLAND (R. T.), CLAYTON (G. W.). — Hereditary congenital non goitrous hypothyroidism. *Am. J. Dis. Child.*, *135*, 568-569, 1981.

[162] WIEDEMANN (H. R.). — Complexe malformatif familial avec hernie ombilicale et macroglossie. Un « syndrome » nouveau? *J. Genet. Hum.*, *13*, 223-232, 1964.

[163] WOLFF (J.), CHAIKOFF (I. L.). — The inhibitory action of excessive iodide upon the synthesis of diiodotyrosine and of thyroxine in the thyroid gland of the normal rat. *Endocrinology*, *43*, 174-179, 1948.

[164] WU (B.), KIKKAWA (Y.), ORZALESI (M. M.), MOTOYAMA (E. K.), KAIBARA (M.), ZIGAS (C. J.), COOK (C. D.). — The effect of thyroxine on the maturation of fetal rabbit lung. *Biol. Neonate*, *22*, 161-168, 1973.

[165] YOKOH (Y.). — The early development of the nervous system in man. *Acta Anat. (Basel)*, *71*, 492-518, 1968.

Adrenal glands

In humans, as in other mammals, the adrenal glands are constituted of two different endocrine entities, an inner portion, the adrenal medulla and an outer layer, the adrenal cortex. These two organs remain functionally separated throughout life, although they are enclosed within a common capsule. No significant direct functional relationship between them is known. Cortex and medulla remain as separate organs (interrenal and suprarenal glands) in lower species, whereas in birds they are inter-dispersed in a single gland.

The medulla secretes catecholamines, the 3 principal ones being epinephrine, norepinephrine and dopamine. The adrenal cortex produces a variety of steroid hormones with diverse effects throughout the body which are broadly classified as gluco-corticoids, mineralocorticoids, progesteroids, androgens and estrogens. During fetal development, various abnormalities in the secretion of androgens may interfere with normal sexual differentiation of the external genitalia. For better understanding of these physiopathological conditions, after reviewing the fetal and neonatal physiology of the adrenal cortex we will present briefly the basic steps of normal sexual differentiation.

NORMAL DEVELOPMENT OF THE ADRENAL GLANDS

ANATOMICAL AND BIOCHEMICAL DEVELOPMENT OF THE HYPOTHALAMIC-HYPOPHYSO-ADRENAL (HHA) AXIS

The adrenal glands
[184, 237, 248, 260, 330, 332]

The two parts of the adrenal gland, cortex and medulla, originate from separate primordia which ultimately fuse to form one gland consisting of two different organs. The cells of the adrenal cortex arise from the proliferation of the cœlomic meso-thelial cells of the posterior abdominal wall and adjacent mesenchymal cells, on either side of the root of the mesentery, medial in position to the upper ends of the mesonephros (Wolffian bodies), in close association with the primordia of the gonads. Because of their common embryologic origin, the adrenal cortex and the gonads have closely related physiological functions, being the sole endocrine glands with the capacity of producing steroid hormones. While differentiating from the gonadal tissue, the mesodermal cells of the adrenal cortex rapidly increase in number and condense into small clusters of acidophilic cells. By 4 post-conceptional weeks, the adrenocortical primordia are separated from the cœlomic epithelium and from the genital ridge, becoming distinct entities on each lateral side of the aorta. The cells of the medulla are ectodermal neurogenic cells, arising from the neural crest to form sympatogonia. Migrating down, they invade the primitive mesodermal anlage at about the 7th embryologic week. Shortly there-after, the sympathetic neural elements become chromaffin cells and by the 8th week will form the adrenal medulla in the center of the adrenal gland. Other ectodermal cells differentiate to form neuro-blasts or sympathoblasts, and latter mature ganglion cells or extramedullary tissue. Throughout fetal life, the adrenal medulla remains inconspicuous and the medullary tissue function is assumed mostly by large paraganglionic masses located along the aorta.

In man and a few subhuman primates, the fetal adrenal cortex is unique in possessing an unusually wide inner cortical zone of large ovoid functional cells, called the "fetal" zone, and a narrow outer zone called the "definitive" cortex, adult zone or neocortex. The latter apparently originates from a second generation of mesenchymal cells, differen-tiating into small basophilic cells which at about 10 weeks progressively surround the earlier clusters.

The fact that during their embryonic development the adrenal glands, the gonads, kidneys and liver arise from the same general area, explains that about 20 % of normal individuals have accessory adreno-cortical tissue or adherent adrenal or cortical ectopic inclusions which are capable of secreting steroid hormones. They may be located from the mediastinum to the scrotum. Small clusters of adrenal cells migrating with gonadal tissue will give rise to ectopic nodules of adrenal cortical tissue within the testis or along the cord in males, near the ovaries in the broad ligaments in the females; tumors developing from ectopic nodules may be observed in the liver or in the lower pole of the kidney. Conversely, inclusion of cells from the genital ridge into the adrenal cortex may be responsible for the occurence of androgenic or œstrogenic tumors in the adrenal cortex in later life. In contrast, true accessory adrenal glands, made up of both medullary and cortical tissues, are very rare and usually found in the cœliac plexus or the renal cortex. Accessory medullary tissue is occasionally found in the bladder and wherever sympathetic nervous tissue is located, in the sympathetic nerve ganglia and plexus along the aorta and in the organ of Zuckerkandl at the lower end of the aorta.

During the 3-4th months, the adrenal glands are very large exceeding the kidney in size and this large size is mainly due to the prominent fetal zone. At six months' gestation the adrenals are about half the size of the kidney and are still one-third as large at birth. Although decreasing in size relative to the other organs, the most rapid growth of the adrenals (3-4 fold) occurs during the last trimester of gestation. At term, the average combined weight of both adrenals is about 9 g [330], representing 0.5 % of the body weight and the fetal zone still occupies 80 % of the cortex.

At birth, or just before birth, rapid degenerative changes begin in the fetal zone which results in a 50 % decrease in the weight of the adrenals during the first month of life. The fetal zone cells become rapidly indistinct and vascular engorgement, marked necrosis, fragmentation of cells, hemorrhage and narrowing of the fetal zone occur to such a degree that the cortex may appear to an unwary pathologist as abnormal adrenal hemorrhage. The adult zone is now about 50 % of the cortex. By 6 weeks of age only fibrous tissue remains between the medulla and the adult zone of the cortex [184, 248, 249, 260, 314, 332]. It is not known when exactly the "fetal zone" disappears completely nor when the "adult zone" finally differentiates into the classical histological zones described by Arnold in 1866 in adult adrenal cortex (peripheral zona glomerulosa, inner zona fasciculata and innermost zona reticularis), but the process appears to be completed by 2-3 years of age. At birth, the medulla is relatively underdeveloped and attains maturation during the first 3 years of life [204]. The abundant ganglion cells and catecholamine-secreting chromaffin cells atrophy during the second year of life, although their main aggregation remains detectable for some years as the organ of Zuckerkandl [352].

From about 18 months of life adrenal weight increases again, gradually in good correlation with body size, with a more rapid increase at puberty, until the combined weight of 8-14 g is attained ($\sim$ 30 % less in females than in males). In fact, in the adult the medulla occupies only a portion of the gland, the head and the body, while the tail is all cortex.

Each adrenal gland is located at the upper pole of the kidney, usually surrounded by the perizonal fat, in a fascial compartment, the Gerota's fascia, preventing the glands from descending with the kidney when they are displaced. For its size, the adrenal is one of the most vascular organs in the body, In adults, the blood flow is about 5 ml per minute. Twenty to fifty arterial branches with very variable pattern and number between individuals, arise from 3 major sources, the superior one from the inferior phrenic artery, the middle one coming directly from the aorta and the inferior from the renal artery. The arterial branches spread over the adrenal capsule, pierce it and organize into a sub-capsular plexus at the cortico-medullary junction. There they form a type of portal circulation, which sends small arterial twigs toward the medulla with capillary loops going back to the cortex, draining the relatively few veins through the medulla to a single central vein. The right adrenal drains to the inferior cava but the left drains into the left renal vein. This peculiar vascular arrangement may play a role in the secretion of adrenal hormones: Corticosteroids must go through the medulla and their high concentration in the efferent blood is thought to be necessary for the activation of the methyltransferase converting norepinephrine into epinephrine [356]. Conversely the high concentration of the latter in the retrograde loops may influence the secretion of cortical steroids.

Although the zonation of the adrenal cortex relies only on histological characteristics, the terms have persisted and attempts to correlate histological appearance and secretory function have been made. The *zona glomerulosa* cells, usually grouped in poorly defined clusters are rounded and small, with large nuclei. The *zona fasciculata* is the largest one, representing about 75 % of the total cortex. It is made of polyhedral cells with a central nucleus, a foamy cytoplasm and abundant lipids. These types of cells gradually blend into the inner zona, the *reticularis* which contains identical cells and smaller, darker cells with very little lipid and a deep staining nucleus. These cells form an anastomosing network. In fact, the adrenal cortex has a continuous "cord-like" structure, in the sense that cords of 10-15 cells extend from the capsule to the medulla in a continuum surrounded by a capillary network. All cells have an ultrastructure similar to other steroid secreting cells with numerous mitochondria and abundant smooth endoplasmic reticulum (SER). The mitochondria are elongated with marked cristae in the zona glomerulosa and are more round and flat in the two other inner zones. The SER is the most prominent feature of all zones, forming a network of anastomosing tubules. The total lipids represent 20 % of the adult adrenal weight but only 4 % in the newborn. Despite the lack of a strict histological delineation, the 3 zonae of the adrenal cortex have relatively defined steroidogenic functions (see review in [265]). Only the glomerulosa cells, which lack 17α-hydroxylase activity, are responsible for mineralocorticoid synthesis (mainly aldosterone, but also corticosterone) under the control of angiotensin and potassium. They are little influenced by adrenocorticotrophic hormone (ACTH). Glucocorticoids (C21-steroids) originate mainly from the fasciculata zone whereas androgens (C19-steroids) and estrogens (C18-steroids) as well as glucocorticoids are made in the reticularis. However 17β-hydroxylase activity is normally very weak even if present, and 17β-estradiol and testosterone are practically not secreted [306]. Because of their "mixed" steroidogenic capacity and because they are both under the control of ACTH for both growth and steroidogenic stimulation the fasciculata and reticularis zones are, in modern concepts, considered as a single functional unit [234-236].

The histological development of the fetal adrenal has been studied in detail [248]. Only immature adrenocortical cells are found in 10-15 mm fetuses (about 6 weeks). By the 20 mm stage (7-8 weeks), there is first evidence of two zones: an outer zone of immature cells and an inner zone showing evidence of functional differentiation. During the first trimester of gestation, an agranular reticulum and the Golgi apparatus develop and the number of mitochondria with vesicular cristae increase in the large eosinophilic cells with pale staining nuclei that are the cells of the inner "fetal" zone. These intracellular organelles develop further during the 2nd trimester and lipid droplets accumulate in mid-pregnancy with a progressive depletion thereafter. The cells of the outer adult zone contain a small cytoplasm and dark staining nuclei. Evidence of active steroidogenic activity does not develop in this zone until the late second trimester of gestation.

Although the fetal adrenal gland can synthesize cholesterol from acetate and hence pregnenolone, it does not possess the complete range of enzymes necessary for the production of all steroids that are made in adults (see below). The fetal adrenals possess a low Δ^5-3β-hydroxysteroid dehydrogenase isomerase (3β-HSD) activity [199, 232] and hence cannot form progesterone from pregnenolone [341]. This classical concept has been recently challenged [284], and for some authors the 3β-HSD would only be inhibited in utero by the high concentration of estrogens of maternal origin, as reproduced by in vitro experiments [354], or by other factors produced by the placenta [346]. The second prominent feature of fetal adrenal steroidogenesis is a high sulfokinase (sulfotransferase) activity, hence the major secretory products of the fetal adrenal are Δ^5-sulfoconjugates, dehydroepiandrosterone sulfate (DHAS), quantitatively the most important, and pregnenolone sulfate [182, 194, 201, 246, 323, 329, 341]. The fetus is also deficient in steroid sulfatase and aromatase but has active C17α-C20 lyase, 16α-hydroxylase. The placenta, which also lacks a number of enzyme activities complements the fetal steroidogenic inabilities: all the enzyme activities cited above which are low in the fetus are highly active in the placenta and vice versa.

DHAS is the principal secretory product of the fetal zone [194, 201-203, 246, 323, 341]. The enzymes necessary for the synthesis of DHA, and sulfokinase activity are detected in both the outer and inner zones, but most of them are found in the fetal zone [199], which in addition is the most functionally active during the first half of pregnancy [202, 203, 341].

The fetal adrenals are also capable of carrying out the complete set of enzymatic steps in the conversion of acetate to cortisol and aldosterone. Hydroxylating enzymatic activity appears sequentially in the cortex, in the order 17α, 11β, 21, and 18 during the second trimester. The adult zone secretes larger quantities of cortisol than of DHAS [191, 194, 315]. Cortisol, the second most important steroid secreted by the fetus, is believed to be confined primarily to the definitive zone [191, 208, 209, 315, 329, 341]. The 3β-HSD which is demonstrable in the fetal adrenal is almost completely localized in the definitive zone, according to histochemical [232, 248, 249] and biochemical [191, 202] studies. Cortisol biosynthesis is identifiable by the 10-15th week [278] and comprises over half of the total steroids produced by cultured adrenal cells in mid-pregnancy [301]. The synthesis of aldosterone has also been demonstrated beginning as early as the 15th gestational week, at about the same time as that of cortisol [214, 290]. Its site of secretion, likely in the adult zone, has not been established with certainty. The fetal kidney contains renin activity and renin substrates [266].

Hypothalamus and pituitary gland

Their embryology and development has been described above. The existence of an hypothalamic corticotropin releasing factor (CRF) had been postulated several years ago, but it is only recently that its structure has been established [338]. Its ontogeny has not yet been studied.

Throughout fetal life, the intermediate lobe which represents less than 20 % of the total pituitary gland, is present as a relatively avascular but well-innervated thin epithelial layer consisting predominantly of one cell type [172]. Immuno- and cytohistochemical studies have shown that these cells are involved in the production of the ACTH/lipotrophin family of peptides [177, 178, 213, 345]. Indeed, it has been recently discovered that ACTH is derived from a large molecule which is also the common precursor for β-lipoprotein (β-LPH). The latter includes within its structure, β-endorphin and γ-LPH itself a precursor of metenkephalin and β-melanotropic-stimulating hormone (β-MSH). ACTH contains the sequences of α-MSH and corticotropin-like inter-mediate lobe peptide (CLIP) (see review in [219]). ACTH and related peptides are located in the intermediate and anterior lobes, not in the posterior lobe of the pituitary. The intermediate lobe shows signs of degeneration after birth in the human, and its role, if any in later life, is not defined.

ACTH was first identified in human fetal pituitaries: Detected by bioassay by 9 week's gestation [291] and by immunocytochemical studies before the 14th week [213]. From both immunocytochemical studies [177, 178] and analysis of pituitary contents [319, 320] it may be concluded that in early gestation (12-18 weeks), ACTH, β-LPH, γ-LPH and β-endorphin are present in substantial amounts whereas α-MSH and CLIP are barely detectable. The latter two are the predominant peptides in mid-gestation. After birth they decrease abruptly while ACTH increases concomitantly.

In anencephalic fetuses the intermediate lobe is underdeveloped or completely absent, α-MSH is lacking [345]. The corticotrophic cells of the anterior lobe are reduced, but still produce β-LPH, endor-phins and ACTH though in much smaller amounts [167, 177, 178, 345].

MATURATION OF THE HHA AXIS

Our knowledge of steroid biosynthesis and of its regulation during fetal life is mostly derived from perfusion studies of the fetus or of the fetoplacental unit, infusions in the fetus in vivo [208, 209, 249, 290, 314, 329, 341] and more recently from in vitro incubations and cultures [191, 194, 203, 214, 246, 301, 315, 354]. It is important to realize that most of these studies have been made in mid-pregnancy. Despite the additional information given by the measurement of steroids in cord blood, we are basically ignorant of the first steps in adrenal fetal biosynthesis and have little information on the events occuring during the third trimester of pregnancy.

Fetal steroidogenesis

As discussed above, the fetus is lacking a number of steroidogenic enzymes. The concept of a materno-feto-placental unit was introduced when it was established that special relationships exist between the fetal adrenals and the placenta for the synthesis of estrogens, and between the mother and the fetus for the supply of glucocorticoids to the fetus [208, 329]. This steroid biosynthesis is complicated and is summarized in Figure VI-32. There is a constant interplay of fetus, placenta and mother to form the bulk of fetal and maternal steroids in pregnancy.

Estriol, the most abundant estrogen excreted as various conjugates by the mother, is formed after 16α-hydroxylation of the DHAS produced by the fetal adrenals. When 16α-hydroxy-DHAS so formed reaches the placenta it is cleaved into 16α-hydroxy-DHA by the active placental sulfatase, and aroma-tized to estriol by the second most active placental enzyme, the aromatase [208, 329]. The placenta through active 3β-HSD, converts DHA of both maternal and fetal origin to Δ⁴-androstenedione, to testosterone and finally to estrone and 17β-estradiol (Fig. VI-32). This is why maternal levels of estriol or estetrol [336] rather than that of estrone-estradiol reflects fetal adrenal activity (synthesis of DHAS and derivatives) and fetal status (liver synthesis of 16α-hydroxy-DHAS).

It seems well established that the fetal adrenal cortex has a very low overall 3β-HSD activity, the enzyme necessary for the conversion of Δ⁵-3β-hydroxysteroid to Δ⁴-3-keto-steroids (e. g. pregne-nolone to progesterone or DHA to Δ⁴-androstene-dione). According to the classical concept, the fetus relies on the placenta for its supply of progesterone, the Δ⁴-3 ketosteroid precursor of cortisol and aldo-sterone biosynthesis (Fig. VI-32). Most of the experi-mental evidence for this pertains to mid-pregnancy. However, it is likely that beyond mid-pregnancy the fetus progressively establishes a system for inde-pendent cortisol biosynthesis since at birth, when the

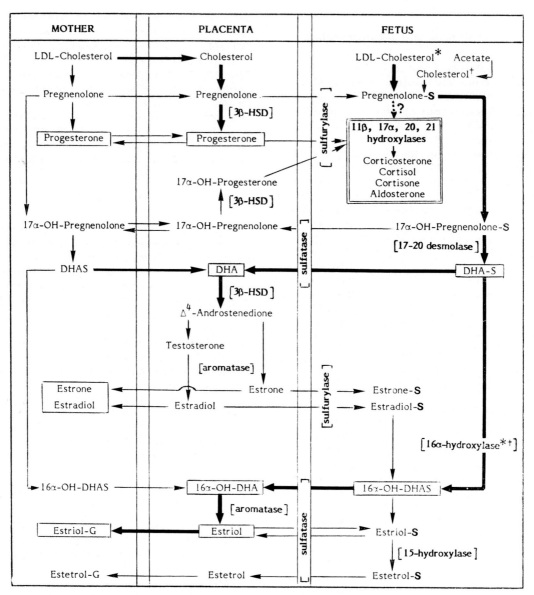

*Primarily in the liver, + to a limited extent in the fetal adrenal.
Abbreviations : S for sulfate, G for glucuronide, OH for hydroxy.

FIG. VI-32. — *Steroid biosynthesis in the materno-feto-placental unit* [182, 193, 196, 210, 312, 336].

supply of progesterone is abruptly withdrawn, the newborn is capable of cortisol biosynthesis whatever its gestational age. Indirect but strong evidence that placental progesterone is not the primary substrate for fetal cortisol biosynthesis in late pregnancy comes from the observation of fetuses with congenital deficiency in 3β-HSD who develop congenital adrenal hyperplasia (see below), or from the observation of reduced fetal plasma cortisol

levels, increased cholesterol in cord blood [168] but no evident change in placental progesterone after administration of synthetic glucocorticoids to the mother [168].

The classical concept that circulating pregnenolone synthetized by the placenta was the primary source of substrate for fetal steroidogenesis has also to be revised. Indeed, it now emerges that fetal cholesterol serves as the principal precursor for the biosynthesis of both DHAS and cortisol in the fetal adrenal gland [196]. From various in vitro and in vivo studies reviewed by Carr and Simpson [193] it appears that neither the amount of pregnenolone delivered to the adrenals by the placenta, nor that of cholesterol synthetized de novo in the fetal adrenal are sufficient precursors for fetal steroidogenesis. Low density lipoprotein (LDL) serves as a major source (about 70 %) of cholesterol utilized by the fetal adrenal. LDL receptors are present in high concentration on adrenal cell membranes of both fetal and definitive zones. The number of LDL-binding sites and the rate of de novo cholesterol biosynthesis are higher in the fetal zone than in the neocortex, but are stimulated in both tissues by ACTH [355]. Once the cholesterol side-chain cleavage system is fully activated by ACTH (as in the adult) the supply of cholesterol to the mitochondria becomes rate-limiting for steroidogenesis [193]. The concentration of LDL in fetal plasma, inversely correlated to that of DHAS, appears to be regulated by the rate of fetal steroidogenesis and by the rate of LDL biosynthesis. The factors controlling cholesterol and LDL synthesis occuring presumably in fetal liver or other fetal tissues are still unknown. On the other hand, the major substrate for steroidogenesis in the placenta is maternal LDL-cholesterol [353] (Fig. VI-32).

Control of fetal adrenal development and fetal steroidogenesis

It has for long been accepted that during the first half of pregnancy the development of the adrenal cortex was dependent on placental factors, becoming ACTH dependent only in the second part of gestation. It has been proposed that hCG might be the trophic agent for the adrenal cortex during early gestation [183]. This concept is mainly derived from the observation that the adrenal glands of anencephalic fetuses which are normally developed until 20 weeks, subsequently become atrophic [183] due to the low plasma levels of ACTH in these fetuses [167, 335]. Normally ACTH levels are detected in fetal plasma by the 12th week of gestation, remain high until 34 weeks with a significant fall in late gestation [355], being higher at all gestational ages than in normal children or adults [166, 274]. As discussed above the fetal zone of the adrenal cortex develops first, growing throughout gestation and the neocortex matures and grows only late in gestation. It has been known for a long time that the atrophy of the adrenal cortex of anencephalic fetuses results mostly in the almost complete absence

of the fetal zone [183]: Progressive disappearance or lack of development? This is not established. However, more recent studies have shown that the adrenals of anencephalic abortuses are small with reduced fetal zones as early as 15 weeks gestation [233], a time when hCG is abundant, that they are producing little DHAS and mainly cortisol in response to ACTH but not to hCG [195]. In these adrenals, the number of LDL binding sites is reduced probably because the lack of an ACTH trophic effect on the LDL-receptors and only de novo cholesterol biosynthesis is stimulated by ACTH [196]. This is strong evidence that ACTH is the main trophic factor for both fetal and definitive zones of the fetal adrenal cortex in vivo. Prolactin, hGH, α-MSH, other ACTH-related peptides and even estradiol have been proposed as possible trophic factors for the fetal adrenal at specific gestational ages. From the review [193] of the conflicting data in the literature there is no evidence that any of these hormones have by themselves an important influence, trophic or steroidogenic, on the human fetal adrenal.

ACTH is also clearly the main factor which stimulates steroidogenesis [191, 194, 322] in both zones of the fetal adrenal cortex, inducing LDL receptors [195] (thus cholesterol uptake), the activity of 3-hydroxy-3-methyl glutamyl Coenzyme A reductase [193] (thus the rate of de novo cholesterol biosynthesis). Because ACTH induces the activities of 3β-HSD [322, 354], 21- and 11β-hydroxylases [171] in the fetal zone cells in vitro, it is believed that opposing factors may prevent ACTH from inducing these enzyme activities in the fetal zone in vivo [322]. However, the ultimate factor(s) responsible for the development and maintenance of two distinct zones in the fetal adrenal cortex as well as the mechanism(s) by which they exhibit a distinct steroidogenic pattern in utero are still unknown.

Maturation of the control mechanism of ACTH secretion

In adults, the secretion of CRF thus that of ACTH and adrenocortical secretions is normally regulated by 3 major mechanisms, a negative feedback system between the hypothalamus, the pituitary gland and the adrenals, circadian variations likely due to neurotransmitter modulation of CRF secretion, and stress (Fig. VI-33). Very little is known about the maturation of these mechanisms in the fetus or newborn infant.

However, it is clear that negative feedback is operating at least in late gestation: maternal administration of various glucocorticoids suppress the

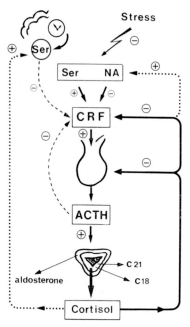

FIG. VI-33. — *Mechanisms regulating the function of the hypothalamic-pituitary-adrenal axis.*

1) Cortisol, cortisone, synthetic glucocorticoids but not androgens have a suppressive effect on the pituitary secretion of ACTH by the pituitary and on that of CRF in the median eminence (long feed-back loops). There is also evidence of a short feed-back control whereby ACTH itself can alter its own secretion (short loop). Part of the negative retroaction of glucocorticoids on ACTH secretion is likely mediated by the activation of serotonin (Ser) and Noradrenaline (NA) which inhibit CRF secretion (···).

2) ACTH and cortisol secretion are normally episodic and cyclic. The profound circadian rhythm, independent of plasma cortisol levels, may be modulated by serotoninergic mechanisms.

3) Stress, whatever its cause (acute hypoglycemia, pyrogens, surgery, pain, fear, anger or frustation) can override the other controlling factors, opening the negative feed-back loops and stimulating ACTH secretion.

levels of ACTH, DHAS and cortisol in cord blood [168, 173] and decrease maternal estriol secretion before delivery [287]. The diminution of fetal plasma ACTH during the last trimester of gestation and during the first postnatal week [355] may reflect an increasing sensitivity of the hypothalamo-pituitary complex to circulating glucocorticoids. The same data may also be suggestive of increased sensitivity of the neocortex to ACTH resulting in higher cortisol production (see below) and subsequent inhibition of ACTH secretion. In newborn infants beyond 3-6 months of age the response to exogenous ACTH is strikingly

higher than later in life [221]. We do not however know the factors controlling the apparent changes in pituitary-adrenal sensitivity.

Circadian rhythms are apparently not mature in the fetus. In newborn infants only unsynchronized fluctuations in cortisol levels are observed [360]. Circadian rhythm of adrenocortical function may develop to the adult type pattern during early infancy [340] and not at 1-3 years of age as classically suggested.

Data in sheep suggest that stress-induced release of ACTH matures in late gestation [302]. The ability of the human fetus to respond to stress in utero is likely operative near term although still a matter of controversy. A significant increase in maternal estriol excretion has not been observed in association with any form of presumed fetal stress, but the evidence is rather indirect and metabolic processes might blunt the fetal adrenal response. Fetal serum ACTH levels are not higher in infants delivered after spontaneous labor than after cesarian section [355], but in this work blood samplings were not repeated in the same subjects. When fetal scalp blood is obtained during labor, ACTH levels increase as labor progresses [169]. Similarly levels of 11-hydroxysteroids in the amniotic fluid are higher during labor in spontaneous vaginal delivery than during cesarian section [339].

MATERNO-FETAL RELATIONSHIPS

It appears well established that maternal ACTH does not cross the placenta [166, 216, 274]. Fetal levels of ACTH are normally higher than in the mother throughout pregnancy [355] and abnormally high ACTH levels in the mother do not influence fetal ACTH levels [166]. Thus the fetus has to rely on its own pituitary function in utero. Fetal adrenal function is in contrast influenced by maternal adrenal function but does not participate significantly in maternal adrenal function. Indeed, in contrast to thyroid hormones, steroid hormones can cross the placental barrier (Table I). The maternal-fetal transfer of cortisol is of physiological importance for the fetus. The fraction of maternal cortisol that crosses the placenta without being converted to cortisone contributes substantially to fetal plasma cortisol (25-50 % near term) [181]. The major portion of maternal cortisol which crosses the placenta (> 80 %) is however converted to cortisone during placental transfer [181, 283]. The fetus also possesses active oxidative pathways and converts cortisol to cortisone [179] or prednisolone to prednisone in particular in the lung [281]. The binding of cortisol (or related glucocorticoids such as prednisolone) to corticosteroid binding globulin (CBG, or transcortin), the levels of which are high during pregnancy, is another factor limiting the maternal transfer of cortisol to the fetus. Because synthetic glucocorticoids do not bind CBG and are not readily metabolized by the fetus, they reach high concentrations in the fetus. Therefore one must remember that when treating the mother with various glucocorticoids the suppressive effect on fetal adrenal function is not only dependent upon the dose given to the mother but also upon the nature of the drug: maternal-fetal gradients in blood levels are about 10 to 1 for cortisol or prednisolone [179], 3 to 1 for betamethasone [173] and 1 to 1 for dexamethasone [289].

The chorioamniotic membranes are able to convert cortisone to cortisol in vitro [279]. This suggests that they might be an additional source of cortisol for the fetus, the importance of which has not been determined in vivo.

The production of cortisol and aldosterone by the fetal adrenal appears to increase from 15 to 36 weeks' gestation, as reflected by amniotic fluid or fetal levels [282, 288, 321, 326]. However, the rise in these hormone levels might also result from concomitant changes in metabolic clearance rate (MCR) or in metabolism. Indeed, the MCR of cortisol is likely high in the fetus because of low fetal plasma CBG concentrations and high unbound cortisol levels, higher than in the mother [321], but is low with a prolonged half-life during the first weeks of life [186]. Moreover, the direct measurement of the MCR of cortisol in the Rhesus monkey shows that it is 4 fold higher in the fetus than in the newborn or adult animal [273]. Among the metabolic changes possibly occuring in late gestation, two are well documented, the decrease in cortisol to cortisone conversion and thus in cortisone/cortisol ratio [282], and the increase in sulfo-derivatives of cortisol [280], normally contemporary with the enzymatic maturation of the synthesis of pulmonary surfactant as shown by the increasing lecithin/sphingomyelin (L/S) ratio. We have however no insight as to the factors controlling these changes in glucocorticoid metabolism.

ADAPTATION
TO EXTRAUTERINE LIFE

Glucocorticoid function

After birth, rapid morphologic changes occur in the adrenal gland, and placental and maternal contri-

butions to fetal steroidogenesis and/or steroid pools are abruptly withdrawn. All these factors contribute to the rapid fall of steroids present in large amounts in umbilical cord blood: progesterone, estrogens, DHAS and its 16α-derivatives, pregnenolone sulfate and its 16α- and 17α-derivatives. Estrogens, among which estriol is the most prominent one as a sulfoconjugate, fall rapidly within the first day of life; disappearance of unconjugated estriol takes less than one day, that of estriol conjugates 10 days [299].

Despite the rapid involution in the fetal zone of the adrenal cortex and a post-natal decrease in plasma levels, Δ^5-3β-hydroxysteroids are still produced in substantial amounts for the first month of life; DHAS, pregnenolone sulfate and their 16α-hydroxy-derivatives decline thereafter more progressively over the first 6 months of life [299]. This is against the hypothesis that œstrogen inhibition of 3β-HSD activity in utero might explain the pattern of secretion of the fetal adrenal cortex. We do not know the factors responsible for the involution of the fetal zone: ACTH levels decline by 75 % during the first week of life [355] exhibiting no further significant changes thereafter. The newborn infant responds normally to ACTH although this response is blunted during the first 24-36 hours of life [185]; reincreasing thereafter it is significantly higher in the first few months of life than later on for both cortisol [221], C_{21} precursors and Δ^5-androgens [226]. Despite a rapid post-natal fall, significant secretion of DHA and DHAS extends beyond the time of extensive fetal zone atrophy and is believed to persist in the border of the remaining fetal zone and permanent zone for several months [202].

Most adrenocorticosteroid hormone levels decline after birth. These changes are now rather well documented and summarized in Table VIII. The blood levels indicate that the neonate is well prepared to respond to the stress of birth and does not physiologically show a period of adrenal insufficiency. Cortisol is indeed the predominant glucocorticoid. However, there continues to be greater cortisol to cortisone conversion in the early neonatal period because of active 11-dehydrogenase activity in the neonate. The ratio cortisone to cortisol declines from 2-3 at birth to less than 0.7 only after the first month of life [300]. Cortisol metabolism is also different in the newborn [211, 316]: There is relative prominence of 6β-hydroxy-cortisol and immaturity of glycuronyl transferase activity. For the first 5 days of life, plasma levels of conjugated 17-hydroxysteroids (17-OHCS) are low and urinary excretion of 17-OHCS/m^2 of body surface area is lower than later in life; urinary 17-ketosteroids (17-KS) are

TABLE VIII. — Post-natal changes in mean levels of adrenocorticoid hormones

Age	P ng/dl	DOC μg/dl	B μg/dl	Aldo * ng/dl	S μg/dl	Cortisol μg/dl	Cortisone μg/dl	OHP ng/dl	DHAS μg/dl	DHA ng/dl	Δ⁴ ng/dl
Maternal vein .	12,000	0.29	3.6	37		54.8	6.1	1,100	60	363	249
Cord vein . .	27,100	0.63	1.1	250		7.0	13.8	3,300	133	649	90
2 h . . .	5,700	0.55	0.9	300		10.4	8.3	890			200
6 h . . .	4,600	0.30	0.28	350	0.82	2.8	7.5	400	140	920	150
24 h . . .	1,250	0.12	0.08	340	0.85	2.7	4.1	90			111
4 days . .	90	0.01	0.19	210	0.73	5.7	2.3	80- 94			40
7 days . .	50	0.005	0.05	87	0.66	3.5	2.2	91-115			36
2-4 weeks. .	5	0.002	0.03	64	0.39	7.5	2.3	80-138	27	287	34
2-5 years . .	5-10	<0.001	0.01	29	<0.5	10.5	<1	26	2.3	25	10
Conversion factor to SI units ×... =nmoles/l. .	0.0318	30.26	28.86	0.0277	28.86	27.6	27.74	0.0302	25.6	0.0347	0.0349

P = Progesterone; DOC = Deoxycorticosterone; B = Corticosterone; Aldo = Aldosterone (in supine position); S = 11-deoxycortisol; OHP = 17α-hydroxyprogesterone; Δ⁴ = Androstenedione
(Combined data from references [180, 221, 224, 292, 293, 300, 324, 325] and personal data).

elevated for the first 2-4 weeks of life up to 2 mg/24 h, declining to less than 2 mg after 1 month and remaining so until about 5 years of age.

Mineralocorticoid function

Three well-defined control mechanisms for aldosterone secretion exist: The renin-angiotensin system (RA), potassium and ACTH [207, 277]. The effect of ACTH is transient. The two other control mechanisms may be of equal importance. Potassium can directly modulate aldosterone secretion (negative feedback), independently of the RA system. The latter is the major system regulating extracellular fluid volume.

Renin and its substrate do not cross the placenta [333] and both are found in the fetal kidney. The RA-aldosterone system is very active in the newborn [211]. At birth, plasma renin activity (PRA) is very high [211, 307]. Neonatal plasma levels of aldosterone are also high and not related to gestational age [180, 211], but urinary excretion and secretion rates are low for the first week of life [349] suggesting a diminished MCR of aldosterone at this age. Fetal aldosterone secretion (as reflected by cord blood levels) is influenced by maternal sodium intake [180, 318, 349]. It is thus likely that the RA system plays a role in the sodium homeostasis of the neonate. Both PRA and aldosterone

(Table VIII) levels decrease progressively in early infancy. This inverse relationship between PRA and aldosterone levels observed with age [211, 307] is believed to reflect the increasing maturity of the proximal nephron with less dependence on distal tubular sodium reabsorptive function [331].

Premature infants frequently develop a transient hyponatraemia during the first two weeks of life apparently related to low sodium intake and excess natriuresis [317], recovering in association with increasing aldosterone production [242]. The sodium wastage in premature infants is likely due to increased superficial nephron perfusion with an inadequate compensatory RA-aldosterone system response [331] possibly associated with a relative insensitivity of the renal tubules to aldosterone [242].

OUTLINE
OF NORMAL SEXUAL DIFFERENTIATION

In normal clinical practice, sex is identified at birth according to the anatomy of the external genitalia of the newborn infant. Indeed, the neonate has already developed through a series of 4 ontogenic stages of sex development in an orderly fashion: (*a*) the genetic sex, as defined by the sex chromosome complement X or Y (chromosomal sex) and the sex-determining genes (genic sex); (*b*) structural and functional differentiation of the gonad (gonadal sex); (*c*) differentiation of the genital ducts and urogenital sinus into internal and external genitalia (somatic sex); (*d*) differentiation of the central nervous system (neuroendocrine sex). However, after birth sexual differentiation continues including the method of rearing (legal sex), the individual's own sexual identity (psychological sex), the development of secondary sex characteristics (phenotypic sex) and sexual comportment (behavioral sex).

As proposed by Jost 35 years ago and confirmed by numerous studies (see reviews in [223] and by Josso in [A]), fetal sexual differentiation is an asymmetrical process: male differentiation must be actively imposed by genetic, and subsequent endocrine mechanisms at "appropriate" critical periods of fetal development, whereas female differentiation of the genital structures is purely "passive".

Genetic sex is determined at the time of fertilization. The embryo's sexual genotype is of paramount importance in determining the sexual orientation of the primitive gonad. Testicular differentiation is governed by a testis organizing gene on the Y chromosome coding for the H-Y antigen, the function of which is controlled by regulatory gene(s) located on the X chromosome and possibly on autosomes. Differentiation of the primitive gonad into an ovary does not appear to be conditioned by the presence of two X chromosomes, but full differentiation requires the presence of a meiotic inducing substance, the genetic control of which is unknown. Absence of the second sex chromosome or genetic mosaicism leads to abnormal or no gonadal differentiation (various forms of gonadal dysgenesis). The testis differentiates rapidly and early in gestation (7-8 weeks) whereas ovarian organogenesis is delayed, slower and progressive (9-24th weeks).

Once differentiated, the fetal testis conditions all the male sex differentiation of the genital tract through the secretion and independent action of

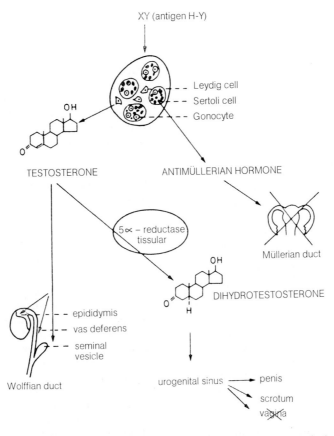

FIG. VI-34. — *Hormonal factors orienting the differentiation of the genital tract towards the male morphotype. Their absence or abnormal function results in a female morphotype.*
Adapted from Josso, in Ref. [A], p. 88, with permission.

two discrete substances, a glycoprotein, anti-Müllerian hormone (AMH) produced by the Sertoli cells, and testosterone produced by the fetal Leydig cells (Fig. VI-34). AMH ipsilaterally triggers the regression of the Müllerian ducts during a short period of development up to 8 weeks' gestation in the human. In the female, devoid of AMH secretion, Müllerian ducts further develop into tubes, uterus and the upper portion of the vagina.

Testosterone, directly or indirectly via its intracellular metabolism into dihydrotestosterone (DHT) in specific target cells, is responsible for the virilization of internal and external genitalia. Testosterone itself will "stabilize" the Wolffian ducts at a critical period, about the 8-9th week, when renal function has been taken over by the definitive kidney [297]. Afterwards, testosterone is no longer necessary for maintenance but is needed for subsequent differentiation into the male accessory organs, epididymis, vas deferens and seminal vesicles, which is achieved by 12 weeks. In the female Wolffian ducts disappear at 5-6 weeks except for residual structures. The action of testosterone on the stabilisation of the Wolffian duct requires high local testosterone concentrations and cannot be reproduced by systemic testosterone administration.

It is DHT and not testosterone which acts on the urogenital sinus to induce the formation of the male urethra, prostate, and to shape the urogenital tubercle and the genital swellings into glans, penile shaft and scrotum. Masculinization of external genitalia begins at about the 10th week (43-45 mm). Male phenotype, i. e. closing of the urethra on the shaft of the penis and fusion of the labio-scrotal swellings in the mid-line is largely accomplished by 12-14 weeks' gestation. After this period the urogenital sinus is no longer androgen-sensitive and labioscrotal fusion does not occur. Complete organogenesis of the penis, prostate and scrotum require an additional month. Further growth of the penis occurs until term.

Both DHT and testosterone exert their action by binding to a cytosolic receptor specified by an X-borne gene, transfer of the androgen-receptor complex to the nucleus where it interacts with chromatin on the target genome to activate gene transcription and increases specific protein synthesis [200]. Androgen-receptors and 5α-reductase activity are present in the female as well as in male primordia. Virilization in the male results from the higher circulating levels of testosterone which are concentrated and metabolized into target cells.

Subjects with ambiguous genitalia are classified according to the genetic sex whether or not the gonad is fully differentiated or functional. Male pseudo-hermaphroditism usually results from either inadequate testicular secretions (either testosterone or AMH, or both), deficiency in 5α-reductase activity, or qualitative or quantitative abnormalities in androgen receptors. Female pseudohermaphroditism results from the exposure to abnormally high levels of androgens in utero, most commonly due to abnormal fetal adrenal biosynthesis or less frequently to maternal transfer. In these genetic females, the ovary and the internal genitalia differentiate normally; Wolffian ducts are not maintained even in cases where it can be shown that the virilizing substance reached the fetus very early in gestation; the only abnormality lies in the virilization of the urogenital sinus to an extent which depends upon both the precocity and the intensity of the androgen exposure (see above).

DISORDERS OF THE ADRENAL IN THE NEONATAL PERIOD

Disordered adrenal function in the newborn results predominantly from adrenal hypofunction whereas adrenal hyperfunction is extremely rare in infancy. Decreased function (which includes hormonal secretion, metabolism and action) of the adrenal cortex may be complete or dissociated resulting in inadequate secretion of glucocorticoids, mineralocorticoids or both, associated or not with androgen over- or underproduction. The causes of hypoadrenalism, listed in Table IX, are numerous. Not all of them are seen in the newborn in whom the early expression of congenital defects is prominent.

ADRENOCORTICOHYPOFUNCTION
GENERAL ASPECTS

Adrenocorticoid hormones have numerous physiological functions amongst which metabolic and vascular effects are prominent [176, 244]. Accordingly, they are classified into 2 groups: gluco- and mineralocorticoids. However, the major natural glucocorticoid cortisol, has mild mineralocorticoid effect, whilst the more potent, mineralocorticoid, naturally secreted, aldosterone, has mild glucocorticoid effect. This dual action is observed for all natural hormones with a variable predominance of either effect. Corticosterone secretion rate is normally 1/10th that of cortisol. When secreted in larger quantities this compound exerts significant gluco-

TABLE IX. — Etiology of adrenal cortical hypofunction

Primary adrenal hypofunction

A. *Complete adrenocortical insufficiency* (decreased or absent production of glucocorticoids, mineralocorticoids and androgens):
  1. Congenital hypoplasia or aplasia of the adrenal gland
     — autosomal recessive
     — X-linked recessive
  2. Congenital adrenal hyperplasia due to defects in cholesterol 20-22 desmolase (lipoid adrenal hyperplasia)
  3. Adrenal necrosis following adrenal vein thrombosis, anticoagulant therapy, fulminating infections, or adrenal hemorrhage
  4. Chronic adrenal insufficiency: Addison's disease due to tuberculosis, syphilis, mycosis (blastomycosis, histoplasmosis, coccidiomycosis) or parasitoses
  5. Autoimmune adrenalitis (also named adrenocortical retraction or so-called idiopathic Addison's disease)
     — isolated
     — associated with multiple endocrinopathies (Schmidt's syndrome, Whitaker's syndrome, diabetes mellitus, hyperthyroidism) and/or vitiligo, pernicious anemia
  6. In the course of other chronic diseases
     — primary familial xanthomatosis (Wolman's syndrome)
     — adrenoleukodystrophy (Schilder's disease)
  7. Iatrogenic
     — surgical (bilateral adrenalectomy)
     — metabolic or toxic effect of drugs (antibiotics, antimitotics, synthetic inhibitors of the early steps in steroid biosynthesis, aminoglutethimide)

B. *Selective adrenocortical insufficiency in:*
  1. Gluco- and mineralocorticoids (increased androgens)
     — Congenital adrenal hyperplasia (CAH) due to deficiency in
       . Δ^4-3β-hydroxysteroid dehydrogenase-isomerase
       . 11β-hydroxylase (hypertensive form)
       . 21-hydroxylase (Debré-Fibiger syndrome)
     — Iatrogenic (drugs such as Danazol: pseudoadrenogenital syndrome)
  2. Glucocorticoids
     — isolated glucocorticoid deficiency (ACTH unresponsiveness)
     — respiratory distress syndrome?
  3. Mineralocorticoids
     — congenital deficiency in 18-hydroxylase or 18-hydroxysteroid dehydrogenase
     — end organ unresponsiveness to salt retaining hormone (pseudohypoaldosteronism)
  4. Androgen deficiency in 17-20 desmolase (lyase) dysfunction

Secondary to insufficient ACTH secretion due to

  1. Pituitary agenesis or destruction (anencephaly, congenital pituitary aplasia or hypoplasia, tumors)
  2. Isolated ACTH deficiency
  3. Hypopituitarism (idiopathic or associated with multiple malformations) (see Table II)
  4. Hypothalamic dysfunction: — primary hypothalamic defect, septooptic malformations
                              — malnutrition, anorexia nervosa
  5. Iatrogenic: — due to cessation of glucocorticoid therapy
                 — infants born to steroid treated mothers

---

and mineralo-activities resulting in suppression of both the ACTH and RA system, increased blood volume and hypertension. 11-Deoxycorticosterone (DOC), 11-deoxycortisol (compound S), 18-hydroxydeoxycorticosterone and 18-hydroxycortisone all have significant mineralocorticoid actions when present in large amount, but probably do not in physiological conditions because of their low secretion rates.

The fundamental role of mineralocorticoid hormones is to maintain sodium homeostasis by stimulating active sodium reabsorption and sodium-potassium transfer across the membranes of many epithelial tissues. The major site of action is the distal tubule of the renal nephron where they facilitate the reabsorption of sodium and the secretion of potassium [244]. Mineralocorticoids as well as the other classes of steroid hormones exert their action through specific receptor proteins in the target cells [200, 240, 334]. Understanding of the mechanism(s) of action of aldosterone or sodium transfer is still theoretical (see review in [A] and Chapter by Oh et al. in this volume).

Glucocorticoids play a key role in the homeostasis of glucose and in the body defense to stress. They stimulate gluconeogenesis and glycogenolysis, and increase protein and fatty acid catabolism. They also inhibit glycolysis in peripheral tissues. In all these actions, which are delayed a few hours before the steroid effect is manifest, they oppose the rapid action of insulin and glucagon. Glucocorticoids also increase blood pressure and glomerular filtration by facilitating catecholamine activity (enhancing the vasoconstrictive action of norepinephrine). The role of the adrenocortical response to stress is unclear, but *glucocorticoids alone have this effect*, and an increase in plasma cortisol is essential for man to withstand severe stress.

Whatever its cause, a deficiency in either mineralo- or glucocorticoids will give clinical manifestations that are highly similar: vasomotor collapse, apneic spells, seizure, inability to withstand stress, ketotic hypoglycemia, polyuria, anorexia, result from glucocorticoid deficiency: hyponatremia, urinary salt wasting, hyperkalemia, hypovolemia, extracellular dehydration, metabolic acidosis result from mineralocorticoid deficiency; however, hypotension, vomiting, dehydration, shock may result from either one or both.

TABLE X. — CAUSES OF ADRENAL HYPOFUNCTION IN THE NEWBORN IN DECREASING FREQUENCY

Prevalent cause
 — Congenital adrenal hyperplasia due to one of the 6 inborn defects of steroid biosynthesis

Rare but not uncommon
 — Iatrogenic, secondary to glucocorticoid therapy
 — Adrenal hemorrhage
 — Congenital adrenal hypoplasia
 — All causes of congenital hypopituitarism

Very rare
 — Pseudohypoaldosteronism
 — Congenital hypoaldosteronism (defect in last step of aldosterone biosynthesis)
 — Isolated glucocorticoid deficiency

Extremely rare
 — Isolated ACTH deficiency (2 cases)
 — Iatrogenic: pseudoadrenogenital syndrome (Danazol) (1 case)

The most common cause of adrenal hypofunction in the newborn infant is due to a defect in steroid biosynthesis (Table X). Whilst the normal adrenal gland does not play a role in normal sexual differentiation, an excessive production of adrenal androgens will masculinize a female fetus (see above). On the other hand, a number of enzymatic defects affecting the adrenal cortex also affect testicular steroidogenesis. In these conditions, deficient testosterone production results in incomplete masculinization of the male genitalia. Thus the various forms of congenital adrenal hyperplasia may be associated with the same range of ambiguity of the external genitalia in both sexes, although it is more commonly observed in females. A prompt and precise etiological diagnosis is essential for proper therapy but also for the proper choice of sex rearing, long-term outlook and genetic counselling.

CONGENITAL ADRENAL HYPERPLASIA (CAH)

Etiology and pathogenesis

The normal biosynthesis of adreno-corticosteroid hormones is depicted in Figure VI-35. Except for some enzyme activities (18-, 21- and 11-hydroxylase) the biosynthetic scheme is the same in the testis and the ovary. There are several forms of CAH, each caused by the deficiency of one of the enzymes necessary for the biosynthesis of cortisol (step 1 to 4 and 7 in Figure VI-35). All have been described. They all result in an inadequate cortisol production, thus in an overproduction of ACTH, and subsequently lead to hyperplasia of the adrenal glands. Deficiencies in all the enzymes involved in the biosynthesis of aldosterone (step 5, 6 in Figure VI-35) and androgens (steps 8, 9, 10 in Figure VI-35) are also known to exist. Because neither aldosterone nor androgens are involved in the negative feedback control of ACTH, these situations do not result in adrenal hyperplasia but in specific hormone deficient states: salt loosing state in both sexes in the first instance, male pseudo-hermaphroditism in genetic males in the second.

Congenital adrenal hyperplasias are inborn errors of steroid biosynthesis with autosomal recessive inheritance. Both sexes are affected. Because one is accustomed to think of CAH in term of 21-hydroxylase deficiency, a lack of knowledge of the other 4 types of CAH has probably led to underestimation of their frequency. We do not know the ultimate biochemical defect leading to decreased enzyme activities. The degree of deficiency is variable, although never complete, and a wide spectrum of clinical situations ensues. As a practical approach to understanding of the hormonal and clinical disturbances, all steroids below a given enzymatic

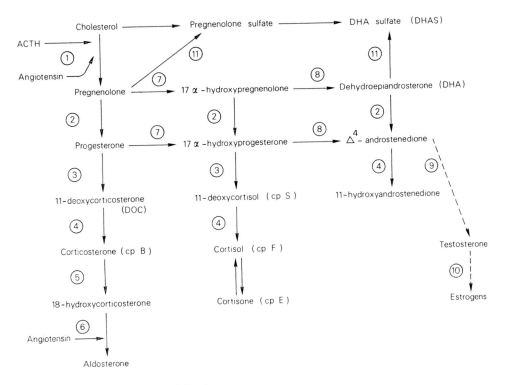

The figures inside the circles relate to the following enzymes:

1   Cholesterol side chain cleaving system (20-22 desmolase)
2   3β-hydroxysteroid dehydrogenase Δ^5-Δ^4 isomerase (3β-ol)
3   Steroid 21-hydroxylase
4   Steroid 11β-hydroxylase
5   Steroid 18-hydroxylase (corticosterone methyloxidase I)
6   18-hydroxysteroid dehydrogenase (corticosterone methyloxidase II)
7   Steroid 17α-hydroxylase
8   Steroid 17α,20-lyase (or desmolase)
9   17β-hydroxysteroid deshydrogenase (17-ketoreductase)
10 Aromatase
11 Sulphotransferase

cp for compound-old denomination
The dashed arrows represent minor enzyme activities in the normal adrenal gland, which may increase to a great extent in pathological conditions such as adrenal tumors.

FIG. VI-35. — *Simplified outline of adrenal steroid biosynthesis.*

block are reduced, while there is an overproduction of the steroids above the blocked step, as well as of steroids of other pathways depending on the site of blockade in steroidogenesis.

Deficiency in cholesterol side-chain cleavage enzyme activity. — This rare defect was first described as "lipoid adrenal hyperplasia" [296] because of a considerable lipid accumulation in both the adrenals and the gonads. The impaired transformation of

cholesterol to pregnenolone (step 1 in Figure VI-35) was originally attributed to a 20-22 desmolase deficiency. The entire side-chain cleavage of cholesterol—20α-hydroxylase, 22α-hydroxylase, and 20,22-desmolase—represents a series of enzyme reactions which may all be affected [252]. Because of the early site in steroid biosynthesis the inability to produce any class of steroids also applies to the gonads, and genetic males may present as phenotypic females. The syndrome is usually incompatible with life, but a few survivors have been reported [257]. The above biological pattern can be reproduced by aminoglutethimide, a drug which acts by inhibiting the desmolase system. Few hormonal studies have been made: urinary excretions of 17OHCS and 17KS or other metabolites are very low or undetectable, that of cholesterol elevated. In one surviving child detectable amounts of 17KS have led to the suggestion of a metabolic pathway of cholesterol to DHA, bypassing 22α-hydroxylation [257]. Differentiation of the enzyme defect from congenital adrenal hypoplasia can be made, when adrenal steroids are absent but gonadal steroids are normal.

3β-HSD deficiency (190). — The lack of 3β-HSD prevents the conversion of Δ^5 steroids to Δ^4 steroids, thus affecting glucosteroid, mineralosteroid and sex steroid pathways (step 2 in Figure VI-35). The defect is also present in testes [311] or ovaries [358]. This is the only form of CAH in which ambiguous genitalia are found in both male and female subjects. This results from two different pathogenic situations. In the male the 3β-HSD defect leads to inadequate testosterone production by the fetal testis and thus to incomplete masculinization of the genitalia. In the female, peripheral conversion of Δ^5 steroids to Δ^4 androgens is mediated by an intact hepatic 3β-HSD which is under a different genetic control than that of the adrenal and gonadal enzyme [190, 259, 311]. The excessive amounts of 17-hydroxypregnenolone and DHA, already produced in utero, are converted respectively into 17-hydroxyprogesterone and Δ^4-androstenedione, then to testosterone which eventually induces clitoral hypertrophy and slight labial fusion in genetic females. Normal 3β-HSD activity in the liver also explains the apparently paradoxical elevation of plasma 17-hydroxyprogesterone, Δ^4-androstenedione and testosterone which has been observed later in life [294] and might erroneously lead to the diagnosis of 21-hydroxylase deficiency [311]. All boys so far reported who have reached puberty developed gynecomastia: Failure to suppress the breast anlage in utero or high estrogen/androgen ratio via peripheral conversion of DHA to estrogens and insufficient testicular secretion of testosterone? This defect is also characterized by a greater accumulation of $C21-\Delta^5$ steroids (17-hydroxypregnenolone) than of $C19-\Delta^5$ steroids (DHA); this is believed to be due to substrate inhibition of the 17-20 desmolase enzyme [294, 303]. There are marked gradations in the severity of the enzyme defect, emphasizing the clinical heterogeneity in this syndrome. Classically incompatible with life [229], the syndrome may either be not apparent in females [190, 229, 358], or detected by

systematic endocrine studies in males with pseudohermaphroditism but no clinical salt loss [294]. The enzyme deficiency also appears to improve with increasing age [255, 311]. With improving means of diagnosis this enzyme defect does not appear to be as rare as was first believed [229, 294].

17α-hydroxylase deficiency (188). — This rare enzyme defect (only a score of reported cases) prevents the formation of any 17α-hydroxylated compounds, thus the formation of cortisol as well as the formation of all sex steroids, but does not affect the biosynthesis of mineralocorticoids (step 7 in Figure VI-35). The enzyme defect is also shared by the gonads; all males will present with pseudohermaphroditism, poor masculinization [335] to complete female phenotype [188]. Females do not have ambiguous genitalia but never develop sexually, despite increasing gonadotropin secretion at the age of puberty [220]. The most common feature of this enzyme defect is its late diagnosis, Indeed, except in ambiguous males, diagnosis is usually made at puberty (impuberism) or in adulthood, when hypertension with hypokalemic alkalosis complicates the disease. The production of 17-deoxysteroid C21 compounds such as pregnenolone, progesterone, DOC and corticosterone is greatly enhanced. Despite low cortisol levels, the patients do not have clinical glucocorticoid deficiency because the usually enormous rise in corticosterone compensates for the lack of cortisol, and is also able to keep ACTH levels in a not too far above normal range.

Aldosterone levels and PRA are subnormal or low, suggesting that salt, water retention and volume expansion is assumed by DOC which also suppresses the renin-angiotensin-aldosterone system. The very slow return to normal of aldosterone secretion, up to 6 months after initiation of glucocorticoid therapy [187], has erroneously been attributed to a combined defect in 18-hydroxylase [347]. Inhibition of the activity of the latter enzyme is potassium dependent [220], becoming reversible when potassium depletion is corrected [305].

11β-hydroxylase deficiency (217). — Referred to as the hypertensive form of CAH, it represents 3 to 7 % of the patients with CAH [271, 350]. This defect prevents the conversion of 11-deoxycortisol (compound S) to cortisol in the glucocorticoid pathway and that of DOC to corticosterone thus to aldosterone in the mineralocorticoid pathway (step 4 in Figure VI-35). DOC and compound S are thus markedly elevated, as are their urinary tetrahydro metabolites, THDOC and THS [A, 327, 357]. As the latter contains the 17,21-dihydroxy, 20-keto group reacting in the classical Porter and Silber reaction, it is measured in the 17-hydroxycorticosteroid (17-OHCS) assay. This is the only form of CAH in which urinary 17-OHCS are normal or elevated. The hormonal pattern described above is reproduced when metyrapone, an inhibitor of 11β-hydroxylation, is used in standard tests of adrenal function.

The androgen pathway is not affected. As a result of ACTH overstimulation, excessive production of androgens in fetal life leads to ambiguous genitalia in females but not in males. In both sexes, post-natal virilization progresses in the absence of proper therapy leading to pseudoprecocious puberty and advanced bone age. Because of the enzymatic block, Δ⁴-androstenedione is also deviated from its normal inactivation as 11β-hydroxyandrostenedione in the adrenals. Accumulation of Δ⁴-androstenedione provides increased substrate for its peripheral conversion to testosterone, the most potent androgen.

As discussed above, the overproduction of cortisol precursors explains the usual absence of clinical signs of glucocorticoid deficiency. Hypertension is an additional finding in many but not all patients [357] and often develops late in childhood. Hypertension and lack of salt wasting symptoms are thought to result from the excessive production of DOC, despite low corticosterone and aldosterone levels [A, 327]. A selective deficiency of the 11β-hydroxylation of the glucocorticoids in the fasciculata with normal 11β-hydroxylation of the mineralocorticoids in the glomerulosa [263] would explain a return to normal aldosterone secretion after instituting glucocorticoid replacement therapy. Clinical salt loss symptoms may however occur in two instances: in the newborn, when the dietary salt intake is too low for the infant's needs and the production of DOC not high enough, and at the time of instituting therapy [241, A].

21-hydroxylase deficiency (190, 271). — This is by far the commonest form of CAH, 80 to 90 % according to most series [A, 231, 350]. The prevalence apparently varies among populations, 1 : 11,000 to 1 : 40,000 live births in the United States, 1 : 5,000 in Switzerland and 1 : 282 in Yupik Eskimos [A, 289 *ter*]. The estimate of the gene frequency for heterozygocity in the european population is about 1 in 35 to 1 in 100.

A defect at this enzyme step blocks the conversion of progesterone to DOC, that of 17α-hydroxyprogesterone to 11-deoxycortisol (step 3 in Figure VI-35). Plasma and urinary cortisol and aldosterone as well as their metabolites are reduced. There is no accumulation of glucocorticoid precursors to compensate for the lack of cortisol, but a marked increase in progestagens, progesterone, 16α-hydroxyprogesterone, and above all of 17α-hydroxyprogesterone. The urinary metabolites of the latter, pregnanetriol and 11-ketopregnanetriol (pregnanetriolone) are markedly increased [245, 271] and measured in the ketogenic steroid (KGS) assay. In the normal newborn, because of the delay in glucuronidation (see above), this measurement underestimates the cortisol production (KGS are normally 1 mg/m²/24 h in the first 5 days of life or 2 to 6 mg/m²/24 h when corrected by gram of urinary creatinine). Later, in affected infants the measurement of urinary KGS and 17-ketosteroids (17KS) does not estimate cortisol production as it does normally because of the abnormally large contribution of 17-hydroxyprogesterone metabolites in the former and of androgens in the latter. In this disease the androgenic biosynthetic pathway is normal and the marked increase in their production results from an ACTH overdrive. As in the case of a defect in 11β-hydroxylase, female fetuses affected with 21-hydroxylase deficiency are virilized in utero but affected male fetuses have normal genitalia.

Virilization and salt-loss are the prominent features in this form of CAH. Because of the apparent great variability in the degree of severity of the enzyme deficiency a wide spectrum is seen both in the degree of virilization and salt-loss manifestations. It is classical to describe a simple virilizing form and a salt-wasting form of 21-hydroxylase deficiency. The existence of two isoenzymes controlling 21-hydroxylation in either the cortisol or the aldosterone pathway has been proposed [351]. The reality of 2 distinct biochemical defects remains however to be demonstrated and appears unlikely. Indeed, recent studies have emphasized the disturbances in the renin-angiotensin-aldosterone system which are found in over 90 % of the patients whether the salt-loosing state is clinically expressed or not. The modern concept is rather that of uniformity in the pathophysiological mechanisms, with variable expression. Despite a rise in PRA which is seen in all, but a few patients, aldosterone cannot be formed in adequate amounts or is lower than expected in regard to PRA levels; thus there is a diminished aldosterone/PRA ratio [A, 218, 254, 258, 337, 343] demonstrating the precariousness of the sodium homeostasis even in the absence of clinical symptoms. Precipitation from this "compensated" state to clinical salt loss can be seen at all ages, particularly in stress conditions. Several factors contribute to aggravate the salt-loss and to create a "vicious cycle". The rise in ACTH may dramatically increase the levels of progesterone, 17-hydroxy progesterone which competitively inhibit the actions of aldosterone in the kidney [A, 253], thus increasing the wastage of sodium. This in turn, via hypovolemia, stimulates the renin angiotensin system but aldosterone is not formed in a sufficient amount. In addition hypovolemia and angiotensin II stimulate ACTH secretion [243, 298, 308]; thus the increased production of the salidiuretic progestagens. The loop of the "vicious cycle" is closed.

In the newborn, delay in the clinical manifestation of severe salt loss is explained by the low MCR of aldosterone (see above) contributing to the maintenance of higher blood levels for a few days [180, 211, 258, 271, 318, 343, 349]. The classical improvement of the salt-wasting syndrome with age is only apparent. Improved sodium homeostasis results from both an increasing sodium dietary intake and a more efficient reabsorption of sodium and bicarbonate in the renal tubule with age [286], while aldosterone production does not change [218].

The allelic variant of CAH due to 21-hydroxylase deficiency, the so-called "late onset" form [272] is not a problem in the neonatal period, since it only becomes apparent later in life.

Clinical expression of the various forms of CAH

From the discussion of the physiopathogenic mechanisms in the various forms of CAH, it is evident that 2 types of clinical manifestation may be seen with variable association according to the different enzymatic blocks: virilization or abnormal development of the genitalia and salt-loss.

Aspects of genitalia at birth.

In the female. — Pseudohermaphroditism (FPH) is a major problem. Virilizing CAH is indeed by all odds the most frequent cause of FPH, and is pathognomonic of a defect in 21-hydroxylase deficiency in genetic females. The degree of abnormality in the external genitalia varies to a great extent. The classical grading in five stages (Prader stages [295]) is commonly used to describe the morphological state of intersexuality (Fig. VI-36). There is however no clearcut separation between the successive stages and assignment of a Prader stage (particulary between P-III and P-IV and P-IV and P-V) may be difficult [206] or might vary according to the observer. On the other hand, there is no correlation between the degree of hypertrophy of the clitoris and the extent of labioscrotal fusion (Fig. VI-37). Except for the site of opening of the vagina, the internal genitalia are completely normal. Pigmentation of the labioscrotal folds is usually seen (Fig. VI-37) reflecting the ACTH and accompanying MSH overproduction. The degree of virilization in 21-hydroxylase deficiency, is variable among patients and within the same family. Prader stages III-IV are the most frequently encountered situations

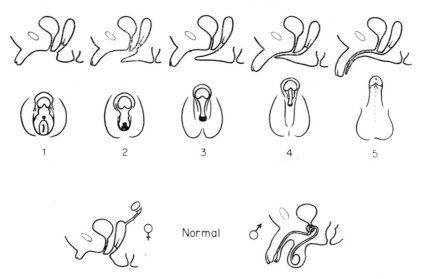

FIG. VI-36. — *Configuration of the genitalia in the various stages of masculinization seen in female pseudohermaphroditism caused by congenital adrenal hyperplasia (top). In stage 1 there is only an enlargement of the clitoris; in stages 2 to 4 there are various degrees of fusion of the labia majora with formation of a urogenital sinus. In stage 5, there is a penile urethra. Configuration in the normal male (right) and females (left) is shown in the bottom.* From PRADER, Ref. [295], with permission.

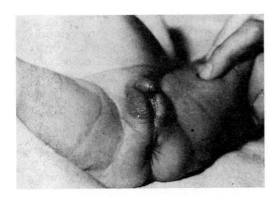

FIG. VI-37. — *Appearance of the external genitalia in a genetic female newborn with CAH due to 21-hydroxylase deficiency: female pseudohermaphroditism, stage 2 of Prader.* Note the marked pigmentation of the genitalia, and the large peno-clitoral organ but the mild posterior fusion of the labia majora.

(60-70 %) [206]. The masculinization may be so profound that a complete penile urethra mimicking the normal male phenotype may be observed (15 % in our series) [206]. The scrotum is however empty. Although, there is no correlation between the Prader stages and the severity of the enzyme block, stage V is more often seen in salt-losing patients. The ambiguity of the genitalia may also be completely ignored, and the correct diagnosis has been occasionaly made late in life in patients with male phenotype, cryptorchidism or infertility.

FPH is also a feature of 11β-hydroxylase deficiency. Usually this enzyme defect causes marked virilization. However, the occurence of mild forms with appearance of signs of virilization late in life but no FPH, is apparently more frequent than classically believed [198].

Few cases of 3β-HSD have been reported in female newborns in association with FPH. The degree of virilization is never pronounced and normal genitalia can also be seen with an evidently affected steroid biosynthesis [358].

External genitalia are normal in the last two forms of CAH (cholesterol side-chain cleavage and 17α-hydroxylase deficiencies) and virilization doesn't occur because of the impaired biosynthesis of the adrenal androgens.

In the male. — Male pseudohermaphroditism (MPH) is observed in the three variants of CAH in which the enzyme defect also involves testicular biosynthesis, *i. e.* the defects in cholesterol side chain cleavage; 17α-hydroxylase or 3β-HSD. The block in the first two enzymes is usually so severe that there is a complete lack of virilization and most genetic males present with a complete female

phenotype. In such patients flith 17α-hydroxylase defects, diagnosis is usually delayed until puberty because there is no salt loss and because the onset of hypertension is usually delayed or ignored until late in life [335].

MPH is a common feature in 3β-HSD deficiency. The degree of ambiguity of the external genitalia also varies among patients [303], between patients of the same family (Fig. VI-38), and is neither related

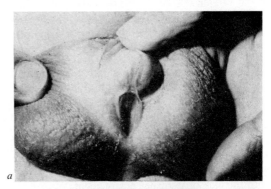

a

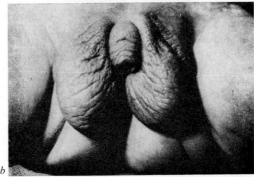

b

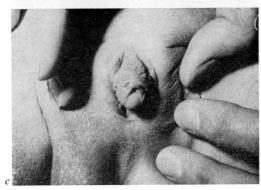

c

FIG. VI-38. — *Male pseudohermaphroditism in 3 patients with CAH due to 3β-HSD deficiency.*

Variations in clinical expression. Patients *a* and *b* were two brothers with severe neonatal salt loss and similar hormonal patterns; the lack of virilization is more pronounced in patient *a* than *b*; despite a mild enzyme defect, and no clinical salt loss, there is a markedly impaired virilization in patient *c*.

to the severity of the salt loss nor to the extent of the enzymatic block [294]. Because cryptorchidism is often associated, male infants with 3β-HSD may resemble the virilized female with 21-OH deficiency.

In all cases, testicular differentiation occurs normally. AMH is normally secreted thus there is a normal regression of the Müllerian ducts and no uterus. When a urogenital orifice is present, it ends in a prostatic utricle of variable size. Classification of the varying degree of "hypospadias" in stages 1 to 5, similar to that of Prader is usually made on the appearance of the external genitalia.

Signs of virilization are rather modest in the male newborn affected with either 11β- or 21-hydroxylase deficiency in whom sex differentiation is completely normal. In the severe forms with clinical salt loss, hyperpigmentation of the external genitalia is suggestive of the disease. In untreated subjects, signs of virilization develop further leading to pseudo-precocious puberty: Appearance of pubic hair, progressive penile enlargement, increased growth velocity and bone maturation, contrasting with the lack of testicular enlargement.

Salt-loss syndrome. — This is the name often used to describe the findings revealing adrenal insufficiency in the neonate. As discussed earlier, features of gluco- and mineralocorticoid insufficiency are both present but the latter predominate in the neonatal period. The affected newborn babies usually have poor appetite, excessive postnatal weight loss and failure to thrive. Acute adrenal crisis usually occurs at 5 to 8 days of life (see above for the pathogenesis). Vomiting, diarrhea, dehydratation are the major signs, often mistaken for pyloric stenosis. If not treated, cardiovascular collapse will occur. Cardiac arrest caused by hyperkalemia may be the cause of death. Disturbances in serum and urinary electrolytes are characteristic of adrenal insufficiency: Hyponatremia, hypernatriuria, low serum chloride and bicarbonate along with hyperkalemia. In contrast, pyloric stenosis leads to hypokalemic alkalosis with no salt wastage in the urine.

Infants of both sexes have an equal risk to present as an acute crisis, when affected with either one of the CAH forms except 17α-hydroxylase deficiency. However, as discussed above salt loss iss eldom seen or is transient in neonates with 11β-hydroxylase deficiency.

Diagnostic approach

CAH should be suspected in any newborn with ambiguous genitalia, presenting with a salt-losing

crisis, difficulties to thrive in the neonatal period or collapse under stress, i. e. during a surgical operation, in bilateral cryptorchidism and also in children coming from families where there is a history of unexplained sudden death in early infancy. The recognition of the condition is essential not only because of the life-saving effect of proper therapy but also because early and appropriate sex assignment is mandatory to permit appropriate sex rearing and gender identification.

The diagnostic approach should include the recognition of adrenal insufficiency, relating it to an inborn error in steroid biosynthesis, identifying the genetic sex, and establishing the anatomical status of the urogenital sinus.

(a) When suspected, the *diagnosis of adrenal insufficiency* is relatively easy to make, provided there is an appropriate choice of investigations and a proper knowledge of the methods used, together with a knowledge of the variations with age in the normal hormonal levels (Table VIII). Determination of serum and urinary electrolytes compared to the sodium intake will demonstrate the loss of sodium in the urine; the findings of high plasma renin activity together with low or inappropriately elevated aldosterone levels (decreased aldosterone/PRA ratio) will demonstrate that the salt loss is the result of mineralocorticoid insufficiency. One should remember that PRA levels are physiologically very elevated in the newborn and influenced by sodium intake and posture. Standard reference figures have been published [258, 343] but may vary between laboratories. Glucocorticoid insufficiency is best demonstrated by the rise in ACTH (and β-LPH) levels. Determination of the plasma level of cortisol is of little help for 2 reasons: they are often normal as the result of excessive endogenous ACTH stimulation; in most laboratories the methods routinely used to estimate "cortisol" are not specific (competitive binding assay using CBG, or radioimmunoassay using nonspecific antibodies both without prior purification): thus when cortisol precursors are markedly raised they are measured in addition to cortisol. The same applies to the measurement of urinary free cortisol levels.

(b) The diagnosis of the responsible adrenal enzyme deficiency is made on the study of androgens and of cortisol precursors in both the plasma and urine (see below).

(c) Genetic sex is identified by either buccal smear or blood karyotype. Because the former presents technical difficulties in early life, the latter

TABLE XI. — CLINICAL AND LABORATORY DATA
IN THE VARIOUS FORMS OF CONGENITAL ADRENAL HYPERPLASIA

| Enzyme deficiency | Ambiguous genitalia | | Salt loss | HTA | PRA | Prominent increase | | 17KS | 17-OHCS |
	Males	Females				Precursor	Metabolite		
Cholesterol desmolase	Yes	No	Yes	No	? ↗	None	None	∼ 0	∼ 0
3β-HSD	Yes	Yes	Yes	No	↗ ↗	17OH-Pregnenolone DHA	Pregnenetriol	↗	↘
17α-hydroxylase	Yes	No	No	Yes	↘	Progesterone, B	Pregnenediol	↗ ↗	↘ ↘
11β-hydroxylase	No	Yes	Rare transient	Yes	↘	DOC, cp S	THDOC, THS	↗	↗
21-hydroxylase	No	Yes	Yes variable	No	↗ ↗	OHP	Pdiol, Ptriol, Pregnanetriolone	↗ ↗	↘ ↘

HTA = hypertension; PRA = plasma renin activity; B = corticosterone; DOC = deoxycorticosterone; cp S = 11-deoxycortisol; OHP = 17α-hydroxyprogesterone; Pdiol = Pregnanediol; Ptriol = Pregnanetriol; TH = Tetrahydroderivative; 17KS = urinary 17-ketosteroids; 17-OHCS = urinary 17-hydroxysteroids (Porter Silber).

is prefered for an unequivocal answer, and also because of its usefulness in differential diagnosis.

(*d*) In infants with ambiguous genitalia *genitography* [251] associated or not with cystography should be performed to establish the exact anatomical connections between the urethra and the opening of either the vagina or the prostatic utricle. This is a necessary step prior to adequate plastic surgery.

Etiological diagnosis

Establishing a precise etiological diagnosis has implications for the supervision of treatment, but also for correct sex assignment and genetic counselling (see below). Diagnosis of the given enzymatic block is oriented by typical associations in the clinical findings but is fully established only on characteristic hormonal abnormalities, which are summarized in Table XI.

Diagnosis should be made before any hormonal therapy which, once instituted, is given for life. In case of severe salt loss, the child should be infused with saline only (1 g of NaCl/kg of body weight per day) for the period of time necessary to obtain biological samplings (blood and 24 hour urine collection). This approach will take care of the immediate problem of the salt loss, and because salt supplementation does not interfere with steroid biosynthesis, it will allow some time for etiological diagnosis.

In current practice, determination of the usual urinary metabolites and that of the plasma concentrations of ACTH, PRA, aldosterone, 17α-hydroxyprogesterone, Δ⁴-androstenedione, testosterone, DHA and DHAS will permit a positive diagnosis of adrenal insufficiency and detect the site of the enzymatic defect.

The levels of 17α-hydroxyprogesterone (OHP) have a fundamental orienting value [225]. When OHP is drastically elevated (more than 10,000 ng/dl or 300 nmoles/l) it is practically diagnostic of a 21-hydroxylase deficiency (the most frequent one). Levels of OHP are abnormal but usually less elevated (1,000-3,500 ng/dl or 30-100 nmoles/l) in 11β-hydroxylase deficiency (where Δ⁴-androstenedione levels are also very high and are always more elevated than that of OHP in our experience) and in 3β-OHD (in which the concomitant rise in DHA and DHA-S is then diagnostic). In the two latter enzymatic defects etiological diagnosis will be established by the respective determinations of the plasma levels of compound S or of 17α-hydroxypregnenolone [294]. Urinary metabolites are also of help in the diagnosis (Table IX).

One should be aware of the fact that hormonal, abnormalities may be *quantitatively* very modest during the first days of life even in the case of 21-hydroxylase deficiency. This situation is most often encountered in newborns with intersex problems but no salt loss and sometimes in those born after cesarean section. Close surveillance in a specialized ward, and repeated hormonal testing are recommended. On occasion, an ACTH stimulation test may be necessary for a definite etiological diagnosis but it should be made under saline infusion because of a risk of precipitating the child into an acute crisis of adrenal insufficiency. Two protocols for ACTH stimulation are currently used: A *short stimulation test* consisting of the injection flush of 0.25 mg of synthetic $ACTH_{1-24}$ (Synacthen) and blood sampling 5' or 15', 30' and 60' later; or *a long stimulation test* consisting of six IM injections of 0.5 mg/m² of depot Synacthen at 12 h intervals, daily urine collections and a single blood sampling 12 h after the last injection. Exogenous ACTH stimulation amplifies the biosynthetic hormone abnormalities and usually gives a definite answer. It also has some implications for the differential diagnosis (see below).

Determination of testosterone levels confirms the fetal origin of virilization and is helpful for differentiating it from the other causes of sexual ambiguity. The determination of the plasma levels of pregnenolone, 17α-hydroxypregnenolone or pregnenolone sulfate, also very useful for the etiological diagnosis of 3β-OHD, is not routinely available but can be obtained later. The estimation of progesterone and corticosterone levels is important for the recognition of 17α-hydroxylase deficiency. This diagnosis, rarely seen in the neonatal period in a genetic male with ambiguous genitalia but no salt-loss, should be considered last, after exclusion of all the other causes of CAH.

Whether or not presenting evident symptoms, a newborn from a family in which a previous sibling is affected with CAH due to any enzymatic defect should be tested, but the investigations kept to the essential minimum. Only the hormone characteristic of the given enzymatic defect should be measured because the occurence of two discrete enzyme defects has not yet been observed in the same family.

Differential diagnosis

From a practical stand point the problem is that of ambiguous genitalia not associated with salt loss or that of salt-loss not associated with intersex.

Indeed, the association of ambiguous genitalia with salt losing symptoms is only encountered in CAH.

Differential diagnosis of intersex. — Because a genetic male may present a complete female phenotype and vice versa, the presence of ambiguous genitalia is not the only condition in which abnormal sex differentiation might occur. This is why the precise determination of the genetic sex is mandatory.

(*i*) *The buccal smear is positive and the karyotype is 46,XX in all instances of female pseudohermaphroditism* (FHP), the various causes of which are detailed in Table XII. This represents the most easily diagnosed condition. The most frequent cause of sexual ambiguity is fetal virilization in utero by its own adrenal androgens. The diagnosis of CAH is made by the hormonal studies described above. A fetal adrenal tumor is exceptional.

When hormonal studies reveal normal plasma levels, a maternal source of androgen hyperproduction is then suspected. The proof is obtained by hormonal studies in the mother which, however, are informative only during the few days post partum in the case of a luteoma of pregnancy or Krukenberg's tumor. Indeed the androgenic production of these ovarian tumors decreases very rapidly with the withdrawal of placental hCG. An iatrogenic cause can be discovered by careful history. Despite the report of about a hundred cases of in utero virilization of a feminine fetus due to maternal ingestion of progestins, androgens or other drugs during pregnancy (Table XII), the direct pathogenic relationship is variable and is questioned for some compounds. Iatrogenic FPH is however increasingly rare since the administration of all the above drugs is nowadays theoretically prohibited in pregnant women. Hormonal levels will be normal in both the mother and the child. Diagnosis of the various causes of "malformative" FPH is based on the association of typical malformations (Table XII). Again hormonal studies will be normal.

Because it is extremely rare, the diagnosis of idiopathic FPH is accepted only after careful studies including an ACTH-stimulation test.

In all etiologies of FPH, the degree of virilization may vary considerably. A complete male phenotype in a genetic female is not exclusively due to virilizing CAH (stage V of Prader). This situation has been observed in FPH due to maternal adrenal tumor or in iatrogenic FPH. Therefore an early and precise etiological diagnosis is of paramount importance in any newborn with apparently normal male genitalia but no palpable gonads. Echography or laparo-

TABLE XII. — Etiology of female pseudo-hermaphroditism (FPH)

A. *Androgen-dependent*

1. *Fetal androgens*
   a) Inborn errors of cortisol biosynthesis (CAH, cf. Table XI)
   b) Other causes: — adrenal adenoma
   — congenital nodular adrenal hyperplasia

2. *Maternal androgens*
   a) Preexistant maternal ovarian or adrenal tumor
   b) Krukenberg tumor (ovarian metastasis, carcinoma of the digestive tract, hCG-dependent)
   c) Luteoma of pregnancy (hyperplasia of thecal cells, benign and regressive)

3. *Iatrogenic*
   a) Maternal therapy (from early in gestation on) with:
   — progestins (norethynodrel, norethindrone, 17α-ethinyl testosterone, 19 nor-17α-ethinyl testosterone, medroxy-progesterone, Danazol [197], (OPH or P?)
   — aminoglutethimide
   b) Accidental maternal ingestion of testosterone

B. *Non-endocrine disturbances*

1. *Part of dysmorphic syndromes of:*
   — Seckel (dwarfism and microcephaly)
   — Silver-Russel (in utero dwarfism; asymetrical development)
   — Robert (phocomelia, cleft palate)
   — Zellweger (cerebro-hepato-renal)
   — Beckwith (macroglossia, exomphalos)
   — Donohue (leprechaunism)
   — Beradinelli (lipodystrophy)
   — Meldenhall (acanthosis, insulin resistance)

2. *Associated with abnormal renal and cloacal development*

C. *Unexplained or idiopathic* (very rare): increased androgen sensitivity?

D. *Pseudo-FPH*

1. Enlargement of the clitoris due to local lesions in neurofibromatosis (Recklinghausen disease) or due to lipoma or haemangioma, cysts [270]

2. Prominent clitoris, appearing falsely enlarged because of the underdevelopment (premature) or hypoplasia (pterigium syndrome) of the labia

3. Labial adhesions (occasionally familial) usually seen in children and not in neonates

---

tomy, will confirm the presence of female internal genitalia which are then normal, as in any case of FPH.

(ii) Buccal smear is negative and the karyotype is 46, XY in all cases of male pseudohermaphroditism (MPH). — In practice, this is the most frequent differential diagnosis to make in newborns presenting ambiguous genitalia, but no palpable gonads and no particular clinical symptoms (the most frequently encountered situation during the first week of life in all etiologies of CAH). When the karyotype reveals a male genotype, all other causes of MPH must be excluded (Table XIII). Two testes are present (often cryptorchid orun descended), the aspect of external genitalia is variable and the etiological diagnosis is made by identifying the factor responsible (Table XIII). The differential diagnosis may be difficult with an enzyme deficiency in the last two steps

of testosterone biosynthesis, *i. e.* a deficit in either 17,20-desmolase (step 8 in Figure VI-35) or 17-keto-reductase (step 9 in Figure VI-35). In the latter, ACTH and cortisol biosynthesis are normal as are salt and water homeostasis. However, a defect in 17,20-desmolase affects adrenal androgen biosynthesis and causes an accumulation in progestagens (OHP in particular) which may be misleading. Diagnosis of such an enzymatic defect is made on the concomitant and marked decrease in all adrenal and testicular androgens under basal conditions and the amplification of these inverse abnormalities following ACTH and hCG stimulation [224 *bis*]. The eventuality of a defect in 17-keto-reductase is occasionally suspected in the neonate. The natural history of this disease is such that the diagnosis is practically made on clinical grounds, but is delayed (a female phenotype at birth, intense virilization at puberty) and then easily confirmed by the findings

TABLE XIII. — Etiology and differential diagnosis in male pseudo-hermaphroditism (MPH)

Cause	External genitalia	Clue to diagnosis
1) Selective Leydig cell hypoplasia (absence of LH-receptors likely)	Feminine or slight clitoral hypertrophy	No response at all to hCG stimulation, high LH, normal FSH. Absence of Leydig cell. No Müllerian structures
2) Inborn errors in testicular biosynthesis (*)		
— 17,20-desmolase (lyase)	Hypospadias	OHP $\nearrow$; all androgens $\searrow$
— 17β-hydroxysteroid dehydrogenase (17-keto-reductase)	Feminine or slightly virilized	T $\pm$ N; androstenedione and estrone $\nearrow\nearrow$, LH $\pm \nearrow$. Profound virilization at puberty
— other enzymes involved in cortisol biosynthesis:	Variable	Cf. Table XI
3) Abnormal testosterone metabolism: deficit in 5α-reductase (**)	Various degrees of hypospadias. Bifid scrotum	$\nearrow$ T/DHT ratio; small prostate; spermatogenesis may be normal
4) Androgen insensitivity syndrome (**) (syndrome of Morris; feminizing testis):		Normal response to hCG test
— complete	Completely feminine	Androgen receptors absent
— incomplete	Varying degree of masculinisation	Androgen receptors decreased or abnormal. Virilization may progress at puberty
5) Persistent Müllerian structures (**): abnormal secretion or action of AMH (hernia uteri inguinale)	Normal masculine	Casual discovery at surgery for either cryptorchidism or hernia inguinalis in which a uterus and Fallopian tubes are found. Normal response to hCG.
6) Iatrogenic	Hypospadias	Maternal progestagen therapy during pregnancy
7) Associated with a large number of dysmorphic syndromes among which are:	Hypospadias	Frequent cryptorchidism associated with:
— Opitz syndrome		— hypertelorism
— Meckel syndrome		— encephalocoele; cleft palate, microphthalmia
— Smith-Lemli-Opitz syndrome		— microcephaly, cleft palate
— brachio-skeletal-genital syndrome		In all cases the cause of incomplete virilisation is unknown
8) Associated with: — renal abnormalities — Wilm's tumour	Hypospadias	Anatomopathological studies

Familial, autosomal recessive (*); X-linked (**). A vagina of variable size is seen in most degrees of hypospadias; there is no uterus except in 5 and there is normal development of Wölffian ducts except in 4.

of subnormal T levels, high LH, and very high levels of Δ^4-androstenedione (greater than that of T) further increasing after hCG stimulation but not suppressible by dexamethasone.

(iii) Buccal smear is of limited value when abnormal gonadal differentiation is the cause of an intersex problem. — One should not be satisfied with the findings of a positive buccal smear, the presence of a uterus and/or a vagina at genitography or echography and repeat hormonal studies which have been normal at first testing. Diagnosis relies on karyotype analysis of blood lymphocytes, skin fibroblasts and both gonads, on histo-pathological examination of the gonads and morphological study of the internal genitalia (Table XIV). Laparotomy is preferred to cœlioscopy in the newborn for gonadal biopsy and eventual castration.

TABLE XIV. — DIFFERENTIAL DIAGNOSIS OF ABNORMAL GONADAL DIFFERENTIATION

	Karyotype	External genitalia	Müllerian ducts (vagina-uterus)	Wölffian ducts	Gonads	Risk of neoplasia ***
True hermaphroditism	46, XX (60 %) 46, XX/46, XY or 46, XY	Ambiguous	Usually present	Variable	Testis **/ ovary ovotestis × 2 ovotestis + ovary or testis	Occasional
Pure gonadal dysgenesis or Swyer syndrome *	46, XY	Feminine	Present	Absent	Streak + streak	High
Turner's syndrome	45, XO or 45, XO plus 45, XO/46, XY	Feminine rarely ambiguous	Present	Absent	Streak + streak	Very rare except if Y present
Mixed gonadal dysgenesis associated or not with autosomal abnormalities	46, XY/45, XO or various mosaics trisomy (13, 18)	Ambiguous and asymetric	Present	Variable	Streak + testis ** Tumor + testis	High
Testicular regression — early in utero (agonadism)	46, XY	Feminine to ambiguous	± present	Variable	Absent	None
— later in utero (rudimentary testis)		Micropenis	Absent	Under-developed	Rudimentary	Unknown
— after birth (vanishing testis)		Masculine	Absent	Present	Absent	None
XX males	46, XX	Masculine or hypospadias	Absent	Present	Testis + testis **	That of cryptorchidism
Klinefelter syndrome	47, XXY and various mosaics	Masculine rare hypospadias	Absent	Present	Testis + testis	Low

* Often familial, probably X-linked recessive; ** Frequently undescended; *** Most commonly benign gonadoblastoma or malignant dysgerminoma.

Differential diagnosis of a salt-losing state. — There are many causes of impaired salt homeostasis in the neonate or the infant (Table XIV). CAH is responsible in about two thirds of the cases. Whatever the cause of the urinary sodium wastage, there is an increase in PRA. Diagnosis of primary hypoaldosteronism (in which aldosterone levels are low and OHP levels normal) is indicated by the plasma ACTH levels before any treatment: They are normal in isolated hypoaldosteronism, elevated in any cause of complete adrenocortical hypofunction (see also below).

The findings of paradoxically high levels of aldosterone but normal ACTH, OHP and cortisol levels are suggestive of pseudo-hypoaldosteronism [285] (see below for more details). The rise in aldosterone is relatively proportional to that of PRA in other causes of salt loss when the renin-aldosterone axis is normal. Careful clinical, biochemical [333] and radiological (pyelogram) studies will permit recognition of a morphological or structural abnormality of the kidney or the urinary tract.

Measurements of urinary and plasma potassium help to distinguish endocrine and renal causes of salt

TABLE XV. — Etiology of salt-losing states

1. *Adrenal:* All causes of primary adrenal insufficiency (complete or selective in mineralocorticoids) (cf. Table IX)
2. *Renal*
   — Structural underdevelopment of the kidney (dysplasia)
   — Obstructive uropathy (urethral valves)
   — Renal tubular disease (cystinosis is the most frequent)
   — Bartter's syndrome
3. *Pseudohypoaldosteronism*
4. *Inappropriate secretion of antidiuretic hormone* (ADH), in association with:
   — Birth injury
   — CNS disease, head injury, meningitis, brain tumors
   — Respiratory disorders
   — Secondary to drug administration (opiates, carbazepine, vincristine)
5. *Part of osmotic diuresis* (diabetes mellitus)
6. *Iatrogenic:* Diuretic administration (therapeutic or accidental)

loss. Tubular sodium loss is characterized by concomitant hypokalaemia and urinary potassium loss. Renal tubular diseases may be associated with and secondary to hyperaldosteronism (see for more details the chapters by Guignard and Torrado and by Oh et al.). The presence of amino-aciduria, proteinuria, glycosuria, phosphaturia and disturbances in acid-base homeostasis are typical features of a Fanconi syndrome (most commonly due to cystinosis). However, some of these abnormalities may also be observed in renal dysplasia or in Bartter's syndrome.

Hypokalaemia (~ 2 mEq/l) and hyperkaliuria are particularly impressive in Bartter's syndrome, associating hyponatremia, hypochloremic alkalosis and juxtaglomerular cell hyperplasia. Clinical features, consisting of failure to thrive, marked growth failure, mental retardation, repeated episodes of dehydratation, vomiting, constipation, may be observed from early in infancy. The disease is however more commonly suspected by the end of the first year of life. A typical facies and familial incidence have been described. The rise in aldosterone levels is usually less than expected in comparison to that of PRA. Blood pressure is consistently normal, but a deficiency in magnesium, abnormal electrolyte transport in red cells and muscles, hypercalciuria, nephrocalcinosis, rickets and progressive renal failure complicate the natural history of this disease. The precise pathogenesis is not understood: arterial unresponsiveness to the vasoconstric-

tive action of renin resulting in a decrease in effective blood volume responsible for increased renin secretion with secondary hyperaldosteronism, or a defect in chloride reabsorption in the ascending portion of the loop of Henlé where it is normally reabsorbed passively together with sodium and potassium have been proposed as alternate hypotheses. More recently it has been thought that an excess production of prostaglandins (known vasodilatory and natriuretic agents) in the reno-medullary cells of the kidney was responsible for the renal tubular abnormalities and this concept has revolutionized the treatment of this disease. Dissociation between clinical and biochemical results and the findings of increased bradykinin plasma levels have thrown some doubt on the excess prostaglandin production being the primary cause of the disease. The current hypothesis is that a vasoactive hormonal imbalance, with a hyperfunctioning of the medullo-surrenal sympathetic system has a role in this syndrome [266 *bis*].

Nevertheless, the only current effective therapeutic management is to utilize prostaglandin synthetase inhibitors (indomethacin) which suppress PRA, plasma aldosterone, bradykinin, catecholamines and more variably decrease urinary prostaglandins and improve potassium loss and clinical signs. Potassium supplementation remains necessary. Unfortunately, this treatment is not always successful [211 *bis*], nor well tolerated (peptic ulceration).

Transient hyponatraemia due to a transient hypoaldosteronism state which may be observed in the neonatal period (most commonly in premature infants) is generally of an earlier onset than in infants affected with CAH. Its pathogenesis has been discussed above, in the physiology section. Except for a relatively increased activity of the renin-angiotensinaldosterone axis [242] there are no endocrine abnormalities. Its management simply requires salt supplementation for a few days.

There is a situation where a clear diagnosis may be difficult: in premature newborns with respiratory distress, elevated OHP levels, low cortisol levels and salt wastage may be observed. Stressful conditions are suspected on clinical grounds and because of moderately elevated ACTH levels. Also plasma OHP levels usually do not rise above 1,000 ng/dl (30 nmoles/l) [280 *bis*]. Repetition of hormonal studies are necessary to eliminate a still clinically asymptomatic or a mild form of CAH [293 *bis*].

Treatment

This has two components: reinstituting normal hormonal balance (substitutive therapy) and correcting the ambiguity of the genitalia when present.

Management of an intersex problem. — This should be recognized at birth by careful clinical examination: aspects and/or pigmentation of the external genitalia, presence or not of intra-scrotal testis in a newborn with complete male phenotype. In any situation where a sexual ambiguity is suspected, *sex assignment must be postponed untill the precise diagnosis is established* (this is perfectly legal in many countries). Indeed, it is both laborious and stressfull for the parents to go through the administrative procedure of changing legal sex. On the other hand, such situations are always extremely difficult for the parents. Their "psychological trauma" is undoubtly influenced by the first declarations of the physicians. They will better understand that the real sex is not evident because of hormonal problems during pregnancy than to have to accept that the first medical assignment of sex was wrong or to cope with the statement that the child is neither a boy nor a girl which is too often abruptly made. Once the decision of sex is finally made, the family should be informed of the practical consequences, of the reasons for and timetable of the surgical steps and of the reproductive potential of their child. Hormonal treatment should be explained. One should keep in mind that from the very first day on, parents need continuous psychological support.

In the most frequent eventuality of CAH due to either 11β-hydroxylase or 21-hydroxylase deficiency, only girls present a sexual ambiguity. The current possibilities of plastic surgery lead to satisfactory results in the forms II to IV of Prader. This is why, once the diagnosis is made, the assignment of female sex should no longer be delayed. The parents must then be given clearcut explanations, that is to say that the baby is indeed a girl with normal ovaries and uterus, and a normal reproductive future, providing she undergoes surgical correction and life long hormonal treatment.

In the attempt to insure a more complete sexual function, clitoridoplasty is now preferred to clitoridectomy but cannot be performed satisfactorily before 6-12 months of age. Perineoplasty and vaginoplasty are usually done at the same time. The pediatric urologist is best competent to decide when to undertake these surgical procedures at the earliest time possible. This will decrease the frequency of urinary infections which often complicate the disease, and the correction of the external genitalia to a female appearance will assure the parents of the sex identity of their daughter. A definitive vaginoplasty remains however often necessary and is best done at the time of puberty. The form V of Prader is still a major problem: Theoretically the only logical attitude would be to conform the

child to the female sex by surgical correction of the external genitalia. But the latter is extremely difficult. There is often no vaginal opening and plastic surgery may be hampered by a high risk of compromising urethral function. This is why male sex assignment may be more reasonable: In this case, male urethral function is always normal but castration and hysterectomy will be necessary. These relatively easy surgical procedures may however be delayed until puberty, but fertility is definitively sacrificed.

Genetic females affected with 3β-OHD are usually slightly virilized and surgical repair is not too difficult. Management will be as explained above.

In genetic males affected with either 3β-OHD, 17α-hydroxylase deficiency or the more exceptional defect in 20-22 desmolase, the ambiguity of the genitalia is often a major problem. A judicious choice of the sex of rearing should be guided, as in any other cause of MPH, by the anatomy of the genitalia and of the urethra; by the estimation of the sexual functional possibilities in adulthood and not by the presence of testis and/or of a Y-chromosome. When the urethral opening is in a perineal position and the phallus so small that any surgical repair will obviously be laborious and bound to fail, the presence of a vaginal cavity is an additional reason for orienting the child to the female sex, despite the certain loss of fertility. Castration and vaginoplasty need to be performed before puberty. On the other hand, when reconstructive surgery of the phallus and male urethra seems feasible (in 3β-OHD, but only rarely in 17α-hydroxylase deficiency), male sex assignment appears a rational choice, because androgen receptivity is normal and because testicular biosynthesis of testosterone seems to improve with age [215, 311].

In any case, it is mandatory not to undertake any surgical procedure without appropriate hormone treatment (see below).

Substitutive hormonal therapy.

(*i*) *Adrenal insufficiency.* — Whatever the etiology of CAH, the therapeutic scheme is similar: administration of glucocorticoid and mineralocorticoid hormones together with salt supplements when needed. Natural glucocorticoid hormones are prefered to synthetic glucocorticoids such as dexamethasone or prednisone. Cortisol (hydrocortisone) is given orally at physiological dosages (*i.e.* 15-20 mg/m² per day, divided into three doses equally spaced). Cortisone is also used, a slightly higher dosage being required (18-30 mg/m²/day). In contrast, the synthetic compound, 9α-fluorohydroxycortisone

(Florinef, Fluorocortisone) is the mineralocorticoid of choice. The daily requirement is about 100 $\mu g/m^2$ (in 2 oral doses). Mineralocorticoid treatment is effective only when salt intake is sufficient. This is why salt supplementation (1 to 2 g per day of sodium chloride) is given to newborns whose dietetic salt intake is usually low. Salt supplements are no longer required in children or adults. Treatment should start as soon as the diagnosis is firmly established and will be continued orally except in the case of vomiting, intercurrent illness or stress. Cortisol should then be administered intramuscularly and the dose doubled or tripled. The aim of the treatment described above, *maintenance therapy*, is to restore physiological levels of cortisol, to suppress ACTH oversecretion and androgen hyperproduction to normal levels, and to maintain salt homeostasis. It is therefore necessary to adjust the therapeutic dosages to each individual's needs and to avoid overtreatment as well as undertreatment. The former will induce overweight, hypertension, growth failure but normal bone maturation and eventually lead to iatrogenic adrenal atrophy, while the latter will be responsible for failure to thrive, hypotension, dehydration, excessive growth rate and accelerated bone maturation. Brusque oscillations between over- and undertreatment should also be avoided because both situations may have tragic consequences and both contribute to growth abnormalities and to ultimate short stature which is a major long-term concern in the treatment of these diseases. Optimal control remains difficult to achieve and in practice such treatments cannot be assumed properly without the long-term assistance of a specialized laboratory and the advice of an experienced pediatric endocrinologist.

The control of treatment includes both clinical and laboratory assessments. The general scheme is to estimate weight, height and blood pressure every 3 months until age two, then every 6 months, and bone maturation twice a year. Hormonal studies can be made at the same times, but must also be repeated 2-4 weeks after any therapeutic alteration.

The urinary excretions of 17-CS, KGS, pregnanediol or pregnanetriol have for long been the only laboratory criteria used. In addition to the difficulties of an accurate urine collection in newborns, these techniques include the measurement of the metabolites of the drug (cortisol or cortisone) administered. Moreover, they cannot give any clue to a selective need for either mineralocorticoid or glucocorticoid hormones. Preference is nowadays given to the measurement of more specific blood parameters.

The efficiency of the mineralocorticoid treatment is, in all etiologies of CAH, assessed by measuring PRA. As long as PRA is not brought back to the limits of normal, there is undertreatment. Recognition of a slight mineralocorticoid over treatment may be more difficult. The ratio of PRA/aldosterone and a decreased kalemia may be indicative. Overt overtreatment leads to hypertension.

The adequacy of the glucocorticoid treatment is followed by different parameters according to the etiology of CAH. In patients, with 21-OH hydroxylase deficiency, the determination of the plasma levels of ACTH, OHP and adrenal androgens is helpful. The time of blood sampling is important in interpreting the results, because of the large circadian diurnal variations of all these hormones [225, 310]. Plasma levels of OHP are best at 8.00 and 16.00 hrs. A level less than 100 ng/dl (3 nmoles/l) together with a loss of circadian variation is indicative of overtreatment. When the morning level of OHP is above 800 ng/dl (25 nmol/l) there is undertreatment. For some authors, the plasma levels of Δ^4-androstenedione (maintained to less than 50 ng/dl or 2 nmoles/l) best reflect the state of adrenal activity [117, 289 *bis*], but until puberty they are in good correlation with OHP levels [293 *bis*]. The best indicator of androgenic exposure, hence of the risk of accelerated bone maturation is still, in girls at any age and in prepubertal boys, the measurement of the plasma levels of testosterone, although they are poorly correlated with that of OHP. Plasma testosterone should be less than 15 ng/dl (0.5 nmol/l) before age 10, less than 30 ng/dl (1 nmol/l) thereafter. Finally plasma OHP and ACTH levels and PRA are highly correlated [243]. The determination of DHA or DHAS is of no help in the therapeutic control of children with 21-hydroxylase deficiency because their blood levels are usually drastically lowered as soon therapy is instituted, even in well-controlled situations. In contrast, in patients with 3β-OHD, DHA/DHAS are the blood parameters of choice to follow glucocorticoid therapy. The latter can be controlled by the measurement of the plasma levels of both compound S and Δ^4-androstenedione in patients with 11β-hydroxylase deficiency and by that of corticosterone in 17α-hydroxylase deficiency.

When the patient does not appear well controlled on clinical and biological grounds, the treatment should be modified without delay, but the following basic principles must be adhered to: First, only one of the two therapeutic components (mineralo- or glucocorticoid) is changed at any one time (to be able to judge the specific effect). Second, salt loss must be corrected (*i. e.* PRA should be brought back to normal) *before* deciding to increase the dosage of glucocorticoid even if the latter seems needed. This brings us back to the concept (discussed above) of one or two forms (pure virilizing form, salt losing form) of CAH due to 21-OH deficiency. In fact, it is now well recognized that PRA is elevated in most, if not all, patients and that systematic mineralocorticoid treatment has permitted us to decrease the average glucocorticoid requirements and thus to improve the ultimate height of these children [247, A].

It is also important to recognize an intercurrent stress or illness and not to perform hormonal studies at that time. Laboratory studies should be made at least 2 weeks after the child has recovered.

(*ii*) *Gonadal insufficiency*. — Treatment with sex hormones, androgens or estrogens, according to classical schemes, is mandatory in castrated patients (see above) to insure the development of secondary sex characteristics (induced puberty). Bone maturation and elevation of LH/FSH are both useful guidelines for determining the optimal age at which such treatments will be initiated.

Treatment of acute adrenal crises. — A state of acute adrenal insufficiency may reveal the disease or supervene at any time during even trivial illnesses or stress. The onset is usually very abrupt: Vomiting, diarrhea, dehydration, fever, vascular collapse, hypothermia, coma. Electrolyte disturbances are characteristic, hypoglycemia may be associated. Whatever the age or the factor responsible, treatment is an emergency. When the diagnosis has been previously established, hydrocortisone (50-100 mg IM or IV) or cortisone (75 mg IM) is administered without delay *before* sending the child to the hospital. Whether or not the child is known as a "salt-loser", the immediate treatment must consider the underlying salt-loss: 11-deoxy-corticosterone acetate (DOCA) is administered intramuscularly (1 to 5 mg according to age). Infusion with 5 % glucose containing 150 mEq of Na/l and 20-150 mg of hydrocortisone hemisuccinate is immediately started. One fourth of the daily requirement (100-200 ml/kg if the child weighs less than 20 kg, 75 ml/kg over this weight) is infused within the first two hours. An intercurrent illness must not be ignored and its specific treatment instituted. Hormonal treatment is thereafter guided by the laboratory findings.

Preventive treatment. — This form of therapy is mandatory in the case of anesthesia, or surgerye ven though it might be judged benign. Elective surgery should only be planed in well-treated patients. For the first 2 days before surgery the child should be given an intramuscular injection of 20 mg/m^2 of cortisone acetate (or 37.5 mg/m^2 of cortisol)

every twelve hours. On the day of surgery, in addition to doubling the IM dosages, an infusion of 5 % glucose containing 100 mg of hydrocortisone hemisuccinate should be instituted before surgery and continued until after the child has recovered from anesthesia. Intramuscular injections of cortisone acetate are continued every 12 hours at a dose of 20 mg/m^2 the day after surgery, then at a half-dose the following day. In the absence of complication, oral replacement therapy can then be resumed.

Mineralocorticoid treatment is advisable in all cases. It should however be limited to a daily IM injection of 1-2 mg of DOCA the day before, the morning of, and the day after surgery, because overtreatment is to be avoided with its risk of sudden hypertension, pulmonary œdema and cardiac failure.

The family should be instructed about the increased needs of cortisol (hydrocortisone) in the case of any intercurrent benign sickness or intense physical effort. Doubling the oral dose is usually sufficient. In case of high fever ($\geqslant 39°$ C) an IM injection of cortisone acetate (25 to 50 mg according to age) should be given.

Genetics. Antenatal diagnosis

All enzyme deficits of adrenal steroid biosynthesis are inborn disorders with an autosomal recessive inheritance. The parents are heterozygote carriers and healthy. The disease is only expressed in the homozygous subjects, even though the biochemical abnormalities (increased OHP levels) may be identified but not associated with clinical symptoms in the mild form of 21-hydroxylase deficiency [A]. Because of the pressing demand of the families endocrinologists have for the last 2 decades searched for a laboratory test for detecting heterozygote carriers. A short ACTH stimulation test with varying protocols [348] is the only test capable of detecting a minor biochemical abnormality: In heterozygous subjects the response of OHP is greater than in homozygous normal subjects but there is an overlap between the two groups. This hormonal test for heterozygosity does not always give a clear cut answer particularly in males [348].

The discovery [215] of a close genetic linkage between the locus for 21-hydroxylase deficiency and the histocompatibility antigen complex (HLA) located on the short arm of chromosome 6, has opened a new method of investigating the heredity of this disease. Recombination data in affected families, have demonstrated that the 21-hydroxylase deficient gene segregates within the HLA-A to B interval and is very close to the locus HLA-B [215], and have also brought evidence for another gene within the HLA-D for the glyoxylase I (GLO) complex. These studies suggest either that the 21-hydroxylase enzyme has 2 chains each coded by a distinct locus, or that one locus codes for a gene of structure, the other for a gene of regulation, both being necessary for the normal activity of the enzyme.

There is also a genetic linkage disequilibrium in this disease with a positive association with HLA, BW 47, a negative association with HLA, B8 in the congenital form and an increased frequency of B14 and DR W-1 HLA haplotypes in the late onset form.

HLA groups can thus be used as markers of the disease. They are helpful for the detection of heterozygous carriers, genetic counselling and antenatal diagnosis, in the absence of recombination (rare). However, the determination of the genetic linkage between a given HLA haplotype and a 21-hydroxylase deficient gene, will only be possible if a prior determination of the HLA groups of an affected subject (homozygous) in a family has been made (Fig. VI-39). It does not permit systematic studies of a population.

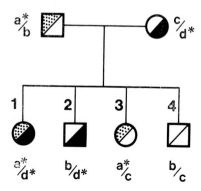

FIG. VI-39. — *Example of HLA typing in subjects of CAH families.*

From the determination of the HLA haplotypes in the CAH affected subject n° 1 (homozygous for 21-OH deficiency), the HLA haplotype carrying the defective gene is identified in the heterozygous parents. Subjects 2 and 3 will be heterozygous carriers as are the parents, while subject 4 escapes from the defective gene (homozygous normal).

Antenatal diagnosis of CAH has been a matter of discussion on ethical grounds because the disease is neither lethal nor disabling. This diagnosis is possible, reliable and is made at the pressing demand of the parents who want to know the sex of the fœtus and whether or not it will be affected. The practice of antenatal diagnosis of 21-OHD has not led to an increased demand for "medical" abortions but on the contrary to a decreased number of systematic "legal" abortions which would have been made because of fear or ignorance of the issue of the pregnancy. Antenatal diagnosis is able to provide precise information to the family and hence has undoubtfully a valuable psychological aspect. Antenatal diagnosis includes the determination of the karyotype and the HLA groups of cultured fetal amniotic cells and the measurement of OHP levels in amniotic fluid (16-17 weeks of pregnancy). The latter is very reliable, providing there is prior establishment of reference standard values [227] and the use of specific techniques, but is does not detect heterozygous carriers. HLA typing is a more difficult technique highly specialized, not widely available, still not free of either technical limitation or recombination [228]. It is useless in a family at risk in whom an affected sibling has died in early infancy and whose HLA groups are unknown.

There is no genetic linkage to the HLA groups for the other enzyme deficiencies responsible for the other forms of CAH. A successful antenatal diagnosis of 11β-hydroxylase has been made on the determination of the amniotic fluid levels of compound S [313]. That of 3β-OHD is theoretically feasible on the hormonal content of the amniotic fluid.

Neonatal mass-screening for CAH

The need for such programs may be discussed. However, the mortality rate in infancy is particularly high in CAH families. Neonatal screening could decrease this mortality and also the morbidity by the early detection of the disease in genetic males in whom the diagnosis is always delayed and often made in life-threatening circumstances, or in genetic females with the form V of Prader. The incidence of the disease appears, however, highly variable among populations (cf. above) and the cost/benefit ratio of such screenings remains difficult to establish. The neonatal mass-screening of 21-OHD is feasible by measuring OHP levels on dried blood specimens taken on filter paper on day 5 of life at the time of other neonatal screens such as PKU. Pilot studies have recently been started and have detected one case out of 7,500 live births in Japan [316 *bis*], none in 18,476 male newborns tested in Lyon, France [212 *bis*] or shown a prevalence of 1 : 5,600 in Italy, 1 : 13,733 in the caucasian population of

Alaska but of 1 : 282 in Yupik Esquimos [289 *ter*]. In all studies, the recall rate has been very low (0.05-0.94 %) and has mainly involved premature infants with or without respiratory distress. The possibility of false negative results is not yet totally excluded.

ISOLATED HYPOALDOSTERONISM

Congenital hypoaldosteronism

This results from enzymatic deficiencies in the two last steps of aldosterone biosynthesis, in 18-hydroxylase (step 5 in Figure VI-35) or in 18-dehydrogenase (step 6 in Figure VI-35). The mitochondrial hydroxylation in position 18 of corticosterone to give aldosterone or that of DOC in 18-OH-DOC, as any other hydroxylation, rather implies a multiple enzymatic complex named "oxidase with mixed function". Indeed, for some authors, 18-hydroxylase is a single enzyme with two discrete activities. This is why the nomenclature of corticosterone methyloxidase (type I or II CMO I or CMO II) as proposed by Ulick is now utilized to designate this enzymatic complex.

These enzyme deficiencies are familial and hereditary due to an autosomal recessive mutant gene. Deficiency in CMO type I [344] appears less frequent than that of type II, of which about 30 cases have been reported. The precise site of the defect is identified by the measurement of the urinary metabolites of 18-hydroxycorticosterone (THB, THA), which are decreased in type I but elevated in type II. Because the metabolites of 18-hydroxycorticosterone are measured in the Porter-Silber assay, urinary excretion of 17OH-CS is thus elevated in type II. In both forms, aldosterone biosynthesis is impaired, plasma aldosterone levels do not rise following ACTH stimulation (normally there is a 3 fold rise). In contrast, the exaggerated production of corticosterone, and to a lesser extent of DOC, is not suppressible by Dexamethasone. Cortisol and ACTH secretion are entirely normal.

Clinical symptoms present a varying degree of severity. Fatal outcome in untreated patients has been reported [344]. However, the isolated salt losing state is often moderately severe or latent because of either the compensatory mineralocorticoid activity of the precursors of aldosterone or the presence of partial enzymatic blocks. Consequently the clinical features are mainly an unexplained

failure to thrive, vomiting, hypotonia, hyponatraemia, hyperkaelemia. Association with juvenile onset diabetes mellitus or idiopathic hypoparathyroidism has been reported [222]. Treatment includes the oral administration of mineralocorticoid and salt supplementation. Clinical symptoms of salt loss appear to improve with age but the enzymatic deficiency does not. It is therefore advisable to maintain the mineralocorticoid supplementive therapy to prevent the impaired growth, consequent to chronic hypoaldosteronism (hypovolemia). Long term prognosis is good.

Pseudohypoaldosteronism

This condition is not "stricto sensu" an adrenal disease, but is an end organ defect, due to renal tubular unresponsiveness to salt-retaining hormones. However, its clinical manifestation is that of an isolated functional insufficiency in mineralocorticoid hormones. Its pathogenesis is still debated but several studies support the concept of multiple target organ involvement that is to say abnormal or absent mineralocorticoid receptors, not only in the renal tubules but also in the skin, colon, sweat and salivary glands [285]. Although most of the 40-50 reported cases are sporadic, the disease may be familial with an autosomal inheritance, either dominant or recessive.

Diagnosis is suspected in a newborn presenting a salt-wasting state usually severe and of an early onset, but refractory to mineralocorticoid therapy. It is easily confirmed on the findings of both elevated PRA and extremely high levels (5 to 10 times normal) of plasma aldosterone and urinary tetrahydroaldosterone, together with normal glucocorticoid and renal function. Plasma levels of aldosterone a re occasionally found within the limits of normal [304].

The only treatment necessary is relatively simple: it consists of salt replacement. The daily sodium requirement is often surprisingly large (10-25 mEq/kg) and the dose is guided by normalized natremia, kalemia, PRA and weight gain. Clinical symptoms seem to improve with age and classically the need for sodium supplementation diminishes after age 2 (< 10 mEq/day) and many patients can manage without treatment. Except for the life-threatening risk of the salt-wastage in early infancy, the long term prognosis appears good. Hypercalciuria, nephrocalcinosis, or other signs of proximal tubular insufficiency may however complicate the course of the disease.

CONGENITAL ADRENOCORTICAL INSUFFICIENCY

Congenital adrenal hypoplasia

This term is used to designate complete adrenal insufficiency due to either the aplasia (very rare) or a structural abnormality of the adrenal glands (early embryologic malformations). Numerous sporadic cases have been reported but it would appear that those conditions are genetically transmitted. Two types are recognized:

The "cytomegalic" form, affects only males and its inheritance is X-linked recessive [267]. The atrophic adrenal cortex shows abnormal architecture. The cortex is poorly differentiated, filled with abnormally large and clear cells resembling the giant cells occasionally found in the normal fetal zone.

The autosomic recessive form. — Both sexes are affected. The adrenal morphology ressembles that found in anencephalic fetuses: small glands in which the fetal zone is markedly reduced while the definitive, adult, zone is relatively conserved with normal differentiation into three zones.

The deficient organogenesis only affects the adrenal glands and the gonads, testes or ovaries, are normal. Sexual differentiation is normal and there are no abnormalities in the development of external genitalia. However, the association with hypothalamic hypogonadotrophic hypogonadism, only suspected at pubertal age, now appears to be a frequent, if not constant, feature of the cytomegalic form [239, 268].

Delivery is usually normal. Clinical features are those of complete and severe adrenal insufficiency which manifests very early in life (< 72 h of age), or even at birth. There is a high mortality rate in the absence of a rapid diagnosis and immediate treatment. In some cases however, the clinical onset may be delayed. Hyperpigmentation is a constant finding. The diagnosis is made on the pathognomonic association of hyponatremia, hyperkalemia, metabolic acidosis, raised PRA and ACTH levels. The extremely low levels of all adrenal hormones exclude any form of CAH except the deficit in 20-22d esmolase. The latter diagnosis is suspected in genetic males presenting with ambiguous genitalia and may be identified in both sexes by the findings of marked hypertrophy of the adrenals at echotomography. A careful history and morphological studies will be helpfull in the diffe-

rential diagnosis from adrenal hemorragic cysts.

Substitution therapy consists of the administration of glucocorticoid and mineralocorticoid hormones at physiological dosages. The risks of an acute adrenal crisis precipitated by any trauma, stress or intercurrent disease are particularly high in these diseases. The treatment of the acute adrenal insufficiency and all forms of preventive therapy are as discussed above in the case of CAH. The therapeutic management of congenital adrenal hypoplasia is usually easier than that of CAH. The adaptation of hormonal dosages to each individual's needs is guided by clinical findings, disappearance of melanodermia, normal thriving and growth and determination of PRA. One should not try to bring ACTH levels back to normal at any price, because marked fluctuations in ACTH secretion persist even in well-controlled patients.

Because of the poor prognosis of the disease in the postnatal period, many authors have studied the possibilities of an antenatal diagnosis of the condition, particularly in pregnant women who have previously lost a child from sudden or unexplained death. One of the positive propositions was to follow the evolution of the maternal levels of œstrogens, estriol levels in particular, which reflect fetal adrenal androgen production. Such an antenatal diagnosis has been successfully made on the observation of low maternal œstrogen levels (cf. review in [222]). However, such findings are not pathognomonic of congenital adrenal hypoplasia: maternal levels of estriol are also low in placental sulfatase deficiency [192] in glucocorticoid treated mothers, in eclamptic toxemia, or in the exceptional case of an isolated ACTH deficiency of the fœtus [359]. Nevertheless, measurement of maternal œstrogens is highly advisable in families at risk for the disorder. The method is simple and not invasive. It may permit one to suspect the diagnosis and to take adequate measures for appropriate investigation and treatment at the time of birth. Deficiency in placental sulfatase is only observed in pregnancy carrying a male fetus. The fetus himself is normal and does not require therapy; the diagnosis is confirmed by enzymatic studies of the placenta.

Dissociated forms of hypoadrenocorticism

Two syndromes have been described, "adrenocortical unresponsiveness to ACTH" [271] and "familial glucocorticoid insufficiency" (see review in [222]), which are both characterized by a selective glucocorticoid deficiency, raised ACTH levels and normal mineralocorticoid function. The incidence is higher in males, but both sexes are affected. It is familial with probably an autosomal recessive inheritance. Associations with achalasia or deficient lacrimation have been reported. In the atrophic adrenals glands, the fasciculata and reticularis zones are almost absent but some clusters of glomerulosa cells may persist. There is no lymphocyte infiltration nor any adrenal antibodies as seen in autoimmune adrenal disorders.

The pathogenesis of the disease is unclear: For some authors, it is the consequence of a congenital abnormality in the action of ACTH at the receptor level or beyond the formation of cyclic adenosine monophosphate (cAMP) [271], for others it results from an inheritable progressive degenerative disorder, not due to autoimmunity but to an unknown cause. In favor of this view is the rather late onset of clinical signs for a congenital defect, and the progressive impairment of mineralocorticoid function in a number of patients.

There are often no problems in early infancy. The first symptoms usually appear at about 2-3 years of age often revealed by an intercurrent illness. Episodes of convulsions preceed the signs of glucocorticoid insufficiency: typical features are the association of hyperpigmented skin and severe hypoglycaemia. Serum and urinary electrolytes are normal as is aldosterone secretion. The differential diagnosis is practically only that of chronic adrenal insufficiency due to autoimmune adrenalitis (Addison's disease). There may be dissociation in timing of the onset of gluco- and mineralocorticoid failure in Addison's disease as well, but the clinical onset is usually later in life in the latter.

Treatment will only require the administration of physiological doses of hydrocortisone (see above). Prolonged follow-up and repeated testing are necessary to provide evidence of no mineralocorticoid dysfunction.

Hypoadrenocorticism associated with cerebral degeneration: neurolipidoses

Two syndromes are known: Wolman's disease [269] and Schilder's disease [275]. In the former, adrenal insufficiency is associated with primary familial xanthomatosis. Both are believed to result from a deficiency of the lysosomal enzyme, cholesterol esterase, which normally hydrolyses the cholesterol esters stored in lipids droplets. Not only is complete

steroidogenesis deficient because of the inability to form free cholesterol, but esterified cholesterol accumulates in all tissues including the brain. The affected child fails to thrive, presents signs of malnutrition, hepatosplenomegaly and extensive adrenal calcifications. The evolution is usually fatal before 1 year of life.

"Bronzed Schilder's" disease, also named diffuse cerebral sclerosis or more recently adrenoleukodystrophy (ALD), is also familial with an X-linked recessive inheritance [275], associating chronic adrenal insufficiency with a progressive demyelinisation of the cerebral white matter of the CNS. Characteristic cytoplasmic striated inclusions are found in the brain and in the adrenal cortex but also in the skin, connective tissues, peripheral nerves and striated muscles. Studies in cultured skin fibroblasts of affected subjects have demonstrated the accumulation of saturated very long chain fatty acids, particularly hexacosanoic acid (C26 : 0) and an increased ratio of C26 : 0 to C22 : 0 fatty acids. It is now recognized that ALD is a lipid storage disorder due to the impaired capacity to oxidize very long chain fatty acids; but the specific biochemical abnormality is not yet established.

The primary adrenal insufficiency is "metabolic", being likely the consequence of the fact that the cholesterol esters with long-chain fatty acids are poor substrates for the cholesterol esterase. As a result the adrenal cells are depleted in free cholesterol. Most commonly, the disease has a delayed onset and manifests between the ages of 4-8 and 20 years but there appears to be a neonatal form of ALD [275]. Adrenal insufficiency is the first manifestation of the disease, followed by symptoms of neurological or mental deterioration, which aggravate inexorably. This is why ALD should be suspected in male children affected with chronic adrenal insufficiency, particularly when there is a familial incidence of associated neurological disorders. The diagnosis involves a familial history, careful and repeated neurological testing, the search for optic nerve, peripheral nerve or spinal cord involvement, skin biopsy and cerebral tomodensitometry [307 bis]. Recent progress in biochemical studies of cultured cells have provided a means of making the diagnosis before the onset of any clinical evidence of the disease, and also of detecting heterozygous carriers. The antenatal diagnosis of ALD has recently been successfully made by Moser et al. [276] on the fatty acid content of cultured amniocytes. In both neurolipidoses, hormonal substitutive therapy (see above) may control the adrenal insufficiency but the prognosis is that of a progressive and fatal neurological deterioration.

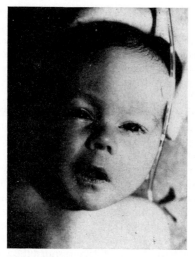
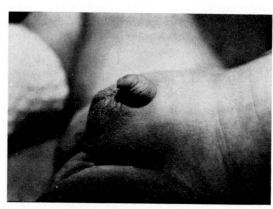

a   *b*

FIG. VI-40. — *Male newborn affected with congenital hypopituitarism.*
a) The low nasal bridge attests to fetal hypothyroidism.
b) Typical aspect of the external genitalia: hypoplastic scrotum, cryptorchidism, underdevelopped phallus (courtesy of
Dr. M. BETHENOD, Hôpital Debrousse, Lyon).

Secondary adrenal insufficiency

Neonatal adrenal insufficiency may result from congenital impaired hypothalamic-pituitary function. Most frequent is the adrenal hypoplasia secondary to anencephaly [64], holoprosencephaly [81], arhinencephaly or associated with midline cleavage malformations [112, 120]. The diagnosis is pathogenetically obvious and the poor prognosis is that of the impaired vital functions. Congenital hypoplasia [132, 150] or aplasia [101] of the pituitary gland leads to a similar form of adrenal insufficiency, the "anencephalic" form [183]. All the above developmental defects may be familial and a genetic autosomal recessive predisposition has been suggested [27, 132]. Even in the rare instances in which an hereditary trait has been clearly shown [309] the great majority of insufficiencies of the anterior pituitary are not associated with recognizable anatomic lesions and the specific etiology is unknown. However, the high incidence (20-40 %) of fetal or neonatal anoxia or traumatic deliveries [205] associated with hypothalamic-pituitary dysfunction is well established.

In idiopathic pituitary insufficiency, impairment of corticotropin function is by far the least frequent one (GH > TSH > ACTH); clinical symptoms are not manifest for several years and are usually rather modest, the defect being partial. A congenital form of isolated ACTH deficiency has however been described, but it is very rare.

A clinical entity of congenital pituitary insuffi-

ciency has recently been described in male newborns [265 *bis*]: micropenis, cryptorchidism, hypoglycemia, hypothyroidism and adrenal insufficiency (Fig. VI-40). The panhypopituitarism is believed to be secondary to hypothalamic dysfunction. Only sporadic cases have been reported.

NEONATALLY ACQUIRED HYPOADRENOCORTICISM

Adrenal hemorrhage

This is not uncommon in the newborn. It is widely admitted that the pathogenic factor is birth trauma and/or anoxia. Its incidence is higher in difficult or prolonged labour, after too vigorous rescucitating manipulations, but it can occur after apparently uneventful deliveries, particularly in premature babies [189]. There is an early onset of clinical symptoms (2-7 days of life). But they are most often nonspecific: palor, cyanosis, tachycardia, acute shock, respiratory distress, intense and prolonged jaundice, microscopic hematuria, resulting primarily from blood loss. Attention may be alerted when palpable masses are discovered in the flank, but when unilateral it can be mistaken for a renal tumor. Indeed, adrenal hemorrhage can be unilateral or bilateral. Variable in intensity, it may extend to the adjacent organs, causing intestinal obstruction [189], compression of the renal vessels or be complicated by renal vein thrombosis. Hypertension may be a complication when an intra-adrenal hematoma ruptures into the renal capsule. There may be a need for urgent surgical decompression of the renal artery. The occurence of gross hematuria or proteinuria is symptomatic of renal vein thrombosis. As the hematoma resolves, adrenal calcifications may be visible as early as the 5th day of life, several months later or they may never occur. On the other hand, adrenal hemorrhage may be totally unrecognized and suprarenal calcifications discovered fortuitously later in life [256].

Adrenal insufficiency is in fact a relatively rare complication, occuring only in bilateral adrenal hemorrhage [189, 328]. The clinical picture is that of a severe adrenal crisis (acute shock, salt wastage). Early diagnosis and treatment are mandatory (see above). Abdominal echotomography may be very helpful [261] in differentiating adrenal from renal hematomas. In neonates recovering from the acute phase of shock and or widespread bleeding, the evolution is often favorable. The adrenal gland has a great capacity for regeneration and adrenal hypofunction manifesting soon after the critical period has elapsed, is most often transient. Adreno-cortical function completely recovers in a few weeks or months. It may however partially persist. Dynamic testing of adrenal function (ACTH test) should be repeated at intervals to discontinue unnecessary treatment in case of full recovery.

Waterhouse-Friderichsen syndrome

This name has been given to the clinical syndrome associating overwhelming sepsis, circulatory collapse, extensive purpura associated with sudden onset of adrenal failure due to bilateral adrenal vasculitis. It is more severe and more constantly observed in invasive meningococcemia (purpura fulminans) than in other forms of sepsis. It may occur in pneumococcal, streptococcal or other infections. The adrenal hemorrhage is due to the extension of the generalized hemorrhagic diathesis and the circulatory collapse is probably the result of severe toxaemia rather than being primarily due to acute adrenal failure. Treatment with high doses of glucocorticoids has not improved the prognosis which is still very poor (cf. review in [222]).

Infants born to glucocorticoid-treated mothers

Corticosteroid therapy is given to pregnant women in two different circumstances: either the mother is affected with a disorder requiring such therapy even during pregnancy or she has received gluco-corticoid treatment at the end of her pregnancy with the aim of promoting pulmonary maturation and preventing neonatal respiratory distress. As discussed above, glucocorticoid hormones crossing the placenta are able to suppress ACTH secretion and adrenal function in the fetus [174, 287]. In the first situation this transplacental transfer is not desirable and in the light of our knowledge of feto-placental pharmacology (see above), the mother should be preferably treated with cortisone, hydro-cortisone, prednisone or prednisolone, of which only about 10 % reach the fetus. Apart from a very uncommon association between cleft palate and maternal glucocorticoid treatment during the first trimester, teratogenic defects have not been observed.

In the second situation, glucocorticoid treatment is addressed to the fetus via the maternal ingestion of synthetic glucocorticoids such as dexamethasone or betamethasone which concentrate more actively in the fetus [173, 289].

In both situations, the suppression of the hypophyso-adrenal axis is only transient, since ACTH secretion resumes normally shortly after birth. Plasma cortisol and DHAS levels usually return to normal within the first 7-10 days of life [175]. Mineralocorticoid function is normal, as ACTH has little influence on aldosterone regulation. Nevertheless, these newborns should be followed closely because of the risk of presenting hypoglycemic episodes during the phase of recuperation. In this case treatment should only be symptomatic (glucose infusion at the dose and for the time necessary to maintain normal glycemia). One should resist the temptation of instituting inopportune glucocorticoid therapy which is of no benefit but will delay the recovery of pituitary and adrenal functions.

ADRENOCORTICAL HYPERFUNCTION: NEONATAL CUSHING SYNDROME

Cushing's syndrome is very rare in children in whom it is usually due to an adrenal tumor. It is not unknown in newborn infants since 63 cases have been reported: 48 adrenal tumors (carcinomas and adenomas), 11 nodular adrenal hyperplasias, 2 ectopic ACTH syndromes and 2 cases secondary to a pituitary adenoma [212, 230, 264]. The incidence is about 3 times higher in females. Familial occurence has been observed [170, 212].

Classically, clinical signs do not manifest in the immediate newborn period [230], but the disease may develop in utero and the features of the syndrome, may be present at birth [212]. An early clinical onset is most often associated with bilateral hyperplasia of the adrenal glands. Nodularity of such glands is a striking and virtually constant feature. The clinical picture associates signs of hypercortisolism (trunculo-facial obesity, worsening extremely rapidly, plethoric face (Fig. VI-41), large fontanelles, severe growth failure, delayed bone maturation, systolic hypertension) and signs of hyperandrogenism (greasy skin, acne, abundant hair, hirsutism, pubic hair). Clinical symptoms always evolve rapidly. Signs of virilization may not have had time to appear by the time of diagnosis. This is made on increased plasma and urinary levels of both glucocorticoids and androgens not suppressible by dexamethasone. Determination of plasma ACTH levels is a useful guide to the etiological diagnosis: those levels are undetectable in the case of micronodular hyperplasia [212], extremely high in cases of ectopic ACTH syndrome.

Near-normal ACTH levels may lead one to suspect the possibility of a pituitary adenoma although it is extremely rare at this period of life [264]. Such a diagnosis may be achieved by radiological investigations and cranial tomodensitometry. When an abdominal tumor is palpable, echography is helpful in visualizing the hypertrophied adrenal gland, but above all in localizing the side of a unilateral tumor prior to surgery.

Investigations must be kept to the essential minimum because these newborns are extremely fragile. Because of the severity and the rapid evolution of the symptoms, a therapeutic decision must not be delayed. Whatever the type (adrenal, ectopic ACTH secreting tissue) a tumor must be removed as promptly as possible. In the other instances, bilateral adrenalectomy is the only therapy capable of rapidly removing the child from the life threatening effects of hypercortisolism.

In general, the prognosis has been poor in neonatal Cushing's syndrome. Adequate treatment with high doses of glucocorticoid hormones (see preventive treatment of CAH at the time of surgery, described above) before, during and after surgery is necessary in all cases, to avoid an immediate post operative crisis of adrenal insufficiency. Lifelong subsequent replacement therapy with both gluco- and mineralocorticoid is needed in cases of bilateral adrenalectomy. Because of atrophy of the contralateral gland and complete inhibition of hypothalamic-pituitary function patients with unilateral tumors have no capacity to cope with stress and may also present with complete adrenal insufficiency as soon as the tumor is removed. Withdrawal from glucocorticoid therapy must be progressive, over several weeks or months, until complete recovery of pituitary and adrenal function (as assessed by ACTH and metyrapone tests). Although adrenal tumors usually have a low degree of malignancy they may invade the kidney or give lung or kidney metastases. A close follow-up (clinical, radiological, laboratory) should be continued for several years.

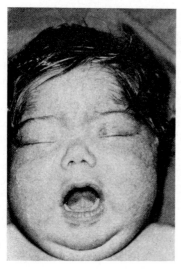

FIG. VI-41. — *Female newborn with congenital Cushing's syndrome due to bilateral nodular adrenal hyperplasia: appearance at 1 week of age* (reproduced from DONALDSON et al., Ref. [212], with permission).

Neonatal hypoglycemia and endocrine disease

The neonate tolerates rather well the immediate postnatal fall in blood glucose concentration to around 40 mg/dl (2.2 nmol/l). However, repeated or prolonged episodes of hypoglycemia lead to permanent neurological lesions and eventually to profound mental retardation. Thus, not only the immediate treatment of hypoglycemic episodes but also the recognition of the factor responsible is of great importance in avoiding this tragic consequence.

Extrapancreatic endocrine abnormalities are responsible for about one third of the neonatal hypoglycemias. These abnormalities are essentially due to glucocorticoid insufficiency, whatever the cause, or to deficient growth hormone (GH) secretion. Hypoglycemia is diagnosed on the occasion of severe clinical manifestations (convulsions, coma), less evident signs (brief apneic spells, palor, cyanosis, tremors, clonic spasms, abnormal cry) or may be apparently asymptomatic leading progressively to feeding problems, and delay in somatic and mental development. Hypoglycemia may be ignored, because it is not a constant feature, in patients known to have adrenal insufficiency who present with an acute adrenal crisis. It may be the revealing symptom of a glucocorticoid insufficiency presenting either as coma, or as repeated episodes of hypoglycemia (recurrent form) of early postnatal onset, possibly associated with cholestasis [262] but not with salt-loss. Because it is relatively frequent (all etiologies considered) cortisol deficiency must be considered in any newborn with spontaneous hypoglycemia, particularly when it appears unexplained or when ketosis is associated.

GH deficiency is not uncommon. Its prevalence varies among studies: from 1 : 30,000 to 1 : 4,000 live births with a predominance in the masculine sex [342].

Hypopituitarism associated with neonatal hypoglycemia is mainly due to developmental defects (aplasia or hypoplasia of the pituitary gland, mide-line defects) [250]. Pituitary deficiency is already manifest in utero: ACTH deficiency is constant, GH deficiency is observed in about half of the patients. The hypoglycemic syndrome is very severe and manifests within the first hours or days of life. Hypoglycemia is one of the cardinal symptoms of congenital panhypopituitarism associating micropenis, deficiency in ACTH and GH [265 *bis*] (Fig. VI-40). The tendency to hypoglycemia is increased when both deficits are present. Spontaneous hypoglycemia is not a constant feature of isolated GH deficiency (11-17 %). Its incidence is higher in young children or after starvation and seems to decrease with age. The pathogenesis of hypoglycemia due to GH deficiency is not well understood (for more details see chapter by Schwartz). In infants affected with multiple congenital deficiencies in pituitary hormones, treatment of the neonatal onset recurrent hypoglycemia is an emergency. Hypoglycemia is not controlled by the correction of the adrenal insufficiency alone (supplementary cortisol therapy, even at high dosage). Combined GH therapy

is required. Treatment with *daily* IM injections of human GH (1-2 mg) must be instituted as soon as possible. Such treatment is mandatory to avoid tragic mental deterioration. In addition it seems to have a beneficial trophic effect on the development of the phallus.

Acknowledgements. — This work was supported by INSERM. The expert and faithfull secretarial assistance of Miss Joëlle Bois is greatfully acknowledged.

REFERENCES

III. *Adrenal.*

[166] ALLEN (J. P.), COOK (D. M.), KENDALL, (J. W.) & McGILVQA, (R.). — Maternal-fetal ACTH relationship in man. *J. Clin. Endocrinol. Metab.*, 37, 230-234, 1973.

[167] ALLEN (J. P.), GREER (M. A.), McGIVRA (R.), CASTRO (A.), FISCHER (D. A.). — Endocrine function in anencephalic infant. *J. Clin. Endocrinol. Metab.*, 38, 94-98, 1974.

[168] ANDERSON (G. E.), FRIIS-HANSEN (B.). — Cord serum lipid and lipoprotein values in normal and betamethasone-treated newborns of varying gestational age. *Acta Paediat. Scand.*, 66, 355-360, 1977.

[169] ARAI (K.), YANAIHARA (T.), OKINAGA (S.). — Adrenocorticotrophic hormone in human fetal blood at delivery. *Am. J. Obstet. Gynecol.*, 125, 1136-1140, 1976.

[170] ARCE (B.), LICEA (M.), HUNG (S.), PADRON (R.). — Familial Cushing's syndrome. *Acta Endocrinol.*, 87, 139-147, 1978.

[171] BAIRD (A. C.), BRISSON (G.), KAN (K. W.), DUGUID (W. C.), SOLOMON (S.). — Control of steroid synthesis in human fetal adrenals in monolayer culture. *Can. J. Biochem.*, 56, 577-584, 1978.

[172] BAKER (B. L.), JAFFE (R. B.). — The genesis of cell types in the adenohypophysis of the human fetus as observed by immunocytochemistry. *Am. J. Anat.*, 143, 137-162, 1975.

[173] BALLARD (P. L.), GRANDBERG (P.), BALLARD (R. A.). — Glucocorticoid levels in maternal and cord serum after prenatal betamethasone therapy to prevent respiratory distress syndrome. *J. Clin. Invest.*, 56, 1548-1554, 1975.

[174] BALLARD (P. L.), GLUCKMAN (P. D.), LIGGINS (G. C.), KAPLAN (S. L.), GRUMBACH (M. M.). — Steroid and growth hormone levels in premature infants after prenatal betamethasone therapy to prevent respiratory distress syndrome. *Ped. Res.*, 14, 122-127, 1980.

[175] BALLARD (P. L.), BALLARD (R. A.), GRANBERG (J. P.), SNIDERMAN (S.), GLUCKMAN (P. D.), KAPLAN (S. L.), GRUMBACH (M. M.). — Fetal sex and prenatal betamethasone therapy. *J. Ped.*, 97, 451-454, 1980.

[175 *bis*] BARTTER (F. C.), PRONOVE (P.), GILLO (J. R.), MacCARDLE (R. C.). — Hyperplasia of the juxtaglomerular complex with hyperaldosteronism and hypokaliemic alkalosis. *Am. J. Med.*, 33, 811-828, 1962.

[176] BAXTER (J. D.), FORSHAN (P. H.). — Tissue effects of glucocorticoids. Am. J. Med., 53, 573-589, 1972.

[177] BEGEOT (M.), DUBOIS (M. P.), DUBOIS (P. M.). — Growth hormone and ACTH in the pituitary of normal and anencephalic human fetuses: immunocytochemical evidence for hypothalamic influences during development. Neuroendocrinology, 24, 208-220, 1977.

[178] BEGEOT (M.), DUBOIS (M. P.), DUBOIS (P. M.). — Immunologic localization of α and β-endorphins and β-lipotropin in corticotropic cells of the normal and anencephalic fetal pituitaries. Cell Tissue Res., 193, 413-422, 1978.

[179] BEITINS (I. Z.), BAYARD (F.), ANCES (I. G.), KOWARSKI (A.), MIGEON (C. J.). — The transplacental passage of prednisone and prednisolone in pregnancy near term. J. Pediatr., 81, 936-945, 1972.

[180] BEITINS (I. Z.), BAYARD (F.), LEVITSKY (L.), ANCES (I. G.), KOWARSKI (A.), MIGEON (C. J.). — Plasma aldosterone concentrations at delivery and during the newborn period. J. Clin. Invest., 51, 386-394, 1972.

[181] BEITINS (I. Z.), BAYARD (F.), ANCES (I. G.), KOWARSKI (A.), MIGEON (C. J.). — The metabolic clearance rate, blood production, interconversion and transplacental passage of cortisol and cortisone in pregnancy near term. Ped. Res., 7, 509-519, 1973.

[182] BELISLE (S.), FENCL (M.), OSATHANONDH (R.), TULCHINSKY (D.). — Sources of 17α-hydroxy-pregnenolone and its sulfate in human pregnancy. J. Clin. Endocrinol. Metab., 46, 721-728, 1978.

[183] BENIRSCHKE (K.). — Adrenals in anencephaly and hydrocephaly. Obstet. Gynecol., 8, 412-418, 1956.

[184] BENNER (M. C.). — Studies on the involution of the fetal cortex of the adrenal cortex. Am. J. Path., 16, 787-798, 1940.

[185] BERTRAND (J.), GILLY (R.), LORAS (B.). — Neonatal adrenal function: free and conjugated plasma 17-hydroxysteroids in the newborn during the first 5 days of life. Effect of hydrocortisone and ACTH administration. In: The Human Adrenal Gland, CURRIE (A. R.), SYMINGTON (T.), GRANT (J. L.) (Eds.), Williams and Wilkins, Baltimore, 608-623, 1962.

[186] BERTRAND (J.), LORAS (B.), GILLY (R.), CAUTENET (B.). — Contribution à l'étude de la sécrétion et du métabolisme du cortisol chez le nouveau-né et le nourrisson de moins de 3 mois. Pathol. Biol., 11, 997-1022, 1963.

[187] BIGLIERI (E. G.). — Mechanisms establishing the mineralocorticoid hormone patterns in the 17α-hydroxylase deficiency. J. Steroid Biochem., 11, 653-657, 1979.

[188] BIGLIERI (E. G.), HERRON (M. A.), BRUST (N.). — 17-hydroxylation deficiency in man. J. Clin. Invest., 45, 1946-1954, 1966.

[189] BLACK (J.), WILLIAMS (D. I.). — Natural history of adrenal haemorrhage in the newborn. Arch. Dis. Child., 48, 183-190, 1973.

[190] BONGIOVANNI (A. M.), EBERLEIN (W. R.), GOLDMAN (A. S.), NEW (M.). — Disorders of adrenal steroid biogenesis. Rec. Prog. Horm. Res., 23, 375-449, 1967.

[191] BRANCHAUD (C. T.), GOODYER (C. G.), HALL (C. St. G.), ARATO (J. S.), SILMAN (R. E.), GIROUD (C. J. P.). — Steroidogenic activity of hACTH and related peptides on the human neocortex and fetal

[192] BRAUSTEIN (G. D.), ZIEL (F. H.), ALLEN (A.), VAN DE VELDE (R.), WADE (M. E.). — Prenatal diagnosis of placental steroid sulfatase deficiency. Am. J. Obstet. Gynecol., 126, 716-719, 1976.

[193] CARR (B. R.), SIMPSON (E. R.). — Lipoprotein utilization and cholesterol synthesis by the human fetal adrenal gland. Endocr. Rev., 2, 306-326, 1981.

[194] CARR (B. R.), PARKER (C. R. Jr.), MILEWICH (L.), PORTER (J. C.), MACDONALD (P. C.), SIMPSON (E. R.). — Steroid secretion by ACTH-stimulated human fetal adrenal tissue during the first week in organ culture. Steroids, 36, 563-574, 1980.

[195] CARR (B. R.), OHASHI (M.), MACDONALD (P. C.), SIMPSON (E. R.). — Human anencephalic adrenal tissue: low-density lipoprotein metabolism and cholesterol synthesis. J. Clin. Endocrinol. Metab., 53, 406-411, 1981.

[196] CARR (B. R.), OHASHI (M.), SIMPSON (E. R.). — Low density lipoprotein binding and de novo synthesis of cholesterol in the neocortex and fetal zones of the human fetal adrenal gland. Endocrinology, 110, 1994-1998, 1982.

[197] CASTRO-MAGANA (M.), CHERUVANKY (T.), COLLIPP (P. J.), GHAVAMI-MAIBODI (Z.), ANGULO (M.), STEWART (C.). — Transient adrenogenital syndrome due to exposure to Danazol in utero. Am. J. Dis. Child., 135, 1032-1034, 1981.

[198] CATHELINEAU (G.), BRÉRAULT (J. L.), FIET (J.), JULIEN (R.), DREUX (C.), CANIVET (J.). — Adrenocortical 11β-hydroxylation defect in adult women with post-menarchial onset of symptoms. J. Clin. Endocrinol. Metab., 51, 287-291, 1980.

[199] CAVALLERO (C.), MAGRINI (U.). — Histochemical studies on 3β-hydroxysteroid dehydrogenase and other enzymes in the steroid-secreting structures of human fœtus. Excerpta Medica Int. Cong. Ser., 132, 667-672, 1967.

[200] CHAN (L.), O'MALLEY (B. W.). — Mechanism of action of the sex steroid hormones. N. Engl. J. Med., 294, 1322-1328, 1372-1381, 1430-1437, 1976.

[201] CHANG (R. J.), BUSTER (J. E.), BLAKELY (J. L.), OKADA (D. M.), HOBEL (C. J.), ABRAHAM (G. E.), MARSHALL (J. R.). — Simultaneous comparison of Δ5-3β-hydroxysteroid levels in the fetoplacental circulation of normal pregnancy in labor and not in labor. J. Clin. Endocrinol. Metab., 42, 744-751, 1976.

[202] COOKE (B. A.), TAYLOR (P. D.). — Site of dehydroepiandrosterone sulfate biosynthesis in the adrenal gland of the previable fetus. J. Endocrinol., 51, 547-556, 1971.

[203] COOKE (B. A.), SHIRLEY (I. M.), DOBBIE (J.), TAYLOR (P. D.). — Metabolism of pregnenolone and dehydroepiandrosterone by homogenized tissue from the separated zones and whole adrenal glands from newborn anencephalic infants. J. Endocrinol., 51, 533-546, 1971.

[204] COWARD (R. E.). — The natural history of the chromaffin cells. Longmans, Greens and Co, London, 1965.

[205] CRAFT (W. H.), UNDERWOOD (L. E.), VAN WYK (J. J.). — High incidence of perinatal insult in children with idiopathic hypopituitarism. J. Pediatr., 96, 397-402, 1980.

[206] DAVID (M.), MOLLARD (P.), DAUDET (M.), LAURAS (B.). — L'ambiguïté sexuelle dans le pseudo-

hermaphrodisme féminin. A propos de 61 observations. *Pédiatrie*, 27, 871-885, 1972.

[207] DAVIES (J. O.), FREEMAN (R. H.). — Mechanisms regulating renin release. *Physiol. Rev.*, 56, 1-56, 1976.

[208] DICZFALUSY (E.). — Steroid metabolism in the human fœto-placental unit. *Acta Endocrinol. (Kbh)*, 61, 649-664, 1969.

[209] DICZFALUSY (E.). — Endocrine functions of the human fetus and placenta. *Am. J. Obstet. Gynecol.*, 119, 419-433, 1974.

[210] DICZFALUSY (E.). — Steroid metabolism in the feto-placental unit. In: *The Fœto-Placental Unit*. PECILE (A.) and FINZI (C.) (Eds.). Excerpta Medica International Congress Series n° 183, 65-109. Excerpta Medica Foundation, Amsterdam, 1979.

[211] DILLON (M. T.), GILLON (M. E. A.), RYNESS (J. M.), DE SWIET (M.). — Plasma renin activity and aldosterone concentration in the human newborn. *Arch. Dis. Child.*, 51, 537-540, 1976.

[211 bis] DILLON (M. J.), SHAH (V.), MITCHELL (M. D.). — Bartter's syndrome: 10 cases in childhood. Results of long-term indomethacin therapy. *Quarterly J. Med.*, 48, 429-446, 1979.

[212] DONALDSON (M. D. C.), GRANT (D. B.), O'HARE (M. J.), SHACKLETON (C. H. L.). — Familial congenital Cushing's syndrome due to bilateral nodular adrenal hyperplasia. *Clin. Endocrinol.*, 14, 519-526, 1981.

[212 bis] DORCHE (C.), BOZON (D.), DAVID (M.), ROLLAND (M. O.). — Systematic neonatal screening for congenital adrenal hyperplasia: a report on 18476 tests. *International Meeting on Neonatal Screening, Tokyo*, 16-21 August 1982, VI-4, 109.

[213] DUBOIS (P. M.), VARGUES-REGAIRAZ (H.), DUBOIS (M. P.). — Human fetal anterior pituitary: immunofluorescent evidence for corticotropin and melanotropin activities. *Z. Zellforsch.*, 145, 131-143, 1973.

[214] DUFAU (M. L.), VILLEE (D. B.). — Aldosterone biosynthesis by human fetal adrenal *in vitro*. *Biochim. Biophys. Acta*, 176, 637-640, 1969.

[215] DUPONT (B.), SMITHWICK (E. M.), OBERFIELD (S. E.), LEE (T. D.), LEVINE (L. S.). — Close genetic linkage between HLA and congenital adrenal hyperplasia (21-hydroxylase deficiency). *Lancet*, ii, 1309-1311, 1977.

[216] DUPOUY (J. P.), CHATELAIN (A.), ALLAUME (P.). — Absence of transplacental passage of ACTH in the rat: direct experimental proof. *Biol. Neonate*, 37, 96-102, 1980.

[217] EBERLEIN (W. R.), BONGIOVANNI (A. M.). — Congenital adrenal hyperplasia with hypertension: unusual steroid pattern in blood and urines. *J. Clin. Endocrinol. Metab.*, 15, 1531-1539, 1955.

[218] EDWIN (C.), LANES (L.), MIGEON (C. J.), LEE (P. A.), PLOTNICK (L. P.), KOWARSKI (A. A.). — Persistence of the enzymatic block in adolescent patients with salt-losing congenital adrenal hyperplasia. *J. Pediatr.*, 95, 534-537, 1979.

[219] EIPPER (B. A.), MAINS (R. E.). — Structure and biosynthesis of adrenocorticotropin, endorphin and related peptides. *Endocr. Rev.*, 1, 1-27, 1980.

[220] FEIT (J. P.), DAVID (L.), PATRICOT (M. C.), MACABEO (V.), LEBACQ (E.), FRANÇOIS (R.). — Le déficit en 17-hydroxylase : une cause de croissance et puberté retardées chez la fille. A propos d'une observation. *Arch. Fr. Péd.*, 35, 395-405, 1978.

[221] FOREST (M. G.). — Age-related response to plasma testosterone, Δ⁴-androstenedione and cortisol to adrenocorticotropin in infants, children and adults. *J. Clin. Endocrinol. Metab.*, 47, 931-937, 1978.

[222] FOREST (M. G.). — Adrenal steroid deficiency states. In: *Clinical Paediatric Endocrinology*. BROOK (C. G. D.) (Ed.). Blackwell Scientific Publications, Oxford, 396-428, 1981.

[223] FOREST (M. G.). — Development of the male reproductive tract. In: *Aspects of Male Infertility*, Vol. 4. DE VERE WHITE (R.) (Ed.). Williams and Wilkins, Baltimore, 1-60, 1982.

[224] FOREST (M. G.), CATHIARD (A. M.). — Ontogenic study of plasma 17α-hydroxyprogesterone in the human. I. Postnatal period. Evidence for a transient ovarian activity in infancy. *Ped. Res.*, 12, 6-11, 1978.

[224 bis] FOREST (M. G.), LECORNU (M.), PERETTI (E. DE). — Familial male pseudohermaphroditism due to 17-20 desmolase deficiency. I. *In vivo* endocrine studies. *J. Clin. Endocrinol. Metab.*, 50, 826-833, 1980.

[225] FOREST (M. G.), PERETTI (E. DE), BERTRAND (J.). — Plasma androgens in the newborn, the infant and the prepubertal child in normal and pathological conditions. In: *Convegno Internazionale di Endocrinologia Pediatrica*. Pasini, Pisa, 15-48, 1976.

[226] FOREST (M. G.), PERETTI (E. DE), BERTRAND (J.). — Age-related shifts in the response of plasma Δ⁴ and Δ⁵ androgens, their C₂₁ precursors and cortisol to ACTH from infancy to puberty. In: *Pathophysiology of Puberty*, CACCIARI (E.) and PRADER (A.) (Eds.). Academic Press, London, 137-155, 1980.

[227] FOREST (M. G.), PERETTI (E. DE), LECOQ (A.), CADILLON (E.), ZABOT (M. T.), THOULON (J. M.). — Concentration of 14 steroid hormones in human amniotic fluid of mid-pregnancy. *J. Clin. Endocrinol. Metab.*, 51, 816-822, 1980.

[228] FOREST (M. G.), BETUEL (H.), BOUÉ (A.), COUILLIN (P.). — Antenatal diagnosis of congenital adrenal hyperplasia (CAH) due to 21-hydroxylase deficiency by steroid analysis in the amniotic fluid of mid-pregnancy: comparison with HLA typing in 17 pregnancies at risk for CAH. *Prenat. Diagnosis*, 1, 197-208, 1981.

[229] GENDREL (D.), CHAUSSAIN (J. L.), ROGER (M.), JOB (J. C.). — L'hyperplasie surrénale congénitale par bloc de la 3β-hydroxystéroïde déshydrogénase. *Arch. Fr. Péd.*, 36, 647-655, 1979.

[230] GILBERT (M. G.), CLEVELAND (W. W.). — Cushing's syndrome in infancy. *Pediatrics*, 46, 217-229, 1970.

[231] GILLET (P.), DAVID (M.), SASSARD (J.), BERTRAND (J.), JEUNE (M.), FRANÇOIS (R.). — Intérêt clinique des dosages d'activité rénine, testostérone, 17α-hydroxyprogestérone et ACTH au cours de la surveillance des hyperplasies congénitales des surrénales par déficit en 21-hydroxylase. *Arch. Fr. Péd.*, 34 (Suppl.), 139-153, 1977.

[232] GOLDMAN (A. S.), YAKOVAC (W. C.), BONGIOVANNI (A. M.). — Development of activity 3β-hydroxysteroid dehydrogenase in human fetal tissue and in two anencephalic newborns. *J. Clin. Endocrinol. Metab.*, 26, 14-22, 1966.

[233] GRAY (E. S.), ABRAMOVICH (D. R.). — Morphologic features of the anencephalic adrenal gland in early pregnancy. *Am. J. Obstet. Gynecol.*, 137, 491-495, 1980.

[234] GRIFFITHS (K.), CAMERON (E. H. D.). — The adrenal cortex. In: *The Cell in Medical Science: Cellular*

Specialization, Vol. 3. BECK (F.) and LLOYD (J. B.) (Eds.). Academic Press, London, 155-191, 1973.

[235] GRIFFITHS (K.), CAMERON (E. H. D.). — Steroid biosynthetic pathways in the human adrenal. In: *Advances in Steroid Biochemistry and Pharmacology*, Vol. 2. BRIGGS (M. H.). (Ed.) Academic Press, New York, 223-265, 1970.

[236] GWYNNE (J. T.), NEY (P. L.). — The adrenal cortex. In: *The Year in Endocrinology, 1977*. INGBAR (Ed.). Plenum Press, 161-189, 1978.

[237] HAMILTON (W. J.), BOYD (J. D.), MOSSMAN (H. W.). — *Human embryology*. W. Heffer and Sons, Ltd, Cambridge, 1962.

[238] HARKNESS (R. A.), TAYLOR (N. F.), BOWMAN (P. R.), GORDON (H.), CUMMINS (M.), VALMAN (H. B.). — The causes of low œstrogen secretion in pregnancy: the development of diagnostic methods for the antenatal detection of familial congenital adrenocortical hypoplasia. *Clin. Endocrinol.*, 12, 453-460, 1980.

[239] HAY (I. D.), SMAIL (P. J.), FORSYTH (C. C.). — Familial cytomegalic adrenocortical hypoplasia: an X-linked syndrome of pubertal failure. *Arch. Dis. Childh.*, 56, 715-721, 1981.

[240] HIGGINS (S. J.), GEHRING (U.). — Molecular mechanisms of steroid hormone action. *Adv. Cancer Res.*, 28, 313-397, 1978.

[241] HOLCOMBE (J. H.), KEENAN (B. S.), NICHOLS (B. L.), KIRKLAND (R. T.), CLAYTON (G. W.). — Neonatal salt loss in the hypertensive form of congenital adrenal hyperplasia. *Pediatrics*, 65, 777-781, 1980.

[242] HONOUR (J. W.), VALMAR (H. B.), SHACKLETON (C. H. L.). — Aldosterone and sodium homeostasis in pre-term infants. *Acta Paediat. Scand.*, 66, 103-109, 1977.

[243] HORNER (J. M.), HINTZ (R. L.), LUETSCHER (J. A.). — The role of renin and angiotensin in salt-losing, 21-hydroxylase deficient congenital adrenal hyperplasia. *J. Clin. Endocrinol. Metab.*, 48, 776-783, 1979.

[244] HORTON (R.). — Aldosterone: review of its physiology and diagnostic aspects of primary aldosteronism. *Metabolism*, 22, 1525-1545, 1973.

[245] HUGHES (I. A.), WINTER (J. S. D.). — The relationship between concentration of 17OH-progesterone and other serum and urinary steroids in patients with congenital adrenal hyperplasia. *J. Clin. Endocrinol. Metab.*, 46, 98-104, 1978.

[246] HUHTANIEMI (I.). — Studies on steroidogenesis and its regulation in human fetal adrenals and testis. *J. Steroid Biochem.*, 8, 491-497, 1977.

[247] JANSEN (M.), WIT (M.), VAN DEN BRANDE (J. L.). — Reinstitution of mineralocorticoid therapy in congenital adrenal hyperplasia. *Acta Paediat. Scand.*, 70, 229-233, 1981.

[248] JOHANNISSON (E.). — Fetal adrenal cortex in human; its ultrastructure at different stages of development and in different functional states. *Acta Endocrinol.*, 58, Suppl. 130, 7-107, 1968.

[249] JOHANNISSON (E.). — Aspects of the ultrastructure and function of the human fetal adrenal cortex. *Contribution to Gynecol. Obstet.*, 5, 109-130, 1979.

[250] JOHNSON (J. D.), HANSEN (R. C.), ALBRITTON (W. L.), WERTHEMANN (V.), CHRISTIANSEN (R. O.). — Hypoplasia of the anterior pituitary and neonatal hypoglycemia. *J. Pediatr.*, 82, 634-641, 1973.

[251] JOSSO (N.), FORTIER-BEAULIEU (M.), FAVRE (C.). — Genitography in intersexual states: a review of 86 cases with new criteria for the study of the urogenital sinus. *Acta Endocrinol. (Kbh)*, 62, 165-180, 1969.

[252] KAZUMI (S.), KYOYA (S.), MIYAWAKI (T.), KIDANI (H.), FUNABASHI (T.), NAKASHIMA (H.), NAKANUMA (Y.), OHTA (G.), ITAGAKI (E.), KATAGIRI (M.). — Cholesterol side-chain cleavage enzyme activity and cytochrome P-450 content in adrenal mitochondria of a patient with congenital lipoid adrenal hyperplasia (Prader disease). *Clin. Chim. Acta*, 77, 301-306, 1977.

[253] KEENAN (B. S.), HOLCOMBE (J. H.), KIRKLAND (R. T.), POTTS (V. E.), CLAYTON (G. W.). — Sodium homeostasis and aldosterone secretion in salt losing congenital adrenal hyperplasia. *J. Clin. Endocrinol. Metab.*, 48, 430-436, 1979.

[254] KEENAN (B. S.), HOLCOMBE (J. H.), WILSON (D. P.), KIRKLAND (R. T.), POTTS (E.), CLAYTON (G. W.). — Plasma renin activity and the response to sodium depletion in salt-losing congenital adrenal hyperplasia. *Ped. Res.*, 16, 118-122, 1982.

[255] KENNY (F. M.), REYNOLDS (J. W.), GREEN (O. G.). — Partial 3β-hydroxysteroid dehydrogenase (3β-HSD) deficiency in a family with congenital adrenal hyperplasia: evidence for increasing 3β-HSD activity with age. *Pediatrics*, 48, 756-765, 1971.

[256] KHURI (F. J.), ALTON (D. J.), HARDY (B. E.), COOK (G. T.), CHURCHILL (B. M.). — Adrenal hemorrhage in neonates: report of 5 cases and review of the literature. *J. Urol.*, 124, 684, 1980.

[257] KIRKLAND (R. T.), KIRKLAND (J. L.), JOHNSON (C. M.), HORNING (M. G.), LIBRIK (L.), CLAYTON (G. W.). — Congenital lipoid adrenal hyperplasia in an eight year-old phenotypic female. *J. Clin. Endocrinol.*, 36, 488-496, 1973.

[258] KOSCHIMUZU (T.). — Plasma renin activity and aldosterone concentration in normal subjects and patients with salt-losing type of congenital adrenal hyperplasia during infancy. *Clin. Endocrinol.*, 10, 515-522, 1979.

[259] LAATIKAINEN (T.), PERHEENTUPA (J.), VIHKO (R.), MAKINO (I.), SJORVALL (J.). — Bile acids and hormonal steroids in bile in a boy with 3β-hydroxysteroid dehydrogenase deficiency. *J. Steroid Biochem.*, 3, 715-724, 1972.

[260] LANMAN (J. T.). — The adrenal gland in the human fetus. *Pediatrics*, 27, 140-158, 1961.

[261] LAWSON (E. E.), LITTLEWOOD (T. R.). — Diagnosis of adrenal hemorrhage by ultrasound. *J. Ped.*, 92, 423-426, 1978.

[262] LEBLANC (A.), ODIEVRE (M.), HADCHOUEL (M.), GENDREL (D.), CHAUSSAIN (J. L.), RAPPAPORT (R.). — Neonatal cholestasis and hypoglycemia: possible role of cortisol deficiency. *J. Ped.*, 99, 577-580, 1981.

[263] LEVINE (L. S.), RAUH (W.), GOTTESDIENER (K.), CHOW (D.), GUNCZLER (P.), RAPPAPORT (R.), PANG (S.), SCHNEIDER (B.), NEW (M. I.). — New studies of the 11β-hydroxylase and 18-hydroxylase enzymes in the hypertensive form of congenital adrenal hyperplasia. *J. Clin. Endocrinol. Metab.*, 50, 258-263, 1980.

[264] LEVY (S. R.), WYNNE (C. V.), LORENTZ (W. B.). — Syndrome de Cushing secondaire à un adénome hypophysaire chez le nourrisson. *Am. J. Dis. Child., J. Pédiat.*, 2, 627-629, 1982.

[265] LIDDLE (G. W.). — The adrenals. Part I: The adrenal cortex. In: *Textbook of Endocrinology.*

WILLIAMS (R. D.). (Ed.). W. B. Saunders Company, Philadelphia, 233-322, 1974.

[265 bis] LOVINGER (R. D.), KAPLAN (S. L.), GRUMBACH (M. D.). — Congenital hypopituitarism and microphallus: four cases secondary to hypothalamic hormone deficiencies. J. Pediat., 87, 1171-1181, 1975.

[266] LJUNGQVIST (A.), WAGERMARK (J.). — Renal juxtaglomerular granulation in the human fetus and infant. Acta Pathol. Microbiol. Scand., 67, 257-266, 1966.

[266 bis] McGIFF (J. C.). — Bartter's syndrome results from an unbalance of vasoactive hormones. Ann. Intern. Med., 87, 369-372, 1977.

[267] MAMELLE (J. C.), DAVID (M.), RIOU (D.), GILLY (J.), TROUILLAS (J.), DUTRUGE (J.), GILLY (R.). — Hypoplasie surrénalienne congénitale de type cytomégalique. Forme récessive liée au sexe. Arch. Fr. Péd., 32, 139-159, 1975.

[268] MAREK (J.). — Gonadotrophin deficiency and adrenocortical insufficiency in children. Brit. Med., J., 2, 828, 1977.

[269] MARSHALL (W. C.), OCKENDEN (B. G.), FORSBROOKE (A. S.), CUMINGS (J. N.). — Wolman's disease. Arch. Dis. Child., 44, 331-341, 1969.

[270] MERLOB (P.), BAHARI (C.), LIBAN (E.), REISNER (S. H.). — Cysts of the female external genitalia in the newborn infant. Am. J. Obstet. Gynecol., 132, 607-610, 1978.

[271] MIGEON (C. J.). — Diagnosis and treatment of adrenogenital disorders. In: Endocrinology, Vol. 2. DeGROOT (L. J.) (Ed.). Grune and Stratton, New York, 1203-1224, 1978.

[272] MIGEON (C. J.), ROSENWAKS (Z.), LEE (P. A.), URBAN (M. D.), BIAS (W. B.). — The attenuated form of congenital adrenal hyperplasia as an allelic form of 21-hydroxylase deficiency. J. Clin. Endocrinol. Metab., 51, 647-649, 1980.

[273] MITCHELL (B. F.), SERRON-FERRÉ (M.), HESS (D. L.), JAFFE (R. B.). — Cortisol production and metabolism in the late gestation Rhesus monkey fetus. Endocrinology, 108, 916-924, 1981.

[274] MIYAKAWA (I.), IKEDA (I.), MAEYAMA (M.). — Transport of ACTH across human placenta. J. Clin. Endocrinol. Metab., 39, 440-442, 1976.

[275] MOSER (H. W.), MOSER (A. B.), KAWANURA (N.), MIGEON (B.), O'NEILL (B. P.), FENSELAU (C.), KISHIMOTO (Y.). — Adrenoleucodystrophy: studies of the phenotype, genetics and biochemistry. J. Hopkins Med., J., 47, 217-224, 1980.

[276] MOSER (H. W.), MOSER (A. B.), POWERS (M.), NITOWSKY (H. M.), SCHAUMBURG (H. H.), NOREIM (R. A.), MIGEON (B. R.). — The prenatal diagnosis of adrenoleukodystrophy. Demonstration of increased hexacosanoic acid levels in cultured amniocytes and fetal adrenal gland. Ped. Res., 16, 172-175, 1982.

[277] MULLER (J.). — Regulation of Aldosterone Biosynthesis. Springer-Verlag, New York, 1971.

[278] MURPHY (B. E. P.). — Steroid arteriovenous differences in umbilical cord plasma: evidence of cortisol production by the human fetus in early gestation. J. Clin. Endocrinol. Metab., 36, 1037-1038, 1973.

[279] MURPHY (B. E. P.). — Chorionic membrane as an extra-adrenal source of fetal cortisol in human amniotic fluid. Nature, 266, 179-181, 1977.

[280] MURPHY (B. E. P.) — Conjugated glucocorticoids in amniotic-fluid and fetal lung maturation. J. Clin. Endocrinol. Metab., 47, 212-215, 1978.

[281] MURPHY (B. E. P.). — Cortisol production and inactivation by the human lung during gestation and infancy. J. Clin. Endocrinol. Metab., 47, 243-248, 1978.

[282] MURPHY (B. E. P.). — Cortisol and cortisone in human fetal development. J. Steroid Biochem., 11, 509-513, 1979.

[283] MURPHY (B. E. P.), CLARK (S. J.), DONALD (I. R.), PINSKY (M.), VEDALY (D.). — Conversion of maternal cortisol to cortisone during placental transfer to the human fetus. Am. J. Obstet. Gynecol., 118, 538-542, 1974.

[284] NIEMI (M.), BAILLIE (A. H.). — 3β-hydroxysteroid dehydrogenase activity in the human fetal adrenal cortex. Acta Endocrinol., 48, 423-428, 1965.

[285] OBERFIELD (S. E.), LEVINE (S.), CAREY (R. M.), BEJAR (R.), NEW (M. I.). — Pseudohypoaldosteronism: multiple target organ unresponsiveness to mineralocorticoid hormones. J. Clin. Endocrinol. Metab., 48, 228-234, 1979.

[286] OETIKER (O. H.), ZURBRUG (R. P.). — Renal regulation of fluid, electrolyte and acid-base homeostasis in the salt losing syndrome of congenital adrenal hyperplasia (SL-CAH). ECF volume: a compensating factor in aldosterone deficiency. J. Clin. Endocrinol. Metab., 46, 543-551, 1978.

[287] OHRLANDER (S.), GENNSER (G.), GRENNERT (L.). — Impact of betamethasone load given to pregnant women on endocrine balance of fetal-placental unit. Am. J. Obstet. Gynecol., 123, 228-236, 1975.

[288] OHRLANDER (S.), GENNSER (G.), ENEROTH (P.). — Plasma cortisol levels in human fetus during parturition. Obstet. Gynecol., 48, 381-387, 1976.

[289] OSATHANONDH (R.), TULCHINSKY (D.), KAMALI (H.), FENCL (M.), TAENSCH (H. W.). — Dexamethasone levels in treated pregnant women and newborn infants. J. Pediatr., 90, 617-620, 1977.

[289 bis] PANG (S.), LEVINE (L. S.), CHOW (D. M.), FAIMAN (C.), NEW (M. I.). — Serum androgen concentrations in neonates and young infants with congenital adrenal hyperplasia due to 21-hydroxylase deficiency. Clin. Endocrinol., 11, 575-584, 1979.

[289 ter] PANG (S.), MURPHEY (W.), LEVINE (L. S.), SPENCE (D. A.), LEON (A.), LAFRANCHI (S.), SURVE (A. S.), NEW (M. I.). — A pilot newborn screening for congenital adrenal hyperplasia in Alaska. J. Clin. Endocrinol. Metab., 55, 413-420, 1982.

[290] PASQUALINI (J. R.), WIQVIST (N.), DICZFALUSY (E.). — Biosynthesis of aldosterone by human fetuses perfused with corticosterone at mid-term. Biochim. Biophys. Acta, 121, 430-431, 1966.

[291] PAVLOVA (E. B.), PRONINA (T. S.), SKEBELSKAYA (Y. B.). — Histostructure of adenohypophysis of human fetuses and contents of somatotrophic and adrenocorticotropic hormones. Gen. Comp. Endocrinol., 10, 269-276, 1968.

[292] PERETTI (E. DE), FOREST (M. G.). — Unconjugated dehydroepiandrosterone plasma levels in normal subjects from birth to adolescence in human: the use of a sensitive radio-immunoassay. J. Clin. Endocrinol. Metab., 43, 982-991, 1976.

[293] PERETTI (E. DE), FOREST (M. G.). — Pattern of plasma dehydroepiandrosterone sulfate levels in human from birth to adulthood: evidence for testicular production. J. Clin. Endocrinol. Metab., 47, 572-577, 1978.

[293 bis] PERETTI (E. DE), FOREST (M. G.). — Pittfalls in the etiological diagnosis of congenital adrenal hyperplasia in the early neonatal period. *Horm. Res.*, *16*, 10-22, 1982.

[294] PERETTI (E. DE), FOREST (M. G.), FEIT (J. P.), DAVID (M.). — Endocrine studies in two children with male pseudohermaphroditism (MPH) due to 3-hydroxysteroid-dehydrogenase deficiency. In: *Adrenal Androgens.* GENAZZANI (A. R.), THIJSSEN (J. H. H.) and SIITERI (P. K.) (Eds.). Raven Press, New York, 141-144, 1980.

[295] PRADER (A.). — Störungen der Geschlechtsdifferenzierung (Intersexualität). In: *Klinik der Inneren Sekretion,* 3. Auflage. LABHART (A.) (Ed.). Springer-Verlag, Berlin, 1978.

[296] PRADER (A.), SIEBENMANN (R. E.). — Nebennieren insuffizienz bei Kongenitalenlipoidhyperplasie der Nebennieren. *Helv. Paediat. Acta,* *12*, 569-595, 1957.

[297] PRICE (D.), ZAAIJER (J. J. P.), ORTIZ (E.), BRINK-MANN (A. O.). — Current views on embryonic sex differentiation in reptiles, birds and mammals. *Ann. Zool.,* *15*, Suppl. 1, 173-195, 1975.

[298] RAYYIS (S. S.), HORTON (R.). — Effect of angiotensin II on adrenal and pituitary function in man. *J. Clin. Endocrinol. Metab.,* *32*, 539-546, 1971.

[299] REYNOLDS (J. W.). — Fetal and neonatal steroid metabolism. In: *Problems in Pediatric Endocrinology.* LA CAUZA (C.) and ROOT (A. W.) (Eds.). Academic Press, London, 239-251. 1980.

[300] ROKICKI (W.), BERTRAND (J.). — The glucocorticoids in normal premature and small for dates newborn infants throughout the neonatal period. In: *Intensive Care of the Newborn,* II. STERN (L.), SALLE (B.) and FRIIS-HANSEN (B.). (Eds.). Masson, New York, 325-342, 1981.

[301] ROOS (B. A.). — Effect of ACTH and cAMP on human adrenocortical growth and function *in vitro. Endocrinology,* *94*, 685-690, 1974.

[302] ROSE (J. C.), MACDONALD (A. A.), HEYMANN (M. A.), RUDOLF (A. M.). — Developmental aspects of the pituitary adrenal axis response to hemorrhagic stress in lamb fetuses *in utero. J. Clin. Invest.,* *61*, 424-432, 1978.

[303] ROSENFIELD (R. L.), RICH (B. H.), WOLFSDORF (J. I.), CASSORLA (F.), PARKS (J. S.), BONGIOVANNI (A. M.), WU (C. H.), SHACKLETON (C. H. L.). — Pubertal presentation of congenital Δ^5-3β-hydroxysteroid dehydrogenase deficiency. *J. Clin. Endocrinol. Metab.,* *51*, 345-353, 1980.

[304] ROSLER (A.), THEODOR (R.), GAZIT (E.), BIOCHIS (H.), RABINOVITZ (D.). — Salt wastage, raised plasma-renin activity and normal or high plasma aldosterone: a form of pseudo-aldosteronism. *Lancet,* *1*, 959-961, 1973.

[305] ROVNER (D. R.), CONN (J. W.), COHEN (E. L.), BERLINGER (F. G.), KEIN (D. C.), GORDON (D. L.). — 17α-hydroxylase deficiency. A combination of hydroxylation defect and reversible blockade in aldosterone biosynthesis. *Acta Endocrinol. (Kbh),* *90*, 490-504, 1979.

[306] SAEZ (J. M.), DAZORD (A.). — Source, métabolisme et rôle des œstrogènes chez l'homme. In: *Les œstrogènes* (XIVe réunion des Endocrinologistes de Langue Française). Masson, Paris, 161-180, 1977.

[307] SASSARD (J.), SANN (L.), VINCENT (M.), FRANÇOIS (R.), CIER (J. F.). — Plasma renin activity in normal subjects from infancy to puberty. *J. Clin. Endocrinol. Metab.,* *40*, 524-525, 1975.

[307 bis] SAUTAREL (M.), FONTAN (D.), COQUET (M.), BIOULAC (P.), GUIBERT (F.), SANDLER (B.), DECHARTRE (C.). — A propos d'une nouvelle observation d'adrénoleucodystrophie. Intérêt diagnostique des biopsies neuromusculaires et cutanées et de l'examen tomodensitométrique. *Pédiatrie,* *36*, 43-53, 1981.

[308] SCHAISON (G.), COUZINET (B.), GOURMELEN (A.), ELKIK (F.), BOUGNERES (P.). — Angiotensin and adrenal steroidogenesis: study of 21-hydroxylase deficient congenital adrenal hyperplasia. *J. Clin. Endocrinol. Metab.,* *51*, 1390-1394, 1980.

[309] SCHIMKE (R. N.), SPAULDING (J. J.), HOLLOWELL (J. G.). — X-linked congenital panhypopituitarism. *Birth Defects,* *7*, 21-23, 1971.

[310] SCHNAKENBURG (W. K.), BIDLINGMAIER (F.), KNORR (D.). — 17-hydroxyprogesterone, androstenedione and testosterone in normal children and in prepubertal patients with congenital adrenal hyperplasia. *Eur. J. Ped.,* *133*, 259-267, 1980.

[311] SCHNEIDER (G.), GENEL (M.), BONGIOVANNI (A. M.), GOLDMAN (A. S.), ROSENFIELD (R. S.). — Persistent testicular Δ^5-isomerase-3β-hydroxysteroid dehydrogenase (Δ^4-3β-HSD) deficiency in Δ^5-3β-HSD form of congenital adrenal hyperplasia. *J. Clin. Invest.,* *55*, 681-690, 1975.

[312] SCHUBERT (K.), SCHADE (K.). — Placental steroid hormones. *J. Steroid Biochem.,* *8*, 359-365, 1977.

[313] SCHUMERT (Z.), ROSENMANN (A.), LANDAU (H.), ROSLER (A.). — 11-deoxycortisol in amniotic fluid: prenatal diagnosis of congenital adrenal hyperplasia due to 11β-hydroxylase deficiency. *Clin. Endocrinol.,* *12*, 257-260, 1980.

[314] SEELY (J. R.). — The fetal and neonatal adrenal cortex. In: *Metabolic, Endocrine and Genetic Disorders of Children.* KELLEY (V. C.) (Ed.). Harper and Row, New York, 225-243, 1974.

[315] SERRON-FERRÉ (M.), LAWRENCE (C. C.), SIITERI (P. K.), JAFFE (R. B.). — Steroid production by definitive and fetal zones of the human fetal fetal adrenal gland. *J. Clin. Endocrinol. Metab.,* *47*, 603-609, 1978.

[316] SHACKLETON (C. H. L.), HONOUR (J. W.), TAYLOR (N. F.) — Metabolism of fetal and neonatal adrenal steroids. *J. Steroid Biochem.,* *11*, 523-529, 1979.

[316 bis] SHIMOZAWA (K.), SAITO (N.), SAKURADA (N.), YATA (J.), HIKITA (Y.), TAKEHIRO (A.), WAVVANA-MI, IGARASHI (Y.), OKADA (K.), ITO (Y.), IRIE (M.). — A pilot neonatal mass-screening study for congenital adrenal hyperplasia due to 21-hydroxylase deficiency in Japan. *International Meeting on Neonatal Screening,* Tokyo, 16-21 August 1982, VI-3, p. 109.

[317] SIEGEL (S. R.), OH (W.). — Renal function as a marker to fetal maturation. *Acta Paediat. Scand.,* *65*, 481-485, 1976.

[318] SIEGEL (S. R.), FISHER (D. A.), OH (W.). — Serum aldosterone concentrations related to sodium balance in the newborn infant. *Pediatrics,* *53*, 410-413, 1974.

[319] SILMAN (R. E.), CHARD (T.), LOWRY (P. J.), SMITH (I.), YOUNG (I. M.). — Human fetal pituitary peptides and parturition. *Nature,* *260*, 716-718, 1976.

[320] SILMAN (R. E.), CHARD (T.), LANDON (J.), LOWRY (P. J.), SMITH (I.), YOUNG (J. M.). — ACTH and

MSH peptides in the human adult and fetal pituitary gland. *Front. Horm. Res.*, 4, 179-187, 1977.

[321] SIMMER (H. H.), FRANKLAND (M. V.), GREIPEL (M.). — Unbound unconjugated cortisol in umbilical cord and corresponding maternal plasma. *Gynecol. Invest.*, 5, 199-221, 1974.

[322] SIMONIAN (M. H.), GILL (G. N.). — Regulation of the fetal adrenal cortex: effects of adrenocorticotropin on growth and function of monolayer cultures of fetal and definitive zone cells. *Endocrinology*, 108, 1769-1779, 1981.

[323] SIMPSON (E. R.), CARR (B. R.), PARKER (C. R. Jr.), MILEWICH (L.), PORTER (J. C.), MACDONALD (P. C.). — The role of lipoproteins in steroidogenesis by the human fetal adrenal cortex. *J. Clin. Endocrinol. Metab.*, 49, 146-148, 1979.

[324] SIPPEL (W. G.), BECKER (H.), VERSMOLD (H. T.), BIDLINGMAIER (F.), KNORR (D.). — Longitudinal studies of plasma aldosterone, corticosterone, deoxycorticosterone, cortisol and cortisone determined simultaneously in mother and child at birth and during the early neonatal period. I. Spontaneous delivery. *J. Clin. Endocrinol. Metab.*, 46, 971-985, 1978.

[325] SIPPELL (W. G.), DÖRR (H. G.), BIDLINGMAIER (F.), KNORR (D.). — Plasma levels of aldosterone, corticosterone, 11-deoxycorticosterone, progesterone, 17-hydroxyprogesterone, cortisol and cortisone during early infancy and childhood. *Ped. Res.*, 14, 39-46, 1980.

[326] SIPPELL (W.G.), MÜLLERHOLVE (W.), DÖRR (H.G.), BINDLINGMAIER (F.), KNORR (D.). — Concentration of aldosterone, corticosterone, 11-deoxycorticosterone, progesterone, 17-hydroxyprogesterone, 11-deoxycortisol, cortisol and cortisone determined simultaneously in human amniotic fluid throughout gestation. *J. Clin. Endocrinol. Metab.*, 52, 385-392, 1981.

[327] SIZONENKO (P. C.), RIONDEL (A. M.), KOHLBERG (I. J.), PAUNIER (L.). — 11β-hydroxylase deficiency: steroid response to sodium restriction and ACTH stimulation. *J. Clin. Endocrinol. Metab.*, 35, 281-287, 1972.

[328] SMITH (J. A. Jr.), MIDDLETON (R. G.). — Neonatal adrenal haemorrhage. *J. Urol.*, 122, 674-677, 1979.

[329] SOLOMON (S.), BIRD (C. E.), LING (W.), IWAMIYA (M.), YOUNG (P. C. M.). — Formation and metabolism of steroids in the fetus and placenta. *Rec. Prog. Horm. Res.*, 23, 297-347, 1967.

[330] SPECTOR (W. S.). — *Handbook of Biological Data*. Saunders (W. B.), Philadelphia, 1956.

[331] SPITZER (A.). — Renal physiology and functional development. In: *Pediatric Kidney Disease*. EDELMAN (C. M.). (Ed.), Little Brown, Boston, 25-128, 1978.

[332] SYMMINGTON (T.). — *Functional pathology of the human adrenal gand*. Livingstone (E. S.), Ltd, London, 1969.

[333] SYMONDS (E. M.), FURLER (I.). — Plasma renin levels in the normal and anephric fetus at birth. *Biol. Neonate*, 23, 133-138, 1973.

[334] THOMPSON (E. B.), LIPPMAN (M. E.). — Mechanism of action of glucocorticoids. *Metabolism*, 23, 159-202, 1974.

[335] TOURNIAIRE (J.), AUDI-PARERA (L.), LORAS (B.), BLUM (J.), CASTELNOVO (P.), FOREST (M. G.). — Male pseudohermaphroditism with hypertension due to 17α-hydroxylation deficiency. *Clin. Endocrinol.*, 5, 53-61, 1976.

[336] TULCHINSKY (D.), FRIGOLETTO (F. D. Jr.), RYAN (K. J.), FISHMAN (J.). — Plasma estetrol as an index of fetal well-being. *J. Clin. Endocrinol. Metab.*, 40, 560-567, 1975.

[337] ULICK (S.), GANTIER (E.), VETTER (K. K.), MARKELLO (J. R.), JAFFE (S.), LOWE (C. V.). — An aldosterone biosynthesis defect in salt-losing disorder. *J. Clin. Endocrinol. Metab.*, 24, 669-672, 1964.

[338] VALE (W.), SPIESS (J.), RIVIER (C.), RIVIER (J.). — Characterization of a 41-residue ovine hypothalamic peptide that stimulates secretion of corticotropin and β-endorphin. *Science*, 213, 1394-1396, 1981.

[339] VERMES (I.), KAJTAR (I.), SZABÓ (E.). — Changes of maternal and fetal pituitary-adrenocortical functions during human labour. *Horm. Res.*, 11, 213-217, 1979.

[340] VERMES (I.), DOHANICS (J.), TÓTH (G.), POUGRÁCZ (J.). — Maturation of the circadian rhythm of the adrenocortical functions in human neonates and infants. *Hormone Res.*, 12, 237-244, 1980.

[341] VILLEE (D. B.). — The development of steroidogenesis. *Am. J. Med.*, 53, 533-544, 1972.

[342] VIMPANI (G. V.), VIMPANI (A. F.), LIDGARD (G. P.), CAMERON (E. H. D.), FARQUHAR (J. W.). — Prevalence of severe growth hormone deficiency. *Brit. Med. J.*, 2, 427-429, 1977.

[343] VINCENT (M.), DESSART (T.), ANNAT (G.), SASSARD (J.), FRANÇOIS (R.), CIER (J. F.). — Plasma renin activity, aldosterone and dopamine beta-hydroxylase activity as a function of age in normal children. *Ped. Res.*, 14, 894-895, 1980.

[344] VISSER (H. K. A.), COST (W. S.). — A new hereditary defect in the biosynthesis of aldosterone: urinary C21-corticosteroid in three related patients with a salt-losing syndrome, suggesting an 18-oxidation defect. *Acta Endocrinol. (Kbh)*, 47, 589-612, 1964.

[345] VISSER (M.), SWAAB (D. F.). — α-MSH in the human pituitary. *Front. Horm. Res.*, 4, 42-45, 1977.

[346] VOUTILAINEN (R.), KAHRI (A. I.). — Placental origin of the suppression of 3β-hydroxysteroid dehydrogenase in the fetal zone cells of human fetal adrenals. *J. Steroid Biochem.*, 13, 39-43, 1980.

[347] WALDHAUSL (W.), HERKNER (K.), NOWOTNY (P.), BRATUSCH-MARRAIN (P.). — Combined 17α- and 18-hydroxylase deficiency associated with complete male pseudohermaphroditism and hypoaldosteronism. *J. Clin. Endocrinol. Metab.*, 46, 236-246, 1978.

[348] WEIL (J.), BIDLINGMAIER (F.), SIPPEL (W. G.), BUTENANDT (O.), KNORR (D.). — Comparison of two tests for heterozygosity in congenital adrenal hyperplasia (CAH). *Acta Endocrinol. (Kbh)*, 91, 109-121, 1979.

[349] WELDON (V. V.), KOWARSKI (A.), MIGEON (C. J.). — Aldosterone secretion rates in normal subjects from infancy to adulthood. *Pediatrics*, 39, 713-723, 1967.

[350] WERDER (E. A.), SIEBENMANN (R. E.), KNORR-MURSET (G.), ZIMMERMANN (A.), SIZONENKO (P. C.), THEINTZ (P.), GIRARD (J.), ZACHMANN (M.), PRADER (A.). — The incidence of congenital adrenal hyperplasia in Switzerland. A survey of patients born in 1960 to 1974. *Helvet. Paediat. Acta*, 35, 5-11, 1980.

[351] WEST (C. D.), ATCHESON (J. B.), STOMCHFIELD

(J. B.), RALLISON (M. L.), CHAVRE (V. J.), TYLER (F. H.). — Multiple or simple 21-hydroxylases in congenital adrenal hyperplasia. *J. Steroid Biochem.*, *11*, 1413-1419, 1979.

[352] WEST (G. B.), SHEPHERD (D. M.), HUNTER (R. B.), MacGREGOR (A. R.). — The functions of the organs of Zuckerkandl. *Clin. Sci.*, *12*, 317-325, 1953.

[353] WINKEL (C. A.), SNYDER (J. M.), MacDONALD (P. C.), SIMPSON (E. R.). — Regulation of cholesterol and progesterone synthesis in human placental cells in culture by serum lipoproteins. *Endocrinology*, *106*, 1054-1060, 1980.

[354] WINTER (J. S. D.), FUJIEDA (K.), FAIMAN (C.), REYES (F. I.), THLIVERIS (J.). — Control of steroidogenesis by human fetal adrenal cells in tissue culture. In: *Adrenal Androgens.* GENAZZANI (A. R.), THIJSSEN (J. H. H.) and SIITERI (P. K.) (Eds.). Raven Press, New York, 55-62, 1980.

[355] WINTERS (A. J.), OLIVER (C.), COLSTON (C.), MacDONALD (P. C.), PORTER (J. C.). — Plasma ACTH levels in the human fetus and neonate as related to age and parturition. *J. Clin. Endocrinol Metab.*, *39*, 269-273, 1974.

[356] WURTMAN (R. J.). — Control of epinephrine synthesis in the adrenal medulla by the adrenal cortex: hormonal specificity and dose response characteristics. *Endocrinology*, *79*, 608-614, 1966.

[357] ZACHMANN (M.), VOLLMIN (J. A.), NEW (M. I.), CURTIUS (H. C.), PRADER (A.). — Congenital adrenal hyperplasia due to deficiency of 11β-hydroxylation of 17α-hydroxylated steroids. *J. Clin. Endocrinol. Metab.*, *33*, 501-508, 1971.

[358] ZACHMANN (M.), FOREST (M. G.), PERETTI (E. DE). — 3β-hydroxysteroid dehydrogenase deficiency. Follow-up study in a girl with pubertal bone age. *Horm. Res.*, *11*, 292-302, 1979.

[359] ZACHMANN (M.), GIRARD (J.), DUC (G.), ILLIG (R.), PRADER (A.). — Low urinary estriol during pregnancy caused by isolated fetal ACTH-deficiency. *Acta Paediat. Scand., Suppl. 277*, 27-31, 1979.

[360] ZURBRÜGG (R. P.). — Hypothalamic-pituitary-adrenocortical regulation. A contribution to its assessment, development and disorders in infancy and childhood with special reference to plasma cortisol circadian rhythm. *Monogr. Pediatr.*, Vol. 7. Karger, Basel, 1976.

7

Nephrology and urology

41

Neonatal renal function and disease

Jean-Pierre GUIGNARD and Antonio TORRADO

RENAL PHYSIOLOGY

The human kidney is formed by two distinct zones: the cortex and the medulla [179]. Each kidney is composed of 1.2 million functional units called nephrons (Fig. VII-1). Each functional unit is formed by a glomerulus and a tubule. The tubule is divided into several segments: the proximal tubule, the loop of Henle, the distal tubule and the collecting duct. An adult nephron measures 20-44 mm length. The diameter of the glomerulus varies from 200 to 350 μ. Eighty percent of the glomeruli are located in the superficial cortex. Deeply located nephrons, the juxtamedullary nephrons, have longer loops of Henle, which penetrate deeply into the renal papillae. In the cortex, the interstitial tissue is isotonic to plasma, whereas it is highly hypertonic in the medullary zone. The concentration gradient between these two zones is 1 : 4.

The kidney has several functions [169]:

(a) regulation of body homeostasis
(b) acid-base regulation
(c) excretion of the end-products of nitrogen metabolism
(d) control of blood pressure
(e) hormonal secretion

Blood supply
[27]

One fifth of the cardiac output perfuses the kidney, i. e. 1,200 ml/min. Blood flow is mainly distributed within the renal cortex. Medullary blood flow represents only 10 % of total renal blood flow. As there is auto-regulation (a myogenic effect) renal blood flow remains constant with arterial perfusion pressures ranging between 80 and 200 mm Hg.

The autonomic nervous system and two hormonal systems share the control of renal blood flow: the renin-angiotensin system and the prostaglandins. Pathophysiologic situations that induce vasoconstriction, such as hypoxemia, acute ischemia, hypercapnia, acidosis and hypovolemic shock, can modify renal blood flow.

Glomerular filtration
[26, 148]

Glomerular filtration represents the first step in urine formation: 20 % of the plasma passing through the glomerular capillaries, i. e. 120 ml/min, enters Bowman's space to form an ultrafiltrate. Glomerular filtration occurs through pores of 70-100 Å width and 400-600 Å length within the capillary wall. The largest normally filtrable molecule has a molecular weight of 70,000. The total filtration area is about 1 m²/kidney. The effective filtration pressure (EFP) is determined by the difference between hydrostatic and oncotic pressures across the glomerular membrane:

$$EFP = GP - (OP + TP)$$

where:

GP = hydrostatic pressure within the glomerular capillaries
OP = oncotic pressure of plasma proteins
TP = hydrostatic tubular pressure

Normally,

$$EFP = 90 - (30 + 15) = 45 \text{ mm Hg}$$

Effective filtration pressure depends on systemic blood pressure, on resistances in afferent and efferent arterioles, on oncotic pressure of plasma proteins and on pressure within the renal tubules.

Solute transport
[30, 49, 85]

In the *proximal tubule*, 65 to 80 % of the glomerular filtrate is reabsorbed, mostly by an active mechanism. This reabsorption is isotonic, *i. e.* the osmolality of the filtrate does not change.

In the *loop of Henle*, urine is concentrated by a countercurrent mechanism. The descending portion of the loop of Henle is highly permeable to water, while its ascending portion is impermeable to water. In the descending limb, there is no active transport. The thin segment of the ascending limb is highly permeable to urea and NaCl. It is not the site of any active transport. The thick portion of the ascending limb is only slightly permeable to urea and sodium. Here, chloride is transported by an active mechanism and sodium passively reabsorbed as its accompanying cation. In the *distal* and *collecting tubules* there is two-way movement of solute (*i. e.* reabsorption and secretion). Proximal reabsorption is regulated by several factors: the state of extracellular fluid volume expansion, the peritubular oncotic pressure, and parathyroid hormone (PTH). The cortical portion of the collecting duct responds to aldosterone. Its papillary portion is highly permeable to urea. The antidiuretic hormone system controls the permeability of the collecting duct to water.

Sodium [111]. — 99 % of the filtered sodium is reabsorbed in the tubules as follows: 65-80 % in the proximal tubule; 20-25 % in the ascending limb of the loop of Henle; the remainder is reabsorbed in the distal and collecting tubules. Extracellular volume expansion inhibits the proximal transport of sodium, whereas aldosterone promotes its reabsorption in the collecting duct by exchange with hydrogen and potassium.

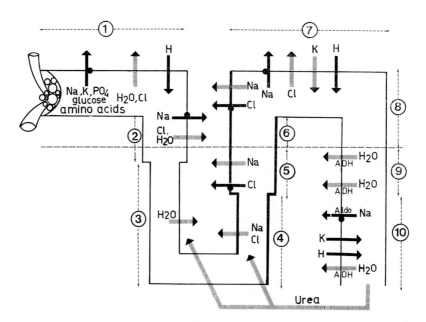

FIG. VII-1. — *Diagram of the nephron indicating the major sites of solute transport.*

Potassium [38]. — This ion is completely reabsorbed in the proximal tubule. Potassium excreted in urine results from distal tubular secretion, which, in turn depends on potassium concentration within the tubular cells. Aldosterone promotes the exchange between sodium and potassium.

Calcium. — Calcium reabsorption parallels sodium reabsorption in the proximal tubule and in the ascending limb of the loop of Henle. Parathyroid hormone promotes distal calcium reabsorption.

Phosphorus. — Phosphate is filtered and reabsorbed in the proximal tubule. Proximal phosphate reabsorption is inhibited by parathyroid hormone. Chronic reduction in GFR is accompanied by phosphate retention.

Hydrogen [146, 177]. — Protons are secreted in the proximal, the distal and the collecting tubules. Proximal hydrogen secretion is highly linked to sodium reabsorption. Most of the secreted protons are utilized in the reabsorption of filtered bicarbonate. The remaining protons are eliminated as ammonium, acid phosphate (titratable acidity), or as free hydrogen ions. Proton secretion is dependent upon the plasma CO_2 tension, the state of extracellular volume expansion, the level of body potassium stores and the activity of carbonic anhydrase. The relationship between PTH, calcium, phosphate and hydrogen transport is still unclear.

Bicarbonate [146]. — The reabsorption of this ion is linked to the secretion of protons and to the reabsorption of sodium. It is subject to the same influences which regulate proton secretion.

Chloride. — Chloride reabsorption is linked to that of sodium. While it is passively reabsorbed in the proximal, distal and collecting tubules, it probably undergoes active reabsorption in the ascending limb of the loop of Henle.

Urea. — Urea is excreted by glomerular filtration and tubular diffusion. It plays an important role in the countercurrent mechanism: its concentration in the interstitium, together with that of sodium chloride is responsible for the generation of the osmotic corticomedullary gradient.

Other solutes. — Glucose and amino-acids are actively and completely reabsorbed in the proximal tubule.

Regulatory functions

Concentration [96, 105]. — Urine concentration takes place in the loop of Henle and the collecting duct. Through the differences in relative permeability of the tubule to water, urea and NaCl, the countercurrent mechanism generates an osmotic cortico-medullary gradient by passive (urea) or active (NaCl) accumulation of solutes in the medullary interstitium. In the presence of vasopressin, water diffuses from the collecting duct into the hypertonic medullary interstitium. The concentrating mechanism is compromised when the deposition of solutes in the medulla is impaired (inhibition of the chloride pump by diuretics, low urinary concentration of urea, as in the normal newborn or in malnutrition) or in the case of cortico-medullary gradient washout (osmotic diuresis, sickle cell disease). Urine concentrating ability is also impaired when the collecting duct epithelium is insensitive to vasopressin (nephrogenic diabetes insipidus, hypercalcemia, hypokalemia) or when there is a lack of circulating vasopressin (central diabetes insipidus).

Urine dilution [105]. — The active reabsorption of NaCl in the ascending limb of the loop of Henle and in the distal tubule lowers urine osmolality and in the absence of ADH leads to the excretion of free water. Any condition lowering the distal reabsorption of NaCl or the volume of glomerular filtrate delivered to the distal tubule, interferes with the formation and excretion of free water. This is the case during the administration of tubular diuretics or when the volume of glomerular filtrate delivered to the distal tubule is decreased, as seen in acute renal failure, adrenal hypofunction, decompensated nephrotic syndrome or cardiac failure.

Acid-base regulation [146]. — Acid-base regulation is maintained by the regeneration of the filtered bicarbonate and the excretion of fixed (non-volatile) acids as ammonium and titratable acidity. The urinary pH is influenced by the plasma bicarbonate concentration and varies between 4.5 and 8.0. At pH values lower than 7.0 urine contains a negligible quantity of bicarbonate. The renal bicarbonate threshold is defined as the plasma concentration at which bicarbonate appears in urine. This threshold, maintained at 24-26 mmol/l, is lowered in certain conditions (in the normal newborn, in proximal renal tubular acidosis, during extracellular volume expansion). In contrast, the renal bicarbonate threshold is raised by extracellular volume contraction (dehydration, administration of diuretics).

Elimination of the end-products of nitrogen metabolism. — The end-products of nitrogen metabolism such as urea, uric acid, ammonium, creatinine and other "uremic toxins" are excreted by glomerular filtration and tubular secretion. They accumulate in blood when there is an acute or chronic lowering of glomerular filtration rate.

Endocrine functions [170]. — Active products such as erythropoietin, renin, 1,25 dihydrocholecalciferol and the prostaglandins are synthetized by the kidney:

(a) *Erytropoietin* is a glycoprotein that promotes hematopoiesis. It is probably produced by cortical cells, in response to hypoxia.

(b) *Renin* is a proteolytic enzyme produced by the juxtaglomerular apparatus. It interacts with angiotensinogen, an α_2-globulin synthetized in the liver, to form angiotensin I, a decapeptide with little intrinsic activity. Angiotensin I is converted by angiotensin converting enzyme to the potent vasoactive octapeptide, angiotensin II.

(c) *1,25 dihydrocholecalciferol* is produced by the 25-hydroxylation of vitamin D_3 in the liver and subsequent 1α-hydroxylation in the kidney. The enzyme 25-OH-D_3-1α-hydroxylase is present only in the mitochondria of the renal cortex.

(d) *Prostaglandins* are synthetized by specialized interstitial cells of the renal medulla from fatty acid precursors. Several vasoactive derivatives are presently identified: PGE_2, PGD_2, PGI_2, $PGF_{2\alpha}$.

MATURATION OF RENAL FUNCTION
[80, 131, 169]

Development of the human kidney goes through three stages: the pronephros, the mesonephros and the metanephros.

Pronephros appears at about the third week of intra-uterine life and disappears during the fourth week.

Mesonephros appears at the fourth week and disappears between the 12th and 16th gestational weeks, forming in the male the epididymus, the vas deferens and the bulbourethral glands, and in the female the Gartner ducts.

Metanephros, from which the definitive kidney derives, appears around the fifth week of intra-uterine life. During intra-uterine life homeostasis is maintained by the placenta; growth of the fetal kidney does consequently not relate to functional requirements.

Fetal life

Throughout fetal life, nephrogenesis occurs in a centrifugal pattern, *i. e.* deep nephrons are the first to be formed. In the human, nephrogenesis is complete by the 35th gestational week. Subsequently, each kidney contains 1.2 million nephrons. The human fetal kidney is able to produce urine as early as the 10-12th week. The urine output of the fetus has been estimated to be 12 ml/hour at the 32nd week, increasing to 28 ml/hour shortly before birth [33]. At the same time, fluid exchange between mother and fetus is about 3,500 ml/hour [153]. Urination is not essential for fetal survival, as demonstrated by the birth of newborns with bilateral renal agenesis. During fetal life, kidney weight increases proportionaly to gestational age, body weight and body surface area [161].

Glomerular filtration rate (GFR) and renal plasma flow (RPF). — Glomerular filtration rate as determined by inulin clearance, increases rapidly between the 28th and 35th gestational weeks (Fig. VII-2) [60]. PAH clearance behaves in a similar way. The appearance of new nephrons during this period is probably responsible for the

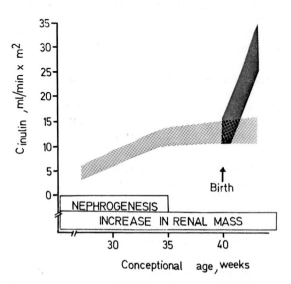

Fig. VII-2. — *Development of glomerular filtration rate in relation to gestational age and postnatal age.*

rapid increases in GFR and RPF. From the 35th week on, the rate of increase abates. During this period GFR per m^2 body surface area remains fairly constant. Progressive increases in blood pressure (Fig. VII-3) and decreases in renal vascular resistance [155] are responsible for the augmentation of GFR and RPF.

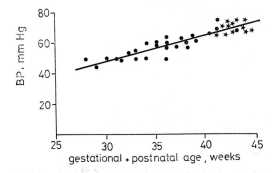

FIG. VII-3. — *Systolic blood pressure in relation to gestational age and postnatal age.*

● Values measured on the first day of life.
∗ Values measured during the first 4 weeks of life.

Tubular transport. — Experimental studies reveal that several mechanisms of tubular transport are operative well before birth. Hydrogen ion as well as glucose tubular transport mechanisms are effective in the fetal animal. The development of tubular transport follows the maturation of enzymatic systems such as Na-K-ATPase or carbonic anhydrase. Renin production appears quite early, as shown by the presence of renin-containing granules in the juxta-glomerular apparatus as early as the 17th gestational week [113].

Urine dilution and concentration. — The ability of the fetus in many mammals to produce a hypotonic urine indicates that the mechanisms of urine dilution are effective early in intra-uterine life. In contrast concentrating ability remains poorly developed throughout fetal life, despite the fetus' ability to synthesize vasopressin.

Postnatal life

After birth, the kidney assumes up all the homeostatic responsibilities handled previously by the placenta. The nature of the remarkably efficient stimulus which follows the termination of placental circulation is unknown (Fig. VII-2). The normal values of renal function observed during the neonatal period are summarized in Table I.

Glomerular filtration rate and renal plasma flow [60, 77, 92]. — The maturation of GFR which slows throughout the last weeks of gestation, accelerates again during the very first days of extra-uterine life. Its value is about 10 ml/min per m^2 at birth, doubling during the first 2 weeks of life (Fig. VII-4). PAH clearance behaves in the same fashion. During the neonatal period, functional maturation is much more rapid than growth of the renal mass. Although GFR at birth is lower in the premature newborn of less than 35 weeks gestational age, the postnatal maturation is comparable to that of the normal newborn [60, 175] (Fig. VII-4).

Hemodynamic and morphological changes seem to be responsible for this rapid maturation of renal function [92]:

— The rapid improvement in renal plasma flow is linked to a lowering of the renal vascular resistance [75].

TABLE I. — NORMAL VALUES OF RENAL FUNCTION IN THE NEONATAL PERIOD

Function	Age of infant				
	Premature infant 1st day	Term infant 1st day	2 weeks	8 weeks	1 year
Glomerular filtration rate (ml/min per m^2)	7	10	25	45	70
Concentrating ability (mOsm/kg H_2O)	480	800	900	1,200	1,400
Daily excretion of urine (ml/24 h)	1-3 ml/kg per hour	15-60 ml/kg per day	250-400	250-400	500-600

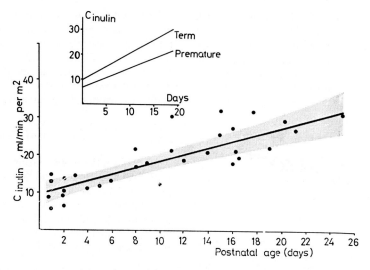

FIG. VII-4. — *Development of glomerular filtration rate (C_{inulin}) during the first 3 weeks of life.*
Regression lines and the 95 % confidence limits. The inset shows the postnatal maturation of the glomerular filtration rate in premature and term neonates.

— Postnatal elevation of systemic blood pressure (Fig. VII-3), probably followed by a similar increase in filtration pressure in the glomerular capillaries, promotes ultrafiltration.

— Finally, the rapid growth of the glomeruli considerably increases the filtration area.

Tubular transport of solutes. — Renal tubules in the newborn are less developed than the glomeruli. Nevertheless, their different segments—proximal, loop of Henle, distal and collecting—are quite functional as far as the mechanisms of solute transport are concerned (sodium, potassium, hydrogen, phosphate and glucose). The hormonal systems, such as aldosterone and PTH, which control these transport mechanisms are also functional. Other transport mechanisms such as those for organic acids develop progressively under the stimulation of exogenous substrates [91].

Urine dilution ability. — Like the adult, the newborn is able to excrete urine with an osmolality as low as 40 mOsm/kg H_2O. Nevertheless, the response to water overload is not comparable to that of the adult as the diuretic response fades before the excretion of all of the water load [118]. Factors other than renal immaturity may be responsible for this phenomenon.

Urine concentrating ability. — Whereas the capacity to concentrate urine is poorly developed in the fetus, in the newborn it is still less than that of the

adult. During dehydration, the maximum urinary osmolality is 700 mOsm/kg H_2O, versus 1,200 mOsm/ kg H_2O in the adult [55]. There are probably several causes for this deficiency [55, 97, 98]:

(*a*) a low cortico-medullary osmotic gradient because the quantity of urea available for concentration in the medulla is limited in the newborn in a high anabolic state;

(*b*) a decreased formation of cyclic AMP in response to ADH stimulation;

(*c*) an inhibition of the ADH-cyclic AMP system by endogenous prostaglandins.

As soon as the newborn is fed a high protein regime, this concentration defect is corrected. This diet provides a source of urea which is utilized in the creation of the necessary cortico-medullary gradient.

Acidification ability. — From the very first days of life the newborn kidney is able to excrete the fixed acids, which derive from oxidation of metabolic substrates, and also to reabsorb the filtered bicarbonate. It can acidify urine in the presence of metabolic acidosis (Fig. VII-6). Minimal values of urinary pH are reached during the second week of life. Because of a low bicarbonate threshold, the plasma concentration of this ion is maintained at values close to 18-20 mmol/l in the preterm infant, and 20-22 mmol/l, in the term neonate, *i. e.* 4-6 mmol/l lower than in the adult. The lower threshold in the neonate does not seem to result from an inability

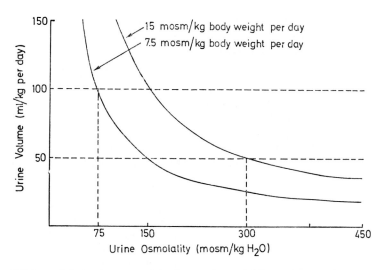

FIG. VII-5. — *Relation between urine volume, urine osmolality and urine solute excretion.*
Isopleths describe daily urine solute excretion of either 15 or 7.5 mosm/kg body weight per day. Adapted from RAY and SINCLAIR [153].

to secrete protons, nor from deficient carbonic anhydrase activity. It is likely that the great heterogenity of nephrons and the relative expansion of extracellular volume in the newborn are responsible for the depressed bicarbonate threshold [149]. During exogenous acid loading, ammonium excretion does not attain that of the adult [56]. However, as soon as the newborn is fed a diet rich in phosphates (cow's milk), this deficit is compensated for by a rise in the excretion of protons as titratable acids. On the whole, acidification capacity in the newborn is essentially normal.

Regulation of sodium balance. — Sodium plays a primary role in the maintenance of extracellular fluid volume. Its excretion is carefully controlled by the kidney. In fact the balance between sodium filtration and reabsorption is remarkably well maintained in the newborn as well as in the adult. The glomerular predominance found in the newborn makes this balance even more striking [63]. The mechanisms controlling sodium excretion are present in the newborn but their efficiency is not the same as that in the adult. Thus sodium balance is often negative in the low birth-weight newborn, who behaves as a salt loser [58, 154] and may present with transient hyperatremia. This is due to a low proximal and distal sodium reabsorption which occurs despite high concentrations of aldosterone [173]. Partial resistance to aldosterone has been suggested [6]. The response of the term newborn to a salt load is also less effective than that of the

adult [5, 46]. In the latter case, natriuresis is achieved by inhibition of proximal transport of sodium. The same mechanism is present in the newborn, but it is masked by active distal reabsorption of sodium [126] probably in response to high plasma aldosterone concentrations.

Hormonal maturation.

Renin-angiotensin-aldosterone. — Plasma concentrations of renin, angiotensin and aldosterone are high in the newborn [15, 29, 48, 68, 106]. They decrease progressively through the first weeks and months of life (Table II). The activity of plasma

TABLE II. — MEAN RENIN, ANGIOTENSIN II AND ALDO-STERONE LEVELS, IN RELATION TO POSTNATAL AGE.

Age	Renin ng/ml × h	Angio-tensin II pmol/l	Aldo-sterone ng/dl
Cord blood	10	180	96
2-3 days	12	81	106
4-11 days.	—	58	—
3-12 months	6	—	60
Adult	⩽2.5	34	14

Modified from C. HOLLERMANN, p. 197 [88].

renin varies proportionally to sodium excretion and inversely to Na balance [172]. The reason for the stimulation of the renin-angiotensin-aldosterone system at this age is not totally clear.

Prostaglandins. — In the premature newborn, the excretion of PGE_2 is rather high and that of $PGF_{2\alpha}$ rather low [174]. The urinary $PGE_2/PGF_{\alpha2}$ ratio decreases progressively throughout the first weeks of life. The relationship between urinary prostaglandin excretion, renal blood flow maturation, blood pressure elevation and urine concentrating ability has not been elucidated.

Conclusion

Renal function in the newborn is well adapted to the usual needs of extra-uterine life. It is more vulnerable to unexpected deprivations or to inappropriate loading. In addition, the newborn is liable to develop toxic drug levels because of the low glomerular filtration rate and the immaturity of certain transport systems, such as that of organic acids, which have not yet been stimulated. Thus the relative immaturity of the newborn kidney must always be kept in mind whenever one prescribes a medication, a dosage schedule or a fluid regimen.

SIGNS OF RENAL DISEASE
IN THE NEWBORN

Historical information concerning gestation, clinical findings and/or laboratory investigations may be suggestive of renal pathology.

Gestational history

Whenever oligohydramnios is present, renal disease, such as renal agenesis, renal hypoplasia, renal dysplasia or severe obstruction of the urinary tract must be considered. Polyhydramnios may indicate an esophageal atresia. It has been shown that about 50 % of patients with esophageal atresia or tracheo-esophageal fistula suffer from renal malformations. Polyhydramnios may also reveal a nephrogenic diabetes insipidus. Perinatal asphyxia

and obstetrical trauma are major threats to renal functional integrity in the first days of life.

Delayed micturition
[127, 163]

About one third of all newborns pass urine at or soon after birth. 92 % of newborns pass urine within the first 24 hours and 99 % within the first 48 hours. Renal pathology must be suspected whenever the infant has had no diuresis by 48 hours of life. Moreover, if by 72 hours of life diuresis does not occur, there is little doubt that a renal cause is incriminated (Table III). A secondary oliguria due to dehydration is the most frequent cause of micturition delay. If the state of hydration is good, the presence of oliguria points to a congenital (renal bilateral agenesis) or acquired (renal vein thrombosis, cortical necrosis) renal pathology.

TABLE III. — DELAYED MICTURITION
IN NEONATE

---

1. *Failure of urine formation
in the immediate newborn period*

Postnatal intravascular hypovolemia
Restriction of oral fluid
Bilateral renal agenesis
Cortical necrosis
Tubular necrosis
Bilateral renal vein thrombosis
Congenital nephrotic syndrome
Congenital pyelonephritis
Congenital nephritis

2. *Obstruction to urine flow
in the immediate newborn period*

Imperforate prepuce
Urethral strictures
Urethral diverticulum
Hypertrophy of the vera montanum
Neurogenic bladder
Ureterocele

Quality of the urinary stream

It is important to observe the newborn passing urine. If the stream is weak or interrupted, an abnormality of the urinary tract is likely (severe vesicoureteral reflux, urethral valves, mega-bladder). The bladder size must always be estimated. It is important to search for residual bladder urine by

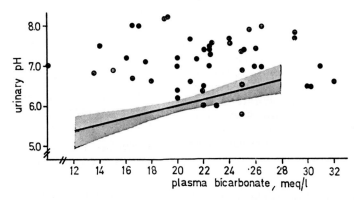

FIG. VII-6. — *Relation between urine pH and the plasma bicarbonate concentration during the first 3 days of life in premature newborn infants.*

The regression line illustrates the values obtained in control neonates and the 95 % confidence limits. The dots (●) represents the values observed in neonates with respiratory distress syndrome (RDS).

palpation and supra-pubic percussion with further confirmation by ultrasonography.

Urine flow rate

The normal infant is able to adjust renal water losses in accordance with the intake of fluid and solute, and with variable extrarenal fluid losses. The relationship between urine volume, urine solute excretion and osmolality is shown in Figure VII-5.

The average infant excretes 15-60 ml of urine per 24 hours during the first 2 days of life, and 240-400 ml/day during the next 4 weeks (Table I). Oliguria is defined as a urine output of less than 0.5 ml/kg per hour [95].

Visible or palpable abdominal mass

Most palpable abdominal tumors in the newborn are renal in origin. An asymetry is sometimes apparent. Careful abdominal palpation is fundamental to their identification. Abdominal palpation is part of the clinical evaluation, at birth and upon discharge from the maternity ward. Several techniques have been described [86, 130]. Bimanual palpation remains the method of choice for identification of an abdominal mass. The left kidney is often palpable in the newborn without any particular significance. Abdominal palpation reveals renal masses in 0.5-0.8 % of children [130]. This clinical finding requires confirmation by ultrasonography. The most common diagnoses are: horseshoe kidney, hydronephrosis, renal tumor, renal vein thrombosis and polycystic disease.

Dysmorphic signs commonly associated with renal malformations

A renal malformation is often found in infants presenting one of the following dysmorphic signs:

— single umbilical artery,
— Potter facies (flat nose, low implantation of the ears, epicanthus, recession of the chin,
— pre-auricular appendage,
— abnormal or low implantation of the ears,
— Prune-Belly syndrome [37, 142].
— VATER syndrome (vertebral abnormalities, anal atresia, tracheo-esophageal fistula, radial dysplasia, renal dysplasia) [144],
— imperforate anus,
— trisomy (see Table IV),
— myelomeningocele.

TABLE IV. — RENAL ANOMALIES IN TRISOMY SYNDROMES

Trisomy	Renal anomaly
11	Dysplastic multicystic kidneys
13-15	Bilateral hydronephrosis
	Renal cysts
16-18	Horseshoe kidneys
	Hydronephrosis
	Dysplastic multicystic kidneys
	Renal cortical cysts
	Abnormal nodule of renal blastema
21	Agenesis/hypoplasia

Modified from C. HOLLERMANN, p. 373 [88].

Urine color

Urine may present different colors. Hematuria must be suspected whenever the urine is red. For the distinction between hematuria and hemoglobinuria urine analysis must be performed on a fresh urine specimen. Red urine may be a sign of excessive urate excretion, red napkin syndrome (infection produced by *Serratia marcescens*) or of cutaneous absorption of a dye, such as eosin.

Macroscopic hematuria

Normal values of the urinary sediment are given in Table V. Causes of macroscopic hematuria in the newborn are:

(*a*) Vascular; asphyxia, hypoxia, vascular disorders, renal vein thrombosis, blood hyperviscosity, cortical and medullary necrosis.

(*b*) Malformations; hydronephrosis, polycystic disease, renal cysts, renal dysplasia.

TABLE V. — Examination of the urine sediment: normal values

---

1. *Qualitative examination*

$<$ 3 red cells
$<$ 5 white cells } per high power field ($\times$ 400)
$<$ 1 hyaline cast

Hemastix: positive when the sediment contains more than 3 red cells per high power field

2. *Semi-quantitative examination* (*Fuchs-Rosenthal counting chamber*)

$<$ 3 red cells/mm³
 (3-10 red cells/mm³ = suspicion, test to be repeated)
$<$ 25 white cells/mm³ (male)
$<$ 50 white cells/mm³ (female)

3. *Quantitative examination* (*Addis count*)

$<$ 1,000 red cells/min
$<$ 1,000 white cells/min

Edema in the newborn
[110]

The relative immaturity of excretory and regulatory functions, as well as the sudden changes inherent to the adaptation to extra-uterine life, explain the high prevalence of fluid imbalance in the newborn [64, 119]. This is often manifested by edema.

Definition. — Edema is defined as an excessive accumulation of interstitial fluid, originating from plasma ultrafiltration. Edema may be caused by:

(*a*) Increased formation of interstitial fluid, itself secondary to increases in:

— hydrostatic capillary pressure,
— capillary permeability,
— capillary ultrafiltration.

(*b*) Decreased mobilization of interstitial fluid because of a decrease in:

— lymphatic drainage,
— plasma oncotic pressure,
— hydrostatic pressure.

In the newborn edema can be classified in a schematic fashion according to etiology (Table VI) [110].

TABLE VI. — Conditions associated with edema in the newborn

---

1. Physiologic
2. Cardiac
3. Renal
4. Miscellaneous:
 — Hypoxia in utero
 — Hyaline membrane disease
 — Erythroblastosis fetalis
 — Umbilical vein thrombosis
 — Lymphedema
 — Congenital ascites (chylous ascites, cirrhosis, peritonitis)
 — Vitamin E deficiency
 — Hypomagnesemia and hypocalcemia
 — Cystic fibrosis
 — Hypoparathyroidism
 — Turner's syndrome

Physiological edema. — Physiological edema appears on the 2nd day of life and disappears on the 7th day. Its pathogenesis is unknown. Renal immaturity may contribute to a transient saline retention, responsible for the extracellular volume changes. Treatment is unnecessary.

Cardiac edema. — Several congenital cardiopathies can provoke edema in the newborn. Fluid and salt retention are due to a decrease in cardiac output with increases in central venous and capillary pressures. The decrease in effective circulating volume causes a decrease in glomerular filtration. This promotes a greater reabsorption of sodium under the influence of aldosterone. The aim of treatment is to restore cardiac output.

Edema of renal origin. — Two principal mechanisms are implicated in the pathogenesis of renal edema.

(*a*) Renal failure (obstructive uropathy, severe hypoxemia, renal vein thrombosis) may cause a decrease in glomerular filtration rate with consequent fluid and salt retention.

(*b*) Decreased plasma oncotic pressure secondary to proteinuria is observed in such diseases as microcystic disease (Finnish nephrotic syndrome), congenital syphilis, Nail-Patella syndrome, congenital toxoplasmosis, cytomegalovirus infections, nephroblastoma, renal vein thrombosis and mercury intoxication. Any of these situations may lead to an increased glomerular permeability and an exaggerated proteinuria. Edema formation results from decreased plasma oncotic pressure.

In the newborn inappropriate secretion of ADH of central origin may be the cause of edema due to exaggerated free water retention.

Other causes of edema. — Edema may be observed in various other pathological conditions (Table VI).

Hydrops fetalis [66]. — Congenital nephrotic syndrome (microcystic disease, syphilis, toxoplasmosis, cytomegalovirus inclusion disease) is a renal cause of hydrops fetalis. This fetal edema is provoked by a decrease in plasma oncotic pressure due to the severe proteinuria.

Ascites

Ascites in the newborn is generally extra-renal in origin (severe hemolytic anemia, intestinal malformation with perforation, intra-uterine infection). Renal causes include obstructive uropathy and congenital nephrotic syndrome.

Nonspecific clinical signs

Renal disease often presents with atypical symptomatology. Symptoms may be referred to the digestive system (feeding refusal, unexplained weight loss sometimes followed by dehydration, vomiting and diarrhea) or to the central nervous system (irritability, fever, convulsions with or without hypocalcemia, hyponatremia or hypomagnesemia).

LABORATORY SCREENING

Urine and blood analyses are suitable for confirmation of renal disease.

Urinalysis

Proteinuria. — Temporary proteinuria often presents during the first 3 days of neonatal life and disappears before the 5th day. From then on, as in the adult, proteinuria is normally less than 4 mg/m^2 per hour or 0.13 mg/kg per hour. Proteinuria varies with gestational age (Table VII) [10] and with post-natal age (Table VIII) [100].

TABLE VII. — Proteinuria
in relation to gestational age

Gestational age (weeks)	Proteinuria (mg/m^2 per h)
< 28	0.86 (0.2-1.33)
30	2.08 (0-9.40)
32	2.32 (0-5.22)
34	2.48 (0-13.07)
36	1.27 (0-4.60)
40	1.29 (0-6.14)

Proteinuria: mean (range).
From B. S. Arant [10].

Microscopic hematuria. — Normal values of red cell urinary excretion are given in Table V. A microscopic hematuria can accompany glomerular or vascular nephropathies, malformative uropathies, urinary tract infections, asphyxic and respiratory distress syndromes and coagulopathies.

Leucocyturia. — Table V gives the values of normal leucocyturia. Pathologic leucocyturia is observed in febrile patients, during severe infectious episodes and in renal parenchymal diseases. Pyuria is often associated with urinary tract infection.

Glucosuria. — The urine of the healthy term normoglycemic neonate contains only trace amounts of glucose. A congenital tubular disorder should be suspected if glucosuria is present and the plasma glucose concentration is not rised. Because of the low glucose renal threshold in low birth-weight infants, significant glucosuria may be observed at a plasma concentration of 150 mg/dl (8.3 mmol/l) [28]. A few premature neonates may even present with glucosuria at plasma concentrations below 100 mg/dl (5.5 mmol/l), a finding that probably reflects heterogeneity of immature nephrons.

Density and osmolality. — There is a linear correlation between urinary osmolality and urinary density, estimated by refractometry (Fig. VII-7). This correlation may be altered by the presence of proteins, glucose or radiologic contrast substances. In the newborn, the urine osmolality varies between 40-700 mOsm/kg H_2O. Pyelonephritis, renal failure, hypokalemia and hypercalcemia are frequent causes of disturbance in urinary concentrating ability. Disturbances in dilutional capacity are observed in the syndrome of inappropriate secretion of ADH, in hypoaldosteronism, in hyperthyroidism, in renal failure and during distal diuretic administration.

Urinary pH. — In the newborn the urine pH will vary between 4.5 and 8.0. Most newborns have a urinary pH of 6.0 during the first few days of life. Urinary pH must always be interpreted in relation to the plasma bicarbonate concentration (Fig. VII-6) [168, 180]. An alkaline urine concomitant with a metabolic acidosis suggests the diagnosis of renal tubular acidosis.

Blood examinations

Plasma creatinine. — Creatinine is produced at a constant rate, as a result of tissue protein catabolism, and is eliminated by glomerular filtration. Thus plasma creatinine concentration reflects the efficacy of its renal excretion. Plasma creatinine concentration which is quite stable in infants and

TABLE VIII. — URINARY CONCENTRATION OF PROTEINS IN SINGLE URINE SPECIMENS IN RELATION TO POSTNATAL AGE

Age days	Total protein mg/l	Albumin mg/l	α_2-microglobulin mg/l	Alpha-amino N mg α-amino N/l	Creatinine mmol/l
1	494 (103-2,360)	143 (14-1,510)	0.28 (0.02-3.69)	172 (75-399)	4.1 (0.8-22)
5	176 (39-798)	21 (4-97)	1.04 (0.07-16.30)	110 (36-335)	2.5 (0.5-14)
15	55 (10-324)	6 (1-33)	0.34 (0.02-6.16)	51 (20-133)	0.5 (0.1-3)
43	46 (12-185)	4 (1-18)	0.13 (0.01-1.61)	46 (17-125)	0.5 (0.09-3)

Mean (Range).
From F. A. KARLSON et al. [100].

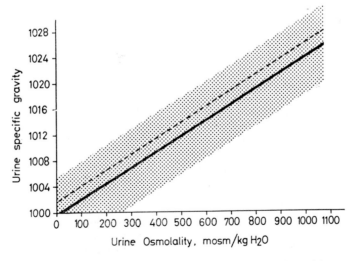

FIG. VII-7. — *Relation between urine specific gravity and osmolality with the 95 % confidence limits.*

The broken line indicates the relation between specific gravity and osmolality in urine containing protein (3 g/liter).

adults, changes considerably during the first days of life. Its concentration is high at birth, decreasing progressively throughout the first days or weeks of life (62, 171). The highest values at birth are found in the most premature infants (Fig. VII-8).

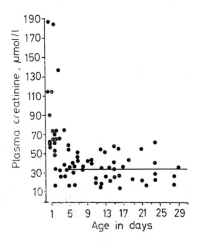

FIG. VII-8. — *Plasma creatinine during the first month of life of newborn infants with different gestational ages. Creatinine measured by the kinetic method* [62].

Plasma urea. — At birth urea concentration is below 40 mg % (7.0 mmol/l). A progressive rise in this parameter during the first days of life, may indicate a renal lesion (functional or organic).

Sodium [109, 140]. — Sick newborns, particularly premature ones, may often present with hyponatremia. According to the circumstances the treatment consists of fluid reduction or sodium administration.

A search for an etiologic diagnosis is essential.

(a) *Dilutional hyponatremia:* this situation can supervene whenever there is:

— Inappropriate administration of a hypotonic solution overwhelming the renal capacity to eliminate free water. This is the most frequent cause of hyponatremia in a healthy newborn.

— Inappropriate secretion of ADH (ISADH) as a consequence of purulent meningitis or cerebral injury due to asphyxia or hemorrhage [124, 129].

— Adrenal failure characterized by a disorder in dilutional capacity.

— Pre-renal failure secondary to cardiac insufficiency or a congenital nephrotic syndrome.

— ISADH as a consequence of drug administration (barbiturates, isoproterenol).

All of these conditions are accompanied by a considerable increase in extra-cellular fluid volume. The treatment consists of fluid restriction with close monitoring of body weight, plasma sodium, plasma and urine osmolality.

(b) *Hyponatremia due to salt wasting:* Salt wasting is possible in situations such as:

— Prematurity: an exaggerated salt wasting is often observed in the low birth-weight infant (< 1.3 kg) during the first weeks of life, leading to a late hyponatremia. Salt wasting is explained by the immaturity of the reabsorptive function of the kidney. This hyponatremia responds to the administration of NaCl in doses of 3 mEq/kg per day. It is transient and disappears in a few weeks [154].

— Adrenogenital syndrome with salt wasting as a consequence of aldosterone deficiency [24, 99]. The diagnosis is usually clear by the 4th to 10th day [107]. Hyponatremia is here associated with hyperkalemia and hypotension.

— Diuretic administration to the mother before birth, or to the newborn [140]: While diuretics can induce hyponatremia by multiple mechanisms, their interference with the dilutional mechanism is at least as important as sodium depletion.

— Extrarenal losses: For example vomiting and diarrhea. As the conditions cited above are characterized by a decrease in extracellular fluid volume, the first aim of treatment is to compensate for the losses by administration of isotonic saline solution.

Bicarbonate. — Renal regulation of acid-base balance is achieved by reabsorption of filtered bicarbonate and by fixed acid excretion. The integrity of glomerular and tubular function is fundamental to this regulation. Any of these functions may be disturbed in the newborn. A metabolic acidosis of renal origin can be secondary to the natural phenomenon of maturation, without any pathologic renal cause.

(a) *Physiological acidosis in the newborn.* — As the renal threshold for bicarbonate excretion is rather low in the newborn, plasma bicarbonate concentration stays at subnormal levels of about 20 mmol/l. In fact there is no acid retention since an effective compensatory elimination of fixed acids occurs. No treatment is needed.

(b) *Late metabolic acidosis.* — Throughout the first weeks of life, the newborn of less than 1,500 g may manifest a metabolic acidosis, accompanied by alkaline urine excretion. This is probably due to a lowering of the renal threshold for bicarbonate excretion, perhaps as an effect of extracellular volume expansion. This condition is temporary and needs no treatment.

(c) *Acidosis due to decrease in renal mass.* — A severe decrease in glomerular filtration rate leads to a metabolic acidosis consequent to a decrease in excretion of ammonium and in the reabsorption of filtered bicarbonate [146].

(d) *Renal tubular acidosis.* — A primary or secondary disturbance in tubular secretion of protons leads to metabolic acidosis:

— because of a decrease in bicarbonate reabsorption and a consequent bicarbonaturia (proximal tubular acidosis),
— by decreasing the excretion of fixed acids (distal tubular acidosis).

In both cases metabolic acidosis is characterized by inappropriate alkalinity of the urine relative to the plasma bicarbonate concentration [168].

EVALUATION OF RENAL FUNCTION

Definitions

Renal function may be estimated by determination of certain laboratory parameters.

Clearances. — The clearance of a substance (x) is defined as the smallest volume of plasma from which the kidney can obtain that quantity of the substance (x) excreted in urine, per minute:

$$C_x = \frac{U_x \cdot V}{P_x}$$

where

C_x = clearance of the substance x,
U_x = urinary concentration of x,
V = urine output expressed in ml/min,
P_x = plasma concentration of x.

Urinary excretion threshold. — This value indicates the plasma concentration of a substance above which that substance appears in urine.

Fractional excretion. — Fractional excretion (Fe) is expressed in % and defines the relationship between the excreted substance x and the filtered substance x

$$Fe_x = \frac{\text{Excreted quantity of } x}{\text{Filtered quantity of } x} = \frac{U_x \cdot V}{P_x \cdot GFR}$$

where

Fe_x = fractional excretion of a substance x,
V = urinary output in ml/min,
GFR = glomerular filtration rate.

Fractional excretion can also be calculated by the formula:

$$Fe_x = \frac{U_x}{P_x} \times \frac{P_{creatinine}}{U_{creatinine}}$$

Filtration fraction (FF). — This term refers to that fraction of renal plasma flow which is filtered by the glomerulus:

$$FF = \frac{\text{Glomerular filtration rate}}{\text{Renal plasma flow}}$$

Titratable acidity. — Means the quantity of acid equivalents present in urine as buffers, mainly phosphate. It is measured by the alkaline titration of urine to the pH of the blood.

Tm. — Tm defines the maximal quantity of a substance which can be reabsorbed in a minute.

Renal blood flow

Para-amino-hippuric acid (PAH) clearance permits the estimation, in adults, of the renal blood flow. As the extraction rate is scanty and variable in newborns [31], PAH clearance is not a reliable index of renal blood flow in the neonatal period.

Glomerular filtration rate
[77, 80, 102, 148]

Glomerular filtration rate can be estimated through the measurement of clearances of products eliminated exclusively (inulin) or mainly (creatinine) by glomerular filtration. It can be estimated by indirect methods, without urine collection or by the observation of the accumulation of endogenous products normally excreted mainly by glomerular filtration (such as creatinine and urea).

Inulin clearance. — Inulin is infused at a constant IV rate for 3 hours. After equilibration of inulin for one hour in its distribution space, urine is collected for 3 to 4 periods and plasma inulin concentration determined in the middle of each period. Inulin clearance, $\frac{UV}{P}$, is an exact index of glomerular filtration.

Objections to this method are:

— need for infusion of an exogenous substance,
— carefully timed urine collection is necessary,
— fastidious chemical determinations of inulin concentration are necessary.

Single injection method. — After a bolus injection of inulin into the blood stream, the marker diffuses into its distribution space and is then eliminated from the body by glomerular filtration. The rate of its plasma concentration decline gives an indirect estimation of its elimination constant [158], which is a function of glomerular filtration rate. In the newborn, this method significantly overestimates GFR [61].

Indirect method by continuous infusion. — With a stable plasma concentration of an exogenous marker (inulin) the excreted quantity must balance the infused quantity. Clearance may then be calculated by the formula:

$$C = \frac{\text{infusion rate of the marker}}{\text{plasma concentration of the marker}}$$

While this indirect method is attractive, it is not very accurate [80]. It can be improved by constantly infusing inulin for at least 24 h.

Creatinine clearance. — Due to the considerable variations of plasma creatinine in the first days of life, estimation of its clearance may give unreliable results [162]. The possible reabsorption of creatinine by the very immature kidney may falsely decrease creatinine clearance.

Urine dilution and concentration ability
[185]

Urine osmolality and urine specific gravity must always be interpreted as a function of the clinical condition of the patient and of the plasma osmolality. In fact, urinary concentration and dilution can appear normal without being appropriate to the clinical condition of the neonate (see p. 952).

Acid-base balance

Urinary pH depends on plasma bicarbonate concentration (Fig. VII-6). An alkaline urine concomitant with a metabolic acidosis, can be due to failure of the renal acidification mechanism. Renal acidification capacity be can approximated by determination of urine pH, ammonium excretion and titratable acidity after loading with NH_4Cl (75 to 150 mmol/m²). Acid excretion must increase within the 5 hours following NH_4Cl administration, urine pH droping below 5.2, NH_4^+ excretion rising to 33 mmol/min/m² (range 24-46) and titratable acidity to 36 mmol/min/m² (range 25-64) [56]. This test is seldom utilized in the newborn.

Urinary electrolytes

Measurement of sodium concentration in urine is suitable for the diagnosis of renal failure and/or salt wasting conditions. Fractional excretion of Na permits the appreciation of disturbances in tubular function associated with acute renal failure. The K/Na ratio is sometimes utilized as an index of aldosterone activity.

Regulation of blood pressure

Pathologic values of blood pressure (Table XI) may signal renal disease. The kidney participates in the regulation of blood pressure through:

— sodium balance,
— the renin-angiotensin-aldosterone system,
— the prostaglandins.

Normal values for the renin-angiotensin-aldosterone system are included in Table II.

RADIOGRAPHIC, RADIOISOTOPIC AND ULTRASONIC EXAMINATIONS

Intravenous urography
[70]

The intravenous injection of 3.0-5.0 ml/kg of an iodinated contrast agent (370 g iodine per liter) is followed by renal excretion of the agent via glomerular filtration and tubular secretion. There are two distinct phases to the examination: 1) nephrography, 2) pyelography. The first phase defines the borders of the renal parenchyma, whereas the second phase demonstrates the calyces, the pelvis and the excretory ducts. The image may be improved by the use of tomography. Intravenous urography is of limited value during the first two weeks of life. It is important that the newborn be well hydrated before the examination because of the high osmotic load which the contrast agent carries (Table IX). The complications observed include ischemia of the renal cortex, papillary or medullary necrosis, and pulmonary edema. Anaphylactic reactions are rare (1/100,000).

TABLE IX. — OSMOLALITY
OF SOME RADIOGRAPHIC CONTRAST MEDIA

Agent	Trade mark	Osmolality (mOsm/ kg H_2O)
Na-Acetotrizoate	Urovist 65 %	1,446
Na-Acetotrizoate	Vasurix 75 %	1,574
Na-Amidotrizoate	Hypaque 45 %	1,360
Na-Amidotrizoate	Urovison	1,464
Meglumine Na-amido-trizoate	Urografin 76 %	1,660
Meglumine Na-amido-trizoate	Angiografin 65 %	1,508
Meglumine Ca-metro-zoate	Ronpacon 280	1,300
Meglumine Ca-metro-zoate	Ronpacon 440	1,940
Iopamidol	Iopamiro 200	413
Iopamidol	Iopamiro 370	796
Na Ioxaglate and me-glumine	Hexabrix	600

Excretory cystography
[70, 121]

The contrast agent, at a concentration of 70 g iodine per liter, is introduced into the bladder under sterile conditions, either through a catheter (Argyl No. 5) or by suprapublic bladder puncture.

Fluid is introduced in the bladder by gravity to produce an urge to urinate. Films are taken during and after micturition, to detect the presence of vesico-ureteral reflux, bladder or urethral malformations, or a residual bladder volume. Excretory cystography is indicated in all newborns presenting with urinary tract infection. The examination may also be performed using a radioisotope marker such as 99m Tc pertechnetate, at a dose of 500 μCi.

Radioisotopic scintigraphy

The rapid injection of a marker isotope (131-I-orthoiodohippurate, 99m-Tc-glucoheptonate or 99m-

Tc-gluconate) permits estimation of renal perfusion and function. There are three phases to this examination: 1) vascular, 2) parenchymal, and 3) excretory. Radioisotopic scintigraphy is indicated whenever renal vascular problems, a renal mass, renal agenesis, hydronephrosis or megabladder is suspected. A major advantage of this method is the very small radiation dose. This examination is frequently complementary to intravenous urography.

Ultrasonography
[23, 157, 166]

Ultrasound examination, using a 5.0 megahertz transducer, is a relatively new technique which can be important in the identification of renal anomalies in the newborn. For example:

— visualization of a non-functioning kidney,
— visualization of a hydronephrosis, of renal cysts or of renal vein thrombosis,
— detection of an obstructive malformation of a ureter or of the urethra,
— detection of an extra-renal abdominal mass,
— detection of a megabladder.

The technique is not invasive and does not involve ionizing radiation, but does require prior sedation of the neonate. It is possible to use this technique at the patient's bedside. The technique may also be used in the prenatal period for detection of certain renal malformations [125].

ARTERIAL HYPERTENSION

Methods
for measuring arterial blood pressure in the newborn

Three different techniques can be utilized for measuring blood pressure in the newborn:

— Flush method
— Sphygmomanometric method
— Doppler technique.

While it is easily applied, **the flush method** gives only approximate results [71, 128]. A 5 cm blood pressure cuff is generally used. Severe anemia, edema or hypothermia give false results [182].

The sphygmomanometric method, with palpation or auscultation, is more difficult to carry out, but also gives more reliable results.

The best method is that utilizing **the Doppler effect** [21, 104, 176]. This method gives an accurate estimate of the systolic pressure, but is less precise for determination of diastolic pressure. The mean pressures obtained by these three methods correlate quite well with those obtained by a direct intra-arterial method [53]. The mean values obtained by indirect and direct methods in low birth-weight newborns are given in Table X.

TABLE X. — MEASUREMENT OF BLOOD PRESSURE IN THE NEONATE

	Umbilical artery (intraarterial) mm Hg	Brachial artery (Doppler) mm Hg
Systolic arterial BP. . .	55 ± 9	60 ± 10
Diastolic arterial BP . .	34 ± 9	40 ± 9

Modified from H. S. DWECK et al. [53].

Physiological factors affecting arterial blood pressure
[29]

There is a progressive rise in blood pressure throughout the last gestational weeks and the first weeks of extrauterine life and a significant correlation exists between systolic blood pressure and gestational age (Fig. VII-3). In the neonate blood pressure values are affected by the feeding schedule and the state of arousal. Table XI shows the mean values of blood pressure during the first week and at 6 weeks of extrauterine life. It is likely that the same factors which affect blood pressure in adults, namely hormonal systems (renin-angiotensin-aldo-sterone, prostaglandins, catecholamines), sodium load, and hereditary factors, play a role in the newborn.

Etiology of arterial hypertension

Hypertension may be due to renal or extra-renal causes:

Renal causes

Renal artery thrombosis
Renal artery embolism
Renal artery stenosis
Obstructive nephropathy
Neuroblastoma

Extra-renal causes

Coarctation of the aorta
Adrenal dysfunction or hemorrhage

Renal artery thrombosis. — Renal artery thrombosis may occur as a complication of umbilical artery catheterization [3, 141]. Any newborn submitted to catheterization of the umbilical artery must be followed prospectively. The resultant hypertension is often unresponsive to antihypertensive agents and carries a poor prognosis. If the thrombosis is unilateral, nephrectomy can normalize the blood pressure. Diagnostic suspicion is elicited by an appropriate history and the diagnosis is confirmed by angiographic and scintigraphic examinations.

Renal artery embolism. — Ductus arteriosus thrombosis can sometimes be the site of origin of

TABLE XI. — BLOOD PRESSURE IN RELATION TO POSTNATAL AGE AND LEVEL OF CONSCIOUSNESS

State of animation	Days						Weeks
	3	4	5	6	7	8-10	6
Awake	72 ± 6	74 ± 9	77 ± 10	77 ± 10	82 ± 9	88 ± 17	96 ± 11
Asleep	68 ± 7	70 ± 8	72 ± 8	72 ± 9	72 ± 9	75 ± 9	89 ± 11
P95 awake		95					113

Arterial systolic blood pressure (X ± SD) measured by the Doppler technique.
P95: 95 percentile.
Modified from M. DE SWIETT et al. [176].

renal artery embolism [52]. Diagnosis is confirmed by renal scintigraphy and renal arteriography. Since in this case the arterial hypertension is renin-dependant, nephrectomy of the involved kidney will cure the condition.

Renal artery stenosis [150, 112]. — An intrinsic stenosis or extrinsic compression of a renal artery can be responsible for a renin-dependant arterial hypertension. Renal scintigraphy and early urographic pictures confirm the diagnosis. High plasma renin levels are difficult to interpret in this age group (Table II).

Obstructive nephropathy [34]. — An obstructive nephropathy, for example stenosis of the pyelo-ureteral junction, may be responsible for arterial hypertension with or without accompanying hyper-reninemia.

Coarctation of the aorta [72]. — Tight coarctation of the aorta may be responsible for severe hypertension in the newborn. When manifest at birth, it is usually proximal to the ductus arteriosus. Plasma renin is sometimes elevated. Surgical treatment can normalize this situation.

Hypertension due to adrenal dysfunction. — Although rare in newborns, an endogenous or exogenous excess of mineralocorticoids or gluco-corticoids may be responsible for high blood pressure [134].

Differential diagnosis

Diagnosis is made with the help of laboratory, radiologic, radioisotopic and ultrasonographic investigations.

Laboratory. — The following laboratory examinations are important in the establishment of an etiological diagnosis of hypertension in the newborn: urine chemistry, urinary sediment, ionogram, plasma urea and creatinine concentrations, catecholamines and urinary 17-ketosteroids (Table XII) [134]. Peripheral plasma renin concentration is also important, but difficult to interpret at this age because of the large individual variations.

Radiologic, scintigraphic and ultrasonographic examinations. — Intravenous urography is suitable for the diagnosis of obstructive uropathies. Ultrasonography is also very helpful in these cases. In a newborn where a renovascular etiology is suspected, aortography is indicated. Renal scintigraphy permits an evaluation of the functional state of the kidneys.

TABLE XII. — NORMAL VALUES
FOR URINARY 17-KETOSTEROIDS

Postnatal age (days)	17-ketosteroids (mg/24 h)
< 7	2.0-2.5
7-90	0.5

Modified from *Amer. Clin. Chemists*, Normal values for Pediatric Clinical Chemistry, Aug. 74, p. 1.

Treatment. — The treatment of a hypertensive newborn is difficult and must consequently be instituted in the hospital. In so far as possible it will be directed at the cause of the hypertension. Symptomatic treatment consists of diuretics and antihypertensive drugs administered in the dosages indicated in Table XIII. Beta-blocking agents seem to be well tolerated during the neonatal period, but their long term effects are unknown. Newborn hypertensive crises may require the administration of diazoxide, sodium nitroprusside or captopril. Experience with the use of these agents in the newborn period is scanty.

TABLE XIII. — ANTIHYPERTENSIVE AGENTS

	Route of administration	Dosage (mg/kg per 24 h)
Hydrochlorothiazide . .	0	1-3
Furosemide	0, IV	1-3
Hydralazine	0, IV	1-4
α-Methyldopa	0, IV	5-40
Diazoxide	IV	2-5
Propranolol	0, IV	0.5-2.0
Na-nitroprusside . . .	IV	2-5
Captopril	0	0.1-0.5

ACUTE RENAL FAILURE
[4, 12, 42, 44, 79, 83]

Definitions

Acute renal failure is characterized by a sudden decrease in glomerular filtration rate, which leads to disturbances in water and electrolyte homeostasis and in acid-base balance, and to the accumulation of nitrogen end-products. It is usually associated with oliguria.

Etiology

As is shown in Table XIV, renal failure may have pre-renal, renal, and post-renal components. In the newborn acute renal failure is often secondary to potentially reversible pre-renal causes. Some of these causes are easily preventable, as for instance:

(*a*) Inadequate administration of fluids during vomiting or diarrhea.

(*b*) Excessive fluid loss via sweating during phototherapy or excessive environmental temperatures [139, 184].

If not corrected, pre-renal causes may lead to intra-renal failure due to ischemic injury of the renal parenchyma.

TABLE XIV. — Etiology of acute renal failure in the neonate.

1. *Prerenal:* Hypovolemia, hypotension and hypoxemia are responsable for a decrease in renal perfusion.
   A) Dehydration: inadequate intake, vomiting, diarrhea, phototherapy, high environmental temperature.
   B) Blood loss, clamping of the aorta during cardiac surgery, hypovolemia secondary to nephrotic syndrome.
   C) Perinatal anoxia, severe respiratory distress.
   D) Congestive cardiac failure.

2. *Intrarenal:* Glomerular, tubular and vascular structures are injured.
   A) Vascular disorders: renal vein or renal artery thrombosis.
   B) Acute renal necrosis: cortical, medullary or papillary secondary to renal ischemia, nephrotoxic agents, hemoglobinuria or myoglobinuria.
   C) Congenital nephropathies: bilateral renal agenesis, bilateral renal hypoplasia, infantile polycystic disease, congenital nephrotic syndrome.
   D) Acute pyelonephritis.

3. *Postrenal:* The condition is secondary to obstructive uropathies:
   — urethral valve,
   — imperforate prepuce,
   — urethral stricture,
   — urethral diverticulum,
   — ureterocele,
   — hypertrophy of the vera montanum,
   — neurogenic bladder,
   — renal tumors.

Pathogenesis of acute pre-renal failure

Disturbances such as hypovolemia, hypotension or hypoxemia which lead to renal vasoconstriction with consequent renal hypoperfusion may lead to acute renal failure (Fig. VII-9). Hypoperfusion associated with vasoconstriction predominantly in the afferent arterioles, induces a decrease in glomerular filtration rate. It is possible that stimulation of the renin-angiotensin system, or of adenosine, is responsible for a decrease in renal blood flow and also a redistribution of flow within the kidney. This may decrease the glomerular filtration rate through alteration of glomerular arteriolar resistance. Decreasing renal plasma flow leads to ischemic reactions at the cellular level, with consequent edema of the vascular and tubular cells. Decreasing glomerular filtration disturbs the urinary dilutional mechanism, favoring oliguria and the advent of a hyponatremic state. As long as renal ischemic lesions do not occur, the renal failure is reversible.

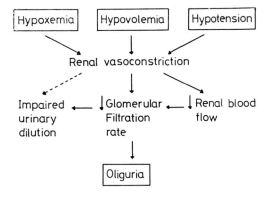

Fig. VII-9. — *Pathogenesis of acute renal failure.*

Clinical diagnosis

The clinical signs of acute renal failure are non-specific. One must bear this diagnosis in mind in any patient who presents with shock, dehydration, severe anemia, sepsis or an associated malformation syndrome. Oliguria, defined as a urine output of less than 0.5 ml/kg per hour [95] is usually the first sign of acute renal failure. Azotemia soon follows the oliguria. In any newborn with a history of acute fetal distress, pre-renal failure should be suspected.

Laboratory diagnosis
[95, 136]

Laboratory examinations permit the confirmation of acute renal failure and may aid in the elucidation of its origin.

Azotemia is characterized by:

Plasma urea > 500 mg/l = 8.3 mmol/l,
Plasma creatinine > 10 mg/l = 88.4 µmol/l,
and also by daily increases above:
Urea: 100 mg/l per day = 1.7 mmol/l per day,
Creatinine: 2.0 mg/l per day = 17 µmol/l per day.

Urine. — Urinalysis can contribute to the differential diagnosis between acute renal failure of pre-renal vs. intra-renal origin. Analysis must be performed as early as possible and prior to diuretic administration. A small number of parameters are utilized in the newborn or infant for the establishment of an etiology for the acute renal failure (Table XV). The usefulness of these parameters in the newborn is controversial [136], and only U/P osm and sodium fractional excretion seem to have a practical value. Caution should be exercised when applying these indices to very premature neonates.

TABLE XV. — Diagnosis
of type of acute renal failure (ARF)

Index	Functional ARF (prerenal)	Acute tubular necrosis (intrarenal)
U-Sediment	Hyaline casts	Granular casts and epithelial cells
U-Specific gravity	> 1,014	< 1,011
U-Na	< 20	> 40
U-Osm	> 500	< 400
U/P Osm	> 2	< 1.1
Fe Na	< 1	> 3
Duration of oliguria	Less than 2 days	More than 2 days
Response to mannitol	Present	Absent

U-specific gravity, U-Na, U-Osm: urine specific gravity, Na and osmolality.
U/P Osm: ratio of the urine over plasma osmolality.
Fe Na: fractional excretion of Na.

Blood chemistry. — Electrolyte disturbances are characterized by a tendency toward hyponatremia, hypocalcemia, hypomagnesemia, hyperphosphatemia and hyperkalemia. Metabolic acidosis is also often present.

Indications for imaging studies

Uroradiologic, scintigraphic, radioisotopic and ultrasonic studies are often helpful. These investigations permit:

(*a*) visualization of both kidneys,
(*b*) estimation of the size and functional state of the kidneys,
(*c*) detection of hydronephrosis or a renal or extrarenal tumor mass,
(*d*) detection of a megabladder.

Voiding cystourethrogram is indicated whenever a vesico-ureteral reflux, or a urethral malformation is suspected.

Intravenous urography is of doubtful value during the first two weeks of life. The osmotic load of the contrast medium (Table IX) is a definite risk for the patient with renal insufficiency.

Renal scintigraphy is the primary mode of investigation used in evaluation of the functional state of the kidneys.

Ultrasonography is the method of choice for confirmation of a diagnosis of urinary tract obstruction, or for identification and localization of a tumor mass.

Treatment of acute renal failure
(Fig. VII-10)

After exclusion of obstruction as the cause of the failure, other factors which may be operative, such as hypovolemia, hypotension, and hypoxemia, must be corrected. Initially any intravascular or interstitial volume deficit which exists must be recognized and corrected as soon as possible.

Rehydration. — The first measure taken consists of the administration of 20-40 ml/kg over two hours of a solution whose composition depends upon the nature of the dehydration [50, 89, 153]. If the cause of renal failure is pre-renal, diuresis should begin in the next few hours.

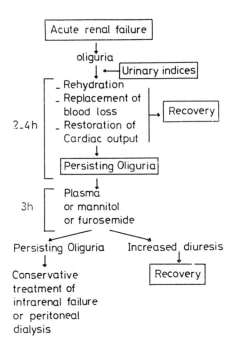

Acute renal failure
↓
oliguria
↓ ← Urinary indices
┌ – Rehydration
│ – Replacement of
│   blood loss   → Recovery
2-4h│ – Restoration of
│   Cardiac output
│   ↓
└ Persisting Oliguria
          ↓
┌ Plasma
3h │ or mannitol
│ or furosemide
└
Persisting Oliguria   Increased diuresis
↓   ↓
Conservative   Recovery
treatment of
intrarenal failure
or peritoneal
dialysis

Fig. VII-10. — *Definition and treatment of acute renal failure in the newborn infant.*

Confirmation of the type of renal failure. — If following fluid administration diuresis does not ensue, and if some doubt persists as to the nature of the renal failure, the following manoeuvres must be tried:

(*a*) if any doubt persists concerning the state of hydration, administration of a circulating volume expanding agent such as plasma or 20 % albumin at a rate of 20 ml/kg over 2 hours is indicated;

(*b*) if the state of hydration is satisfactory, 20 % mannitol in a dosage of 2.5 ml/kg IV or furosemide 1-3 mg/kg IV is given. In the case of acute pre-renal failure, a diuretic response must be evident during the following three hours and the urine output must attain a rate of at least 2-3 ml/kg per hour. Otherwise persistent oliguria indicates the presence of a renal parenchymal lesion. Hypertonic mannitol should not be given to the premature neonate because of the cerebral risk of an acute rise in plasma osmolality.

Conservative treatment of intra-renal failure:

(a) *Fluid administration* [95, 140, 153]. — The aim of fluid administration is to maintain fluid balance. Insensible losses, as well as apparent renal and extra-renal losses must be taken into account.

Body weight is the best guide to the state of fluid balance. The newborn should be weighed every 8 hours. As caloric needs of the newborn cannot be attained, a daily loss of 0.2 to 1.0 % of body weight is expected. If body weight remains stable, iatrogenic fluid overload must be suspected. Insensible fluid osses are estimated as follows [95]:

Term newborn: 0.7-1.0 ml/kg per hour.
Pre-term newborn: 2.0-2.5 ml/kg per hour.

If the infant is subjected to phototherapy, 0.6-0.8 ml/kg per hour must be added to these volumes. If oral feeding is not feasible a 10 % glucose solution (555 mmol/l) is indicated.

(b) *Sodium.* — In the majority of cases the hyponatremia accompanying acute renal failure is a dilutional hyponatremia. Thus, it must not be compensated for by sodium administration, but rather by fluid restriction. However, if a salt-wasting situation is documented, sodium must be replaced as isotonic sodium chloride or isotonic sodium bicarbonate.

(c) *Potassium.* — The electrocardiogram is the best indicator of hyperkalemia. Whenever cardiac rythm disturbances accompany hyperkalemia the potassium level must be corrected quickly. The aims of treatment are:

(1) Control of the cardiac effects of hyperkalemia by either:

— slow intravenous administration of a 10 % calcium gluconate solution at a rate of 0.5-1.0 ml/kg for 2-4 minutes under E. C. G. surveillance. This potassium-lowering effect is transient;

— correction of metabolic acidosis by administration of an 8.4 % Na bicarbonate solution, in a dose of 2 ml/kg. The effect is also transient;

— administration of a 25 % glucose solution IV, 4 ml/kg to drive K into the cells.

(2) Production of negative potassium balance:

— administration of an ion-exchange resin (Kayexalate) in a dose of 1 g/kg, either "per os" or "per rectum", every six hours. The resin is diluted in 10 ml of 70 % sorbitol. This is the only method available for effective extraction of potassium from the body.

(d) *Convulsions.* — These are generally secondary to an electrolyte imbalance, e. g. hyponatremia, hypocalcemia, hypomagnesemia, or secondary to arterial hypertension. Anticonvulsive therapy consists of the administration of intravenous phenobarbital (6 mg/kg) or diazepam, IV or per rectum (0.3 mg/kg).

(e) *Arterial hypertension.* — The primary cause of arterial hypertension is iatrogenic fluid overload. The treatment is symptomatic (see p. 958). If the situation is not alleviated peritoneal dialysis is indicated.

(f) *Acidosis.* — Symptomatic metabolic acidosis must be treated by the administration of sodium bicarbonate. First of all hypocalcemia must be corrected to prevent the decrease in ionized calcium which will follow correction of acidosis. Great care must be taken during sodium bicarbonate administration because of the threat of cerebral hemorrhage or cardiac overload.

(g) *Infections.* — Infections are frequent in infants presenting with oligo-anuria. They should be treated with antibiotic agents corresponding to sensitivity testing. Dosage must be carefully adapted to the degree of renal failure [47].

INDICATIONS FOR PERITONEAL DIALYSIS [122]. — Most situations will respond to conservative therapy. However peritoneal dialysis is indicated in the following conditions:

(*a*) clinical: cardiac overload with pulmonary edema or congestive heart failure, water intoxication or persistent renal failure with uremic syndrome;

(*b*) laboratory: association of two or more of the following:

plasma urea concentration > 3 g/l (> 50 mmol/l),
plasma bicarbonate concentration < 12 mmol/l,
plasma potassium concentration > 8 mmol/l.

Peritoneal dialysis [178, 187].

(a) *Technique.* — The bladder must first be emptied, then the abdominal skin is carefully disinfected and draped. Following local anesthesia, a specially designed infant catheter is introduced into the abdominal cavity, 2 cm below the umbilicus in the median line. It is then fixed to the abdominal wall.

(b) *Fluids.* — A dialysate solution at a volume of 30-50 ml/kg is introduced by gravitational flow into the peritoneal cavity. It should be previously heated to 37° C. Dialysis cycles are usually of one hour duration: 10 minutes for loading, 40 minutes for exchange and 10 minutes for drainage. The dialysate must be cultured every day or whenever the outflow is cloudy.

(c) *Solution composition.* — Generally a solution containing sodium (134 mmol/l), chloride (103.5 mmol/l), lactate (35 mmol/l), calcium (1.75 mmol/l) and magnesium (0.5 mmol/l) is used for the first cycles. Glucose is added to the dialysate if water is to be extracted from the body. Glucose concentration in the dialysate must not exceed 5 %. Potassium in a concentration of 1.5-2.5 mmol/l is added to the solution after correction of hyperkalemia.

(d) *Complications:*

— drainage difficulties are frequent and may necessitate replacement of the catheter;

— hemorrhage may occur secondary to trauma or to a coagulopathy;

— peritonitis is more frequent when dialysis lasts longer than 24 hours. Cultures are mandatory whenever the dialysate becomes turbid, when the patient has pertinent physical findings or when there is unexplained fever. Peritonitis can be treated with intra-abdominal and/or systemic antibiotics (gentamicin, 8 mg/l dialysate, cloxacillin, 100 mg/l dialysate, tobramycin, 8 mg/l dialysate cephalotine, 250 mg/l dialysate). Prophylactic administration of antibiotics is not recommended;

— intestinal or bladder perforation;

— abdominal distension causing respiratory embarrassment;

— hyperglycemia with the use of hypertonic glucose solutions;

— hypoproteinemia: due to the fact that the peritoneal membrane is permeable to proteins a progressive protein depletion is often observed.

Evolution

In cases of acute tubular necrosis, the oliguric phase is often followed by an isosthenuric polyuric phase. Electrolyte and fluid losses must be compensated and fluid balance assessed hourly. The polyuric phase is preceded by a decrease in renin production and a rise in glomerular filtration rate.

Prognosis of acute renal failure

Pre-renal failure has an excellent prognosis if the predisposing factors are quickly and easily corrected. However intra-renal failure may have a poor outcome, the degree of recovery of renal function being dependent on the nature of the parenchymal lesion. Post-renal failure has a favorable prognosis whenever the obstruction is corrected early and before parenchymal injury occurs.

CONGENITAL NEPHROPATHIES

Congenital nephrotic syndrome

The nephrotic syndrome, characterized by massive proteinuria, hypoalbuminemia and generalized edema, with or without ascites, is rare in newborns. The proteinuria is secondary to an idiopathic injury to the basal membrane (congenital nephrotic syndrome of the Finnish type) or to infectious, toxic or vascular factors (Table XVI).

TABLE XVI. — ETIOLOGY
OF THE NEPHROTIC SYNDROME IN THE NEWBORN

1. Idiopathic: Finnish type (microcystic disease).

2. Secondary:
   — Infectious: syphilis, toxoplasmosis, cytomegalic inclusion disease.
   — Vascular: renal vein thrombosis.
   — Toxic: heavy metals.

Microcystic disease or Finnish type nephrotic syndrome. — This is an autosomal recessive disease observed mostly in Finland (10-12 cases/100,000 live births) [84]. The pathogenesis is unknown. A congenital error in metabolism has been suggested. The total number of glomeruli per kidney is often elevated.

(a) *Clinical.* — The congenital nephrotic syndrome is often associated with placental hypertrophy, in which the weight of the placenta may attain 40 % of the weight of the newborn. Prematurity is frequent, and 3/4 of the patients present with fetal distress [93]. The short stature and pallor of the newborn are striking. Edema and ascites appear in the first week of life in half of the sick neonates who survive. They often present respiratory distress with hypoxemia and hypotension.

(b) *Laboratory.* — The massive proteinuria is usually selective. Plasma protein electrophoresis is characteristic, with diminished levels of albumin and immunoglobulin G, and elevated levels of the alpha-2-macroglobulins. Total lipids and cholesterol are already elevated in the neonatal period. Hypocalcemia and hypokalemia occur frequently. Prenatal diagnosis may be suggested by an elevation of alpha-fetoprotein in the mother's blood or in the amniotic fluid [183].

(c) *Prognosis and treatment.* — The congenital nephrotic syndrome is fatal, with death generally occuring in the course of the first year, due to either infection or other undetermined causes. Treatment is symptomatic. Resistance to corticosteroids and immunosuppressive agents is the rule. Attempts at renal transplantation generally meet with failure.

Congenital tubular defects

Bartter's syndrome [14]. — The syndrome is probably transmitted in an autosomal recessive pattern. The pathogenesis may be related to disturbed prostaglandin synthesis. It is characterized by hyperplasia of the juxtaglomerular apparatus, hyperreninemia, hyperaldosteronemia, hypokalemia with metabolic alkalosis, and hyposthenuria. Arterial blood pressure is normal. The clinical manifestations which may appear shortly after birth include failure to thrive and polyuria which may lead to episodes of severe dehydration. The treatment consists of the administration of potassium and abundant liquids, along with the use of inhibitors of prostaglandin synthesis such as indomethacin and aspirin [135, 181].

A congenital alkalosis of renal origin without hyperplasia of the juxtaglomerular apparatus, has been recently described [32].

Nephrogenic diabetes insipidus [159]. — This disease is transmitted via a dominant gene linked to the X chromosome, with variable penetrance in the female heterozygote. It is characterized by a lack of response of the collecting tubule to the action of antidiuretic hormone. Polyhydramnios may be present during gestation. Diabetes insipidus may present as an unexplained fever or as hypernatremic dehydration secondary to unrecognized polyuria. The diagnosis rests on the simultaneous determination of plasma and urinary osmolalities. A vasopressin test will confirm the diagnosis. The treatment consists of the administration of adequate quantities of liquids, a diminution of the oral osmotic load, and the use of diuretics such as the thiazides [54]. The prognosis depends upon an early diagnosis and the proper management of the hyperosmolar state [65, 160].

Other tubular defects. — Numerous congenital problems are associated with perturbations of the renal reabsorption of solutes. The diagnosis of these conditions is generally established after the neonatal period, unless there is a known hereditary pattern. The accumulation of endogenous toxic products, or the excessive loss of solutes is generally responsible for the symptomatology. Among these conditions are the following:

— Proximal tubular acidosis
— Distal tubular acidosis
— Hereditary fructose intolerance
— Wilson's disease
— Galactosemia
— Familial hypophosphatemic rickets
— The glycogenoses
— Cystinosis
— Cystinuria.

Polycystic kidney disease

The cystic kidney diseases form a group with heterogeneous etiologies, morphologies and prognoses. Numerous classifications have been proposed. These diseases are generally not diagnosed until after the neonatal period. Only the infantile type of polycystic disease will be discussed in this chapter, since the expression of adult types within the neonatal period is very rare [164].

Infantile polycystic disease [19, 20, 147]. — This is an hereditary disease transmitted in an autosomal recessive fashion [117]. It is distinct from the adult type which follows an autosomal dominant pattern. Infantile polycystic disease is frequently accompanied by oligohydramnios, a Potter type facies and pulmonary hypoplasia. The volume of the renal masses may produce difficulty during delivery. Prenatal diagnosis is sometimes possible based upon ultrasonic examination. The cysts correspond to dilatations of distal tubules and collecting ducts. There are areas of normal tissue. The disease may present in two different forms during the neonatal period:

Perinatal form. — The abdominal cavity is occupied by two immense cystic renal masses. In this form practically all of the tubules are dilated. The infants are frequently still-born or succumb shortly after birth, either from renal insufficiency, or from respiratory difficulty due to pulmonary hypoplasia, or from respiratory difficulty secondary to diaphragmatic compression. The hepatic injury (fibrous or cystic) is generally of little importance.

Neonatal form. — This manifests as palpable abdominal masses found upon the first clinical examination of the newborn. The evolution of the disease is characterized by the appearance of proteinuria, hematuria and hypertension, followed by oliguria and progressive renal insufficiency. Death occurs during the first month of life and is usually secondary to renal or pulmonary insufficiency.

Differential diagnosis. — Differential diagnosis depends upon a family history and upon the presence of associated congenital malformations. Other causes of an abdominal mass must be excluded: hydronephrosis, bilateral tumors, renal vein thrombosis. Ultrasound is the examination of choice, along with intravenous urography. Treatment is symptomatic for the renal insufficiency.

Renal hypoplasia and dysplasia
[40, 59, 90]

These two distinct situations are often associated [18, 20]. Simple hypoplasia, or that accompanied by oligomeganephronia, is rarely diagnosed in the neonatal period. Renal dysplasia comprises a heterogenous group of malformations. The affected kidneys may contain cysts of variable shape and form. In 90 % of cases renal dysplasia is associated with ureteral, urethral or bladder malformations. Many situations may be associated with renal dysplasia: congenital cardiopathies (ventricular septal defect, coarctation of the aorta), duodenal, esophageal or rectal stenosis, central nervous system malformations (Arnold-Chiari disease).

Malformation syndromes with renal involvement

A certain number of malformation syndromes are accompanied by renal problems:

Hereditary onycho-osteodysplasia (Nail-Patella syndrome) [165]. — This syndrome, transmitted in an autosomal dominant pattern, is characterized by hypoplasia and dysplasia of the nails and iliac spines, by malformation of the radial head and by hypoplasia of the patella. Thirty to 40 % of the patients present with a renal injury characterized by proteinuria, with or without accompanying nephrotic syndrome. Progressive evolution toward renal insufficiency is observed in 25 % of the cases. The etiology of the renal involvement seems to concern the basal glomerular membrane.

Ehlers-Danlos syndrome (cutis hyperelastica) [94]. — This disease is inherited in an autosomal dominant mode, or in a recessive sex-linked mode. It is characterized by connective tissue weakness with articular hyperlaxity, exaggerated cutaneous elasticity and a tendency toward hematoma formation. The renal involvement may consist of hematuria, hypoplastic kidneys, infantile polycystic disease and a distal tubular acidosis.

Cerebro-hepato-renal syndrome (Zellweger's syndrome) [25, 43]. — This syndrome is transmitted in an autosomal recessive pattern. The pathogenesis seems to involve a defect in fetal iron metabolism. The syndrome, whose features partially resemble those of Down syndrome, is characterized by hypotonia, hypertelorism, a high forehead, Brushfield spots, transverse palmar creases, an epicanthal fold, hepatomegaly, skeletal and cardiac malformations. Renal cysts are frequently present. Death within the first months of life generally occurs secondary to respiratory insufficiency, convulsions and hemorrhage.

Oculo-cerebro-renal syndrome (Lowe's syndrome) [1]. — Transmitted in a recessive sex-linked mode, this syndrome is characterized by ocular anomalies (cataracts, glaucoma, buphthalmos), cerebral problems with severe mental retardation, hypotonia, hyporeflexia, and abnormalities in renal function. The renal problems consist of a Fanconi syndrome with hyperaminoaciduria, phosphaturia, glucosuria and bicarbonaturia. Treatment is symptomatic.

Fetal alcohol syndrome [143, 167]. — Anomalies of renal morphogenesis have been described in the fetal alcohol syndrome. The anomalies include renal hypoplasia and dysplasia, malformative uropathies and horseshoe kidneys.

ACQUIRED DISEASES

Urinary tract infection (UTI)

The importance of urinary tract infection in the neonate is explained by (a) the relatively high incidence of infection, (b) the immediate risk posed by its frequent association with septicemia, (c) the long term risk posed by its association with urologic malformations, and (d) the efficacy of therapeutic measures in preventing the destruction of renal parenchyma.

Definitions. — Urine in the bladder is normally sterile. The appearance of bacteria in the bladder is by definition a bacteriuria. One must distinguish between (a) lower urinary tract infection with bacteria only in the excretory channels, and (b) pyelonephritis in which bacteria are growing in the renal parenchyma. The latter is often associated with septicemia.

Incidence. — The frequency of UTI in the neonate is rather high; it has been found to be 0.7 % in normal newborns at term, 2.9 % in premature newborns [57], 2.2 % among high-risk newborns, and 3.4 % among post-mature neonates [120]. Boys are affected more often than girls in a proportion of 5 : 1.

Presentation [2, 17, 120]. — The presentation of urinary tract infection (UTI) in the neonate is highly variable (Table XVII). The UTI may range from a simple asymptomatic bacteriuria to the local manifestation of a septicemia. The most frequent mode of presentation is as poor feeding and failure to thrive (42-61 %). UTI may also present with vomiting (31-37 %), diarrhea (14-20 %), or fever (21-44 %). Other symptoms which may be present include lethargy, irritability and even convulsions. Dehydration, icterus or cyanosis may be found on physical examination, and the kidneys will be palpable in 10-20 % of cases.

TABLE XVII. — SYMPTOMS
OF NEONATAL URINARY TRACT INFECTION

	Total number	%
Total number of neonates .	1,762	
Infected neonates. . . .	43	2.4
Symptomatic infections . .	34	1.9
Asymptomatic infections .	9	0.5

Incidence of symptoms in infected neonates

Vomiting	16	37
Weight loss, dehydration. .	13	30
Fever	9	21
Diarrhea	6	14
Palpable kidneys	6	14
Poor feeding	5	12
Jaundice	16	37
Metabolic acidosis . . .	9	21
Miscellaneous	15	35

Diagnosis. — Only the demonstration of bacteria in a properly collected specimen can assure the diagnosis of a urinary tract infection. UTI is proven when a midstream urine specimen contains more than 100,000 bacteria/ml. In the neonatal population where special urine collection bags are utilized, any sample which contains more than 10^4 bacteria/ml is suspect. The diagnosis is confirmed by suprapubic puncture. If this is performed correctly, the growth of even a single colony on the culture plates is proof of UTI [101].

URINE COLLECTION BAGS. — The urine is collected by spontaneous micturition into a plastic bag fixed to the genitals, following disinfection of the perineal region using a solution such as chlorhexidine or more simply soapy water with a sterile water rinse. If micturition does not occur within one hour, the procedure must be repeated. After collection the urine is immediately placed on a dipslide with two culture plates [82]. The slide is read after 24 hours at room temperature.

TECHNIQUE OF SUPRAPUBIC BLADDER PUNCTURE. — This technique has been described in detail [13, 133]. It is performed within an hour following the ingestion of liquids by the infant. The bladder must be percussed to assure the presence of urine.

(a) The infant is placed in the dorsal decubitus position and held in place by an assistant.

(b) The skin on the abdomen is cleansed with chlorhexidine or 70 % alcohol.

(c) The puncture is performed in the median umbilico-pubic line, 1 cm above the symphysis using a 2 cm No. 21 needle. The urine is aspirated into a sterile 5 cm³ syringe.

(d) After aspiration the urine is immediately placed on the culture plate.

BLADDER CATHETERIZATION. — This method should not be used unless there is no alternative because of the danger of iatrogenic infection [78].

TABLE XVIII. — BACTERIOLOGY
OF NEONATAL URINARY TRACT INFECTION

	No of cases	
Organisms	43	%
E. coli	29	67
Klebsiella-Aerobacter	9	21
Proteus	1	2
E. coli + Proteus	2	5
E. coli + Klebsiella	1	2
E. coli + Enterococcus	1	2

Bacteriology [2, 120]. — E. coli is the organism most frequently encountered in UTI of the newborn (Table XVIII). Klebsiella-Aerobacter usually is in second place. A combination of two organisms, which is a sign of contamination in older children, is occasionnally found in neonates [120].

Urinary sediment. — Pyuria is frequently associated with bacteriuria. However, pyuria is not pathognomonic of UTI; it is simply a sign of urinary tract inflammation. Hematuria is not rare among neonates presenting with UTI.

Malformations of the urinary tract associated with infection [17, 51, 120]. — UTI in the newborn is often associated with urologic malformations or dysfunctions such as vesico-ureteral reflux or obstructive uropathy. These malformations are found in 42-55 % of infected neonates. They govern the treatment of UTI in this age group and affect its prognosis. Vesico-ureteral reflux is foremost among these uropathies.

VESICO-URETERAL REFLUX (VUR). — Reflux as found in newborns is frequently not pathological, and may disappear spontaneously in the first years of life. This is probably related to the maturation of the trigone of the bladder. As it matures, the path of the ureter through the wall elongates producing an effective anti-reflux mechanism. In other cases the reflux is a direct consequence of the UTI. It disappears with relief of the edema caused by the infection. Finally, certain cases of reflux are due to a congenital malformation of the terminal ureters. These will disappear only after surgical intervention. Whatever the cause, the VUR may be more or less severe. It may be limited to the lower ureter (stage 1) or it may ascend into the pyelo-calyceal system (stage 2) and even cause dilatation (stage 3). VUR, like obstructive uropathy, threatens the integrity of the renal parenchyma. However only infected VUR associated with intra-renal reflux can provoke parenchymal scarring [145, 151].

INTRA-RENAL REFLUX [87, 145, 151]. — In the majority of cases VUR is limited to the pyelo-calyceal system. Intra-renal or pyelo-renal reflux, on the contrary, presents with opacification of the renal parenchyma on excretory cystography. The incidence of intra-renal reflux is small. Its importance resides in the fact that it is a prerequisite to the occurence of atrophic scarring. Recent experimental work has elucidated the pathogenesis of reflux-related pyelonephritis [87, 145]. Refluxing papillae are present in 2/3 of infants. They permit reflux of infected urine into the parenchyma thus initiating progressive destruction. Such destruction appears early in life. If is thus essential to diagnose the condition very early in order to give the infants the benefit of prophylactic antibiotic therapy.

Radiographic and ultrasonic examinations. — All newborns with proven UTI should be investigated, following sterilization of their urine, by such methods as:

— intravenous urography (at the beginning of the third week of life),

— excretory cystography,

— ultrasonography.

Ultrasonography is the method of choice, particulary when the examination will need to be repeated, as in studying the evolution of a hydronephrosis.

Therapy.

URINARY TRACT INFECTION DURING THE COURSE OF SCEPTICEMIA. — If the UTI is associated with a state of scepticemia, therapy consists of the administration of gentamicin 2-7.5 mg/kg per day, along with ampicillin 100-200 mg/kg per day or amoxicillin 50-100 mg/kg per day. The course of treatment should last 10 days.

URINARY TRACT INFECTION AND PYELONEPHRITIS. — If the infection is limited to the urinary tract and renal parenchyma, therapy should consist of intravenous ampicillin 50-100 mg/kg per day in 3 or 4 doses, or amoxicillin 20-50 mg/kg per day in 3 or 4 doses for a total of 10 days. If the treatment is effective, the urine should be sterile by the third day.

INFECTION ASSOCIATED WITH AN OBSTRUCTIVE MALFORMATION OF THE URINARY TRACT. — It is necessary that the obstruction be relieved after the shortest possible delay. Indeed, the integrity of the renal parenchyma depends upon early intervention [123].

URINARY TRACT INFECTION ASSOCIATED WITH REFLUX. — Patients presenting with UTI who are found to have reflux should be given the benefit of long-term prophylactic therapy. This generally consists of amoxicillin p. o. in one dose of 10-20 mg/kg per day or sulfonamides 50 mg/kg per day.

Cortical necrosis and medullary necrosis [45, 108, 138]

These two conditions, frequently found in association with one another, are most often secondary to a severe, prolonged episode of ischemia. They are observed with serious asphyxia, septic shock, hemorrhagic shock, severe anemia, erythroblastosis fetalis, placental hemorrhage and disseminated intravascular coagulation (DIC). The pathogenesis of the resultant renal necrosis is shown in Figure VII-11.

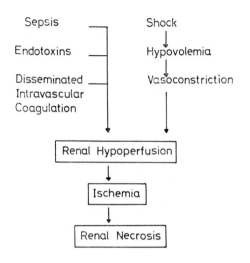

FIG. VII-11. — *Pathogenesis of renal necrosis.*

Cases of renal medullary necrosis have been described following the administration of hypertonic contrast agents (angiography) and also in cases of severe hyperbilirubinemia. This is a result of a direct toxic effect of unconjugated bilirubin on the medullary tissue.

Presentation. — Renal necrosis manifests itself by oliguric or anuric renal insufficiency. The kidneys are palpable. A constant hematuria appears early in the course, frequently accompanied by proteinuria. Medullary necrosis may be accompanied by a concentrating defect and sodium wasting. A thrombosis of the renal vein may complete the picture.

Differential diagnosis. — The clinical examination does not permit the differentiation between cortical and medullary necrosis. It is also difficult to rule out renal vein thrombosis or arterial embolization. Necrotic cortical tissue becomes calcified, producing a ring of opacification around the kidneys on X ray, thus permitting a retrospective diagnosis. A nephrogram with prolonged opacification of the pyramids is observed with medullary necrosis. Deformation of the pyelocalyceal system caused by sloughed necrotic tissue may also be seen.

Upon recovery, the oliguric phase is followed by an isosthenuric diuretic phase. This concentrating defect is sometimes permanent. Progressive renal insufficiency may also ensue.

Therapy and prognosis. — The treatment is symptomatic (see Acute Renal Failure). The prognosis is poor. Progressive renal insufficiency may appear. Bilateral cortical necrosis is most often fatal.

Papillary necrosis
[36, 156]

This condition is rare among newborns. It has been described in hyperosmolar states (dehydration) and in serious hyperbilirubinemia. The kidneys are palpable. Microscopic or macroscopic hematuria is the rule. Death generally occurs in several weeks due to progressive renal insufficiency. A salt-wasting syndrome has sometimes been seen in survivors. This may be due to destruction of juxta-medullary nephrons.

Renal vein thrombosis
[11, 16]

Renal vein thrombosis is a serious condition when seen in the neonatal period. 75 % of cases occur during the first months of life. Boys are affected more often than girls.

Pathogenesis. — Renal vein thrombosis is frequently secondary to a pre- or post-natal insult. In the newborn it is associated with a state of dehydration, asphyxia or hypoxemia. It is more frequent in infants of diabetic mothers. It may occur as a complication of angiography, if the infant is not sufficiently hydrated. The thrombosis generally begins in the peripheral renal veins (interlobular veins, vasa recta), then extends to the renal veins, suprarenal veins, and even to the inferior vena cava. The thrombosis may be unilateral or bilateral.

Clinical signs. — Thrombosis of the renal veins is characterized by large, hemorrhagic kidneys in 2/3 of patients, and also by oliguria. If the episode is severe, progressive renal insufficiency will follow. 30 % of the patients are anemic and 90 % thrombocytopenic [11]. One often sees elevated levels of the products of degradation of fibrin and low levels of

fibrinogen, factor V, and plasminogen. Disturbances in plasma electrolytes, uric acid and creatinine levels are a function of the severity of the renal insufficiency.

Diagnosis. — The differential diagnosis is that of large, hemorrhagic kidneys, i. e. nephroblastoma, hydronephrosis, cortical necrosis, medullary necrosis, papillary necrosis. The presence of hematologic signs of a disseminated coagulopathy confirm the diagnosis. The examination of choice is ultrasonography, which permits the visualization of non-functioning, non-cystic kidneys. Intravenous urography, in cases where it has been utilized, is abnormal in around 90 % of cases.

Therapy. — Treatment is that of serious renal insufficiency (see p. 960). The use of heparin has been recommended [11]. The dosage used is an initial bolus of 100 IU/kg followed by 25 IU/kg per hour. This is adjusted to maintain the activated partial thromboplastin time 1.5 to 2.0 times above normal. The treatment is continued until the thrombocyte count and coagulation factors have normalized. There is no indication for surgery during the acute phase. If the kidney is non-functional by the age of 4-6 months, nephrectomy should be considered to avoid the hypertension which may follow.

Prevention. — The administration or ingestion of hyperosmolar solutions must be avoided, and states of dehydration treated rapidly. Infants of diabetic mothers, and those presenting with cyanotic congenital cardiopathies must be watched closely.

Prognosis. — The prognosis is grave. The outcome is frequently fatal.

DRUGS AND THE NEWBORN KIDNEY

From the pharmacokinetic point of view, the newborn is distinguished from the adult by:

— The space of distribution of drugs
— The protein binding of drugs
— Hepatic elimination of drugs
— Renal elimination of drugs.

The dosage of medications given to neonates must be determined with these factors in mind. It must also be adjusted frequently, as rapid changes may occur in all these parameters.

Diuretics
[49, 114, 115, 116]

In the neonate the most frequently used diuretics are the loop diuretics (furosemide, ethacrynic acid), osmotic diuretics (mannitol), and occasionally the potassium-sparing diuretics (spironolactone, amiloride).

The loop diuretics. — Furosemide and ethacrynic acid inhibit resorption of sodium chloride in the ascending limb of the loop of Henle, producing a maximal natriuresis of 20-25 % of the filtered load. These diuretics impair the mechanism of concentration and, in the adult, the effectiveness of the mechanism of dilution. In the newborn, the infant, or the edematous adult, these diuretics are able to bring about an increase in the clearance of free-water [115]. They also have a non-specific potassium-wasting effect, secondary to the increased distal sodium load which is available at the Na/K-H exchange sites in the collecting duct. The excretion of calcium is increased. These diuretics also produce renal vasodilatation and perhaps an augmentation in venous capacitance, which may account for their rapid effect when used in the treatment of pulmonary edema.

In the newborn, the use of intravenous furosemide produces an effect within an hour [186]. The maximum effect occurs three hours after injection, and the duration of action is six hours. A dose of 1 mg/kg administered to six low-weight infants (1,490 g) aged 10-57 days, produced a net loss averaging 28 ml/kg of water, 3.6 mmol/kg Na, and 0.3 mmol/kg of K, with an increase in excretion of free-water [152].

Distal potassium-sparing diuretics. — These relatively weak diuretics provoke the retention of potassium by inhibiting Na/K-H exchange at the level of the collecting duct. They act by inhibition of the action of aldosterone (spironolactone) or by inhibition of the distal diffusion of sodium (amiloride). Their natriuretic effect is additive to that of loop diuretics.

Osmotic diuretics. — Mannitol, which is freely filtered at the glomerulus, inhibits the passive reabsorption of water in the proximal tubule and the loop of Henle. It is chiefly used in states of incipient prerenal failure.

Filtration diuretics. — Aminophylline, the glucocorticoids, the cardiac glycosides and other inotropic agents such as isoproterenol and dopamine may effect a diuresis via their augmentation of renal perfusion and the consequent increase in glomerular filtration rate.

Resistance to treatment. — In order for the loop diuretics and the potassium-sparing diuretics to be effective, it is necessary that a significant proportion of the glomerular filtrate reach their sites of action. Their effectiveness decreases with any significant lowering of glomerular filtration, or with exaggerated proximal reabsorption (diminution of effective extracellular volume). Primary or secondary hyperaldosteronism also diminishes the effect of loop diuretics, by increasing reabsorption of Na in the collecting tubule.

Side effects of diuretics. — The most common side effects are the depletion of extracellular fluid volume and total body potassium stores. Hyponatremia may occur as a consequence of the inhibition of free-water clearance, or of Na wasting. Metabolic alkalosis secondary to hypokalemia or to the contraction of the extracellular fluid space is sometimes observed.

Nephrotoxic agents or drugs which may alter renal function
[41]

Antibiotics [7, 8, 9]. — The nephrotoxicity of gentamicin, cotrimoxazole and the cephalosporins is well established in adults. It is probably identical for newborns, although proof is lacking:

— gentamicin: acute tubular necrosis,
— kanamycin: acute renal tubular necrosis,
— cephalosporins: acute renal tubular necrosis, interstitial nephritis,
— cotrimoxazole: acute renal tubular necrosis, interstitial nephritis.

Anticonvulsants. — The intravenous administration of diazepam may provoke a transient decrease in renal blood flow and glomerular filtration in the infant [76].

Vasodilators. — Tolazoline, an alpha-sympatholytic agent used as a pulmonary vasodilator for persistent fetal circulation [69] with pulmonary hypertension, may induce renal vasoconstriction and consequent oliguria [132].

Indomethacin. — A transient yet significant decrease in glomerular filtration and urine flow has been observed after the administration of indomethacin, a prostaglandin inhibitor used for pharmacologic closure of the ductus arteriosus in the premature infant with persistant fetal circulation [35, 37].

Disinfectants. — The mercury present in certain disinfectant preparations may attain nephrotoxic concentrations in the blood. It may provoke renal ischemia with acute tubular necrosis.

Contrast agents [67, 74]. — Major side effects have been described with radiographic examinations (angiography) which utilize hypertonic contrast agents: renal vein thrombosis, medullary necrosis, ischemia, hypoperfusion and renal insufficiency. These products must be used with prudence and only after adequate hydration of the infant. The use of non-ionic contrast agents with osmolalities around 450 mosm/kg H_2O markedly reduces the risk of toxicity in neonates. The osmolality of certain products employed in radiology is indicated in Table IX.

REFERENCES

[1] ABBASSI (V.), LOWE (C. U.), CALCAGNO (P. L.). — Oculo-cerebro-renal syndrome: a review. *Amer. J. Dis. Child.*, *115*, 145-168, 1968.

[2] ABBOTT (G. D.). — Neonatal bacteriuria, the value of bladder puncture in resolving problems of interpretation arising from voided urine specimens. *Austr. Paediatr. J.*, *14*, 83-86, 1978.

[3] ADELMAN (R. D.). — Neonatal hypertension. *Pediatr. Clin. North Am.*, *25*, 99-110, 1978.

[4] ANAND (S. K.), NORTHWAY (J. D.), CRUSSI (F. G.). — Acute renal failure in newborn infants. *J. Pediatr.*, *92*, 985-988, 1978.

[5] APERIA (A.), BROBERGER (O.), THODENIUS (K.), ZETTERSTRÖM (R.). — Renal response to an oral sodium load in newborn full term infants. *Acta Paediat. Scand.*, *61*, 670-676, 1972.

[6] APERIA (A.), BROBERGER (O.), HERIN (P.), ZETTERSTRÖM (R.). — Sodium excretion in relation to sodium intake and aldosterone excretion in newborn pre-term and full-term infants. *Acta Paediat. Scand.*, *68*, 813-817, 1979.

[7] APPEL (G. B.), NEU (H. C.). — The nephrotoxicity of antimicrobial agents. I. *New Engl. J. Med.*, *296*, 663-670, 1977.

[8] APPEL (G. B.), NEU (H. C.). — The nephrotoxicity of antimicrobial agents. II. *New Engl. J. Med.*, *296*, 722-728, 1977.

[9] APPEL (G. B.), NEU (H. C.). — The nephrotoxicity of antimicrobial agents. III. *New Engl. J. Med.*, *296*, 784-787, 1977.

[10] ARANT (B. S. Jr.). — Developmental patterns of renal functional maturation compared in the human neonate. *J. Pediatr.*, *92*, 705-712, 1978.

[11] ARNEIL (G. C.), MACDONALD (A. M.), MURPHY (A. V.), SWEET (E. M.). — Renal venous thrombosis. *Clin. Nephrol.*, *1*, 119-131, 1973.

[12] ASCHINBERG (L. C.), ZEIS (P. M.), HAGEMAN (J. R.), VIDYASAGAR (D.). — Acute renal failure in the newborn. *Crit. Care Med.*, *5*, 36-42, 1977.

[13] BAILEY (R. R.), LITTLE (P. J.). — Suprapublic bladder aspiration in diagnosis of urinary tract infection. *Brit. Med. J.*, *1*, 293-294, 1969.

[14] BARTTER (F. C.), PRONOVE (P.), GILL (J. R. Jr.), MACCARDLE (R. C.). — Hyperplasia of the juxtaglomerular complex with hyperaldosteronism and hypokalemic alkalosis: a new syndrome. *Amer. J. Med.*, *33*, 811-828, 1962.

[15] BEITINS (I. Z.), BAYARD (F.), LEVITSKY (L.), ANCES (I. G.), KOWARSKI (A.), MIGEON (C. J.). — Plasma aldosterone concentration at delivery and during the newborn period. *J. Clin. Invest.*, *51*, 386-394, 1972.

[16] BELMAN (A. B.). — Renal vein thrombosis in infancy and childhood. A contemporary survey. *Clin. Pediat.*, *15*, 1033-1044, 1976.

[17] BERGSTRÖM (T.), LARSON (H.), LINCOLN (K.), WINBERG (J.). — Studies of urinary infections in infancy and childhood: XII. Eighty consecutive patients with neonatal infection. *J. Pediatr.*, *80*, 858-866, 1972.

[18] BERNSTEIN (J.). — The morphogenesis of renal parenchymal maldevelopment. (renal dysplasia). *Pediatr. Clin. North Am.*, *18*, 395-407, 1971.

[19] BERNSTEIN (J.). — Heritable cystic disorders of the kidney: the mythology of polycystic disease. *Pediatr. Clin. North Am.*, *18*, 435-444, 1971.

[20] BERNSTEIN (J.). — The classification of renal cysts. *Nephron*, *11*, 91-100, 1973.

[21] BLACK (I. F. S.), KOTRAPU (N.), MASSIE (H.). — Application of Doppler ultrasound to blood pressure measurement in small infants. *J. Pediatr.*, *81*, 932-935, 1972.

[22] BLAUFOX (M. D.), FREEMAN (L. M.). — Radionuclide techniques for the evaluation of diseases of the urinary tract in children. *Semi. Nucl. Med.*, *3*, 27-53, 1973.

[23] BOINEAU (F. G.), ROTHMAN (J.), LEWY (J. E.). — Nephrosonography in the evaluation of renal failure and masses in infants. *J. Pediatr.*, *87*, 195-201, 1975.

[24] BONGIOVANNI (A. M.), ROOT (A. W.). — The adrenogenital syndrome. *New Engl. J. Med.*, *268*, 1283-1289, 1963.

[25] BOWEN (P.), LEE (C. S. N.), ZELLWEGER (H.). — A familial syndrome of multiple congenital defects. *John Hopkins Med. J.*, *114*, 402-414, 1964.

[26] BRENNER (B. M.), HUMES (H. D.). — Mechanics of glomerular ultrafiltration. *New Engl. J. Med.*, *297*, 148-154, 1977.

[27] BRENNER (B. M.), BEEUWKES (R.). — The renal circulations. *Hospital Practice*, *7*, 35-46, 1978.

[28] BRODEHL (J.), FRANKEN (A.), GELLISSEN (K.). — Maximal tubular reabsorption of glucose in infants and children. *Acta Paediat. Scand.*, *61*, 413-420, 1972.

[29] BROUGHTON-PIPKIN (F.), SMALES (O. R. C.). — A study of factors affecting blood pressure and angiotensin II in newborn infants. *J. Pediatr.*, *91*, 113-119, 1977.

[30] BURG (M. B.). — The nephron in transport of sodium, amino acids, and glucose. *Hospital Practice*, *10*, 99-109, 1978.

[31] CALCAGNO (P. L.), RUBIN (M. I.). — Renal extraction of para-aminohippurate in infants and children. *J. Clin. Invest.*, *42*, 1632-1639, 1963.

[32] CALCAGNO (P. L.). — A short communication. Congenital renal alkalosis. *Pediat. Res.*, *13*, 1379-1381, 1979.

[33] CAMPBELL (S.), WLADIMIROFF (J. W.), DEWHURST (C. J.). — The antenatal measurement of fetal urine production. *J. Obstet. Gynaec. Br. Comm.*, *80*, 680-686, 1973.

[34] CARELLA (J. A.), SILBER (I.). — Hyperreninemic hypertension in an infant secondary to pelviureteric obstruction treated successfully by surgery. *J. Pediatr.*, *88*, 987-989, 1976.

[35] CATTERTON (Z.), SELLERS (B.), GRAY (B.). — Inulin clearance in the premature infant receiving indomethacin. *J. Pediatr.*, *96*, 737-739, 1980.

[36] CHRISPIN (A. R.), HULL (D.), LILLIE (J. G.), RIDSON (R. A.). — Renal tubular necrosis and papillary necrosis after gastroenteritis in infants. *Brit. Med. J.*, *1*, 410-412, 1970.

[37] CIFUENTES (R. F.), OLLEY (P. M.), BALFE (J. W.), RADDE (I. C.), SOLDIN (S. J.). — Indomethacin and renal function in premature infants with persistent patent ductus arteriosus. *J. Pediatr.*, *95*, 583-587, 1979.

[38] COHEN (J. J.). — Disorders of potassium balance. *Hospital Practice*, *1*, 119-128, 1979.

[39] COLODNY (A. H.), GRISCOM (N. T.). — Clue to diagnosis of neonatal urinary ascites. Relative radiolucency of liver shadow. *Urology*, *11*, 295-299, 1978.

[40] CROCKER (J. F. S.), BROWN (D. M.), VERNIER (R. L.). — Developmental defects of the kidney. *Pediatr. Clin. North Am.*, *18*, 355-376, 1971.

[41] CURTIS (J. R.). — Drug-induced renal disease. *Drugs*, *18*, 377-391, 1979.

[42] DANIEL (S. S.), JAMES (L. S.). — Abnormal renal function in the newborn infant. *J. Pediatr.*, *88*, 856-858, 1976.

[43] DANKS (D. M.), TIPETT (P.), ADAMS (C.), CAMPBELL (P.). — Cerebro-hepato-renal syndrome of Zellweger. *J. Pediatr.*, *86*, 382-387, 1975.

[44] DAUBER (I. M.), KRAUSS (A. N.), SYMCHYCH (P. S.), AULD (P. A. M.). — Renal failure following perinatal anoxia. *J. Pediatr.*, *88*, 851-855, 1976.

[45] DAVIES (D. J.), KENNEDY (A.), ROBERTS (C.). — Renal medullary necrosis in infancy and childhood. *J. Pathol.*, *99*, 125-130, 1969.

[46] DEAN (R. F. A.), McCANCE (R. A.). — The renal responses of infants and adults to the administration of hypertonic solutions of sodium chloride and urea. *J. Physiol. Lond.*, *109*, 81-97, 1949.

[47] DETTLI (L.). — Drug dosage in patients with impaired renal function. *Progress in Pharmacology*, vol. 1, *4*, Fischer, Stuttgart, New York, 1978.

[48] DILLON (M. J.), GILLIN (M. E. A.), RYNESS (J.), DE SWIET (M.). — Plasma renin activity and aldosterone concentration in the human newborn. *Arch. Dis. Childh.*, *51*, 537-540, 1976.

[49] DIRKS (J. H.). — Mechanisms of action and clinical uses of diuretics. *Hospital Practice*, *9*, 99-110, 1979.

[50] DRESZER (M.). — Fluid and electrolyte requirements in the newborn infant. *Pediatr. Clin. North Am.*, *24*, 537-546, 1977.

[51] DREW (J. H.), ACTON (C. M.). — Radiologic findings in newborn infants with urinary infection. *Arch. Dis. Childh.*, *51*, 628-630, 1976.

[52] DURANTE (D.), JONES (D.), SPITZER (R.). — Neonatal renal arterial embolism syndrome. *J. Pediatr.*, *89*, 978-981, 1976.

[53] DWECK (H. S.), REYNOLDS (D. W.), CASSADY (G.). — Indirect blood pressure measurement in newborns. *Amer. J. Dis. Child.*, *127*, 492-494, 1974.

[54] EARLEY (L. E.), ORLOFF (J.). — The mechanism of antidiuresis associated with administration of hydrochlorothiazide to patients with vasopressin-resistant diabetes insipidus. *J. Clin. Invest.*, *41*, 1988-1997, 1962.

[55] EDELMANN (C. M. Jr.), BARNETT (H. L.). — Role of the kidney in water metabolism in young infants. Physiologic and clinical considerations. *J. Pediatr.*, *56*, 154-179, 1960.

[56] EDELMANN (C. M.Jr.), SORIANO (J. R.), BOICHIS (H.), GRUSKIN (A. B.), ACOSTA (M. I.). — Renal bicarbonate reabsorption and hydrogen ion excretion in normal infants. *J. Clin. Invest.*, *46*, 1309-1317, 1967.

[57] EDELMANN (C. M. Jr.), OGWO (J. E.), FINE (B. P.), MARTINEZ (A. B.). — The prevalence of bacteriuria in full-term and premature newborn infants. *J. Pediatr.*, *82*, 125-132, 1973.

[58] ENGELKE (S. C.), SHAH (B. L.), VASAN (U.), RAYE (J. R.). — Sodium balance in very low-birth-weight infants. *J. Pediatr.*, *93*, 837-841, 1978.

[59] FARKAS (A.), FIRSTATER (M.), JOHNSTON (J. H.). — Neonatal solitary renal cysts associated with posterior urethral valves. *J. Pediatr. Surg.*, *14*, 132-137, 1979.

[60] FAWER (C. L.), TORRADO (A.), GUIGNARD (J. P.). — Maturation of renal function in full-term and premature neonates. *Helv. Paediat. Acta*, *34*, 11-21, 1979.

[61] FAWER (C. L.), TORRADO (A.), GUIGNARD (J. P.). — Single injection clearance in the neonate. *Biol. Neonate*, *35*, 321-324, 1979.

[62] FELDMAN (H.), GUIGNARD (J. P.). — Plasma creatinine in the first month of life. *Archiv. Dis. Child.*, *57*, 123-126, 1982.

[63] FETTERMAN (G. H.), SHUPLOCK (H. A.), PHILIPP (F. J.), GREGG (H. S.). — The growth and maturation of human glomeruli and proximal convolutions from term to adulthood. Studies by microdissection. *Pediatrics*, *35*, 601-619, 1965.

[64] FRIIS-HANSEN (B.). — Body composition during growth. *Pediatrics*, *47*, 264-274, 1971.

[65] GAUTIER (E.), SIMPKISS (M.). — The management of nephrogenic diabetes insipidus in early life. *Acta Paediat.*, *46*, 354-370, 1957.

[66] GIACOIA (G. P.). — Hydrops fetalis (Fetal edema). *Clin. Pediat.*, *19*, 334-339, 1980.

[67] GILBERT (E. F.), KHOURY (G. H.), HOGAN (G. R.), JONES (B.). — Hemorrhagic renal necrosis in infancy: relationship to radiopaque compounds. *J. Pediatr.*, *76*, 49-53, 1970.

[68] GODARD (C.), GEERING (J. M.), GEERING (K.), VALLOTON (M. B.). — Plasma renin activity related to sodium balance, renal function and urinary vasopressin in the newborn infant. *Pediat. Res.*, *13*, 742-745, 1979.

[69] GOETZMAN (B. W.), SUNSHINE (P.), JOHNSON (J. D.), WENNBERG (R. P.), HACKEL (A.), MERTEN (D. F.), BARTOLETTI (A. L.), SILVERMANN (N. H.). — Neonatal hypoxia and pulmonary vasospasm: response to tolazoline. *J. Pediatr.*, *89*, 617-621, 1976.

[70] GOLDMANN (H. S.), FREEMANN (L. M.). — Radiographic and radioisotopic methods of evaluation of the kidneys and urinary tract. *Pediatr. Clin. North Am.*, *18*, 409-434, 1971.

[71] GOLDRING (D.), WOHLTMANN (H.). — Flush method for blood pressure determinations in newborn infants. *J. Pediatr.*, 40, 285-289, 1952.

[72] GOLDRING (D.). — Treatment of the infant and child with coarctation of the aorta. *Pediatr. Clin. North Am.*, 25, 111-118, 1978.

[73] GREENHILL (A.), GRUSKIN (A. B.). — Laboratory evaluation of renal function. *Pediatr. Clin. North Am.*, 23, 661-679, 1976.

[74] GRUSKIN (A. B.), OETLIKER (O. H.), WOLFISH (N. M.), GOOTMAN (N. L.), BERNSTEIN (J.), EDELMANN (C. M. Jr.). — Effects of angiography on renal function and histology in infants and piglets. *J. Pediatr.*, 76, 41-48, 1970.

[75] GRUSKIN (A. B.), EDELMANN (C. M. Jr.), YUAN (S.). — Maturational changes in renal blood flow in piglets. *Pediat. Res.*, 4, 7-13, 1970.

[76] GUIGNARD (J. P.), FILLOUX (B.), LAVOIE (J.), PELET (J.), TORRADO (A.). — Effect of intravenous diazepam on renal function. *Clin. Pharmacol. Ther.*, 18, 401-404, 1975.

[77] GUIGNARD (J. P.), TORRADO (A.), DA CUNHA (O.), GAUTIER (E.). — Glomerular filtration rate in the first three weeks of life. *J. Pediatr.*, 87, 268-272, 1975.

[78] GUIGNARD (J. P.), FAWER (C. L.), KROENER (A.), QUELOZ (J.), LANDRY (M.). — Infections urinaires après cystographie mictionnelle par sondage. *Schweiz. Med. Wschr.*, 105, 1654-1656, 1975.

[79] GUIGNARD (J. P.), TORRADO (A.), MAZOUNI (S. M.), GAUTIER (E.). — Renal function in respiratory distress syndrome. *J. Pediatr.*, 88, 845-850, 1976.

[80] GUIGNARD (J. P.), TORRADO (A.), FELDMAN (H.), GAUTIER (E.). — Assessment of glomerular filtration in children. *Helv. Paediat. Acta*, 35, 437-447, 1980.

[81] GUIGNARD (J. P.). — Renal function in the newborn infant. *Pediatr. Clin. North Am.*, 29, 777-790, 1982.

[82] GUTTMAN (D.), NAYLOR (G. R. E.). — Dipslide: an aid to quantitative urine culture in general practice. *Brit. Med. J.*, 3, 343-345, 1967.

[83] HAFTEL (A. J.), EICHNER (J.), MALING (J.), WILSON (M. L.). — Myoglobinuria renal failure in a newborn infant. *J. Pediatr.*, 93, 1015-1016, 1978.

[84] HALLMAN (N.), NORIO (R.), RAPOLA (J.). — Congenital nephrotic syndrome. *Nephron*, 11, 101-110, 1973.

[85] HAYS (R. M.). — Principles of ion and water transport in the kidney. *Hospital Practice*, 9, 79-88, 1978.

[86] HENDERSON (K. C.), TORCH (E. M.). — Differential diagnosis of abdominal masses in the neonate. *Pediatr. Clin. North Am.*, 24, 557-578, 1977.

[87] HODSON (J.). — Reflux nephropathy. *Med. Clin. N. Amer.*, 62, 1201-1221, 1978.

[88] HOLLERMAN (C. E.). — *Pediatric Nephrology*, Hans Huber Publishers, Bern, 1979.

[89] HOLLIDAY (M. A.), SEGAR (W. E.). — The maintenance need for water in parenteral fluid therapy. *Pediatrics*, 19, 823-832, 1957.

[90] HOLLIDAY (M. A.). — Developmental abnormalities of the kidney in children. *Hospital Practice*, 6, 101-112, 1978.

[91] HOOK (J. B.), WILLIAMSON (H. E.), HIRSCH (G. H.). — Functional maturation of renal PAH transport in the dog. *Can. J. Physiol. Pharmacol.*, 48, 169-175, 1970.

[92] HORSTER (M.), VALTIN (H.). — Postnatal development of renal function: micropuncture and clearance studies in the dog. *J. Clin. Invest.*, 50. 779-795, 1971.

[93] HUTTUNEN (N. P.). — Congenital nephrotic syndrome of Finnish type: study of 75 patients. *Arch. Dis. Childh.*, 51, 344-348, 1976.

[94] IMAHORI (S.), BANNERMAN (R. M.), GRAF (C. J.), BRENNAN (J. C.). — Ehlers-Danlos syndrome with multiple arterial lesions. *Amer. J. Med.*, 47, 967-977, 1969.

[95] JAIN (R.). — Acute renal failure in the neonate. *Pediatr. Clin. North Am.*, 24, 605-618, 1977.

[96] JAMISON (R. L.), MAFFLY (R. H.). — The urinary concentrating mechanism. *New Engl. J. Med.*, 295, 1059-1067, 1976.

[97] JOPPICH (R.), SCHERER (B.), WEBER (P. C.). — Renal prostaglandins: relationship to the development of blood pressure and concentrating capacity in pre-term and full-term healthy infants. *Europ. J. Pediatr.*, 132, 253-259, 1979.

[98] JOPPICH (R.), KIEMANN (U.), MAYER (G.), HÄBERLE (D.). — Effect of antidiuretic hormone upon urinary concentrating ability and medullary cAMP formation in neonatal piglets. *Pediat. Res.*, 13, 884-888, 1979.

[99] KAPLAN (S. A.). — Diseases of the adrenal cortex II: congenital adrenal hyperplasia. *Pediatr. Clin. North Am.*, 26, 77-90, 1979.

[100] KARLSSON (F. A.), HARDELL (L. I.), HELLSING (K.). — A prospective study of urinary proteins in early infancy. *Acta Paediat. Scand.*, 68, 663-667, 1979.

[101] KASS (E. H.). — Asymptomatic infections of the urinary tract. *Trans. Ass. Amer. Physicians*, 69, 56-63, 1956.

[102] KASSIRER (J. P.). — Clinical evaluation of kidney function. Glomerular filtration. *New Engl. J. Med.*, 285, 385-389, 1971.

[103] KASSIRER (J. P.). — Clinical evaluation of kidney function. Tubular function. *New Engl. J. Med.*, 285, 499-502, 1971.

[104] KIRKLAND (R. T.), KIRKLAND (J. L.). — Systolic blood pressure measurement in the newborn infant with the transcutaneous Doppler method. *J. Pediatr.*, 80, 52-56, 1972.

[105] KOKKO (J. P.). — Renal concentrating and diluting mechanisms. *Hospital Practice*, 2, 110-116, 1979.

[106] KOTCHEN (T. A.), STRICKLAND (A. L.), RICE (T. W.), WALTERS (D. R.). — A study of the renin-angiotensin system in newborn infants. *J. Pediatr.*, 80, 938-946, 1972.

[107] KOTOYAN (N.). — Aspects of perinatal endocrinology. *Pediatr. Clin. North Am.*, 24, 529-535, 1977.

[108] LEONIDAS (J. C.), BERDON (W. E.), GRIBETZ (D.). — Bilateral renal cortical necrosis in the newborn infant: roentgenographic diagnosis. *J. Pediatr.*, 79, 623-627, 1971.

[109] LEVIN (M. L.). — Hyponatremic syndromes. *Med. Clin. North Amer.*, 62, 1257-1272, 1978.

[110] LEWY (J. E.), MOEL (D. I.). — Pathogenesis and management of edema in the newborn. *Clin. Perinatol.*, 2, 117-123, 1975.

[111] LEWY (M.). — The pathophysiology of sodium balance. *Hospital Practice*, 11, 95-106, 1978.

[112] LJUNGQVIST (A.), WALLGREN (G.). — Unilateral renal artery stenosis and fatal arterial hyper-

tension in a newborn infant. *Acta Paediatr.*, *51*, 575-584, 1962.

[113] LJUNGQVIST (A.), WAGERMARK (J.). — Renal juxtaglomerular granulation in the human fœtus and infant. *Acta Path. Microbiol. Scand.*, *67*, 257-266, 1966.

[114] LOGGIE (J. M. H.), KLEINMAN (L. I.), VAN MAANEN (E. F.). — Renal function and diuretic therapy in infants and children. Part I. *J. Pediatr.*, *86*, 485-496, 1975.

[115] LOGGIE (J. M. H.), KLEINMAN (L. I.), VAN MAANEN (E. F.). — Renal function and diuretic therapy in infants and children. Part II. *J. Pediatr.*, *86*, 657-669, 1975.

[116] LOGGIE (J. M. H.), KLEINMAN (L. I.), VAN MAANEN (E. F.). — Renal function and diuretic therapy in infants and children. Part III. *J. Pediatr.*, *86*, 825-832, 1975.

[117] LUNDIN (P. M.), OLOW (I.). — Polycystic kidneys in newborns, infants and children. A clinical and pathological study. *Acta Paediat.*, *50*, 185-200, 1961.

[118] McCANCE (R. A.), NAYLOR (N. J. B.), WIDDOWSON (E. M.). — The response of infants to a large dose of water. *Arch. Dis. Childh.*, *29*, 104-109, 1954.

[119] MACLAURIN (J. C.). — Changes in body water distribution during the first two weeks of life. *Arch. Dis. Childh.*, *41*, 286-291, 1966.

[120] MAHERZI (M.), GUIGNARD (J. P.), TORRADO (A.). — Urinary tract infection in high-risk newborn infants. *Pediatrics*, *62*, 521-523, 1978.

[121] MAJD (M.), BELMAN (A. B.). — Nuclear cystography in infants and children. *Urol. Clin. North Am.*, *6*, 395-407, 1979.

[122] MANLEY (G. L.), COLLIPP (P. J.). — Renal failure in the newborn. Treatment with peritoneal dialysis. *Amer. J. Dis. Child.*, *115*, 107-110, 1968.

[123] MAYOR (G.), GENTON (N.), TORRADO (A.), GUIGNARD (J. P.). — Renal function in obstructive nephropathy: long-term effect of reconstructive surgery. *Pediatrics*, *56*, 740-747, 1975.

[124] MENDOZA (S. A.). — Syndrome of inappropriate antidiuretic hormone secretion (SIADH). *Pediatr. Clin. North Am.*, *23*, 681-690, 1976.

[125] MENDOZA (S. A.), GRISWOLD (W. R.), LEOPOLD (G. R.), KAPLAN (G. W.). — Intrauterine diagnosis of renal anomalies by ultrasonography. *Amer. J. Dis. Child.*, *133*, 1042-1043, 1979.

[126] MERLET-BENICHOU (C.), DE ROUFFIGNAC (C.). — Renal clearance studies in fetal and young guinea pigs: effect of salt loading. *Amer. J. Physiol.*, *232*, 178-185, 1977.

[127] MOORE (E. S.), GALVEZ (M. B.). — Delayed micturition in the newborn period. *J. Pediatr.*, *80*, 867-873, 1972.

[128] MOSS (A. J.). — Indirect methods of blood pressure measurement. *Pediatr. Clin. North Am.*, *25*, 3-14, 1978.

[129] MOYLAN (F. M. B.), HERRIN (J. T.), KRISHNAMOORTHY (K.), TODRES (I. D.), SHANNON (D. C.). — Inappropriate antidiuretic hormone secretion in premature infants with cerebral injury. *Amer. J. Dis. Child.*, *132*, 399-402, 1978.

[130] MUSELES (M.), GAUDRY (C. L.), BASON (W. M.). — Renal anomalies in the newborn found by deep palpation. *Pediatrics*, *47*, 97-100, 1971.

[131] NASH (M. A.), EDELMANN (C. M. Jr.). — The developing kidney: immature function or inappropriate standard? *Nephron*, *11*, 71-90, 1973.

[132] NAUJOKS (S.), GUIGNARD (J. P.). — Renal effects of tolazoline in rabbits. *Lancet*, *2*, 1075-1076, 1979.

[133] NELSON (J. D.), PETERS (P. C.). — Suprapubic aspiration of urine in premature and term infants. *Pediatrics*, *36*, 132-134, 1965.

[134] NEW (M. I.), LEVINE (L. S.). — Adrenocortical hypertension. *Pediatr. Clin. North Am.*, *25*, 67-81, 1978.

[135] NORBY (L.), LENTZ (R.), FLAMENBAUM (W.), RAMWELL (P.). — Prostaglandins and aspirin therapy in Bartter's syndrome. *Lancet*, *2*, 604-606, 1976.

[136] NORMAN (M. E.), ASADI (F. K.). — A prospective study of acute renal failure in the newborn infant. *Pediatrics*, *63*, 475-479, 1979.

[137] NUNN (I. N.), STEPHENS (F. D.). — The triad syndrome: a composite anomaly of the abdominal wall, urinary system and testes. *J. Urol.*, *86*, 782-794, 1961.

[138] OGATA (E. S.), GOODING (C. A.), PHIBBS (R. H.). — Angiographic and ultrasonographic appearance of renal cortical and medullary necrosis in the newborn. *Pediat. Radiol.*, *3*, 226-229, 1975.

[139] OH (W.), KARECKI (H.). — Phototherapy and insensible water loss in the newborn infant. *Amer. J. Dis. Child.*, *124*, 230-232, 1972.

[140] OH (W.). — Disorders of fluid and electrolytes in newborn infants. *Pediatr. Clin. North Amer.*, *23*, 601-609, 1976.

[141] PLUMER (L. B.), KAPLAN (G. W.), MENDOZA (S. A.). — Hypertension in infants. A complication of umbilical artery catheterization. *J. Pediatr.*, *89*, 802-805, 1976.

[142] PRAMANIK (A. K.), ALTSHULER (G.), LIGHT (I. J.), SUTHERLAND (J. M.). — Prune-belly syndrome associated with Potter (renal non-function) syndrome. *Amer. J. Dis. Child.*, *131*, 672-674, 1977.

[143] QASI (Q.), MASAKAWA (A.), MILMAN (D.), McGANN (B.), CHUA (A.), HALLER (J.). — Renal anomalies in fetal alcohol syndrome. *Pediatrics*, *63*, 886-889, 1979.

[144] QUAN (L.), SMITH (D. W.). — The Vater association. Vertebral defects, Anal atresia, T-E fistula with esophageal atresia, Radial and Renal dysplasia: a spectrum of associated defects. *J. Pediatr.*, *82*, 104-107, 1973.

[145] RANSLEY (P. G.), RISDOM (R. A.). — Reflux and renal scarring. *Brit. J. Radiol.*, suppl. *14*, 1-35, 1978.

[146] RECTOR (F. C.), COGAN (M. G.). — The renal acidoses. *Hospital Practice*, *4*, 99-111, 1980.

[147] REILLY (K. B.), RUBIN (S. P.), BLANKE (B. G.), YEH (M. N.). — Infantile polycystic kidney disease: a difficult antenatal diagnosis. *Amer. J. Obstet. Gynec.*, *133*, 580-582, 1979.

[148] RENKIN (E. M.), ROBINSON (R. R.). — Glomerular filtration. *New Engl. J. Med.*, *290*, 785-792, 1974.

[149] ROBILLARD (J. E.), SESSIONS (C.), BURMEISTER (L.), SMITH (F. G.). — Influence of fetal extracellular volume contraction on renal reabsorption of bicarbonate in fetal lambs. *Pediatr. Res.*, *11*, 649-655, 1977.

[150] ROBSON (A. M.). — Special diagnostic studies for the detection of renal and renovascular forms of hypertension. *Pediatr. Clin. North Am.*, *25*, 83-98, 1978.

[151] ROLLESTON (G. L.), MALING (T. M. J.), HODSON (C. J.). — Intrarenal reflux and the scarred kidney. *Arch. Dis. Childh.*, *49*, 531-539, 1974.

[152] ROSS (B. S.), POLLAK (A.), OH (W.). — The pharmacologic effects of furosemide therapy in the low-birth-weight infant. *J. Pediatr.*, *92*, 149-152, 1978.

[153] ROY (R. N.), SINCLAIR (J. C.). — Hydration of the low-birth-weight infant. *Clin. Perinatol.*, *2*, 393-417, 1975.

[154] ROY (R. N.), CHANCE (G. W.), RADDE (I. C.), HILL (D. E.), WILLIS (D. M.), SHEEPERS (J.). — Late hyponatremia in very low-birth-weight infants. *Pediat. Res.*, *10*, 526-531, 1976.

[155] RUDOLPH (A. M.), HEYMANN (M. A.). — The circulation of the fetus *in utero*. Methods for studying distribution of blood flow, cardiac output and organ blood flow. *Circulat. Res.*, *21*, 163-184, 1967.

[156] SALM (R.), VOYCE (M. A.). — Renal papillary necrosis in a neonate (with an hypothesis as to its aetiology). *Brit. J. Urol.*, *42*, 277-283, 1970.

[157] SANDERS (R. C.). — Renal ultrasound. *Radiol. Clin. North Am.*, *13*, 417-434, 1975.

[158] SAPIRSTEIN (L. A.), VIDT (D. G.), MANDEL (M. J.), HANUSEK (G.). — Volumes of distribution and clearances of intravenously injected creatinine in the dog. *Amer. J. Physiol.*, *181*, 330-336, 1955.

[159] SCHOEN (E. J.). — Renal diabetes insipidus. *Pediatrics*, *26*, 808-816, 1960.

[160] SCHRAGER (G. O.), JOSEPHSON (B. H.), FINE (B. F.), BERGER (G.). — Nephrogenic diabetes insipidus presenting as fever of unknown origin in the neonatal period. *Clin. Pediat.*, *15*, 1070-1072, 1976.

[161] SCHULZ (D. M.), GIORDANO (D. A.), SCHULZ (D. H.). — Weights of organs of fetuses and infants. *Arch. Path.*, *74*, 244-250, 1962.

[162] SERTEL (H.), SCOPES (J.). — Rates of creatinine clearance in babies less than one week of age. *Arch. Dis. Childh.*, *48*, 717-720, 1973.

[163] SHERRY (S. N.), KRAMER (I.). — The time of passage of the first stool and the first urine by the newborn infant. *J. Pediatr.*, *46*, 158-159, 1955.

[164] SHOKEIR (M. H. K.). — Expression of « adult » polycystic renal disease in the fetus and newborn. *Clin. Genet.*, *14*, 61-72, 1978.

[165] SIMILÄ (S.), VESA (L.), WASZ-HÖCKERT (O.). — Hereditary onycho-osteodysplasia (the Nail-Patella syndrome) with nephrosis-like renal disease in a newborn boy. *Pediatrics*, *46*, 61-65, 1970.

[166] SLOVIS (T. S.), PERLMUTTER (A. D.). — Recent advances in pediatric urological ultrasound. *J. Urol.*, *123*, 613-620, 1980.

[167] SMITH (D. W.). — The fetal alcohol syndrome. *Hospital Practice*, *10*, 121-128, 1979.

[168] SORIANO (J. R.). — The renal regulation of acid-base balance and the disturbances noted in renal tubular acidosis. *Pediatr. Clin. North Am.*, *18*, 529-545, 1971.

[169] SPITZER (A.). — Renal Physiology: impact of recent developments on clinical nephrology. *Pediatr. Clin. North Am.*, *18*, 377-393, 1971.

[170] STEIN (J. H.). — Hormones and the kidney. *Hospital Practice*, *7*, 91-105, 1979.

[171] STONESTREET (B. S.), OH (W.). — Plasma creatinine levels in low-birth-weight infants during the first three months of life. *Pediatrics*, *61*, 788-789, 1978.

[172] SULYOK (E.), NEMETH (M.), TENYI (I.), CSABA (I. F.), VARGA (F.), GYÖRY (E.), THURZO (V.). — Relationship between maturity, electrolyte balance and the function of the renin-angiotensin-aldosterone system in newborn infants. *Biol. Neonate*, *35*, 60-65, 1979.

[173] SULYOK (E.), VARGA (F.), GYÖRY (E.), JOBST (K.), CSABA (I. F.). — Postnatal development of renal sodium handling in premature infants. *J. Pediatr.*, *95*, 787-792, 1979.

[174] SULYOK (E.), ERTL (T.), CSABA (I. F.), VARGA (F.). — Postnatal changes in urinary prostaglandin E excretion in premature infants. *Biol. Neonat.*, *37*, 192-196, 1980.

[175] SVENNIGSEN (N. W.). — Single injection polyfructosan clearance in normal and asphyxiated neonates. *Acta Paediat. Scand.*, *64*, 87-95, 1975.

[176] SWIET DE (M.), FAYERS (P.), SHINEBOURNE (E. A.). — Systolic blood pressure in a population of infants in the first year of life: the Brompton study. *Pediatrics*, *65*, 1028-1035, 1980.

[177] TANNEN (R. L.). — Control of acid excretion by the kidney. *Annu. Rev. Med.*, *31*, 35-49, 1980.

[178] TENCHKOFF (H.). — Peritoneal dialysis today: a new look. *Nephron*, *12*, 420-436, 1974.

[179] TISHER (C. C.). — Functional anatomy of the kidney. *Hospital Practice*, *5*, 53-65, 1978.

[180] TORRADO (A.), GUIGNARD (J. P.), PROD'HOM (L. S.), GAUTIER (E.). — Hypoxaemia and renal function in newborns with respiratory distress syndrome (RDS). *Helv. Paediat. Acta*, *29*, 399-405, 1974.

[181] VERBERCKMOES (R.), VAN DAMME (B.), CLEMENT (J.), AMERY (A.), MICHIELSEN (P.). — Bartter's syndrome with hyperplasia of renomedullary cells: successfull treatment with indomethacin. *Kidney Int.*, *9*, 302-307, 1976.

[182] VIRNIG (N. L.), REYNOLDS (J. W.). — Reliability of flush blood pressure measurements in the sick newborn infant. *J. Pediatr.*, *84*, 594-598, 1974.

[183] WIGGELINKUIZEN (J.), NELSON (M. M.), BERGER (G. M. B.), KASCHULA (R. O. C.). — Alpha-fetoprotein in the antenatal diagnosis of the congenital nephrotic syndrome. *J. Pediatr.*, *89*, 452-455, 1976.

[184] WILLIAMS (P. R.), OH (W.). — Effects of radiant warmer on insensible water loss in newborn infants. *Amer. J. Dis. Child.*, *128*, 511-514, 1974.

[185] WINBERG (J.). — Determination of renal concentration capacity in infants and children without renal disease. *Acta Paediat. Scand.*, *48*, 318-328, 1959.

[186] WOO (W. C. R.), DUPONT (C.), COLLINGE (J.), ARANDA (J. V.). — Effects of furosemide in the newborn. *Clin. Pharmacol. Ther.*, *23*, 266-271, 1978.

[187] ZAMORA (J.), MARTINEZ (F.), MENDIZABAL (S.), SIMON (J.). — Diálisis peritoneal en el recien nacido. *An. Esp. Pediat.*, *13*, 477-486, 1980.

42

Urologic disorders of the newborn

J. PREVOT and M. SCHMITT

Neonatal urology is traditionally divided into two parts, including deformities obvious to external inspection and deformities of the inner urinary tract. We need to add those demonstrated at antenatal ultrasonography which raise new questions about diagnosis, management before birth and neonatal care.

External malformations are easily recognized by the physician; the neonatalogist and the pediatric urologist will have to answer the parent's request about the methods and the time of surgical correction.

Among the anomalies of the inner urinary tract, obstructive uropathy is the most important to take into account on two grounds:

— the newborn's kidney ability to grow is significant unless the development of the renal parenchyma is impeded;

— obstructive uropathy creates an excess of pressure and thus permanent lesions within the renal parenchyma especially if the urine is infected. Early relief of the cause of obstruction, before infection occurs, allows for renal growth.

Diagnosis is facilitated by antenatal ultrasonographic studies. The obstruction can be found at any level of the urinary tract. Lesions within the urethral tract have bilateral repercussions and induce renal failure.

Early, effective diversion of urine is the essential principle in the management of obstructive uropathy. If a primary radical surgical correction is impossible because of a too precarious state, one should obtain temporary drainage. Still catheter drainage runs a high risk of infection and urinary diversion without drainage renders delayed correction difficult.

DIAGNOSIS AND INVESTIGATION OF UROLOGICAL DISORDERS IN THE NEWBORN

Diagnosis

The diagnosis of malformations of the urinary tract in the newborn is based upon:

— physical and functional examination,
— general signs,
— special investigations, sometimes guided by in utero ultrasonography.

Physical and functional examination comes first. In every neonate, one must palpate the lumbar region; the supra-pubic region should be normal and supple. Free peritoneal ascites, marked by dullness on percussion and transmitting light at transillumination, almost always reflects obstructive uropathy.

In the male, the external parts must be carefully examined: the testes are easily felt because the cremasteric muscles are relaxed; the urethra, urinary meatus and foreskin should be inspected closely. In the female, the vulva should not be fused and there should not be any abnormal cystic structures.

In both, urination must be studied: 92 % of newborns micturate within 24 hours; 99 % by 48 hours. The character of the urine stream is noted, especially in boys. Total absence of micturition is of great importance, especially if occuring with drop by drop discharge at the urinary meatus.

General signs may go with malformations not obvious to external inspection but are not specific (growth retardation, diarrhoea, loss of appetite). Fever is not common. All these findings require close physical examination and further investigations.

Special investigations are justified whenever there are local abnormalities or a general disorder after a questionable ultrasonographic study performed before birth. Other indications include children with a congenital malformation or a prior diagnosed deformity, especially in the following cases:

— Other anomalies of the urogenital region except balanic hypospadias.
— Imperforate anus (especially high or supralevator lesions), vertebral and thoracic defects, œsophageal atresia which together form an association of congenital defects known by the acronym V. A. T. E. R.
— Cardiac malformations.
— The "Prune Belly syndrome".
— Hermaphroditism.
— Single umbilical artery (27 % associated renal deformities).
— Spina bifida (72 % of cases).
— Anomalies of the urinary tract may also occur in infants with ear malformations.

Special investigations

The neonate's kidney is immature, has a low urinary concentrating power and secretion can be affected by the disorder or malformation considered.

Hence, intravenous pyelography does not have the same benefit as in adults or older children.

Ultrasonography is the examination of choice. Even in renal failure, ultrasonographic imaging gives information about the presence and the shape of the kidney and the urinary tract. If a lumbar mass is felt on palpation, ultrasonography can determine the origin, limits and nature of the tumor: solid tumors can mimic either renal vein thrombosis, medullary renal necrosis or nephroblastoma; liquid tumors can correspond to polycystic kidneys or hydronephrosis, already diagnosed before birth.

The second most important investigation is voiding **cystography** performed through a suprapubic bladder puncture. This procedure can show evidence of vesicoureteral reflux and hence gives information about the state of the ureter and renal pelvis and calyces. Additionally, the condition and quality of the bladder are visualized and finally, the permeability and function of the urethra are demonstrated.

Intravenous pyelography gives further specific information when the infant has survived more than 72 hours, is not infected and has a steady metabolic balance.

Instrumental investigations require a qualified pediatric urologist. They include:

— endoscopic examination with miniaturized cold light equipment which permits ureteral catheterization,
— antegrade pyelography through a percutaneous needle puncture into the renal pelvis,
— the test devised by Whitaker which records the pressure in the urinary system and permits the documentation of outflow resistance.

Catheter arteriography through the umbilical artery is justified only if the diagnosis of a lumbar mass cannot be made by the above investigations. This procedure is easily performed and carries few complications.

Radionucleide renal imaging using 99m Tc DTPA and DMSA or hippurate are useful to document urinary obstruction in difficult cases.

Laboratory studies consist of urinalysis (sediment, erythrocyte and leukocyte count, Gram stain) of the urine obtained with a plastic collecting device removed after 3 hours. If the urine seems

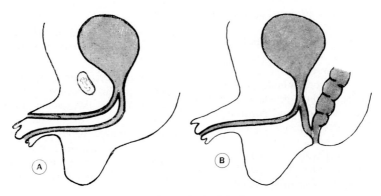

FIG. VII-14. — *Urethral duplication.*

A) Epispadial duplication.
B) Hypospadial duplication.

creating a dorsal penile curvature. Duplication is rarely complete, but can be functional if complete. Most often, the accessory urethra is blind, ending near the pubic bones; if not, it joins the normally positioned urethra behind the corpora cavernosa.

In hypospadial duplication, the superior urethra has a normally positioned meatus that is usually stenotic. Voiding occurs through the inferior urethra where the meatus opens into a perineal or anal position.

Epispadial duplication requires complete excision of the dorsal channel.

In hypospadial duplication, dilatation of the dorsal channel is unsuccessful. The patient has severe hypospadias and hence requires adequate surgical repair early in childhood; the dorsal channel may best be neglected. In the neonate, an intravenous pyelography demonstrates the quality of bladder voiding and the condition of the upper urinary tract. Associated abnormalities should be recognized.

Bifid penis or diphallia. — This malformation is characterized by a duplicated glans with two fused corporal bodies. Each glans has its urethra, but only one is functional. In minor forms, the glans is bilobular. Associated abnormalities are common, either urinary or extra-urinary.

These deformities require reconstruction around the age of 2 years.

Megalo-urethra. — Megalo-urethra is a flabby deformity of the penis expanding during micturition. Stephens (1963) describes 2 types:

— in the scaphoid type, the corpora cavernosa are present but elongated; excision of the redundant tissues is satisfactory, restoring normal function;

— in the fusiform type, there is an absence of both corpora cavernosa, and no solid tissue allowing reconstruction. The malformation is commonly associated with abdominal musculature deficiency (Prune Belly syndrome).

II. — HIDDEN ANOMALIES

Obstructive urethral valves

Valves are classified by Young into three types: those distally from the vera montanum (the most frequently encountered), those arising from the vera montanum, and the diaphragm. They are congenital and may be hypertrophic folds of the vera montanum.

Their disposition explains how and why they obstruct the urethra and why severe hydro-uretero-nephrosis often develops during intra-uterine life.

At birth, the lesions usually worsen because of an impaired urine stream and infection.

The most typical clinical feature is the absence of true spontaneous micturition. Urine is emitted drop by drop; the patient constantly wets himself. On palpation, the bladder is distended and sometimes, a fluctuating lumbar mass is found, on one or both sides.

The infant may present with urinary ascites. Prognosis is not necessarily bad, but diagnosis must be made quickly.

Ultrasonography is helpful; voiding cysto-urethrogram performed by supra-pubic puncture is diagnostic. The bladder appears thickened and there are more or less frank diverticula circling the bladder like a halo.

Hydro-uretero-nephrosis is present, mostly bilateral, but not necessarily symetrical.

If no vesico-ureteral reflux is demonstrated, intravenous urography is of importance; in that case the lesions are less severe.

The urethra is best seen on oblique view films showing dilatation of the proximal prostatic urethra, and a decreased stream in the distal perineal and balanic urethra. The valve appears as a sharply defined lucency.

Management involves nephrologic relief, antibiotic administration and bladder drainage through a promptly inserted supra-pubic tube. Renal function should be evaluated.

If upper urinary tract lesions are limited, especially if there is no vesico-ureteral reflux, the valves can be destroyed endoscopically either by fulguration or resection. In case of severe distension of the urinary tract, drainage of the obstruction by pyelostomy or ureterostomy for a prolonged period should be advocated. Prognosis of these patients depends on renal recovery and on vesical sphincter function.

Urethral diverticulum

Diverticula of the anterior urethra are small segmented dilatations, creating a valve mechanism with a distally normal urethra. They have the same effect as anterior urethral valves. Diagnosis is made by ultrasonography; management is carried out by endoscopic unroofing of the obstructive distal fold; followed by urethral catheter drainage. It is stressed that this approach should be done promptly as soon as the diagnosis is made.

Diverticula of the posterior urethra, are usually diverticula of the prostatic utricle. They may not present symptomatically at this age.

Congenital urethral polyps

They are attached to the urethra in the vicinity of the vera montanum; their degree of obstruction is variable. The diagnosis is suggested by cysto-urethrography and confirmed by endoscopy. Removal is necessary, either via endoscopy or open excision.

Urethral atresia

Urethral atresia is the most severe urethral malformation and is frequently associated with the Prune Belly syndrome. Renal dysplasia and patent urachus may also be found in this context.

Congenital fistula and imperforate anus

In boys with a high imperforate anus, the rectum opens into the posterior urethra through a recto-urethral fistula. Meconium discharge through the meatus is highly diagnostic. The catheter inserted into the urethra enters the rectum and drains no urine. As a consequence of the rectourethral fistula, urinary infection occurs. Complete temporary bowel diversion is the rule (Fig. VII-15).

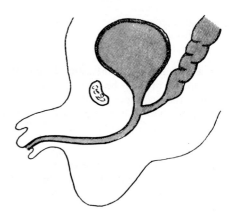

FIG. VII-15. — *Congenital fistula with anal atresia.*

ABNORMALITIES AND OBSTRUCTION OF THE URETHRA IN GIRLS

Some deformities found in boys, have the same clinical feature in girls, *i. e.* vesico-urethral duplication or urethral diverticula. But, there are also specific anomalies of the female urethra.

Urogenital sinus. — There is a single urogenital orifice due to the absence of development of the vesicovaginal wall. An inserted catheter usually ends up inside the bladder. This anomaly may be unique or associated with congenital adrenal hyperplasia.

Hypospadias and epispadias. — Also exist in the female. Their diagnosis is difficult, but they are rarely severe. In the neonate, they are usually asymptomatic.

Fused labia minora. — Are anecdotal rather than actually pathologic. The mucosa of the labia minora is fused closing the vulva except for a small anterior opening where urine discharges.

Despite its appearance, this anomaly is harmless. Easy unsticking with a probe requires no general anesthesia. This procedure should be performed as soon as possible in order to avoid urinary reflux into the vagina.

Cystic tumors. — At the vulva accounts for three disorders: paraurethral cysts, hydrocolpos and ureterocele:

— the paraurethral cyst, which is a rare disorder, should be drained and excised,

— hydrocolpos is a collection of whitish fluid developing because of imperforate hymen,

— ectopic insertion of an ureterocele is also possible.

In the latter, puncture of the cyst must be followed by injection of contrast material into the cavity to visualize its precise shape.

THE PRUNE BELLY SYNDROME

This condition is due to a mesenchymal developmental arrest. The syndrome combines a triad of lesions: cryptorchidism, urinary tract anomalies and absence of the abdominal musculature. The disease does not seem to be hereditary though it occurs essentially in boys. Girls are very rarely affected.

Before birth, the syndrome can be diagnosed by ultrasonography showing oligohydramnios, increase in the abdominal perimeter and urinary tract dilatation. At birth, the bulky abdomen is restricted to a flaccid abdominal wall formed of wrinkled skin and peritoneum. The movements of the bowel are easily seen and the dilated urinary tract is felt on palpation.

The extent of the malformation of the abdominal wall is variable. Prognosis depends on associated anomalies (cardiac deformities, malrotation of the gut) and on the kind of uropathy. In severe instances there is urinary tract dilatation with renal parenchymal dysplasia, creating fatal renal failure. In minor forms, there is dolichomegaureter with normal renal function.

Surgical intervention to create early urinary diversion is necessary if the urologic condition is debilitating. When possible, spontaneous evolution may lead to recession of the dilatation. If urologic conditions are satisfying, reconstruction of the abdominal wall is possible by plication or muscle transposition.

REFERENCES

General reading

BLACKWELL (B.), EVANS (M. D.). — Obstructive uropathy in the neonate. *Clinics in Perinatology, Vol 8, n° 2,* 273-286.
KELALIS (P. P.), KING (L. R.). — *Clinical pediatric urology.* Saunders, 1976.
RAVITCH (M. M.) et coll. — *Pediatric surgery.* 3e édition 1979. Year Book medical publishers, Chicago. Tome 2.
WILLIAMS (D. I.), JOHNSTON (J. H.). — *Pediatric urology,* second edition. Butterworths, 1982.
STEPHENS (F. D.). — *Congenital malformations of the rectum anus and genitourinary tracts.* Edited by R. Webster, Livingstone, Edinburgh, 1983.

Anomalies of the kidney

MARSHALL (F. F.), JEFF (R. D.), SMOLEV (J. K.). — Neonatal bilateral ureteropelvic junction obstruction. *J. Urol., 123,* 107-109, 1980.
PERLMUTTER (A. D.), KROOVAND (R. L.), WENLAI (Y.). — Management of ureteropelvic obstruction in the first year of life. *J. Urol., 123,* 535-537, 1980.
THOMPSON (D. P.), LYNN (M. B.). — Congenital anomalies associated with solitary kidney. *Mayo Clinic Proc., 41,* 538-548, 1966.

Anomalies of the ureter

BONDONNY (J. M.). — Les urétérocèles chez l'enfant : tentative de classification et de schéma thérapeutique. *Ann. Urol., 15,* 120-123, 1981.
WHITTAKER (R. M.). — Methods of assessing obstruction in dilated ureters. *Brit. Jrnl. Urol., 45,* 15-22, 1973.
GONZALES (J.). — Le développement du haut appareil urinaire du fœtus au cours du 3e trimestre de la grossesse. *Bull. Ass. Anat., 64,* 391-398, 1980.
HENDREN (W. H.). — Pathologie de la jonction urétérovésicale. *Chir. Pediatr., 20,* 229-299, 1979.
PRÉVOT (J.), SCHMITT (M.). — L'urétérocèle orthotopique simple du nourrisson. *Ann. Urol., 9,* 89-94, 1975.

Anomalies of the bladder

MOLLARD (P.), SARKISSIAN (J.), LORAS (O.). — Reconstruction vésicale pour exstrophie. *J. Urol. Nephrol., 87,* 199-207, 1981.
Symposium « Exstrophie vésicale ». *Ann. Chir. Inf., 12,* 359-483, 1971.

Anomalies of the urethra

CENDRON (J.), MELIN (Y.). — L'épispadias (108 cas). *Ann. Urol., 13,* 207-213, 1979.
KURTH (K. H.), ALLEMAN (E. R. J.), SCHRODER (E. H.). — Major and minor complications of posterior urethral valves. *J. Urol., 126,* 517-519, 1981.

MOLLARD (P.), SARKISSIAN (J.), TOSTAIN (J.). — Traitement des lésions du haut appareil en amont des valves de l'urètre postérieur. *Chir. Pediatr.*, *22*, 411-415, 1981.

Symposium « Hypospadias ». DUCKETT (J. W.) guest editor, In *Urol. Clin. North Am.*, *8*, 3, 371-591, 1981.

YOUNG (M. H.), McKAY (R. W.). — Congenital valvular obstruction of prostatic urethra. *Surg. Gyn. Obstet.*, *48*, 509-515, 1929.

The Prune Belly syndrome

RANDOLPH (J.), CAVETT (C.), ENG (Gloria). — Surgical correction and rehabilitation for children with « Prune Belly » syndrome. *Ann. Surg.*, *193*, 757-762, 1981.

8

Digestive
and surgical pathology

43

Intestinal adaptation, maturation and related disorders

Claude C. ROY

INTRODUCTION

The functional immaturity of the intestinal tract, liver and pancreas during the first few weeks of life has important clinical implications:

(*a*) The low birth weight infant is more vulnerable to malnutrition with its adverse short-term and long-term repercussions on growth and development because of the following factors:

— LBW infants have greater caloric needs in relationship to their surface area and a very high rate of protein synthesis and turnover.

— The extent of possible dietary manipulations is limited by metabolic and neurologic immaturity.

— Fecal sequestration of ingested nutrients is more extensive than in the full term infant and is compounded by a restricted gastric capacity and the frequent occurrence of gastro-esophageal reflux.

(*b*) As a result of congenital structural defects requiring surgery, the immature remaining bowel must adapt and compensate for the smaller surface area of the absorptive apparatus.

This work was supported in part by the Medical Research Council of Canada and the Canadian Cystic Fibrosis Foundation.

(*c*) The immature gastrointestinal tract of the neonate is uniquely sensitive to a certain number of enteric disorders with a high morbidity and sometimes life-threatening consequences.

This chapter provides an overview of the biochemical physiologic and ontogenic determinants in neonatal gastrointestinal development. In-depth coverage of these various aspects can be found in recent reviews [41, 67, 74]. It attracts attention to the functional limitations which should be recognized for the optimal nutritional management of the newborn. Finally, some perinatal disorders either related to feeding or with serious repercussions on nutrition will be discussed.

MATURATION OF DIGESTIVE AND ABSORPTIVE FUNCTION

Only a modest number of studies are available, comparing the digestibility and absorption of macro- and micronutrients to the functional development of the liver, the pancreas, the stomach and the intestinal tract in the neonate. This section attempts to correlate the development of gastrointestinal function [41] with the capacity to digest and absorb carbohydrates, proteins and fats in the hope of providing a physiological background for current feeding regimens and practices.

I. — CARBOHYDRATE DIGESTION AND ABSORPTION

Carbohydrates account for 1/3 to 1/2 of the total energy ingested by breast-fed or formula-fed neonates. Although a premature infant's brain represents only 12 % of body weight, it may account for more than 50 % of basal energy expenditures [52].

Intraluminal and mucosal hydrolysis of polysaccharides.

— Carbohydrates in breast milk and in formulas, mainly lactose, sucrose and glucose polymers (maltodextrins) are essentially unaltered when they reach the small intestine. However, native and modified starches found as stabilizers in infant formulas and in most baby foods must be attacked by alpha-amylases from salivary and pancreatic secretions and/or by gluco-amylase of the brush border [75] (Fig. VIII-1). Both salivary and pancreatic amylase are detectable early during the second half of gestation. Salivary amylase is abundant in the neonate but is rapidly inactivated by gastric HCl and pepsin while pancreatic amylase is essentially absent in fasting duodenal juice [146, 46] and fails to respond to pancreozymin-secretin stimulation during the first 3 months of life [46]. Amylase activity found in the duodenal juice of newborns appears to be of salivary origin [91]. The role of brush border glucoamylase which breaks down alpha-1,4 linkages between glucose molecules has not been established in the overall digestion of starch. It hydrolyzes amylose (α-1,4, linked glucose units) more rapidly than amylopectin which is made up of both α-1,4 and α-1,6 linked glucose molecules (Fig. VIII-1) but exerts its optimal hydrolytic activity on oligo-saccharides of 5 to 9 glucose units. Glucoamylase activity in one month old infants is comparable to that observed in older children [72].

Starch intolerance.

— That starch digestibility is limited in neonates was demonstrated by a slow and small increase of blood glucose in response to the gastric administration of a starch solution as compared to an equicaloric amount of glucose [54]. Up to 6 months of age, the hydrolysis of amylo-pectin is incomplete and dextrins are found in large amounts in the jejunum [6]. Severe diarrhea can

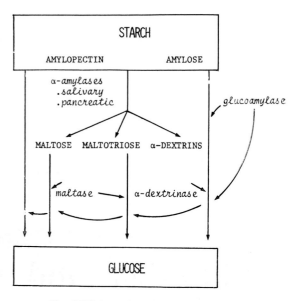

FIG. VIII-1. — *Overall hydrolysis of starch.*

The narrow line and arrow between amylopectin and glucose indicates that glucoamylase is less active against that substrate than against amylose, the other constituent of starch. Modified after LEE P.C. et al. [75].

result if starch is fed as a 6 % solution (40 g/day) in a one month old [25]. Although not a clinical problem of recognized significance, limitations in the capacity of newborns and young infants to digest starch have been found. Iatrogenic diarrhea can be caused by large amounts of cereals offered to neonates in a "thickened feeding" regimen to reduce gastroesophageal reflux. A recent study [72] shows that glucoamylase activity decreases with increasing severity of villus atrophy. However, the degree of depression tends to parallel maltase activity rather than the more severe decreases in lactase, sucrase and alpha-dextrinase. Thus, a relative degree of starch intolerance may be seen in three circumstances:

— Normal developmental delay in pancreatic alpha-amylase.
— Diseases associated with severe mucosal damage.
— Infants with sucrase-isomaltase deficiency.

Mucosal hydrolysis of disaccharides.

— A study of the intrauterine development of disaccharidases in fetal intestinal mucosa shows that sucrase, maltase and alpha-dextrinase are already present at 10 weeks of gestation [4]. By the 32nd week of gestation, these enzymes have 70 % of the activity found in the full term newborn while lactase represents only about 30 % of that found in term babies [3]. In contrast to sucrase, maltase and alpha-dextrinase, lactase is a non-adaptable enzyme. It cannot be induced by feeding its substrate [37].

Disaccharide intolerance. — Disacchari-

dase activity is higher in the jejunum and proximal ileum than in the duodenum and distal ileum and is dependent on the presence of mature, well differentiated epithelial cells [42]. Epithelial cells in the crypts are immature and do not have a microvillous structure. As they migrate up the villus they acquire the machinery for the hydrolysis and transport of carbohydrates. Findings associated with disaccharide intolerance have been well described [78] and occur in the following circumstances:

(a) Feeding of excessively large amounts of disaccharides, i. e., lactose > 10 g/dl.

(b) Intestinal hurry or shortening of the small bowel preventing the adequate exposure of disaccharides to the brush border enzymes.

(c) Disorders associated with brush border damage usually lead to lactose intolerance because lactase is present in concentrations lower than the other disaccharidases. Several months may be seen between histologic repair and the return of normal lactase activity.

(d) Congenital disaccharidase deficiencies need to be considered in the differential diagnosis of diarrhea in the newborn. Congenital lactase deficiency is a rarity while sucrase-isomaltase deficiency is much more common. Administration of formulas containing sucrose and glucose polymers leads to onset of symptoms shortly after birth.

Temporary lactose malabsorption has been well identified in neonates, especially in prematures but generally does not lead to problems unless lactose concentration exceeds 10 g/dl. However, lactose breath tests are positive in most prematures up to 50 days of age and studies suggest that two thirds of ingested lactose may reach the colon [83]. Although reducing substances can be found in the stools in up to 50 % of formula-fed and breast-fed neonates, the concentration rarely exceeds 0.5 % when tested by Clinitest tablets. A recent study in prematures found no difference in the fecal excretion of carbohydrate-derived energy in response to two formulas containing either 100 % lactose or 50 % lactose and 50 % glucose polymers as its carbohydrate source [63].

Absorption of monosaccharides. —

Active transport of glucose and galactose occurs as early as 10 weeks of gestation and increases only in the jejunum during the following 8 weeks creating the jejunoileal transport difference observed after birth [8]. However, the rate of glucose absorption from the perfused jejunum of young infants is much lower than in adults. The rate of glucose transport does not go beyond 4.5 g/hour whereas in adults it is 30 g/hour (Fig. VIII-2). This difference cannot be accounted for by the surface area of the absorptive apparatus since the Km (the affinity of glucose for its carrier) is three times lower than in adults [144]. In vitro work suggests that glucose is absorbed more rapidly if it is administered as a disaccharide or as an oligosaccharide. Recent studies provide evidence that brush border oligosaccharidase and disaccharidase enzymes are topographically located so that they can bind disaccharides and efficiently deliver their products of hydrolysis to the monosaccharide transport system of the cell [42]. Replacing lactose in a formula with an osmolality of 290-300 mOsm/kg increases the osmotic load by 200 mOsm/kg. Each gram of glucose/100 ml of formula augments the osmolality of the formula by 58 mOsm/kg [15]. As young infants have been shown to be very sensitive to hyperosmolar formulas in terms of fluid shifts [90], the replacement of 50 % of lactose by glucose polymers, a mixture of medium-chain length glucose polymers with minimal branching (1,6 glucose linkages) represents an advance in the design of formulas designed for LBW infants. These glucose polymers require neither α-amylase nor lactase, most of the molecular bonds are 1,4 glucose linkages.

Malabsorption of monosaccharides. —

Primary monosaccharide malabsorption is a rare disorder characterized by the absence of the carrier-mediated transport system for glucose and galactose [30]. The acquired type is frequent and is secondary to a number of conditions:

— Infectious gastroenteritis (rotavirus particularly).
— Necrotizing enterocolitis.
— Intractable diarrhea of early infancy.
— Neonatal surgery of the G. I. tract.
— Contaminated small bowel syndrome.

The pathogenesis is sometimes obscure. Microbial proliferation leading to the presence of large amounts of free bile acids known to interfere with intestinal transport of monosaccharides is often implicated [39]. In most cases with intractable diarrhea of early infancy, the inability to absorb monosaccharides is caused by a severe decrease in effective absorptive surface. A recent report has

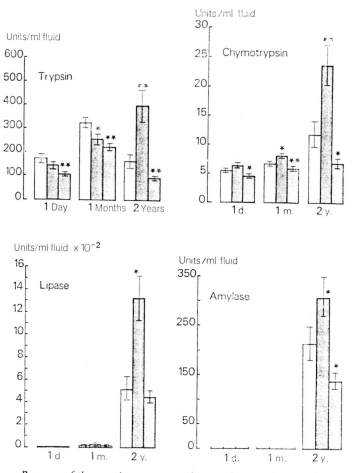

Fig. VIII-2. — *Response of the exocrine pancreas to hormonal stimulation as a function of age.*
Open bars correspond to basal values, full bars to enzyme activities following cholecystokinin-pancreozymin and hatched
  bars to activities after secretin.
Asterisk: $p < .05$.   Double asterisk: $p < .005$.
(Modified from LEBENTHAL E. and LEE P. C., *Pediatrics*, 66, 556-560, 1980).

shown that the surface area can be reduced to as little as 10 % of normal during the acute stage of the disease [65].

II. — PROTEIN DIGESTION AND ABSORPTION

In the period of life during which anabolic activity is at its highest level, providing the proper amount of high biologic value proteins is critical for the synthesis and accretion of proteins. Determination of the protein needs of preterm infants is being studied intensely through the use of several methods which all have their limitations. To determine protein requirements in adults, graded amounts of a high quality protein source are fed along with an adequate energy intake. The linear relationship between protein intake and nitrogen retention flattens out as one reaches the optimal protein intake [108]. However, this occurs only at protein intakes of 9 g/kg/day in neonates [123], who are known to develop abnormal amino acid patterns under regimens providing half of that amount of protein [35].

The metabolic and neurological immaturity of the neonate needs to be taken into account in the determination of the optimal source and form of protein which should be fed to LBW infants. To optimize nitrogen retention, energy needs need to be met by appropriate carbohydrate and lipid intakes. A high energy intake enhances amino acid re-utilization for protein synthesis. Attention to protein quality also has benefit in terms of nitrogen retention since it reduces protein breakdown[94].

Gastric proteolysis. — As with HCl, there is a transient high production of pepsin during the first few days of life with a return to low levels before a steady but slow increase over a period of several months. Studies in neonates have shown that 3 to 4 hours after a feeding of cow milk or breast milk, the proteins are still not hydrolyzed in the stomach [85, 44]. The explanation for failure of peptic digestion in the stomach is that gastric pH never falls to the low levels necessary for peptic hydrolysis to take place.

Pancreatic proteolytic enzymes. — Secreted as inactive precursors, they are activated in the duodenum by the activation of trypsinogen by the duodenal peptidase, enterokinase. This enzyme is found in the duodenal mucosa by 26 weeks of gestation [3]. The endopeptidases trypsin and chymotrypsin are found earlier (17 weeks) in human fetuses than lipase which is present only at 34 weeks while amylase is essentially absent [74]. Proteolytic activity is detectable in the meconium of fetuses as small as 500 g [77]. This may explain why even small prematures generally do well on a whole protein such as that which is provided by human milk or a milk base formula. Postnatally substantial concentrations of trypsin and chymotrypsin are found in the fasting state as opposed to the essential absence of lipase and amylase. An interesting observation is that there is no response to cholecystokinin (CCK-PZ) during the first month of life (Fig. VIII-2). Diet modifies the developmental pattern of pancreatic enzymes. Feeding premature infants a high starch diet for 30 days results in the appearance of a low level of amylase activity whereas feeding a high protein diet leads to higher trypsinogen and lipase concentrations. Surprisingly a high fat diet does not lead to a change in exocrine pancreatic enzymes [146]. The source of protein was shown to influence pancreatic function when prematures fed a soy base formula showed a greater trypsin and lipase concentration in response to CCK-PZ and secretin than those fed a cow milk base formula [73].

Brush border and cytoplasmic peptidases. — Dietary and endogenous proteins are hydrolyzed in the intestinal lumen into large amounts of small peptides and relatively small quantities of free amino acids transported by an active sodium-dependent process similar to the one described for glucose. Peptides undergo further hydrolysis by brush border peptidases or else are taken up as di- and tripeptides by enterocytes in which specific intracellular peptidases are responsible for their final breakdown into amino acids.

Although peptidase activity is found in fetuses as young as 8 weeks after conception and has been shown to be present in the jejunum, ileum and colon, the results of a number of studies recently compiled are difficult to interpret. Their relevance to the ability of the small intestine to deal with peptides in its lumen or to hydrolyse absorbed peptides remains to be determined [67]. It has been estimated that the bulk of di- and tripeptidase activity is due to cytoplasmic enzymes which hydrolyse dipeptides and tripeptides which have entered the enterocyte through a transport system of broad specificity [5]. Of interest however, is the observation that small peptides made up of either dicarboxylic amino acids (glutamic acid and aspartic acid) or amino acids (proline, hydroxyproline and glycine) undergo little hydrolysis at the brush border and are preferentially taken up as peptides [115]. This is of interest in view of the observations that these two classes of amino acids have a much slower rate of absorption in the perfused human jejunum than branched-chain amino acids (leucine, isoleucine and valine) [112].

As pointed out above, brush border hydrolysis of di- and tripeptides is relatively modest relative to the hydrolysis which takes place in the cytosol. However, brush border peptidases are able to hydrolyze oligopeptides and even polypeptides such as the B-chain of insulin [5]. In conditions where there is brush border damage or shortening of the small intestine leading to a reduced absorptive surface area, experimental work suggests that administration of peptides has significant advantages over a mixture of amino acids. Furthermore, a recent study showing differences in the absorption of two different protein hydrolysates confirms the presence of specific peptide-transport systems for dipeptides and tripeptides [31].

III. — FAT DIGESTION AND ABSORPTION

At birth, the newborn has to adjust to a rapid transition from his or her high in utero carbohydrate diet to the high fat (40 % to 50 % of total calories) diet of human milk and formulas. Not only is fat the major source of energy in the diet of the small infant but it is also the vehicle for fat-soluble vitamins. In addition, several fatty acids are constituents of membranes and of brain structural lipids. Linoleic acid cannot be synthesized de novo. It is essential for normal growth and for the synthesis of prostaglandins, ubiquitous 20-carbon unsaturated fatty acids with widespread, diversified and essential roles in most organ systems [34].

Compared to adults, the digestion and absorption of fat are relatively inefficient in newborns and more so in prematures [67]. Only the normal full term neonate on breast milk can achieve a normal ($\geqslant 95$ %) coefficient of fat absorption. In the LBW neonate, figures of 75 % to 85 % obtained on human milk drop to between 45 % and 60 % when cow's milk is given. Substituting vegetable oils for butterfat leads to a significant improvement. Formula fed LBW's usually absorb 70 % to 85 % of ingested fat. Further improvement is noted when 40 % to 50 % of dietary triglycerides are medium chain triglycerides (MCT). Complete correction ($\geqslant 95$ %) has been noted when 80 % of the lipid source is MCT [103]. However, problems with GI tolerance and worry about an insufficient intake of linoleic acid has disqualified such a formula for prematures.

The digestive phase defect. —

Fat digestion is a prerequisite for its subsequent absorption. It involves chemical events taking place in the stomach (hydrolysis of ingested fat by lingual lipase) and duodenum (hydrolysis of dietary fat and biliary phospholipids by the pancreatic lipase-colipase system and by phospholipase A_2). This is followed by physical events leading to the micellar dispersion of lipolytic products by bile acids. Some insoluble lipids such as cholesterol are not altered chemically during digestion but micellar solubilization is required for their absorption. In contrast, lipids such as medium chain triglycerides require only chemical hydrolysis as the digestive products are water-soluble.

Gastric and lingual lipase. —

Fat digestion is initiated in the stomach by a gastric [76] and a lingual lipase [50] active at the acid pH of the stomach. The end-products of this lipolysis mainly di- and monoglycerides are thought to be essential to maintain fat droplets in an emulsion which will then allow the next step to take place namely, hydrolysis by pancreatic lipase. Animal and clinical studies suggest that lingual and gastric lipases are of physiological importance in situations such as the newborn period where lipolytic mechanisms are stressed by a high fat intake and a low pancreatic lipase activity [49].

Pancreatic lipase. —

Duodenal fluid contains inadequate amounts of pancreatic lipase [146, 73] and there is no response to CCK-PZ during the first months of life [73]. A large percentage of fat in the feces of newborn infants is in the neutral lipid fraction with triglycerides representing a significant proportion [133]. This confirms the presence of a lipolytic phase defect.

Bile acids. —

Duodenal concentrations of bile acids are low in neonates particularly in LBW infants, and increase with age. In preterm babies weighing less than 1,300 g, concentrations of bile acids after a feeding are generally below the one required to solubilize the products of lipolysis [62]. This deficiency of bile salts correlates well with the degree of steatorrhea [111]. A reduction of the pool size of bile acids and an increase in fecal loss account for the low intraluminal concentrations. The size of the cholate pool corrected for surface area in full-term and premature newborns corresponds to 48 % and 22 % of adult values respectively [134]. On an 80 % MCT formula, the fecal loss of bile acids was decreased by more than 40 % as the % of fat absorption increased from 78 % to 95 % [103]. An in vitro study has shown the absence of an ileal mechanism for the active transport of taurocholate in fetuses and neonates [23]. There is also a possibility that a significant proportion of intraluminal bile acids could be reabsorbed passively in the jejunum. This untimely (too early) reabsorption documented in young animals could further compromise the micellar phase of fat digestion [9].

The absorptive phase. —

In discussing fat uptake from the lumen, five individual steps need to be recognized (Fig. VIII-3).

Diffusion through the unstirred water layer. —

In any situation in which a biological membrane or cell surface is immersed in a solution there exist concentric layers of water extending out from the aqueous lipid interface. Since the effective surface area of the unstirred water layer in the small bowel is small in relationship with the greater surface area of the underlying villi and microvilli, the unstirred water layer constitutes an important diffusion barrier. In fact, the diffusional resistance of the unstirred water layer to absorption is greater than that of the protein lipid membrane because of the poor aqueous diffusibility of lipolytic products [114]. The major physiological function of the bile acid micelle is to overcome unstirred water layer resistance [135]. Fatty acids of medium chain length (MCFA) are absorbed nearly as well in the absence

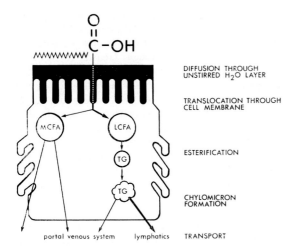

DIFFUSION THROUGH
UNSTIRRED H₂O LAYER

TRANSLOCATION THROUGH
CELL MEMBRANE

ESTERIFICATION

CHYLOMICRON
FORMATION

TRANSPORT

FIG. VIII-3. — Uptake of long-chain (LCFA) and medium-chain fatty acids (MCFA). Five well-individualized steps are recognized for LCFA. The two intracellular events esterification and chylomicron formation are bypassed by MCFA. After extrusion from the enterocyte LCFA are transported mainly through the lymphatics, whereas that of MCFA occurs through the portal venous system. (From ROY, C. C.: *In* LEBENTHAL, E., editor: Textbook of gastroenterology and nutrition in infancy, New York, 1981, Raven Press).

as in the presence of bile acid micelles. As the chain length is increased the fatty acids (LCFA) become progressively more dependent upon the presence of bile acid micelles. In the case of a very hydrophobic compound such as cholesterol, no absorption occurs in the absence of bile acids.

The thickness of the unstirred water layer has not been measured in neonates. In any case diffusion through this layer is handicapped because of the low concentrations of bile acids available for the formation of micelles.

Translocation through the cell membrane. — Penetration of lipid molecules does not occur through aqueous channels but by diffusion through the structured protein-lipid membrane as monomers. Micellar aggregates break up at the surface, the component molecules partition between the unstirred aqueous layer and the cell membrane and then diffusion takes place. There is evidence that a protein in the cytosol of the enterocyte may facilitate the transport of fatty acids to the endoplasmic reticulum and thereby reduce the resistance to translocation [92]. Of interest is the observation that a diet high in unsaturated fat increases the fatty acid binding protein (FABP) in the distal small bowel which constitutes a reserve area for absorption in

situations such as in the newborn period during which fat intake is considerable and the digestive phase is impaired. Values following MCT feeding suggest that FABP is not involved in the transport of MCFA in the cell cytosol.

Esterification. — Fatty acids and monoglycerides are largely resynthesized to triglycerides after having been taken up by the enterocytes. Activation of fatty acids by the microsomal fatty acid CoA lipase is an essential step prior to esterification. The levels of both activating and esterification enzymes are higher in the jejunum than in the ileum. Jejunal and ileal esterification respectively reach their peak during weaning and adulthood. Luminal contents (oral intake and pancreaticobiliary secretions) appear to be important in the development and maintenance of intestinal fatty acid esterification. Although it is difficult to extrapolate animal data to humans, the information currently available suggests that fatty acid activation and esterification does not appear to be a limiting step in the process of fat absorption, even in unfavorable situations such as the newborn period [53].

Chylomicron formation. — The intracellular event which follows the resynthesis of triglycerides is the formation of intestinal chylomicrons. The bulk of dietary lipids (triglycerides and cholesterol) are transported as chylomicrons. Very low density lipoproteins (VLDL) are also formed post-prandially but play only a minor role. In the fasting state, VLDL predominate and are responsible for the transport of endogenous lipids (intestinal and biliary). Nascent high density lipoproteins (N-HDL) are also synthesized by the intestine. They mainly transport cholesterol but also LCFA and in contrast to chylomicrons and VLDL, they are released not only in lymph but also in the portal venous system.

There are still few studies on the efficiency of chylomicron formation in the newborn period. Chylomicrons are not observed post-prandially during the first week of life. Of interest is the fact that gestational age does not seem to influence the appearance of chylomicrons, nor their size or number. These data do not necessarily suggest that poor formation of chylomicrons may be a limiting step in the overall scheme of fat uptake by the enterocyte. It is possible that a high turnover rate of absorbed lipids could explain these results [67]. In circumstances where the absorptive capacity of the small bowel is challenged by large fat loads, the distal segments have been shown to accumulate more fat than the proximal segments. This has been attributed to the limited capacity of the ileum for chylomicron synthesis or secretion [143]. Since the lower bowel is called upon as a reserve area for absorption in the newborn period when the fat load is considerable in the face of a digestive phase defect, it is possible that a limited ability to synthesize chylomicrons could contribute to fat malabsorption.

Transport in the lymphatics or in the portal venous system. — The final step in the uptake of fat from the lumen is its transport within the cell and its exocytosis. Although the bulk of LCFA are exported in the lymphatics, a certain % is transported in the portal venous system (Fig. VIII-3). They can be bound to albumin and enter the systemic circulation as monomers or else enter into the formation of nascent HDL [121]. The proportion of LCFA transported in the portal vein varies with the amount of fat presented to the absorptive apparatus and the solubility of the perfused fatty acids [82]. The importance of this finding in the context of the better coefficient of fat absorption associated with unsaturated LCFA feeding of infants remains unknown. MCFA absorption in lymph is negligible and occurs almost entirely in the portal vein in their nonesterified form bound to albumin.

NUTRITIONAL MANAGEMENT

The preceding section has provided some physiological background helpful for the design and development of optimal nutritional management programs. However, much of the data available on nutrient needs, tolerance and long term effects is fragile or incomplete [101]. Moreover, as recently pointed out, definition of optimal post-natal growth has not been clearly established. Long term goals for growth of low birth weight infants need to be defined with the understanding that a compromise may be necessary between the ideal and what is functionally and maturationally attainable [116].

The following will examine benefits and hazards of current feeding practices in terms of macronutrient composition and concentration as well as in terms of present methods of alimentation. The role and the place of parenteral nutrition will not be discussed as it is beyond the framework of this chapter.

Macronutrient composition and concentration

Carbohydrates. — Natural milks, human or bovine, contain lactose. In attempts to either increase caloric content or to improve tolerance and digestibility formulas have been designed by substituting or adding glucose, fructose or more recently, glucose polymers. Although lactose levels only reach mature levels close to term, no significant differences in the utilization of maltose, sucrose and lactose were demonstrated in 2 weeks old LBW infants [58]. LBW formulas in which 50 % of lactose is replaced by glucose polymers have a theoretical advantage. A greater caloric density can be fed without the increase in osmolality inherent to the use of disaccharides. However, a recent study has shown that the fetal sequestration of carbohydrate-derived energy does not differ from that of an isocaloric formula containing 100 % lactose [63]. Furthermore, studies have yet to confirm that small bowel water and electrolyte homeostasis is favored.

Proteins. — Protein synthesis is the key process in the production of all new cell structures and for this, an optimal availability of aminoacids is required. If a mixture of aminoacids is of inferior biologic value, the aminoacids which are lowest in concentration in proportion to their requirement will control the rate of synthesis for the proteins coded to contain these aminoacids. Protein quality is therefore critical but to a certain extent it can be made up by quantity. However, protein overloading of the premature who is biochemically immature may cause metabolic imbalances and undue stresses which may have deleterious effects on brain development and later intellectual performance [35].

Milk base formulas with a whey/casein ratio of 18/82 at a daily intake of 3.0 g/kg lead to abnormal aminoacid patterns as well as to a certain degree of azotemia and hyperammonemia which is much more discrete in low birthweight infants fed a whey predominant (whey/casein: 60/40) formula [98]. Nutritional benefits of whey predominant formulas have been reported in terms of % nitrogen absorption [136]. Our own data also shows a greater nitrogen retention whether expressed as mg/kg/day or as mg/kg/kcal. A further argument aga250st the use of casein predominant formulas can be mounted from the recent epidemiological survey suggesting that the presence of casein as the predominant protein seems to be related to the formation of lactobezoars which have been reported with increasing frequency over the past few years [106].

In view of the poor response of pancreatic proteolytic enzymes to stimulation during the first few months of life, it would be expected that hydrolysed proteins would be advantageous. A casein hydrolysate formula improves % nitrogen absorption but does not enhance nitrogen retention. Although soybean isolate formulas are satisfactory in terms of nitrogen balance, they are contraindicated in LBW infants. Hypophosphatemia from lowered phosphorus absorption may lead to phosphorus deficiency rickets [109].

The optimal protein intake for the LBW infant has not been precisely defined even though a number of studies have been carried out relating protein intake to weight gain and growth [122] to nitrogen balance studies [95] and to protein accretion rates of the "reference fetus" [145]. Current recommendations of the American Academy of Pediatrics for protein intake in LBW infants are 2.25 to 5.0 g/kg/day. In view of the close interrelation between protein metabolism and energy needs, an adequate energy intake of 110 to 150 kcal/kg/day is essential. The concentration of proteins in mature milk cannot meet the needs of the LBW neonate. However, milk produced during the first 4 to 6 weeks post-partum by mothers who have delivered preterm infants contains substantially higher concentrations of protein, fat and energy [2]. A recent study has shown that feeding with either milk from mothers of preterm infants or a whey base formula is more appropriate for growth than feeding with pooled milk from mothers of term infants [45].

Lipids. — As alluded to previously, fat provides about half of the calories in human milk and in formulas. The source of fat in formulas is vegetable oil. Although more soluble than animal fat and requiring lower concentrations of bile salts to form micelles, the unsaturated fatty acids of vegetable oil are somewhat less efficiently absorbed than those of human milk. This has to do with the structure of breast milk triglycerides, wherein a large proportion of the less-soluble saturated fatty, palmitic acid, is in the 2-position of the glycerol molecule rendering it more soluble as a monoglyceride than as a free fatty acid and therefore more completely absorbed after lipolysis [32]. A further advantage of breast milk is that it contains bile-salt stimulated lipase [51]. In addition, it is known that human milk triglycerides are very vulnerable to gastric lipolysis affected to some extent by gastric lipase but more extensively by swallowed lingual lipase [59].

Medium chain triglycerides (MCT) are well absorbed since they are easily hydrolyzed and MCFA do not need to form micelles since they are water soluble. There is no evidence that they facilitate the absorption of long chain fatty acids (LCFA). Most studies tend to show that at a concentration of 40 % to 50 % of total lipids, they tend to improve fat absorption but this has not been confirmed by others [102]. An important observation on the role

of MCT is that their use is associated with a greater absorption of calcium in preterm infants [105].

In summary, there is evidence that preterm breast milk meets most of the nutrient needs of the LBW infant and is the source of nutrients which is most consonant with its gastrointestinal and metabolic immaturity. There are still conflicting views as to the appropriate composition of formulas for LBW neonates. There is evidence that they have distinct advantages and can promote retention rates of nutrients comparable to fetal accretion rates [110]. However, indirect calorimetry studies do not confirm this and suggest that the accretion rate of fat is much greater and that of protein is smaller than what occurs in utero and in human milk fed neonates [21].

Methods of alimentation

Nutritional depletion and support has become an important aspect of the care of the critically ill newborn. Much of the success in the increased survival rate for very LBW infants comes from a more organized and intensive approach to nutrition. Various methods are available for the delivery of nutrients, each with specific indications or associated problems. These can be summarized as follows:

(a) Parenteral

— Central vein catheter,
— Peripheral vein.

(b) Enteral by bolus or on a continuous basis

— Oral
— Intragastric,
— Duodenal or jejunal.

Parenteral nutrition is beyond the framework of this chapter and will not be discussed. Oral or nipple feeding is indicated for neurologically intact infants without significant anomalies. This route is generally not possible for preterms of less than 32 to 34 weeks gestation. In the case of smaller neonates, a combination of intragastric and oral routes is necessary to insure that by the first week, at least 110 kcal/kg are fed. The keystone for feeding ill or very LBW infants is tube feeding.

A large study [137] comparing nasojejunal (NJ) to nasogastric (NG) feeding in LBW infants has shown a mean incremental weight velocity which was significantly less on NJ feeding than on NG. Trans-pyloric feeding has been claimed to result in better growth owing to the tolerance for more calories and a reduction in the incidence of pulmonary aspiration [130]. However, another group documented a significantly greater fecal wastage of calories on NJ than on NG feedings and correspondingly a faster weight gain [104]. Finally, a more recent study failed to show an advantage of NJ over NG feeding [26].

Delivery of formula or human milk into the duodenum or upper jejunum bypasses a certain % of the absorptive surface but more importantly, it short circuits digestive processes initiated in the stomach (gastric and lingual lipase) and duodenum (bile-salt stimulated lipase of human milk). Furthermore, some complications need to be contended with namely, tube dislodgement, abdominal distension, ileus and intestinal perforation [96].

For these reasons, it is advocated that NJ feedings be reserved for exceptional circumstances where the risk of aspiration is particularly great.

Bolus feeding appears to have theoretical advantages over continuous feeding. Bolus gastric feeding of newborn infants has been shown to induce secretion of enteric hormones [81] which have local and possibly trophic effects on the bowel. It has also been postulated that continuous infusion of milk or formula might influence the acquisition of the enterohormonal responses to feeding and affect functional intestinal maturation. However, two studies have failed to elicit differences in blood levels of fat or carbohydrate metabolites, insulin and enteroglucagon between bolus and continuous gastric feeding [80] or between continuous gastric and jejunal feeding [86]. Disadvantages of bolus feeding include delayed gastric emptying secondary to volume and osmolality, risk of aspiration, bradycardia and impaired ventilation [93].

DISORDERS AND DISEASE ENTITIES

The following section briefly discusses some of the more frequent and challenging gastrointestinal problems developing in the newborn period.

I. — THE SHORT-BOWEL SYNDROME

The short bowel syndrome is the result of alterations of gastrointestinal motility, secretion, digestion, and absorption that occur after extensive small bowel resection [69]. The most common clinical conditions that require the removal of significant lengths of the small intestine occur in the neonatal period.

Short bowel syndrome in neonates:

— Intestinal malrotation with volvulus and bands.
— Jejunoileal atresias.
— Meconium ileus.
— Omphalocele and gastroschisis with volvulus.
— Duplications and other abdominal tumors.
— Internal hernias.
— Congenitally short small bowel.

Differences
between the jejunum and ileum

A brief recall of the structural and functional differences between the jejunum and ileum is essential to understand the physiopathology of the short bowel syndrome.

Anatomic differences. — The small intestine of the neonate measures about 250 cm. There is no specific anatomic structure that marks the end of the jejunum and the beginning of the ileum. The proximal two fifths is the jejunum, and the rest is the ileum. However, the structural and functional differences between the two are important and significantly modify the severity, treatment, and prognosis of the short bowel syndrome. The diameter of the proximal jejunum is twice that of the distal ileum; its surface area is greatly increased by the circular folds (plicae circulares), which are sparser and smaller in the ileum. These folds are covered by mucosa that, throughout the small intestine, is composed of villi, crypts, lamina propria, and muscularis mucosae. A further anatomic advantage of the jejunum over the ileum in terms of surface area relates to the fact that its villi are taller.

Functional differences. — The inner layer of the mucosa consists of a continuous sheet of a single layer of columnar epithelial cells lining both the crypts and the villi. Crypt epithelium is largely made up of undifferentiated cells that will acquire absorptive properties as they travel up the villi to replace senescent enterocytes coming off the tip of the villi. The luminal surface of each absorptive cell (mature enterocyte) is increased thirty-fold by great numbers of microvilli that in turn are covered by a surface coat of glycoprotein. The microvilli not only are responsible for absorption but also participate in the digestion of carbohydrates and proteins because they are the site of several enzymes hydrolyzing these substrates. Microvilli are also endowed with specific receptor sites that play an important role in the absorption of vitamin B_{12}-intrinsic factor complex, calcium, iron, and perhaps also conjugated bile acids. The surface-coat glycoprotein ("fuzz") provides a unique micro-environment where dietary constituent molecules are trapped and may come into contact with adsorbed pancreatic enzymes and with the apical plasma membranes of microvilli. The duodenum and jejunum are responsible for the absorption of most dietary constituents except vitamin B_{12} and bile acids. With regard to fat absorption, experimental studies suggest that the capacity of the ileum to form chylomicrons is limited when compared to that of the jejunum.

Capacity of adaptation of the small intestine. — The ileum compensates for its smaller surface area by a slower transit time. It has a very effective functional reserve capable of taking over for the resected jejunum. The latter has a limited capacity to adapt to and compensate for the absorptive function of the ileum. This is attributable partly to the more rapid transit through the jejunum and partly to the lack of specific receptors for vitamin B_{12} and conjugated bile acids on the microvillous membrane of the jejunum.

Adaptation of the remaining small bowel plays an important role in the prognosis, but there have been few measurements of the residual small bowel in man. Roentgenographic studies invariably show dilatation of the remaining small bowel loops and

eventually elongation over a certain period of time. Examination of biopsy specimens shows a true increase in villous size, the result of expansion of the proliferative zone (crypt size). As a result of this adaptive hyperplasia, which takes place over a period of several months, there is an increased surface area available for absorption and a corresponding improvement in absorption.

Intestinal growth is controlled by a feedback mechanism that is governed by exogenous (diet) and a number of endogenous agents [139]. From animal studies, several mechanisms have been suggested which mediate adaptation after small bowel resection (Fig. VIII-4).

Luminal contents. — Animals maintained on total parenteral nutrition after intestinal resection do not undergo adaptation. Gastric infusion of a polymeric diet is more effective than a monomeric diet [17]. Fat, with the exception of medium-chain triglycerides, appears to be the most effective dietary component to stimulate adaptation [89]. It is not yet clear whether the effect of these nutrients is direct or is mediated by bile and pancreatic secretions, which have been shown to stimulate mucosal growth in the ileum.

Gastrointestinal hormones. — After gut resection there follows a compensatory adaptation of the

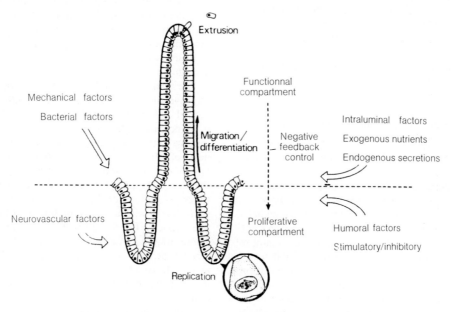

FIG. VIII-4. — *Intestinal cell turnover in the small intestine.*

Enterocytes possess a feedback control whereby cell division in the proliferative compartment (the crypts) is regulated by the number of cells in the functional compartment. Exogenous and endogenous factors listed are discussed in the text. (From WILLIAMSON R. C. N., *N. Engl. J. Med.*, 298, 1445, 1978).

remaining intestine. There is good evidence that these changes are humorally mediated. Raised plasma levels of gastrin, motilin, pancreatic polypeptide and enteroglucagon have been documented in adults [12]. These peptides may possibly represent the circulating mediators of such adaptive responses. It would therefore be of great interest to confirm these findings in infants and correlate intestinal histology, mucosal cell kinetics and absorptive function with circulating gut hormones.

Dilatation and stasis of the remaining gut may enhance functional adaptation. Neurovascular changes that occur after resection may contribute to adaptive hyperplasia though evidence in this regard is still fragmentary.

Physiopathology

Gastrointestinal motility. — Factors that lead to alterations in gastrointestinal motility include the following:

(a) Gastric hypersecretion has been documented.

(b) The extent of the decrease in surface area available for absorption is a critical factor. The absorptive capacity of the remaining bowel is influenced by the presence or absence of the ileocecal valve as well as of the colon.

(c) Bacterial contamination of the upper bowel is almost always present in the early phase after a wide resection. Through the production of phenols and amines bacterial overgrowth may affect motility.

(d) Deconjugated (free) and dehydroxylated (secondary) bile acids, as well as hydroxylated fatty acids, are potent cathartics.

Impairment of digestion. — Factors leading to impairment of digestion include the following:

(a) Pancreatic function is impaired whenever malnutrition is present.

(b) Micellar solubilization is defective because of a decrease in conjugated bile acids. Newborn and premature infants constitute the majority of pediatric patients with the short bowel syndrome. As previously discussed they already have a significant degree of fat malabsorption during the first month of life because of low intraduodenal concentrations of conjugated bile acids. After an ileal resection, losses in the feces often exceed the capacity of the liver to maintain critical micellar concentrations [113]. There is invariably a very high predominance of glycine over taurine conjugated bile acids (G/T) ratio as a result of large fecal losses. Because of

their low pK_a, glycoconjugates may be precipitated if the duodenum is acidic and therefore may not be available for solubilization of fat. Furthermore, in the common situation in which the small bowel is contaminated, the bile acids are deconjugated and therefore cannot form micelles with the products of lipolytic digestion.

(c) Digestion of disaccharides and peptides is reduced because of accelerated transit and brush-border changes through bacterial contamination.

Absorptive defects. — All nutrients, including water, electrolytes, fat, protein, carbohydrate, and all vitamins, are absorbed subnormally after massive resection of the small intestine. The degree of malabsorption varies with the type of resection. Long segments of mid-small bowel can be resected without many problems. However, when a much shorter segment of the proximal or distal small intestine is removed, severe symptoms can develop.

Clinical findings

The clinical picture produced by massive small bowel resection is one of starvation and diarrhea [14]. Appetite is invariably voracious unless there is a significant degree of abdominal distention. The latter is an indication that the continuity of the bowel or its motility is compromised or, more frequently, that unabsorbed nutrients are undergoing bacterial breakdown in the colon, thus producing large amounts of gas. Vomiting suggests stenosis or stricture at the anastomotic site or the formation of a stagnant loop.

The diarrhea is often intractable but tends to improve as compensatory changes take place. In fact, it has been clinically demonstrated that there is an increase in the absorptive surface of the remaining small intestine by increases in diameter and thickness of the wall and concomitant widening of villi with increased arborizations. Furthermore, there is a gradual decrease in the gastric hypersecretion and in the motility of the stomach and small bowel with a corresponding increased absorptive capacity for fat, proteins, and carbohydrates. These adaptive changes may gradually modify the clinical picture, but they occur more frequently in the ileum after proximal resection than in the jejunum when the distal small bowel has been removed.

There is usually a rapid weight loss with muscle wasting and decreased body fat. Excessive water and electrolyte losses lead to dehydration and a strong craving for salt. Anorexia and vomiting may occur when there is a significant degree of metabolic acidosis.

Anemia and hypoproteinemia are constant features. Manifestations of impaired protein absorption are low levels of serum proteins and hypoalbuminemia. Low serum carotene and cholesterol values associated with steatorrhea reflect the diminished absorption of fat. As a consequence of fat malabsorption, there is commonly evidence of vitamin D deficiency and malabsorption of calcium. Hypocalcemia is more likely to develop when the ileocecal valve has been resected. Magnesium balance tends to parallel that of calcium. Tetany may occur during the early phase, and osteomalacia develops in longstanding cases. Iron deficiency is likely to develop if the upper bowel has been removed, and vitamin B_{12} deficiency if the ileum was resected. Purpura and generalized bleeding reflects impaired coagulation caused by malabsorption of vitamin K. Hyperoxaluria and its complication, nephrolithiasis may occur [129].

X-ray findings

The transit time from mouth to anus measured with a nonabsorbable marker such as carmine red can be as short as 12 minutes. Roentgenographic studies should be done for assessment of the length of the remaining bowel, and for ascertaining that it is of reasonably normal caliber throughout and is emptying itself of its contents.

Management

The infant with a massive small bowel resection presents a challenging management problem. It is impossible to plan for proper care unless the clinician establishes close contact with the surgeon to determine the areas and length of small bowel resected, the presence or absence of the ileocecal valve, the type of anastomosis, the presence or absence of adhesions or peritonitis, and, most important, the percentage and appearance of the remaining small bowel.

Diet. — Small amounts (10 ml/kg) of a dilute formula (0.33 kcal/ml) administered every 3 hours should be started promptly. We favor Pregestimil, and gradually increase the volume before increasing the caloric density to 0.50 kcal/ml and eventually to full strength (0.67 kcal/ml). An increased stool output with the appearance of fecal reducing substances is an indication that tolerance limits have

been exceeded [40]. A 24 to 48-hour period of fasting is then indicated before resumption of the formula at a lower caloric density.

There is now considerable experience with the use of continuous enteral feeding [100]. It represents a significant advantage. A large number of calories (up to 180 cal/kg/day), water (up to 275 ml/kg/day), and electrolytes can be provided while low-osmolality feedings are used. Although elemental diets have theoretical disadvantages (amino acids, monosaccharides, absence of fat, high osmolality) in terms of tolerance and capacity to induce adaptive changes in the remaining bowel, they are used with success by some groups.

Parenteral alimentation. — The degree of panmalabsorption is usually severe, and parenteral alimentation is necessary to supplement insufficient oral calories. Even if oral calories are practically negligible, the oral route should be maintained, since experimental evidence suggests that maintenance of a normal mucosa and adaptation are dependent to some extent on luminal nutrition. In the event that oral intake is totally impossible because of excessively large water and electrolyte losses, or there is less than 80 cm of bowel left, a central catheter is used. Total parenteral nutrition may be necessary for extended periods.

Prognosis

The outcome after a wide intestinal resection is mainly dependent on the following:

— Extent of the resection.
— Area of small bowel (jejunal or ileum) resected.
— Function of the remaining bowel.
— Preservation of the ileocecal valve.
— Ability of the shortened intestine to adapt.

In a survey of 50 infants who had an extensive resection before the age of 2 months, less than 5 % of cases with 38 to 75 cm of remaining small bowel died. The mortality was 50 % in those who had between 15 and 38 cm of small bowel left. The presence of the ileocecal valve was critical. There were no survivors in 11 patients who were left with 40 cm or less of small intestine and in whom the ileocecal valve had been resected [14].

The presence of associated anomalies or of extreme prematurity adds to the risk. Significant as a poor prognostic factor is the appearance of distention, anorexia, or vomiting, since chances are that a further resection will be necessary [99, 140]. Parenteral nutrition has remarkably improved the prognosis of the short bowel syndrome by ensuring survival while compensatory changes occur in the remaining small bowel. Since there are isolated cases of survival in infants who had less than 15 to 20 cm of remaining small bowel after surgery, the physician cannot "close the door" on young infants with massive resections.

II. — NECROTIZING ENTEROCOLITIS

Necrotizing enterocolitis (NEC) in the newborn infant is an acute fulminating disease associated with focal or diffuse ulceration and necrosis of the lower small bowel and of the colon [16]. The ileum is the most common site of the disease. In close to three fourths of cases there are lesions in the colon, with the following distribution in decreasing order of frequency; ascending colon, cecum, transverse colon, and rectosigmoid. The stomach and upper small bowel are rarely affected. In the past decade it has become a notorious major illness. There is no seasonal pattern and both sexes are equally affected. Necrotizing enterocolitis may complicate a lower bowel obstruction (Hirschsprung's disease or meconium ileus). There are now reports of necrotizing enterocolitis occurring after major surgery [1], as after open-heart surgery, correction of gastroschisis, and imperforate anus.

Pathogenesis

There is no single etiologic factor. NEC is primarily seen in low birth weight newborns. More than 50 % of cases occur in babies weighing less than 1,500 g.

Exchange transfusions, umbilical arterial catheters, perinatal asphyxia, respiratory distress syndrome, polycythemia and congenital heart disease are known risk factors. However, studies have shown that birth weight, gestational age, Apgar scores, respiratory distress syndrome, and other perinatal risk factors do not differ from those of control groups.

Ischemia. — The decrease in mesenteric flow as a concomitant of asphyxia in animals and the histologic findings of ulceration and necrosis have given strong support to a selective circulatory ischemia of the gut wall as an essential component of the disease [126]. The decrease in perfusion observed with asphyxia is attributable to actual physiologic shunting of blood away from the gastrointestinal tract and toward more vital areas. This phenomenon is similar to the "diving reflex" seen in aquatic mammals. It could account not only for the postnatal development of acute NEC but also for congenital segmental stenoses and atresias of the gastrointestinal tract, the likely result of intrauterine asphyxia.

The role of both arterial and venous umbilical catheters in disruption of the hemodynamics of the splanchnic circulation is difficult to assess. The relationship of NEC to umbilical vein catheterization and exchange transfusion is irrefutable. The catheter residing in the portal vein increases portal vein pressure. The role of arterial catheters is less certain.

Infection. — There is abundant evidence that altered intestinal function and an injured mucosa through ischemia do not by themselves lead to NEC. Intestinal bacteria play an important role [117]. Clinical studies have long documented outbreaks of NEC [131]. In some epidemics no microorganisms have been found, whereas in others, they have been associated with coronavirus [20], coxsackie virus B_2, *Klebsiella*, *Salmonella*, pathogenic *Escherichia coli*, and *Clostridium* [19]. The normal gram negative flora in the bottle-fed neonate *(E. coli)* may play a secondary role by invading the gut wall [11], producing an infection that in turn leads to the typical accumulation of gas, which dissects the bowel wall (pneumatosis) and mesentery and may invade the portal vein. Decreased mucosal resistance through lack of mucosal immunity may be a compounding factor accounting for systemic invasion of the sick infant by his own normal flora. Close attention to hand-washing technique before one handles neonates at risk and isolation of cases of NEC are believed to be wise precautions until more is known of the relationship between infection and NEC.

Nutrition. — Most babies (97 %) developing NEC have been fed either clear fluids or formula before developing symptoms [16]. In 80 % the initial symptoms of NEC occur within the first 3 days of initiation of oral feeding and more than a third are symptomatic within 24 hours. Infants who develop the disease within the first week have generally been fed earlier. Feeding a premature infant within the first 48 hours after birth seems to be an important risk factor. The volume and the type of feeding have also been the subject of some scrutiny. One group found those premature infants on daily formula increments of 20 to 50 ml/kg more at risk than those on a 10 ml/kg schedule. This needs further examination. That the immune properties (humoral antibodies and cellular components) of human milk and its low pH protect against proliferation of gram negative pathogens and invasion are well known. However, at least two studies [64, 87] have failed to show a demonstrable protective effect. Additional studies are necessary in this important area as the relationship between feeding and NEC has not been confirmed by all groups. Nevertheless it seems prudent to delay enteral feeding, to give small amounts, and, if possible, to offer human milk to babies at risk.

TABLE I. — CLINICAL COURSE OF NECROTIZING ENTEROCOLITIS

	Perinatal period	*Latent period*	*Acute illness*	*Late symptoms*
Premature infant	Respiratory distress Apnea Asphyxia Exchange transfusion	24 hours to 3 weeks	Abdominal distention Vomiting Rectal bleeding Perforation Peritonitis Sepsis, shock	Strictures in ileum or colon

Modified from TOULOUKIAN (J.), POSCH (J. N.), SPENCER (R.), *J. Pediatr. Surg.*, 7, 194-209, 1972.

Clinical course and findings

Classically, symptoms are noted within the first 5 days of life, though they may occur as early as the first day and as late as the fourth week after birth (Table I). An early onset of disease tends to be more severe and more acute. However a recent study has not been able to confirm this and suggests that there is no difference in the relative frequency of maternal and perinatal events related to the development of NEC [141]. Feedings are poorly tolerated. Regurgitation and vomiting are followed by abdominal distension and bloody stools. Diarrheal stools are not frequent (25 %) during the initial stage of the disease, since obstructive phenomena predominate. Within a few hours, there is evidence of perforation and peritonitis. Lethargy, severe acidosis, sepsis, disseminated intravascular coagulation, and shock rapidly supervene. In other cases, the course is not so fulminating, the baby is lethargic and feeds poorly, mild abdominal distention is noted, and bloody diarrhea is usually seen, followed by ileus. A few days later, intestinal perforation and peritonitis are detected, or there is gradual clearing of the symptoms.

Initially physical findings are most often dominated by the overall picture of a sick-looking baby with a moderately distended but soft abdomen. Fullness may be palpated in one area of the abdomen, and it may be tender. A purplish discoloration in one area of the abdomen, usually around the umbilicus, is indicative of an intraperitoneal hemorrhage. In certain cases, the abdominal wall may become ecchymotic and necrotic. This is an indication of an underlying perforation with peritonitis.

In some cases, it is likely that the disease has run its course before birth. Perforation is then diagnosed within a few hours after birth. In others, the first symptoms are those of a partial obstruction in the distal small bowel or colon which may occur later in the neonatal period or after a few months.

X-ray diagnosis

The classic findings in advanced cases include the presence of the bubbly or of the linear type of pneumatosis intestinalis, the demonstration of gas in the portal system, and free air in the peritoneal cavity. Early roentgenographic diagnosis that may confirm a clinical picture compatible with incipient or mild NEC is of great help. Progress has been made in that direction. In one series [66], 87 % presented with early roentgen features before definitive diagnosis. These features include ileus with moderate distention, irregular and scattered bowel loops, loss of bowel-wall definition through edema, and finally the presence of fluid-filled loops and peritoneal fluid.

Treatment

As soon as the diagnosis of NEC is entertained, oral feedings should be withheld, and nasogastric suction and intravenous fluids should be started before a roentgenogram is taken. Parenteral antibiotics are indicated. Since the intestinal flora is clinically and experimentally an important pathogenic factor, oral antibiotics have been used in addition to the systemic antibiotics, but they have generally not been shown to be useful. Flat films of the abdomen are recommended every 8 to 12 hours for the first few days to detect early perforation and to follow the roentgenologic course of the disease. Nasogastric suction is discontinued when roentgenograms no longer demonstrate pneumatosis and when the gastric return is small and clear-colored.

Feedings are resumed gradually after a period of about 10 days of medical therapy.

Any evidence of rapid clinical deterioration (acidosis and thrombocytopenia), intestinal perforation (free air), or peritonitis (tenderness, rigidity, edema, and discoloration of the abdominal wall) constitutes an indication for immediate surgery [118].

Total parenteral nutrition is not infrequently needed for the small infant who requires an ileostomy. After discharge, neonates with NEC must be followed closely for signs of perforation or partial obstruction. These complications can occur as late as 3 to 5 months after an acute bout of NEC.

In terms of prevention, the following recommendations are made:

— Delay oral feedings for 5 to 7 days in low birth weight newborns with a history of perinatal asphyxia.

— Hypertonic (hypercaloric) formulas are not recommended in sick newborns.

— In the presence of significant polycythemia (hematocrit over 75 %), consider a small phlebotomy and exchange transfusion with plasma by way of a peripheral vein.

— Encourage mothers of low birth weight newborns to provide fresh breast milk.

— Arterial umbilical catheters should lie in the aorta below the takeoff point of the renal arteries.

— Venous umbilical catheters should not be positioned in the portal vein for an exchange transfusion.

Complications

Acute. — Sepsis is said to be present in 60 % of cases. Peritonitis is an acute complication that occurs in the 20 % to 30 % who develop an intestinal perforation. Abscesses, meningitis, and disseminated intravascular coagulation [55] are other complication related to infection. Shock with metabolic complications such as hypoglycemia and acidosis is usual in the severe forms of the disease.

Chronic. — The incidence of strictures or atresias after acute NEC is said to be between 18 % and 25 % [107]. The time interval is variable and may be as long as a year. However, in most cases, the condition becomes detectable within 60 days. The majority (60 %) occur in the left colon. All patients treated for NEC should have a barium enema 3 weeks after reinstitution of feedings.

Prognosis

In a large survey of 31 intensive care units in the USA and Canada the overall death rate in 798 cases seen between 1975 and 1977 was 29.3 %. It is estimated that 1 in 100 to 1 in 200 deaths probably result from NEC annually in the USA.

The prognosis is adversely affected by the degree of prematurity and ongoing problems with ventilation. Neonatologists in our hospital [125] have attracted attention to the fact that early-onset NEC is associated with a much poorer prognosis than the late-onset (more than 7 days) form of the disease. The mortality was 32 % in the former group versus 12 % in the latter. The rate of survival is much better in full-term infants [124] and in those whose disease has been triggered by an exchange transfusion.

III. — INTRACTABLE DIARRHEA

Diarrhea in young infants is usually a self-limited disease responsive to supportive care. However, from time to time, the physician is confronted with a patient whose diarrhea is severe and rapidly leads to life-threatening fluid, electrolyte, protein disorders and malnutrition. A wide variety of disorders are responsible for the intractable diarrhea syndrome. There are two forms of the syndrome, a primary form called nonspecific enterocolitis and a secondary form under which a number of disease entities are grouped:

Entities responsible for intractable diarrhea

Anatomical:

— Hirschprung's disease.
— Short bowel syndrome.
— Congenital or acquired stenosis.
— Malrotation.
— Contaminated small bowel syndrome.
— Intestinal lymphangiectasia.

Enteric infections and infestations:

— *Salmonella enteritis.*
— *Escherichia coli enteritis.*
— *Shigella enteritis.*
— *Campylobacter enteritis.*
— *Yersinia enteritis.*
— *Staphylococcus enteritis.*
— *Rotavirus enteritis.*
— *Giardiasis.*
— *Coccidiosis.*
— *Candidal enteritis.*

Extraintestinal infection:
— Urinary tract infection.
— Sepsis.

Acquired sugar intolerance:
— Lactose intolerance.
— Monosaccharide intolerance.

Acquired protein intolerance:
— Cow's milk protein intolerance.
— Soybean protein intolerance.

Cystic fibrosis

Congenital absorption defects:
— Sucrase-isomaltase deficiency.
— Glucose-galactose malabsorption.
— Congenital chloride diarrhea.
— Primary bile acid malabsorption.
— Congenital lactase deficiency.

Inflammatory bowel disease:
— Necrotizing enterocolitis.
— Ulcerative colitis.
— Granulomatous colitis.
— Pseudomembranous enterocolitis.

Tumors:
— Neuroblastoma.
— Ganglioneuroma.
— VIP (vasoactive intestinal polypeptide)-secreting tumors.

Endocrine disorders:
— Adrenal insufficiency.
— Adrenogenital syndrome.
— Thyrotoxicosis.

Milcellaneous:
— Cœliac disease.
— Abetalipoproteinemia.
— Acrodermatitis enteropathica.
— Enterokinase deficiency.
— Defects of chylomicron formation and secretion.
— Wolman's disease.
— Immunodeficiency states.

Nonspecific enterocolitis

Nonspecific enterocolitis is the most common cause of intractable diarrhea. Avery and his colleagues [7] established certain criteria; diarrhea lasting more than 2 weeks during the first 3 months of life in the absence of any clinical, laboratory, or roentgenographic evidence of an identifiable disease entity. The pathophysiologic mechanisms responsible for the primary form of intractable diarrhea of early infancy are poorly understood. The primary event appears to involve damage to the mucosa of the small intestine, but the nature of the aggressor remains unknown. A workable hypothesis is that an undetected infection favors a hypersensitivity reaction to foreign proteins. The diarrhea rapidly becomes self-perpetuating through a combination of factors such as (1) loss of absorptive surface and diminution of brush-border enzymes, (2) injurious effect of undigested dietary antigens or of bacterial antigens on an inflamed mucosa that has lost its autodefense mechanisms, (3) bacterial overgrowth leading to invasion of the bowel wall, impaired monosaccharide transport, and bile salt deconjugation, and (4) pancreatic insufficiency and depressed local immune mechanisms, well known complications of starvation and malnutrition.

Clinical features. — Although the average age of onset in most series is between 3 and 5 weeks, there are patients presenting as late as 4 to 5 months. The initial phase can masquerade as a feeding problem. There is no fever and no signs of toxicity, and the diarrhea may appear to respond transiently after a formula change or a brief period of intravenous fluid therapy. In most cases, however, the symptoms are those of an infectious gastroenteritis [120].

The diarrhea is severe and profuse. It may respond favorably to a period of fasting or use of clear fluids orally, but it will begin again with the reintroduction of formula. More often, the diarrhea is secretory and will continue unabated despite discontinuation of all oral intake.

Gastrointestinal symptoms other than diarrhea were initially considered to be relatively rare by our group. In retrospect, vomiting (70 %) and abdominal distention (50 %) are surprisingly common.

Systemic manifestations are most impressive. The clinical picture is dominated by dehydration, acidosis, and malnutrition. The majority of our own cases were below birth weight when first seen.

The feeding history is of interest in that invariably affected infants have been and are being formula-fed when the symptoms begin. We have seen only one breast-fed baby with nonspecific enterocolitis.

Extraintestinal infections and administration of antibiotics can be documented by history in half the cases.

Laboratory, X-ray and histologic findings. — A constant finding is hypoalbuminemia. Air-fluid levels are especially evident in those infants with abdominal distention. Mild to severe inflammatory changes with mucosal alterations in the small bowel are present. The histologic features of the upper small bowel do not correlate well with the severity of the symptoms or with the degree of malnutrition [43]. However, a form of nonspecific enterocolitis with a particularly bad prognosis is associated with small bowel biopsy specimens showing almost complete lack of recognizable mucosal architecture [22]. They may be milder in the jejunum than in the ileum. Inflammatory changes are also occasionally noted in the colon.

Diagnosis. — The young infant with diarrhea that lasts for more than 2 weeks and shows continued loss of weight should be considered as having intractable diarrhea of infancy once results of stool examinations have indicated that pathogenic microorganisms (bacteria and viruses) are not present.

Stool pH and tests for reducing substances will permit detection of a primary or secondary disaccharidase deficiency. Stools should also be checked for the presence of occult blood; milk colitis, allergic gastroenteropathy, and nonspecific enterocolitis may be seriously considered if stools are positive for blood. A barium enema and an upper gastrointestinal examination should be done early in the investigation. A rectoscopic examination and rectal biopsy should be carried out. A small bowel biopsy is important for the diagnosis, especially since a few entities responsible for the secondary form of intractable diarrhea give rise to specific biopsy features. Because the duodenum is intubated for the small bowel biopsy, duodenal fluid can be collected through separate tubing for aerobic and anaerobic cultures and quantitation of pancreatic enzymes. Results of a sweat test and determination of stool chymotrypsin should help to rule out the possibility of cystic fibrosis. Malnutrition readily brings about exocrine pancreatic insufficiency; the associated hypoproteinemia and edema may give rise to falsely low sweat chloride values. The serum electrolyte abnormalities seen in chloride diarrhea or the adrenogenital syndrome can be easily noted. Measurements of immunoglobulins and cellular immunity tests will rule out an immune defect. Evaluation of stool volume and electrolyte concentration and measurement of bile acid excretion [10] should be obtained. Catecholamine, vasoactive intestinal peptide (VIP), gastrin, and calcitonin assays will rule out tumors associated with diarrhea.

Treatment of nonspecific enterocolitis. — Emergency therapy should be aimed at restoring blood volume and acid-base and electrolyte abnormalities. Because all these patients are severely malnourished, caloric deficits are high [47]. Peripheral parenteral nutrition is initiated during the initial period of observation and testing. A short period of bowel rest is recommended as part of the work-up, since it will provide the physician with an opportunity to see what effect it has on the stool output. Continuing severe diarrhea (more than 50 ml/kg/day) in the absence of any oral intake indicates a secretory type of intractable diarrhea, which will prove more difficult to control.

We attempt refeeding with Pregestimil (casein hydrolysate, long-chain and medium-chain triglycerides, and glucose polymer) given in small amounts at a concentration of 0.33 kcal/ml (10 kcal/30 ml). If tolerance is good, increasing quantities and concentrations are offered and the infant is discharged on this formula for the next few months. In the absence of a good response, a low concentration and a small volume of the same formula is given continuously through a small nasogastric silicone rubber tube. During this period most of the calories are provided by the peripheral intravenous route. Infants with intractable diarrhea are very sensitive to hyperosmolar solutions. Consequently, we suggest that solutions exceeding 285 mOsm/kg of water should not be given. On the other hand, the volume can often be increased up to a range of 200 to 250 ml/kg/day. Tolerance is monitored by stool volume rather than by the number of evacuations [84]. Stool pH and reducing substances are checked regularly. Elemental diets are used by some groups; however, their high osmolality is a distinct disadvantage. Dilute breast milk has also been used successfully.

Unfortunately, significant amounts of calories are poorly tolerated by a certain number of infants fed by either the intermittent oral or the continuous nasogastric route, and they have to be discontinued. A severe form of secretory diarrhea with 24-hour stool volumes of 100 to 300 ml/kg/day precludes enteral feedings. A central catheter, is then necessary [61, 79, 56]. Attempts at reintroduction of oral feedings are made at monthly intervals.

Antibiotics have not been helpful. Corticosteroids have been used in some cases with severe atrophy and absence of signs of regeneration of the mucosa, however, they have not been shown to be effective. Antidiarrheal medications are useless and probably harmful. Cholestyramine is said to be effective in cases where large fecal bile acid losses are documented, yet we have had no success with this drug. Temporary improvement has been reported with cimetidine [33] and cyclophosphamide [128].

Prognosis. — The outcome of this severe and challenging affection has changed dramatically with the advent of parenteral nutrition [71]. The mortality has dropped from 75 % to 10 %. However, the morbidity is high and the course is often unpredictable. A lethal familial protracted form has been reported [18]. After the patient is discharged from a lengthy hospitalization, persisting diarrhea and failure to thrive are seen in a few patients whose small bowel histologic condition shows evidence of ongoing severe damage. Fortunately, the majority of infants with nonspecific enterocolitis exhibit catch-up growth and eventually follow normal developmental milestones.

Cow milk protein intolerance

Intolerance to cow milk proteins has been the subject of much study over the past several years [13, 24, 36]. Better definition, stricter application of diagnostic criteria, and critical evaluation of certain immunologic correlates have significantly contributed to a better understanding and a greater awareness of the entity.

Pathogenesis. — Different immunologic mechanisms have been shown to be abnormal, but it is still not clear whether they cause the symptoms or are secondary phenomena [29].

Metabolic abnormality. — On the basis of a series of studies, the loss of blood and albumin in stools was shown to be substantially greater when susceptible infants ingest homogenized milk instead of a heat-processed formula. A heat-labile toxic protein has been suggested to explain these findings. The possibility that whole proteins or large peptides could exert a direct toxic effect on a genetically predisposed intestinal mucosa or one that is immature or injured (by gastroenteritis) is likewise a plausible explanation.

Hypersensitivity reaction. — Betalactoglobulin, absent from breast milk, is the protein with the greatest antigenicity; lactalbumin, casein, and bovine serum albumin are less potent. Intestinal transport of macromolecules is especially important during the early months of life when the immune system cannot as effectively prevent the absorption of antigens and neutralize the ones gaining access to the circulation [27, 127]. Besides the qualitative properties and the size of the antigen load, three other factors may enhance the absorption of macromolecules:

— Decreased intraluminal proteolytic activity a frequent complication of malnutrition.
— Defective mucosal barrier secondary to immaturity or injury.
— Relative deficiency of secretory IgA from decreased synthesis in the neonate.

Humoral response to milk proteins. — Antibodies to ingested proteins found in the serum (circulating antibodies) and in intestinal secretions (coproantibodies) are of doubtful significance, since there is a wide overlap with normal controls. A recent study shows that all infants given either a milkbase or a soybase formula develop a prompt rise in hemagglutinins, in contrast to those fed a casein hydrolysate formula [28]. Low titers also reported in breast-fed infants suggest that proteins vary in their antigenic potential.

Since IgG and IgM antibodies to milk are present, they would be expected to react in the presence of an antigen excess and lead to complement activation. One study showing a decrease in complement on oral challenge could not be confirmed by another group. The case is therefore very weak for an Arthus type of delayed reaction in milk hypersensitivity.

The immunologic basis for an immediate hypersensitivity reaction is not more securely established though clinically anaphylactic reactions are well known. The role of reaginic IgE antibodies is supported by the presence of IgE milk antibodies and by the observation that symptoms can be prevented by disodium cromoglycate (cromolyn sodium). However, there is no objective proof that IgE antibodies are fixed to mast cells and induce the release of mediators. By use of the RAST technique, titers of IgE antibodies have been found to be higher in milk sensitive children and increased mucosal IgE cells have been found after a challenge with milk. However, the RAST test to milk proteins may also be positive in atopic patients. Increased IgE plasma cells have been found in conditions such as celiac disease and gastroenteritis.

Is cell-mediated immunity involved? The only indication that cell-mediated immunity could be involved comes from the observation that lymphocytes from patients with milk intolerance may undergo blast transformation when cultured in the presence of cow milk antigens. There are currently several groups examining the in vitro response of mucosal explants to milk antigens in terms of release of chemical mediators that induce inflammatory changes. Preliminary results are encouraging.

Incidence. — Cow milk protein intolerance is overdiagnosed when the diagnosis rests only on the symptomatic improvement of digestive disturbances after removal of milk from the diet. Even reliance on the strict criteria of Goldman [38] may not be appropriate to determine the incidence. The three recommended clinical remissions and exacerbations do not necessarily occur within 48 hours of elimination and reintroduction of milk. A conservative figure for the incidence of milk protein intolerance can probably be set at 0.5 % with a predominance in males.

The incidence is greatly increased in children from families having allergies (asthma, rhinitis, urticaria, atopic dermatitis). Atopy is found in 47 % to 80 % of families of affected infants. It is said to be more frequent in cases of selective IgA deficiency. A few studies indicate that breast feeding may protect infants born to atopic families from eczema and asthma, but this will require confirmation. There are no data on the protective effect of exclusive breast feeding during the first 4 to 6 months against the development of cow milk protein intolerance. We believe that breast feeding during the first 2 to 3 months is not protective.

Clinical features. — A wide range of symptoms and signs affecting the gastrointestinal tract, the respiratory system, and the skin are described.

Clinical manifestations associated with cow milk protein intolerance:

Acute forms of the disease:

— Anaphylactic reaction,
— Gastroenteritis,
— Intractable diarrhea,
— Necrotizing enterocolitis,
— Acute colitis;

Chronic syndromes:

— Wilson-Heiner-Lahey syndrome,
— Allergic gastroenteritis,
— Celiac-like syndrome,
— Infantile colic?

Acute manifestations. — The disease may be acute and manifest itself as an anaphylactic reaction. A role in the sudden infant death syndrome has been suggested. In other cases, the onset is characterized by a bout of gastroenteritis from which the infant fails to convalesce. Whether such patients who can go on to "intractable diarrhea", represent complications of infectious gastroenteritis remains to be determined. Necrotizing enterocolitis (NEC) could be an acute and catastrophic manifestation of cow milk and soy protein intolerance. It has been described in several low birth weight infants, but cow milk protein intolerance may be a complication of necrotizing enterocolitis rather than its cause. Acute cow milk- or soy protein-induced colitis is an occasional mode of presentation. It occurs

within the first week or two. Clinical, roentgenographic, endoscopic and histologic findings do not differ from those of an infectious colitis or a chronic ulcerative colitis. Prompt remission usually occurs after elimination of milk- or soy-based formulas.

Wilson-Heiner-Lahey syndrome. — Chronic intestinal blood loss is common in cow milk protein intolerance. It is usually occult, will go unnoticed for long periods, and may result in profound iron-deficiency anemia and hypoalbuminemia [142].

Allergic gastroenteritis. — An abnormal response of the gastrointestinal tract to cow milk often leads to significant losses of proteins. The syndrome was originally described as "allergic gastroenteropathy" [132]. It involves infants with eosinophilia and varying degrees of eczema, asthma, or allergic rhinitis and who, on milk ingestion, develop vomiting, diarrhea, peripheral edema with hypoalbuminemia, occult blood in the stools with hypochromic anemia, and failure to thrive. Steatorrhea and jejunal mucosal changes are not features of this condition. Further characterization of this syndrome reveals striking gastric mucosal changes and only modest patchy jejunal histologic abnormalities. A satisfactory response to milk withdrawal has been obtained in the three patients we have seen with this syndrome. However, this has not been the experience of others [60] who report failure of response to milk withdrawal and the need for corticosteroids in the majority of patients.

Celiac-like syndrome. — This clinical entity consists of chronic diarrhea with some vomiting and a variable degree of fat malabsorption. The symptoms may go unnoticed until failure to thrive and eventual malnutrition attracts attention. D-xylose absorption is invariably abnormal and the intestinal biopsy shows an enteropathy of variable severity [70]. The lesion may be indistinguishable from the one seen in celiac disease, but generally the atrophy is less severe and is patchy. Disaccharidase activity correlates well with the severity of the histologic changes.

Infantile colic. — Generally speaking, paroxysmal fussing is not helped by dietary manipulations and it occurs as frequently on breast milk as on milk-based formulas. A recent paper showing that elimination of cow milk from the diet of lactating mothers had a favorable effect on infantile colic [57] awaits confirmation.

Diagnosis. — Close attention to the dietary history is essential, especially in infants who, for variable periods, have been breast fed. The feeding of supplements is important to document; adverse reactions to cow milk proteins tend to occur within a few days after their introduction, and remission of symptoms after their elimination is usually rapid. However response to a milk challenge may take much longer following a long period on a milk free diet. Although there is solid clinical evidence of a cause-and-effect relationship between the ingestion of milk proteins and the symptoms described above, the immunologic correlates are weak and cannot be used to confirm or rule out the diagnosis. Some workers have suggested that routine histological examination of small intestinal biopsy specimens before and after a cow milk challenge is useful. Others suggest that jejunal biopsies are not necessary because symptomatic children invariably have histologic changes [119].

The 1-hour blood-xylose test is a reliable index of small bowel mucosal function. It has proved to be a valuable means of validating the diagnosis [88], particularly in infants who do not develop symptoms or who have an equivocal response during the few days after a milk challenge. The diagnosis can be validated safely and noninvasively by the following approach:

— History and symptoms compatible with the diagnosis while the child is on a milk-based formula.
— Good clinical progress on a milk-free diet.
— Normal 1-hour blood-xylose level 4 to 10 weeks after clinical recovery.
— Significant drop of the 1-hour blood-xylose level with or without symptoms 4 days after reintroduction of cow milk proteins in a hospital setting.

Treatment. — In most cases, milk elimination results in a rapid amelioration of symptoms and nutritional rehabilitation. Nutramigen is a casein hydrolysate formula that can be used as a milk substitute. Pregestimil is a formula which we have found very helpful, particularly in young infants. Intolerance to soy is present or develops in 30 % to 40 % of infants with cow milk protein intolerance. Soy formulas are therefore contraindicated during the first few weeks in view of the fact that response to the initial period of milk withdrawal is crucial for confirmation of the diagnosis. The cost acceptability of casein hydrolysate formulas warrant the use of a soy formula on a long-term basis. Reintroduction of cow milk and bovine proteins is best carried out in the context of a carefully monitored challenge after the age of 12 months.

Prevention. — Breast feeding is strongly advocated as the sole article of nutrition for the first 6 months, especially in infants with a family history of atopy. A casein hydrolysate formula would appear to have some benefits in terms of milk hemagglutinins, but there is no information on the protection it may confer against intestinal manifestations of cow milk protein intolerance. A recent paper suggests that breast feeding offers no protection against the development of extra-intestinal manifestations such as atopic dermatitis and asthma [68].

The presence of cow milk proteins in breast milk and of antibodies to cow milk in cord blood warrants the recommendation that women with a family history of allergy abstain from large quantities of milk during pregnancy and lactation.

Soy protein intolerance

Soy formulas account for more than 10 % of commercial formula sales. They are recommended for a wide variety of infantile gastrointestinal disorders such as paroxysmal fussing, regurgitation, vomiting, diarrhea, galactosemia, lactose intolerance and cow milk protein intolerance.

Although the antigenicity of present-day heat-processed soy protein-isolate formulas is less than soy flour, there are still concerns with regard to the high incidence (about 30 %) of milk-sensitive infants who are intolerant for soy protein. Although most infants with soy protein intolerance have concomitant cow milk intolerance, there are some cases where soy protein sensitivity appears to be primary and not facilitated by a preceding injury to the mucosal barrier. A variety of adverse responses have been reported: anaphylactic reactions, necrotizing enterocolitis, colitis and enterocolitis with a flat mucosa [97, 48, 138].

REFERENCES

[1] AMOURY (R. A.), GOODWIN (C. D.), McGILL (C. W.) et al. — Necrotizing enterocolitis following operation in the neonatal period. J. Pediatr. Surg., 15, 1-8, 1980.
[2] ANDERSON (G. H.), ATKINSON (S.), BRYAN (M. H.). — Energy and macronutrient content of human milk during early lactation from mothers giving birth prematurely and at term. Amer. J. Clin. Nutr., 34, 258-265, 1981.
[3] ANTONOWICZ (I.), LEBENTHAL (E.). — Developmental pattern of small intestinal enterokinase and disaccharidase activities in the human fetus. Gastroenterology, 72, 1299-1303, 1977.
[4] ANTONOWICZ (I.), MILUNSKY (A.), LEBENTHAL (E.) et al. — Disaccharidase and lysosomal enzyme activities in amniotic fluid, intestinal mucosa and meconium. Biol. Neonate, 32, 280-289, 1977.

[5] AURICCHIO (S.). — Developmental aspects of brush border hydrolysis and absorption of peptides. In *Textbook of Gastroenterology and Nutrition in Infancy*. Edited by E. LEBENTHAL. Raven Press, New York, 1981, 375-384.

[6] AURICCHIO (S.), DELLA PIETRA (D.), VEGNENTE (A.). — Studies on intestinal digestion of starch in man. II. Intestinal hydrolysis of amylopectin in infants and children. *Pediatrics*, 39, 853-862, 1967.

[7] AVERY (G. B.), VILLAVICIENCIO (O.), LILLY (J. R.) et al. — Intractable diarrhea in early infancy. *Pediatrics*, 41, 712-722, 1968.

[8] BACK (P.), ROSS (K.). — Identification of 3 beta-hydroxy-5-cholenic acid in human meconium. *Hoppe-Seyleris Z-Physiol. Chem.*, 354, 83-89, 1973.

[9] BALISTRERI (W. F.). — Fat maldigestion: a reflection of immaturity of the enterohepatic circulation. In *Feeding the Neonate Weighing less than 1 500 grams, Nutrition and Beyond*. Edited by P. L. SUNSHINE. Report of the 79th Ross Conference on Pediatric Research. Ross Laboratories, Columbus, Ohio, 17-22, 1980.

[10] BALISTRERI (W. F.), PARTIN (J. C.), SCHUBERT (W. K.). — Bile acid malabsorption: a consequence of terminal ileal dysfunction in protracted diarrhea of infancy. *J. Pediatr.*, 89, 21-28, 1977.

[11] BELL (M. J.), FEIGIN (R. D.), TERNBERG (J. L.). — Changes in the incidence of necrotizing enterocolitis associated with variation of the gastrointestinal flora in neonates. *Am. J. Surg.*, 138, 629-631, 1979.

[12] BESTERMAN (H. S.), ADRIAN (T. E.), MALLISON (C. N.) et al. — Gut hormone release after intestinal resection. *Gut*, 23, 854-862, 1983.

[13] BHANA (S. L.), HEINER (D. S.). — Cow's milk allergy: pathogenesis, manifestations, diagnosis and management. *Adv. Pediatr.*, 25, 1-37, 1978.

[14] BOHANE (T. D.), HAKA-IKSE (K.), BIGGAR (W. D.) et al. — A clinical study of young infants after small intestinal resection. *J. Pediatr.*, 94, 552-558, 1979.

[15] BRANS (Y. W.). — Meeting carbohydrate needs. In *Feeding the Neonate weighing less than 1,500 grams, Nutrition and Beyond*. Edited by P. L. SUNSHINE. Report of the 79th Ross Conference on Pediatric Research. Ross Laboratories, Columbus, Ohio, 1980, 23-32.

[16] BROWN (E. G.), SWEET (A. Y.), edit. — *Neonatal necrotizing enterocolitis*, New York, 1980, Grune and Stratton.

[17] BUTS (J. P.), MORIN (C. L.), LING (V.). — Influence of dietary components on intestinal adaptation after small bowel resection in rats. *Clin. Invest. Med.*, 2, 59-66, 1979.

[18] CANDY (D. C. A.), LARCHER (V. F.), CAMERON (D. J. S.) et al. — Lethal familial protracted diarrhea. *Arch. Dis. Child.*, 56, 15-23, 1981.

[19] CASHORE (W. J.), PETER (G.), LAUERMANN (M.) et al. — Clostridia colonization and clostridial toxin in neonatal necrotizing enterocolitis. *J. Pediatr.*, 98, 308-311, 1981.

[20] CHANY (C.), MOSCOVICI (O.), LEBON (P.) et al. — Association of coronavirus infection with neonatal necrotizing enterocolitis. *Pediatrics*, 69, 209-214, 1982.

[21] CHESSEX (P.), REICHMAN (B.), VERELLEN (G.) et al. — Quality of growth in premature infants fed their own mothers' milk. *J. Pediatr.*, 102, 107-112, 1983.

[22] DAVIDSON (G. P.), CUTZ (E.), HAMILTON (J. R.) et al. — Familial enteropathy: a syndrome of protracted diarrhea from birth, failure to thrive, and hypoplastic villus atrophy. *Gastroenterology*, 75, 783-790, 1978.

[23] DE BELLE (R. C.), VAUPSHAS (V.), VITULLO (B. B.) et al. — Intestinal absorption of bile salts: immature development in the neonate. *J. Pediatr.*, 94, 472-476, 1979.

[24] DELÈSE (G.), NUSSLÉ (D.). — L'intolérance aux protéines du lait de vache chez l'enfant. *Helv. Paediat. Acta*, 30, 135-149, 1975.

[25] DE VIZIA (B.), CICCIMARRA (F.), DE CICCO (N.) et al. — Digestibility of starches in infants and children. *J. Pediatr.*, 86, 50-55, 1975.

[26] DREW (J. H.), JOHNSTON (R.), FINOCCHIARO (C.) et al. — A comparison of nasojejunal with nasogastric feedings in low birth weight infants. *Aust. Paediat. J.*, 15, 98-100, 1979.

[27] EASTHAM (E. J.), LICHAUCO (T.), GRADY (M. I.) et al. — Antigenicity of infant formulas: role of immature intestine on protein permeability. *J. Pediatr.*, 93, 561-564, 1978.

[28] EASTHAM (E. J.), LICHAUCO (T.), PANG (K.) et al. — Antigenicity of infant formulas and the induction of systemic immunological tolerance by oral feeding: cow's milk versus soy milk. *J. Pediatr. Gastroenterol. Nutr.*, 1, 23-29, 1982.

[29] EASTHAM (E. J.), WALKER (W. A.). — Effect of cow's milk on the gastrointestinal tract: a persistent dilemma for the pediatrician. *Pediatrics*, 60, 477-481, 1977.

[30] FAIRCLOUGH (P. D.), CLARK (M. L.), DAWSON (A. M.). — Absorption of glucose and maltose in congenital glucose-galactose malabsorption. *Pediat. Res.*, 12, 1112-1114, 1978.

[31] FAIRCLOUGH (P. D.), HEGARTY (J. E.), SILK (D. B. A.) et al. — Comparison of the absorption of two protein hydrolysates and their effects on water and electrolyte movements in the human jejunum. *Gut*, 21, 829-834, 1980.

[32] FILER (L. J. Jr.), MATTSON (F. H.), FOMON (S. J.). — Triglyceride configuration and fat absorption by the human gut. *J. Nutr.*. 99, 293-299, 1969.

[33] FISHER (S. E.), BOYLE (J. T.), HOLTZAPPLE (P.). — Chronic protracted diarrhea and jejunal atrophy in an infant. *Dig. Dis. Sci.*, 26, 181-186, 1981.

[34] FRIEDMAN (Z.). — Polyunsaturated fatty acid metabolism in infants. In *Textbook of Gastroenterology and Nutrition in Infancy*. Edited by E. LEBENTHAL. Raven Press, New York, 1981, 521-551.

[35] GAULL (G. E.), RASSIN (D. K.), RAIHA (N. C. R.) et al. — Milk protein quantity and quality in low-birth-weight infants. *J. Pediatr.*, 90, 348-355, 1977.

[36] GERRARD (J. W.), MACKINZIE (J. W. A.), GOLUBOFF (N.) et al. — Cow's milk allergy: prevalence and manifestations in a unselected series of newborns. *Acta Paediatr. Scand.*, *(Suppl.)* 234, 1-21, 1973.

[37] GILAT (T.), DILIZKY (F.), GELMAN-MALACHI (E.) et al. — Lactase in childhood: a non adaptable enzyme. *Scand. J. Gastroenterol.*, 9, 395-398, 1974.

[38] GOLDMAN (A. S.), ANDERSON (D. W.), SELLERS (W. A.) et al. — Milk allergy: oral challenge

with milk and isolated milk proteins in allergic children. *Pediatrics*, *32*, 425-443, 1963.

[39] GRACEY (M.), BURKE (V.). — Sugar-induced diarrhea in children. *Arch. Dis. Child.*, *48*, 331-336, 1973.

[40] GRACEY (M.), BURKE (V.), OSHIN (A.) *et al.* — Bacteria, bile salts and intestinal monosaccharide malabsorption. *Gut*, *12*, 683-692, 1971.

[41] GRAND (R. J.), WATKINS (J. B.), TORTI (F. M.). — Development of the human gastro-intestinal: a review. *Gastroenterology*, *70*, 790-810, 1976.

[42] GRAY (C. M.). — Carbohydrate digestion and absorption. *N. Engl. J. Med.*, *293*, 1225-1230, 1975.

[43] GREENE (H. L.), McCABE (D. R.), MERENSTEIN (G. B.). — Protracted diarrhea and manutrition in infancy: changes in intestinal morphology and disaccharidase activities during treatment with total intravenous nutrition or oral elemental diets. *J. Pediatr.*, *87*, 695-704, 1975.

[44] GRIEDER (H. R.), DENTAN (E.). — Pelargon « 80:20 ». *Praxis*, *60*, 310-316, 1971.

[45] GROSS (S. J.). — Growth and biochemical response of preterm infants fed human milk or modified infant formula. *N. Engl. J. Med.*, *308*, 237-241, 1983.

[46] GRYBOSKI (J. D.), THAYER (W. R.), SPIRO (H. M.). — Esophageal motility in infants and children. *Pediatrics*, *31*, 382-395, 1963.

[47] GUNN (T.), BROWN (R. S.), PENCHARZ (P.) *et al.* — Total parenteral nutrition in malnourished infants with intractable diarrhea. *Can. Med. Assn. J.*, *117*, 357-360, 1977.

[48] HALPIN (T. C.), BYRNE (W. J.), AMENT (M. E.). — Colitis, persistent diarrhea and soy protein intolerance. *J. Pediatr.*, *91*, 404-407, 1977.

[49] HAMOSH (M.). — A review. Fat digestion in the newborn: Role of lingual lipase and preduodenal digestion. *Pediatr. Res.*, *13*, 615-622, 1979.

[50] HAMOSH (M.), SCANLON (J. W.), GANOT (D.) *et al.* — Fat digestion in the newborn: characterization of lipase in gastric aspirates of premature and term infants. *J. Clin. Invest.*, *67*, 838, 1981.

[51] HERNELL (O.), BLACKBERG (L.), FREDRIKZON (B.) *et al.* — Bile salt stimulated lipase in human milk and lipid digestion during the neonatal period. In *Textbook of Gastroenterology and Nutrition in Infancy*. Edited by E. LEBENTHAL. Raven Press, New York, 1981, 465-471.

[52] HOLLIDAY (M. A.). — Metabolic rate and organ size during growth from infancy to maturity and during late gestation and early infancy. *Pediatrics*, *47*, 169-178, 1971.

[53] HOLTZAPPLE (P. G.), SMITH (G.), KOLDOVSKY (O.). — Uptake, activation, and esterification of fatty acids in the small intestine of the suckling rat. *Pediatr. Res.*, *9*, 786-791, 1975.

[54] HUSBAND (J.), HUSBAND (P.), MALLINSON (C. N.). — Gastric emptying of starch meals in the newborn. *Lancet*, *2*, 290-292, 1970.

[55] HUTTER (J. J. Jr.), HATHAWAY (W. E.), WAYNE (E. R.). — Hematologic abnormalities in severe neonatal necrotizing enterocolitis. *J. Pediatr.*, *88*, 1026-1031, 1976.

[56] HYMAN (C. J.), REITER (J.), RODNAN (J.) *et al.* — Parenteral and oral alimentation in the treatment of the nonspecific protracted diarrheal syndrome in infancy. *J. Pediatr.*, *78*, 17-29, 1971.

[57] JAKOBSSON (I.), LINGBERG (T.). — Cow's milk as a cause of infantile colic in breast-fed infants. *Lancet*, *1*, 437-439, 1978.

[58] JARNETT (E. C.), HOLMAN (G. H.). — Lactose absorption in premature infants. *Arch. Dis. Child.*, *41*, 525-527, 1966.

[59] JEVSEN (R. G.), CLARK (R. M.), DE JONG (F. A.) *et al.* — The lipolytic triad: human lingual, breast milk and pancreatic lipases: physiological implications of their characteristics in digestion of dietary fats. *J. Pediatr. Gastroenterol. Nutr.*, *1*, 243-257, 1982.

[60] KATZ (A. J.), GOLDMAN (H.), GRAND (R. J.). — Gastric mucosal biopsy in eosinophilic (allergic) gastroenteritis. *Gastroenterology*, *73*, 705-709, 1977.

[61] KEATING (J. P.), TERNBERG (J. L.). — Amino-acid hypertonic glucose treatment for intractable diarrhea in infants. *Am. J. Dis. Child.*, *122*, 226-228, 1971.

[62] KATZ (L.), HAMILTON (J. R.). — Fat absorption in infants of birth weight less than 1,300 gm. *J. Pediatr.*, *85*, 608-614, 1974.

[63] KIEN (C. L.), SUMMERS (J. E.), STETINA (J. S.) *et al.* — A method for assessing carbohydrate energy absorption and its application to premature infants. *Amer. J. Clin. Nutr.*, *36*, 910-916, 1982.

[64] KLIEGMAN (R. M.), PITTARD (W. B.), FANAROFF (A. A.). — Necrotizing enterocolitis in neonates fed human milk. *J. Pediatr.*, *95*, 450-453, 1979.

[65] KLISH (W. J.), UDALL (J. N.), RODRIGUEZ (J. T.). — Intestinal surface area in infants with acquired monosaccharide intolerance. *J. Pediatr.*, *92*, 566-571, 1978.

[66] KOGUTT (M. S.). — Necrotizing enterocolitis of infancy: early roentgen patterns as a guide to prompt diagnosis. *Radiology*, *130*, 367-370, 1979.

[67] KOLDOVSKY (O.). — Digestion and absorption. In *Perinatal Physiology*. Edited by U. STAVE. Plenum Press, 2nd edition, 1978, 317-356.

[68] KRAMER (M.), MOROZ (B.). — Do breast-feeding and delayed introduction of solid foods protect against subsequent atopic eczema? *J. Pediatr.*, *98*, 546-550, 1981.

[69] KREJS (G. J.). — The small bowel. I. Intestinal resection. *Clin Gastroenterol*, *8*, 373-386, 1979.

[70] KUITUVEN (P.), RAPOLA (J.), SAVILAHTI (E.) *et al.* — Response of the jejunal mucosa to cow's milk in the malabsorption syndrome with cow's milk intolerance. *Acta Paediatr. Scand.*, *62*, 585-595, 1973.

[71] LARCHER (V. F.), SHEPHERD (R.), FRANCIS (D. E. M.) *et al.* — Protracted diarrhea in infancy: analysis of 82 cases with particular reference to diagnosis and management. *Arch. Dis. Child.*, *52*, 597-605, 1977.

[72] LEBENTHAL (E.), LEE (P. C.). — Glucoamylase and disaccharidase activities in normal subjects and in patients with mucosal injury of the small intestine. *J. Pediatr.*, *97*, 389-393, 1980.

[73] LEBENTHAL (E.), LEE (P. C.). — The development of pancreatic function in premature infants after milk-based and soy-based formulas. *Pediatr. Res.*, *15*, 1240-1244, 1981.

[74] LEBENTHAL (E.), LEE (P. C.). — Review article. Interactions of determinants in the ontogeny of the gastrointestinal tract: a unified concept. *Pediatr. Res.*, *17*, 19-24, 1983.

[75] LEE (P. C.), NORD (K. S.), LEBENTHAL (E.). — Digestibility of starches in infants. In *Textbook of Gastroenterology and Nutrition in Infancy*. Edited by E. LEBENTHAL. Raven Press, New York, 1981, 423-433.

[76] LEVY (E.), GOLDSTEIN (R.), FREIER (S.) et al. — Characterization of gastric lipolytic activity. BBA 666, 316-326, 1981.

[77] LIEBERMAN (J.). — Proteolytic enzyme activity in fetal pancreas and meconium. *Gastroenterology*, 50, 183-190, 1966.

[78] LIFSHITZ (F.). — Carbohydrate problems in pediatric gastroenterology. *Clin. Gastroenterol.*, 6, 415-429, 1977.

[79] LLOYD-STILL (J. D.), SHWACHMAN (H.), FILLER (R. M.). — Protracted diarrhea of infancy treated by intravenous alimentation. *Am. J. Dis. Child.*, 125, 364, 365-368, 1973.

[80] LUCAS (A.), BLOOM (S. R.), AYNSLEY-GREEN (A.). — Metabolic and endocrine events at the time of the first feed of human milk in preterm and term infants. *Arch. Dis. Child.*, 53, 731-736, 1978.

[81] LUCAS (A.), BLOOM (S. R.), AYNSLEY-GREEN (A.). — Development of gut hormone responses to feeding in neonates. *Arch. Dis. Child.*, 55, 678-682, 1980.

[82] McDONALD (G. B.) WEIDMAN (M.). — Does palmitic acid alter the route of transport of other fatty acids from the intestine? *Gastroenterology*, 76, 1199, 1979 (Abstract).

[83] MACLEAN (W. C. Jr), FINK (B. B.). — Lactose malabsorption by premature infants: magnitude and clinical significance. *J. Pediatr.*, 97, 383-388, 1980.

[84] MACLEAN (W. C.), LOPEZ DE ROMANA (G.), MASSA (E.) et al. — Nutritional management of chronic diarrhea and malnutrition, primary reliance on oral feeding. *J. Pediatr.*, 97, 316-323, 1980.

[85] MASON (S.). — Some aspects of gastric function in the newborn. *Arch. Dis. Child.*, 37, 387-391, 1962.

[86] MILNER (R. D. G.), MINOLI (I.), MORO (G.) et al. — Growth and metabolic and hormonal profiles during transpyloric and nasogastric feeding in preterm infants. *Acta Paediatr. Scand.*, 70, 9-13, 1981.

[87] MORIARTEY (R. R.), FINER (N. N.), COX (S. F.) et al. — Necrotizing enterocolitis and human milk. *J. Pediatr.*, 94, 295-296, 1979.

[88] MORIN (C. L.), BUTS (J. P.), WEBER (A.) et al. — One hour blood xylose test in diagnosis of cow's milk protein intolerance. *Lancet*, 1, 1102-1104, 1979.

[89] MORIN (C. L.), LING (V.). — Adaptation of the small bowel after resection in response to intraluminal lipid. *Gastroenterology*, 74, 1070, 1978 (Abstract).

[90] MILLA (P.), HARRIES (J. T.). — Development of water and electrolyte secretion, absorption and their requirements during the neonatal period. *Second International symposium on Infant Nutrition, Intermediary metabolism and the development of the gastrointestinal tract*. Niagara Falls June 1982.

[91] NORMAN (A.), STRANVIK (B.), DJAMAE (O.). — Bile acids and pancreatic enzymes during absorption in the newborn. *Acta Paediatr Scand*, 61, 571-576, 1972.

[92] OCKNER (R. K.), MANNING (J. A.). — Fatty acid binding protein in small intestine: identification, isolation and evidence for its role in cellular fatty acid transport. *J. Clin. Invest.*, 54, 326-328, 1974.

[93] PATEL (B. D.), DINWIDDIE (R.), KUMAR (S. P.) et al. — The effects of feeding on arterial blood gases and lung mechanisms in newborn infants recovering from respiratory disease. *J. Pediatr.*, 90, 435-438, 1977.

[94] PENCHARZ (P. B.). — The protein needs of preterm infants. In *Meeting nutritional goals for low birth weight infants*. Ross Clinical Research Conference, 1980, Columbus, Ohio.

[95] PENCHARZ (P. B.), COCHRAN (W.), SCRIMSHAW (N. S.) et al. — Protein metabolism in human neonates: 1. Nitrogen balance studies and estimated obligatory N losses. *Clin. Sci. Mol. Med.*, 52, 485-490, 1977.

[96] PEREZ RODRIGUEZ (J.), QUERO (J.), FRIAS (E. G.). — Duodenal perforation by a tube of silicone rubber during transpyloric feeding. *J. Pediatr.*, 92, 113-116, 1978.

[97] POWEL (G. K.). — Enterocolitis in low birth weight infants associated with milk and soy protein intolerance. *J. Pediatr.*, 88, 840-844, 1976.

[98] RAÏHÄ (N. C. R.), HEINONEN (K.), RASSIN (D. K.) et al. — Milk protein quantity and quality in low birth weight infants. 1. Metabolic responses and effects on growth. *Pediatrics*, 57, 659-684, 1976.

[99] RICKHAM (P. P.). — Subtotal intestinal resection in the newborn. *Ann. Chir. Infant*, 18, 173-182, 1977.

[100] RICOUR (C.), DUHAMEL (J. F.), NIHOUL-FEKETE. — Nutrition entérale à débit constant chez l'enfant. *Arch. Franç. Pédiatr.*, 34 (2), 154-170, 1977.

[101] ROY (C. C.), DARLING (P.). — Pitfalls in the design and manufacture of infant formulas. *J. Pediatr. Gastroenterol. Nutr.*, 2, S282-S292, 1983.

[102] ROY (C. C.), LEPAGE (G.), CHARTRAND (L.) et al. — Early postnatal nutrition and later growth of low birth weight newborns. *Pediatr. Res.*, 13, 407, 1979 (Abstract).

[103] ROY (C. C.), SAINTE-MARIE (M.), CHARTRAND (L.) et al. — Correction of the malabsorption of the preterm infant with a medium-chain triglyceride formula. *J. Pediatr.*, 446-450, 1975.

[104] ROY (R. N.), POLLNITZ (R. P.), HAMILTON (J. R.) et al. — Impaired assimilation of nasojejunal feeds in healthy low birthweight newborn infants. *J. Pediatr.*, 90, 431-434, 1977.

[105] SANTERRE (J.). — Calcium and phosphorus retention in preterm infants. In STERN (L.), OH (W.), FRIIS-HANSEN (B.) editors, *Intensive care in newborn*. Masson Publ. USA, New York, 1979, 205-210.

[106] SCHREINER (R. L.), BRADY (M. S.), ERNST (J. A.) et al. — Lack lactobezoars in infants given predominantly whey protein formulas. *Am. J. Dis. Child.*, 136, 437-439, 1982.

[107] SCHWARTZ (M. Z.), RICHARDSON (C. J.), HAYDEN (C. K.) et coll. — Intestinal stenosis following successful medical management of necrotizing enterocolitis. *J. Pediatr. Surg.*, 15, 890-899, 1980.

[108] SCRIMSHAW (N. S.). — An analysis of past and present recommended dietary allowances for protein in health and disease. *N. Engl. J. Med.*, 294, 136-142, 1976.

[109] SHENAI (J. P.), JHAVERI (B. M.), REYNOLD (J. W.) et al. — Nutritional balance studies in very low birthweight infants: role of soy formula. *Pediatrics*, 67, 631-637, 1981.

[110] SHENAI (J. P.), REYNOLDS (J. W.), BALSON (S. G.). — Nutritional balance studies in very low birthweight infants: enhanced nutrient retention rates by an experimental formula. *Pediatrics*, 66, 233-238, 1980.

[111] SIGNER (E.), MURPHY (G. M.), EDKINS (S.) *et al.* — Role of bile salts in fat malabsorption of premature infants. *Arch. Dis. Child.*, 49, 174-180, 1974.

[112] SILK (D. B. A.), CHUNG (Y. C.), BERGER (K. L.) *et al.* — Comparison of oral feeding of peptide and amino acid meals to normal human subjects. *Gut*, 20, 291-299, 1979.

[113] SILVERMAN (A.), ROY (C. C.). — *Pediatric Clinical Gastroenterology*. 3rd Edition CV Mosby, St Louis, 1983, 287-294.

[114] SIMMONDS (W. J.). — Lipid absorption. In *Biochemical and Clinical Aspects*, edited by K. ROMMEL, H. GOEBELL and R. BÖHMER. MTP Press Lancaster, England, 51-65.

[115] SLEISENGER (M. H.), KIM (Y. S.). — Protein digestion and absorption. *N. Engl. J. Med.*, 300, 659-663, 1979.

[116] STERN (L.). — Early postnatal growth of low birthweight infants: What is optimal? *Acta Paediatr. Scand., Suppl. 296*, 6-13, 1982.

[117] STEIN (H.), BECK (J.), SOLOMON (A.) *et al.* — Gastroenteritis with necrotizing enterocolitis in premature babies. *Brit. Med. J.*, 2, 616-619, 1972.

[118] STEVENSON (J. K.), OLIVER (T. K.), GRAHAM (B.) *et al.* — Aggressive treatment of neonatal necrotizing enterocolitis: 38 patients with 25 survivors. *J. Pediatr. Surg.*, 6, 28-35, 1971.

[119] SUMITHRAN (E.), IYNGKARAN (N.). — Is jejunal biopsy really necessary in cow's milk protein intolerance? *Lancet*, 2, 1122-1123, 1977.

[120] SUNSHINE (P.), SINATRA (F. R.), MITCHELL (C. H.). — Intractable diarrhea of infancy. *Clin. Gastroenterol.*, 6, 445-461, 1977.

[121] SURAWICZ (C. M.), FILLERY (J.), SAUNDERS (D. R.) *et al.* — Human jejunal absorption of long-chain fatty acid (LCFA) without chylomicron formation. *Gastroenterology*, 76, 1256, 1979 (Abstract).

[122] SVENNINGSEN (N. W.), LINDBROTH (M.), LINDQUIST (B.). — A comparative of varying protein intake in low birthweight infants. *Acta Paediatr. Scand., Suppl. 296*, 28-31, 1982.

[123] SYNDERMAN (S. E.), BOYER (A.), KOGUT (M. D.) *et al.* — The protein requirement of the premature infant. I. The effect of protein intake on the retention of nitrogen. *J. Pediatr.*, 74, 872-880, 1969.

[124] TAKAYANAGI (K.), KAPILA (L.). — Necrotizing enterocolitis in older infants. *Arch. Dis. Child.*, 56, 486-471, 1981.

[125] TEASDALE (F.), LE GUENNEC (J. C.), BARD (H.) *et al.* — Neonatal necrotizing enterocolitis: The relation of age at the time of onset to prognosis. *Can. Med. Ass. J.*, 123, 387-390, 1980.

[126] TOULOUKIAN (R. J.), POSCH (J. N.), SPENCER (R.). — The pathogenesis of ischemic gastroenterocolitis of the neonate: selective gut mucosal ischemia in asphyxiated neonatal piglets. *J. Pediatr. Surg.*, 7, 194-205, 1972.

[127] UDALL (J. N.), WALKER (W. A.). — The physiologic basis and pathologic for the transport of macromolecules across the intestinal tract. *J. Pediatr. Gastroenterol. Nutr.*, 1, 295-301, 1982.

[128] UNSWORTH (J.), HUTCHINS (P.), MITCHELL (J.) *et al.* — Flat small intestinal mucosa and autoantibodies against the gut epithelium. *J. Pediatr. Gastroenterol. Nutr.*, 1, 503-513, 1982.

[129] VALMAN (H. B.), OBERHOLZER (V. G.), PALMER (T.). — Hyperoxaluria after resection of ileum in childhood. *Arch. Dis. Child.*, 49, 171-173, 1974.

[130] VAN CAILLIE (M.), POWELL (G. K.). — Nasoduodenal versus nasogastric feeding in the very low birthweight infant. *Pediatrics*, 56, 1065-1072, 1975.

[131] VIRNIG (N. L.), REYNOLDS (J. W.). — Épidemiological aspects of neonatal necrotizing enterocolitis. *Am. J. Dis. Child.*, 128, 186-190, 1974.

[132] WALDMAN (T. A.), WOCHNER (R. D.), LASTER (L.), GORDON (R. S.). — Allergic gastroenteropathy. *N. Engl. J. Med.*, 276, 761-769, 1967.

[133] WATKINS (J. B.), BLISS (C. M.), DONALDSON (R. M.) *et al.* — Characterization of newborn fecal lipid. *Pediatrics*, 53, 511-515, 1974.

[134] WATKINS (J. B.), SZCZEPANIK (P.), GOULD (J. B.) *et al.* — Bile salt metabolism in the human premature infant. *Gastroenterology*, 69, 706-713, 1975.

[135] WESTERGAARD (H.), DIETSCHY (J. M.). — The mechanism whereby bile acid micelles increase the rate of fatty acid and cholesterol uptake into the intestinal mucosal cell. *J. Clin. Invest.*, 58, 97-108, 1976.

[136] WHARTON (B. A.), SCOTT (P. H.), BERGER (H. M.). — Dietary protein for low birthweight babies. *Acta Paediatr. Scand., Suppl. 296*, 32-37, 1982.

[137] WHITFIELD (M. F.). — Poor weight gain of the low birthweight infant fed nasojejunally. *Arch. Dis. Child.*, 57, 597-601, 1982.

[138] WHITINGTON (P. F.), GIBSON (R.). — Soy protein intolerance: four patients with concomitant cow's milk intolerance. *Pediatrics*, 59, 730-732, 1977.

[139] WILLIAMSON (R. C. N.). — Intestinal adaptation. *N. Engl. J. Med.*, 298, 1393-1402, 1443-1450, 1978.

[140] WILMORE (D. W.). — Factors correlating with a successful outcome following extensive intestinal resection in newborn infants. *J. Pediatr.*, 80, 88-95, 1972.

[141] WILSON (R.), KANTO (W. P.), MCCARTHY (B. J.) *et al.* — Age at onset of necrotizing entero-colitis. *Am. J. Dis. Child.*, 136, 814-816, 1982.

[142] WOODRUFF (C. W.), CLARKE (J. L.). — The role of fresh cow's milk in iron deficiency. I. Albumin turnover in infants with iron deficiency anemia. I. Comparison of fresh cow's milk with a prepared formula. *Am. J. Dis. Child.*, 124, 18-30, 1972.

[143] WU (A. L.), BENNETT-CLARK (S.). — Resistance of intestinal triglyceride transport capacity in the rat to adaptation to altered luminal environment. *Am. J. Clin. Nutr.*, 29, 157-168, 1975.

[144] YOUNOSZAI (M. K.). — Jejunal absorption of hexose in infants and adults. *J. Pediatr.*, 85, 446-448, 1974.

[145] ZEIGLER (E. E.), O'DONNELL (A. M.), NELSON (S. E.) *et al.* — Body composition of the reference fetus. *Growth*, 40, 329-341, 1976.

[146] ZOPPI (G.), ANDREOTTI (G.), PAJNO-FERRA (F.) *et al.* — Exocrine pancreas function in premature and full term neonates. *Pediatr. Res.*, 6, 880-886, 1972.

44

Hepato-biliary disease in the newborn

Mervin SILVERBERG

INTRODUCTION

During the 1950's, extrahepatic biliary atresia, gram negative septicemia, and idiopathic "neonatal hepatitis" accounted for over 90 % of all cases of prolonged neonatal mixed hyperbilirubinemia. In the 1980's extrahepatic biliary atresia is still the single most common cause of neonatal cholestasis [36, 29], however, very few cases are due to unknown causes, and even less are due to bacterial sepsis. About one-third of these infants have liver disease due to infections with known microorganisms, and about one-quarter of the cases are due to genetic-metabolic disorders. The development of excellent anesthesiology practices and surgical techniques has made it possible to operate on newborns with minimal morbidity and mortality. The early exclusion of surgically correctible causes of neonatal cholestasis, therefore, is of paramount importance.

CLINICAL APPROACH TO HEPATOBILIARY DISEASE IN THE NEWBORN

Hepatobiliary disease in the newborn is usually characterized by hepatomegaly and cholestasis *i. e.* mixed hyperbilirubinemia, with the conjugated fraction exceeding 2 mg/dl. The infant's skin takes on a greenish hue, the urine darkens and soon after decreased stool pigmentation is noted. Although the degree of ductal obstruction anywhere along the biliary collecting system correlates well with the degree of acholic stools, this cannot be relied upon, completely. Modest amounts of pigment may be added to the stool via enteric secretions and sloughed enterocytes, even in the presence of total extrahepatic biliary atresia. A choledochal cyst or stricture may permit variable amounts of bile to enter the stool.

Inherited conjugated hyperbilirubinemia (Dubin-Johnson or Sprinz-Nelson Syndromes, Constitutional Hepatic Dysfunction) is a pigment excretory defect which should be differentiated from parenchymal disease of the liver. About half of these parents are consanguinous and both autosomal recessive and autosomal dominant inheritance patterns have been reported. The diagnosis is usually confirmed by liver biopsy which reveals a grossly black liver due to granular melanin-like brown pigment particularly in the centrilobular hepatocytes. *Rotor syndrome*, is a variant which has no hepatic pigment although supposedly has a similar metabolic defect. It has been reported in some of the same families with Dubin-Johnson syndrome. A lethal variant, including arthrogryposis, has been reported in a family of North African descent [29].

Last but not least, selected secondary hepatic disorders present with neonatal cholestasis and should be excluded early in the diagnostic work up. These include severe hemolytic disease of the newborn and gram negative sepsis.

Generally, poor feeding and failure to thrive may be noted by the second week of life. This is more common in metabolic disorders and with infectious etiologies. Hepatomegaly is variable, and is most marked in metabolic disorders. The liver is small and enlarges progressively in extrahepatic biliary atresia. Splenomegaly is usually minimal in the latter condition, although the spleen is small in the early stages of almost all but a few storage diseases e. g. Gaucher, Type 2.

A variety of clinical features have been found to be useful in the differential diagnosis. Infectious causes have often been associated with skin lesions, chorioretinitis, and central nervous system disorders. The increased association of hepatocellular disease with trisomy 13, 18 and 21 may be inferred by the presence of multiple congenital anomalies. Situs inversus occurs in a small proportion of infants with extrahepatic biliary atresia and the polysplenia syndrome. Finally, an unusual facies has been reported in the syndromatic variety of paucity of

the intrahepatic bile ducts and in Zellweger's syndrome (see Fig. VIII-5).

DIAGNOSTIC APPROACH TO NEONATAL HEPATOBILIARY DISEASE

The highest priority is to differentiate those conditions that require immediate treatment. These include certain infectious causes, such as gram negative septicemia and urinary tract infections [4], toxoplasmosis, syphilis, listeriosis, and herpes simplex. Appropriate antimicrobial agents should be administered as soon as possible. Selected metabolic disorders may be brought under control quickly by dietary alterations and these include hereditary tyrosinemia, galactosemia and hereditary fructose intolerance. This triad of metabolic diseases cause very similar clinical features involving severe hepatocellular and renal tubular dysfunction. An accurate sweat test with sweat chloride values in excess of 70 mEq will permit early intervention in cases of cystic fibrosis. Disorders of coagulation are common to many hepatobiliary diseases and require immediate diagnosis and correction with parenteral blood products.

Standard blood liver function tests such as

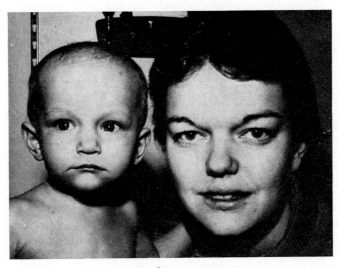
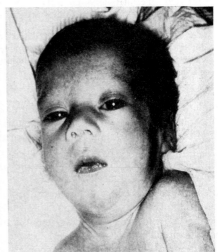

a *b*

FIG. VIII-5.

a) Syndromatic paucity of intrahepatic bile ducts (arterio-hepatic dysplasia). One month old who had neonatal cholestasis and no extrahepatic bile ducts were found at laparotomy at age 5 weeks. Age 3 months, following an unsuccessful portoenterostomy, the typical facial features were noted *i. e.* triangular facies, deep set eyes with hypertelorism and prominent forehead. Note mother has similar features. Skull X-rays in both mother and child reveal a small facial structure and a flat face.

b) Cerebro-hepato-renal syndrome (Zellweger syndrome). One month old infant with marked hypotonia. Mongoloid facies; high forehead, flattened face. (Courtesy of Dr. S. GOLDFISCHER).

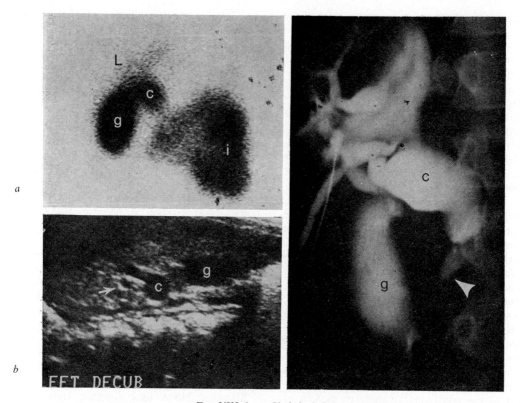

FIG. VIII-6. — *Choledochal cyst.*

Upper left: Technetium-99-m HIDA [N, α, (2,6-dimethyl-acetanilide)] iminodiacetic acid cholescintigraphy at 90 minutes post injection: gallbadder (*g*), choledochal cyst (*c*) and passage of the dye into the intestine (*i*) are evident; L = liver.
Lower left: sonogram showing the dilated common bile duct abutting the choledochal cyst (*c*) and the gallbladder (*g*). The arrow points to the inferior vena cava. Right: Transhepatic cholangiogram demonstrating the choledochal cyst (*c*) and the dilated common bile duct proximal to an area of stricture (arrow). (Courtesy of Dr. I. ZANZI).

aminotransferases, total proteins, albumin, alkaline phosphatase, 5′ nucleotidase, and gamma-glutamyl transpeptidase are useful markers of hepatocellular function. However, they are of no value in differentiating between extrahepatic and intrahepatic causes of neonatal cholestasis. This lack of specificity also applies to newer biochemical tests such as serum alpha-fetoprotein [20] and lipoprotein-x [34], serum [19] and urine bile acids, and Vitamin E and riboflavin absorption tests [28].

Anecdotal reports of endoscopic retrograde cholangiopancreatography [50], percutaneous transhepatic cholangiography [9] and laparoscopy [47] suggests the need for further evaluation of these techniques in neonatal cholestasis, if the appropriate equipment and expertise is available. Some of these invasive techniques await the development of more miniaturized instrumentation which would permit better visualization in these small infants.

Ultrasonography is an ideal non-invasive modality which has sophisticated two dimensional capabilities that may be helpful in selected patients [9]. It has been useful in the diagnosis of choledochal cysts (Fig. VIII-6), but has had limited application in extrahepatic biliary atresia.

Three diagnostic studies still appear to be most useful together in differentiating between intrahepatic and extrahepatic cholestasis:

(*a*) **Duodenal intubation and analysis of the duodenal aspirate for bile pigment** is a simple inexpensive way of confirming the patency of the extrahepatic biliary ducts [13]. The intubation is performed under fluoroscopic control and the fluid is collected by gravity drainage for 24 hours; two-hour aliquots are examined. Ten to 15 ml of 25 % magnesium sulfate instillations may be required to stimulate adequate bile secretion. A negative test is of little

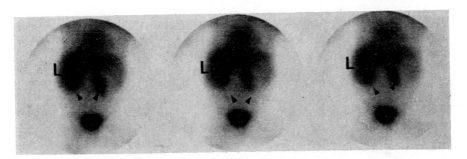

FIG. VIII-7. — *Radionuclide imaging with technetium-99m-PIPIDA* [*N, α-isopropyl acetanilide iminodiacetic acid*] *in a two and a half month old male patient with total extrahepatic biliary atresia.*

Images are shown at 35, 40 and 45 minutes after the intravenous tracer injections, and were obtained following the administration of phenobarbital for 3 days. The gallbladder and bile ducts are not visible, unlike normals. Abundant tracer activity is noted in the liver (L), kidneys (arrows), bladder and cardiac pools. (Courtesy of Dr. I. ZANZI).

value, but the presence of bile pigment, even by direct visualization, excludes the diagnosis of biliary atresia.

(*b*) **Hepatobiliary radionuclide imaging.** — The use of ^{131}I rose-bengal (RB) in the evaluation of biliary excretion disorders has been available for scintigraphic studies for many years [41]. Despite its accuracy of 80-90 %, the main disadvantages are the relatively high beta emission radiation dose required, the long half life (8 days) and the relatively poor resolution of the images. Measurement of excreted ^{131}I-RB in stool has been useful, however the procedure is tedious and the meticulous separation of urine from stool may be an exercise in frustration.

The development of a new class of imaging agents, the N-substituted iminodiacetic acid analogues (IDA) with a technetium-99m (^{99m}Tc) (half-life, 6 hours) label has provided the clinician with an opportunity to obtain excellent gamma camera imaging of very high resolution and low radiation [22] (Fig. VIII-7). The main disadvantage is that the short half life does not permit delayed imaging beyond 24 hours after injection and those infants with marked intrahepatic cholestasis may not be diagnosed correctly. The combined use of ^{131}I-RB and ^{99m}Tc-IDA agents or the use of Ruthenium-97 (half life 2.9 days) may circumvent this problem. Others have shown that pre-treatment of the affected infant by hepatic microsomal induction using phenobarbital (5 mg/kg body weight/day) for 3-5 days will enhance and accelerate biliary excretion of ^{99m}Tc-IDA [26], if the ducts are patent. The few cases of false negatives that are truly due to intrahepatic disease, may be diagnosed correctly by detecting the poor hepatic extraction.

(*c*) **Liver biopsy.** — The examination of liver biopsies obtained during laparotomy or by the percutaneous route has provided a high degree of accuracy in the differential diagnosis. The examiner must have extensive experience and the specimen should contain an adequate number of portal triads (see Fig. VIII-10).

Concurrently, serological and culture studies should be performed to exclude cytomegalovirus, hepatitis B, adenovirus, rubella and coxsackie viruses. The remaining metabolic-genetic disorders should be considered and excluded, when appropriate. Foremost among these are the sweat test for cystic fibrosis and the serum alpha-1-antitrypsin and Pi-typing for the definitive phenotype. It should be noted that the serum level of the protease inhibitor (Pi) may be falsely elevated in the presence of inflammation, since it is an acute phase reactant.

Specific tests for metabolic disorders should be pursued if there is a suggestive family history or the parents are consanguinous. Multi-system involvement is also more common in this group of diseases.

LIVER DISEASE IN THE NEWBORN ASSOCIATED WITH ABNORMALITIES OF THE BILE DUCTS

EXTRAHEPATIC BILIARY ATRESIA (EHBA)

The single most common cause of prolonged progressive neonatal cholestasis is extrahepatic biliary atresia (EHBA). The incidence varies from 1 in 8,000 to 1 in 20,000 live births. There are claims that the incidence is higher in the Far East.

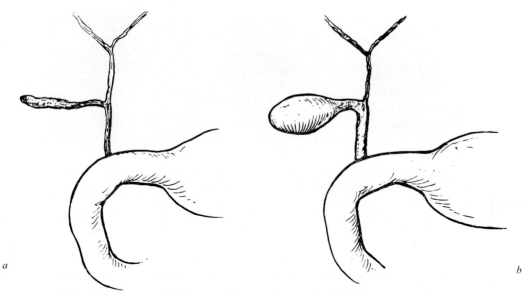

a   *b*

FIG. VIII-8. — *Extrahepatic biliary atresia.*

The two variants represent the most common findings after careful dissection of the porta hepatis at surgery. A portoenterostomy is required in both situations. These lesions were previously referred to as "inoperable" or "non-correctible". (Modified from reference [16]).

In the North American and Japanese experiences, females predominate and compared to males they are more likely to have *inoperable* lesions (Fig. VIII-8). Familial cases are very rare. In the non-operated patient the course is characterized by inexorable biliary cirrhosis and death before the fourth year of life.

Etiology and pathogenesis

The exact etiology, indeed whether or not there is more than one cause, is unclear. A number of facts are more or less agreed upon by most workers in this field:

(*a*) Despite the emphasis on the extrahepatic aspect of the biliary system, it is likely that the causal factor(s) affects the hepatic parenchyma, as well. This accounts for the difficulties often found in differentiating intrahepatic disorders from EHBA. Additionally, it may explain the frequent progression of liver disease that occurs despite successful surgical correction of EHBA.

(*b*) Embryonic maldevelopment, although the oldest proposed etiology, has gained very few adherents over the many years. The only support comes from the fact that there is an association with minor and major congenital malformations in 10-25 % of cases e. g. vascular anomalies, poly-

splenia syndrome etc. (see below). On the other hand, these malformations may be secondary to other toxic or infectious agents which may be the major underlying factor. Other facts that oppose this hypothesis include the extreme rarity of the lesion in stillborns and premature infants and the delayed onset of cholestasis *after* birth in the vast majority of cases. Meconium is almost always normal in color and the youngest infant noted to have acholic stools was 3 days of age. Finally, cholangiography in some patients, and examination of the porta hepatis in most cases reveals evidence of pre-existing patency and normal development of the bile ducts.

(*c*) The most popular etiological possibility is that it is a perinatally acquired disorder which progresses postnatally with an obliterative cholangiopathic process of unknown origin. Some cases have occurred in the same family with neonatal hepatitis or evidence of hepatitis in the mother [42]. In others, rubella virus, cytomegalovirus, listeria and hepatitis B surface antigenemia have all been found in affected infants. Experimentally, reovirus 3 has been implicated [3].

Clinical features

The clinical signs and symptoms are usually indistinguishable from the many other varieties of the neonatal cholestatic syndrome. The earliest sign within the first 4 weeks of life is that of a greenish hue discoloration of skin and sclerae in association with darkening of the urine. Although the loss of pigment in the stool fluctuates initially, acholic (clay-colored) stools develop eventually in most, but not in all cases. The infants are usually born full term with appropriate birth weight and nutrition. Hepatomegaly is progressive, involving both lobes of the liver, and splenomegaly is noted in 75 % of all patients within a few weeks, but may not be noted at the initial examination. Signs of portal hypertension and cirrhosis including hypersplenism, ascites, edema and gastrointestinal bleeding rarely occur before 6 months of age, and pruritis becomes a very distressing sign with persistant cholestasis after 3 months of age.

Laboratory features

Hyperbilirubinemia is of the mixed type and increases progressively. The conjugated fraction usually is more than 50 % of the total level. Fluctuations in serum bilirubin and lower levels of conjugated bilirubin may be found, during the first month of the disease. Although the vast majority of patients have total serum bilirubins under 15.0 mg/dl, occasional values in excess of 20.0 mg/dl have been reported. Other tests of liver function also tend to become progressively more deranged, however, no diagnostic pattern can be delineated. Using the three diagnostic modalities *i. e.* analysis of duodenal fluid, radionuclide imaging, and a percutaneous liver biopsy, pre-operative diagnosis of EHBA can be made in over 95 % of cases.

Early liver biopsy cases may show an accumulation of bile pigment in hepatocytes and Kupfer cells, and bile plugs in canaliculi. An inflammatory reaction occurs in the portal connective tissue and mild fibrosis may extend along the perilobular septa. At this stage, the correct diagnosis may be difficult to make. In the infant progressing to total EHBA as opposed to intrahepatic cholestasis, bile ductular proliferation in all the portal areas is the most characteristic feature (Fig. VIII-9*a, b*). Focal areas of bile extravasation may form "bile lakes". These findings are not pathognomonic of EHBA since they may also be found in choledochal cysts and strictures, as well as in rare cases of alpha-1-antitrypsin deficiency. Giant cell transformation (Fig. VIII-10), hypertrophy of intrahepatic arterioles, and inflammatory infiltration are all not helpful in the differential diagnosis.

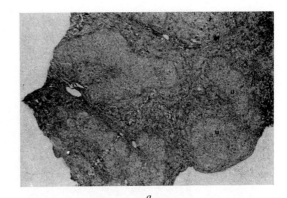

a

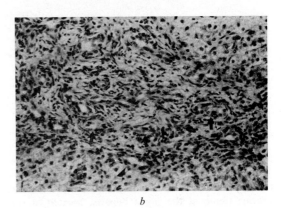

b

Fig. VIII-9. — *Biliary atresia.*

a) Biliary cirrhosis. Regenerative nodules (*n*) surrounded by broad strands of fibrous connective tissue with marked ductular proliferation. Hematoxylin-eosin × 10.

b) Higher magnification depicting a portal space with pronounced ductular proliferation (arrows). Hematoxylin-eosin × 150.

Treatment

Medical management. — Medical therapy is of minor importance in most cases of EHBA in whom the diagnosis has not been unduly delayed. Exceptions are related to their susceptibility to infection, which should be treated aggressively. Disorders of vitamin deficiencies and malnutrition are later developments.

Surgical management. — Although Kasai and his Japanese colleagues devised the first corrective hepatoportoenterostomy in the mid 1950's for "non-correctable" lesions (Fig. VIII-8), it took about two decades before pediatric surgeons outside Japan *i. e.* United States, France, Australia, Italy and Britain, were able to perfect their techniques

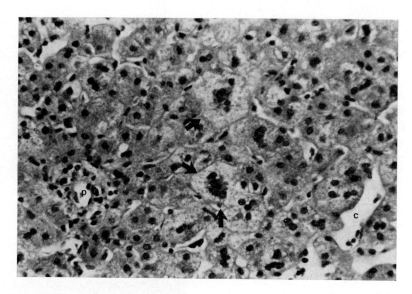

FIG. VIII-10. — *Giant cell transformation is found in many neonatal hepatic disorders.*
Note the multinucleated giant cells with abundant vacuolated cytoplasm (arrows). (*p*) portal space; (*c*) central vein. Hematoxylin-eosin × 500. (Courtesy of Dr. E. KAHN).

and modifications in order to simulate the impressive Japanese results [21]. The basis for the operation is the demonstration by Kasai and others that within fibrous tissue at the porta hepatis, located at the bifurcation of the portal vein, there are microscopically patent bile channels which are in continuity with the intrahepatic bile ducts (Fig. VIII-11). These channels are almost invariably present during the first 60 days of life, thereafter, they are progressively obliterated by an unknown process, so that after the 12th week of life very few are patent and bile flow after a portoenterostomy is very unlikely. No patient has ever had bile flow when surgery was performed after 5 months of age.

Unfortunately, bile flow is not synonymous with "cure", even if the infant becomes anicteric. As many as half of these patients develop signs and symptoms of progressive biliary cirrhosis and portal hypertension. According to the American Academy of Pediatrics Surgical Section Biliary Atresia Registry report in 1981 (a 10 year review of the American experience), there has been an overall postoperative mortality of 30 %, most of which occurred during the first 12 months after surgery.

About 20 % of EHBA are considered "correctable" lesions with patency of one or both of the proximal hepatic ducts. Bile flow occurs in virtually all of these infants, post-operatively, although many still show progression to severe chronic biliary cirrhosis. When the gall bladder and distal ducts are

patent, a hepatoportocholecystostomy is the procedure of choice.

Prognosis

The Japanese results are encouraging. They report an overall 5-year survival rate of about 40 %; considering only those cases operated upon with newer techniques since 1977, the results may be twice that rate.

The post-operative course and prognosis correlate with (*a*) *age at time of surgery,* as noted, above, (*b*) *histological classification of the resected fibrous remnant* [8, 40] of the extrahepatic bile ducts in the portahepatis (Fig. VIII-11). *Type I ducts:* lumina measuring more than 150 microns in diameter, with or without ductular epithelial lining; *Type II ducts:* lumina from 30-150 microns; *Type III ducts:* no epithelial lined structures visible. Virtually all patients with Type I ducts will drain bile, and only a rare case with Type III ducts will drain successfully; (*c*) *hepatic histology.* Although the Japanese report a correlation between good results and degree of hepatic fibrosis at the time of surgery, others claim this feature does not correlate well; (*d*) long term good results are affected by thep revalence or absence of the common complication of *cholangitis.* The solution to this serious post-operative problem has been elusive. Reconstruction of the intestinal

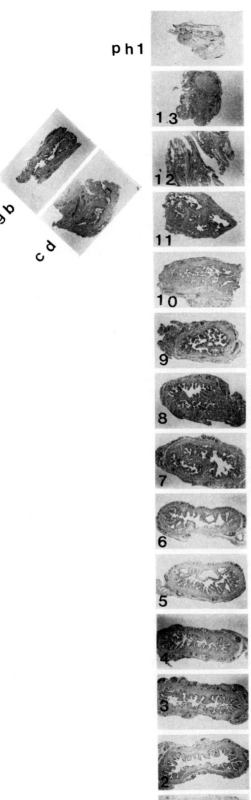

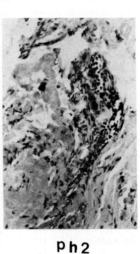

ph2

Fig. VIII-11.

Proximal extrahepatic biliary atresia. Serial sections of the extrahepatic ducts. Both the common duct in the center (figs n° 1-11) and the cystic duct (*cd*) are patent. Hypoplasia of the gallbladder (*gb*) is evident. The hepatic duct (figs n° 12-13) is hypoplastic. Note the markedly distorted ducts seen following frozen sections of the porta-hepatis (*ph 1, ph 2*), which measured up to 207 microns. Hematoxylin-eosin × 150 (Courtesy of Dr. E. KAHN).

conduit with more than ten different operations plus various prophylactic antimicrobial regimens have reduced, but have not eliminated this major pitfall.

Hepatic transplantation, when available, had produced dismal one year survival figures of less than 40 %. With the advent of the use of cyclosporin A, survival rates have more than doubled; however, the latter are still based on small numbers.

CHOLEDOCHAL CYST [23]

The choledochal cyst is the second most common anomaly of the extrahepatic biliary system. The pathogenesis is unknown. Cystic transformation may involve any portion of the common bile duct and in the newborn the cyst volume varies from 5-300 ml. The common duct distal to the cyst is usually narrowed or totally obstructed in the young infant and the clinical picture is similar to most cases of prolonged neonatal cholestasis. The condition is more common in females and there appears to be a higher incidence among orientals. The triad, cholestasis, mass and fever, seen in older children, is rarely found in the young infant.

Histologically, there is ductular proliferation and bile stasis, identical to extrahepatic biliary atresia, which is reversible with early and appropriate surgical intervention.

The diagnosis can be made by radionuclide, or ultrasound studies, or by operative cholangiogram (Fig. VIII-6). The treatment of choice is excision of the cyst with a Roux-en-Y-jejunal anastomosis; when technically unfeasable, a cystojejunostomy is performed. Unfortunately, in all operated cases the incidence of recurrent ascending cholangitis is 10-65 %.

CONGENITAL STENOSIS
OF THE DISTAL COMMON BILE DUCT

Congenital stenosis of the distal common bile duct is a rare condition in the newborn and presents with prolonged neonatal cholestasis. It may be a variant of the choledochal cyst. The diagnosis has been made only with an intraoperative cholangiogram and a by-pass procedure is usually curative.

SPONTANEOUS PERFORATION
OF THE EXTRAHEPATIC BILE DUCT

Bile peritonitis due to a spontaneous perforation of the extrahepatic bile duct system is rare but usually occurs during the first month of life. In most cases, the perforation is at the junction of the cystic and common hepatic duct, which may be associated with a congenital weakness in this region. In fact, the etiology is unclear in most cases. The bile duct system is usually otherwise normal or reveals distal abnormalities such as strictures, gallstones, or mucus plugs. Neonatal cholestasis is mild, although the degree of acholic stools and dark urine is disproportionately severe. Inguinal and umbilical hernias, as well as hydroceles are not uncommon accompanying findings.

The diagnosis is made by the finding of bile peritonitis and the rapid appearance of high radioactivity levels in the ascitic fluid following radionuclide administration [41].

Treatment varies with the associated bile duct abnormalities. Cholangiography during laparotomy will demonstrate the bile leak and a simple repair is indicated in an otherwise normal duct system. Strictures, choledochal cysts and biliary atresia are associated findings which require definitive surgery.

PAUCITY OF INTERLOBULAR BILE DUCTS
(INTRAHEPATIC BILIARY HYPOPLASIA) [51]

Neonatal cholestasis has been noted with 2 main types of decreased numbers of interlobular bile ducts. The *"syndromatic"* variety, often referred to as *arterio-hepatic dysplasia* [46], is associated with a number of malformations. In order of frequency, these include stenosis of major arterial blood vessels, particularly, peripheral pulmonary stenosis, a typical facies (Fig. VIII-5a), skeletal and eye anomalies [35]. Hepatic parenchymal disease is variable, but is usually mild. Progressive liver disease occurs with no obvious contributing factors (see Fig. VIII-12a, b). A significant number of these infants have very small extrahepatic bile ducts which are grossly indistinguishable from extrahepatic biliary atresia. These cases when subjected to a hepatic portoenterostomy have no bile flow postoperatively, and may be adversely affected by the surgery [27].

The *non-syndromatic* variety of paucity of interlobular bile ducts is associated with more severe

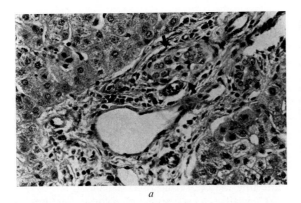

a

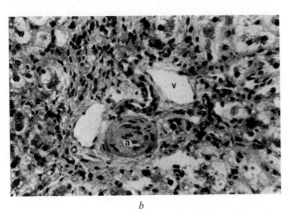

b

FIG. VIII-12. — *Arteriohepatic dysplasia.*

a) At 5 weeks of age. Portal space with evolving destruction characterized by solid clustering and pyknosis of bile duct epithelium (arrows). Hematoxylin-eosin × 200.

b) At 27 weeks of age. Portal space without interlobular bile ducts; (*v*) vein, (*a*) thickened small artery. Hematoxylin-eosin × 200. (Courtesy of Dr. E. KAHN).

and progressive liver disease. Occasionally, these infants have had the PiZ phenotype, and 2 siblings have been described with excess amounts of the cholic acid precursor, trihydroxycoprostanic acid in the blood and urine [16].

FIBROPOLYCYSTIC DISEASES OF THE LIVER [43]

In the absence of a known etiology, fibropolycystic diseases are described according to the specific morphological features in each child. Included in this category in the newborn are congenital hepatic fibrosis and childhood polycystic disease of the liver and kidney. Other terms that are used are

biliary dysplasia, fibroadenomatosis, fibrocholangiomatosis, and cystic fibroangioadenomatosis. The term *fibropolycystic* emphasizes the 2 most important pathological features *i. e.* fibrosis and intrahepatic cysts. Common to all varieties, both in the newborn and in older children are the features of mild hepatocellular dysfunction, mendelian inheritance, and in over 50 % of the infants, immature fibrous tissue and cystic changes are found in the kidneys.

CHILDHOOD FIBROPOLYCYSTIC DISEASE

Familial cases follow a recessive form of inheritance. The infants present with a protuberant abdomen due to bilateral renal enlargement, which often causes respiratory distress, as well. Renal insufficiency can be noted early. The liver is mildly enlarged, with normal or minimal abnormalities of liver function. Jaundice may be exaggerated by neonatal sepsis.

The diagnosis can be established by intravenous pyelography, abdominal ultrasound, computerized tomographic studies and liver or kidney biopsies. The hepatic lesions involve the portal region which reveal increased fibrous tissue and numerous abnormally dilated bile ducts lined by cuboidal epithelium (Fig. VIII-13*a*, *b*).

Treatment is directed at management of renal and cardiac insufficiency, and early detection of infection.

CONGENITAL HEPATIC FIBROSIS

Congenital hepatic fibrosis is inherited in an autosomal recessive manner and rarely presents in the neonate. It is characterized by dense swathes of non-inflammatory, periportal fibrous tissue containing numerous atypical dilated bile ducts. The duct spaces are occasionally referred to as *Meyenberg complexes* or microhamartomas. Parenchymal cell function and morphology is usually normal. Associated disorders include infantile polycystic disease (Fig. VIII-13*a*), Meckel's syndrome, Ivemark's familial dysplasia, medullary sponge kidney, and nephronophthisis. The high incidence of portal hypertension due to abnormal portal veins, is rarely seen in the first month of life.

In the absence of the late findings of portal hypertension and cholangitis, treatment is limited to the management of renal insufficiency whenever it is present in the early cases.

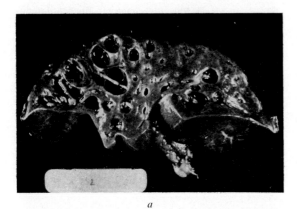

a

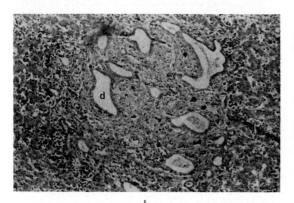

b

FIG. VIII-13. — *Infantile polycystic disease in a 3 day old newborn.*

a) Liver; gross appearance of the liver with marked cystic dilatation of the bile ducts.

b) Congenital hepatic fibrosis in the same patient. Portal fibrosis with expansion of the portal space and increase in number of dilated interlobular bile ducts (*d*). Note the sharp delineation between portal spaces and normal hepatic parenchyma. Hematoxylin-eosin × 10. (Courtesy of Dr. E. KAHN).

LIVER DISEASE IN THE NEWBORN ASSOCIATED WITH INFECTIONS

CYTOMEGALOVIRUS NEONATAL HEPATITIS

Cytomegalovirus (CMV) is a member of the herpes group of DNA viruses which has unusual characteristics of latency, persistance, and specific clinical patterns [44]. The isolation of CMV has been confusing at times due to the impression that it often is present as an opportunistic invader.

Transmission is usually during intrauterine life, but may also occur during delivery, via breast feeding or from blood transfusions. With increased use of CMV screening of newborns for suspected infectious disease, it has become obvious that this virus is very common in congenital infections in developed countries *i. e.* 0.2 to 2.0 % of all live births. The prevalence of maternal carriers of CMV is higher in lower socioeconomic populations. Although most of these infected infants do not have the typical stigmata at birth, up to 15 % eventually develop evidence of clinical disease, most often affecting the central nervous system.

Clinically, a spectrum of typical features is associated with CMV infections (see Table I). Although anecdotal cases have been noted with biliary atresia, this etiological relationship is rare. A liver biopsy demonstrating inclusion bodies (see Fig. VIII-14), may be very suggestive, however, it is most important to document the presence of the virus infection by serological techniques. Viruria has been noted for years after infection. Giant cell transformation and a reduction in the number of intrahepatic bile ducts are not uncommon. Transfer factor and antiviral agents have been used to treat some of these infants with variable success. A vaccine is being developed.

HERPES SIMPLEX VIRUS (HSV) NEONATAL HEPATITIS

Herpes simplex virus (HSV) infections in the newborn are relatively rare and most cases of hepatitis are associated with disseminated overwhelming infection. The number of cases due to HSV-1 has been increasing during the past decade, however, HSV-2 still outnumbers the former by a ratio of 2 to 1. The mortality rate is high and extensive acute necrosis of the liver is usually found. It is noteworthy that there is a relative absence of inflammatory reactions in the liver.

The typical clinical stigmata are noted in only half of the affected infants (see Table I).

HEPATITIS A (HAV) OR B (HBV) VIRUS NEONATAL HEPATITIS

No case of neonatal hepatitis-A has ever been reported, although the widespread use of HAV markers has been limited. HBV infection in the newborn is an uncommon cause of clinical disease in this age period [37]. In developed countries verti-

TABLE I. — Liver disease in the newborn associated with infectious disorders

Infection	Clinical findings	Laboratory features	Treatment
Cytomegalovirus	Cholestasis, hepatitis, petechiae-ecchymosis, hepatosplenomegaly, encephalopathy.	Hepatic dysfunction. Thrombocytopenia, periventricular intracranial calcification, viruria, abnormal serology.	None.
Herpes simplex (disseminated)	Cholestasis, hepatomegaly, encephalopathy, vesicular eruption; very lethal.	Abnormal serology, virus cultured from lesions.	Acyclovir.
Hepatitis B	Cholestasis, hepatosplenomegaly; mothers have hepatitis B. Minimal to mild disease in most cases.	Hepatic dysfunction, abnormal serology after 4 weeks of age; maternal "e" antigenemia.	Passive immunization with HBIG plus vaccine.
Rubella	Hepatosplenomegaly, intrauterine growth retardation, eye and heart malformations, encephalopathy, purpura.	Virus cultured from tissues and body fluids; abnormal serology.	None.
Coxsackie B	Hepatosplenomegaly, myocarditis, meningoencephalitis	Hepatic dysfunction, abnormal serology.	None.
Syphilis	Cholestasis, hepatosplenomegaly, hemolytic anemia, rashes, rhinitis.	Hepatic dysfunction, bone lesions on X-ray, abnormal serology.	Penicillin.
Toxoplasmosis	Cholestasis, hepatosplenomegaly, encephalopathy, chorioretinitis, microcephaly.	Hepatic dysfunction, intracranial calcification, organisms in CSF, abnormal serology.	Sulfonamide preparations, Pyrimethamine, ? corticosteroids. Spiramycin

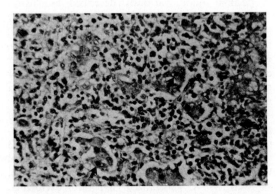

Fig. VIII-14. — *Cytomegalovirus.* Portal space with marked mononuclear infiltration and intranuclear inclusions in ductal epithelium (arrows). Hematoxylin-eosin × 500. (Courtesy of Dr. E. Kahn).

cal transmission occurs predominantly in situations where the mother has acute hepatitis-B during the 3rd trimester and rarely with a maternal carrier state. In contrast, in high prevalence developing countries, as many as 40 % of offspring of chronic carrier hepatitis-B mothers develop antigenemia. Transmission is predominantly during delivery and is greatly enhanced by the presence of high complement fixing hepatitis B surface antigen titers and "e" antigen in the infected mother. Serial blood studies in these offspring reveal that the vast majority develop antigenemia after the age of 6 weeks. Most infants become carriers, with a smaller proportion developing mild hepatitis; severe hepatitis is rare. The infected infants may be an important pool epidemiologically in later life for carrier incidence, chronic liver disease and hepatoma. Due to these late risk factors, passive and active immunization against hepatitis-B in selected newborns is considered very important.

RUBELLA VIRUS NEONATAL HEPATITIS

The association of neonatal cholestasis with multiple congenital anomalies, particularly involving the heart, eyes and hearing should suggest congenital rubella infection. In addition, signs of acute congenital rubella may be present (see Table I).

Less frequently, hepatitis may be the only feature of congenital rubella infection and is clinically indistinguishable from many other causes of neonatal cholestasis. Giant cell transformation, bile duct paucity and the rare association with extrahepatic biliary atresia have all been reported.

The correct diagnosis is confirmed by serological studies in both mother and newborn.

COXSACKIE VIRUS NEONATAL HEPATITIS

Coxsackie virus neonatal hepatitis is rare and may occur as the only manifestation of the infection. More often, signs of systemic involvement of the heart and central nervous system are evident (see Table I). Giant cell transformation of hepatocytes is common.

SYPHILITIC NEONATAL HEPATITIS

Syphilitic neonatal hepatitis occurs as part of an in utero infection and is usually accompanied by the various stigmata of congenital syphilis (see Table I). The liver biopsy reveals extensive intralobular fibrosis with mononuclear cell infiltration and cirrhosis may be present on the initial specimen.

TOXOPLASMOSIS NEONATAL HEPATITIS

Toxoplasmosis neonatal hepatitis is associated with characteristic clinical features (Table I), but less commonly may cause neonatal cholestasis alone. Liver function and liver biopsy studies are not helpful in the differential diagnosis. A positive dye test confirms the diagnosis.

TUBERCULOUS NEONATAL HEPATITIS

Tuberculous neonatal hepatitis may be acquired by aspiration of infected amniotic fluid or via the neonate's respiratory tract. Caseated granuloma are found in the liver and the infant is usually critically ill.

LIVER DISEASE IN THE NEWBORN ASSOCIATED WITH METABOLIC-GENETIC DISORDERS
(Table II)

HEREDITARY TYROSINEMIA

Hereditary tyrosinemia is the only hereditary metabolic disorder involving tyrosine that is associated with significant neonatal liver damage and infantile cirrhosis. The condition has been known by various names, including tyrosinosis, congenital tyrosinosis, tyrosinemia, tyrosyluria and hypermethioninemia.

A wide variety of clinical abnormalities have been reported usually varying with the age of the patient (see Table II). In the newborn, acute manifestations include: hepatosplenomegaly, jaundice, failure to thrive and vomiting with diarrhea. In the more severely affected infants, evidence of severe hepatic necrosis is evident i. e. a hemorrhagic diathesis due to a deficiency of liver coagulation factors and generalized edema and ascites, due to hypoalbuminemia and portal hypertension. Bouts of vomiting, diarrhea and abdominal distension may be cyclic and are often associated with febrile episodes. A peculiar odor, variously described as "fishy" "mousy" or "cabbagy", has been noted in some very sick infants, probably associated with excretion of methionine breakdown products, e. g. alpha-keto-gamma methiobutyrate. Hypoglycemia may occur at any time particularly if the infant is fasting for more than four hours at a time and hepatic coma may ensue.

Laboratory studies reveal marked elevations of aminotransferases, mixed hyperbilirubinemia, prolonged prothrombin time, hypoalbuminemia, and thrombocytopenia. Most patients have demonstrated very high plasma levels of tyrosine and methionine, as well as a generalized hyperaminoacidemia. Urinary aminoacids reflect the same abnormalities noted in the blood, and many tyrosyl derivatives are found in the urine i. e. p-OH-phenylpyruvic acid, p-OH-phenyllactic acid, p-OH-phenylacetic acid, etc. A high urinary excretion of delta-amino levulinic acid, succinylacetone and succinlyacetoacetone has been reported in a number of patients [14].

The basic biochemical defect is uncertain. The most recent speculations are focused on a deficiency of hepatic fumaryl acetoacetate hydrolase and maleylacetoacetate isomerase [25]. Abnormalities

TABLE II. — PROGRESSIVE LIVER DISEASE IN THE NEWBORN ASSOCIATED WITH METABOLIC DISORDERS

Inborn error of metabolism	Enzyme deficiency	Inheritance	Common clinical manifestations	Laboratory data
A. Carbohydrate metabolism 1. Heriditary fructose intolerance	Fructose-1-phosphate aldolase (liver)	Aut. Rec.	Vomiting, jaundice, hepatomegaly * Rx-fructose-sucrose-free diet.	↓ glucose, ↓ PO$_4$, ↓ uric acid, ↑ SGOT/SGPT, renal tubular dysfunction, liver biopsy-cholestasis, pseudotubular formation, fat accumulation.
2. Galactosemia	Galactose-1-phosphate uridyl transferase (erythrocytes, liver)	Aut. Rec.	Vomiting, jaundice, hepatomegaly, failure to thrive, neonatal sepsis, cataracts. Rx-galactose free diet.	↓ Glucose, ↑ reducing substances in the urine, abnormal liver function tests, renal tubular dysfunction; liver biopsy-cholestasis, pseudotubular formation, fat accumulation.
3. Glycogen storage disease type IV	α-1,4-glucan 6-glycosyl transferase (Brancher enzyme) (liver and leucocytes)	Aut. Rec.	Vomiting, diarrhea, failure to thrive, hepatosplenomegaly. Rx-frequent feedings, high protein diet.	Abnormal liver function tests, acidosis, liver biopsy-fatty, and excess glycogen (amylopectin).
B. Aminoacid metabolism Hereditary tyrosinemia	? fumaryl acetoacetate hydrolase and ? maleyl-acetoacetate isomerase (liver)	Aut. Rec.	Failure to thrive, jaundice, hepatosplenomegaly, Fanconi's syndrome. Rx-low phenylalanine and low tyrosine diet.	Abnormal liver function tests ↑ serum and urine tyrosine and methionine, positive ferric chloride tests, renal tubular dysfunction, ↑ urine succinylacetone and succinylacetoacetone; liver biopsy-fatty, necrosis.
C. Lipid metabolism 1. Wolman's disease	Acid lipase (leucocytes & liver)	Aut. Rec.	Vomiting, diarrhea, hepatosplenomegaly, failure to thrive, cholestasis. Rx-none.	Symetrical calcification of adrenals, anemia, vacuolation of lymphocytes, deposition of triglycerides and cholesterol esters in selected organs.
D. Bile acid metabolism 1. Familial tri-OH-co-prostanic acid (THCA) syndrome	THCA → cholic acid defect (? 24 hydroxylating enzyme)	?Aut. Rec.	Cholestasis, hepatomegaly; Rx-cholestyramine & phenobarbital.	Mixed bilirubinemia, ↓ cholic acid ↑ THCA; liver biopsy-fibrosis, paucity of intrahepatic bile ducts.
2. Byler's fatal familial cholestasis	Unknown defect	Aut. Rec.	Cholestasis, hepatosplenomegaly, steatorrhea, Pruritis, failure to thrive. Rx-cholestyramine & phenobarbital.	↑ Serum bile acids; occasionally ↑ lithocholic acid; liver biopsy-fibrosis.
E. Unclassified 1. Alpha-1-antitrypsin deficiency	Unknown defect	Co. Dom.	Cholestasis, hepatomegaly, portal hypertension. Rx-? liver transplant; ? anabolic agents, ? IV alpha-1-antitrypsin.	↓ Serum alpha-1-antitrypsin, phenotypes: PiZZ, ? PiSZ; liver biopsy-PAS positive, diastase resistant globules in periportal hepatocytes.

* Rx = Treatment

TABLE II (Continued).

Inborn error of metabolism	Enzyme deficiency	Inheritance	Common clinical manifestations	Laboratory data
2. Cystic fibrosis	Unknown defect	Aut. Rec.	Pancreatic insufficiency pulmonary infections and complications, cholestasis, hepatomegaly. Rx-extensive supportive treatment and pancreatic replacement.	↑ Sweat Cl, steatorrhea, may have abnormal liver function tests; liver biopsy-ductal proliferation, cholestasis, & focal inflammation. Inspissated intrahepatic and choledochal secretions.
3. Zellweger's syndrome (cerebro-hepato-renal syndrome)	? Mitochondrial defect	Aut. Rec.	Characteristic facies, CNS disorders, hypotonia, cholestasis, hepatomegaly. Rx-none.	↑ Precursors of cholic and chenodeoxycholic acid, ↑ serum and tissue iron, abnormal and ↑ tissue lipids, hyperpipecolaturia, skeletal abnormalities, asymptomatic renal cortical cysts; liver biopsy-fibrosis, excessive iron, abnormal mitochondria.
4. Neonatal iron storage disease	Unknown defect	?Aut. Rec.	Small for gestational age, cholestasis, hepatosplenomegaly, death occurs within 6 months of age. Rx-none.	Mild to severe disturbances of liver function tests and coagulation; liver biopsy-massive iron deposition in liver and pancreas.

in tyrosine and methionine metabolism are probably secondary rather than primary phenomena.

The liver in the newborn is usually smooth and of variable size. Hepatocytes may be transformed into a pseudoacinar pattern, and these tubular structures may encircle small plugs of bile. Fatty changes within hepatic parenchymal cells is generalized and glycogen is depleted. Evidence of giant cell transformation may be noted but inflammation is not common. Progressive fibrosis with regenerative nodules results in early micro and macronodular cirrhosis.

Hereditary tyrosinemia appears to be inherited as an autosomal recessive disorder. The best genetic studies have come from investigations of a French Canadian isolate in Quebec, Canada [38].

GALACTOSEMIA [39]

Galactosemia is one of the earliest known metabolic disorders, described about 75 years ago. It is inherited as an autosomal recessive disorder. Classical galactosemia has an incidence varying between 1 in 25,000 to 1 in 187,000 live births, and the chance frequency is estimated to be about 1.25 % of the population. The basic defect is believed to be due to a deficiency of galactose-1-phosphate-uridyl transferase, a liver enzyme necessary for the metabolism of galactose-1-phosphate. There are at least six variants of the enzyme, although the liver is affected only in the "classic" variant.

Galactosemic infants are normal at birth and do not develop signs or symptoms until they are fed galactose (as contained in lactose). Failure to thrive, recurrent bouts of vomiting and diarrhea, jaundice, anemia and a hemorrhagic diathesis are common findings. Lenticular cataracts may be present at birth, having developed during fetal life with maternal exposure to galactose. Neonatal prolonged cholestasis and sepsis are not uncommon presenting manifestations, and unexplained death associated with septicemia should give rise to suspicion of this condition.

Pathologically, the livers of affected newborns show panlobular fatty metamorphosis, portal ductular proliferation and cholestasis. Pseudoglandular or pseudoacinar transformation of hepatocytes is usually mild at this stage and the lobular architecture is intact. Giant cell transformation of hepatocytes has also been noted.

Laboratory studies reveal the presence of galactose in the urine, when the child is on a galactose containing diet. The definitive diagnostic test is the determination of erythrocytic galactose-1-phosphate-uridyl transferase, which will be less than 50 % of normal. Use of a liver biopsy for enzyme analysis is usually unnecessary.

The accumulation of galactose-1-phosphate is suspected as the important pathogenic factor. Galactose itself is not toxic systemically and the intermediate metabolite is suspected of interfering with protein synthesis and inhibiting the conversion of glycogen into glucose. The same mechanism causes the accumulation of the sugar alcohol, galactitol, in the lens, which leads to cataract formation.

HEREDITARY FRUCTOSE INTOLERANCE [10]

Hereditary fructose intolerance is due to a deficiency of fructose-1-phosphate aldolase, presumably within the liver. It is inherited as an autosomal recessive disorder and its frequency has been assessed at about 1 in 30,000 births. This disorder characteristically has a dramatic onset with the introduction of fructose containing foods. This is becoming less usual in newborns, since sucrose containing formulas are used mainly in special circumstances and it is also less common to find solid foods containing sucrose (fructose/glucose) introduced during the first month of life. Unlike older children, most affected infants do not develop a distaste for sucrose and therefore anorexia is uncommon. Protracted vomiting, hepatomegaly, jaundice and failure to thrive may be noted. Hypoglycemia has been reported in rare cases. When sucrose is used as a sweetener for baby milks, as is common in some areas in Europe, earlier and more severe manifestations may be noted. Evidence of renal tubular dysfunction may be noted at a very young age.

The hepatic pathology is similar to that of hereditary tyrosinemia and galactosemia. Significant fatty metamorphosis of hepatocytes is noted and cholestasis which is both hepatocellular and canalicular may be found. Pseudoacinar transformation is noted even at an early stage. Practically all of these early abnormalities disappear with the removal of fructose from the diet.

The basic defect in hereditary fructose intolerance is a deficiency or absence of the enzyme fructose-1-phosphate aldolase. Although the accumulation of fructose-1-phosphate has always been considered to be the toxigenic factor, there is no evidence to support this claim. Another proposed mechanism for the toxic effects, particularly the hepatogenic hypoglycemia, is the rapid phosphorylation of fructose to fructose-1-phosphate which results in a relative deficiency of adenosinetriphosphates.

The diagnosis is usually made by the demonstration of fructose in the urine when the patient is on a fructose containing diet. Fructose-1-phosphate aldolase may be directly assayed from a needle biopsy of liver tissue. The use of a fructose tolerance test may cause hypoglycemia and is therefore not recommended for diagnosis, except in unusual circumstances. Exclusion of fructose-containing foods from the diet in the affected newborn will prevent liver damage. Newborns in families with affected siblings should be on the diet from birth and tested for the defect at 2-3 months of age.

ALPHA-1-ANTITRYPSIN DEFICIENCY

Alpha-1-antitrypsin (alpha-1-AT) deficiency has long been known for its association with young adult familial emphysema. Fortuitously, an etiological relationship between infantile cirrhosis and this protease inhibitor was established [24]. Today, a variety of related hepatic disorders are documented, with the majority of infants presenting with prolonged neonatal cholestasis.

Alpha-1-AT is a glycoprotein which constitutes 90 % of the alpha-1-globulin fraction of serum. It is synthesized in hepatocytes and genetic polymorphism can be demonstrated by starch gel electrophoresis with or without isoelectric focusing. At least 24 different alleles can be documented using protease inhibitor (Pi) genotyping and they have been labelled with the letters of the alphabet, according to their electrophoretic mobility. PiM is the most common allele, contributing 50 % of the normal protease level, while PiZ, which is most often associated with hepatic and lung disease, contributes only 15-20 %. A rare Pi- (or Pi null) produces no alpha-1-AT. The inheritance pattern is codominant. Virtually, all affected pediatric patients are of the PiZZ genotype, although liver disease in adult PiZ heterozygotes has been recorded. In western populations the incidence of PiZZ is about 1 in 2,000 [32], with lesser frequency in blacks, making it a relatively common genetic disorder.

The exact mechanism of damage to the liver in patients with alpha-1-AT is unknown. The accumulation of the eosinophilic intracytoplasmic globules is not injurious, since they are found in about 10 %

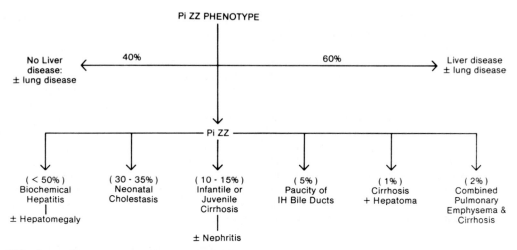

FIG. VIII-15. — *Alpha-1-antitrypsin deficiency PiZZ phenotypes.* Only 60 % of PiZZ develop liver disease, and in children 2 % of these have combined hepatic and pulmonary manifestations. PiZZ infants constitute one-quarter of all cases of neonatal cholestasis.

of PiZ homozygotes and heterozygotes without any evidence of liver disease, at any time.

The majority of PiZZ infants present with typical prolonged neonatal cholestasis (see Fig. VIII-15). Occasionally, the infants may demonstrate evidence of hypoprothrombinemia and ascites. The various liver function tests are not helpful, including radionuclide scintigraphy, Some infants appear to lose their jaundice after a few weeks, however, the prognosis should be guarded since slowly progressive liver disease may ensue. As a matter of fact, children who present with cirrhosis and a neonatal history of transient cholestasis will be alpha-1-AT deficient in more than 80 % of cases.

The liver biopsy is usually helpful but experience is necessary, since some features of extrahepatic biliary atresia or paucity of intrahepatic bile ducts may be present. The finding of intracytoplasmic globules in the periportal cells is diagnostic. These globules are best distinguished by their periodic-acid-schiff staining, resistant to diastase treatment (Fig. VIII-16). During the first 1-2 months of life the globules may only be detected by electron microscopic examination. The accumulated globules can be verified as probable precursors of alpha-1-AT by immunofluorescence. Membrano-proliferative glomerulonephritis, chronic active hepatitis, cirrhosis and hepatomas have been noted in older children, but have never been seen in the neonatal period.

Treatment has been mainly symptomatic and supportive. A successful liver transplant was performed in a sixteen year old with end stage cirrhosis [17]. Intravenous alpha-1-AT has been tried

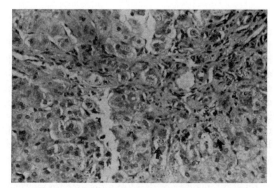

FIG. VIII-16. — *Alpha-1-antitrypsin deficiency.* Note the PAS positive diastase resistant globular inclusions in the periportal hepatocytes (arrows). D-PAS stain × 500. (Courtesy of Dr. E. KAHN).

with poor results and recently investigators have attempted to stimulate alpha-1-AT production by the use of anabolic non-virilizing agents.

CEREBRO-HEPATO-RENAL SYNDROME (CHRS) OR ZELLWEGER'S SYNDROME

The cerebro-hepato-renal syndrome (CHRS) describes a familial congenital disorder which has metabolic overtones. Most infants present in the newborn period with generalized hypotonia, a mongoloid facies (Fig. VIII-5b), cerebral dysfunction, mild to progressive liver disease, and numerous skeletal anomalies, the most common being chondral calcifications. Asymptomatic renal cortical cysts have been found in all autopsied cases. Liver histology includes fatty metamorphosis and periportal fibrosis. Excessive iron deposition is often seen in the hepatocytes and Kupfer cells. Neonatal cholestasis is rare. Metabolic abnormalities include pipecolic aciduria, excess trihydroxycoprostanic acid in the blood, and abnormal peroxisome and mitochondrial functions [11].

WOLMAN'S DISEASE
(VISCERAL XANTHOMATOSIS)

Wolman's disease is due to a deficiency of lysosomal acid lipase resulting in an accumulation of cholesterol ester and triglycerides in tissues throughout the body associated with a high cholesterol turnover e. g. adrenal, intestinal mucosa, liver and spleen [33]. An autosomal recessive inheritance has been documented.

The infants present during the first month of life with diarrhea, failure to thrive and cholestasis. Progressive hepatosplenomegaly is noted and calcifications and bilateral enlargement of the adrenal glands are the hallmarks of this disorder. The disease is progressive and uniformly fatal before the age of 6 months. Ante-natal diagnosis is possible by amniotic fluid analysis.

CHOLESTASIS WITH PERIPHERAL LYMPHATIC AND HEMANGIOMATOUS ABNORMALITIES (AAGENAES SYNDROME)

A number of kindreds, mainly of Norwegian ancestry, have been described with a history of prolonged familial neonatal cholestasis [1]. Defective peripheral and hepatic lymphatics have been demonstrated by lymphangiography. The development of lymphedema of the lower extremities occurs after 5 years of age in most cases, but has been noted in the newborn. A number of patients and unaffected family member have cutaneous lymphangiomas and hemangiomas.

Liver biopsies usually reveal normal or proliferating bile ducts often with giant cell transformation. Steatorrhea and hypoprothrombinemia are commonly found. Cirrhosis is rare.

FAMILIAL HEPATIC STEATOSIS

A variety of familial clinical syndromes have been reported in newborn and young infants with severe hepatic steatosis [46]. The onset is usually sudden and almost all have died after a very short illness. Of the 24 cases in the literature, there is no sexual predilection and the inheritance is probably an autosomal recessive. Clinical evidence of liver disease may be absent, particularly in apparently normal newborns dying within a few days of onset of the illness.

Histologic evidence of widespread fatty metamorphosis has been noted in the liver, myocardium and kidneys. However, the degree and organ involvement varies in different siblings. Microscopically, the fat consists of both fine and coarse vacuoles and histochemical analysis is also variable *i. e.* neutral fat, fatty acids, etc.

CYSTIC FIBROSIS

Cystic fibrosis is the most common lethal hereditary disease among the Caucasian population.

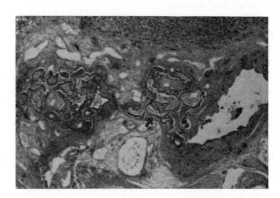

FIG. VIII-17. — *Cystic fibrosis.* Large portal space with inspissated eosinophilic material contained within dilated bile ducts (arrows). Hematoxylin-eosin × 10. (Courtesy of Dr. E. KAHN).

If affects one child in every 2 500 live births and is inherited in an autosomal recessive fashion. Liver disease in older infants and children is very common, however, in the newborn period rare cases present with prolonged neonatal cholestasis [29]. Many of these do not have the more traditional pulmonary or gastrointestinal manifestations, although meconium ileus is common. Liver biopsy may reveal focal inflammation and eosinophilic concretions in the interlobular bile ducts (Fig. VIII-17). The common hepatic duct may be obstructed by thick viscid secretions. Milder cases clear spontaneously or with choleretics.

SYNDROMATIC PAUCITY
OF INTRAHEPATIC BILE DUCTS
(see p. 1020)

INFANTILE IRON STORAGE DISEASE

An infantile form of iron storage disease affects the liver, pancreas, heart, endocrine and exocrine glands [12]. The onset of jaundice associated with cirrhosis and giant cell transformation may occur in the first few days of life. Excessive iron deposition in the hepatic parenchymal cells differentiates this condition from transfusion hemosiderosis in which iron is found predominantly in the reticuloendothelial cells. This disorder must be separated from the cerebrohepatorenal syndrome and hereditary tyrosinemia where a similar iron storage may be noted. There appears to be an autosomal recessive type of inheritance, however, there is no overlap with the idiopathic hemochromatosis seen in older children and adults.

Infants with *Niemann-Pick, Gaucher, Glycogenosis type IV, Fucosidosis, Mannosidosis* and *Cholesterol-ester* and *Urea cycle disorders* rarely show serious newborn liver damage (see Table III). Hepatomegaly is common, however, cholestasis and severe hepatic dysfunction, if they occur at all, are usually delayed until after the first month of life.

TABLE III. — MILD LIVER DISEASE
IN THE NEWBORN ASSOCIATED WITH METABOLIC DISORDERS *

1. *Storage diseases*
   a) Glycogenesis types I, II, III, VI.
   b) Gm-1 Gangliosidosis.
   c) Gaucher's disease.
   d) Niemann-Pick disease.
   e) Mucopolysaccharidosis.
   f) Sandhoff's disease.
   g) Mucolipidosis
   h) Fucosidosis.
   i) Mannosidosis.
   j) Cholesterol ester storage disease.

2. *Fatty livers*
   a) Reye's Syndrome.
   b) A-beta-lipoproteinemia.
   c) Excessive fat ingestion.
   d) Diabetes mellitus.
   e) Urea cycle disorders.
   f) Aminoacidopathies e. g. homocystinuria, methylmalonic aciduria, familial protein intolerance, etc.

* Most commenty found in other infants and children.

LIVER DISEASE IN THE NEWBORN
DUE TO TUMORS

VASCULAR TUMORS

Primary neoplasms of the liver are common during the first year of life, but most categories do not surface clinically in the neonatal period. The main exceptions are vascular tumors (hemangiomas), consisting of infantile hemangioendotheliomas, or the more common cavernous hemangioma.

Hemangiomas are congenital vascular malformations containing fibrous tissue and variably sized vascular channels. They are the commonest benign tumors of infants [15]. In some reports the ratio of females to males is 2 to 1.

Hepatomegaly is the most common presenting sign, sometimes associated with an audible bruit. Liver function tests are usually within normal limits, however, some cases present with neonatal cholestasis and diffusely abnormal liver function tests. Many infants have elevated alpha-fetoprotein. Florid congestive heart failure due to arterio-venous shunting is not uncommon. Other serious complications include rupture, disseminated intravascular coagulopathy and a hemrorrhagic diathesis due to hypoprothrombinemia or thrombocytopenia (Kassabach-Merritt Syndrome). These coagulopathies are associated with consumption and sequestration, respectively. More than half the patients also have benign cutaneous hemangiomata.

Non-invasive ultrasonography may be diagnostic and will determine the extent of the lesion. These hypervascularized lesions are amenable to angiographic studies. In the newborn, umbilical arteriography may clearly define the tumor mass. Venous angiography can also provide excellent details of the vascularity of the tumor.

Although the hepatic hemangiomas decrease with time, the reduction in size is often not as complete or rapid as the cutaneous lesions. On the other hand, the infant with signs of heart failure or coagulopathy requires urgent intervention. Radiation therapy, 400 to 600 rads over a 10-14 day period, and prednisone 20 mg daily or every other day have been associated with rapid regression in most but not all cases. In those infants who do not respond, ligation of the hepatic artery is indicated, although the results are variable.

HEPATOBLASTOMA

Hepatoblastoma, although rare, is the most commonly reported primary malignant neoplasm of the liver, accounting for 5-10 % of these tumors [18]. It usually presents with asymptomatic hepatic enlargement and normal liver function tests except for an elevated serum alpha-fetoprotein. Hepatoblastomas show a male predilection and are occasionally associated with hemihypertrophy and widespread hemangiomata. The diagnosis is made by sonography and angiographic studies. Resection of these malignant tumors is the treatment of choice, however, with a very large tumor mass, pretreatment with radiation and chemotherapy is indicated. Except with complete resection, the prognosis must be guarded.

PELIOSIS HEPATIS

Peliosis hepatis is a congenital lesion of unknown etiology which is characterized by blood filled spaces in the parenchyma of the liver associated with areas of necrosis [31]. Hepatomegaly with normal to mild disturbances of liver function tests are the usual presenting manifestations.

METASTATIC NEOPLASMS

Neuroblastoma is the commonest congenital malignant neoplasm. In the newborn, almost 20 % are found to have hepatic metastases at the time of the original diagnosis (Pepper syndrome). Giant hepatomegaly is frequently noted occuring over a relatively short period of time. Liver function tests are usually normal and jaundice is uncommon. The primary lesion may be visualized in the abdomen with an intravenous pyelogram, but it may also be extra-abdominal. Serum catecholamines are elevated in most cases. This metastatic type of neuroblastoma responds dramatically to a short course of irradiation and chemotherapy. The general approach to management is conservative, since infants without bone metastases have a relatively good survival rate. Spontaneous regression is not uncommon.

A blind liver biopsy is contraindicated, since the incidence of post-biopsy hemorrhage is high.

LIVER DISEASE ASSOCIATED WITH HEPATOTOXIC AGENTS

A wide variety of potentially hepatotoxic agents are prescribed or otherwise given either to the mother at term or to the vulnerable newborn. The hepatic reaction is often similar to any other neonatal cholestatic syndrome and should be differentiated early. The toxicity may be due to effects on only one metabolic function e. g. 17-alpha-alkyl-substituted steroids on bile flow, or more severe hepatocellular injury e. g. antithyroid drugs, antipyretics [7] and antibiotics [6].

Pyrrolizidine alkaloids are found in a variety of plant species, particularly crotolaria and senecio. *Venoocclusive disease* causing endophlebitis in the central veins in the liver has been recorded in young infants and children in Jamaica exposed to "bush-tea" or maternal milk containing the alkaloids [45].

Intravenous alimentation has been associated with cholestasis and progressive liver damage [48]. These abnormalities are probably due to a number of agents in the intravenous solutions affecting the vulnerable host who is usually a malnourished newborn infant. Putative factors include amino acids, hyperamonemia and fatty acids. One-third of infants treated in this manner for more than 2 weeks develop some form of hepatic abnormality. The majority respond to discontinuing or modifying the therapy e. g. rate of administration.

REFERENCES

[1] AAGENAES (O.), VANDERHOGAN (C. V.), REFSUM (S.). — Hereditary recurrent intrahepatic cholestasis from birth. *Arch. Dis. Childh.*, 43, 646-657, 1968.
[2] ALTMAN (R. P.). — Biliary atresia: Current perspectives in surgical treatment. In: *Clinical Disorders in Pediatric Gastroenterology and Nutrition.* Edited by F. LIFSHITZ, Marcel DEKKER, Inc., New York and Basel, 89-99, 1980.
[3] BANGARU (B.), MORECKI (R.), GLASER (J. H.), GARTNER (L. M.), HOROWITZ (M. S.). — Comparative studies of biliary atresia in the human newborn and reovirus-induced cholangitis in mice. *Lab. Investig.*, 43, 456-462, 1980.
[4] BERNSTEIN (J.), BROWN (K.). — Sepsis and jaundice in early infancy. *Pediatrics*, 29, 873-882, 1962.
[5] BERNSTEIN (J.), CHANG (C. H.), BROUGH (A. J.), HEIDELBERGER (K. P.). — Conjugated hyperbilirubinemia in infancy associated with parenteral alimentation. *J. Pediatr.*, 90, 361-367, 1977.

[6] BISTRITZER (R.), BARILAY (Z.), JONAS (A.). — Iso-niazid-rifampin induced fulminant liver disease in an infant. *J. Pediatr.*, 97, 480-482, 1980.

[7] BULUGAHAPITIYA (D. T.), HEBRON (B.), BECK (P. R.). — Salicylate hepatitis with acidosis in an infant. *Lancet*, 1, 1295-1296, 1979.

[8] CHANDRA (R. S.), ALTMAN (R. P.). — Ductal remnants in extrahepatic biliary atresia: a histo-pathological study with clinical correlation. *J. Pediatr.*, 93, 196-200, 1978.

[9] DOUILLET (P.), BRUNNELL (F.), CHAUMONT (P.) et al. — Ultrasonography and percutaneous cholangiography in children with dilated bile ducts. *Am. J. Dis. Child.*, 135, 131-133, 1981.

[10] GITZELMAN (R.), STEINMANN (B.), VANDENBER-GHE (G.).— *Hereditary fructose intolerance in The Metabolic Basis of Inherited Disease*. Ed. J. B. STAN-BURY, J. B. WYNGAARDEN, D. S. FREDRICKSON, J. GOLDSTEIN and M. BROWN. 5th Edition, McGraw-Hill, New York, 124-132, 1982.

[11] GOLDFISCHER (S.), MOORE (V. L.). — Peroxisomal and mitochondrial defects in the cerebro-hepato-renal syndrome. *Science*, 182, 62-64, 1973.

[12] GOLDFISCHER (S.), GROTSKY (H. W.), CHANG (C. H.), BERMAN (E. L.), RICKERT (R. R.), KARMARKER (S. T.), ROSKAMP (J. O.), MORECKI (R.). — Idio-pathic neonatal iron storage involving the liver, pancreas, heart and endocrine and exocrine glands. *Hepatology*, 1, 58-64, 1981.

[13] GREENE (H. L.), HELINEK (G. L.), MORAN (R.), O'NEILL (J.). — A diagnostic approach to prolonged obstructive jaundice by 24 hour collection of duo-denal fluid. *J. Pediatr.*, 95, 412-414, 1979.

[14] GRENIER (A.), LESCAULT (A.), LABERGE (C.) et al. — Detection of succinylacetone and the use of its measurement in mass screening for hereditary tyrosinemia. *Clin. Chim. Acta*, 123, 93-99, 1982.

[15] GRUNER (M.), JABLONSKI (J. P.). — Angiomes du foie. *Ann. Chir. Infant.*, 17, 408, 1976.

[16] HANSON (F.), ISENBERG (J.), NEVIN (J.), WILLIAMS (G.) et al. — The metabolism of 3,7,12 trihy-droxy-5 Cholestan-26-Oic acid in two siblings with cholestasis due to intrahepatic bile duct anomalies. *J. Clin. Invest.*, 56, 557-587, 1975.

[17] HOOD (J. M.), KOPE (L. J.), PETERS (R. L.) et coll. — Liver transplantation for advanced liver disease with alpha-1-antitrypsin deficiency. *N. Engl. J. Med.*, 302, 272-275, 1980.

[18] ISHAK (K. G.), GLUNZ (P.). — Hepatoblastoma and hepatic carcinoma in infancy and childhood: report of 47 cases. *Cancer*, 20, 396-422, 1967.

[19] JAVITT (N. B.), MORRISSEY (K. P.), STIEGEL (E.) et al. — Cholestatic syndromes in infancy: dia-gnostic value of serum bile acid pattern and choles-tyramine administration. *Pediat. Res.*, 7, 119-125, 1973.

[20] JOHNSTON (D. I.), MOWAT (A. P.), ORR (H.), KOHN (J.). — Alpha-fetoprotein in the diagnosis of obstructive jaundice. *Acta Pediatr. Scand.*, 65, 633-629, 1976.

[21] KASAI (M.), SUZJKI (H.), OHSHAHI (E.), OHI (R.), CHIBA (T.), OKAMOTO (A.). — Technique and result of operative management of biliary atresia. *World J. Surg.*, 2, 571-580, 1978.

[22] KLINGENSMITH III (W. C.), FRITZBERG (A. R.), SPITZER (V. M.) et al. — Clinical comparison of 99 m technetium diethylida and 99m technetium PAPIDA for evaluation of the hepatobiliary sys-tems. *Radiology*, 134, 195-199, 1980.

[23] KOBAYASHI (A.), OHBE (Y.). — Choledochal cyst in infancy and childhood: analysis of 16 cases. *Arch. Dis. Child.*, 52, 121-128, 1977.

[24] LATIMER (J. S.), SHARP (H. L.). — Alpha-1-anti-trypsin deficiency in childhood. In: *Current Problems in Pediatrics*, 11 ed. GLUCK (L.), Chicago Year Book Medical Publishers, 1980.

[25] LINDBLAD (B.), LINDSTEDT (S.), STEEN (G.). — On the defects in hereditary tyrosinemia. *Proc. Natl. Acad. Sci. USA*, 74, 4641-4645, 1977.

[26] MAJD (M.), REBA (R. C.), ALTMAN (R.P.). — Hepa-tobiliary scintigraphy with technetium 99 PAPIDA in the evaluation of neonatal jaundice. *Pediatrics*, 76, 140-145, 1981.

[27] MARKOWITZ (J.), DAUM (F.), KAHN (E.) et al. — Arteriohepatic Dysplasia. I. Pitfalls of Diagnosis and Management. *Hepatology*, 3, 74-76, 1983.

[28] MELHORN (D. K.), GROSS (S.), IZANT (R. J..) Jr. — The red cell hydrogen peroxide hemolysis test and vitamin E absorption in the differential diagnosis of jaundice in infancy. *J. Pediatr.*, 81, 1082-1087, 1972.

[29] MOWAT (A. P.). — *Liver Disorders in Childhood*. Butterworths, London, 1979.

[30] NEZELOF (C.), DUPARAT (H. C.), JOUBARD (T. F.), ELISCHAR (E.). — A lethal familial syndrome asso-ciating arthrogryposis multiplex congenita, renal dysfunction and a cholestatic and pigmentary liver disease. *J. Pediatr.*, 94, 258-260, 1979.

[31] NUERNBERGER (S. P.), RAMOS (C. V.). — Peliosis hepatis in an infant. *J. Pediatr.*, 87, 424-426, 1975.

[32] O'BRIEN (M.), BURST (N.), MURPHY (W.). — Neo-natal screening for alpha-1-antitrypsin deficiency. *J. Pediatr.*, 92, 1006-1010, 1978.

[33] PATRICK (A. D.), LAKE (B. D.). — Deficiency of acid lipase in Wolman's disease. *Nature*, 222, 1067-1068, 1969.

[34] POLEY (J. R.), SMITH (E. J.), BOON (D. J.) et al. — Lipoprotein-x and the double 131 I-Rose Bengal test in the diagnosis of prolonged obstructive jaundice. *J. Ped. Surg.*, 7, 660-669, 1972.

[35] RIELY (C.), COTILIER (E.), JENSEN (P.) et al. — Arteriohepatic dysplasia: a benign syndrome of intrahepatic cholestasis with multiple organ invol-vement. *Ann. Int. Med.*, 91, 520-527, 1979.

[36] ROY (C. C.), SILVERMAN (A.), COZZETTO (F. J.). — *Pediatric Clinical Gastroentrology*. 2nd edition, C. V. Mosby Co., St. Louis, 1975.

[37] SCHWEITZER (I. L.). — Infection of neonate and infants with hepatitis B virus. *Prog. Med. Virol.*, 20, 27-48, 1975.

[38] SCRIVER (C. R.), LAROCHELLE (J.), SILVERBERG (M.). — Hereditary tyrosinemia and tyrosyluria in a French Canadian isolate. *Am. J. Dis. Child.*, 113, 41-46, 1967.

[39] SEGAL (S.). — Disorders of galactose metabolism. In: *The Metabolic Basis of Inherited Disease*. Eds. J. B. STANBURY, J. B. WYNGAARDEN, D. S. FREDRICKSON, J. GOLDSTEIN and M. BROWN. 5th ed., McGraw-Hill, New York, 167-191, 1982.

[40] SHEBA (T.), KASAI (M.), SASANO (N.). — Histo-pathological studies on intrahepatic bile ducts in the vicinity of porta hepatis in biliary atresia. *J. Ped. Surg.*, 16, 152, 1981.

[41] SILVERBERG (M.), ROSENTHALL (L.), FREEMAN (L.). — Rose Bengal excretion studies as an aid in the differential diagnosis of neonatal jaundice. In: *Pediatric Nuclear Medicine*. Ed. L. M. FREEMAN and D. M. BLAUFOX, Grune & Stratton, New York, 151-162, 1975.

[42] SILVERBERG (M.), CRAIG (J.), GELLIS (S. S.). — Problems in the diagnosis of biliary atresia. *Am. J. Child.*, *11*, 574-584, 1960.

[43] SILVERBERG (M.). — Chronic liver disease in children. In: *The Liver and Biliary System in Infants and Children*. Ed. R. K. CHANDRA. Churchill Livingstone, Edinburgh, London and New York, 174-195, 1979.

[44] STARR (S. E.). — Cytomegalovirus. *Pediatr. Clin. N. Am.*, *26*, 283-293, 1979.

[45] STUART (K. L.), BRAS (G.). — Veno-occlusive disease of the liver. *Quart. J. Med.*, *26*, 291-315, 1957.

[46] SUPRUN (H.), FREUNDLICH (E.). — Fatal familial steatosis of myocardium, liver and kidneys. *Acta Paediatr. Scand.*, *70*, 247-252, 1981.

[47] TAKADI (H.), MIURA (K.), YAMAGATA (S.). — Peritoneoscope: present status in Japan. In: *Advances in Gastrointestinal Endoscopy*. Padna Piccia, 393-397, 1972.

[48] TOULOUKIAN (R. J.), SEASHORE (J. H.). — Hepatic secretory obstruction with total parenteral nutrition in the infant. *J. Ped. Surg.*, *10*, 353-360, 1975.

[49] WATSON (G. H.), MILLER (V.). — Arteriohepatic dysplasia: familial pulmonary arterial stenosis with neonatal liver disease. *Arch. Dis. Child.*, *48*, 459-466, 1973.

[50] WAYE (J. D.). — Endoscopic retrograde cholangiopancreatography in an infant. *Am. J. Gastroenterol.*, *65*, 461, 1976.

[51] WITZLEBEN (C. L.). — Bile duct paucity (intrahepatic atresia). In: *Perspectives in Pediatric Pathol.* Ed. H. S. ROSENBERG and J. BERNSTEIN, Masson Publishing USA, Inc., New York, 7, 185-201, 1982.

[52] LILLY (J. R.), STELLIN (G.), PAU (C. L. M.), OHI (R.). — Historical background of the biliary atresia registry. In: *Extrahepatic Biliary Atresia* F. DAUM and S. E. FISCHER, Marcel DEKKER Pub., New York and Basel, 73-77, 1983.

45

Surgical problems of the newborn

Pierre-Paul COLLIN, M. D.

with the collaboration of

Arié L. Bensoussan, M. D., Jacques C. Ducharme, M. D., Frank M. Guttman, M. D., Alain Ouimet, M. D., Hervé Blanchard, M. D. and Sami Youssef, M. D.

Lesions of the neck

Alain OUIMET, M. D.

CYSTIC HYGROMA

Etiology. — The embryology of this tumor like malformation resides in the arrest of maturation of primary lymphatic sacs and of their union with the venous system.

Localisation. — These masses are found mainly in the neck and are rarely so invasive as to cause symptoms. Cystic hygromas are either on the right or the left of the midline sometimes extending into the floor of the mouth or the superior mediastinum. The most frequent primary site is the posterior triangle of the neck.

Symptomatology and diagnosis. — A mass in the neck of soft consistency is most often seen shortly after birth but can be discovered a few months later. These masses are covered with thinned skin and are mainly whithish in color. Redness and pain will be present if infection complicates the lesion; if traumatized, a bluish tint will appear signifying blood inside the cysts. Hemangiomatous elements can also give a blue color.

Localisation, consistency and evolution are the main diagnostic features of cystic hygroma. The laboratory does not contribute to the diagnosis and radiologic imaging can be used to show extension and compression.

Pathology. — Macroscopic examination shows multiple cystic spaces of varied volumes containing clear or milky fluid. Histological slides show angiomatous epithelium bordering large empty spaces. Inflammatory cells are present if infection complicates the evolution and hemangiomatous elements are defined when present. Malignant degeneration has not been reported.

Treatment. — Surgery is the only effective treatment. Infection contra-indicates surgery and antibiotics are the treatment of choice followed by a drainage procedure when needed. Definitive surgery may be postponed indefinitely as involution sometime follows an inflammatory reaction.

Surgery is usually a simple excisional procedure when extension and adhesions to nervous and vascular structures are limited. It should not be delayed after the diagnosis has been made and should be done as an elective procedure when not complicated by compression and respiratory distress.

General anesthesia is mandatory and a transverse cervical approach is preferred. This approach should be modified where the floor of the mouth or the mediastinum are to be explored. Mutilating surgery is not justified. As many cystic spaces should be excised as possible leaving vital structures intact.

Complications and prognosis. — Hematoma and recurrence are rare with meticulous surgery and the use of aspirating drains under the skin flaps. Antibiotics are used regularly in newborn and young infants. Deaths are usually associated with lesions so extensive that vital prognosis was guarded from the beginning.

HEMANGIOMA

Hemangiomas in the neck are related to the skin and the parotid glands. They may be of a capillary or mixed type and involution is the natural process. When the diagnosis is in doubt, especially as relates to parotid lesions, biopsy can be done using careful hemostasis.

Different approches are used when involution does not occur or when enlargement produces local complications. Steroids have been used either locally or systemically to induce involution or to treat secondary complications due to size. Radiotherapy may be helpful in localized lesion but long term complications especially in the head and neck region render the use of this therapy exceptional. Surgery can be performed but is not without complications as permanent facial nerve lesions can be seen in up to 25 % of cases. Nerve grafting procedures as used today would probably lower this percentage.

INFLAMMATORY MASSES

Inflammatory masses, adenitis and absceses, in the neck are related to contamination either in the nursery or at home by direct contact. Adenitis leading to abscess formation is rarely caused by bacteria other than staphylococcus in the newborn period. Latent periods of up to 90 days have been reported. Antibiotics are used in the pre-abscess phase but drainage is the usual procedure when the abscess is established. Culture is mandatory.

Parotitis, mostly staphylococcal, is rarely seen in the newborn period. These children are often severely sick, dehydrated and prone to infection. Rehydration, buccal hygiene and antibiotics form the basis of treatment. Prognosis is related to prematurity and associated malformations.

SUGGESTED READING

[1] CONLEY (John). — *Salivary glands and the facial nerve.* Georg Thieme, Publishers, 1975.

Tracheal anomalies of the newborn

Alain OUIMET, M. D.

TRACHEOMALACIA

Respiratory distress of varying severity can be caused by tracheomalacia. It can be diagnosed by tracheoscopy when observing rhythmic occlusion of the trachea with each inspiration. Immature car-tilagenous rings are the anatomic feature of this lesion. Dyspnea, with or without cyanosis, intercostal and supraclavicular tugging and decreased alveolar breath sounds at auscultation are the main findings suggesting this condition. Newborns with severe symptoms require prolonged tracheal intubation as a supportive measure but most will have moderate to mild symptoms, when treated with good respiratory care. Tracheomalacia is usually a self correcting disease as maturation of the tracheal rings increases with age. Surgery has been used with success in severe and longstanding cases. Recurrent respiratory infection is the commonest complication.

TRACHEAL STENOSIS

Tracheal stenosis is usually an acquired lesion. Prolonged tracheal intubation in premature and term newborns is the usual cause.

The stenosis is sub-glottic in most cases and the severity of symptoms is related to the residual internal diameter of the trachea. Treatment is determined by the degree of stenosis and the associated symptoms. In patients with mild to moderate stenosis and few symptoms, tracheoscopy at regular intervals will assess tracheal growth and determine the necessity for additional treatment. In moderate to severe stenosis with severe symptoms, surgery is the treatment of choice, either as an endotracheal procedure or as a resection and anastomosis procedure. The experience of the surgeon is an important determinant in the success of surgery. Tracheal stenosis can be congenital and requires urgent

treatment as these newborns present with severe neonatal asphyxia. Tracheostomy following endoscopy (when possible) is the treatment of choice since tracheal intubation will not be possible. Definitive surgery is planned when the child is older.

TRACHEAL CYSTS AND ANGIOMAS

Tracheal cysts and angiomas are rare lesions. Recurrent upper respiratory tract infection is the usual form of presentation. Diagnosis is established by endoscopy and surgical treatment is advisable.

VOCAL CORD PARALYSIS

Vocal cord paralysis is rare in the newborn. The etiology other than traumatic is unknown. We have seen a single case where compression of the recurrent laryngeal nerve by a large pericardial cyst was treated by removal of the cyst followed by normal vocal cord function.

SUGGESTED READING

[1] BLUESTONE (Charles D.), STOOL (Sylvan E.). — Ed. W. B. SAUNDERS, Publishers, 1983.

Esophageal atresia

Jean-Gauthier DESJARDINS

INTRODUCTION

Prior to 1940, esophageal atresia, was always a lethal condition. The first patients to survive this condition were operated on by Leven and Ladd in 1939 using a multi-stage technique: closure of the distal fistula, cervical esophagostomy, gastrostomy and later esophageal replacement.

In 1941, Dr Cameron Haight was the first to successfully treat this anomaly by closure of the fistula and primary anastomosis of the esophagus.

Since that time, the survival rate of these patients has improved and is reported to be between 63 and 90 % [33].

INCIDENCE

Esophageal atresia is reported to occur from 1 per 2,500 to 1 per 6,800 births [34].

EMBRYOLOGY

The primitive intestine, which at the beginning is a tube-like structure, will give rise to the esophagus from its posterior wall formed by stratified epithelium and to the trachea from its anterior wall formed by cylindrical ciliated epithelium. Laterally, on each side, these epithelial cells proliferate toward the inside of the primitive intestine and fuse together in the midline to create the two tubes: the trachea and the esophagus. These cells will degenerate and be replaced by mesenchymatous tissue. A fault in this process of epithelialisation will result in esophageal atresia and/or tracheo-esophageal fistula.

CLASSIFICATION

Many classifications have been proposed to describe these anomalies. Ladd's classification which appears to be the one most widely known, has been used in our series of 100 cases observed at Ste-Justine Hospital, during a ten year period (1962-1971).

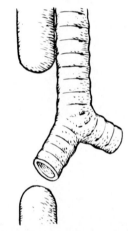

Fig. VIII-18. — *Œsophageal atresia.*

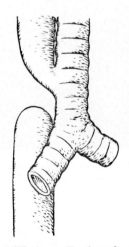

Fig. VIII-19. — *Œsophageal atresia with a proximal tracheo-œsophageal fistula.*

Type I (Fig. VIII-18): Esophageal atresia without fistula; 17 patients (17 %).

Type II (Fig. VIII-19): Esophageal atresia with a proximal tracheo-esophageal fistula; 0 patient (0 %).

Type III and IV (Fig. VIII-20): Esophageal atresia with a distal tracheo-esophageal fistula; 80 patients (80 %).

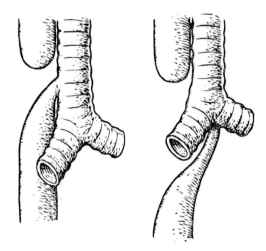

Fig. VIII-20. — *Œsophageal atresia with a distal tracheo-œsophageal fistula.*

Type V (Fig. VIII-21): Esophageal atresia with a proximal and distal tracheo-esophageal fistula; 1 patient (1 %).

Type VI (Fig. VIII-22): Tracheo-esophageal fistula without esophageal atresia; 2 patients (2 %).

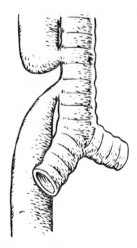

Fig. VIII-21. — *Œsophageal atresia with a proximal and a distal tracheo-œsophageal fistula.*

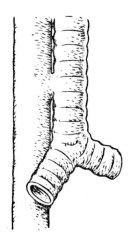

FIG. VIII-22. — *Tracheo-œsophageal fistula*
(H type).

CLINICAL PRESENTATION

Esophageal atresia can be suspected and identified at birth [12, 22, 24, 36]. The clinical signs most often observed are: Excessive salivation, cyanotic spells, respiratory distress and dysphagia.

In patients with esophageal atresia, the swallowing mechanism is impaired. The saliva accumulates in the proximal esophageal pouch and pharynx, and causes cyanotic spells and respiratory distress when it overspills into the trachea.

If these infants are fed, they will choke, cough and develop cyanosis. When the buccopharyngeal secretions are aspirated they immediately become pink and normal.

Esophageal atresia must then be immediately suspected when a newborn presents excessive secretions and the esophageal patency must be determined.

A distal tracheo-esophageal fistula may be suspected in a newborn who presents with abnormal abdominal distention. The fistula will allow air to reach the stomach and small intestines, giving rise to intestinal distention. The fistula will also allow reflux of gastro-intestinal contents up into the trachea, causing a chemical pneumonitis. When there is no fistula, the abdomen is scaphoid and soft.

DIAGNOSIS

When esophageal atresia is suspected, the diagnosis can rapidly be confirmed by inserting a catheter down the esophagus. This catheter must be rigid

and also the largest that can pass through the nostril of the infant, otherwise if it is small and soft it can curl in the proximal esophagus, wrongly suggesting that it has gone down into the stomach.

If the catheter blocks abruply at 9 or 10 cm from the nostril, the diagnosis is virtually made. A chest film is taken, antero-posterior and lateral, to confirm the diagnosis and determine the level of obstruction in regard to the thoracic vertebrae. This X-ray can be done with or without contrast media and should include the lungs and the abdomen to verify the absence or presence of air in the digestive tract and to eliminate associated pulmonary pathology.

If contrast media is employed it is important to delicately inject the minimum amount necessary (1 to 2 cc) to establish the diagnosis and localisation of the proximal esophageal pouch. After the X-ray has been taken it is also imperative to aspirate all the contrats media back into the syringe. This test is also usefull to visualise a tracheo-esophageal fistula at this level (Fig. VIII-23, VIII-24).

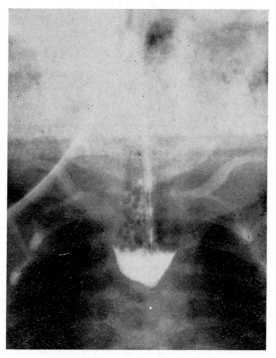

FIG. VIII-23. — *Proximal esophageal pouch:
frontal view (A. P.).*

When no contrast media is used, the paediatric radiologist can make the diagnosis by observing a distention of the proximal esophageal pouch by secretions and air which compress the trachea.

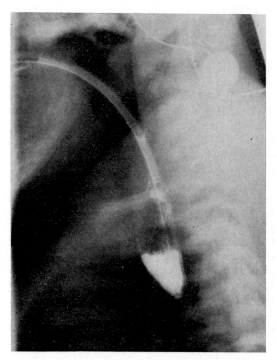

FIG. VIII-24. — *Proximal esophageal pouch: lateral view.*

The presence of a right upper lobe atelectasis or pneumonitis may also lead one to the diagnosis as it is frequently associated with this pathology.

PRE-OPERATIVE TREATMENT

The diagnosis of esophageal atresia is most often made during the first hours or days of life. The pre-operative treatment will thus depend upon the time at which the diagnosis is made, on the absence or presence of associated pulmonary pathology, on the absence or presence of associated congenital anomalies and the degree of prematurity.

This anomaly must be surgically treated as soon as the diagnosis is made, but good pre-operative preparation is essential to improve the surgical risk. Generally, these infants are placed in an isolette with 100 % humidity and oxygen if needed. The head is slightly elevated to 30° to prevent the reflux of gastric acid from the stomach into the trachea. A Replogle catheter under suction is placed in the upper esophageal pouch to prevent aspiration of saliva into the trachea. Pre-operative prophylactic antibiotics are started. If needed, respiratory physiotherapy and intravenous fluids are given. A gastrostomy may also be necessary to reduce and prevent

the reflux of gastric contents into the trachea if a respiratory infection is present and if the pre-operative treatment must be prolonged.

TREATMENT

The treatment will vary according to the presence or absence of a tracheo-esophageal fistula. But in all cases the treatment must achieve two major goals:

(*a*) Prevent pulmonary aspiration:

— by maintaining a continuous suction in the upper esophageal pouch or by creating a cervical esophagostomy in type I (atresia without a fistula),
— by closure of the fistula in all other types.

(*b*) Restore the integrity of the digestive tract.

Treatment of esophageal atresia (type I)

This pathology may be managed by two different protocols of treatment:

First, a cervical esophagostomy and a gastrostomy are done soon after birth and a definitive procedure is performed around one year of age: retro-sternal colic, jejunal or gastric transposition.

The second protocol of treatment assumes that the two esophageal segments will grow within weeks and that an anastomosis between the two segments will be possible around 8 or 12 weeks of life. Some authors mechanically dilate the two esophageal segments with that goal in mind [9].

A gastrostomy is done soon after birth and a catheter is placed under suction in the upper esophageal segment. At 8 or 12 weeks an opacification of the two segments is made to determine whether the distance between them will allow an anastomosis. A right thoracotomy and an end to end esophageal anastomosis is then performed.

If the two segments seem too far apart to permit an anastomosis, a cervical esophagostomy is then performed and the definitive procedure is done at the age of one year.

Treatment of esophageal atresia with a distal tracheo-esophageal fistula (types III and IV)

The treatment of this anomaly consists in the closure of the fistula and an esophago-esophageal anastomosis through an extra-pleural right postero-lateral thoracotomy soon after birth. The extra-pleural approach offers less morbidity and better survival than the trans-pleural approach. If a leak at the anastomosis should develop soon after the operation an esophago-cutaneous fistula will form and should eventually close itself spontaneously. In contrast, if the trans-pleural route is employed, the leak will cause a tension pneumothorax and a pyopneumothorax which can be fatal. The mortality and morbidity are higher. For these reasons, the extra-pleural approach is favored.

Treatment of types II and V

When a fistula is present at the level of the upper esophageal segment the diagnosis is difficult and rarely made at birth. Even at operation, for a presumptive type III, the fistula is often missed when the upper esophageal pouch is dissected from the trachea, because the fistula can be very high in the neck [2, 7, 19].

When the diagnosis is made, usually because of respiratory complications, the treatment is closure of the fistula through a cervical approach.

RESULTS OF TREATMENT

Results in the treatment of esophageal atresia depend on pre-, per- and post-operative factors.

Pre-operative factors.

(*a*) *Early diagnosis.* — The diagnosis of esophageal atresia at birth is relatively simple with the passage of a catheter into the stomach and analysis of the pH of the aspirated secretions. Early diagnosis will accelerate the treatment and help prevent the pre-operative complications that are frequently seen in these patients when the diagnosis is delayed: Right upper lobe atelectasis, aspiration pneumonia or diffuse emphysema. Early diagnosis reduces mortality and morbidity.

(*b*) *Prematurity and low birth weight.* — Prematurity and low birth weight e. g. an infant with a birth weight of less than 2.27 kg is associated with a high mortality [1, 37]. With esophageal atresia prematurity is present in approximately 25 to 40 %. It is, indeed a major factor in the prognosis of esophageal atresia. In our series, at Ste-Justine Hospital in Montreal, 40 % of the cases of eso-

phageal atresia were premature, with a mortality rate of 44 %.

(*c*) *Associated congenital anomalies.* — Associated congenital anomalies are reported to be present in between 30 to 50 % of cases. In our series 60 % presented with associated congenital anomalies; of these, 38 % were major, lethal congenital anomalies and the mortality rate in this group of patients was 52 %. The major anomalies encountered were: cardio-vascular, digestive, urinary, nervous system, pulmonary and soft tissue anomalies.

Operative factors. — The surgical approach will influence the survival of these patients. The extra-pleural approach results in less mortality and less morbidity. The one stage procedure equally shows less mortality and morbidity, the multiple stage technique being reserved most often for the less fortunate cases. The single layer end to end anastomosis is the one most often employed but unfortunately the one which will give rise to the most leaks. Haight's anastomosis, in two layers will reduce the percentage of leaks but will produce a higher percentage of stenoses [8, 19, 24, 26, 34, 39].

The presence of a gastrostomy will not reduce the incidence of anastomotic complications [19, 34]. Many authors [14, 22, 35] report major complications with the use of a gastrostomy. Gastrostomy should be reserved for selected cases with complications: pre-operative pneumonia, leaks or severe stenosis.

Post-operative factors.

(*a*) *Pulmonary complications.* — Broncho-pneumonia and atelectasis are frequent post-operative complications [2, 13, 27]. In our series, 50 % of our patients had pulmonary complications in their long term evolution, mostly related to bronchial aspiration.

(*b*) *Anastomotic complications.* — The esophageal anastomosis is sometimes the site of a stenosis which may require one or several sessions of bouginage [19, 34]. In our series, 30 % developed a stenosis, but only 10 % required more than two sessions of bouginage. Many of these stenoses will recur in spite of good medical treatment because they are associated with significant gastro-esophageal reflux [4, 15, 28]. When the esophageal reflux is corrected the stenosis will respond to medical treatment and disappear.

An anastomotic leak is the most serious complication in the treatment of this anomaly. The mortality and morbidity depend on the trans or extra-pleural approach employed which will give rise to a generalized empyema or a localised infection (esophago-cutaneous fistula) [34]. The incidence of this complication in our patients was 16 %. In the literature the incidence of this complication is directly related to the type of anastomosis employed, being 10 % with the two layer anastomosis and 20 % with the one layer anastomosis [23]. The recurrence of a tracheo-esophageal fistula is also a most serious complication, occuring in up to 6 % of cases [2, 4, 37].

(c) *Anomalies of esophageal motricity.* — Many authors have reported anomalies of esophageal motricity following the repair of an esophageal atresia [6, 10, 15, 25, 27]. In our series, anomalies of esophageal motricity have been observed and were responsible for long term complications occuring in these patients: Aspiration pneumonia and dysphagia. Some authors believe that this anomaly in the motricity of the esophagus is caused by a congenital innervation anomaly of the esophagus [23, 27, 32].

In our series, X-ray study and clinical observation indicate that if the dissection of the lower esophageal segment is held to the very minimum necessary to divide and suture the fistula, the long term results are much better, with much less aspiration pneumonia and dysphagia. We have even observed normal esophageal peristalsis post-operatively in some of these patients.

These results lead us to believe that the anomalies of esophageal motricity observed in these patients are the result of excessive dissection of the lower esophagus.

ANALYSIS OF RESULTS

Results in the treatment of esophageal atresia depend on the degree of prematurity, the association of severe congenital malformations and pulmonary complications.

Most centers use the pre-operative prognostic classification of David Waterston based on these factors:

Type A: Birth weight of 2.5 kg or more and an excellent general condition without associated congenital anomalies.

Type B:

— Birth weight between 1.8 and 2.5 kg and an excellent general condition.

— Birth weight of 2.5 kg or more but with moderate pulmonary complications and associated congenital anomalies.

Type C:

— Birth weight of less than 1.8 kg.
— Birth weight of more than 1.8 kg but with severe pulmonary complications and associated congenital malformations.

As reported by T. H. Holder of Kansas City [23], in analysing various series in 1979, the survival rate of patients in group A is 94 to 100 %, patients in group B, 80-96 %, and patients in group C, 37-76 %, for an over all survival rate of 63 to 90 %.

In our series of 80 patients the over all survival rate is 70 %. However, if we eliminate the premature babies (40 %) where the mortality rate is 44 %, and the severe associated congenital malformations (38 %), where the mortality rate is 52 %, the survival rate for the remaining group A patients is 100 %.

LONG TERM RESULTS

In a study reported from the Boston Children's Hospital [23], on 42 patients followed for 5 to 25 years, most of these patients lead a normal life but many of them present with occasional dysphagia and 10 % have frequent problems. In our series, after 5 years of follow up, no stenosis could be found. A post-operative stenosis, if correctly treated, will not affect esophageal function. However, the esophageal motricity is often disturbed in most of these patients and is responsible, most of the time, for the chronic pulmonary complications and dysphagia observed in them.

REFERENCES

[1] ABRAHAMSON (J.), SHANDLING (B.). — Esophageal Atresia in an Underweight Baby: A challenge. *J. Pediatr. Surg.*, 7, 608-611, 1972.
[2] ANDRIEU-GUITRANCOURT (J.), TYCHYJ (J.), ENSEL (J.), DEHESDIN (D.). — Troubles respiratoires et de déglutition après cure chirurgicale de l'atrésie de l'œsophage. *Ann. Oto-Laryng.*, 95, 445-459, 1978.
[3] ASCHCRAFT (K. W.), HOLDER (T. M.). — The story of Esophageal Atresia an Tracheoesophageal Fistula. *Surgery*, 65, 332-340, 1969.
[4] ASCHCRAFT (K.W.), GOODWIN (C.), AMOURY (R. A.), HOLDER (T. M.). — Early recognition and Aggressive Treatment of Gastroesophageal Reflux Following Repair of Esophageal Atresia. *J. Pediatr. Surg.*, 12, 317-321, 1977.

[5] BUCKER (R. H.), COX (W. A.), PAULING (F. W.), SEITTER (G.). — Complications of Congenital Tracheoesophageal Fistula. *Am. J. Surg., 124,* 705-710, 1972.

[6] BURGESS (J. N.), CARLSON (H. E.), ELLIS (F. H.). — Esophageal Function after successful Repair of Esophageal Atresia and Tracheoesophageal Fistula. *J. Thorac. Cardiovasc. Surg., 56,* 667-673, 681-682, 1968.

[7] CLOUD (D. T.). — Anastomotic Technic in Esophageal Atresia. *J. Pediatr. Surg., 3,* 561-564, 1968.

[8] CORAN (A. G.). — One-stage Repair of Esophageal Atresia in the High-risk Neonate. *Ann. Thorac. Surg., 21,* 470, 1976.

[9] DE LORIMIER (A. A.), HARRISON (M. R.). — Long GAP Esophageal Atresia Primary anastomosis after Esophageal Elongation by Bougrenage and Esophagomyotomy. *J. Thorac. Cardiovasc. Surg., 79,* 138-141, 1980.

[10] DESJARDINS (J. G.), STEPHENS (C. A.), MOES (C. A. E.). — Results of Surgical Treatment of Congenital Tracheoesophageal Fistula with a note on Cine-Fluorographic Findings. *Ann. Surg., 160,* 141-145, 1964.

[11] DESJARDINS (J. G.), TASSÉ (D.). — Étude expérimentale de la dysphagie postopératoire observée chez les cas d'atrésie de l'œsophage. *Union Méd. Can., 95,* 598-600, 1966.

[12] DUCHARME (J. C.), COLLIN (P. P.), MAALOUF (H.). — L'atrésie de l'œsophage. *Union Méd. Can., 93,* 409-414, 1964.

[13] DUDLEY (N. E.), PHELAN (P. D.). — Respiratory Complications in long-term Survivors of Esophageal Atresia. *Arch. Dis. Child., 51,* 279-282, 1976.

[14] DURANCEAU (A.), DESJARDINS (J. G.), COLLIN (P. P.). — L'atrésie de l'œsophage : Résultats du traitement dans un centre de Chirurgie Infantile. *Union Méd. Can., 102,* 1720-1725, 1973.

[15] DURANCEAU (A.), FISHER (S. R.), FLYE (M. W.) et al. — Motor Function of the Esophagus after Repair of Esophageal Atresia and Tracheoesophageal Fistula. *Surgery, 82,* 116-123, 1977.

[16] FONKALSRUD (E. W.). — Gastroesophageal Fundoplication for Reflux Following Repair of Esophageal Atresia. *Arch. Surg., 114,* 48-51, 1979.

[17] GERMAN (J. C.), MAHOUR (G. H.), WOOLEY (M. M.). — Esophageal Atresia and Associated Anomalies. *J. Pediatr. Surg., 11,* 299-306, 1976.

[18] GOODWIND (C. D.), ASCHCRAFT (K. W.), HOLDER (T. M.) et al. — Esophageal Atresia with double tracheoesophageal Fistula. *J. Pediatr. Surg., 13,* 269-273, 1978.

[19] HAIGHT (C.). — Congenital Atresia of the Esophagus. *Postgrad. Med., 36,* 463-469, 1964.

[20] HAYS (D. M.), WOOLEY (M. M.), SYNDER (W. H.). — Esophageal Atresia and Tracheoesophageal Fistula : Management of the Uncommon Types. *J. Pediatr. Surg., 1,* 240-252, 1966.

[21] HOLDER (T. M.), ASCHCRAFT (K. W.). — Esophageal Atresia and Tracheoesophageal Fistula. *Curr. Probl. Surg.,* 1-68, 1966.

[22] HOLDER (T. M.), CLOUD (D. T.), LEWIS (J. E.), PILLING (G. P.). — Esophageal Atresia and Tracheoesophageal Fistula. *Pediatrics, 34,* 542-549, 1964.

[23] HOLDER (T. M.). — Esophageal Atresia: A Follow up Study, Presentation at the *Pediatric Surgical Symposium, Pittsburgh,* Sept. 1979. (Not published).

[24] JOHNSONBEAUGH (R. E.). — A new Diagnostic Procedure for Evaluating Esophageal Atresia. *Am. J. Dis. Child., 116,* 175-178, 1968.

[25] KIRKPATRICK (J. A.), CRESSON (S. L.), PILLING (G. P.). — The motor Activity of the Esophagus in Association with Esophageal Atresia and Tracheoesophageal Fistula. *Am. J. Roentgenol., 86,* 884-887, 1961.

[26] LEIX (F.), SCHWAB (C. E.). — End to Side Operative Technic for Esophageal Atresia with Tracheoesophageal Fistula. *Am. J. Surg., 118,* 225-235, 1969.

[27] LIND (J. F.), BLANCHARD (R. J.), GUYDA (H.). — Esophageal Motility in Tracheoesophageal Fistula and Esophageal Atresia. *Surg. Gynecol. Obst., 123,* 557-564, 1966.

[28] PARKER (F. A.), CHRISTIE (D. L.), CAHILL (J. L.). — Incidence and Significance of Gastroesophageal Reflux Following Repair of Esophageal Atresia and Tracheoesophageal Fistula and the Need for Anti-reflux Procedures. *J. Pediatr. Surg., 14,* 5-8, 1979.

[29] PIERRETTI (R.), SHANDLING (B.), STEPHENS (C. A.). — Resistant esophageal Stenosis Associated with Reflux after Repair of Esophageal Atresia. *J. Pediatr. Surg., 9,* 355-357, 1974.

[30] ROMSDAHL (M. M.), HUNTER (J. A.), GROVE (W. J.). Tracheoesophageal Fistula and Esophageal Atresia. *J. Thorac. Cardiovasc. Surg., 52,* 571-578, 1966.

[31] SHAFIE (M. E.), KLIPPEL (C. H.), BLAKEMORE (W. S.). — Congenital Esophageal Anomalies: A plea for using Anatomic Descriptions rather than Classifications. *J. Pediatr. Surg., 13,* 355, 1978.

[32] SHEPARD (R.), FENN (S.), SEIBER (W. K.). — Evaluation of Esophageal Function in Postoperative Esophageal Atresia and Tracheoesophageal Fistula. *Surgery, 59,* 608-617, 1966.

[33] STRODEL (W. E.), CORAN (A. G.), KIRSH (M. M.) et al. — Esophageal Atresia a 41 year experience. *Arch. Surg., 114,* 523-527, 1979.

[34] SWENSON (O.). — *Pediatric Surgery,* 3e éd. Appleton Century Crafts, New York, 1969.

[35] TYSON (K. R. T.). — Primary Repair of Esophageal Atresia without Staging or Preliminary Gastrostomy. *Ann. Thorac. Surg., 21,* 378-381, 1976.

[36] WAYSON (E. E.), GARNJOBST (W.), CHANDLER (J. J.), PETERSON CLARE (G.). — Esophageal Atresia with Tracheoesophageal Fistula. *Am. J. Surg.,* 110-112, 162-167, 1965.

[37] WOOLEY (M. M.). — Prematury Additional Malformations, *International Symposium, Œsophageal Atresia, Bremen,* Supplément Zu Bd. 17/Z. Kinderch., 47, 1975.

[38] YOUNG (D. G.). — Successful Primary Anastomosis in Œsophageal Atresia after Reduction of a Long Gap between the Blind Ends by Bouginase of the Upper Pouch. *Br. J. Surg., 54,* 321-329, 1967.

[39] YOUNG (D. G.), DRAINER (I. K.). — Esophageal Atresia. *Br. J. Hosp. Med., 7,* 629-636, 1972.

Congenital broncho-pulmonary anomalies

Pierre-Paul COLLIN

Some congenital pulmonary anomalies may require surgical treatment during the first few months of life. These are divided into two major groups, depending upon the predominant anlage affected: Those originating in the primitive foregut and its derivative, the lung bud (broncho-pulmonary or foregut anomalies), and those arising from the sixth embryonic arch and its derivative, the pulmonary vasculature.

The first group includes pulmonary sequestration, congenital bronchial cysts, adenomatoid malformation of the lung and congenital lobar emphysema. Anomalies of the second group are mainly cardiovascular and will be discussed in the chapter dealing with congenital heart disease.

Factors responsible for most major developmental anomalies of the lung must exert their effects between the 25th and 40th day of embryonic life.

BRONCHO-PULMONARY SEQUESTRATION

Pulmonary sequestration is characterized by a precise anatomical triad: It is a mass of aberrant lung tissue that has no normal connection with the bronchial tree nor with the pulmonary artery. It is supplied by an anomalous artery arising from the aorta. Its venous drainage is via either the azygos system, the pulmonary veins or the inferior vena cava. The anomaly may be intralobar or extralobar: the former lies contiguous to normal lung parenchyma and within the same visceral pleural envelope, the latter is enclosed within its own pleural sheath, usually in close proximity to the lung parenchyma, but sometimes within or below the diaphragm.

The embryologic origin of this malformation is well established, but its pathogenesis remains unclear [1, 2].

In over 60 % of cases, the lesion will be found in the posterior basal segment of the left lobe, the next most frequent site being the right lower lobe. Right lower lobe sequestrations are usually associated with other pulmonary and vascular abnormalities such as pulmonary hypoplasia, and an abnormal partial pulmonary venous return below the diaphragm. This is the condition known as "scimitar syndrome". In most cases, there is a systemic artery arising from the lower thoracic or upper abdominal aorta and supplying the right lower lobe.

Extralobar sequestration is mostly asymptomatic, but such is not the case with the intralobar variety. Recent reports tend to show that this lesion not only is more frequent than previously thought but is symptomatic in most cases. The left lower lobe sequestration is liable to cause respiratory problems, while in the scimitar syndrome the symptomatology may be respiratory but will mainly be cardiovascular, due to the presence of a more or less significant left to right shunt. In a series of 21 cases treated in our institution, all had been symptomatic before the age of 10 and 3 underwent surgery during the first year of life. Although not reported in neonates at necropsy, sporadic reports have appeared of the anomaly becoming manifest in infants less than 3 months old and even in newborns of 3 and 7 days old [4, 5].

The roentgen appearance of the lesion will vary according to the severity and frequency of previous episodes of infection. Fistulization into the airways of contiguous lung tissue may result from infection and will show radiograms highly suggestive of bronchiectasis, a pulmonary abscess or even a diaphragmatic hernia (see Fig. VIII-25).

Presumptive diagnosis is usually made, however, on a simple chest film, when it shows a suspected shadow in the lower portion of the lung. Tomograms and bronchograms can be useful but the definitive diagnosis depends upon the opacification of the anomalous vessel by angiography. Preoperative diagnosis by aortography is important, in view of the hazards involved in severing the anomalous systemic vessel during surgical resection [7].

Treatment is essentially surgical and consists of a lobectomy or a segmental resection. Local excision is usually satisfactory in the extralobar type. The prognosis is excellent.

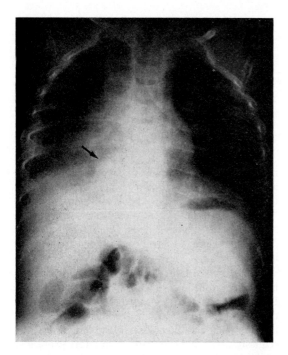

FIG. VIII-25. — *Typical aspect of "scimitar syndrome" with blurred and slightly smaller right lung field.* There is also a pseudotumor in the right lower mediastinal area, which proved to be aberrant hepatic tissue, herniating through the diaphragm.

CONGENITAL BRONCHIAL CYSTS

The congenital bronchial cyst although relatively uncommon is certainly the most frequent in this clinical group of anomalies. It results from an abnormality of budding or branching of the tracheo-bronchial tree during embryonic development. Intrathoracic foregut cysts are usually classified into three categories [8], from their etiology: (1) the posterior mediastinal cyst (also called neurenteric or archenteric) (2) the intramural oesophageal cyst or esophageal duplication, (3) the bronchial cyst proper.

Neurenteric cyst

Histologically, the cyst wall contains both neural and gastrointestinal elements and is lined by digestive epithelium. The presence of ciliated columnar epithelium is not uncommon and is in harmony with the normal evolution of the foetal esophagus. This should not be construed as evidence of a bronchogenic cyst. The cyst is generally close to the thoracic spine, which often shows

vertebral anomalies. It may also be connected by a stalk to the gastrointestinal tract. Communication with the esophagus is rare, but quite frequent with the stomach and duodenum, when the cyst extends within the abdomen.

The roentgenologic appearance is of a sharply defined round or oval lobulated mass of homogeneous density. Air in the cyst suggests a communication with the digestive tract and can be confirmed by a barium meal.

Neurenteric cysts are rarely asymptomatic. They very often cause pain, may grow very large and give rise to compression atelectasis, thereby leading to respiratory distress.

Gastroenteric cyst

Also known as esophageal duplication or intramural esophageal cyst, the gastroenteric cyst results from a failure of complete vacuolation of the originally solid esophagus. Its histology, as well as its roentgenologic appearance are similar to that of a neurenteric cyst. It is rarely symptomatic unless complicated by peptic ulceration [8].

Bronchial cyst

Bronchial cysts develop in the pulmonary parenchyma or the mediastinum with a fairly equal incidence. The anomaly appears to have a predilection for males and also for yemenite jews. These thin-walled cysts are lined with respiratory epithelium and usually filled with mucoid material. Their wall may contain mucous glands, cartilage, elastic tissue and smooth muscle.

In the parenchyma, there is a predilection for the lower lobes. The typical roentgenologic appearance is of a sharply circumscribed solitary round or oval shadow of uniform density, usually in the medial third of the lung. When the embryonic defect occurs at a later stage in intra-uterine development, it will often produce multiple peripheral cysts, sometimes communicating with the parent bronchus. These cysts are lined with columnar epithelium and usually contain no mucous glands. The wall rarely contains cartilage; they often show much elastic tissue but no muscle fibres [10].

In the mediastinum, bronchial cysts are found mainly in the paratracheal, carinal, hilar and paraesophageal regions. There have been some rare reports of bronchial cysts in the pericardium [11]. The majority are situated in the vicinity of the carina, often attached by a stalk to one of the major airways; in this location, even a small cyst can cause symptoms by putting pressure on surrounding structures. In infants particularly, the intimate relationship of these cysts to the trachea and major bronchi may cause respiratory embarrassment and sometimes severe respiratory distress [12].

How then, should we deal with an intrathoracic cystic lesion? In the 50's some people [13] used to think that spontaneous regression without surgical removal was the rule for pulmonary cysts, even when they were demonstrated during the first weeks and months of life. Experience of the past 25 years has shown the fallacy of that assertion. Repeated bouts of infection and severe episodes of respiratory distress are indisputable surgical indications. Another motivation for surgery lies in the fact that malignant tumors have been shown to develop in association with pulmonary cystic lesions. Many recent reports have pointed out that a relationship may exist between congenital cystic lesions and sarcomas of the lungs in young children. Surgical removal of those cystic lesions carries very little morbidity and an excellent prognosis, and should not be unduly delayed [14].

CYSTIC ADENOMATOID MALFORMATION OF THE LUNG

Much more rarely does one come upon the anomaly known as congenital cystic adenomatoid malformation of the lung. Fontanus, in 1638, is said to have made the original description of the disease in a 5 month old baby. Since then, numerous reports have brought the number of published cases over the 500 mark. However, the histologic findings in some of those cases are more consistent with a diagnosis of congenital cystic bronchiectasis or some variety of bronchogenic cysts, so that cystic adenomatoid malformation is probably not as common as the literature might lead one to believe. During the past 25 years, we have only had 7 cases at Ste-Justine Hospital. In each of them, the anomaly was limited to one lobe. Lobectomy was done in the early days of life in 3 of them and between the age of 4 and 6 months in the other four. All had a normal recovery.

In this anomaly, the embryonic insult occurs at a later stage than in sequestration or bronchogenic cyst; that is around the 35th day, which corresponds to the secondary broncho-pulmonary bud stage. At certain points, the distal lobular branchings fail to canalize. Beyond those areas, the process of cavitation progresses normally, leaving isolated hollow segments, lined by a normal mucosa. As the mucous secretions cannot be evacuated nor reabsorbed, there is fluid accumulation and cyst formation. At birth, dilatation of the lungs cause the cysts to rupture into the bronchi and their fluid content is replaced by air. These cystic cavities rapidly increase in size, because their opening into the bronchus is tangential to the circumference of the cyst and acts as a valve, allowing air in but not out [15]. These cysts have a normal bronchial or alveolar wall, lined by cuboidal and ciliated columnar cells. This epithelium may show excessive proliferation giving the lesion an adenomatous look, whence the term cystic adenomatoid malformation (Fig. VIII-26).

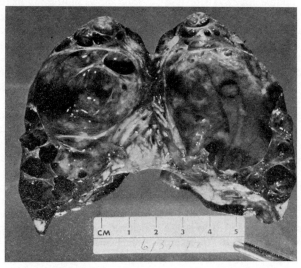

FIG. VIII-26. — *Cross section of a pulmonary lobe showing typical aspect of adenomatoid malformation.*

Although some cases have been described in older children, the anomaly is usually found in newborns and babies. In a series of 50 cases published in 1972, 46 were term newborns and 21 premature babies [16]. Holder also reported that the anomaly is often discovered at necropsy of stillborn babies. Hydramnios and anasarca are said to occur in 20 to 50 % of cases.

The clinical picture is similar to congenital lobar emphysema, except that the onset of respiratory distress is more rapid and more precocious. The roentgenologic appearance of the chest is also different showing irregular clear areas within a dense mass. The lesion is usually well defined and rarely affects more than one lobe. The heart and mediastinum are displaced by this overdistended mass, which increases in size with each inspiration, rapidly leading to a state of respiratory distress. Emergency surgery is usually needed.

CONGENITAL LOBAR EMPHYSEMA

Congenital lobar emphysema in infants belongs to the same clinical group, although there are differences in embryology and histopathology. The condition is characterized by severe overinflation of one or several segments of a pulmonary lobe, usually causing severe respiratory distress.

There is a distinct predilection for the left upper lobe and a slightly lesser one for the middle and right upper lobes. There is bilateral involvement in a small percentage of cases. Out of 30 cases observed at Ste-Justine since 1962, we only had 3 involving the left upper and right middle lobes. There is a male-female ratio of 3 to 1 and it is almost non existent in coloured people.

The usual clinical picture is progressive respiratory distress, starting a few weeks after birth and sometimes not recognized until the fourth or fifth month of life.

Several different mechanisms are said to be at the origin of this abnormality. It is usually classified into three groups:

In the first one, the bronchial obstruction is due to absence or dysplasia of bronchial cartilage. However, this is rarely clearly demonstrated in resected specimens, probably because, in many cases, the abnormal bronchus is left in situ as the bronchial stump.

The second group includes cases where the bronchial obstruction is produced by pressure from an abnormal vessel, such as a large patent ductus arteriosus or an anomalous pulmonary vessel. Less than 10 % of cases belong in that group.

The third category, designated as idiopathic, is the largest, including all those where no particular cause can be identified. The notion of a polyalveolar lobe, recently described by Hislop and Reid brings an attractive pathogenic explanation to a good number of those cases. These investigators made a morphometric and pathologic study of surgical specimens resected from infants showing the classic clinical and roentgenographic features of infantile lobar emphysema. They found a considerable increase in the number of alveoli, and, in some cases, not only were the alveoli increased in number but also in size. The study also showed that this alveolar giantism often was limited to some segments of a lobe. In 6 of our cases where emphysema was located in the left upper lobe a segmental resection could be done instead of a lobectomy. Taffer and Schuster recently reported 10 cases of polyalveolar lobes in the last 31 cases of congenital lobar emphysema treated at the Boston Children's Medical Center.

The roentgenographic manifestations of infantile lobar emphysema are distinctive and usually there is little difficulty in diagnosis. The cardinal features are overinflation and air-trapping, manifested by a markedly increased volume of the affected lobe, producing compression atelectasis of the lung's other lobes. Identification of vascular markings in the radiolucent area is important, permitting differentiation from congenital air cysts, post-pneumonic pneumatocele and loculated pneumothorax. Air-trapping is manifested by the fluoroscopic evidence of the mediastinal swing of paradoxical respiration. Infrequently, the overinflated lobe shows uniformily increased density rather than translucency. This is explained by a pathophysiologic impairment of fluid drainage probably secondary to bronchial obstruction. The foetal lung normally is filled with fluid; some is squeezed out as the infant passes through the birth canal, and the remainder is cleared by the pulmonary lymphatics and veins and perhaps by the airways themselves. Generally speaking, the diagnosis can easily be made from the plain roentgenogram. However, in some cases of associated cardiovascular anomalies, angiocardiography may be required to confirm a doubtful roentgenologic diagnosis, revealing anomalous vessels compressing the bronchi.

Bronchoscopy may be justified where aspiration of a foreign body is suspected, but under no circumstances should bronchography be done, for fear of dangerously aggravating the respiratory distress.

Surgical resection of the affected lobe or segment

is mandatory and is very often an emergency operation. To us, watchful waiting does not appear justified, in view of the hazards involved for the patient and the relatively low morbidity attached to that procedure. One small detail is worth mentioning. Since anesthesia is almost always endotracheal and respiration is assisted, it is important for the surgeon to proceed quickly in opening the chest in order to relieve as rapidly as possible the pressure exerted on the normal parenchyma.

REFERENCES

[1] BOYDEN (E. A.). — Developmental anomalies of the lungs. *Amer. J. Surg.*, *89*, 79-89, 1955.
[2] PRYCE (D. M.). — Lower accessory pulmonary artery with intralobar sequestration of lung: a report of seven cases. *J. Path. Bact.*, *58*, 457-467, 1946.
[3] COLLIN (P. P.), BRAUN (P.). — The many faces of pulmonary sequestration. Présentation au *Congrès du Collège Royal des Chirurgiens du Canada*, Ottawa, 1980.
[4] JENSEN (F. O.), McLEAN (A. D.). — Intralobar sequestration of the lung with tension cysts: an unusual presentation of 2 cases with clinical and radiological evidence of tension phenomena. *Australas. Radiol.*, *14*, 269, 1970.
[5] LANE (S. D.), BURKO (H.), SCOTT (H. W.). — Congenital bronchopulmonary foregut malformation. *Radiology*, *101*, 291, 1971.
[6] ZALEFSKY (M. N.), JANIS (M.), BERNSTEIN (R.). — Intralobar bronchopulmonary sequestration with bronchial communication. *Chest*, *59*, 266-270, 1971.
[7] BRAUN (P.), COLLIN (P. P.). — Séquestration pulmonaire chez l'enfant. *Med. Hyg.*, *33*, 309-310, 1976.
[8] KIRWAN (W. O.), WALBAUM (P. R.), McCORMACK (R. J. M.). — Cystic intrathoracic derivatives of the foregut and their complications. *Thorax*, *28*, 424, 1973.
[9] BAUM (G. L.), RACZ (I.) et coll. — Cystic disease of the lung: report of 88 cases with an ethnologic relationship. *Ann. J. Med.*, *40*, 578, 1966.
[10] SPENCER (H.). — *Pathology of the lung*. 2nd edition, Oxford, Pergamon press, 1968.
[11] STEINBERG (I.). — Angiocardiography in the differential diagnosis of pericardial and mediastinal tumors. *Ann. J. Ræntgen.*, *84*, 409, 1960.
[12] STORER (J.), KIRAGUS (C.). — Considerations on an unrecognized mediastinal cyst. *J. Pediatr.*, *51*, 194, 1959.
[13] CAFFEY (J.). — On the natural regression of pulmonary cysts during early infancy. *Pediatrics*, *11*, 48-63, 1953.
[14] WEINBERG (A. G.) et coll. — Mesenchymal neoplasia and congenital pulmonary cysts. *Ped. Rad.*, *9*, 179-182, 1980.
[15] COLLIN (P. P.), CLERMONT (J.). — Maladie kystique congénitale du poumon. *Can. J. Surg.*, *9*, 66-71, 1966.
[16] HALLORAN (L. G.), SILVERBERG (S. G.), SALZBERG (A. M.). — Congenital cystic adenomatoid malformation of the lung. *Arch. Surg.*, *104*, 715, 1972.
[17] HOLDER (T. M.), CHUSTY (M. G.). — Cystic adenomatoid malformation of the lung. *J. Thorac. Card. Vasc. Surg.*, *47*, 590, 1964.
[18] BENSOUSSAN (A. L.), BRAUN (P.), BLANCHARD (H.), COLLIN (P. P.). — Emphysème lobaire congénital : traitement médical ou chirurgical ? *Union Méd. Can.*, *104*, 735-739, 1975.
[19] HISLOP (A.), REID (L.). — New pathological findings in emphysema of childhood: 1. Polyalveolar lobe with emphysema. *Thorax*, *25*, 682-690, 1970.
[20] TAFFER (D.), SCHUSTER (S.) et coll. — Polyalveolar lobe: anatomic and physiologic parameters and their relationship to congenital lobar emphysema. *J. Pediatr. Surg.*, *15*, 931-937, 1980.

Diaphragmatic hernia (excluding hiatus hernia)

Alain OUIMET

EMBRYOLOGY AND PATHOGENESIS

The diaphragm results from the fusion of several elements: septum transversum, dorsal mesentery and pleuro-peritoneal folds. At the third embryonic week, the septum transversum will form the ventral portion of the diaphragm separating the heart from the abdominal viscera. The posterior part of the diaphragm will develop from the dorsal mesoderm at 4 weeks. Pleuro-peritoneal folds then form on each side, extending laterally and posteriorly to complete the separation of the thoracic and peritoneal cavities.

There exist during this development two lateral foramina by which peritoneal and pleural cavities communicate. The cervical myotomes then migrate to form the muscular elements between the two serosa at the 8th week.

During that time, the primitive (intestinal) gut developing in the cœlomic cavity will re-enter the peritoneal cavity at the 10th week.

Anomalies in diaphragmatic development or

in the return of the primitive gut into the abdominal cavity can result in diaphragmatic hernia which can be of 3 types:

(a) Postero-lateral hernia (Bochdalek),
(b) Anterior hernia (Morgagni),
(c) Diaphragmatic eventration.

Three simultaneous anomalies explain the formation of a postero-lateral hernia:

(a) Premature return of the primitive gut into the peritoneal cavity.
(b) Delayed closure of one or both lateral foramina
(c) Delayed migration of the muscular element[s] in between the pleuro-peritoneal folds.

The anterior hernia (Morgagni) is situated in the retro-sternal region. It is the result of an absence of tissue, the non-fixation of the anterior portion of diaphragmatic structures or non-migration of muscular elements. The severity of the defect can amount to total absence of structures formed by the septum transversum and result in a peritoneo-pericardial cavity.

Diaphragmatic eventration is an elevation of the diaphragm without protrusion of peritoneal contents into the pleural space. It can be congenital secondary to total absence of muscle fibers in the diaphragm. It can be seen in the newborn and the fetus by ultrasound examination. It can also be acquired and secondary to obstetrical or surgical trauma causing diaphragmatic atrophy.

INCIDENCE

The postero-lateral hernia is the most frequent and affects males and females equally. Those children with postero-lateral hernias will present early in the neonatal period and those with anterior or with diaphragmatic eventration will present later or will be discovered by chance.

Other malformations are frequently associated with postero-lateral hernia but rarely with anterior hernia and exceptionally with eventration. The most frequent malformations are those of the digestive tract, in particular, anomalies of fixation, and of the cardiopulmonary system.

CLINICAL FINDINGS

Respiratory distress syndrome is the usual presentation of a postero-lateral hernia. The measurement of blood gases will evaluate the severity of the distress and also serve to establish guidelines for prognosis.

The triad of respiratory distress, scaphoid abdo-

men and dextrocardia is characteristic of postero-lateral hernia.

Children with anterior hernia (Morgagni) or diaphragmatic eventration usually present with repeated respiratory tract infections or are completely asymptomatic.

MANAGEMENT

Early diagnosis of a congenital diaphragmatic hernia in patients with respiratory distress and pre-operative resuscitation are essential to obtain good results. Pre-operative evaluation is based on radiology and the measurement of blood gases (pO_2, pCO_2, pH).

Plain radiographs of good quality in the anterio-posterior and the lateral views will show the typical appearance of air-distended segments of bowel in the thoracic cavity (see Fig. VIII-27). In rare instances where cystic diseases of the lungs, either primary or secondary can mimic this appearance, barium studies are indicated.

Supportive measures must start at the refering hospital. Nasogastric and endotracheal intubation are essential. Resuscitation with a bag and mask is not acceptable as it will result in blowing up the stomach and further compromise of an already impaired pulmonary system. Adequate ventilation with supplemental oxygen, a secure intravenous line and transportation within a heated incubator accompanied by qualified personnel are required.

SURGERY

The abdominal approach is prefered by many surgeons. It gives direct access to correct associated intestinal malformations, facilitates decompressive technique (abdominal contents) when needed, prevents accidental intestinal mishandling and gives a good view for dissection of the posterior fold of the diaphragm. This approach can be used for a postero-lateral or anterior hernia. Diaphragmatic eventration should be corrected in symptomatic patients by an abdominal or thoracic approach.

PROGNOSIS

Success in the treatment of diaphragmatic hernia (postero-lateral) depends in a large part on the rapidity of diagnosis and of initiating resuscitative measures. Antenatal diagnosis on routine ultrasonography is now increasingly noted. Deaths are secondary to pulmonary hypoplasia or to associated malformations, mainly cardiac. Pro-

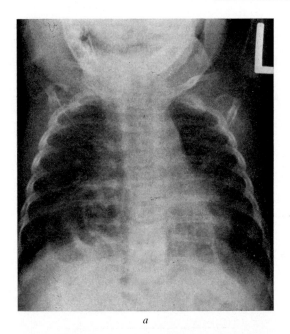

a

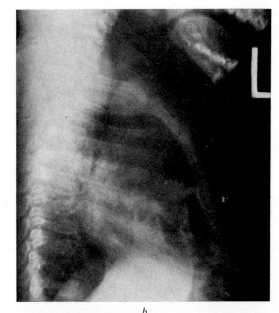

b

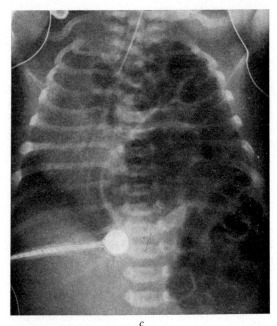

c

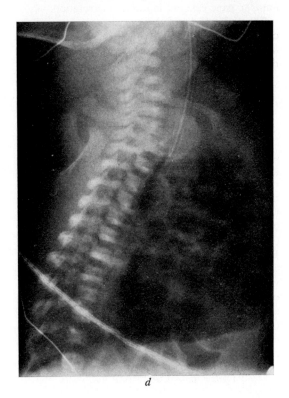

d

FIG. VIII-27.

a, b) Antero-posterior and lateral views. Hernia of Morgagni.

c, d) Antero-posterior and lateral views. Hernia of Bochdalek.

Typical appearance of left-sided hernia with left thorax full of intestinal loops and displacement of mediastinum. Note presence of endotracheal tube. ECG leads and cutaneous pO_2 monitor are present.

gnosis in anterior hernia or in eventration is excellent except in cases associated with malformations incompatible with life.

REFERENCES

[1] GERBAUX (J.), COUVREUR (J.), TOURNIER (G.). — Pathologie respiratoire de l'enfant. 2ᵉ édition, Flammarion, Paris, 1979.

[2] RAFFENSPERGER (J.). — Swenson's Pediatric Surgery. 4ᵉ édition. Appleton-Century-Crofts, New York, 1980.

[3] RAVITCH (M.), WELCH (K.), BENSON (C. D.), ABERDEEN (E.). — Pediatric Surgery. 3ᵉ édition. Year Book Medical Publishers, New York, 1979.

[4] RICKHAM (P. P.), LISTER (J.), IRVING (I. M.). — Neonatal Surgery. 2ᵉ édition. Butterworths, London, 1978.

[5] PELLERIN (D.), BERTIN (P.). — Techniques de chirurgie pédiatrique. Masson édit., Paris, 1978.

Congenital duodenal obstruction

Jacques-Charles DUCHARME and Pierre BOUDROS GHOSN

In the neonatal period the duodenum can be the site of obstruction caused by atresia, stenosis, annular pancreas and intestinal malrotation.

The embryology of this area is complex and the causes of these malformations are not well known [2, 3]. The obstruction usually occurs distal to the ampulla of Vater.

CLINICAL DATA

Since obstruction is usually virtually complete and distal to the ampulla of Vater, these babies generally present within the first few days of life with bilious vomiting. In the rare case where obstruction is proximal to the ampulla, the diagnosis is not as obvious. Our case material consists of 28 babies operated between January 1970 and December 1979 (Table I). Fourteen had a history of polyhydramnios. Fourteen were seen within 24 hours after birth and 23 within 72 hours (Table II). Twenty-five babies vomited green material. Five babies had incomplete obstruction (stenosis or intraluminal diaphragm) and presented somewhat later. The majority (25 of 28) passed normal meconium. The abdominal examination was usually normal. Occasional gastric

TABLE I. — CONGENITAL DUODENAL OBSTRUCTION

Stenosis or atresia	21 cases
Annular pancreas (with or without atresia or diaphragm)	7 cases

TABLE II. — AGE AT DIAGNOSIS

1 day	14 cases
1-2 days	7 cases
2-3 days	2 cases
+ 3 days	5 cases

peristaltic waves were observed, as they are in pyloric stenosis. The presence of these waves in the newborn baby who vomits green material strongly suggests duodenal obstruction. Babies presenting after three days of life had the usual signs of dehydration.

DIAGNOSIS

A plain film of the abdomen in the upright position is sufficient to establish the diagnosis. The double bubble with a fluid level in the stomach and first portion of the duodenum is typical (Fig. VIII-28). If the obstruction is complete there will be no gas in the distal bowel. If the obstruction is partial, as in stenosis or intraluminal diaphragm, some gas will be visible in the distal bowel. In this case a barium swallow may be necessary to show the stenosis or diaphragm. The barium enema is less useful since there is no microcolon in duodenal obstruction.

ASSOCIATED MALFORMATIONS

Sixty-eight percent (19 out of 28) of our patients had associated malformations (Table III!). In a

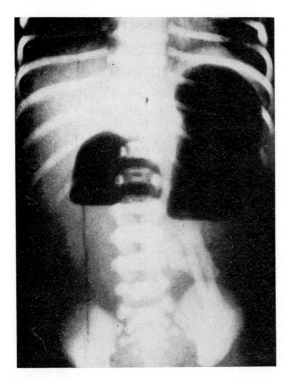

FIG. VIII-28. — *Plain film of the abdomen in the upright position AP showing double bubble in stomach and duodenum.*

TABLE III. — ANOMALIES
ASSOCIATED WITH DUODENAL OBSTRUCTION

	Number	%
Mongolism	4	14
Esophageal atresia	4	14
Imperforate anus	4	14
Malrotation	3	9.5
Cardiac anomalies	3	9.5
Meckel's diverticulum	2	7
Situs inversus	2	7
Clubbed feet	1	3.5
Cataract	1	3.5
Urethral valve	1	3.5
Total	28	

survey by the American Academy of Pediatrics this percentage was found to be 48 % [2].

Down syndrome was present in 4 patients (14 %). In other series its incidence has been as high as 30 % [2]. The diagnosis is confirmed by chromosome studies, usually completed within a day or two.

TREATMENT

The baby is kept in a warm and humidified incubator, in the neonatal unit, a nasogastric tube with intermittent suction prevents aspiration of vomitus. Dehydration and metabolic alkalosis are corrected before surgery.

TABLE IV. — ANATOMOSES

Side-to-side duodeno-duodenostomy.	16
Side-to-side duodeno-jejunostomy	10
End-to-end duodeno-duodenostomy	2
Total	28

A transverse incision in the right upper quadrant will allow the surgeon to see the nature of the obstruction: atresia or annular pancreas. There are important structures in this area and one should refrain from useless and even dangerous dissection. To insure patency of the distal bowel, saline should be injected into the bowel and visually followed down to the rectum. Although we did not encounter multiple atresias in this particular group of patients, most authors recommend this maneuver [4]. Both duodenal atresia and annular pancreas are treated by bypassing the site of obstruction. We have used 3 types of anastomoses (Table IV). A gastrostomy was constructed in 21 patients. Normal duodenal transit was frequently slow to return. The shortest postoperative period was 17 days. If the anastomosis is not functional after 5 or 6 days, parenteral alimentation (usually through a peripheral vein) is started. Some of our anastomoses have taken as long as 60 and one 72 days to attain adequate function. For this reason some surgeons in our group insert a silastic feeding catheter through the anastomosis down to the jejunum, and bring it out through the gastrostomy opening. This allows enteral feeding while waiting for the anastomosis to function. The gastrostomy keeps the stomach empty. We had 3 intraluminal diaphragms (windsock) in our series. They are more difficult to recognise at surgery [6]. Insertion of a foley catheter through the gastrostomy down through the duodenum helps to find them. Resection of the diaphragm is done through a duodenotomy. The ampula of Vater is often located between the mucosal layers [6] of the diaphragm. It must be looked for and protected.

The association of esophageal atresia and tracheo-

TABLE V. — SUMMERY OF 5 DEATHS

Associated conditions	Operations	Time of death	Cause of death
Imperforate anus Hypoglycemia Prematurity	Colostomy Duodeno-jejunostomy	3 days post-op	Atelactasis + acidosis
Esophageal atresia Malrotation	Duodeno-duodeno-stomy Gastrostomy Gastric-transsection	8 days post-op	Kernicterus
Prematurity Esophageal atresia Imperforate anus Meckel diverticulum	Duodeno-jejunostomy Gastrostomy Colostomy	3 days post-op	Hyaline membrane disease
Mongolism VSD	Duodeno-duodeno-stomy	21 days post-op	Pneumonia
—	Duodeno-duodeno-stomy Gastrostomy Appendectomy	61 days post-op	Wound dehissence; meningitis

esophageal fistula with duodenal atresia is particularly dangerous. Mortality rates up to 76 % have been reported [2]. One must first correct the duodenal atresia and do a gastrostomy, followed by section and closure of the tracheo-esophageal fistula. The esophageal anastomosis can be done at the same time or postponed, depending on the condition of the baby.

RESULTS

Five of our 28 babies did not survive (Table V). Four of these had associated anomalies. Once over the initial phase surviving babies had a satisfactory course.

REFERENCES

[1] BERDON (W. E.). — Micro-colon in newborn infants with intestinal obstruction. *Radiology*, 90, 878-885, 1968.
[2] FONKALS RUD (E. W.), DELORIMIER (A. A.), HAYS (D. M.). — Congenital atresia and stenosis of the duodenum. *Pediatrics*, 43, 79-83, 1969.
[3] GRAY (S. W.), SKANDALADIS (J. E.). — *Embryology for surgeons*. W. B. Saunders, Philadelphia, 129, 1972.
[4] LYNN (H. B.). — *Pediatric Surgery*. Year book medical publishers, Inc., Chicago, 911-912, 1979.
[5] SWENSON (O.). — *Pediatric Surgery*, Appleton-Century-Crofts, New York, 1969.
[6] RICHARDSON (W. R.), MARTIN (L. W.). — Pitfalls in the surgical management of the incomplete duodenal diaphragm. *J. Pediatr. Surg.*, 4, 303-312, 1969.

Pyloric stenosis

Jacques-Charles DUCHARME

Pyloric stenosis is one of the most common surgical diseases of the neonate. In a pediatric hospital with 15,000 surgical admissions/year we see approximately 50 patients with this disease in contrast to 2 or 3 malrotations and 3 duodenal atresias a year.

ETIOLOGY

The etiology of hypertrophic pyloric stenosis remains obscure despite extensive research. Dodge [1] has succeeded in producing hypertrophic pyloric stenosis in the dog after prolonged antenatal maternal stimulation with pentagastrin. Janik's [2] results seem to contradict Dodge's work. From his work with rabits and dogs Janik concluded that *a*) pentagastrin does not cause pyloric stenosis, *b*) human gastrin does not cross the canine placental barrier, *c*) gastrin has no documented role in the etiology of pyloric stenosis.

Spitz [3] using optical microscopy, reported a diminution in the number and a change in the structure of ganglion cells of the pylorus. Jona [4] described normal neurons, interstitial plexus and smooth muscular fibers of the pylorus at electron microscopy.

PRESENTATION

In a recent series of 100 consecutive cases treated at Ste-Justine Hospital and reviewed for this chapter, the familial incidence was 8 %. It was often a first born (35 %) and a male (89 to 11 females), in comparison with the usually reported 4:1 male: female ratio. Rarely symptoms were present at birth, as early as the 4th or 5th day of life, or as late as 5 months, but the average in our experience was 3 weeks. Vomiting is always present, contains ingested food, and is never green. Early on the baby may only vomit once or twice a day. As the obstruction progresses, vomiting becomes more frequent and projectile. In 5 % of the cases the vomitus is brownish because it contains blood, usually thought to be due to secondary esophagitis.

If the symptoms last more than 10 days the weight curve is fairly typical: birth weight, the highest weight reached by the baby, and the admission weight form a triangle that we have found in 34 % of our patients. With time the baby voids less and the urine is more concentrated. Constipation was present in 47 of our patients. Nowadays it is rare to see these long thin, dehydrated babies that we saw in the past after 4, 5 or 6 weeks of evolution.

Two patients presented with icterus. This is due to a rise in the indirect bilirubin [5] secondary either to a diminution of the activity of the hepatic enzyme glucuronyl-transferase, or to increased entero-hepatic reabsorption of bilirubin sequestered in the G. I. tract.

DIAGNOSIS

Physical examination is important. One should sit on the left side of the bed. With some patience and sugar water to relax the baby, one can often see gastric peristaltic waves going from left to right in the upper abdomen. They were seen in 42 % of our patients. By flexing the right thigh of the baby on the abdomen, one can then relax the abdominal wall muscles and easily palpate the hypertrophic pylorus (Fig. VIII-29). The percentage of palpated olives increases with patience, gentleness and experience. In this series, the surgeons felt the olive in 83 % of cases. The diagnosis can be made with certainty on clinical grounds alone. In the rare case where physical examination is inconclusive, an upper G. I. series is done. A long pyloric canal, violent gastric waves and delayed emptying are typical (Fig. VIII-30).

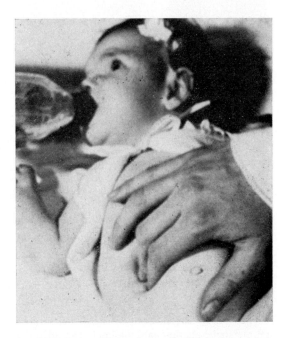

Fig. VIII-29. — *After relaxing the baby with a nipple, and by standing on the baby's left, the fingers can feel the pylorus under the rectus muscle.*

This examination also helps to rule out gastro-esophageal reflux which sometimes presents with symptoms similar to pyloric stenosis.

If symptoms have persisted more than a week, hypochloremic metabolic alkalosis will be present. The potassium is usually normal. If it is above

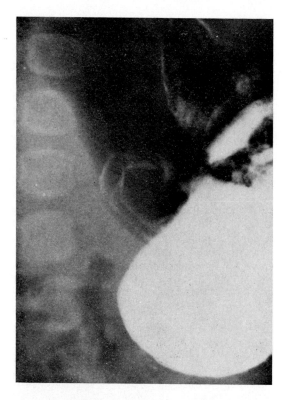

FIG. VIII-30. — *Typical X-ray appearance of pyloric stenosis; elongated, stenotic and curved upward pyloric canal.*

normal, one should consider the possibility of adrenal hyperplasia with sodium loss. This pathology may also present at that age with vomiting and dehydration. We have noted a good correlation between the severity of hypochloremia and the degree of obstruction.

TREATMENT

When these babies present early, dehydration and metabolic alkalosis are minimal. The operation can be carried out after a few hours of I. V. therapy with 5 % dextrose and NaCl 0.2 %. If the alkalosis is more significant (*i. e.* $CO_2 > 30$ mEq) we use 5 % dextrose NaCl 0.45 % at the rate of 20-25 cm³ per hour. We add KCl (3 mEq/100 cm³) after the first voiding. The baby is ready for surgery when he or she has gained about 100 grams, voided 5 or 6 times and when the CO_2 has come down to about half the excess value. This usually takes 24 to 48 hours. We do not consider these babies as sur-

gical emergencies, and operate on them within the regular operating room schedule.

If the baby has esophagitis, nasogastric suction is put in place on admission. Otherwise the baby is kept N. P. O. and the nasogastric tube placed on suction a few hours before surgery in order to drain the stomach before anesthesia. The nasogastric tube is removed moments before anesthesia to prevent gastro-esophageal reflux during induction of anesthesia. The pyloromyotomy is carried out either through a transverse incision through the right rectus muscle or through a gridiron incision. The operation is simple and completed in less than 30 minutes (Fig. VIII-31, VIII-32).

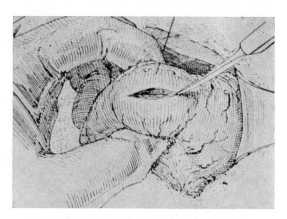

FIG. VIII-31. — *The pylorus must be pulled out of the abdomen. Incision on the serosa.*

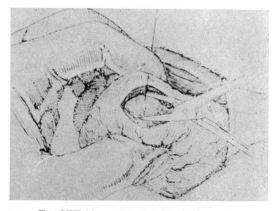

FIG. VIII-32. — *Completed pyloromyotomy. The mucosa is bulging between the pyloric muscle.*

A Levin tube is kept under suction for 6 hours after surgery. It is important, in order to prevent closure of the pylorus muscle, to have liquids pass through the pylorus. This is why oral feeding is begun early, on the first day.

The feedings are increased in volume 30, 60, 90 ccs every 2-3-4 hours in the following days. In most instances the baby is back on a regular diet by the 4th or 5th day.

Only 30 % of patients with pyloric stenosis stop vomiting immediately after surgery. The others do continue vomiting although much less than before surgery, for a period of up to 15 days. If the parents are told of this fact, the baby can be sent home early even if he or she is still vomiting. Our average post-op stay is 3.7 days.

RESULTS

They are excellent. We have not had a surgical death since 1963. The only complications in this series were a 9 % infection rate which is high, and one reoperation for revision of an incomplete pyloromyotomy.

REFERENCES

[1] DODGE (J. A.). — Production of duodenal ulcers and hypertrophic pyloric stenosis by administration of pentagastrin to pregnant and new born dogs. *Nature*, 225, 284-285, 1970.
[2] JANIK (J. S.), AKBAR (A. M.), BURRINGTON (J. D.), BURKE (G.). — The role of gastrin in congenital hypertrophic pyloric stenosis. *J. Pediatr. Surg.*, 13, 151-154, 1978.
[3] SPITZ (L.), KAUFMANN (C. E.). — The neuropathological changes in congenital hypertrophic pyloric stenosis. *S. Afr. J. Surg.*, 13, 239-242, 1975.
[4] JONA JUDA (Z.). — Electron microscopic observations in infantile hypertrophic pyloric stenosis. *J. Pediatr. Surg.*, 13, 17-20, 1978.
[5] WOOLEY (M. M.), FELSHER (B. F.), ASCH (M. J.), CARPIO (N.), ISAACS (H.). — Jaundice. Hypertrophic pyloric stenosis. Hepatic glucuronyl-transferase. *J. Pediatr. Surg.*, 9, 359-363, 1974.
[6] BENSON (Cl.). — *Pediatric Surgery*. Year book medical publishers Inc., Chicago, 891-894, 1979.

Intestinal obstruction: overview

Frank M. GUTTMAN

Although newborn babies may vomit once or twice, bile stained vomitus is the cardinal sign of intestinal obstruction. It should arouse immediate concern for a surgical cause of the obstruction. Some neonatologists advocate intubation of the stomach at birth. If more than 20 ml of gastric

TABLE I. — CAUSES OF NEONATAL VOMITING

1. *Medical*	2. *Surgical*
(*a*) Cerebral	(*a*) Intrinsic lesions
— Hemorrhage-increased intra-cranial pressure	— Atresia or stenosis (anywhere in the intestinal tract)
— Meningitis	— Hirschsprung's disease
(*b*) Sepsis	— Duplication
— Peritonitis	— Necrotizing enterocolitis
— Meningitis	— Esophago-gastric chalasia
— Pyelonephritis	(*b*) Intraluminal obstruction
— Septicemia	— Meconium ileus; uncomplicated and complicated
(*c*) Gastric irritation	— Meconium plug obstruction
— Drugs (maternal)	— Small left colon syndrome
— Swallowed blood	(*c*) Extrinsic lesions
(*d*) Prematurity	— Malrotation-volvulus
— Hypothermia	— Hernia
	— Adhesions
	— Preduodenal portal vein
	— Annular pancreas
	— Diaphragmatic hernia (late)
	— Hiatal hernia

aspirate is found, intestinal obstruction is probably present. The multiple medical and surgical causes of vomiting in the neonatal period are outlined in Table I. A variety of clinical states give rise to vomiting. The most frequent ones are: (*a*) sepsis, of the peritoneum, of the meninges, the kidney, and septicemia, giving rise to ileus, (*b*) intestinal obstruction, and (*c*) increased intracranial pressure.

There are two other so-called cardinal signs of intestinal obstruction. These are abdominal distension and failure to pass meconium. Both are irregular and depend on other factors for their appearance. Abdominal distension is seen least as the level of obstruction is higher in the gastrointestinal tract. With lower obstruction it becomes a prominent feature of the clinical picture. Failure to pass meconium is frequently seen in intestinal obstruction. However, because meconium passage *may occur once or several times* even with complete intestinal obstruction, e. g. ileal atresia, *it is extremely important not to rule out intestinal obstruction based on the passage of stool.* The onset of the important sign of bile-vomitus must engender an immediate alarm signal to investigate for surgical intestinal obstruction. Resuscitation and maintenance during clinical and radiological assessment is essential.

Some of the conditions will be dealt with individually. The most urgent conditions in neonatal surgery are diaphragmatic hernia (Bochdalek) and malrotation. Diaphragmatic hernia gives rise mainly to respiratory distress and only later to frank intestinal obstruction as more of the gut dilates, especially when a nasogastric tube is not used immediately. In malrotation, the danger is that because of the abnormally narrow and long root of the mesentary, volvulus will occur and there will be loss of intestine through infarction.

During the period of clinical and radiological investigation it is essential to maintain homeostasis-warmth, fluids, electrolytes and oxygenation, and prevent further gastrointestinal dilatation with proper naso-gastric drainage (not a Nr 4 feeding tube!). A newborn of normal weight should have a Nr 12 French red rubber catheter with several extra holes cut, placed into the stomach, or the newly available pediatric size gastric sump tubes. In our experience at Ste-Justine Hospital as well as in the literature, fully 25 % of neonatal intestinal obstruction is caused by Hirschsprung's disease. This is important to keep in mind since the enterocolitis of Hirchsprung's disease can be disastrous.

Neonatal peritonitis

Frank M. GUTTMAN

Neonatal peritonitis may occur associated with septicemia. It may develop from umbilical stump sepsis, or as a complication of neonatal intestinal perforation, necrotizing enterocolitis, and meconium ileus. Early features are vomiting with distension and sometimes diarrhea. Free intraperitoneal fluid may be seen on X-ray as may the signs of the other distinctive syndromes. In complicated meconium ileus (cystic fibrosis) one may see the soap bubble appearance of the meconium, with calcifications. This may be further complicated by ileal atresia. Peritonitis consequent on necrotizing enterocolitis or idiopathic perforation may show free air on the abdominal films.

TREATMENT

Usually laparotomy is indicated after massive wide-spectrum antibiotics are begun. If no perforation is found, the abdomen should be washed and may be closed without drainage. Neonatal ascites (urine, chyle or bile) may be differentiated from peritonitis by the absence of serious clinical signs and symptoms, other than distension and intraperitoneal fluid, although vomiting may be present. The X-ray will not show intestinal distension. An abdominal paracentesis will give the diagnosis by examination of the aspirate.

Primary peritonitis is usually seen in infants and small children. The organism is often streptococcus, or pneumococcus, which is seen much more frequently in girls (Mason Brown) suggesting that the source of entry may be vaginal.

Necrotizing enterocolitis

Frank M. GUTTMAN

This clinical entity had been reported with increasing frequency during the 1960's and 70's presumably concomittant with the increase in survival of premature babies. It has been called in the past, colonic perforation secondary to exchange transfusions; ischemic perforation of the gut; neonatal necrotizing enterocolitis; and neonatal peritonitis. N. E. C. is seen primarily in premature infants where some major stress has occurred. N. E. C. is not present where ischemic injury is found consequent on the distension of neglected atresia, in Hirschsprung's disease, in volvulus or hernia, in pseudomembranous enterocolitis or inflammatory bowel disease.

INCIDENCE

Neonatal intensive care especially the cardio-respiratory care of the premature neonate has improved enormously over the past twenty years. The incidence of N. E. C. has increased dramatically during this period and has been estimated to be from 1-7 % of newborn admissions. The current trend to concentrate high risk pregnancies in tertiary centers, with rapid safe transport systems, results in a high incidence of the disease in specialized I. C. U.'s. The increase is also due to the increased use of intensive care monitoring procedures through the umbilicus and the increased awareness of this entity.

ETIOLOGY

The etiology of this illness is not clear, however its pathogenesis seems to be involved in vascular insufficiency. It has been suggested that this entity is similar to non-occlusive intestinal vascular insufficiency in the elderly. Other concomitant factors suggested have been hyperosmolar feedings, altered or immature intestinal immunity, and infection.

Lloyd emphasized the high incidence of peritoneal stress in spontaneous perforation of the gut [1]. He suggested that the selective redistribution of blood flow away from the gut was the etiological factor and likened this to the "diving reflex" of swimming mammals. Touloukian has demonstrated this selective ischemia in the neonatal piglet by radioisotopic examination [2]. He showed that hypoxia will result in a pattern of ischemia similar to that found in N. E. C.

An increase in the incidence of N. E. C. is certainly seen in numerous low-flow states i. e. myocardial insufficiency reduced perfusion pressure, elevated portal pressure, and increased vascular resistance. Touloukian et al. have also shown that the reason exchange transfusion is associated with an increased incidence of N. E. C. may be the demonstrated acute rise in portal pressure during the exchange [3]. Autopsy examination of infants dying from N. E. C. shows evidence of ischemia of other organs (except for the essential-heart, lungs, brain) i. e. the kidneys, liver, adrenals, muscle and skin.

Clinical sepsis is often seen with N. E. C. and is considered secondary to loss of the mucosal barrier and invasion by the normal enteric pathogens. Because this disease entity occurs in epidemic-like spurts, some have suggested that infectious agents are primarily responsible. It has also been suggested (Barlow et al. [4]) that the newborn's normal host immune defense mechanisms are wanting. Barlow showed that newborn rats were protected from hypoxic ischemic damage by breast milk feedings. The protective factor in breast milk was presumably macrophages and possibly IgA.

Most believe that the etiology of N. E. C. is multifactorial. The final pathway seems to be mesenteric vascular insufficiency with loss of mucosal integrity and invasion of the bowel wall by the normal intestinal flora. The process of damage is accentuated by early hyperosmolar feedings. Although the illness has been reported in breast-fed babies, it is possible that breast milk may have a protective effect. Prophylaxis with total gut rest, and parenteral alimentation in high risk babies seems to have reduced the onset of the more serious forms of this illness in several nurseries [5]. At Ste-Justine Hospital this program of identification of high risk infants and a go-slow feeding plan has reduced the annual rate of N. E. C. from 30/year to 4/year over the past three years [6].

PATHOLOGY

The pathological picture in this disease process is varied, with different degrees of ischemic damage. Macroscopically one may see a clean-cut perforation on the antimesenteric border in otherwise normal appearing bowel. The more common finding is hemorrhagic infarction which may or may not be associated with perforation. Microscopic changes show edema of the submucosa, and in the mucosa with all stages of ischemic injury showing hemorrhage and necrosis.

DIAGNOSIS

The important factor in the diagnosis of N. E. C. is recognition and close observation of infants at risk. We have dealt with most of these factors in the section on etiology. They are; birth weight and prematurity, respiratory distress syndrome, congenital heart disease, sepsis, prolonged labor and placenta praevia giving fetal distress. The typical history will be that of a premature or stressed infant with a low Apgar score at birth, presenting with abdominal distension, irritability, temperature instability, vomiting and loose seedy stools which may have bloody streaks. These signs usually present at 5-10 days after birth, but a fulminating picture may be present at either end of this period. Indeed, a full term breast fed baby may present with the syndrome although this is not typical. The physical examination will reveal the abdominal distension and tenderness. Rectal examination may reveal blood or bloody stools. Clinically one must assess whether perforation or peritonitis are present. Frank perforation will be suggested by the absence of liver dullness, and the general abdominal tympanic response to percussion. The abdominal wall may be reddened by cellulitis and the amount of tenderness and rebound tenderness can be assessed with practice. Occasionally a mass may be felt.

Laboratory investigation should include a CBC, and platelet count, electrolytes, blood gases, bili-

rubin and a coagulogram. Thrombocytopenia is generally an indication of severe gram-negative sepsis and may be used to monitor the evolution. It is not however, entirely reliable. Santulli et al. [1] point out that they have had several patients with perforation without a drop in platelets. Homeostasis of these factors is required. Stools should be examined regularly for occult blood. Blood, urine, stool, and umbilical cultures should be taken. X-ray studies are essential and include the chest and abdomen with an upright or a lateral shoot-through to have two views of the abdomen. Intestinal distension is seen initially and then pneumatosis intestinalis (Fig. VIII-33). A barium enema should not be done. It is essential to do sequential 6-8 hour. films and repeated clinical evaluations of the baby. Catastrophic events occur rapidly in this disease and it is essential to operate early with a complication but to withhold surgery when not required. The air in the bowel wall is usually bubbly. When present as a halo around the gut lumen, intestinal necrosis may be presumed. Portal vein air is a serious sign but not inevitably fatal as it is in the adult (Fig. VIII-44). The differential diagnosis of pneumoperitoneum itself includes traumatic perforation by a thermometer in the rectum, and that, seen more often today, consequent on pneumo-

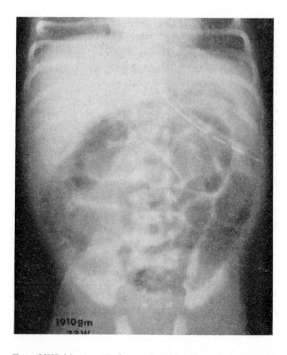

Fig. VIII-33. — *Radiograph of a premature neonate with intestinal pneumatosis. This is especially evident in the ascending colon and transverse colon.*

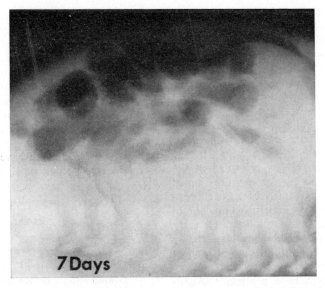

FIG. VIII-34. — *Necrotizing enterocolitis with perforation seen anteriorly in lateral shoot-through.*
Note also gas in the portal venous system.

mediastinum in infants on a ventilator. A fixed loop of small bowel remaining distended for over 24 hours is often a sign of intestinal infarction.

TREATMENT

Since this disease has a range of severity, there is a place for non-operative as well as operative management with close and repeated clinical and radiological examination. Concomitant disease- e. g. respiratory distress syndrome, congenital heart disease etc., must be treated. Fluid replacement is necessary. Transfusion as required. The essential elements of prophylaxis and treatment of early uncomplicated patients are gut rest and antibiotics. An adequate nasogastric catheter is passed and proper care given to the suction system. Systemic and enteric antibiotics are given.

The choice of antibiotics relates to the sensitivities of the bacteria involved in the various parts of the world. The most common agents are *E. coli* and *Klebsiella*. Coverage should begin with a newer generation of cephalosporins (e. g. cefoxitin) which covers gram positive cocci, oral anaerobes, *E. coli*, *Klebsiella* and *B. fragilis*; associated with an aminoglycoside, e. g. gentamycin, covering *proteus*, *enterobacter*, *pseudomonas*, *Klebsiella*, *E. coli*, *serratia* and *staphylococcus*. If laparotomy is carried out specific cultures and sensitivities should be obtained. Some authors recommend intra-abdominal (through the N. G. tube), antibiotics, kanamycin or gentamycin or both. In the presence of ileus, it is unlikely that the antibiotics would progress down the intestinal tract.

Peripheral parenteral nutrition is begun. We keep the central route for use after failure of the peripheral route which can last, with rotation, for several months.

The abdomen should be palpated for increasing tenderness, masses or tympanism. The X-rays will demonstrate increasing intra-mural gas or its disappearance. Measurement of abdominal girth regularly, will also give an appreciation of change.

The clinical picture will determine when to begin gradual reduction of these measures. If all progresses satisfactorily after 6-10 days with lessening of distension, lessening of aspirate, and passage of stool; nasogastric suction is discontinued. Enteric feedings of glucose water are begun very slowly and increased progressively. Dilute simplified formulas are indicated with simple sugars, shorter peptides and medium-chain triglycerides, because of malabsorption which follows ischemia.

Successful management of the non-operated form of this illness, is sometimes followed by late sequellae of colonic ischemic stenosis. It is recommended that a barium enema be carried out 2-3 months following established N. E. C. in all patients to rule out stricture formation.

Operation is indicated by increasing irritability, instability of the patient associated with continued sepsis over 48 hours. Frank peritonitis, abdominal tender mass or perforation will lead to laparotomy. Changes in the abdominal wall, edema, erythema, and cellulitis are also signs that laparotomy should be carried out. The extent of this disease in the gut is variable. It may extend to the entire superior mesenteric arterial circulation. Frequently only the terminal ileum is involved. However when extensive resection will result in a short gut syndrome (duodenorectal) it has been our policy to close the abdomen with no or a little resection of the worst part and to return again in 36-48 hours.

Occasionally more bowel has recovered at the second laparotomy to allow for a more limited resection. In volvulus, this maneuver is more successful. We sometimes close without resection, not to return. In general, it has been our policy not to carry out a primary anastomosis, although this certainly could be feasible when there is little intra-abdominal sepsis and when the proximal ostomy will be closer to the ligament of Treitz. Here, a primary anastomosis may contribute to more rapid recuperation. Prior to reconstruction at 6-9 months, barium studies must be done to evaluate stricture formation. We have seen the occasional patient who was reconstructed too early and presented with stricture formation distal to the anastomosis.

RESULTS (Table II)

The long term results of N. E. C. have recently been reviewed by Santulli et al. [7]. They reported that there was a definite dramatic improvement in survival of all groups comparing 1955-1974 and 1975-1978. This was especially evident for the medical group (16 % to 78 %) whereas the surgically treated group improved from 30 to 40 %.

Late stricture formation occurred in 21 % of both earlier and later series. They note that these strictures became apparent in 10-42 days following the onset of the disease. Malabsorption may be a problem depending on the extent of the resection. Death is most often due to sepsis and peritonitis.

In Santullis' series follow-up has been for 1-5 years in 23 patients and in 8, over 5 years [7]. In general all these children are doing well. One child 8 years of age is mildly mentally retarded. Two younger and two older children have an increased number of daily bowel movements.

REFERENCES

Neonatal peritonitis

[1] MASON BROWN (J. J.). — *Surgery of Childhood.* Edward Arnold (Publishers) Ltd., 811, 1962.

Necrotizing enterocolitis

[1] LLOYD (J. R.). — The etiology of Gastrointestinal Perforation in the Newborn. *J. Pediatr. Surg.*, 4, 77, 1969.
[2] TOULOUKIAN (R. J.), POSCH (J. N.), SPENCER (R.). — The Pathogenesis of Ischemic Gastroenterocolitis of the Neonate. *J. Pediatr. Surg.*, 7, 194, 1972.
[3] TOULOUKIAN (R. J.), KADAR (A.), SPENCER (R. P.). — The Gastrointestinal Complications of Neonatal Umbilical Venous Exchange Transfusion. *Pediatrics*, 51, 36, 1973.
[4] BARLOW (B.), SANTULLI (T. V.), HEIRD (W. C.) et al. — An experimental Study of Acute Neonatal Enterocolitis. The Importance of Breast Milk. *J. Pediatr. Surg.*, 9, 587, 1974.
[5] PHILIPPART (A. I.), RECTOR (F. E.). — *Necrotizing Enterocolitis in Pediatric Surgery.* Ed. RAVITCH M. M., 975, vol. 2, 3rd édit. Year Book Publ., 1979.
[6] TEASDALE (F.), LeGUENNEC (J. C.), BARD (H.) et al. — *Neonatal Necrotizing Enterocolitis* (in press).

TABLE II. — SURVIVAL IN NECROTIZING ENTEROCOLITIS

Authors	No. cases	Period	Survival med TT	Survival surgical TT
TOULOUKIAN et al. [2]	25	1955-1966	2/10 (20 %)	4/15 (27 %)
WILSON & WOOLEY [8]	16	1958-1968	1/7 (14 %)	3/9 (33 %)
STEVENSON et al. [9]	38	1962-1969	13/19 (68 %)	12/19 (63 %)
DUDGEON et al. [10]	63	1970-1972	26/44 (59 %)	5/19 (26 %)
BELL et al. [11]	23	1970-1972	11/14 (78 %)	4/9 (44 %)
WAYNE et al. [12]	30	1971-1974	—	21/30 (70 %)
SANTULLI et al. [15]	64	1955-1974	6/37 (16 %)	8/27 (30 %)
ROBACK et al. [13]	69	1970-1973	13/27 (47 %)	14/42 (33 %)
O'NEILL et al. [14]	52	1970-1974	22/32 (69 %)	12/20 (60 %)
PHILIPPART & RECTOR [5]	73	1974-1976	30/41 (73 %)	26/32 (81 %)
SANTULLI et al. [7]	46	1975-1978	28/36 (78 %)	4/10 (40 %)

[7] SCHULLINGER (J. N.), SANTULLI (T. V.), MOLLITT (D. L.) et al. — Necrotizing Enterocolitis in Long-Term Follow-up in Congenital Anomalies. *Pediatric Surg. Symposium*, September 14-15, Pittsburgh, Pa., 75, 1979.

[8] WILSON (S. E.), WOOLLEY (M. M.). — Primary Necrotizing Enterocolitis in Infants. *Arch. Surg.*, 99, 563, 1969.

[9] STEVENSON (J. K.), OLIVER (T. K.), GRAHAM (C. B.) et al. — Aggressive Treatment of Necrotizing Enterocolitis: 38 Patients with 25 Survivors. *J. Pediatr. Surg.*, 6, 28, 1971.

[10] DUDGEON (D. L.), CORAN (A.), LAOPE (F. A.) et al. — Surgical Management of Acute Necrotizing Enterocolitis in Infancy. *J. Pediatr. Surg.*, 8, 607, 1973.

[11] BELL (M. J.), KOSLOSKE (A. M.), BENTON (C.) et al. — Neonatal Necrotizing Enterocolitis. Prevention of Perforation. *J. Pediatr. Surg.*, 8, 601, 1973.

[12] WAYNE (E. R.), BARRINGTON (J. D.), HUNTER (J.). — Neonatal Necrotizing Enterocolitis. *Arch. Surg.*, 110, 476, 1975.

[13] ROBACH (S. A.). — Necrotizing Enterocolitis. *Arch. Surg.*, 109, 314, 1974.

[14] O'NEILL (J. A.), STOHLMAN (M. T.), MENG (H. C.). — Necrotizing Enterocolitis in the Newborn. *Ann. Surg.*, 182, 274, 1975.

[15] SANTULLI (T. V.), SCHULLINGER (J. N.), HEIRD (N. C.) et al. — Acute Necrotizing Enterocolitis in Infancy. A review of 64 cases. *Pediatrics*, 55, 376, 1975.

Intestinal atresia

Frank M. GUTTMAN

Atresia and stenosis of the small intestine are among the common causes of intestinal obstruction in the newborn. During the past 20 years, the early recognition, understanding and treatment of this problem have undergone marked improvement. However, the pathogenesis of this entity is still not understood. None of the current theories and experimental evidence correlates with the possible pathogenesis of hereditary multiple atresia, as described by Guttman and his associates [9], which occurs throughout the intestinal tract from the antrum to the rectum.

INCIDENCE

A large survey of members of the Surgical Section of the American Academy of Paediatrics was reported by de Lormier et al. [7]. The site of obstruction was proximal jejunum 31 %, distal jejunum 20 %, proximal ileum 13 %, and distal ileum 36 %. In our own series from Ste-Justine Hospital, we found an almost equal division of duodenal atresia and jejunoileal atresia, which is contrary to most reported series where jejunoileal atresia is 2:1 more common than duodenal atresia. The overall incidence has been estimated as 1:330 live births to 1:1,500 live births [8].

TYPES OF INTESTINAL ATRESIA

These have been well described by Bland-Sutton [4] and elaborated on by the work of Louw [13], and of Nixon [17]. Included in these is the diaphragm which is a stenosis in that it is a partial obstruction with an eccentric perforation resulting in incomplete intestinal obstruction. This is rare in the jejunoileal region but occurs more frequently in the duodenal area.

In type I stenosis, there is a complete diaphragm. From the outside, it is difficult to see where the obstruction is located. In type II, the bowel is an atretic band for a variable distance. One of the patients in our series had an atretic band replacing almost the entire small bowel. Here, the mesentery is intact. Type III has discontinuous bowel with a breach in the mesentery. A special form of this, which Touloukian classifies as type 3b occurs where the defect in the mesentery is so extensive that the bowel folds around it in the typical "apple peel" or "christmas tree" deformity [21].

Type IV comprises multiple atresias which prior to our report in 1973 was thought not to be located in the duodenum and the jejunoileal region in the same patient, or be jejunoileal and colonic in the same patient. We found several patients who had multiple atresias throughout the intestinal tract, most of which were of a hereditary form but several were not associated with consanguinity.

PATHOGENESIS

Bland-Sutton [4], who first proposed the accepted classification of intestinal atresia, suggested that atresia occurs at the site of predilection of embryologic events or where excessive reabsorption of the vitelline duct might explain ileal atresia. The theory of the solid stage of intestinal growth and subsequent vacuolization was proposed by Tandler [20]. This theory has been challenged by indirect and direct study. The presence of lanugo, squamous epithelial cells and bile distal to the obstruction, as shown by Louw [13] and by Santulli and Blanc [19], is evidence against Tandler's theory because of the discrepancy in the embryologic calendar of events.

On direct study, Lynn and Espinos [14] found occlusion in some human embryos, but in most, there was none. Moutsouris [15] also found no significant solid proliferative stage of growth in the jejunum or ileum. Although there was an intense proliferative stage in the duodenum, nowhere could he demonstrate obvious complete obliteration. Thus, it would seem that other factors are required to explain atresia of the small intestine. Mechanical events, such as hernia into the umbilicus, strangulation and intussusception have been reported as possible etiologic factors. Laufman and his colleagues [11] produced types 2 and 3 atresia by devascularizing intestinal segments in a sterile peritoneum. Louw and Barnard [13] demonstrated the direct effect of interruption of blood supply to the intestine in the fetal dog and were able to produce all three types of atresia. In some patients, Nixon and Tawes [17] were able to disprove this cause through arteriography, which demonstrated patent vessels to the atretic segment. Nonetheless, in some patients, it would seem that the vascular accident theory is attractive. Experimentally, the work of Barnard [13], carried out in the dog, has been confirmed by Santulli and Blanc [19] in the rabbit and by Abrams [1] in the lamb.

Louw and Barnard [13] suggested that the rapid proliferative stage of growth in the duodenum leads to susceptibility to hypoxia. Courtois [5] demonstrated that intestinal perforation produced in fetal rabbits may heal without a trace or with a residual stenosis or atresia. A recent careful microscopic study by Tsujimoto and his associates [22] demonstrated that the atresia and stenosis produced by interruption of the fetal mesenteric vessels in rabbits shows rapid liquefaction and resolution of the infarcted intestine, with little exudate or adhesions and minimal fibrosis. Perforation of the intestine was common in these experiments, suggesting

perhaps a relationship to neonatal perforation of the intestine of non apparent origin. Rittenhouse and his group [18] have recently suggested that current theories do not explain the less common type 1 multiple septums with multiple atresia. We recently have reported on the widespread association of lesions, from the stomach to the rectum, in hereditary multiple atresia [9]. Here, the presence of atresia in the stomach, duodenum, jejunum, ileum, colon and rectum together in five patients points to some unknown mechanism of a genetic nature. Since this report, we have seen two more newborns with the same clinical tableau coming from the same region. Thus, we are left with no tenable single theory as to the pathogenesis of all types of intestinal atresia.

RELATIONSHIP OF BIRTH WEIGHT AND GESTATIONAL AGE

In most reports of congenital anomalies in infants, only the incidence of low birth weight has been recorded; no differentiation was made between those with low birthweight due to short gestational age and those who were small for dates and had intrauterine growth retardation. Battaglia and Lubchenco [2] introduced the classification of newborn infants by weight and gestational age, which we have used to assess the association between intestinal atresia and intrauterine development. Until 1970, we based our estimate of gestational age on menstrual history only. Thereafter, we included patients in whom there was a good correlation between menstrual history and clinical evaluation. Only 27 infants in our series were at term and of normal weight. Four infants born at term were small for date babies. A total of 22 babies were preterm, and 19 of these were of appropriate weight for gestational age. The mortality rate is about the same for the preterm and term groups when the weight is appropriate. In this series, it was demonstrated that intestinal atresia is a congenital malformation associated with a high incidence of preterm babies but with a low incidence of intrauterine growth retardation. This is in contrast to the findings of Cozzi and Wilkinson [6] in anorectal and esophageal anomalies, but since clinical examination concerning gestational age was only systematically carried out in our hospital since 1970, we cannot be certain that the gestational age is correct. There has been a gradual improvement in the survival rate. Sixteen of 24 infants survived in the first period and 26 of 29 patients in the second period. The over-all survival rate for the 12 year period was 79 %.

ASSOCIATED ANOMALIES

Associated malformations were found in 34 of the 59 patients in our series [10]. Duodenal atresia is associated primarily with Down syndrome, cardiac anomalies, esophageal atresia and imperforate anus. In contrast, jejunoileal atresia is associated with anomalies of the abdominal wall or abdominal cavity with the exception of intestinal malrotation, which was more common in duodenal atresia. However, in only eight patients with jejunoileal atresia could the probable cause, such as malrotation, volvulus or meconium peritonitis, be identified during the surgical procedure.

DIAGNOSIS

It has become possible to diagnose intestinal obstruction antenatally. Polyhydramnios is common (about 50 %) in babies with proximal bowel obstruction. When present, amniofetography may be carried out as well as ultrasonography which is non-invasive. Touloukian has used this to diagnose in utero diaphragmatic hernia and atresia [21]. In the newborn, abdominal distention is present depending on the level of the obstruction. Bile vomitus is the cardinal sign. Passage of meconium at several times is not uncommon in small bowel atresia. Radiologic investigation is imperative.

ROENTGENOGRAPHIC STUDIES

Supine and upright roentgenographic views of the abdomen presenting two air filled cavities with fluid levels (double bubble sign), will usually establish a diagnosis of duodenal atresia. The diagnosis of jejunal and ileal obstruction may be more difficult. A contrast study of the large intestine is often helpful. It sometimes will permit one to eliminate other causes of obstruction, such as aganglionosis, malrotation or the meconium plug syndrome. Microcolon, or unused colon, often found in ileal atresia is suggested by Berdon and his colleagues as pathognomonic of ileal atresia. We have found this not to be so as it was present in only nine of 13 patients with ileal atresia when the study was carried out [10]. At the jejunal level, we found

microcolon present in three of four patients. Thus, the presence of microcolon per se does not limit the site of obstruction, and we would agree with the final remarks of Berdon and his co-workers [3]: "microcolon is not a simple unused colon but a complex situation due to multiple factors operating in the fetus and probably in the mother as well".

TREATMENT

The treatment has been well described by Nixon & Tawes [17] and by Louw who emphasized the necessity of excision of the proximal bulb prior to anastomosis. Preoperative management includes fluid, electrolyte and thermal correction. Nasogastric suction is required especially if transport for several hours is necessary. The decision as to how to connect bowel or not to connect will depend on the type of atresia I, II, III, on the multiplicity of obstruction and on the level of the obstruction. When the obstruction is high, every effort should be made to restore bowel continuity rather than do a temporary ostomy. In general, an end-to-end connection is best, the distal bowel often must be fish-mouthed so that the final anastomosis is a back-to-back one. Occasionally, a Bishop-Koop or a Santulli end-to-side anastomosis with a chimney for decompression is the wisest course. When proximal dilatation extends over a large portion of the bowel, a tailoring tapering of the proximal end may be used with the GIA stapling device to bring the ends to a better fit.

Results are currently good with a survival rate reported from 80-94 % in various studies.

REFERENCES

[1] ABRAMS (J. S.). — Experimental intestinal atresia. *Surgery*, 64, 185, 1968.
[2] BATTAGLIA (F. C.), LUBCHENCO (L. O.). — A practical classification of newborn infants by weight and gestational age. *J. Pediatr.*, 71, 159, 1967.
[3] BERDON (W. E.), BAKER (D. H.), SANTULLI (T. V.). — Microcolon in newborn infants with intestinal obstruction. *Radiology*, 90, 878, 1968.
[4] BLAND-SUTTON (J.). — Imperforate ileum. *Am. J. Med. Sci.*, 98, 457, 1889.
[5] COURTOIS (B.). — Les origines fœtales des occlusions congénitales du grêle dites par atrésie. *J. Chir.*, 78, 405, 1959.
[6] COZZI (F.), WILKINSON (A. W.). — Intrauterine growth rate in relation to anorectal and œsophageal anomalies. *Arch. Dis. Child.*, 44, 59, 1969.
[7] DE LORMIER (A. A.), FONKALSRUD (E. W.), HAYS (D. M.). — Congenital atresia and stenosis of the jejunum and ileum. *Surgery*, 65, 819, 1969.
[8] GROSFELD (J. L.). — *Atresia and stenosis of the*

jejunum and ileum in paediatric surgery. Yearbook Medical Publ. Inc., Chicago, London, 3rd Edition, 933, 1979.

[9] GUTTMAN (F. M.), BRAUN (P.), GARANCE (P. H. A.) et al. — Multiple intestinal atresia and a new syndrome of hereditary multiple atresia involving the gastrointestinal tract from stomach to rectum. *J. Pediatr. Surg.*, 8, 565, 1973.

[10] GUTTMAN (F. M.), BRAUN (P.), BENSOUSSAN (A. L.) et al. — The pathogenesis of intestinal atresia. *Surg. Gynecol. Obstet.*, 141, 203, 1975.

[11] LAUFMAN (H.), MARTIN (W. B.), METHOD (H.) et al. — Observations in strangulation obstruction. — II. Fate of sterile devascularized intestine in peritoneal cavity. *Arch. Surg.*, 59, 550, 1949.

[12] LOUW (J. H.). — Resection and end-to-end anastomosis in the management of atresia and stenosis of the small bowel. *Surgery*, 62, 940, 1967.

[13] LOUW (J. H.), BARNARD (C. N.). — Congenital intestinal atresia, observations of its origin. *Lancet*, 2, 1065, 1955.

[14] LYNN (H. B.), ESPINOS (S.). — Intestinal atresia; an attempt to relate location to embryologic processes. *Arch. Surg.*, 79, 357, 1959.

[15] MOUTSOURIS (C.). — The "solid stage" and congenital intestinal atresia. *J. Pediatr. Surg.*, 1, 446.

[16] NIXON (H. H.). — Intestinal obstruction in the newborn. *Arch. Dis. Child.*, 30, 13, 1955.

[17] NIXON (H. H.), TAWES (R.). — Etiology and treatment of small intestinal stresia; analysis of a series of 127 jejunoileal atresias and comparison with duodenal atresias. *Surgery*, 69, 41, 1970.

[18] RITTENHOUSE (E. A.), BECKWITH (J. B.), CHAPPELL (J. S.). — Multiple septa of the small bowel. *Surgery*, 71, 714, 1970.

[19] SANTULLI (T. V.), BLANC (W. A.). — Congenital atresia of the intestine. *Ann. Surg.*, 154, 939, 1961.

[20] TANDLER (J.). — Zur Entwicklungsgeschichte des menschlichen Duodenum in frühen embryonals Toden. *Morph. Jahrb.*, 29, 187, 1900.

[21] TOULOUKIAN (R. J.). — *Intestinal atresia and stenosis in paediatric surgery.* W. B. Saunders, Philadelphia, London, Toronto, 331, 1980.

[22] TSUJIMOTO (K.), SHERMAN (F.), RAVITCH (M. M.). — Experimental intestinal atresia in the rabbit fetus; segmental pathological studies. *Johns Hopkins Med. J.*, 131, 287, 1972.

Volvulus of the newborn

Jacques-Charles DUCHARME

Intestinal volvulus in the newborn is usually secondary to another anomaly of the digestive tract, such as small bowel atresia, meconium ileus, duplication, mesenteric cyst and patent omphalomesenteric duct. The most common cause is intestinal malrotation [1]. Rarely volvulus may occur in an otherwise normal newborn [2].

PRESENTATION

When volvulus is a complication of small bowel atresia or meconium ileus, it frequently occurs in utero. If the volvulus occurs after birth, the baby presents symptoms of bowel obstruction, rapidly followed by a worsening of his or her general condition.

In the absence of the above mentioned previous anomalies, the baby has normal bowel function in the first hours of life. Bowel obstruction is heralded by the sudden onset of bilious vomiting. Blood appears in the stool, caused by infarction of the bowel. Vascular collapse occurs. Within a few hours, if the situation is not corrected, the compromised

venous return is followed by necrosis of the bowel, shock and death, often within 24 to 36 hours of the onset of symptoms.

DIAGNOSIS

The short history and rapidly progressive deterioration are typical. Abdominal distension is mild since the obstruction is usually high. The abdomen feels doughy.

Abdominal X-rays show signs compatible with high small bowel obstruction with an unusually small amount of intestinal gas in the abdomen. In a baby who has been previously well this picture is almost pathognomonic (Fig. VIII-35). A barium swallow occasionally will opacify the first few abdominal loops forming a spiral (Fig. VIII-36) or corkscrew appearance.

TREATMENT

This is a surgical emergency. Shock should be treated simultaneously with preparation for surgery,

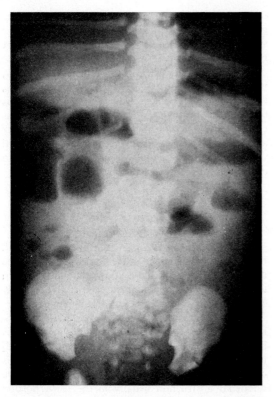

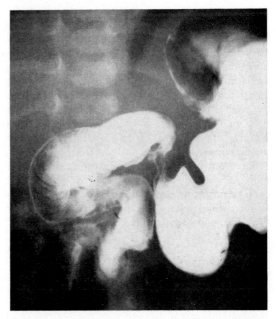

FIG. VIII-36.— *Spiral of intestinal loops above a volvulus of the small bowel secondary to malrotation.*

FIG. VIII-35. — *36 hour old baby. Abdominal X-rays showing a small accumulation of gas in several proximal bowel loops, with fluid levels visible in the upright position. There is practically no gas in the colon.*

induction of anesthesia and surgery. The volvulus is usually clockwise. The small bowel is exteriorised and untwisted counter clockwise.

Intestinal viability is often difficult to evaluate. If the volvulus involves a long segment of bowel and its viability is doubtful, detorsion followed by a second laparotomy 24 hours later, will often allow conservation of more bowel length than thought possible at first encounter.

If only a short segment of bowel is resected the prognosis is excellent. When resection is extensive, hyperalimentation for a few months, has allowed us to rehabilitate babies who had, as little as 15 cm of jejunum, with an intact ileocaecal valve.

REFERENCES

[1] DONNELLAN (W. L.), SWENSON (O.). — *Pediatric Surgery*. Appleton-Century-Croft, New York, 1969.
[2] PELLERIN (D.), BERTIN (P.). — *Ann. Chir. Inf.*, 13, 83-94, 1972.

Intestinal malrotation

Jacques-Charles DUCHARME, Pierre BOUDROS GHOSN

This section is based on 25 cases of intestinal malrotation, treated at Ste-Justine Hospital between January 1970 and December 1979. We have excluded from this series patients with diaphragmatic hernia, gastroschisis and omphalocele. Because the latter, even if always accompagnied by malrotation, differ in presenting symptoms, treatment and prognosis.

Bowel rotation is a complex embryological phenomenon [1]. The malformation is produced by an arrest of rotation at any stage before its termination. Many variations of the anomaly are therefore possible, but usually peritoneal (Ladd's band) press on the duodenum. The caecum is in the right upper quadrant and the mesentery is not fixed to the posterior abdominal wall. The small bowel is supported only by the pedicle of the superior mesenteric artery.

Seven out of our 25 cases presented with one or more associated anomalies: two of these were rather benign: a preduodenal portal vein and a double gallbladder. The other five were major (Table I), affecting treatment and prognosis.

TABLE I. — Major associated malformations (25 patients)

Imperforate anus	2
Duodenal diaphragm	1
Jejunal atresia	1
Caecal stenosis	1
ASD	1
Esophageal atresia	1
Patent ductus arteriosus	1

PRESENTATION

Intestinal malrotation generally presents as an intermittent high intestinal obstruction during the first month of life (17 of our 25). The baby vomits green material but keeps passing meconium or stools. Clinical examination of the abdomen is not remarkable. Distension is absent (16/25 patients).

Because of the deficient fixation of the mesentery, volvulus is common (6/25 patients) when it occurs, the abdomen becomes distended; bloody stools follow. The baby's general condition worsens rapidly: ashen color and tachycardia accompany a floppy baby with a doughy abdomen. Any clinical work-up must be completed rapidly since only an emergency operation can save the baby's life.

INVESTIGATION

Plain films of the abdomen are frequently normal. If Ladd's bands exert extreme pressure on the duodenum, one may find a double bubble of gas in the stomach and duodenum, as seen is any virtually complete duodenal obstruction in the newborn.

Intestinal malrotation is the only neonatal intestinal obstruction where an upper G. I. series is indicated. It is now accepted as being more useful [3] than a barium enema for the diagnosis of this condition. It will demonstrate (*a*) an incomplete duodenal obstruction usually in the third portion of the duodenum (Fig. VIII-37), (*b*) an abnormal position of the angle of Treitz, (*c*) the first jejunal loops to the right of the midline.

The barium enema is less reliable as a diagnostic tool since the presence of the caecum in the right upper quadrant is not always associated with

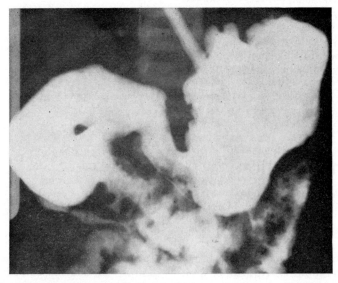

Fig. VIII-37. — *26 hour old baby: the duodenum is dilated to its third portion.*

symptoms. In addition, barium may rapidly fill the distal ileum masking the caecum and making diagnosis impossible.

If a volvulus is also present, plain films of the abdomen are often difficult to interpret (Fig. VIII-38). However, an unusually small amount of intestinal air and some fluid levels suggest a volvulus. As noted above the history of intermittent green vomitus, followed by bloody stools, a distended and painful abdomen and altered general condition in a neonate strongly suggest the diagnosis.

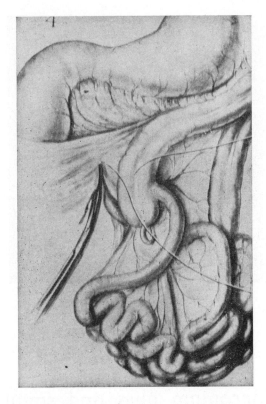

FIG. VIII-39. — *The scissors are cutting Ladd's bands obstructing the duodenum.*

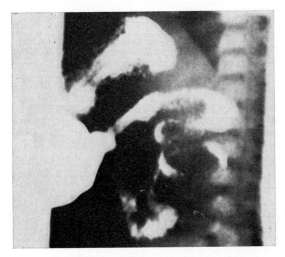

FIG. VIII-38. — *Midgut volvulus secondary to malrotation.*

TREATMENT

Once the diagnosis is confirmed, surgery must be done within a few hours. The effects of midgut volvulus with possible bowel necrosis are so rapid and so dangerous that no time should be wasted.

Preparation for surgery consists of nasogastric suction, correction of fluid and electrolyte imbalance and monitoring of vital signs to detect an impending volvulus. Surgical repair consists of sectioning Ladd's bands obstructing the duodenum (Fig. VIII-39). At the completion of the operation, the colon is on the left side of the abdomen and the small bowel in the right paracolic gutter. Appendectomy is usually done to avoid delays in diagnosis in case of possible later appendicitis in a patient with a cæcum in an abnormal position. If a volvulus in also present, the bowel will be found twisted clockwise. Correction is achieved by a counter-clockwise movement. If normal color and pulsation returns the problem is solved. If viability of the intestine is

doubtful, it is preferable not to excise the bowel unless there is perforation. The abdomen is closed after correction of the volvulus [2]. After 24 to 36 hours of supportive treatment with I. V. solutions, dextran and antibiotics, the abdomen is reopened. In most instances one will find that a much smaller portion of the intestine than previously thought, will need to be resected.

Because of the possibility of an intraluminal diaphragm (Fig. VIII-40), the permeability of the duodenum is tested: a nasogastric tube or a Foley catheter inserted via a gastrostomy is threaded through the entire duodenum.

RESULTS

Symptoms consistently disappear after the operation. Our series includes 3 patients with delayed return to normal: one patient with a stenosis at the level of the caecum had a 60 day delay before return of normal intestinal transit. Another patient with

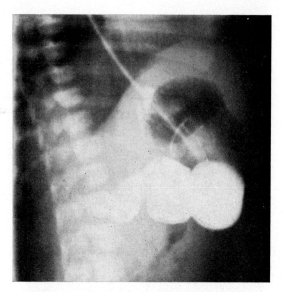

FIG. VIII-40. — *Upper G. I. series*
establishing the presence of a duodenal diaphragm
in a patient with malrotation.

a 360 degree volvulus suffered from intestinal obstruction due to adhesions a few days after surgery. A third patient, who had not had an appendectomy, had a wound infection.

Two of our 25 operated patients died. The first had associated jejunal atresia and died of peritonitis. The other death occurred in a baby with imperforate anus and an interatrial septal defect, who died of septicema on the third post-operative day. The other 23 patients were cured.

REFERENCES

[1] BILL (A. H.). — The malrotation of intestine. *Pediatric Surgery*, Year-book medical publishers, Inc., Chicago, 912, 1979.
[2] KRASNA (I. H.). — Low molecular weight dextran an re-exploration in the management of ischemic midgut volvulus. *J. Pediatr. Surg.*, 13, 480-843, 1978.
[3] THOMSON (A. J.). — Rœntgendiagnosis of midgut malrotation: value of upper gastrointestinal radiographic study. *J. Pediatr. Surg.*, 7, 243-252, 1972.

Meconium plug and small left colon syndrome

Jacques-Charles DUCHARME

The meconium plug syndrome was described in 1956 by Clatworthy [1]. In this syndrome, a cylinder of hardened meconium obstructs the lumen of the colon and rarely the ileum [2]. Obstructive symptoms disappear when this hardened meconium is expulsed. These babies have a normal sweat test. A deficiency in trypsin was initially suspected as the etiology but this was later disproved [3]. It is presently believed that a temporary anomaly of colonic motility [4] is involved. Intramural ganglion cells are normal. This anomaly allows more water to be reabsorbed from the meconium, causing the formation of a dry and hardened plug. The syndrome is similar to the small left colon syndrome described by Davis [5], which occurs, in a high percentage of cases, in babies of diabetic mothers.

From 1975 to 1979 10 patients were diagnosed as having meconium plug at Ste-Justine Hospital. All these babies presented in the neonatal period with abdominal distension, severe enough in some cases to cause increased collateral circulation of the abdominal wall. Nine babies did not pass meconium in the first 24 hours of life. The other baby had passed a small cylinder of gray meconium. Green vomitus was the rule. Abdominal X-rays showed diffuse intestinal distension. Air-fluid levels were often present (Fig. VIII-41).

Radiopaque enema with a water soluble material is essential. Occasionally meconium debris is scattered throughout the colon. In 9 of our cases a meconium plug was identified, with proximal distension, and a distal microcolon (Fig. VIII-42). This transitional zone is usually located at the left splenic flexure or in the descending colon (8 cases out of 10). This image is almost identical to congenital megacolon (Hirschsprung's disease). In our 10 cases the water soluble enema was followed by prompt evacuation of the meconium plug, and relief of symptoms.

Because clinically and radiologically the meconium plug syndrome closely mimics Hirschsprung's disease, all babies in whom such a plug is found should have either a rectal biopsy or rectal manometry. Out of our 10 babies with the initial diagnosis

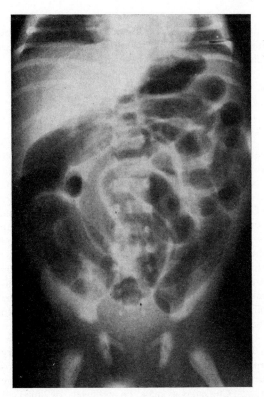

FIG. VIII-41. — *Diffuse intestinal distension proximal to a meconium plug.*

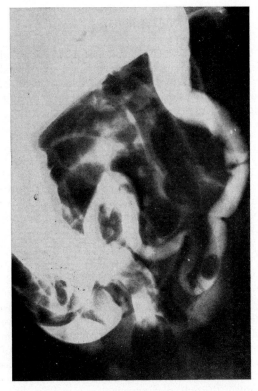

FIG. VIII-42. — *Meconium plug obstructing the descending colon. Note caliber difference at the level of the splenic flexure resembling congenital megacolon.*

of meconium plug, one baby was proven to have a congenital megacolon by biopsy. Caecal perforation has been reported with the meconium plug syndrome. We have not encountered it among our patients.

REFERENCES

[1] CLATWORTHY (H. W.), HOWARD (W. H. R.), LLOYD (J.). — The meconium plug syndrome. *Surgery, 39,* 131-142, 1956.

[2] SHIGEMOTO (H.). — Neonatal meconium obstruction in the ileum without mucoviscidosis. *J. Pediatr. Surg., 13,* 475-479, 1978.

[3] ELLIS (D. G.), CLATWORTHY (H. W.). — The meconium plug syndrome revisited. *J. Pediatr. Surg., 1,* 54-61, 1966.

[4] BENSON (C.), ADELMAN (S.). — *Meconium plug and small left colon syndrome.* Year-book medical publishers, Inc., p. Chicago, 1033, 1979.

[5] DAVIS (W. S.), CAMPBELL (J. B.). — Neonatal small left colon syndrome. *Am. J. Dis. Child., 129,* 1024, 1975.

Biliary atresia

Hervé BLANCHARD, Arié L. BENSOUSSAN

Atresia of the biliary tract represents the most frequent cause of mortality for infants with hepatic diseases. Before the introduction by Kasai of early surgical drainage of the bile ducts life expectancy was limited to between 8 and 24 months.

DEFINITION

Biliary atresia: a combination of destruction and degeneration of the biliary tract leading to partial or total obstruction. Cholestasis, biliary cirrhosis, portal hypertension and hepatic insufficiency subsequently develop.

INCIDENCE

Reported rates vary between 1:14 to 25,000. In our 29 patient series, 70 % were female. Contrary to popular belief there is no greater frequency of the disease in Asia.

ETIO-PATHOGENESIS

DEVELOPMENTAL THEORY. — Failure of development, especially of channeling of the primitive biliary tract. Biliary atresia is seldom found in still-births or early deaths. However up to 25 % of cases of biliary atresia have associated abnormalities: preduodenal vena cava, hepatic artery abnormalities, the polysplenic syndrome.

INFECTION THEORY. — None of the bacterial or viral agents suspected has yet satisfied Koch's criteria.

VASCULAR THEORY. — This involves ischemia as the basis of atresia in an analogous fashion to intestinal atresia. Okamoto and Okasora succeeded, by interruption of the vascularization of the biliary tract of young pups, in producing a form of biliary atresia similar to human biliary atresia, both macro- and microscopically.

EXTENSION OF HEPATITIS FROM THE PARENCHYMA TO THE INTRA- AND EXTRA-HEPATIC BILIARY TRACT. — The biliary tract lesions in biliary atresia would correspond to the lesions of the cells in hepatitis. Against this theory is the fact that premature and S. G. A. infants account for only a small fraction of biliary atresia (10 % in our series) while they are more frequently represented in neonatal hepatitis.

PROGRESSIVE INFLAMMATORY THEORY. — Systematic histologic studies show the disease to result from a progressive sclerosing inflammatory process occuring before or after birth. This leads to (1) progressive degeneration of the biliary tract with partial or complete obstruction, (2) partial or complete destruction of the biliary tract.

Ito, Sugito and Shimofi produced a necrotizing cholangitis similar to human biliary atresia by injecting Sporidesmin, a product of Pithomyces Chartorum, into foetal or newborn rabbits.

CLASSIFICATION OF BILIARY ATRESIA

Atresia of the extra-hepatic biliary tract. — A correctable variety (10-15 %), a non-correctable variety (85-90 %). Non-correctable forms: This denomination was used, before the introduction of porto-enterostomy by Kasai, to designate cases of biliary atresia with absence of a permeable common hepatic duct or a cystic one, so that there is no communication between the hilar plate and the intra-hepatic biliary tract. Correctable forms: Here the distal biliary tract is atretic. Proximally it ends blindly or in a cystic pouch but it communicates freely with the intra-hepatic portion of the biliary tract. This allows surgical drainage into the G. I. tract.

Hypoplasia of intra- and extra-hepatic biliary tract. — Gross inspection or intra-operative cholangiography reveal a very small diameter biliary tract. Cholestasis may be relieved by medical treatment alone. Despite an early disappearance of jaundice, some patients with this syndrome ultimately develop cirrhosis.

CLINICAL ASPECTS

The bile retention syndrome is characteristic: muco-cutaneous jaundice, light stools, dark urine and pruritus. One must distinguish between early and late events (when the disease is allowed to run its natural course).

Early events: prolonged physiologic jaundice with dark urine. In 20 % of cases, jaundice begins after the first 2 weeks of life.

Although occuring early, light stools are often noted only late. About 50 % of cases show hepatomegaly within the first week of life. The liver consistency is firm to hard. The spleen is increased in size in 10 % of cases but is not clinically palpable before the 6th to 8th week of life. The children look otherwise to be in good heatlh during the first six months.

Late events or natural evolution: after six months major complications begin to occur; cirrhosis, malabsorption, delayed growth, muscular wasting, osteoporosis. Every body liquid and tissue becomes jaundiced. Intestinal secretions may even give acholic stools a yellow tint. The skin is yellow-green. There is abdominal distention with hepato-splenomegaly and ascites. Intense pruritus may lead to extensive scratch lesions. Death occurs between the 8th and 24th month usually secondary to G. I. hemorrhage, chronic hepatic insufficiency or systemic bacterial infection.

BIOLOGY

Early phase. — Direct (conjugated) hyperbilirubinemia (50-70 %). Serial monitoring of bilirubinemia may show misleading fluctuations. Alkaline phosphatase, SGOT, leucine amino-peptidase and 5-nucleotidase serum levels are increased. Albumin; proteins and their ratio are within normal limits. Prothrombin and thromboplastin times are normal. Vitamin K will correct an increased prothrombin time occuring in 5 to 10 % of cases. A search for bile pigments in the stools will be negative if properly done: *i. e.* a digital extraction with the child in ventral decubitus so as to prevent urinary contamination of the specimen. Lipoprotein-x levels are elevated in biliary atresia while they will be absent or low in neonatal hepatitis.

Late phase. — Enzymes levels are markedly elevated. Albumin levels are decreased, globulins are increased, the albumin/globulin ratio is reversed. Coagulation tests, especially vitamin K dependant ones, are disturbed. Anemia, leucopenia and thrombocytopenia are secondary to hypersplenism.

DIAGNOSIS

Every newborn, more than two weeks of age, with jaundice should be suspected of having biliary atresia until proven otherwise. Early diagnosis, before 2 months, is necessary for good surgical results to be obtained. Both clinical and biological investigations can lead to a diagnosis of biliary atresia. Among the best diagnostic means are:

(1) Iodine-131 tagged Rose Bengal fecal excretion test. A fecal elimination of less than 10 % of the administered dose after 72 hours is compatible with biliary atresia.

(2) Technicium-99 tagged HIDA (N[N′(2-6 dimethyl phenyl) carbamoyl methyl] iminodiacetic acid) excretion test. The absence of excretion of Tc

99 PIPIDA or DISIDA after phenobarbital stimulation for four days is even more in favor of biliary atresia.

(3) Japanese investigators report very good results with duodenal intubation under fluoroscopic control in proving the absence of bilirubin in the duodenal secretions.

(4) Percutaneous liver biopsy although non specific, may reveal portal space widening, neoductal proliferation with biliary thrombi, varying degrees of fibrosis and lymphangiectasia of the portal space.

(5) Abdominal ultrasound. Some associated abnormalities may be found: preduodenal portal vein, multiple spleens, inferior vena cava malformations.

A positive diagnosis is made by laparotomy and per-operative cholangiography. As an alternative translaparoscopic cholangiography followed by laparotomy as needed has been suggested.

DIFFERENTIAL DIAGNOSIS

To establish the correct etiology for conjugated hyperbilirubinemia during the first two months of life is difficult because multiple causes overlap in their clinical and laboratory presentations (Table I).

An elevated level of direct bilirubin in the newborn or the young infant warrants an early appropriate investigation because in the case of biliary atresia surgical correction before 60 days of age is essential if good results are to be obtained. Biochemical and nuclear medecine tests used for distinguishing biliary atresia and neonatal hepatitis are based on indirect evaluation of biliary tract flow. Results should thus be interpreted with caution.

We have adopted the following diagnostic work-up in evaluating infants with elevated conjugated bilirubin.

(1) Admission to hospital and physical examination.

(2) Rule-out viral (Torch) or bacterial infection.

(3) Alpha$_1$, antitrypsin level.

(4) Look for reducing substances in urine.

(5) Ultrasound to eliminate a common bile duct cyst.

(6) Duodenal intubation during 24 hours for direct visualization of bile.

(7) Hepato-biliary scan with Tc 99 PIPIDA or DISIDA.

The absence of bile in the duodenum and a negative hepato-biliary scan mandate an exploratory laparotomy with cholangiography and open liver

Medical	*Surgical*
1. *Infectious hepatitis* a) Toxoplasmosis b) Rubella } Torch c) Cytomegalovirus d) Herpes simplex e) Hepatitis B f) Coxsackie virus g) Echovirus h) Syphilis i) Bacterial infection	1. *Biliary obstruction* a) Extra-hepatic — atretic biliary tract — biliary plug — congenital stenosis of the common bile duct — duodenal atresia b) Intra-hepatic — atresia of the intra-hepatic biliary tract
2. *Idiopathic hepatitis*	
3. *Toxic hepatitis* a) Total parenteral nutrition	
4. *Metabolic and genetic diseases* a) Rotor syndrome b) Dubin-Johnson syndrome c) Alpha$_1$ antitrypsin deficiency d) Tyrosinemia e) Hypermethionemia f) Trisomy 18	
5. *Biliary obstruction* a) Hypoplasia of intra- or extra- biliary tract b) Alagille's syndrome	

biopsy. The golden rule: early diagnosis and early surgical correction = best results in surgical treatment of biliary atresia.

TREATMENT

Essentially surgical, it is undertaken as soon as proof of complete irreversible cholestasis has been established. The exploration must be made before two months of age for good results to be obtained.

Exploration and biliary deviation are performed according to the principles enunciated by Kasai. Pre-operatively, parenteral vitamin K is given 24 hours before surgery. At our institution antibiotics (cephalosporin) are began 12 hours before the operation.

The exploration: between the years 1965 and 1980, 33 infants had surgical exploration of their biliary tree at Ste-Justine Hospital. Three of those had hypoplasia of the biliary tract. Twenty-nine had

a non-correctable form of atresia. One patient had neonatal hepatitis.

The procedure: the borders of a surgical incision at the hepatic hilum are anastomosed to a jejunal loop (hepatico-porto-enterostomy) or to the gall bladder (hepatico-porto-cholecystotomy) when the gall bladder and common bile duct are not obstructed.

ANATOMO-PATHOLOGY

Macroscopy: the hepatico-duodenal ligament shows variable degrees of inflammation. The porta hepatis is usually more severely involved. Fibrosis varies from mild to marked.

The liver is increased in size with a yellow to olive-green tint. A firm to ligneous consistency is usual with a smooth surface or one with micronodules. Glisson's capsule sometimes shows an extensive venous pattern.

Microscopy: *Porta hepatis:* bile ducts with diameters from 100 to 200 microns have been observed in 30 % of our cases. Similar cellular and inflammatory lesions to those of the intra-hepatic canalicules have been found for the endothelium of small bile ducts of the porta hepatis. The canalicular architecture is distorted by intra or pericanalicular fibrous nodules.

Liver: hepato-cellular focal degeneration, necrosis, giant cells are signs of liver cells toxicity. Widening and fibrosis of portal spaces, neoductal proliferation and neoductal biliary thrombi are also seen.

RESULTS

Among the seventeen patients who had biliary deviation and had a follow-up period ranging from 9 months to 5 years, 9 had bile excretion. For three of those patients excretion stopped at between 2 and 6 weeks after operation: two of these patients had a second operation performed and one had subsequent bile excretion. Among the patients with bile excretion 5 have bilirubin levels under 1 mg % and 2 have levels of about 3 mg % and are jaundiced. In Japan, cure rates with bile excretion and absence of jaundice vary from 29 to 55 %.

COMPLICATIONS

Major complications associated with surgery of biliary atresia include: (1) ascending cholangitis:

84 %; (2) portal hypertension: 40-85 %; (3) hepatic fibrosis or cirrhosis: 50 %. Recurrent cholangitis because of associated hepatic fibrosis and canalicular obstruction is of poor prognosis.

PROGNOSIS

The immediate prognosis for patients treated for biliary atresia depends on (1) the age at which surgery is done, (2) the degree of hepatic parenchymatous alteration, (3) the presence of bile canaliculi in the porta hepatis fibrous tissue, (4) the surgical procedure, (5) the incidence of postoperative ascending cholangitis.

Our experience leads us to be cautious in not giving false hope to parents in discussing prognosis even if immediate results from surgery show partial or complete regression of jaundice.

FUTURE TREATMENTS

Liver transplantation may be considered for patients where bile excretion did not occur or subsequently arrested.

REFERENCES

[1] KASAI (M.), KIMURA (S.), ASAKURA (Y.), SUZUKI (H.), TAIRA (Y.), OHASHI (E.). — Surgical treatment of biliary atresia. *J. Pediatr. Surg.*, 3, 665, 1968.
[2] DANKS (D. M.), CAMPBELL (P. E.), CLARKE (A. M.), JONES (P. G.), SOLOMON (J. R.). — Extra-hepatic biliary atresia. The frequency of potentially operable cases. *A. M. J. Dis. Child.*, 128, 684, 1974.
[3] CHIBA (T.), KASAI (M.), SASANO (N.). — Reconstruction of intrahepatic bile ducts in congenital biliary atresia. *Tohoku J. Exp. Med.*, 115, 99, 1975.
[4] CHIBA (T.), KASAI (M.), SASANO (N.). — Histopathological studies on intrahepatic bile duct in the vicinity of the porta hepatis in biliary atresia. *Tohoku J. Exp. Med.*, 118, 199, 1976.
[5] ODIEVRE (M.), VALAYER (J.), RASEMON PINTA (M.), HABIB (E. C.), ALAGILLE (D.). — Hepatic portoenterostomy or cholecystostomy in the treatment of extrahepatic biliary atresia. *J. Pediatr.*, 88, 774, 1976.
[6] BILL (A. H.), HAAS (J. E.), FOSTER (G. L.). — Biliary atresia: histopathologic observations and reflections upon its natural history. *J. Pediatr. Surg.*, 12, 977, 1977.
[7] GAUTHIER (M.), JEHAN (P.), ODIEVRE (M.). — Histologic study of biliary fibroses remnants in 48 cases of extrahepatic biliary atresia: correlation with postoperative bile flow restoration. *J. Pediatr.*, 89, 704, 1976.
[8] KASAI (M.), SUZUKI (H.), OHASHI (E.), OHI (R.), CHIBA (T.), OKAMOTO (A.). — Technique and results of operative management of biliary atresia. *World J. Surg.*, 2, 581, 1978.
[9] LILLY (J. R.), HITCH (D. C.). — Postoperative ascending cholangites following portoenterostomy for biliary atresia: measures for control. *World J. Surg.*, 2, 581, 1978.
[10] HIRSIG (J.), KARA (O.), RICKHAM (P. P.). — Experimental investigation into the etiology of cholangitis following operation for biliary atresia. *J. Pediatr. Surg.*, 13, 55, 1978.
[11] CARCASSONNE (M.), BENSOUSSAN (A. L.). — Long-term results in treatment of biliary atresia. *Progr. Pediatr. Surg.*, 10, 151, 1977.
[12] OKAMOTO (E.), OKASORA (T.) et al. — An experimental study on the etiology of congenital biliary atresia. *Cholestasis in infancy its pathogenesis, diagnosis and treatment.* Univ. of Tokyo Press, 217-224, 1980.
[13] ITO (T.), SUGITO (T.), SHIMOJI (H.). — Obstructive jaundice produced by Sporidesmin, a product of Pithomyces Chartarum: Experimental studies in the pathogenesis of biliary atresia in rabbits. *Cholestasis in infancy its pathogenesis, diagnosis and treatment.* Univ. of Tokyo Press, 225-239, 1980.

Congenital megacolon

Sami YOUSSEF

This is an intestinal obstruction due to absence of intramural ganglia in the distal bowel.

Hirschsprung first described the disease in 1887. In 1920, Dalla Valle of Naples recognized the aganglionosis and familial nature of the disease; but it remained to Swenson in 1948 to prove that the dilatation of the proximal colon in this disease was due to the absence of peristaltic movement in the distal narrow aganglionotic segment on which he based his curative rectosigmoidectomy operation.

PATHOLOGY

There is an aganglionic segment of bowel involving the rectum and extending proximally for a varying distance.

(*a*) Short segment Hirschsprung:

— rectum only involved,
— rectum and lower sigmoid.

(*b*) Long segment Hirschsprung:

— proximal to sigmoid,
— total colonic.

Histological examination of the diseased bowel shows, (1) a total absence of ganglion cells in both Auerbach's and Meissener's plexus, (2) increase in size and number of nerve bundles in the plexus, (3) markedly increased acetylcholinesterase activity.

ETIOLOGY AND EMBRYOLOGY

There is an interruption in the caudal migration of the ganglion cells in the intestinal tube. There is a hereditary factor, with a definite familial incidence. A significant association with Down syndrome has been reported.

INCIDENCE

The disease occurs in one in 10,000 births.

In short segment Hirschsprung the male to female ratio is 4:1, but the sex ratio is equal in long segment disease.

In short segment, there is a 1/20 risk that brothers will have it and a 1/100 risk for sisters. In long segment, the risk to siblings is one in 10.

CLINICAL FEATURES

The infants are usually full term with normal birth weight. In the great majority, the symptoms appear in the first week of life.

— Vomiting. Most common: 90 %. It is bile-stained and may be fecal.
— Abdominal distension.
— Failure to pass meconium in the first 24-48 hours.
— Reluctance to feed.

— Diarrhea is a late sign and is usually due to enterocolitis.
— Rectal examination. Empty rectum with explosive passage of flatus and meconium when the finger is withdrawn.

INVESTIGATIONS

— *X-ray:* A-P upright of the abdomen. May show multiple loops of distended bowel with air-fluid levels, and absence of air in the rectum.

— Barium enema. Shows the transition zone; except that it may be absent in about half of the time in the first week of life; 24 hour film is important to show delayed evacuation of barium.

— Anorectal manometry. There is a failure of relaxation of the internal sphincter after rectal distension. A normal reflex should be present after 40 weeks of gestation; this is unreliable in the neonatal period.

— Rectal biopsy is the only test that provides definitive diagnosis. Currently, the common technique is to do suction biopsy of the mucosa and submucosa 3 and 5 cm above the dentate line, for histology and acetylcholinesterase estimation.

DIFFERENTIAL DIAGNOSIS

— Lower ileal and colonic atresia. Barium enema.

— Meconium plug syndrome may be a presentation of Hirschsprungs, in 20 %. The subsequent behaviour of the child allows for the differentiation between the two.

— Meconium ileus. Due to fibrocystic disease. X-rays and sweat test later.

— Malrotation. Barium studies.

— Colonic inertia. Seen with prematurity and hypoglycemia.

TREATMENT

Myomectomy. — For the rare ultra-short segment that involves the internal sphincter.

Treatment in the neonatal period:

(*a*) *Non-operative:* daily enemas with normal saline. Never inject under pressure for fear of perforation. This treatment is also used for children who present with enterocolitis, and is continued for a few days until they improve clinically, when a colostomy is performed.

(b) *Colostomy:* most surgeons prefer a colostomy upon the diagnosis of Hirschsprung's disease. It should be done with minimum of delay; otherwise there is an increase in the incidence of enterocolitis and septicemia. There is, though, a variation in opinion as to the site of the colostomy. Some do it at the transition zone; but many, do it in the right transverse colon as protection when the corrective procedure is done.

Definitive surgery. — Done at age 6-12 months, when morbidity and mortality is lower. Recently, some surgeons recommend earlier intervention, so that the child will have an earlier psychological adaptation to learn to defecate.

The operation is a pull-through recto-sigmoidectomy. A variety of operations exist. They are named after their chief protagonist:

Swenson. — Who was the first to describe definitive surgery for this disease. It is a sound operation and consists of resection of the aganglionic segment down to the anal canal. The normal colon is brought down and an anastomosis is done.

Soave. — A popular operation. An endorectal pullthrough. It's advantage is to eliminate the pelvic dissection.

Duhamel. — The bowel is resected to the peritoneal reflection, and the rectum is closed. The normal colon is then brought down in a tunnel behind the rectum and an end-to-side anastomosis is done between the rectum and normal colon. It is a good operation in total colonic aganglionosis.

RESULTS AND PROGNOSIS

This has changed dramatically in the last 25 years. The mortality from the definitive operation is $< 5 \%$, but about 20 % have residual symptoms. The mortality in the neonatal period remains very high, 15-20 %, due largely to delay in diagnosis and in the recognition of enterocolitis.

Ano-rectal anomalies

Sami YOUSSEF

A group of congenital anomalies in the formation of the terminal gut. In the great majority, there is a small abnormal outlet for the bowel, either on the surface of the perineum or vulva or internally as a "fistula" into the urethra in the male, or the vagina in the female.

PATHOLOGICAL ANATOMY

Best considered in relationship to its classification of which there are about 27 varieties. The international classification was established in Melbourne in 1970. The central factor in it, is the relationship of the termination of the bowel to the muscular floor of the pelvis (and in particular to the puborectalis sling). The lesions are high, if the bowel terminates cranial to the sling; or low, if it terminates caudal to the sling. An intermediate group is when the fistula is in the sling, but the bowel proper terminates above it.

Male

(a) *High malformations.* — The commonest deformity in this group is anorectal agenesis with recto-urethral fistula. Ano-rectal agenesis with recto-vesical fistula is rare. In 20 %, there is no fistula. In this group, is also contained rectal atresia which is rare.

(b) *Intermediate.* — Anal agenesis with or without a rectobulbar fistula. A rare ano-rectal stenosis, belongs to this group.

(c) *Low:*

— At normal anal site: covered anus, anal stenosis;

In 1965-1969, the surgical section of the American Academy of Pediatrics surveyed 1,142 patients:

Males (661)	% 58	*Females* (481)	% 42
Low		*Low*	
(a) *At normal site*		(a) *At normal site*	
— Anal stenosis	5	— Anal stenosis	3
— Covered anus	5	— Covered anus	1
(b) *At perineal site*		(b) *At perineal site*	
— Anocutaneous fistula	25	— Anocutaneous fistula	5
— Anterior perineal anus	8	— Anterior perineal anus	22
Intermediate		*Intermediate*	
(a) *Anal agenesis*		(a) *Anal agenesis*	
— Without fistula	6	— Without fistula	2
— With fistula	1	— With fistula	
(b) *Anorectal stenosis*	1	— rectovestibular	8
		— rectovaginal (low)	15
High		(b) *Anorectal stenosis*	1
(a) *Anorectal agenesis*			
— Without fistula	10	*High*	
— With fistula		(a) *Anorectal agenesis*	
— rectourethral	29	— Without fistula	3
— rectovesical	9	— With fistula	
(b) *Rectal atresia*	1	— rectovaginal (high)	9
		— rectocloacal	5
Total	100	— rectovesicular	1
		(b) *Rectal atresia*	
		(c) *At vulvar site*	
		— Anovulvar fistula	8
		— Anovestibular	10
		— Vestibular anus	7

— At perineal site: anterior perineal anus, ano-cutaneous fistula (most common form of this group).

Female

(*a*) *High.* — These are less common than in boys. Most of these, have a fistula opening into the upper vagina or to a cloaca. The pubo-rectalis sling here surrounds the vagina below the fistula.

(*b*) *Intermediate.* — The most common form here is anal agenesis with a low vaginal fistula. The rest are rare and include an agenesis without a fistula, or with a recto-vestibular fistula, and ano-rectal stenosis. In this intermediate form, the pubo-rectalis is in normal relationship to the bowel.

(*c*) *Low.* — These are more frequent in the female than high lesions. The anterior perineal anus is the most common here, where the sphincter muscles are usually all present and the function of the anus is normal.

ASSOCIATED ANOMALIES

These are common, over 60 % of ano-rectal malformations have associated anomalies. They are more common (73 %) and more severe in the high type than in the low type (35 %).

Hasse, reviewed 1,420 patients with ano-rectal malformations and noted this incidence of associated anomalies:

	%
Urogenital	19.7
Extremities and spine	13.1
Cardiovascular	7.9
Gastrointestinal	6.0
Esophageal atresia	5.6
Abdominal wall defects	1.9
Cleft palate	1.5
Mongolism	1.5
Meningomyelocele	0.4
Miscellaneous	8.0

Some of these anomalies tend to be associated together, as seen in the syndrome of Vater.

ETIOLOGY

(*a*) *Genetic factors.* — Most cases are sporadic. Genetic factors may be more important in some forms than others, and a few cases of autosomal inheritance have been described.

(*b*) *Environmental factors.* — Maternal ingestion of thalidomide and oral contraceptives have been implicated. Folic acid deficiency and inhibitors could theoretically cause multiple system anomalies. Mechanical factors in the excessive ventral folding of the embryo may be a factor. Intrinsic muta-genesis: random mutations due to errors of DNA replication could explain its occurence, especially with the association of other anomalies.

INCIDENCE

Occurs in about 1 in 5,000 births with variations from 1/1,800: 1/10,000. Boys (58 %) are more affected than girls (42 %). High anomalies are more common in boys, while low anomalies are more common in girls.

CLINICAL FEATURES

Most infants are of good birth weight. In most instances, the lesion is noticed immediately after birth. Abdominal distension is marked, if there is no fistula or if the fistula doesn't decompress the bowel. Inspection and probing in the perineum is very important to determine the presence of a fistula. Urine should be examined for meconium or squamous cells to identify a fistula with the urinary tract. Simple X-ray with the child inverted in the true lateral view may help to locate the level of the anomaly. The child should be 18-24 hours old and should be held in that position for 3 minutes before the X-ray is taken. In the female, perineal inspection is essential:

— One orifice: cloaca and lesion is high.
— Two orifices: either high or intermediate lesion.
— Three orifices: low lesion.

TREATMENT

The central aim is to produce a continent child. The principles of the methods to achieve this aim are:

— Maximal use of the pubo-rectalis sling.
— Effective employment of the external sphincter.
— Minimal disturbance of pelvic sensation.
— Best use of perineal skin.

In the neonatal period, the main responsibility is to distinguish between the high and the low lesions:

(*a*) Low lesions with fistula are treated by a cut-back procedure, followed a week later by dilatation untill it is no longer necessary.

(*b*) Anal stenosis is treated by dilatation only.

(*c*) Ectopic anus requires no treatment except in the presence of stenosis.

(*d*) Intermediate and high lesions are treated by a defunctioning colostomy in the neonate. The distal colon should be washed out to prevent enterocolitis in it and, or urinary tract infection. Following the colostomy, cystourethrography and an IVP should be done.

Definitive surgery is deferred till the age of 6-9 months. Stephens described his technique of identifying the pubo-rectalis sling and pulling the bowel through it. The endorectal pullthrough modi-fication avoids injury to the levator sling and to pubic nerves. Intermediate lesions can be repaired through a sacral approach only, or via an added abdomino-perineal approach, by an anterior peri-neal approach just posterior to the scrotum.

RESULTS

Low mortality rate in low types, but about 30 % in high lesions; which is mainly due to asso-ciated anomalies.

As for functional results, when simple cutback or dilatation is done the results are very good. As for high lesions, the ultimate results vary and full success is about 50 % in our studies. The over-whelming importance of the pubo-rectalis sling should be re-emphasized.

Omphalocele and gastroschisis

Salam YAZBECK and Arié L. BENSOUSSAN

OMPHALOCELE

An omphalocele is an anomaly of the abdominal wall characterised by the protrusion of the intra-abdominal organs at the base of the umbilical cord. It is covered by a non-vascularised and transparent membrane called the amniotic sac.

EMBRYOLOGY

According to Duhamel, an omphalocele is the result of abnormal morphogenesis. In the 1.5 to 3 mm embryo, there are four folds: one cephalic, one caudal, and two lateral folds. These folds will extend toward each other in order to form the future umbilical ring. A malformation of the cephalic fold leads to an epigastric abdominal wall defect which is referred to as "epigastric omphalocele". This entity may be associated with lower thoracic malformations, anterior diaphragmatic defects and cardiac anomalies.

A failure in the formation of the caudal fold leads to a lower abdominal wall defect or "hypogastric omphalocele". This entity may be associated with imperforate anus and/or extrophy of the urinary bladder.

Failure of normal folding and fusion at the level of the lateral folds prevents the abdominal wall from closing completely. The umbilical ring will remain widely open. This entity is referred to as "omphalocele" or "hernia in the cord" depending on the size of the defect.

DIAGNOSIS

Omphalocele is a rare condition occuring at the rate of 1 in 1,860 to 1 in 6,600 births. Only 50% of these patients will be candidates for surgical treatment because of the high incidence of severe associated anomalies observed in these patients.

Between 1954 and 1976, 56 patients with ompha-

loceles were treated at l'Hôpital Sainte-Justine de Montréal. 33 were males and 23 females. Prematurity or low birth weight was noted in 30 % of the cases. This is in accordance with the figures reported in the literature.

The diagnosis is usually evident at birth (Fig. VIII-43). However in the patients with a small omphalocele or hernia in the cord, the anomaly may be easily missed. For this reason clamping of the umbilical cord close to the abdominal wall can enclose a bowel segment and cause intestinal obstruction or infarction.

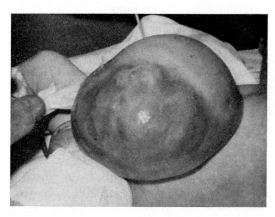

FIG. VIII-43. — *Omphalocele:*
the umbilical cord is inserted on the amniotic sac.
The liver and the intestines herniate into the sac.

The size of the abdominal wall defect will determine the degree of difficulty which will be encountered with the surgical treatment. An abdominal wall defect greater than 5 cm usually indicates the presence of a "giant" omphalocele containing a large portion of the liver; this implies more difficulties in the fascial closure. Usually during the first hours of life the amniotic sac is transparent and the content of the omphalocele can be examined easily.

In some patients the amniotic sac is already ruptured at birth or ruptures shortly after birth. This was the case in 23 % of our patients. During the first physical examination associated anomalies should be looked for very carefully. They are present in 2/3 of the cases according to the literature (60 % in our series).

ASSOCIATED ANOMALIES

Digestive	15
(Duodenal obstruction or intestinal atresia)	
Neurological	3
Cardiovascular	1
Genito-urinary	2
Diaphragmatic hernia	1
Beckwith-Wiedemann syndrome	1
Chromosomal	5
Multiple anomalies.	6
Total	34/56

Laboratory investigation is rapid and kept to a minimum. An antero-posterior X-ray of the abdomen and the chest will show the cardiac silhouette, the lungs and the gas pattern in the abdomen. Blood is drawn for cross matching, blood count, electrolytes, blood gases, calcium and glucose. The latter is very important because of the frequent association with the Beckwith-Wiedemann syndrome and its accompanying hypoglycemia.

GASTROSCHISIS

Gastroschisis is a congenital abdominal wall anomaly characterized by the evisceration of bowel loops through a paraumbilical defect. The eviscerated bowel must be separated from the umbilical cord by a bridge of skin; there is no amniotic sac over the herniated intra-abdominal content.

EMBRYOLOGY

The embryology of gastroschisis is still speculative. Duhamel thought that gastroschisis might be due to "a relatively early teratogenic action which may prevent the differentiation of the embryonic mesenchyme forming the framework of the somatopleure with subsequent resorption of the ectoblastic layer of the somatopleure in the region of the lateral fold".

The most attractive theory has been advanced by Shaw, who considers that gastroschisis results from the rupture of a hernia in the cord. The rupture

occurs at the site of the involuted right umbilical vein with subsequent evisceration of the bowel.

DIAGNOSIS

The incidence of gastroschisis varies according to the series. Between 1954 and 1976 twenty patients were treated in our institution, compared to 56 omphaloceles. But even with the decrease in birth rate, this trend seems to be reversing. There were 12 females and 8 males. Prematurity is common in all series (60 to 85 %).

The diagnosis is evident at birth (Fig. VIII-44). Usually the major part of the small bowel and the colon are eviscerated. Frequently the stomach is also eviscerated but this is rarely the case for the gallbladder, the bladder or the internal genitalia.

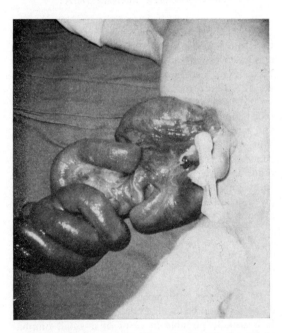

FIG. VIII-44. — *Gastroschisis: the umbilical cord is normally inserted, the small intestine and the colon herniate through a small abdominal wall defect situated to the right of the umbilical cord, there is no covering membrane on the herniated viscera; the small bowel looks thickened adherent and shortened.*

Because of the prolonged exposure of the viscera to the amniotic fluid, the bowel frequently looks thick, matted and covered with a gelatinous matrix. It also looks shortened and the peritoneal cavity is relatively small. The small size of the abdominal wall defect, when compared to the amount of bowel eviscerated, may be a major factor in compromising the blood supply to the herniated bowel resulting in engorgement and even necrosis of part of the herniated bowel.

Hypothemia is frequently noted because of the heat loss through the eviscerated bowel and the frequent association of prematurity.

In 20 to 40 % of patients associated anomalies are encountered (9/20 in our series). The majority of these anomalies concern the alimentary tract *i. e.* malrotation and atresia.

MANAGEMENT OF GASTROSCHISIS AND OMPHALOCELES

PREOPERATIVE MANAGEMENT

The preoperative management is identical for both omphalocele and gastroschisis and is aimed at keeping the infant warm and adequatly hydrated. Nasogastric decompression is instituted at birth and the child is placed in a sterile plastic bag which should be tied loosely below the shoulders. Warm moist gauzes are placed on the abdominal defect and warm saline introduced into the plastic bag. This will allow for an easy inspection of the eviscerated viscera of the hernia content. Intravenous fluids are started immediately at birth as are broad spectrum antibiotics and 1 mg of vitamin K is given. The infant is brought to the operating room as soon as possible.

OPERATIVE TECHNIQUE

In the cases of omphaloceles, primary fascial closure should be the first choice whenever possible. It is usually possible in cases of a small omphalocele (defect < 5 cm). The amniotic sac is excised and the content of the abdominal cavity is carefully inspected in search of associated anomalies. When the omphalocele is larger, primary closure is sometimes still possible and implies a forceful stretching of the abdominal cavity to accommodate the hernial content. Frequently primary closure may lead to an unacceptable level of intra-abdominal pressure with a subsequent compression of the inferior vena cava and the diaphragm. In these cases, a staged closure is preferred, using either skin flaps (ventral hernia as described by Gross) or the silastic chimney as described by Schuster. The

latter will allow for complete closure over a period of 7 to 10 days.

If the omphalocele is ruptured, it should be managed as for gastroschisis.

In the case of gastroschisis, it is usually mandatory to enlarge the size of the defect in order to inspect the entire length of the digestive tract. If there is an infarcted bowel segment, it should be resected and a primary anastomosis performed only if the bowel walls are not too thick. In this case as in the cases of associated atresia, it is preferable to postpone the anastomosis until the time of the definitive closure. A cautious attempt to evacuate the intestinal content proximally and distally may be very helpful.

A primary closure must not be attempted if it excessively increases the intra-abdominal pressure because of the possible compression of the vena cava and the diaphragm. A staged procedure may then be used, as described in the case of omphalocele.

The utilisation of a silastic pouch allows for a definitive closure within a period of 7 to 10 days, but it is associated with an increased risk of infection, entero-cutaneous fistula and dislocation of the silastic sheaths. Some authors have advised the systematic use of a gastrostomy with this technique but it is being increasingly abandoned because of the high rate of infection reported under these conditions. In our series 50 % of the patients showed a wound infection when the silastic pouch was associated with a gastrostomy. On the other hand, out of 31 cases of omphalocele or gastroschisis closed without a gastrostomy, only 7 presented a wound infection.

RESULTS AND PROGNOSIS

Dramatic advances and progress have been made in general neonatal care, anesthesia, fluid management and methods of mechanical ventilation. This has led to better definitive results but the postoperative course is frequently complicated.

Paralytic ileus is frequently prolonged in cases of gastroschisis or ruptured omphacele. The patients should receive total parenteral nutrition until normal peristalsis resumes. In our series, 18 patients presented a prolonged paralytic ileus; in 6 patients the ileus period lasted between 3 and 24 weeks after the definitive closure. In three patients death occured after six months of paralytic ileus. Transitory malabsorption and diarrhea are frequently observed at the resumption of normal peristalsis. Entero-cutaneous fistulæ are regularly reported especially when the silastic pouch is used.

The mortality rate of the patients with ompha-locele is still very high, around 40 % in the literature and 36 % in our series. It is directly related to the serious associated anomalies frequently encountered in these cases. The mortality associated with gastro-schisis is lower, around 13 % in most recent series.

RECOMMENDED READINGS

[1] RICKMAN (P. P.), LISTER (J.), IRVING (I. M.). — Neo-natal surgery. Ed. Butterworths, 2nd edition, 309-328, 1978.
[2] JONES (P. G.). — Clinical pediatric surgery. Blackwell Scientific Publication, 2nd edition, 119-123, 1976.
[3] DUHAMEL (B.). — Morphogenèse pathologique. Masson, édit., Paris, 57-93, 1966.
[4] RAVITCH (M. M.) et al. — Pediatric surgery. Year-Book Medical Publication, 3th edition, 778-801.
[5] SHAW (A.). — The myth of gastroschisis. J. Pediatr. Surg., 10, 235, 1975.

Sacro-coccygeal teratoma

Hervé BLANCHARD and Arié L. BENSOUSSAN

This is the most common variety of teratoma found in the child (47 %). Contrary to previous theories, the S. C. T. is a true tumor with constituents derived from all three embryonic layers (chordo-mesoblastic, ectoblastic and endoblastic). Those constituents of the tumor are not normally found in the sacro-coccygeal region.

EPIDEMIOLOGY

One case of S. C. T. for every 35 to 40,000 births, girls out-number boys by 3: 1 in our series of 30 patients. Previous twin pregnancies vary from 9 to 50 %. Ashcraft and Holder described cases of familial S. C. T.

ASSOCIATED ABNORMALITIES

These are rare, except in the series of Izant which reports a rate of 33 %.

PHYSIO-PATHOLOGY

The greater incidence of S. C. T. in girls could imply a relationship between S. C. T. and the appearance and migration of germinal cells. These cells arise from the urogenital fold around the fourth week in the male and between the fifth and seventh week in the female. For some authors, this would allow for a wider dissemination of germinal cells and thus the larger number of girls with S. C. T.

The precocity, the localization, the structure and mode of development of S. C. T. indicate that they arise from totipotential embryonal foci that have eluded the "primary organizer" during embryonal development. The teratomatous primordium, while differentiating produces a variety of ectopic tissue. If these tissues develop synchronously with the host tissue the teratoma will be benign; if the tera-matous tissues do not mature but continue to grow as embryonal tissues, a malignant embryonal tera-toma will result.

SYMPTOMS AND DIAGNOSIS

The newborn with a S. C. T. will have an obvious sacro-coccygeal or para-coccygeal mass. Their size may constitute a praevia obstacle and require a caesarian section. In our series we had a 15 % rate of caesarian section.

Internal or external hemorrhage may lead to shock and death. Hypothermia threatens the newborn because of the high radiant energy loss from the large surface area involved. The thin epithelium is also readily ulcerated and, with cuta-neous necrosis, allows for bacterial infection.

In most cases the tumor will alter the shape of the buttocks, perineum, or sacro-coccygeum to a variable extent, the anus is displaced both caudally and anteriorly.

In many cases the S. C. T. with buttock involvement shows pre-sacral extension. A rectal exam is mandatory for all newborns with a S. C. T. While of less spectacular presentation, presacral teratomas are more ominous.

Presenting symptoms may be (*a*) digestive: low obstruction or rectal compression, (*b*) urinary: reduced urine output or anuria by urethral compression, (*c*) vascular: edema of the lower extremities secondary to compromised venous return, (*d*) neurological by compression of the pelvic nerves.

Careful examination will reveal a posterior shift of the sacro-coccygeum and a surging perineum. The rectal exam will reveal a rectum displaced forward by the mass.

Early diagnosis is important for the following reasons (1) only 5 % of these tumors are malignant when diagnosed in the neonatal period, (2) between the 2nd and 5th month, 30-40 % are malignant, (3) at one year of age the malignancy rate is 50 % and approaches 100 % at 5 years.

INVESTIGATIONS

Abdominal and pelvic X-ray films are helpfull in evaluating C. S. T. Signs include anterior displacement of the rectum and calcified spots in 50-60 % of cases. An IVP, a cystography and a recto-sigmoid barium enema may be usefull.

DIFFERENTIAL DIAGNOSIS

To be made against an epitheliazed myelo-meningocele, a pelvic or perineal neurogenic tumor or a rectal duplication. A hemangioma, cystic lymphangioma, a fibroma or a lipoma of the buttock region should also be ruled-out. A high degree of suspicion is essential for the diagnosis of S. C. T. to be made because it may appear as a cutaneous sinus or as a slightly raised bluish area analogous to an hemangioma.

TREATMENT

This requires a radical excision continuous with the coccyx. The coccyx must be resected, otherwise recurrence rates are 30-40 %. It is imperative that the levator ani muscles be meticulously reconstructed after excision if anal incontinence is to be avoided. Sacral nerves should be carefully preserved.

ANATOMO-PATHOLOGY

Macroscopically: although usually large, some S. C. T.'s are rather small (1-15 cm). The altered skin is thin, raised by underlying cysts and abnormal vessels run their course under it. There may be ulcerated or necrotic areas. Cysts, always present in these lesions, are often multiple and of varying size.

Microscopically: elements from all three embryonal layers may be found. These derived elements may exist in their fœtal, embryonal or adult form.

The most frequent tumors, with a wide degree of differentiation, are: the skin and its glandular annex, the teeth and their precursors, the respiratory and the intestinal tissues with their associated glands or central nervous tissue:

— neuroglial tissue with or without ependymal cavities, with or without nervous cells,

— choroidal-lined cavities,

— immature nervous tissue which although very frequent is of no clinical malignant character in the young child,

— retinal tissue derived cells forming a thin wrinkled layer of pigmented epithelium,

— peripheral nervous tissue composed of sympathetic nerves and ganglia, immature neuroblastic tissue and Pacini corpuscules.

Next are mesenchymatous derived tissues: From adipose and cartilaginous to osseous and muscular, striated or smooth. Less frequently found tissues include gastric, pancreatic, hepatic or pulmonary endodermal derivatives.

PROGNOSIS

This is a function of the precocity of diagnosis and of proper initial treatment for either the pre- or retro-sacral S. C. T. All 10 patients in our series whom we operated on before 4 months of age are alive with a follow-up period between 10 and 20 years. In 4 of them immature nervous tissue was found.

The patients should be regularly followed for the first 6 months and then every 6 months for 3 years. An early diagnosis of local recurrence is possible by close examination of the perineal space and by performing a rectal exam for the pre-sacral space.

OTHER TERATOMAS

As Budd points out, their distributions seem to indicate that teratomas take their origin from embryonal tissues next to the primitive axis. In the child, by order of frequency are found: ovarian (30 %), testicular (8.6 %), retroperitoneal (5.6 %), mediastinal (4.2 %), cranio-facial (3.2 %) and cervical (2.3 %) tumors.

Clinically they commonly present as very slow growing masses. In contrast a cervical or anteromediastinal mass may cause great respiratory distress which commands quick surgical relief; moreover because of their great malignant potential, they warrant both an early diagnosis and early treatment.

REFERENCES

[1] WILLIS (R. A.). — *Embryonic tumors and teratomas.* Chap. 11, p. 410-454. The borderland of embryology and pathology. Butterworths and Co. Ltd., London, 1958.
[2] BLANCHARD (H.), COLLIN (P. P.), GUÉRIN (R.), PERREAULT (G.), CLERMONT (J.), GARANCE (P.). — Tératome sacro-coccygien chez l'enfant, étude clinique et artériographique. *Union Méd. Can.*, 100, 1311, 1971.
[3] ASHLEY (D. J. B.). — Origin of teratomas. *Cancer*, 32, 390, 1973.
[4] ASHCRAFT (K. W.), HOLDER (T. M.). — Hereditary presacral teratoma. *J. Pediatr. Surg.*, 9, 691, 1974.
[5] BERRY (G. L.), KEELING (J.), HILTON (C.). — Teratoma in infancy and childhood: a review of 91 cases. *J. Pathol.*, 98, 241, 1967.
[6] ALTMAN (R. P.), RANDOLPH (J. G.), LILLY (J. R.). — Sacrococcygeal teratoma. American Academy of Pediatrics, Surgical section survey, 1973. *J. Pediatr. Surg.*, 9, 389, 1974.
[7] MAHOUR (G. H.), WOOLEY (M. M.), TRIVEDI (S. N.), LANDING (B. H.). — Sacrococcygeal teratoma, a 33 year experience. *J. Pediatr. Surg.*, 10, 183, 1975.
[8] WOOLEY (M. M.). — Malignat teratoma in infancy and childhood world. *J. Surg.*, 4, 39, 1980.
[9] IZANT (R. J.) Jr. — Sacrococcygeal teratoma. *Pediatric surgery*. Chicago. Yearbook Medical Publishers 859, 1962.

Abdominal mass in the newborn and older child

Frank M. GUTTMAN

An abdominal mass presenting in childhood is likely to be hepatosplenomegaly of lymphoma, leukemia or portal hypertension. Of the retroperitoneal masses, hydronephrosis is most common especially in infancy. Nephroblastomas and neuroblastoma are fairly common in the lower age groups. In *the neonatal age range*, most retroperitoneal masses will be benign, either hydronephrosis, polycystic or multicystic disease, or mesoblastic nephroblastoma (Bolande tumour). True Wilms is rare in the neonate but neuroblastoma may occur although it has a good prognosis. In the infant from 1 year on more than 50 % of abdominal masses will be retroperitoneal malignancy.

CLINICAL FINDINGS

The mode of presentation is often fortuitous since symptoms are not frequent. Occasionally fever may be present or the child presents with fatigue. Often, it is a parent, who, during a bath will palpate the mass, and sometimes a pediatrician will note the mass on routine physical examination. Occasionally we have seen slight trauma give rise to an acute bleed into a renal neoplasm. Abdominal palpation must be carried out with gentleness and patience. The kidneys can be readily palpated in the infant. The surface of multicystic kidneys will be appreciated. Currently a high-intensity light source may be used to transilluminate cystic lesions. A Wilms tumour is generally smoother than a neuroblastoma where the surface is usually nodular. The neuroblastoma may extend past the midline whereas this is unusual in Wilms. Careful examination of the liver, the pelvis by rectal examination and the existance of lymphadenopathy is important. Horner's syndrome or aniridia are signs of stellate ganglion involvement and of Wilms tumour. In neuroblastoma skin nodules may be present. In addition to the usual laboratory tests, urinary VMA should be tested.

X-RAY INVESTIGATION

In addition to plain films of the abdomen and chest films, the initial essential test is the intravenous pyelogram. In some centers it is routine to inject the dye into a foot vein with a tourniquet in place. Release of the tourniquet results in an inferior venocavogram and then an I. V. P. Calcification in the plain films suggests neuroblastoma, although more rarely Wilms, adrenal tumour or teratomas may show calcification. The main features on I. V. P. are either an extrarenal mass pushing the kidney downwards or an intrarenal lesion of hydronephrosis or tumour with distortion of the pyelocaliceal system. Late films are sometimes required. Bone surveys should be done in all patients if hydronephrosis has been ruled out. Routine arteriography is not recommended. Ultrasound has added much since it is non-invasive and will give an accurate appreciation of the solidity or fluidity of the mass.

Occasionally paraspinal neuroblastoma will give rise to neurological symptoms. Oblique views of the spine should be then obtained to assess enlargement of the neural foramina. If enlarged, myelography should be carried out. Liver-spleen scanning has a role in extra-renal masses, but not in renal or pararenal tumours. Again in extrarenal sites, ultrasound has proven to be a very useful tool to differentiate liver, spleen, intestinal duplication, and teratomas. In liver tumours, angiography may be useful. When hydronephrosis has been ruled out, a bone marrow should be done pre-operatively although this may also be done per-operatively.

9

Hereditary
and congenital disorders

46

Genetic and teratologic anomalies

Luc LARGET-PIET and Annick LARGET-PIET

It is known at present that 3 % of the newly born present with malformations. Two thirds of these are due to genetic problems, representing only a minority when compared to the many perturbations caused by the presence of an abnormal genetic coding that may exist as early as in the ovum. About 70 % of spontaneous abortions are due to chromosomal anomalies that are usually incompatible with the progress of pregnancy.

In spite of the considerable progress in the therapeutics of infantile diseases, only a few pathological problems of congenital origin may benefit from any effective therapy. This has probably raised the interest in such areas, as diminution in the frequency of such anomalies may be anticipated when there is an organized system for their prevention.

The birth of a malformed child may raise several questions concerning both the patient and the possible intrafamilial repercussions, such as:

— What is the etiology of the malformation?
— Is it an isolated malformation?
— Could it benefit from treatment?
— Is there a risk of recurrence?

The understanding of the mechanisms of occurence of congenital anomalies may bring an answer to such questions. These mechanisms may be genetic (involving genes or chromosomes) or non genetic.

Transmission of hereditary pathological characteristics

One should distinguish the transmission of monogenic characteristics that obey Mendel's laws from multifactorial heredity that associates genetic and environmental factors [19, 38].

HEREDITY
OF MONOFACTORIAL CHARACTERISTICS

AUTOSOMAL LINKED HEREDITY

Dominant heredity. — Heredity is said to be autosomal when the pair of the allele genes responsible for the characteristic is situated on one of the 22 pairs of autosomes. A dominant characteristic (A) express itself in the heterozygous state (A*a*). The gene (*a*) is normal and recessive. The homozygous state (AA) may be ignored. It is probable that a characteristic different from the heterozygote would arise and the malformation in this case may be fatal.

Autosomal dominant heredity may be defined according to the following criteria:

— the transmission of a pathological characteristic is "vertical" when one of the patient's parents

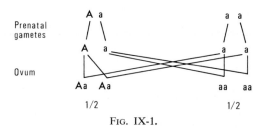

Prenatal gametes

Ovum

1/2   1/2

FIG. IX-1.

is affected, and half of the patient's children are affected,

— the disease affects both sexes equally,

— a healthy subject comes from healthy descendants,

— among the patient's brothers, one in two is affected.

In Figure IX-1, the patients are born from the marriage of an affected heterozygote (A*a*) and a homozygous normal (*aa*). The subject carrying the anomaly will produce two types of gametes in equal numbers. (A and *a*). All the gametes of the partner will be (*a*). Half of the descendants will be affected and the other half will be normal.

The healthy subjects are in fact homozygous for the normal gene (*a*). Their children would be healthy in case of marriage with a normal homozygote. Numerous disease are transmitted in an autosomal dominant way, such as Von Recklinghausen's neurofibromatosis (Fig. IX-2), facio-scapulo-humeral myopathy of Landouzy Dejerine, Steinert's myotonia, aniridia, achondroplasia (Fig. IX-3), Huntington's chorea, osteogenesis imperfecta (Fig. IX-4,) microspherocytosis of Minkowski Chauffard, Bourneville tuberous sclerosis and Franceschetti's syndrome (Fig. IX-5).

Exceptions to the rule of autosomal dominance. — A dominant gene does not always manifest itself among its carriers. A subject may seem normal

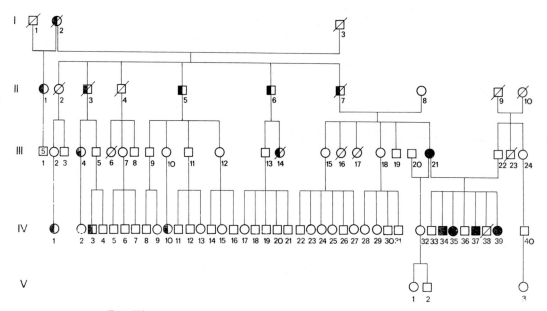

FIG. IX-2. — *Autosomal dominant heredity; Von Recklinghausen's disease.*

■ Examined subjects.
□ Non examined subjects,

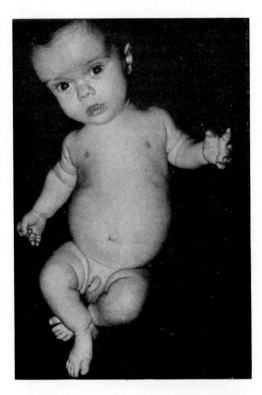

FIG. IX-3. — *Achondroplasia. Phenotype.*

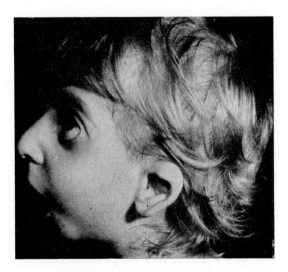

FIG. IX-5. — *Franceschetti's syndrome. Phenotype.*

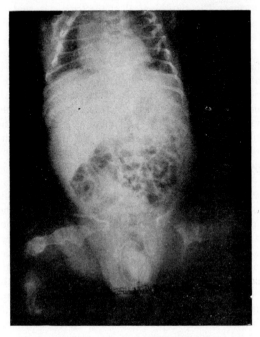

FIG. IX-4. — *Porak and Durante's disease (osteogenesis imperfecta).* Radiological aspect.

but in fact be heterozygous for the diseased gene, since geneological investigations may prove that one of his parents is affected, or one of his children. Thus a skip of a generation may take place. To explain these facts some notions on penetration and expressivity may be reviewed.

The penetration of a gene is the percentage of the subjects expressing the disease out of the number of individuals carrying the diseased gene. The penetration of a gene may therefore be incomplete. In general, the gene may express itself in a variable percentage among its carriers.

The expressivity in itself can also be variable, *i. e.*, the genetic disease may present clinically with different symptomatology in the same family or from one family to another. Thus osteogenesis imperfecta for example may begin prenatally (Porak and Durante disease) or at a later stage (Lobstein's disease).

The clinical signs may vary according to the sex of the subject. "Alport's syndrome" that associates chronic haematuric nephropathy and perception deafness more frequently affects males. However, 5 % of affected females may present with a grave form of the disease.

The penetration and expressivity of a gene do not depend only on the diseased gene but also on the rest of the genome as well as on the environment. The existence of allelic gene modifications is possible. Figure IX-6 shows that first cousin patients have a one in two probability of having received the same modifier ($a2$) or ($a3$) and therefore resemble each other. In contrast, the diseased parent (A$a1$) could

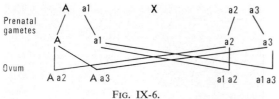

FIG. IX-6.

transmit either (A) or (a1), hence the absence of clinical identity between himself and his affected children.

The gene modification could be non allelic and occupy different loci: Investigating blood groups of the ABO system may provide an example.

An apparent exception to the rule of dominance is the sudden appearance of a diseased subject in a seemingly intact family. If the gene shows complete penetration it is then a mutation. Out of ten cases of achondroplasia, eight are mutants. Their descendants will have the disease in 50 % of cases.

RECESSIVE HEREDITY

The recessive gene (a) will show itself in the homozygous state (aa). The genotypes (AA) and (Aa) correspond to a normal phenotype.

Infantile polycystic disease is transmitted in this way. It usually involves perinatal death. The kidneys are of large size and features of the face are usually abnormal (Potter syndrome). Nevertheless, some cases may show a prolonged evolution. The disease may also present with later onset between 5 and 10 years of age. Its prognosis then largely depends on the associated biliary fibro-adenomatosis.

The union which is more commonly encountered is that of two heterozygotes (Aa×Aa). Irrespective of sex, 25 % of children are affected (Fig. IX-7) while 75 % are clinically normal. However, 2 out of 3 are heterozygotes for the diseased gene, like their parents.

It is impossible to prove that one of the genes (a) transmitted by one of the parents could result from a recent mutation. It is therefore considered that the heterozygous parents have themselves

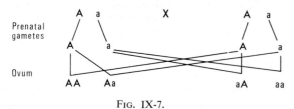

FIG. IX-7.

received the diseased gene from one of their own parents. The union of a heterozygote with a normal homozygote (Aa × AA) may result in the birth of normal babies, but 50 % of them will be heterozygous (Fig. IX-8).

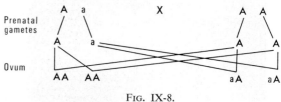

FIG. IX-8.

On the other hand, in some case of perception deafness for example, the union of a homozygous affected (aa) with a homozygous normal (AA) would give rise to descendants entirely heterozygous (Aa).

The descendants of a couple composed of one heterozygote (Aa) and the other homozygous (aa), will be 50 % heterozygous and 50 % affected homozygous. In such a case, investigating the family pedigree is of prime importance in view of a dominant heredity that may involve the transmission of a recessive trait, i. e., pseudo-dominance.

Nevertheless, the vast majority of infants presenting with a disease of recessive autosomal transmission, are born from parents phenotypically normal. The pathological characteristic is said to be "horizontal" when the subjects affected belong to the same generation.

However, because of the small size of human families, it is frequent that only one subject is affected in each generation of a family investigated across several generations. The existence of one unique patient does not therefore permit the elimination of a disease of genetic origin. Thus the risk of recurrence is particularly difficult to estimate when a first child is suffering from isolated perception deafness.

There are numerous diseases transmitted in an autosomal recessive manner. Most of the metabolic diseases obey this mode of transmission. Of particular interest are those related to the metabolism of amino-acids, carbohydrates and lipids. Examples of these are phenylketonuria, the glycogenoses, mucopolysaccharidosis (Fig. IX-9 and IX-10), oligosaccharidosis and neurolipidosis. Moreover, the congenital nephrotic syndrome of the Finnish type, mucoviscidosis, and Friedreich's ataxia have an identical mode of transmission. Figures IX-11 and IX-12 show malformations characteristic of diastrophic dwarfism [39].

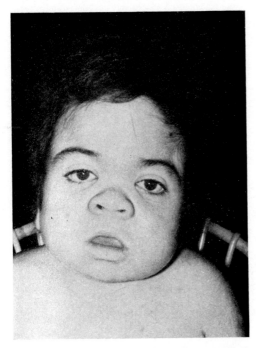

FIG. IX-9. — *Mucopolysaccharidosis of type I (Hurler).*
Phenotype.

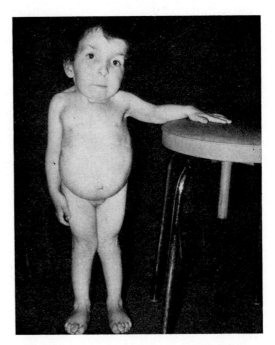

FIG. IX-11. — *Diastrophic dwarfism.* Phenotype.

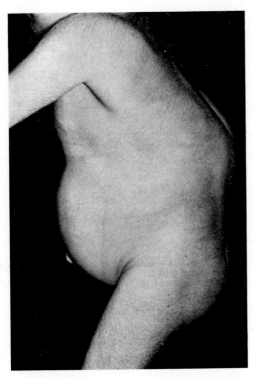

FIG. IX-10. — *Mucopolysaccharidosis of type I (Hurler).*
Dorsal kyphosis.

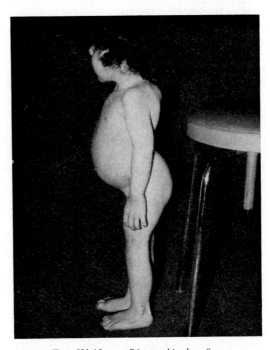

FIG. IX-12. — *Diastrophic dwarfism.*
Lateral aspect.

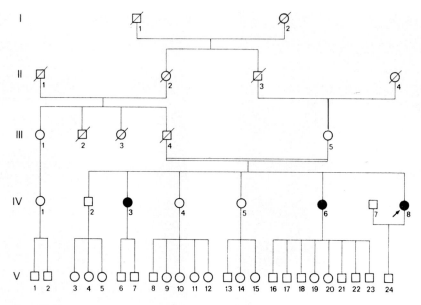

FIG. IX-13. — *Autosomal recessive heredity.* Deafness after consanguinous marriage.

CONSANGUINITY

The notion of consanguinity may involve two elements; the marriage of two related persons and the children born from this marriage. A consanguinous union increases the risk of having a diseased child born with an autosomal recessive trait and carrying two identical genes (Fig. IX-13). In fact, according to Hardy and Weinberg's law, if p corresponds to the frequency of the gene (A) and q to the frequency of the gene (a), the population is composed of three groups of individuals: $p2$ homozygous for the normal gene (AA), $2pq$ heterozygous (Aa) and $q2$ homozygous for the recessive gene (aa). In the general population, the probability for a subject to be heterozygous is equal to $2pq$. It is the same probability for the other partner for the same gene ($2pq \times 2pq$). If

$$q = \frac{1}{100}, 2pq = 2 \times \frac{1}{100} \times \frac{99}{100} = \frac{1}{50}.$$

The frequency of such unions is therefore

$$\frac{1}{50} \times \frac{1}{50} = \frac{1}{2,500}.$$

The risk of having a child born affected is $\frac{1}{10,000}$ for the considered disease within the general population where unions are at random, *i. e.* a wide range of mixtures. In contrast, if an individual is married to his first cousin, the probability that the latter is heterozygous for the same gene is $\frac{1}{8}$. The probability that the two partners, are heterozygous for the same gene is therefore $\frac{1}{400}$. The frequency of affected subjects is $\frac{1}{1,600}$. So the risk is highly elevated.

In fact if the individual III$_1$ is married to his first cousin III$_2$, the probability that III$_1$ would be heterozygous for a gene is $2pq$, and $\frac{1}{50}$ for a considered disease. There is one chance out of two for this gene to be passed to him from his father II$_1$. The subject II$_1$ has also one chance out of two to have received the same gene from his father. The latter may have transmitted the same gene to his son II$_2$ who could transmit it with one chance out of two, to his daughter III$_2$. The sum of these probabilities is $\frac{1}{16}$. The explanation may be identical if the gene is transmitted by ancestor I$_2$ (Fig. IX-14).

The probability that III$_2$ would be heterozygous for the gene (a) if III$_1$ is himself heterozygous for the same gene is

$$\frac{1}{8}\left(\frac{1}{16} + \frac{1}{16} = \frac{1}{8}\right).$$

In general the probability that two first cousins

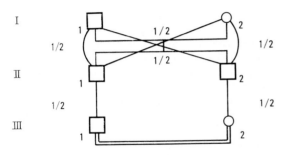

Consanguinous union

FIG. IX-14.

would be heterozygous for the same gene received from a common ancestor is

$$2pq \times \frac{1}{8} = \frac{pp}{4}.$$

The degree of relationship between two individuals can be estimated by considering the coefficients of relationship (r) and the consanguinity (F).

The relationship coefficient (r) is defined as the probability that two persons possess one or more genes in common from the same ancestor. It is $\frac{1}{8}$ for first cousins.

The consanguinity coefficient (F) is the probability that one individual had received the two alleles of one pair from an ancestor. In the case of marriage between first cousins, the consanguinity coefficient is $\frac{1}{16}$.

The consanguinity coefficient is always half the relationship coefficient (Fig. IV-15).

	Consanguinity coefficient (F)	Relationship coefficient (r)
Father daughter. . .	1/4	1/2
Uncle niece	1/8	1/4
Cousins 1st degree. .	1/16	1/8
Cousins 2nd degree. .	1/64	1/32
Cousins 3rd degree. .	1/256	1/128

FIG. IX-15. — *Coefficients of consanguinity* (F) *and relationship* (r).

INTERMEDIATE HEREDITY

In this form of heredity the heterozygous subject for a recessive gene (*a*) presents with biological or clinical and biological signs that are different from that of a homozygote. In the former case the disease is not entirely symptomless. In thalassemia, for example, the homozygote suffers from Cooley's disease, the heterozygote may present with discrete signs, such as anaemia, subicterus and splenomegaly (Rietty, Greppi-Michelli syndrome) or some blood abnormalities such as moderate polyglobulinemia associated with hypochromia and normal sideremia (Silvestroni Bianco's syndrome).

SEX CHROMOSOME LINKED HEREDITY

The individuality of the laws of transmission of characters linked to sex chromosomes is essentially due to the existence of the Y chromosome in males, whose size on the one hand and its genic concents on the other hand do not correspond to the X chromosome. Consequently, if there is a mutant gene on the X chromosome in a male subject, the disease will manifest itself if this gene is recessive, *i. e.* not masked by a normal gene of the homologous chromosome.

Recessive heredity linked to an X chromosome

Most diseases linked to sex chromosomes are transmitted in this way. This is the case in certain forms of myopathies, particularly "Duchenne de Boulogne" and "Becker" myopathies.

— "Duchenne de Boulogne" myopathy (DDB I) is a progressive disabling muscular dystrophy that is usually fatal between 15 and 18 years of age. The onset is before the age of 3 years, in the form of difficulty in walking. Gowers maneuver (difficulty in rising from the floor) is characteristic of the disease. The muscular atrophy involves the pelvic girdle and the quadriceps. This is complicated by thoracic scoliosis and other deformities.

Females do not suffer clinically, but carriers of the pathologic gene (*a*) are heterozygous or transmitters of (A*a*). The descendants of their union with a normal male are composed of clinically normal daughters, but one in two is heterozygous like her mother. Half of the sons are diseased while the other half are genetically intact and therefore healthy (Fig. IX-16).

— "Becker" myopathy (DDB II): males suffering from this late onset myopathy, transmit the disease to their daughters who will all be obligatory trans-

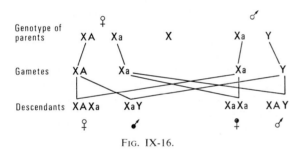

FIG. IX-16.

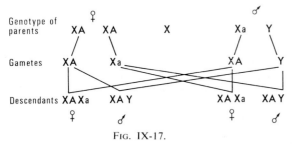

FIG. IX-17.

mitters of the disease. All sons will be normal (Fig. IX-17). In the first generation all children will then be clinically normal. In practice, examinations to search for heterozygous characteristics among the daughters are not useful since they are obligatory transmitters.

A male suffering from X-linked recessive disease, has received the abnormal gene from his mother, who as a female carrier, may have received the X chromosome carrying the pathologic gene, either from her father or from her mother (Fig. IX-18).

— In theory, an affected female is born as the descendant of an affected male and a female carrier (Fig. IX-19).

Half of the daughters will be affected, the other half will be carriers. Half of the sons will be affected and the other half will be normal.

The existence of an affected daughter necessitates the elimination of Turner's syndrome from the diagnosis, as her complement is 45,X where the single X

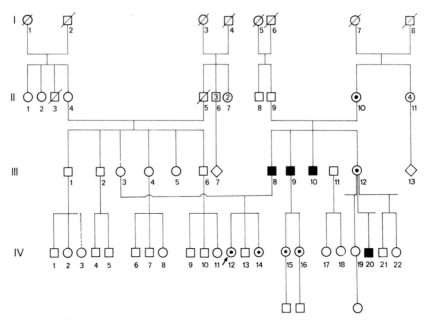

FIG. IX-18. — X-linked recessive heredity. Genealogy of Becker's myopathy.

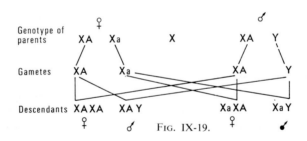

FIG. IX-19.

carries the mutation. This is also the case in "testicular feminization syndrome" whose chromosome formula is 46,XY.

Well known X-linked recessive diseases other than the myopathies, are: haemophilia A and B, daltonism, Hunter's disease (Fig. IX-20) or mucopolysaccharidosis type II, and anhydrotic ectodermal dysplasia.

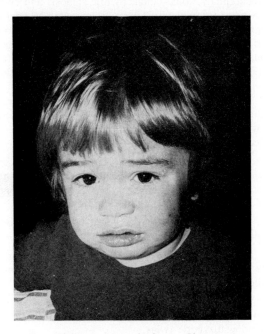

FIG. IX-20. — *Hunter's disease.* Phenotype.

Figure IX-21 shows the X linked transmission of Hunter's disease.

Dominant heredity linked to the X chromosome

This is more rare. A form of familial rickets that is hypophosphataemic and vitamin resistant seems to be transmitted in this way. This may also be the case in pigmenta incontinenta. An affected male XAY will give rise in his descendants to affected daughters and healthy sons. The transmission is therefore father-daughter (Fig. IX-22).

Within the descendants of an affected heterozygous mother and a normal father, half of the daughters and half of the sons will suffer from the disease (Fig. IX-23).

The mode of transmission of the "oro-facio-digital" syndrome of Papillon-Leage and Psaume should be pointed out here. This is transmitted in a dominant X-linked form, but is fatal in the homozygotes (Fig. IX-24).

It may be seen in the descendants of an affected mother, that among daughters one in two is diseased, but there is never a diseased son except if the latter presents with Klinefelter's syndrome 47,XXY.

Y-linked or "holanderic" heredity

Nowadays, only hypertrichosis of the ears is considered to be linked to a gene localised on

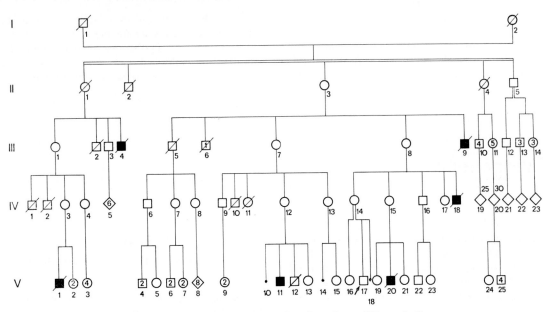

FIG. IX-21. — *X-linked recessive heredity.* Genealogy of Hunter's disease.

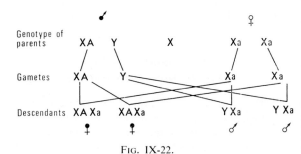

FIG. IX-22.

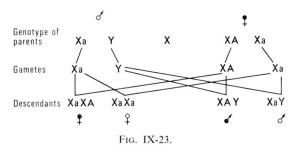

FIG. IX-23.

♀ \ ♂	Xa	Y
XA	XA Xa	XA Y fatal
Xa	Xa Xa	Xa Y

FIG. IX-24.

the Y chromosome. It affects males, who also transmit it. All the daughters will be healthy but all the sons will be affected.

MULTIFACTORIAL AND POLYGENIC HEREDITY

Among numerous malformations that are commonly seen; those such as hare-lip and cleft palate, anencephaly, spina-bifida, pyloric stenosis and club foot, are not transmitted in accordance with Mendel's laws of heredity. However, intrafamilial accumulation of such anomalies is known. The causes of these malformations are said to be multifactorial, *i. e.* associated in their etiology with the influence of the environment and genic or polygenic factors.

The principal characteristics of this type of heredity were defined by Carter. When a child is affected by one of this type of malformations, the risk of recurrence is estimated to be about 5 %.

— The risk seems to vary from one family to another. If two babies present with hare-lip, the probability of recurrence is 10 %. It is the same if one parent and one child are affected.

— The risk of recurrence is greater if the malformation is more serious.

— The risk for the relatives of the affected person is proportionally less high if the frequency among the general population is a significant one.

— The occurence of the anomaly in monozygous twins is greater in comparison to the occurence among dizygotic twins.

— The consanguinity ratio is sometimes increased.

If a child is suffering from pyloric stenosis that affects the female sex at a frequency of 5 $\%_{oo}$, the risk of recurrence for a first degree relative is multiplied by 10. It is multiplied by 5 for a second degree relative and by 1.5 for a third degree relative.

Cytogenetics

In 1956, Tijo and Levan [52] showed that the number of chromosomes in the human species is 46. In 1959, Lejeune, Gautier and Turpin discovered the trisomy 21 characteristic of mongolism [32]. Thus chromosomal pathology was born and the etiology of numerous malformation syndromes was identified.

METHODS OF OBTAINING HUMAN CHROMOSOMES

The study of human chromosomes may be undertaken from cells in interphase, meiosis or mitosis.

Cells in interphase. — When a genomic pathology is suspected, cells in interphase can be utilised to determine the number of X or Y chromosomes of the subject.

Barr [1] had shown that in females at the level of the nucleus, there are rounded or triangular condensations at the nuclear membrane. He called them Barr corpuscules. These correspond to the inactivated X according to the hypothesis of Mary Lyon [37]. A correlation therefore exists between the number of X chromosomes of the individual and the number of Barr corpuscles in each cell. In the human there are as many chromatin corpuscles as X chromosomes minus one. Thus a normal female possesses one Barr corpuscle while a normal male has a one negative chromatin number (Fig. IX-25).

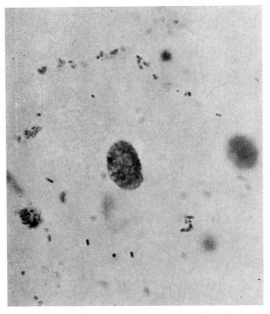

FIG. IX-25. — *Two Barr bodies, in a 47, XXX subject.*

As regards the study of the Y chromosome, quinacrine treatment before observation in fluorescent light may be sufficient. There are as many fluorescent corpuscles as the Y content in the cell [46].

Cells in meiosis. — These are not commonly utilised. A testicular biopsy in used or more rarely, an ovarian one. They may be employed in particular cases as in sterility or in genosomic mosaicism [36].

Cells in mitosis. — All tissue that can multiply in vitro is utilizable. The general principle

is to obtain the cellular division blocked at the metaphase stage during which the chromosomes are well individualized. There are many variants that follow the chosen tissue in relation to the diagnostic possibilities [55].

The culture of cutaneous fibroblasts is particularly useful in cases of mosaicism, *i. e.* when in the same individual colonies. The numbers of chromosomes differ over several cellular colonies. The usefulness of such techniques is invaluable in establishing banks of cells or in quantifying fibroblastic enzymes.

The bone marrow gives a good deal of information and will confirm hemopathologic diagnosis and follow up of the case.

The study of amniotic cells allows for chromosomal and biochemical investigations of the foetus.

The blood lymphocyte, however remains, the prefered element. The culture technique is relatively simple and cellular growth is rapidly observed within 72 hours. Transport of the obtained material should be done at ambient temperature. A delay of more than 48 hours before culturing is to be avoided.

Irrespective of the technique utilized for cell culture, cells are placed in an incubator at 37° C in an appropriate nutrient material (e. g., TC 199, RPMI, etc.) for a variable period of time according to the tissue. When colchicine is added to lymphocyte cultures from the beginning, it blocks the cells in metaphase (Fig. IX-26). The use of hypotonic solutions leads to rupture of the nucleus. The stained preparations are then examined microscopically and mitotic profiles are photographed. Prints are

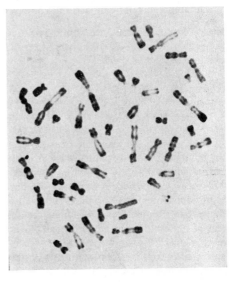

FIG. IX-26. — *Dispersed cells in metaphase.*

then enlarged, chromosomes are cut out and assembled together resulting in a chromosome map or karyotype of the subject.

Until 1970, staining techniques such as "Giemsa staining" used to result in a uniformity of colour of chromosomes. The only criteria to be relied on for classification, therefore, were the size of the chromosome and the position of its centromere. Fifteen years ago, modifications in the banding technique allowed the exact identification of every pair of chromosomes and the recognition of intra- or inter-chromosomal changes that are not visible by standard techniques. Banding techniques also provided a better demonstration of different variants such as secondary constrictions or satellite formation.

After treatment, the chromosomal structure shows alterations of dark zones and clear zones, named differently according to the obtained observations.

— Q bands correspond to results obtained after the action of mustard on quinacrine following Casperson's method [5], with ultraviolet microscopy. This technique is particularly reserved for the study of the Y chromosome which is intensely fluorescent at the distal parts of its long arms.

— G bands (Giemsa) are demonstrated either by denaturation or by enzymatic digestion (e. g. trypsin) followed by Giemsa staining [11].

— R bands (Reverse) are obtained after denaturation by heat. They represent the counter type of bands observed by techniques used for G bands [10].

— C bands (centromeres) correspond to specific staining of the centromeric regions and the secondary constrictions of chromosomes 1, 9 and 16.

— T bands are used to study the telomeric regions which are impregnated with acridine orange [12].

Such diverse techniques are complementary and have considerably increased the information obtained in investigating human cells.

HUMAN KARYOTYPING

The human species contains 46 chromosomes that are divided into 44 common chromosomes or autosomes in both sexes and two sex chromosomes or gonosomes as XX in the female and XY in the male. Every pair of chromosomes includes an element of maternal origin and another of paternal origin (Fig. IX-27).

The classification of chromosomes that obtained after the Denver Convention [9] in 1960 was reviewed in London [35] in 1963 and then in Chi-

cago [6] in 1966. The nomenclature of denaturation was defined at the Paris Conference [44] in 1971. This classification involved on the one hand, length from the biggest to the smallest chromosome and on the other hand the role of the centromeric index that was defined as

$$\frac{p}{p+q}\left(\frac{\text{lenght of short arms}}{\text{total lenght}}\right).$$

According to the position of the centromere,

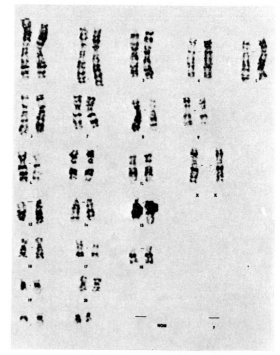

FIG. IX-27. — *Normal karyotype.*

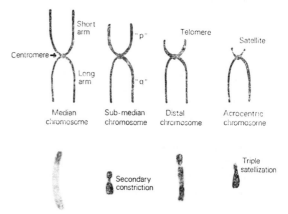

FIG. IX-28. — *Classification and function of the position of the centromere.*

chromosomes are designated as median, submedian, and distal or acrocentric (Fig. IX-28). The part of the chromosome above the centromere is called the short arm and is designated as "*p*" while the part below the centromere is called the long arm and designated as "*q*". The distal part of the long arm and of the short arm is called the telomere. The acrocentric chromosomes are practically lacking short arms. Their centromeres are positioned as satellites that could be in the form of double or triple satellites, making what is described as physiologic variants. In fact it may be possible though not yet demonstrated, that these bands, as a result of their repositioning or reshuffling, could themselves induce one form or another of real pathology.

Besides the variability of satellite formation, the heterochromic zones which are said to be secondary constrictions in chromosomes 1, 9 and 16, should be pointed out. The polymorphism of the Y chromosome is well known and depends principally on racial factors.

The autosomes arranged in pairs are designated from 1 to 22. The genosomes are always designated as X or Y. Because of the difficulty in precisely identifying the different pairs when using standard techniques, a literal classification in groups from A to G is also used. The correlation between the numerical and the literal classification is shown as follows (Table I):

TABLE I

Name of the group	Number of the pair	Structure of chromosomes
A	1, 2, 3	1 and 3 → medians 2 ⟶ submedians
B	4, 5	Distals
C	6, 7, 8, 9, 10, 11, 12, X	8, 10, 12 ⟶ distals 6, 7, 9, 11, X → submedians
D	13, 14, 15	Acrocentrics
E	16, 17, 18	16 → median 17 → submedian 18 → distal
F	19, 20	Medians
G	21, 22, Y	Acrocentrics (the long arms of the Y are parallels)

THE CHROMOSOMAL ANOMALIES. DEFINITIONS

A chromosomal error may involve the structure or the number of chromosomes, whether autosomes or genosomes [24].

STRUCTURAL ANOMALIES

The chromosomal structure may be altered following a break in either one or several chromosomes. This leads to intra- or interchromosomal modifications.

Intrachromosomal modifications (Fig. IX-29)

Deletions. — The loss of a fragment may be more or less important than the loss of a chromosome. This can be detected by the current techniques, that may demonstrate an extensive fragment of a chromosome.

The ring. — If the deletion takes place at the extremities of the short arms and of the long arms, a new chromosome will be formed as a result of fusion of the free ends, *i. e.* making a ring. This form is unstable. Therefore the chromosomal formula of the subjects carrying the "ring" is usually of mosaicism.

Isochromosomes. — The formation of isochromosomes is caused by abnormal division of the centromere, that takes place transversely and not longitudinally. This results in two new median chromosomes, one is composed of two short arms and the other of two long arms. Thus there is duplication of one arm and a lack of the other. Such a phenomenon is observed particularly in chromosome X.

The inversions. — These result from the upside down inversion (180°) of a chromosome fragment that lies between two breaks. The inversion is called peri- or paracentral as the inverted fragment may or may not contain the centromeric region.

Interchromosomal modifications (Fig. IX-30). — Translocations are the consequence of breaks affecting several chromosomes inside the same cell. They may be defined as a transfer of a chromosome of a chromosomal segment into another chromosome. When a translocation is accompanied by neither loss nor gain of material, *i. e.* the full chromosomal

INTRACHROMOSOMAL MODIFICATIONS

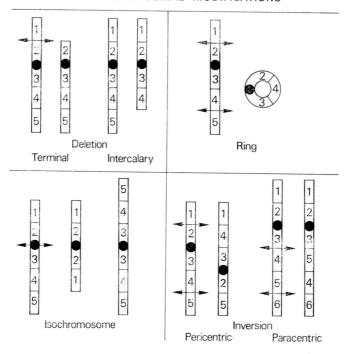

FIG. IX-29.

complement is preserved, no alteration of the phenotype is expected; this is called balanced translocation. There are several types of translocation to be distinguished.

Simple translocation. — This is the transfer of a fragment of a chromosome into the distal part of another chromosome. Therefore such chromosomes do not keep their centromeric index.

Reciprocal translocations. — This corresponds to exchange of terminal chromosomal fragments between two chromosomes that are non homologous. If the exchanged segments are of identical size, the resulting new chromosomes keep their initial form. This can be demonstrated by denaturation (banding) techniques.

Translocation by central fusion: "Robertsonian translocation". — This is fusion of two acrocentric chromosomes at the level of the centromeric region. One chromosome keeps its centromere, the break takes place in its short arm while in the other chromosome the break is just underneath its centromere. This results in a new median or submedian chromosome depending on whether the translocation has taken place in two chromosomes of the same group

or of two different groups. The existence of a balanced translocation may lead to the formation of abnormal gametes after meiotic malsegregation.

NUMERICAL ANOMALIES

These occur as a consequence of non-disjunction of paired chromosomes at the time of the 1st or 2nd meiotic division, or at the time of mitosis.

In the normal state in man, the gametes contain a haploid number "n" of 23 chromosomes, while the somatic cells are characterised by the haploid number "$2n$" of 46. Multiples of "n" are euploid, "$3n$" and "$4n$" correspond to triploids and tetraploid respectively (Fig. IX-31). In general, these polypoids are not viable and are constantly found in abortion material. No doubt they are caused by the fertilization of the ovum by two sperms, or by non-expulsion of the polar globule. Tetraploids take place at the time of a mitotic error, inhibiting the first division of the zygote.

In the aneuploid, the numerical error is not in multiples of "n". The commonest form is hyperploid (for example: $2n + 1$), or hypoploid (for example: $2n - 1$).

INTERCHROMOSOMAL MODIFICATIONS

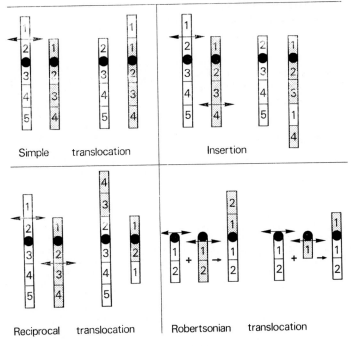

Simple   translocation

Insertion

Reciprocal   translocation

Robertsonian   translocation

FIG. IX-30.

Trisomy. — A trisomy is characterized by the presence of three identical copies of one chromosome. Of the 3 chromosomes in such a case one is often individualised in relation to the others, *i. e.* a free form. The total number of chromosomes in the cell is therefore $2n + 1 = 47$. The trisomy is generally due to meiotic error but could also be the result of a mitotic nondisjunction. If it takes place as an error during the first blastomeric division, all cells of the individual will be trisomic. If the error takes place at a later stage, two clones would remain in the same subject resulting in mosaicism.

The supernumerary element may be found translocated on another chromosome. The total number of chromosomes remain unchanged but the abnormal configurations may help the diagnosis. It is therefore a trisomy due to translocation. In half the cases, this has taken place as a direct consequence of prenatal balanced translocation and in the other half it occurs "de novo".

Monosomy. — This is characterized by the absence of one chromosome in a given pair. In the human species, total autosomic monosomy is usually not viable and may be demonstrated in abortion material. Only the X gonosomic monosomy is viable and leads to Turner's syndrome.

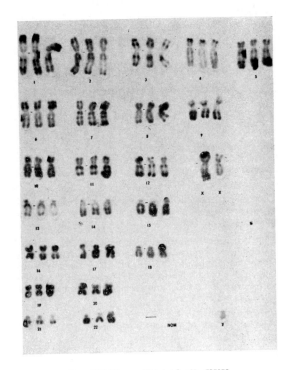

FIG. IX-31. — *Triploidy 69, XXY.*

INTERNATIONAL NOMENCLATURE OF CHROMOSOMAL ANOMALIES

The present nomenclature was established and approved at the Paris Conference in 1971. The following table includes the principal formulas used in cases of numerical and structural aberrations.

NUMERICAL ABERRATIONS

Gonosomic aberrations	Turner's syndrome ———→ 45,X Klinefelter's syndrome → 47,XXY "Double Y" ————————→ 47,XYY
Autosomic aberrations	Signs { + in front of the supernumerary chromosome { − in front of the subnumerary chromosome Trisomy 21 in a boy ———→ 47,XY,+21 Monosomy 21 in a girl ——→ 45,XX,−21 Triploidy ————————→ 69,XYY

Mosaicism →	The different clones come from the same zygote (the abbreviation "mos" is facultative)
	. Two clones —→ 45,X/46,XX
	            or mos 45,X/46,XX
	    . → 46,XY/47,XY,+21
	. Three clones → 45,X/46,XX/47,XXX

Chimerism →	The different clones come from two or more zygotes . Chi 46,XX/46,XY

STRUCTURAL ABERRATIONS

Symbols used

p = short arm; *q* = long arm; *cen* = centromere; *s* = satellite; *h* = secondary constriction; *ter* = distal extremity of an arm; (:) = break; (::) = break-reunion; →: until *a*; *mar* = marker.

The sign (+) or (−) placed after *q*, *p*, *s* or *h* indicates an increase or a decrease in length of the considered region.

Every chromosomal arm is divided into regions that are numbered from 1 to 4 at maximum. Every region is subdivided into bands, coded from 1 to 9. Certain bands contain sub-bands. The codes (1) designate the juxtacentromeric zones. A point given on a chromosome is therefore indicated by:

— the number of the chromosome,
— the symbol of the concerned arms,
— the number of the region,
— the number code of the band, and consequently the sub-band.

Examples

(*a*) Intrachromosomal shuffling

Deletion = (del)	*Terminal deletion* of a long arm at 9. Point of break region 3 band 1
	    46,XX,del (9) (*q*31)
	or 46,XX,del (9) (*pter* → *q*31)
	Intercalary deletion on the long arm of 9. Point of break region 1, band 2 and region 3, band 1. Disappearance of the segment between these two regions
	    46,XX,del (9) (*q*12 *q*31)
	or 46,XX,del (9) (*pter* → *q*12 :: *q*31 → *qter*)

Ring = r	*Ring of chromosome* X, reunion of the arms *p* and *q* after breaks at *p*21 and *q*21 46,X,*r* (X) (*p*21 *q*21) or 46,X,*r* (X) (*p*21 → *q*21)
Isochromosome = i	*Isochromosome* for the short arms of chromosome 17 46,XX,*i* (17*p*) or 46,XX,*i* (17*p*) (*pter* → *cen* → *pter*)

Inversion = inv	*Pericentric inversion* of chromosome 9. The inverted segment is between two break points: region 1, band 3 of *p* and region 3, band 1 of *q*
	    46,XY,*inv* (9) (*p*13 *q*31)
	or 46,XY,*inv* (9) (*pter* → *p*13 :: *q*31 → *p*13 :: *q*31 → *qter*)
	Paracentric inversion of the long arms of chromosome 9. Points of break: region 1, band 3 and region 3, band 1
	    46,XY,*inv* (9) (*q*13 *q*31)
	or 46,XY,*inv* (9) (*pter* → *q*13 :: *q*31 → *q*13 :: *q*31 → *qter*)

(*b*) Interchromosomal reshuffling

Reciprocal translocation = t or rcp	*Between two autosomes*, the smaller number is to be given first. Exchange of distal fragments between chromosomes 4 and 12. Points of break: region 2, band 4 for the long arms of 4 and region 2, band 3 for the long arms of 12
	    46,XX,*t* (4; 12) (*q*24; *q*23)
	or 46,XX,*rcp* (4; 12) (*q*24; *q*23)
	or 46,XX,*t* (4; 12) (4 *pter* → 4 *q*24 :: 12 *q*23 → 12 *qter*; 12 *pter* → 12 *q*23 :: 4 *q*24 → 4 *qter*)
	Between autosomes and gonosomes, the gonosome is designated first. Exchange of distal fragments between chromosome X and 4. Points of break: region 2, band 1, for the long arms of X; region 2, band 4, for the long arms of 4
	    46,XX,*t* (X; 4) (*q*21; *q*24)
	or 46,XX,*t* (X; 4) (X *pter* → X *q*21 :: 4 *q*24 → 4 *qter*; 4 *pter* → 4 *q*24 :: X *q*21 → X *qter*)

| Robert-
sonian
trans-
location
= t
or rob | Centromeric fusion between chromosome D and chromosome G
(a) If the origin of the centromere is unknown
45,XX,t (13q 21q)
or 45,XX,rob (13q 21q)
or 45,XX,rob (13; 21) (13q → cen → 21q)
(b) If the origin of the centromere is known
45,XX,t (13q 21q) (p11; q11)
or 45,XX,t (13; 21) (13 qter → 13 q11 :: 21 q11 → 21 qter) |

(c) Consequences of parental reshuffling

Abnormal chromosome

Transmitted directly by malsegregation

Transmitted after aneusomy of recombination

Symbolised by (der)

Symbolised by (rec)

— The symbols (der) or (rec) are followed by the number corresponding to the centromere of the reconstituted chromosome.

— The paternal or maternal origin of the chromosome is designated by pat or mat.

(a) *Malsegregation*

Examples:
A balanced paternal translocation
46,XY,t (1; 13) (q43; q13)
may result in two abnormal chromosomes
der (1) and der (13)
By malsegregation, two non balanced karyotypes may lead to
46,XX (ou XY), der (1) pat
or 46,XX (ou XY), der (13) pat

(b) *Aneusomy of recombination*

A parental pericentric inversion may include a deficient duplication, after crossing-over in the inversion pathway
A mother → 46,XX,inv (3) (p14 q21)
may give
46,XX,rec (3) dup p, inv (3) (p14 q21)
or 46,XX,rec (3) dup q, inv (3) (p14 q21)

EXAMPLES
OF CHROMOSOMAL PATHOLOGY

AUTOSOMAL ABERRATIONS

Autosomal chromosome pathology is dominated by three major syndromes; the trisomies 21, 18 and 13. The discovery of new entities has demonstrated the existence of aberrations at the level of each of the autosomes. However, total trisomies are rare. The commonest trisomies are those carried on the short or on the long arms. The identification of such cases helps precise genetic counselling and the establishment of a genetic history.

Trisomy 21

In 1959, the first disease of chromosomal origin was reported [32] to be due to the presence of three copies of the chromosome 21. The term "trisomy 21" was then used to indicate "mongolism". This syndrome represents the commonest problem seeking genetic advice. Its incidence is approximately 1/650 live births. All races are subject to the disease and there is no sex ratio.

Maternal age is an undisputable etiologic factor. The possibility of having an infant affected by the disease is significantly higher with an older aged mother. The curve representing occurence of the disease with maternal age shows in fact two peaks, the first around the age of 28 years and the second near the age of 37 years. The first peak includes sporadic or inherited translocations representing half the number of cases and corresponding to the maximum number of births. The risk of having a child born with the disease is 1 in 2,000 at a maternal age of 20 years, 1 in 500 at 35 years, 1 in 100 at 40 years and 1 in 50 at the age of 45 years [40]. The existence of chromosome 21 markers permits the demonstration of about 60 % of the nondisjunctions during gametogenesis in the mother.

The role of infectious agents and ionizing radiation as etiological factors, is uncertain.

The phenotype in trisomy 21 is suggestive, though sometimes debatable in the neonatal period. Hypotonia is a constant sign. The skull is spheroidal with brachycephaly and absence of the occipital bosses. The face is lunar (Fig. IX-32), the palpebral fissures are oblique and elevated laterally. The internal angle of the eye is masked by epicanthus and the pupils are sometimes eccentric. At birth, brushfield spots are commonly observed in the iris. Strabismus is not uncommon and the eyelids often show belpharitis. The nose shows wide nostrils, flat tip and flat nasal bridge; a misleading appearance of hypertelorism.

The mouth opening is small and is usually half opened with a protruding thick and foliated tongue. The inferior lip is everted and the palate is highly arched. The teeth may appear later than normal and display an irregular fashion. The ears are small, the superior edge and the helix are markedly bent

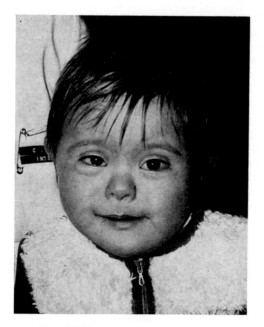

FIG. IX-32. — *Trisomy 21: phenotype.*

type: 92.5 % of cases correspond to free forms
with an accidental non-disjunction (Fig. IX-33)
and 4.8 % of cases are due to a translocation

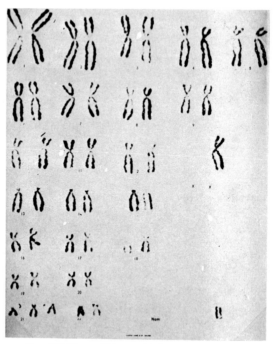

FIG. IX-33. — *Trisomy 21 free: 47, XX + 21.*

forwards, the lobules are malformed and the auditory canal is narrow. The hair is fine, scanty and
tough. The neck is short with an excess of skin.

In the extremities, rhizomelic brevity may be
noticed. The hands are short, massive and bulky.
The thumb is implanted high. Clinodactyly of the
5th finger and brachymesophalangia are frequent.
A transverse palmar crease (simian crease) is uni-
or bilateral, the axial triradius ends in t'' and the
index of transversality is increased. The feet are
short and flat. The skin is dry, rough and mottled.

With respect to internal malformations, cardiopathies such as atrio-ventricular malformations are
the most common and encountered in 40 % of cases.

Next in frequency of occurence are dudenal
stenosis and malformations of the urogenital
system. Bone anomalies are typical, particularly
the presence of a small pelvis. Genu valgum is
frequent.

Mental retardation is constantly present and the
intellectual quotient according to Gauss's curve is
between 30 and 70, around 50 in average. Sociability
and affection in these infants are preserved. The
height remains limited and puberty is normal.
These patients look older than their real age. Life
expectancy is affected by the presence of cardiac
malformations, respiratory infections and the occurence of leukemia. From 25 % to 30 % die during
the first year and 50 % before the age of 5 years.

Genetic counselling depends on the cytogenetic

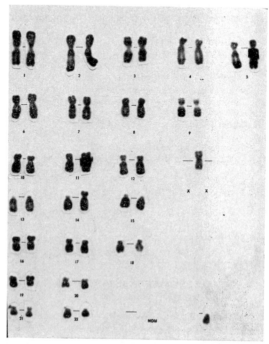

FIG. IX-34. — *Trisomy 21 by translocation:*
46, XY, t (14q; 21q).

(Fig. IX-34). Half of the cases of trisomy 21 are linked to a translocation that happened "de novo", 2.7 % present with mosaicism [21]. It is also known that cases of trisomy 21 may be associated with gonosomic aneuploidy (Fig. IX-35). The explanation of such an association is uncertain.

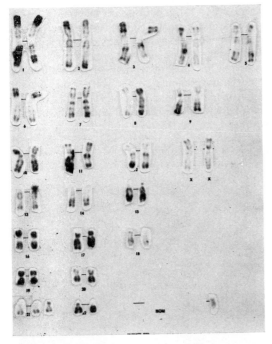

FIG. IX-35. — *Trisomy 21
associated with Klinefelter's syndrome: 48, XXY + 21.*

Trisomy 18

Trisomy 18 or "Edward's syndrome" was first described in 1960 [13]. The frequency of occurence is 1/5,000 births and affects girls three or four times as often as boys [7]. The rate of occurence of the disease in relation to maternal age has two peaks, the first around the age of 25 years and the second around the age of 40 years. The occurence of trisomy 18 seems to have a seasonal character. Pregnancy is usually complicated by hydramnios. Fœtal movements are weakly perceived. Development of the placenta is reduced and there is usually one umbilical artery. The infant is hypotrophic and looks post-mature.

The presenting dysmorphia is suggestive of the disease. The skull is small with scaphocephaly, large fontanelles, fine nose and small horizontal palpebral fissures. The mouth is small with a narrow arched palate and micrognathia. The ears are cha-

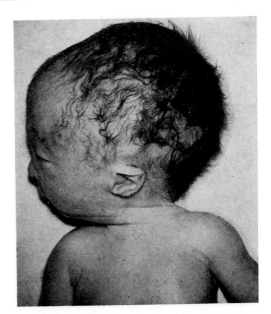

FIG. IX-36. — *Trisomy 18.* Phenotype.

racteristic; implanted lower than normal with an acute angle at the junction of the superior and posterior borders of the helix (Fig. IX-36). There is a short neck with cervical webs. The sternum is short with reduced points of ossification. The nipples are rudimentary and markedly separated apart. Hernias are frequent because of the weak musculature. The narrow pelvis is a constant sign. The upper limbs are very characteristic where the arms are in a beseeching position, the fingers are always flexed with overriding of the index finger on the middle one and the little finger over the ring finger (Fig. IX-37). This may render it difficult to study the dermatoglyphics in such cases. Sometimes the arches are highly elevated, a transverse palmar crease is not rare and the axial triradius may be found as t''. Hypoplasia of the nails, subluxation of the hips and Rocker-bottom foot usually associate with the preceeding picture.

In boys, cryptorchism must be sought for and so should hypoplasia of the labia majora in girls. As regards visceral involvement, cardiac problems present in more than 95 % of cases, mostly in the form of interventricular defects or a ductus arteriosus. Next come urinary malformations (such as horse-shoe kidney, ectopic kidney and double ureter), pulmonary anomalies (such as abnormal segmentation or absence of a lobe of the lung), digestive, skeletal and cerebral anomalies. Mental retardation is usually severe. Life expectancy is in general short although some adolescents have been

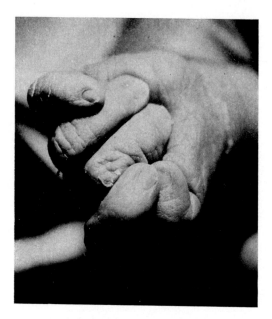

FIG. IX-37. — *Trisomy 18.*
Anomalies of the fingers.

Trisomy 13

This was described in 1960 by Patau [45]. The frequency is variable, one in 7,000 births on average. There is some predominance among girls. The average maternal age differs according to the cyto-genetic type; 32 years of age in the free form and 24 years in the translocations. Pregnancy proceeds normally, labour may be slightly premature and the birth weight of the baby is around 2,500 g. The pathology in cases of trisomy 13 is dominated by three pathognomonic signs; wolf's face that displays hare lip, microphtalmia and hexadactyly (Fig. IX-39). In the head one notices microcephaly with absence of frontal bosses, large fontanelles, depressed temporal regions and ulceration of the vertex (Fig. IX-40).

reported. The trisomy is free and homogenous in most cases (Fig. IX-38). Sometimes it is also in the form of mosaicism or partial trisomy.

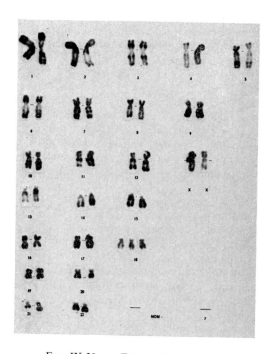

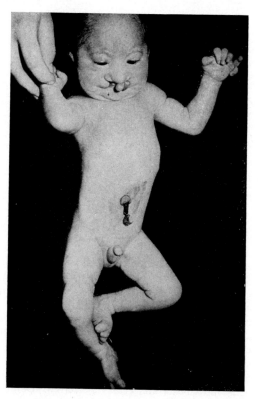

FIG. IX-39. — *Trisomy 13.* Phenotype.

FIG. IX-38. — *Trisomy 18: karyotype.*

Ocular manifestations vary from microphtalmos to coloboma of the iris, retinal dysplasia and anophtalmia or cyclopia. Hemangioma commonly involves the eye lids and may be seen in the frontal or in the temporal regions. The ears are

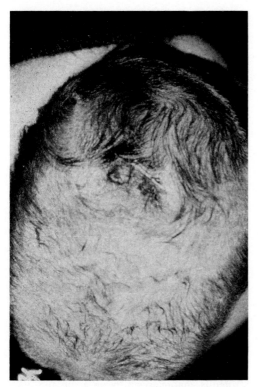

FIG. IX-40. — *Trisomy 13.*
Ulceration of the vertex.

implanted lower than normal with malfolding of the helix. The hare-lip is uni- or bilateral and accompanied by cleft palate. Aplasia of the face may extend to cebocephaly.

Cerebral malformations are typical, particularly arrhinencephaly or the absence of the olfactory bulb and tract. Median facial cleft may arise from a developmental error affecting the precordial plate during the third week. Ocular anomalies and malformations of the frontal part of the brain may also result from the same error.

The skeleton shows several malformations such as hypoplasia of the lower ribs, spina bifida and rocker-bottom feet with backward protruding heels. The fingers are flexed and hexadactyly is frequent and always on the ulnar side. The nails are small and hyperconvexed. Regarding the genital system there is cryptorchism in boys and bicornate uterus in girls.

Cardiac anomalies present in 80 % of cases, in the form of interauricular or interventricular septal defects, ductus arteriosus and sometimes dextrocardia. In 30 % of cases, urinary malformations present as polycystic kidney, horseshoe kidney, hydronephrosis or double ureter. Anomalies of the digestive system, such as colon malformations, Meckel's diverticulum and omphalocele are rare.

The dermatoglyphics in trisomy 13 are characterized by the presence of a transverse palmar crease, increased radial arches and loops and a highly elevated axial triradius. Embryonic hemoglobin (Gower 2) persists throughout the gestational period. Neutrophils show peculiar nuclear projections. Average life expectancy is 130 days.

Cytogenetic studies show a free homogenous form in 80 % of cases. There are also forms of mosaicism and de novo translocations or translocations inherited from a parent. Generally, translocation takes place with another chromosome of group D and with a preference for 14. In familial translocation (13q 14q) the risk of early abortion is about 20 %.

Cases of partial trisomy 13 are less well known but two distinct categories seem to exist. Trisomies for the distal portion in which there is polydactyly and persistence of the embryonic hemoglobin and trisomies for the proximal portion with hare lip cleft palate and modified neutrophils.

Trisomy 9p

This was be identified with the discovery of banding (denaturation) techniques, mainly because of the secondary constrictions [30, 49]. It is characterized by microcephaly, large anterior fontanelle, slight hypertelorism, globular nose, small eyes deeply embedded in the orbit with strabismus. The ears are large and protruding. Cheeks are chubby, mouth angles are drooping and the lower lip is everted. The chin is marked by a horizontal depression. These signs collectively give the appearance of a state of anxiety (Fig. IX-41). The neck is large and short. The nipples are widely apart. In the hands, there are long palms contrasting with brachymesophalangia, clinodactyly of the fifth finger and marked irregularity of the flexion creases. The transverse palmar crease, the absence or the fusion of the triradius subdigitals b and c, and the excess of digital arches are the principal dermatoglyphic signs in trisomy 9p. There is no particular visceral anomaly. Intellectual retardation is constant with an IQ around 50. Instability and agitation are frequent. Cases in adults have been published.

Usually trisomy 9p associates a proximal trisomy of the long arms or partial trisomy or monosomy of another chromosome. It is sometimes a consequence of malsegregation of a familial translocation (Fig. IX-42 and IX-43).

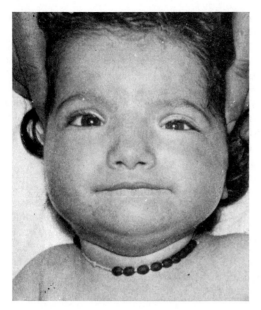

FIG. IX-41. — *Trisomy 9p*. Phenotype.

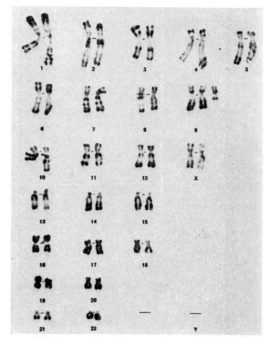

FIG. IX-43. — *Trisomy 9p: karyotype.*

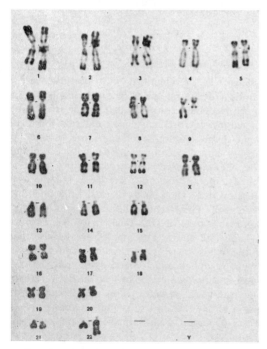

FIG. IX-42. — *Maternal balanced translocation*
46, XX, t (9; 22) (q13; q13).

Monosomy 5p

This was described in 1963 under the name of "cri du chat" (or cat's cry) syndrome [33]. This

syndrome is characterized by an acute and painful cry, like the mew of a cat. This is mainly due to a reduced larynx size without major structural changes. The cry disappears at the age of about 3 years, but the voice remains with an acute tone.

In addition to such pathognomonic signs, some dysmorphic features also exist, such as microcephaly, hypertelorism which is quite pronounced, micrognathia, rounded face, apparent metopic suture, epicanthic fold, descending obliquity of the palpebral fissures, divergent strabismus and pretragal tubercle (Fig. IX-44). Cardiac, cerebral and renal anomalies are reported.

The dermatoglyphic appearance in trisomy 5p most commonly shows a distal flexion crease interrupted near the second interdigital space. The body weight at birth is below 2,500 g and there is persistent staturoponderal hypotrophy. Hypotonia or hypertonia may be present. Mental deficiency is constant and severe. The frequency of trisomy 5p is disputable but ranges around one in 50,000 births. It occurs de novo in 80 % of cases (Fig. IX-45), the rest are the consequence of parental rearrangement, pericentric inversion of the fifth, maternal translocation or mosaicism. The genes characteristic of the syndrome are situated in zone 5p 14 and 5p 15.

The notion of the type and contra type [34] may be permitted when comparing the clinical signs of monosomy 5p with those of trisomy 5p.

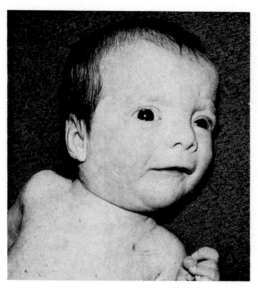

FIG. IX-44. — *Monosomy 5p: phenotype.*

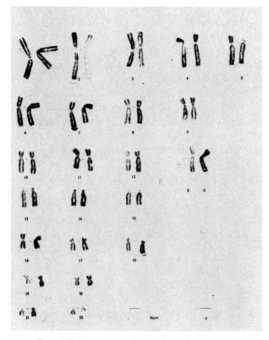

FIG. IX-45. — *Syndrome 5p⁻: karyotype.*

GONOSOMAL ABERRATIONS

Turner's syndrome

This was described by Turner [54] in 1938, the chromosomal origin of the disease was demonstrated by Ford [17] in 1959 who showed a karyotype 45,X in affected females.

This anomaly is the only viable gonosomal monosomy in man. The frequency is about one in 2,500 newly born females. This estimate is 50 times higher in foetal waste (abortion material) as 97-98 % of such conceptions are eliminated by abortion. Full term birth and the age of the parents are average. The chromosome X left over is of maternal origin in 75 % of cases.

The diagnosis may be suspected in the foetus when there is voluminous lymphoedema of the neck and arms. Newly born females are small in length (46 cm) and are relatively underweight (2,500 g). They may present with lymphoedema of the back, hands and feet. This is associated with the presence of a cervical web and marked laxity of the skin (Fig. IX-46). Such a highly suggestive form is similar to "Bonnevie-Ullrich" syndrome, which is not very specific, as only 30 % of such cases are of Turner's syndrome. However, more than 70 % of cases of Turner's syndrome present with lymphoedema.

In infancy, dwarfism is associated with dysmorphic signs. The retarded growth is accentuated, and there is no pubertal increase. Growth is slow and is prolonged in its course because of late fusion of the developing cartilage. Dysmorphic signs in Turner's syndrome are variable in number and in intensity. They are usually non specific when taken individually, their diagnostic value lies in their association.

The face looks triangular, palpebral fissures are oblique downwards and laterally with apparent epicanthus and ptosis. The palate is highly arched. Anomalies of the temporo-mandibular joint such as retrognathism may be noted. The ears are implanted low and malfolded. There is also a low and irregular hair line. In 25 to 50 % of cases the neck is short with a webbed appearance. The chest is rounded and the nipples are distantly apart. The biachromial dimension is greater than the intertrochanteric. In 75 % of cases abundance of naevi is noted. Cubitus valgus is frequent and so is bradymetacarpia. The intellectual quotient is normal in the majority of cases. In adolescents there is primary amenorrhea.

Cardiac anomalies are present in more than 20 % of cases, particularly coarctation of the aorta.

Renal manifestations are present in more than 50 % of cases but are often clinically silent. Intravenous pyelography may reveal a duplicated kidney, horseshoe kidney, renal agenesis or hypoplasia and hydronephrosis.

Sensory manifestations are partly auditory and partly visual. The former is due to perception deaf-

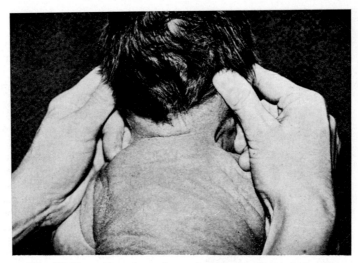

FIG. IX-46. — *Turner's syndrome: Pterygium colli (cervical web).*

ness in 50 % of cases, and the latter include myopia and cataract.

Radiography of the skeleton may explain the shortness of the neck as there is hypoplasia of the upper cervical vertebrae, and may confirm other signs as those in the wrist and hand (elevated lunate and shortness of the 4th metacarpal) and an effaced internal tibial condyle in the knee (Kosowicz sign).

Dermatoglyphic signs are mainly represented by

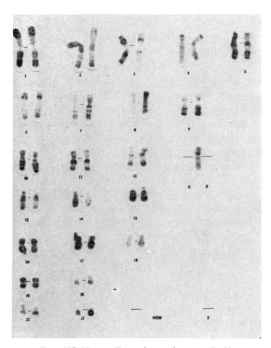

FIG. IX-47. — *Turner's syndrome: 45, X.*

the position of the axial triradius as t' or t'' with termination of the line T as 11; the triradius b is deviated towards the ulnar side. The index of transversality is lowered while the total number of crests of the digital pulps is increased with a frequent increase in whorls. There is also an increase in the number of hypothenar figures.

Cytogenetic studies demonstrate varying karyotypic numbers. The classic form of 45,X (Fig. IX-47) is present in more than half of cases. Barr corpuscles are absent in interphasic nuclei. A positive sex chromatin may accompany forms of mosaicism or anomalies of structure such as isochromosomes, deletion of an X chromosome or an X chromosome in a ring (Fig. IX-48).

"Noonan's" syndrome is used to designate a male or female subject, clinically identified as Turner's syndrome with a normal karyotype [43].

X-Polysomies in females

The karyotype 47,XXX was described in 1959 [25]. This anomaly is quite frequent but does not correspond to a clinical entity.

The constitutions 48,XXXX and 49,XXXXX are rare. The anomaly 48,XXXX was reported in 1961 [4]. The cranio-facial dysmorphia gives an appearance similar to that of trisomy 21 (Fig. IX-50). The intellectual quotient ranges between 50 and 70.

The chromosomal complement 49,XXXXX (Fig. IX-51) was first noted and published in 1963 [28]. The patient presents a coarse appearance with hypertelorism, radio-cubital synostosis and mental retardation [52].

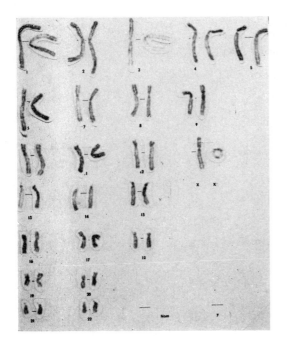

FIG. IX-48. — *Turner's syndrome: 46, X, r (X)*.

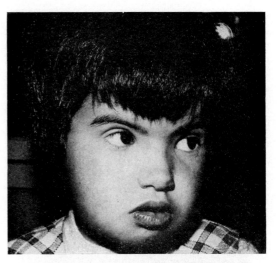

FIG. IX-50. — *Syndrome 48, XXXX*. Phenotype.

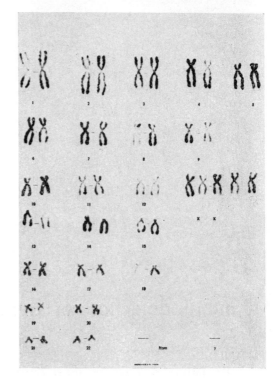

FIG. IX-51. — *Karyotype: 49, XXXXX*.

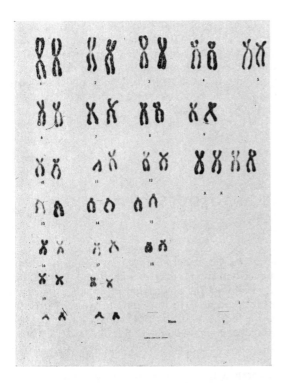

FIG. IX-49. — *Karyotype: 48, XXXX*.

X-Polysomies in males

Klinefelter syndrome was described in 1942 [29]. It associates gynaecomastia and testicular atrophy in which there is azoospermia without atrophy of the Leydig cells. The abnormal karyotype 47,XXY was discovered in 1959 [26]. Its frequency is 1.18 per 1,000 male births. The diagnosis is not commonly made in young infants in spite of the presence of ectopic testes, hypospadias or hypoplasia of the penis and the scrotum. Gynaecomastia may appear around the age of 12 years.

At puberty, hormonal secretions are not altered. The intellectual development is normal in general. However, there may be some degree of mental disability and psychiatric problems are noted.

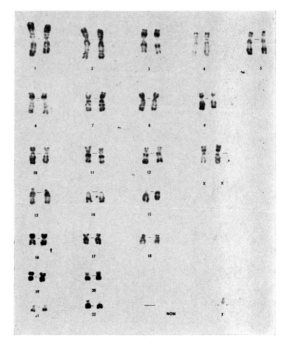

Fig. IX-53. — *Klinefelter's syndrome.* Karyotype 47, XXY.

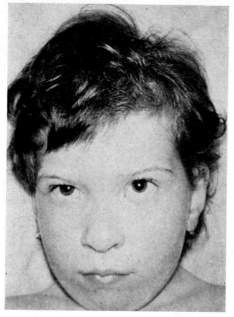

Fig. IX-52. — *Syndrome 49, XXXXX.* Moderate facial dysmorphy.

The karyotype is 47,XXY homogenous in 80 % of cases (Fig. IX-53). The karyotype 48,XXXY and 49,XXXXY are accompanied by mental debility. Clinically, symptoms are similar to Klinefelter's syndrome in those of 48,XXYY. Similarity to trisomy 21 is found among patients possessing the karyotype 49,XXXXY.

Antenatal detection of genetic disorders

Since the early observations on foetal karyotypes [51] utilizing amniotic fluid obtained in the 17th week of pregnancy, numerous publications have emerged [14, 41, 42]. Thus, an accurate approach has developed permitting prenatal detection of certain genetic disorders.

The rapid increase of knowledge in this area appears to be due to three main factors. Firstly, prenatal diagnosis could radically transform genetic counselling in a good number of incurable genetic problems. Secondly, improvement in puncture techniques and the rapidity of establishing a diagnosis have allowed the application of amniotic puncture more frequently. Thirdly, the discovery in 1972 [3] of the high level of the alpha-1-foeto-protein in the amniotic fluid when there is a neural tube defect in the foetus, has permitted the application of amniocentesis in families with high genetic risks. Moreover, research activities currently taking place seem to be promising.

PROTOCOL
OF PRENATAL DIAGNOSIS

The approach nowadays seems to be well known. It is composed of six steps: genetic consultation, obstetric consultation, amniotic puncture, study of the amniotic fluid, follow up of pregnancy and examination of the newly born. It is therefore a combination of clinical and laboratory efforts [2].

Genetic consultation should be done either before pregnancy or at the earliest possible time during pregnancy. This aims at performing genetic investigations and establishing a complete genetic tree. During the consultation, the possibility of amniocentesis should be raised and the limits and risks of such a procedure should be explained to the patient. The question of the possibility of interruption of pregnancy should also be considered and discussed. It is useful to determine the couple's wish to know (or not) the sex of the fetus. However, performing prenatal karyotyping for sex determination does not seem to be justified except in the case of a known sex-linked anomaly.

When prenatal investigations aim at the detection of a metabolic disease, it is necessary to find evidence of some enzymatic deficit in the fetus. When investigating the possibility of recurrence of a neural tube defect, the alpha-1-foeto-protein (AFP) level should be measured in the maternal serum in the fifteenth week of pregnancy.

It is preferable that the first four steps in the protocol be carried out in the same centre. Synchronization between the involved teams is important. The amniotic fluid must be maintained during transport in ambient temperature, in 30 ml flasks of the Falcon type. A delay more than 24 hours between the time of puncture and the beginning of culture, is not desirable. We usually ask the father himself to bring the flask to the laboratory.

When a fetal anomaly is found at abortion, verifying the diagnosis may be difficult because of the intra-amniotic injection of hypertonic saline. Anatomical examination of the foetus may confirm the diagnosis, particularly chromosomal anomalies and neural tube defects.

It is important to analyse the progress and evolution of pregnancy after amniocentesis, as well as the state of the infant at birth. For this purpose, a form is given to the parents with the results of the examination. The obstetric and the pediatric reports should be sent back after the birth of the infant.

TECHNIQUES

Cell culture and chromosome preparations. — Prenatal diagnosis of chromosomal and metabolic disorders requires culture of fetal cells. This can be carried out using cells from the skin of from the urinary system of the fetus and from the amniotic membrane. From 10 to 15 ml of liquid are placed in glass Petri dishes for culture and kept in an incubator at 37° C, containing an atmosphere of 95 % air and 5 % CO_2. The pH of the medium should be 7.3.

Chromosome preparations should be made, not before the 11th day, on glass cover slips. Twenty hours earlier, the medium should be replaced by a fresh one. Such a period of growth in culture permits finding ample mitotic profiles.

Measuring alpha-1-foeto-protein. Enzymatic studies. — This is carried out by a radioimmunologic technique using the serum of the mother, by radioimmunologic technique or by radial immunodiffusion of Mancini using the amniotic fluid. However, the latter method does not permit the detection of an AFP level if it is less than 1 mg/ 100 ml. Measuring the AFP level should be routine whatever the indication for amniotic puncture is.

Prenatal detection of metabolic diseases necessitates obtaining large quantities of cells. If the heterozygote possesses an enzymatic expression, it is important to know their activities before performing amniocentesis. The diagnosis is made on the fetal cells by direct measurement of their enzymatic activity or by measuring the metabolic activity after the introduction of a precursor marked by radioactive elements. In parallel to the fetal cells under investigation, control cells should be cultured. Because of the variety and also rarity of detectable diseases, national and international cooperation is required, and samples under investigation may be sent to a laboratory which is specialized in the suspected disease.

INDICATIONS AND RESULTS

From the technical point of view, detection of the fetal karyotype is performed over a period 13 days on average. A period of 22 days may be encountered

TABLE II. — Chromosomal indications for early amniocentesis [20]

Indications for chromosomal examinations	European experience		American experience	
	Investigated pregnancies	Affected foetuses	Investigated pregnancies	Affected foetuses
Maternal age	2,269	63 (2.8 %)	3,012	79 (2.6 %)
Recurrence of trisomy 21.	1,047	14 (1.3 %)	1,924	23 (1.2 %)
Parental translocation.	179	12 (6.7 %)	293	29 (9.9 %)
Risk of X-linked affection. . . .	280	♂=124 (44.3 %)	433	♂=200 (46.2 %)

when investigating some metabolic diseases. If the fluid is bloody, it should be diluted in several Petri dishes, thus allowing growth of some cellular clusters. However, the presence of blood may lead to failure of culture in 2 % of cases. Another puncture is then required, 12-15 days after the first one. It seems wise to suggest another amniocentesis when no cells are observed by the 8th day of culture.

The detection of mosaicism in culture remains a delicate problem to be solved. When detected in a Petri dish in a cellular population, it appears logical to consider the in vitro origin of the mutation. On the other hand, if mosaicism is found in many Petri dishes, it is then essential to repeat the puncture. If there is association of two clones, one normal and the other trisomic (13) and then monosomic (13) at the second puncture, it may be thought that such mosaicism is of recent appearance and the fetus is normal. Confirmation of this hypothesis becomes clear at birth of the infant.

CHROMOSOMAL INDICATIONS
(Table II)

The search for a chromosomal anomaly is the most common indication for amniocentesis, representing 70 %-92 % of all indications according to statistics. Variations may be explained by the relative interest and specialization of different units in the field of prenatal diagnosis. However, results obtained in our laboratory are similar to those of other centres (Table III).

Parents without chromosomal anomalies.

Maternal age. — The risk of a chromosomal anomaly after the age of 40 years is about 3.4 %. It is estimated as 1.5 % in females between 35 and

40 years. Maternal age is the most common indication for amniocentesis.

Chromosomal anomalies detected in samples of amniotic fluid, vary from 2.6 % to 5.5 %. In more than half of the observations, trisomy 21 is the detected anomaly. It should be pointed out however, that certain anomalies are incompatible with life and are not always diagnosed at birth.

On the other hand, the number of chromosome imbalances diagnosed in utero in the same age group (35-40 years) is about 1 %. In western Europe, public health programmes consider amniotic puncture for all females above the age of 38 years if they wish. Though the risk of chromosomal disorders is 0.69 % in infants of mothers less than 19 years of age, amniocentesis is at present not considered for them.

Past history of trisomy 21. — When there is a past history of trisomy 21, the case may be considered for prenatal diagnosis. Such an indication does not need to be accepted for psychological reasons only. The frequency of recurrence is almost 1 % and this in itself justifies amniocentesis.

Abnormal course of pregnancy. — When pregnancy is associated with clinical and laboratory signs that could lead to threatened abortion, the case may be considered for amniocentesis. This is also the case when there is a history of recurrent spontaneous abortion.

When one of the parents is a carrier of a chromosomal structural anomaly. —
In most statistics, amniocentesis indicated after the discovery of familial translocation, represents a small percentage, less than 5 %. Parental chromosomal anomalies are composed of equal parts of reciprocal translocation and of Robertsonian translocation. Apart from Dq Dq translocations, 90 % are translocations of 13q 14q.

TABLE III. — INDICATIONS FOR AND RESULTS OF EARLY AMNIOCENTESIS
FROM OUR PERSONAL EXPERIENCE [31]

Indications	Number	% genic chromosome	% total	% affected fœtus
Chromosomal				
(a) *Maternal age*				
— Above 40 years	301	27.8	22.6	10 (3.3)
— From 35 to 40 years	208	19.2	15.6	1
(b) *Structural anomalies*				
— Translocations	64	5.9	4.8	8 (12.5)
— Others	29			
(c) *History of*				
— Trisomy 21	290	26.8	21.8	3 (1)
— Others	60			
(d) *Miscellaneous*	127	11.7	9.5	
Total	1,079	100.0	81	22 (2)
Genic				
(a) *Monofactorial heredity*				
— X linked recessive	40	15.9	3	12 (30)
— Autosomal recessive metabolic	21	19.4	1.5	5 (23.8)
— Others	8			
— Autosomal dominant	1			
(b) *Multifactorial heredity*				
— Spina bifida	100			3 (1.7)
— Anencephaly	75	70	13.2	
— Pregnancy with abnormal course	6	2.3	0.4	5
Total	251	100.0	19	25
	1,330			47

In our study, the number of affected fetuses was 5.3 % in cases of Robertsonian translocation and 13.1 % when the translocation was reciprocal.

The risk appears to be higher in maternal translocation than in paternal translocation.

Genic diseases of monofactorial transmission.

— Among diseases of autosomal recessive transmission, metabolic disorders represent the majority of indications for early amniocentesis. However, the number of cases examined in most centres is about 2 % of the total indications. Nowadays, it is quite possible to establish prenatal diagnosis in about 100 metabolic disorders.

The majority of these diseases lead to early death of the infant, or present with a grave clinical picture associated with mental retardation. Metabolic disorders of lipids and mucopolysaccharidosis represent 70 % of the indications. Among metabolic disturbances related to glucose, glycogenosis type II is the most frequent. In contrast, there are fewer indications in the aminoacidopathies. Rapid death during the neonatal period without an established diagnosis, would probably explain this phenomenon. The hope that comes from attempted dietetic treatment in certain aminoacidopathies is probably overestimated. These two factors explain to an extent, the lack of genetic counseling in relation to the family. The number of diseased fetuses at theoritical risk is one in four.

— Among diseases of autosomal transmission not accompanied by an enzymatic anomaly, a small number may be diagnosed by early amniocentesis. This is mainly by the estimation of alpha-1-fœtoprotein in the maternal serum and in the amniotic fluid. Examples of this are the congenital nephrotic syndrome of the Finnish type [47] and Meckel's syndrome [50]. The latter associates occipital meningocele, polycystic kidney and polydactyly.

Genic diseases of multifactorial transmission. — It is now more common to perform prenatal diagnosis for detecting neural tube defects (Fig. IX-54 and IX-55). This as an indication, represents a variable percentage (from 2.9 % to 41 %) of total indications, according to the geographic locale of different centres. In our centre, detection of central nervous system anomalies represents more than 13 % of indications for prenatal diagnosis. The frequency of such anomalies varies from one region to another. In Northern Ireland and Scotland it is from 6 to 8 in every 1,000 births. It is above 3 % in certain regions in the West of France. In the United States it varies from 1.4 to 3.1 %. The risk of recurrence is in general 1-5 %. Figure IX-56 shows the abortion material at the 19th week in such a case. Amniotic puncture was indicated because of a history of fraternal spina bifida.

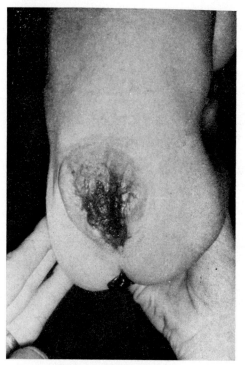

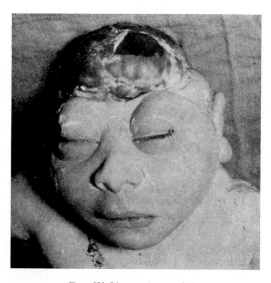

FIG. IX-55. — *Spina-bifida.*

FIG. IX-54. — *Anencephaly.*

Results should be interpreted with caution. A high level of A. F. P. in the amniotic fluid does not seem to persist when the neural tube lesion is closed. This is also the case in certain encephaloceles, and in spina bifida with meningocele. These malformations represent about 10 % of neural tube anomalies. Moreover, false positive results have been reported. This is probably due to mixing of fetal blood with the amniotic fluid. Isolated elevations of A. F. P. have been described with other malformations; omphalocele, œsophageal atresia, duodenal atresia, hydrocephaly, Turner's syndrome, trisomy 13 and sacro-coccygeal teratoma.

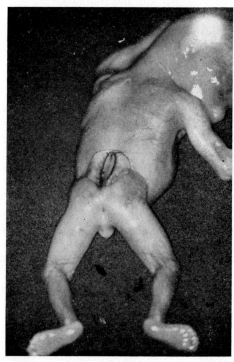

FIG. IX-56. — *Aborted material after prenatal diagnosis of neural tube anomaly* (AFP 9 mg/100 ml in the amniotic cavity).

However, prenatal diagnosis of anomalies of the neuro-ectodermal pouch should be considered in families with high genetic risk and not only among females who previously gave birth to an affected child. Also sisters of the mother should be considered, in view of possible matrilinear transmission. Such considerations could lead to a 10 % diminution in the number of patients.

NEW APPROACHES
TO ANTENATAL DIAGNOSIS

Beside techniques that are commonly utilized there are four groups of special methods currently practised.

— Fetal blood obtained under fetoscopic control allows the diagnosis of hemoglobino-pathies and hemophilia [16]. However, the presence of a percentage of 5 % of abortions necessitated the search for better techniques.

— Molecular genetic techniques permit the diagnosis of errors at the level of DNA. Early work has been done on hemoglobinopathies using bacterial endonucleases. The use of DNAC radio-active probing obtained a copy of the RNA messenger gene with the use of reverse transcriptase [27].

— The use of a "genetic link" during pregnancy to diagnose congenital adrenal hyperplasia which results from deficiency of 21 hydroxylase [8]. The link with the locus HLA-B situated on the short arm of chromosome 6 is a narrow one.

— Fine analysis of fetal proteins has become possible by the use of specific antisera. The technique of cellular hybridization (hybridomes) represents a promising step in this area.

To conclude, it seems necessary to consider the problem of prenatal diagnosis in two aspects:

— Quantitative aspect: At present, there are two important indications. First is the maternal age as the risk of meiotic malsegregation increases considerably from the age of 38 years. This has increased the rate of amniocentesis in that age group. Second, is the detection of anomalies of the neuroectodermal pouch despite the limited methods of detection. This has become a more frequent indication for prenatal diagnosis.

— Qualitative aspect: This is related to the possible risk. Diseases of recessive autosomal transmission, recessive X-linked diseases and to a lesser extent familial translocations, represent a few disorders with high genetic risk.

Genetic counseling

The genetic counselor is an individual whose aim is to estimate the risk of appearance or recurrence of a genetic disease in a family. This approach is clinical in the first place, but should rest however, on complementary laboratory investigations which are usually complex.

— The investigation should include all information concerning the history of pregnancy; absorption of drugs, the existence of infectious elements, eruptions, exposure to X-ray and metrorrhagia. The circumstances of labour should be specified, as should the state of the newly born and its neuro-motor and staturo-ponderal development.

— The genealogic information should be recorded. This should concern first of all the fraternal history of an affected child and particularly a search for a past history of abortion or still-birth. Concerning the father, the investigation should include his age at the time of birth of the affected child, place of birth, origin, consanguinity with the partner and clinical examination if indicated. A list of the brothers and sisters of the father and their descendants should be obtained and the grand-parents and their fraternal relations should be included. The same is identically applied to the mother. Sometimes such investigations are inadequate and medical files or further investigations may be needed.

Giving genetic advice to the consulting couple should take into consideration the following points:

— The notion of statistical risk should be made clear and the psychological aspect should be evaluated. This may entail the number of affected children, the degree of the problem, whether or not it is fatal in the long or short term, whether associated or not with mental retardation, and the chances of an effective treatment. This would certainly require assessment of the psychological capabilities of the couple and their intellectual level. The value of prenatal diagnosis is an important element for the couple in view of their decision to consider another pregnancy.

— Moreover, the genetic advice should not be only directive but also informative. The couple should have the freedom to make a decision after having received objective information. It is therefore important to explain the mechanisms leading to the appearance of the disease. This should not lead one partner to feel responsible for the occurence of the anomaly in their child. The existence of familial translocation and finding of evidence of a transmitted characteristic in recessive X linked diseases, are a difficult psychological problem for the one who is carrying the characteristic. Couples or families may split apart as a result.

In practice, the detection and prevention of genetic disorders is approached in different circumstances that we have grouped into four categories. Prompt genetic counseling after the detection of a genetic disorder is in fact an item of a protocol of prevention.

> **Situation 1:** This is concerned with the prevention of chromosomal diseases on the one hand and genic diseases on the other hand, in the absence of the affected infant or the related person.

Chromosomal disorders.

Detection of balanced translocations. — The frequency of balanced translocations in the general population is one in 250 couples. The progress in techniques of chromosomal investigations that have demonstrated the pericentric inversions, is in fact suggestive of a higher frequency of structural anomalies.

At present, genetic counseling seems to be essential, in the face of a past history of two early spontaneous abortions. When investigating the case, the obstetrical history may bring to light some information about the possible etiology of the repeated abortions, and so permits distinguishing abortions due to zygotic causes from abortions due to maternal causes. In abortions due to zygotic disorders, retention of uterine contents is prolonged and the development of the embryo does not correspond to the period of gestation. The ovum is usually clear and the embryo is punctiform and usually macerated. In such a case, when searching for anomalies of chromosome structure, the karyotype of the parents should be performed systematically. Chromosomal anomalies are found in about 6 % of cases. It is usually a reciprocal or Robertsonian translocation (Fig. IX-57 and IX-58), pericentric inversion or chromomomes markers $Gp+$, $Dp+$. The risk for the descendants is variable depending on the type of the detected anomaly. It is estimated as 5 % in the case of translocation $t(21q\ 22q)$. It is also different according to the sex of the parent carrier of the anomaly, for translocation $t(Dq/Gq)$: the risk is 10 % if the mother is responsible and 4 % if the father is the carrier. The risk is 100 % in the case of translocations $t(21q\ 21q)$ and $t(22q\ 22q)$. In the latter case, the genetic counselor can not offer more than suggesting adoption, or artificial insemination if the father is carrying the anomaly. In the other types of translocation, early amniocentesis can be proposed to the couple who would keep trying, knowing that early miscarriage should be kept is mind.

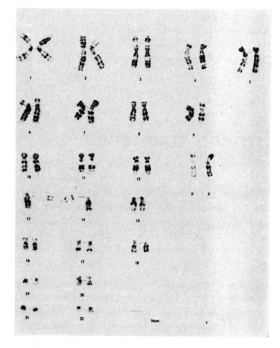

FIG. IX-57. — *Maternal balanced translocation.*
45, XX, t (13q; 14q).

Prenatal prevention of chromosomal aberrations linked to maternal age. — It is acceptable nowadays that prenatal detection of chromosomal aberrations by amniocentesis should be proposed for all pregnant

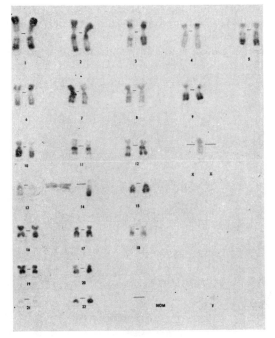

Fig. IX-58. — *Trisomy 13 by translocation.*
Karyotype.

women above the age of 38 years even when there is no particular past history suggestive of a problem (see above).

Genic affections.

Genetic counseling and consanguinity. — Premarital genetic advice must be envisaged in the case of future consanguinous union. Risks are variable according to the degree of parental relationship and are usually considered in view of recessive autosomal transmission. In practice, unions between individuals of a consanguinity coefficient greater than 1/16 are not advised.

Prevention of neural tube disorders by measuring the alpha-1-fœto-protein in the maternal serum during pregnancy. — Detection of neural tube anomalies by amniocentesis has led to a decrease of 10 % in the number of cases of spina bifida and anencephaly. The prenatal diagnosis in such cases was performed only in families where a previous child was affected. Therefore, 90 % of anomalies of the neural tube could not be detected by that approach. Measuring the A. F. P. in the maternal serum during pregnancy has been thus proposed for those at high risk [48].
The technique is principally radio-immunological.

The concentration of A. F. P. varies during pregnancy reaching a maximum between the 30th and 35th weeks of pregnancy. It is preferable to carry out the test between the 16th and the 18th weeks of pregnancy. The percentage of neural tube anomalies varies according to different statistics, from 80 % to 96 % for anencephaly and from 55 % to 80 % for spina bifida [15].

However, increased maternal A. F. P. is not specific for an anomaly of the neural tube. Maternal causes such as hepatitis or tumours and fetal causes such as necrosis and twins may be responsible for an increased level of maternal A. F. P. Moreover, around 3 % of those tested have shown an increase in the level of A. F. P. In this group, the risk that the fetus would present with spina bifida remains, around 1/20. A detection program as such, necessitates informing the public about the importance of genetic consultation between the 16th and the 18th weeks. Detection of these anomalies appears to be justifiable among populations where the risk is above 3 %.

Systematic neonatal detection of phenylketonuria. — This anomaly of mental retardation is transmitted as a recessive autosomic character. Guthrie [23] has proposed the systematic detection of this disease, that has a frequency of 1/10,000. The detection technique is relatively simple, facility of transport, reliability of results, non expensiveness of the test and efficient dietetic therapy, are important modifying factor.

> **Situation 2:** A child of a consulting couple is suspected of a genetic disorder.

The birth of a malformed child. —
Two situations are encountered in practice:

The child is stillborn or died in the neonatal period. — Complete inquiry about the familial past history and the character of pregnancy must be carried out. All particulars about birth, such as date and place and any other relevant information should be obtained. A detailed clinical examination should be performed to include all external malformations including dermatoglyphic variations. The latter may be difficult to study because of immaturity of the crests, particularly in the premature. If diagnosis can not be established clinically, it is important to obtain a blood sample or skin biopsy for karyotyping. It is necessary to take photographs of the infant and also radiographs. All such information must be recorded and filed. If there is occipital meningocele, polycystic kidney must be sought for even in the absence of hexadactyly. Meckel's syndrome of autosomal recessive transmission may lead to modifying the genetic advice. Further to the above investigations, several possibilities may be encountered:

manner. Unfortunately, the information is frequently insufficient, one or more elements are usually missing from the files. The association of retarded intra-uterine growth with signs of malformation may be suggestive of a chromosomal aberration. The exis-tence of previous spontaneous abortions reinforces

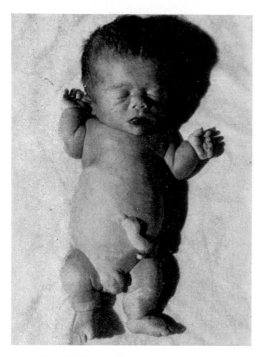

FIG. IX-59. — *Thanatophoric dwarfism.*
Phenotype.

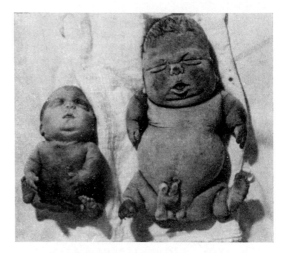

FIG. IX-60. — *Achondrogenesis*
in two cousins.

— The diagnosis is made. Figure IX-59 shows a newborn who died a few minutes after birth. The clinical examination suggested thanatophoric dwarfism and lethal genotypic chondroplasia. The diagnosis was confirmed by X-ray. Genetic coun-seling in this case was reassuring. A dominant autosomal mutation is the likelihood in such a case. Figure IX-60 and IX-61 illustrate the clinical and radiological signs of achondrogenesis which is of autosomal recessive transmission.

— If a diagnosis cannot be made in spite of available complete recorded files, it is difficult to reach a conclusion. Culture of cutaneous fibro-blasts may be conserved in liquid nitrogen as cell lines in view of possible later application of new techniques for cytogenetic study. It seems necessary that the genetic counselor should put forward the risk of recurrence, as certain phenocopies of trisomy 18 appear to be transmitted in an autosomal recessive

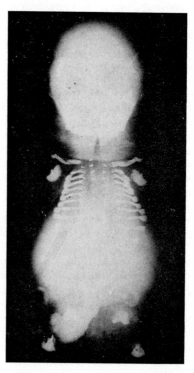

FIG. IX-61. — *Achondrogenesis:*
radiological aspect.

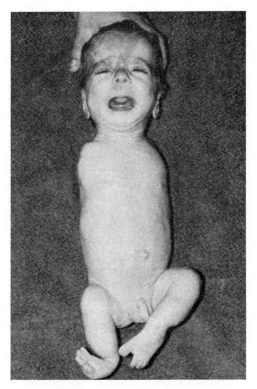

FIG. IX-62. — *Amelia.*

this hypothesis. Studying the karyotype of the parents is essential with a view to searching for translocation or another structural anomaly such as pericentric inversion. With neonatal death of an infant considered to have achondroplasia, the diagnosis must be discussed even in the abence of radiographic documents. For the poorly informed observer, confusion with another genotypic chondrodystrophy is readily possible.

If the infant is alive. — The diagnostic approach should rest on the most complete information. This comprises not only full investigations but also study of the post-natal development of the child, the evolution of the staturo-ponderal curve, the cephalic measurements and the neuro-motor development. The prognosis of a malformation depends largely on the presence of associated intellectual retardation. In spite of the reluctance of the parents, hospitalization of the child may prove necessary from a diagnostic and prognostic point of view.

The diagnosis and the extent of the malformations should be considered only after complete assessment of the child, searching particularly for associated external and internal malformations. When there is mixed deafness in two families, presenting in a

parent and in two children in association with pre-auricular or cervical fistulæ, renal malformations should be sought for. A demonstrated hypoplasia permits the diagnosis of branchio-oto-renal (B.O.R.) dysplasia, of autosomal dominant transmission.

The existence of isolated or associated malformations does not sum up the total of neonatal genetic pathology. For example in metabolic disorders such as aminoacidopathies and glucopathies the clinical picture is entirely different, and may show no structural changes at all.

Situation 3: One partner in a couple is affected by a genetic disorder.

The application of the laws of transmission of monofactorial characteristics permits precise genetic counseling in most cases.

The descendants from a patient affected by hemophilia or by Becker's myopathy will be healthy only at the first generation. The diseased gene is carried by the X chromosome, e. g. fixed perception deafness. The risk for the descendants is essentially linked to the frequency of the gene in the general population. This is calculated by the application of the law of Hardy and Weinberg. If the frequency of patients aa is $\frac{1}{3,600}$, that of the gene a is $\frac{1}{60}$. The frequency of heterozygotes $2pq$ is $\frac{1}{30}$. The risk for a patient of having a diseased child is in the region of $\frac{1}{120}$. The genetic advice is therefore reassuring in the majority of cases.

Precise evaluation of risk is rather more delicate when a dominant autosomal gene has an incomplete penetration. In the case of Von Recklinghausen's disease, the probability of an affected descendant from a diseased subject is perhaps less than 50 %.

In the case of multifactorial heredity, it seems more difficult to benefit from genetic advice, where both genetic and environmental factors are involved. Genetic counseling in this respect is based on statistical results and not on the application of known mechanisms of transmission. This is the case in labiopalatine fissure, congenital dislocation of the hip and some metabolic disorders such as gout and diabetes. When one of the parents has a cleft palate, the risk of having an affected child is estimated according to statistics as 5-7 %.

Situation 4: A relative of the patient, not the parents, seeking genetic advice.

Chromosomal disorders. — It is relatively frequent nowadays that a brother or a sister of a patient with a chromosomal anomaly wishes to know the risk concerning his or her own descendants. The answer is essentially dependent on the existence or the absence of a balanced translocation in the person seeking the advise. This is the case in trisomy 21, furthermore, if such a person has no chromosomal anomalies the risk remains as that in the general population essentially dependent on maternal age.

Genic disorders: Detection of heterozygotes. — One of the very delicate situations encountered in genetic counseling is the case of sisters of a patient suffering from an X-linked recessive disorder like Duchenne and Becker myopathy or hemophilia. The initial risk for one of these sisters having an affected child is 12.5 % in addition to the risk that one in two of them will be transmitter, a probability one in two of having a boy and a probability one in two that the latter will be affected. The problem is however the non reliability of the techniques of detection of heterozygotes. About 75 % of transmitters of Duchenne myopathy can now be detected by measuring the creatine phosphokinase (CPK), electromyography and histological, histochemical and electronic investigations made on biopsy. These measures are valuable when positive. Moreover, the elevation of CPK which is non specific, is diminished in the heterozygotes after the tenth year. It seems preferable therefore to do this in infancy. The same problems are posed with Becker's myopathy whose evolution is much slower and compatible with reproduction.

The detection of transmitters of hemophilia A is possible in about 90 % of cases by measuring the anti-hemophilic factor.

In the case of diseases of autosomal recessive transmission, the genetic advice for the relatives, apart from consanguinous marriage, is generally reassuring. The risk essentially depends on the frequency of heterozygotes for the considered disorder in the general population. The frequency of Tay Sachs disease among Ashkenazi Jews is 1/3,600, the frequency of heterozygotes is 1/30. In the United States, a program of systemic detection of heterozygotes based on measuring the level of hexosaminidase A has been carried out initially with serum in populations of high risk. Genetic counseling and amniocentesis are thus proposed to a couple who are heterozygotes for the disease.

The detection of heterozygote forms of hemoglobinopathies is the essential preventive measure in such hereditary disease. Concerning thalassemia, two million heterozygotes are known to exist in Italy. In this detection priority is given to the relatives of a detected child in a family. Electrophoresis of hemoglobin is employed, the A_2 fraction of hemoglobin is elevated in heterozygotes of thalassemia. The existence of polycythemia associated with hypochromia and normal sideremia may assist in the diagnosis. The detection of a heterozygote must be accompanied by examining the partner. The marriage of two heterozygotes is not advised and contraception should be arranged. Nevertheless, antenatal diagnosis is considered as a last solution if pregnancy is envisaged by the couple.

Teratogenesis

Well protected in the uterus, the human embryo remains vulnerable to teratogenic agents. These could be defined as exogenous processes capable of producing malformations or increasing the frequency of an anomaly in the population.

The embryo is composed of cells that are in a process of evolution. At any particular moment, cells in active proliferation may be observed and also others in differentiation. During the latter stage, there is the possibility that some undifferentiated cells may acquire new characteristics that sketch out the features of a defined organ.

Normal morphogenesis is strictly programmed for cellular proliferation and tissue formation. These processes result in the different tissues and organs of the human being.

Embryonic development is controled by genetic and environmental factors. The latter are largely composed of exogenous factors that cross the placenta. Some malformations may be induced if the environment is altered by the action of a noxious agent.

— During gametogenesis, a noxious agent does not induce malformations at the level of the gonads, but may cause sterility.

TABLE IV. — Calendar showing periods of sensitivity
of principal organs to teratogenic agents

The organ	The critical period in weeks	Period of least sensitivity in weeks
Central nervous system	The end of the 2nd week → beginning of the 6th week	6th week → neo-natal period
Heart	2 1/2 weeks → 5 1/2 weeks	5 1/2 weeks → the end of the 8th week
Arms and legs	3 1/2 weeks → the end of the 7th week	8th week
Eyes	3 1/2 weeks → 7 1/2 weeks	7 1/2 weeks → term
Ear	3 1/2 weeks → 11 1/2 weeks	11 1/2 weeks → beginning of the 20th week
Teeth	The end of the 6th week → the end of the 8th week	The end of the 8th week → the end of the 16th week
Palate	The end of the 6th week → beginning of the 12th week	12th week
External genital organs	6 1/2 weeks → the end of the 12th week	The end of the 12th week → term

TABLE V

Drugs		Malformations
Thalidomide		Amelia, phocomelia (Fig. IX-62)
Anti-epileptics — Trimethadione — Diphenylhydantoin — Paramethadione — Phenobarbital		Facial dysmorphia, cardiac malformations, digital malformations
Antibiotics — Tetracycline		Hypoplasia of the enamel and yellow colouration of teeth
Hormones	*Androgens* — Ethisterone, Norethisterone, Pregnenolone	Masculinization of female fœtus
	Œstrogen — Diethylstilbesterol (DES)	Vaginal adenocarcinoma in young girls
	Antithyroid and iodine drugs — Potassium iodide — Propylthiouracil	Goitre
Cytotoxic drugs (anti-tumor drugs)	*Anti-metabolites* ⟨ Aminopterin	Central nervous system
	Methotrexate	Skeletal problems
	Alkylating agents — Busulfan	Skeletal malformations, palatine fissure and visceral disorders

— During the stage of segmentation, lesions are either severe and fatal or mild and reversible.

— Embryonic periods correspond to periods of maximal teratogenic sensitivity: Every organ has its own period of differentiation. This vulnerable period may begin unassociated with any visible development. This is due to the fact that biochemical differentiation preceeds morphological differentiation (Table IV). A noxious agent may induce several malformations which could develop simultaneously. The same agent can result in different effects depending on the stage of morphogenesis during which it interferes [18, 56].

EXAMPLES OF TERATOGENIC AGENTS IN MAN

Drugs. — Some drugs are known to possess specific teratogenic effect [53]. Representative ones and their effects are summarized in Table V.

Infectious agents. — Rubella is responsible in utero for cataracts, cardiac anomalies, mental retardation and deafness. If the mother is infected during the first month, congenital malformations will be present in 50 % of cases. The frequency does not exceed 20 % if the infection takes place during the second or third month. Toxoplasmosis and diseases in which there are cytoplasmic inclusions may equally perturb embryonic development. These diseases can result in cerebral and ocular disorders (such as microcephaly, hydrocephaly and microphtalmia).

Ionizing radiation. — *I. e.* strong doses of X-ray or exposure of the mother to radio-active material or to atomic radiation. The most vulnerable period is between the 3rd and the 8th week. There is no teratogenic risk for a dose below 10 rads. The risk starts at about 30 rads and is certain at a dose of 100 rads. The nervous system and the eye represent the most sensitive organs.

Other possible factors. — Other factors such as nutritional disturbances or ectopic implantation of the ovum may induce teratogenic effects. Mechanical factors are suggested as are immunological ones, by the presence of anti-tissue antibodies.

In fact not all congenital malformations are due to a unique exogenous factor that has exerted its effect during the sensitive period of embryogenesis. More common is a complex interaction that involves genetic factors. Better knowledge of teratogenic agents is necessary in order to understand the mechanism of embryopathies and their prevention.

REFERENCES

[1] BARR (M. L.), BERTRAM (E. G.). — A morphological distinction between neurones of the male and female and the behaviour of the nucleolar satellite during accelerated nucleoprotein synthesis. *Nature, 163,* 676-677, 1949.

[2] BOUÉ (J.). — Conseil génétique en vue du diagnostic prénatal des anomalies chromosomiques. In: *Diagnostic prénatal,* Ed. A. Boué. Inserm, Paris, 23-38, 1976.

[3] BROCK (D. J. H.), SUTCLIFFE (R. G.). — Alpha-fœto-protein in the antenatal diagnosis of anencephaly and spina-bifida. *Lancet, II,* 197-199, 1972.

[4] CARR (D. H.), BARR (M. L.), PLUNKETT (E. R.). — An XXXX sex chromosome complex in two mentally defective females. *Canad. Med. Ass. J., 84,* 131-137, 1961.

[5] CASPERSSON (T.), ZECH (L.), JOHANSSON (C.), MODEST (E. J.). — Identification of human chromosomes by DNA binding fluorescent agents. *Chromosoma, 30,* 215-227, 1970.

[6] CHICAGO CONFERENCE. — Standardization in human cytogenetics. *Birth defects,* II, 2, 1966.

[7] CONEN (P. E.), ERKMAN (B.). — Frequency and occurrence of chromosomal syndromes. II. E trisomy. *Amer. J. Hum. Genet., 18,* 387-398, 1966.

[8] COUILLIN (P.), NICOLAS (H.), BOUÉ (J.), BOUÉ (A.). — HLA typing of amniotic fluid cells applied to prenatal diagnosis of congenital adrenal hyperplasia. *Lancet, 1,* 1076, 1979.

[9] DENVER CONFERENCE. — On the nomenclature of human mitotic chromosomes. *Ann. Hum. Genet., 24,* 319-325, 1960.

[10] DUTRILLAUX (B.), LEJEUNE (J.). — Sur une nouvelle technique d'analyse du caryotype humain. *C. R. Acad. Sci. (Paris),* 2638-2640, 1971.

[11] DUTRILLAUX (B.), GROUCHY (J.) DE, FINAZ (C.), LEJEUNE (J.). — Mise en évidence de la structure fine des chromosomes humains par digestion enzymatique (pronase en particulier). *C. R. Acad. Sci. (Paris),* 273, 587-588, 1971.

[12] DUTRILLAUX (B.). — Nouveau système de marquage chromosomique : les bandes T. *Chromosoma, 41,* 395-402, 1973.

[13] EDWARDS (J. H.), HARNDEN (D. G.), CAMERON (A. H.), CROSSE (V. M.), WOLFF (O. H.). — A new trisomic syndrome. *Lancet, i,* 787-790, 1960.

[14] EPSTEIN (C. G.), GOLBUS (M. S.). — The prenatal diagnosis of genetic disorders. *Ann. Rev. Med., 29,* 117-128, 1978.

[15] FERGUSON-SMITH (M. A.), RAWLINSON (H. A.), MAY (H. M.) and coll. — Avoidance of anencephalic and spina-bifida births by maternal serum alfa-fetoprotein screening. *Lancet, 1,* 1330-1333, 1978.

[16] FIRSHEIN (S. I.), HOYER (L. W.), LAZARCHICK (J.), FORGET (B. G.), HOBBINS (J. C.), CLYNE (L. P.), PITLICK (F. A.), MUIR (W. A.), MERKATZ (I. R.),

MAHONEY (M. J.). — Prenatal diagnosis of classic hemophilia. *N. Engl. J. Med.*, *300*, 937-941, 1979.

[17] FORD (C. E.), JONES (K. W.), POALNI (P. E.), ALMEIDA (J. C.) DE, BRIGGS (J. H.). — A sex chromosomal anomaly in a case of gonadal dysgenesis (Turner's syndrome). *Lancet, i*, 711-713, 1959.

[18] FRAZER (F. C.), McKUSICK (V. A.). — *Congenital malformations*. Excerpta Medica, New York, 1970.

[19] FREZAL (J.), FEINGOLD (J.), TUCHMANN-DUPLESSIS (H.). — *Génétique, maladies du métabolisme, embryopathies*. Flammarion, Paris, 1971.

[20] GALJAARD (H.). — European experience with prenatal diagnosis of congenital disease: a survey of 6,121 cases. *Cytogenet. Cell., Genet.*, *16*, 453-467, 1976.

[21] GIRAUD (F.), MATTEI (J. F.). — Aspects épidémiologiques de la trisomie 21. *J. Génét. Hum.*, *23*, 1-30, 1975.

[22] GROUCHY (J.) DE, TURLEAU (C.). — *Atlas des maladies chromosomiques*. Expansion Scientfique, Paris, 1977.

[23] GUTHRIE (R.), SUSI (A.). — A simple phenylalanine method for detection of phenylketonuria in large population of newborn infants. *Pediatrics*, *32*, 338, 1963.

[24] HAMERTON (J. L.). — *Human cytogenetics*. Vol. I, General cytogenetics. Vol. II, Clinical cytogenetics. Academic Press, Inc., New York, 1971.

[25] JACOBS (P. A.), BAIKIE (A. G.), COURT BROWN (W. N.), MACGREGOR (T. N.), MACLEAN (N.), HARDNEN (D. G.). — Evidence for the existence of the human superfemale. *Lancet, ii*, 423-425, 1959.

[26] JACOBS (P. A.), STRONG (J. A.). — A case of human intersexuality having a possible XXY sex determining mechanism. *Nature*, *183*, 302-303, 1959.

[27] KANY (W.), DOZY (A. M.). — Antenatal diagnosis of Sickle cell anemia by DNA analysis of amniotic fluid cells. *Lancet*, *2*, 910-912, 1978.

[28] KESAREE (N.), WOOLLEY (P. V.). — A phenotypic female with 49 chromosomes, presumably XXXXX. *J. Pediat.*, *63*, 1099-1103, 1963.

[29] KLINEFELTER (H. F.), REIFENSTEIN (E. C.), ALBRIGHT (F.). — Syndrome characterized by gynecomastia, aspermatogenesis without a leydigism and increased excretion of follicle stimulating hormone. *J. Clin. Endocr.*, *2*, 615-627, 1942.

[30] LARGET-PIET (L.), PENNEAU (M.). — Trisomie partielle pour les bras courts d'un chromosome 9. *Ouest Méd.*, *19*, 1238-1241, 1969.

[31] LARGET-PIET (L.), LARGET-PIET (A.). — Détection des anomalies fœtales par examen du liquide amniotique (expérience de 1 330 diagnostics). *Mises à jour en gynécologie et obstétrique*, Éd. Vigot, Paris, 217-226, 1980.

[32] LEJEUNE (J.), GAUTIER (M.), TURPIN (R.). — Étude des chromosomes somatiques de neuf enfants mongoliens. *C. R. Acad. Sci. (Paris)*, *248*, 1721-1722, 1959.

[33] LEJEUNE (J.), LAFOURCADE (J.), BERGER (R.), VIALATTE (J.), BOESWILLWALD (M.), SERINGE (P.), TURPIN (R.). — Trois cas de délétion partielle du bras court d'un chromosome 5. *C. R. Acad. Sci. (Paris)*, *257*, 3098-3102, 1963.

[34] LEJEUNE (J.), LAFOURCADE (J.), BERGER (R.), RÉTHORÉ (M. O.). — Maladie du cri du chat et sa réciproque. *Ann. Génét.*, *8*, 11-16, 1965.

[35] LONDON CONFERENCE. — On the normal human karyotype. *Cytogenetics*, *2*, 264-268, 1963.

[36] LUCIANI (J. M.). — Les chromosomes méiotiques de l'homme. I. La méiose normale. *Ann. Génét.*, *13*, 101-111, 1970.

[37] LYON (M. F.). — Sex chromatin and gene action in the mammalian X chromosome. *Amer. J. Hum. Genet.*, *14*, 135-148, 1962.

[38] McKUSICK (V. A.). — Mendelian inheritance in Man. *Catalogs of Autosomal Dominant Recessive and X-Linked Phenotypes*. Fifth edition. Johns Hopkins University Press, Baltimore, 1979.

[39] MAROTEAUX (P.). — *Maladies osseuses de l'enfant*. Flammarion, Paris, 1974.

[40] MIKKELSEN (M.). — The effect of maternal age on the incidence of Down's syndrome. *Human Genet.*, *16*, 141-146, 1972.

[41] MILUNSKY (A.). — *Genetic disorders and the fetus*. Plenum Press, New York, 1979.

[42] MURKEN (J. D.). — *Prenatal diagnosis*. Enke, Stuttgart, 1979.

[43] NOONAN (J. A.), EHMKE (D. A.). — Associated non-cardiac malformations in children with congenital heart disease. *J. Pediat.*, *63*, 468, 1963.

[44] PARIS CONFERENCE. — Standardization in human cytogenetics. *Birth Def.*, *8*, 7, 1972.

[45] PATAU (K.), SMITH (D. W.), THERMAN (E.), INHORN (S. L.), WAGNER (H. P.). — Multiple congenital anomaly caused by an extra-autosome. *Lancet, i*, 790-793, 1960.

[46] PEARSON (P. L.), BOBROW (M.), VOSA (C. G.). — Technique for identifying Y chromosomes in human interphase nuclei. *Nature*, *226*, 78-80, 1970.

[47] RAPOLA (J.), AULA (P.), HUTTUNTEN (N. P.), SEPPALA (M.). — Antenatal diagnosis of congenital nephrosis. *Lancet, I*, 89-90, 1975.

[48] REPORT of the U. K. Collaborative Study on Alpha-fetoprotein in relation to neural tube defects. Maternal serum alpha-fetoprotein measurement in antenatal sreening for anencephaly and spinabifida in early pregnancy. *Lancet*, *1*, 1323-1332, 1977.

[49] RETHORE (M. O.), LARGET-PIET (L.), ABONYI (D.), BOESWILLWALD (M.), BERGER (R.), CARPENTIER (S.), CRUVEILLER (J.), DUTRILLAUX (B.), LAFOURCADE (J.), PENNEAU (M.), LEJEUNE (J.). — Sur quatre cas de trisomie pour le bras court du chromosome 9. Individualisation d'une nouvelle entité morbide. *Ann. Génét.*, *13*, 217-232, 1970.

[50] SELLER (M. J.). — Meckel syndrome and the prenatal diagnosis of neural tube defects. *J. Med. Genet.*, 462-465, 1978.

[51] STEELE (M. W.), BREG (W. R. Jr.). — Chromosome analysis of human amniotic fluid cells *Lancet*, *1*, 383-386, 1966.

[52] TIJO (J. H.), LEVAN (A.). — The chromosome number of man. *Hereditas*, *42*, 1-6, 1956.

[53] TUCHMANN-DUPLESSIS (H.), VENCHELY (C.). — *Tératogenèse médicamenteuse*. Ed. Flammarion, Paris, 53-64, 1974.

[54] TURNER (H. H.). — A syndrome of infantilism, congenital webbed neck and cubitus valgus. *Endocrinology*, *23*, 566-574, 1938.

[55] TURPIN (R.), LEJEUNE (J.). — *Les chromosomes humains*. Gauthier-Villars, Paris, 1965.

[56] WARKANY (J.). — *Congenital malformations*. Notes and comments. Year Book Medical Publishers, Inc. Chicago, 1971.

47

Inborn errors of metabolism

Michel VIDAILHET and Alain MORALI

Introduction

The number of currently known hereditary metabolic disorders is considerable surpassing 200 in all. However, when considered separately, many of these diseases occur only rarely or even exceptionally. Their number is further multiplied by the occurence of multiple enzymatic variants accounting for the extreme genetic heterogeneity observed. Considering only the disorders for which a precise enzyme deficiency has been proven, Stanbury, Wyngaarden and Fredrickson [333] in 1978, listed 147 different diseases. To this list, one can add disorders resulting from deficiencies in intestinal absorption and renal tubular reabsorption, genetic disorders of non enzymatic proteins (transport proteins and structural proteins), and metabolic disorders for which the precise mechanisms remain uncertain (cystinosis, cystic fibrosis, etc.). In addition, since 1978, new enzyme disorders have been discovered in the area of the hyperphenylalaninemias due to biopterin deficiency [17, 68, 69, 185], organic acidemias [135, 148], and mucolipidoses with the discovery of the sialidoses [103, 146, 209]. We shall not discuss the genetic disorders of specific metabolism such as: endocrine diseases resulting from disorders in hormonogenesis, hematological and

immunological diseases resulting from erythrocyte and leukocyte enzyme disorders, certain connective tissue diseases such as Marfan's syndrome and Ehler Danlos syndrome, or the metabolic myopathies. Diseases of carbohydrate metabolism such as the glycogenoses, congenital galactosemia, fructose intolerance, and enzyme disorders of gluconeogenesis are discussed in the chapter on Glucose metabolism.

One can schematically distinguish three categories of hereditary metabolic disorders according to their causal mechanism:

— Enzyme disorders altering the intermediate metabolisms of amino acids, carbohydrates, or lipids.

— Hereditary transport system disorders altering the intestinal absorption and renal tubular reabsorption of various metabolites.

— Lysosomal disorders of varying complexity. More than 40 lysosomal disorders have been identified, most of them corresponding to a precise enzyme deficiency. One of these, type II mucolipidosis, represents a model of deficiency in posttranslational enzyme modification. Others, such as cystinosis, Salla's disease [5] and type IV mucolipidosis, result from more uncertain mechanisms.

Genetic basis of hereditary metabolic diseases. Expression of genetic abnormalities

All these diseases are transmitted according to mendelian principles, most often as autosomal recessive traits, frequently as X-linked recessive or dominant traits, and only rarely as autosomal dominant traits. The first description of an hereditary metabolic disease is attributed to Garrod, in 1908. He described alcaptonuria, constituting the model on which he created the concept of inborn errors of metabolism. The concept "one gene-one enzyme-one disease" or even "one gene-one enzyme" is no longer acceptable. An enzyme's activity can be genetically modified in a variety of manners:

— The enzyme can be quantitatively altered when the genetic abnormality inhibits the synthesis of the enzymatic protein. This can result from a mutation in a regulatory gene inhibiting the protein synthesis or from a "nonsense" mutation in a structural gene blocking the synthesis of the polypeptide chain.

— The enzyme is often qualitatively altered by a nucleotide sequence modification in a structural gene, resulting in the synthesis of a protein with abnormal amino acid sequences; this structural alteration can create a decrease in the enzyme's activity of varying severity depending on the amino acids implicated and the location of the abnormality in relation to the molecule's active site.

The multiplicity of possible alterations has been extensively studied in the globin chains of hemoglobin and in certain erythrocyte enzymes which are easily amenable to detailed analysis such as glucose-6-phosphate-dehydrogenase (G6PD) and hypoxanthine-guanine-phosphoribosyl-transferase (HGPRT). Over a hundred different variants have been discovered for G6PD. This concept of distinct alterations and enzymatic variants is most crucial. It accounts for the fact that one enzyme disorder can express itself with varying degrees of severity. This is the case in numerous amino acid disorders [186, 308, 350], organic acidemias, and lysosomal disorders in which "infantile", "juvenile" and even "adult" forms have been distinguished. In a given individual, a combination of 2 alleles coding for different enzymatic variants results in

so called "heterozygote compounds". This further increases the possibility for heterogeneity. As we have seen, the "one gene-one enzyme" concept is refutable since several genes, regulatory and structural, intervene in the synthesis of one protein. It is also refuted by the existence of enzymes comprised of distinct polypeptide subunits, each under the dependence of a different structural gene. Conversely, distinct enzymes can contain one or more identical subunits. Hence, a mutation involving the structural gene for this subunit would simultaneously affect different enzymes. Such is the case in Sandhoff's disease (type 2 GM_2 gangliosidosis) in which two hexosaminidases, "A" and "B" are inactive. Both these hexosaminidases contain a β chain. "A" hexosaminidase contains α and β chains, while "B" hexosaminidase contains only β chains. In Sandhoff's disease, a modification in the β subunit causes an alteration in both hexosaminidases. In contrast, in Tay-Sachs disease (type "B" GM_2 gangliosidosis), only the "A" hexosaminidase is inactive since the alteration concerns only the α chain [332]. The existence of regulatory genes and the discovery of enzymes composed of subunits coded by different genes has led to replacement of the "one gene-one enzyme" concept by the "one cistron-one polypeptide" concept. However even this newer formulation, better adapted to modern genetics, has become inexact. Other alterations can occur after transcription and translation: After ribosomal elaboration, the enzymatic protein can undergo post-translational modifications indispensable for it's activity and intracellular transport. For example, before being able to penetrate lysosomes, several lysosomal enzymes, such as hexosaminidase, α-glucosidase, and cathepsin D, must undergo shortening of their polypeptide chains and phosphorylation of their oligosaccharide fractions yielding mannose-6-phosphate, an indispensible marker for pinocytosis and cellular recapturing of these enzymes. An abnormality during this post-translational phase appears to be implicated in type 2 mucolipidosis or "I cell disease" [162, 163]. An equally important concept is that of vitamin dependency. Many enzymatic reactions require coenzymes derived from vitamins B_1, B_6, B_{12}, folic acid, and others. It has been known for some time that lack of these vitamins and their corresponding cofactors can result in serious metabolic disorders. In addition to these dietary deficiencies, there exist a number of enzymatic disorders that are partially or totally corrected by continuous administration of large doses of these vitamins [2, 83, 187, 291, 293, 296, 346]. The physiopathology of the "vitamin dependent" disorders is not always identical. Cofactor deficiency can result from altered intestinal absorption of the vitamin, altered transport due to carrier protein deficiency, alterations in an enzyme necessary for coenzyme activation, or abnormalities in the binding of an apoenzyme to a coenzyme [232, 291]. Related, yet distinct from these cofactor disorders, are disorders involving a number of non enzymatic protein factors that activate the catabolism of certain sphingolipids, such as gangliosides, by their corresponding lysosomal enzymes. These activators, called cohydrolases, seem essential for the interaction between the hydrosoluble enzyme and its glycolipid substrate. Cohydrolase deficiency is responsible for the "AB" variant of GM_2 gangliosidosis [61] and possibly for Niemann-Pick disease type C [53].

Prenatal diagnosis

The history of prenatal diagnosis of hereditary metabolic diseases parallels that of prenatal diagnosis of chromosomal aberrations. The finding that fœtal cells were easily accessible in amniotic fluid for culturing and karyotyping soon led to the study of their other characteristics and enzymatic machinery. Amniotic fluid samples initially contain a composite of different cell types (amniotic epithelial cells, epitheliomorphic cells, and fibroblastic type cells). During culturing, the fibroblastic type cells divide more actively, quickly becoming the predominant and subsequently unique cell population. Concomitant studies demonstrated that enzymatic activities present in cultured cutaneous fibroblasts were also present in cultured amniotic cells. This finding made possible the prenatal diagnosis of those hereditary diseases for which biochemical proof could be obtained from fibroblast cultures. Currently, it is possible to diagnose prenatally a substantial number of disease (Table I). This does not mean that prenatal diagnostic measures are often indicated. Most hereditary metabolic diseases occur rarely, some extremely so. At the present time, two of the most frequent disorders, cystic fibrosis and phenylketonuria, are not amenable to prenatal diagnosis. However, recent evidence suggests that these 2 diseases may become so in the near future [387, 392, 390]. Initial studies in prenatal diagnosis date back to more than 12 years ago [231]. Even so, prenatal diagnosis of hereditary metabolic diseases remains in many respects a delicate undertaking demanding a thorough understanding of its technical, biochemical, ethical and psychological difficulties. A detailed understanding of the suspected metabolic disorder, discussion with the parents as completely and honestly as possible, and a rigorous realisation of the various diagnostic stages, are indispensable for maximizing the chances of success. There is no room for improvisation. Prenatal diagnostic procedures should be carefully planned beforehand. Amniocentesis should not be done too early. Before 15 weeks of gestation, the insufficient quantity of amniotic fluid (less than 200 ml) [29, 231] and insufficient content of viable amniotic cells, lower the chances of success and render fœtal and maternal risks excessive. If performed after 17 weeks of gestation, the additional 3 weeks necessary for biochemical analysis would place the results at a time when termination of the pregnancy may be too late. Hence, the best time for amniocentesis is during the 16th or 17th week of gestation. Techniques utilized for amniocentesis and cell culture are the same as those employed for cytogenetic studies. Ultrasonic visualisation is necessary for localising the placenta, eliminating the possibility of twins, and identifying the best site for sampling. Amniocentesis is done under local anesthesia and strictly aseptic conditions, using needles such as those used for spinal taps. Twenty milliliters of fluid are removed. To be sure of it's amniotic origin, several drops are deposited on reactive strips (albumin, glucose, pH). One ml should be reserved for systematic $\alpha 1$-fœto-protein analysis (screening for anencephaly and myelomeningocele) [231]. The remaining 19 ml are used for culturing. The culture time necessary for obtaining a sufficient quantity

TABLE I. — HEREDITARY METABOLIC DISEASES WITH AVAILABLE ANTENATAL DIAGNOSIS

Disease	Enzymatic or other assays	Disease	Enzymatic or other assays

Lipidoses

Disease	Enzymatic or other assays	Disease	Enzymatic or other assays
Familial hypercholesterolemia	Lipoprotein cell surface receptors	Krabbe's leukodystrophy [20]	Galactocerebroside galactosidase
Fabry's disease [78]	α-Galactosidase	Metachromatic leukodystrophy [191]	Arylsulfatase A (C. A. C.), metabolism of ^{35}S sulfatide
Farber's disease [233]	Ceramidase	Mucosulfatidose [6]	Arylsulfatases A, B and C
Gaucher's disease [231]	β-Glucosidase	Niemann - Pick disease [32, 161] (types A, B and C)	Sphingomyelinase
G.M.1. gangliosidosis [180]	β-Galactosidase	Refsum's disease [88]	Phytanic hydroxylase
G.M.2. gangliosidosis [248]		Tangier's disease [164]	
Tay-Sachs type	Hexosaminidase A		
Sandhoff type	Hexosaminidases A and B		
Wolman's and cholesterol ester storage diseases [55, 256]	Acid esterase	Hyperglycerolemia [151]	Glycerol-kinase

Mucopolysaccharidoses [231]

Disease	Enzymatic or other assays	Disease	Enzymatic or other assays
Hurler's disease (M. P. S. I. H.)	α-L-Iduronidase ^{35}S sulfate incorporation	San Filippo's disease, type C (M. P. S. III C)	α-Glucosamine-N-acetyl transferase ^{35}S sulfate incorporation
Scheie's disease (M. P. S. I S)	α-L-Iduronidase ^{35}S sulfate incorporation	San Filippo's disease, type D (M. S. P. III D)	N-Acetyl-glucosamine 6-sulfate sulfatase ^{35}S sulfate incorporation
Hunter's disease (M. P. S. II)	Sulfo-iduronate sulfatase ^{35}S sulfate incorporation	Morquio disease, type A (M. S. P. IV A)	Galactosamine 6-sulfate sulfatase
San Filippo's disease, type A (M. P. S. III A)	Heparan sulfate sulfatase ^{35}S sulfate incorporation	Morquio disease, type B (M. P. S. IV B)	β-Galactosidase
San Filippo's disease, type B (M. P. S. III B)	N-acetyl-α-D-glucosaminidase ^{35}S sulfate incorporation	Maroteaux-Lamy disease (M.P.S. VI)	Arylsulfatase B ^{35}S sulfate incorporation
Mucopolysaccharidosis, type VII (M. P. S. VII)	β-Glucuronidase ^{35}S sulfate incorporation		

Mucolipidoses, Oligosaccharidoses

Disease	Enzymatic or other assays	Disease	Enzymatic or other assays
Fucosidosis [355]	α-L-Fucosidase	Mucolipidosis, type III [190]	Lowered cellular acid hydrolases Elevated A. F. hydrolases
Mannosidosis [214]	α-D-Mannosidase	Mucolipidosis, type IV [7, 192]	^{35}S sulfate incorporation, ultrastructural study of A. C.
Mucolipidosis, type I [41]	Neuraminidase	Aspartyl - glucosaminuria [268]	Aspartyl-glycosamine-amido-hydrolase
Mucolipidosis, type II (I cell disease) [4, 174]	Lowered cellular acid hydrolases Elevated A. F. hydrolases		

A. C.: Amniotic fluid cells; A. F.: Amniotic fluid; M. U.: Maternal urine.

TABLE I (continued)

Disease	Enzymatic or other assays	Disease	Enzymatic or other assays
Carbohydrate disorders			
Galactosemia [1, 231]	Galactose-1-PO$_4$-uridyl transferase	Galactokinase deficiency [1, 231]	Galactokinase
Glycogenosis, type II [62, 231]	Acid maltase	Glycogenosis, type III [62, 231]	Amylo 1-6-glucosidase
Glycogenosis, type IV [172]	Branching enzyme		
Amino-acid disorders			
Argininosuccinic aciduria [105]	Arginino-succinase ^{14}C citrulline metabolism	Maple syrup urine disease [231]	Branched ketoacid decarboxylases
Citrullinemia [105]	Arginino-succinate synthetase ^{14}C citrulline metabolism	Hyperlysinemia [231]	Lysine-ketoglutarate reductase
Argininemia [213]	Erythrocytic arginase (F. E.)	Ornithinemia (retinal gyrate atrophy) [323]	Ornithine-transaminase
Cystinosis [305 b]	[35]S cystine incorporation	Phenylalaninemia due to dihydropteridine reductase deficiency [185]	Dihydropteridine-reductase
Classical homocystinuria [109]	Cystathionine-synthetase	Tyrosinosis, type II [106]	Tyrosine amino-transferase
Methylene tetra-hydrofolate reductase deficiency [160]	Methylene TF$_4$ reductase	Sulfite-oxidase deficiency [317]	Sulfite oxidase
Histidinemia [120, 177]	Histidase	Hypervalinemia [231]	Valine transaminase
Organic acidemias			
Isovaleric acidemia [25]	Isovaleryl-CoA-dehydrogenase	Glutaric acidemia, type I [138]	Glutaryl-CoA-dehydrogenase Glutaric acid (A. F.)
β-Methyl-crotonyl-glycinuria	β-Methyl-crotonyl-CoA-carboxylase	Glutaric acidemia, type II, [137]	Acyl-CoA-dehydrogenases
Methyl malonic acidemia [2, 239]	Methyl-malonyl-CoA-mutase, or racemase or adenosyl B 12 ^{14}C propionate incorporation Methyl malonic acid (A. F. and U. M.)	Multiple carboxylase deficiency [296]	Propionyl, β-methyl crotonyl acetyl-CoA and pyruvate, carboxylases
Propionic acidemia [132]	Propionyl-CoA-carboxylase ^{14}C propionate incorporation Methyl citric acid (A. F.)	Methyl acetoacetic aciduria [74]	β-Ketothiolase [14]C Isoleucine oxidation
Glyceric acidemia (type I) [36]	Glycerate dehydrogenase	Hydroxy-methyl-glutaric-aciduria [93]	3-Hydroxy-3-methyl-glutaryl-CoA-lyase 3-Hydroxy-3-methyl-glutaric acid (A. F. and M. U.).

A. C.: Amniotic fluid cells; A. F.: Amniotic fluid; M. U.: Maternal urine.

TABLE I (continued)

Disease	Enzymatic or other assays	Disease	Enzymatic or other assays
		Organic acidemias	
Lactic acidosis with pyruvate carboxylase deficiency [221]	Pyruvate carboxylase	Pyroglutamic aciduria [225]	Glutathione synthetase (C.A.C.)
Lactic acidosis with pyruvate dehydrogenase deficiency [287]	Pyruvate dehydrogenase E_1, E_2, E_3		
		Miscellaneous disorders	
Lesch-Nyhan disease [189]	Hypoxanthine-guanine-phosphoribosyl transferase (H. G. P. R. T.)	Congenital erythropoietic porphyria [80]	Cosynthetase Uroporphyrin I (A. F.)
Adenosine deaminase deficiency [122]	Adenosine deaminase	Hypophosphatasia [237]	Alkaline phosphatase Fetal echography
Acid phosphatase deficiency [231]	Acid phosphatase	Congenital adrenal hyperplasia (21-hydroxylase deficiency) [266]	H. L. A. group
Menkes disease [171]	^{64}Cu incorporation	C_4 deficiency [267]	H. L. A. group

A. C.: Amniotic fluid cells; A. F.: Amniotic fluid; M. U.: Maternal urine.

of cells for enzyme analysis is at least 3 or 4 weeks. Several complications are possible; unsuccessful tapping requiring further attempts, fluid contamination by maternal blood, infection of the yolk sac, needle damage to the fetus, or abortion. The procedure should be performed by a trained obstetrician [29]. Failure of the culture to grow is rare but possible as it occurs in 0.5 to 3 % of cases [231]. The occurence of maternal cells contaminating the sample can lead to diagnostic errors.

Most of the technical difficulties are related to enzyme analysis. Although the activities of certain enzymes are easily mesurable, others, such as branched keto-acid decarboxylases, methylmalonyl coenzyme A mutase, pyruvate carboxylase, pyruvate dehydrogenase and several lysosomal enzymes, etc., can only be analysed by highly specialised laboratories. The extreme genetic heterogeneity and multitude of possible abnormal alleles account for the variety of phenotypes observed. Correct diagnosis requires a thorough understanding of the enzymatic system involved and enzymatic activites encountered in normal subjects, patients and heterozygotes. The

diagnosis cannot be approximate. Different enzyme deficiencies can yield the same set of apparently individualised clinical, biological and pathological findings. An example of this is San Filippo's disease (type III mucopolysaccharidosis), for which there exist four distinct forms (A, B, C, D) resulting from alterations in four distinct enzymes (Table I). Conversely, an alteration in the same enzyme can give clinical presentations of extremely variable severity according to the impact of the qualitative or quantitative abnormality on the enzyme's activity. As we have seen, this applies to a number of metabolic disorders including phenylketonuria, M. S. U. D., urea cycle enzyme disorders, organic acidemias, sphingolipidoses, mucopolysaccharidoses, etc. The severity of enzymatic deficiency evaluated "in vitro" frequently does not reflect these clinical differences. For example, in Scheie's disease (M. P. S. type I S), α-L-iduronidase deficiency appears to be as profound in vitro as in Hurler's disease (M. P. S. type I H) even though it's clinical presentation is much less severe. Prenatal diagnosis has been most successful when the suspected disorder is one for which precise studies have previously been done and enzyme activity has been analysed in normal fibroblasts and amniotic cells, and if possible, in fibroblasts of both the propositus and obligatory heterozygotes.

To illustrate the importance of parental studies, it is known that certain heterozygotes for diseases including metachromatic leukodystrophy [191], Tay-Sachs disease [240], and Sandhoff's disease [86], present with very low enzyme activities similar to those of homozygous patients when using standard substrates. In spite of this enzyme deficiency, apparently identical to that in homozygous patients, these heterozygous subjects have no symptoms. In such cases, only studies of amniotic cell uptake and their hydrolysis of labeled natural substrate allow differentiation of the affected fetus from heterozygotes [191]. The problems associated with cell culture and enzyme analysis have stimulated the search for other diagnostic methods. Attempts at directly evaluating enzyme activity in non cultured amniotic fluid cells have been disappointing; the cellular pleiomorphism and the large percentage of dead cells explain the low percentage of results. For most enzyme determinations, the direct use of amniotic fluid is inaccurate. Enzyme activities so measured do not accurately reflect those in fetal serum because of the presence of other tissues (maternal tissues, placenta, membranes, fœtal urine, etc.). Certain laboratory determinations, on the other hand, may be of considerable help. In addition to α1-fœto-protein and acetylcholinesterase, for which the diagnostic importance in neural tube abnormalities is well known, one can include the analysis of certain organic acids including methylmalonic, methylcitric, glutaric, and 3-hydroxy-3-methylglutaric acids. These acids are found in elevated concentrations in the amniotic fluid of fœtuses suffering from the corresponding organic acidemias (methylmalonic, propionic, glutaric and 3-hydroxy-3-methylglutaric acidemias). Another promising method is the ultrastructural study of amniotic cells. These studies can reveal characteristic inclusions in a number of lysosomal diseases such as Pompe's disease[231], Wolman's disease [367], or type IV mucolipidosis [192]. More often, however, all these methods are too uncertain to allow dispensing with enzyme analysis. More recently, four different techniques have been added to the growing list of prenatal diagnostic tests [89, 315]. The first technique requires sampling of fœtal blood by fœtoscopy [213] effected at 18 to 20 weeks of gestation. An endoamnioscope of reduced caliber (1.7 to 2 mm) equipped with a needle, allows puncture of a fœtal vein in the chorionic plate and aspiration of one

or two milliliters of fœtal blood. After purification of the placental blood from maternal blood contaminants (Orskov-Jacobs-Stewart technique), various studies can be carried out. In diagnosing hemoglobin disorders such as thalassemia, hemoglobin synthesis is studied using a radioactive precursor. A simpler technique consists of separating the hemoglobins by isoelectric focusing [89]. Analysis of fetal blood also permits the antenatal diagnosis of hemophilia and familial septic granulomatosis. In the future it should allow for the diagnosis of argininemia (by erythrocyte arginase determination) and various congenital immune disorders [213]. In practice, this technique of fetal blood sampling is extremely delicate and is much more hazardous than amniocentesis. The second technique stems from the exciting new advances in molecular genetics in the field of genetic "engineering". It consists of isolating the DNA of amniotic cells and it's molecular hybridisation with radioactive mRNA (or with a copy of DNA, c-DNA, reconstructed from the mRNA using reverse transcriptase). This technique pinpoints quantitative or qualitative abnormalities in DNA sequences constituting the structural genes of globin chain synthesis. These methods, introduced by Kan [181 b] and Orkin [251], have already been extended to the antenatal diagnosis of X linked (Duchenne muscular dystrophy, O. T. C. deficiency) or autosomic disorders (phenylketonuria) [390, 392, 393]. Another technique takes advantage of the close genetic linking possible between the genes responsible for the suspected disease and the genes responsible for identifiable tracers on amniotic cells. In the case of congenital adrenal hyperplasia due to 21-hydroxylase deficiency, studies have shown that, in a given sibship, every time two or more of the siblings were affected, their HLA group was identical. This finding has allowed for prenatal diagnosis in such cases [266]. In the same manner, fraction C4 complement deficiency can also be diagnosed prenatally [267]. Lastly fetal tissue sampling by chorion biopsy around 10 weeks of gestation led to an important improvement permitting antenatal diagnosis much more early in gestation. Direct enzymatic assays or D. N. A. analysis already permit early prenatal diagnosis of a growing number of metabolic diseases. The advantages of early sampling and diagnosis are numerous to physicians and patients. However sampling failure and spontaneous abortion rates are respectively around 4 and 6 % [394, 395, 396]. At present, the prenatal diagnosis of hereditary metabolic disorders is of little therapeutic interest, except for particular diseases (vitamin dependent forms of certain organic acidemias such as methylmalonic acidemia). Confirmation of a diagnosis can only result in an interruption of pregnancy. This solution is seldom questioned when dealing with seriously debilitating diseases, leading to severe mental deterioration and death within several months or years regardless of therapeutic efforts. In contrast, other metabolic diseases result in only minor handicaps and are amenable to therapy providing that they are treated early and followed closely. For certain metabolic disorders such as histidinemia, it has not been proven that the disorder is directly responsible for the clinical abnormalities (Table I). Indications for prenatal diagnosis should be decided according to the nature of the disease, the effectiveness of possible therapeutic

measures, and the physical, psychological and emotional consequences of the disease and it's treatment for the child and his or her family. Parents who look forward to pregnancy often are very anxious during this period and can benefit from psychological counseling. If the prenatal diagnosis is positive, abortion can be very traumatic for the mother. Even though interruption of the pregnancy might have been initially accepted, it sometimes happens that the parents refuse this otherwise logical alternative when abortion is indeed proposed. It is obvious that their decision should be respected. Although these situations occur rarely, they emphasize the importance of repeated, tactful, and honest discussion with the parents.

Neonatal screening

We shall not discuss the screening procedures for "high risk" newborns whose family history indicates the possibility of a metabolic disorder. This chapter discusses the routine neonatal screening of certain metabolic disorders. The importance of routine screening became apparent after Bickel's demonstration of the effectiveness of phenylalanine restricted diets in phenylketonuria [21]. Initial methods based on verifying excess phenylpyruvic acid in the urine were shown to be inaccurate. It was only after methods detecting hyperphenylalaninemia were perfected that phenylketonuria screening became generalised [363]. The method described by Guthrie permitted systematic screening of this disease in industrialised nations as early as the 1960's. Since then other techniques such as chromatography and automatic fluorimetric analysis have been proposed. The screening test is effected as follows: 3 to 7 days after initiation of milk feeding, several drops of the newborn's blood are obtained by micropuncture and deposited on a special filter paper labeled with the appropriate identification (infant's name; physician, and hospital). The sample is sent by mail to a screening center where phenylalanine analysis is carried out by one of the above mentioned methods. If the test is positive, complementary determinations (phenylalanine, tyrosine, ortho-hydroxyphenylacetic and phenylpyruvic acids, urinary biopterins) are necessary to confirm the diagnosis and specify the type of hyperphenylalaninemia. This confirmational stage is critical for several

reasons. Moderate transient hyperphenylalaninemias and immaturity tyrosinemias are frequent and require no treatment. Conversely, moderate increases in phenylalanine should not be falsely reassuring since the eventuality of a biopterin deficiency, though rare, must be eliminated because of the particular treatment it imposes. Besides routine screening for phenylketonuria, screening for other metabolic diseases has been proposed. These include the various amino acids disorders (histidinemia, homocystinuria, M. S. U. D.) and galactosemia. As in phenylalaninemia, increases in the other aminoacids can also be detected by paper chromatography techniques. Guthrie adapted his bacteriological test to other metabolites including leucine, methionine, histidine, lysine, tyrosine and galactose, by using different inhibiters and bacterial strains. Table II indicates the major diseases and several corresponding tests. Because of cost considerations, the indications for systematic neonatal screening of disorders other than phenylketonuria should be carefully examined. A given screening test is readily justifiable when it can be done on the same blood sample used for phenylketonuria testing and when it's corresponding disorder is relatively frequent and effectively treatable. This is true for the systematic screening of congenital hypothyroidism by TSH analysis: The disease incidence is appropriate (approximately 1/3,500 births), the screening test is sensitive and specific, and early initiation of treatment limits the severity of the resulting mental disorders.

TABLE II. — Hereditary metabolic diseases
for which systematic neonatal screening has been recommended

Disease	Screening methods		Screening time	Treatment
Phenylketonuria	Guthrie (PhA) Chromatography Fluorimetry	Blood	4 to 7 days	Phenylalanine restricted diet *
Maple syrup urine disease	Guthrie (Leu) Chromatography	Blood	2 to 4 days	Branched aminoacid restricted diet *
Homocystinuria	Guthrie (Meth) Brand Chromatography	Blood Urines	4 to 7 days	Methionine restricted diet *
Histidinemia	Guthrie (Hist) Chromatography	Blood	4 to 7 days	Histidine restricted diet
Galactosemia	Beutler Guthrie (Gal) Paigen	Blood	Birth or 4 to 7 days	Galactose
Cystic fibrosis	B. M. Test (Meconium)		First meconium	Treatment of respiratory and digestive complications
	Immunoreactive Trypsin	Blood	4 to 7 days	
Hypothyroidism **	T. S. H.	Blood	4 to 7 days	Replacement therapy (L. thyroxine)

* Several types are treated with cofactors or corresponding vitamins.
** Disease which in most cases is not genetic.

During the Heidelberg symposium in 1978 [22], several recommendations were made:

— Four diseases, for which there exist reliable tests applicable on a large scale, should receive priority in screening due to the urgency of their treatment. They include phenylketonuria, congenital hypothyroidism, galactosemia and maple syrup urine disease.

— Three diseases, tyrosinemia, homocystinuria and histidinemia, cannot be considered for priority screening, even though they all have routine screening tests, because they either have important clinical variants that can escape testing (homocystinuria, tyrosinemia) or because their treatment is not proven to be effective (histidinemia).

— The other amino acid diseases, the organic acidurias, the transport disorders, and cystic fibrosis cannot be considered for routine screening. In the case of cystic fibrosis tests should be improved to eliminate the excessive number of false positive and false negative results. Moreover, it has not been shown that early diagnosis and initiation of treat-

ment in this disease significantly improves its long term prognosis.

— Screening of hemoglobin disorders and hemolytic anemias resulting from erythrocyte abnormalities can only be proposed for high risk groups. Hyperlipidemias should only be screened in high risk families.

These recommendations are not definitive and will probably evolve in the future. Even their present formulation can be the subject of discussion, especially when it comes to the systematic screening of congenital galactosemia and M. S. U. D. The screening of these two diseases four days after initiation of milk feeding added to the necessary postal laboratory delays yields test results at a time when the newborn infant is already suffering either from apparent hepatic malfunction, or from neurological symptoms with characteristic abnormal odor. Congenital galactosemia screening can be justified by its moderately high incidence (1/50,000 births) and the relative success of dietary therapy. To be truly effective, screening would necessitate sampling of umbilical cord blood immediately after birth for enzyme analysis (either Beutler's or Paigen's technique). As for M. S. U. D. which occurs in 1/300,000 births, the early appearance and severity of neurological symptoms, and the impossibility of screening before the fourth day after birth, whereas clinical symptoms appear 3 or 4 days later, combine to render screening illusory. Published results confirm this conclusion [242]. Limited by socioeconomic considerations, supplemental increase in work load, and required handling of the newborn, routine laboratory screening of hereditary metabolic diseases can only be proposed in our opinion, under the following conditions:

— The causal relationship between the metabolic disorder and clinical symptoms (most often encephalopathy) should be firmly established.

— The disease to be screened should be amenable to effective treatment.

— The disease's detection should be realizable by methods that are simple, sensitive, fairly specific, economical and applicable on a large scale.

— Parallel with the existence of screening centers, centers capable of confirming the diagnosis and assuring treatment are necessary.

— Lastly, the disease's incidence should be high enough to warrant financial support. Representing a part of the public health and prevention program, neonatal screening should be supported only if it's development does not threaten the financing of more urgent programs.

Guidelines to neonatal diagnosis

Certain neonatal clinical and laboratory findings such as persistent acidosis, hyperammonemia and hypoglycemia with hepatomegaly can alert the physician to the possibility of a metabolic disorder. When symptoms are less specific, the family history and circumstances leading to the disease's onset are of capital importance [301 b].

Family history. — A precise study of the genealogy is necessary. The discovery of consanguinity is an argument in favor of an autosomal recessive disorder. When male cousins or uncles are affected, an X-linked disorder should be suspected. It is important to study the medical history of siblings for the occurence of neonatal deaths or neonatal abnormalities even if the latter were supposedly acquired disorders such as septicemia, anoxia, or subarachnoid hemorrhage. Their childhood history should also be studied for evidence of hypoglycemia, acute encephalopathy, ataxia, metabolic acidosis, hepatomegaly, or acute episodes labelled "intoxication", "acetonemic vomiting", or Reye's syndrome.

Circumstances leading to the disease's onset. — An important negative finding is the absence of fetal or perinatal distress that might explain the observed abnormalities. In general, metabolic disorders are characterised by a latent interval during which the neonate is apparently normal. This latent interval is of variable duration. In Wilson's disease, symptoms appear only in childhood or adolescence. On the other hand, the latent interval can be very short (5 to 6 days in maple syrup urine disease (M.S.U.D.), or even several hours in pyruvate carboxylase deficiency). The symptomatology can take on an intermittent or cyclic character (periodic ketosis).

Orienting clinical findings. — Certain clinical findings are suggestive of a hereditary metabolic disorder. These include neurological manifestations, such as alterations in consciousness (lethargy, alternating hyperexcitability and somnolence), hypertonia, convulsions, abnormal movements of the eyes or extremities, and feeding problems. Other suggestive findings include vomiting, hepatomegaly, jaundice, splenomegaly, abnormal breath or urine odor, and a hemorrhagic syndrome. For example, the association of severe hypotonia, myoclonia, and a pseudo-periodic EEG tracing is very suggestive of glycine encephalopathy. The association of hepatomegaly, jaundice (with conjugated and unconjugated hyperbilirubinemia) and hepatic cytolysis is suggestive of galactosemia or tyrosinosis in it's acute infantile form. Severe bone demineralization is suggestive of type II mucolipidosis or hypophosphatasia. The principal causes of abnormal

TABLE III. — ABNORMAL ODORS
AND THEIR CAUSAL DISORDERS

Abnormal odor (urine, breath, skin, feces)	Disorder
Musty odor	Phenylketonuria
Maple syrup like odor (curry, burnt caramel)	Maple syrup urine disease
Hops odor (dried celery)	Methionine intestinal absorption deficiency (oast-house syndrome)
Boiled cabbage odor	Hypermethioninemias hypertyrosinemias severe hepatic failure
Fishy odor	Trimethylaminuria
Cheese odor (sweaty feet)	Isovaleric acidemia HMG-CoA lyase deficiency, type II glutaric aciduria
Cat's urine odor	Methyl crotonyl glycinuria HMG-CoA lyase deficiency

TABLE IV. — ABNORMAL URINE COLORS
AND THEIR CAUSAL DISORDERS

Abnormal urine color	Disorder
Blackening (after exposure to light, air or after alkalinisation)	Alcaptonuria
Indigo blue	Blue-diaper syndrome (tryptophan malabsorption)
Port wine	Porphyria

urine odor or color are indicated in Tables III and IV.

Orienting laboratory findings. — A number of simple laboratory tests can be diagnostically helpful in newborns thought to have a hereditary metabolic disorder. Glycemia and ketonemia can be measured immediately using reactive strips. Laboratory blood determinations should include glycemia, acid-base equilibrium and ammonemia. Other useful determinations include the blood count, prothrombin

consumption time, fibrinogen, calcemia, azotemia, transaminases, lactic acid, β-OH-butyrate and thin layer chromatography of amino acids. Several simple urinary tests are helpful, including determinations of ketones *(Acetest)*, reducing sugars *(Clinitest)*, glucose *(Clinistix)*, and phenylpyruvic acid *(Phenistix)*. Laboratory analysis of fresh urine should include the 2-4 DNPH test for α-keto-acids, Brand's test for sulfur-amino acids, and thin layer chromatography of urinary amino acids. When a metabolic disorder is suspected, it is important to set aside a small quantity of blood and urine for eventual testing. Several urine samples should be obtained and frozen. Five to ten ml of heparinized blood should be centrifuged and the plasma placed in several tubes and frozen.

Associations of clinical and laboratory findings. — Neurological manifestations can be isolated or associated with acidosis, ketosis, hypoglycemia, hyperammonemia, or alkalosis. Other associations include hypoglycemia with or without ketosis, severe acidosis with or without hematological manifestations, pancytopenia, or hepatic insufficiency. The etiologies corresponding to these situations are indicated in Tables V, VI, VII,

TABLE V. — POSSIBLE CAUSES OF KETOTIC
OR NON-KETOTIC HYPOGLYCEMIA IN NEONATES

Hypoglycemia
Ketotic Abnormalities in gluconeogenesis: — Type I glycogenosis (moderate ketosis) * — Fructose 1-6 diphosphatase deficiency * — Phosphoenolpyruvate carboxykinase deficiency * Glycogen synthetase deficiency * Methylmalonic acidemia Propionic acidemia Pyruvate carboxylase deficiency ** Multiple carboxylase deficiency * Type II glutaric aciduria (and type I during crises) * +
Non-ketotic Type II glutaric aciduria (and type I during crises) * HMG-CoA lyase deficiency * Non-ketotic C6-C10 dicarboxylic aciduria * Systemic carnitine deficiency * Hereditary fructose intolerance * Congenital galactosemia *

* Hepatomegaly; ** Intermittent hypoglycemia; + Slight or intermittent ketosis; HMG-CoA, hydroxymethyl-glutaryl coenzyme A.

TABLE VI. — Possible causes of severe non-ketotic metabolic acidosis with or without neurologic manifestations in neonates.

Severe non-ketotic metabolic acidosis

With neurologic manifestations
Type II glutaric aciduria
HMG-CoA lyase deficiency
Non-ketotic C6-C10 dicarboxylic aciduria (moderate acidosis)
Systemic carnitine deficiency (acidosis during crises)
Congenital hyperlactacidemias

Without neurologic manifestations
Type II D glyceric aciduria
Pyroglutamic aciduria caused by glutathione synthetase deficiency

---

HMG-CoA, hydroxymethyl-glutaryl coenzyme A.

TABLE VII. — Hereditary metabolic disorders that can cause pancytopenia in neonates (predominantly neutropenia).

Pancytopenia

Methylmalonic acidemia
Propionic acidemia
Isovaleric acidemia
Beta-ketothiolase deficiency
Multiple carboxylase deficiency (anemia, thrombocytopenia)
Familial protein intolerance with lysinuria
Type IB Glycogenosis

TABLE VIII. — Hereditary metabolic disorders that can cause neonatal hepatocellular insufficiency.

Hepatocellular insufficiency

Congenital galactosemia
Hereditary fructose intolerance
Tyrosinosis (type I)
Reye's like syndrome (deficits in β-oxidation):
— systemic carnitine deficiency
— hepatic carnitine palmityl transferase deficiency
— type II glutaric aciduria
— non-ketotic dicarboxylic aciduria
— HMG-Coa lyase deficiency

HMG-CoA, hydroxymethyl-glutaryl coenzyme A.

VIII and IX. Depending on the suspected etiology more specialised testing can be undertaken, such as ion exchange or gas chromatography of blood and urinary amino acids, gas chromatography of urinary organic acids coupled to mass spectrometry, and determinations of pyruvicemia, glucosemia, erythrocyte galactose-1-phosphate and urinary oligo- and mucopolysaccharides. Enzyme analysis can be carried out in blood cells, hepatocytes, or cultured skin fibroblasts. Finally, a positive response to treatment can provide an additional diagnostic finding. For example, in congenital galactosemia, the clinical and biological status improves rapidly after galactose removal. Although a given hereditary metabolic disorder can be suspected in the circum-

stances described above, diagnosis should not be made prematurely. Ancillary tests are sometimes necessary to confirm the diagnosis and avoid errors. For instance, galactosuria can be observed in newborns without it necessarily being caused by galactosemia or galactokinase deficiency.

Increases in certain amino acids such as phenylalanine, tyrosine and methionine, can be observed in various hepatic disorders or in immature newborns receiving an excessive protein intake. Severe hyperammonemia is not always caused by a specific enzyme deficiency [10, 129]. Severe neonatal hypoglycemia should first direct attention to the possibility of hyperinsulinism, especially when there is no ketosis. Since we are speaking of genetic disorders, the affirmation or exclusion of a hereditary metabolic disorder is of major importance for the family of the patient. For this reason, it is important that the diagnosis be accurate, even if specific identification can only be made after the patient's death. At the patient's death, a number of samples should be obtained immediately: skin samples (placed in isotonic saline at room temperature) for fibroblast cultures and enzyme analysis; blood and urine samples (placed in a series of tubes and frozen at − 30° C) for eventual biochemical analyses; liver, renal, cerebral or muscle needle biopsy when necessary for ultrastructural studies (immediate fixation) or enzyme analysis (frozen at − 60° C). The occurence of autopsy delay may make ultrastructural studies much less significant and enzyme analysis impossible. Samples taken during autopsy do, on the other hand, allow customary histopathological studies to be performed.

TABLE IX. — Possible hereditary metabolic disorders causing neonatal neurologic distress

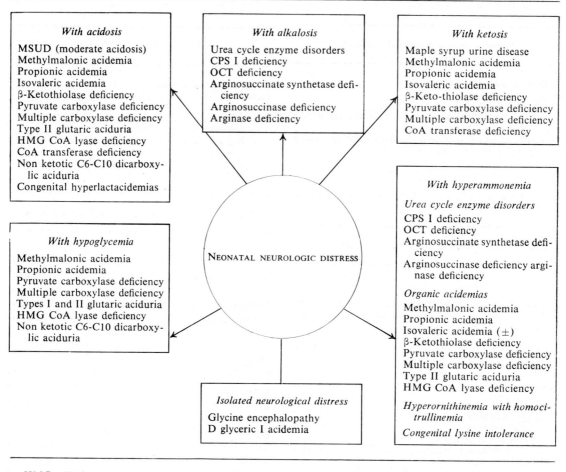

With acidosis

MSUD (moderate acidosis)
Methylmalonic acidemia
Propionic acidemia
Isovaleric acidemia
β-Ketothiolase deficiency
Pyruvate carboxylase deficiency
Multiple carboxylase deficiency
Type II glutaric aciduria
HMG CoA lyase deficiency
CoA transferase deficiency
Non ketotic C6-C10 dicarboxy-
    lic aciduria
Congenital hyperlactacidemias

With alkalosis

Urea cycle enzyme disorders
CPS I deficiency
OCT deficiency
Arginosuccinate synthetase defi-
    ciency
Arginosuccinase deficiency
Arginase deficiency

With ketosis

Maple syrup urine disease
Methylmalonic acidemia
Propionic acidemia
Isovaleric acidemia
β-Keto-thiolase deficiency
Pyruvate carboxylase deficiency
Multiple carboxylase deficiency
CoA transferase deficiency

With hypoglycemia

Methylmalonic acidemia
Propionic acidemia
Pyruvate carboxylase deficiency
Multiple carboxylase deficiency
Types I and II glutaric aciduria
HMG CoA lyase deficiency
Non ketotic C6-C10 dicarboxy-
    lic aciduria

NEONATAL NEUROLOGIC DISTRESS

With hyperammonemia

Urea cycle enzyme disorders
CPS I deficiency
OCT deficiency
Arginosuccinate synthetase defi-
    ciency
Arginosuccinase deficiency argi-
    nase deficiency

Organic acidemias
Methylmalonic acidemia
Propionic acidemia
Isovaleric acidemia (±)
β-Ketothiolase deficiency
Pyruvate carboxylase deficiency
Multiple carboxylase deficiency
Type II glutaric aciduria
HMG CoA lyase deficiency

*Hyperornithinemia with homoci-
    trullinemia*

Congenital lysine intolerance

Isolated neurological distress

Glycine encephalopathy
D glyceric I acidemia

HMG : Hydroxymethylglutaric.
CPS : Carbamyl phosphate synthetase.

OCT   : Ornithine carbamyl transferase.
MSUD : Maple syrup urine disease.

Disorders of amino acid metabolism

In this section we shall discuss only amino acid disorders in the strict sense—that is to say, the disorders involving abnormalities in the amino acids themselves. Certain enzyme disorders affecting amino acid catabolism after the initial steps of transamination and decarboxylation and resulting in accumulation of organic acids will be discussed in the following section on organic acidemias. There are several types of hereditary amino acid disorders. The first type is represented by only one disease; cystinosis. This lysosomal disease results from intralysosomal accumulation of cystine, by a mechanism that is still poorly understood. The second type of amino acid disorder includes the specific deficiencies in one of the intestinal absorption and/or renal tubular reabsorption systems and affects one or more amino acids. Numerous disorders of this type have been identified, the most common being cystinuria-lysinuria. The third type of amino acid disorder, by far the most important due to the large number of diseases belonging to this group, includes the enzyme disorders affecting amino acid metabolism. Although there are approximately only twenty amino acids, the number of these disorders is considerably higher due to the multitude of reactions amino acids can undergo (hydroxylation, oxidation, transamination, methylation, coupling, etc.).

PHENYLKETONURIA

Definition and generalities. — Phenylketonuria (P. K. U.) can no longer be defined as phenylpyruvic oligophrenia, owing to the success of dietary measures in preventing the appearance of mental deficiency in this disease. P. K. U. is a hereditary metabolic disorder transmitted as an autosomal recessive trait, and arises from the permanent inactivity of hepatic phenylalanine hydroxy-

lase. It is characterised by phenylalaninemia exceeding 25 mg/100 ml (1,500 μmol/l), normal tyrosinemia, and urinary excretion of phenylpyruvic and orthohydroxyphenylacetic acids (P. P. A. and O. OH. P. A.) when normal protein dietary conditions exist (3 g/kg/day in the neonatal period). It was Fölling in 1934 who discovered P. K. U.; Jervis in 1947 who demonstrated the deficiency in phenylalanine's hepatic hydroxylation, and Mitoma, Udenfriend and Kaufman who studied the enzyme system responsible for it's hydroxylation (Fig. IX-63). This system involves an enzyme complex comprised of phenylalanine hydroxylase, dihydropteridine reductase, and the cofactors NADH and tetrahydrobiopterin [186]. In true P. K. U., phenylalanine hydroxylase itself is inactive, showing less than 1 % of it's normal activity. Two important advances were made in the treatment of this disorder when Bickel in 1954 demonstrated the efficacy of a low phenylalanine diet, and when Guthrie, in 1961, proposed a simple neonatal screening procedure that was accurate and economical. The implementation of this screening method has permitted the diagnosis of true P. K. U. as well as the diagnosis of the other hyperphenylalaninemias, discussed in the differential diagnosis.

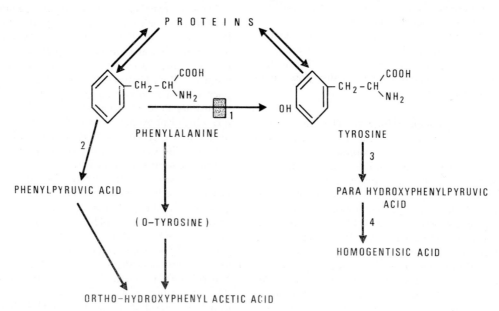

1 . PHENYLALANINE HYDROXYLASE
2 . PHENYLALANINE TRANSAMINASE
3 . TYROSINE AMINOTRANSFERASE
4 . PARA–HYDROXY PHENYLPYRUVATE OXIDASE

FIG. IX-63. — *Simplified scheme of phenylalanine metabolism.*

Genetics and epidemiology. — This disorder is the most common of the hereditary metabolic encephalopathies. It's real incidence differs with the country and population studied, varying from 1/4,500 births in Northern Ireland to 1/61,800 births in Japan. In France, the incidence is 1/15,000 births and is approximately the same in the U. S. A. [363]. It is transmitted as an autosomal recessive trait and affects male and female newborn alike. The type of genetic mutation responsible for the enzyme's inactivation remains uncertain and is probably variable; in several studies, failure to demonstrate material cross-reacting with "antiphenylalanine hydroxylase" antibodies might suggest a block in the enzyme's polypeptide chain synthesis or absence of an enzymatic protein resulting from a mutation in a regulatory gene. Other studies indicate the presence of a functionally inactive protein resulting from mutations in a structural gene [154, 186]. Different mutations would be responsible for different mutant alleles, explaining the existence of more or less severe enzymatic variants. The existence of heterozygote compounds (that is, subjects having 2 different mutant alleles for phenylalanine hydroxylase) would explain the multiplicity of observed phenotypes. In effect, in addition to classical P. K. U., one can observe "atypical P. K. U." and "persistent moderate hyperphenylalaninemias" in which the deficit in phenylalanine hydroxylase is less severe. Güttler has published a very complete study fo the genetic hypotheses explaining the 3 principal phenotypes in phenylalanine hydroxylase deficiency [154].

Clinical presentation. — The clinical presentation of non treated P. K. U. has been well defined. The infant seems completely normal at birth and during the neonatal period. In some cases, digestive problems and vomiting are noted in the first weeks, leading to a false diagnosis of pyloric stenosis. A delay in psychomotor development and even regression becomes evident after several months; convulsive episodes are noted in 25 % of cases, some of them corresponding to West syndrome with hypsarrythmia. Other findings include a depigmentation of hair and irises, abnormal urine odor described as a "musty odor" and frequent eczematous cutaneous lesions. In 96 % to 98 % of cases, mental deficiency is severe with an IQ below 50. The infants are constantly agitated and show abnormal movements; unceasing movements of their hands and fingers, violent antero-posterior contorsions of the trunk. They are restless, sometimes agressive, and often manifest a total affective indifference that can be qualified as psychotic.

Neurological examination reveals hypertonia, exaggerated tendon reflexes, and trembling of the extremities. When walking is acquired, it remains clumsy, rigid and jerky. Microcephaly is common. When treated early and properly followed, P. K. U. has an excellent prognosis and mental deficiency is avoidable. Long term statistical studies comparing affected children and their non affected siblings none-the-less demonstrate a slightly lower IQ in P. K. U. infants, even when treated early [282]. In the early school years, deficiencies in language [228], fine motricity, and temporo-spatial organisation can handicap the child [278].

Diagnosis. — The diagnosis of P. K. U. is biochemical, consisting of analysis of plasma phenylalanine and tyrosine levels, and analysis of urinary excretion of certain metabolites including phenylpyruvic acid (P. P. A.) and ortho-hydroxy-phenylacetic acid (O. OH. P. A.). On a normal protein diet, a severe deficiency in phenylalanine hydroxylation can be confirmed by phenylalaninemia exceeding 25 mg/100 ml, normal tyrosinemia (lower than 5 mg/100 ml), urinary O. OH. P. A. exceeding 10 mcg/ml and the presence of P. P. A. in the urine (easily identified by the ferric chloride test or "Phenistix" reactive strips). Frequently, immaturity in phenylalanine's transamination reaction can delay the excretion of P. P. A. For this reason, urine tests have been abandoned and preference is given to tests measuring phenylalaninemia, as does Guthrie's Test. Conversely, one can observe hyperphenylalaninemias caused by "immaturity", or true "transitory P. K. U." characterised by phenylalanemia which can exceed 25 mg/100 ml, normal tyrosinemia, and excretion of P. P. A. and O. OH. P. A. All these disorders eventually normalize despite the return to a normal protein diet. The possibility of immaturity and enzymatic "variants" [283] necessitates systematic verification of the diagnosis of true P.K.U. at 3 or 6 months of age. An oral phenylalanine loading test (100 mg/kg/24 h during 5 days) can distinguish between true P. K. U., atypical P. K. U., and transient hyperphenylalaninemia. It is also necessary to systematically eliminate the possibility of hyperphenylalaninemia due to tetrahydrobiopterin deficiency whether it results from a deficiency in dihydrobiopteridine reductase (D. H. P. R.) or in biopterin synthesis. Diagnosis has been facilitated by recent improvements in techniques evaluating the activities of phenylalanine hydroxylase and D. H. P. R. from several milligrams of liver obtained by needle biopsy. Urinary biopterin studies and D. H. P. R. determinations in fibroblasts, leucocytes, or platelets [69] can also be helpful. We shall discuss the other types of hyperphenylalaninemia in a separate section. The diagnosis of heterozygous states remains a delicate problem. Enzyme analysis cannot be routinely proposed since it requires liver biopsy. Thus, the diagnosis of heterozygous states depends on phenylalanine and tyrosine assays after fasting and after loading tests. Even though there are significant differences between obligatory heterozygotes and normal subjects, due to overlapping in the two populations; one can only indicate the probability of heterozygotism without proving it with certainty [81].

Treatment. — The treatment of P. K. U. is based on dietary restriction of phenylalanine. However, since phenylalanine is an essential amino acid, the residual intake must remain sufficient (approximately 250-300 mg/24 hours). Phenylalanine "tolerance" varies according to the infant and the severity of the enzyme deficiency. Plasma phenylalanine levels are customarily maintained slightly higher than normal (2 to 6 mg/100 ml) in order to avoid the risks associated with deficiency. These risks, including anemia, growth retardation, cutaneous lesions, and mental deficiency, can be as detrimental as those caused by excess intake. The level at which the phenylalaninemia should be maintained remains a subject of discussion. This type of restricted diet can be achieved using protein hydrolysates low in phenylalanine (Lofenalac, P. K. U. diät, Albumaid XP) or mixtures of pure amino acids lacking phenylalanine (Aminogran, P. K. aid) (see Table X). These products should

always be given along with natural protein sources (small quantities of milk for example) to assure a minimal intake of phenylalanine. Follow-up of treated P. K. U. infants necessitates periodic clinical and biochemical control: growth and weight gain, psychomotor development and phenylalaninemia levels. The diet should be adapted to age and laboratory findings (introduction of green vegetables, fruits, and special low protein foods; flours, noodles, bread, low protein cookies, etc.). The dietician, psychologist, and biochemist should work along with the pediatrician in treating these children. Except for diet restrictions, the life of these children should be as normal as possible (family life, peer contact, schooling, etc.). The majority of authorities advise discontinuation of dietary restrictions at the age of 6 or 7 years. Here again, uncertainties persist. A growing number of workers, including Bickel, advocate continuation of strict dietary restriction until the age of 12. A problem which will become increasingly important in the years to come is that of P. K. U. mothers. It has conclusively been proven that children of non-treated P. K. U. mothers suffer from intra-uterine growth retardation, microcephaly, mental deficiency, and cardiac malformations. According to Lenke [206], the risks are increased when phenylalaninemia levels exceed 15 mg/100 ml. Restricted diets, initiated before pregnancy and maintaining phenylalaninemia below 8 mg/100 ml, may improve the outlook for the birth of normal infants. Komrower has outlined the practical difficulties of initiating and maintaining such diets in many cases, and has em-

TABLE X. — COMPOSITION OF SEVERAL LOW PHENYLALANINE PRODUCTS

Product name	Phenylalanine mg/100 g	Protein g/100 g	Lipid g/100 g	Carbohydrate g/100 g	Cal kcal/100 g	Vitamins	Minerals
Lofenalac	80	15	18	57	450	+	+
Albumaid XP	0	30	0	55	370	+ Except lipid soluble	+
P. K. U. Diät	0	40	0	48	352	+	+
Aminogran	0	100 *	0	0	400	0	0 **
P. K. Aid	0	100 *	0	0	400	0	0 **

* Mixture of pure amino acids.
** Marketed with a special mineral additive.

phasized the need for prospective studies in this poorly understood area [195].

HYPERPHENYLALANINEMIAS OTHER THAN PHENYLKETONURIA

Routine neonatal screening has revealed the existence of hyperphenylalaninemias other than phenylketonuria. These types of hyperphenylalaninemia should be identified either because they require no

treatment at all or because they require a different therapeutic approach. Several classifications have been proposed [19, 26]. Güttler has [154] published a comprehensive review on this subject. We have adopted the simpler classification proposed by Tourian and Sidbury and illustrated in Table XI [357].

"Atypical" and "moderate" phenylketonurias.

— These terms are used to designate the partial deficiencies of phenylalanine hydroxylase activity characterised by phenylalaninemias lower than 25 mg/100 ml for normal protein diets. This

TABLE XI. — SCHEMATIC TABLE OF DIFFERENT HYPERPHENYLALANINEMIAS

Disease	Clinical presentation	Basic defect	Phenyl-alaninemia (mg/ 100 ml)	Tyro-sinemia (mg/ 100 ml)	Urinary metabolites (P. P. A. and O. OH. P. A.)*	Treatment
Classical phenylketonuria	Severe mental retardation	PhA ** hydroxylase inactivity	⩾ 25	⩽ 5	+ + +	PhA ** restricted diet
Atypical phenylketonuria	Normal or moderate mental retardation	Reduced PhA hydroxylase (1 to 3 %)	15 to 25	⩽ 5	+	PhA ** restricted diet (debatable)
Mild hyperphenylalaninemia	Normal	Reduced PhA hydroxylase (5 to 7 %)	5 to 15	⩽ 5	0	None
Transient hyperphenylalaninemia	Normal	Immaturity or enzymatic variant of PhA hydroxylase	Elevated	⩽ 5	+ or 0	None or temporary PhA restricted diet
Hyperphenylalaninemia due to defective PhA transaminase	Normal	Defective transamination of PhA	4 to 30	⩽ 5	0	None
Dihydropteridine reductase deficiency	Mental retardation + seizures	Dihydropteridine reductase deficiency	⩾ 4	⩽ 5	+ + or 0 $\frac{Biopterins}{BH_4} = \nearrow$	PhA restricted diet + DOPA + 5 OH TRYPT
Defective biopterin synthesis	Mental retardation + seizures	Biopterin synthesis deficiency	⩾ 4	⩽ 5	+ + or 0 $\frac{Neopterin}{Biopterins} = \nearrow$	PhA restricted diet + DOPA + 5 OH TRYPT
Transient tyrosinemia	Prematurity+protein rich diet	P. OH. phenylpyruvate oxidase immaturity	4 to 25 (transient)	5 to 50 (transient)	Tyrosyluria	Normal protein diet + vitamin C
Tyrosinosis	Cirrhosis, rickets, tubulopathy	Fumaryl-aceto-acetase deficiency	4 to 6	⩾ 5	Tyrosyluria	Restricted PhA and TYR diet + glutathione

* PPA: Phenylpyruvic acid; O. OH. P. A.: Orthohydroxyphenylacetic acid.
** PhA: Phenylalanine.

25 mg limit is arbitrary. Some investigators have adopted 20 mg/100 ml as a limit [154], others 30 mg/100 ml. Urinary excretion of P.P.A. and O.OH.P.A. depends not only on phenylalanine plasma levels, but also on phenylalanine transaminase activity, often immature in newborns. Excessive excretion of P. P. A. occurs when phenylalaninemia exceeds 15 mg/100 ml. Within this group, it is common to distinguish two subgroups the "atypical P. K. U". in which phenylalanine levels are from 15 to 25 mg/100 ml, and the "moderate P. K. U." or "moderate hyperphenylalaninemias" for which phenylalaninemia ranges from 5 to 15 mg/100 ml. For some authorities, the limit between these two groups is considered to be 10 mg/100 ml and their distinction depends on their differences in tolerance to phenylalanine intake and loading tests. The importance of distinguishing between these two subgroups arises from practical considerations. The moderate P. K. U. or hyperphenylalaninemias necessitate no treatment and the psychomotor prognosis for these infants is excellent. In atypical P. K. U., the mental prognosis is still under discussion. Because of contradictions in published results, it seems wise for the moment to prescribe dietary restrictions for these infants [154]. During the neonatal period, the biochemical findings can be similar to those in true P. K. U. Therefore, diagnosis should be verified by loading tests at 3 or 6 months of age. These atypical and moderate P. K. U.'s are also transmitted as autosomal recessive traits. The type of deficiency observed is most often identical in a given sibship. Enzyme analysis of liver biopsies demonstrates a residual activity of phenylalanine hydroxylase corresponding to 2 to 7 % of normal values.

Transient hyperphenylalaninemias and phenylketonurias.

— This type of hyperphenylalaninemia is caused by a hydroxylation deficiency that spontaneously corrects itself within several weeks. In reality, in certain cases, the normalization is only apparent since IV phenylalanine loading tests demonstrate the persistence of abnormal kinetics causing an inhibition of the hydroxylation system by elevated concentrations of phenylalanine [283]. In such cases, phenylalaninemia can be considerably elevated during the neonatal period with excretion of P. P. A. The existence of these cases confirms the necessity of verifying the diagnosis of true P. K. U. at 3 months of age to avoid pursuing dietary restrictions unnecessarily [250].

Hyperphenylalaninemias caused by transaminase deficiency.

— This type is very rare. Phenylalaninemia is elevated without excretion of P. P. A. or O. OH. P. A. after protein rich diets. Phenylalanine loading provokes an increase in tyrosinemia. Phenylalanine normalizes under a normal protein diet.

Hyperphenylalaninemias caused by tetrahydrobiopterin (BH₄) deficiency.

— In 1975, Kaufman [185] first reported a case of P. K. U. from D. H. P. R. deficiency in an infant suffering from severe mental deficiency despite dietary restrictions that were initiated early and correctly followed. Since BH_4 acts as a cofactor in other hydroxylation systems (tyrosine hydroxylase and tryptophan hydroxylase) necessary for the synthesis of neurotransmitters (DOPA, norepinephrine, serotonin), it was proposed that DOPA, CarbiDOPA, and 5-OH-tryptophan be added to the phenylalanine restricted diet [68]. Two types of BH_4 deficiencies can be distinguished:

Hyperphenylalaninemias caused by D. H. P. R. deficiency. — The deficiency in D. H. P. R. can be demonstrated in a variety of tissues. In contrast to phenylalanine hydroxylase deficiency, it can also be demonstrated in cultured fibroblasts. This deficiency is transmitted in an autosomal recessive manner. The parents of patients exhibit D. H. P. R. activities that are reduced to 50 % of normal values. Prenatal diagnosis of this disorder is possible by the measurement of D. H. P. R. activity in cultured amniotic cells.

Hyperphenylalaninemias caused by dihydrobiopterin synthesis deficiency. — In 1977, another type of "malignant" hyperphenylalaninemia was described, characterised by tetraplegia, myoclonic crises and death despite early dietary restriction even though phenylalanine hydroxylase and D. H. P. R. activities remain normal. Several case studies since then have shown that a deficiency in dihydrobiopterin synthesis is at fault. This deficiency can result from a number of distinct disorders affecting the synthesis of dihydrobiopterin. As in D. H. P. R. deficiency, the phenylalaninemia can exceed 20 mg/100 ml or be only slightly elevated. Unlike D. H. P. R. deficiency, these biosynthesis abnormalities are not amenable to prenatal diagnosis at the present time.

Diagnosis of hyperphenylalaninemias caused by BH_4 deficiency. — Although hyperphenylalaninemias caused by disorders in biopterin metabolism are relatively rare (1 case for 100 cases of true P. K. U.), their pejorative evolution and successful treatment by DOPA and 5-OH-tryptophan justify their routine screening in cases of neonatal hyperphenylalaninemia due to hydroxylation deficiency. Several methods have been proposed, including [17]:

— Analysis of the urinary metabolites of serotonin (5-hydroxyindol-acetic acid) and the catecholamines (homovanillic and vanillylmandelic acid) after normalization of phenylalaninemia by dietary restriction. Under these conditions, low titers of these metabolites indicate BH_4 deficiency.

— A therapeutic test with BH_4 (2 mg/kg) which causes a fall in phenylalaninemia when its excess is due to a deficiency in BH_4.

— Determinations of phenylalanine hydroxylase, D. H. P. R. activity and BH_4 concentrations in liver biopsies.

— The most promising method, both precise and non aggressive, appears to be the assay of reduced and oxidized biopterins in the urine, combined with a blood D. H. P. R. assay.

Other causes of neonatal hyperphenylalaninemia.

— In addition to the transient neonatal tyrosinemias listed in Table XI, hyperphenylalaninemia can be observed in the following circumstances:

— in newborns of P. K. U. mothers. Phenylalaninemia can remain elevated for 5 to 7 days after birth;

— in infants with renal failure and especially acute hepatic failure: Tyrosine elevation is accompanied by elevations in other amino acids;

— in newborns treated with pyrimethamine [64] or with the association of trimethoprim-sulfamethoxazole [142].

TYROSINEMIA AND TYROSINOSIS

We shall here discuss three disorders: transient neonatal tyrosinemia, tyrosinosis with hepato-renal involvement (type I tyrosinemia) and Richner-Hanhart syndrome (type II tyrosinemia). However it must be kept in mind that any form of severe hepatic failure, whether it be viral, toxic or metabolic (galactosemia, fructose intolerance) in origin, is frequently accompanied by an elevation in tyrosine, phenylalanine and methionine. This elevation is a direct consequence of hepatic failure. We shall not discuss the hereditary disorders of tyrosine metabolism without hypertyrosinemia. These include albinism, alkaptonuria and the enzyme disorders of thyroid hormone synthesis.

Transient neonatal tyrosinemia.

— This disorder was frequently observed in premature babies prior to 1975 due to the use of excessive dietary protein (5 to 6 g/day) from artificial milks with a high protein content. The disorder has become much less frequent with the increasing use of humanized milk and breast feeding. It's incidence has fallen from 1 % in 1972 (3.6 % of infants weighing less than 2,500 g) to 0.2 % in 1978 [157]. This disorder apparently results from an immaturity in para-hydroxyphenylpyruvate oxidase. Associated with elevated serum tyrosine levels is an elevated urinary excretion of tyrosyl derivatives (parahydroxyphenyl-pyruvic, lactic and acetic acids). Treatment with ascorbic acid and reduction of dietary protein normalizes the tyrosinemia and the often associated hyperphenylalaninemia. La Du and Gjessing [198] noted that the immaturity also affects tyrosine amino-transferase. According to most studies, this hypertyrosinemia apparently causes no pathological manifestations and leaves no sequelæ. Even though several investigators have reported lower intellectual performances 7 to 8 years after transient tyrosinemia, it is not certain whether this difference is directly related to the tyrosine excess or to other associated transient metabolic abnormalities [157, 198].

Type I hereditary tyrosinosis.

— Type I tyrosinosis is particularly frequent in the Scandinavian countries (1/100,000 births in Norway, 1/120,000 births in Sweden) and in Quebec in a population of French Canadian Origin living in the Chicoutimi region [198]. Transmitted as a hereditary autosomal recessive disorder, characteristic findings include cirrhosis, tubular nephropathy and vitamin D resistant rickets. Two forms can be distinguished:

— an acute form, dominated by a rapidly progressing cirrhosis that is usually fatal within several months [147];

— a subacute form, evolving less rapidly and characterized by rickets, complex tubulopathy and cirrhosis that may secondarily transform into a hepatoblastoma.

Biochemical hallmarks include moderate tyrosinemia (6-12 mg/100 ml), hypermethioninemia, elevated tyrosyluria (tyrosine and its parahydroxy-phenyl, lactic, pyruvic and acetic derivatives), excessive urinary delta aminolevulinic acid, and an increase in serum alpha-1-fœto-protein. Glycosuria, hyperaminoaciduria, and hyperphosphaturia occur secondary to renal tubular damage. The deficiency in hepatic parahydroxyphenylpyruvate oxidase accounts for the elevated tyrosinemia and tyrosyluria, and the relative therapeutic success of dietary reduction in phenylalanine and tyrosine. However, it does not explain the totality of the clinical findings, in particular the hepatic and renal lesions. Parahydroxyphenylpyruvate oxidase deficiency appears more likely to be the consequence rather than the cause of the primary metabolic deficiency. A more plausible explanation for these findings would be a deficiency in fumaryl-aceto-acetase, as proposed by Fallstrom [101]. The addition of cystine and glutathione supplements to the phenylalanine and tyrosine restricted diet might improve therapeutic results.

Type II tyrosinosis: Richner-Hanhart syndrome.

Type II tyrosinosis: Richner-Hanhart syndrome. — In 1969, Wadman [368] determined that the Richner-Hanhart syndrome was caused by a disorder in tyrosine metabolism. The major symptoms include a bilateral pseudo-herpes keratitis appearing in the first weeks after birth, followed by a painful hyperkeratosis of the hands and feet. Psychomotor deficiency is observed in 50 % of cases. Laboratory findings include hypertyrosinemia, normal or slightly elevated phenylalaninemia [205] and, excessive urinary excretion of tyrosine and parahydroxyphenyl acetic acids. The responsible enzyme deficiency seems to involve cytosolic tyrosine amino-transferase while mitochondrial tyrosine amino-transferase appears to maintain normal activity [130]. Several mechanisms have been proposed to explain the seemingly paradoxical increase in the urinary excretion of parahydroxyphenyl pyruvic, lactic and acetic acids [106, 130, 205]. An important point to note is the remarkable efficacy of phenylalanine and tyrosine restricted diets in avoiding ocular and cutaneous lesions.

MAPLE SYRUP URINE DISEASE (M. S. U. D.)

In 1954, Menkes [229 b] reported this disorder in four newborns of the same sibship all suffering from a rapidly fatal encephalopathy. Their urines gave off a strong maple syrup odor. In 1957, Westall [372 b], linked this disease to a metabolic disorder of the branched amino acids causing elevations in the plasma levels of leucine, isoleucine and valine. In 1959, Menkes, Dancis and MacKenzie simultaneously pinpointed the disorder to an enzyme deficiency in the decarboxylation of the branched alpha-keto-acids. Subsequently, clinical forms that where less severe and also less frequent

than the classical form were identified. They were classified as the subacute, moderate, intermittent, and thiamine-sensitive forms. Other enzyme deficiencies were soon discovered at other levels in branched amino acid catabolism. They included hypervalinemia caused by valine transaminase deficiency (see Fig. IX-64), and especially the various organic acidemias (see Table XVI) enumerated in the section devoted to the organic acidemias.

Clinical and laboratory findings.

The classical acute form. — The incidence of this form is estimated at 1/300,000 births. Cases have been noted in all races. The infant appears normal at birth, with symptoms appearing after an interval of 4 to 10 days (most often the 5th or 6th day after birth). Attention is drawn by refusal to eat, vomiting, difficulties in breast feeding, and crying. Neurological symptoms progress rapidly. Most often there is hypertonia interspaced with occasional paroxysms of opisthotonus following minor stimulation. Less frequently, generalized hypotonia or alternating hyper- and hypotonia can be observed. The state of consciousness degenerates to lethargy, then coma. Convulsive episodes are relatively rare, but abnormal limb movements are frequent, resembling crawl strokes in the upper limbs and pedaling movements in the lower limbs. A clinical finding of major diagnostic value is the perception of a maple syrup odor emitted by the infants skin and urine. In general, death ensues within a matter of weeks, precipitated by respiratory distress, apnea, or food inhalation. This hereditary disease is transmitted in an autosomal recessive manner. From a laboratory standpoint, the plasma and urine branched amino acids are normal at birth, but increase in the first few days after birth. Plasma leucine levels attain extremely high values (30-40 mg/100 ml in comparison to the normal 0.75-2.35 mg/100 ml) while valine and isoleucine levels rarely exceed 15-20 mg/100 ml. One notes the presence of allo-isoleucine, an isomer of isoleucine normally absent in the blood and urine. This increase in branched amino acids can be easily and rapidly confirmed by unidimensional thin layer chromatography. More precise determinations, necessary for therapeutic equilibration, require ion exchange or gas chromatography techniques. Concomitantly, one notes the existence of acidosis, ketosis and occasionally hypoglycemia and abnormal excretion of alpha-ketoacids easily demonstrated by the 2.4. D. N. P. H. test. Thin layer chromatography or more precise gas chromatography of the alpha-ketoacids reveals a plasma and urinary accumulation of the branched

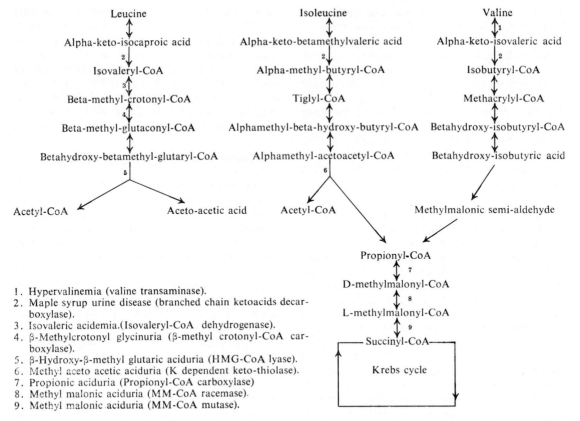

1. Hypervalinemia (valine transaminase).
2. Maple syrup urine disease (branched chain ketoacids decarboxylase).
3. Isovaleric acidemia.(Isovaleryl-CoA dehydrogenase).
4. β-Methylcrotonyl glycinuria (β-methyl crotonyl-CoA carboxylase).
5. β-Hydroxy-β-methyl glutaric aciduria (HMG-CoA lyase).
6. Methyl aceto acetic aciduria (K dependent keto-thiolase).
7. Propionic aciduria (Propionyl-CoA carboxylase)
8. Methyl malonic aciduria (MM-CoA racemase).
9. Methyl malonic aciduria (MM-CoA mutase).

FIG. IX-64. — *Hereditary disorders of branched chain amino acids.*

alpha-ketoacids. The prenatal diagnosis of this disease is made possible by analysis of branched alpha-keto-acid decarboxylases in cultured amniotic cells. Dancis [68 b] demonstrated that in this classical acute form, enzyme activity was practically absent, ranging form 0 to 2 % of the normal values.

Other clinical forms [367 b]. — Besides the classical acute form, less severe forms have been identified, all genetically distinct and most often corresponding to less serious enzyme deficiencies [68 b]:

The subacute form. — The first symptoms appear only after 3 or 4 weeks, sometimes even later. The spontaneous evolution of the disease is longer but it is usually fatal within the first year. However, there are exceptions. In the case reported by Donnell, the patient was thirteen years old and presented with microcephaly, severe mental deficiency, spastic paraplegia and epilepsy. One can include here a moderate form reported by Schulman [307 b] in a female infant suffering only from moderate mental deficiency at 20 months of age. In these subacute

and moderate forms, enzyme activity attains only 2 to 8 % of the normal values.

The intermittent form. — The first cases of this form were reported by Norris [231 b]. It evolves in a cyclic manner with episodes triggered by infections, surgery or protein excess. The episodes are characterised by ataxia, disorders in tonus, and alterations in consciousness ranging from obtundation to profound coma. In many instances, these crises can be fatal. Between crises, the infant appears normal except in several cases in which psycho-motor deficiencies have been noted. During episodes, one notes the characteric abnormal urine odor and plasma and urine elevations in branched amino and alpha-keto-acids. These findings disappear between crises. Enzyme activity ranges from 8 to 15 % of normal values.

The thiamine sensitive form. — This form was identified by Scriver 1971 [308 b] in an 11 month old infant suffering from severe psycho-motor deficiency. Excess doses of vitamin B_1 administered in a continuous manner corrected the biological abnormalities.

Treatment. — Symptoms appear when plasma levels of the amino acids and their corresponding alpha-keto-acids become elevated, particularly when leucine levels exceed 10-12 mg/100 ml. Treatment consists of maintaining the branched amino acid titers at approximately normal values by implementing diets low in leucine, isoleucine, and valine. Since these three essential amino acids are necessary for normal protein synthesis, a minimal quantity of leucine, isoleucine, and valine must be present in the diet. It is advisable to maintain the plasma levels of these three amino acids between 2 and 5 mg/100 ml, slightly higher than the normal values. In the classical acute form, depending on the infant, leucine tolerance is between 200 and 600 mg/day. All alimentary proteins contain substantial quantities of branched amino acids. Therefore, dietary restriction necessitates the utilization of semi-synthetic diets in which protein requirements are essentially provided by amino acid mixtures lacking the three branched amino acids. Natural proteins must be strictly limited to quantities corresponding to the infant's tolerance to branched amino acids. Requirements in water, mineral salts, trace elements, vitamins, fats, and carbohydrates must not be neglected. In the initial phase of treatment or during periods of decompensation, excessively high levels of branched amino acids (especially leucine), should be rapidly lowered to less than 10 mg/100 ml. Peritoneal dialysis has been shown to be the most effective technique—even more effective than exchange transfusion. Dialysis sessions should not exceed 48 hours. When treatment is initiated early enough (within the first 10 days after birth), and when a satisfactory equilibrium is rapidly obtained and maintained, results tend to be excellent with normal intellectual development. The best results are obtained when there is a previous family history of M. S. U. D. In these cases, the diagnosis is usually made much earlier, before the appearance of clinical symptoms. Such was the case in 3 of 6 of our cases. In the subacute and moderate forms, branched amino acid tolerance is considerably higher than in the classical acute form. Leucine tolerance ranges from 900 to 1,200 mg/day. In some patients, a simple low protein diet is adequate therapy. In the intermittent forms, normal protein diets can be maintained provided that protein intake is diminished or abolished during periods of infection or stress causing excessive catabolism.

CONGENITAL HYPERAMMONEMIAS

Since the description of arginino-succinic aciduria by Allan in 1958, numerous enzyme disorders affecting the different stages of the urea cycle have been identified [105]: Mitochondrial carbamyl-phosphate synthetase deficiency (C. P. S. I).; ornithine carbamyl transferase (O. C. T.) deficiency; argininosuccinate synthetase deficiency responsible for citrullinemia; argininosuccinate lyase (A. S. L.) deficiency, responsible for argininosuccinic aciduria; arginase deficiency responsible for argininemia. More recently there has been discovered a deficiency in N-acetylglutamate synthetase, the enzyme necessary for the synthesis of N-acetylglutamate which, in turn, activates C. P. S. I. All these urea cycle disorders are hereditary and transmitted in an autosomal recessive manner. O. C. T. deficiency, the most frequent of them is an exception since it is transmitted as a dominant sex linked trait. Urea cycle disorders are not the only metabolic disorders capable of causing severe hyperammonemia. Other hereditary metabolic disorders are frequently accompanied by hyperammonemia even in the complete absence of hepatic failure. This is the case in methylmalonic, propionic, isovaleric and methylacetoacetic acidemias, as well as in pyruvate carboxylase deficiency [366]. Different mechanisms have been proposed to explain the abnormalities in ureogenesis and the hyperammonemia encountered in these diseases [65]. Whatever the mechanism, when hyperammonemia is paradoxically associated with metabolic acidosis and ketosis (more often it is associated with respiratory alkalosis), investigations should be oriented towards the organic acidemias. Other disorders can also give hyperammonemia:

— congenital protein intolerance with hyperlysinuria caused by abnormalities in the transport of basic amino acids [320] (see p. 1161);
— hyperammonemia with hyperornithinemia and homocitrullinuria [316] (Table XII);
— congenital lysine intolerance [59] (Table XII).

Enzyme disorders affecting the urea cycle. — For each of the enzyme disorders affecting the urea cycle, clinical forms of varying degrees of severity have been reported. Each corresponds to one of the different enzyme variants in which enzyme activity can be absent or merely diminished.

General clinical presentation and treatment.

(*a*) *Neonatal forms.* — The neonatal forms are the most severe and are often rapidly fatal. After

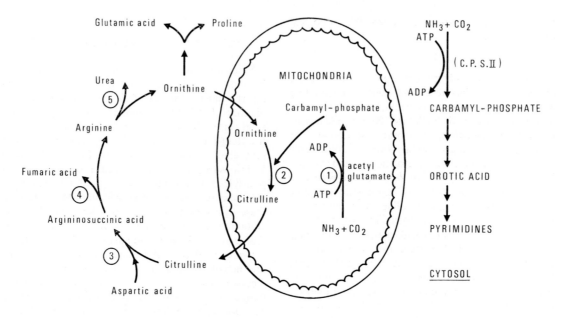

1. Carbamyl-phosphate synthetase I (C.P.S.I)
2. Ornithine-carbamyl transferase (O.C.T.)
3. Argininosuccinate-synthetase
4. Argininosuccinate-lyase
5. Arginase

FIG. IX-65. — *Schematic representation of the urea cycle.*

a symptom free interval of from one to several days after birth, the infant begins showing lack of appetite, vomiting, progressive alterations in consciousness from lethargy to coma, tonus alterations, convulsions, and abnormal movements. Laboratory determinations reveal considerable ammonemia, at levels substantially higher than those observed in severe hepatic failure, and often surpassing 1,000 μg/100 ml. At the same time, glutaminemia is always elevated, while glutamic acid and alanine are occasionally elevated. Blood urea remains at normal levels despite decreased synthesis of urea. Hepatic steatosis is a common finding. Occasionally one observes an increase in transaminases and a decrease in coagulation factors of hepatic origin. Alkalosis is present more often than ketosis or metabolic acidosis. The E. E. G. shows non specific diffuse alterations. The treatment of these acute neonatal forms classically includes elimination of nitrogen intake, limitation of intestinal ammoniogenesis by antibiotic therapy and enemas, and peritoneal dialysis to which exchange transfusion can be coupled. Once protein intake is resumed, it should be limited to 0.8 to 1 g protein/kg/day. Recently,

the utilization of keto analogues of the essential amino acids has been suggested. However, their limited efficacy and elevated cost are arguments against their use. More promising are the use of sodium benzoate (250-350 mg/kg/day IV during the acute phase) and phenylacetic acid. These two substances stimulate urinary nitrogen elimination in the form of hippuric acid (benzoic acid+glycine) and phenylacetylglutamine (phenylacetic acid+glutamine), greatly decreasing the level of hyperammonemia [39]. Administration of urea cycle intermediaries such as arginine (200-700 mg/kg/day) in the treatment of citrullinemia and argininosuccinic acidemia, arginine or citrulline in the treatment of O. C. T. deficiency, seem equally promising. Administration should be continued after the acute phase combined with a low protein diet.

(b) Subacute forms. — In addition to the acute neonatal form, there exists a subacute form affecting newborns and infants. This form is characterized by psychomotor deficiency, neurological disorders of varying types and degrees, convulsions, vomiting, growth deficiency, and aversion to protein-rich

TABLE XII. — Aᴍɪɴᴏ ᴀᴄɪᴅ ᴅɪsᴏʀᴅᴇʀs ᴡɪᴛʜ ʜʏᴘᴇʀᴀᴍᴍᴏɴᴇᴍɪᴀ (see also organic acidurias)

Disease	Clinical forms	Biological findings	Basic defect	Genetics
Carbamyl - phosphate synthetase deficiency [105]	Acute neonatal ⎫ subacute ⎬ Forms intermittent ⎭	Hyperammonemia Glutaminemia	C. P. S. I deficiency (liver, leucocyte)	Autosomal recessive
Ornithine-transcarbamylase deficiency [105, 318]	Acute neonatal ⎫ subacute ⎬ Forms intermittent ⎭	Hyperammonemia Glutaminemia Orotic aciduria + +	O.T.C. deficiency (liver, jejunal mucosa)	X-linked dominant
Citrullinemia [352, 364]	Acute neonatal ⎫ subacute ⎬ Forms intermittent ⎭	Hyperammonemia Citrullinemia Glutaminemia Orotic aciduria +	Arginino-succinate synthetase deficiency (liver, fibroblasts)	Autosomal recessive
Arginino-succinic aciduria [58, 105, 308]	Acute neonatal ⎫ subacute ⎬ Forms intermittent ⎭ Trichorrhexis nodosa	Hyperammonemia Arginino - succinic aciduria Citrullinemia Glutaminemia Orotic aciduria +	Arginino-succinate-lyase deficiency (liver, leucocytes, fibroblasts)	Autosomal recessive
Argininemia [46, 105]	Subacute form Mental retardation, paraplegia	Hyperammonemia Argininemia	Arginase deficiency (liver, erythrocytes)	Autosomal recessive
N - Acetyl - glutamate synthetase deficiency [8]	Acute neonatal form	Hyperammonemia Glutaminemia	N-Acetyl-glutamate synthetase deficiency (liver)	Autosomal recessive (?)
Hyperammonemia with ornithinemia and homocitrullinemia [316]	Mental retardation, periodic crisis of lethargy, ataxia, seizures, protein intolerance	Hyperammonemia Ornithinemia Homocitrullinuria	Probable intramitochondrial ornithine transport defect	Autosomal recessive
Protein intolerance with lysinuria [274, 320]	Vomiting, diarrhoea, hypotrophy, protein aversion, hepato-splenomegaly, neutropenia, thrombocytopenia, inconstant mental retardation	Hyperammonemia Dibasic amino-aciduria Lysinuria hypo-ornithinemia Hypolysinemia Hypoargininemia	Dibasic amino acid transport defect	Autosomal recessive
Congenital lysine intolerance [59, 252]	Coma, seizures, hypotrophy mental retardation, spasticity	Hyperammonemia Lysinemia	Partial deficiency in lysine N. A. D. oxido-reductase	?

foods. The clinical state can rapidly deteriorate after infection or stress, as evidenced by continuous vomiting, dehydration, coma, and sometimes even death.

(*c*) *Intermittent forms.* — The last clinical type, the intermittent form, evolves in acute episodes separated by periods of apparent normality. The crises are precipitated by excessive protein intake, or by excessive protein catabolism occuring after infections or surgical procedures. These episodes are characterized by headaches and vomiting followed by alterations in consciousness, convulsions, and coma that can occasionally be fatal.

Diagnosis. — When confronted with extreme hyperammonemia without jaundice or hepatitis, a urea cycle enzyme deficiency can be suspected.

It is confirmed by determination of blood and urine amino acids levels, urinary orotic acid levels and enzyme analysis. These tests confirm the deficiency and specify it's type. In the diagnosis of intermittent forms, protein loading tests are often helpful. Palmer and Oberholzer stressed the diagnostic value of urinary ammonia nitrogen to urea nitrogen ratios exceeding 0.15 and ammonia excretion exceeding 1.5 g/g creatinine [253].

(a) *Differential diagnosis.* — In the differential diagnosis, one must exclude the hyperammonemias associated with severe viral or metabolic hepatitis, organic acidemias accompanied by ketoacidosis, certain intoxications (salicylates), and hypoglycemia. One must not forget the transient hyperammonemias, occuring in premature infants with idiopathic respiratory distress syndrome or perinatal asphyxia [10, 129]. These transient hyperammonemias are not related to any congenital enzyme deficiency and their cause remains poorly understood. Lastly, hyperammonemia can be a finding in cases of Reye's syndrome. Although the clinical and biochemical findings in Reye's syndrome are normally rather characteristic, the existence of "intermittent" variants can pose some diagnostic confusion. Recurrences should draw attention to this possibility. Protein loading tests and enzyme analysis carried out between episodes are helpful in diagnosing these intermittent forms [350].

(b) *O. C. T. deficiency.* — O. C. T. deficiency is the most frequent of the urea cycle enzyme disorders. Transmitted as a dominant sex-linked trait, this disorder is generally fatal in boys but less severe in girls. There are exceptions to this rule, since less severe cases have been reported in boys, while serious clinical manifestations have been reported in certain heterozygous girls and women [318]. Enzyme analysis has demonstrated considerable genetic heterogeneity in this disease, as well as a large number of enzymatic variants. Amino acid studies are not able to precisely locate the metabolic block. Ornithine levels are not elevated. On the other hand, urinary orotic acid is considerably increased, since excess carbamyl-phosphate is directed towards pyrimidine synthesis. Urinary orotic acid levels have been proposed as a means of neonatal diagnosis for this disease [257] and have been shown to be of value in diagnosing heterozygous states in females. Enzyme analysis can be performed on liver or intestinal biopsy. Prenatal diagnosis requires fetal liver biopsy or direct gene analysis.

(c) *Carbamylphosphate synthetase I deficiency (C. P. S. I).* — Mitochondrial C. P. S. I deficiency is very rare, having been reported in only a dozen families. Of varying severity, this disorder can cause acute manifestations in newborns or even infants and young children. It is distinguishable from O.C.T. deficiency by the absence of elevation in urinary orotic acid. However, it's confirmation necessitates C. P. S. I determinations in liver biopsies or leukocytes. For the moment, it's prenatal diagnosis is not available.

(d) *Citrullinemia, argininosuccinic aciduria and argininemia.* — These disorders are easily identifiable by blood and urinary amino acid determinations. They also present forms of varying severity. For the first two disorders, acute, subacute, and intermittent forms have been reported. The most frequent of the three disorders is argininosuccinic aciduria, with an estimated incidence of 1/70,000 births [208]. Characteristic alterations are present in the hair of affected patients. Hairs are short, dry, fragile, and present trichorrhexis nodosa. The least frequent of these three disorders is argininemia, having been reported in only a handful of cases. All these diseases are transmitted as autosomal recessives. Prenatal diagnosis is possible for argininosuccinic aciduria and citrullinemia. Arginase deficiency on the other hand, cannot be demonstrated in fibroblasts or amniotic cells. It's antenatal diagnosis would require erythrocyte arginase determinations after sampling of fetal blood [231].

(e) *N-Acetylglutamate synthetase deficiency.* — This deficiency is related to the urea cycle disorders, and more specifically to C. P. S. I deficiency. N-Acetylglutamate is a potent physiological activator of C. P. S. I. A recent publication reported three severe neonatal cases in the same sibship [8]. As in C. P. S. I deficiency, there is no increase in any one particular amino acid, nor in urinary orotic acid. It is interesting to note the efficacy of treatment with carbamylglutamate (1.7 nmol/kg/day) associated with arginine supplements.

GLYCINE ENCEPHALOPATHY

Most neonatalogists are familiar with this condition because of the rapid onset of symptoms and it's severity. The designation "glycine encephalopathy" is preferred over "hyperglycinemia without ketosis", initially proposed to contrast this disorder with the "hyperglycinemias with ketosis". The latter is synonymous with several organic acidemias such as propionic and methylmalonic acidemia.

In glycine encephalopathy, hyperglycinemia can be moderate or even absent even though glycine levels in C. S. F. are increased from 10 to 30 times normal values. In contrast, in the hyperglycinemias with synthetase, the enzyme necessary for converting glycine to serine (Fig. 1X-66). Perry [264] demonstrated that cerebral glycine synthetase was also inactive and that cerebral glycine levels were extremely elevated. The disease's severity probably stems from glycine's inhibitory role on synaptic transmission.

$$\text{Glycine} + FH_4 + NAD$$
$$\overset{1}{\rightleftharpoons} FH_4CH_2OH + NH_3 + CO_2 + NADH$$

$$\text{Glycine} + FH_4CH_2OH + NAD$$
$$\overset{2}{\rightleftharpoons} \text{Serine} + FH_4 + NADH$$

1: Cleavage enzyme system of glycine (inactive in glycine encephalopathy).
2: Serine-hydroxy-methyltransferase.

Fig. IX-66. — *Conversion of 2 moles of glycine to serine.*

This disorder is transmitted as an autosomal recessive trait. Pregnancy and delivery are normal. It is only after an interval of 2 or 3 days after birth that severe neurological symptoms appear: extreme hypotonia, lethargy and irregular superficial respirations. Respiratory failure often requires ventilatory assistance. The only other metabolic abnormalities include hyperglycinuria, moderate hyperglycinemia ranging from 6-14 mg/100 ml (N = 1.5 ± 0.3 mg/100 ml), and extreme increases in C. S. F. glycine levels ranging from 1-2 mg/100 ml (N = 0.06 ± 0.01 mg/100 ml). The ratio C. S. F. glycine/glycinemia is approximately 10 times higher than normal. A major element in the diagnosis is the E. E. G., demonstrating a flat tracing interrupted periodically by bursts of sharp wave activity. Even though such tracings are not pathognomonic in themselves, they are of extreme diagnostic value when they occur at this age and in the clinical context described above. The prognosis is not favorable. Should the infant survive the initial period of respiratory failure thanks to modern methods of ventilatory assistance, severe mental deficiency with microcephaly and convulsions are nonetheless unavoidable. E. E. G. findings secondarily evolve towards hypsarrythmia. Different therapeutic approaches have been tried unsuccessfully, such as diets lacking glycine and serine, or administration of benzoic acid to facilitate glycine elimination in the form of hippuric acid. Treatment with strychnine, a specific antagonist of the glycinergic system in the C. N. S., as proposed by Gitzelmann [127], has given better results even though it does not prevent the occurrence of mental deficiency [371]. Glycine synthetase deficiency can be demonstrated in liver and brain cells, but not in cultured fibroblasts and amniotic cells. A minor form of this disease, attributed to a partial deficiency in glycine's cleavage enzyme, has been reported [113]. Other metabolic diseases, that should be eliminated in the differential diagnosis, include the organic acidemias presenting with hyperglycinemia such as propionic and methylmalonic acidemias. Acidosis, ketosis, and urinary organic acid determinations are helpful in directing the diagnosis. As reported by Brandt [36], it is much more difficult to eliminate the possibility of D-glyceric acidemia. The clinical E. E. G. and laboratory findings (hyperglycinemia, C. S. F. elevations in glycine, and absence of acidosis and ketosis) are similar to those found in glycine encephalopathy caused by glycine synthetase deficiency. However, in D-glyceric acidemia, neurological symptoms appear later and more progressively. Between the 8th day and the 2nd month after birth, the infant presents with myoclonia, episodes of hypertonia and hypotonia. The diagnosis is confirmed by chromatography of urinary organic acids, which reveals the massive excretion of D-glyceric acid (1.5-2.5 g/24 hours).

HISTIDINEMIA

Histidinemia is an autosomal recessive disorder that is relatively frequent, occuring in 1/11,000 to 1/17,000 births. In Japan, the incidence has been reported as 1/10,000 [177]. This disorder results from a deficiency in histidase, the enzyme catalyzing histidine's deamination to urocanic acid. In addition to increases in serum and urinary histidine, one observes a decrease in formiminoglutamic acid and an increase in histidine's transamination products (imidazole pyruvic, imidazole lactic, and imidazole acetic acids). Imidazole pyruvic acid gives a characteristic green coloration to ferric chloride and phenistix reactive strips. Histidase activity can be measured in liver biopsy and in the epidermal stratum corneum. Prenatal diagnosis of this disorder is possible. Essential clinical findings in histidinemia include language deficiencies, moderate mental deficiency and behavioral problems. The severity of the disorder is quite variable. For example, some brothers and sisters of affected infants present no clinical symptoms even though they have the same metabolic disorder. However, Ghadimi [120] maintains that these individuals only appear normal on routine examination and after customary methods of psychometric evaluation. When studied with more accurate methods, they are indeed shown to have language deficiencies and behavioral abnormalities. This would justify routine neonatal screening, and appropriate treatment of all diagnosed cases. Low histidine diets effectively control the disorder [328].

DISORDERS IN THE METABOLISM OF SULFUR-CONTAINING AMINO ACIDS

Abnormalities in methionine and cysteine metabolism can be caused by genetic disorders, most often of autosomal recessive inheritance. Furthermore, transient disorders can be caused by enzymatic immaturity, certain drugs, or associated diseases. In the genetic disorders, routine or directed screening and sometimes prenatal diagnosis is possible even though most of these disorders are of relatively later onset, provided that the neonatalogist is familiar with the disease's characteristics.

We shall discuss the homocystinurias, the hypermethioninemias, the cystathioninurias, sulfite oxidase deficiency, and cystinosis. Disorders in sulfur containing amino acid transport such as cystinuria-lysinuria will be discussed in the following section.

The homocystinurias. — The term "homocystinuria" is generally used to designate the disorder resulting from a deficiency in cystathionine synthetase. Since other causes of homocystinuria are known, this definition can lead to confusion. Thus, it seems more logical to speak of "the homocystinurias" as a group of disorders with different causes.

"Classic" homocystinuria, due to cystathionine synthetase deficiency. — No clinical manifestations are present in the neonatal period. Some workers

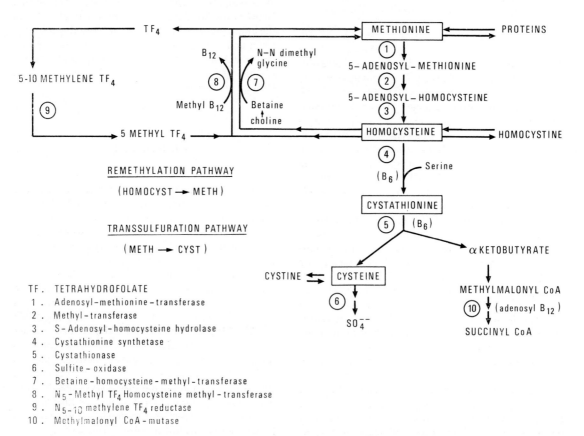

FIG. IX-67. — *Sulfur containing amino acid metabolism.*

maintain that this disorder should be routinely screened for, especially in cases where there exists a family history of the disease. Treatment is effective in certain cases. The disorder in homocysteine metabolism (Fig. IX-67) is caused by a complete or partial deficiency in the hepatic enzyme cysta-thionine-β synthetase, necessary for catalyzing the condensation of homocysteine and serine into cystathionine (provided that the cofactor pyridoxal phosphate is present).

Principal manifestations include luxation of the lens (after 2 years of age), myopia, a Marfan-like appearance (dolichostenomelia, arachnodactyly, scoliosis, thoracic deformities, and osteoporosis), mental retardation, "Charley Chaplin" gait, and arterial and venous thromboses that can be fatal (50 % of patients die before 20 years of age).

A qualitative diagnosis can be made using Brand's reaction (potassium cyanide-sodium nitroprusside) which reveals the presence of sulfur containing amino acids in the urine. This test should be performed two weeks after birth to avoid false negative results [312]. The reaction is also positive in cystinuria. However, cystinuria differs in that amino acid chromatography demonstrates an increased excretion of arginine, ornithine and lysine (see: "Disorders in amino acid transport"). On the other hand, Marfan's disease shows none of these biochemical abnormalities. When Brand's test is positive, a homocysteine specific test (Spaeth and Barber test) should be done. High voltage electrophoresis and especially amino acid column chromatography are also useful. In cystathionine synthetase deficiency, chromatography demonstrates homocystinuria (normally absent) that can attain levels of 300 mg/24 hours (1.12 mmol/24 hours) [235]. Cysteine is absent in the blood and urine while cysteine-homocysteine mixed disulfide is abnormally present. Methioninemia is generally elevated and homocystine becomes detectable in plasma (up to 54 mg/l or 200 μmol/l). In homozygotes, oral methionine loading tests (100 mg/kg or 670 μmol/kg) give prolonged elevations in plasma methionine but no urinary increase in organic sulfates. In heterozygotes, hypermethioninemia is not always present.

Cystathionine synthetase activity can be measured in liver cells, brain cells, and cultured skin fibroblasts or amniotic cells. Prenatal diagnosis is possible [109]. Circulating lymphocytes stimulated by phytohemagglutinin can also be used [131]. Routine neonatal screening for hypermethioninemia or homocystinuria has been proposed by some investigators. Results obtained have been variable. The disease incidence is approximately 1/45,000 births. This disorder is of autosomal recessive inheritance, but presents considerable genetic heterogeneity. Vitamin B_6 is effective in treating about half of the cases [77]. It is administered orally at doses of 25 to 1,200 mg/day. Occasionally, resistance to vitamin B_6 develops, in which case folic acid (at least 10 mg/day) or betaine (9.6 g/day taken in 6 doses) should be given [327]. The diet should be low in methionine and enriched in cysteine by using protein substitutes such as methionaid (Milner Laboratories) [360]. These therapeutic measures should be initiated as soon as possible in order to avoid clinical manifestations. Lastly, antiaggregant drugs have also been proposed in treating this disorder.

Other causes of homocystinuria. — The other causes of homocystinuria are less frequent. Among these causes, of considerable interest are deficits in the remethylation of homocysteine to methionine (Fig. IX-67) by decreased activity of N-5-methyl-tetrahydrofolate-homocysteine methyltransferase (for which methyl B_{12} is a coenzyme). Biochemical findings common to all these disorders include a normal or lowered methioninemia, normal or increased levels of cystathionine in the plasma and urine, and an increased urinary excretion of sulfates after methionine loading tests (as in normal subjects).

Remethylation deficiencies can be caused by genetic abnormalities in vitamin B_{12} metabolism such as defective formation of methyl B_{12} or defective vitamin B_{12} absorption. These disorders are characterized by methylmalonic acidemia caused by proximal disorders in vitamin B_{12} metabolism [236, 298]. The clinical presentation is different than that in the "classic" form of methylmalonic acidemia (as caused by racemase deficiency, for example). In vitamin B_{12} disorders, convulsions, growth deficiencies, cerebellar and posterior column symptoms are noted. There is no ketoacidosis, and megaloblastic anemia can be present.

Early prescription of vitamin B_{12} in massive doses (1 mg/day I. M. or 10 mg/day P. O.) can correct the biochemical abnormalities and halt the clinical progression [13].

A deficiency in 5-10 methylene tetrahydrofolate reductase [160] (Fig. IX-67) can also block the remethylation pathway. The neonatal form of this disorder leads to a progressive neurological deterioration that is most often fatal. Laboratory findings include those cited above plus a hypofolicemia caused by the deficiency in 5-methyl tetrahydrofolate, the principal form of folate in blood and cells. Prenatal diagnosis can be performed by enzyme assay in cultured amniotic cells. Treatment should be started as early as possible with oral administration of methionine and pyridoxine and intramuscular administration of folinic acid and vitamin B_{12}.

Hypermethioninemias [235].

— Except for protein synthesis, the majority of methionine's metabolic pathways start off by it's conversion to S-adenosyl methionine catalysed by adenosyl-methionine transferase (AMT) or synthetase. Further transformations occurring in the transulfuration pathway yield cysteine (Fig. IX-67). A number of congenital or acquired abnormalities in this pathway can cause hypermethioninemia.

The "specific" hypermethioninemias. — These disorders are infrequent. Gaull [115] individualised three types of hypermethioninemia according to the presence of AMT deficiency or myopathy. Type I is caused by hepatic AMT deficiency. Type II presents a myopathy but AMT activity is normal. Type III presents without AMT deficiency or myopathy.

(a) *Type I: adenosyl methionine transferase deficiency*. — The diagnosis can be made after routine screening of the hypermethioninemias [116]. Methioninuria is elevated. There are no other abnormalities in the sulfur containing amino acids nor in hepatic function and most often, clinical abnormalities are absent. Extrahepatic AMT activity is generally normal when measured in erythrocytes, cultured fibroblasts or lymphocytes. However, one case has been reported in which the infant presented feeding problems, hypotrophy and a strong permanent odor suggestive of "boiled cabbage" [141] in the first two months after birth. Treated with a low methionine diet, his development was normal at age six.

(b) *Type II: hypermethioninemia associated with a myopathy* [115]. — This disorder has been reported only recently. The muscular involvement is proximal and symmetrical. Ultrastructural examination of muscle reveals numerous myelin figures.

The other hypermethioninemias. — Cystathionine-synthetase deficiency has already been discussed with the homocystinurias. Hypermethioninemia is frequently noted in severe hepatic failure (methioninemia is an indicator of hepatic failure); aromatic amino acid levels are often increased in the serum, while branched chain amino acid levels are decreased (Fisher's ratio). Hypermethioninemia is also a common finding in type I tyrosinosis, with hepatic lesions being partly responsible (see under: Tyrosinemia).

Transient neonatal hypermethioninemia is frequent when protein intake is excessive (6 to 7 g/kg/day) because of non-adapted milk or unbalanced formulas. One of the mechanisms responsible for this hypermethioninemia is the hepatic immaturity in AMT, cystathionine-synthetase, and cystathionase in premature infants [338].

Cystathioninurias.

— Abnormal urinary excretion of cystathionine is encountered in a number of different circumstances.

Primary cystathioninuria caused by cystathionase deficiency (Fig. IX-67). — Primary cystathioninuria is transmitted as an autosomal recessive trait and shows considerable genetic heterogeneity [255]. No clinical manifestations are noted. Cystathioninuria varies from 0.4 to 26.8 μmol/mg of creatinine. In the urine, one notes the presence of cystathionine derivatives such as N-acetylcystathionine. Normally undetectable, plasma cystathionine shows increases of 0.01 to 0.08 μmol/ml and parallel increases in CSF and other tissues (liver, brain). Enzyme activity can be measured in liver cells or cultured lymphoid cells. The disease incidence ranges from approximately 1/18,000 to 1/78,000 births. Vitamin B_6 dependant forms have been reported, effectively treated orally with 100 to 500 mg of vitamin B_6 /day.

The other cystathioninurias. — Cystathionase is absent in the fœtal liver [338] and appears only several weeks after birth. Before this date, cystathioninuria is increased (up to 0.11 μmol/mg of creatinine or 25 μg/mg of creatinine), especially in premature infants. Vitamin B_6 deficiency can also cause cystathioninuria since pyridoxal phosphate is a coenzyme for cystathionine synthetase and cystathionase (Fig. IX-67). Severe hepatic lesions are accompanied by cystathionase deficiency. Lastly cystathioninuria has been reported in certain tumors such as neuroblastomas and hepatoblastomas (45 % of cases) [117].

Sulfite oxidase deficiency.

— Sulfite oxidase (SO) is an enzyme necessary for the conversion of sulfite to inorganic sulfate (Fig. IX-68). Although rare, this deficiency gives severe neurological manifestations in neonates: convulsions, hemiplegia, choreo-athetotic movements, pseudo-encephalitis, and lens luxation [317]. The urine contains large quantities of S-sulfo-L-cysteine, sulfite, taurine and thiosulfate, but little or no sulfate (5-50 % of total urinary sulfur is excreted as inorganic sulfate instead of the normal 75-95 %). Sulfite oxidase deficiency can be combined with a xanthine oxidase (XO) deficiency [361]. In these cases, additional findings include hypouricemia, hypouricosuria and increased

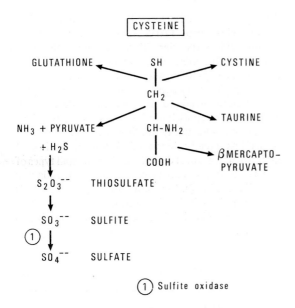

1 Sulfite oxidase

FIG. IX-68. — *Cysteine metabolism.*

xanthine and hypoxanthine in the blood and urine. XO and SO can be measured in liver cells, and XO in jejunal mucosal cells. Both enzymes are flavoproteins containing molybdenum. It has been postulated that this deficiency is due either to an abnormality in the protein transporting molybdenum or an abnormality in molybdenum's incorporation in the enzymes.

Cystinosis. — This disease of autosomal recessive inheritance, results in a tissue accumulation of cystine and it's crystals. An adult, juvenile and infantile form can be distinguished.

The adult form, or benign cystinosis, has an excellent prognosis. Cystine crystals are often accidentally discovered in the cornea or bone marrow. The cystine content of leukocytes is increased to up to 30 times the normal values [306 *b*].

Juvenile cystinosis, or the intermediate form, is characterised by partial tubular and glomerular lesions. Cystine crystals can be found in the cornea, conjunctiva and bone marrow. Retinopathy and hypotrophy can be present. Cystine levels are intermediate between those observed in the adult and infantile forms.

The infantile form is the most severe form of cystinosis [306]. It is characterised by eye involvement and a complex tubulopathy (Fanconi syndrome) that eventually leads to terminal renal failure. The disorder becomes evident at about 6 months of age with water reabsorption abnormalities including polyuria, polydypsia, and vulnerability to dehydration. At about one year of age, patients manifest vitamin D resistant rickets and growth retardation. The disease is sometimes discovered much later by the presence of proteinuria. Patients have blond hair and fair skin. The vitamin resistant rickets progresses despite prescription of preventive doses of vitamin D. Growth retardation becomes more accentuated, eventually leading to dwarfism. Slit lamp examination shows refractile opacities in the cornea and conjunctiva after 3 months of age. Photophobia is sometimes present. Peripheral retinopathy is an early finding [305 *b*]. As the disease progresses, the rickets and growth retardation become more serious. Repeated infections lead to hepatosplenomegaly and terminal chronic renal failure.

Laboratory findings reflect the proximal tubular insufficiency of De Toni Debre Fanconi syndrome. Associated glomerular lesions progress leading to renal insufficiency. Birefractory cystine crystals are noted in the bone marrow. Free cystine levels are extremely elevated in leukocytes (80 to 100 times normal values) and in cultured fibroblasts. Determination of leukocyte cystine content in umbilical blood can be used for neonatal diagnosis in high risk families. Prenatal diagnosis is possible [305 *b*, 333 *b*].

Cystinosis is characterised by marked intracellular accumulation of free cystine. It is stored in the lysosomes. The exact mechanism responsible for this remains uncertain.

Symptomatic treatment of cystinosis is directed at equilibrating renal function by providing adequate water, sodium, potassium, phosphorus and bicarbonate. Growth retardation can be limited by constant rate enteral feeding providing a regular intake of protein and energy sources in large quantities [153]. Any thyroid insufficiency should be treated. Terminal renal failure occurs in 6 to 12 years, and necessitates hemodialysis or renal transplantation. There is no recurrence of the disease in the renal transplant, but diffuse lysosomal storage persists.

Specific therapy is aimed at combating cystine accumulation. Diets low in methionine and cysteine have been abandoned. B. A. L. and D-penicillamine are also no longer used. Recent attempts at using dithiothreitol (D. T. T.) and ascorbic acid in elevated doses have been unsuccessful. It is known that cysteamine lowers leukocyte cystine content and can improve creatinine clearance [385]. The utilization of liposomes as vectors for these substances is currently being studied [73].

DISORDERS
IN RENAL AND INTESTINAL TRANSPORT
OF AMINO ACIDS

The kidneys and intestines play a major role in the regulation of amino acid intake and output. By means of active transport systems, they insure jejunal absorption and proximal tubular reabsorption of amino acids. These transport systems are specific for one substrate or for a group of substrates. For the latter, five types of transport systems have been distinguished, each corresponding to a class of amino acids: dicarboxylic amino acids (Glu, Asp),

dibasic amino acids (Lys, Arg, Orn) and cystine, imino acids (Pro, OHPro) and glycine, neutral amino acids (Ala, Ser, Thr, Val, Leu, Ile, Phe, Tyr, Try, His, Gln, Asn, Met, Cys) and β-amino acids (β-Ala, β-aminoisobutyric acid, Tau).

The carrier substances are macromolecular proteins whose structure is genetically determined, allowing for repression of synthesis or alterations in structure. Our understanding of transport mechanisms has greatly increased following studies of amino acid transport disorders. The principal types of transport disorders are listed in Table XIII (adapted from Scriver [313]). We shall only discuss Hartnup's disease, imino-glycinuria, cystinuria-lysinuria, and familial protein intolerance with dibasic amino aciduria.

TABLE XIII. — Hereditary disorders in amino acid transport

Disorder	Amino acids involved	Transmission	Organs involved	Symptoms
Disorders involving a group of amino-acids				
Cystinuria-lysinuria	Cystine, Lys, Orn, Arg	AR (and AD)	Kidneys-intestine *	Renal stones
Dibasic amino-aciduria	Lys, Orn, Arg	AR	Kidneys-intestine	Hypotrophy ± mental retardation
Familial protein intolerance with hyperammonemia (syn: congenital lysinuria, dibasic hyperaminoaciduria)	Lys, Orn, Arg, peptide	AR	Kidneys-intestine	Growth deficiency, vomiting, diarrhea, convulsions, distaste for proteins, hypotonia, hepatomegaly, neutropenia, thrombocytopenia
Hartnup's disease	Neutral AA except iminoglycine	AR	Kidneys-intestine	Pellagroid rash, cerebellar ataxia, mental retardation, indoluria
Iminoglycinuria	Pro, OH-Pro, Gly	AR (and AD)	Kidneys-intestine *	0
Dicarboxylic acidurias I and II	Glu, Asp	AR (?)	Kidneys-intestine *	Mental retardation, hypotrophy, hypoglycemia
Disorders involving one A. A.				
Cystinuria	Cystine	AR	Kidneys	0
Glycinuria	Gly	AR (and AD)	Kidneys	Renal stones
Lysinuria	Lys	AR	Kidneys	0
Hydroxylysinuria	OH-Lys	AR	Kidneys	Mental retardation, myoclonia, tremors, convulsions
Tryptophan malabsorption [311] (blue diaper syndrome)	Try	AR (?)	Intestine	Blue diapers, hypercalcemia, nephrocalcinosis
Tryptophanuria	Try	AR	Intestine	Growth retardation
Methionine malabsorption [169] (oast-house disease)	Met	AR	Intestine	Blond hair, convulsions, psychomotor retardation, hops or dried celery odor, diarrhea
Histidinuria	His	AR	Kidneys-intestine	Mental retardation

* Indicates that the intestine is only involved in certain forms of the disorders but not in others (genetic heterogeneity). AR: Autosomal recessive; AD: Autosomal dominant.

Disorders in neutral amino acid transport.

— There exists a principal and specific transport system for the neutral amino acids. Hartnup's disease is caused by abnormalities in this system. There also exist systems that are specific for one of the neutral amino acids (Try, Met) and these too can be deficient.

Hartnup's disease.

— This rare disorder is caused by an autosomal recessive mutation [311] affecting the intestinal and renal transport of neutral amino acids (except Pro, OHPro, and Gly). Clinical manifestations are solely due to tryptophan malabsorption and defective nicotinamide synthesis. The intestinal abnormality only affects the absorption of free amino acids; the dipeptides participating in other transport systems are absorbed normally [207]. The tryptophan not absorbed by the intestines is transformed by colonic bacteria into indoles and scatoles; substances that are absorbed, conjugated and then excreted (increased indoluria and indicanuria). Hyperaminoaciduria is a constant finding and is essential for the diagnosis (10 fold increase in Ala, Ser, Thr, Val, Leu, Ile, Phe, Tyr, Try and His). Tubular and glomerular functions remain normal. Amino acid transport in other tissues (sweat, saliva, fibroblasts and leukocytes) remain normal, demonstrating the multiplicity of transport systems in different tissues.

Detection of heterozygotes is only possible by in vitro studies of intestinal transport. The disease incidence is estimated at 1/20,000 births. Clinical symptoms occur in "attacks" often precipitated by fever, stress, solar exposure, and sulfonamides. A pigmented rash resembling that seen in pellagra appears on skin surfaces exposed to the sun. Neurological manifestations are variable [207]: Cerebellar ataxia with nystagmus, intentional tremor, and hypotonia are possible but are usually only transient. Mental retardation is noted in 15 % of the cases.

Marked improvement occurs after treatment with nicotinamide (40 to 250 mg/day) and avoidance of exposure to the sun. Temporary colonic decontamination with neomycin also seems beneficial.

Disorders in the transport of imino acids and glycine: familial iminoglycinuria.

— Iminoglycinuria is generally discovered during aminoacidopathy screening programs. It shows no specific clinical findings. Its importance stems from its genetic heterogeneity and the progress it has made possible in the study of imino acid and glycine transport systems. At least three systems have been identified: a high capacity and low affinity system, common to all 3-amino acids (but with

more affinity for iminoacids), a low capacity glycine-specific system, and a low capacity imino-acid specific system. Furthermore, glycine shares a common renal transport system with other amino acids (neutral, dibasic, etc.).

The genetic transmission of iminoglycinuria is an autosomal recessive. It's incidence is estimated at 1/20,000 births. At least 4-allelic mutations have been incriminated for the phenotypes observed [314]. Although the cases first reported presented mental retardation, patients with iminoglycinuria are most often clinically normal. Diagnosis of homozygous states is readily confirmed by paper chromatography which reveals the presence of free proline and hydroxyproline in the urine after 6 months.

In the differential diagnosis, one should eliminate type I and II hyperprolinemias and hydroxyprolinemia. In the latter, iminoglycinuria is present but is associated with increased blood levels of proline and hydroxyproline. Fanconi syndrome also presents with iminoglycinuria, but is associated with a global deficiency in tubular function. Newborns normally present a physiological iminoglycinuria that persists until 3 months of age; after 6 months, all iminoacidurias are considered pathological regardless of their intensity. As for glycinuria, it is considered pathological when exceeding 150 mg/24 hours or 160 μmol/g of total urinary nitrogen [314].

Isolated hyperglycinuria without iminoaciduria can be seen in certain heterozygous states for certain phenotypes of iminoglycinuria, or in the "K*m*" variant of the homozygous state. De Vries also reported hyperglycinuria with renal lithiasis of autosomal dominant transmission [79]. This might be a heterozygous form of familial iminoglycinuria. Lastly, a dominantly transmitted glucoglycinuria often associated with hypophosphatemic ricketts has been reported [314].

Disorders in the transport of basic amino acids and cystine.

Cystinuria-lysinuria.

— Cystinuria-lysinuria is characterized by the urinary precipitation of cystine, the least soluble amino acid, and an increased urinary excretion of lysine, arginine, ornithine and mixed disulfur cystein-homocysteine. It is caused by a hereditary abnormality in the intestinal and renal transport systems of these amino acids, and is transmitted in an autosomal recessive manner.

It's incidence varies: 1/20,000 in England, 1/15,000 in the U. S. A., 1/100,000 in Sweden [351]. Both sexes are equally affected and manifestations generally appear in the second or third decades.

Patients present with renal colic (abdominal pain and hematuria) that is often complicated by urinary infections, anuria, and eventually chronic renal failure and high blood pressure. The calculi are radiopaque showing up as multiple round opacities located in the pelvis and calices of both kidneys. Cystine stones are amber-yellow, waxy, smooth or granular. Microscopic examinations of urinary sediment after centrifugation and acidification demonstrates hexagonal and flat crystals. Brand's reaction (potassium cyanide and sodium nitroprusside), identifies excessive urinary levels of sulfur-containing amino acids such as cystine. The reagent turns redish-purple when urinary concentrations of cystine exceed 200 mg/l (or 75-125 mg/g of creatinine). Homozygous stone formers usually excrete more than 250 mg/g of creatinine. This test is positive for all sulfhydril substances. Sullivan's reaction (napthoquinone and sodium sulfonate) is more sensitive, giving a red coloration for concentrations exceeding 70 mg/l. Precise quantitative or qualitative analysis of urinary amino acids necessitates ion-exchange or gas chromatography.

The pathogenesis of this disorder is complex. The intestinal absorption of cystine, arginine, lysine, and ornithine is deficient. The corresponding diamines are found in the urine (agmatine, cadaverine, putrescine). There is no abnormality in cysteine transport, thus demonstrating the independence of the intestinal and renal transport systems of cystine and cysteine. The intestinal absorption deficiency was demonstrated "in vivo" by jejunal perfusion of dibasic amino acids. Howe-

ver, since the transport of dipeptides (lysylglycine, for example) is normal, there are no nutritional deficiencies. The intestinal deficiency can be partial or complete for the different amino acids. Lysine and cystine mutually inhibit each other's intestinal absorption, but not renal absorption. A more recent study [57] showed that the lysine transport defect occured at the brush border. This is different than that which occurs in familial protein intolerance with lysinuria [275, 294] where an L-lysine transport defect occurs at the baso-lateral membrane.

Renal abnormalities involve only cystine and the 3-dibasic amino acids. According to Dent and Rose, a common transport system for these 4 amino acids is deficient. This still remains to be proven since separate deficiencies are possible (isolated cystinuria, isolated dibasic amino aciduria). It seems more probable that these are separate transport systems with common affinities. In cystinuria-lysinuria, the urinary excretion of other amino acids is moderately increased (glycine, methionine, cystathionine, homocysteine-cysteine mixed disulfide).

Combined intestinal and renal studies permitted Rosenberg [290, 351] to propose a classification into 3 distinct genetic types (Table XIV). Cystinuria was redefined as a genetic disorder of complex recessive inheritance resulting from 3 allelic mutations. Differentiation of the 3 types of cystinuric homozygotes required in vitro intestinal transport studies of all 4 amino acids.

Treatment is aimed at decreasing the excretion of cystine and increasing it's solubility (precipitation

TABLE XIV. — CLASSIFICATION OF CYSTINURIAS (ROSENBERG)

Analysis	Type I	Type II	Type III
Intestine			
— In vitro transport	Cystine, Lys, Arg = 0 Cys = N	Lys = 0 ↘ Cystine	↘ Cystine (sometimes N) ↘ Lys (of variable degree)
— Oral cystine loading	No plasma cystine ↗	No plasma cystine ↗	Slow plasma cystine
Kidney			
— In vitro transport	Cys, Cystine = N ↘ Lys		Cystine = N ↘ Lys
— Urinary amino acid excretion	↗ Cystine, Lys, Arg Orn	↗ Cystine, Lys, Arg, Orn	↗ Cystine, Lys, Arg, Orn
— Urinary amino acid excretion in heterozygotes	N	↗ Cystine, Lys	↗ Cystine, Lys

N = Normal.

TABLE XV. — Amino acid disorders not described in the text

Disease	Clinical symptoms	Laboratory findings	Basic defect
Lysine metabolism			
Hyperlysinemia [119]	Inconstant mental retardation	Hyperlysinemia (uria)	Lysine keto-reductase
Hyperlysinemia with periodic ammonia intoxication[59]	Seizures, coma after high protein intake, mental retardation	Intermittent hyperlysinemia, argininemia, ammonemia (after lysine loading)	Possible deficiency in lysine-NAD oxidoreductase
Saccharopinuria [42, 47]	Inconstant mental retardation	Hyperlysinemia (uria), saccharopinuria	Saccharopine-dehydrogenase (lysine ketoreductase may be reduced)
Pipecolic acidemia [353]	Mental retardation, hypotonia, hepatomegaly, amblyopia	Hyperpipecolatemia (uria)	Unknown
Alpha-aminoadipic aciduria, type I [148, 271]	Mental retardation	Hyperamino adipatemia (uria), alpha-keto adipaturia	Alpha-keto adipate dehydrogenase
Alpha-aminoadipic aciduria, type II [45, 216]	Inconstant mental retardation, hypotonia seizures, immunologic deficiency (1 case)	Hyperamino adipatemia (uria) without alpha-keto adipaturia	Possible defect of mitochondrial alpha-amino adipate transaminase
Amino acid metabolism			
Prolinemia, type I [111, 309]	Mental retardation, seizures, deafness nephropathy, several subjects normal	Hyperprolinemia (uria), iminoglycinuria	Proline oxidase
Prolinemia, type II [309, 359]	Mental retardation, seizures, several subjects normal	Hyperprolinemia (uria), iminoglycinuria; delta-1 pyrroline-5-carboxylic aciduria	Delta-1-pyrroline 5-carboxylate dehydrogenase
Hydroxyprolinemia [289, 309]	Mental retardation, growth retardation, several subjects normal	Hydroxyprolinemia (uria), iminoglycinuria	Hydroxyproline, oxidase
Iminodipeptiduria [269]	Chronic otitis and sinusitis; dermatosis; splenomegaly	Iminodipeptiduria	Prolidase
Disorders affecting the gamma-glutamyl cycle			
Glutathioninuria [307, 384]	Mental retardation	Brand test positive, glutathioninuria	Gamma-glutamyl transpeptidase
Glutathion deficiency with gamma-glutamyl cysteine synthetase deficiency [285]	Anemia; spino-cerebellar degeneration; peripheric neuropathy; myopathy	Hemolytic anemia; glutathione deficiency, hyperamino aciduria	Gamma-glutamyl cysteine synthetase
5-oxoprolinuria with glutathion synthetase deficiency [28, 225]	Anemia, mental retardation when enzyme deficiency is generalized	Hemolytic anemia; metabolic acidosis; 5-oxoprolinuria; glutathione deficiency	Glutathione-synthetase
5-oxoprolinuria with 5-oxoprolinase deficiency [201, 202]	Vomiting, diarrhea, abdominal pain, urinary lithiasis (oxalate)	5-oxoprolinuria	5-oxoprolinase
Disorders in tryptophan metabolism			
Tryptophanemia [299]	Growth and mental retardation; ataxia; pellagroid dermatosis	Tryptophanemia (uria), indole-acetic aciduria	Probable defect of tryptophane pyrrolase

TABLE XV (continued)

Disease	Clinical symptoms	Laboratory findings	Basic defect
Disorders in tryptophan metabolism			
Xanthurenic aciduria [194, 346]	Diarrhea, stomatitis, mental retardation, pellagroid dermatosis	Hemolytic anemia; xanthurenic aciduria; hydroxy-kynureninuria	Kynureninase
Miscellaneous enzyme disorders			
Hyperornithinemia with retinal gyrate atrophy [322, 323]	Night blindness; chorioretinal degeneration; loss of peripheral vision; amyotrophy	Hyperornithinemia; hyperornithinuria; hypolysinemia	Ornithine keto acid transaminase
Formimino - glutamic aciduria [261]	Inconstant speech deficiencies; inconstant mental retardation	Megaloblastic anemia, formimino glutamic aciduria	Formimino-transferase
Carnosinemia (alpha-alanyl-histidine) [204, 238, 262]	Mental retardation; seizures (several subjects normal)	Carnosinemia (uria), anserinuria	Carnosinase
Sarcosinemia (N-methyl glycine) [118, 370]	Mental retardation (great heterogeneity among reported cases)	Sarcosinemia (uria)	Sarcosine-dehydrogenase
Beta-alaninemia [310]	Neonatal onset lethargy seizures, hypotonia	Beta-alaninemia (uria), beta-amino aciduria, elevation of GABA (blood, urine)	Possible defect in beta-alanine transaminase
Threoninemia [280]	Growth retardation convulsions	Hyperthreoninemia, hyperthreoninuria	Unknown
Beta-mercaptolactate cystine disulfiduria [235]	May be asymptomatic	Urinary excretion of mixed disulfide of cystine and beta-mercaptolactate	Beta-mercapto-pyruvate sulfur-transferase

occurs at urinary concentrations exceeding 300 mg/l). Low methionine diets are dangerous and of little use; it suffices to simply avoid excessive methionine intake. Diuresis should be achieved so as to decrease urinary cystine concentration; a cystinuric adult excreting up to 1 g of cystine per day should drink at least 3 to 4 liters of water daily. Since the risk of cystine supersaturation is highest at night when urine flow is at its lowest, the importance of drinking 1 or 2 glasses of water before sleep and at 3 o'clock in the morning must be stressed. These measures can prevent renal stones from forming in 2/3 of the patients. In order to increase cystine's solubility, the urine should be alkalinized to a pH greather than 7 by the use of sodium bicarbonate (for adults 5 to 10 g per day spread out over regular intervals and at night). Urine sterility, calciuria, and digestive tolerance should be controlled regularly. In uncomplicated cases, the increase in water intake and urine alkalinization is generally adequate in treating these patients.

When these measures fail or one kidney is removed because of cystine stones, D-penicillamine (1 to 2 g/day in adults) has been shown to be effective. This drug chelates cystine yielding the mixed disulfide of cysteine-penicillamine, 50 times more soluble than cystine. However, intolerance can develop to this drug. Even more troublesome is the frequent development of side-effects that can be serious. Allergic reactions occur in 50 % of cases (fever, rash, arthralgia). For this reason, D-penicillamine should be introduced in progressively increased doses over a 1 to 2 month period. Other side effects include hypogueusia, increase in zincuria and cupruria, pyridoxine deficiency, hematological disorders (pancytopenia, eosinophilia, neutropenia), epidermolysis, nephrotic syndrome, Goodpasture's syndrome, and lupus. Other drugs can be substituted including N-acetyl D-penicillamine (2 to 4 g/day in adults) which is as effective, yet less dangerous than D-penicillamine. The drug 2-mercapto-propionylglycine can prevent stone formation and has few side effects. Diazepoxide has also been used.

Surgical stone removal should be reserved for

cases in which drug therapy has been ineffective after several months.

Familial protein intolerance with lysinuria. — This rare autosomal recessive disorder is particularly prevalent in Finland where its incidence is estimated at 1/60,000 to 80,000 births [320]. Clinical abnormalities become noticeable at weaning: the introduction of cow's milk causes vomiting and diarrhea. Older children demonstrate a dislike of protein rich foods. Ingestion of proteins can result in convulsions and coma. Later findings include growth deficiencies, hypotonia, amyotrophy, hepatomegaly, and occasionally splenomegaly and diffuse osteoporosis. Mental retardation may also be noted. Laboratory findings include hyperammonemia after protein ingestion, excessive urinary orotic acid excretion, neutropenia, and often increased transaminase, aldolase and lacticdehydrogenase.

This disorder is caused by an abnormality in the intestinal and renal transport of dibasic amino acids, resulting in an excessive urinary excretion of lysine, arginine, and ornithine and a decreased intestinal absorption of these amino acids. More precise studies have demonstrated that the primary disorder is a block in lysine's transport out of enterocytes, hepatocytes and renal tubular cells. The resulting intracellular accumulation creates a competitive inhibition for arginine and ornithine uptake [275]. Ornithine deficiency causes a functional disturbance in the urea cycle and hyperammonemia; this is immediately corrected by arginine administration. For long term treatment, it is more effective to administer an amino acid whose absorption is not limited by lysine's intracellular accumulation. Citrulline has been shown to be the most effective for this purpose (2 to 3.5 g/day) [274] and should be associated with a low protein diet.

OTHER DISORDERS
OF AMINO ACID METABOLISM

Because of their number, we cannot detail all the disorders of amino acid metabolism. Table XV lists the amino acid disorders caused by enzyme deficiencies.

Organic acidemias

DEFINITION AND GENERALITIES

The term "organic acid" is ordinarily used to designate the water soluble carboxylic acids not reacting with ninhydrin [348]. The definition includes the short chain fatty acids. According to this definition, the organic acidemias also encompass the amino acid disorders in which increases in alphaketoacids are associated with increases in the corresponding amino acids. These disorders, previousely discussed in the section devoted to amino acid disorders, can be diagnosed by amino acid analysis. In the same manner, certain disorders in glycogenolysis and gluconeogenesis (fructose-1-6-diphosphate deficiency, type I glycogenosis, and phosphoenolpyruvate carboxykinase deficiency), will be discussed with the enzyme disorders of carbohydrate metabolism elsewhere in this book even though they present with pathological organic acidemia. From a practical standpoint, the organic acidemias constitue a well differentiated group of enzyme disorders with similar clinical and laboratory manifestations. They are diagnosed by the same methods. Discovered in 1966, they have stimulated increasing interest. The separation, identification, and quantification of organic acids has been made possible by developments in gas chromatography coupled with mass spectrography (GC/MS). Even so, our understanding is far from complete, as is illustrated by the fact that a large number of peaks obtained in normal urine, by the high resolution of capillary column chromatography, still have not been identified. Isovaleric acidemia was the first disorder to be identified [349]. Almost each year since then, new diseases have been discovered or additional information collected concerning already known diseases. Discoveries concern not only the more prevalent organic acidemias involving branched chain amino acid metabolism (Fig. IX-64), but also disorders involving the metabolism of other amino acids, long chain fatty acids, ketone bodies, pyruvate, the Krebs cycle and the respiratory chain. Certain enzyme deficiencies, whether they are vitamin dependent or not, can simultaneously involve different metabolic responses. For example, holocarboxylase synthetase deficiency affects the carboxylation of pyruvate, acetyl, propionyl and 2-methyl crotonyl coenzyme A; acyl-coenzyme A dehydrogenase deficiency simultaneously alters the oxidation of fatty acids, glutamyl coenzyme A, and branched short chain fatty acids; dihydrolipoyl-dehydrogenase deficiency simultaneously affects the decarboxylation of pyruvate, 2-oxoglutarate and branched chain alpha-keto-acids.

STUDY METHODS

Plate chromatographic techniques have been proposed for diagnosing urinary increases in organic acids or acyl-glycine derivatives [3, 85]. For a number of reasons, these techniques are insufficient [178, 348]. Accurate diagnosis necessitates gas chromatography of the urinary organic acids, according to proven techniques, When abnormal peaks are present, further analysis by mass spectrography is required to precisely identify the metabolites in excess. Unfortunately, abnormal peaks can be caused by numerous sources of error including plastic substances, used in manufacturing urine receptacles, chemicals used to conserve urine, and substances originating form foods or drugs. As discussed by Jellun [178], other artifacts can include organic acids resulting from urinary bacterial proliferation, and 4-hydroxyphenylacetic acid excreted in the course of intestinal infections. Urine samples should be collected without addition of preservatives and analysed immediately or frozen at $-20°$ C if immediate analysis is not possible. Organic acid analysis can also be performed on plasma, C. S. F. or amniotic fluid [239, 377]. Interpretation of results should take into account the age of the subject, since urinary organic profiles are different in newborns, infants and adults [24, 149]. In some cases, interpretation is made difficult by the elimination of a number of metabolic byproducts originating above the metabolic block and their acyl-glycines and hydroxylated derivates. For example, in isovaleric acidemia, the major urinary metabolites are isovalerylglycine and 3-hydroxyisovaleric acid. On the other hand, isovaleric acid is only present in minute quantities in the urine, even during acute episodes at which time it accumulates in the blood. In 3-hydroxymethylglutaric acidemia, the urinary

excretion of this acid is accompanied by the excretion of 3-methylglutaric and 3-methylglutaconic acids probably derived from 3-methylglutaconyl CoA, a metabolite originating above the block. The complexity of interpreting organic acidemias is most noted in disorders in which a multiple enzyme deficiency is incriminated. The best example of this is type II glutaric aciduria. Reported cases of this disease have been very inconsistant, with each report mentioning the discovery of another abnormal urinary metabolite such as glutaric, butyric, ethylmalonic, isovaleric, isobutyric and 2-methylbutyric acids. This explains the multitude of nomenclatures given to this disorder. This disorder has also been referred to as type II glutaric aciduria, ethylmalonic and adipic aciduria [217], and multiple deficiency in acyl CoA dehydrogenases [137].

CLINICAL FINDINGS

Except for several exceptions, the different organic acidemias present similar clinical manifestations.

Acute neonatal forms. — Neonatologists should be familiar with these forms since their spontaneous prognosis is poor, and they are often fatal if treatment is not rapidly initiated. In many cases, the diagnosis is suspected only after several deaths occur in the same sibship. Frequently, the diagnosis is confused with that of neonatal infections or septicemia because of the presence of vomiting, metabolic acidosis and occasional thrombocytopenia or hepatic findings (hepatomegaly and increase in transaminases). This disorder is frequently mistaken for pyloric stenosis even though the presence of metabolic acidosis is extremely uncharacteristic of the latter. Other enzyme disorders can also be unjustly incriminated. For example, the presence of marked hyperammonemia can logically lead to suspicion of urea cycle enzyme disorders. Confronted with such hyperammonemias, one should consider the possibility of methylmalonic acidemia, propionic acidemia, or pyruvate carboxylase deficiency, especially if the hyperammonemia is accompanied by acidosis. Several findings can suggest an organic acidemia. Characteristically, pregnancy and delivery evolve normally without incident. It is only after an asymptomatic interval of 24 to 48 hours after birth (sometimes shorter or longer) that symptoms appear: feeding problems, vomiting, hypo- or hypertonia, dyspnea with polypnea, grunting, lethargy, seizures, then progressive deterioration to coma and death. Other findings that can suggest the diagnosis are metabolic acidosis (which quickly relapses after correction), ketonuria (uncommon in newborns), hyperlactacidemia and abnormal odor.

Intermittent forms. — This form is characterized by acute episodes most often triggered by an increase in catabolism after infections, surgery, fasting, or excessive intake of precursors of involved metabolites (for example, protein rich meals in the case of isovaleric, propionic or methylmalonic acidemias). Initial symptoms include repeated vomiting, polypnea, ataxia, followed by alterations in consciousness and seizures leading to coma. Rehydration with glucose solutions often reverses the symptomatology even though the diagnosis has not been established or limited to an "episode of acetonemic vomiting". Between episodes, the infant is often completely normal, or sometimes suffers from neurological manifestations such as ataxia or choreo-athetosis. During acute episodes, besides metabolic acidosis, diagnostically useful findings include ketosis, hypoglycemia, hyperlactacidemia, hyperammonemia, and abnormal breath and urine odor (Tables III-IX). The absence of ketosis during hypoglycemic episodes without hyperinsulinemia and despite increases in free fatty acids, should cause one to suspect a deficiency in fatty acid beta-oxidation, as in carnitine deficiency or deficiencies in ketone body synthesis (3-hydroxy-3-methyl-glutaric aciduria).

Chronic forms with neurological symptoms. — These are the most misleading forms, since clinical manifestations appear progressively and do not suggest a perturbation in intermediate metabolism. Extreme hypotonia, resembling that seen in Werdnig-Hoffman's disease, can be present, as in 3-methylcrotonylglycinuria [335]. When manifestations include progressive dystonia, choreo-athetosis, dysarthria, and absence of apparent metabolic abnormalities, only analysis of urinary organic acids can diagnose the possibility of type I glutaric aciduria. Clinical findings may resemble Friedreich's syndrome, Charcot-Marie syndrome, or certain hereditary ataxias if the studies of Blass, Kark and others concerning pyruvate dehydrogenase deficiency are confirmed [27, 183].

Organic acidurias lacking characteristic clinical manifestations. — In several organic acidurias, it has been impossible to discern any logical or consistant clinical pattern for the given biochemical abnormality. This is the case for

D-2-hydroxyglutaric aciduria, as described by Chalmers in a child suffering from an exudative enteropathy [48]. Another example was reported by Truscott in a child suffering from strabismus and mental deficiency who presented with an abnormal urinary excretion of deoxyribose metabolites including deoxyerythropentonic acid and 2-deoxyribitol [358]. A final example that can be cited is that of D-lactic aciduria without lactic acidosis [92].

THE PRINCIPAL ORGANIC ACIDEMIAS

Only isovaleric, methylmalonic and propionic acidemia, beta-methylorotonyl-glycinuria and beta-ketothiolase deficiency will be discussed. The other organic acidurias are indicated in Table XVI.

Isovaleric acidemia. — More than twenty cases of this disorder have been reported. It is caused by a deficiency in isovaleryl CoA dehydrogenase and the accumulation of isovaleric acid, a metabolite of L-leucine (Fig. IX-64). Two forms can be distinguished:

The acute neonatal form manifests itself 48-72 hours after birth with feeding difficulties, repeated vomiting, polypnea, lethargy, convulsions, then coma and a very strong disagreable odor described as one of cheese or sweaty feet. The resemblance of this odor to that of short chain fatty acids, led Tanaka et al. [349] to analyse the organic acids by gas chromatography. Their studies revealed the presence of isovaleric acid. Two previous case studies reported by Sidbury as "sweaty feet syndrome" were retrospectively found to correspond to authentic isovaleric acidemia. This very characteristic odor is not always present. Leukopenia or even pancytopenia are possible associated findings [188]. In this acute neonatal form, of poor prognosis, the infant dies rapidly if not treated effectively. Death and even mental deficiency can be avoided by peritoneal dialysis, administration of elevated doses of glycine (250 mg/kg/day) (aimed at accelerating conversion to the less toxic and more rapidly excreted isovaleryl-glycine), and a restricted leucine diet [302] or simply a low protein diet (1.5 g/kg/day). Acute episodes of decompensation can occur if treatment is not correctly followed or during periods of increased catabolism secondary to infections or other forms of stress.

TABLE XVI. — Hereditary organic acidurias

Disease	Essential symptoms	Urinary organic acids	Basic defect
Carnitine deficiency [49, 126, 184, 279]	Acute crises simulating Reye's syndrome: vomiting, coma, hypoglycemia, hypertransaminasemia, hyperammonemia, progressive muscular weakness	(Inconstant) dicarboxylic aciduria: adipic, sebacic, suberic acids	Carnitine deficiency (exact basic defect still unknown)
Dicarboxylic aciduria without ketosis [149 b, 241]	Hypoglycemic crises with lethargy, coma, metabolic acidosis without ketosis	3-Hydroxy-isovaleric, 3-hydroxy-isobutyric, 5-hydroxyhexanoic, adipic sebacic, suberic acids, hexanoyl glycine	Defective fatty acid beta-oxidation
Glutaric aciduria, type I [35, 110, 134, 203, 374]	Severe and progressive dyskinetic syndrome with dysarthria, choreoathetosis. Possibility of acute episodes mimicking Reye's syndrome	Glutaric, glutaconic, 3-hydroxy-glutaric acids	Glutaryl CoA-dehydrogenase deficiency
Glutaric aciduria, type II [97, 137, 217, 270, 344]	Acute crises with acidosis, hypoglycemia without ketosis; severe neonatal forms: vomiting, coma, acidosis, hypoglycemia, hyperammonemia, possible sweaty-feet odor. Rapid death	Adipic, ethyl-malonic, glutaric, 2-hydroxy-butyric, 2-hydroxy-isovaleric, hexanoic, isobutyric, isovaleric, lactic, propionic, sebacic, suberic acids	Multiple acyl CoA dehydrogenases deficiency
Glyceric acidemia, type I [36, 145, 193]	Severe hypotonia, seizures, rapid death, hyperglycinemia without ketosis and without acidosis	D-Glyceric acid	Glycerate-dehydrogenase deficiency
Glyceric acidemia, type II [369]	Mental retardation, hypotrophy, chronic acidosis, normoglycinemia	D-Glyceric acid	Unknown
Hydroxy-methyl-glutaric aciduria [93, 135, 288]	Severe hypoglycemic crises with metabolic acidosis, hyperammonemia mimicking Reye's syndrome. Neonatal forms possible	3-hydroxy-3-methyl-glutaric, 3-methyl-glutaconic, 3-hydroxy-isovaleric, 3-methyl-glutaric acids	3-hydroxy-3-methyl-glutaryl, CoA lyase deficiency
Isovaleric acidemia [25, 56, 94, 188, 302]	Vomiting, lethargy, coma, sweaty-feet smell, acidosis, ketosis, severe neonatal and acute intermittent forms	Isovaleric, 3-hydroxy-isovaleric acids, isovaleryl-glycine	Isovaleryl CoA dehydrogenase deficiency
α-Keto adipic aciduria [271]	Psychomotor retardation	2-Keto adipic, 2-hydroxy adipic, 2-amino adipic, 1,2-butene dicarboxylic acids	Unknown
Lipoamide dehydrogenase deficiency [27, 287]	Infantile forms: psychomotor deterioration, persistent metabolic acidosis, occasional hypoglycemia; death in first year, juvenile forms with Friedreich's ataxia (disputed)	Lactic, pyruvic, 2-oxoglutaric acids	Deficiency of E_3 (third component of pyruvate oxyglutarate and branched chain ketoacid dehydrogenases)
Methyl-acetoacetic aciduria [71, 166, 286, 301]	Acute crises with vomiting, tachypnea, dehydration, ketosis, acidosis, hypoglycemia, coma. Forms of different severity	2-Methyl-acetoacetic, acetoacetic, 2-methyl-3-hydroxybutyric, 3-hydroxybutyric acids, tiglyl-glycine	3-Keto-thiolase deficiency
3-Methyl crotonyl-glycinuria [133, 335]	Vomiting, acidosis, ketosis, particular cat urine smell. Cases mimicking Werdnig-Hoffman disease	3-Methyl-crotonic, methyl-citric, 3-hydroxy-isovaleric, 3-hydroxy propionic acids; 3-methyl-crotonyl glycine, tiglyl-glycine	Methyl crotonyl CoA carboxylase (biotin responsive and unresponsive types)

TABLE XVI (continued)

Disease	Essential symptoms	Urinary organic acids	Basic defect
Methylmalonic aciduria, type I (mutase deficiency) [38, 140, 246, 336]	Acute neonatal forms: vomiting, dyspnea, coma Severe metabolic acidosis, ketosis, hypoglycemia, hyperammonemia, hyperglycinemia, osteoporosis, neutropenia, mental retardation Intermittent forms: acute crises with vomiting, ketosis, acidosis and coma	Methylmalonic, methylcitric, propionic, lactic acids	Methylmalonyl CoA mutase deficiency
Methylmalonic aciduria, type III (adenosyl B_{12} deficiency) [187, 232]			Defective synthesis of adenosyl B12
Methylmalonic aciduria, type IV (racemase deficiency) [182]			Methyl-malonyl CoA racemase deficiency
Methylmalonic aciduria with deranged sulfur metabolism, type II [83, 139]	Mental retardation, abnormal cerebellar and spinal cord function. Inconstant anemia; absence of ketosis and of acidosis; homocystinuria, cystathioninuria	Methylmalonic acid	Defective synthesis of adenosyl and methyl-cobalamins
Multiple carboxylase deficiency [135, 296, 389, 397]	Hypotonia, mental retardation, cutaneous rash, alopecia, immunodeficiency, metabolic crises with acidosis, ketosis	Pyruvic, lactic, propionic, 3-methylcrotonic acids and their metabolites	Holocarboxylase - synthetase (neonatal form) or Biotinidase (infantile form) deficiency
Orotic aciduria [324]	Megaloblastic anemia-neutropenia	Orotic acid	Orotate phosphoribosyl transferase or orotidine 5-phosphate decarboxylase deficiency
Primary oxaluria, type I	Nephrocalcinosis, nephrolithiasis, extrarenal oxalate deposits; renal failure	Oxalic, glycolic, glyoxylic acids	2-Oxyglutarate - glyoxylate-carboxy ligase deficiency
Primary oxaluria, type II		Oxalic, L-glyceric acids	D-Glyceric dehydrogenase deficiency
Propionic acidemia [63, 132, 343, 383]	Vomiting, coma, acidosis, ketosis, hyperammonemia, hyperglycinemia, pancytopenia, severe neonatal and acute intermittent forms	Propionic, 3-hydroxypropionic, methylcitric, 3-hydroxybutyric, 3-hydroxy-3-methylglutaric, 2-methyl-3-oxy valeric acids	Propionyl CoA carboxylase deficiency; biotin responsive and unresponsive types
Pyroglutamic aciduria [28, 201, 202]	Chronic hemolytic anemia, metabolic acidosis	Pyroglutamic acid	Glutathione-synthetase deficiency
Pyruvate carboxylase deficiency [366, 221]	Neonatal forms: metabolic acidosis, ketosis, hypoglycemia, hyperammonemia, rapid death. Infantile forms with Leigh's encephalopathy	Pyruvic, lactic acids	Pyruvate carboxylase deficiency
Pyruvate decarboxylase deficiency [27, 102]	Neonatal forms with metabolic acidosis, encephalopathy, death in first year. Juvenile cases with chronic ataxia (debated)	Pyruvic, lactic, 2-oxyglutaric acids	Deficiency of E_1 (first component of pyruvate dehydrogenase complex)

The second clinical form, called the chronic form, is characterised by episodes of vomiting, ketoacidosis, abnormal odor, and coma occuring after infections or protein ingestion. Between episodes, the infant may be normal [94] or can present with mental deficiency. Often, he or she spontaneously manifests a profound dislike of protein rich foods.

The accumulation of isovaleric acid is caused by a deficiency in isovaleryl CoA dehydrogenase, the enzyme necessary for the conversion of isovaleryl CoA to 3-methylcrotonyl CoA. This enzyme deficiency can be demonstrated in leukocytes, cultured fibroblasts or amniotic cells, thus making possible the prenatal diagnosis of this disorder [25]. Except during acute phases, the system conjugating isovaleric acid and glycine is very effective, since almost all of the non-metabolised isovaleryl CoA is excreted in the form of isovaleryl-glycine. Because of this fact and because of it's stability, isovaleryl-glycine has become the essential metabolite for diagnosis. During acute phases, the conjugating system is overloaded causing an increase in plasma and urinary levels of isovaleric acid, as well as 3-hydroxy-isovaleric acid. The latter probably derives from the omega-1 oxidation of isovaleric acid.

Methylmalonic acidemia. — Methylmalonic acidemia is the most frequent and most thoroughly studied organic acidemia. Since it's simultaneous discovery by Stokke [336] and Ober-

holzer [246] in 1967, almost fifty cases have been reported. The metabolic cause of this disorder is a deficiency in the conversion of methylmalonyl CoA (MMCoA) to succinyl CoA. This conversion occurs in two steps: transformation of D-MMCoA to succinyl CoA by the action of a mutase (Fig. IX-69). Three different types of deficiencies have been reported:

— deficiency in methylmalonyl CoA racemase [182],

— deficiency in methylmalonyl CoA apomutase, for which a number of enzymatic variants have been identified,

— deficiency in 5'-deoxyadenosyl B_{12}, an apomutase cofactor derived from vitamin B_{12}. This last type of deficiency can be subdivided into a number of distinct disorders. One of these disorders involves a deficiency in two cofactors, adenosyl B_{12} and methyl B_{12}, both derived from vitamin B_{12}. The generally moderate methylmalonic acidemia is accompanied by hypomethioninemia due to defective remethylation of homocysteine into methionine. A second type of disorder involves only adenosyl B_{12} and is caused by deficiency in one of the reductases or in adenosyltransferase, all necessary for it's synthesis (Fig. IX-68). A final disorder involves a binding deficiency between the apoenzyme and it's coenzyme [232].

Deficiencies in racemase, apomutase, or adenosyl B_{12} can all give similar clinical findings. These

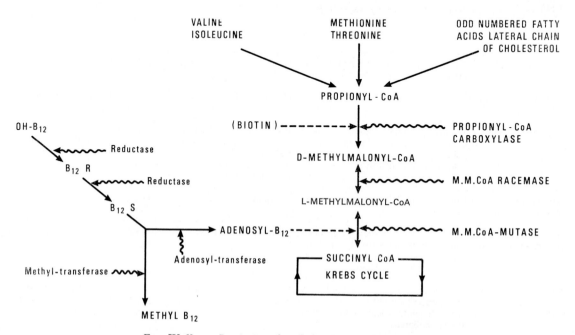

Fig. IX-69. — *Propionic and methyl malonic acid metabolism.*

deficiencies most often present as acute neonatal syndromes characterized by dyspnea, vomiting, hypotonia and alterations in consciousness. Laboratory findings include severe metabolic acidosis, ketosis and hyperglycinemia. Hypoglycemia, hyperammonemia, neutropenia, thrombopenia, or even pancytopenia are frequent associated findings. If the infant should survive, later manifestations can include psychomotor deficiency, failure to thrive, and osteoporosis. Intercurrent infections can cause acute relapses characterised by vomiting and eventual coma or death. Hyperuricemia is frequent and chronic tubulo-interstitial nephropathy can develop [38]. Besides this classical form, other clinical types have been reported including intermittent forms, characterized by episodes of vomiting, polypnea, lethargy and ketosis, and relatively benign adult forms [124].

Shortly after the discovery of methylmalonic acidemia, it was noted that some forms were insensitive to vitamin B_{12}, while others were sensitive to high doses of continuously administered B_{12}. The sensitive forms are caused by a deficiency in adenosyl B_{12} synthesis or in it's binding to the apoenzyme. However, results obtained "in vitro" with cultured skin fibroblasts did not necessarily parallel "in vivo" findings. Certain forms that were vitamin B_{12} sensitive "in vitro" were not so "in vivo" [187]. The diagnosis of methylmalonic acidemia is confirmed by MMA determinations in the blood and especially urine. MMA urinary excretion is extremely elevated, often exceeding several grams daily. Gas chromatography shows associated increases in propionic acid, and, during acute episodes, increases in ketone bodies and various metabolites [140]. Long chain neutral ketonuria (butanone, pentanone and hexanone) is also present. Forced diuresis and dialysis techniques are necessary in the management of acute crises. Outside of these acute periods, treatment consists of lowering protein intake. Some investigators prefer the use of amino acid substitutes lacking the principal MMA precursors (leucine, valine, threonine and methionine) given along with small quantities of natural proteins. In vitamin sensitive forms, in addition to daily administration of vitamin B_{12} (1 mg/24 hours IM or 10 mg/24 hours per os) it is necessary to prescribe a low protein diet since B_{12} sensitivity is usually incomplete. Prenatal diagnosis of the different types of MMA is possible [378]. Cultured amniotic cells can be used for enzyme analysis or for studies of ^{14}C incorporation into protein using labelled propionate. MMA levels are elevated in amniotic fluid and even maternal urine. Several investigators have treated vitamin B_{12} sensitive forms "in utero" by administration of massive doses of vitamin B_{12}

to the mother during the last 9 weeks of pregnancy.

Clinically very different from methylmalonic acidemia, is a syndrome associating methylmalonic aciduria, homocystinuria and hypomethioninemia. It's clinical manifestations include growth deficiency, convulsions and symptoms of cerebellar and posterior column lesions. Megaloblastic anemia can be present. Urinary excretion of methylmalonic acid and homocystine is considerably lower than in the classical forms of methylmalonic acidemia or homocytinuria. Before implicating a genetic abnormality serum B_{12} levels should be determined to eliminate the eventuality of a vitamin deficiency or absorption abnormality [379].

Propionic acidemia. — Propionic acidemia was first reported in 1968 in a newborn with severe metabolic acidosis who died on the 5th day of life. The cases presenting hyperglycinemia and ketosis reported by Childs [51] were secondarily shown to be propionic acidemias. Propionyl CoA carboxylase deficiency was demonstrated by several investigators [132, 173]. As in many organic acidemias, forms of varying severity have been described [63]; severe neonatal forms, intermittent forms, and even benign forms [258]. A less constant finding was reported by Wolf [383] who noted forms of different severity in the same sibship despite apparently similar "in vitro" enzyme deficiency. Complementary studies have demonstrated the genetic heterogeneity and the existence of numerous enzymatic variants [382]. Of particular interest are biotin sensitive forms which simultaneously involve other carboxylases requiring biotin as a cofactor; 3-methylcrotonyl-CoA carboxylase, acetyl CoA carboxylase, and pyruvate carboxylase [303]. Two distinct forms of biotin responsive multiple carboxylase deficiency are now recognized: an acute severe neonatal form due to holocarboxylase deficiency and a subacute form, due to biotinidase deficiency associating dermatologic (alopecia, dermatitis, chronic moniliasis) with neuro-psychic symptoms [389, 397].

During acute phases, characteristic findings include metabolic acidosis, ketosis, hyperammonemia, hyperlactacidemia, hyperglycinemia, and urinary excretion of long chain neutral ketone bodies. Pancytopenia can dominate the clinical picture [343].

Diagnosis depends on demonstrating the excess in propionic acid by chromatography of the volatile acids [263], and excesses in 3-hydroxypropionic acid, propionylglycine and methylcitric acid by G.C./M.S. Enzyme analysis can be done on leukocytes [132], fibroblasts [373], or amniotic cells, thus permitting the prenatal diagnosis of this disorder. During severe acute phases, in addition to peritoneal dialysis and exchange transfusion, treatment consists of administering sodium citrate [50] and glycine in elevated doses to encourage detoxification and renal elimination of propionic acid in the form of methyl-citrate and propionyl glycine. The existence of biotin sensitive forms justifies the systematic administration of biotin in large doses (20 mg/24 hours). Treatment during non acute periods is aimed at limiting intake of the principal propionic acid precursors (isoleucine, valine, threonine, and methionine) either by limiting protein intake to 1-1.5 g/kg/day, or by administering amino acid substitutes lacking these precursors along with a limited quantity of natural protein. Continuation of glycine administration appears justified.

Beta-ketothiolase deficiency. — This disorder in isoleucine metabolism was first reported by Hillman and Keating [166], then by Daum [71]. Forms of varying severity have been identified:

— severe forms characterized by continuous vomiting, hypotrophy, ketoacidosis and intolerance to normal protein intake,

— intermittent forms, evolving in episodes triggered by infections or surgery [301]. The clinical findings can be falsely attributed to salicylate intoxi-

cation, especially since excess amounts of methylace-toacetate and acetoacetate can interfere with sali-cylate determination [286]. Organic acid analysis shows excretion of 2-methylacetoacetate, as well as 2-methyl-3-hydroxybutyric acid and tiglic acid. The latter two are intermediary metabolites in isoleucine's breakdown to 2-methylacetoacetate (Fig. IX-64).

Hillman [166] also noted the presence of hyper-glycinemia and excretion of long chain neutral ketones bodies (butanone and to a lesser degree pentanone and hexanone). Robinson et al. [286] showed that the beta-ketothiolase deficiency (K^+ dependent) not only affected the beta-oxidation of 2-methylacetoacetate, but also that of acetoacetate and short chain beta-ketoacids produced during the final stages of fatty acid beta-oxidation. The accumulation of ketone bodies during acute episodes can be attributed to the insufficient conversion of acetoacetyl CoA to acetyl CoA. A deficiency in a slightly different type of acetoacetyl CoA thiolase has also been reported [74]. The treatment of acute episodes consists of alkalinizing and rehydrating with glucose solutions. After these episodes, protein restriction alone is sufficient. Part of the protein intake can be given in the form of amino acid substitutes lacking isoleucine.

Disorders of lipid metabolism

GENETIC DEFECTS IN THE BETA-OXIDATION OF FATTY ACIDS

In recent years a number of hereditary metabolic disorders affecting beta-oxidation have been reported. They are characterized by vomiting, alterations in consciousness, metabolic acidosis, severe hypoglycemia without ketosis, and hepatic and muscular lipid accumulation. These disorders present acute neonatal forms, fatal within several days (as in certain cases of type 2 glutaric aciduria), or intermittent forms in which clinical, laboratory, and histological findings resemble those found in Reye's syndrome [243].

Type 2-glutaric aciduria [137, 270]. — Also termed ethylmalonic aciduria [217], this disorder

is caused by a deficiency in acyl CoA dehydrogenases which simultaneously affect the catabolism of fatty acids derived from branched amino acids (isovaleric, isobutyric, alpha-methylbutyric acids) and trypto-phan (glutaric acid), as well as from long chain fatty acids (butyric acid, with excretion of adipic and ethylmalonic acid). The manifestations in this organic aciduria are very similar to those observed in Jamaican vomiting disease, caused by hypogly-cine, a vegetal toxin that inhibits the activity of the same acyl CoA dehydrogenases [348]. Type 2-glutaric aciduria presents either as a severe neonatal form with vomiting, coma, "sweaty feet" odor, hypoglycemia, hyperammonemia, and metabolic acidosis [137, 270, 344], or as an intermittent form evolving into episodes of hypoglycemia without ketosis [97].

Generalised carnitine deficiency [98, 126, 184]. — This disorder manifests itself in a similar manner, with episodes of acute encephalopathy, vomiting, lethargy, coma, hepatic failure, metabolic acidosis, hypoglycemia without ketosis, hepatic steatosis, and lipid myopathy. During acute episodes, findings resemble those of Reye's syndrome. Muscular weakness and predominantly proximal amyotrophy can be present. These abnormalities are due to a severe deficiency in carnitine, a substance to which long chain fatty acids are bound to allow their transport across the internal membrane of mitochondria where they undergo beta-oxidation. Another finding, although inconstant, is dicarboxylic aciduria with adipic, suberic, and sebacic acid, excretion [49, 126, 184]. Uncertainty still exists as to the origin of the carnitine deficiency [279].

C_6-C_{10}-dicarboxylic aciduria without ketosis.

— This entity clinically manifests itself as episodes of lethargy or coma with hypoglycemia. It is also due to a disorder in beta-oxidation of fatty acids [149 b, 241].

Carnitine-palmityl transferase (C.P.T.) deficiency [11, 84].

— In the forms generally observed in adults [84], this disorder is characterised primarily by muscular abnormalities including muscular pain, cramps, and myoglobinuria after strenuous physical activity. In the more commonly cited adolescent or adult forms the deficiency appears only to affect skeletal muscle while leaving other metabolic systems intact. Recently, Bougneres [31] reported an infant suffering from hepatic CPT deficiency responsible for fasting hypoglycemia and hypoketonemia. Mention should also be made of three cases reported by Hermier [165] in which an encephalopathy of undetermined origin was associated with CPT deficiency.

REFSUM'S DISEASE

Reported in 1945 as "heredopathia atactica polyneuritiformis", Refsum's disease appears in the second decade of life but occasionally between 5-10 years of age. Initial manifestations include visual abnormalities (hemeralopia) loss of equilibrium and motor deficiency, Schematically, clinical manifestations include [88, 334]:

— retinitis pigmentosa with hemeralopia and narrowing of the visual field,
— polyneuritis with hypertrophy of major nerves,

— cerebellar ataxia,
— perceptional deafness,
— anosmia,
— ichthyosis,
— epiphyseal dysplasia,
— cardiomyopathy,
— elevated C.S.F. protein levels without increases in the C. S. F. cell count.

The disease evolves in acute episodes interspersed with remissions of varying duration. Death can occur during these acute phases or unexpectedly during remission. Acute episodes can be triggered by infections or other stress by increasing endogenous catabolism liberating phytanic acid. Post mortem lipid studies in various tissues have demonstrated that in certain tissues (liver and kidney), phytanic acid constitutes more than half of the total fatty acid content. Serum levels of phytanic acid reach 50 to 500 times the normal level (N = 2 mg/ml) and thus provide an excellent means of diagnosis. The accumulation of phytanic acid is secondary to a deficiency in phytanate hydroxylase. This deficiency can be demonstrated in tissues and cultured fibroblasts or amniotic cells. Treatment is based on diets lacking phytanic acid (intake of less than 20 mg or if possible 10 mg/day). In practice, realization of such diets is difficult. Gibberd [121] emphasized the efficacy of associating plasma exchanges with these dietary measures.

Recently an infantile form of phytanic acid storage disease has been described associated with facial dysmorphy, hypotonia, deafness, retinitis pigmentosa, mental retardation, hepatomegaly hypocholesterolemia, and phytanic oxidase deficiency [388]. This disease has marked similarity to neonatal adrenoleukodystrophy, pipecolic acidemia, cerebrohepato-renal syndrome of Zellweger and contributes to the newly opened chapter of genetic peroxisomal disorders [391].

SPHINGOLIPIDOSES

Sphingolipidoses are lysosomal diseases resulting from deficiency in one of the lysosomal enzymes. Sphingolipids contain a ceramide portion composed of one molecule of sphingoside linked by an amide bond to one fatty acid molecule. The ceramide in its turn is bound to a phosphorylcholine radical (sphingomyelin) or to a carbohydrate chain which differs for each sphingolipid (Fig. IX-70).

Gangliosidoses [248]. — These disorders manifest themselves in infants as progressive encephalopathies, associating psychomotor deterioration, retinal lesions and a particular neuronal alteration called Schaffer-Spielmeyer utricular degeneration. Gangliosides are sphingolipids containing one or several molecules of N-acetylneuraminic acid (NANA). The different types of gangliosides are distinguished by the number of sialic acids and the length of the carbohydrate chain.

GM_1 gangliosidoses. — These disorders are caused by deficiencies in beta-galactosidase responsible for GM_1 breakdown in the CNS (Fig. IX-70).

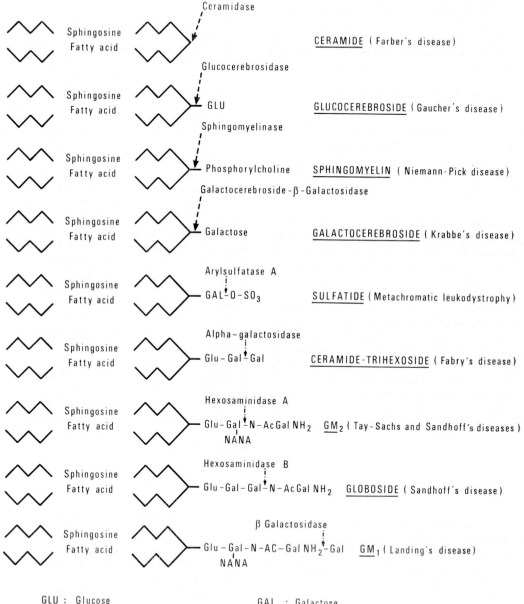

FIG. IX-70. — *Schematic representation of the enzyme deficiencies and accumulated sphingolipid in various sphingolipidoses.*

Other beta-galactosidases act on different substrates. In GM_1 gangliosidosis, the beta-galactosidase deficiency is responsible for the accumulation of GM_1 in the brain and retina, and the accumulation of other beta-galactosides in particular a polysaccharide resembling keratan-sulfate in the viscera. This explains the analogies noted between Landing's disease and certain mucopolysaccharidoses such as Hurler's disease.

(a) *Generalised GM_1 gangliosidosis type 1.* — Also called Landing's disease [200, 295], this disorder appears in the first weeks after birth. Initially, one notes neonatal edema affecting the face and extremities, and occasionally ascites. After several months, facial dysmorphism becomes evident, with enlarged skull, large forehead, coarse facial features, flattened nose, low-set ears, macroglossia, and hypertelorism. These physical features resemble those found in Hurler's disease. Progressive psychomotor deterioration is a constant finding. The infant is hypoactive and hypotonic. Episodes of muscular contraction and myoclonia are frequent. Hepatosplenomegaly is almost always present. The infant is often blind and deaf. Respiratory infections are frequent and death generally ensues in 2 or 3 years.

In half of the cases, cherry red spots are seen on ophthalmoscopic examination. The cornea is sometimes opalescent. Radiologically, one notes a hypoplasia of the antero-superior portions of one or two lumbar vertebrae similar to that seen in Hurler's disease. The long bones, metacarpals, and phalanges are short and thick. Lymphocytes are vacuolated. Histological studies provide evidence of the storage abnormalities in a variety of organs. Electron microscopy of cells from most organs reveals voluminous vacuoles containing a low density granular substance. These vacuoles are identical to those observed in the mucopolysaccharidoses. In nerve cells, membranous cytoplasmic bodies, similar to those in Tay-Sach's disease are present. Biochemical analysis shows the mixed nature of the storage material. GM_1 accumulates in the brain and, to a lesser degree, in the viscera while a mucopolysaccharide resembling keratan-sulfate accumulates only in the viscera. Beta-galactosidase deficiency can be demonstrated in serum, leukocytes, fibroblasts, and amniotic cells. Prenatal diagnosis is possible [180]. This disorder is transmitted in an autosomal recessive manner. Heterozygous states can be detected by enzyme analysis.

(b) *GM_1 gangliosidosis type 2: juvenile form* [215, 248]. — Type 2 is very rare. It can be distinguished from Landing's disease by it's later onset (6 to 20 months), absence of dysmorphism, and presence of visceral and ophthalmologic symptoms. It presents as a progressive mental deterioration with hypotonia followed by spastic quadriplegia and convulsions. Death occurs in a context of decerebration in 3 to 10 years. The enzyme deficiency is severe, although less so than in Landing's disease. Prenatal diagnosis is possible, as is the diagnosis of homozygous and heterozygous states.

(c) *Later forms of beta-galactosidase deficiency.* — These forms are characterized by ataxia, myoclonia, pyramidal and extrapyramidal symptoms, retinal red spot, and coarse facial features. Their differential diagnosis from the sialidoses can be difficult. The sialidoses present an absence of neuraminidase activity in addition to the partial deficiency in beta-galactosidase (see section on mucolipidoses).

GM_2 gangliosidoses.

(a) *Tay-Sachs disease (GM_2 gangliosidosis, type 1).* — This disorder is caused by a deficiency in hexosaminidase A as demonstrated in the serum, tears, leukocytes, fibroblasts or amniotic cells. GM_2 accumulates in the neurons of the CNS, retina, and Auerbach's plexus (diagnostic value of rectal biopsies). The disease is much more prevalent among Ashkenasi Jews, with an incidence of 1/3,600 births, whereas the incidence in other populations is only 1/360,000 births. Symptoms appear 3 to 6 months after birth and include psychomotor deficiency, hypotonia, convulsions, and exaggerated reactions to noise. Audiogenic myoclonia, often mistaken for hyperacousis, are very characteristic. Deglutitional complications and infections eventually lead to death by 2 to 5 years of age. Ophthalmoscopic examination reveals an infiltrated cream-colored macula with a central cherry-red spot. Transaminase and LDH levels are elevated. Characteristic cytologic alterations can be noted in the brain, retinal ganglion cells and Auerbach's plexus after rectal biopsy. The utricular neurons present dilated perikaryons containing a storage material that stains with PAS and lipid stains. Electron microscopy reveals the presence of membranous cytoplasmic bodies (M. C. B.) composed of a central core of variable density surrounded by concentric layers. This disorder is inherited in an autosomal recessive manner. Prenatal diagnosis and diagnosis of heterozygote states are possible. Some heterozygote individuals can show apparently complete enzyme deficiency when artificial substrates (such as methylumbelliferyl-N-acetyl-β-D-glucosaminide) are used. In such circumstances labelled natural substrate (e. g. ganglioside GM_2 tritiated in its Gal NAC portion) should be used to distinguish, enzymatically, heterozygotes from affected homozygotes. For this reason, accurate prenatal diagnosis requires prior enzyme analysis of the parents [240].

(b) *Sandhoff's disease: GM₂ gangliosidosis, type 2.* — Sandhoff's disease is caused by a deficiency in hexosaminidase A and B resulting from an abnormality in the "beta" subunit common to both enzymes [332]. In addition to the GM_2 accumulation in the brain and retina there is a visceral accumulation (liver, spleen, and kidneys) of a ganglioside termed globoside [297]. Sandhoff's disease presents the same clinical manifestations as Tay-Sach's disease. Histological studies (liver biopsy), biochemical analysis (excess globoside in the serum, urine, and tissues), and enzyme analysis are necessary to differentiate these two diseases [365]. Prenatal diagnosis and diagnosis of heterozygous states are possible. However, here again, prior enzyme analysis of the parents is necessary to eliminate the possibility of an apparent total deficiency in heterozygotes [86]. There is no ethnic predisposition for this disease.

(c) *GM₂ gangliosidosis AB variant.* — Reported by Sandhoff [297] and more recently by De Baecque [72], this disorder presents manifestations very similar to those in Tay-Sach's disease, although somewhat less severe. Despite the accumulation of GM_2 in the brain and retina, the activity of both hexosaminidases remains normal when determined with ordinary artificial substrates. The cause of this disorder is an abnormality in a nonenzymatic protein necessary for the interaction between the water soluble enzyme and its glycolipid substrate [61].

(d) *Juvenile form of GM₂ gangliosidosis.* — Less severe than the preceding forms, this form becomes apparent at 2 to 10 years of age. Findings include ataxia, spasticity, progressive mental deterioration and blindness. Death usually follows at 5 to 15 years of age. This disorder results from a deficiency either in hexosaminidase A (type III [37]) or in hexosaminidase A and B (type IV [211]).

(e) *Adult form of GM₂ gangliosidosis.* — Reported by Rapin, then Kaback, this form clinically resembles spinocerebellar degeneration [277] or amyotrophic lateral sclerosis [181].

GM₃ gangliosidosis. — Clinically distinct from the preceding gangliosidoses, this disorder has been termed GM_3 sphingolipodystrophy [222] or cerebral spongiosis with GM_3 gangliosidosis [347]. Manifestations are first noted at birth and include hypotonia,

convulsions and dysmorphism characterised by macroglossia, hypertrophic gums, thickened skin, and hirsutism. The infant generally dies in several months. Autopsy reveals a spongiosis of the white matter similar to that reported by Van Bogaert and Bertrand, as spongious degeneration. Sphingolipid analysis shows a considerable increase in GM_3 ganglioside while the GM_1 and GM_2 analogues are absent. These abnormalities are not caused by defective catabolism, but rather by a disorder in the biosynthesis of GM_2 and GM_1 from GM_3 by deficiency in N-acetylgalactosaminyl transferase [222]. Thus, contrary to the other gangliosidoses, this disorder is not lysosomal.

Niemann-Pick disease [32]. — Even more so than the other sphingolipidoses, Niemann-Pick disease cannot be considered a single entity but as a group of separate diseases (Table XVII). In 1960, Croker [66] distinguished four distinct types according to differences in age of onset, rate of progression and neurological symptoms. Initially individualized by the presence of characteristic foam cells termed Pick cells, this disorder is now defined as an autosomal recessive hereditary disease with sphingomyelin accumulation. Sphingomyelin is a sphingolipid present in a variety of tissues since it is a normal constituent of cell membranes and myelin. It is composed of a sphingosine portion (ceramide) bound to phosphorylcholine by a phosphodiester bond. Lipids other than sphingomyelin can also be present in excessive quantities, including cholesterol, lysobiphosphatidic acid, and other sphingolipids.

Type A Niemann-Pick disease. — In type A, accumulation of sphingomyelin in the viscera and nervous system results from a severe deficiency in sphingomyelinase (0 to 9 % of normal activity). Sphingomyelinase is a lysosomal enzyme that catalyses sphingomyelin's breakdown to ceramide and phosphorylcholine. Occasionally, symptoms are already present at birth (jaundice or generalized edema). After several weeks, neurological and visceral involvement becomes evident, with hepatosplenomegaly, hypotonia, psychomotor deterioration, feeding difficulties, and cachexia. Cherry-red spots are sometimes seen on ophthalmoscopic examination. The disease progresses rapidly and is usually fatal before 3 years of age. Labelled sphingomyelin or an artificial chromogenic analogue of sphingomyelin can be used for determining sphingomyelinase activity in leukocytes, skin fibroblasts, or cultured amniotic cells [32, 231]. Heterozygous states can be diagnosed by enzyme analysis.

TABLE XVII. — Different types of Niemann-Pick's disease

Disease	Age of first symptoms	Clinical symptoms	Survival	Basic defect
Niemann-Pick Type A	Before 6 months	Occasionally jaundice and ascites in neonates; hepatomegaly, splenomegaly, cachexia, severe mental regression	Less than 3 years	Sphingomyelinase (0 to 9 %)
Niemann-Pick Type B	Variable (infancy to adulthood)	Hepato-splenomegaly; reticulo-micronodular pulmonary infiltrate; absence of neurological symptom	Very long	Sphingomyelinase (15 to 20 %)
Niemann-Pick Type C Classical form	1 to 2 years	Neurological dysfunction: seizures myoclonia, spasticity; mental regression: mild hepato-splenomegaly	5 to 15 years	? Sphingomyelinase (exact defect still debated)
Niemann-Pick Type C Infantile form	Neonate	Neonatal cholestatic jaundice; hepato-splenomegaly; cachexia; absent or mild neurological symptoms	About 3 months	? Sphingomyelinase (exact defect still debated)
Niemann-Pick Type D	2 to 4 years	Mental deterioration; ataxia; seizures; mild hepato-splenomegaly	12 to 20 years	? Perhaps similar to type C
Niemann-Pick Type E	Adulthood	Mild hepato-splenomegaly	Long	?

Type B Niemann-Pick disease. — Individuals presenting type B show no signs of neurological involvement. Visceral manifestation include hepato-splenomegaly, an interstitial pulmonary infiltrate, predisposition to respiratory infections, and repeated episodes of pneumothorax. The disease is discovered at various ages, often during adolescence or adulthood. The diagnosis is confirmed by the presence of Pick cells in the myelogram, characteristic inclusions in various tissues studied by electron microscopy, accumulation of sphingomyelin in cultured cells and sphingomyelinase deficiency. The enzyme deficiency (15-20 % of normal values) is less severe than in type A. A possible explanation for the absence of neurological involvement in type B might be the existence of two distinct isoenzymes; isoenzyme A which provides 30-40 % of the cerebral "sphingomyelinase" activity, and isoenzyme B, which provides nearly all of the hepatic "sphingomyelinase" activity. Analogous to what has been demonstrated in GM_2 gangliosidosis, it is probable that isoenzymes A and B are both deficient in type A while only isoenzyme B is deficient in type B.

Type C Niemann-Pick disease. — In type C or the "subacute" form of Niemann-Pick disease,

symptoms first appear at 3-4 years of age, represented by convulsions, myoclonia, and spasticity. Hepatosplenomegaly is more moderate than in type A and B. Death usually occurs at 5 to 15 years of age. Sphingomyelin, cholesterol and lysobiphosphatidic acid accumulation is less severe than in type A and B, and sphingomyelinase activity in tissues is often paradoxically normal. Sphingomyelinase activity in fibroblasts can be decreased to a variable extent, thus allowing for prenatal diagnosis in certain cases [161]. As indicated by Christomanou's studies [53], this disorder appears to be caused by a deficiency in a non-protein activator, as in the AB variant of GM_2 gangliosidosis. This non-protein activator is probably a co-hydrolase necessary for the enzyme's interaction with it's lipid substrate. The individualization of type C according to age of onset or prognostic criteria is debatable, as indicated in a recent study by Guibaud [152]. From two personal observations and similar reported cases, these investigators identified a rapidly fatal cholestatic form of type C Niemann-Pick disease presenting as jaundice and hepatosplenomegaly. Neurological symptoms are absent or appear only secondarily. Biochemical and enzymatic findings are the same as in type C.

Type D Niemann-Pick disease. — Cases of type D were initially reported among French Canadians living in Nova Scotia. Neurological symptoms are discovered at 2 to 3 years of age and progress to quadriplegia and dementia by age 12 to 20. Type D is very similar to type C and to various other cases reported by Dunn, Holland, Kornfeld, Neville, Norman, and most recently Wenger [372]. These cases showed discretely or moderately elevated cholesterol and sphingomyelin levels in the tissues studied, and a normal or moderately decreased sphingomyelinase activity, thus making their biological phenotypes indistinguishable from that of type C. Occasionally, "sea-blue" histiocytes are observed instead of Pick cells [372].

Type E Niemann-Pick disease. — This fifth type was added to the classification by Fredrickson and Sloan to include adult cases that could not be classified with the other types. Moderate hepatosplenomegaly, discrete hepatic and renal increases in sphingomyelin content, and normal or moderately decreased sphingomyelinase activities have been reported in cases of this type [32].

Gaucher's disease [33]. — Biochemically characterised by the accumulation of glucocerebroside due to a deficiency in lysosomal glucocerebrosidase, Gaucher's disease is divided into three genetically distinct forms, all of autosomal recessive inheritance.

Type I. — This form, also termed the adult form or chronic form, is the most frequent. Major clinical manifestations include hepatosplenomegaly, anemia, thrombocytopenia, bone lesions including rarefaction of the cortex and episodes of aseptic osteomyelitis caused by focal vascular necrosis, yellow-brown pigmentation of the skin, and pulmonary interstitial infiltrates. There is no nervous system involvement. Patients with this diseases can live long lives. A diagnostically orienting laboratory finding is an increased serum acid phosphatase level. Histological examination of bone marrow and other tissues demonstrates the presence of Gaucher's cells identified by their filamentous cytoplasm. Characteristic tubular inclusions are seen on ultrastructural examination. The enzyme deficiency (12 to 45 % of normal) can be demonstrated using artificial substrates in either leukocytes, fibroblasts or cultured amniotic cells. Test conditions must be carefully controlled in order to accurately analyse the deficient isoenzyme (optimal activity at pH 4) [273]. This is particularly true for the diagnosis of heterozygotes and for prenatal diagnosis.

Type II. — Also termed the acute infantile form, type II is distinguished from the other forms by the severity of the nervous system involvement. Symptoms become evident at 4 to 6 months of age, and include abdominal distension, voluminous hepatosplenomegaly, rapid mental deterioration, and spastic quadriplegia with opisthotonus. Patients generally die before 1 year of age. Gaucher's cells are present in the viscera and bone marrow. Serum acid phosphatase activity is elevated. Beta-glucosidase activity is decreased in leukocytes, cultured fibroblasts and amniotic cells. The enzyme deficiency is more severe than in the adult form [33].

Type III. — Type III represents a more heterogeneous group including older children with hepatosplenomegaly and neurological abnormalities. In most cases, neurological involvement is limited to convulsions or EEG alterations. In some cases, hypertonia, tremor, walking and coordination abnormalities and mental deficiency have been noted. Beta-glucosidase activity ranges from 6 to 15 % of normal values when determined with natural substrates and from 15 to 45 % with artificial substrates [342].

Metachromatic leukodystrophy (MLD). — Biochemically, this disease is characterised by the lysosomal accumulation of sulfatides in the nervous system caused by a deficiency in cerebroside sulfatase (also known as arylsulfatase A). MLD (or sulfatidosis) is of autosomal recessive inheritance. Neuropathologically, this disorder is characterized by myelin degeneration in the central and peripheral nervous system, with accumulation of metachromatic granules, corresponding to sulfatides, in the cytoplasm of oligodendrocytes, Schwann cells, and macrophages. Ultrastructural studies show a characteristic prism and herring-bone arrangement to these inclusions. MLD is commonly divided into 4 types according to the age of onset and rate of progression.

Congenital form of MLD. — This form is extremely rare. It is fatal within several days after birth [40].

Late infantile form of MLD. — This form is the most frequent, with it's incidence estimated at 1/40,000 births [91]. Symptoms appear at age 1 to 4, and involve the peripheral nervous system: hypotonia, muscular deficiency and decreased tendon reflexes. These findings generally precede manifestations of central nervous system involvement including pyramidal symptoms and mental deterioration. Occasionally however, initial symptoms can include diplegia or spastic paraplegia. The disease progresses rapidly with aggravation of neurological symptoms, mental deterioration leading to quadriplegia, blindness and death.

Juvenile form of MLD. — This form becomes apparent between 5 and 21 years of age. Initial findings most often include motor and language deficiencies, hand tremor, and coordination abnormalities. The disease progressively leads to mental deterioration, convulsions, spastic tetraplegia, bulbar involvement, and death within several years. In some cases, despite early onset and severe mental retardation in the first years of life, the disease progresses more slowly than in the classical late infantile form with additional neurological symptoms appearing only 9 to 10 years later [156].

Adult forms of MLD. — This form is defined to include the cases appearing after 21 years of age. Symptoms resemble schizophrenia or organic dementia. Neurological findings such as motor abnormalities, ataxia, convulsions, and pyramidal and extrapyramidal signs appear much later. Diagnostically helpful laboratory findings include increased CSF protein levels, decreased nerve conduction velocity, and abnormal sulfatiduria. Histochemical and ultrastructural studies on biopsied peripheral nerves demonstrate their metachromatic nature and characteristic inclusions. Decreases in arylsulfatase A activity are easily demonstrated with artificial substrates in leukocytes and cultured fibroblasts. Despite major differences in their clinical presentation, the four types of MLD demonstrate approximately identical enzyme activities [90, 91, 156]. Heterozygotes are identified by the partial nature of their enzyme deficiency. However, since certain heterozygotes demonstrate very low enzyme activity despite the absence of any clinical manifestations, prenatal diagnosis can only be considered after identification of obligatory heterozygotes.

Mucosulfatidosis [6, 91]. — This fifth type of MLD is very different from the previous types. In mucosulfatidosis, the three arylsulfatases (A, B and C) are inactive. The inactivity of B arylsulfatase is responsible for the associated mucopolysaccharide accumulation. Symptoms appear before two years of age. In addition to the neurological manifestations of MLD, mucosulfatidosis is characterised by coarse facial features, hepatosplenomegaly, Adler-Reilly inclusions, in leukocytes, and bone lesions similar to those seen in mucopolysaccharidosis. Excess quantities of dermatan and keratan sulfates are

found in the urine. This disease is also of autosomal recessive inheritance. Prenatal diagnosis and diagnosis of heterozygous states are possible.

Krabbe's disease: globoid leukodystrophy. — Krabbe's disease is characterised by severe diffuse demyelination in the central and peripheral nervous system. Giant multinucleated cells called globoid cells are present in the white matter. Ultrastructural studies of peripheral nerve biopsies show characteristic inclusions in the globoid cells as well as in Schwann cells [210]. In the white matter, a major decrease in sulfatide content is contrasted with a relatively conserved cerebroside content, suggesting a deficit in galacto-cerebroside catabolism. Suzuki [339] demonstrated that the deficit was due to a deficiency in galacto-cerebroside beta-galactosidase.

Classical acute form. — Symptoms are first noted at 1 to 6 months and include vomiting, irritability, and psychomotor regression. Mental deterioration, spasticity, and episodes of hypertonia with opisthotonus usually lead to decerebrate rigidity. Occasionally, peripheral nerve lesions can result in hypotonia. Additional manifestations can include blindness, convulsions, respiratory infections, and cachexia. Death occurs at 6 months to 3 years of age. Diagnostically helpful findings include elevated CSF protein levels, decreased nerve conduction velocity, and optic nerve atrophy. Ultrastructural studies of peripheral nerve biopsies and enzyme analysis confirm the diagnosis. The enzyme deficiency can be demonstrated in serum, leukocytes, and cultured fibroblasts. Prenatal diagnosis is possible [340]; in heterozygotes, cerebroside beta-galactosidase activity is intermediate between normal and homozygote values. The use of artificial substrates has facilitated enzyme analysis [20].

Juvenile form. — This form has a later onset and progresses much more slowly. Major clinical findings include pyramidal symptoms, optic nerve atrophy and mental deterioration. Peripheral neuropathy and CSF protein elevations can be absent [67]. In the few cases reported, cerebroside beta-galactosidase activity was extremely low [339].

Fabry's disease. — Also known as "angiokeratoma corporis diffusum universale", this genetic disorder is transmitted as an incomplete recessive (intermediate) X-linked trait. It is characterized by an accumulation of ceramide trihexoside (galactosyl-galactosyl-glucosyl-ceramide) and dihexosyl ceramide (digalactosylceramide) resulting from a deficiency in alpha-galactosidase A [78]. This accumulation is found in the walls of blood vessels located in the skin, kidneys, heart, and nervous system. Vacuolated cells contain a glycolipid storage material in the cytoplasm and characteristic dense, osmiophilic, lamellar inclusions.

Clinical manifestations are consequences of the glycolipid accumulation in the tissues. They include acroparesthesia and a chronic burning sensation in the hands and feet. Periodic crises of severe pain are accompanied by moderate fever and increase in sedimentation rate. Since these manifestations appear during childhood or adolescence before the appearance of characteristic cutaneous lesions, diagnostic confusion is frequent. The presence of angiokeratomas is very characteristic. Generally, they slowly develop between the umbilicus and knees as clusters of small red or blue-black angiectasies that are flat or slightly elevated and discretely hyperkeratotic. These angiokeratomas are not absolutely pathognomonic since they are also seen in alpha-L-fucosidase deficiency [100]. As the patient ages, the diffuse vascular lesions become more severe and can lead to vascular accidents such as myocardial infarction or stroke. Progressive renal involvement is a constant finding, initially presenting as proteinuria, polyuria and a tubulopathy. Renal insufficiency and death are inevitable unless hemodialysis and kidney transplant are carried out. The cardiac, pulmonary, digestive, muscular and bone lesions in this disorder give rise to a number of clinical findings. Eye manifestations are frequent and are of considerable diagnostic value. Abnormalities such as tortuous retinal and conjunctival blood vessels, and characteristic corneal opacities consisting of whorled opaque bands are of help in diagnosis even though they are not specific for this disorder (amodiarone and chloroquine therapy can give similar findings). Manifestations are often observed in heterozygous females; corneal dystrophy, cutaneous lesions, crises of pain in the extremities, and even renal lesions have been noted [150]. However, these female heterozygous forms can be asymptomatic, or on the contrary, as severe as the male hemizygous forms. From a laboratory standpoint, diagnosis is confirmed by the abnormal urinary excretion of di- and trihexoxylceramides and by enzyme analysis. In hemizygous males, the activity of alpha-galactosidase (measured with natural substrates or even more easily with artificial substrates) is greatly decreased in serum, leukocytes, cultured fibroblasts and amniotic cells. Enzyme analysis is possible in heterozygous females [108]. Diphenylhydantoin and carbamazepine are the most effective drugs for treating the periodic crises of excruciating pain in the extremities. Renal allografts have given satisfactory results in patients with severe renal failure [265]. Recently, Brady et al. [34] have reported promising results with injections of alpha-galactosidase purified from human placenta by a method they had previously used in Gaucher's disease. Touraine [356] has proposed fetal liver transplants.

Farber's disease. — This autosomal recessive disorder is characterised by a generalised accumulation of ceramide in tissues. It is caused by a deficiency in lysosomal acid ceramidase. In the severe form, findings include periarticular and subcutaneous nodules, limitation of joint movement, hoarseness, pulmonary infiltrates, mental deficiency and cachexia. Death occurs by the age of 2 years. In the less severe variant, hoarseness and mental deficiency may be absent. Survival is prolonged to adolescence or adulthood [233, 259]. The diagnosis of heterozygous states and prenatal diagnosis are possible by enzyme analysis.

WOLMAN'S DISEASE
AND CHOLESTEROL ESTER
STORAGE DISEASES

Wolman's disease is an autosomal recessive disorder caused by a generalized accumulation of triglycerides and cholesterol esters due to the inactivity of lysosomal acid lipase [114]. Manifestations are first noticed a few weeks after birth and include vomiting, diarrhea, marked hypotrophy, abdominal distension and hepatosplenomegaly. In a few cases, jaundice and persistent fever have been noted. Death generally occurs before 6 months of age. The most suggestive finding is an adrenal enlargement characterised by it's regularity and the presence of small calcifications. These calcifications are present in almost [304] all patients and are easily seen on X-rays. Massive lipid accumulation is observed in the adrenal glands, intestinal lamina propria, mesenteric lymph nodes, liver and kidneys. Electron microscopy demonstrates the presence of lipid droplets and crystals of cholesterol in the vacuolated cytoplasm. Characteristic lysosomal inclusions containing neutral fats and cholesterol crystals are observed in cultured fibroblasts [367]. Acid lipase inactivity can be demonstrated in tissues, leukocytes, cultured fibroblasts and amniotic fluid cells. As in all hereditary lysosomal disorders, there exists a relatively benign variant of this disorder, caused by a deficiency in acid esterase. Initially reported by Lageron and by Infante et al. [176, 199], this form presents with hepatomegaly, hepatic accumulation of triglycerides and cholesterol, hyperlipemia, splenomegaly, portal hypertension, infiltration of the intestinal mucosa by lipid containing histiocytes, and premature atherosclerosis. The enzyme deficiency is demonstrable in the various tissues, leukocytes, and cultured fibroblasts. Forms that are intermediate between Wolman's disease and hepatic cholesterol ester storage disease have been reported [14, 114].

LIPOPROTEIN DISORDERS

Familial lipoprotein deficiencies. — Three genetic disorders have been distinguished in which one or several classes of lipoproteins are absent in the plasma or are present in abnormally low concentrations. Abetalipoproteinemia was the first disorder reported and is characterised by absence of chylomicrons, V. L. D. L. and L. D. L. The second disorder is hypobetalipoproteinemia characterised by extremely low L. D. L. levels, and the third is Tangier's disease characterised by H. D. L. deficiency.

Abetalipoproteinemia. — Other synonyms for this rare disorder include Bassen-Kornzweig's disease, acanthocytosis, and congenital absence of β-lipoproteins or L. D. L. The hallmarks of this disorder are: abetalipoproteinemia, fat malabsorption, acanthocytosis, pigmented retinitis and ataxia. The steatorrhea noted soon after birth is associated with a malabsorption of the fat soluble vitamins (A, D, E, K) that also results in hypotrophy. On histological examination the cytoplasm of the enterocytes is vacuolised with lipid droplets and there is hepatic steatosis without fibrosis. Psychomotor retardation is a later finding. There is a progressive spino-cerebellar syndrome associating posterior column and cerebellar findings with skeletal abnormalities (hollow foot, kyphoscoliosis or hyperlordosis). Eye involvement is constant as evidenced by a pigmented retinitis (seconde decade), decreased visual acuity, nystagmus and ophthalmoplegia.

Acanthocytes are present in the blood (50-70 %). These are erythrocytes of decreased half life that have a characteristic sea-urchin shape and whose sodium pumping mechanism is defective [107]. Anemia becomes severe early in childhood.

Abetalipoproteinemia yields severe disturbances in plasma lipids, with concentrations lowered to less than 50 %. Triglycerides are often undetectable, phospholipids are lowered by 75 %, and cholesterolemia is often lower than 0.25 g/l. No beta-lipoproteins are found on lipoprotein electrophoresis. Analytic ultra-centrifugation demonstrates an absence of L. D. L., chylomicrons, and V. L. D. L. Apolipoprotein B (apo B) is absent in the plasma.

The primary defect is probably a disorder in apo B synthesis [164]. The endoluminal phase of fat digestion is most likley normal. In enterocytes, triglycerides do not receive their normal apoprotein envelope and cannot be transported into Golgi bodies for use as lipoprotein precursors. Lipoproteins are not synthesized and therefore do not enter the lymphatic channels.

Abetalipoproteinemia is of autosomal recessive inheritance and affects males more than females. More than a quarter of the cases published involve Ashkenazi Jews. Obligatory heterozygotes present no detectable clinical or biological abnormalities in contrast to that which is seen in hypobetalipoproteinemia.

Symptomatic treatment essentially consists of early initiation of dietary measures: prescription of medium chain triglycerides (MCT) using products such as Triceme, Liprocil or Pregestimil, supplementation of fat soluble vitamins, and a decrease or elimination of long chain triglycerides. Long term utilization of MCT necessitates surveillance of possible hepatic changes. These dietary measures improve digestion and can prevent retinal and neurological effects (especially long term administration of vitamin E).

Hypobetalipoproteinemia. — Hypobetalipoproteinemia is an extremely rare disorder inherited as an autosomal dominant trait. It is characterized by severe hypocholesterolemia and hypotriglyceridemia. Beta-lipoproteins (L. D. L.), pre-beta-lipoproteins (V. L. D. L.), and apo B are all absent in the plasma [164]. Heterozygote forms require no treatment. Homozygous forms are treated with supplemental administration of fat soluble vitamins.

Although quite similar, abetalipoproteinemia and hypobetalipoproteinemia are considered as distinct disorders by the majority of authors. A major difference is that hypobetalipoproteinemia heterozygotes cannot maintain normal L. D. L. levels, while in abetalipoproteinemia no clinical or biochemical abnormalities are present in heterozygotes.

Tangier's disease. — This extremely rare autosomal recessive disorder is characterised by severe plasma H. D. L. deficiency and an accumulation of cholesterol esters in a variety of tissues. Homozygotes present a marked hypocholesterolemia with normal or elevated triglyceridemia, and a characteristic hypertrophy of the tonsils which are covered with yellow-orange bands. These esters also accumulate in other organs including the spleen, thymus, intestinal mucosa, skin, liver and lymphatic ganglia. A peripheral neuropathy is sometimes noted. Heterozygotes have lowered plasma H. D. L. levels (50 % of normal) but no tissue accumulation. H. D. L. deficiency causes the formation of abnormal chylomicron residues which can be phagocytized by histiocytes explaining the presence of cholesterol esters in these cells. The primary defect seems to be an abnormality in apolipoprotein A_1 which results in hypercatabolism of H. D. L. constituents. Other kinds of apolipoprotein A_1 abnormalities have been observed in H. D. L. deficient states.

The hyperlipoproteinemias.

— The hyperlipoproteinemias (HLP) are characterised by plasma increases in either cholesterol or triglycerides or both. They can be classified into primary or secondary hyperlipoproteinemias. Most often, they are secondary to other diseases—a possibility that should be systematically excluded in all children with hyperlipidemia. Hepato-biliary diseases such as intra- or extrahepatic cholestasis can result in hypercholesterolemia. Other less frequent causes include endocrine disorders (myxedema, Cushing's syndrome), pancreatic disorders (acute or chronic pancreatitis), type I glycogenosis, diabetic ketosis, nephrotic syndrome, lupus erythematosus and terminal renal failure. Primary hyperlipoproteinemias [114 *b*] are less frequent. They are classified according to biochemical criteria (De Gennes), electrophoretic migration patterns (Fredrickson), or their apoproteins (Alaupovic). The different types of HLP are indicated in Table XVIII. We shall only discuss types I and II since they are the principal forms encountered in children.

Type I hyperlipoproteinemia.

— Synonyms: essential fat induced hyperlipemia, familial hypertriglyceridemias, hyperchylomicronemia, Burger-Grutz disease, familial lipoprotein-lipase deficiency. Extremely rare during childhood, this disorder is characterised by a marked increase in plasma triglycerides (from 10 to 100 g/l). Most often the disorder is accidently discovered due to the serum's lactescent appearance; the chylomicrons float spontaneously to the top after several hours of decantation at + 4° C forming a cream layer on top of a clear plasma infranatant layer. Occasionally the disorder is discovered as a glyceridemic syndrome; abdominal

pain, pancreatitis, eruptive xanthomatosis, hepatomegaly, steatosis, splenomegaly, fatigue and postprandial sleepiness. Ophtalmoscopic examination may show retinal lipemia. Foam cells are seen in the bone marrow. X-rays reveal characteristic bone lesions (filling defects, rarefaction of the matrix, or densification). The major complication is acute hemorrhagic pancreatitis. Atherogenesis is not usual.

The serum is lactescent because of the severe hypertriglyceridemia. Plasma cholesterol levels are normal or slightly elevated and the triglyceride/cholesterol ratio is greater than 2.5. Electrophoresis demonstrates a hyperchylomicronemia and a 25 % reduction in HDL and LDL. Apoproteins A_I and A_{II} are decreased as well as apo B to a lesser degree [284]. Apo C_{II}, an activator of lipoprotein lipase, is increased. This last finding is of interest since type I HLP is supposedly caused by a deficiency in lipoprotein lipase (or more precisely, extrahepatic triglyceride lipase). The increase in apo C_{II} may be a compensatory mechanism. Heterozygous subjects demonstrate enzyme activity that is intermediate between that found in homozygotes and normal subjects. Variants have been reported in which enzyme activity is only deficient on natural substrates but not on artificial substrates. These cases illustrate the genetic heterogeneity of this disorder. Finally, cases have been reported in which an apo C_{II} deficiency was found along with extremely low lipoprotein lipase activity.

Type I HLP seems to be transmitted in an autosomal recessive manner.

Treatment basically consists of dietary measures. Fat intake should be lowered according to test results. Care should be taken not to induce a highly atherogenic secondary hyperlipemia by excessive carbohydrate intake, which can transform type I HLP to type V. The use of MCT helps in avoiding this possibility. Treatment is aimed at maintaining triglyceridemia below 10 g/l. Transfusion of fresh blood, plasma, and purified apo C_{II} has also been proposed.

Type "II_a" hyperlipoproteinemia.

— Synonyms: familial hypercholesterolemia, essential hypercholesterolemia with or without tendon xanthomatosis, and familial hyper-β-lipoproteinemia.

This is the most frequent form of primary HLP. It rarely gives clinical manifestations in children, but affects 0.1 to 0.5 % of the general population.

This autosomal disorder is either of incomplete dominant or intermediate inheritance. The serum is always clear. It's main characteristic is hypercholesterolemia without hypertriglyceridemia; the cholesterol/triglyceride ratio exceeds 2.5. The pri-

TABLE XVIII. — CLASSIFICATION OF HYPERLIPOPROTEINEMIAS (ADAPTED FROM FREDRICKSON, WHO)

Types	Disease	Cholesterol	Serum, triglycerides	Increased LP fraction	Lipoproteins apoproteins	Pathogenesis	Heredity	Clinical symptoms	Treatment
I	Essential hyperlipemia (syn: hyperchylomicronemia, exogenous hyperglyceridemia or Burger Gruts disease)	N	Lactescent TG/C > 2.5	Chylomicrons	↗ Chylomicrons ±↘ Apo CII	Extra-hepatic LP lipase deficiency	AR	Abdominal pain Xanthomas Pancreatitis Hepatomegaly No atheromas	↘ Fat MCT
IIa	Familial hypercholesterolemia (syn: familial hyper-βLP)	↗↗	Clear N C/TG > 2.5	β	↗ LDL ↗ Apo B	Deficiency in LDL cell receptors	AD or intermediate	Atheroma ++ Xanthomas ++ CV accidents Early death	↘ C and satured fat ↗ Polyinsatured fat Cholestyramine Fenofibrate Surgery; PE
IIb	Mixed hyperlipemia (II +IV) (syn: hyper-β and pre-βLP)	↗↗	↗↗	Pre-β+β	↗ LDL +VLDL ↗ Apo CIII-B	?	?	Atheroma ++ Obesity CV accidents	Hypocaloric feedings ↗ Carbohydrates
III	Broad βLP (syn: dys βLP)	↗↗	Opalescent ↗↗	(broad β) pre-β	↗ IDL ↗ LDL ↗ Apo E ↗ Apo E III	Deficient catabolism of LP remnants Abnormal Apo E	AD with variable expression	Atheroma ++ Lipid deposits Palmar xanthomas Hyperuricemia GIT	↗ Carbohydrates ↗ Animal fat ± hypolipemiant drugs
IV	Hyper pre-βLP (syn: sugar induced endogenous familial hyperglyceridemia)	N	Opalescent ↗↗ TG/C > 2.5	Pre-β	↗ VLDL ↗ Apo B-CIII	?	AD	Obesity CV accidents Xanthomas Abdominal pain Hepatomegaly Hyperuricemia GIT	Hypocaloric feeding ↘ Rapidly absorbed carbohydrates
V	Mixed endogenous and exogenous hyperglyceridemia (fat and carbohydrate dependent)	N	Opalescent or lactescent ↗↗ TG/C > 2.5	Chylomicrons + pre-β	↗ Chylomicrons + VLDL	Abnormal Apo E or Apo CIII	?	Abdominal pain Pancreatitis Xanthomas Hepatomegaly Obesity, GIT	Hypocaloric intake ↗ Carbohydrates ↗ Animal fat ± Hypolipemiant drugs
	Hyper-α-lipoproteinemia (syn: hypercholesterolemia) (6 bis)	↗	N	α	↗ HDL	?	AD	No CV accidents No obesity	—

LP: Lipoprotein (EMIA), N: Normal, TG: Triglyceride, C: Cholesterol, PE: Plasma exchange, AR: Autosomal recessive, AD: Autosomal dominant, MCT: Medium chain triglycerides, CV: Cardio-vascular, GIT: Glucose intolerance.

mary defect is an abnormality in LDL metabolism, due to a deficiency in LDH uptake by extrahepatic membrane receptors. Because of this, LDL cannot be metabolized in these cells thus causing an increase in cholesterolemia. In heterozygous patients, cholesterolemia ranges from 7 to 13 mmol/l (2.7 to 5 g/l). Apoprotein B levels are almost double that seen in normal subjects. Clinical manifestations are usually not observed until adulthood, at which time, tendon xanthomas, and xanthelasma can be noted. 50 % of male patients present with heart attacks before 50 years of age.

In homozygous patients, cholesterolemia ranges from 15 to 25 mmol/l (6 to 10 g/l). A finding specific to homozygotes are tuberous xanthomas which appear in the first three years or are occasionally present at birth. Arcus corneum is an early finding. Cardiovascular complications generally lead to death prior to age 20. Both parents of homozygous patients are necessarily heterozygous for this disorder.

Two types of mutation have been reported. The first is an "Rbo" mutation ("negative receptors") that totally incapacitates LDL receptors. The second is an "Rb"-mutation ("defective receptor") usually causing a 90 % reduction in fixation capacity (although this percentage is variable). Both mutations are allelic. Rbo-Rb-compound heterozygotes have been reported. A third allele is suspected of hindering receptor assembly during LDL internalization. "Pseudo-homozygotes" have been reported. They respond well to treatment and their parents are apparently normal.

Forms of polygenic heredity have also been reported; in these forms, cholesterol is only slightly elevated (6 to 8 mmol/l or 2.3 to 3 g/l) and cardiovascular disease is more frequent than in the general population. The treatment of type II_a HLP is dietary and medical. Diets should be low in cholesterol (200 mg/day) and low in saturated fats (eggs, animal fat). Drug therapy includes the administration of cholestyramine (600 to 1,500 mg/kg/day), nicotinic acid (80 to 90 mg/kg/day) and fenofibrate (Lipanthyl: 300 mg/day), the latter being preferred over Lipavlon. When these measures are insufficient in homozygotes, surgery can be considered. Ileo-ileal by-pass (Buchwald) is poorly tolerated in children. Porto-caval shunts (Starzl) should only be used for homozygous patients in whom medical treatment is ineffective. It has been proposed [381] that severe forms be treated by repeated plasma exchange.

Screening for type II_a HLP [284]. — At one time, it was considered possible to systematically screen all newborns for this condition. Total blood cholesterol studies on blood taken from the umbilical cord were shown to be of little help. The same was true of LDL studies. Additional screening criteria such as a family history of hypercholesterolemia in three generations and xanthomatosis in one family member were proposed without success. Interpretation of cholesterol levels before 1 year of age is problematic. After age one, the diagnostic value of cholesterolemia is more certain, but the number of false positive and false negative results remains high. It therefore seems unadvisable to screen for type II HLP in unselected populations. On the other hand, screening of high-risk families or groups is justified, even though the true benefit of diet and drug therapy has not been completely established. Prenatal screening of homozygous forms is possible after the 16th week of gestation (Brown and Goldstein).

CEROID-STORAGE DISEASES

Also known as cerebro-retinal degeneration with accumulation of lipid pigments, "ceroid lipofuscinosis", and Batten's disease [386], the ceroidoses correspond to the various forms of amaurotic idiocy in which non specific lipid accumulation is present: neonatal form (Santavuori's disease), infantile form (Bielschowsky-Jansky disease), juvenile form (Batten-Spielmeyer-Vogt disease), and adult form (Kuf's disease). Histochemical, ultrastructural, and immunofluorescent studies demonstrate the accumulation of lipid pigments of the ceroid or lipofuscin type, identified by the following criteria: positive staining with Soudan Black, autofluorescence, and insolubility in lipid solvents. The exact nature of these lipid pigments remains unknown. The most thoroughly studied is lipofuscin, a yellow-brown pigment that accumulates in various tissues (especially nervous and cardiac) with aging. Abnormal accumulation of lipid pigments (called ceroid) can occur under a variety of pathological circumstances including vitamin E deficiency, hepatic disorders, and specific storage diseases such as metachromatic leukodystrophy, Refsum's disease and gangliosidosis. Ceroids appear to be polymers produced by the auto-oxidation of unsaturated lipid precursors [386]. In Santavuori's disease, the most precocious and severe form of ceroidosis, Svennerholm demonstrated an accumulation of polyunsaturated fatty acids in the liver, serum, and cerebral cortex [341]. In serum lecithin, ara-

TABLE XIX. — Neuronal ceroid lipofuscinoses.

	Infantile type (Santavuori)	Late juvenile type (Jansky-Bielschowski)	Juvenile type (Batten, Spielmeyer-Vogt)	Adult form (Kufs)
Onset	1 year	2-5 years	5-10 years	After 12 years
Survival	1 to 3 years	1 to 4 years	11 years (mean)	5 to 35 years
Mental deterioration	++ rapid	++	Slow	Very slow
Ataxo-pyramidal syndrome	++	++	+	+
Visual deterioration	++	+	++	0
Optic fundi	Diffuse hypopigmentation	Macular degeneration	Macular degeneration	Normal
Microcephaly	++	+	0	0
E. R. G.	++	++	++	0
Cerebral atrophy	Very severe	Severe	Function of duration	Moderate

chidonic acid (20 : 4, n = 6) is abnormally elevated, while linoleic acid (18 : 2, n = 6) is decreased. In the juvenile form, Pullarkart observed a considerable decrease in docosahexanoic acid [272]. The ceroid accumulation observed in amaurotic idiots is ultrastructurally very characteristic; it occurs as "fingerprint" or "curvilinear" deposits as well as very dense granules. Ceroidoses are hereditary diseases transmitted in an autosomal recessive manner. The principal clinical findings are listed in Table XIX. In general, the sooner the onset of the disease, the more severe and rapid the progression, resulting within a matter of months or years in a state of cerebral decortication. Certain ancillary procedures are helpful in making the diagnosis. Fundoscopic examination shows initial alterations in the macula with a loss of the foveal reflex followed by retinal depigmentation and pigment changes spreading to the periphery. Early in the disease, electroretinograms show evidence of malfunction of first the cones and then the rods. Subsequently the tracing rapidly flattens substantiating the preferential involvement of the external retinal strata. EEG's show a slow diffuse dysrythmia; photic stimulation gives exceedingly amplified spikes after a shortened latent period. Vacuolated lymphocytes and neutro-philic granulocytes with numerous azurophilic granulations are observed in blood smears; however, these cytological modifications are not always present. Electron microscopy of skin, conjunctival, and rectal mucosal biopsies demonstrate characteristic ceroid accumulation. CSF determinations and nerve conduction rates remain normal. As for the treatment, understanding of the pathogenesis of this disorder has led to attempts at using antioxidizing agents and vitamin E in elevated doses without apparent success.

HYPERGLYCEROLEMIA

Guggenheim [151] reported 2 brothers presenting with moderate psychomotor deficiency, spasticity, impaired growth, osteoporosis, adrenal insufficiency, and non-specific myopathy. Metabolic studies demonstrated hyperglycerolemia and hyperglyceroluria. Enzyme analysis showed a glycerolkinase deficiency in leukocytes and cultured fibroblasts. It will probably be possible to demonstrate this deficiency in cultured amniotic cells.

Disorders of carbohydrate metabolism

Omitted from this chapter are the carbohydrate disorders resulting in hypoglycemia since they are discussed in the chapter on glucose metabolism. These disorders include glycogenoses of type I, III and VI, glycogen synthetase deficiency, fructose and galactose intolerance, and enzyme disorders affecting gluconeogenesis such as fructose 1-6-diphosphatase deficiency. Furthermore certain enzyme disorders of amino acid metabolism and fatty acid beta-oxidation can give severe hypoglycemia. They are discussed in the sections entitled "Organic acidemias" and "disorders of lipid metabolism".

GLYCOGENOSIS [62]

Table XX lists the various glycogenoses and their essential findings. We shall only discuss type II and type IV glycogenosis.

Type II glycogenosis [98]. — The clinical manifestations of this lysosomal disorder sharply contrast to those of other hepatic or muscular glycogen storage diseases. This disorder does not affect cytosolic glycogen nor glycemic regulation. It is characterised by a lysosomal accumulation of glycogen in most tissues and is caused by acid maltase (alpha 1-4-glucosidase) deficiency.

Classic infantile form: Pompe's disease. — This disease is usually fatal before age one due to irreversible cardiac failure. Although they can occur neonatally, clinical manifestations generally appear during the third or fourth months. Cardiac failure is the most frequent finding. Occasionally, attention is drawn by abnormal hypotonia or macroglossia. Hepatomegaly is always observed. Thoracic X-rays show considerable cardiomegaly. Echocardiography shows the myocardium to be enlarged. ECG findings include deep narrow Q waves indicative of septal hypertrophy, signs of left ventricular hypertrophy, and marked shortening of the P-R interval. Diagnosis

TABLE XX. — GLYCOGENOSES

Type	Affected organs	Enzyme deficiency	Essential features
I (Von Gierke)	Liver, kidney, intestine	Glucose-6-phosphatase (Ia) or translocase (Ib)	Hepatomegaly, stunted growth, infections (Ib), hypoglycemia, hyperlipemia, acidosis
II (Pompe)	Generalized	α-1-4-glucosidase (acid maltase)	Severe form: asystole, muscle weakness, hepatomegaly, macroglossia, cardiomegaly. Mild form: ressembles limb girdle dystrophy
III (Forbes-Cori)	Liver, muscle	Amylo-1-6-glucosidase (debranching enzyme)	Hepatomegaly, hypoglycemia, muscular hypotonia; sometimes cardiomyopathy
IV (Andersen)	Generalized	Amylo-1-4, 1-6-transglucosidase (branching enzyme)	Severe infantile cirrhosis
V (McArdle)	Muscle	Myophosphorylase	Intolerance to exercise: muscle cramps, fatigue, myoglobinuria
VI (Hers)	Liver	Phosphorylase or phosphorylase kinase	Hepatomegaly, hypoglycemia
VII (Tarui)	Muscle, erythrocytes	Phosphofructokinase	Intolerance to exercise: muscle cramps, fatigue, myoglobinuria, hemolytic anemia

is confirmed by the almost complete inactivity of acid maltase on enzyme assay in leukocytes, cultured fibroblasts, and various tissues. Since results are often discordant when using leukocytes, it is preferable to use lymphocytes for enzyme assays [23]. Histochemical and ultrastructural studies confirm the lysosomal glycogen accumulation in various tissues. No effective treatment is presently known for this disorder. It's prenatal diagnosis is possible.

Juvenile and adult forms. — These forms are less severe and demonstrate no myocardial involvement. In the juvenile form, difficulties in walking and a progressive decrease in muscular force are the first symptoms noted. In the adult form, symptoms are absent until the second, third or fourth decade of life. One initially notes a myopathy of the lower extrimeties that progresses at a variable rate. Cases have been reported in patients over 60 years old. In the cases reported by Reuser [281], residual acid maltase activity ranged from 7 % to 22 % of normal values. Immunological studies suggest a considerable heterogeneity in this deficiency [23, 281]. Several workers have reported cases in which clinical, pathological, and biochemical findings were typical without any apparent decrease in acid maltase activity [70].

Type IV glycogenosis: Andersen's disease [62]. — This peculiar disorder was first reported by Andersen. The storage material is a glycogen of abnormal structure that Cori identified to be the polysaccharide amylopectin. It's accumulation and structure is caused by a deficiency in the branching enzyme (alpha-1,4-glucan: alpha-1,4-glucan 6-glycosyl transferase) in all tissues but predominantly in the liver where it is associated with a rapidly progressing cirrhosis. The child is normal at birth, then rapidly develops hepatosplenomegaly, abdominal distension, and portal hypertension before 6 months of age. Moderate jaundice may be present. Laboratory findings reflect the progressive cirrhosis; increases in transaminases and bilirubin, and abnormalities in serum protein electrophoresis are noted. On the other hand, hypoglycemia is not present and tests normally used to diagnose hepatic glycogenoses (glucagon and galactose tests) remain normal. There is no increase in circulating lipids or lactate levels. Liver biopsy orients the diagnosis by demonstrating the polysaccharide accumulation. The enzyme deficiency can be diagnosed in leukocytes or cultured skin fibroblasts and prenatal diagnosis is possible [172]. The disease is usually fatal before 2 years of age. In addition to Andersen's disease, another adult form has been reported in several patients presenting as progressive neurological involvement characterized by severe muscular deficiency, sensory deficits, and dementia. The implicated polysaccharide closely resembles amylopectin [260]. It is also appropriate here to mention myoclonic epilepsy with Lafora's bodies in which the storage material has been shown to be a polysaccharide.

MUCOPOLYSACCHARIDOSES

Mucopolysaccharidoses are hereditary disorders of autosomal recessive inheritance, with the exception of Hunter's disease which is recessive X-linked. They are characterised by the lysosomal accumulation of acid mucopolysaccharides also termed glycosaminoglycans (G. A. G.). This accumulation results from a deficiency of enzymes involved in the catabolism of glycosaminoglycans such as keratan sulfate (K. S.) in Morquio's disease, dermatan sulfate (D. S.) and heparan-sulfate (H. S.) in the other mucopolysaccharidoses. The breakdown of G. A. G. normally occurs in successive stages starting from the non reductor end of the molecule. Inactivity of an enzyme necessary for this catabolism causes a lysosomal accumulation of the non-catabolised mucopolysaccharide.

The mucopolysaccharidoses have been clearly differentiated from the mucolipidoses (also termed oligosaccharidoses). Most of the mucolipidoses are characterized by an abnormal tissue accumulation and urinary excretion of oligosaccharides while G. A. G. excretion remains normal. In certain sphingolipidoses such as GM_1 gangliosidosis and mucosulfatidosis the sphingolipid accumulation is associated with an accumulation and urinary excretion of G. A. G.

Except for Morquio's disease, which is considered separately because of it's distinct clinical manifestations, the mucopolysaccharidoses and mucolipidoses are all characterised by facial abnormalities and associated bone involvement of varying severity. In Hurler's disease (M. P. S. type I. H.) and the classic form of Hunter's disease, major facial abnormalities and bone lesions are noted soon after birth. On the other hand, these symptoms are only moderate and appear much later in Scheie's disease (M. P. S. type I. S.), SanFilippo's disease, and the moderate form of Hunter's disease. Mental deficiency is also variable according to the disease; it is severe in San Filippo's disease and Hurler's disease, while absent in Scheie's disease and Maro-

TABLE XXI. — Essential clinical and biochemical features of mucopolysaccharidoses

Disease		Enzymatic defect	Urinary glycosamino-glycans	Clinical presentation	Genetics
Type I	Hurler Type I-H	α-L-Iduronidase	Dermatan-sulphate and heparan-sulphate	Severe dysmorphy and dysostosis, hepato-splenomegaly, hernia, deafness, dwarfism, corneal clouding, articular involvement, mental retardation, cardiac involvement, death before adolescence	Autosomal recessive
	Scheie Type I-S (previousely called, type V)			Corneal opacities, hypoacousia, articular involvement, aortic valve involvement, death in adulthood	
Type II Hunter	Hunter (severe type)	Iduronate-2-sulfate sulfatase	Dermatan-sulphate and heparan-sulphate	Marked dysmorphy and dysostosis, nanism, deafness Absence of corneal opacities, mental retardation, death durring adolescence	X linked recessive
	Hunter (mild type)			Mild dysmorphy and dysostosis, absence of corneal opacities, hypoacousis, moderate mental retardation, survive longer than 30 years	
Type III San Filippo	Type III$_A$	Heparan-N-sulfatase	Heparan-sulphate	Mild dysmorphy and dysostosis Severe mental retardation	Autosomal recessive
	Type III$_B$	N-Acetyl-α-D-glucosaminidase			
	Type III$_C$	α-Glucosamine N-acetyl-transferase			
	Type III$_D$	N-Acetyl-glucosamine-6-sulfate-sulfatase			
Type IV Morquio	Type IV$_A$	N-Acetyl-galactosamine-6-sulfate-sulfatase	Keratan-sulphate	Spondylo-epiphyseal dysplasia (platyspondyly, sternal protrusion, odontoid hypoplasia) Articular laxity, corneal opacities, normal IQ, long life	Autosomal recessive
	Type IV$_B$	β-Galactosidase			
Type VI Maroteaux-Lamy	Type VI Severe form	Arylsulfatase B	Dermatan-sulphate	Major dysostosis, dwarfism, corneal and cardiac involvement Normal intelligence	Autosomal recessive
	Type VI Mild form			Bone lesions, corneal opacities	
Type VII Sly		β-Glucuronidase	Dermatan-sulphate and heparan-sulphate	Variable severity, multiple dysostoses, hepatomegaly, splenomegaly, variable mental retardation	Autosomal recessive

teaux-Lamy disease. The presence of corneal clouding also depends on the disease. Table XXI lists the essential clinical findings in these various disorders. Since mucopolysaccharide accumulates in most tissues, frequent findings include hepatomegaly, splenomegaly, macroglossia, myocardial and valvular lesions, and even a cutaneous accumulation that causes a thickening of the skin and coarse facial features. The abnormal mucopolysacchariduria can be screened by the acetylpyridinium chloride test and toluidine blue or alcian blue tests. However, these simple tests can sometimes give falsely positive or negative results. Direct determination of urinary mucopolysaccharide levels and chromatography are more accurate. Blood smears demonstrate characteristic vacuolated lymphocytes (Mittwoch cells) and vacuolated lymphocytes containing metachromatic granulations (Gasser cells). G. A. G. accumulation occurs in parenchymal and mesenchymal cells. Ultrastructurally, the lysosomes are abundant and distended by a finely granular substance. Specific enzyme deficiencies can be demonstrated in various tissues, leukocytes and cultured fibroblasts or amniotic cells. Curiously enough, the same phenotype can be caused by different enzyme deficiencies (San Filippo's disease, for example). Conversely, distinct phenotypes can be caused by a deficiency in the same enzyme (Hurler's disease and Scheie's disease are both caused by a deficiency in α-L-iduronidase). Manifestations in Scheie's disease are moderate, probably due to some residual enzyme activity, although this has never been demonstrated in "in vitro" enzyme studies. Forms of intermediate severity corresponding to compound heterozygotes or "double heterozygotes" have been reported.

Currently, there exists no truly effective treatment for these disorders. Plasma and leukocytes transfusions have given unsatisfactory results. Recent attempts at transplanting bone marrow have been undertaken.

MUCOLIPIDOSES

The mucolipidoses represent a somewhat confusing group of disorders because of their more recent individualization, the utilisation of conflicting terminology, and the persistence of biochemical uncertainties for several of these disorders. The name mucolipidoses was initially proposed to emphasize the often heterogeneous nature of storage material (composed of oligosaccharides, polysaccharides,

and complex lipids). This group of disorders includes relatively well understood diseases with accumulation of both sphingolipids and glycoproteins (GM_1 gangliosidosis, mucosulfatidosis, and fucosidosis) diseases in which the exact nature of the storage material and enzyme deficiencies remain uncertain (mucolipidoses I, II, III and IV) and diseases demonstrating no lipid accumulation (mannosidosis and aspartylglycosaminuria).

Later, the term "oligosaccharidoses" was proposed to emphasize the abnormal accumulation and urinary excretion of oligosaccharides [218]. Major contributions to the biochemical understanding of these disorders were made by Strecker [337], who proposed the term "sialidoses" to differentiate those disorders in which the accumulated and excreted oligosaccharides were sialyl-oligosaccharides or sialosides. In this group [103], were included the mucolipidoses I, II and III, the "myoclonia-cherry red spot" syndrome, and nephrosialidosis. However, according to Lowden and O'Brien [209], the term sialidosis should only be used for diseases in which the sialidase (neuraminidase) deficiency appears to be primary (with a partial deficiency in heterozygotes), as in type I mucolipidosis and "myoclonia-cherry red spot syndrome". On this basis, they excluded from the sialidoses type I and II mucolipidosis since their neuraminidase deficiency is probably secondary (Table XXII). Further biochemical and enzyme studies will no doubt lead to a better classification of these disorders. When mucolipidosis is suspected clinically, a number of ancillary procedures are helpful in confirming the diagnosis. Urinary glycosaminoglycan (G. A. G.) determinations can rule out the diagnosis of mucopolysaccharidosis. Oligosaccharide chromatography can be performed by relatively simple methods [175]. Analysis of lysosomal, serum and leukocyte enzymes (fucosidase, mannosidase, N-acetyl-hexosaminidase, neuraminidase, etc.) should be suggested by the clinical manifestations and the type of oligosacchariduria. When the clinical presentation is atypical, a complete study of urinary oligosaccharides should be carried out. Recent observations have shown that it is sometimes difficult to establish an accurate diagnosis. Urinary oligosaccharide analysis and complementary genetic studies can be helpful in these cases [146].

Type I mucolipidosis (type II sialidosis in O'Brien's classification). — Reported in 1968 as lipomucopolysaccharidosis [330], this disorder is characterised by clinical and radiological findings similar to those in Hurler's disease (facial abnormalities, gum hypertrophy, macroglossia, dor-

sal kyphosis, stiffening of joints, hernias, corneal clouding, and deafness). Associated neurological findings are suggestive of sphingolipidosis (mental deterioration, myoclonia, choreo-athetotic movements, ataxia, and cherry-red spots). Symptoms appear in the first years of life and progress slowly.

Patients generally die before reaching adulthood. Of the lysosomal enzymes, only N-acetyl-neuraminidase (sialidase) is decreased in fibroblasts and leukocytes [41]. Sialosides accumulate in tissues and in the urine. Enzyme activity in heterozygotes is reduced to half of normal values. The prenatal

TABLE XXII. — MUCOLIPIDOSES
(MUCOSULFATIDOSIS AND GM$_1$ GANGLIOSIDOSIS ARE DISCUSSED WITH THE LIPIDOSES)

Disease	Clinical presentation	Enzymatic defect	Oligosacchariduria	
Mucolipidosis, type I (1968)	Onset in first years, dysmorphy and dysostosis, degenerative encephalopathy, macular cherry red spot	Neuraminidase inactivity; sometimes decreased β-galactosidase activity	X 500 to 1,000 Sialosides	
Nephrosialidosis (1978)	Onset in first months, severe encephalopathy, proteinuria, renal insufficiency, dysmorphy and disostosis, macular cherry red spot, rapid death	Neuraminidase inactivity	X 400 Sialosides	
Macular cherry red spot-myoclonus syndrome (1978)	Onset in adolescence, myoclonus macular cherry red spot, long survival	Neuraminidase deficiency	Sialosides ↗	
Mucolipidosis, type II, I-cell disease (1967)	Onset in first weeks, major dysmorphy and dysostosis, hepatosplenomegaly, corneal opacities, mental deterioration, death before 4 years	N-acetylglucosaminyl-phosphotransferase deficiency	X 40 to 120 Sialosides	
Mucolipidoses, type III, Hurler pseudo-polydystrophy (1966)	Onset in first years, mild dysmorphy and dysostosis, articular involvement Absent or mild mental retardation long survival	N-acetylglucosaminyl-phosphotransferase deficiency	X 10 to 20 Sialosides	Oligosacchari-doses
Mannosidosis (1967)	Onset in first years, dysmorphy and dysostosis less severe than in Hurler's disease, deafness, mental retardation, long survival	α-D-mannosidase deficiency	Mannosyl-oligosaccharides	
Fuco-sidosis (1967) Type I	Onset in first year, dysmorphy and dysostosis of Hurler type, mental retardation, death before 4 years	α-L-Fucosidase deficiency	Fucosyl-oligosaccharides	
Type II	Mild dysmorphy and dysostosis, diffuse angiokeratosis, prolonged survival			
Aspartyl-glycosaminuria (1966)	Hurler type dysmorphy and dysostosis, mental retardation, long survival	Aspartyl-glycosamine hydrolase	Aspartyl-glucosamine and glyco-asparagines	
Mucolipidosis, Type IV (1974)	Mental retardation, corneal clouding	?	Normal	
Salla disease (1979)	Mental retardation, gross facial features, long survival	?	Normal	

diagnosis of this disorder is possible by sialidase determination in amniotic fluid cells. A juvenile form has been reported, mainly by investigators in Japan. A partial deficiency in beta-galactosidase can be associated with the neuraminidase deficiency [170, 380].

Myoclonia-Cherry-Red spot syndrome (type I sialidosis in O'Brien classification).

— Described by Rapin [276], this syndrome appears at 8 to 15 years of age and is characterized by a decrease in visual acuity and myoclonus of the limbs triggered by the patient's emotions or movements. Mental retardation and facial abnormalities are not present. Vacuolated lymphocytes and storage cells containing a glycoprotein storage material have been noted [354].

Type II mucolipidosis.

— De Mars and Leroy described this disorder in 1967 [76] under the name of "I cell disease" because of the presence of numerous bifringent inclusions in the perinuclear cytoplasm of cultured fibroblasts. This is the most frequent of the mucolipidoses and most original of the lysosomal diseases. It is usually fatal within several years. Clinically, the patients present with facial abnormalities similar to those in Hurler's disease except that they appear earlier and are more severe. Dwarfism, cutaneous infiltration, gum hypertrophy and hernias are also noted several weeks after birth. Associated bone lesions progressively evolve into a Hurler-type multiple dysostosis; however, radiological findings differ in that they appear much earlier and demonstrate severe bone demineralization in the neonatal period. Similar demineralization is noted in infants with fetal calcium deficiency born to mothers with hypoparathyroidism or vitamin D deficiency. The most striking feature is noted on analysis of lysosomal enzymes. Except for acid phosphatase and beta-glucosidase, these enzymes show decreased activity in cells (cultured fibroblasts, for example) but greatly increased activity in biological fluids (serum, amniotic fluid, and culture media). This particular enzymatic pattern is caused by alterations in identifying sites on the enzyme's hydrocarbon chains. These sites are necessary for lysosomal penetration. This has been explained by a deficiency of N-acetylglucosaminylphosphotransferase which precludes the generation of the common phosphomannosyl recognition marker of lysosomal enzymes [162, 163]. This autosomal recessive disorder can be readily diagnosed by assay of lysosomal enzymes (demonstrates a 10 or 100 fold increase in activity), and by

studying the morphology and enzymes of cultured skin fibroblasts. Prenatal diagnosis has been possible in a number of cases [4, 174].

Type III mucolipidosis.

— Described by Maroteaux and Lamy as Hurler's pseudo-polydystrophy [219], this disorder closely resembles type II mucolipidosis in it's clinical similarities and by similar though less severe lysosomal enzyme abnormalities in serum, urine, and fibroblasts. It can be distinguished by it's later onset, lesser degree of severity and slower progression [190]. Cellular deficiencies in beta-galactosidase and neuraminidase are less marked than in type II mucolipidosis.

Nephrosialidosis.

— Maroteaux [220] first described this disorder in 1978. It is classified as a mucolipidosis, and more specifically as a sialidosis since it is biochemically characterized by abnormal excretion of oligosaccharides with terminal sialic acid molecules (sialosides) and by a deficiency in alpha-2,6-neuraminidase. Clinical findings include facial abnormalities, hernias, hepatosplenomegaly, skeletal abnormalities, similar to those in Hurler's disease and severe mental retardation. This form of sialidosis is characterized by the presence of renal failure that is responsible for death within several years. Associated findings can include cherry-red spots, large numbers of vacuolated lymphocytes, and foam cells resembling Pick cells on bone marrow examination.

Type IV mucolipidosis.

— Herman [18] reported this autosomal recessive disorder in 1974 in a Jewish population of Ashkenazi origin. Corneal clouding is noted several weeks after birth, followed by progressive mental deterioration, retinal changes with degeneration, and optic nerve atrophy. Facial features are heavy without being coarse. Pyramidal symptoms, hypotonia, and ataxia may be noted. Abnormal mucopolysacchariduria and oligosacchariduria are not present, even though tissue accumulation of gangliosides and mucopolysaccharides is noted. This storage abnormality is easily demonstrable in tissues, especially by ultrastructural studies of conjunctival biopsies [143]. Kohn [192] proposed the prenatal diagnosis of this disorder on purely ultrastructural criteria based on the degree of lysosomal accumulation evidenced by fibrillo-granular inclusions and concentric lamellar bodies. The demonstration of cellular accumulation of mucopolysaccharides (especially hyaluronic acid) GM_3 and GD_3 explains this disease's present classification among the mucolipidoses [7].

Salla's disease. — Reported in Finland by Aula [5], in 1979, this disease is characterized by gross facial features, mental retardation, dysarthria, difficulties in walking, and the presence of vacuolated lymphocytes. Bone lesions are minimal. There is no corneal clouding nor visceral involvement. Ultrastructural studies demonstrate the lysosomal storage abnormalities. No abnormalities are noted on analysis of mucopolysaccharides, oligosaccharides and lysosomal enzymes. The only finding is excessive urinary excretion of sialic acid.

Mannosidosis. — Ockermann described this autosomal recessive disorder in 1967 [249]. It is characterised by an accumulation of mannose terminal oligosaccharides due to a deficiency in lysosomal alpha-D-mannosidase. Patients present with facial abnormalitites [329], dysostosis similar to but less severe than that in Hurler's disease, deafness, and mental retardation. Hernias, corneal and lens clouding, hepatosplenomegaly, and recurrent infections have also been noted [104]. Diagnosis is confirmed by determinations of alpha-D-mannosidase levels in serum, leukocytes, and fibroblasts, and chromatography of oligosaccharides. The lysosomal storage abnormalities are readily demonstrated by ultrastructural studies of liver or conjunctival biopsies. Prenatal diagnosis is possible [214].

Fucosidosis. — Fucosidosis was first described by Durand et al. in 1967 [95, 96]. Two types can be distinguished.

Type I fucosidosis. — Symptoms appear about one year after birth and include respiratory infections, cutaneous infiltrates, Hurler type facial abnormalitites of varying severity, and dysostosis mainly affecting the vertebrae. Marked neurological involvement is noted, characterized by severe psychomotor deterioration and hypotonia followed by spastic quadriplegia. Patients die in a context of decerebration between ages 4 and 6.

Type II fucosidosis. — Mental degeneration begins at the same age as in type I but progresses more slowly. Neurological symptoms are less severe and include hypo- or hypertonia, and convulsions. Hurler-type facial abnormalities, predominantly vertebral dysostosis, and dwarfism appear progressively. A particular type of cutaneous lesion resembling the angiokeratomas of Fabry's disease may be noted. Survival is generally long [100].

Although the delineation of fucosidosis into two types demonstrates the heterogeneity of clinical findings, the distinction is somewhat arbitrary [355]. Intermediate forms exist and are difficult to classify. Furthermore, both types have been observed in the same sibship. Laboratory findings are similar in both types; presence of vacuolated lymphocytes, inactivity of alpha-L-fucosidase, and fucosyl oligosacchariduria. Lysosomal accumulations are readily seen by ultrastructural studies of skin, conjunctiva, liver, and rectal biopsies.

Aspartyl glycosaminuria. — This disease was discovered in Finland by Palo during a systematic study of aminoaciduria in mentally retarded patients. Palo noted that 11 patients with similar clinical manifestations presented with an identical peptide abnormality. Detailed biochemical studies showed that the disorder is caused by accumulation of 2-acetamido-1-(beta-L-aspartimido) 1,2-dideoxy-beta-D-glucose (A. A. D. G.) and glycoasparagines of higher molecular weight [179]. Clinical manifestations appear several months after birth and included diarrhea, recurrent infections, facial abnormalities, dwarfism, Hurler-type multiple dysostosis, and mental retardation. This disease results from a deficiency in a lysosomal enzyme named aspartyl glucosamine-amidohydrolase. The lysosomal storage abnormalities are seen on electron microscopy [155]. Abnormal urinary excretion of aspartyl-glycosamine can be demonstrated by electrophoresis or chromatography of amino acids and chromatography of oligosaccharides. This autosomal recessive disease occurs almost exclusively in Finland where it's incidence has been estimated at 1/26,000 births. Heterozygous states can be diagnosed by plasma enzyme assay. The prenatal diagnosis of this disorder will probably be possible [268].

Hereditary disorders of purine metabolism

(Fig. IX-71)

DEFICIENCY
IN HYPOXANTHINE-GUANINE
PHOSPHORIBOSYL TRANSFERASE
(H. G. P. R. T.)

The importance of the purine recovery pathway in purine metabolism was made evident by the description of the Lesch-Nyhan syndrome in 1964 [189, 245]. This disorder is caused by an inactivity of H. G. P. R. T. and is of recessive X-linked inheritance. It causes an overproduction of purines and uric acid explaining findings such as hyperuricemia, hyperuricuria, uric acid lithiasis and tophi. Lesch-Nyhan syndrome is further characte-

rized by a severe encephalopathy with choreo-athetosis, spastic paralysis, and behavioral abnormalities including aggressiveness and self-mutilation. The exact cause of this encephalopathy remains mysterious. Lesch-Nyhan syndrome is not extremely rare since more than a hundred cases have been reported. For the moment, all attempts at treating this disorder have been unsuccessful [189]. In addition to this classic form in which H.G.P.R.T. activity is practically absent, other clinical forms and numerous enzymatic variants have been reported [9]. In boys and adult males, a partial deficiency in H. G. P. R. T. is responsible for an overproduction of uric acid and renal lithiasis. In one out of five cases, neurological symptoms are present but are

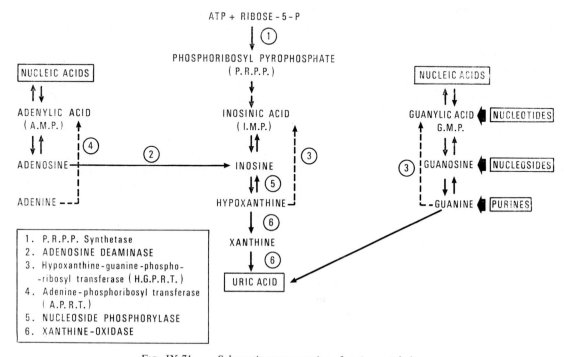

FIG. IX-71. — *Schematic representation of purine metabolism.*

not as severe as in Lesch-Nyhan syndrome. Enzyme activity can attain 50 % of normal values. No precise correlations have been found between the severity of clinical findings and the in vitro enzyme activity or type of enzyme variant. Diagnosis is confirmed by the presence of hyperuricemia, hyperuricosuria, and decreased H. G. P. R. T. activity in erythrocytes, leukocytes, fibroblasts and amniotic cells. Prenatal diagnosis is possible.

ADENINE PHOSPHORIBOSYL TRANSFERASE (A. P. R. T.) DEFICIENCY [44]

Since it's original description in 1974 about a dozen cases have been reported. The disease is characterised by the appearance of severe renal lithiasis in young children. The kidney stones are composed of 2,8-dehydroxyadenine (2,8-DHA) resulting from adenine's oxidation by xanthine oxidase. These calculi are easily mistaken for uric acid calculi because of their similar appearance and staining with common stains such as murexide. They can however be distinguished by more sophisticated analyses such as liquid chromatography, mass spectrometry, X-ray diffraction, and erythrocyte A. P. R. T. determinations. In A. P. R. T. deficiency blood and urinary uric acid levels are normal. It is of autosomal recessive inheritance, and heterozygotes can be identified by enzyme assay. Treatment is based on increasing fluid intake, limiting purine intake, and inhibiting xanthine oxidase with allopurinol (15 mg/kg/24 hours). Xanthine oxidase is responsible for the transformation of adenine (highly soluble) to 2,8-DHA (extremely insoluble).

PHOSPHORYL PYROPHOSPHATE (P. R. P. P.) SYNTHETASE HYPERACTIVITY [15]

Most often affecting adults, P. R. P. P. synthetase hyperactivity causes an overproduction of purines and uric acid and gives all the manifestations of gout. Patients with this disorder show no neurological manifestations, except for one case of encephalopathy reported in a young child.

XANTHINURIA: XANTHINE OXIDASE DEFICIENCY [43]

When xanthine oxidase is inactive, purine catabolism is blocked at the level of hypoxanthine and xanthine, resulting in hypouricemia, hypouricuria and xanthine lithiasis. The disorder is most often discovered by the finding of hypouricemia (10-13 mg/l). Occasionally, urinary lithiasis is the initial finding; in this case, the concomitant hypouricemia and hypouricuria distinguishes these calculi from uric acid lithiasis. Xanthinuria is generally a benign disorder and xanthine calculi are not always present. The sole treatment consists of maintaining an increased diuresis. A particular form of xanthinuria with severe encephalopathy is caused by a combined deficiency in xanthine oxidase and sulfite oxidase (see p. 1154).

PURINE METABOLISM, ENZYME DISORDERS AND IMMUNE DEFICIENCIES

Giblett [122] first described adenosine deaminase deficiency in children with a severe immune deficiency simultaneously affecting T and B lymphocyte function. Later, the same workers [123] and others [158], reported a nucleoside phosphorylase deficiency in children with T lymphocyte deficiency. Several theories were proposed to explain the immune deficiencies in these enzyme disorders: a secondary deficiency in pyrimidine synthesis [305], an accumulation of purine nucleotides in the lymphocytes altering DNA synthesis and energy pathways; perturbations in S-adenosyl-methionine metabolism and methylation reactions, and other hypotheses have been proposed. Whatever the mechanism, the enzyme deficiency is a valuable marker of the causal disease and makes possible it's prenatal diagnosis.

HYPOURICEMIA OF RENAL ORIGIN [75, 112]

In addition to the hypouricemias secondary to certain drug treatments or to complex tubular defects such as De Toni-Debre-Fanconi syndrome, several cases have been reported in which the urinary loss of uric acid was caused by a renal deficiency in uric acid reabsorption. This abnormality seems to be genetic and of autosomal recessive inheritance. The disorder can be asymptomatic or result in uric acid lithiasis. In several cases, hypercalciuria was associated with the hyperuricuria.

Disorders of pyrimidine metabolism

OROTIC ACIDURIA

In addition to abnormal excretion of orotic acid (also seen in certain congenital hyperammonemias such as O. C. T. deficiency), orotic aciduria presents at least 2 genetic alterations in pyrimidine biosynthesis (Fig. IX-72) which clinically manifest themselves as megaloblastic anemia, leucopenia, growth deficiency, and an excessive urinary excretion of orotic acid. Until now eight cases of orotic aciduria have been reported [324]. Because patients with this disorder cannot synthetise pyrimidine, this essential substance must be provided in the diet. In seven of the eight cases, two enzyme activities were deficient: orotate phosphoribosyl transferase and orotidine 5′-phosphate decarboxylase. In the eighth case only orotidine 5-phosphate decarboxylase was inactive. In addition to orotic acid, orotidine was present in the urines. Administration of uridine (2-4 g/d) is effective in treating these disorders.

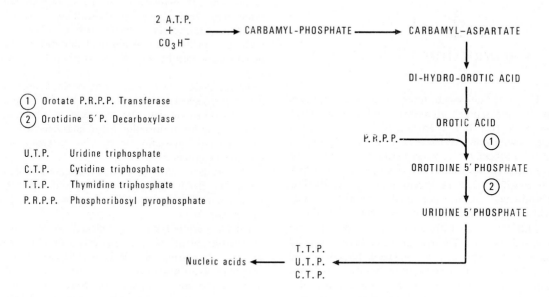

FIG. IX-72. — *Schematic representation of pyrimidine biosynthesis.*

Hereditary disorders in the metabolism of trace elements

Our understanding of the metabolism and physiological role of trace elements has been rapidly increasing. A number of pathological entities have been attributed to trace element disorders, essentially involving iron, iodine, zinc, copper, selenium, and chromium. The role of other trace elements such as cadmium, vanadium, molybdenum, and manganese has also received attention recently. Trace elements intervene in various areas including hematopoiesis, thyroid hormones, metalloenzymes, oxydation-reduction and glycoregulation.

We shall discuss only three hereditary disorders in trace element metabolism: acrodermatitis enteropathica involving zinc, Wilson's disease and Menkes' disease involving copper [300].

ACRODERMATITIS ENTEROPATHICA

This rare autosomal recessive disorder appears in the first months after birth and is fatal when untreated [12]. It is characterised by chronic diarrhea, hypotrophy, alopecia, and a periorificial and distal erythematosquamous dermatitis. Zinc levels are usually low in the blood, erythrocytes, and hair follicles [234]. The metalloenzymes such as alkaline phosphatase are also decreased. Several rare cases without hypozincemia have been reported [197].

Oral treatment with zinc-sulfate (100 mg/day) is rapidly effective. The treatment should be continued indefinitely, especially in pregnant patients since zinc deficiency can cause abortion and malformations. Zinc acetate, gluconate and pantothenate can also be administered orally at doses of 1 mg of zinc/kg/day [144].

Similar clinical findings have been reported after hypozincemias caused by excessive intestinal loss (chronic diarrhea) or dietary insufficiency (parenteral feeding). The treatment is the same, and is just as effective.

WILSON'S DISEASE

Also called hepatolenticular or hepatocerebral degeneration, this rare autosomal recessive disorder is characterised by an accumulation of copper responsible for hepatic cirrhosis and lesions in the brain, eyes, and kidneys [300, 319]. The incidence of the homozygous form is 1/200,000 births. Cox distinguished three genetic forms: the classic juvenile form, the adult form and an atypical juvenile form; the classic juvenile form generally appears at age 10 to 16 (never before age 4). Hepatic lesions are most often the initial manifestations, represented by cirrhosis, chronically progressive hepatitis, or acute liver failure with hemolysis. Neurological involvement is manifested by an extrapyramidal syndrome, tremor, writing difficulties, scholastic difficulties, unexpressive facies, behavioral abnormalities, and passivity. Additional findings include hepatosplenomegaly and Kayser-Fleischer corneal rings.

The adult form is first noted at 19 to 35 years of age. Neurological findings dominate the symptomatology and include lenticular degeneration. There also exists an atypical juvenile form characterised by lowered ceruloplasmin levels in heterozygotes (genetic heterogeneity).

The primary defect in Wilson's disease is a deficiency in hepatocyte copper excretion into the biliary canaliculi, probably of lysosomal origin (Sternlieb).

Plasma ceruloplasmin is reduced to less than 10 mg/100 ml in 80 % of patients, but is normal in 4 % of patients with Wilson's disease. Plasma copper levels are also lowered (N $= 108 \pm 10$ μg/ml). The proportion of copper not bound to ceruloplasmin (albumin, amino acids) is increased. Urinary copper levels rapidly increase to more than 200 μg/24 hours (normally less than 70 μg/24 hours). Liver biopsy shows that hepatic copper content is increased to almost 100 times the normal values, accumulating in the lysosomes. In homozygotes and most heterozygotes, oral or venous Cu 67 loading shows a deficiency in ceruloplasmin copper uptake, increased liver uptake, lowered biliary excretion, and increased urinary excretion.

D-Penicillamine is the treatment of choice. It causes regression of neurological manifestations and prevents the appearance of clinical symptoms in asymptomatic forms discovered in high risk families. It's utilization can cause a variety of complications, including cutaneous, hematological (neutropenia, anemia, aplasia), renal (nephrotic syndrome), and systemic (lupus, dermatomyositis, myasthenia) manifestations.

MENKES' DISEASE

Also termed Kinky-hair or steely-hair syndrome, Menkes' disease is a recessive X-linked disorder of copper metabolism [128, 300]. Soon after birth, patients present with convulsive encephalopathy, hair alterations (pili torti), hypothermia, growth deficiencies, facial abnormalities, and bone lesions. These patients are very susceptible to infection. The copper deficiency is caused by it's abnormal intestinal absorption. Plasma levels of copper and ceruloplasmin are low, as is hepatic copper content. Treatment is based on parenteral administration of copper. It is most effective when initiated soon after birth. Prenatal diagnosis is possible [171] by determining sex and Cu 64 uptake in cultured amniotic cells, the latter being increased in affected hemizygotes.

REFERENCES

[1] ALLEN (J. T.), HOLTON (J. B.) et coll. — Gas liquid chromatographic determination of galactitol in amniotic fluid for possible use in prenatal diagnosis of galactosaemia. Clin. Chim. Acta, 110, 59-63, 1981.

[2] AMPOLA (M. G.), MAHONEY (M. J.) et coll. — Prenatal therapy of a patient with vitamin B12-responsive methylmalonic acidemia. N. Engl. J. Med., 293, 314-317, 1975.

[3] ANDO (T.), NYHAN (W. L.). — A simple screening method for detecting isovalerylglycine in urine of patient with isovaleric acidemia. Clin. Chem., 16, 420-422, 1970.

[4] AULA (P.), RAPOLA (J.) et coll. — Prenatal diagnosis and fetal pathology of I-cell disease (mucolipidosis type II). J. Pediat., 87, 221-226, 1975.

[5] AULA (P.), AUTIO (S.) et coll. — « Salla disease ». A new lysosomal storage disorder. Arch. Neurol., 36, 88-94, 1974.

[6] AUSTIN (J. H.). — Studies in metachromatic leukodystrophy. XII. Multiple sulfatase deficiency. Arch. Neurol., 28, 258-264, 1973.

[6 b] AVOGARO (P.), CAZZOLATO (G.) et coll. — Familial hyper-alphalipoproteinemia, further studies on serum lipoproteins and some serum enzymes. Clin. Chim. Acta, 77, 139-145, 1977.

[7] BACH (G.), ZIEGLER (M.) et coll. — Mucopolysaccharide accumulation in cultured skin fibroblasts derived form patients with mucolipidosis. IV. Amer. J. Hum. Genet., 29, 610-618, 1977.

[8] BACHMANN (C.), KRÄHENBÜHL (S.) et coll. — N-acetylglutamate synthetase deficiency: a disorder of ammonia detoxication. N. Engl. J. Med., 304, 543, 1981.

[9] BAKAY (B.), NISSINEN (E.) et coll. — Utilization of purines by an HPRT variant in an intelligent, non mutilative patient with features of the Lesch-Nyhan syndrome. Pediatr. Res., 13, 1365-1370, 1979.

[10] BALLARD (R. A.), VINOCUR (B.) et coll. — Transient hyperammonemia in the preterm infant. N. Engl. J. Med., 299, 920-925, 1978.

[11] BANK (J. W.), DI MAURO (S.) et coll. — A disorder of muscle lipid metabolism and myoglobinuria. Absence of carnitine palmitoyl-transferase. N. Engl. J. Med., 292, 443-449, 1975.

[12] BAUDON (J. J.), FONTAINE (J. L.) et coll. — Acrodermatitis enteropathica. Étude anatomoclinique de deux cas familiaux traités par le sulfate de zinc. Arch. Fr. Pediat., 35, 63-73, 1978.

[13] BAUMGARTNER (E. R.), WICK (H.) et coll. — Congenital defect in intracellular cobalamin metabolism resulting in homocystinuria and methylmalonic aciduria. II. Biochemical investigations. Helv. Paediat. Acta., 34, 483-496, 1979.

[14] BEAUDET (A. L.), FERRY (G. D.) et coll. — Cholesterol ester storage disease: clinical, biochemical and pathological studies. J. Pediat., 90, 910-914, 1977.

[15] BECKER (M. A.), MEYER (L. J.) et coll. — Gout with purine overproduction due to increased phosphoribosylpyrophosphate synthetase activity. Amer. J. Med., 55, 232-242, 1973.

[16] BERARD (M.), TOGA (M.) et coll. — Pathological findings in one case of neuronal and mesenchymal storage disease. Its relationship to lipidoses and mucopolysaccharidoses. Pathol. Europ., 3, 172-183, 1968.

[17] BERLOW (S.). — Progress in phenylketonuria: defects in the metabolism of biopterin. Pediatrics, 65, 837-839, 1980.

[18] BERMAN (E. R.), LIVNI (N.) et coll. — Congenital corneal clouding with abnormal systemic storage bodies: a new variant of mucolipidosis. J. Pediat., 84, 519-526, 1974.

[19] BERRY (H. K.), SUTHERLAND (B. S.) et coll. — Interpretation of results of blood screening studies for detection of phenylketonuria. Pediatrics, 37, 102-106, 1966.

[20] BESLEY (G. T. N.), GATT (S.). — Spectrophotometric and fluorimetric assays of galactocerebrosidase activity, their use in the diagnosis of Krabbe's disease. Clin. Chim. Acta, 110, 19-26, 1981.

[21] BICKEL (H.), GERRARD (J.) et coll. — Influence of phenylalanine intake on the chemistry and behavior of a phenylketonuric child. Acta Paediat., 43, 64-77, 1954.

[22] BICKEL (H.). — Rationale of neonatal screening for inborn errors of metabolism. In: Neonatal screening for inborn errors of metabolism. H. BIC-

KEL, R. GUTHRIE, G. HAMMERSEN, eds., Springer-Verlag, Berlin, 1-6, 1980.

[23] BIENVENU (J.), MATHIEU (M.) et coll. — Étude immuno-chimique de l'alpha 1,4-glucosidase acide chez sept malades atteints de glycogénose de type II. *Pediatrie* (Lyon), *34*, 659-676, 1979.

[24] BJÖRKMAN (L.), MCLEAN (C.) et coll. — Organic acids in urine from human newborns. *Clin. Chem.*, *22*, 49-52, 1976.

[25] BLASKOVICS (M. E.), NG (W. G.) et coll. — Prenatal diagnosis and a case report of isovaleric acidaemia. *J. Inher. Metab. Dis.*, *1*, 9-11, 1978.

[26] BLASKOVICS (M. E.), SCHAEFFLER (G. E.) et coll. — Phenylalaninemia. Differential diagnosis. *Arch. Dis. Child.*, *49*, 835-843, 1974.

[27] BLASS (J. P.), AVIGAN (J.) et coll. — A defect in pyruvate decarboxylase in a child with an intermittent movement disorder. *J. Clin. Invest.*, *49*, 423-432, 1970.

[28] BOIVIN (P.), GALAND (C.) et coll. — Déficit en glutathion synthétase avec 5-oxoprolinurie. Deux nouveaux cas et revue de la littérature. *Nouv. Presse Méd.*, *7*, 1531-1535, 1978.

[29] BOUE (A.). — Le risque fœtal de l'amniocentèse précoce. *Nouv. Presse Méd.*, *8*, 2947-2958, 1979.

[30] BOUE (J.), MORER (I.) et coll. — Diagnostic prénatal : résultats de 1 532 ponctions amniotiques et étude prospective de 1 023 cas. *Nouv. Presse Méd.*, *8*, 2949-2953, 1979.

[31] BOUGNERES (P. F.), SAUDUBRAY (J. M.) et coll. — Fasting hypoglycemia resulting from hepatic carnitine palmitoyl transferase deficiency. *J. Pediat.*, *98*, 742-746, 1981.

[32] BRADY (R. O.). — Sphingomyelin lipidosis: Niemann-Pick disease. In: *The metabolic Basis on inherited Diseases*. J. B. STANBURY, J. B. WYNGAARDEN , D. S. FREDRICKSON, eds. McGraw-Hill, New York, 718-730, 1978.

[33] BRADY (R. O.). — Glycosyl ceramide lipidosis: Gaucher's disease. In: *The metabolic Basis of inherited Diseases*, J. B. STANBURY, J. B. WYNGAARDEN, D. S. FREDRICKSON, eds. McGraw-Hill, New York, 731-746, 1978.

[34] BRADY (R. O.), TALLMAN (J. F.) et coll. — Replacement therapy for inherited enzyme deficiency: use of purified ceramide trihexosidase in Fabry's disease. *N. Engl. J. Med.*, *289*, 9-14, 1973.

[35] BRANDT (N. J.), GREGERSEN (N.) et coll. — Treatment of glutaryl CoA dehydrogenase deficiency (glutaric aciduria). *J. Pediat.*, *94*, 669-673, 1979.

[36] BRANDT (N. J.), RASMUSSEN (K.) et coll. — D-Glyceric acidemia and non ketotic hyperglycinemia. Clinical and laboratory findings in a new syndrome. *Acta Paediat. Scand.*, *65*, 17-22, 1976.

[37] BRETT (E. M.), ELLIS (R. B.) et coll. — Late onset GM2 gangliosidosis: clinical, pathological and biochemical studies on 8 patients. *Arch. Dis. Child.*, *48*, 775-785, 1973.

[38] BROYER (M.), GUESRY (P.). — Acidémie méthylmalonique avec néphropathie hyperuricémique. *Arch. Fr. Pédiat.*, *31*, 543-552, 1974.

[39] BRUSILOW (S.), TINKER (J.) et coll. — Aminoacid acylation: a mechanism of nitrogen excretion in inborn errors of urea synthesis. *Science*, *207*, 659-661, 1980.

[40] BUBIS (J. J.), ADLESBERG (L.). — Congenital metachromatic leukodystrophy. *Acta Neuropath.*, *6*, 298-302, 1966.

[41] CANTZ (M.), GEHLER (J.) et coll. — Mucolipidosis I: increased sialic acid content and deficiency of an alpha-N-acetylneuraminidase in cultured fibroblasts. *Biochem. Biophys. Res. Commun.*, *74*, 732-738, 1977.

[42] CARSON (N. A. J.), SCALLY (B. G.) et coll. — Saccharopinuria: a new inborn error of lysine metabolism. *Nature*, *218*, 679, 1968.

[43] CARTIER (P.), PERIGNON (J. L.). — Xanthinurie. *Nouv. Presse Med.*, *7*, 1381-1390, 1978.

[44] CARTIER (P.), HAMET (M.) et coll. — Lithiase urinaire de l'enfant ; possibilité d'un déficit héréditaire en adénine phosphoribosyltransférase. *Nouv. Presse Méd.*, *9*, 1767-1770, 1980.

[45] CASEY (R. E.), ZALESKI (W. A.) et coll. — Biochemical and clinical studies of a new case of alpha-aminoadipic aciduria. *J. Inher. Metab. Dis.*, *1*, 129-135, 1978.

[46] CATHELINEAU (L.). — L'hyperammoniémie dans la pathologie pédiatrique. *Arch. Fr. Pediat.*, *36*, 724-735, 1979.

[47] CEDERBAUM (S. D.), SHAW (K. N. F.) et coll. — Hyperlysinemia with saccharopinuria due to combined lysine-ketoglutarate reductase and saccharopine dehydrogenase deficiencies presenting as cystinuria. *J. Pediatr.*, *95*, 234-238, 1979.

[48] CHALMERS (R. A.), LAWSON (A. M.) et coll. — D-2-Hydroxyglutaric aciduria: case report and biochemical studies. *J. Inher. Metab. Dis.*, *3*, 11-15, 1980.

[49] CHAPOY (P.), ANGELINI (S.). et coll. — Déficit systémique en carnitine. Place dans le syndrome de Reye. *Nouv. Presse Méd.*, *10*, 499-502, 1981.

[50] CHEEMA-DHADLI (S.), LEZNOFF (C. C.) et coll. — Effect of 2 methylcitrate on citrate metabolism: implication for the management of patients with propionic acidemia and methylmalonic aciduria. *Pediat. Res.*, *9*, 905-908, 1975.

[51] CHILDS (B.), NYHAN (W. L.) et coll. — Idiopathic hyperglycinemia and hyperglycinuria, a new disorder of amino-acid metabolism. *Pediatrics*, *27*, 522-538, 1961.

[52] CHOOK (H.), COTTON (R. G. H.) et coll. — Observations indicating the nature of the mutation in phenylketonuria. *J. Inher. Metab. Dis.*, *2*, 79-84, 1979.

[53] CHRISTOMANOU (H.). — Niemann-Pick disease type C: evidence for the deficiency of an activating factor stimulating sphingomyelin and glucocerebroside degradation. *Hoppe-Seyler's Z. physiol. Chem.*, *361*, 1489-1502, 1980.

[54] CLAYTON (B. C.). — The principles of treatment by dietary restriction as illustrated by phenylketonuria in *The Treatment of Inherited Metabolic Disease*. D. N. RAINE, ed., Medical and technical Publishing, Lancaster, 1-32, 1975.

[55] COATES (P. M.), CORTNER (J. A.) et coll. — Prenatal diagnosis of Wolman disease. *Amer. J. Med. Genet.*, *3*, 397-407, 1978.

[56] COHN (R. M.), YUDKOFF (M.) et coll. — Isovaleric acidemia: use of glycine therapy in neonates. *N. Engl. J. Med.*, *299*, 996-999, 1978.

[57] COICADAN (L.), HEYMAN (M.) et coll. — Cystinurie: reduced lysine permeability at the brush border of intestinal membrane cells. *Pediatr. Res.*, *14*, 109-112, 1980.

[58] COLLINS (F. S.), SUMMER (G. K.) et coll. — Neonatal argininosuccinic aciduria. Survival after early diagnosis and dietary management. *J. Pediat.*, *96*, 429-432, 1980.

[59] COLOMBO (J. P.), BURGI (W.) et coll. — Congenital lysine intolerance with periodic ammonia intoxication. A defect in L-lysine degradation. *Metabolism*, 16, 910-925, 1967.

[60] COMMITTEE CN NUTRITION, AMERICAN ACADEMY CF PEDIATRICS. — Special diets for infants with inborn errors of amino-acid metabolism. *Pediatrics*, 57, 783-792, 1976.

[61] CONZELMANN (E.), SANDHOFF (K.). — AB variant of infantile GM2 gangliosidosis: Deficiency of a factor necessary for stimulation of hexosaminidase A-catalyzed degradation of ganglioside GM2 and glycolipid GA2. *Proc. nat. Acad. Sci. U. S.*, 75, 3979-3983, 1978.

[62] CORNBLATH (M.), SCHWARTZ (R.). — *Disorders of carbohydrate metabolism in infancy.* 1 vol. 2nd ed., W. B. Saunders Cy. Philadelphia, 1976.

[63] COSTIL (J.), DEBARD (A.) et coll. — Acidémie propionique. A propos de deux observations. *Sem. Hôp. (Paris)*, 56, 22-27, 1980.

[64] COSTIL (J.), RICHARDET (J. M.) et coll. — Hyperphénylalaninémie induite par la pyriméthamine. *Nouv. Presse Méd.*, 5, 26-27, 1976.

[65] COUDE (F. X.), SWEETMAN (L.) et coll. — Inhibition by propionyl Coenzyme A of N-acetyl-glutamate synthetase in rat liver mitochondria. A possible explanation for hyperammonemia in propionic and methylmalonic acidemia. *J. Clin. Invest.*, 64, 1544-1551, 1979.

[66] CROCKER (A. C.). — The cerebral defect in Tay-Sachs and Niemann-Pick disease. *J. Neurochem.*, 7, 69-80, 1961.

[67] CROME (L.), HANEFELD (F.) et coll. — Late onset globoid leukodystrophy. *Brain*, 96, 841-848, 1973.

[68] CURTIUS (H. Ch.), NIEDERWIESER (A.) et coll. — Atypical phenylketonuria due to tetrahydrobiopterin deficiency. Diagnosis and treatment with tetrahydrobiopterin, dihydrobiopterin and septiapterin. *Clin. Chim. Acta*, 93, 251-262, 1979.

[68 b] DANCIS (J.), HUTZLER (J.) et coll. — Enzyme activity in classical and variant forms of maple syrup urine disease. *J. Pediat.*, 81, 312-320, 1972.

[69] DANKS (D. M.), COTTON (R. G. H.). — Early diagnosis of hyperphenylalaninemia due to tetrahydrobiopterin deficiency (malignant hyperphenylalaninemia). *J. Pediat.*, 96, 854-856, 1980.

[70] DANON (M. J.), OH (S. J.) et coll. — Lysosomal glycogen storage disease with normal acid maltase. *Neurology*, 31, 51-57, 1981.

[71] DAUM (R. S.), LAMM (Ph.) et coll. — A new disorder of isoleucine catabolism. *Lancet*, 2, 1289-1290, 1971.

[72] DE BAECQUE (C. M.), SUZUKI (K.) et coll. — GM2 gangliosidosis, AB variant. *Acta Neuropath.*, 33, 207-226, 1975.

[73] DE BROHUN-BUTLER (J.), TIETZE (F.) et coll. — Depletion of cystine in cystinotic fibroblasts by drugs enclosed in liposomes. *Pediat. Res.*, 12, 46-51, 1978.

[74] DE GROOT (C. J.), HAAN (G. L.) et coll. — A patient with severe neurologic symptoms and aceto acetyl CoA thiolase deficiency (Abst.). *Pediat. Res.*, 11, 1112, 1977.

[75] DELLAS (J. A.). — Hypouricémie d'origine rénale. A propos d'un cas. *Sem. Hôp. (Paris)*, 56, 475-476, 1980.

[76] DE MARS (R.), LEROY (J. G.). — The remarkable cells cultured from a human with Hurler's syndrome; an approach to visual selection for *in vitro* genetic studies. *In vitro*, 2, 107-118, 1967.

[77] DESBOIS (J. C.), CHARPENTIER (C.). — Homocystinuries sensibles à la vitamine B6. Étude à long terme de la sensibilité à la pyridoxine. In: *Journées Parisiennes de Pédiatrie.* Flammarion, Paris, 212-226, 1979.

[78] DESNICK (R. J.), KLIONSKY (B.) et coll. — Fabry's disease (alpha-galactosidase A deficiency) In: *The metabolic Basis of inherited Diseases.* J. B. STANBURY, J. B. WYNGAARDEN, D. S. FREDRICKSON, eds. McGraw-Hill, New York, 810-840, 1978.

[79] DE VRIES (A.), KOCHWA (S.) et coll. — Glycinuria, a hereditary disorder associated with nephrolithiasis. *Amer. J. Med.*, 23, 408-415, 1957.

[80] DEYBACH (J. Ch.), GRANDCHAMP (B.) et coll. — Prenatal exclusion of congenital erythropoietic porphyria (Gunther's disease) in a fetus at risk. *Hum. Genet.*, 53, 217-221, 1980.

[81] DHONDT (H. L.), FARRIAUX (J. P.). — Diagnostic des hétérozygotes de la phénylcétonurie par l'épreuve de charge orale en phénylalanine. *J. Génét. Hum.*, 27, 145-156, 1979.

[82] DI FERRANTE (N.), HYMAN (B. H.) et coll. — Mucopolysaccharidosis VI (Maroteaux-Lamy disease). Clinical and biochemical study of a mild variant case. *J. Hopkins Med. J.*, 135, 42-54, 1974.

[83] DILLON (M. J.), ENGLAND (J. M.) et coll. — Mental retardation, megaloblastic anemia, methylmalonic aciduria and abnormal homocysteine metabolism due to an error in vitamin B12 metabolism. *Clin. Sci. Mol. Med.*, 47, 43-61, 1974.

[84] DI MAURO (S.), DI MAURO (P. M. M.). — Muscle carnitine palmityl transferase deficiency and myoglobinuria. *Science*, 182, 929-931, 1973.

[85] DREYFUS (P. M.), DUBE (V. E.). — The rapid detection of methylmalonic acid in urine. Sensitive index of vitamin B12 deficiency. *Clin. Chim. Acta*, 15, 525-528, 1967.

[86] DREYFUS (J. C.), POENARU (L.) et coll. — Absence of hexosaminidase A and B in a normal adult. *N. Engl. J. Med.*, 292, 61-63, 1975.

[87] DRUMMOND (K. N.), MICHAEL (A. F.) et coll. — The blue diaper syndrome; familial hypercalcemia with nephrocalcinosis and indicanuria. *Amer. J. Med.*, 37, 928-948, 1964.

[88] DRY (J.), DELPORTE (M. P.) et coll. — La maladie de Refsum. *Sem. Hôp. Paris*, 52, 1683-1690, 1976.

[89] DUBART (A.), GOOSSENS (M.) et coll. — Le diagnostic prénatal dans les hémoglobinopathies humaines. *Reprod. Nutr. Develop.*, 20, 523-537, 1980.

[90] DUBOIS (G.), TURPIN (J. C.) et coll. — Arylsulfatases A and B in leukocytes: a comparative statistical study of the late infantile and juvenile forms of metachromatic leukodystrophy and controls. *Biomedicine*, 33, 2-4, 1980.

[91] DULANEY (J. T.), MOSER (H. W.). — Sulfatide lipidosis: metachromatic leukodystrophy. In: *The metabolic Basis of inherited Diseases.* J. B. STANBURY, J. B. WYNGAARDEN, D. S. FREDRICKSON, McGraw-Hill, New York, 770-809, 1ᵗ¹⁸

[92] DURAN (M.), VAN BIERVLIET (J. P. G. M.) et coll. — D-Lactic aciduria, an inborn error of metabolism. *Clin. Chim. Acta*, 74, 297-300, 1977.

[93] DURAN (M.), SCHUTGENS (R. B. H.) et coll. — 3-hydroxy-3-methylglutaryl coenzyme A lyase deficiency: post-natal management following pre-

natal diagnosis by analysis of maternal urine. *J. Pediat.*, 95, 1004-1006, 1979.

[94] DURAN (M.), VAN SPRANG (J. F.) et coll. — Two sisters with isovaleric acidaemia. Multiple attacks of keto-acidosis and normal development. *Europ. J. Pediat.*, 131, 205-211, 1979.

[95] DURAND (P.), PHILIPPART (M.) et coll. — Una nuova malattia da accumulo di glycolipidi (ceramidi tetraosidi). *Minerva Pediat.*, 19, 2187-2196, 1967.

[96] DURAND (P.), BORRONE (C.) et coll. — On genetic variants in fucosidosis. *J. Pediat.*, 89, 688-690, 1976.

[97] DUSHEIKO (G.), KEW (M. C.) et coll. — Recurrent hypoglycemia associated with glutaric aciduria type II in an adult. *N. Engl. J. Med.*, 301, 1405-1409, 1979.

[98] ENGEL (A. G.), GOMEZ (M. B.) et coll. — The spectrum and diagnosis of acid maltase deficiency. *Neurology*, 23, 95-106, 1973.

[99] ENGEL (A. G.), ANGELINI (C.). — Carnitine deficiency of human skeletal muscle with associated lipid storage myopathy. *Science*, 179, 899-902, 1973.

[100] EPINETTE (W. W.), NORINS (A. L.) et coll. — Angiokeratoma corporis diffusum with alpha-L-fucosidase deficiency. *Arch. Dermatol.*, 107, 754-757, 1973.

[101] FALLSTROM (S. P.), LINDBLAD (B.) et coll. — Hereditary tyrosinemia. Fumarylacetoacetase deficiency (Abst.). *Pediatr. Res.*, 13, 78, 1979.

[102] FARREL (D. F.), CLARK (A. F.) et coll. — Absence of pyruvate decarboxylase activity in man: a cause of congenital lactic acidosis. *Science*, 187, 1082-1084, 1975.

[103] FARRIAUX (J. P.), STRECKER (G.). — La mucolipidose II ("I cell disease"). Une sialidose? *Arch. Fr. Pediatr.*, 36, 225-234, 1979.

[104] FARRIAUX (J. P.). — La mannosidose. In: *Les oligosaccharidoses.* FARRIAUX (J. P.), ed., Crouan et Roques, Lille, 89-98, 1976.

[105] FARRIAUX (J. P.). — *Le cycle de l'urée et ses anomalies.* 1 vol., 263 p., Doin, Paris, 1978.

[106] FAULL (K. F.), GAN (I.) et coll. — Metabolic studies on two patients with non hepatic tyrosinemia using deuterated tyrosine loads. *Pediat. Res.*, 11, 631-637, 1977.

[107] FEIT (J. P.), DAVID (M.) et coll. — L'abêtalipoprotéinémie. Étude clinique, génétique, endocrinienne et métabolique d'une nouvelle observation familiale. *Pédiatrie (Lyon)*, 32, 753-780, 1977.

[108] FENSOM (A. H.), BENSOM (P. F.) et coll. — Fibroblast alpha-galactosidase A activity for identification of Fabry's disease heterozygotes. *J. Inher. Metab. Dis.*, 2, 9-12, 1979.

[109] FLEISHER (L. D.), LOWGHI (R. C.) et coll. — Homocystinuria: investigations of cystathionine synthase in cultured fetal cells and the prenatal determination of genetic status. *J. Pediat.*, 85, 677-680, 1974.

[110] FLORET (D.), DIVRY (P.) et coll. — Acidurie glutarique. Une nouvelle observation. *Arch. Fr. Pediatr.*, 36, 462-470, 1979.

[111] FONTAINE (G.), FARRIAUX (J. P.) et coll. — L'hyperprolinémie de type I. Étude d'une observation familiale. *Helv. Paediat. Acta*, 25, 165-176, 1970.

[112] FRANCK (M.), MANY (M.) et coll. — Familial renal hypouricemia: two additional cases with uric acid lithiasis. *Brit. J. Urol.*, 51, 88-91, 1979.

[113] FRAZIER (D. M.), SUMMER (G. K.) et coll. — Hyperglycinuria and hyperglycinemia in two siblings

with mild developmental delays. *Amer. J. Dis. Child.*, 132, 777-781, 1978.

[114] FREDRICKSON (D. S.), FERRANS (V. J.). — Acid cholesteryl ester hydrolase deficiency (Wolman's disease and cholesteryl ester storage disease). In: *The metabolic Basis of inherited Diseases.* J. B. STANBURY, J. B. WYNGAARDEN, D. S. FREDRICKSON, ed. McGraw-Hill, New York, 670-687, 1978.

[114 b] FREDRICKSON (D. S.), GOLDSTEIN (J. L.) et coll. — The familial hyperlipoproteinemias. In: *The metabolic Basis of inherited Diseases.* J. B. STANBURY J. B. WYNGAARDEN, D. S. FREDRICKSON, ed. McGraw-Hill, New York, 4th ed., 604-655, 1978.

[115] GAULL (G. E.), BENDER (A. N.). et coll. — Methioninemia and myopathy: a new disorder. *Ann. Neurol.*, 9, 423-432, 1981.

[116] GAULL (G. E.), TALLAN (H. H.) et coll. — Hypermethioninemia associated with methionine adenosyl transferase deficiency: clinical, morphologic and biochemical observations on four patients. *J. Pediat.*, 98, 734-741, 1981.

[117] GEISER (C. F.), SHIH (V. E.). — Cystathioninuria and its origin in children with hepatoblastoma. *J. Pediat.*, 96, 72-75, 1980.

[118] GERRITSEN (T.), WAISMAN (H. A.). — Hypersarcosinemia in the *Metabolic Basis of Inherited Disease.* STANBURY J. B., WYNGAARDEN J. B., FREDRICKSON D. S., ed. McGraw-Hill, New York, 514-517, 1978.

[119] GHADIMI (H.). — The hyperlysinemias in *The Metabolic Basis of Inherited Disease.* STANBURY J. B., WYNGAARDEN J. B., FREDRICKSON D. S., ed. McGraw-Hill, New York, 387-396, 1978.

[120] GHADIMI (H. K.). — Histidinemia. Biochemistry and behavior. *Amer. J. Dis. Child.*, 135, 210-211, 1981.

[121] GIBBERD (F. B.), PAGE (N. G. R.) et coll. — Heredopathia atactica polyneuritiformis (Refsum's disease) treated by diet and plasma exchange. *Lancet*, 1, 575-578, 1979.

[122] GIBLETT (E. R.), ANDERSON (J. E.) et coll. — Adenosine deaminase deficiency in two patients with severely impaired cellular immunity. *Lancet*, 2, 1067-1069, 1972.

[123] GIBLETT (E. R.), AMMAN (A. J.) et coll. — Nucleoside phosphorylase deficiency in a child with severely defective T-cell immunity and normal B cell immunity. *Lancet*, 1, 1010-1013, 1975.

[124] GIORGIO (A. J.), TROWBUDGE (M.) et coll. — Methylmalonic aciduria without vitamin B12 deficiency in an adult sibship. *N. Engl. J. Med.*, 295, 310-313, 1976.

[125] GIORGIO (A. J.), PLAUT (G. W. E.). — A method for the colorimetric determination of urinary methylmalonic acid in pernicious anemia. *J. Lab. Clin. Med.*, 66, 667-676, 1965.

[126] GLASGOW (A. M.), ENG (G.) et coll. — Systemic carnitine deficiency simulating recurrent Reye syndrome. *J. Pediat.*, 96, 889-891, 1980.

[127] GITZELMANN (R.), STEINMANN (B.) et coll. — Non ketotic hyperglycinemia treated with strychnine, a glycine receptor antagonist. *Helv. Paediat. Acta*, 32, 517-525, 1977.

[128] GODDON (R.), FREYCON (M. T.) et coll. — Une nouvelle observation de maladie de Menkes. *Pediatrie (Lyon)*, 34, 336-341, 1979.

[129] GOLDBERG (R. N.), CABAL (L. A.) et coll. — Hyperammonemia associated with perinatal asphyxia. *Pediatrics*, 64, 336-341, 1979.

[130] GOLDSMITH (L. A.). — Molecular biology and molecular pathology of a newly described molecular disease. Tyrosinemia type II (The Richner-Hanhart Syndrome). *Exp. Cell. Biol.*, *46*, 96-113, 1978.

[131] GOLDSTEIN (J. L.), CAMPBELL (B. K.) et coll. — Homocystinuria: heterozygote detection using phytohemagglutinin-stimulated lymphocytes. *J. Clin. Invest.*, *52*, 218-221, 1973.

[132] GOMPERTZ (D.), STORRS (C. N.) et coll. — Localization of enzymic defect in propionic acidemia. *Lancet*, *1*, 1140-1144, 1970.

[133] GOMPERTZ (D.), DRAFFAN (G. H.) et coll. — Biotin responsive beta-methylcrotonyl aciduria. *Lancet*, *2*, 22-24, 1971.

[134] GOODMAN (S. I.), MARKEY (S. P.) et coll. — Glutaric aciduria; a "new" disorder of aminoacid metabolism. *Biochem. Med.*, *12*, 12-21, 1975.

[135] GOODMAN (S. I.), MARKEY (S. P.). — *Diagnosis of organic acidemias by gas chromatography-mass spectrometry*. 1 vol. R. LISS, New York, *1*, 1981.

[136] GOODMAN (S. I.), NORENBERG (M. D.) et coll. — Glutaric aciduria: biochemical and morphologic considerations. *J. Pediat.*, *90*, 746-750, 1977.

[137] GOODMAN (S. I.), MCCABE (E. R. B.) et coll. — Multiple acyl-CoA dehydrogenase deficiency (glutaric aciduria type II) with transient hypersarcosinemia and sarcosinuria: possible inherited deficiency of an electron transfer flavoprotein. *Pediat. Res.*, *14*, 12-17, 1980.

[138] GOODMAN (S. I.), GALLEGOS (D. A.) et coll. — Antenatal diagnosis of glutaric acidemia. *Amer. J. Hum. Genet.*, *32*, 695-699, 1980.

[139] GOODMAN (S. I.), MOE (P. G.) et coll. — Homocystinuria with methylmalonic aciduria: two cases in a sibship. *Biochem. Med.*, *4*, 500-515, 1970.

[140] GOODMAN (S. I.), MCCABE (E. R. B.) et coll. — Methylmalonic/beta-hydroxy-*n*-valeric aciduria du to methylmalonyl CoA mutase deficiency. *Clin. Chim. Acta*, *87*, 441-449, 1978.

[141] GOUT (J. P.), SERRE (J. C.) et coll. — Une nouvelle cause d'hyperméthioninémie de l'enfant : le déficit en S-adénosyl méthionine synthétase. *Arch. Fr. Pédiatr.*, *34*, 416-423, 1977.

[142] GOUTET (J. M.), AYMARD (P.) et coll. — Hyperphénylalaninémie provoquée par le triméthoprim sulfaméthoxazole chez un nourrisson hétérozygote de phénylcétonurie. *Nouv. Presse Méd.*, *8*, 4045-4046, 1979.

[143] GOUTIERES (F.), ARSENIO-NUNES (M. L.) et coll. — Mucolipidosis IV. *Neuropädiatrie*, *10*, 321-331, 1979.

[144] GORDON (E. F.), GORDON (R. C.) et coll. — Zinc metabolism: basic, clinical and behavioral aspects. *J. Pediat.*, *99*, 341-349, 1981.

[145] GRANDGEORGE (D.), FAVIER (A.) et coll. — L'acidémie D-glycérique. A propos d'une nouvelle observation anatomo-clinique. *Arch. Fr. Pediatr.*, *37*, 577-584, 1980.

[146] GRAVEL (R. A.), LOWDEN (J. A.) et coll. — Infantile sialidosis: a phenocopy of type I GM1 gangliosidosis. *Amer. J. Hum. Genet.*, *31*, 669-679, 1979.

[147] GRAY (R. G. F.), PATRICK (A. D.) et coll. — Acute hereditary tyrosinaemia type I: clinical, biochemical and haematological studies in twins. *J. Inher. Metab. Dis.*, *4*, 37-40, 1981.

[148] GRAY (R. G. F.), O'NEILL (E. M.) et coll. — Alphaaminoadipic aciduria: chemical and enzymatic studies. *J. Inher. Metab. Dis.*, *2*, 89-92, 1979.

[149] GREGERSEN (N.), INGERSLEV (J.) et coll. — Low molecular weight organic acid in the urine of the newborn. *Acta Paediat. Scand.*, *66*, 85-89, 1977.

[149 *b*] GREGERSEN (N.), ROSLEFF (F.) et coll. — Non ketotic C6-C10 dicarboxylic aciduria: biochemical investigations of two cases. *Clin. Chim. Acta*, *102*, 179-180, 1980.

[150] GUBLER (M. C.), LENOIR (G.) et coll. — Early renal changes in hemizygous and heterozygous patients with Fabry's disease. *Kidney Intern.*, *13*, 223-235, 1978.

[151] GUGGENHEIM (M. A.), MCCABE (E. R. B.) et coll. — Glycerol kinase deficiency with neuromuscular skeletal and adrenal abnormalities. *Ann. Neurol.*, *7*, 441-449, 1980.

[152] GUIBAUD (P.), VANIER (M. T.) et coll. — Forme infantile précoce, cholestatique, rapidement mortelle de la sphingomyélinose, type « C ». *Pédiatrie*, *(Lyon)*, *34*, 103-114, 1979.

[153] GUILLOT (M.), BROYER (M.) et coll. — Nutrition entérale à débit constant en néphrologie pédiatrique. *Arch. Fr. Pédiat.*, *37*, 497-505, 1980.

[154] GÜTTLER (F.). — Hyperphenylalaninemia: Diagnosis and classification of the various types of phenylalanine hydroxylase deficiency in childhood. *Acta Paediat. Scand. Suppl.*, *280*, 74, 1980.

[155] HALTIA (M.), PALO (J.) et coll. — Aspartylglycosaminuria: a generalized storage disease. Morphological and histochemical studies. *Acta Neuropath.*, *31*, 243-255, 1975.

[156] HALTIA (M.), PALO (J.) et coll. — Juvenile metachromatic leukodystrophy. Clinical, biochemical and neuropathologic studies in nine new cases. *Arch. Neurol.*, *37*, 42-46, 1980.

[157] HALVORSEN (S.). — Screening for disorders of tyrosine metabolism. In: *Neonatal screening for inborn errors of metabolism*. H. BICKEL, R. GUTHRIE, G. HAMMERSEN eds., Springer Verlag, Berlin, 45-57, 1980.

[158] HAMET (M.), GRISCELLI (C.) et coll. — A second case of inosine phosphorylase deficiency with severe T cell abnormalities. *Adv. Exp. Med. Biol.*, *76*, 477-480, 1977.

[159] HANSEN (S.), PERRY (T. L.) et coll. — Urinary bacteria: potential source of some organic aciduria. *Clin. Chim. Acta*, *39*, 71-74, 1972.

[160] HARPEY (J. P.), ROSENBLATT (D. S.) et coll. — Homocystinuria caused by 5, 10 methylenetetrahydrofolate reductase deficiency: a case in an infant responding to methionine, folinic acid, pyridoxine and vitamin B12 therapy. *J. Pediat.*, *98*, 272-278, 1981.

[161] HARZER (K.), SCHLOTZ (W.) et coll. — Neurovisceral lipidosis compatible with Niemann-Pick disease, type C: morphological and biochemical studies of a late infantile case and enzyme and lipid assays in a prenatal case of the same family. *Acta Neuropath.*, *43*, 97-104, 1978.

[162] HASILIK (A.), NEUFELD (E. F.). — Biosynthesis of lysosomal enzymes in fibroblasts. Synthesis as precursors of higher molecular weight. *J. Biol. Chem.*, *255*, 4937-4945, 1980.

[163] HASILIK (A.), WAHEED (A) et coll. — Enzymatic phosphorylation of lysosomal enzymes in the presence of U. D. P.-N-acetylglucosamine: absence of activity in I-cell fibroblasts. *Biochem. Biophys. Res. Commun.*, *98*, 761-767, 1981.

[164] HERBERT (P. N.), GOTTO (A. M.) et coll. — Familial lipoprotein deficiency. In: *The metabolic Basis of inherited Diseases* J. B. STANBURY, J. B.

WYNGAARDEN, D. S. FREDRICKSON, ed. McGraw-Hill, New York, 544-588, 1978.

[165] HERMIER (M.), CARRIER (H.) et coll. — Hypotonie et encéphalopathie convulsivante avec myopathie lipidique et déficit en palmityl carnitine transférase (P. C. T.). Entité nouvelle? *Pédiatrie (Lyon)*, 34, 503-518, 1979.

[166] HILLMAN (R. E.), KEATINE (J. P.). — Beta-keto-thiolase deficiency as a cause of the "ketotic hyperglycinemia syndrome". *Pediatrics*, 53, 221-226, 1974.

[167] HIRSCHHORN (R.), BERATIS (N.) et coll. — Adenosine-deaminase in a child diagnosed prenatally. *Lancet*, 1, 73-75, 1975.

[168] HOEFNAGEL (D.), POMEROY (J.). — Hydroxylysinuria. *Lancet*, 1, 1341, 1970.

[169] HOOFT (C.), TIMMERMANS (J.) et coll. — Methionine malabsorption syndrome. *Ann. Paediat.* (Basel), 205, 73-84, 1965.

[170] HOOGEVEN (A. T.), VERHEIJEN (F. W.) et coll. — Genetic heterogeneity in human neuraminidase deficiency. *Nature*, 285, 500-502, 1980.

[171] HORN (N.). — Copper incorporation studies on cultured cells for prenatal diagnosis of Menke's disease. *Lancet*, 1, 1156-1158, 1976.

[172] HOWELL (R. R.), KABACK (M. M.) et coll. — Type IV glycogen storage disease: branching enzyme deficiency in skin fibroblasts and possible heterozygote detection. *J. Pediat.*, 78, 638-642, 1971.

[173] HSIA (Y. E.), SCULLY (K. J.) et coll. — Inherited propionyl CoA carboxylase deficiency in ketotic hyperglycinemia. *J. Clin. Invest.*, 50, 127-130, 1971.

[174] HUIJING (F.), WARREN (R. J.) et coll. — Elevated activity of lysosomal enzymes in amniotic fluid of a fetus with mucolipidosis II (I-cell disease). *Clin. Chim. Acta*, 44, 453-455, 1973.

[175] HUMBEL (R.), COLLART (M.). — Oligosaccharides in urine of patients with glycoprotein storage disease. I. rapid detection by thin layer chromatography. *Clin. Chim. Acta*, 60, 143-147, 1975.

[176] INFANTE (R.), POLONOVSKI (J.) et coll. — Polycorie cholestérolique de l'adulte. II. Étude biochimique. *Presse Méd.*, 75, 2829-2832, 1967.

[177] ITO (F.), AOKI (K.) et coll. — Histidinemia. Biochemical parameters for diagnosis. *Amer. J. Dis. Child.*, 135, 227-229, 1981.

[178] JELLUM (E.). — Profiling of human body fluids in healthy and diseased states using gas chromatography and mass spectrometry with special reference to organic acids. *J. Chromatogr.*, 143, 427-462, 1977.

[179] JENNER (F. A.), POLLITT (R. J.). — Large quantities of 2-acetamido-1-(beta-L-aspartamido) 1,2-dideoxy-glucose in the urine of mentally retarded siblings. *Biochem. J.*, 103, 48 p., 1967.

[180] KABACK (M. M.), SLOAN (H. R.) et coll. — GM1 gangliosidosis type 1: in utero detection and fetal manifestations. *J. Pediat.*, 82, 1037-1041, 1973.

[181] KABACK (M.), MILES (J.) et coll. — Hexosaminidase A deficiency in early adulthood: a new type of GM2 gangliosidosis. *Abst. Am. Soc. Hum. Genet.*, 29th Ann. Meet. Vancouver, 1978.

[181 b] KAN (Y. W.), TRECARTIN (R. F.) et coll. — Prenatal diagnosis of beta-thalassemia and sickle cell anemia. Experience with 24 cases. *Lancet*, 1, 268-271, 1977.

[182] KANG (E. S.), SNODGRASS (P. J.) et coll. — Methyl-malonyl-Coenzyme A racemase defect: another cause of methylmalonic aciduria. *Pediat. Res.*, 6, 875-879, 1972.

[183] KARK (R. A. P.), RODRIGUEZ-BUDELLI (M.). — Pyruvate dehydrogenase deficiency in spinocerebellar degenerations. *Neurology*, 29, 126-131, 1979.

[184] KARPATI (G.), CARPENTIER (S.) et coll. — The syndrome of systemic carnitine deficiency: clinical, morphologic, biochemical and pathophysiologic features. *Neurology*, 25, 16-24, 1975.

[185] KAUFMAN (Z.), HOLTZMAN (N. A.) et coll. — Phenylketonuria due to a deficiency of dihydropteridin-reductase. *N. Engl. J. Med.*, 293, 785-790, 1975.

[186] KAUFMAN (S.). — The phenylalanine hydroxylating system in phenylketonuria and its variants. *Biochem. Med.*, 15, 42-54, 1976.

[187] KAYE (C. I.), MORROW (G.) et coll. — In vitro "responsive" methylmalonic aciduria: a new variant. *J. Pediat.*, 85, 55-59, 1974.

[188] KELLEHER (J.), YUDKOFF (M.) et coll. — The pancytopenia of isovaleric acidemia. *Pediatrics*, 65, 1023-1027, 1980.

[189] KELLEY (W. N.), WYNGAARDEN (J. B.). — The Lesch-Nyhan syndrome. In: *The metabolic Basis of inherited Diseases*. 4th ed; J. B. STANBURY, J. B. WYNGAARDEN, D. S. FREDRICKSON, ed. McGraw-Hill, New York, 1011-1036, 1978.

[190] KELLY (T. E.), THOMAS (G. H.) et coll. — Mucolipidosis III (pseudo-Hurler polydystrophy): clinical and laboratory studies in a series of 12 patients. *John Hopkins Med. J.*, 137, 156-175, 1975.

[191] KIHARA (H.), HO (C. K.) et coll. — Prenatal diagnosis of metachromatic leukodystrophy in a family with pseudoarylsulfatase A deficiency by the cerebroside sulfate loading test. *Pediat. Res.*, 14, 224-227, 1980.

[192] KOHN (G.), LIVNI (N.) et coll. — Prenatal diagnosis of mucolipidosis IV by electron microscopy. *J. Pediat.*, 90, 62-66, 1977.

[193] KOLVRAA (S.), CHRISTENSEN (E.) et coll. — Studies of the glycine metabolism in a patient with D-glyceric acidemia and hyperglycinemia. *Pediat. Res.*, 14, 1029-1034, 1980.

[194] KOMROWER (G. M.), WESTALL (R.). — Hydroxy-kynureninuria. *Amer. J. Dis. Child.*, 113, 77-80, 1967.

[195] KOMROWER (G. M.), SARDHARWALLA (I. B.) et coll. — Management of maternal phenylketonuria: an emerging clinical problem. *Brit. Med. J.*, 1, 1383-1387, 1979.

[196] KRESS (B. C.), MILLER (A. L.). — Altered serum α-D-mannosidase activity in mucolipidosis II and mucolipidosis III. *Biochem. Biophys. Res. Comm.*, 81, 756-763, 1978.

[197] KRIEGER (I.), EVANS (G. N.) et coll. — Acrodermatitis enteropathica without hypozincemia: therapeutic effect of a pancreatic enzyme preparation due to a zinc binding ligand. *J. Pediat.*, 96, 32-35, 1980.

[198] LA DU (B. N.), GJESSING (L. R.). — Tyrosinosis and tyrosinemia in *The Metabolic Basis of Inherited Disease*. STANBURY (J. B.), WYNGAARDEN (J. B.), FREDRICKSON (D. S.), ed. McGraw-Hill, New York, p. 256-267, 1978.

[199] LAGERON (A.), CAROLI (J.) et coll. — Polycorie cholestérolique de l'adulte. I. — Étude clinique électronique, histochimique. *Presse Méd.*, 75, 2785-2790, 1967.

[200] LANDING (B. H.), SILVERMAN (F. N.) et coll. — Familial neurovisceral lipidosis. *Amer. J. Dis. Child.*, *108*, 503-522, 1964.

[201] LARSSON (A.), MATTSSON (B.) et coll. — 5-oxoprolinuria due to hereditary 5-oxoprolinase deficiency in two brothers. A new inborn error of the gamma-glutamyl cycle. *Acta Paediat. Scand.*, *70*, 301-308, 1981.

[202] LARSSON (A.), ZETTERSTRÖM (R.) et coll. — Pyroglutamic aciduria (5-oxoprolinuria) an inborn error in glutathione metabolism, *Pediat. Res.*, *8*, 852-856, 1974.

[203] LEIBEL (R. L.), SHIH (V. E.) et coll. — Glutaric aciduria; a metabolic disorder causing progressive choreo-athetosis. *Neurology*, *30*, 1163-1168, 1980.

[204] LEININGER (M. L.), CHAPOY (P.) et coll. — La carnosinémie, première observation française. *Pédiatrie (Lyon)*, *35*, 341-345, 1980.

[205] LEMONNIER (F.), CHARPENTIER (C.) et coll. — Tyrosine aminotransferase isoenzyme deficiency. *J. Pediat.*, *94*, 931-932, 1979.

[206] LENKE (R. R.), LEVY (H. L.). — Maternal phenylketonuria and hyperphenylalaninemia. *N. Engl. J. Med.*, *303*, 1202-1208, 1980.

[207] LEONARD (J. V.), MARRS (T. C.). — Intestinal absorption of amino-acids and peptides in Hartnup disorder. *Pediat. Res.*, *10*, 246-249, 1976.

[208] LEVY (H. L.), COULOMBE (J. T.) et coll. — Newborn urine screening. In: *Neonatal screening for inborn errors of metabolism.* BICKEL (H.), GUTHRIE (R.), HAMMERSEN (G.), ed. Springer Verlag, Berlin, 83-103, 1978.

[209] LOWDEN (J. A.), O'BRIEN (J. S.). — Sialidosis: a review of human neuraminidase deficiency. *Amer. J. Hum. Genet.*, *31*, 1-18, 1979.

[210] LYON (G.), JARDIN (L.) et coll. — Étude au microscope électronique d'un nerf périphérique dans un cas de leucodystrophie de Krabbe. *J. Neurol. Sci.*, *12*, 263-274, 1971.

[211] MACLEOD (P. M.), WOOD (S.) et coll. — Progressive cerebellar ataxia, spasticity, psychomotor retardation, and hexosaminidase deficiency in a 10 year old child: juvenile Sandhoff disease. *Neurology*, *27*, 571-573, 1977.

[212] MACE (J. W.), GOODMAN (S. I.). — The child with an unusual odor. *Clin. Pediat.*, *15*, 57-62, 1976.

[213] MAHONEY (M. J.), HOBBINS (J. C.). — Fetoscopy and fetal blood sampling. In: *Genetic Disorders and the Fetus.* A. MAHONEY ed., Plenum Press, New York, 501-526, 1979.

[214] MAIRE (I.), HERMIER (M.) et coll. — A propos d'une étude familiale de mannosidose. Intérêt de l'étude pour le diagnostic prénatal. In: *Les oligosaccharidoses.* FARRIAUX (J. P.), ed. Crouan et Roques, Lille, 149-158, 1976.

[215] MAMELLE (J. C.), VANIER (M. T.) et coll. — Étude clinique, ultrastructurale et biochimique d'un cas de gangliosidose à GM2 de type 2. *Arch. Fr. Pediat.*, *32*, 925-940, 1975.

[216] MANDERS (A. J.), OOSTROM (C. G. V.) et coll. — Alpha-amino-adipic aciduria and persistance of fetal haemoglobin in an oligophrenic child. *Eur. J. Pediat.*, *136*, 51-55, 1981.

[217] MANTAGOS (S.), GENEL (M.) et coll. — Ethylmalonic-adipic aciduria. *In vivo* and *in vitro* studies indicating deficiency of activities of multiple acyl-CoA dehydrogenases. *J. Clin. Invest.*, *64*, 1580-1589, 1979.

[218] MAROTEAUX (P.), HUMBEL (R.). — Les oligosaccharidoses. Un nouveau concept. *Arch. Fr. Pédiatr.*, *33*, 641-643, 1976.

[219] MAROTEAUX (P.), LAMY (M.). — La pseudopolydystrophie de Hurler. *Presse Méd.*, *74*, 2889-2892, 1966.

[220] MAROTEAUX (P.), HUMBEL (R.) et coll. — Un nouveau type de sialidose avec atteinte rénale : la néphrosialidose. I. — Étude clinique, radiologique et nosologique. *Arch. Fr. Pédiatr.*, *35*, 819-829, 1978.

[221] MARSAC (C.), AUGEREAU (Ch.) et coll. — Antenatal diagnosis of pyruvate carboxylase deficiency. *Lancet*, *1*, 675, 1981.

[222] MAX (S. R.), MACLAREN (N. K.) et coll. — GM3 (hematoside) sphingolipodystrophy. *N. Engl. J. Med.*, *291*, 929-931, 1974.

[223] MCARDLE (B.). — Myopathy due to a defect in muscle glycogen breakdown. *Clin. Sci.*, *10*, 13-35, 1951.

[224] MCKUSICK (V. A.), HOWELL (R. R.) et coll. — Allelism, non allelism and genetic compounds among the mucopolysaccharidoses. *Lancet*, *1*, 993-996, 1972.

[225] MEISTER (A.). — 5-oxoprolinuria (pyroglutamic aciduria) and other disorders of glutathione biosynthesis. In *The Metabolic Basis of Inherited Disease.* STANBURY (J. B.), WYNGARRDEN (J. B.), FREDRICKSON (D. S.), ed. McGraw-Hill, New York, 328-335, 1978.

[226] MEISTER (A.). — On the enzymology of amino-acid transport. *Science*, *180*, 33-39, 1973.

[227] MELANÇON (S. B.), DALLAIRE (L.) et coll. — Dicarboxylic amino-aciduria: an inborn error of amino-acid conservation. *J. Pediat.*, *91*, 422-427, 1977.

[228] MELNICK (C. R.), MICHALS (K. K.) et coll. — Linguistic development of children with phenylketonuria and normal intelligence. *J. Pediat.*, *98*, 269-272, 1981.

[229] MENKES (J. H.). — Idiopathic hyperglycemia: isolation and identification of three previously undescribed urinary ketones. *J. Pediat.*, *69*, 413-421, 1966.

[229 b] MENKES (J. H.), HURST (P. L.) et coll. — A new syndrome: progressive familial infantile cerebral dysfunction associated with an unusual urinary substance. *Pediatrics*, *14*, 462-466, 1954.

[230] MILSTEIN (S.), KAUFMAN (S.) et coll. — Hyperphenylalaninemia due to dihydropteridine reductase deficiency: diagnosis by measurement of oxidised and reduced pterins in urine. *Pediatrics*, *65*, 806-810, 1980.

[231] MILUNSKY (A.). — Genetic disorders and the fetus. Diagnosis, prevention and treatment. MILUNSKY ed., 1 vol., 703 p. Plenum Press, New York, 1979.

[231 b] MORRIS (M. B.), FISCHER (D. A.) et coll. — Late onset branched chain keto-aciduria (Maple syrup urine disease). *Lancet*, *2*, 149-152, 1966.

[232] MORROW (G.), REVSIN (B.) et coll. — A new variant of methylmalonic acidemia. Defective coenzyme-apoenzyme binding in cultured fibroblasts. *Clin. Chim. Acta*, *85*, 67-72, 1978.

[233] MOSER (H. W.). — Ceramidase deficiency: Farber's lipogranulomatosis. In: *The metabolic Basis of inherited Diseases.* J. B. STANBURY, J. B. WYNGAARDEN, D. S. FREDRICKSON, ed. McGraw-Hill, New York, 707-717, 1978.

[234] MOYNAHAN (E. J.). — Acrodermatitis entero-pathica: a lethal inherited human zinc deficiency disorder. *Lancet, II*, 339-400, 1974.

[235] MUDD (S. H.), LEVY (L. H.). — Disorders of transsulfuration. In: *The metabolic Basis of inherited Diseases.* J. B. STANBURY, J. B. WYNGAAR-DEN, D. S. FREDRICKSON, ed. McGraw-Hill, New York, 408-503, 1978.

[236] MUDD (S. H.), LEVY (H. L.) et coll. — A derange-ment in B12 metabolism leading to homocysti-nuria, cystathioninemia and methylmalonic aci-duria. *Biochem. Biophys. Res. Commun., 35*, 121-126, 1969.

[237] MULIVOR (R. A.), MENNUTI (M.) et coll. — Pre-natal diagnosis of hypophosphatasia: genetic, biochemical and clinical studies. *Amer. J. Hum. Genet., 30*, 271-282, 1978.

[238] MURPHEY (W. H.), LINDMARK (D. G.) et coll. — Serum carnosinase deficiency concomitant with mental retardation. *Pediat. Res., 7*, 601-606, 1973.

[239] NAKAMURA (E.), ROSENBERG (L. E.) et coll. — Microdetermination of methylmalonic acid and other short chain dicarboxylic acids, by gas chromatography: use in prenatal diagnosis of methylmalonic acidemia and in studies of isovaleric acidemia. *Clin. Chim. Acta, 68*, 127-140, 1976.

[240] NAVON (R.), PADEH (B.) et coll. — Apparent deficiency of hexosaminidase A in healthy members of a family with Tay-Sachs disease. *Amer. J. Hum. Genet., 25*, 287-293, 1973.

[241] NAYLOR (E. W.), MOSOVICH (L. L.) et coll. — Intermittent non-ketotic dicarboxylic aciduria in two siblings with hypoglycemia/an apparent defect in beta-oxidation of fatty acids. *J. Inher. Metab. Dis., 3*, 19-24, 1980.

[242] NAYLOR (E. W.). — Newborn screening for maple syrup urine disease (branched chain ketoaciduria). In: *Neonatal Screening for inborn errors of meta-bolism.* H. BICKEL, R. GUTHRIE, G. HAMMERSEN, ed. Springer-Verlag, Berlin, 19-28, 1980.

[243] NEIMANN (N.), VIDAILHET (M.) et coll. — Insuffi-sance hépatique aiguë de l'enfant avec stéatose viscérale et encéphalopathie (syndrome de Reye). *Ann. Pediat. (Paris), 22*, 195-202, 1975.

[244] NEUFELD (E. F.), LIEBAERS (I.) et coll. — The Hunter syndrome in females: is there an auto-somal recessive form of iduronate sulfatase defi-ciency. *Amer. J. Hum. Genet., 29*, 455-461, 1977.

[245] NYHAN (W. L.). — Clinical features of the Lesh-Nyhan syndrome. *Arch. Intern. Med., 130*, 186-192, 1972.

[246] OBERHOLZER (V. G.), LEVIN (B.) et coll. — Methyl-malonic aciduria: an inborn error of metabolism leading to chronic metabolic acidosis. *Arch. Dis. Child., 42*, 492-504, 1967.

[247] O'BRIEN (J. S.), GUGLER (E.) et coll. — Spondylo-epiphyseal dysplasia, corneal, clouding, normal intelligence and acid beta galactosidase deficiency. *Clin Genet., 9*, 495-504, 1976.

[248] O'BRIEN (J. S.). — The gangliosidoses. In: *The metabolic Basis of inherited Diseases.* J. B. STANBU-RY, J. B. WYNGAARDEN, D. S. FREDRICKSON, ed. McGraw-Hill, New York, 841-865, 1978.

[249] OCKERMANN (P. C.). — A generalised storage disorder resembling Hurler's syndrome. *Lancet, 2*, 239-241, 1967.

[250] O'FLYNN (M.), HOLTZMAN (N. A.) et coll. — The diagnosis of phenylketonuria. A report from the collaborative study of children treated for phenylketonuria. *Amer. J. Dis. Child., 134*, 769-774, 1980.

[251] ORKIN (S. H.), ACTER (B. P.) et coll. — Application of endonuclease mapping to the analysis and pre-natal diagnosis of thalassemia caused by globin gene deletion. *N. Engl. J. Med., 229*, 166-172, 1978.

[252] OYANAGI (K.), SOGAWA (H.) et coll. — Clinical and biochemical studies on periodic hyperammonemia with hyperlysinemia and homocitrullinuria. *Tohoku J. Exp. Med., 120*, 105-112, 1976.

[253] PALMER (T.), OBERHOLZER (V. G.). — Diagnosis of urea cycle disorders. *Ann. Clin. Biochem., 14*, 136-138, 1977.

[254] PALO (J.). — Prevalence of phenylketonuria and some other metabolic disorders among mentally retarded patients in Finland. *Acta Neurol. Scand., 43*, 573-579, 1967.

[255] PASCAL (T. A.), GAULL (G. E.) et coll. — Cysta-thionase deficiency: evidence for genetic hetero-geneity in primary cystathioninuria. *Pediat. Res., 12*, 125-133, 1978.

[256] PATRICK (A. D.), WILLCOX (P.) et coll. — Prenatal diagnosis of Wolman's disease. *J. Med. Genet., 13*, 49-51, 1976.

[257] PAUL (T. D.), NAYLOR (E. W.) et coll. — Urine screening for metabolic disease in newborn infants. *J. Pediat., 96*, 653-656, 1980.

[258] PAULSEN (E. P.), HSIA (Y. E.). — Asymptomatic propionic acidemia: variability of clinical expres-sion in a Mennonite kindred. *Amer. J. Hum. Genet., 26*, 66 a, 1974.

[259] PAVONE (L.), MOSER (H. W.) et coll. — Farber's lipogranulomatosis: ceramidase deficiency and prolonged survival in three relatives. *John Hopkins Med. J., 147*, 193-196, 1980.

[260] PERESS (N. S.), DI MAURO (S.) et coll. — Adult polysaccharidosis: clinicopathological, ultrastruc-tural and biochemical features. *Arch. Neurol., 36*, 840-845, 1979.

[261] PERRY (T. L.), APPLEGARTH (D. A.) et coll. — Metabolic studies of a family with massive formi-mino-glutamic aciduria. *Pediat. Res., 9*, 117-122, 1975.

[262] PERRY (T. L.), HANSEN (S.) et coll. — Carnosine-mia. A new metabolic disorder associated with neu-rologic disease and mental defect. *N. Engl. J. Med., 227*, 1219-1227, 1967.

[263] PERRY (T. L.), HANSEN (S.) et coll. — Volatile acids in normal human physiological fluids. *Clin. Chim. Acta, 29*, 369-374, 1970.

[264] PERRY (T. L.), URQUHART (N.) et coll. — Non ketotic hyperglycinemia. Glycine accumulation due to an absence of glycine cleavage in brain. *N. Engl. J. Med., 292*, 1269-1273, 1975.

[265] PHILIPPART (M.), FRANKLIN (S. S.) et coll. — Reversal of an inborn sphingolipidosis (Fabry's disease) by kidney transplantation. *Ann. Intern. Med., 77*, 195-200, 1972.

[266] POLLACK (M. S.), MAURER (D.) et coll. — Prenatal diagnosis of congenital adrenal hyperplasia (21-hy-droxylase deficiency) by HLA typing. *Lancet, 1*, 1107-1108, 1979.

[267] POLLACK (M. S.), OCHS (H. D.) et coll. — HLA typing of cultured amniotic cells for the prenatal diagnosis of complement C4 deficiency. *Clin. Genet., 18*, 197-200, 1980.

[268] POLLITT (R. J.). — Aspartylglycosaminuria. In: *Les oligosaccharidoses.* FARRIAUX (J. P.), ed. Crouan et Roques, Lille, 59-65, 1977.

[269] POWELL (G. F.), KUROSKY (A.) et coll. — Prolidase deficiency: report of a second case with quantitation of the excessively excreted amino-acids. *J. Pediat.*, *91*, 242-246, 1977.

[270] PRZYREMBEL (H.), WENDEL (U.) et coll. — Glutaric aciduria type II: report on a previously undescribed metabolic disorder. *Clin. Chim. Acta*, *66*, 227-239, 1976.

[271] PRZYREMBEL (H.), BACHMAN (D.) et coll. — Alpha-ketoadipic aciduria, a new inborn error of lysine metabolism: biochemical studies. *Clin. Chim. Acta*, *58*, 257-269, 1975.

[272] PULLARKAT (R. K.), PATEL (V. K.) et coll. — Leukocyte docosahexaenoic acid in juvenile form of ceroid-lipofuscinosis. *Neuropädiatrie*, *9*, 127-130, 1978.

[273] RAGHAVAN (S. S.), TOPOL (J.) et coll. — Leukocyte beta-glucosidase in homozygotes and heterozygotes for Gaucher disease. *Amer. J. Hum. Genet.*, *32*, 158-173, 1980.

[274] RAJANTIE (J.), SIMELL (O.) et coll. — Lysinuric protein intolerance: a two year trial of dietary supplementation therapy with cirrulline and lysine. *J. Pediat.*, *97*, 927-932, 1980.

[275] RAJANTIE (J.), SIMELL (O.) et coll. — Basolateral-membrane transport defect for lysine in lysinuric protein intolerance. *Lancet*, *1*, 1219-1221, 1980.

[276] RAPIN (I. S.), GOLD-FISCHER (A.) et coll. — The cherry red spot-myoclonus syndrome. *Ann. Neurol.*, *3*, 224-242, 1978.

[277] RAPIN (I. S.), SUZUKI (K.) et coll. — Adult (chronic) GM2 gangliosidosis: atypical spinocerebellar degeneration in a Jewish sibship. *Arch. Neurol.*, *33*, 120-130, 1976.

[278] RAPOPORT (D.), SAUDUBRAY (J. M.) et coll. — Étude psychologique de 20 enfants phénylcétonuriques traités tôt. *Ann. Pediat. (Paris)*, *22*, 509-516, 1975.

[279] REBOUCHE (C. J.), ENGEL (A. G.). — In vitro analysis of hepatic carnitine biosynthesis in human systemic carnitine deficiency. *Clin. Chim. Acta*, *106*, 295-300, 1980.

[280] REDDI (O. S.). — Threoninemia a new metabolic defect. *Pediatrics*, *93*, 814-816, 1978.

[281] REUSER (A. J. J.), KOSTER (J. F.) et coll. — Biochemical, immunological and cell genetic studies in glycogenosis type II. *Amer. J. Hum. Genet.*, *30*, 132-143, 1978.

[282] REY (J.), REY (F.). — Phénylcétonurie et développement mental : un problème mal posé. *Arch. Fr. Pediatr.*, *35*, 3-10, 1978.

[283] REY (F.), LEEMING (R. J.) et coll. — La phénylcétonurie « transitoire ». Un déficit permanent. *Arch. Fr. Pediatr.*, *36*, 48-55, 1979.

[284] REY (J.), FARRIAUX (J. P.) et coll. — Les hyperlipoprotéinémies et la prévention de l'althérome chez l'enfant. In: *16e Congrès Ass. Pediat. Langue Franç. Toulouse*, 30 juin-6 juillet 1981, 1 volume, 227-291.

[285] RICHARDS (F.), COOPER (M. R.) et coll. — Familial spino-cerebellar degeneration haemolytic anemia and glutathione deficiency. *Arch. Intern. Med.*, *134*, 534-537, 1974.

[286] ROBINSON (B. H.), SHERWOOD (W. G.) et coll. — Aceto-acetyl CoA-thiolase deficiency: a cause of severe ketoacidosis in infancy simulating salicylism. *J. Pediat.*, *95*, 228-233, 1979.

[287] ROBINSON (B. H.), TAYLOR (J.) et coll. — Deficiency of dihydrolipoyl dehydrogenase (a component of the pyruvate and alpha-ketoglutarate dehydrogenase complexes): a cause of congenital lactic acidosis in infancy. *Pediat. Res.*, *11*, 1198-1202, 1977.

[288] ROBINSON (B. H.), OEI (J.) et coll. — Hydroxymethylglutaryl-CoA lyase deficiency: features resembling Reye syndrome. *Neurology*, *30*, 714-718, 1980.

[289] ROESEL (R. A.), BLANKENSHIP (P. R.) et coll. — Hydroxyproline metabolism in two sisters with hydroxyprolinemia. *Hum. Hered.*, *29*, 364-370, 1979.

[290] ROSENBERG (L. E.), DOWNING (S.) et coll. — Cystinuria: biochemical evidence for three genetically distinct diseases. *J. Clin. Invest.*, *45*, 365-371, 1966.

[291] ROSENBERG (L. E.). — Disorders of propionate methylmalonate and cobalamin metabolism. In: *The metabolic Basis of inherited Diseases*. J. B. STANBURY, J. B. WYNGAARDEN, D. S. FREDRICKSON, ed. McGraw-Hill, New York, 411-429, 1978.

[292] ROSENBLATT (D. S.), ERBE (R. W.). — Methylenetetrahydrofolate reductase in cultured human cells. II. Genetic and biochemical studies of methylenetetrahydrofolate reductase deficiency. *Pediat. Res.*, *11*, 1141-1143, 1977.

[293] ROWE (P. B.). — Inherited disorders of folate metabolism. In: *The metabolic Basis of inherited Diseases*. J. B. STANBURY, J. B. WYNGAARDEN, D. S. FREDRICKSON, ed. McGraw-Hill, New York, 430-457, 1978.

[294] RUBINO (A.). — Function of the intestinal brush border membrane in health and disease. E. S. P. A. G. N. Bern, Sept. 23-26, 1981, Abst. in *Pediat. Res.*, *15*, 1173-1178, 1981.

[295] SACREZ (R.), JUIF (J. G.) et coll. — La maladie de Landing; idiotie amaurotique infantile précoce avec gangliosidose généralisée de type GM1. *Pediatrie (Lyon)*, *22*, 143-162, 1967.

[296] SANDER (J. E.), MALAMUD et coll. — Intermittent ataxia and immunodeficiency with multiple carboxylase deficiencies: a biotin responsive disorder. *Ann. Neurol.*, *8*, 544-547, 1980.

[297] SANDHOFF (K.), HARZER (K.) et coll. — Enzyme alterations and lipid storage in three variants of Tay-Sachs disease. *J. Neurochem.*, *18*, 2469-2489, 1971.

[298] SANN (L.), DIVRY (P.) et coll. — L'acidurie méthylmalonique sensible à la vitamine B12. *Pediatrie (Lyon)*, *35*, 205-212, 1980.

[299] SARDHAWALLA (I. B.), FOWLER (B.). — Tryptophanaemia. Observations on four cases. *Intern. Symp. Inborn errors of metabolism*, Interlaken, Sept. 2-5, 1980.

[300] SASS-KORTSAK (A.), BEARN (A. G.). — Hereditary disorders of copper metabolism (Wilson's disease and Menkes' disease). In: *The metabolic Basis of inherited Diseases*, J. B. STANBURY, J. B. WYNGAARDEN, D. S. FREDRICKSON, ed. McGraw-Hill, New York, 1098-1125, 1978.

[301] SAUDUBRAY (J. M.), LABOUREAU (J. P.) et coll. — Coma acidocétosique post-appendicectomie: déficit héréditaire en bêta-cétothiolase. *Arch. Fr. Pediatr.*, *32*, 671-672, 1975.

[301 *b*] SAUDUBRAY (J. M.). — Les acidoses métaboliques d'origine héréditaire. Orientation diagnostique générale et principales étiologies. *Rev. Praticien (Paris)*, *25*, 2621-2639, 1975.

[302] SAUDUBRAY (J. M.), SORIN (M.) et coll. — Acidémie isovalérique. Étude et traitement chez trois frères. *Arch. Fr. Pediatr.*, *33*, 795-808, 1976.

[303] SAUNDERS (M.), SWEETMAN (L.) et coll. — Biotin responsive organic aciduria. Multiple carboxylase defects and complementation studies with propionicacidemia in cultured fibroblasts. *J. Clin. Invest.*, *64*, 1695-1702, 1979.

[304] SCHAUB (J.), JANKA (G. E.) et coll. — Wolman's disease; Clinical, biochemical and ultrastructural studies in an unusual case without stricking adrenal calcification. *Eur. J. Pediat.*, *135*, 45-53, 1980.

[305] SCHMALSTIEG (F. C.), NELSON (J. A.) et coll. — Increased purine nucleotides in adenosine deaminase-deficient lymphocytes. *J. Pediat.*, *91*, 48-51, 1977.

[305 b] SCHNEIDER (J. A.), VERROUST (F. M.) et coll. — Prenatal diagnosis of cystinosis. *N. Engl. J. Med.*, *290*, 878-882, 1974.

[306] SCHNEIDER (J. A.), SCHULMAN (J. D.) et coll. — Cystinosis and the Fanconi syndrome. In: *The metabolic Basis of inherited Diseases*. J. B. STANBURY, J. B. WYNGAARDEN, D. S. FREDRICKSON, ed. McGraw-Hill, New York, 1660-1682, 1978.

[306 b] SCHNEIDER (J. A.), BRADLEY (K.) et coll. — Increased cystine in leukocytes from individuals homozygous and heterozygous for cystinosis. *Science*, *157*, 1321-1322, 1967.

[307] SCHULMAN (J. D.), GOODMAN (S. I.) et coll. — Glutathioninuria: inborn error of metabolism due to tissue deficiency of gamma-glutamyl transpeptidase. *Biochem. Biophys. Res. Commun.*, *65*, 68-74, 1975.

[307 b] SCHULMAN (J. D.), LUTSBERG (T. J.) et coll. — A new variant of maple syrup urine disease (branched chain ketoaciduria). *Amer. J. Med.*, *49*, 118-124, 1970.

[308] SCHUTGENS (R. B. H.), BEEMER (F. A.) et coll. — Mild variant of argininosuccinic aciduria. *J. Inher. Metab. Dis.*, *2*, 13-14, 1979.

[308 b] SCRIVER (C. R.), MACKENZIE (S.) et coll. — Thiamine responsive maple syrup urine disease. *Lancet*, *1*, 310-312, 1971.

[309] SCRIVER (C. R.). — Disorders of proline and hydroxyproline and 5-oxoproline metabolism. In: *The Metabolic Basis of Inherited Disease*. STANBURY (J. B.), WYNGAARDEN (J. B.), FREDRICKSON (D. S.), ed. McGraw-Hill, New York, 336-361, 1978.

[310] SCRIVER (C. R.), PUESCHEL (S.) et coll. — Hyperbeta-alaninemia associated with beta-amino-aciduria and gamma-aminobutyric aciduria, somnolence and seizures. *N. Engl. J. Med.*, *274*, 635-643, 1966.

[311] SCRIVER (C. R.), ROSENBERG (L. E.). — Nature and disorders of neutral amino-acid transport. In: *Aminoacid metabolism and its disorders*. Saunders publ., Philadelphia, 187-196, 1973.

[312] SCRIVER (C. R.), ROSENBERG (L. E.). — Sulfur aminoacids. In: *Aminoacid metabolism and its disorders*. Saunders publ., Philadelphia, 207-233, 1973.

[313] SCRIVER (C. R.). — The human biochemical genetics of amino-acid transport. *Pediatrics*, *44*, 348-357, 1969.

[314] SCRIVER (C. R.). — Familial iminoglycinuria. In: *The Metabolic Basis of Inherited Disease*. STANBURY (J. B.), WYNGAARDEN (J. B.), FREDRICKSON (D. S.), ed. McGraw-Hill, New York, 1593-1606, 1978.

[315] SEALE (T. W.), RENNERT (O. M.). — Prenatal diagnosis of thalassemias and hemoglobinopathies. *Ann. Clin. Lab. Sci.*, *10*, 383-394, 1980.

[316] SHIH (V. E.), EFRON (M. L.) et coll. — Hyperornithinemia, hyperammonemia and homocitrullinuria. A new disorder of amino-acid metabolism associated with myoclonic seizures and mental retardation. *Amer. J. Dis. Child.*, *117*, 83-92, 1969.

[317] SHIH (V. E.), ABROMS (I. F.) et coll. — Sulfite oxidase deficiency. Biochemical and clinical investigations of a hereditary metabolic disorder in sulfur metabolism. *N. Engl. J. Med.*, *297*, 1022-1028, 1977.

[318] SHORT (E. M.), CONN (H. O.) et coll. — Evidence of X Linked dominant inheritance of ornithine transcarbamylase deficiency. *N. Engl. J. Med.*, *288*, 7-12, 1973.

[319] SICOT (Ch). — La maladie de Wilson. *Conc. Méd. (Paris)*, *96*, 3990-3994, 1974.

[320] SIMELL (O.), PERHEENTUPA et coll. — Lysinuric protein intolerance. *Amer. J. Med.*, *59*, 229-240, 1975.

[321] SIMELL (O.). — Diamino acid transport into granulocytes and liver slices of patients with lysinuric protein intolerance. *Pediat. Res.*, *9*, 504-508, 1975.

[322] SIMELL (O.), TAKKI (K.). — Raised plasma ornithine and gyrate atrophy of the choroid and retina. *Lancet*, *1*, 1031-1033, 1973.

[323] SIPILA (I.), SIMELL (I.). — Gyrate atrophy of the choroid and retina with hyperornithinemia. *J. Clin. Invest.*, *66*, 684-687, 1980.

[324] SMITH (L. H.). — Pyrimidine metabolism in man. *N. Engl. J. Med.*, *288*, 764-771, 1973.

[325] SMITH (I.), WOLFF (O.). — Natural history of phenylketonuria and influence of early treatment. *Lancet*, *2*, 540-543, 1974.

[326] SMITH (I.), CLAYTON (B. E.) et coll. — New variant of phenylketonuria with progressive neurological illness unresponsive to phenylalanine restriction. *Lancet*, *1*, 1108-1110, 1975.

[327] SMOLIN (L. A.), BENEVENGA (N. J.) et coll. — The use of betaine for the treatment of homocystinuria. *J. Pediat.*, *99*, 467-472, 1981.

[328] SNYDERMAN (S. E.), SANSARICQ (C.) et coll. — The nutritional therapy of histidinemia. *J. Pediat.*, *95*, 712-715, 1979.

[329] SPRANGER (J.), GEHLER (J.) et coll. — The radiographic features of mannosidosis. *Radiology*, *119*, 401-407, 1976.

[330] SPRANGER (J.), WIEDEMANN (H. R.) et coll. — Lipomucopolysaccharidose. *Z. Kinderheilk.*, *103*, 285-290, 1968.

[331] SPRANGER (J.), CANTZ (M.) et coll. — Mucopolysaccharidosis II (Hunter disease) with corneal opacities. *Eur. J. Pediat.*, *129*, 11-16, 1978.

[332] SRIVASTAVA (S. K.), WIKTOROWICZ (J. E.) et coll. — Interrelationship of hexosaminidases A and B: confirmation of the common and the unique subunit theory. *J. Biol. Chem.*, *249*, 2054-2057, 1974.

[333] STANBURY (J. B.), WYNGAARDEN (J. B.) et coll. — Inherited variation and metabolic abnormality. In: *The metabolic Basis of inherited Diseases*. J. B. STANBURY, J. B. WYNGAARDEN, D. S. FREDRICKSON, ed. McGraw-Hill, New York, 2-32, 1978.

[333 b] STATES (B.), BLAZER (B.) et coll. — Prenatal diagnosis of cystinosis. *J. Pediat.*, *87*, 558-562, 1975.

[334] STEINBERG (D.), MIZE (C. E.) et coll. — Phytanic acid in patients with Refsum's syndrome and response to dietary treatment. *Arch. Intern. Med.*, *125*, 75-87, 1970.

[335] STOKKE (O.), ELDJARN (L.) et coll. — Beta-methyl-crotonyl-CoA carboxylase deficiency: a new metabolic error in leucine degradation. *Pediatrics*, *49*, 726-735, 1972.

[336] STOKKE (O.), ELDJARN (L.). — Methylmalonic acidemia: a new inborn error of metabolism which may cause fatal acidosis in the neonatal period. *Scand. J. Clin. Lab. Invest.*, *20*, 313-328, 1967.

[337] STRECKER (G.), MICHALSKI (J. C.). — Biochemical basis of six different types of sialidosis. *Febs Letters*, *85*, 20-24, 1978.

[338] STURMAN (J. A.), GAULL (G. E.) et coll. — Absence of cystathionase in human fetal liver: is cystine essential? *Science*, *169*, 74-76, 1970.

[339] SUZUKI (K.), SUZUKI (Y.). — Galactosyl ceramide lipidosis: globoid cell leukodystrophy (Krabbe's disease). In: *The metabolic Basis of inherited Diseases*. J. B. STANBURY, J. B. WYNGAARDEN, D. S. FREDRICKSON, ed. McGraw-Hill, New York, 747-769, 1978.

[340] SUZUKI (K.), SCHNEIDER (E. L.) et coll. — In utero diagnosis of globoid cell leukodystrophy (Krabbe's disease). *Biochem. Biophys. Res. Commun.*, *45*, 1363-1366, 1971.

[341] SVENNERHOLM (L.), HAGBERG (B.) et coll. — Polyinsaturated fatty acid lipidosis. II: lipid biochemical studies. *Acta Paediat. Scand.*, *64*, 489-496, 1975.

[342] SVENNERHOLM (L.), HAKANSSON (G.) et coll. — Assay of the beta-glucosidase activity with natural labelled and artificial substrats in leukocytes from homozygotes and heterozygotes with the Norrobottnian type (type 3) of Gaucher disease. *Clin. Chim. Acta*, *106*, 183-193, 1980.

[343] SWEETMAN (L.), NYHAN (W. L.) et coll. — Propionic acidaemia presenting with pancytopenia in infancy. *J. Inher. Metab. Dis.*, *2*, 65-69, 1979.

[344] SWEETMAN (L.), NYHAN (W. L.) et coll. — Glutaric aciduria type II. *J. Pediat.*, *96*, 1020-1026, 1980.

[345] TADA (K.), ITO (H.) et coll. — Congenital tryptophanuria with dwarfism (« H » disease-like clinical features without indicanuria and generalized amino-aciduria): a probably new inborn error of tryptophan metabolism. *Tohoku J. Exp. Med.*, *80*, 118-134, 1963.

[346] TADA (K.), YOKOYAMA (Y.) et coll. — Vitamin B6 dependent xanthurenic aciduria. *Tohoku J. Exp. Med.*, *95*, 107-114, 1968.

[347] TANAKA (J.), GARCIA (J. H.) et coll. — Cerebral sponginess and GM3 gangliosidosis: ultrastructure and probable pathogenesis. *J. Neuropath. Exper. Neurol.*, *34*, 249-262, 1975.

[348] TANAKA (K.). — Disorders of organic acid metabolism. In *Biology of Brain Dysfunction*. 3. GAULL (G. E.), ed. Plenum Press, N. Y., 145-214, 1975.

[349] TANAKA (K.), BUDD (M. A.) et coll. — Isovaleric acidemia: a new genetic defect of leucine metabolism. *Proc. Nat. Acad. Sci.*, *56*, 236-242, 1966.

[350] THALER (M. M.), HOOGENRAAD (N. J.) et coll. — Reye's syndrome due to novel protein tolerant variant of ornithine transcarbamylase deficiency. *Lancet*, *2*, 438-440, 1974.

[351] THIER (S. O.), SEGAL (S.). — Cystinuria. In: *The Metabolic Basis of Inherited Disease*. STANBURY (J. B.), WYNGAARDEN (J. B.), FREDRICKSON (D. S.), ed. McGraw-Hill, New York, 1578-1592, 1978.

[352] THOENE (J.), BATSHAW (M.) et coll. — Neonatal citrullinemia: treatment with keto-analogues of essential aminoacids. *J. Pediat.*, *90*, 218-224, 1977.

[353] THOMAS (G. H.), HASLAM (R. H. A.) et coll. — Hyperpipecolic acidemia associated with hepatomegaly, mental retardation, optic nerve dysplasia and progressive neurological disease. *Clin. Genet.*, *8*, 376-382, 1975.

[354] THOMAS (P. K.), ABRAMS (J. D.) et coll. — Sialidosis type I: cherry red spot-myoclonus syndrome with sialidase deficiency and altered electrophoretic mobilities of some enzymes known to be glycoproteins. *J. Neurol. Neurosurg. Psychiat.*, *42*, 873-888, 1979.

[355] TONDEUR (M.). — La fucosidose. In: *Les oligosaccharidoses*. FARRIAUX (J. P.), éd. Crouan et Roques, Lille, 43-49, 1977.

[356] TOURAINE (J. L.), MALIK (M. C.) et coll. — Maladie de Fabry: deux malades améliorés par la greffe des cellules de foie fœtal. *Nouv. Presse Méd.*, *8*, 1499-1503, 1979.

[357] TOURIAN (A. Y.), SIDBURY (J. B.). — Phenylketonuria. In: *The metabolic Basis of inherited Diseases*. J. B. STANBURY, J. B. WYNGAARDEN, D. S. FREDRICKSON, ed. McGraw-Hill, New York, 240-255, 1978.

[358] TRUSCOTT (R. J. W.), HALPERN (B.) et coll. — Abnormal deoxyribose metabolites in the urine of a child with a possible new inborn error of metabolism. *Biomed. Mass. Spectrom.*, *6*, 453-459, 1979.

[359] VALLE (D.), GOODMAN (S. I.) et coll. — Type II hyperprolinemia. Δ-1-pyrroline-5-carboxylic dehydrogenase deficiency in cultured skin fibroblasts and circulating lymphocytes. *J. Clin. Invest.*, *58*, 598-603, 1976.

[360] VALLE (D.), SHASHIDHAR (P. G.) et coll. — Homocystinuria due to cystathionine synthetase deficiency: clinical manifestations and therapy. *John Hopkins Med. J.*, *146*, 110-117, 1980.

[361] VAN DER HEIDEN (J. C.), BEEMER (F. A.) et coll. — Simultaneous occurrence of xanthine oxidase and sulfite oxidase deficiency. A molybdenum dependent inborn error of metabolism. *Clin. Biochem.*, *12*, 206-208, 1979.

[362] VANNEUVILLE (F. J.), LEROY (J. G.) et coll. — Prenatal diagnosis of hypophosphatasia. *Arch. Intern. Physiol. Biochem.*, *88*, B 300, 1980.

[363] VEALE (A. M. O.). — Screening for phenylketonuria. In: *Neonatal Screening for inborn errors of metabolism*. BICKEL (H.), GUTHRIE (R.), HAMMERSEN (G.), eds. Springer Verlag, Berlin, 7-18, 1980.

[364] VIDAILHET (M.), LEVIN (B.) et coll. — Citrullinémie. *Arch. Fr. Pédiatr.*, *28*, 521-532, 1971.

[365] VIDAILHET (M.), NEIMANN (N.) et coll. — Maladie de Sandhoff (gangliosidose à GM2 de type 2). *Arch. Fr. Pediatr.*, *30*, 45-60, 1973.

[366] VIDAILHET (M.), LEFEBVRE-LEPOIRE (E.) et coll. — Congenital lactic acidosis with pyruvate carboxylase inactivity. *J. Inher. Metab. Dis.*, *4*, 131-132, 1981.

[367] VIDAILHET (M.), HATIER (R.) et coll. — Étude ultrastructurale d'un cas de maladie de Wolman (déficit en estérase acide). *Biol. Cell. (Paris)*, *32*, 3 a, 1978.

[367 b] VIDAILHET (M.), BROCARD (O.) et coll. — Aspects électro-cliniques des leucinoses. *Rev. E. E. G. Neurophysiol.*, *8*, 61-70, 1978.

[368] WADMAN (S. K.), VAN SPRANG (F. J.) et coll. — An exceptional case of tyrosinosis. *J. Ment. Def. Res.*, *12*, 269-281, 1969.

[369] WADMAN (S. K.), DURAN (M.) et coll. — D-glyceric acidemia in a patient with chronic metabolic acidosis. *Clin. Chim. Acta*, *71*, 477-484, 1976.

[370] WAISMAN (H. A.), GERRITSEN (T.). — Hypersarcosinemia. *Amer. J. Dis. Child.*, *113*, 134-137, 1967.

[371] WARBURTON (D.), BOYLE (R. J.) et coll. — Non ketotic hyperglycinemia. Effects of therapy with strychnine. *Amer. J. Dis. Child.*, *134*, 273-275, 1980.

[371 b] WELNER (D.), MEISTER (A.). — A survey of inborn errors of aminoacid metabolism and transport in man. *Ann. Rev. Biochem.*, *50*, 911-968, 1981.

[372] WENGER (D. A.), BARTH (G.) et coll. — Nine cases of sphingomyelin lipidosis, a new variant in Spanish-American children. *Amer. J. Dis. Child.*, *131*, 955-960, 1977.

[372 b]. WESTALL (R. G.), DANCIS (J.) et coll. — Maple syrup urine disease. *Amer. J. Dis. Child.*, *94*, 571-572, 1957.

[373] WEYLER (W.), SWEETMAN (L.) et coll. — Deficiency of propionyl-CoA carboxylase in a patient with methylcrotonylglycinuria. *Clin. Chim. Acta*, *76*, 321-328, 1977.

[374] WHELAN (D. T.), HILL (R.) et coll. — L-glutaric acidemia: investigation of a patient and his family. *Pediatrics*, *63*, 88-93, 1979.

[375] WIEGAND (C.), THOMPSON (T.) et coll. — The management of life threatening hyperammonemia: a comparison of several therapeutic modalities. *J. Pediat.*, *96*, 142, 1980.

[376] WILCKEN (B.), SMITH (A.) et coll. — Urine screening for aminoacidopathies: is it beneficial. *J. Pediatr.*, *97*, 492-497, 1980.

[377] WILKINSON (S. P.), NIVEN (S. E.) et coll. — Quantitationof organic acids in amniotic fluid by gas chromatography. *Clin. Chim. Acta*, *99*, 241-245, 1979.

[378] WILLARD (H. F.), AMBANI (L. M.) et coll. — Rapid prenatal and postnatal detection of inborn errors of propionate, methylmalonate and cobalamin metabolism: a sensitive assay using cultured cells. *Hum. Genet.*, *34*, 277-283, 1976.

[379] WILLIAMS (A. J.), IRELAND (J. T.). — Neonatal acidosis associated with transient methylmalonic aciduria and vitamin B12 deficiency. *Acta Paediat. Scand.*, *66*, 117-119, 1977.

[380] WINTER (R. M.), SWALLOW (D. M.) et coll. — Sialidosis type 2 (acid neuraminidase deficiency): clinical and biochemical features of a further case. *Clin. Genet.*, *18*, 203-210, 1980.

[381] WITZUM (J. L.), WILLIAMS (C. J.) et coll. — Successful plasmapharesis in a 4 year old child with homozygous familial hypercholesterolemia. *J. Pediat.*, *97*, 615-618, 1980.

[382] WOLF (B.). — Reassessment of biotin-responsiveness in "unresponsive" propionyl CoA carboxylase deficiency. *J. Pediat.*, *97*, 964-966, 1980.

[383] WOLF (B.), PAULSEN (E. P.) et coll. — Asymptomatic propionyl CoA carboxylase deficiency in a 13 year old girl. *J. Pediat.*, *95*, 563-564, 1980.

[384] WRIGHT (E. C.), STERN (J.) et coll. — Glutathionuria: gamma-glutamyl transpeptidase deficiency. *J. Inher. Metab. Dis.*, *2*, 3-7, 1979.

[385] YUDKOFF (M.), FOREMAN (J. W.). — Effects of cysteamine therapy in nephropathic cystinosis. *N. Engl. J. Med.*, *304*, 141-145, 1981.

[386] ZEMAN (W.), DYKEN (P.). — Neuronal ceroid lipofuscinosis (Batten's disease) : relationship to amaurotic family idiocy. *Pediatrics*, *44*, 570-583, 1969.

[387] BROCK (D. J. H.), BEDGOOD (D.) et coll. — Prenatal diagnosis of cystic fibrosis by assay of amniotic fluid microvillar enzymes. *Hum. Genet.*, *65*, 248-261, 1984.

[388] BUDDEN (S. S.), KENNAWAY (N. G.). — Dysmorphic syndrome with phytanic acid oxidase deficiency, abnormal very long chain fatty acids, and pipecolic acidemia: studies in four children. *J. Pediat.*, *108*, 33-39, 1986.

[389] BURRI (B. J.), SWEETMAN (L.) et coll. — Heterogeneity of holocarboxylase synthetase in patients with biotin-responsive multiple carboxylase deficiency. *Am. J. Hum. Genet.*, *37*, 326-337, 1985.

[390] LIDSKY (A. S.), GUTTLER (F.) et coll. — Prenatal diagnosis of classic phenylketonuria by D. N. A. analysis. *Lancet*, *1*, 549-551.

[391] MOSER (H. W.). — Peroxisomal disorders. *J. Pediat.*, *108*, 89-91, 1986.

[392] NEWMARK (P.). — Testing for cystic fibrosis. *Nature*, *318*, 309, 1985.

[393] OLD (J. M.), BRIAND (P. L.) et coll. — Prenatal exclusion of ornithine transcarbamylase deficiency by direct gene analysis. *Lancet*, *1*, 73-75, 1985.

[394] POENARU (L.), CASTELNAU (L.) et coll. — First trimester prenatal diagnosis of mucolipidosis II (I cell disease) by chorionic biopsy. *Am. J. Hum. Genet.*, *36*, 1379-1385, 1984.

[395] SIMONI (G.), BRAMBATTI (B.) et coll. — Diagnostic application of first trimester trophoblast sampling in 100 pregnancies. *Hum. Genet.*, *66*, 252-259, 1984.

[396] STOUT (J. T.), JACKSON (L. C.) et coll. — First trimester diagnosis of Lesh-Nyhan syndrome: applications to other disorders of purine metabolism. *Prenat. Diagn.*, *5*, 183-189, 1985.

[397] WOLF (B.), GRIER (R. E.) et coll. — Deficiency biotinidase activity in late-onset multiple carboxylase deficiency. *N. Engl. J. Med.*, *208*, 161, 1983.

Index